IMMUNOLOGY OF RHEUMATIC DISEASES

IMMUNOLOGY OF RHEUMATIC DISEASES

Edited by

Sudhir Gupta, M.D., F.R.C.P.(C), F.A.C.P.
University of California College of Medicine
Irvine, California

and

Norman Talal, M.D.
University of Texas Health Science Center
San Antonio, Texas

PLENUM MEDICAL BOOK COMPANY
New York and London

Library of Congress Cataloging in Publication Data

Main entry under title:

Immunology of rheumatic diseases.

Includes bibliographies and index.
1. Rheumatism—Immunological aspects. I. Gupta, Sudhir. II. Talal, Norman.
[DNLM: 1. Rheumatism—immunology. WE 544 I337]
RC927.I495 1985 616.7'23 85-19090
ISBN-13: 978-1-4612-9509-9 e-ISBN-13: 978-1-4613-2493-5
DOI: 10.1007/ 978-1-4613-2493-5

233 Spring Street, New York, N.Y. 10013

Plenum Medical Book Company is an imprint of Plenum Publishing Corporation

Dedicated to
Abha Gupta, Ankmalika Gupta, Marilynn Talal,
Andrew Talal, and Melissa Talal

Contributors

Robert Ader • Division of Behavioral and Psychosocial Medicine, Department of Psychiatry, University of Rochester School of Medicine and Dentistry, Rochester, New York 14642

M. Teresa Aguado • Department of Immunology, Scripps Clinic and Research Foundation, La Jolla, California 92037

Margaret A. Alspaugh • Department of Medicine and Pathology, University of Missouri-Columbia, School of Medicine and Cancer Research Center, Columbia, Missouri 65201

J. F. Bach • INSERM U 25, Hopital Necker, 75015 Paris, France

Harry G. Bluestein • Division of Rheumatology, Department of Medicine, University of California Medical Center, San Diego, California 92103

Gian Franco Bottazzo • Department of Immunology, Middlesex Hospital Medical School, London W1P 9PG, England

Dennis A. Carson • Department of Basic and Clinical Research, Scripps Clinic and Research Foundation, La Jolla, California 92037

M. Dardenne • INSERM U 25, Hopital Necker, 75015 Paris, France

Deborah Doniach • Department of Immunology, Middlesex Hospital Medical School, London W1P 9PG, England

Anthony S. Fauci • Laboratory of Immunoregulation, National Institute of Allergy and Infectious Diseases, National Institutes of Health, Bethesda, Maryland 20205

Marc Feldmann • ICRF Tumour Immunology Unit, Department of Zoology, University College London, London WC1E 6BT, England

Sherman Fong • Department of Basic and Clinical Research, Scripps Clinic and Research Foundation, La Jolla, California 92037

Øystein Førre • Oslo Sanitetsforenings Rheumatism Hospital, Oslo, Norway

A. E. Gharavi • Rheumatology Unit, Royal Postgraduate Medical School, The Hammersmith Hospital, London W12 OHS, England

Sudhir Gupta • Department of Medicine, Division of Basic and Clinical Immunology, University of California, Irvine, California 92717

Bevra H. Hahn • Department of Medicine, Division of Rheumatology, University of California, Los Angeles, California 90024

John A. Hansen • The Fred Hutchinson Cancer Research Center, the Puget Sound Blood Center, and the University of Washington School of Medicine, Seattle, Washington 98121

E. N. Harris • Rheumatology Unit, Royal Postgraduate Medical School, The Hammersmith Hospital, London W12 OHS, England

Evelyn V. Hess • Department of Medicine, University of Cincinnati Medical Center, Cincinnati, Ohio 45267

Torstein Hovig • Institute of Pathology, Electron Microscopic Laboratory, Rikshospitalet, The National Hospital, Oslo, Norway

J. Eugene Huffstutter • Department of Medicine, Division of Rheumatology and Immunology, Medical University of South Carolina, Charleston, South Carolina 29425

G. R. V. Hughes • Rheumatology Unit, Royal Postgraduate Medical School, The Hammersmith Hospital, London W12 OHS, England

J. R. Kalden • Institut und Poliklinik für Klinische Immunologie, und Rheumatologie der Universität Erlangen-Nürnberg, D-8520 Erlangen, Federal Republic of Germany

Allen P. Kaplan • Division of Allergy, Rheumatology, and Clinical Immunology, Department of Medicine, The State University of New York at Stony Brook, Health Sciences Center, Stony Brook, New York 11794

Paul Katz • Department of Medicine, Georgetown University School of Medicine, Washington, D.C. 20007

Brian L. Kotzin • Department of Medicine, University of Colorado Health Sciences Center, and Rheumatology Section, Veterans Administration Medical Center, Denver, Colorado 80220

E. Carwile LeRoy • Department of Medicine, Division of Rheumatology and Immunology, Medical University of South Carolina, Charleston, South Carolina 29425

Allen Litwin • Department of Medicine, University of Cincinnati Medical Center, Cincinnati, Ohio 45267

Daniel J. McCarty • Department of Medicine, Medical College of Wisconsin, Milwaukee, Wisconsin 53226

Michael L. Miller • National Institutes of Health, National Institute of Arthritis, Diabetes, and Digestive and Kidney Diseases, Arthritis, and Rheumatism Branch, Cellular Immunology Section, Bethesda, Maryland 20205

Gerald T. Nepom • Genetic Systems Corporation, and the University of Washington School of Medicine, Seattle, Washington 98121

Marilyn C. Pike • Department of Medicine, Massachusetts General Hospital, Boston, Massachusetts 02115

Ken D. Pischel • Division of Rheumatology, Department of Medicine, University of California Medical Center, San Diego, California 92103

Gerard Renoux • Laboratoire d'Immunologie, Faculté de Médecine, F-37032 Tours Cedex, France

Micheline Renoux • Laboratoire d'Immunologie, Faculté de Médecine, F-37032 Tours Cedex, France

Frank R. Schmid • Department of Medicine, Section of Arthritis-Connective Tissue Diseases, Northwestern University Medical School, Chicago, Illinois 60611

Peter H. Schur • Division of Rheumatology and Immunology, Brigham and Women's Hospital, Harvard Medical School, Boston, Massachusetts 02115

Gordon C. Sharp • Department of Medicine and Pathology, University of Missouri-Columbia, School of Medicine and Cancer Research Center, Columbia, Missouri 65201

Richard M. Silver • Department of Medicine, Medical University of South Carolina, Charleston, South Carolina 29403

Ralph Snyderman • Laboratory of Immune Effector Function, Howard Hughes Medical Institute, and Division of Rheumatic and Genetic Diseases, Department of Medicine, Duke University Medical Center, Durham, North Carolina 27710

Alfred D. Steinberg • National Institutes of Health, National Institute of Arthritis, Diabetes, and Digestive and Kidney Diseases, Arthritis and Rheumatism Branch, Cellular Immunology Section, Bethesda, Maryland 20205

Samuel Strober • Department of Medicine, Division of Immunology, Stanford University Medical Center, Stanford, California 94305

Norman Talal • Clinical Immunology Section, Audie L. Murphy Memorial Veterans Administration Hospital, and Department of Medicine, The University of Texas Health Science Center at San Antonio, San Antonio, Texas 78284

Argyrios N. Theofilopoulos • Department of Immunology, Scripps Clinic and Research Foundation, La Jolla, California 92037

Jørn Thoen • Institute of Immunology and Rheumatology, Rikshospitalet, The National Hospital, Oslo, Norway

David E. Trentham • Department of Medicine, Harvard Medical School, and Department of Rheumatology and Immunology, The Brigham and Women's Hospital, Boston, Massachusetts 02115

John H. Vaughan • Department of Basic and Clinical Research, Scripps Clinic and Research Foundation, La Jolla, California 92037

Kristian Waalen • Institute of Immunology and Rheumatology, Rikshospitalet, The National Hospital, Oslo, Norway

Ralph C. Williams, Jr. • Department of Medicine, University of New Mexico School of Medicine, Albuquerque, New Mexico 87131

Nathan J. Zvaifler • Department of Medicine, School of Medicine, University of California, San Diego, California 92103

Preface

Recent developments in basic science and clinical rheumatology make it appropriate at this time to create a volume devoted to the immunology of rheumatic diseases. The impact of molecular biology, gene cloning, and new technologies for establishing hybridomas and T-cell lines in the laboratory is now beginning to be felt in clinical medicine. There is a general air of excitement and a feeling that we stand on the threshold of a new era in molecular medicine and clinical science. It is this excitement that we have tried to capture in this book.

This volume is divided into five sections entitled Basic Mechanisms, Autoimmunity, Classical Concepts of Rheumatic Diseases, Pathogenetic Mechanisms, and Therapy. This is not an arbitrary arrangement but represents our belief that from an understanding of basic mechanisms of disease pathogenesis will come new and more successful forms of treatment for the sufferers of rheumatic disorders. We have tried in the selection of authors to choose internationally recognized experts who have both a scientific and a clinical orientation to their subjects. We believe the marriage of clinical and basic disciplines represents the best hope for rapid knowledge transfer from the laboratory to the clinic, where such knowledge can be used to improve patient health.

The section on Basic Mechanisms emphasizes our belief that rheumatic diseases are fundamentally disorders of immunologic regulation based on properties of immune response genes. The five chapters proceed from analysis of the heterogeneity and structure of immune response genes through discussions of their role in immunologic networks, resulting in lymphocyte stimulation, and the production of soluble factors such as the interleukins and interferons. The importance of T-cell subpopulations and natural killer cells is emphasized.

The second section on Autoimmunity focuses on newer aspects of humoral and cellular responses to autoantigens. The selection of topics is based on those responses that appear to have pathogenetic importance and in the study of which the impact of molecular biology is most clearly evident. Four of these chapters primarily concern autoantibodies commonly seen in systemic lupus erythematosus, an indication of the importance of this disorder for understanding autoimmunity in general. Rheumatoid arthritis is represented by new information about rheumatoid factor and the immune response to collagen. The role of Ia molecules in endocrine autoimmunity is also considered in this section.

The third section concerns Classical Concepts of Rheumatic Diseases and is introduced by a consideration of infectious agents and the various ways that they can directly or indirectly lead to rheumatic disorders. Molecular mimicry and the cross-relatedness of antigens are demonstrated using rheumatic fever as a model. New developments in gout and scleroderma research are considered from the clinical point of view. Consideration of the importance of vasculitis and immune complexes in rheumatic diseases rounds out this section.

Specific Pathogenetic Mechanisms are next considered focusing on events that follow upon the abnormalities of the basic immunoregulatory mechanisms discussed in the first section. Rheumatoid arthritis serves as a model for abnormal immune interactions involving macrophages and dendritic cells, leading to abnormalities of T cells and T-cell factors. The inflammatory cascade and the neutrophil are considered from the standpoint of complement abnormalities, vasomotor lability, and mechanisms of tissue necrosis. The ability of drugs to induce rheumatic syndromes is examined, as is the very important area of psychoneuroimmunology, with its implications for the role of stress in disease mechanisms.

The final section attempts to synthesize all that has preceded it in focusing on new approaches to immunotherapy. These approaches include both immunostimulation and immunosuppression through drugs, plasmapheresis, and total lymphoid irradiation. Obviously, many different experimental approaches are being tried. We are still far from our goal of an established, rational, and specific immunotherapeutic approach to rheumatic diseases based on sound pathophysiological principles. It is to be hoped that this collection of papers on the immunology of rheumatic diseases will mark a beginning and point the way toward a time, not too distant, when this goal will be achieved.

We hope this volume will serve as a source of references to current literature on various aspects of the basic and clinical immunology of rheumatic diseases for immunologists, rheumatologists, physicians, and pediatricians, whether they be academicians or practicing clinicians.

Irvine, California Sudhir Gupta
San Antonio, Texas Norman Talal

Contents

IMMUNOLOGY OF RHEUMATIC DISEASES

I

Basic Mechanisms

1

Human Immune Response Genes

Gerald T. Nepom and John A. Hansen

I. INTRODUCTION

The generation of an immune response is a complex process requiring multiple interactions and cellular events. The genetic elements participating in immune recognition and response appear to serve as permissive signals, the "green lights" of the immune network. Their interaction provides the basis for coordinated immune function. We summarize here recent information on the nature of these inherited elements and discuss the implications of these findings for genetically determined disease susceptibility.

II. GENETICS OF IMMUNE RESPONSE

The discovery that genetically disparate strains of rodents respond differently to challenge with particular antigens dates from the early and mid-1960s and is the subject of a recent comprehensive review (Benacerraf, 1981). The early observations in guinea pigs and mice were later extended to rats and nonhuman primates and led to the general concept that certain distinct genes were critical for expression of specific immune responses. The basic observations consisted of the demonstration that challenge of one strain or individual with a particular antigen might lead to a positive immune response whereas challenge of a different strain with the same antigen would not. In animal models, backcrossing of selected strains was successfully utilized to map the "responder" phenotype. In this way, the putative genes that controlled the immune responses were localized. Many of these have been mapped to a closely linked family of genes known as the major histocompatibility complex (MHC) (Benacerraf, 1981; McDevitt, 1980; Dorf, 1981).

Gerald T. Nepom • Genetic Systems Corporation, and the University of Washington School of Medicine Seattle, Washington 98121 *John A. Hansen* • The Fred Hutchinson Cancer Research Center, the Puget Sound Blood Center, and the University of Washington School of Medicine, Seattle, Washington 98121.

III. THE HUMAN MAJOR HISTOCOMPATIBILITY COMPLEX: HLA

A. Structure of the HLA System

The human MHC is known as the human leukocyte antigen (HLA) system (Dauset, 1981). As in other species, the MHC in humans is a multigene family controlling a series of cell surface glycoproteins. These structures are readily detectable because of the profound effects they cause when presented as foreign antigen to another individual. The reaction that may follow this stimulation is called an alloimmune response. Evidence of alloimmune responses occurs when transplant patients reject grafts from other individuals or when transfused patients produce antibodies to their blood product donors.

Dausset was the first to demonstrate (Dausset and Nenna, 1952; Dausset 1954) that leukoagglutinating antibodies occurred as an immunologic response to transfusion. This was followed by the demonstration of Payne and Rolfs (1958) and van Rood *et al.* (1958) that leukocyte antibodies could also be found in the sera of multiparous women. Eventually, these alloantibodies were shown to recognize a series of highly polymorphic antigens controlled by three closely linked genes known as HLA-A,B,C. The products of the HLA-A,B,C loci are therefore said to be serologically defined. The MHC can also be defined by an *in vitro* assay known as the mixed lymphocyte culture reaction (MLR).

In the MLR, coculture of lymphocytes from different individuals results in blast transformation and cell proliferation. The MLR was found to be nonreactive between monozygotic twins, but MLR between dizygotic twins was usually positive (Bain and Lowenstein, 1964). Almost all reactions between unrelated individuals are positive, but MLR between sibling pairs can be positive or negative (Bach and Hirschhorn, 1964), suggesting that some genetic factor(s) responsible for stimulation in MLR segregate in families. Further family studies revealed that the MLR-stimulating factor(s) were linked to HLA (Amos and Bach, 1968; Albertini and Bach, 1968; Eijsvoogel *et al.*, 1970). The possibility that MLR stimulation might be controlled by a separate locus closely linked to HLA-A,B,C was suggested by Yunis and Amos (1971). Studies in HLA recombinant families established the concept that a "single distinct locus," which they named the MLR-stimulating (MLR-S) locus, was responsible for controlling T-cell recognition in MLR. The MLR-S locus is now referred to as the HLA-D region.

The HLA system is located on the short arm of chromosome 6 approximately 15 centimorgans from the centromere (Fig. 1). Four loci are formally recognized. The genes for these are designated HLA-A, B, C, and D (Teresaki, 1980). The HLA-A,B,C genes control the expression of three very similar structures known as class I products. In both humans and rodents, class I molecules are noncovalently linked heterodimers that separate under reducing conditions to one heavy chain and one light chain. The heavy chain is a glycoprotein with a relative molecular weight (M_R) of approximately 44,000, and the light chain is a polypeptide with a M_R of approximately 12,000. The gene for the class I heavy chain is located on chromosome 6, whereas the gene for the light chain known as β_2-microglobulin is found on chromosome 15. Class I gene products are expressed by virtually all nucleated cells including mature blood platelets.

B. Genes of the HLA-D Region

The HLA-D region, first known as the MLR-S locus, is homologous with the I region of H-2. Both the I region and the D region contain genes that control serologically defined

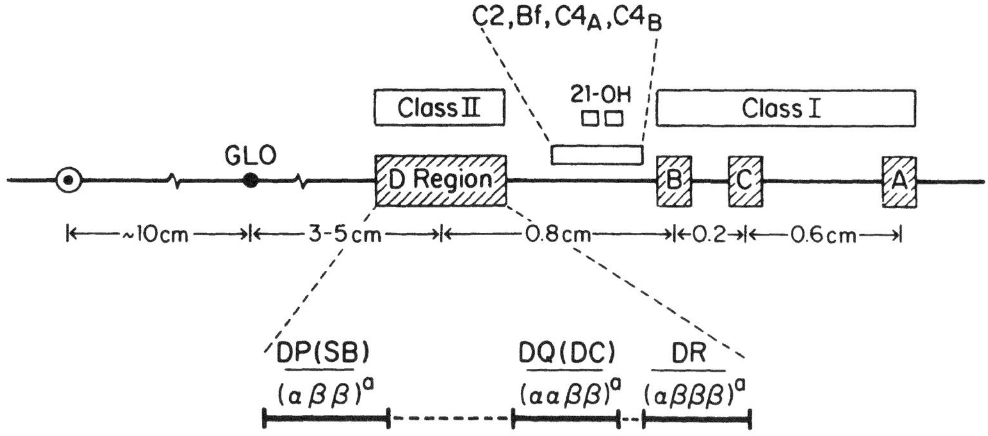

Figure 1. Genetic map of the HLA region. A tentative arrangement of α and β genes encoding class II molecules is shown mapping within the HLA-D region. [a]Exact number and linear order of α and β genes are not known.

cell surface structures referred to as class II antigens. In the mouse these are known as I-region-associated (Ia) antigens, and in humans they have been called "Ia-like," "B cell alloantigens," or D-region-associated (HLA-DR) alloantigens (Winchester and Kunkel, 1979). The latter have been classified using selected alloantisera and association analyses defining distinct specificity groups or clusters representing 14 alloantigens designated DR1 through DRw14.

1. Distinct D-Region Loci Designated DR, DQ, and DP

Studies of the HLA-D region with DNA probes have indicated the presence of at least three gene loci. These have been called DR, DQ, (previously DS or DC), and DP (previously SB) (Bodmer *et al.*, 1984). In the mouse, two I-region gene loci called I-A and I-E have been defined (Klein and Figueroa, 1981; Snell, 1981). Both human and mouse class II structures are heterodimers consisting of one heavy chain (α chain) and one light chain (β chain) (Springer *et al.*, 1977). In the mouse, the I-A locus contains at least three different genes (Aα, Aβ, Eβ), and the I-E locus at least one gene (Eα) (Jones *et al.*, 1978; Hood *et al.*, 1983). Alpha genes encode glycoproteins with M_R of approximately 34,000, which are only slightly polymorphic from one haplotype to another; when variation from allele to allele occurs, it primarily involves scattered codon and amino acid substitutions (Wake *et al.*, 1982; Larhammar *et al.*, 1982). Beta chains are glycoproteins with M_R of approximately 29,000. In mouse and man, these are highly polymorphic and contain the predominant antigenic specificities recognized by alloantiserums (Kaufman and Strominger, 1982; Walker *et al.*, 1983).

Within the HLA-D region, the DR, DQ, and DP loci contain a total of approximately five α genes and seven β genes (Shackelford *et al.*, 1982). Molecular analysis indicates that although the fundamental structures of human α and β polypeptides are very similar to each other, each locus (DR, DQ, or DP) retains some uniqueness compared to the others, reflected in conservation of particular amino acid sequences (Allison *et al.*, 1978; Bono and Strominger, 1982; Corte *et al.*, 1981; Goyert *et al.*, 1982; Hurley *et al.*, 1982). The α and β polypeptides assort intracytoplasmically in concert with a third polypeptide called the invariant chain (Day and Jones, 1983; Kvist *et al.*, 1982). Eventually one α chain and one β chain form a heterodimer that is exported to the cell membrane. The carboxy-terminal ends of both polypeptides remain intracytoplasmic, a hydrophobic portion of each passes through the plasma membrane, and the amino-terminal ends are extracellular. Thus, both α and β chains possess elements that can potentially interact with intracellular molecules or with other cells, receptors, or antigens outside the cell. A schematic model for two class II heterodimers, one DR molecule and one DQ molecule, is illustrated in Fig. 2. Each of the three D-region loci (DR, DQ, DP) contains two, three, or more genes coding for α and β chains. Thus, considerable variation can occur by selection expression of individual class II genes or by rearrangements of α and β chain combinations.

As is outlined below, such structural variations in Ia expression form the basis for polymorphic recognition among cells of the immune system. Ia molecules are produced constitutively by B cells and monocyte-macrophages. Stimuli of various sorts dramatically increase the amounts and possibly the types of Ia molecules expressed. In addition, some T cells can be induced to express Ia molecules on activation. It is the interplay among cells of these various types that determines the nature and strength of normal immune

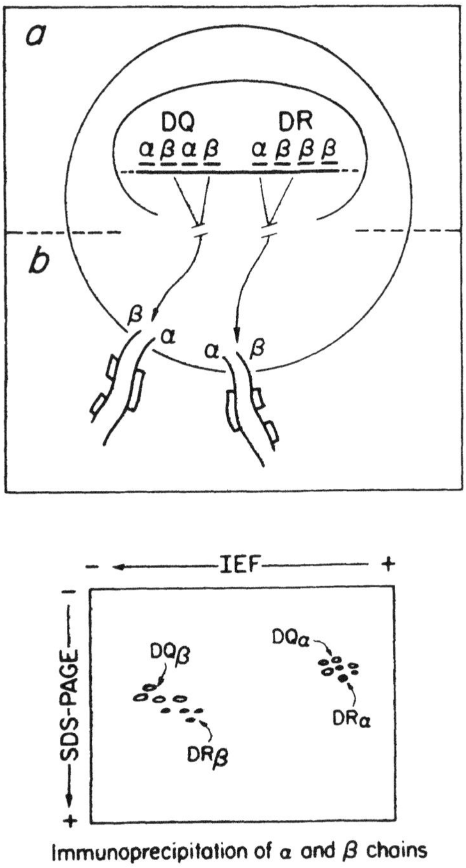

Figure 2. Schematic illustration of class II molecular synthesis and expression. Two prototype α genes and two β genes are shown (a), which encode class II polypeptides forming the heterodimers DRα DRβ and DQα DQβ. Only two such molecules are shown, but more are actually expressed in most human B cells (see text). Each αβ molecule is found on the cell surface after assembly, where it serves as a regulatory element and as a target for alloreactivity (b). One method of characterizing these molecules is illustrated in the bottom panel. Each polypeptide chain is electrophoretically distinct and will migrate with a characteristic pattern on analytic gel electrophoresis. Shown is a typical two-dimensional polyacrylamide gel separating the prototype α and β polypeptides. (Adapted from Nepom *et al.*, 1984a,b and O'Farrell *et al.*, 1977.)

response, and it is in this context that the expression of various Ia molecules by communicating lymphoid cells serves the system as a regulatory signal.

2. T-Cell Function and D-Region Products: Expression of Immune Response and Immune Suppression Phenomena

An example of how this "works" is provided by the study of immune T cells, which have a twofold specificity, for specific antigen and for the genetic element functioning as a permissive signal. This functional "dual recognition" presumably operates as specific membrane-associated receptor-mediated events among collaborating cells of the immune network. Multiple levels of interactions between different cells are involved, including T-cell–monocyte, T-cell–B-cell, and T-cell–T-cell dependent events (Neiderhuber and Frelinger, 1976; Rosenthal, 1978). When the outcome of recognition of the immune response (Ir) gene-encoded products is permissive, the immune system responds, involving many additional activition cascades. When the outcome of the interaction is negative, the immune response does not occur either simply for lack of responsive cells or because of generation of suppressor cells (Benacerraf, 1981). When suppressor cells are induced, the responsible Ir gene is often called an Is gene, for "immune suppression." In the case of MHC-linked Ir genes, some of the molecular mechanisms for these regulatory events have been intensively studied, and these form the basis for current hypotheses relating human disease and autoimmunity to specific Ir gene function.

C. Genetic Mechanisms of HLA-D Diversity

In the following sections we approach the problem of understanding Ir gene function by analyzing the mechanisms by which diversity occurs within the HLA-D region. Each of the four mechanisms discussed involves information about Ia molecular structure, which leads to some insight into expression of the Ir gene phenomenon in man.

1. Polymorphisms Exist at Multiple HLA-D Region Loci

A glance at the map of the HLA-D region illustrates the complexity of potential allelic variation. For each expressed gene locus present in an outbred population, molecular variation within that gene among different individuals translates into structural heterogeneity and potential antigenic polymorphism. The β genes of the human D region exemplify this situation. Although only a few β genes have actually been isolated and clearly identified by determination of their DNA structure, it is already apparent that the variability in primary DNA sequence is a source of considerable diversity. Substitution of individual DNA bases within the first and second extracellular coding regions translates into altered amino acids in the expressed polypeptide, so that, for example, the DR2 β sequence differs from that of the homologous β chain from a DR6 haplotype (Larhammer *et al.*, 1983; Long *et al.*, 1983; Kratzin *et al.*, 1983).

Diversity extends well beyond a comparison of the conventional DR specificities HLA-DR1 through DRw14. In a recent study of β chains expressed on cell lines derived from HLA-D homozygous donors, we have identified variation within HLA-DR4-associated haplotypes for β chains controlled by genes of at least two separate loci, DR and DQ (Nepom *et al.*, 1984a). Thus, among a series of HLA-DR4 individuals, we have identified six distinct electrophoretic β-chain variants, apparently representing allelic variation within a single β-chain locus. Each of the expressed β chains presumably shared some structural features common to all, since they all came from cells typing as DR4, yet they were clearly different gene products. Similar observations have been made for DR2 and DRw8 haplotypes (Nepom *et al.*, 1984b; Baldwin *et al.*, 1985). These studies demonstrate that multiple distinct β chains can be expressed in different individuals who carry identical serologic HLA-DR specificities. The implication of this finding for diversity and Ir genes is clear. The HLA specificities DR1 through DRw14 represent statistically defined clusters derived from the reactivity patterns of alloimmune sera. These clusters, however, do not necessarily comprise a homogeneous set of genes. The DR4 haplotype, for example, can be subdivided by HLA-D (HTC) typing and by biochemical analysis into at least six variants. From our studies of the DR4, DR2, and DR8 haplotype families, we estimate that there are at least 50 or more DR β-chain allelic variants in the population.

An additional complexity is contributed by the knowledge that more than one β chain is expressed in each individual. Indeed, most cells analyzed to date express from three to four distinct Ia molecules (Andrews *et al.*, 1982; Bohme *et al.*, 1983; de Kretser *et al.*, 1982; Karr *et al.*, 1982a; Markert and Cresswell, 1980; Shackelford *et al.*, 1983), the products of genes within the DR, DQ, and the DP loci. We have studied the allelic variants of an expressed DQ β chain within the DR4 family of haplotypes (Nepom *et al.*, 1984a). Here again, we found additional, unexpected variation. At least three distinct electrophoretic β-chain variants of DQ were expressed among cells that typed as DR4 homozygous.

Allelic variation as a source of diversity, then, is far more than contrasting DR specificities such as DR2 and DR4. The standard DR1 through DRw14 antigens actually represent public serologic determinants that define clusters of similar but not necessarily identical haplotypes. These "DR-defined" haplotypes may have evolutionary significance, but they do not describe unique D-region polymorphisms. As a consequence, conventional HLA-DR serologic specificities are not necessarily appropriate markers for specific Ir genes. Some other determinants such as more selective serologic markers, biochemical analysis, or cellular typing by MLC may provide informative means for identifying and analyzing functionally relevant molecular variants within the HLA-D region.

2. *Epitopes Define Structural and Functional Properties of Human Class II Molecules*

An epitope is a name given by immunologists to that portion of a target structure ("antigen") that is complementary to the binding site of a ligand (antibody molecule or T-cell receptor). Each class II gene product is a complex polypeptide with multiple epitopes, which may function in cell interactions. Whenever the structure of a particular D-region α or β chain is altered so that a particular epitope is changed, it becomes a molecule with potentially altered function.

The variable expression of particular epitopes, then, is a source of functional diversity for Ir genes. This is not, however, the same mechanism as allelic variation mentioned above. Each of the serologically defined specificities, including the standard HLA-DR1 through DRw14, may be expressed on one or more HLA-encoded Ia molecules. As indicated by the + symbols in Table I, for instance, the DR4 specificity represents an

Table 1. HLA Class II Epitopes Mapped to Specific HLA-D Region Loci: A Partial Epitope Map Illustrating the Relationship Between HLA-DR/DQ Specificities and Specific HLA-Encoded Molecules[a]

	Dw4		Dw5		Dw7		Dw10		Dw15	
Serologic specificities	DR	DQ	DR	DQ	DR	DQ	DR	DQ	DR	DQ
Epitopes defined by alloantisera										
DR4[b,c]	+	–	–	–	–	–	+	–	+	–
DR5[d]	–	–	+	±	–	–	–	–	–	–
DRw52[d]	–	–	+	+	–	–	–	–	–	–
DQw3	–	+	–	+	–	–				
DQw1	–	–	–	–	–	–	–	–	–	–
Unique epitopes defined by monoclonal antibodies										
17.15[b]	?	+	?	+					–	–
IVD12[f]	?	+								
SG465[b,e]	–	+	–	+	–	+	–	+	–	+
109d6[e]	–	+			+	–				

[a] Each DR or DQ locus may encode more than one class II molecule.
[b] Nepom *et al.* (1984a), and unpublished data.
[c] Maeda and Hirata (1984).
[d] Karr *et al.* (1982b, 1983).
[e] Goyert and Silver (1983); Goyert *et al.* (1983).
[f] Giles *et al.* (1983).

epitope present on Ia molecules encoded within the DR locus of cells which constitute the HLA-D defined clusters Dw4, Dw10 and Dw15. In fact, six different haplotypes including these two have been identified which contain Ia molecules bearing the DR4 specificity (Nepom, *et al.*, 1983; Groner, *et al.*, 1983). The assignment of a particular serologic specificity to a unique epitope sometimes demonstrates unexpected relatedness between loci: for instance, the epitope defining the allospecificity HLA-DR5 has been detected on products of both the DR and DQ loci (Karr, *et al.*, 1983). Similarly, the supratypic specificity DRw52 (MT2), found on haplotypes positive for DR2, DR3 and DR5, is detected on both DR- and DQ-encoded molecules derived from DR5 haplotypes (Karr, *et al.*, 1982b). The DQw3 (MT4) supratypic specificity has been detected on DQ-encoded molecules derived from either DR4 or DR5 haplotypes (Goyert and Silver, 1983). Even when two molecules share a particular epitope, as in the case of DQw3 on some DR4 and DR5 haplotypes, these molecules are distinct and differ from each other in various portions of their structures.

These examples clearly indicate extensive complexity of molecular diversity among Ir genes both at the haplotype level and at the level of individual D-region loci (DR, DQ, DP, etc.), and they demonstrate that a specific gene or epitope identified on one haplotype may occur at a different locus on another haplotype.

Since Ir gene-mediated events primarily represent interactions between cells, the most relevant functional epitopes are not necessarily those recognized by alloimmume sera. It is more likely that those epitopes recognized by T cells are the functional elements related to Ir phenomena. Any particular HLA class II molecule can potentially display several distinct epitopes, some of which may be recognized serologically, although others may only be recognized by immune T cells (Table 2).

Table 2. HLA Class II Molecules Contain Multiple Functional Epitopes

A. Alloimmune response epitopes
 1. Defined serologically
  DR specificities
  DQ specificities
 2. Defined by T-cell recognition
  HLA-D specificities
  DP/PLT specificities
B. Normal immune response epitopes
 1. Defined by HLA-restricted T-cell responses
  Antigen-specific T helper cell responses/proliferation
  Antigen-specific cytotonic T-cell (CTL) responses
 2. Defined by response to particular antigens

T cells recognizing allogeneic Ia molecules are considered representative of normal antigen-responsive T cells, since many antigen-specific T-cell clones also display alloreactivity (Benacerraf and Burakoff, 1978). This has led to the concept that recognition of alloantigen is essentially equivalent to the recognition of autologous Ia and foreign antigen ("self + *X*").

It has been observed for several years that alloimmune T cells recognize specificities distinct from the DR serologic specificities. In other words, some cells sharing the same DR specificity express different D antigens (Fuller *et al.*, 1978; Suciu-Foca *et al.*, 1981; Reinsmoen and Bach, 1982; Nose *et al.*, 1982; Mickelson *et al.*, 1983). In our analysis of the differing HLA-D antigens expressed by cells of the DR4 haplotype, we found a striking correlation between expression of a particular polymorphic DR β chain and the HLA-D specificities associated with DR4 (Nepom *et al.*, 1983). Our interpretation of these findings was that the HLA-D specificity reflects an epitope recognized by T cells that is expressed on multiple β-chain variants. Evidence to support this hypothesis comes from a similar study of the DR2 specificity, where two DR β chains were identified, only one of which varied with HLA-D type and therefore probably carried the D-specific epitope (Nepom *et al.*, 1984b).

In the case of antigen-specific T-cell responses, Ia recognition is also likely to be epitope specific. Recent analyses using human T-cell clones have shown that antigen recognition can be restricted to Ia epitopes similar to or identical with serologically defined specificities. Ball and Stastny (1984) have described a mumps-antigen-specific T-cell clone that only reacted with MT-3 positive antigen-presenting cells. Other investigators have described antigen-specific T-cell clones that appear to subdivide serologically defined specificities (Jacobsen *et al.*, 1985).

3. Heterozygous Individuals May Express Unique Epitopes with Combinatorial Determinants

Conceptually, epitopes should be regarded as "three-dimensional" elements and thus as conformation dependent. This model is consistent with the observations mentioned above for alloimmune T-cell responses, which appear to be functionally analogous to the conventional immune recognition occurring when immuno T cells recognize specific antigens in a process that requires simultaneous recognition of "self." When extended to consideration of Ir gene-regulated events, the notion of conformation-dependent epitopes has one additional feature. Since each Ia molecule is a heterodimer consisting of one α and one β chain, differential assortment of distinct α chains with the same β chain (or vice versa) might create novel combinatorial determinants, which potentially could function as distinct epitopes (Fig. 3).

There is evidence from experimental animals that novel determinants presumably arising from a combinatorial mechanism can operate to generate genetic diversity within heterozygous individuals. In this model, α chains genetically derived from one parent and β chains from the other assort within the offspring to generate novel heterodimers expressing unique antigenic determinants. These combinatorial epitopes have been recognized both serologically by monoclonal antibodies (LaFuse *et al.*, 1980a,b) and functionally by T cell clones (Beck *et al.*, 1982).

It is not known whether this phenomenon also exists in humans. There are, however, two examples of HLA–disease associations in which this kind of gene complementation may occur. Type I insulin-dependent diabetes mellitus (IDDM) has been associated in various populations with two different HLA specificities, HLA-DR3 and DR4. The relative risk for individuals positive for both DR3 and DR4 is greater than the relative risk for DR3,3 or DR4,4 homozygotes (Svejgaard and Ryder, 1981). A second example of this phenomenon occurs in children with seropositive juvenile rheumatoid arthritis. This disease, like rheumatoid arthritis in adults, is associated with HLA-DR4. The frequency of DR4 in the childhood form is 85% (Nepom *et al.*, 1984c). More strikingly, the frequency

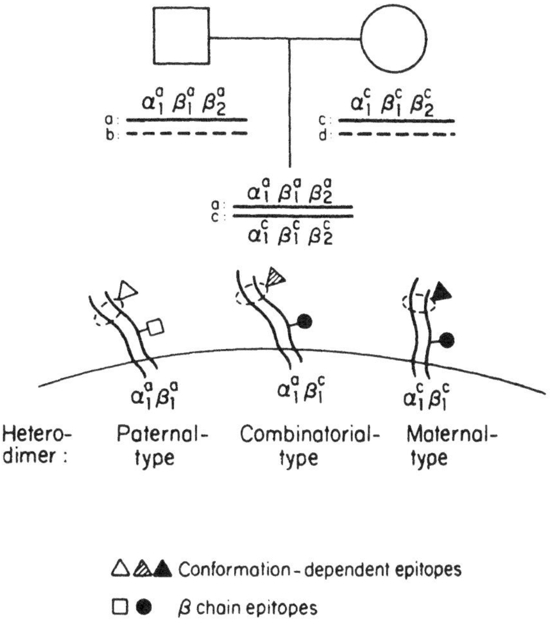

Figure 3. Combinatorial epitopes associated with class II molecules. The association between α and β chains potentially forms conformation-dependent epitopes, as shown schematically for one α:β heterodimer formed in the progeny of two HLA-disparate parents. Other combinatorial epitopes (not shown) could also be expressed in the same offspring, such as those associated with an $\alpha_1^c\ \beta_1^a$ heterodimer.

of DR4 homozygotes among the patients was 54% compared to 3% for normal controls. When the DR4 homozygotes were studied in detail, however, it was apparent that most were actually heterozygous for two distinct DR4 variants known as Dw4 and LD"40." The presence in these patients of one Dw4 haplotype and one LD"40" is a further example of how gene complementation for D-region products may be functionally significant and in this case confer increased disease risk. This example is also potential evidence that combinatorial mechanisms may play a role in generating D-region diversity, thereby contributing to immune function.

We should repeat the point that combinatorial mechanisms in humans have not been proven. There are alternative explanations for the heterozygous disease associations mentioned above, such as the presence of complementary or *trans*-acting genetic elements that are expressed when two haplotypes are present (Fathman *et al.*, 1981; Gladstone and Pious, 1980). Furthermore, the model requires sufficient polymorphism among α chains so that the probability for combinatorial associations with β chains would be high.

IV. THE EXPRESSION OF PARTICULAR HLA-D EPITOPES VARIES ON CELLS OF DIFFERENT ORIGIN

An additional mechanism that could contribute significantly to the role that D-region products might play as receptors for Ir or Is function has recently been described as a result of observations demonstrating unexpected or altered Ia expression on various cell types. Human Ia molecules have generally been found on β cells, monocytes, activated T cells, some bone marrow cells, and some leukemic cells. Several recent investigations, however, have reported unexpected variations in Ia expression. Shipp *et al.*, (1983) have described a unique "Ia-like" antigen that appears to be distinct from other D-region molecules. This antigen was found on mature B cells and B-lymphoblastoid cell lines but not on monocytes or activated T cells. Biochemical studies identified this putative B-cell-specific molecule as a distinct "Ia-like" product. These findings are similar to the observations of Torok-Storb *et al.* (1983), who demonstrated the expression of a DR4 β chain, defined by monoclonal antibody 17.15, on B cells and B-lymphoblastoid cell lines but not on monocytes or hematopoietic precursor cells (BFU-E). In contrast to the previous observation, however, the 17.15 epitope was also expressed on activated T cells.

A growing number of investigators have now described additional Ia antigens or molecules that are expressed only after cell activation. Newman *et al.* (1983) and Wang *et al.* (1983) have found that DQ molecules are expressed at greatly enhanced levels on T cells and precursor B cells following activation. Concomitant changes in DR antigens were not observed. Since DQ expression normally appears to be low on immature cells, the quantitative increase is seen after activation might be functionally significant. Fuggle *et al.* (1983) have described a similar observation using a monoclonal antibody that recognizes Ia-like molecules only on activated but not on resting B cells. These authors suggest that additional determinants or epitopes may be expressed on preexisting Ia molecules during the activation process, presumably as a result of conformational changes. The mechanisms by which such diverse expression might affect lineage-specific functions are, at this point, entirely obscure.

V. EVIDENCE FOR GENETIC CONTROL OF IMMUNE RESPONSE IN HUMANS

A. Association and Linkage of Immune Response Genes to HLA

The first evidence that immune responsiveness in humans was related to HLA came from studies demonstrating that among unrelated individuals statistical associations exist between responsiveness to certain antigens and HLA. These observations have been made for a series of antigens (see Table 3), testing responses *in vivo* to vaccines by assaying specific antibody titers or responses *in vitro* by assaying T cell proliferation. The association analysis eventually focused on the HLA-D region from the demonstration that responses to specific antigens, such as tetanus toxoid and schistosomal worm antigen, were associated with certain HLA-D antigens (Table 3). Low responsiveness to schistosomal worm antigen *in vitro* was associated with DR2,Dw12 in Japanese (Sasazuki *et al.*, 1980a), and low responsiveness to tetanus toxoid was associated with the Japanese HLA-D specificity DHO (Sasazuki *et al.*, 1978b).

The demonstration that Ir genes were actually linked to HLA, however, required family studies. The first such studies reported (Table 3) described results of immune response testing *in vitro* to measles antigens (Haverkorn *et al.*, 1975) streptococcal

Table 3. Association and Linkage of Immune Responses with HLA

Antigen[a]	Reference
HLA association studies	
In vitro responses	
Streptococcal antigen	Greenberg *et al.* (1975)
Vaccinia virus	de Vries *et al.* (1977)
Tetanus toxoid	Sasazuki *et al.* (1978b)
In vivo responses	
Influenza A vaccine	Spencer *et al.* (1976)
Rubella vaccine	Kato *et al.* (1978)
HLA-D association studies	
In vitro responses	
Tetanus toxoid: low Responses associated with HLA-Dw12(LD"DHO")	Sasazuki *et al.* (1978b)
SWA: low responses associated with DR2, Dw12	Sasazuki *et al.* (1980a)
HLA linkage studies	
In vitro responses	
Measles antigen	Haverkorn *et al.* (1975)
Streptococcal antigen	Greenberg *et al.* (1980)
SCW antigen	Sasazuki *et al.* (1980b)
(T,G)-A—L	Hsu *et al.* (1981)

[a] SWA, schistosomal worm antigens; SCW, streptococcal cell wall; (T,G)-A—L, synthetic polypeptide copolymer containing tyrosine, glutamine, alanine, and lysine.

antigens (Greenberg *et al.*, 1980), and the synthetic polypeptide (T,G)–A—L (Hsu *et al.*, 1981), all of which suggested the existence of HLA-linked Ir genes. This type of linkage analysis was extended by Sasazuki *et al.* (1980b), who analyzed not only the mode of inheritance but also the cellular mechanisms involved. With streptococcal cell wall (SCW) antigen-specific T-cell proliferation used as a model, "high" and "low" responders were defined by a frequency distribution analysis of the response (the natural logarithm of the counters per minute). Each member of the 23 families tested was then assigned either "high" or "low" for responder phenotype. Many "high" responder children were found in families where both parents were "low" responders, leading to the hypothesis that "low" responsiveness to SCW antigen is controlled by a single recessive gene. When all informative "backcross" families were analyzed, two genetic models remained tenable: (1) simple inheritance of a recessive "high" responder gene; or (2) simple inheritance of a dominant "low" responder gene.

B. Linkage of Immune Suppressor Genes to HLA

Further examination of informative families suggested a very close linkage between HLA and "low" responsiveness (maximum lod score = 4.311 was obtained at $\theta = 0.00$), and a population study among Japanese revealed a frequency for the HLA-linked "low" responder gene of 0.235 (Sasazuki *et al.*, 1983). Association analysis revealed that the gene for "low" responsiveness to SCW antigen was in linkage disequilibrium with HLA-MT1, a supratypic HLA-D specificity. By separating T cells into helper (T_H) and suppressor (T_S) subsets, it was shown that proliferative responses to SCW antigen were mediated by T_H cells, whereas "low" responses to SCW antigen were mediated by T_S cells (Nishimura and Sasazuki, 1983). T cells from "low" responders failed to respond even in the presence of monocytes from "high" responders, whereas T cells from "high" responders responded well even if "low"-responder monocytes were used as the antigen presenting cells (APC). Therefore, the dominant human gene for "low" responsiveness to SCW antigen is analogous to the immune suppressor (Is) genes described in the mouse (Dorf, 1981). These genes control immune responsiveness by inducing T_S cells, which in turn inhibit the responses of T_H cells.

These examples of population studies provide the best evidence that control over immune responses to certain antigens resides within the HLA-D region. The mechanisms for this control are apparently based on the critical recognition by T cells of "antigen + Ia" (on the surface of an antigen presenting cell), a cellular interaction that is presumed to occur *in vivo*. The *in vitro* model for this phenomenon (cited above) is dependent on the recognition by antigen-reactive T cells of the appropriate D-region-encoded class II epitope. In those types of experiments, T cells have been shown to be dependent on recognition of either DR-, DQ-, or DP-encoded molecules (Berle and Thorsby, 1982; Eckels *et al.*, 1983; Gonwa *et al.*, 1983b); thus, it is likely that each of these loci also potentially controls functional Ir-gene products *in vivo*.

VI. CONCLUDING REMARKS

We have tried in this chapter to describe experimental observations that support the hypothesis that human Ir genes exist and are found within the HLA system. Population studies have indicated that certain genetic elements have significant effects on the specific immune responses to a number of antigens. Some of these genetic elements are associated with, and some are linked to, particular HLA specificities. Our ability to recognize distinct HLA class II determinants or epitopes, however, has until recently been very limited. Combined biochemical, serologic, and molecular approaches have enabled us to recognize a number of mechanisms for generating diversity within the D region whereby the expression of certain epitopes might contribute to immune responsiveness. These functionally relevant Ia-encoded epitopes arise from the genetic complexity of the HLA-D region, and eventually knowledge about their interactions with T-cell receptors will provide the basis for understanding Ir and Is gene phenomena as well as normal and abnormal immune responsiveness.

REFERENCES

Albertini, R. J., and Bach, F. H., 1968, Quantitative assay of antigenic disparity of HLA—the major histocompatibility locus in man, *J. Exp. Med.* **128:**639–651.

Allison, J. P., Walker, L. E., Russell, W. A., Pellegrino, M. A., Ferrone, S., Reisfield, R. A., Frelinger, J. A., and Silver, J., 1978, Murine Ia and human DR antigens: Homology of amino-terminal sequences, *Proc. Natl. Acad. Sci. U.S.A.* **74:**5135–5139.

Amos, D. B., and Bach, F. H., 1968, Phenotypic expressions of the major histocompatibility locus in man (HLA): Leukocyte antigens and mixed leukocyte culture reactivity, *J. Exp. Med.* **128:**623–637.

Andrews, D. W., Bono, M. R., and Strominger, J. L., 1982, A homozygous human cell line contains three subsets of HLA-DR-like antigens distinguishable by amino acid sequencing, *Biochemistry* **21:**6625–6628.

Bach, F. H., and Hirschhorn, K., 1964, Lymphocyte interaction: A potential histocompatibility test *in vitro, Science* **143:**813–814.

Bain, B., and Lowenstein, L., 1964, Genetic studies on the mixed leukocyte reaction, *Science* **145:**1315–1316.

Baldwin, G. C., Mickelson, E., Hansen, J. A., Nisperos, B., Antonelli, P., Nepom, B. S., and Nepom, G. T., 1985, Electrophoretic variation between class II molecules expressed on HLA-DRw homozygous typing cells reveals multiple distinct haplotypes, *Immunogenetics* **31:**49–60.

Ball, E. J., and Stastney, P., 1984, Antigen-specific HLA-restricted human T-cell lines, *Immunogenetics* **19:**13–26.

Beck, B. N., Frelinger, J. G., Shigeta, M., Infante, A. J., Cummings, D., Hammerling, G., and Fathman, C. G., 1982, T cell clones specific for hybrid 1-A molecules, *J. Exp. Med.* **156:**1186–1194.

Benacerraf, B., 1981, Role of MHC gene products in immune regulation, *Science* **212:**1229–1238.

Benacerraf, B., and Burakoff, S. J., 1978, The biological significance of alloreactivity, in: *Genetic Control of Autoimmune Disease* (N. Rose, E. Bigazzi, and N. Warner, eds.), Elsevier, Amsterdam, pp. 321–326.

Berle, E., and Thorsby, E., 1982, Both DR and MT Class II HLA molecules may restrict proliferative T-lymphocyte responses to antigen, *Scand. J. Immunol.* **16:**543–547.

Bodmer, J., and Bodmer, W., 1984, Histocompatibility, *Immunol. Today* **5:**251–254.

Bohme, J., Owerback, D., Denaro, M., Lernmark, A., Peterson, P. A., and Rask, L., 1983, Human class II major histocompatibility antigen β chains are derived from at least three loci, *Nature* **301:**82–84.

Bono, M. R., and Strominger, J. L., 1982, Direct evidence of homology between human DC-1 antigen and murine 1-A molecules, *Nature* **299:**836–838.

Corte, G., Calabi, F., Damiani, G., Bargellesi, A., Tosi, R., and Sorrentino, R., 1981, Human Ia molecules carrying DC1 determinants differ in both α- and β-subunits from Ia molecules carrying DR determinants, *Nature* **292:**357–360.

Dausset, J., 1954, Leuco-agglutinins. IV. Leuco-agglutinins and blood transfusion, *Vox Sang.* **4:**190–198.

Dausset, J., 1981, The major histocompatibility complex in man, *Science* **213:**1469–1474.

Dausset, J., and Nenna, A., 1952, Presence d'une leuco-agglutinine dans le serum d'un cas d'agranulocytose chronique, *C. R. Soc. Biol. (Paris)* **146:**1539–1541.

Day, C. E., and Jones, P. O., 1983, The gene encoding the 1a antigen-associated invariant chain (II) is not linked to the H-2 complex, *Nature* **302:**157–159.

de Kretser, T. A., Crumpton, M. J., Bodmer, J., and Bodmer, W. F., 1982, Two-dimensional gel analysis of the polypeptides precipitated by a polymorphic HLA-DR1, 2, w6 monoclonal antibody: Evidence for a third locus, *Eur. J. Immunol.* **12:**600–606.

Dorf, M. E., 1981, Genetic control of immune responsiveness, in: *The Role of the Major Histocompatibility Complex in Immunobiology* (M. E. Dorf, ed.), Garland, New York, pp. 221–254.

Eckels, D., Lake, P., Lamb, J., Johnson, A., Shaw, S., Woody, J., and Hartzkan, R., 1983, SB-restricted presentation of influenza and herpes simplex virus antigens to human T-lymphocyte clones, *Nature* **301:**716–718.

Eijsvoogel, V. P., Schellekens, P. T. A., Breur-Vriesendorp, B., van Leeuwen, A., Koch, C., and van Rood, J. J., 1970, HLA identity and one allelic differences in families and unrelated individuals, in: *Histocompatibility Testing 1970* (P. I. Terasaki, ed.), Munksgaard, Copenhagen, pp. 523–529.

Fathman, C. G., Kimoto, M., Melvold, R., and David, C., 1981, Reconstitution of Ir genes, Ia antigens, and mixed lymphocyte reaction determinants by gene complementation, *Proc. Natl. Acad. Sci. U.S.A.* **78:**1853–1857.

Fuggle, S., Kirkley, J., Ting, A., and Morris, P. J., 1983, A monoclonal antibody recognizing HLA-DR2 on malignant and activated cells, *Immunogenetics* **18:**415–428.

Fuller, T. C., Einarson, M., Pinto, C., Ahern, A., and Yunis, E. J., 1978, Genetic evidence that HLA-DR (Ia) specificities include multiple HLA-D determinants on a single haplotype, *Transplant. Proc.* **10:**781.

Giles, R., Nunez, G., Hurley, C., Nunez-Roldan, A., Winchester, R., Stastny, P., and Capra, J. D., 1983, Structural analysis of a human I-A homologue using a monoclonal antibody that recognizes an MB-3 like specificity, *J. Exp. Med.* **157:**1461–1470.

Gladstone, P., and Pious, D., 1980, Identification of a transacting function regulating HLA-DR expression in a DR-negative cell variant, *Somat. Cell Genet.* **6:**285–298.

Gonwa, T., Peterlin, B. M., and Stobo, J. D., 1983a, Human Ir genes: Structure and function, *Adv. Immunol.* **34:**71–96.

Gonwa, T., Picker, L., Raff, H., Goyert, S., Silver, J., and Stobo, J., 1983b, Antigen-presenting capabilities of human monocytes correlates with their expression of HLA-DS, an Ia determinant distinct from HLA-DR, *J. Immunol.* **130:**706–711.

Goyert, S. M., and Silver, J., 1983, Further characterization of HLA-DS molecules: Implications for studies assessing the role of human Ia molecules in cell interactions and disease susceptibility, *Proc. Natl. Acad. Sci. U.S.A.* **80:**5719–5723.

Goyert, S. M., Shively, J. E., and Silver, J., 1982, Biochemical characterization of a second family of human Ia molecules, HLA-DS, equivalent to murine I-A subregion molecules, *J. Exp. Med.* **156:**550–556.

Goyert, S. M., Moriuchi, J., Winchester, R. J., and Silver, J., 1983, HLA-DS molecules and their relation to supertypic specificities, *Hum. Immunol.* **8:**53–63.

Groner, J. P., Watson, A. J., and Bach, F. H., 1983, Dw/LD-related molecular polymorphism of DR4 β chains, *J. Exp. Med.* **157:**1687–1691.

Greenberg, L. J., Gray, E. D., and Yunis, E. J., 1975, Association of HLA-5 and immune responsiveness *in vitro* to streptococcal antigens, *J. Exp. Med.* **141:**935–943.

Greenberg, L. J., Bradley, P. W., Chopyk, R. L., and Lalovel, J. M., 1980, Immunogenetics of response to a purified antigen from group A streptococci, II Linkage of reponse to HLA, *Immunogenetics* **11:**161–167.

Haverkorn, M. J., Hofman, B., Masurel, N., and van Rood, J. J., 1975, HLA-linked genetic control of immune response in man, *Transplant Rev.* **22:**120–124.

Hood, L., Steinmetz, M., and Malissen, B., 1983, Genes of the major histocompatibility complex of the mouse, *Annu. Rev. Immunol.* **1:**529–568.

Hsu, S. H., Chan, M. M., and Bias, W. B., 1981, Genetic control of major histocompatibility complex-linked immune responses to synthetic polypeptides in man, *Proc. Natl. Acad. Sci. U.S.A.* **78:**440–444.

Hurley, C. K., Shaw, S., Nadler, L., Schlossman, S., and Capra, J. D., 1982, Alpha and beta chains of SB and DR antigens are structurally distinct, *J. Exp. Med.* **156:**1557–1562.

Jacobson, S., Nepom, G. T., Richert, J. R., Biddison, W. E., and McFarland, H. F., 1985, Identification of a specific HLA DR2 Ia molecule as a restriction element for measles virus-specific HLA class II-restricted cytotoxic T cell clones, *J. Exp. Med.* **161:**263–268.

Jones, P. P., Murphy, D. B., and McDevitt, H. O., 1978, Two gene control of the expression of a murine Ia antigen, *J. Exp. Med.* **148:**925–939.

Karr, R. W., Kannapell, C., Stein, J., Fuller, T., Duquesnoy, R., Rodey, G., Mann, D., Gebel, H., and Schwartz, B. D., 1982a, Demonstration of a third structurally distinct human Ia beta chain by two-dimensional gel electrophoresis, *J. Exp. Med.* **156**:652–657.

Karr, R. W., Kannapell, C., Stein, J., Gebel, H., Mann, D., Duquesnoy, R., Fuller, T., Rodey, G., and Schwartz, B. D., 1982b, Molecular relationships of the human B cell alloantigens, MT2, MB3, MT4, and DR5, *J. Immunol.* **128**:1809–1818.

Karr, R., Kannapell, C., Zangara, R., Goyert, S., Silver, J., and Schwartz, B. D., 1983, An HLA-DR5 homozygous cell line expresses two DS (I-A-like) molecules, *J. Exp. Med.* **158**:1374–1379.

Kato, S., Kimura, M., Takahura, I., Sakakibara, T., Inoue, H., and Tsuji, K., 1978, Possible associations between HLA antigens and the immune responsiveness to attenuated rubella vaccine, *Tissue Antigens* **11**:475–478.

Kaufman, J. F., and Strominger, J. L., 1982, HLA-DR light chain has a polymorphic N-terminal region and a conserved 1g-like C-terminal region, *Nature* **297**:694–697.

Klein, J., and Figueroa, F., 1981, Polymorphism of the mouse H-2 loci, *Immunol. Rev.* **60**:23–51.

Kratzin, H., Yang, C., Gotz, H., Thinnes, F. P., Kruse, T., Egert, G., Pauly, E., Kolbel, S., Wernet, P., and Hilschmann, N., 1983, Heterogeneity of class II histocompatibility antigens isolated from a human lymphoblastoid B cell line homozygous at the HLA Loci, *Hum. Immunol.* **8**:65–73.

Kvist, S., Wiman, K., Claesson, L., Peterson, P. A., and Dobberstein, B., 1982, Membrane insertion and oligomeric assembly of HLA-DR histocompatibility antigens, *Cell* **29**:61–69.

LaFuse, W., McCormick, J., Corser, P., and David, C., 1980a, Gene complementations to generate Ia antigens (Ia.23) on hybrid molecules, *Transplantation* **30**:341–346.

LaFuse, W. P., McCormick, J. F., and David, C. S., 1980b, Serological and biochemical identification of hybrid 1a antigens, *J. Exp. Med.* **151**:709–715.

Larhammar, D., Schenning, L., Gustafsson, K., Wiman, K., Claesson, L., Rask, L., and Peterson, P., 1982, Complete amino acid sequence of an HLA-DR antigen-like β chain as predicted from the nucleotide sequence; similarities with immunoglobulins and HLA-A-B and -C antigens, *Proc. Natl. Acad. Sci. U.S.A.* **79**:3687–3691.

Larhammer, D., Andersson, A., Andersson, M., Bill, P., Bohme, J., Claesson, L., Denaro, M., Emmoth, E., Gustafsson, K., Hammarling, V., Heldin, E., Hyldig-Nielsen, J. J., Lind, P., Schenning, L., Servenius, B., Widmark, E., Rask, L., and Peterson, P. A., 1983, Molecular analysis of human class II transplantation antigens and their genes, *Hum. Immunol.* **8**:95–103.

Long, E. Gorski, J., Rollini, P., Wake, C. T., Strubin, M., Rabomdin-Combe, C., and Mach, B., 1983, Molecular Analysis of the genes for human class II antigens of the major histocompatibility complex, *Hum. Immunol.* **8**:113–121.

Maeda, H., and Hirata, R., 1984, Molecular identifications of HLA-DR4, MT3, and TB21 antigens on HLA-DR4 homozygous B cell lines, *J. Immunol.* **132**:574–577.

Markert, M. L., and Cresswell, P., 1980, Polymorphism of human B-cell alloantigens: Evidence for three loci within the HLA system, *Proc. Natl. Acad. Sci. U.S.A.* **77**:6101–6104.

McDevitt, H. O., 1980, Regulation of the immune response by the major histocompatibility system, *N. Engl. J. Med.* **303**:1514–1517.

Mickelson, E. M., Nisperos, B., Layrisse, Z., Kim, S. J., Thomas, E. D., and Hansen, J. A., 1983, Analysis of the HLA-DRw8 haplotype: Recognition by HTC typing of three distinct antigen complexes in Caucasians, Native Americans, and Orientals, *Immunogenetics* **17**:399–410.

Neiderhuber, J. E., and Frelinger, J. A., 1976, Expression of Ia antigens on T and B cells and their relationship to immune-response functions, *Transplant. Rev.* **30**:101–130.

Nepom, B. S., Nepom, G. T., Mickelson, E., Antonelli, P., and Hansen, J. A., 1983, Electrophoretic analysis of human HLA-DR antigens from HLA-DR4 homozygous cell lines: Correlation between β chain diversity and HLA-D, *Proc. Natl. Acad. Sci. U.S.A.* **80**:6962–6966.

Nepom, G. T., Nepom, B. S., Antonelli, P., Mickelson, E., Silver, J., Goyert, S. M., and Hansen, J. A., 1984a, The HLA-DR4 family of haplotypes consist of a series of distinct DR and DS molecules, *J. Exp. Med.* **159**:394–404.

Nepom, G. T., Nepom, B., Wilson, M., Mickelson, E., Antonelli, P., and Hansen, J. A., 1984b, Multiple "Ia-like" molecules characterize HLA-DR2-associated haplotypes which differ in HLA-D, *Hum. Immunol.* **10**:143–151.

Nepom, B. S., Nepom, G. T., Mickelson, E., Schaller, J. A., Antonelli, P., and Hansen, J. A., 1984c,

Specific HLA-DR4-associated histocompatibility molecules characterize patients with juvenile rheumatoid arthritis, *J. Clin. Invest.* **74**:287–291.

Newman, R., Delia, D., Greaves, M., Navarrete, C., Fainboim, L., and Festenstein, H., 1983, Differential expression of HLA-DR and DR-linked determinants on human leukemias and lymphoid cells, *Eur. J. Immunol.* **13**:172–176.

Nishimura, Y., and Sasazuki, T., 1982, HLA-linked immune suppression gene for streptococcal cell wall antigen, *Nature* **302**:67–69.

Nose, Y., Sato, K., Nakagawa, N., Kondoh, K., Inouye, H., and Tsuji, K., 1982, HLA-D clusters associated with DR4 in the Japanese population, *Hum. Immunol.* **5**:199–203.

O'Farrell, P. Z., Goodman, H. M., and O'Farrell, P. H., 1977, High resolution two-dimensional electrophoresis of basic as well as acidic proteins, *Cell* **12**:1133–1142.

Payne, R., and Rolfs, M. R., 1958, Fetomaternal leukocyte incompatibility, *J. Clin. Invest.* **37**:1756–1763.

Reinsmoen, N. L., and Bach, F. H., 1982, Five HLA-D clusters associated with HLA-DR4, *Hum. Immunol.* **4**:249–258.

Rosenthal, A. S., 1978, Determinant selection and macrophage function in genetic control of the immune response, *Immunol. Rev.* **40**:136–152.

Sasazuki, T., Kohno, Y., Iwamoto, I., Tanimura, M., and Naito, S., 1978b, Association between and HLA haplotype and low responsiveness to tetanus toxoid in man, *Nature* **272**:359–360.

Sasazuki, T., Ohta, N., Isohisa, I., Numano, F., and Maezawa, H., 1979a, Association between Takayasu disease and HLA-DHO, *Tissue Antigens* **14**:177–178.

Sasazuki, T., Hayase, R., Iwamoto, I., and Tsuchida, H., 1979b, HLA and acute poststreptococcal glomerulonephritis, *N. Engl. J. Med.* **301**:1184–1185.

Sasazuki, T., Ohta, N., Kaneoka, R., and Kojima, S., 1980a, Association between and HLA haplotype and low responsiveness to schistosomal worm antigen in man, *J. Exp. Med.* **152**:314s–318s.

Sasazuki, T., Kaneoka, H., Nishimura, Y., Kaneoka, R., Hayama, M., and Okhuni, H., 1980b, An HLA-linked immune suppression gene in man, *J. Exp. Med.* **152**:297s–313s.

Sasazuki, T., Nishimura, Y., Muto, M., and Ohta, N., 1983, HLA-linked genes controlling immune response and disease susceptibility, *Immunol. Rev.* **70**:51–75.

Shackelford, D. A., Kaufman, J. F., Korman, A. J., and Strominger, J. L., 1982, HLA-DR antigens: Structure, separation of subpopulations, gene cloning and function, *Immunol. Rev.* **66**:133–187.

Shackelford, D. A., Lampson, L. A., and Strominger, J. A., 1983, Separation of three class II antigens from a homozygous human B cell line, *J. Immunol.* **130**:289–296.

Shipp, M., Schwartz, B., Kannapell, C., Griffith, R., Scott, M., Ahmed, P., David, J. M., and Nahm, M., 1983, A unique DR-related B cell differentiation antigen, *J. Immunol.* **131**:2458–2467.

Snell, G. D., 1981, Studies in histocompatibility, *Science* **213**:172–178.

Spencer, M. J., Cherry, J. D., and Terasaki, P. I., 1976, HLA antigens and antibody response after influenza A vaccination. Decreased response associated with HLA type W16, *N. Engl. J. Med.* **294**:13–16.

Springer, T. A., Kaufman, J. F., Siddoway, L. A., Giphart, M., Mann, D. L., Terhorst, C., and Strominger, J. L., 1977, Chemical and immunological characterization of HL-A-linked B-lymphocyte alloantigens, *Cold Spring Harbor Symp. Quant. Biol.* **41**:387–396.

Suciu-Foca, N., Godfrey, M., Khan, R., Woodward, K., Rohowsky, C., Reed, E., Hardy, M., and Reemtsma, K., 1981, New HLA-D alleles associated with DR1 and DR2, *Tissue Antigens* **17**:294–302.

Svejgaard, A., and Ryder, L. P., 1981, HLA genotype distribution and genetic models of insulin-dependent diabetes mellitus, *Ann. Hum. Genet.* **45**:293.

Terasaki, P. I., ed., 1980, *Histocompatibility Testing 1980*, University of California, Los Angeles Press, Los Angeles.

Torok-Storb, B., Nepom, G. T., Nepom, B. S., and Hansen, J. A., 1983, HLA-DR antigens on lymphoid cells differ from those on myeloid cells, *Nature* **305**:541–543.

van Rood, J. J., Eernisse, J. G., and Van Leeuwen, A., 1958, Leucocyte antibodies in sera from pregnant women, *Nature* **181**:1735–1736.

de Vries, R., Kreeftenberg, H., Loggen, H., and van Rood, J. J., 1977, *In vitro* immune responsiveness to vaccinia virus and HLA, *N. Engl. J. Med.* **297**:692–696.

Wake, C. T., Long, E. O., and Mach, B., 1982, Allelic polymorphism and complexity of the genes for HLA-DR β chains; direct analysis by DNA-DNA hybridization, *Nature* **300**:372–373.

Walker, L. E., Hewick, R., Hunkapiller, M. W., Hood, L. E., Dreyer, W. J., and Reisfeld, R. A., 1983, N-Terminal amino acid sequences of the α and β chains of HLA-DR1 and HLA-DR2 antigens, *Biochemistry* **22:**185–188.

Wang, C., Al-Katib, A., Lane, C., Koziner, B., and Fu, S. M., 1983, Induction of HLA-DC/DS (Leu 10) antigen expression by human precursor B cell lines, *J. Exp. Med.* **158:**1757–1762.

Winchester, R. J., and Kunkel, H. G., 1979, The human Ia system, *Adv. Immunol.* **28:**221–292.

Yunis, E. J., and Amos, D. B., 1971, Three closely linked genetic systems relevant to transplantation, *Proc. Natl. Acad. Sci. U.S.A.* **68:**3031–3035.

2

Lymphocyte Subpopulations

Phenotypic Expression and Functions in Health and Rheumatic Diseases

Sudhir Gupta

I. INTRODUCTION

Since the first delineation of T- and B-lymphocyte systems almost two decades ago, rapid progress has been made in identifying and understanding the functions of various subsets of cells of T- and B-cell lineages. The heterogeneity of T-cell subsets in humans was first defined by the presence of distinct receptors for immunoglobulin isotypes and more recently by the presence of differentiation antigens as defined by monoclonal antibodies. This has led to a better understanding of the complex immune network at both the cellular and molecular levels (Fig. 1). In the past 5 years, studies of immunoglobulin gene rearrangement have provided new insight into differentiation and maturation pathways of B-cell lineage and understanding of their perturbations in disease states, including autoimmune disorders. Therefore, before discussing the lymphocyte responses in rheumatic disease, it would be appropriate to discuss the lymphocytes in general with regard to their surface phenotypes, functions, and activation and proliferation, differentiation, and maturation pathways of T- and B-cell lineage. This brief review highlights the vast heterogeneity of lymphocyte subsets and interactions among themselves and a number of biologically active molecules (cytokines) produced by them and cells of monocyte–macrophage lineage.

Sudhir Gupta • Department of Medicine, Division of Basic and Clinical Immunology, University of California, Irvine, California 92717.

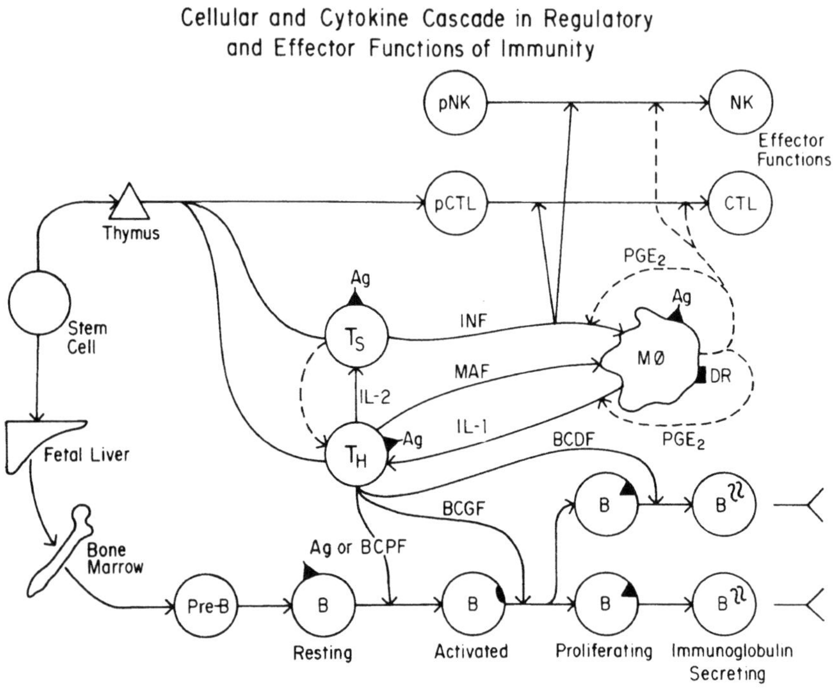

Figure 1. Cellular and molecular network of immune system. T_S, suppressor T cells; T_H, helper T cells; INF, interferon; IL1, interleukin 1; IL. 2, interleukin 2; MAF, macrophage-activating factor; Ag, antigen; PGE_2, prostaglandin E_2; MØ, macrophage; pNK, pre-natural-killer cells; NK, natural killer cells; pCTL, precytotoxic T lymphocytes; CTL, cytotoxic T lymphocytes; BCPF, B-cell-proliferating factor; BCDF, B-cell-differentiating factor; BCGF, B-cell growth factor. Interrupted lines represent negative regulation.

II. PHENOTYPIC CHARACTERISTICS OF MAJOR LYMPHOCYTE SUBPOPULATIONS

A. T-Lymphocyte Lineage

During their journey through the thymus, the committed lymphoid stem cells, after interacting with thymic epithelial cells and a family of thymic factors or hormones, differentiate and mature into the cells of T-cell lineage. These cells express a number of surface antigens, markers, and receptors and acquire different effector and immunoregulatory functions. A list of these markers is shown in Table 1. It is beyond the scope of this chapter to discuss all the markers of lymphocyte subpopulations (including those of T-cell lineage) in detail; these have recently been reviewed (Gupta and Good, 1979a,b, 1980, 1981; Gupta and Kapoor, 1980; Gupta *et al.*, 1980; Ross, 1979; Reinherz and Schlossman, 1980).

T lymphocytes comprise approximately 80% of circulating lymphocytes. At the present time there is no recognizable distinct marker for committed stem cells for T cell lineage. The earliest cells recognizable in this lineage are at the cortical thymocyte level or just prior to it. Terminal deoxynucleotidyl transferase (TdT) enzyme activity is present in high amounts of pre-T cells and immature T cells. Cortical thymocytes also bear

Table 1. Markers/Antigens/Receptors of Human Lymphoid Cells of T-Cell Lineage

Lineage	Marker
Stem cells	? Alloantigen
Pre-T cells (including immature T)	Terminal deoxynucleotidyl transferase (TdT)
	Peanut agglutinin
	OKT10, T10, OK-T6, T6, T9
T cells	SRBC receptors
	IgG Fc receptors (Tγ)
	IgM Fc receptors (Tμ)
	IgA Fc receptors (Tα)
	IgE Fc receptors (Tξ)
	IgD Fc receptors (Tδ)
	OKT4, Leu 3, T4
	OKT8, Leu 2, T8
	CL1.3, 89b1, 38.1, 35.1, 9.6, 4A, UCHT1, T1
	OKT3, Leu 1, T3, T11, Leu 4, Leu 5
	DR antigens (only on activated T cells)
	Tac antigen or IL-2 receptor and T9 (on activated T cells)
	K^+ channels

receptors for peanut agglutinin, and this marker has been used to separate and analyze the functions of cortical and medullary thymocytes. Monoclonal-antibody-defined antigens, T10, T9, and T6, are present on thymocytes, T9 being present on early thymocytes, T6 on common thymocytes, and T10 on all early, common, and mature thymocytes. T9 antigen appears to define the transferrin receptor and is also present on activated mature T cells. Peripheral blood mature T cells have receptors for sheep red blood cells (SRBC) and monoclonal-antibody-defined antigens (T1, T3, Leu 1, Leu 4, Leu 5, 9.6, T11, UCHT 1, 89 bl, 38.1, 4A, 3AI, and CL 1.3). The antigens 9.6, T11, 35.1, and Leu 5 define the receptor for SRBC on T lymphocytes. There are other marker antigens that are present on a subset of distinct immunoregulatory and effector cells, and these are discussed separately in Section IV.

Some of these antigens participate in activation or inhibition of certain functions of T lymphocytes. More recently, human T lymphocytes have been shown to express K^+ channels (De Coursey *et al.*, 1984a; Matteson and Deutsch, 1984; Chandy *et al.*, 1984, 1985; Cahalan *et al.*, 1985). Approximately 300 K^+ channels are present per T lymphocyte. The K^+ channels have been shown to be important in various functions of human T lymphocytes (Chandy *et al.*, 1984), and their abnormality could be related to abnormal T cell functions (De Coursey *et al.*, 1984b; Chandy *et al.*, 1985).

Although it is almost completely lacking on resting T lymphocytes, the majority of antigen- or mitogen-activated T lymphocytes express a receptor (Tac antigen) for interleukin 2 (IL-2) that is required for the proliferation of T lymphocytes (Uchiama *et al.*, 1981a,b). Transferrin receptor is also present on activated peripheral blood T cells and appears to express later than Tac antigen during T cell activation. The expression of transferrin receptor is dependent on the expression of Tac antigen because blocking of

Tac receptor by anti-Tac antibody will block transferrin receptor expression and therefore DNA synthesis and the proliferation of T lymphocytes. HLA-DR is also present on a majority of activated T cells; however, its temporal relationship with Tac antigen and transferrin receptor is not known. The dissociation between Tac and DR antigen expression following tetanus toxoid stimulation (Yokoi *et al.*, 1982) and in primary immunodeficiencies (Gupta, 1984) clearly demonstrates that the DR and Tac antigens are expressed during different stages of T cell activation.

The cell surface glycoproteins present on the T cell surface appear to play an important role in T cell functions. T3 or Leu 4 monoclonal antibodies that recognize the 19 to 22-kd molecule are strongly mitogenic for resting T cells (Van Wauwe *et al.*, 1980). Addition of T3 monoclonal antibody to T-cell cultures causes the release of various T-cell lymphokines including IL-2 and γ interferon (γ-INF) (Palacios, 1982; Chang *et al.*, 1982). In contrast, anti-T3 antibody is known to inhibit mixed lymphocyte culture (MLC) response, helper function, cytotoxic T-lymphocyte (CTL) generation, and CTL effector function (Chang *et al.*, 1981; Reinherz *et al.*, 1980). It has been suggested that the T3 molecule may serve as part of a T-cell recognition unit for antigen (Reinherz *et al.*, 1982a). OKT11 and Leu 5 antibodies, when added to T-cell cultures, inhibit the proliferation of T cells by preventing them from becoming sensitive to IL-2 and by inhibiting the production of IL-2 (Van Wauwe *et al.*, 1980; Palacios and Martinez-Maza, 1982). Anti T1 (Leu 1) monoclonal antibodies enhance B-cell differentiation in a dose-dependent fashion. These observations clearly indicate that some specific T-cell surface glycoproteins are functionally important in a variety of intra- and intercellular processes.

B. B-Lymphocyte Lineage

Until recently, the earliest cell identified along the B-cell lineage was the pre-B cell, which is characterized by the presence of an intracytoplasmic μ heavy chain of immunologlobulin but lacks surface Ig. However, very recently it was demonstrated that when the immunoglobulin gene in the germ line of stem cells is rearranged, the stem cell is committed to B-cell lineage with the rare exception of Ig gene rearrangement in some T-cell leukemias (Korsmeyer and Waldmann, 1984). During the activation and differentiation of B lymphocytes, a number of receptors or antigens are expressed on them (Table 2). These markers have recently been reviewed (Gupta and Good, 1980; McKenzie and Zola, 1983; Gupta and Kapoor, 1980), and, therefore, only a few recent advances are discussed here. In the postnatal period, pre-B cells are present exclusively in the bone marrow and comprise 1% of total mononuclear cells. B lymphocytes constitute 12–15% of peripheral blood lymphocytes. FMC 1 monoclonal antibody defines all surface Ig^+ B lymphocytes. This antigen is lacking in pre-B cells and fully differentiated plasma cells. FMC 7 monoclonal antibody defines only 50% of FMC 1^+ or surface Ig^+ B lymphocytes and appears to mark a more mature B lymphocyte, which could be analogous to the LyB5-negative mouse B lymphocytes (Zola *et al.*, 1984). FMC 7 is a protein that is integrated in the cell membrane. The antigen is rapidly synthesized and turned over, is not cell-cycle dependent, and is relatively resistant to changes induced by cultures in the presence of phorbol ester.

The heterogeneity of B lymphocytes has also been demonstrated by B1 and B2 monoclonal antibodies. B1 antigen is present on a majority of surface Ig^+ B lymphocytes

Table 2. Markers/Antigens/Receptors of Human Lymphoid Cellsof B-Cell Lineage

Lineage	
Stem cells	? Alloantigen
Pre-B cells	Intracytoplasmic μ heavy chain
	EB virus receptor (subpopulation)
	DR antigen (subpopulation)
B cells	Surface immunoglobulin
	MRBC receptors
	Epstein–Barr virus receptor
	IgG Fc receptors
	IgM Fc receptors
	IgA Fc receptors
	IgE Fc receptors
	Complement component receptors
	DR antigen
	Receptor for BCGF, BCDF (activated B cells)
	Tac antigen (activated B cells)
	B1, B2, B4, FMC 1, FMC 7
	Ca^{2+} channels; K^{+} channels

and on all B-cell malignancies except plasma cell myeloma (Stashenko *et al.*, 1980). It is an approximately 30,000-molecular-weight antigen. B1 antigen is also present on EBV-transformed B-cell lines and cell lines from Burkitt's lymphoma. In contrast, B2 antigen is present on only a subset of $B1^{+}$ B cells. It is a 120- to 130,000-molecular-weight antigen, and the anti-B2 antibody has a much more restricted reactivity than anti-B1 antibody. This antibody does not react with cell lines from Burkitt's lymphoma or with cells from Waldenstrom's macroglobulinemia or nodular mixed lymphocytic and diffuse histiocytic lymphoma (Nadler *et al.*, 1981).

Receptors for mouse red blood cells (MRBC) on human B lymphocytes deserve a brief account here because they are discussed again in the context of some rheumatic diseases. The receptor for MRBC is present on a subset of human B lymphocytes (Gupta *et al.*, 1976a) that predominantly carry surface IgM. The MRBC bind to B cells independent of surface Ig, Fc receptor, and complement receptors. Studies of fetal liver (Gupta *et al.*, 1976c) and of leukemia and lymphoma (Gupta and Grieco, 1975; Gupta *et al.*, 1976b) clearly demonstrated that MRBC bind to a relatively immature B lymphocyte.

Interleukin-2 (IL-2) receptor (Tac antigen) had been believed to be expressed exclusively on activated T cells; however, Tsudo *et al.* (1984) have shown the presence of Tac antigen on approximately 25% of normal activated B cells. These activated B cells respond by proliferation in the presence of exogenous IL-2.

Resting B lymphocytes lack receptors for B-cell growth factor (BCGF) and B-cell differentiation factor (BCDF); however, they are present on activated and proliferating and cycling B lymphocytes, respectively (Muraguchi *et al.*, 1984). Since antibodies to receptors have not been developed, the evidence for the presence of BCGF and BCDF is indirect but strong.

C. Third-Population Lymphoid Cells

Approximately 5–6% of peripheral blood lymphoid cells are non-T and non-B cells and have been given several names; e.g., L cells, K cells, null cells, third-population cells, unclassified cells. All of these cells have Fc receptors and are nonphagocytic and esterase negative. The majority of third-population cells are large granular lymphocytes (LGL) in morphology and mediate natural killing (NK) and antibody-dependent cellular cytotoxicity (ADCC) functions. The large granular lymphocytes display a variety of surface markers (Table 3); however, they fail to place these cells in any definite lineage. The LGL have Tac antigen, T8, OKT10, OKM1, Leu 7, Leu 11, GM1, INF receptor, Lyt 3, Leu 5, and low-affinity SRBC receptor. Functional analysis has revealed that the best marker for LGL is Leu 11^+ Leu 7^-. The heterogeneity of LGL has recently been reviewed (Ortaldo and Herberman, 1984).

III. FUNCTIONS OF MAJOR LYMPHOCYTE SUBPOPULATIONS

Cell separation techniques utilizing various surface markers have permitted the analysis of T, B, and third-population lymphoid cells (Table 4). These functions have recently been reviewed (Gupta and Good, 1979a,b, 1980, 1981; Gupta and Kapoor, 1980). Therefore, only the most recent developments are briefly discussed here. Autologous or allogeneic T cells following *in vitro* activation, by virtue of expressing HLA-DR antigens, stimulate in the AMLR (T–T AMLR) or allogeneic mixed lymphocyte reaction (T–T MLR) (Damle and Gupta, 1982b; Gupta, 1983a,b). α-Lymphotoxin, which synergizes the NK function of INF, is produced by T lymphocytes, NK cells and B-cell lines. It has tumor necrosis property. More recently, BCGF and BCDF have been shown to be produced by human and murine T cells. After activation with anti-u, resting B cells enlarge in size and express receptors for BCGF and will respond by proliferation in the presence of BCGF. However, for these cycling B cells to differentiate into immunoglobin secreting cells, another factor, BCDF, is required (Fig. 2). These factors are produced by T cells, most likely by T helper cells. Recently BCGF and BCDF have been produced by T–T hybrids and characterized (Mur-

Table 3. Markers/Antigens/Receptors of Human Lymphoid Cells of Third-Population "Unclassified" Lymphoid Cells (Includes Majority of Large Granular Cells)

IgG Fc receptors (high affinity)
Receptors for EBV (subpopulation)
DR antigen (subpopulation)
Interferon receptor
IL-2 receptor ?
Lyt 3, Leu 5, aGM1, OKM1, OKT10, Leu 7, Leu 11, NK8, OKT8, B73.1
Low-affinity SRBC receptor

Table 4. Functions of Human Lymphocyte Subpopulations[a]

Properties	T cells	B cells	Third-population lymphoid cells
Proliferative responses			
Antigens	+	−	−
Allogeneic cells (R)	+	−	−
Allogeneic cells (S)	+	+	+
Autologous cells (R)	+	−	−
Autologous cells (S)	−	+	+
Epstein–Barr virus	−	+	+ S*
Immunoregulatory functions			
Suppressor	+	−	+
Helper	+	−	− ?
Cytotoxic responses			
Cell-mediated lympholysis	+	−	?
Antibody-dependent cytotoxicity	+ S*	−	+
Natural killer activity	+ S*	−	+
Mitogen-induced cytotoxicity	+	+	+
Lymphokine production			
BCGF, BCDF	+	−	+
Leukocyte migration inhibition factor	+	+	+
Macrophage migration inhibition factor	+	+	+
Blastogenic factor	+	+	+
Lymphotoxin (α)	+	+	+
Interferon (γ)	+	−	+
Interleukin-2	+	−	+
Interleukin-1	−	−	+
Antibody synthesis	−	+	+ S*
Miscellaneous			
Precursors of B cells	−	−	+
Precursors of T cells	−	−	+
Precursors of granulocytes	−	−	+
Precursors of erythrocytes	−	−	+

[a]R, responder; S, stimulator; S*, subpopulation.

aguchi *et al.*, 1984). The BCGF prepared from T–T hybrid has a molecular weight of 18–20,000 with isoelectric point 6.3. It is sensitive to treatment with trypsin or chymotrypsin, distinct from IL-2 and BCDF, stable over a pH range of 4.0–10.0, and actively absorbed by B-cell blasts but not by T-cell blasts. It is likely that there are more than two BCGF (Yoshizaki *et al.*, 1983; Swain *et al.*, 1983). There is recent evidence that human LGL contained in the third population also produce BCGF (Ortaldo and Herberman, 1984). The BCDF produced by T–T hybrid has a molecular weight of 30–35,000 with an isoelectric point of 5.9. It is actively absorbed by CESS cells but not by anti-u-activated B cells. It is distinct from BCGF and IL-2 (Muraguchi *et al.*, 1984). T cells produce BCDF. It is not clear if BCDF is produced by LGL.

Interleukin 1 (IL-1), which is a product of activated macrophages, is also produced by LGL (Ortaldo and Herberman, 1984). Interleukin 2 is produced by T lymphocytes

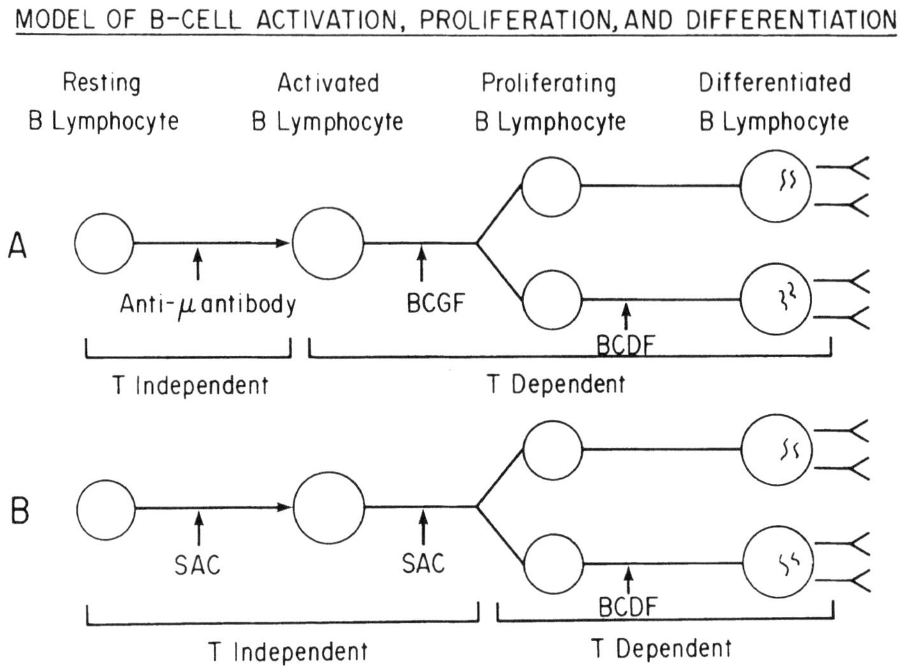

Figure 2. Role of T-cell-derived B-cell growth (BCGF) and differentiation factor (BCDF) in B-cell activation, proliferation, and differentiation. SAC, *staphylococcus* Cowan I.

and LGL; it is known to enhance NK function and support the growth of T cells. It is now clear that IL-2 enhances NK activity by inducing the production of γ-INF, which in turn potentiates NK functions. The gene for IL-2 has been cloned and shown to be located on chromosome 4q. The subject of interleukins is discussed in detail in Chapter 4.

IV. SUBPOPULATIONS OF T LYMPHOCYTES

The two major subpopulations, the helper/inducer and suppressor/cytotoxic T cells, have been identified by the presence of receptors for immunoglobulin isotypes and monoclonal-antibody-defined differentiation antigens.

A. T-Lymphocyte Subsets Defined by Immunoglobulin Isotype Receptors

Human T lymphocytes have been shown to express receptors for all immunoglobulin isotypes; however, two of them, T cells with IgM Fc receptor (Tμ) and T cells with IgG Fc receptor (Tγ), have been extensively studied. Their enzymatic, morphological, kinetic, and immunologic functions have recently been reviewed (Gupta, 1978, 1981; Gupta and Good, 1978a,b, 1980, 1981; Gupta *et al.*, 1980; Moretta *et al.*, 1978) and therefore are only summarized. These two subpopulations are distinct with regard to morphology, RNA content, locomotor properties, electrophoretic mobility, expression of histamine receptor, sensitive to enzymes, and cytotoxic and immunoregulatory functions. Tμ cells include cells with helper/inducer functions, and Tγ cells have cytotoxic/suppressor functions. It became clear, however, that neither of these subsets is functionally mutually exclusive (because Tμ cells also contain precursors of suppression) and the receptors for IgG isotype were unstable. Therefore, data on Tμ and Tγ cells in rheumatic disorders (discussed in Section V) should be interpreted in that context.

B. T-Lymphocyte Subsets Defined with Monoclonal Antibodies

The advent of hybridoma technology has provided a variety of monoclonal antibodies that define differentiation and maturation antigens. Antibodies were developed that were thought to be homogeneous, and defined two major subsets: helper/inducer and suppressor/cytotoxic (Reinherz and Schlossman, 1980). However, it became apparent that the T-cell subsets defined with two major monoclonal antibodies are not homogeneous, and each population contains several distinct functions. OK T or T series of antibodies were initially utilized. These terminologies are used interchangeably in this chapter. Initially, $OKT4^+$ cells were thought to contain helper/inducer functions and $OKT8^+$ cells suppressor/cytotoxic function. Their functions are summarized in Table 5. These functions have recently been reviewed (Reinherz and Schlossman, 1980). In this section, further heterogeneity among $T4^+$ and $T8^+$ populations is discussed. The heterogeneity of im-

Table 5. Functions of Major Subpopulations of Human T Lymphocytes

Functions	$OKT4^+$ (Leu 3^+)	$OKT8^+$ (Leu 2^+)
Proliferative response		
Soluble antigens	+	−
Phytohemagglutinin	+	±
Concanavalin A	+	+
Allogeneic MLC	+	+
Autologous MLC (T–non-T)	+	−
Autologous MLC(T–T)	+	−
Lymphokine production		
Interleukin 2	+	±
Gamma interferon	±	+
Cytotoxicity		
MHC class I specific	−	+
MHC class II specific	+	−
Regulatory functions		
Helper		
T–B interaction	+	−
T–T interaction	+	−
T–Macrophage interaction	+	−
Suppressor		
T–B interaction	+S[a]	+S
T–T interaction	+S	+S

[a]S, subpopulation.

munoregulatory and cytotoxic functions among T4 and T8 populations can be defined by the following:

1. Monoclonal antibodies that define subsets of T4$^+$ and T8$^+$ T cells, e.g., 9.3, Leu 8, 2H4, OKT20, OKT17.
2. Autoantibodies against a subset of T4$^+$ or T8$^+$ cells—juvenile rheumatoid arthritis (JRA) serum.
3. At the clonal level.
4. Radiosensitivity.
5. Concanavalin A (Con A)-inducible suppressor activity.

1. *Functional Heterogeneity of T4$^+$ T Cells*

The initial evidence of functional heterogeneity of T4$^+$ cells (Fig. 3) came from studies of Thomas *et al.* (1980, 1982a,b, 1983), Reinherz *et al.* (1982b) and Damle and Gupta (1982a,b). Thomas *et al.* (1980) showed that when a number of nonirradiated OKT4$^+$ cells were added to pokeweed mitogen (PWM)-driven B-cell cultures, the number of plaque forming cells (PFC) generated did not follow a linear relationship with the number of added cells. At low numbers of T4$^+$ cells, a helper effect was observed, whereas at relatively high numbers of T4$^+$ cells, a decrease in PFC response was observed; however, this decrease in PFC response was not observed when high numbers of irradiated OKT4$^+$ cells were used instead.

These results suggested that within radiosensitive T4$^+$, suppressor cells may be

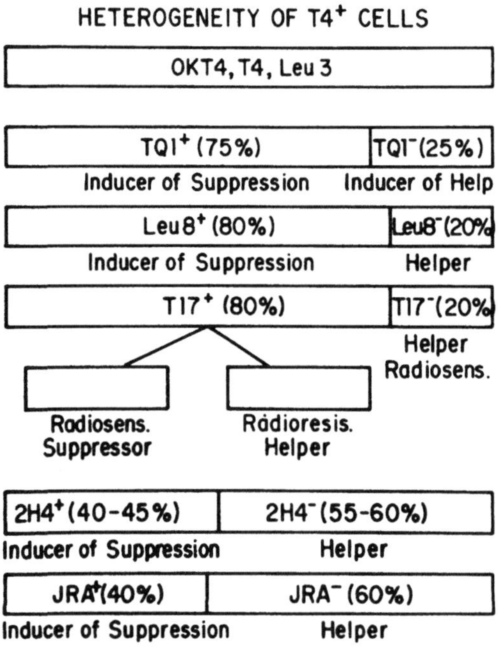

Figure 3. Functional heterogeneity of OKT4$^+$ T cells.

generated. When *in vitro* PWM-activated $T4^+$ cells were added to cultures of B cells and fresh nonirradiated and irradiated T cells in the presence of PWM, it was demonstrated that activated $T4^+$ contain suppressor cell activity that requires interaction with the radiosensitive fresh $T4^+$ cells. These investigators utilized a monoclonal antibody OKT-17 that defines an antigen present on all resting T cells; however, on activation with lectin, a subpopulation of $OKT4^+$ cells loses this antigen. Using this approach, Thomas *et al.* (1983) were able to separate $T4^+$ 17^+ and $T4^+$ 17^- subsets and examine their immunoregulatory functions in PFC assay. They demonstrated that $T4^+$ 17^- (20%) T cells are radiosensitive helpers, whereas $T4^+$ 17^+ cells (80%) contain radioresistant helpers and radiosensitive suppressors.

Reinherz *et al.* (1982b), using a monoclonal antibody TQ1, demonstrated that $T4^+$ $TQ1^-$ (25%) cells were inducers of help. In contrast, $T4^+$ $TQ1^+$ (75%) cells were inducers of suppression and responded in T–non-T AMLR. C. Morimoto (personal communication), using another monoclonal antibody (2H4) that defines a subset of $T4^+$ cells, demonstrated that $T4^+$ $2H4^+$ cells are inducers of suppression, whereas $T4^+$ $2H4^-$ cells were effector helpers.

Damle *et al.* (1984), using a monoclonal antibody (Leu 8) that is totally distinct from $OKT8^+$ and defines a subset of Leu 3^+ $T4^+$ cells, demonstrated that Leu 3^+ Leu 8^- cells are helpers and Leu 3^+, Leu 8^+ cells are inducers of suppression.

Morimoto *et al.* (1981) demonstrated that JRA sera contain anti-T-cell autoantibodies. These sera reacted preferentially with a subset of $T4^+$ cells. By separating $T4^+$ JRA^+ and $T4^+$ JRA^- cells, these investigators reported that JRA^+ $T4^+$ cells are inducers of suppression and that JRA^+ $T4^-$ cells are the helpers in an immunoglobulin synthesis and secretion assay.

Damle and Gupta (1982a) used a different approach to demonstrate suppressor cell activity in $T4^+$ cells. They activated unseparated T cells with Con A for 48 hr and then separated them into $T4^+$ and $T8^+$ cells or activated $T4^+$ and $T8^+$ with Con A and utilized them as regulators against the autologous T-cell response to mitogens or alloantigens. Con-A-inducible suppressor activity was observed in both $T4^+$ and $T8^+$ populations. Furthermore, suppressor activity was radiosensitive. In the AMLR model it was demonstrated that $T4^+$ cells respond to autologous non-T cells (T–non-T AMLR) and express helper activity (Damle and Gupta, 1982b), whereas activated T cells also stimulate $T4^+$ cells (T–T AMLR), but these $T4^+$ cells express suppressor activity (Gupta, 1983a,b), thereby demonstrating functional heterogeneity of $T4^+$ cell.

Biddison *et al.* (1982) presented evidence for possible cytotoxic function of $T4^+$ cells. Meuer *et al.* (1982) developed $T4^+$ and $T8^+$ cytotoxic T-cell clones and demonstrated that $T4^+$ cytotoxic T cells recognize class II antigens of the major histocompatibility complex (MHC) region, whereas $T8^+$ cells recognize class I antigens of the MHC region.

Recently, a lack of T4 antigen but normal proportions of Leu 3 antigen on T cells from certain subjects has been described (Sato *et al.*, 1984). Functional analysis of these $T4^-$ Leu 3^+ cells showed normal proliferative response and helper function. Since these two antibodies were detecting the same epitope, it was evident that the T4 epitope may be genetically polymorphic. Fuller *et al.* (1984), using eight murine anti-T4 monoclonal antibodies, clearly demonstrated that at least five and possibly seven different epitopes can be recognized on the T4 molecule. The T4 reactive epitope variations are common but do not appear related to the stage of T helper cell differentiation. The T4 epitope cannot be unmasked by neuraminidase treatment or T-cell stimulation with lectins, soluble antigens, or allogeneic lymphocytes. The family study suggests that the alterations in OKT4 phenotype are autosomal codominant expression of the T4 gene product. The significance of this polymorphism on the function of T4 cells remains unclear.

In summary, the T4$^+$ cells are heterogeneous (Fig. 2). The resting T4$^+$ cells contain (1) radiosensitive helpers, (2) radiosensitive helpers, (3) radiosensitive inducers of suppression, (4) precursors of suppressors (Con A and T–T AMLR), and (5) precursors of cytotoxic T cells. The activated T4 cells contain (1) effector suppressors, and (2) effectors of cytotoxicity (recognizing class II MHC antigens).

2. *Functional Heterogeneity of T8$^+$ Cells*

Resting T8$^+$ cells require interaction with radiosensitive T4$^+$ cells to exert their suppressor effect on B-cell responses, and the suppressive influence of T8$^+$ cells is radiosensitive (Fig. 4). T8$^+$ cells mediate their suppressive influence by decreasing synthesis and secretion of helper factor by T4$^+$ cells (Thomas *et al.*, 1981, 1983). In contrast to activated T4$^+$ cells, which require radiosensitive fresh T4$^+$ cells to exert their suppressive effect, activated T8$^+$ cells do not require radiosensitive T4$^+$ cells to exert their suppressor influence. This suggests two distinct mechanisms for suppressor function of T4$^+$ and T8$^+$ cells. The heterogeneity of T8$^+$ cells was defined by monoclonal antibodies 9.3 and OKT20. Damle *et al.* (1984) separated Leu 2$^+$ 9.3$^+$ and Leu 2$^+$ 9.3$^-$ T cells and demonstrated that Leu 2$^+$ 9.3$^+$ T cells were cytotoxic and Leu 2$^+$ 9.3$^-$ cells were suppressors. Utilizing Leu 8 monoclonal antibodies, these investigators further subclassified Leu 2$^+$ 9.3$^-$ cells into Leu 2$^+$ 9.3$^-$, Leu 8$^+$ and Leu 2$^+$ 9.3$^+$ Leu 8$^-$ cells. The Leu 2$^+$ 9.3$^-$ Leu 8$^-$ cells were inducers of suppressors, and Leu 2$^+$ 9.3$^-$ Leu 8$^+$ cells were suppressors. Thomas *et al.* (1982b) used OKT20 monoclonal antibody to define

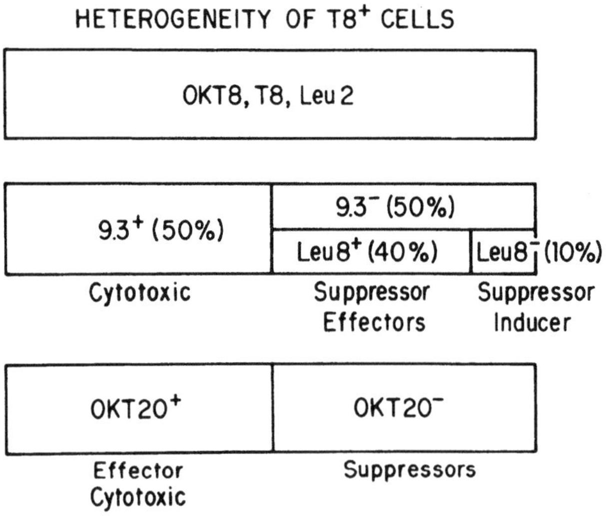

Figure 4. Functional heterogeneity of OKT8$^+$ T cells.

functional heterogeneity of $T8^+$ cells. The antigen defined with OKT20 monoclonal antibody is present on a small percentage of resting lymphocytes but is present in varying proportions on activated T cells. Functional analysis demonstrated that the $T8^+$ $OKT20^+$ cells are cytotoxic effectors and that those with $T8^+$ $OKT20^-$ phenotypes are precursors of cytotoxic cells and suppressor effector cells.

Thomas *et al.* (1983) demonstrated that irradiated activated $T8^+$ cells, in contrast to nonirradiated activated $T8^+$ cells, which consistently suppress B cell responses, when added to a mixture of B cells, fresh $OKT4^+$ T cells, and PWM, amplified the response. This amplifying effect of irradiated activated $T8^+$ cells was highly dependent on the magnitude of the helper activity obtained with fresh $OKT4^+$ cells. It should be stressed, however, that activated $OKT8^+$ cells are not helpers since they do not induce a PFC response in purified B cells. The mechanism(s) of activated T8-cell-mediated enhancement is unclear; one of the possible mechanisms could be that activated $T8^+$ cells could be analogous to murine contrasuppressor inducer with Lyt 1^-2^+ phenotype (Gershon *et al.*, 1981).

At the clonal level, Meuer *et al.* (1982) demonstrated that $T8^+$ clones possess cytotoxic effector functions recognizing class I antigens of the MHC region and lack suppressor activity.

In summary, resting T8 cells contain precursors and effectors of suppressors, inducers of suppressors, and precursors and effectors of cytotoxic functions. The activated $T8^+$ cells under appropriate experimental conditions show an enhancing influence, possibly contrasuppression.

Thus, there is a functional heterogeneity within $T4^+$ and $T8^+$ T cells. This could be interpreted in the following ways: (1) precursors of functionally distinct subsets exist within both $T4^+$ and $T8^+$ cells; or (2) T4 and T8 molecules themselves do not mark distinct subsets but are intimately involved in the function of T-cell subsets they define regardless of type of function. By use of anti-T4A-E monoclonal antibodies, inhibition of helper influence in PFC response and cytotoxic functions against class II antigen targets was observed. Similarly, anti-T8 antibody will block cytotoxic functions of $T8^+$ cells against class I antigen targets. Therefore, T4 and T8 molecules may be part of the recognition units for class II and class I MHC antigens, respectively.

V. LYMPHOCYTES IN RHEUMATIC DISORDERS

A. Rheumatoid Arthritis

Rheumatoid arthritis (RA) is a chronic systemic inflammatory disorder of unknown etiology characterized by articular inflammation of multiple joints; if it continues it usually results in progressive joint destruction and deformity. Extraarticular features such as rheumatoid nodules, arteritis, neuropathy, scleritis, pericarditis, lymphadenopathy, and splenomegaly occur with considerable frequency. These extraarticular manifestations, once considered complications of RA, are now considered integral and systemic manifestations of RA. Quantitative and qualitative analysis of lymphocytes in RA have revealed conflicting results; however, the evidence of B-cell hyperreactivity is almost universally observed.

1. Analysis of Lymphocytes in the Peripheral Blood

a. T Lymphocytes

i. Quantitative Analysis of T Cells. Earlier studies utilized sheep RBC rosette formation as the measure of total T lymphocytes (E-RFC) in patients with rheumatoid arthritis. In general, total T cells in inactive RA or mildly active RA are normal in proportions (Plater-Zyberk *et al.*, 1983; Moutsopoulos *et al.*, 1976; Meijer *et al.*, 1982; Slavin and Strober, 1981; Raeman *et al.*, 1981; Burmester *et al.*, 1978; Keith and Currey, 1973). Froland *et al.* (1973), in a small number of patients with RA studied, showed increased proportions of E-RFC; however, the value of E-RFC in the control group was only 15%. Therefore, it is apparent that their assay was suboptimal in detecting all T cells and was defining only a subset. The E-RFC was found to be decreased, particularly in active RA (Rawson and Huang, 1976; Talal *et al.*, 1974; Williams *et al.*, 1973). Williams *et al.* (1973), using anti-T-cell heteroantiserum, reported decreased proportion of T cells in active RA but observed no difference between inactive RA and a control group. More recently, monoclonal antibodies have been used to analyze T cells in RA. Veys *et al.* (1982b) reported normal proportions and numbers of T cells. Kotzin *et al.* (1983) reported normal proportions but decreased numbers of T cells. In contrast, Raeman *et al.* (1981) observed decreased proportions but normal numbers of monoclonal-antibody-defined T cells in RA. The discrepancies among these studies appear to arise from differences in selection of patients with regard to disease activity and treatment.

ii. Qualitative Analysis of T Cells. Since an early description (Yu and Peter, 1974) of depressed T-cell-mediated immunity in patients with RA, a number of investigators have reported impaired T-cell functions in RA. These have included cutaneous anergy to recall antigens (Andrianakos *et al.*, 1977a) and decreased mitogen-induced (Horwitz and Garrett, 1977; Scheinberg *et al.*, 1978; Rawson and Huang, 1976; Corrigall *et al.*, 1979; Percy *et al.*, 1978; Silverman *et al.*, 1976; Wolinski *et al.*, 1980; Slavin and Strober, 1981) and viral-antigen-induced (Wolf, 1978; Chattopadhyay *et al.*, 1979c) responses. Silverman *et al.* (1976) reported depressed PHA and Con A but normal PWM responses in a subgroup of RA patients with erosive disease. Menard *et al.* (1977) observed a decreased PHA response in RA patients positive for antinuclear antibodies. Using BuDR and light experiments, Rawson and Huang (1976) demonstrated a relative but nonsignificant deficiency of Con-A-responsive cells in RA compared to controls; however, when ratios of PHA/Con A responses were considered, the ratio in RA was significantly decreased compared to controls. These investigators found normal PHA responses in RA (Rawson and Huang, 1976); the binding of lymphocytes from RA to iodinated PHA was, however, less than in controls (Rawson and Huang, 1974b).

A number of other investigators have also observed normal PHA responsiveness in RA (Bernstein *et al.*, 1980; Slavin and Strober, 1981; Dunne *et al.*, 1982; Scheinberg *et al.*, 1978). Bernstein *et al.* (1980) found normal PHA-induced T-cell colony formation in RA. Slavin and Strober (1981) found a normal PHA response in purified E-RFC but a depressed response in a mononuclear cell preparation; serum was shown to be inhibitory in the latter system.

Wolinski *et al.* (1980) reported prostaglandin-mediated depressed PHA responses in RA that were improved by *in vitro* treatment of mononuclear cells with indomethacin. The allogeneic mixed lymphocyte response (MLR) studies have also shown conflicting results. Astorga and Williams (1969) and Rawson and Huang (1974a) have reported depressed MLR when compared to controls, whereas Hasler *et al.* (1983) have found normal MLR in RA patients. More recently, Radon *et al.* (1982) have reported that T cells from patients with RA proliferate in response to IgG rheumatoid factor. Seitz *et al.* (1983) demonstrated that depressed antigen-induced proliferative response in RA was caused by a defect in antigen presentation by monocytes. Production of two major lymphokines in RA has been investigated. Chattopathyay *et al.* (1979c) demonstrated impaired leukocyte migration inhibition factor production on stimulation with PHA. Hasler *et al.* (1983) reported decreased γ-INF production in the autologous mixed lymphocyte reaction but normal γ-INF production in MLR in patients with RA.

b. Immunoregulatory T-Cell Subsets. The putative helper/inducer and suppressor/cytotoxic T lymphocytes have been quantitated using receptors for immunoglobulin isotypes and monoclonal antibodies. As discussed in the general discussion of immunoregulatory T-cell subsets, the T-cell subsets defined by monoclonal antibodies T4 and T8 contain multiple subsets with distinct immunoregulatory and cytotoxic effector functions; therefore, any quantitative changes in T4 and/or T8 T cells might not correlate with the functional alterations.

i. Quantitative Analysis of T-Cell Subsets Defined with Fc Receptors for Immunoglobulin Isotypes. The Tμ cells have been found to be present in normal (Palacios *et al.*, 1981; Doblong *et al.*, 1981) or decreased proportions (Meuer *et al.*, 1982) in patients with RA. Meijer *et al.* (1982) observed decreased proportions and absolute numbers of Tμ cells in active RA compared to inactive RA and control group; however, in the inactive group only the proportions and not the numbers of Tμ cells were decreased when compared to the control group. The proportions of Tγ cells in RA appear to be normal (Mathieu *et al.*, 1981; Meijer *et al.*, 1982; Forre *et al.*, 1982a; Palacios *et al.*, 1981; Doblong *et al.*, 1981; Bellamy *et al.*, 1983; Nilsson and Biberfield, 1982). Meijer *et al.* (1982) found normal numbers of Tγ cells in both active and inactive RA, but the proportions of Tγ cells were significantly increased in inactive RA compared to controls. Non-Tμ, non-Tγ cells have been shown to be increased in both active and inactive RA (Meijer *et al.*, 1982). Several explanations have been suggested for decreased Tμ cells in RA. These include modulation by immune complexes, ecotaxis from peripheral blood to joint fluid or synovium, and presence of cytotoxic antibodies against Tμ cells. None of these possibilities has been tested in great detail. Emmons *et al.* (1983) have demonstrated that IgM RF preferentially modulates binding of IgG-containing complexes to Tμ and Tγ cells and is not different from normal IgM in inhibiting the binding of IgM complexes to Tμ cells. Based on these observations, these investigators have suggested that IgM RF preferentially modulate Tγ cell functions and do not affect Tμ cell functions.

ii. Quantitative Analysis of Monoclonal-Antibody-Defined T-Cell Subsets. The results of analyses of monoclonal-antibody-defined T-cell subsets have also been plagued with conflicting findings. The proportions and numbers of $T4^+$ or Leu 3^+ T cells in RA have been shown to be normal (Burmester *et al.*, 1981; Duke *et al.*, 1983; Nilsson and Biberfield, 1982; Forre *et al.*, 1982a; Egeland *et al.*, 1983; Veys *et al.*, 1982b; Fox *et al.*, 1982c; Bellamy *et al.*, 1983), increased (Verdickt *et al.*, 1983; Veys *et al.*, 1982b; Queiros and Rocha, 1983; Kotzin *et al.*, 1983), or decreased (Haraoni *et al.*, 1984). Similarly $T8^+$ or Leu 2^+ cells have been found to be normal (Fox *et al.*, 1982c; Burmester *et al.*, 1981; Nilsson and Biberfield, 1982; Forre *et al.*, 1982; Egeland *et al.*, 1983; Duke *et al.*, 1983), decreased (Verdickt *et al.*, 1983; Kotzin *et al.*, 1983; Duke *et al.*, 1983; Veys *et al.*, 1982b; Queiros and Rocha, 1983; Raeman *et al.*, 1981; Abe *et al.*, 1984; Bellamy *et al.*, 1983), or increased (Haraoni *et al.*, 1984). Therefore, the ratios of $T4^+$/$T8^+$ cells are normal (Burmester *et al.*, 1981; Nilsson and Biberfield, 1982), increased (Bellamy *et al.*, 1983; Duke *et al.*, 1983; Veys *et al.*, 1982b; Raeman *et al.*, 1981), or decreased (Haraoni *et al.*, 1984). Duke *et al.* (1983) found decreased proportions but normal numbers of $T8^+$ cells. Queiros and Rocha (1983) reported increased proportions of $T4^+$ and decreased proportions of $T8^+$ cells only in active RA; decreased $T8^+$ cells correlated with the circulating IgG complexes. Abe *et al.* (1984) have found a deficiency of $T8^+$ cells in RA with vasculitis when compared to RA without vasculitis. Haraoni *et al.* (1984) analyzed two groups of patients with RA using monoclonal antibodies and found decreased $T4^+$ and increased $T8^+$ cells, resulting in a lower T4/T8 ratio, in anergic RA patients (those who showed poor proliferative response to recall antigens) when compared to unanergic RA patients. The mechanism(s) for T-cell subset abnormality remains unclear.

iii. Quantitative Analysis of Activated T-Cell Subsets. The evidence of *in vivo* activation of T cells in the peripheral blood of RA, as determined by the expression of HLA-DR or Ia antigens, has been examined. Activated T cells in RA are reported to be normal (Duke *et al.*, 1983; Forre *et al.*, 1982a,b) or increased (Harouni *et al.*, 1984; Papadimitriou *et al.*, 1982; Yu *et al.*, 1980; Burmester *et al.*, 1981; Kluin-Nelemans *et al.*, 1984). Burmester *et al.* (1981) observed increased Ia-bearing T cells predominantly in the $T8^+$ population. Similarly, Marouni *et al.* (1984) reported increased Ia^+ T cells in anergic RA patients; 50% Ia^+ T cells were $OKT8^+$, and only 20% were $OKT4^+$ cells. The functional significance of these Ia^+ T-cell subsets in the pathogenesis of RA is unclear.

It would be interesting to examine two other antigens (Tac and transferrin receptors) on T cells from RA since there is a dissociation between Tac and Ia antigens (Gupta, 1984).

iv. Immunoregulatory Functions. Both spontaneous and induced helper and suppressor functions have been studied in RA. Egeland *et al.* (1983) reported a deficiency of Leu $3a^+$ cell helper function (on cell-for-cell basis) in RA compared to normal controls. Bellamy *et al.* (1983) also observed a deficiency of T helper function in RA. They examined immunoglobulin production by peripheral blood B lymphocytes in cultures containing various combinations of B and T cells by a reverse hemolytic plaque-forming cell assay. Responses were markedly increased in controls when T cells were either irradiated or depleted of Tγ cells before coculturing with B lymphocytes. No such enhancement was observed in RA. However, addition of normal allogeneic T replacing factors to RA B cells restored the responses, indicating that in RA there is a defect at the levels of T helper cells and/or their interactions with B lymphocytes. This defect did not correlate with the ratio of $T4^+$/$T8^+$ cells, which was independent of disease activity. In contrast, Patel and Panayi (1984) recently examined helper T-cell functions for spontaneous production of IgM RF *in vitro* in RA. Cocultures of normal B cells with normal autologous or allogeneic T cells failed to synthesize IgM RF. In contrast, RA T cells induced IgM RF production by normal as well as RA B cells. The helper/inducer effect of T cells from RA for RF production was not HLA-DR 4 restricted. Kluin-Nelemans *et al.* (1984) also showed increased helper T-cell activity in RA. It would be of interest to examine the purified activated (Ia^+) T-cell subsets function in RF production in RA. It is possible that active T helper/inducer cells could be responsible for IgM RF in RA.

Egeland *et al.* (1983) demonstrated increased spontaneous suppressor cell activity of $OKT8^+$ cells (on cell-for-cell basis) in RA. The mitogens Con A and PHA have the property of inducing suppressor activity in T cells. Dunne *et al.* (1982) reported normal PHA- and Con-A-induced suppressor activity in RA against a proliferative response of autologous T cells to PHA, Con A, and PWM; however, autologous plasma could abrogate this induced suppressor activity in RA. Palacios *et al.* (1981) and Tsoukas *et al.* (1980) also reported normal mitogen-induced suppressor activity in RA against PWM-induced immunoglobulin synthesis. Abe *et al.* (1984) observed normal Con-A-induced suppressor cell activity in RA without vasculitis, but a deficiency of suppressor function was observed in RA with vasculitis. Tosato *et al.* (1981, 1984), Bardwick *et al.* (1980), and Depper *et al.* (1981) observed a deficiency of suppressor T-cell function regulating Epstein–Barr virus-induced responses in RA. Keystone *et al.* (1980) reported a deficiency of antigen-specific cell activity in RA. Abdou *et al.* (1981) reported a deficiency of suppressor cell activity in patients with RA of less than 6 month's duration. This deficiency of suppressor T-cell function correlated with the presence of antilymphocyte antibody. However, the specificity of these antibodies with regard to monoclonal-antibody-defined T-cell subsets and their functions remains to be determined.

c. Cytotoxic T-Cell Functions. Because lymphocytes from patients with RA become transformed into EBV-infected continuous B cell lines more readily than those from normals, the cytotoxic responses against EBV versus infected target cells were examined in RA (Tsoukas *et al.*, 1982). Cytotoxic cells were generated by two cycles of stimulation with mitomycin-C-treated autologous EBV-infected B cells, and their lytic activity was assessed on [^{51}Cr]-labeled target cells. Patients with RA demonstrated cytotoxicity similar to the control group against autologous EBV-infected targets. The cytotoxicity was mediated by T cells having phenotype characteristic of T cells from normal individuals, i.e., $OKT3^+$, $OKT8^+$. Therefore, it appears that in RA higher EBV-induced transformation of B lymphocytes is not a result of a deficiency of cytotoxic T-cell functions but appears to arise from a deficiency of regulatory (suppressor) T-cell functions.

d. B Lymphocytes

i. Quantitative Analysis of B Lymphocytes. Earlier studies of B-cell quantitation utilized both C3 receptors and surface Ig as markers. Mellbye *et al.* (1972) reported decreased proportions of $C3^+$ receptor and surface Ig^+ B cells in RA. In contrast, several other investigators have found normal proportion of surface Ig^+ B lymphocytes (Slavin and Strober, 1981; Moutsopoulos *et al.*, 1976; Raeman *et al.*, 1981; Williams *et al.*, 1973; Meijer *et al.*, 1982). Williams *et al.* (1973) found normal proportions of surface IgM-, IgA-, and IgG-bearing B cells in RA. However, in the majority of these disorders, no consideration was given to disease activity and type of treatment. Youinou *et al.* (1984) found normal proportions of B lymphocytes in both active and inactive RA, but a significant increase in the ratio of surface IgM^+/surface IgD^+ B cells was observed in very active RA. This was associated with decrease in mouse erythrocyte rosette-forming cells (MRFC). These investigators also observed increased MRFC in inactive RA. Plater-

Zyberk *et al.* (1983) also reported increased proportions of MRFC and normal proportions of surface Ig^{+} B cells in RA. The latter study, however, did not express their data in relation to disease activity or treatment.

Since during activation of B lymphocytes surface IgD is lost (Kuritani and Cooper, 1982), and MRFC appears to be a marker of relatively immature B cells (Gupta *et al.*, 1976a) and to be lost during *in vitro* activation (Forbes *et al.*, 1981), the findings of Youinou *et al.* (1984) could suggest that in active RA, B lymphocytes are activated *in vivo*. The evidence of B-cell activation in RA is also supported by spontaneous DNA synthesis by B lymphocytes (Al-Balaghi *et al.*, 1984). Tosato *et al.* (1984) also reported an increase in spontaneously EBV-infected B cells in RA. Doblong *et al.* (1979) demonstrated the presence of IgM RF idiotype-positive lymphocytes in RA; the majority of idiotype-positive cells were B lymphocytes; however, 7% were T lymphocytes. Idiotype-positive B cells could be the precursors of the plasma cells that are producing RF. The RF idiotype-positive T lymphocytes may explain the positive irrigation inhibition with aggregated IgG in RA. These cells may participate in the immune response to IgG as helper T cells or suppressor T cells and thus modulate the B cell response. Alternatively, the idiotype-positive T lymphocytes might be effector T cells playing an important role in the pathogenesis of the RA.

ii. Quantitative Analysis of Immunoglobulin-Secreting B Cells. Spontaneously Ig-secreting B lymphocytes have been shown to be normal (Palacios *et al.*, 1981; Petersen *et al.*, 1984) or increased (Bell and Pinto, 1984; Pardo and Levinson, 1983; Al-Balaghi *et al.*, 1982). Bell and Pinto (1984) reported a correlation between increased spontaneously Ig-producing B cells and extraarticular manifestations in RA. They concluded that in RA patients whose disease is primarily articular, active Ig synthesis is limited to the synovial compartment, whereas in those with extraarticular features, active Ig-producing B cells also appear in the circulation. Pardo and Levinson (1983), using a reverse hemolytic PFC assay, also reported increased numbers of Ig-secreting cells in RA than in other types of arthritis and healthy controls. These investigators did not find any correlation between increased Ig-secreting cells and disease activity or concomitant corticosteroid treatment; however, patients who were on gold therapy had normal numbers of Ig-secreting B cells. This suggests that the gold could affect the mechanisms controlling *in vivo* B-lymphocyte activation. Al-Balaghi *et al.* (1984) also found increased spontaneously IgM- and IgA-secreting B cells in active RA, whereas the number of IgG-secreting B cells were normal.

A number of cellular and soluble substances derived from T cells regulate B cell activation; therefore, it would be of interest to examine the production and influence of BCPF, BCGF, and BCDF. In fact, Al-Balaghi *et al.* (1984) have reported the presence of a BCGF-like factor in the synovial fluid of RA.

Although EBV-induced Ig-secreting cells are increased in RA (Fong *et al.*, 1982; Tosato *et al.*, 1984), polyclonal-mitogen-stimulated Ig-secreted cells in RA are normal (Bellamy *et al.*, 1983; Palacios *et al.*, 1981; Doblong *et al.*, 1981; Petersen *et al.*, 1984) or decreased (Pardo *et al.*, 1984; Plater-Zyberk *et al.*, 1983). Pardo *et al.* (1984) examined PWM- and peptidoglycan-, the major constituent of the cell wall of grain-positive bacteria, -induced Ig-secreting cells in RA. Pokeweed mitogen-induced Ig-secreting cells were similar in RA and other arthritis groups, but responses were moderately depressed compared to healthy controls. The responses to peptidoglycan were markedly decreased in RA when compared to the other arthritis group and normal control group. The impaired responses were not attributable to aberrant kinetic response, shift in dose–response pattern, decreased cell survival in cultures, or the inability of peptidoglycan to active RA cells. Cell fractionation studies indicated that peptidoglycan-reactive B cells were present in some RA patients, but their reactivity was abrogated by suppressor T cells. More recently, Tac antigen has found on activated B cells. It would be important to examine the B cells from RA for the expression of Tac receptor and their response to IL-2.

iii. Serum Immunoglobulins and Specific Antibodies. Serum Ig levels in RA are essentially normal (Plater-Zyberk *et al.*, 1983; Kapoor *et al.*, 1981). However, increased spontaneous production of IgM RF in RA is well documented (Olsen *et al.*, 1982). Olsen *et al.* (1984) reported the effect of gold and D-penicillamine on the levels of spontaneously produced IgM RF. They suggested that the changes in spontaneous IgM RF constitute a sensitive indicator of disease activity and response to therapy in RA. This effect of D-penicillamine on spontaneous IgM RF could result from its inhibiting influence on T helper cells (Lipsky and Ziff, 1980). Specific antibody responses to *Brucella* antigen, tetanus toxoid, and flagellin in RA have been examined (reviewed by Yu and Peter, 1974). Normal responsiveness, hyporesponsiveness, and hyperresponsiveness have been observed. More recently, Segond *et al.* (1979) examined *in vitro* specific antibody response to trinitrophenyl (TNP) in patients with RA. None of these patients were receiving immunosuppressive drugs or corticosteroid, and none had taken nonsteroidal antiinflammatory agents for at least 72 hr. The mean anti-TNP response of RA patients was significantly lower than that of the other arthritis group and the healthy control group. A follow-up study in a few patients suggested that RA lymphocytes could increase *in vitro* antibody response on treatment.

e. Third-Population Lymphoid Cells. A number of studies have reported results of IgG Fc-receptor-positive lymphocytes in RA. Both increased (Sharpin and Wilson, 1977; Wooley and Panayi, 1978; Hall and Winrow, 1979) and normal proportions (Froland *et al.*, 1975; Brown *et al.*, 1979; Horwitz and Juul-Nielsen, 1977) of Fc-receptor-positive lymphocytes have been found in RA. The ADCC activity in RA has been shown to be increased (Sany *et al.*, 1976), decreased (Froebel *et al.*, 1979; McGill and Twinn, 1977), or unchanged (Panayi and Corrigall, 1977; Rosenberg and Currey, 1979; Diaz-Jouanen *et al.*, 1976; Penschow and MacKay, 1980). Using a different indicator system that defines receptor for the IgG Fc constant region 2 domain, Hall *et al.* (1980) reported an increase in third-population lymphoid cells in RA compared with patients with osteoarthritis, ankylosing spondylitis, and a healthy control group. This population is also responsible for natural killing activity. Natural killing activity is dealt with in detail in Chapter 5.

2. Analysis of Lymphocytes in Synovial Fluid and Synovial Tissue

Compartmentalization of immune response is a well-established phenomenon, a typical example being sarcoidosis, in which local immune response appears to play a major role in the pathogenesis of pulmonary manifestations of the disease. Similarly, it is very likely that the local immune responses are responsible for joint pathology in RA. It is not clear at the present time whether some of these immune cells emigrate from the circulation to the joint cavity or whether some of the systemic manifestations of RA are due to emigration of reactive immune cells from the joint cavity to the peripheral blood. In this section, the local immune responses at the level of synovial tissue and in the synovial fluid of RA are discussed in detail.

a. Qualitative and Quantitative Analysis of T Lymphocytes. The presence of large numbers of T lymphocytes as compared to B lymphocytes both in the synovial fluid and in synovial tissue indicates the important role of the T lymphocytes in the chronic rheumatoid inflammatory reaction. Increased proportions of T lymphocytes defined by E-RFC in synovial fluid (Traycoff *et al.*, 1976; Froland *et al.*, 1973; Sheldon *et al.*, 1974; Utsinger, 1975) and in synovial tissues (Van Boxel and Paget, 1975; Loewi *et al.*, 1975; Abrahamsen *et al.*, 1975; Bankhurst *et al.*, 1976) of RA have been described. More recently, using monoclonal antibodies (OKT3, Leu 1, or Leu 4), several investigators have reported increased proportions of T cells in the synovial fluid (Duke *et al.*, 1983; Nilsson and Biberfield, 1982) and synovial tissue (Kurosaka and Ziffs, 1983; Klareskog *et al.*, 1982) in RA. Klareskog *et al.* (1982) reported that the majority of the T cells in the synovial tissue were adjacent to HLA-DR-expressing cells.

The responses of synovial fluid lymphocytes in RA to mitogenic and antigenic stimulation have been studied by several investigators. These cells respond poorly to PHA, Con A, and PWM compared to peripheral blood lymphocytes (Reynolds and Abdou, 1973; Petersen *et al.*, 1982, 1983; Loewi and Papamichail, 1972; Abrahamsen *et al.*, 1978; Burmester *et al.*, 1978; Ivanyi *et al.*, 1973). Petersen *et al.* (1983) demonstrated no defect in monocyte function in synovial fluid responsible for depressed PHA and Con A responses: addition of blood monocytes to monocyte-depleted synovial fluid lymphocytes did not improve PHA or Con A responses. Incubation of synovial fluid cells with aggregate-free human γ-globulin prior to stimulation elicits an even poorer response (Reynolds and Abdou, 1973), perhaps because of its effect on the receptors on the surface of lymphocytes. Petersen *et al.* (1982, 1983) reported that the responses to *Candida*, PPD, and *E. coli* antigens are normal in synovial fluid mononuclear cells.

More recently, mitogen-induced or spontaneously produced mediators by T cells have been studied in synovial fluids of RA. Interleukin 2 has been found to be increased in RA synovial fluid (Wilkins *et al.*, 1983); IL-2 in rheumatic diseases is discussed in detail in Chapter 4. Al-Balaghi *et al.* (1984) have demonstrated the presence of BCDF-like (helper) factor in synovial fluid of patients with RA. This like factor appears to be produced by DR^+ activated T cells within the joint of RA and causes increased PFC response by peripheral blood mononuclear cells in response to PWM. This differentiation/helper effect was predominantly on IgM PFC response. No correlation was observed between the activity of this factor in the synovial fluid and the serum or synovial fluid IgM RF levels.

b. Quantitative and Qualitative Analysis of Immunoregulatory T-Cell Subsets. Immunoregulatory T cells in synovial fluid and tissue have been quantitated using immunoglobulin isotype receptors and monoclonal antibodies. Forre *et al.* (1982a) found no significant increase in Tγ cells either in the synovial fluid or synovium tissue. In contrast, Nilsson and Biberfield (1982) and Mathieu *et al.* (1981) observed a relative decrease in T cells in RA synovial fluid as compared to the peripheral blood. In the synovial fluid, decreased ratios of $T4^+/T8^+$ T cells have been described by several investigators (Fox *et al.*, 1983; Duclos *et al.*, 1982; Veys *et al.*, 1982a; Lydyard *et al.*,

1982; Duke *et al.*, 1983). Decreased proportions of T4 cells (Nilsson and Biberfield, 1982; Forre *et al.*, 1982a) and decreased (Duke *et al.*, 1983; Nilsson and Biberfield, 1982) or normal proportions (Forre *et al.*, 1982a) of T8 cells in the synovial fluid have been observed.

In the synovial tissue, studies of $T4^+$ and $T8^+$ T cells have been rather conflicting. An increased (Janossy *et al.*, 1981; Duke *et al.*, 1982; Klareskog *et al.*, 1982; Meijer *et al.*, 1982; Kurosaka and Ziff, 1983), a decreased (Egeland *et al.*, 1983), and normal (Forre *et al.*, 1982a) proportions of $T4^+$ cells have been described in the synovial membrane of RA. The majority of $T4^+$ cells were in close contact with HLA-DR-expressing cells. Analyses of $T8^+$ cells in RA synovial tissue have also revealed increased (Fox *et al.*, 1982a; Kurosaka and Ziff, 1983), normal (Forre *et al.*, 1982a), and decreased (Egeland *et al.*, 1983) proportions of $T8^+$ cells. Therefore, the ratios of $T4^+/T8^+$ cells were either increased (Kurosaka and Ziff, 1983; Janossy *et al.*, 1981; Duke *et al.*, 1982; Klareskog *et al.*, 1982; Meijer *et al.*, 1982), decreased (Kurosaka and Ziff, 1983; Burmester *et al.*, 1981; Fox *et al.*, 1982a), or normal (Egeland *et al.*, 1983). These conflicting results appear to be caused by different areas of rheumatoid synovium sampled by different investigators.

To resolve this issue, Kurosaka and Ziff (1983) studied the monoclonal-antibody-defined T-cell subset distribution in RA synovium using an immunoelectron microscopic technique. The perivascular mononuclear cell collections of the RA synovial membrane were variable in composition and size among different patients with RA and within the same patient's tissue. The lympyhocyte-rich areas contained mainly small lymphocytes, whereas transitional areas contained blast cells, macrophages, plasma cells, and lymphocytes. In both areas, 80% of lymphocytes were $OKT3^+$. In lymphocyte-rich areas, $OKT4^+$ cells were the predominant cells, with a high $OKT4^+/OKT8^+$ cell ratio. Macrophagelike cells were seen in small proportions. In contrast, in the transitional areas, $OKT8^+$ were predominant, resulting in lower $OKT4^+/OKT8^+$ cell ratios. $OKT8^+$ cells in this area tended to be large and blastlike as compared to $T8^+$ cells in the lymphocyte-rich area. In the transitional area, abundant macrophagelike cells were seen in close contact with $OKT8^+$ cells.

Duke *et al.* (1984), using a combined immunohistological and histochemical analysis, examined the lymphocyte and macrophage populations in the rheumatoid nodules (RN). This analysis revealed that the RN is composed of strongly $HLA\text{-}DR^+$ and adenosine-triphosphate-negative macrophages that contain large amounts of acid phosphatase. The lymphocytic infiltration was sparse and poorly organized and composed entirely of T cells with a normal proportion of both $OKT4^+$ and $OKT8^+$ T-cell subsets. Therefore, these observations are in contrast with those in rheumatoid synovium.

In addition to quantitative analysis of immunoregulatory T cells, functional analyses have been carried out by some investigators. The helper activity of T cells in the synovial compartment is either decreased (Kluin-Nelemans *et al.*, 1984; Egeland *et al.*, 1983) or normal (Chattopadhyay *et al.*, 1979b). Egeland *et al.* (1983) found a deficiency of Leu 3^+ T cell helper function in synovial tissue eluates from two of three patients with RA. Although a lack of spontaneous or mitogen-induced suppressor cell activity has been described in synovial fluid and tissue in RA (Chattopadhyay *et al.*, 1979a,b; Winchester, 1982), other investigators have reported strong suppressor activity in purified $T8^+$ cells from rheumatoid synovial tissue (Petersen *et al.*, 1984; Egeland *et al.*, 1983). Chattopadhyay *et al.* (1980) also described increased suppressor cell activity in synovial tissue T cells from a patient with X-linked hypogammaglobulinemia with rheumatoid-like arthritis. These investigators proposed that two distinct immunoregulatory phenomena might be operating in classical RA and RA associated with hypogammaglobulinemia. However, this might not be true, especially after the studies of Kurosaka and Ziff (1983), who demonstrated predominance of $T4^+$ or $T8^+$ cells in synovial tissue depending on the area involved. Therefore, variation in the immunoregulatory function could likely arise from different areas of synovial tissue analyzed.

c. Activated T Cells. There is a general agreement that in rheumatoid synovial fluid and synovial tissue, activated T cells as defined by the expression of HLA-DR antigens are increased (Kluin-Nelemans *et al.*, 1984; Burmester *et al.*, 1981; Fox *et al.*, 1982c; Forre *et al.*, 1982a,b; Klareskog *et al.*, 1981; Janossy *et al.*, 1981). Burmester *et al.* (1981) further categorized the $HLA\text{-}DR^+$ T cells in the synovial compartment and observed that the predominant $HLA\text{-}DR^+$ cells were $OKT8^+$ when compared to HLA DR^+ $OKT4^+$ cells. Forre *et al.* (1982b) have also shown that activated T cells in the synovial tissue were as good a stimulator in the mixed lymphocyte reaction as were the non-T cells. Klareskog *et al.* (1982) also demonstrated that activated T cells from synovial fluid were stimulators in the autologous mixed lymphocyte reaction.

d. Quantitative and Qualitative Analysis of B Lymphocytes. B lymphocytes, as determined by surface immunoglobulins or receptors for C3, in the synovial compartment constitute a minor population of total lymphocytes (Abrahamsen *et al.*, 1975; Van Boxel and Paget, 1975).

Immunofluorescence studies of rheumatoid synovial sections have revealed cells with rheumatoid factor, primarily IgM and IgG classes (Mellors *et al.*, 1959; Munthe and Natvig, 1972). Cells secreting IgM RF have been demonstrated in the eluates of cells from synovial membrane (Smiley *et al.*, 1968; Vaughan *et al.*, 1976; Mellors *et al.*, 1959; Egeland *et al.*, 1982a,b). Vaughan *et al.* (1976) also observed increased RF production by bone marrow cells from patients with RA. These investigators suggested that increased RF production by synovial membrane lymphoid cells could result from migration of cells from bone marrow to synovial tissue. More recently, investigators have examined the total immunoglobulin production and numbers of immunoglobulin-producing cells in the synovial compartmental mononuclear cells. There is general agreement that total Ig-producing cells in synovial fluid and synovial tissue from RA are increased (Chattopadhyay, 1979a; Al-Balaghi *et al.*, 1984; Petersen *et al.*, 1984; Sliwinski and Zwaifler, 1970). Among total Ig, IgG is the predominant class of Ig produced by these cells (Al-Balaghi *et al.*, 1984; Petersen *et al.*, 1984). To date there are no studies regarding specific antibody response of B lymphocytes from RA synovial fluid or synovial membrane. Since activated B cells express IL-2 receptor, and IL-2 has been found in the joints of RA, it would be interesting to examine IL-2 receptors on synovial B cells and their response to IL-2.

The results on mitogen-stimulated Ig production by synovial mononuclear cells have revealed conflicting data. Chattopadhyay *et al.* (1979a) reported increased Ig production by PWM-stimulated synovial mononuclear cells. In contrast, Petersen *et al.* (1984) reported depressed Ig production by PWM- and EBV-stimulated synovial fluid mononuclear cells. The difference in the results could reflect differences in the sample tested (synovial membrane versus synovial fluid), patient population, and assay systems. No attempt was made to correlate Ig production with the quantitative and qualitative analysis of immunoregulatory cells, although Petersen *et al.* (1984) suggested that the depressed responses were caused by increased suppressor cell activity.

e. Third-Population Lymphoid Cells. Analysis of IgG Fc-receptor-positive cells in rheumatoid synovial fluid shows reduced expression of Fc receptors (Nakai *et al.*, 1977), reduced levels of T cells (Biberfield *et al.*, 1979), and reduced antibody-dependent cellular cytotoxicity (Diaz-Jouanen *et al.*, 1976; Corrigall and Panayi, 1978). Synovial tissue lymphocytes also display reduced ADCC activity compared to peripheral blood (Abrahamsen *et al.*, 1977). This could be a result of blocking of Fc receptors by antiglobulins and immune complexes present in the sera and synovial fluid of RA (Fink *et al.*, 1977; Nakai *et al.*, 1977). Corrigall and Panayi (1978) reported a lack of blocking factors responsible for reduced ADCC in RA synovial fluid. However, capping of Fc receptors following interaction with immune complexes could account for it.

B. Juvenile Rheumatoid Arthritis

Juvenile rheumatoid arthritis (JRA) is the most common chronic arthritis of childhood, affecting an estimated 60,000–200,000 children in the United States. Overall, the disease may begin at any age during childhood, and girls are more often affected than boys. There are three major types of JRA: (1) systemic onset disease accounts for about 20% of JRA; (2) polyarticular disease without the extraarticular manifestations of systemic onset disease occurs in approximately 40% of children with JRA; and (3) pauciarticular onset JRA affects 40% or more of children with JRA. Immunologic analyses have revealed differences between classical RA and JRA.

1. Qualitative and Quantitative Analysis of T Lymphocytes

Brenner *et al.* (1975) and Strelkauskas *et al.* (1976) have reported decreased proportions of T cells in active JRA. Strelkauskas *et al.* (1976) found no correlation between decreased T cells and treatment with prednisone or nonsteroidal antiinflammatory agents. Hoyeraal *et al.* (1975) reported a reduced delayed hypersensitivity reaction in JRA. Strelkauskas *et al.* (1976) reported a decreased proliferative response of mononuclear cells from JRA by PHA; however, PHA-induced proliferation of purified T cells from JRA was comparable to age and sex-matched normal controls. It is likely that the reduced PHA response in the total mononuclear population reflected a quantitative decrease in T cells. A number of other investigators have found normal responses to mitogens and antigens (Stratton and Peter, 1972; Corrigall *et al.*, 1979; Froebel *et al.*, 1979).

2. Qualitative and Quantitative Analysis of Immunoregulatory T-Cell Subsets

Doblong *et al.* (1981) reported decreased proportions of Tγ cells and normal proportions of Tμ cells in the peripheral blood of patients with JRA. This was associated with the deficiency of Con-A-induced suppressor cell activity for the T-cell proliferative response. In contrast, Forre *et al.* (1982a) reported normal proportions of Tγ cells in the peripheral blood, synovial fluid, and synovial tissue of JRA. A reduced suppressor cell activity in JRA has been reported by Strelkauskas *et al.* (1978a,b) that was considered to result from the presence of antibodies directed against a distinct subset of immunoregulatory T cells. Froelich *et al.* (1981), using a system similar to that described by Strelkauskas *et al.* (1978a,b), failed to demonstrate the presence of anti-T-cell-subset antibodies in JRA sera compared with normal sera. Similarly, Williams *et al.* (1981) failed to demonstrate an anti-T-cell antibody in JRA sera selective against $T\gamma$ cells. The reasons for these discrepancies remain unclear.

Morimoto *et al.* (1981) reported the presence of an anti-T-cell antibody in sera of active JRA patients that preferentially reacted with a subset (40%) of $T4^+$ cells. Borel *et al.* (1984), in a large series of 107 patients with active JRA, using indirect immunofluorescence and a fluorescence-activated cell sorter (FACS), demonstrated presence of anti-T-cell antibody in 75% of those with systemic onset, 70% with a pauciarticular, and 68% of those with a polyarticular onset disease. Longitudinal studies appeared to suggest a correlation with disease activity, particularly in individual patients who were positive for anti-T-cell antibodies, and remission was almost invariably associated with negative anti-T-cell antibodies. It was further demonstrated that JRA sera and T cells contain inducers of suppressors, which would explain the hyperimmunoglobulinemia in active JRA. However, these investigators did not perform simultaneous analysis of $T4^+$ and $T8^+$ cells. Forre *et al.* (1982a) observed normal proportions of Leu 2^+ T cells in blood, synovial fluid, and synovial tissue of JRA and normal proportions of Leu 3^+ T cells in the blood, but their proportion was slightly decreased in synovial fluid of JRA.

In vivo evidence of T-cell activation, as defined by HLA-DR^+ T cells, has been observed in the synovial fluid and synovial tissue but not in the peripheral blood of JRA (Forre *et al.*, 1982a). These investigators have also demonstrated that these HLA-DR^+ T cells stimulate the mixed lymphocyte reaction to a degree similar to the stimulatory capacity of non-T cells (Forre *et al.*, 1982b).

3. *Quantitative and Qualitative Analysis of B Lymphocytes*

The association of hypergammaglobulinemia with active JRA has been well recognized (Goel *et al.*, 1974). An IgA deficiency in association with JRA was first described by Cassidy *et al.* (1966) and Huntley *et al.* (1967). Since then, several investigators have reported IgA deficiency in JRA (Barkley *et al.*, 1979; Bluestone *et al.*, 1975; Cassidy *et al.*, 1977; Panush *et al.*, 1972; Pelkonen *et al.*, 1983). Pelkonen *et al.* (1983) observed two groups of IgA deficiency in JRA: transient and persistent IgA deficiency. Transient IgA deficiency was associated with treatment with gold and antimalarials. The gold-induced IgA deficiency usually developed abruptly soon after institution of gold therapy. In a few cases, low IgA levels returned to normal despite continuing gold therapy. In patients with persistent IgA deficiency, the course is mild and oligoarticular. In contrast, in patients with transient IgA deficiency, the disease is characterized by early onset, a polyarticular course, and prolonged activity.

Strelkauskas *et al.* (1976) reported increased proportions of B lymphocytes in JRA peripheral blood. Fong *et al.* (1982) examined the EBV-induced IgM anti-IgG lymphocytes in JRA. The frequencies of IgM anti-IgG precursor B cells increased with age in normal children. Patients with seropositive JRA had higher precursor frequency than age-matched normal controls. Children with seronegative systemic onset, pauciarticular onset, and hidden RF-seropositive JRA had IgM anti-IgG precursor B cell frequencies comparable to their age-matched controls. However, children with polyarticular onset seronegative JRA, like their adult counterparts, have EBV-induced IgM anti-IgG precursor cell frequencies significantly lower than normals.

4. Third-Population Lymphoid Cells

Strelkauskas *et al.* (1976) reported data on third-population cells in JRA by calculating the sum of T- and B-cell percentages and subtracting it from 100. No definite marker (e.g., IgG Fc receptor) assay was used. Using the negative definition of third population cells, they reported increased proportions in a majority of patients with active JRA. The results were similar when absolute numbers were used. Brenner *et al.* (1975) also observed an increased proportion of "null" cells in active JRA. The NK and ADCC functions were not analyzed.

C. Systemic Lupus Erythematosus

Systemic lupus erythematosus (SLE) is a multisystem and multifactorial disease characterized by a great variety of clinical and serological abnormalities. Lupus is considered a prototype autoimmune disease of the organ-nonspecific type. A number of abnormalities of lymphocytes have been reported. I intend to review in detail the qualitative and quantitative abnormalities of lymphocyte subsets in SLE, both *in vivo* and *in vitro*.

1. Quantitative Analysis of T Lymphocytes

The earlier studies quantifying T-cell proportions and numbers utilized sheep red blood cell rosette formation (E-rosette) as a marker of T cells; however, in the past 4 years, monoclonal antibodies have been used to quantify T cells and T-cell subsets in various disorders, including SLE. In general, most investigators have reported significant lymphopenia in patients with active SLE. Absolute lymphocyte counts are significantly lower in the active stage of the disease than in inactive disease; however, the development of lymphopenia does not precede the active stage of disease (reviewed by Raveche and Steinberg, 1979).

T lymphocytes as determined by E-rosettes tend to be decreased in proportion and absolute numbers (Raveche and Steinberg, 1979; De Horatius *et al.*, 1980; Tsokos and Ballow, 1983). The decrease in the proportions and numbers of E-rosette-forming T cells is more profound in active SLE than in inactive SLE, although even the latter has lower proportions and/or numbers of T cells than healthy controls. "Active" T cells, as defined by high-affinity E-rosette-forming cells (a subset of total T cells), appear to be selectively decreased in SLE. The decrease of this subpopulation of T cells is marked in active SLE (Rivero *et al.*, 1977). Inactive SLE patients are reported to have normal proportions of "active" T cells. The "active" rosette test is subject to technical variation, and, furthermore, the functional significance of "active" T cells is unclear.

More recently, monoclonal antibodies have been utilized to enumerate T cells and T-cell subsets in SLE. The results of the analysis of monoclonal-antibody-defined T cells have been rather conflicting; normal proportions of OKT3$^+$, T3$^+$, Leu 4$^+$, and Leu 1$^+$

(Smolen *et al.*, 1982; Bakke *et al.*, 1983; Kammer *et al.*, 1983; Lipnik *et al.*, 1984) or decreased proportions of Leu 1^+ and $T3^+$ (Morimoto *et al.*, 1980a; Tsokos and Ballow, 1983) cells have been described in active SLE. Bakke *et al.* (1983) reported decreased absolute numbers of $OKT3^+$ T cells in both untreated active SLE and in those treated with prednisone. The T-cell lymphopenia in SLE appears to be caused by anti-T-lymphocyte antibodies that have different specificities for distinct immunoregulatory T cells (discussed below).

2. Quantitative Analysis of T-Cell Subsets

T-cell subsets with presumably distinct immunoregulatory and effector functions, as defined by receptors for immunoglobulin isotypes or the presence of monoclonal-antibody-defined differentiation antigens, have been analyzed in patients with lupus. In general, there is more agreement in the abnormality of T-cell subsets defined with receptors for immunoglobulin isotypes than in those defined by monoclonal antibodies in SLE.

a. T-Cell Subsets Defined with Receptors for Immunoglobulin Isotypes. Several authors have reported a significant reduction in the proportions and absolute numbers of Tγ cells in patients with systemic lupus erythematosus (Fauci *et al.*, 1978; Moretta *et al.*, 1979; Hamilton and Winfield, 1979; Coovadia *et al.*, 1981; Alarcon-Segovia and Ruiz-Arguilles, 1978; Alarcon-Segovia and Palacios, 1981b). In contrast, Matsumoto *et al.* (1980) observed no consistently low levels of Tγ cells in SLE; however, information on disease activity and treatment is lacking from their report. Alarcon-Segovia and Palacios (1981b) observed normal proportion of Tγ cells in patients with diphyenylhydantoin-induced SLE. In spontaneous idiopathic SLE, the levels of Tγ cells appear to correlate with disease activity. Because Tγ cells function as suppressor cells and effectors of ADCC, Moretta *et al.* (1979) examined the functions of a Tγ-cell-enriched population from patients with active SLE. There was no difference in suppressor cell function and ADCC in Tγ cells from active SLE and from healthy controls. These investigators concluded that T-cell defects present in SLE patients are mainly of a quantitative rather than a qualitative type. The decrease of Tγ cells could either be caused by loss of IgG Fc receptor following *in vivo* interactions with antigen–antibody complexes (De Horatius *et al.*, 1980) or result from cytotoxic anti-T-cell antibodies against Tγ cells (Sakane *et al.*, 1979b; Okudaira *et al.*, 1979).

b. T-Cell Subsets Defined with Monoclonal Antibodies. Morimoto *et al.* (1980a) reported a significant reduction in T5/T8 (suppressor/cytotoxic) phenotype T cells in patients with spontaneous and drug-induced active SLE; however, in the latter group, only two patients were studied. Therefore, it is not clear at present if drug-induced lupus has similar T-cell subset abnormalities as idiopathic spontaneous SLE and will require a study of much larger patient sample size. This decrease in the proportion of T5/T8 cells has been explained by the presence of anti-T-cell antibodies selective against T5/T8 cells in active SLE (Morimoto *et al.*, 1980b,c, 1983a). Tsokos and Ballow (1983) described a deficiency of the Leu $2a^+$ (suppressor/cytotoxic) phenotype T cells in patients with SLE but observed no significant difference in the proportion of Leu $3a^+$ (helper/inducer) phenotype T cells. This resulted in significantly elevated Leu $3a^+$/Leu $2a^+$ cell ratios.

When data were critically analyzed for individual patients, three of ten patients also had deficiencies of Leu $3a^+$ cells. When they examined the cytotoxic and Con-A-induced suppressor function, they observed a deficiency in cytotoxic function but normal con-A-inducible suppressor cell function. This would be in contradiction to a number of studies that have reported such a deficiency of suppressor cell function (discussed below). The majority of patients in Tsokos and Ballow's (1983) study were on prednisone, which could have some influence on T-cell subset functions.

Smolen *et al.* (1982) studied 32 patients with SLE using monoclonal antibodies. Abnormalities of Leu $3a^+$ (helper/inducer) phenotype T cells were more common than those of Leu $2a^+$ (suppressor/cytotoxic) phenotype T cells, therefore resulting in a wide range of Leu $3a^+$/Leu $2a^+$ ratios. Three major patterns emerged: (1) a low Leu $3a^+$/Leu $2a^+$ ratio was observed in patients with severe renal disease and thrombocytopenia and onset of SLE by 20 years of age; (2) patients with a high Leu $3a^+$/Leu $2a^+$ ratio had multisystem disease including lymphadenopathy but only rarely renal disease; and (3) patients with normal Leu $3a^+$/Leu $2a^+$ ratios had the most widespread multisystem disease, often involving the kidneys and the central nervous system. The ratio did not correlate, however, with the duration of disease, disease activity, or corticosteroid dosage.

Bakke *et al.* (1983) observed a marked reduction in the proportion and numbers of $OKT4^+$ (helper/inducer) phenotype cells and a relative reciprocal increase in $OKT8^+$ (suppressor/cytotoxic) phenotype T cells, which resulted in a depressed ratio of $OKT4^+$/$OKT8^+$ cells. However, the absolute number of $OKT8^+$ T cells was decreased. The ratio correlated with corticosteroid treatment and certain manifestations of disease activity. These investigators also observed two subgroups, one with low $OKT4^+$/$OKT8^+$ ratio, who were young women with rash, arthritis, and a high serological activity index (based on anti-DNA, anti-DNP, and complement levels), and another group with low serological activity index and borderline $OKT4^+$/$OKT8^+$ ratio.

More recently, Morimoto *et al.* (1984) analyzed the specificity of anti-T-cell antibodies that interfere with suppressor functions. Several patterns emerged: antibodies preferentially reacting with $T8^+$ suppressor effector cell and those reactive with $T4^+$ suppressor inducer subset. Lupus patients with high $T4^+$/$T8^+$ ratios had anti-T-cell antibodies predominantly reactive with the $OKT8^+$ suppressor effector cells. Patients with low $T4^+$/$T8^+$ ratios had antibodies against either the $T4^+$ suppressor inducer or both the $T4^+$ suppressor inducer and $T8^+$ suppressor effector cells. In addition, in another group, anti-T-cell antibodies were reactive with neither functional $T4^+$ suppressor inducer nor functional $T8^+$ suppressor cells. These investigators also observed a significant correlation between the circulating $T4^+$/$T8^+$ ratio of peripheral T cells and the relative ability of their anti-T-cell antibody to kill $T8^+$ cells versus $T4^+$ cells. Yamada *et al.* (1984) also reported anti-T-cell antibody reaction against both $OKT4^+$ and $OKT8^+$ T cells. Therefore, it appears that anti-T-cell antibodies could be responsible for quantitative and qualitative deficiencies of T-cell subsets in at least a subgroup of patients with SLE.

3. Functional Studies of T Lymphocytes

a. Delayed-Type Hypersensitivity. Several investigators have analyzed the delayed-type hypersensitivity (DTH) to recall antigens in patients with SLE. Total anergy, marked depression to all test antigens (Abe and Homma, 1971; Andrianakos *et al.*, 1977b;

Gottlieb *et al.*, 1979; Gordon and Yanagihara, 1977; Horwitz, 1972), selective depression to tuberculin (Hahn *et al.*, 1973; Block *et al.*, 1968), trichophyton (Hahn *et al.*, 1973), and *Candida* (Landry, 1977), and intact DTH (Goldman *et al.*, 1972) have been described. Raveche and Steinberg (1979) found that patients with active disease had depressed DTH, especially to tuberculin. These patients also had lymphopenia and anti-T-cell antibodies. These investigators also observed that DTH returned towards normal following treatment with either cyclophosphamide or azothioprine. Paty *et al.* (1975) also reported that patients with moderate to severe disease activity had a high frequency of anergy and few positive responses to SK-SD and *Candida* antigens, whereas patients with inactive or mildly active SLE had more normal reactions. In contrast, Rosenthal and Franklin (1975) found only minimal improvement in skin reactivity on follow-up study of the initially active patients at a time when disease was less active. Patients with active SLE also have marked impairment in sensitization to dinitrochlorobenzine (Abe and Homma, 1971; Foad *et al.*, 1975; Landry, 1977; Raveche and Steinberg, 1979) and to keyhole limpet hemocyanin (KLH) (Horwitz, 1972). It appears that lymphopenia and anti-T-cell antibodies are perhaps the most important factors responsible for DTH abnormality; however, the possibility of monocyte chemotactic defect has not been explored.

b. Proliferative Response of Lymphocytes to Mitogens, Antigens, and Alloantigens. In a number of different assays, patients with active SLE demonstrate defective T-cell functions. A majority of investigators agree that patients with active SLE have a reduced proliferative response to phytohemagglutinin (Bell, 1978; Glinski *et al.*, 1976; Lockshin *et al.*, 1975; Utsinger and Bluestein, 1974; Utsinger, 1976; Suciu-Foca *et al.*, 1974; Markenson *et al.*, 1978; Nies and Louie, 1978; Horwitz and Garrett, 1977; Utsinger and Yount, 1977; Scheinberg *et al.*, 1978; Ruiz-Arguelles *et al.*, 1979), concanavalin A (Horwitz *et al.*, 1977a; Scheinberg *et al.*, 1978), pokeweed mitogen, a T-cell-dependent B-cell mitogen (Nies and Louie, 1978; Sakane *et al.*, 1978; Fauci *et al.*, 1978; Bobrove and Miller, 1977), and tetanus toxoid (Gottlieb *et al.*, 1979). In general, there is a relationship between depressed response to PHA and disease activity (Glinski *et al.*, 1976; Utsinger and Bluestein, 1974; Utsinger, 1976; Utsinger and Yount, 1977).

Suciu-Foca *et al.* (1974) examined the influence of corticosteroids on PHA response of lymphocytes from SLE and observed no significant difference between steroid-treated lupus patients and untreated patients. Utsinger and Young (1977) reported a deficiency of B-cell helper effect on T-cell proliferative response in patients with active SLE; therefore, the T-cell defect in SLE appears not to be solely an intrinsic T-cell defect. Anti-T-cell antibodies present in the sera of patients with active SLE appear to inhibit T-cell responses to PHA, Con A, soluble antigens, and allogeneic cells (Strelkauskas *et al.*, 1976; Bell, 1978; Rosling *et al.*, 1978). Utsinger and Yount (1977) reported no role of macrophages in deficient PHA-induced T-cell proliferation in SLE; in contrast, Markenson *et al.* (1978) demonstrated correction of PHA response following removal of adherent cells in SLE.

Bernstein *et al.* (1980) examined T-cell colony formation in SLE. They observed a significant reduction in PHA-induced T-cell colony formation in patients with SLE. Colony growth showed a strong correlation with disease activity but did not correlate with responses of blood lymphocytes to PHA in suspension cultures, with the number of circulating T cells, or with serological abnormalities. More recently, Kammer (1983) reported impaired T-cell capping using anti-T3, -T4, and -T8 monoclonal antibodies in patients with active SLE. This suggests an intrinsic disorder of T cells in SLE. Lymphocytes from patients with SLE appear to have an increased proliferative response to nucleosides conjugated to keyhole limpet hemocyanin. The proliferative response of T cells and T-cell subsets in the autologous mixed lymphocyte reaction (AMLR) has been extensively studied in patients with SLE and is discussed in detail in Chapter 3.

c. Cytotoxic Functions in SLE. Ruiz-Arguelles *et al.* (1979) studied PHA-induced cellular cytotoxicity in mononuclear cells from patients with SLE. A diminished lectin-induced cytotoxicity was observed. Sera from patients with active lupus inhibited PHA-induced cytotoxicity. The factor in the serum was not immune complex or immunoglobulins.

Antibody-dependent cytotoxicity (ADCC) has been reported to be normal (Diaz-Jouanen *et al.*, 1976) or decreased (Scheinberg and Cathcart, 1976; Cooper *et al.*, 1978; Gershwin *et al.*, 1977; Feldman *et al.*, 1976) in patients with SLE. The differences in the results could be explained by the different targets used in these studies. Both groups reported normal ADCC against chicken RBC as targets; however, Cooper *et al.* (1978) observed decreased ADCC against Chang liver cells. In contrast, Feldman *et al.* (1976) and Scheinberg and Cathcart (1976) reported reduced ADCC using chicken RBC. Raveche and Steinberg (1979) reported reduced ADCC against Chang cells in active SLE and near normal ADCC against chicken RBC in inactive SLE and in both active and inactive SLE. The effector cell population against Chang liver cells appears to be lymphoid cells, whereas against chicken RBC both lymphoid cells and macrophages could be effectors in ADCC. Kumagai *et al.* (1981) have reported the presence of an anti-T-cell antibody in SLE that can induce ADCC against T cells as targets. Tsokos and Ballow (1981) examined cytotoxic T lymphocyte functions in patients with SLE. The generation of CTL function in MLR was significantly lower than that in normal individuals. No direct correlation was observed between MLR proliferative response and deficient CTL function. Low CTL function correlated with increased disease activity and increased serum DNA binding. Sera from the majority of patients with SLE had no inhibitory effect on the generation of CTL function.

The natural killer (NK) functions (Hoffman, 1980) and cytotoxicity against xenoantigens (Carpentier *et al.*, 1979) have been found to be reduced in SLE. Natural killer functions are discussed in detail in Chapter 5.

d. Functional Analysis of Immunoregulatory T Lymphocytes. There is general agreement among investigators that in active SLE there is a deficiency of spontaneous as well as Con-A-induced suppressor cell activity (Sakane *et al.*, 1978, 1979a,b, 1983; Honda *et al.*, 1982; Morimoto *et al.*, 1979b; Bresnihan and Jasin, 1977; Kammer *et al.*, 1983; Newman *et al.*, 1979; Strelkauskas *et al.*, 1976; Kaufman and Bostwick, 1979; Krakauer *et al.*, 1979; Morimoto *et al.*, 1979a,b; Sagawa and Abdou, 1979; Clough *et al.*, 1980; Tsokos and Barlow, 1983; Fauci *et al.*, 1978; Coovadia *et al.*, 1981; Alarcon-Segovia and Palacios, 1981b; Horowitz *et al.*, 1977). However, few investigators have failed to demonstrate a lack of suppressor defect in SLE (Delfraissy *et al.*, 1980; Nies *et al.*, 1981; Nakamura *et al.*, 1982; Tsokos and Ballow, 1983). Abdou *et al.* (1976) and Sakane *et al.* (1983) demonstrated a lack of helper function and deficiency of suppressor T-cell functions in active SLE. A significant correlation was observed between abnormal DNA binding or serum complement levels and suppressor cell activity. In a later study, Sagawa and Abdou (1979) observed no increase in DNA-binding cells and anti-DNA in supernatants; the number of cells synthesizing Ig and Ig secretions were not increased. However, Kaufman and Bostwick (1979) found no correlation between lack of Con-A-induced suppressor cell activity and organ involvement, drug treatment, anti-DNA antibodies, or thymic hormone levels. Nies *et al.* (1981) have reported normal suppressor as well as helper T-cell function, whereas others have observed only a defect in helper T-cell function (Kumagai *et al.*, 1982; Delfraissy *et al.*, 1980).

These differences in the results of immunoregulatory T-cell defects in patients with SLE appear to arise from (1) different target cell systems used to determine suppressor/helper functions, (i.e., B-cell colony assay, immunoglobulin synthesis, B-cell proliferation, or T-cell proliferation to mitogens or alloantigens); (2) spontaneous versus induced suppressor effector cell assay (Con-A-induced, adenosine-induced, or EBV-induced); (3) use of purified versus unseparated populations of T cells in coculture experiments; (4) active versus inactive SLE; (5) presence or absence of anti-T-cell antibodies; and (6) the nature and duration of treatments. The defective suppressor T-cell function has been explained by the presence of anti-T-cell antibodies against suppressor T cells (Sagawa and Abdou, 1979; Honda *et al.*, 1982; Morimoto *et al.*, 1979, 1980a,b, 1984; Sakane *et al.*, 1979b, 1983; Okudaira *et al.*, 1982; Strelkauskas *et al.*, 1979; DeHoratius *et al.*, 1980; Moretta *et al.*, 1979). Anti-T-cell antibodies against $OKT4^+$ or $T4^+$ T cells (Morimoto *et al.*, 1981) and $OKT8^+$ or $T8^+$ T cells (Morimoto *et al.*, 1980, 1984; Sakane *et al.*, 1983) have been demonstrated. These antibodies with different specificities could explain multiple immunoregulatory defects observed in patients with SLE. Sakane *et al.* (1978) demonstrated that in SLE the defect was in the generation of suppressor signals; the response to suppressor signal was normal.

More recently, Sakane *et al.* (1983), using purified $OKT4^+$ and $OKT8^+$ T-cell subsets from patients with active SLE, have demonstrated a defect in $OKT4^+$ suppressor T cells that is intrinsic to SLE and a defect of $OKT8^+$ effector suppressor cells in SLE that is caused by the presence of anti-$OKT8^+$ T-cell antibodies. Morimoto *et al.* (1984), however, observed the presence of anti-T-cell antibodies in SLE against both $T4^+$ suppressor inducer and $T8^+$ suppressor effector T cells.

e. Mediator Production in SLE. Abnormalities in the production of a number of soluble mediators [including interferon, interleukin 1, interleukin 2, migration inhibition factor (MIF), and Con-A-induced suppressor factor] have been described in patients with active lupus. Interleukins and interferon are discussed in Chapters 4 and 5. Abe *et al.* (1973) examined MIF production by T cells in response to native DNA; the latter was used as antigen because in patients with SLE there are circulating DNA-sensitized lymphocytes. They demonstrated that SLE cells produced MIF in response to native DNA. The results were more positive in active SLE than in inactive SLE. Ilefeld and Krakauer (1980) reported a deficiency of Con-A-induced suppressor factors from lymphocytes from SLE. Kumagai *et al.* (1982) reported deficient PHA-induced "helper" factor production that is required for B-cell colony formation in patients with active SLE.

f. Thymic Factors in SLE. Thymic epithelium produces a family of thymic factors that are capable of differentiating immature or immunoincompetent T cells into immunocompetent cells. It is unclear whether thymic epithelium produces a prohormone (a large molecule) that by some enzymatic cleavage is broken down into a number of biologically active thymic factors or hormones. Several of them have been purified and synthesized, and radioimmunoassays have been developed to measure their levels in the circulation and culture supernatants. The New Zealand black (NZB) mice, a model of human lupus, have defects in the morphology of thymic epithelium (De Vries and Hijman, 1966) with failure to produce thymic hormone (Bach *et al.*, 1973).

Sera from patients with active SLE have been found to be deficient in thymic humoral factor (Bach and Carnand, 1976; Kaufman and Bostwick, 1979). Horwitz *et al.* (1977b) were able to correct the deficient Con-A-inducible suppressor cell activity in patients with SLE by incubating SLE peripheral blood mononuclear cells with thymosin or cultured thymic epithelial cells. However, Kaufman and Bostwick (1979) found no correlation between the levels of thymic hormone and deficient suppressor activity in SLE. Michalevicz *et al.* (1978) demonstrated a significant increase in the number of E-rosette-forming T cells in patients with active SLE following *in vitro* incubation with thymic humoral factor and levamisole. This was in contrast to a lack of response in lymphocytes from patients with inactive SLE and normal controls. Scheinberg *et al.* (1975) also demonstrated a similar increase in the proportion of E-rosette-forming T cells following incubation with thymosin. Palacios and Alarcon-Segovia (1981) reported correction of deficient autologous mixed lymphocyte reaction (AMLR) in SLE with thymic factor *in vitro*.

These studies suggest that the deficiency of thymic hormone secretion might play a role in T-cell lymphopenia and certain abnormalities of immunoregulation in SLE. However, it remains to be determined whether the deficiency of thymic hormone in SLE is a primary or secondary phenomenon and whether the correction of T-cell function by thymic hormone treatment in murine SLE would prevent or retard the progress of autoimmune phenomena and their consequences.

4. Qualitative and Quantitative Analysis of B Lymphocytes in SLE

Systemic lupus erythematosus has been considered a prototype autoimmune disease. It is characterized by production of a large variety of autoantibodies (Tan, 1984), hyperimmunoglobulinemia (Cass *et al.*, 1968; Harvey *et al.*, 1954; Quismorio and Friou, 1970), increased immunoglobulin turnover (Levy *et al.*, 1970), and increased spontaneous immunoglobulin production (Okudaira *et al.*, 1980), the latter including an increase in cells producing autoantibodies, such as anti-DNA (Bankhurst and Williams, 1975, 1976; Bell *et al.*, 1973; Vaughan and Chihara, 1973), and cells producing antibodies with a variety of specificities unrelated to self antigens (Morimoto *et al.*, 1977; Budman *et al.*, 1977). These studies demonstrate the generalized hyperreactivity of B lymphocytes in SLE. A controversy exists whether there is a primary B-cell defect (Nies *et al.*, 1981; Suzuki *et al.*, 1982a,b; Okudaira *et al.*, 1980) or whether B-cell abnormalities are secondary to immunoregulatory T cell abnormalities (Kumagai *et al.*, 1982; Tsokos and Ballow, 1983; Clough *et al.*, 1980; Morimoto *et al.*, 1979a).

Kumagai *et al.* (1982) have examined B cell proliferation using a semisolid agar assay for B-cell colony formation in response to lipopolysaccharide (LPS) and PHA and T cells in patients with SLE. These investigators observed an increased number of B-cell colonies that were formed spontaneously in patients with SLE compared to controls. Following LPS activation, the number of B-cell colonies was further increased, and their numbers were significantly greater than those found in normal controls. When the role of PHA-stimulated T cells ("helper factor") was analyzed, T cells from patients with active SLE were defective in supporting B-cell colony formation. In contrast, Abe *et al.* (1982), using a liquid culture system, observed deficient [^{3}H]thymidine incorporation by non-T cells from patients with SLE when lymphocytes were stimulated with LPS. Furthermore, these investigators did not find any defect in helper T-cell function. The differences between the two studies could be related to the different culture systems used and different patient groups.

Depressed proliferative response to PWM, a helper T-cell-dependent B-cell mitogen, in SLE also suggests a deficiency of helper T cells in SLE. Morimoto *et al.* (1983b) examined the *in vitro* response of SLE lymphocytes to nucleosides conjugated to keyhole limpet hemocyanin (KLH). Nucleosides were selected because they are a part of the nucleic acid antigen and appear to be involved in autoimmunity and they covalently bind to either soluble IgG or cells that have been shown to induce unresponsiveness in mice. A significant proliferative response to nucleoside–KLH conjugate was observed in SLE lymphocytes, and SLE lymphocytes responded specifically to low doses of conjugates and not to carrier KLH alone. The SLE lymphocytes spontaneously produced a high level of antinucleoside antibodies that was further increased by stimulation with nucleoside and KLH conjugates. In contrast, normal control lymphocytes failed to produce antibodies to nucleosides either spontaneously or after antigenic stimulation.

The antibody responses to *in vivo* immunization have given variable results following influenza vaccine immunization of patients with SLE: normal (Brodman *et al.*, 1978; Louie *et al.*, 1978; Ristow *et al.*, 1978) or decreased (Williams *et al.*, 1978) antibody responses have been observed. In the latter study, primary immune response appears to be impaired to a greater extent than the secondary response. In contrast, Clough *et al.* (1980) observed normal IgM anti-DNA antibody production *in vitro* on stimulation with PWM, but a defect in the IgM-to-IgG switchover was observed. This defect appeared to be related to deficient switch T-cell function. However, these differences between *in vivo* and *in vitro* systems could arise from complex interactions between cells and antigens rather than between cells and mitogens. Similar to influenza, antibody responses to *Brucella* antigens have been shown to be normal (Lee *et al.*, 1960) or decreased (Baum and Ziff, 1969). Immunoglobulin G responses were normal; however, IgM responses were impaired (Baum and Ziff, 1969). A deficient IgM but normal IgG response has also been observed following immunization with KLH (Baum and Ziff, 1969).

In SLE normal resting antibody levels of blood group antigens and proteus OX-2 have been observed (Muschel, 1961); however, Zingale *et al.* (1963) observed increased resting antibody levels against blood group antigens. Normal antibody responses to immunization with tetanus toxoid and rickettsiae (Lee *et al.*, 1960; Abe and Homma, 1971) and increased antibody responses to penicillin (Harris and Vaughan, 1960) and a variety of viral antigens (Evans and Rothfield, 1973; Hollinger *et al.*, 1971; Hurd *et al.*, 1972; Phillips and Christian, 1971; Wilson *et al.*, 1973) have been observed in SLE. The resting antibody levels to streptolysin O, influenza, *E. coli*, and *Shigella* have also been observed in SLE (Williams *et al.*, 1978; Muschel, 1961; Baum and Ziff, 1969).

Patients with active SLE have markedly increased IgG and IgA antibody-forming cells but relatively normal numbers of cells producing IgM antibody (Grayson *et al.*, 1979). The degree of increase correlated with disease activity. These observations support the observations that peripheral blood lymphocytes from active SLE produce excessive amounts of antibody of all Ig classes but particularly of the IgG class (Ginsburg *et al.*, 1979). Tsokos *et al.* (1983) examined *in vitro* generation of plaque-forming cell (PFC) response from B cells in SLE infected with Epstein–Barr virus (EBV). They observed that B cells from SLE generated EBV-induced PFC responses similar to those produced by normal B cells infected with EBV within the first 14 days of culture. T cells from SLE patients failed to suppress the EBV-induced PFC response; however, B cells from SLE patients are susceptible to suppression by normal allogeneic T cells. These studies suggested that the B cells in SLE are not intrinsically defective.

Suzuki *et al.* (1982a) reported that B cells from SLE patients are much less susceptible to anti-Fab antibody-mediated suppression than B cells from normal subjects. This group extended their study to examine the effect of anti-IgM and anti-IgD antibodies on the differentiation of B cells in normal subjects, SLE, and rheumatoid arthritis (RA) to investigate the differential sensitivity of B-cell subsets to anti-Ig antibodies (Suzuki *et al.*, 1982a). In normal subjects and patients with RA, the spontaneous development of IgG and IgM secretory cells (measured by reverse PFC assay) was markedly suppressed by anti-IgM or anti-IgD antibodies. More than 50% of peripheral blood B cells were IgD^+ and/or IgM^+ in normals and RA. In SLE patients, however, the suppression of IgG and IgM production by anti-IgM or anti-IgD antibodies was markedly reduced, particularly in active SLE. The proportion of IgD-bearing cells in peripheral blood B cells was significantly reduced. A good correlation was observed between reduced susceptibility of B cells to anti-IgM antibody-mediated suppression and decreased proportion of IgD-bearing B cells in SLE. The decrease in IgD-bearing B cells was not caused by cytophilic antibody or antilymphocyte antibodies.

More recently, Tosato *et al.* (1984) examined the question of whether patients with SLE and RA have more circulating EBV-infected B cells than normals, since in both diseases, *in vitro* regulatory T-cell abnormalities related to EBV have been described. To address this question, they examined the frequency of spontaneously transformed B cells in the peripheral blood of eight normals, 15 patients with RA, and eight patients with SLE. The mean frequency of spontaneously transforming B cells in patients with SLE did not differ from that in normal controls; in contrast, in RA the mean frequency of spontaneously transformed B cells was significantly greater ($10.1/10^6$ B cells) than in normal controls ($2.8/10^6$ B cells).

5. Conclusions

There is general agreement that in active SLE a qualitative and quantitative deficiency of suppressor T cells is present; however, deficiencies of helper T cells, helper factor, and switch T cells also appear to exist. Delayed cutaneous hypersensitivity and proliferative response to PHA are impaired in SLE; however, allogeneic MLR appears to be relatively preserved. The CTL functions are also impaired. The above abnormalities appear to be in part caused by the presence of anti-T-cell antibodies. B lymphocytes in active SLE are in a stage of polyclonal activation as shown by the presence of increased numbers of immunoglobulin-secreting cells, decreased numbers of IgD-bearing cells, and increased spontaneous immunoglobulin production. The response to PWM by B cells for Ig production is impaired in SLE. Few investigators have demonstrated an intrinsic defect of B cells; others have shown a defect in IgM-to-IgG switchover. *In vivo* primary (IgM) antibody response is impaired, whereas IgG response is relatively normal. Thymic factor levels are decreased; however, lack of correlation with disease activity or anti-DNA and measurements of thymic factor levels in subjects over 30 years of age make the interpretation of the result difficult.

In conclusion, multiple immunologic defects, both at T- and B-cell levels, some of them interrelated and others independent, exist in active SLE.

D. Progressive Systemic Sclerosis

Progressive systemic sclerosis (PSS) is a generalized disorder of connective tissue characterized by fibrosis and degenerative changes in the skin, synovium, digital arteries, and in parenchyma and small arteries of certain internal organs, notably the esophagus, intestine, lung, heart, kidney, and thyroid. The origin of PSS is unclear. The demonstration of a variety of cellular and humoral abnormalities indicates that immunologic mechanisms are important in its pathogenesis.

1. T Lymphocytes

Several investigators have reported decreased proportions and absolute numbers of E-rosette-forming T cells in patients with PSS (DeJesus and Clancy, 1975; Horwitz and Garrett, 1977; Gupta *et al.*, 1979; Segond *et al.*, 1982; Whiteside *et al.*, 1983; Inoshita *et al.*, 1981). In contrast, Lockshin *et al.* (1975) reported normal proportions of T cells in four patients with PSS studied. Whiteside *et al.* (1983) and Keystone *et al.* (1982) reported normal proportions of T cells using monoclonal antibodies. It remains to be determined whether sera from PSS contain factors that inhibit binding of T cells with SRBC. T-cell subsets have been enumerated with Ig Fc receptor or by monoclonal-antibody-defined differentiation antigens. Gupta *et al.* (1979) and Alarcon-Segovia *et al.* (1981) reported a deficiency of Tμ cells. The proportion of Tγ cells has been reported to be decreased (Whiteside *et al.*, 1983; Inoshita *et al.*, 1981), normal (Alarcon-Segovia *et al.*, 1981), or increased (Gupta *et al.*, 1979). These discrepancies could be explained by different geographical distribution, sample size, and the treatment that patients were receiving at the time of study. Whiteside *et al.* (1983) reported a normal proportion of OKT4$^+$ T cells but a significantly decreased proportion of OKT8$^+$ cells, resulting in a high OKT4$^+$/OKT8$^+$ ratio in PSS. There was no correlation between Tγ cells and OKT8$^+$ T-cell levels. The group with the high OKT4$^+$/OKT8$^+$ ratio was clinically indistinguishable from the group having a normal OKT4$^+$/OKT8$^+$ ratio. In these two groups of PSS patients, no difference was observed in terms of immunoglobulin levels and frequency of immune complexes or autoantibodies. In contrast, Bakke *et al.* (1983) observed a normal ratio of OKT4$^+$/OKT8$^+$ T cells in PSS.

A number of functional assays have been used to study the immunoregulatory activity in PSS. Inoshita *et al.* (1981), Alarcon-Segovia *et al.* (1981), and Krakauer *et al.* (1981) demonstrated increased helper activity in patients with PSS against PWM-driven B-cell differentiation to immunoglobulin-producing cells. Whiteside *et al.* (1983) observed no difference in short-lived nonspecific suppressor cell function between PSS and controls. Krawitt *et al.* (1982) observed normal Con-A-induced suppressor cell activity against allogeneic MLC in PSS; however, using indomethacin in cultures of mononuclear cells stimulated with PHA, they observed indirect evidence of increased prostaglandin-induced (probably suppressor monocyte-mediated) suppressor activity in PSS. Segond *et al.* (1982) also observed increased suppressor activity in nylon-wool-adherent celor primary antibody response in PSS. Though the distinct immunoregulatory activities can be demonstrated in the system used, it is apparent that in PSS the immunoregulatory system is abnormal.

Patients with PSS have also been shown to have a depressed proliferative response to mitogens and soluble antigens (Whiteside *et al.*, 1981; Salem and Morse, 1976; Horwitz and Garrett, 1977; Hughes *et al.*, 1977). Salem and Morse (1976) reported normal PHA but depressed Con A and PWM responses, whereas Lockshin *et al.* (1975) demonstrated a normal proliferative response to PHA, Con A, and PWM in patients with PSS studied. Bernstein *et al.* (1980) reported normal T-cell colony formation in response to PHA in PSS. Niwa and Kanoh (1979) reported depressed delayed-type hypersensitivity in PSS.

The lymphocytes from patients with PSS have been shown to produce a chemotactic factor and a migration inhibition factor when stimulated *in vitro* with collagen preparations (Currie *et al.*, 1970; Stuart *et al.*, 1976). Kondo *et al.* (1976) also reported production of a lymphokine in response to cutaneous antigen in patients with PSS.

2. B Lymphocytes

Although there is evidence of B-lymphocyte hyperactivity in PSS, the proportions of C3-receptor-bearing B cells (DeJesus and Clancy, 1975) and the proportion and numbers of surface Ig^+ B cells (Gupta *et al.*, 1979) in PSS are comparable to those in a control group. Serum immunoglobulins are modestly elevated (Inoshita *et al.*, 1981). Patients with PSS demonstrate circulating autoantibodies (Davis and Jason, 1976; Malaviya *et al.*, 1980; Husson *et al.*, 1976; Tan *et al.*, 1980; Whiteside *et al.*, 1983), cryoglobulins (Malaviya *et al.*, 1980; Husson *et al.*, 1976), and increased levels of circulating immune complexes (Malaviya *et al.*, 1980). We reported cryoglobulinemia in 11 of 31 patients with PSS (Malaviya *et al.*, 1980). All cryoproteins showed the presence of IgM, IgG, and C3. In three cryoproteins, detailed analysis showed the presence of κ as well as λ light chains both in IgG and IgM.

Segond *et al.* (1982) examined the nonspecific B-cell response in a reverse PFC assay in PSS and found it to be normal; however, the anti-TNP response was depressed. This suggests that patients with PSS have a selective deficiency of primary specific antibody response. Niwa and Kanoh (1979) also reported similar results. However, results on *in vivo* antibody response in PSS have been conflicting (Niwa and Kanoh, 1979; Kallenberg *et al.*, 1981).

Gupta *et al.* (1979) reported normal proportions and numbers of lymphoid cells with IgG Fc receptors (including third-population and B lymphocytes). However, Cooper *et al.* (1978) observed depressed ADCC in patients with PSS. No study has been published regarding phenotypic and functional analysis of NK cells in PSS.

Recently, Roumm *et al.* (1984) have examined the phenotypic expression of skin infiltrates in PSS. Total T cells, T-cell subsets, B cells, and macrophages were enumerated in the skin samples of 21 patients with PSS. The dermal mononuclear infiltrates consisted mostly of activated T lymphocytes with mean $T4^+/T8^+$ ratio of 2.4 ± 1.3. Only a few $B1^+$ and $T6^+$ cells were observed. There was no correlation between the skin or blood $T4^+/T8^+$ ratios and the degree of skin thickening. On histological examination, more than 50% of untreated patients with PSS had predominant dermal mononuclear cell (MNC) infiltration. A significant correlation was observed between MNC infiltration and the degree and progression of skin thickening.

E. Sjogren's Syndrome

Sjogren's syndrome (SS) is a chronic inflammatory disorder characterized by diminished lacrimal and salivary gland secretion resulting in keratoconjunctivitis sicca and xerostomia. The glandular insufficiency also affects other exocrine glands and is associated with lymphocytic and plasma cell infiltration as well as features of autoimmunity. Primary SS (Sicca complex unaccompanied by an associated disorder) may be distinguished from secondary SS (SS occurring with rheumatoid arthritis) clinically, immunogenetically, and serologically (Moutsopoulos *et al.*, 1979). In the following sections I will discuss the analysis of T and B lymphocytes and their subsets in peripheral blood, glandular tissue, and gastric tissue in patients with SS.

1. Qualitative Analysis of T Lymphocytes and Their Subsets

T lymphocytes have been analyzed in peripheral blood, salivary glands, gastric mucosa, and in pseudolymphoma associated with SS. The results of E-rosette-forming T cells have been rather conflicting. In the peripheral blood, E-rosette-forming T cells have been shown to be reduced (Talal *et al.*, 1974; Moutsopoulos *et al.*, 1976) or normal (Moutsopoulos and Fauci, 1980; Strelkauskas *et al.*, 1976). With monoclonal antibodies OKT3, T3, and Leu 1, the percentages and absolute numbers of total T cells in SS are reported to be normal (Fox *et al.*, 1982b, 1983) or decreased (Bakshi *et al.*, 1983; Morimoto *et al.*, 1982a). These differences could be caused by differences in patient group or technical differences. Patients with SS, unlike SLE patients, lack antilymphocyte antibody and therefore could not account for Tγ-cell lymphopenia reported by some investigators.

Moutsopoulos and Fauci (1980) reported an analysis of Tγ cells in patients with SS with or without extraglandular manifestations. A deficiency in the levels of Tγ cells was observed in nine of ten patients with SS with extraglandular manifestations and in three of ten with glandular manifestations. This decrease was explained by the presence of a blocking factor present in the sera of a subset of patients with SS that reversibly blocked the expression of IgG Fc receptor on Tγ cells. This blocking factor was found diffusely in the IgG fraction and not in the IgM fraction. This deficiency of Tγ cells did not correlate with Con-A-induced suppressor activity, which was found to be normal.

More recently, monoclonal antibodies have been utilized to study the T-cell subsets in SS. The majority of investigators agree regarding a quantitative deficiency of $OKT8^+$, $T8^+$, Leu $2a^+$ T cells in the peripheral blood of patients with primary and secondary SS (Morimoto *et al.*, 1982a; Fox *et al.*, 1982c; Bakshi *et al.*, 1983), resulting in increased $T4^+/T8^+$ ratios (Fox *et al.*, 1982c; Morimoto *et al.*, 1982a). This decrease in $OKT8^+$ T cells was not caused by anti-$T8^+$ antilymphocyte antibodies (Fox *et al.*, 1982c; Bakshi *et al.*, 1983). Morimoto *et al.* (1982a) reported increased $T4^+/T8^+$ ratios in ten of 14 patients with SS and decreased ratios in four of 14; however, these investigators did not explain whether their patients had primary or secondary SS. Bakshi *et al.* (1983) observed increased ratios of Leu $3a^+$/Leu $2a^+$ cells only in secondary SS, whereas in primary SS, the ratios were normal. Fox *et al.* (1982c) and Morimoto *et al.* (1982a) found no deficiency of $OKT4^+$, $T4^+$ cells in the blood of SS patients.

There is general agreement that the predominant cell types infiltrating the salivary and lacrimal glands in SS are E-rosette-forming, heteroantiserum-reactive, and monoclonal-antibody-defined T cells (Talal *et al.*, 1974; Tannenbaum *et al.*, 1975; Greenspan *et al.*, 1974; Fox *et al.*, 1982c, 1983; Adamson *et al.*, 1982). Among the T cells, the majority of cells reacted with anti-Ia monoclonal antibodies (and therefore were activated T cells) and were $OKT4^+$ (Fox *et al.*, 1982c, 1983). Fox *et al.* (1983) found no difference in T cells or T-cell phenotypes in salivary glands of patients with or without pseudolymphoma. The findings in pseudolymphoma with T-cell infiltration contradict its B-cell origin reported earlier (Faguet *et al.*, 1978). Kilpi *et al.* (1983) examined lymphocytic infiltrations of gastric mucosa in seven patients with primary or secondary SS. Three had primary SS, and four had secondary SS. The profile of T-cell distribution was similar to that observed in salivary glands: predominant cells were $OKT3^+$, $OKT4^+$, with a high $OKT4^+$/$OKT8^+$ ratio and increased $OKIa^+$ (activated) T cells. These observations clearly suggest that SS is a systemic disease (even primary SS) affecting many organs rather than a disease localized to a single exocrine gland.

2. Functional Analysis of T Cells and Their Subsets

Patients with Sicca syndrome generally show a normal delayed hypersensitivity response to tuberculin and dinitrochlorobenzene (Leventhal *et al.*, 1967; Whaley *et al.*, 1971); however, patients with secondary SS or Sicca syndrome with lymphoma show diminished response to these antigens (Leventhal *et al.*, 1967; Whaley *et al.*, 1971). Michalski and McCombs (1977) reported a normal proliferative response to optimal concentrations of PHA but reduced responsiveness to suboptimal concentrations of PHA in SS. Leventhal *et al.* (1967) and Bakshi *et al.* (1983) reported a decreased proliferative response to PHA and Con A. In contrast, Moutsopoulos and Fauci (1980) reported normal PHA-, Con-A-,and PWM-induced proliferation in untreated patients with SS with or without extraglandular manifestations.

The immunoregulatory functions of T cells in SS demonstrated normal Con-A-induced suppressor cell activity against the PWM-induced plaque-forming cell (PFC) response in allogeneic cocultures (Moutsopoulos and Fauci, 1980). No correlation was observed between Con-A-induced suppressor activity and the levels of $T\gamma$ cells. Fox *et al.* (1982c) reported that in primary SS, as in controls, the Ig production was $OKT4^+$ T cell dependent. In patients with SS with lymphoma, Ig synthesis was independent of $OKT4^+$ help. Studies are required on the function of $OKT8^+$ in the regulation of antibody production in SS.

3. Quantitative and Qualitative Analysis of B Lymphocytes

The proportions and numbers of surface immunoglobulin-bearing (Moutsopoulos *et al.*, 1976; Moutsopoulos and Fauci, 1980; Strelkauskas *et al.*, 1976) and monoclonal-antibody-defined B cells (Morimoto *et al.*, 1982a) are comparable to controls. In contrast,

Bakshi *et al.* (1983) have reported increased proportions of surface immunoglobulin-positive B cells in primary and secondary SS. Van Boxel *et al.* (1973) reported marked increases in the number of B-lymphocyte-carrying multiple-heavy-chain isotypes. This could be interesting in light of the increased susceptibility of SS patients to develop lymphomas. Lymphomas in SS arise from monoclonal expansion of B lymphocytes regardless of their histological features (Zulman *et al.*, 1979). No study of monoclonal antibodies against B-cell differentiation antigen on lymphoma in SS has been published. In gastric mucosa infiltrates in SS, surface Ig-bearing B cells are similar to those in the peripheral blood (Kilpi *et al.*, 1983). Fox *et al.* (1983) examined B lymphocytes in salivary glands of patients of SS with or without pseudolymphoma. The distribution of surface Ig-bearing B cells was similar to that in their peripheral blood. No evidence of monoclonality was observed. Salivary glands in both groups of SS (with and without pseudolymphoma) demonstrated the presence of $B532^+$ B cells, which are lacking in the peripheral blood of controls and patients with SS.

B lymphocytes from SS do not have increased spontaneous immunoglobulin/antibody production (Moutsopoulos and Fauci, 1980; Morimoto *et al.*, 1982a); however, B lymphocytes from patients with SS and lymphoma have increased spontaneous immunoglobulin production (Talal *et al.*, 1970).

Although the primary antibody responses to tetanus toxoid are normal in patients with SS, reduced secondary antibody responses are commonly observed, especially in secondary SS (Whaley *et al.*, 1971). Isohemagglutinin antibody titers (anti-A1, anti-A2, and anti-B) are significantly reduced in Sicca syndrome, whereas only levels of anti-A and anti-A2 antibodies are reduced in SS with RA (Whaley *et al.*, 1971).

Hyperimmunoglobulinemia of polyclonal nature is a common finding in SS (Bloch *et al.*, 1965; Whaley *et al.*, 1973). Although all three major classes of immunoglobulin may be elevated, the elevation is most marked for IgG and least for IgA (Gumpel and Hobbs, 1970; Whaley *et al.*, 1973; Talal *et al.*, 1970). It is perhaps surprising that IgA levels are least affected, as SS is a disease primarily affecting mucosal surfaces. A monoclonal IgG K cryoglobulin has been reported in SS (Zinneman and Caperton, 1977). Macroglobulinemia and cryomacroglobulinemia have also been observed in SS (Talal *et al.*, 1967; Pincus and Dekker, 1970; Anderson and Talal, 1972). Patients with SS associated with malignant lymphoma may be complicated with hypogammaglobulinemia (Talal *et al.*, 1967).

Increased levels of circulating immune complexes and a variety of organ-nonspecific (rheumatoid factor, ANA, anti-DNA, antimitochondrial antibody, anti-smooth-muscle antibody, antiinsulin antibody) and organ-specific antibodies against salivary and pancreatic duct, thyroid, adrenal, parathyroid, pituitary, ovary, gastric parietal cells, and erythrocytes have been described in SS (Whaley and Buchanan, 1980).

4. *Cytotoxicity in SS*

Feldman *et al.* (1976) reported normal ADCC in SS and RA. Bakshi *et al.* (1983) reported an increase in the proportions of null cells; however, they did not use Leu 11 monoclonal antibody, which actually defines the majority of cells in this population. Fox *et al.* (1983) reported a decreased proportion of Leu 7^+ cells in SS associated with decreased ADCC and NK function. Goto *et al.* (1981) also reported deficient NK functions in SS. Fox *et al.* (1983) also reported deficient cytotoxic T-lymphocyte activity in SS. More precise and detailed studies, using monoclonal-antibody-defined populations of effector cells, are needed to study the number and functions of cytotoxic cells in SS.

F. Polymyositis and Dermatomyositis

Polymyositis and dermatomyositis are diffuse inflammatory disorders of striated muscle that cause symmetrical weakness and, to a lesser extent, atrophy of muscles, principally of the limb girdles, neck, and pharynx.

1. T Lymphocytes

Although the exact mechanisms responsible for muscle injury in polymyositis are unknown, there is substantial evidence that suggests that cell-mediated immunity plays a major role. Morphological data indicate that the majority of cells in the infiltrates are lymphocytes and macrophages. Strelkauskas *et al.* (1976) observed a marked reduction in the proportions of circulating T cells in patients with dermatomyositis. In a preliminary immunohistological study of a small sample of polymyositis biopsies, Rowe *et al.* (1981) have shown the presence of T lymphocytes bearing HLA-DR antigen (both defined with monoclonal antibodies), which is indicative of activated T cells. More recently, Rowe *et al.* (1983) have examined biopsy specimens from treated and untreated patients with polymyositis using peroxidase staining with a panel of monoclonal antibodies to human leucocyte antigens. In untreated patients, Leu $3a^+$ T cells were the predominant T cell subsets, and ratios of Leu $3a^+$/Leu $2a^+$ cells in the muscles were similar to those found in the control peripheral blood. These T cells also expressed DR antigens. In the treated group, only few T cells were seen. In muscular dystrophy cases (disease control), the majority of infiltrating cells were dendritic and lacked T cell antigens.

Several investigators have demonstrated that lymphocytes from patients with polymyositis can damage muscle cells in culture in various systems (Currie *et al.*, 1971; Dawkins and Mastaglia, 1973; Haas and Arnason, 1974). *In vitro* treatment of lymphocytes with antilymphocyte serum or *in vivo* treatment of the patients with immunosuppressive drugs reduces this effect. A correlation exists between the activity of the myositis and the cytotoxicity of patient's lymphocytes for cultured muscle cells.

The sensitivity of lymphocytes to muscles from patients with polymyositis is also evident in proliferation and lymphokine production assays. Currie *et al.* (1971) have demonstrated lymphocyte proliferation in response to whole-muscle homogenate. The response is roughly proportional to the activity of the disease. Johnson *et al.* (1972) have demonstrated production of lymphotoxin by lymphocytes from patients with polymyositis when exposed to autologous muscles *in vitro*. The lymphotoxin produced will damage human muscle cells in culture. Lymphotoxin is also released by lymphocytes in cellular infiltrates in muscles from polymyositis. This could be one mechanism for muscle damage in polymyositis. Delayed cutaneous hypersensitivity to recall antigens is normal except in patients who are on immunosuppressive treatment: Lisak and Zweiman (1975) showed essentially normal mitogen-induced proliferation in polymyositis.

2. B Lymphocytes

The evidence for a defect in B-cell immunity in polymyositis is inconclusive. Strelkauskas *et al.* (1976) tested three patients with dermatomyositis and found increased proportions of circulating SIg^+ B cells in two. Serum immunoglobulins have been reported to be reduced (Dawkins and Mastaglia, 1973), normal, or elevated (Barwick and Walton, 1963; Bohan *et al.*, 1977; Lisak and Zweiman, 1976; Logan *et al.*, 1966). Good and Yunis (1974) described an increased frequency of polymyositis and dermatomyositis in patients with congenital hypogammaglobulinemias including those with selective IgA deficiency. The incidence of RF, ANA, and immunoconglutinin is not significantly increased except in those patients with overlap syndrome and other connective tissue diseases (Bohan *et al.*, 1977; Dawkins and Mastaglia, 1973). Antibodies to crude muscle extracts or myosin are found in a frequency similar to that in muscular dystrophy or controls. Attempts to demonstrate antimuscle antibody by immunofluorescent technique have been unrewarding. Immune complexes have also been implicated in the pathogenesis of polymyositis. Antibodies and complement deposition have been demonstrated in walls of blood vessels of skeletal muscles in children with polymyositis (Whitaker and Engle, 1972) but are lacking in adult patients with polymyositis.

Strelkauskas *et al.* (1976) found increased proportions of "null" cells in the blood of three patients with dermatomyositis tested. However, NK and ADCC functions were not tested. It appears that T-cell-mediated immunity may be primarily involved in the pathogenesis of polymyositis and dermatomyositis. The immunologic aberrations (T cell mediated) are likely to be specific (muscles), lacunar (no generalized T-cell defects), and transient.

G. Mixed Connective Tissue Disease

Mixed connective tissue disease (MCTD) is a term for a syndrome characterized by an admixture of clinical features found in systemic lupus erythematosus, progressive systemic sclerosis (PSS), and polymyositis and serologically by high titers of circulating antibodies to nuclear ribonucleoprotein (RNP) antigen. A great deal of controversy exists regarding whether MCTD is a distinct entity or a variant of SLE, PSS, polymyositis, or one aspect of a heterogeneous group of overlap syndrome. There are a limited number of immunologic studies available in MCTD. These patients, like SLE patients, have hyperimmunoglobulinemia. Alarcon-Segovia and Ruiz-Arguelles (1980) examined T cells and T-cell subsets in patients with MCTD. They studied 11 patients with MCTD; however, the patients were not further divided into active and inactive stages. Total T cells were reduced, but a more profound diminution was observed in T cells with low affinity for SRBC and in $T\gamma$ cells. Non-T cells bearing IgG Fc receptors, surface Ig-positive B cells, and myeloperoxidase-positive monocyte macrophages were decreased in MCTD as compared to controls. The percentage of surface Ig-positive B cells in controls in this study was much higher (39%) than those reported in the literature (Gupta and Good, 1980). This could be because of attachment of cytophilic Ig or the reagent anti-Ig *per se* via Fc receptors on non-B, non-T cells. These authors did not use $F(ab')_2$ reagents. Furthermore, it appears that the $Fc\gamma$ receptor assay is not optimal because B cells, null cells, and monocytes all possess Fcγ receptors, and therefore one would have expected a much higher proportion of $Fc\gamma^+$ cells in the non-T-cell fraction than that reported in this study.

Both spontaneous and Con-A-induced suppressor cell activity against antibody production by B cells in a PWM-driven PFC assay were significantly reduced in MCTD. Anti-RNP IgG antibody, when incubated with cells from MCTD or controls, completely abrogated both spontaneous and Con-A-induced suppressor cell activity. Alarcon-Segovia *et al.* (1979a) have shown that anti-RNP IgG from serum of patients with MCTD can penetrate into live human mononuclear cells bearing Fc receptors, including Tγ cells. Penetration of this antibody into Tγ cells causes their deletion and abrogation of suppressor cell function. Similar penetration of antibody into Fc receptor-bearing cells has also been shown to occur *in vivo* in MCTD (Alarcon-Segovia *et al.*, 1979b). Alarcon-Segovia and Palacios (1981b) examined T cells that form rosettes with autologous RBC (Tar cells) in MCTD. Tar cells are postthymic cells. Tar cells were increased in all seven patients with MCTD compared to healthy controls. Despite this, Tγ cells were decreased, and diminished suppressor activity was observed. This activity was not corrected by serum thymic factor but was corrected by the addition of either allogeneic Tμ or mononuclear cells depleted of Tar cells. This lack of correction of suppressor function by thymic factor in MCTD is in contrast to that observed in SLE. Palacios and Alarcon-Segovia (1981) also observed that T cells and Tar cells from patients with MCTD respond poorly in the AMLR, and the deficient AMLR is not corrected by *in vitro* addition of serum thymic factor to the cultures. Studies of monoclonal-antibody-defined T-cell subsets and other immunologic functions at both the cellular and molecular levels are required in MCTD in order to understand its pathogenesis.

H. Ankylosing Spondylitis

The term ankylosing spondylitis (AS) derives from the Greek *ankylos* ("bent" or "crooked") and *spondylos* ("vertebra"). Ankylosing spondylitis affects both sexes, with males having more symptoms and more severe disease; it is a prototype of the seronegative spondylarthopathies, a group of interrelated disorders that includes psoriatic arthritis, Reiter's syndrome, the reactive arthropathies, and juvenile chronic polyarthropathy. All of these disorders are associated with HLA-B27, absence of serum rheumatoid factor, and lack of rheumatoid nodules. There is considerable evidence for immunologic abnormalities in patients with AS.

1. T Lymphocytes

The data on T-cell proportions and numbers in AS are rather conflicting. A relative T-cell lymphopenia has been described in AS (Fan *et al.*, 1977; Bryom *et al.*, 1979; Sotnik, 1979). Sotnik (1979) has suggested that lymphopenia correlates with disease activity and possibly c-reactive protein (CRP) interfering with SRBC rosette formation with T cells. In contrast, Bluestone *et al.* (1975), Christiansen *et al.* (1978), Rosenthal and Muller (1975), Hickling *et a.*, (1982), Nikbin *et al.* (1975), and Nilsson and Biberfield (1980) failed to demonstrate any significant T lymphopenia in patients with AS or any correlation with disease activity. Hickling *et al.* (1982) did not find any factor in the sera of patients with active AS that would inhibit rosette formation between SRBC and T cells. Veys *et al.* (1983) more recently applied monoclonal antibodies to examine T cells and T-cell subsets in patients with AS and reactive synovitis (RS). The proportions and numbers of $OKT3^+$ and $OKT8^+$ cells in both groups were comparable to those of the control group. The proportions of $OKT4^+$ T cells but not the absolute numbers were significantly increased in AS compared to controls. The ratios of $OKT4^+/OKT8^+$ T cells in AS and RS were comparable to healthy controls.

Fan *et al.* (1977) and Kalovidouris and Johnson (1983) reported normal proliferative response to PHA, Con A, and PWM in patients with AS, although Froebel *et al.* (1975) have reported depressed proliferative response to suboptimal dosage of PHA in AS. Kalovidouris and Johnson (1983) also looked for any evidence of *in vivo* sensitization of T lymphocytes to spinal antigens. They examined the proliferative response to small pieces of spinal ligaments, disks, and sacroiliac cartilage by lymphocytes from eight patients with AS and eight healthy controls. No significant proliferative response was observed in either group, indicating a lack of sensitization of T lymphocytes to spinal antigens in patients with AS. These investigators also examined the capacity of AS lymphocytes to produce proliferation inhibitory factor (PIF) in response to spinal antigens and found no PIF production. Trentham *et al.* (1978) failed to observe migration inhibition factor (MIF) production in AS in response to collagen II and III; this was in contrast to MIF production in RA.

2. B Lymphocytes

There is general agreement regarding B-cell hyperactivity in patients with ankylosing spondylitis. Increased proportions of B lymphocytes and immunoblasts have been reported in AS (Sotnik, 1979; Eghtedari *et al.*, 1976; Hickling *et al.*, 1982). The techniques utilized included EAC (complement receptor) rosette formation or surface Ig determination using whole anti-Ig reagents. Furthermore, no precautions have been taken to identify or exclude monocytes from the mononuclear preparations. Therefore, B-cell studies are required using $F(ab')_2$ reagents and monoclonal antibodies directed against B cell differentiation antigens. It would be of interest to examine any evidence of B-cell activation *in vivo,* that is, the response of B cells to BCGF in the absence of prior *in vitro* antigen stimulation.

Increased levels of serum immunoglobulins have been reported in patients with AS (Laurent and Panayi, 1983; Howell *et al.*, 1972; Hickling *et al.*, 1982; Veys and Van Laere, 1973; Kendall *et al.*, 1973; Kinsella *et al.*, 1975; Cowling *et al.*, 1980; Ogryzlo *et al.*, 1959; Eghtedari *et al.*, 1976; Calguneri *et al.*, 1981), the most significant increase being in serum IgA and IgG; the levels of IgM are usually normal (Laurent and Panayi, 1983; Veys and Van Laere, 1973; Kinsella *et al.*, 1973; Cowling *et al.*, 1980). The increased levels are usually correlated with the disease activity, for example, with elevated sedimentation rate and CRP. Veys and Van Laere (1973), however, did not find such correlation between elevated serum IgA and disease activity.

The consistency and highest levels of IgA that are observed in AS have led to the suggestion that this reflects increased intestinal mucosal synthesis in response to gut-derived antigen (Trull *et al.*, 1983). A number of studies have been carried out to identify potentially pathogenic microorganisms in the feces of patients with AS. Ebringer *et al.* (1978), in the largest study, showed that *Klebsiella pneumoniae* (*KP*) is isolated more frequently during episodes of active disease. Trull *et al.* (1983) therefore examined anti-KP IgA antibodies in patients with AS, RA, psoriatic arthritis, and healthy controls. A significantly increased level of anti-KP IgA antibody was observed in patients with AS with elevated sedimentation rate compared to controls or patients with elevated sedimentation rate and RA or psoriatic arthritis. Granfors *et al.* (1980) have also reported high titers of IgA antibodies to *Yersinia* serotype in patients with *Yersinia*-induced reactive arthritis, and the levels correlated with the disease activity. Measurements of levels of secretory IgA antibodies to KP in the saliva or gastrointestinal fluids may provide more conclusive evidence of mucosal immunity to potentially arthritogenic bacteria.

Patients with AS have also been shown to have elevated levels of acute-phase proteins, namely, CRP, fibrinogen, α_1-antitrypsin, and ninth component of complement (Laurent and Panayi, 1983).

I. Polymyalgia Rheumatica

This is a relatively common syndrome in females over 50 years of age and is characterized by severe aching and stiffness in the neck, shoulder girdle, or pelvic girdle muscle areas, which last for a month or longer. The etiology and pathogenesis of this disorder remain unknown. Hazleman *et al.* (1975) reported *in vitro* enhanced proliferative responses of peripheral blood lymphocytes to homologous arterial wall. However, Papaioannou *et al.* (1979) found no such evidence of T-cell sensitization to arterial wall. Circulatory immune complexes are often very high. Benlahrache *et al.* (1983) examined monoclonal-antibody-defined T cells and T-cell subsets in 35 patients with polymyalgia rheumatica. Eleven of 35 patients had no steroid treatment. The proportion of total T cells as measured by E-rosette formation and OKT3 monoclonal antibody was significantly decreased compared to age-matched controls. OKT4$^+$ cells were comparable in the two groups. OKT8$^+$ cells and Tγ cells were significantly reduced in the patient group; however, Con-A-induced suppressor cell function for B-cell response to trinitrophenyl (anti-TNP) in five patients studied was normal. No correlation was observed between monoclonal-antibody-defined T cells and T-cell subsets and steroid treatment, disease activity, or circulating immune complexes. However, a significant correlation was observed between Tγ cells and circulating immune complexes. Studies are required using monoclonal antibodies that further subdivide OKT4$^+$ and OKT8$^+$ T cells into distinct precursor, effector, and inducer populations.

J. Behcet's Syndrome

Behcet's syndrome (BS) is characterized by a triad of recurrent aphthous stomatitis, genital ulcers, and uveitis leading to blindness. The disease has a chronic course with periodic exacerbations and progressive deterioration of the involved tissues. The etiopathogenesis of Behcet's syndrome is unknown. There is some evidence, however, to suggest that the immune system plays an important role in its pathogenesis.

1. T Lymphocytes

Victorino *et al.* (1982) examined T cells and T-cell subsets defined with Ig Fc receptor expression in patients with Behcet's syndrome. Patients included those without treatment and those treated with prednisone or levamisole. No lymphopenia was observed. E-rosette-forming T cells were normal in proportions and numbers. Both the proportions and absolute numbers of $T\mu$ cells were significantly decreased when compared to controls; the $T\gamma$ cell levels were, however, within the range for normal controls. The responses to PHA and Con A were similar to controls except that at 250 μg/ml Con A (supramitogenic dose) and 4 μg/ml PWM, the proliferative response was depressed. After levamisole treatment, the proportions of $T\mu$ cells increased, and response to mitogen returned to control values. A mild reduction in short-lived suppressor cell activity was observed.

More recently, Sakane *et al.* (1982) examined T cells and T-cell subsets using a panel of monoclonal antibodies. They divided the patients into three groups: inactive, preactive, and active. The preactive group included patients with mild clinical manifestations with progressive deterioration and final passage into frank active stage of the disease. The proportion of $OKT4^+$ cells decreased with a concomitant increase in $OKT8^+$, resulting in abnormally low ratios of $OKT4^+/OKT8^+$ T cells in the preactive stage of BS. In the active and inactive stages of BS, the proportions of $OKT4^+$ and $OKT8^+$ T cells were comparable to controls. The proliferative responses to PHA and Con A were essentially normal in all three groups of BS. These investigators also observed deficient AMLR and Con-A-induced suppressor cell activity against T- and B-cell responses in preactive BS. The deficient AMLR was caused by decreased numbers and functions of $OKT4^+$ T cells. This was also associated with a deficiency of autologous rosette-forming T cells after Con A stimulation. These abnormalities were lacking in patients in active and inactive stages of the disease. The allogeneic MLR was also deficient in the preactive stage of BS. These investigators have suggested that these immunologic abnormalities could be prerequisite to active BS.

Lehner (1969), Rogers *et al.* (1974), and Sanefuji (1974) have demonstrated specific T-cell-mediated immunity to mucosal antigens in patients with BS. Sanefugi (1974) demonstrated production of migration inhibition factor by lymphocytes from BS in response to mucosal antigens. Rogers *et al.* (1974) have demonstrated cytotoxicity by BS lymphocytes against homogenates or cultures of oral epithelium.

2. *B Lymphocytes*

The participation of humoral immunity in BS was suggested by Oshima *et al.* (1963), Shimizu *et al.* (1965), and O'Duffy *et al.* (1971), who reported elevated levels of serum immunoglobulins in BS. Antibodies against autologous or fetal mucous membrane have also been demonstrated in BS (Oshima *et al.*, 1963; Shimizu *et al.*, 1965; Lehner, 1967; O'Duffy *et al.*, 1971). Circulating immune complexes are also present in high titers in patients with BS (Williams and Lehner, 1977; Levinsky and Lehner, 1978; Gupta *et al.*, 1978). Abdou *et al.* (1978) have described disturbances in the salivary immunoglobulin secretory system and abnormalities of the coagulation and fibrinolytic systems that may also be of pathogenetic importance.

Thus, it appears that both cell-mediated and humoral immunity (including local immunity) may have an important role in the pathogenesis of BS. This is further strengthened by its association with the HLA-B5 genotype.

VI. CONCLUSION

In this chapter, quantitative and qualitative analyses of lymphocyte subpopulations in various rheumatic disorders are discussed. A detailed account of the heterogeneity of immunoregulatory T cells is presented. Based on the model of B-cell activation, proliferation, differentiation, and interactions with various cytokines, it is evident that in rheumatic disorders there is B-cell activation *in vivo*. Autoimmunity appears to be related to abnormal immunoregulatory T-cell functions and B-cell hyperreactivity, which could be independent of each other. Data on T4 and T8 T cells in rheumatic disorders should be interpreted with caution because each of these subsets is functionally heterogeneous.

ACKNOWLEDGMENTS. Part of the work cited here was supported by grants from U.S. Public Health Services: AG-04361, AI-20717, and AI-21808.

REFERENCES

Abdou, N. I., Sagawa, A., Pascual, E., Hebert, J., and Sadeghee, S., 1976, Suppressor T-cell abnormality in idiopathic systemic lupus erythematosus, *Clin. Immunol. Immunopathol.* 192–199.

Abdou, N. I., Schumacher, H. R., Colman, R. W., Sagawa, A., Hebert, J., Pascual, E., Carroll, E. T., Miller, M., South, M. A., and Abdon, N. L., 1978, Behcets disease: Possible role of secretory component deficiency, synovial inclusions, and fibrinolytic abnormality in the various manifestations of the disease, *J. Lab. Clin. Med.* **91**:409–422.

Abdou, N. I., Lindsley, H. B., Luz, S., Racela, E. P., and Hassanein, K. M., 1981, Suppressor T cell dysfunction and anti-suppressor cell antibody in active early rheumatoid arthritis, *J. Rheumatol.* **8**:9–18.

Abe, T., and Homma, M., 1971, Immunological reactivity in patients with systemic lupus erythematosus (humoral antibody and cellular immune response), *Acta Rheum. Scand.* **17**:35–46.

Abe, T., Hara, M., Yamasaki, K., and Homma, M., 1973, Cell-mediated immune response in systemic lupus erythematosus, *Arthritis Rheum.* **16**:688–694.

Abe, T., Toguchi, T., Takeuchi, T., Kiyotaki, M., and Homma, M., 1982, Mitogenic response to lipopolysacchride by B lymphocytes from patients with systemic lupus erythematosis, *Scand. J. Immunol.* **15**:475–482.

Abe, T., Takeuchi, T., Koide, J., Hosono, O., Homma, M., Morimoto, C., and Yokohari, R., 1984, Suppressor T cell function in patients with rheumatoid arthritis complicated by vasculitis, *Arthritis Rheum.* **27**:752–759.

Abrahamsen, T. G., Froland, S. S., Natvig, J. B., and Pahle, J., 1975, Elution and characterization of lymphocyte from rheumatoid inflammatory tissue, *Scand. J. Immunol.* **4**:823–830.

Abrahamsen, T. G., Froland, S. S., Natvig, J. B., and Pahle, J., 1977, Antibody-dependent cytotoxicity mediated by cells eluted from synovial tissues of patients with rheumatoid arthritis and juvenile rheumatoid arthritis, *Scand. J. Immunol.* **6**:1251–1261.

Abrahamsen, T. G., Froland, S. S., and Natvig, J. B., 1978, *In vitro* mitogen stimulation of synovial fluid lymphocytes from rheumatoid arthritis and juvenile arthritis, *Scand. J. Immunol.* **7**:81–90.

Adamson, T., Fox, R. I., Frisman, D. M., and Howell, F. V., 1982, Immunohistologic analysis of lymphoid infiltrates in primary Sjogren's syndrome using monoclonal antibodies, *J. Immunol.* **130**:203–208.

Alarcon-Segovia, D., and Palacios, R., 1981a, Differences in immunoregulatory T cell circuits between diphenylhydantoin related and spontaneously occuring systemic lupus erythematosus, *Arthritis Rheum.* **24**:1086–1092.

Alarcon-Segovia, D., and Palacios, R., 1981b, Human posthymic precursor cells in health and disease. IV. Abnormalities in immunoregulatory T cell circuits in mixed connective tissue disease, *Arthritis Rheum.* **24**:1486–1496.

Alarcon-Segovia, D., and Ruiz-Arguelles, A., 1978, Decreased circulating thymus-derived cells with receptor for Fc portion of immunoglobulin G in systemic lupus erythematosus, *J. Clin. Invest.* **62**:1390–1394.

Alarcon-Segovia, D., and Ruiz-Arguelles, A., 1980, Suppressor cell loss and dysfunction in mixed connective tissue disease, *Arthritis Rheum.* **23**:314–318.

Alarcon-Segovia, D., Ruiz-Arguelles, A., and Fishbein, E., 1979a, Antibody penetration into living cells. I. Intranuclear immunoglobulin in peripheral blood mononuclear cells in mixed corrective tissue disease and systemic lupus erythematosus, *Clin. Exp. Immunol.* **35**:364–375.

Alarcon-Segovia, D., Ruiz-Arguelles, A., and Llorente, L., 1979b, Antibody penetrating into living cells. II. Anti-ribonucleoprotein IgG penetrates into Tr cells causing their deletion and the absorption of suppressor function, *J. Immunol.* **122**:1855–1863.

Alarcon-Segovia, D., Palacios, R., and Ibanez de Kasep, G., 1981, Human posthymic precursor cells in health and disease. VI. Immunoregulatory circuits of the peripheral blood mononuclear cells from patients with progressive systemic sclerosis, *J. Clin. Lab. Immunol.* **5**:143–148.

Al-Balaghi, S., Strom, H., and Moller, E., 1982, High incidence of spontaneous Ig-producing lymphocytes in peripheral blood and synovial fluid of patients with active seropositive rheumatoid arthritis, *Scand. J. Immunol.* **16**:69–76.

Al-Balaghi, S., Strom, H., and Moller, E., 1984, B cell differentiation factor in synovial fluid of patients with rheumatoid arthritis, *Immunol. Rev.* **78**:7–23.

Anderson, L. G., and Talal, N., 1972, The spectrum of benign to malignant lymphoproliferation in Sjogren's syndrome, *Clin. Exp. Immunol.* **10**:199–221.

Andrianakos, A. A., Sharp, J. T., Person, D. A., Lidsky, M. D., and Duffy, J., 1977a, Cell-mediated immunity in rheumatoid arthritis, *Ann. Rheum. Dis.* **36**:13–20.

Andrianakos, A. A., Tsichlis, P. N., Merikas, E. G., Marketos, S. G., Sharp, J. T., and Merikas, G. E., 1977b, Cell-mediated immunity in systemic lupus erythematosus, *Clin. Exp. Immunol.* **30**:89–96.

Astorga, G. P., and Williams, R. C., 1969, Altered reactivity in mixed culture of lymphocytes from patients with rheumatoid arthritis, *Arthritis Rheum.* **12**:547–554.

Bach, J. F., and Carnand, C., 1976, Thymic factors, *Prog. Allergy* **21**:342–400.

Bach, J. F., Dardenne, M., and Salomon, J., 1973, Studies of thymus products. IV. Absence of serum thymic activity in adult NZB and (NZB × NZW)F_1 mice, *Clin. Exp. Immunol.* **14**:247–256.

Bakke, A. C., Kirkland, P. A., Kitridon, R. C., Quismorio, F. P., Rea, T., Ehresmann, G. R., and Horowitz, D. A., 1983, T lymphocyte subsets in systemic lupus erythematosus. Correlation with corticosteroid therapy and disease activity, *Arthritis Rheum.* **26**:745–750.

Bakshi, A., Miyasaka, N., Kavathas, P., Daniels, T. E., Strand, C. V., Herzenberg, L. A., and Talal, N., 1983, Lymphocyte subsets in Sjogren's syndrome: A quantitative analysis using monoclonal antibodies and the fluorescence-activated cell sorter, *J. Clin. Lab. Immunol.* **10**:63–69.

Bankhurst, A. D., and Williams, R. C. Jr., 1975, Identification of DNA binding lymphocytes in patients with systemic lupus erythematosus, *J. Clin. Invest.* **56**:1378–1385.

Bankhurst, A. D., Husby, G., and Williams, R. C., Jr., 1976, Predominance of T cells in the lymphocytic infiltrates of synovial tissues in rheumatoid arthritis, *Arthritis Rheum.* **19**:555–562.

Bardwick, P. A., Bluestein, H. G., Zvaifler, N. H., Depper, J. M., and Seegamiller, J. E., 1980, Altered regulation of Epstein–Barr virus induced lymphoblast proliferation in rheumatoid arthritis lymphoid cells, *Arthritis Rheum.* **23**:626–632.

Barkley, D. O., Hohermuth, H. J., Howard, A., Webster, A. D. B., and Ansell, B. M., 1979, IgA deficiency in juvenile chronic polyarthritis, *J. Rheumatol.* **6**:219–224.

Barwick, D. D., and Walton, J. N., 1963, Polymyositis, *Am. J. Med.* **35**:646–660.

Baum, J., and Ziff, M., 1969, Decreased 19S antibody response to bacterial antigens in systemic lupus erythematosus, *J. Clin. Invest.* **48**:758–767.

Bell, D. A., 1978, Cell mediated immunity in systemic lupus erythematosus: Observations on *in vitro* cell-mediated immune response in relationship to number of potentially reactive T cells disease activity and treatment, *Clin. Immunol. Immunopathol.* **31**:301–307.

Bell, D. A., and Pinto, J., 1984, Distribution of activated B lymphocytes in the circulation and synovial fluid in rheumatoid arthritis, *Clin. Immunol. Immunopathol.* **31**:272–281.

Bell, D. A., Clark, C., Blomgren, S. E., and Vaughan, S. H., 1973, Anti-DNA antibody production by lymphoid cells of NZB/w mice and human systemic lupus erythematosus (SLE), *Clin. Immunol. Immunopathol.* **1**:293–303.

Bellamy, N., Cairns, E., and Bell, D. A., 1983, Immunoregulation in rheumatoid arthritis: Evaluation of T lymphocyte function in the control of polyclonal immunoglobulin synthesis *in vitro*, *J. Rheumatol.* **10**:19–27.

Benlahrache, C., Segond, P., Auquier, L., and Bouvet, J. P., 1983, Decreased of the OKT8 positive T cell subset in polymyalgia rheumatica. Lack of correlation with disease activity, *Arthritis Rheum.* **26:**1472–1480.

Bernard, A., and Boumsell, L., 1984, Differentiation human leukocyte antigens: A proposed nomenclature, *Immunol. Today* **5:**158–159.

Bernstein, M. L., Winkelstein, A., and Dobson, S. A., 1980, Depressed T cell colony growth in systemic lupus erythematosus, *Arthritis Rheum.* **23:**385–391.

Biberfield, G., Nilsson, E., and Biberfield, P., 1979, T lymphocyte subpopulations in synovial fluid of patients with rheumatic disease, *Arthritis Rheum.* **22:**978–982.

Biddison, W. E., Rao, P. E., Talle, M. A., Goldstein, G., and Shaw, S., 1982, Possible involvement of the OKT4 molecule in T cell recognition of class II HLA antigens, *J. Exp. Med.* **156:**1065–1076.

Bloch, K. J., Buchanan, W. W., Wohl, M. J., and Bunim, J. J., 1965, Sjogren's syndrome. A clinical, pathological and serological studies of sixty-two cases, *Medicine (Baltimore)* **44:**187–231.

Block, S. R., Gibbs, C. B., Stevens, M. B., and Shulman, C. E., 1968, Delayed hypersensitivity in systemic lupus erythematosus, *Ann. Rheum. Dis.* **27:**311–318.

Bluestone, R., Goldberg, L. S., Weisbart, R. M., Morris, R. I., and Holborow, E. S., 1975, Aberrant immunity in (HLA) W 27 positive rheumatic disease, *Ann. Rheum. Dis.* **34**(Suppl. 1):46–48.

Bobrove, A. M., and Miller, P., 1977, Depressed *in vitro* B lymphocyte differentiation in systemic lupus erythematosus, *Arthritis Rheum.* **20:**1326–1333.

Bohan, A., Peter, J. B., Bowman, B. S., and Pearson, C. M., 1977, A computer-assisted analysis of 153 patients with polymyositis and dermatomyositis, *Medicine (Baltimore)* **56:**255–286.

Borel, Y., Morimoto, C., Cairns, L., Mantzouranis, E., Strelkauskas, A. J., and Schlossman, S. F., 1984, Anti-T cell antibody in juvenile rheumatoid arthritis, *J. Rheumatol.* **11:**56–61.

Brenner, A. I., Sheinberg, M. A., and Cathcart, E. S., 1975, Surface characteristics of synovial fluid and peripheral blood lymphocytes, in inflammatory arthritis, *Arthritis Rheum.* **18:**297–303.

Bresnihan, B., and Jasin, H. E., 1977, Suppressor function of peripheral blood mononuclear cells in normal individuals and in patients with systemic lupus erythematosus, *J. Clin. Invest.* **59:**106–116.

Brodman, R., Gilfillan, R., Glass, D., and Schur, P. H., 1978, Influenza vaccine response in systemic lupus erythematosus, *Ann. Intern. Med.* **88:**735–740.

Brown, K. A., Embling, P. H. F., Perry, J. D., and Holborow, E. J., 1979, Electrophoretic behaviour of blood and synovial fluid lymphocytes in rheumatoid arthritis, *Clin. Exp. Immunol.* **36:**272–278.

Budman, D. R., Merchant, E. B., Steinberg, A. D., Doft, B., Gershwin, M. E., Lizzo, E., and Reeves, J. P., 1977, Increased spontaneous activity of antibody-forming cells in the peripheral blood of patients with active SLE, *Arthritis Rheum.* **20:**829–833.

Burmester, G. R., Kalden, J. R., Peter, H. H., Schedel, I., Beck, P., and Wittenbog, A., 1978, Immunological and functional characteristics of peripheral blood and synovial fluid lymphocytes from patients with rheumatoid arthritis, *Scand. J. Immunol.* **7:**405–417.

Burmester, G. R., Yu, D. T. Y., Irani, A. M., Kunkel, H. G., and Winchester, R. J., 1981, Ia^+ T cells in synovial fluid and tissues of patients with rheumatoid arthritis, *Arthritis Rheum.* **24:**1370–1376.

Byrom, N. A., Hobbs, J. R., Timlin, D. M., Campbell, M. A., Dean, A. J., and Webley, M., 1979, T and B lymphocytes in patients with acute anterior uveitis and ankylosing spondylitis, and in their household contacts, *Lancet* **2:**601–603.

Cahalan, M. D., Chandy, K. G., DeCoursey, T. E., and Gupta, S., 1985, A voltage gated K^+ channel in human T lymphocytes, *J. Physiol. (London)* **358:**197–237.

Calguneri, M., Cooke, M., Shinebaum, R., Swinburne, L., and Wright, V., 1981, Secretary IgA, immune defense pattern in ankylosing spondylitis and *Klebsiella, Ann. Rheum. Dis.* **40:**600–604.

Carpentier, B., Carnand, C., and Bach, J. F., 1979, Selector depression of the xernogeneic cell-mediated lympholysis in systemic lupus erythematosus, *J. Clin. Invest.* **64:**351–360.

Cass, R. M., Mogan, E. S., and Jacox-Vaughan, J. H., 1968, Immunoglobulin G, A, and M in systemic lupus erythematosus, *Ann. Intern. Med.* **69:**749–756.

Cassidy, J. T., Burt, A., Sullivan, D. B., and Dickinson, D. G., 1966, Changes in serum immunoglobulins in juvenile rheumatoid arthritis, *Arthritis Rheum.* **9:**850–851.

Cassidy, J. T., Petty, R. E., and Sullivan, D. B., 1977, Occurrence of selective IgA deficiency in children with juvenile rheumatid arthritis, *Arthritis Rheum.* **20**(Suppl):181–183.

Chandy, K. G., DeCoursey, T. E., Cahalan, M. D., and Gupta, S., 1984, Voltage gated potassium channels are required for human T lymphocyte activation, *J. Exp. Med.* **160:**369–385.

Chandy, K. G., DeCoursey, T. E., Cahalan, M. D., and Gupta, S., 1985, Ion channels in lymphocytes, *J. Clin. Immunol.* **5**:1–7.

Chang, T. W., Kung, P. C., Gingras, S. P., and Goldstein, G., 1981, Does OKT3 monoclonal antibody react with antigen recognition structure on human T cells? *Proc. Natl. Acad. Sci. U.S.A.* **78**:1805–1808.

Chang, T. W., Testa, D., Kung, P. C., Perry, L., Dreskin, H. J., and Goldstein, G., 1982, Cellular origin and interactions involved in interferon production induced by OKT3 monoclonal antibodies, *J. Immunol.* **128**:585–589.

Chattopadhyay, C., Chattopadhyay, H., Natvig, J. B., Michaelsen, T. E., and Mellbye, O. J., 1979a, Lack of suppressor-cell activity in rheumatoid synovial lymphocytes, *Scand. J. Immunol.* **10**:309–316.

Chattopadhyay, C., Chattopadhyay, H., Natvig, J. B., and Mellbye, O. J., 1979b, Rheumatoid synovial lymphocytes lack concanavalin-A activated suppressor cell activity, *Scand. J. Immunol.* **10**:479–486.

Chattopadhyay, H., Chattopadhyay, C., and Natvig, J. B., 1979c, Hyporesponsiveness to synovial antigens in rheumatoid synovial and blood lymphocytes using the indirect migration inhibition test, *Scand. J. Immunol.* **10**:585–592.

Chattopadhyay, C., Natvig, J. B., and Chattopadhyay, H., 1980, Excessive suppressor T-cell activity of rheumatoid synovial tissue in X-linked agammaglobulinemia, *Scand. J. Immunol.* **11**:455–459.

Christiansen, F. T., Hawkins, B. R., and Dawkins, R. L., 1978, Immune functions in ankylosing spondylitis and their relatives: Influence of disease and HLA-B 27, *Clin. Exp. Immunol.* **33**:270–275.

Clough, J. D., Frank, S. A., and Calabrese, L. J., 1980, Deficiency of T cell-mediated regulation of anti-DNA production in systemic lupus erythematosus, *Arthritis Rheum.* **23**:24–29.

Cooper, S. M., Harding, B., Mirick, G. R., Schneider, J., Quismorio, F. P., and Friou, G. J., 1978, Selective decrease in antibody-dependent cell-mediated cytotoxicity in systemic lupus erythematosus and progressive systemic sclerosis, *Clin. Exp. Immunol.* **34**:235–240.

Coovadia, H. M., Mackay, I. R., and Dapice, A. J., 1981, Suppressor cells assayed by three different methods in patients with chronic active hepatitis and systemic lupus erythematosus, *Clin. Immunol. Immunopathol.* **18**:268–275.

Corrigall, V. M., and Panayi, G. S., 1978, Lymphocyte studies in rheumatoid arthritis. II. Antibody mediated and mitogen-induced lymphocyte cytotoxicity in synovial fluid and peripheral blood, *Ann. Rheum. Dis.* **37**:410–415.

Corrigall, V., Panayi, G. S., and Laurent, R., 1979, Lymphocyte studies in rheumatoid arthritis III. A comparative study of the responses of peripheral blood and synovial fluid lymphocytes to phytomitogens, *Scand. J. Rheumatol.* **8**:10–16.

Cowling, P., Ebringer, R., and Ebringer, A., 1980, Association of inflammination with reused serum IgA in ankylosing spondylitis, *Ann. Rheum. Dis.* **39**:545–549.

Currie, S., Saunders, M., and Knowles, M., 1970, Immunological aspects of systemic sclerosis. *In vitro* activity of lymphocytes from patients with this disorder, *Br. J. Dermatol.* **84**:400–409.

Currie, S., Saunders, M., Knowles, M., and Brown, A. E., 1971, Immunologic aspects of polymyositis, *Q. J. Med.* **157**:63–84.

Damle, N. K., and Engleman, E. G., 1983, Immunoregulatory T cell circuits in man. Alloantigen-primed inducer T cells activate antigen-specific suppressor T cells in the absence of the initial antigenic stimulus, *J. Exp. Med.* **158**:159–173.

Damle, N. K., and Gupta, S., 1982a, Heterogeneity of concanavalin A-induced suppressor T cell in man defined with monoclonal antibodies, *Clin. Exp. Immunol.* **48**:581–588.

Damle, N. K., and Gupta, S., 1982b, Autologous mixed lymphocyte reaction in man. V. Functionally and phenotypically distinct human T cell subpopulations respond to non T and activated T cells in AMLR, *Scand. J. Immunol.* **16**:59–68.

Damle, N. K., Mohaghehpour, N., and Engleman, E. G., 1984, Soluble antigen-primed inducer T cells activate antigen-specific suppressor T cells in the absence of antigen-pulsed accessory cells: Phenotypic definition of suppressor inducer and suppressor effect cells, *J. Immunol.* **132**:644–650.

Davis, P., and Jason, M. I. V., 1976, Serological changes in progressive systemic sclerosis, *Rheumatol. Rehab.* **15**:45–50.

Dawkins, R. L., and Mastaglia, F. L., 1973, Cell-mediated cytotoxicity to muscle in polymyositis, *N. Engl. J. Med.* **288**:434–438.

DeCoursey, T. E., Chandy, K. G., Gupta, S., and Cahalan, M. D., (1984a), Voltage gated K^+ channel in human T lymphocytes a role in mitogenesis? *Nature* **307**:465–468.

DeCoursey, T. E., Chandy, K. G., Fishbach, M., Talal, N., Cahalan, M. D., and Gupta, S., 1984b, Differences in ion channel expression in T lymphocytes from MLR-lpr and MLR-+/+ mice, *Fed. Proc.* **43**:1736.

DeHoratius, R. J., Tung, K. S. K., and Pincus, T., 1980, Reduced T lymphocyte subsets in systemic lupus erythematosus, *Immunopathology* **17**:245–256.

DeJesus, D. B., and Clancy, R. L., 1975, Circulating T- and B-lymphocytes in progressive systemic sclerosis, *J. Rheumatol.* **2**:336–339.

Delfraissy, J. F., Segond, P., Galanand, P., Wallon, P., Wallon, C., Massias, P., and Dormont, J., 1980, Depressed primary *in vitro* antibody response in untreated systemic lupus erythematosus. T helper cell defect and lack of defective suppressor cell function, *J. Clin. Invest.* **66**:141–148.

Depper, J. M., Bardwick, P. A., Bluestein, H. G., Zvaifler, N. J., and Seegmiller, J. E., 1979, Abnormal regulation of rheumatoid lymphoid cells, *Arthritis Rheum.* **22**:605 (Abstract).

Depper, J. M., Bluestein, H. G., and Zvailer, N. J., 1981, Impaired regulation of Epstein–Barr virus induced lymphocyte proliferation in rheumatoid arthritis is due to a T cell defect, *J. Immunol.* **127**:1899–1902.

De Vries, M. J., and Hijman, W., 1966, A deficient development of the thymic epithelium and autoimmune disease in NZB mice, *J. Pathol. Bacteriol.* **91**:487–494.

Diaz-Jouanen, E., Bankhurst, A. D., and Williams, R. C., 1976, Antibody mediated lymphocytotoxicity in rheumatoid arthritis and systemic lupus erythematosus, *Arthritis Rheum.* **19**:133–141.

Doblong, J. H., Forre, O., Natvig, J. B., and Michaelsen, T. E., 1979, Demonstration of rheumatoid factor idiolypic antigens on peripheral blood B and T lymphocytes from patients with rheumatoid arthritis, *Scand. J. Immunol.* **9**:273–279.

Doblong, J. H., Chattopadhyay, C., Forre, O., Hoyeraal, H. M., and Natvig, J. B., 1981, Con-A-induced suppressor cell activity and T lymphocyte subpopulations in peripheral blood lymphocytes of patients with rheumatoid arthritis and juvenile rheumatoid arthritis, *Scand. J. Immunol.* **13**:367–373.

Duclos, M., Zeidler, H., Liman, W., Pichler, W. J., Rieber, P., and Peter, H. H., 1982, Characterization of blood and synovial fluid lymphocytes from patients with rheumatoid arthritis and other joint diseases by monoclonal antibodies (OKT series) and acid alpha-naphthyl esterase staining, *Rheumatol. Int.* **2**:75–82.

Duke, O., Panayi, G. S., Janossy, G., and Poulter, L. W., 1982, An immunohistological analysis of lymphocyte subpopulations and their microenvironment in the synovial membranes of patients with rheumatoid arthritis using monoclonal antibodies, *Clin. Exp. Immunol.* **49**:22–30.

Duke, O., Panayi, G. S., Janossy, G., Poulter, L. W., and Tidman, N., 1983, Analysis of T cell subsets in the peripheral blood synovial fluid of patients with rheumatoid arthritis by means of monoclonal antibodies, *Ann. Rheum. Dis.* **42**:357–361.

Duke, O. L., Hobbs, S., Panay, G. S., Poulter, L. W., Rasker, J. J., and Janossy, G., 1984, A combined immunohistological and histochemical analysis of lymphocyte and macrophage subpopulations in the rheumatoid nodule, *Clin. Exp. Immunol.* **56**:239–246.

Dunne, J. V., Sengar, D. P. S., Pearson, D., McKendry, R. J. R., and Gardell, D., 1982, Nonspecific suppressor cells in rheumatoid arthritis, *J. Clin. Lab. Immunol.* **9**:99–104.

Ebringer, R. W., Cawdell, D. R., Cowling, P., and Ebringer, A., 1978, Sequential studies in ankylosing spondylitis: Association of *Klebsiella* pneumonia with active disease, *Ann. Rheum. Dis.* **37**:146–151.

Egeland, T., Lea, T., Saari, G., Melloye, O. J., and Natvig, J. B., 1982a, Quantitation of cells secreting rheumatoid factor of IgG, IgA, and IgM class after elution from rheumatoid synovial tissue, *Arthritis Rheum.* **25**:1445–1450.

Egeland, T., Lea, T., Mellbye, O. J., Pahle, J. A., Ottesen, T., and Natvig, B., 1982b, Quantitation of cells secreting immunoglobulins after elution from rheumatoid synovial tissue, *Scand. J. Immunol.* **16**:413–419.

Egeland, T., Lea, T., and Mellbye, O. J., 1983, T cell immunoregulatory functions to rheumatoid arthritis patients, *Scand. J. Immunol.* **18**:355–362.

Eghtedari, A. A., Davis, P., and Bacon, P. A., 1976, Immunological reactivity in ankylosing spondylitis, *Ann. Rheum. Dis.* **35**:155–157.

Emmons, R. P., Davis, D. J. S., and Moretta, L., 1983, The effects of IgM rheumatoid factor on EAM and EAG rosette formation with Fc receptor bearing lymphoid cells, *Arthritis Rheum.* **26**:1098–1103.

Evans, A. S., and Rothfield, N. F., 1973, EB virus and other viral antibodies in systemic lupus erythematosus, *Lancet* **1**:1127–1128.

Faguet, G. B., Webb, H. H., Agee, J. F., Ricks, W. B., and Sharbaugh, A. H., 1978, Immunologically diagnosed malignancy in Sjogren's pseudolymphoma, *Am. J. Med.* **65**:424–429.

Fan, P. T., Clements, P. J., Yu, D. T., Opelz, G., and Blueston, R., 1977, Lymphocyte abnormalities in ankylosing spondylitis, *Ann. Rheum. Dis.* **36**:471–473.

Fauci, A. S., and Montsopoulos, H. M., 1981, Polyclonal triggered B cells in the peripheral blood and bone marrow of normal individuals and in patients with systemic lupus erythematosus and primary Sjogren's syndrome, *Arthritis Rheum.* **24**:577–583.

Fauci, A. S., Steinberg, A. D., Haynes, B. F., and Walen, G., 1978, Immunoregulatory aberrations in systemic lupus erythematosus, *J. Immunol.* **121**:1473–1478.

Faure, G., Kahn, M. F., Bach, M. A., and Bach, J. F., 1982, T cell subsets in the blood of rheumatoid arthritis patients in clinical remission, *Arthritis Rheum.* **25**:1507–1509.

Feldman, J. L., Becker, M. J., Moutsopoulos, H., Fye, K., Blackman, M., Epstein, V., and Talal, N., 1976, Antibody-dependent cell-mediated cytotoxicity in selected autoimmune diseases, *J. Clin. Invest.* **58**:173–179.

Fink, P. C., Schedel, I., Peter, H. H., and Deicher, H., 1977, Inhibition of spontaneous and antibody-dependent cellular cytotoxicity by sera and isolated antiglobulin preparations from rheumatoid arthritis patients, *Scand. J. Immunol.* **6**:173–183.

Foad, B. S., Khuller, S., Freimer, E. H., Kirsher, A. B., and Sheon, R. P., 1975, Cell-mediated immunity in systemic lupus erythematosus: Alterations with advancing age, *J. Lab. Clin. Med.* **85**:133–137.

Fong, S., Miller III, J. J., Moore, T. L., Tsoukas, C. D., Vaughan, J. H., and Carson, D. A., 1982, Frequency of Epstein–Barr virus-inducible IgM anti IgG B lymphocytes in normal children and children with juvenile rheumatoid arthritis, *Arthritis Rheum.* **25**:959–965.

Fontana, A., Hengartner, H., Weber, E., Fehr, K., Grob, P. J., and Cohen, G., 1982, Interleukin 1 activity in synovial fluid of patients with rheumatoid arthritis, *Scand. J. Immunol.* **2**:67–73.

Forbes, I. J., Zalewski, P. D., Valente, L., and Murray, A. W., 1981, Loss of receptor activity for mouse erythrocytes precedes tumor promotor induced maturation of chronic lymphocytic leukemic cells, *Cancer Lett.* **14**:187–192.

Forre, O., Thoen, J., Doblong, J. H., Egeland, T., Kvien, T. K., Mellbye, O. J., and Natvig, H. B., 1982a, Detection of T-lymphocyte subpopulations in the peripheral blood and the synovium of patients with rheumatoid arthritis and juvenile rheumatoid arthritis using monoclonal antibodies, *Scand. J. Immunol.* **15**:221–226.

Forre, O., Doblong, J. H., and Natvig, J. B., 1982b, Augmented numbers of HLA-DR positive T lymphocytes in the synovial fluid and synovial tissue of patients with rheumatoid arthritis and juvenile rheumatoid arthritis, *Scand. J. Immunol.* **15**:227–231.

Fox, R. I., Adamson, T. C., Frisman, D., Royston, I., and Vaughan, J. H., 1982a, Identification of lymphocyte infiltration synovial membrane in rheumatoid arthritis, *Arthritis Rheum.* **25**:S50.

Fox, R. I., Carsten, S. A., Fong, S., Robinson, C. A., Howell, F. V., and Vaughan, J. H., 1982b, Use of monoclonal antibodies to analyze peripheral blood and salivary gland lymphocyte subsets in Sjogren's syndrome, *Rheumatology* **25**:419–426.

Fox, R. I., Fong, S., Sabharwal, N., Carstens, S. A., Kung, P. C., and Vaughan, J. H., 1982c, Synovial fluid lymphocytes differ from peripheral blood lymphocytes in patients with rheumatoid arthritis, *J. Immunol.* **128**:351–354.

Fox, R. I., Adamson, T. C. III, Fong, S., Robinson, C. A., Morgan, E. L., Robb, J. A., and Howell, F. V., 1983, Lymphocyte phenotype and function in pseudo-lymphoma associated with Sjogren's syndrome, *J. Clin. Invest.* **72**:52–62.

Froebel, K., Sturrocck, R. D., Dick, W. C., and MacSween, R. N., 1975, Cell-mediated immunity in the rheumatoid diseases. I. Skin testing and mitogenic responses in sero-negative arthritides, *Clin. Exp. Immunol.* **22**:446–452.

Froebel, K., Sturrock, R. D., Reynolds, P., Grenan, A., Roxburgh, A., and MacSween, R. N. M., 1979, *In vitro* reaction of lymphocytes in rheumatoid arthritis and other rheumatoid disease, *Ann. Rheum. Dis.* **38**:535–543.

Froelich, C., Bankhurst, A. D., Crowe, W. E., Williams, R. C., Warner, N. L., and Levinson, J. E., 1981, Flow cytometry and cytoadherence studies of sera from children with juvenile rheumatoid arthritis and normal controls, *Arthritis Rheum.* **24**:457–463.

Froland, S. S., Natvig, J. B., and Husby, G., 1973, Immunological characterization of lymphocytes in synovial fluids from patients with rheumatoid arthritis, *Scand. J. Immunol.* **2**:67–72.

Froland, S. S., Natvig, J. B., and Wisloff, F., 1975, Lymphocyte subpopulations in rheumatoid arthritis, *Rheumatology* **6**:231–241.

Fuller, T. C., Trevithick, J. E., Fuller, A. A., Colvin, R. B., Cosimi, A. B., and Kung, P. C., 1984, Antigen polymorphism of the T4 differentiation antigen expressed on human T helper/inducer lymphocytes, *Hum. Immunol.* **9**:89–102.

Gershon, R. K., Eardley, D. D., Durum, S., Green, D. R., Shen, F. W., Yamauchi, K., Canton, H., and Murphy, D. B., 1981, Contrasuppression: A novel immunoregulatory activity, *J. Exp. Med.* **153**:1533–1546.

Gershwin, M. E., Glinski, W., Chuset, T., and Steinberg, A. D., 1977, Lymphocyte dependent antibody-mediated cytolysis of DNA-anti-DNA-coated target cells using human and murine SLE effector populations, *Clin. Immunol. Immunopathol.* **8**:280–291.

Ginsburg, W. W., Finkelman, F. D., and Lipsky, P. E., 1979, Circulating and pokeweed mitogen-induced immunoglobulin secreting cells in systemic lupus erythematosus, *Clin. Exp. Immunol.* **35**:76–88.

Glinski, W., Gershwin, M. E., Budman, D. R., and Steinberg, A. D., 1976, Study of lymphocyte subpopulations in normal humans and patients with SLE by fractionation of peripheral blood lymphocyte on a discontinuous Ficoll-gradient, *Clin. Exp. Immunol.* **26**:228–238.

Goel, K. M., Logan, R. W., Barnard, W. P., and Shanks, R. A., 1974, Serum immunoglobulin and BLc/BLa globulin concentrations in juvenile rheumatoid arthritis, *Ann. Rheum. Dis.* **33**:35–38.

Goldman, J. A., Litwin, A., and Adams, L. E., 1972, Cellular immunity to nuclear antigens in systemic lupus erythematosus, *J. Clin. Invest.* **51**:2669–2677.

Good, R. A., and Yunis, E., 1974, Association of autoimmunity, immunodeficiency and aging in man, rabbits, and mice, *Fed. Proc.* **33**:2040–2050.

Gordon, B. L., and Yanagihara, R., 1977, Treatment of systemic lupus erythematosus with a treatment for a minimum period of 4 months, *Ann. Allergy* **39**:227–236.

Goto, M., Tanimoto, K., Chihara, T., and Horiuchi, Y., 1981, Natural cell-mediated cytotoxicity in Sjogren's syndrome and rheumatoid arthritis, *Arthritis Rheum.* **24**:1377–1381.

Gottlieb, A. B., Lahita, R. G., Chiorazzi, N., and Kunkel, H. G., 1979, Immune function in systemic lupus erythematosus. Impairment of *in vitro* T-cell proliferation and *in vivo* antibody response to exogenous antigen, *J. Clin. Invest.* **63**:885–892.

Granfors, K., Vihjanen, M., Tiilikainen, A., and Toivanen, A., 1980, Persistance of IgM, IgG and IgA antibodies to *Yersinia* in *Yersinia* arthritis, *J. Infect. Dis.* **141**:424–429.

Grayson, J., Blaese, R., Steinberg, A. D., Dooley, N. J., and Koski, I. R., 1979, Circulating immunoglobulin secreting cells in patients with systemic lupus erythematosus, *Clin. Res.* **27**:326A.

Greenspan, J., Daniels, T., Talal, N., and Sylvester, R., 1974, The histopathology of Sjogren's syndrome in labial salivary gland biopsies, *Oral Pathol.* **37**:217–228.

Gumpel, J. M., and Hobbs, J. R., 1970, Serum immunoglobulins in Sjogren's syndrome, *Ann. Rheum. Dis.* **29**:681–683.

Gupta, S., 1978, Functionally distinct subpopulations of human T lymphocytes. A brief review, *Clin. Bull.* **8**:100–107.

Gupta, S., 1981, Human T cell subpopulations with receptors for immunoglobulin isotypes, *Clin. Immunol. News Lett.* **2**:51–57.

Gupta, S., 1983a, Cellular interactions in human T–T autologous mixed lymphocyte reaction, *Behr. Inst. Mitt.* **72**:101–106.

Gupta, S., 1983b, Autologous mixed lymphocyte reaction in health and disease states in man, *Vox. Sang.* **44**:265–288.

Gupta, S., 1984, Study of activated T cells in man. I. Discrepancy between Tac antigen and DR antigen on T cells in patients with primary immunodeficiency, *Scand. J. Immunol.* **19**:465–468.

Gupta, S., and Good, R. A., 1979a, Human T lymphocyte subpopulations as defined by Fc receptors, *Thymus* **1**:135–149.

Gupta, S., and Good, R. A., 1979b, Lymphocytes–1979, *Henry Ford Hosp. Med. J.* **27**:224–235.

Gupta, S., and Good, R. A., 1980, Markers of human lymphocyte subpopulations in primary immunodeficiency and lymphoproliferative disorders, *Semin. Hematol.* **17**:1–29.

Gupta, S., and Good, R. A., 1981, Subpopulations of human T lymphocytes: Laboratory and clinical studies, *Immunol. Rev.* **56**:89–114.

Gupta, S., and Grieco, M. H., 1975, Rosette-formation with mouse erythrocytes. Probable marker for human B lymphocytes, *Int. Arch. Allergy Appl. Immunol.* **49**:734–742.

Gupta, S., and Kapoor, N., 1980, Lymphocyte subpopulations: Surface, intracellular, enzymatic markers and functions, in: *Infections Complicating the Abnormal Host* (M. H. Grieco, ed.), Yorke Medical Books, New York, pp. 84–128.

Gupta, S., Good, R. A., and Siegal, F. P., 1976a, Rosette formation with mouse erythrocytes. II. A marker for human B and non T lymphocytes, *Clin. Exp. Immunol.* **25**:319–327.
Gupta, S., Good, R. A., and Siegal, F. D., 1976b, Rosette-formation with mouse erythrocytes. III. Studies in primary immunodeficiency and lymphoproliferative disorders, *Clin. Exp. Immunol.* **26**:204–213.
Gupta, S., Pahwa, R., O'Reilly, R., Good, R. A., and Siegal, F. P., 1976c, Ontogeny of lymphocytes subpopulation in human fetal liver, *Proc. Natl. Acad. Sci. U.S.A.* **73**:919–922.
Gupta, R. C., O'Duffey, J. D., and McDuffie, F. C., 1978, Circulating immune complexes in active Behcet's disease, *Clin. Exp. Immunol.* **34**:213–218.
Gupta, S., Malaviya, A. N., Rajagopalan, P., and Good, R. A., 1979, Subpopulations of human T lymphocytes. IX. Imbalance of T cell subpopulations in patients with progressive systemic sclerosis, *Clin. Exp. Immunol.* **38**:342–347.
Gupta, S., Winchester, R. J., and Good, R. A., 1980, General orientation of human T lymphocytes, in: *Clinical Immunology* Vol. 4 (F. H. Bach and R. A. Good, eds.) Academic Press, New York, pp. 1–31.
Haas, D. C., and Arnason, B. G. W., 1974, Cell-mediated immunity in polymyositis, *Arch. Neurol.* **31**:192–196.
Hahn, B. H., Babgy, M. K., and Osterland, C. K., 1973, Abnormalities of delayed hypersensitivity in systemic lupus erythematosus, *Am. J. Med.* **55**:25–31.
Hall, N. D., and Winrow, V. R., 1979, A new approach to the study of high avidity Fc receptors on rheumatoid lymphocytes, *Ann. Rheum. Dis.* **38**:485 (Abstract).
Hall, N. D., Winrow, V. R., and Bacon, P. A., 1980, Lymphocytes bearing Fc receptors in rheumatoid arthritis. I. An increased subpopulation of cells in RA detected with Fabc rosettes, *Ann. Rheum. Dis.* **39**:554–559.
Hamilton, M. E., and Winfield, J. B., 1979, T cells in systemic lupus erythematosus. Variation with disease activity, *Arthritis Rheum.* **22**:1–6.
Haraoni, B., Wilder, R. L., Malone, D. G., Allen, J. B., Katona, I. M., and Wahl, S. M., 1984, Immune function in severe, active rheumatoid arthritis. A relationship between peripheral blood mononuclear cell proliferation to soluble antigens and mononuclear cell subset profile, *J. Immunol.* **133**:697–701.
Harris, J., and Vaughan, J., 1960, Penicillin antibody in disease, *J. Clin. Invest.* **39**:995 (Abstract).
Harvey, A. M., Schulman, L. E., Tumulty, P. A., Conley, C. L., and Schoenrich, E. H., 1954, Systemic lupus erythematosus review of the literature and analysis of 138 cases, *Medicine (Baltimore)* **33**:291–437.
Hasler, F., Bluestein, H. G., Zvaifler, N. J., and Epstein, L. B., 1983, Analysis of the defects responsible for the impaired regulation of Epstein–Barr virus induced B cell proliferation by rheumatoid arthritis lymphocytes. I. Diminished gamma interferon production in response to autologous stimulation, *J. Exp. Med.* **157**:173–188.
Hazleman, B. L., MacLennan, I. C. M., and Esiri, M. M., 1975, Lymphocyte proliferation to artery antigen as a positive diagnostic test in polymyelgia rheumatica, *Ann. Rheum. Dis.* **34**:122–127.
Hickling, P., Turnbull, L., and Dixon, J. S., 1982, The relationship between disease activity, immunoglobulins and lymphocyte subpopulations in ankylosing spondylitis, *Rheum. Rehab.* **21**:145–150.
Hoffman, T., 1980, Natural killer function in systemic lupus erythematosus, *Arthritis Rheum.* **23**:30–35.
Hollinger, F. B., Sharp, J. T., and Lidsky, M. D., 1971, Antibodies to viral antigens in systemic lupus erythematosus, *Arthritis Rheum.* **14**:1–11.
Honda, M., Sakane, T., Steinberg, A. D., Kotani, H., Tsunematsu, T., Moriyama, K., and Fukase, M., 1982, Studies of immune functions of patients with systemic lupus erythematosus. Antibodies to desialized, rather than intact T cells preferentially bind to and eliminate suppressor effector T cells, *J. Clin. Invest.* **69**:940–949.
Horwitz, D. A., 1972, Impaired delayed hypersensitivity in systemic lupus erythematosus, *Arthritis Rheum.* **15**:353–359.
Horwitz, D. A., and Garrett, M. A., 1977, Lymphocyte reactivity to mitogens in subjects with systemic lupus erythematosus, rheumatoid arthritis and scleroderma, *Clin. Exp. Immunol.* **27**:92–99.
Horwitz, D. A., and Juul-Nielsen, K., 1977, Human blood L lymphocytes in patients with active systemic lupus erythematosus, rheumatoid arthritis and scleroderma: A comparison with T and B cells, *Clin. Exp. Immunol.* **30**:370–378.
Horwitz, D. A., Garrett, M. A., and Craig, A. H., 1977a, Serum effects of mitogenic reactivity in subjects with systemic lupus erythematosus, rheumatoid arthritis and scleroderma. Technical consideration and lack of correlation with anti-lymphocyte antibodies, *Clin. Exp. Immunol.* **27**:100–110.
Horowitz, S., Borcherding, W., Moorthy, A. V., and Goldstein, A. L., 1977, Induction of suppressor T cells in systemic lupus erythematosus by thymosin and cultured thymic epithelium, *Science* **197**:999–1001.

Howell, F. A., Chamberlain, M. A., and Perry, R. A., 1972, IgG anti-globulin levels in patients with psoriatic arthropathy, ankylosing spondylitis and gout, *Ann. Rheum. Dis.* **31**:129–131.

Hoyeraal, H. M., Froland, S. S., and Wisloff, F., 1975, Lymphocyte populations and cellular immune reactions in juvenile rheumatoid arthritis, *Scand. J. Immunol.* **4**:801–803.

Hughes, P., Holt, S., Powell, N. R., Allonby, I. D., and Dodd, J. K., 1977, The relationship of defective cell-mediated immunity to visceral disease in systemic sclerosis, *Clin. Exp. Immunol.* **28**:233–240.

Huntley, C. C., Thorpe, D. P., Lyerly, A. D., and Kelsey, W. M., 1967, Rheumatoid arthritis with IgA deficiency, *Am. J. Dis. Child.* **113**:411–418.

Hurd, E. R., Dowdle, W., Casey, H., and Ziff, M., 1972, Virus antibody levels in systemic lupus erythematosus, *Arthritis Rheum.* **15**:267–274.

Husson, J. M., Druet, P., Contet, A., Fiessinger, J. N., and Camilleri, J. P., 1976, Systemic sclerosis and cryoglobulinemia, *Clin. Immunol. Immunopathol.* **6**:77–82.

Ilfeld, D. N., and Krakauer, R. S., 1980, Suppression of immunoglobulin synthesis of systemic lupus erythematosus patients by concanavalin A-activated normal human spleen cell supernatants, *Clin. Immunol. Immunopathol.* **17**:196–202.

Inoshita, T., Whitehead, T. L., Rodnan, G. P., and Taylor, F. H., 1981, Abnormalities of T lymphocyte subsets in patients with progressive systemic sclerosis (PSS, scleroderma), *J. Lab. Clin. Med.* **97**:264–277.

Ivanyi, L., Lehner, T., and Berry, H. C., 1973, The response of synovial fluid lymphocytes to T and B stimulate *in vitro*, *Immunology* **25**:905–908.

Janossy, G., Panayi, G., Duke, O., Bofill, M., Poulter, L. W., and Goldstein, G., 1981, Rheumatoid arthritis: A disease of T lymphocyte/macrophage immunoregulation, *Lancet* **2**:839–842.

Johnson, R. L., Fink, C. W., and Ziff, M., 1972, Lymphotoxin formation by lymphocytes and muscle in polymyositis, *J. Clin. Invest.* **51**:2435–2449.

Kallenberg, C. G. M., Van Der Voort Beelen, J. M., D'Amaro, J., and The, T. H., 1981, Increased frequency of B8/DR3 in scleroderma and association of the haplotype with impaired cellular immune response, *Clin. Exp. Immunol.* **43**:478–485.

Kalovidouris, A. E., and Johnson, R. L., 1983, Cellular immunity in ankylosing spondylitis. Lack of response to spinal tissue antigens, *J. Rheumatol.* **10**:98–101.

Kammer, G. M., 1983, Impaired T cell capping and receptor regeneration in active systemic lupus erythematosus. Evidence for a disorder intrinsic to the T lymphocytes, *J. Clin. Invest.* **72**:1686–1697.

Kammer, G. M., Birch, R. E., and Polmar, S. M., 1983, Impaired immunoregulation in systemic lupus erythematosus: Defective adenosine-induced suppressor T lymphocyte generation, *J. Immunol.* **130**:1706–1712.

Kapoor, A. K., Khan, I. U., Tuleja, N., Dash, U. C., Jain, U. K., Siddigni, J. S., Singh, M., Bhushan, V., Mehrotra, R. M. L., and Bahuguna, L. M., 1981, Lymphocyte subpopulations and immunoglobulins in blood in rheumatoid arthritis, *Indian J. Med. Res.* **74**:595–599.

Kaufman, D. B., and Bostwick, E., 1979, Defective suppressor T-cell activity in systemic lupus erythematosus, *Clin. Immunol. Immunopathol.* **13**:9–18.

Keith, H. I., and Currey, H. L. F., 1973, Rosette-formation by peripheral blood lymphocytes in rheumatoid arthritis, *Ann. Rheum. Dis.* **32**:202–207.

Kendall, M. J., Farr, M., and Williamson, N., 1973, Serum immunoglobulins in ankylosing spondylitis, *Br. Med. J.* **2**:172.

Keystone, E. C., Gladman, D. D., Buchanan, R., Cane, D., and Poplonski, L., 1980, Impaired antigen specific suppressor cell activity in patients with rheumatoid arthritis, *Arthritis Rheum.* **23**:1246–1250.

Keystone, E. C., Lau, C., Gladman, D. D., Wilkinson, S., Lee, P., and Shore, A., 1982, Immunoregulatory T cell subpopulations in patients with scleroderma using monoclonal antibodies, *Clin. Exp. Immunol.* **48**:443–488.

Kilpi, A., Bergroth, V., Konttinen, Y. T., Murphy, C. P. J., Reitamo, S., and Wegelins, O., 1983, Lymphocyte infiltrations of the gastric mucosa in Sjogren's syndrome, *Arthritis Rheum.* **26**:1196–1200.

Kinsella, T. D., Espino, L., and Vasey, F. B., 1975, Serum complement and immunoglobulin levels in sporadic and familial ankylosing spondylitis, *J. Rheumatol.* **2**:308–313.

Klareskog, L., Forsum, U., Wigren, A., and Wigzell, H., 1982, Relationship between HLA-DR expressing cells and T lymphocytes of different subsets in rheumatoid synovial tissue, *Scand. J. Immunol.* **15**:501–507.

Kluin-Nelemans, H. C., Vander Linden, J. A., Gmelig-Meyling, F. H. J., and Schuurman, H. J., 1984, HLA-DR positive T lymphocytes in blood and synovial fluid in rheumatoid arthritis, *J. Rheumatol.* **11**:272–276.

Koike, T., Kobayashi, S., Yoshiki, T., Itoh, T., and Shirai, T., 1979, Differential sensitivity of functional subsets of T cells to the cytotoxicity of natural T-lymphocytotoxic autoantibody of systemic lupus erythematosus, *Arthritis Rheum.* **22:**123–129.

Kondo, H., Rabin, B. S., and Rodnan, G. P., 1976, Cutaneous antigen stimulating lymphokine production by lymphocytes of patients with progressive systemic sclerosis (scleroderma), *J. Clin. Invest.* **58:**1338–1394.

Konttinen, Y. T., Reitamo, S., Ranki, A., Hayry, P., Kankaanapaa, U., and Wegelins, O., 1981, Characterization of the immunocompetent cells of rheumatoid synovium from tissue sections and eluates, *Arthritis Rheum.* **24:**71–79.

Korsmeyer, S., and Waldmann, T. A., 1984, Immunoglobulin genes: Rearrangement and translocation in human lymphoid malignancy, *J. Clin. Immunol.* **4:**1–11.

Kotzin, B. L., Kansas, G. S., Engleman, E. G., Hoppe, R. T., Kaplan, H. S., and Strober, S., 1983, Changes in T cell subsets in patients with rheumatoid arthritis treated with total lymphoid irradiation, *Clin. Immunol. Immunopathol.* **27:**250–260.

Krakauer, R. S., Clongh, J. D., Frank, S., and Sundeen, J. T., 1979, Suppressor cell function defect in idiopathic systemic lupus erythematosus, *Clin. Immunol. Immunopathol.* **14:**327–333.

Krakauer, R. S., Sundeen, J., Sander, D. N., and Scherbel, A., 1981, Abnormalities of immunoregulation in progressive systemic sclerosis, *Arch. Dermatol.* **117:**80–82.

Krawitt, E. L., Holdstock, G., Bland, J. H., Chastency, B. F., and Albertini, R. J., 1982, Suppressor cell activity in progressive systemic sclerosis, *J. Rheumatol.* **9:**263–267.

Kumagai, S., Steinberg, A. D., and Greur, I., 1981, Antibodies to T cells in patients with systemic lupus erythematosus can induce antibody dependent cell-mediated cytotoxicity against human T cells, *J. Clin. Invest.* **67:**605–614.

Kumagai, S., Sredni, B., House, S., Steinberg, A. D., and Green, I., 1982, Defective regulation of B lymphocyte colony formation in patients with systemic lupus erythematosus, *J. Immunol.* **128:**258–262.

Kurosaka, M., and Ziff, M., 1983, Immunoelectron microscopic study of the distribution of T cell subsets in rheumatoid synovium, *J. Exp. Med.* **158:**1191–1210.

Kwritani, T., and Cooper, M. D., 1982, Human B cell differentiation. II. Pokeweed mitogen-responsive B cells belong to a surface immunoglobulin D negative subpopulation, *J. Exp. Med.* **155:**1561–1566.

Landry, M., 1977, Phagocyte function and cell-mediated immunity in systemic lupus erythematosus, *Arch. Dermatol.* **113:**147–154.

Lanier, L. L., Engleman, E. G., Gatenby, P., Babcock, G. F., Warner, N. L., and Herzenberg, L. A., 1983, Correlation of functional properties of human lymphoid cell subsets and surface marker phenotypes using multiparameter analysis and flow cytometry, *Immunol. Rev.* **74:**143–160.

Laurent, M. R., and Panayi, G. S., 1983, Acute phase proteins and serum immunoglobulins in ankylosing spondylitis, *Ann. Rheum. Dis.* **42:**524–528.

Lee, S. L., Meiselas, L. E., Zingale, S. B., and Richman, R., 1960, Antibody production in systemic lupus erythematosus (SLE) and rheumatoid arthritis (RA), *J. Clin. Invest.* **39:**1005–1006.

Lehner, T., 1969, Characterization of mucosal antibodies in recurrent aphthous ulceration and Behcet's syndrome, *Arch. Oral. Biol.* **14:**843–853.

Leventhal, B. G., Waldorf, D. S., and Talal, N., 1967, Impaired lymphocyte transformation and delayed hypersensitivity in Sjogren's syndrome, *J. Clin. Invest.* **46:**1338–1345.

Levinsky, R. J., and Lehner, T., 1970, Circulating soluble immune complexes in recurrent oral ulceration and Behcet's syndrome, *Clin. Exp. Immunol.* **32:**193–198.

Levy, J., Barett, E. V., MacDonald, N. S., and Klineberg, J. R., 1970, Altered immunoglobulin metabolism in systemic lupus erythematosus, *J. Clin. Invest.* **49:**708–715.

Lipnik, R. N., Balow, J. E., and Tsokos, G. C., 1984, Lymphocyte subpopulations in patients with systemic lupus erythematosus, *Clin. Immunol. Immunopathol.* **31:**181–190.

Lipsky, P. E., and Ziff, M., 1980, Inhibition of human helper T cell function *in vitro* by D-penicillamine and $CuSO_4$, *J. Clin. Invest.* **65:**1069–1076.

Lisak, R. P., and Zweiman, B., 1975, Mitogen and muscle extract induced *in vitro* proliferative responses in myasthenia gravis, dermatomyositis and polymyositis, *J. Neurol. Neurosurg. Psychiatry* **38:**521–524.

Lisak, R. P., and Sweiman, B., 1976, Serum immunoglobulin levels in myasthenia gravis, polymyositis and dermatomyositis, *J. Neurol.* **39:**34–37.

Lockshin, M. D., Eisenhauer, A. C., Kohn, R., Weksler, M., Block, S., and Mushlin, S. B., 1975, Cell-mediated immunity in rheumatic disease. II. Mitogen response in RA, SLE and other illnesses: Correlation with T and B lymphocyte population, *Arthritis Rheum.* **18:**245–250.

Loewi, G., and Papamichail, M., 1972, Studies of mononuclear cells from inflammatory joint effusions, *Int. Arch. Allergy* **45**:285–289.

Loewi, G., Lance, E. M., and Reynolds, J., 1975, Study of lymphoid cells from inflamed synovial membranes, *Ann. Rheum. Dis.* **34**:524–528.

Logan, R. G., Bandera, J. M., Mikkelsen, W. M., and Duff, I. F., 1966, Polymyositis: A clinical study, *Ann. Intern. Med.* **65**:996–1007.

Louie, J. S., Nies, K. M., Shoji, K. T., Fraback, R. C., Abrass, C., Border, W., Cherry, J. D., and Imagaun, D., 1978, Clinical and antibody responses after influenza immunization in systemic lupus erythematosus, *Ann. Intern. Med.* **88**:790–792.

Lydyard, P. M., Hanglow, A., Hartley, I., Young, A., and Roitt, I., 1982, Immunoregulation in patients with rheumatoid arthritis, *Lancet* **1**:799.

Malaviya, A. N., Rajagopalan, P., Gupta, S., and Taneja, R. L., 1980, Cryoglobulinemia and circulating immune complexes in progressive systemic sclerosis, *Indian J. Med. Res.* **72**:359–364.

Markenson, J. A., Morgan, J. W., Lockshin, M. D., Joachim, C., and Winfield, J. B., 1978, Responses of fractionated cells from patients with systemic lupus erythematosus and normals to plant mitogen: Evidence for a suppressor population of monocytes, *Proc. Soc. Exp. Biol. Med.* **158**:5–9.

Mathieu, A., Meren, M. C., and Pisano, L., 1981, T lymphocytes of peripheral blood and synovial fluid in rheumatoid arthritis, *Arthritis Rheum.* **24**:658–661.

Matsumoto, K., Osakalse, K., Ohi, H., Yoshizawa, N., Harada, M., and Halano, M., 1980, Alteration of T lymphocyte subpopulations in primary renal disease and systemic lupus erythematosus, *Scand. J. Immunol.* **11**:187–193.

Matteson, D. R., and Deutsch, C., 1984, K channels in T lymphocytes: A patch clamp study using monoclonal antibody adhesion, *Nature* **307**:468–470.

McGill, P. E., and Twinn, I., 1977, Antibody mediated cytotoxicity in rheumatoid arthritis, *Ann. Rheum. Dis.* **36**:268–270.

McKenzie, I. F. C., and Zola, H., 1983, Monoclonal antibodies to B cells, *Immunol. Today* **4**:10–16.

Meijer, C. J. L. M., Lapeber, G. J. M., Cnossen, J., Damsteeg, M. G. M., and Cats, A., 1982, T lymphocyte subpopulations in rheumatoid arthritis, *J. Rheumatol.* **9**:8–24.

Mellbye, O. J., Messner, R. P., DeBord, J. R., and Williams, R. C., 1972, Immunoglobulin and receptors for C_3 on lymphocytes, *Arthritis Rheum.* **15**:371–381.

Mellors, R. C., Heimer, R., Corcos, J., and Korngold, L., 1959, Cellular origins of rheumatoid factor, *J. Exp. Med.* **110**:875–886.

Mellors, R. C., Nowoslcowski, A., Korngold, L., and Sengston, B. L., 1961, Rheumatoid factor and the pathogenesis of rheumatoid arthritis, *J. Exp. Med.* **113**:475–483.

Menard, H. A., Dion, J., and Richard, C., 1977, Antinuclear antibody: Predictive of lymphocyte response in rheumatoid arthritis, *J. Rheumatol.* **4**:21–26.

Meuer, S. C., Schlossman, S. F., and Reinherz, E. L., 1982, Clonal analysis of human cytotoxic T lymphocytes $T4^+$ and $T8^+$ effector T cells recognize products of different major histocompatibility complex regions, *Proc. Natl. Acad. Sci. U.S.A.* **79**:4395–4399.

Michalevicz, R., Many, A., Ramot, B., and Trainer, N., 1978, The *in vitro* effect of thymic humoral factor and levamisole on peripheral blood lymphocytes in systemic lupus erythematosus patients, *Clin. Exp. Immunol.* **31**:111–115.

Michalski, J. R., and McCombs, C., 1977, Decreased lymphocyte reactivity to a suboptimal concentration of phytohemagglutinin in Sjogren's syndrome, *Arthritis Rheum.* **20**:851–858.

Moretta, L., Ferrarini, M., and Cooper, M. D., 1978, Characterization of human T cell subpopulations as defined by specific receptors for immunoglobulins, *Contemp. Top. Immunobiol.* **8**:19–53.

Moretta, A., Mingari, M. D., Santoli, D., Perlmann, P., and Moretta, L., 1979, Human T-lymphocyte subpopulations: Alterations in systemic lupus erythematosus, *Scand. J. Immunol.* **10**:223–228.

Morimoto, C., Abe, T., Hara, M., and Homma, M., 1977, *In vitro* TNP specific antibody formation by peripheral lymphocytes from patients with systemic lupus erythematosus, *Scand. J. Immunol.* **6**:575–579.

Morimoto, C., Abe, T., Toguchi, T., Kiyotaki, M., and Homma, M., 1979a, Studies of antilymphocyte antibody of patients with active SLE, *Scand. J. Immunol.* **10**:213–221.

Morimoto, C., Abe, T., and Homma, M., 1979b, Altered function of suppressor T lymphocytes in patients with active systemic lupus erythematosus. *In vitro* immune response to autoantigen, *Clin. Immunol. Immunopathol.* **13**:161–170.

Morimoto, C., Reinherz, E. L., Schlossman, S. F., Schur, P. H., Mills, J. A., and Steinberg, A. D., 1980a, Alterations in immunoregulatory T cell subsets in active systemic lupus erythematosus, *J. Clin. Invest.* **66**:1171–1174.

Morimoto, C., Reinherz, E. L., Abe, T., Homma, M., and Schlossman, S. F., 1980b, Characteristics of anti-T cell antibodies in systemic lupus erythematosus: Evidence for selective reactivity with normal suppressor cells defined by monoclonal antibodies, *Clin. Immunol. Immunopathol.* **16**:474–484.

Morimoto, C., Abe, T., Toguchi, T., Kiyotaki, M., and Homma, M., 1980c, Studies of antilymphocyte antibody in patients with active SLE, *Scand. J. Immunol.* **11**:479–488.

Morimoto, C., Reinherz, E. L., Borel, Y., Mantzouranis, E., Steinberg, A. D., and Schlossman, S. F., 1981, Autoantibody to an immunoregulatory inducer population in patients with juvenile rheumatoid arthritis, *J. Clin. Invest.* **67**:753–761.

Morimoto, C., Distaso, J. A., Borel, Y., Schlossman, S. F., and Reinherz, E. L., 1982a, Communicative interactions between subpopulations of human T lymphocytes required for generation of suppressor effector function in a primary antibody response, *J. Immunol.* **128**:1645–1650.

Morimoto, C., Reinherz, E. L., Nadler, L. M., Distaso, J. A., Steinberg, A. D., and Schlossman, S. F., 1982b, Comparison on T- and B-cells markers in patients with Sjogren's syndrome and systemic lupus erythematosus, *Clin. Immunol. Immunopathol.* **22**:270–278.

Morimoto, C., Reinherz, E. L., Borel, Y., and Schlossman, S. F., 1983a, Direct demonstration of the human supressor inducer subset by anti-T cell antibodies, *J. Immunol.* **130**:157–161.

Morimoto, C., Steinberg, A. D., Schlossman, S. F., and Bord, Y., 1983b, *In vitro* nucleoside specific immune response by lymphocytes from systemic lupus erythematosus, *J. Clin. Invest.* **71**:1402–1409.

Morimoto, C., Reinherz, E. L., Distaso, J. A., Steinberg, A. D., and Schlossman, S. F., 1984, Relationship between systemic lupus erythematosus T cell subsets, anti T cell antibodies and T cell functions, *J. Clin. Invest.* **73**:689–700.

Moutsopoulos, H. M., and Fauci, A. S., 1980, Immunoregulation in Sjogren's syndrome. Influence of serum factors on T-cell subpopulations, *J. Clin. Invest.* **65**:519–528.

Moutsopoulos, H. M., Fye, K. H., Sawada, S., Becker, M. J., Goldstein, A., and Talal, N., 1976, *In vitro* effect of thymosin on T lymphocyte rosette formation in rheumatic disease, *Clin. Exp. Immunol.* **26**:563–573.

Moutsopoulos, H. M., Weber, B. L., Vlagopoulos, T. P., Chused, T. M., and Decker, J. L., 1979, Differences in the clinical manifestation of Sicca syndrome in the presence or absence of rheumatoid arthritis, *Am. J. Med.* **66**:733–736.

Munthe, E., and Natvig, J. B., 1972, Immunoglobulin classes, subclasses and complexes of IgG rheumatoid plasma cells, *Clin. Exp. Immunol.* **12**:55–70.

Muraguchi, A., Kehrl, J. H., Butler, J. L., and Fanci, A. S., 1984, Regulation of human B-cell activation, proliferation and differentiation by soluble factors, *J. Clin. Immunol.* **4**:337–347.

Muschel, L. W., 1961, Systemic lupus erythematosus and normal antibodies, *Proc. Soc. Exp. Biol. Med.* **106**:622–625.

Nadler, L., Shashenko, P., Hardy, R., VanAgthoven, A., Terhorst, C., and Schlossman, S. F., 1981, Characterization of a human B cell specific antigen (B_2) distinct from B_1, *J. Immunol.* **126**:1941–1947.

Nakai, H., Morito, T., Tanimoto, K., and Horiuchi, Y., 1977, Reduced Fc receptor bearing cells in peripheral bloods of patients with systemic lupus erythematosus and in rheumatoid synovial fluid, *J. Rheumatol.* **4**:405–413.

Nakamura, Z. I., Asano, T., Yano, K., and Ojuji, T., 1982, Reevaluation of suppressor cell function in systemic lupus erythematosus, *Clin. Immunol. Immunopathol.* **24**:72–82.

Newman, B., Black, S., Lomnitzer, R., Disler, P., and Rabson, A. R., 1979, Lack of suppressor cell activity in systemic lupus erythematosus, *Clin. Immunol. Immunopathol.* **13**:187–193.

Nies, K. M., and Louie, J. S., 1978, Impaired immunoglobulin synthesis by peripheral lymphocytes in systemic lupus erythematosus, *Arthritis Rheum.* **21**:51–57.

Nies, K. M., Stevens, R. H., and Louie, J. S., 1981, Impaired immunoglobulin M synthesis by peripheral blood lymphocytes in systemic lupus erythematosus: A primary B-cell defect, *Clin. Immunol. Immunopathol.* **19**:118–130.

Nikbin, B., Brewerton, D. A., Byron, N., James, O. C. N., Malka, S., McLeod, L., Slater, C., Warren, R. E., and Hobbs, J. R., 1975, Lymphocyte function in ankylosing spondylitis, *Ann. Rheum. Dis.* **34**(Suppl. 1):49–52.

Nilsson, E., and Biberfeld, C., 1980, Subpopulations of T lymphocytes in patients with ankylosing spondylitis, *Ann. Rheum. Dis.* **39**:566–569.

Nilsson, E., and Biberfield, G., 1982, T lymphocyte subpopulations defined by monoclonal antibodies in synorial fluid of patients with rheumatic disease, *J. Clin. Lab. Immunol.* **9**:93–97.

Niwa, Y., and Kanoh, T., 1979, Immune deficiency states and immune imbalance in systemic lupus erythematosus and other autoimmune diseases, *Clin. Immunol. Immunopathol.* **12**:289–300.

O'Duffy, J. D., Carney, J. A., and Deodhar, S., 1971, Behcet's disease: Report of 10 cases, 3 with new manifestations, *Ann. Intern. Med.* **75**:561–570.

Ogryzlo, M. A., Machachlan, M., and Danphrinee, J. A., 1959, The serum proteins in health and disease; filter paper electrophoresis, *Am. J. Med.* **27**:596–616.

Okudaira, K., Nakai, H., Hayakawa, T., Kashiwado, T., Tanimoto, K., Horiuchi, Y., and Juji, T., 1979, Detection of antilymphocyte antibody with two-color method in systemic lupus erythematosus and its heterogeneous specificities against human T cell subsets, *J. Clin. Invest.* **64**:1213–1220.

Okudaira, K., Tanimoto, K., Nakamura, T., and Horiuchi, Y., 1980, Spontaneously enhance *in vitro* immunoglobulin synthesis by B cells in systemic lupus erythematosus, *Clin. Immunol. Immunopathol.* **16**:267–278.

Okudaira, K., Searles, R. P., Tanimoto, K., Horiuchi, Y., and Williams, R. C., Jr., 1982, T lymphocyte interaction with immunoglobulin G antibody in systemic lupus erythematosus, *J. Clin. Invest.* **69**:1026–1038.

Olsen, N., Ziff, M., and Jasin, H. E., 1982, *In vitro* synthesis of immunoglobulins and IgM rheumatoid factor by blood mononuclear cells of patients with rheumatoid arthritis, *Rheum. Int.* **2**:59–66.

Olsen, N., Ziff, M., and Jasin, H. E., 1984, Spontaneous synthesis of IgM rheumatoid factor by blood mononuclear cells from patients with rheumatoid arthritis. Effect of treatment with gold salt or D-penicillanine, *J. Rheumatol.* **11**:17–21.

Ortaldo, J. R., and Herberman, R. B., 1984, Heterogeneity of natural killer cells, *Annu. Rev. Immunol.* **2**:359–394.

Oshima, Y., Shimizu, T., Tokohari, R., Matsumoto, T., Kano, K., Kagami, T., and Nagaya, H., 1963, Clinical studies on Behcet's syndrome, *Ann. Rheum. Dis.* **22**:36–45.

Pachman, L. M., Hafeman, C., and Janor, D., 1977, IgA deficiency and juvenile rheumatoid arthritis, *Arthritis Rheum.* **20**(Suppl.):445–448.

Palacios, R., 1982, Mechanisms of T cell activation: Role and functional relationship of HLA-DR antigens and interleukins, *Immunol. Rev.* **63**:73–110.

Palacios, R., and Alarcon-Segovia, D., 1981, Human posthymic precursor cells in health and disease. VI. Effect of serum thymic factor on the response of cells from patients with systemic lupus erythematosus or mixed connective tissue disease in autologous mixed lymphocyte reaction, *Clin. Immunol. Immunopathol.* **18**:362–367.

Palacios, R., and Martinez-Maza, O., 1982, Is the E-receptor on human T lymphocytes a negative signal receptor? *J. Immunol.* **129**:2479–2485.

Palacios, R., Ruiz-Arguelles, A., and Alarcon-Segovia, D., 1981, Human post-thymic precursor cells in health and disease. IX. Immunoregulatory T cell circuits in peripheral blood of patients with rheumatoid arthritis, *Clin. Exp. Immunol.* **43**:473–477.

Panayi, G. S., and Corrigall, V., 1977, Functional assay of cytotoxic lymphocytes involved in antibody mediated cytotoxicity in normal and rheumatoid subjects, *Ann. Rheum. Dis.* **36**:257–260.

Panush, R. S., Bianco, N. E., Schur, P. H., Rocklin, R. E., David, J. R., and Stillman, J. S., 1972, Juvenile rheumatoid arthritis cellular hypersensitivity and selective IgA deficiency, *Clin. Exp. Immunol.* **10**:103–110.

Papadimitriou, G., Bacon, P. A., and Hall, N. D., 1982, Circulating activated lymphocytes in rheumatoid arthritis. A marker of synovial inflammation, *J. Rheumatol.* **9**:217–223.

Papaioannou, C. C., Hunder, G. G., and McDuffie, F. C., 1979, Cellular immunity in polymyalgia rheumatica and giant cell arteritis. Lack of response to muscle or artery homogenate, *Arthritis Rheum.* **22**:740–745.

Pardo, I., and Levinson, A. I., 1983, Circulating immunoglobulin-secreting cells in rheumatoid arthritis, *Clin. Immunol. Immunopathol.* **29**:29–34.

Pardo, I., Carafa, C., Dziarski, R., and Levinson, A. I., 1984, Analysis of *in vitro* polyclonal B cell differentiation responses to bacterial peptidoglycan and pokeweed mitogen in rheumatoid arthritis, *Clin. Exp. Immunol.* **56**:253–262.

Patel, V., and Panayi, G. S., 1984, Enhanced T helper cell function for the spontaneous production of IgM rheumatoid factor *in vitro* in rheumatoid arthritis, *Clin. Exp. Immunol.* **57**:584–592.

Paty, J. G., Sienknecht, C. W., Townes, A. S., Hanissian, A. S., Miller, J. B., and Masi, A. F., 1975, Impaired cell-mediated immunity in systemic lupus erythematosus, *Am. J. Med.* **59**:769–779.

Pelkonen, P., Savilahti, E., and Makela, A. L., 1983, Persistent and transient IgA deficiency in juvenile rheumatoid arthritis, *Scand. J. Rheumatol.* **12**:273–279.

Penschow, J., and MacKay, I. R., 1980, NK and K cell activity of human blood: Differences according to sex, age and disease, *Ann. Rheum. Dis.* **39**:82–86.

Percy, J. S., Davis, P., Russell, A. S., and Brosson, E., 1978, A longitudinal study of *in vitro* tests for lymphocyte function in rheumatoid arthritis, *Ann. Rheum. Dis.* **37**:416–420.

Petersen, J., Andersen, V., Bendixen, G., Bentzen, K., Kristensen, J. H., Hansen, T. I., and Wiik, A., 1982, Functional characteristics of synovial fluid and blood mononuclear cells in rheumatoid arthritis and tranmatic synovitis, *Scand. J. Rheumatol.* **11**:75–80.

Petersen, J., Andersen, V., Hansen, T. I., Kristensen, J. H., Wiik, A., and Thyssen, J., 1983, Synovial fluid and blood monocyte influence on lymphocyte proliferation in rheumatoid arthritis and traumatic synovitis, *Scand. J. Rheumatol.* **12**:299–304.

Petersen, J., Ingemann-Hansen, T., and Halkjaer-Kristensen, J., 1984, Spontaneous and induced immunoglobulin secretion by synovial fluid B lymphocytes in rheumatoid arthritis, *Ann. Rheum. Dis.* **43**:140–145.

Phillips, P. E., and Christian, C. L., 1971, Virus antibody studies in connective tissue diseases, *Arthritis Rheum.* **14**:180–181.

Pincus, G. S., and Dekker, A., 1970, Benign lymphoepithelial lesion of the parotid glands associated with reticulum cell sarcoma. Report of a case and review of the literature, *Cancer* **25**:121–127.

Plater-Zyberk, C., Clarke, M. F., Lam, K., Memford, P. A., Room, G. R. W., and Mani, R. N., 1983, *In vitro* immunoglobulin synthesis by lymphocytes from patients with rheumatoid arthritis. I. Effect of monocyte depletion and demonstration of an increased proportion of lymphocytes forming rosettes with mouse erythrocytes, *Clin. Exp. Immunol.* **52**:505–511.

Queiros, M. V., and Rocha, B., 1983, T cell subsets in patients with rheumatoid arthritis reduction of cells with Leu 2A phenotype in patients with serum IgG immunocomplex, *Clin. Exp. Immunol.* **54**:509–514.

Quismorio, F. P., and Friou, G. J., 1970, Serological factors in systemic lupus erythematosus and their pathogenetic significance, *CRC Crit. Rev. Clin. Lab. Sci.* pp. 639–683.

Radon, N., Cleveland, R. P., and Leon, M. A., 1982, Peripheral T lymphocytes from rheumatoid arthritis patients recognize determinants on light chains and/or Fab fragments of immunoglobulin G, *J. Clin. Invest.* **70**:329–334.

Raeman, F., DeCock, W., Debenkelaar, T., Decree, J., and Verhaegen, H., 1981, Enumeration of T cells and T lymphocyte subsets in autoimmune disease using monoclonal antibodies, *Clin. Exp. Immunol.* **45**:475–479.

Raveche, E. S., and Steinberg, A. D., 1979, Lymphocyte and lymphocyte functions in systemic lupus erythematosus, *Semin. Hematol.* **16**:344–370.

Rawson, A. J., and Huang, T. C., 1974a, Lymphocytes in rheumatoid arthritis. I. Response to allogeneic cells and to phytomitogens, *Clin. Exp. Immunol.* **16**:41–46.

Rawson, A. J., and Huang, T. C., 1974b, Lymphocytes in rheumatoid arthritis. II. Quantitative binding of phytomitogens, *Clin. Exp. Immunol.* **16**:47–52.

Rawson, A. J., and Huang, T. C., 1976, Lymphocyte populations in rheumatoid arthritis, *Arthritis Rheum.* **19**:720–724.

Reinherz, E. L., and Schlossman, S. F., 1980, The differentiation and function of human T lymphocytes, *Cell* **19**:821–827.

Reinherz, E. L., Meuer, S., Fitzgerald. K., Hussey, R. E., Levine, H., and Schlossman, S. F., 1982a, Antigen recognition by human T lymphocytes is linked to surface expression of the T_3 molecular complex, *Cell* **30**:735–743.

Reinherz, E. L., Morimoto, C., Fitzgerald, K., Hussey, R. E., Daley, J. F., and Schlossman, S. F., 1982b, Heterogeneity of human $T4^+$ inducer T cells defined by a monoclonal antibody that delineates two functional subpopulations, *J. Immunol.* **128**:463–468.

Reinherz, E. L., Hussey, R. E., and Schlossman, S. F., 1980, A monoclonal antibody blocking human T cell function, *Eur. J. Immunol.* **10**:758–762.

Reynolds, M. D., and Abdou, N. I., 1973, Comparative study of the *in vitro* proliferative responses of blood and synovial fluid leukocytes of rheumatoid arthritis patients, *J. Clin. Invest.* **52**:1627–1631.

Ristow, S. C., Douglas, R. C., and Condemi, J. J., 1978, Influenza vaccination of patients with systemic lupus erythematosus, *Ann. Intern. Med.* **88**:786–789.

Rivero, S. J., Llorente, L., Diaz-Jouanen, E., and Alarcon-Segovia, D., 1977, T-lymphocyte subpopulations in untreated SLE variations with disease activity, *Arthritis Rheum.* **20**:1169–1173.

Rogers, R. S., Sam, W. M., and Shorter, R. G., 1974, Lymphocytotoxicity in recurrent aphthous stomatitis. Lymphocytotoxicity for oral epithelial cells in recurrent aphthous stomatitis and Behcet's syndrome, *Arch. Dermatol.* **109**:361–363.

Room, G. R. W., Plater-Zyberk, C., Clarke, M. F., and Maini, R. N., 1982, B lymphocyte subpopulation which forms rosettes with mouse erythrocytes increased in rheumatoid arthritis, *Rheumatol. Int.* **2**:175–180.

Rosenberg, J. N., and Currey, H. L. F., 1979, Antibody dependent and PHA-induced cellular cytotoxicity in rheumatoid arthritis, *Ann. Rheum. Dis.* **38**:347–350.

Rosenthal, C. J., and Franklin, E. C., 1975, Depression of cellular-mediated immunity in systemic lupus erythematosus, *Arthritis Rheum.* **18**:207–217.

Rosenthal, M., and Muller, W., 1975, Lymphocyte subpopulation normals and patients with rheumatoid arthritis and ankylosing spondylitis, *J. Rheumatol.* **2**:355–358.

Rosling, A. E., Rhodes, E. L., and Watson, B., 1978, Removal of a blocking factor from the sera of patients with systemic lupus erythematosus with levamisole, *Clin. Exp. Dermatol.* **3**:39–42.

Ross, G. D., 1979, Identification of lymphocyte subpopulations by surface marker analysis, *Blood* **53**:799–811.

Roumm, A. D., Whiteside, T. L., Medsger, Jr., T. A., and Rodnan, G. P., 1984, Lymphocytes in the skin of patients with progressive systemic sclerosis quantification, subtyping and clinical correlation, *Arthritis Rheum.* **27**:645–653.

Rowe, D. J., Isenbergh, D. A., McDougall, J., and Beverley, P. C. L., 1981, Characterization of myositis infiltrates using monoclonal antibodies to human leukocyte antigens, *Clin. Exp. Immunol.* **45**:290–298.

Rowe, D., Isenberg h., D. A., and Beverley, P. C. L., 1983, Monoclonal antibodies to human leukocyte antigens in polymyositis and muscular dystrophy, *Clin. Exp. Immunol.* **54**:327–336.

Ruiz-Arguelles, A., Diaz-Jonanen, E., and Alarcon-Segovia, D., 1979, PHA-induced cellular cytotoxicity inhibition by a non-immunoglobulin factor present in sera from patients with active systemic lupus erythematosus, *Arthritis Rheum.* **22**:59–65.

Sagawa, A., and Abdou, N. I., 1979, Suppressor-cell antibody in systemic lupus erythematosus. Possible mechanism for suppressor-cell dysfunction, *J. Clin. Invest.* **63**:536–539.

Sakane, T., Steinberg, A. D., and Green, I., 1978, Studies of immune functions of patients with systemic lupus erythematosus. I. Dysfunction of suppressor T-cell activity related to impaired generation of rather than response to suppressor cells, *Arthritis Rheum.* **21**:657–664.

Sakane, T., Steinberg, A. D., Reeves, J. P., and Green, I., 1979b, I. Studies of immune functions of patients with systemic lupus erythematosus. T cell subsets and antibodies to T cell subsets, *J. Clin. Invest.* **64**:1260–1269.

Sakane, T., Kotani, H., Takada, S., and Tsunematsu, T., 1982, Functional aberration of T cell subsets in patients with Behcet's disease, *Arthritis Rheum.* **25**:1343–1351.

Sakane, T., Kotani, H., Takada, S., Murakawa, Y., and Ueda, Y., 1983, A defect in the suppressor circuits among $OKT4^+$ cell population in patients with systemic lupus erythematosus occurs independently of a defect in the $OKT8^+$ suppressor T cell function, *J. Immunol.* **131**:753–761.

Salem, N. B., and Morse, J. H., 1976, Lymphocyte response to mitogens in progressive systemic sclerosis, *Arthritis Rheum.* **19**:875–882.

Sanefuji, M., 1974, Cell-mediated immunity in uveitis. 3. Leucocyte migration inhibition test in Behcet's disease, *Acta Soc. Ophthalmol. Jpn.* **78**:408.

Sany, J., Clot, J., Freitas, M., Charmasson, E., and Serre, H., 1976, Antibody-dependent cell cytotoxicity (ADCC) of rheumatoid arthritis blood lymphocytes, *Rev. Rhum. Mal. Osteoartic.* **43**:333–338.

Sato, M., Hayashi, Y., Yoshida, H., Yanagawa, T., and Yura, Y., 1984, A family with hereditary lack of $T4^+$ inducer/helper T cell subsets in peripheral blood lymphocytes, *J. Immunol.* **132**:1071–1073.

Scheinberg, M. A., and Cathcart, E. S., 1976, Antibody-dependent direct cytotoxicity of human lymphocytes, *Clin. Exp. Immunol.* **24**:317–322.

Scheinberg, M. A., Cathcart, E. S., and Goldstein, A., 1975, Thymosin-inducer reduction of "null cells" in peripheral blood lymphocytes of patients with SLE, *Lancet* **1**:424–426.

Scheinberg, M. A., Santos, L., Mendez, N. F., and Musatti, C., 1978, Decreased lymphocyte response to PHA, ConA and calcium ionophore (A-23187) in patients with RA and SLE and reversal with levamisole in rheumatoid arthritis, *Arthritis Rheum.* **21**:326–329.

Segond, P., Delfraissy, J. F., Galanand, P., Wallon, C., Massias, P., and Dormont, J., 1979, Depressed primary *in vitro* antibody response in rheumatoid arthritis, *Clin. Exp. Immunol.* **37**:196–204.

Segond, P., Salliere, D., Galanand, P., Desmottes, R. M., Massias, P., and Fiessinger, J. N., 1982, Impaired primary *in vitro* antibody response in progressive systemic sclerosis patients: Role of suppressor monocytes, *Clin. Exp. Immunol.* **47**:147–154.

Seitz, M., Vogt, P., Muller, W., Hunstein, W., and Gemsa, D., 1983, Characterization of blood mononuclear cells of rheumatoid arthritis patients. II. Depressed PPD presentation by monocytes to T lymphocytes, *Clin. Immunol. Immunopathol.* **29**:242–253.

Sharpin, R. K. C., and Wilson, J. D., 1977, Increased EA rosette-formation by lymphocytes from patients with rheumatoid arthritis, *Clin. Exp. Immunol.* **29**:205–212.

Sheldon, P. J., Papamichael, M., and Holborow, E. J., 1974, Studies on synovial fluid lymphocytes in rheumatoid arthritis, *Ann. Rheum. Dis.* **33**:509–514.

Shimizu, T., Katsuta, Y., and Oshima, Y., 1965, Immunological studies on Behcet's syndrome, *Ann. Rheum. Dis.* **24**:494–499.

Silverman, H., Hohnson, J., Vaughan, J., and McGlamory, J., 1976, Altered lymphocyte reactivity in rheumatoid arthritis, *Arthritis Rheum.* **3**:509–515.

Slaughter, L., Carson, D. A., Jansen, F. C., Holdbrook, T. L., and Vaughan, J. H., 1978, *In vitro* effects of Epstein–Barr virus on peripheral blood mononuclear cells from patients with rheumatoid arthritis and normal subjects, *J. Exp. Med.* **148**:1429–1434.

Slavin, S., and Strober, S., 1981, *In vitro* T cell mediated function in patients with active rheumatoid arthritis, *Ann. Rheum. Dis.* **40**:60–63.

Sliwinski, A. J., and Zvaifler, N. J., 1970, *In vivo* synthesis of IgG by rheumatoid synovium, *J. Lab. Clin. Med.* **76**:304–310.

Smiley, J. D., Sachs, C., and Ziff, M., 1968, *In vitro* synthesis of immunoglobulin by rheumatoid synovial membrane, *J. Clin. Invest.* **47**:624–632.

Smolen, J. S., Chused, T. M., Leiserson, W. M., Reeves, J. P., Alling, D., and Steinberg, A. D., 1982, Heterogeneity of immunoregulatory T-cell subsets in systemic lupus erythematosus. Correlation with clinical features, *Am. J. Med.* **72**:783–790.

Sotnik, D. T., 1979, T cells in ankylosing spondylitis, *Ann. Rheum. Dis.* **38**:199–200.

Stashenko, P., Nadler, L. M., Hardy, R., and Schlossman, S. F., 1980, Characterization of a B lymphocyte specific antigen, *J. Immunol.* **125**:1678–1685.

Stratton, J. A., and Peter, J. B., 1972, Response of synovial fluid and peripheral blood lymphocytes to *in vitro* stimulation, *Arthritis Rheum.* **15**:457.

Strelkauskas, A. H., Schauf, V., and Dray, S., 1976, Alterations in T, B and null cells in children with autoimmune disease, *Clin. Immunol. Immunopathol.* **6**:359–368.

Strelkauskas, A. J., Schauf, V., Wilson, B. S., Chess, L., and Schlossman, S. F., 1978a, Isolation and characterization of naturally occurring subclasses of human peripheral blood T cells with regulatory functions, *J. Immunol.* **120**:1278–1282.

Strelkauskas, A. J., Callery, R. T., McDowell, J., Borel Y., and Schlossman, S. F., 1978b, Direct evidence of loss of human suppressor cells during active autoimmune disease, *Proc. Natl. Acad. Sci. U.S.A.* **75**:5150–5154.

Strelkauskas, J. A., Callery, R. T., Borel, Y., and Schlossman, S. F., 1979, Functional characteristics of human T-lymphocyte subsets identified by sera from patients with systemic lupus erythematosus, *Clin. Immunol. Immunopathol.* **14**:47–55.

Stuart, J.M., Postlethwaite, A. F., and Kang, A. H., 1976, Evidence for cell-mediated immunity to collagen in progressive systemic sclerosis, *J. Lab. Clin. Med.* **88**:601–607.

Suciu-Foca, N., Buda, J. A., Thiem, T., and Reemtsmu, K., 1974, Impaired responsiveness of lymphocytes in patients with systemic lupus erythematosus, *Clin. Exp. Immunol.* **18**:295–301.

Suzuki, H., Sakurami, T., and Imura, H., 1982a, Relationship between reduced B cell susceptibility to IgM antibodies and reduced IgD bearing B cells in patients with systemic lupus erythematosus, *Arthritis Rheumat.* **25**:1451–1459.

Suzuki, H., Sakurami, T., and Imura, H., 1982b, Reduced susceptibility to anti-Fab antibodies of B cells in patients with systemic lupus erythematosus, *Int. Arch. Allergy Appl. Immunol.* **69**:296–301.

Swain, S. L., Howard, M., Kappler, J., Marrack, P., Watson, R., Booth, R., Wetzel, G., and Dutton, R. W., 1983, Evidence for 2 distinct classes of murine B cell growth factor with activities indifferent functional assays, *J. Exp. Med.* **158**:822–935.

Talal, N., Sokoloff, L., and Barth, W. F., 1967, Extrasalivary lymphoid abnormalities in Sjogren's syndrome (reticulum cell sarcoma, "pseudolymphoma," macroglobulinemia), *Am. J. Med.* **43**:50–65.

Talal, N., Asofsky, R., and Lightbody, P., 1970, Immunoglobulin synthesis by salivary gland lymphoid cells in Sjogren's syndrome, *J. Clin. Invest.* **49**:49–54.

Talal, N., Sylvester, R. A., Daniels, T. E., Greenspan, J. S., and Williams, R. C. , Jr., 1974, T and B lymphocytes in perpheral blood and tissue lesions in Sjogren's syndrome, *J. Clin. Invest.* **53**:180–189.

Tan, E. M., 1984, Antinuclear antibodies in diagnosis and management, in: *The Biology of Immunologic Disease* (F. J. Dixon and D. W. Fisher, eds.), Sinauer Associates, Sunderland, Massachusetts, pp. 319–324.

Tan, E. M., Rodnan, G. P., Garcia, I., Moroi, Y., Fritzler, M. J., and Peebles, C., 1980, Diversity of antinuclear antibodies in progressive systemic sclerosis anticentromere antibody and its relationship to CREST syndrome, *Arthritis Rheum.* **23**:617–625.

Tannenbaum, H., Pincus, G. S., Anderson, L. G., and Schur, P. H., 1975, Immunologic characterization of the mononuclear cell infiltrates in rheumatoid synovia, in rheumatoid nodules, and in lip biopsies from patients with Sjogren's syndrome, *Arthritis Rheum.* **18**:305–314.

Thomas, Y., Sosman, J., Irigoyen, O., Friedman, S. M., Kung, P. C., Goldstein, G., and Chess, L., 1980, Functional analysis of T cell subsets defined by monoclonal antibodies. I. Collaborative T-T interactions in the immunoregulation of B cell differentiation, *J. Immunonal.* **125**:2402.

Thomas, Y., Rogozinski, L., Irigoyen, O., King, P. C., Goldstein, G., and Chess, L., 1981, Functional analysis of human cell subsets defined by monoclonal antibodies. III. Regulation of helper factors produced by T cell subsets, *J. Immunol.* **126**:1948–1951.

Thomas, Y., Rogozinski, L., Irigoyen, O. H., Shen, H. H., Talle, M. A., Goldstein, G., and Chess, L., 1982a, Functional analysis of human T cell subsets defined by monoclonal antibodies. V. Suppressor cells within the activated $OKT4^+$ population belong to a distinct subset, *J. Immunol.* **128**:1386–1390.

Thomas, Y., Rogozinski, L., Rothman, P., Rabbani, L. E., Andrews, S., Irigoyen, O. H., and Chess, L., 1982b, Further dissection of the functional heterogeneity within the $OKT4^+$ and $OKT8^+$ human T cell subsets, *J. Clin. Immunol.* **2**(Suppl. 1):85–145.

Thomas, Y., Rogozenski, L., and Chess, L., 1983, Relationship between human T cell functional heterogeneity and human T cell surface molecules, *Immunol. Rev.* **74**:113–128.

Tosato, G., Steinberg, A. D., and Blaese, R. M., 1981, Defective EBV-specific suppressor T cell function in rheumatoid arthritis, *N. Engl. J. Med.* **305**:1238–1243.

Tosato, G., Steinberg, A. D., Yarchoan, R., Heilman, C. A., Pike, S. E., DeSeau, V., and Blaese, R. M., 1984, Abnormally elevated frequency of Epstein–Barr virus infected B cells in the blood of patients with rheumatoid arthritis, *J. Clin. Invest.* **73**:1789–1795.

Traycoff, R. B., Pascual, E., and Schumalher, H. R., 1976, Mononuclear cells in human synovial fluid: Identification of lymphoblasts in rheumatoid arthritis, *Arthritis Rheum.* **19**:743–748.

Trentham, D. E., Dynesius, R. A., and Rocklin, R. E., 1978, Cellular sensitivity to collagen in rheumatoid arthritis, *N. Engl. J. Med.* **299**:327–332.

Trull, A. K., Ebringer, R., Panayi, G. S., Colthrope, D., James, D. C. O., and Ebringer, A., 1983, IgA antibodies to *Klebsiella* pneumonia in ankylosing spondylitis, *Scand. J. Rheumat.* **12**:249–253.

Tsokos, G. C., and Ballow, J. E., 1981, Cytotoxic responses to alloantigens in systemic lupus erythematosus, *J. Clin. Immunol.* **1**:208–216.

Tsokos, G. C., and Ballow, J. E., 1983, Phenotype of T lymphocytes in systemic lupus erythematosus: Decreased cytotoxic/suppressor subpopulation is associated with deficient allogeneic cytotoxic responses rather than with concanavalin A-induced suppressor cells, *Clin. Immunol. Immunopathol.* **26**:267–276.

Tsokos, G. C., Margrath, I. T., and Ballow, J. S., 1983, Epstein Barr virus induced normal B cell responses but defective suppressor T cell responses in patients with systemic lupus erthematosus, *J. Immunol.* **131**:1797–1801.

Tsoukas, C. D., Carson, D. A., Fong, S., Pasquali, J. L., and Vaughan, J. H., 1980, Cellular requirements for pokeweed mitogen-induced autoantibody production in rheumatoid arthritis, *J. Immunol.* **125**:1125–1129.

Tsoukas, C. D., Carson, D. A., Fong, S., Slovin, S. F., Fox, R. I., and Vaughan, J. H., 1982, Lysis of autologous Epstein–Barr virus infected B cells by cytotoxic T lymphocytes of rheumatoid arthritis patients, *Clin. Immunol. Immunopathol.* **24**:8–14.

Tsudo, M., Uchiama, T., and Uchino, H., 1984, Expression of Tac antigen on activated normal human B cells, *J. Exp. Med.* **160**:612–617.

Uchiama, T., Broder, S., and Waldmann, T. A., 1981a, A monoclonal antibody (anti-Tac) reactive with activated and functionally mature human T cells. I. Production of anti-Tac monoclonal antibody and distribution of Tac(+) cells, *J. Immunol.* **126:**1393–1397.

Uchiama, T., Nelson, D. L., Fleisher, T. A., and Waldmann, T. A., 1981b, A monoclonal antibody (anti-Tac) reactive with activated and functionally mature human T cells. II. Expression of Tac antigen on activated cytotoxic killer T cells, suppressor cells and one of two types of helper T cells, *J. Immunol.* **126:**1398–1403.

Utsinger, P. D., 1975, Synovial fluid lymphocytes in rheumatoid arthritis, *Arthritis Rheum.* **18:**595–602.

Utsinger, P. D., 1976, Lymphocyte responsiveness in systemic lupus erythematosus, *Arthritis Rheum.* **19:**88–92.

Utsinger, P. D., and Bluestein, H. G., 1974, Sequential studies of T and B lymphocytes in RA and SLE, *J. Rheumatol.* **1**(Suppl.):75.

Utsinger, P. D., and Yount, W. J., 1977, Phytohemagglutinin response in systemic lupus erythematosus. Reconstitution experiments using highly purified lymphocyte subpopulations and monocytes, *J. Clin. Invest.* **60:**626–638.

Van Boxel, J. A., and Paget, S. A., 1975, Predominatly T cell infiltrate in rheumatoid synovial membranes, *N. Engl. J. Med.* **293:**517–520.

Van Boxel, J. A., Hardin, J. A., Green, I., and Paul, W. E., 1973, Multiple heavy chain determinants on individual B lymphocytes in the peripheral blood of patients with Sjogren's syndrome, *N. Engl. J. Med.* **289:**823–827.

Van Wauwe, J. P., DeMey, J. R., and Goosen, J. G., 1980, OKT3: A monoclonal antihuman T lymphocyte antibody with potent mitogenic properties, *J. Immunol.* **124:**2708–2713.

Vaughan, J. H., and Chihara, T., 1973, Lymphocyte function in rheumatic disorders, *Arch. Intern. Med.* **135:**1324–1328.

Vaughan, J. H., Chichara, T., Moore, T. L., Robbins, D. L., Tanimoto, K., Johnson, J. J., and McMillan, R., 1976, Rheumatoid factor producing cells detected by direct hemolytic plaque assay, *J. Clin. Invest.* **58:**933–941.

Verdickt, W., DeQueker, J., Ceuppens, J. L., Stevens, E., Gantama, K., and Vermylen, C., 1983, Effect of lymphoplasmapherisis on clinical indices and T cell subsets in rheumatoid arthritis. A double blind controlled study, *Arthritis Rheum.* **26:**1419–1425.

Veys, E. M., and Van Laere, M., 1973, Serum IgG, IgM and IgA levels in ankylosing spondylitis, *Ann. Rheum. Dis.* **32:**493–496.

Veys, E. M., Hermanns, P., Verbruggen, G., Schindler, J., and Goldstein, G., 1982a, Evaluation of T cell subsets with monoclonal antibodies in synovial fluid in rheumatoid arthritis, *J. Rheumatol.* **9:**821–826.

Veys, E. M., Hermanns, P., Schindler, J., Kung, P. C., Goldstein, G., Symoens, J., and Van Wauwe, J., 1982b, Evaluation of T cell subsets with monoclonal antibodies in patients with rheumatoid arthritis, *J. Rheumatol.* **9:**25–29.

Veys, E. M., Verbruggen, G., Hermanns, P., Mielants, H., VanBruwaene, P., DeBrabanter, G., DeLandsheere, D., and Immesoette, C., 1983, Peripheral blood T lymphocyte subpopulations in HLA-B27 related rheumatic diseases: Ankylosing spondylitis and reactive synovitis, *J. Rheumatol.* **10:**140–143.

Victorino, R. M. W., Ryan, P., Hughes, G. R. V., and Hodgson, H. J. F., 1982, Cell-mediated immune functions and immunoregulatory cells in Behcet's syndrome, *Clin. Exp. Immunol.* **48:**121–128.

Whaley, K., and Buchanan, W. W., 1980, Sjogren's syndrome and associated diseases, in: *Clinical Immunology* (C. W. Parker, ed.), W. B. Saunders, Philadelphia, pp. 632–666.

Whaley, K., Glen, A. C. A., MacSween, R. N. M., Deodhar, S., Dick, W. C., Huki, G., Williamson, J., and Buchanan, W. W., 1971, Immunological responses in Sjogren's syndrome and rheumatoid arthritis, *Clin. Exp. Immunol.* **9:**721–731.

Whaley, K., Webb, J., McAvoy, B. A., Hughes, G. R. C., Lee, P., MacSween, R. N. M., and Buchanan, W. W., 1973, Sjogren's syndrome. 2. Clinical associations and immunological phenomena, *Q. J. Med.* **42:**513–548.

Whitaker, J. N., and Engel, W. K., 1972, Vascular deposits of immunoglobulin and complement in diopathic inflammatory myopathy, *N. Engl. J. Med.* **286:**333–338.

Whiteside, T. L., Kumagai, B., Medsger, T. A., Jr., and Rodnan, G. P., 1981, Descrepancies between *in vitro* responses to *Candida* antigen in patients with progressive systemic sclerosis (PSS, scleroderma), *J. Clin. Immunol.* **1:**250–256.

Whiteside, T. L., Kumagai, Y., Roumm, A. D., Almendinger, R., and Rodnan, G. P., 1983, Suppressor cell function and T lymphocyte subpopulations in peripheral blood of patients with progressive systemic sclerosis, *Arthritis Rheum.* **26:**841–847.

Wilkins, J. A., Warrington, R. J., Signrdson, S. L., and Rutherford, W. J., 1983, The demonstration of an interleukin-2-like activity in the synovial fluid of rheumatoid arthritis patients, *J. Rheumatol.* **10:**109–113.

Williams, B. D., and Lehner, T., 1977, Immune complexes in Behcet's syndrome and recurrent oral ulcerations, *Br. Med. J.* **1:**1387–1389.

Williams, G. W., Steinberg, A. D., Reinertsen, J. L., Klassen, C. W., Decker, J. L., and Dolan, M. D., 1978, Influenza immunization in systemic lupus erythematosus. A double blind trial, *Ann. Intern. Med.* **88:**729–734.

Williams, R. C., Jr., DeBoard, J. R., Mellbye, O. H., Messner, R. P., and Lindstrom, F. D., 1973, Studies of T- and B- lymphocytes in patients with connective tissue diseases, *J. Clin. Invest.* **52:**283–295.

Williams, R. C., Froelich, C. J., Kilpatrick, K., Crowe, W. E., and Levinson, J. E., 1981, T cell subset specificity of lymphocyte reactive factors in juvenile rheumatoid arthritic and system lupus erythematosus sera, *Arthritis Rheum.* **24:**585–591.

Wilson, C. B., Dixon, F. J., Evans, A. S., and Glassock, R. J., 1973, Antiviral antibody responses in patients with renal diseases, *Clin. Immunol. Immunopathol.* **2:**121–132.

Winchester, R. J., 1982, Applications of monoclonal antibodies to the analysis of synovial tissues of patients with rheumatoid arthritis, *Scand. J. Rheumatol. (Suppl.)* **45:**3.

Winchester, R. J., Winfield, J. B., Siegal, F., Wernet, P., and Bentwich, Z., 1974, Analysis of lymphocytes from patients with rheumatoid arthritis and systemic lupus erythematosus, *J. Clin. Invest.* **54:**1082–1092.

Winkelstein, A., Rodnan, G. P., and Heilman, D., 1972, Cellular immunity in progressive systemic sclerosis (scleroderma), *Ann. Rheum. Dis.* **31:**126–128.

Wolf, R. E., 1978, Hyporesponsive of lymphocytes to viral antigens in rheumatoid arthritis, *Arthritis Rheum.* **21:**238–241.

Wolinsky, S. I., Goodwin, J. S., Messner, R. P., and Williams, R. C., Jr., 1980, Role of prostaglandin in the depressed cell-mediated immune response in rheumatoid arthritis, *Clin. Immunol. Immunopathol.* **17:**31–37.

Wood, D. D., Ihrie, E. J., Dinarello, C. A., and Cohen, P. L., 1983, Isolation of an interleukin-1-like factor from human joint effusions, *Arthritis Rheum.* **26:**975–983.

Wooley, P. H., and Panayi, G. S., 1978, Studies of lymphocytes in rheumatoid arthritis. I. uptake of ^{125}I heat aggregated human IgG by Fc receptor bearing lymphocytes, *Ann. Rheum. Dis.* **37:**343–346.

Yamada, A., Shah, R., Cohen, P. L., and Winfield, J. B., 1984, T cell subset specificity of anti-lymphocyte antibodies in systemic lupus erythematosus (SLE). Absence of preferential cytotoxicity for cells bearing the OKT8 phenotype, *Arthritis Rheum.* **27**(Suppl.)**:**S84.

Yokoi, T., Miyawaka, T., Yachie, A., Ohzeki, S., and Taniguchi, N., 1982, Descrepancy in expression ability of Tac antigen and Ia determinations defined by monoclonal antibodies on activated or cultured cord blood T lymphocytes, *J. Immunol.* **129:**1441–1445.

Yoshizaki, K., Nakagawa, T., Fukunaga, K., Kaieda, T., Maruyama, S., Kishimoto, S., Yamamura, Y., and Kishimoto, T., 1983, Characterization of human B cell growth factor (BCGF) from cloned T cells or mitogen stimulated T cells, *J. Immunol.* **139:**1241–1246.

Youinou, P. Y., Irving, W. L., Shipley, M., Hayes, J., and Lydyard, P. M., 1984, Evidence for B cell activation in patients with active rheumatoid arthritis, *Clin. Exp. Immunol.* **55:**91–98.

Yu, D. T. Y., and Peter, J. B., 1974, Cellular immunological aspects of rheumatoid arthritis, *Semin. Arthritis Rheum.* **4:**25–52.

Yu, D. T. Y., Winchester, R. J., Fu, S. M., Gibofsky, A., Ko, H. S., and Kunkel, H. G., 1980, Peripheral blood Ia positive T cells. Increases in certain diseases and after immunization, *J. Exp. Med.* **151:**91–100.

Zingale, S. B., Sanchez, A. J. C., Andrada, J. A., Stringa, S., and Manni, J. A., 1963, Appearance of anticoagulant factors and certain autoimmune antibodies following antigenic stimulation with blood group substances in patients with systemic lupus erythematosus, *Arthritis Rheum.* **6:**581–598.

Zinneman, H. H., and Caperton, E., 1977, Cryoglobulinemia in a patient with Sjogren's syndrome, and factors of cryoprecipitation, *J. Lab. Clin. Med.* **89:**483–487.

Zola, H., Moore, H. A., Hohmann, A., Hunter, I. K., Nikolontsopoulos, A., and Bradley, J., 1984, The antigen of mature human B cell detected by the monoclonal antibody FMC7: Studies on the nature of the antigen and modulation of its expression, *J. Immunol.* **133:**321–326.

Zulman, M., Jaffe, R., and Talal, N., 1979, Evidence that malignant lymphoma of Sjogren's syndrome is a monoclonal B cell neoplasm, *N. Engl. J. Med.* **299:**1215–1218.

3

The Autologous Mixed Lymphocyte Reaction

Sudhir Gupta

I. INTRODUCTION

At the turn of the century, Ehrlich (1957) proposed that the immunity to autologous antigen is highly abnormal and would result in a disease process. At midcentury, Burnet (1959) proposed his immunologic theory of clonal selection, which included deletion of autoreactive clones during ontogeny. According to this theory, autoantibodies and other autoimmune reactions are the result of the appearance of forbidden clones secondary to somatic mutation. However, in the last 15 years, there has been increasing evidence that immune reactions are driven by recognition of both self and nonself antigens. A number of major histocompatibility complex (MHC)-restricted immune reactions demonstrated the requirement of identity at the MHC loci for interactions between lymphocytes and macrophages. Thus, lymphocyte receptors for autologous MHC determinants play a crucial role in the recognition and effector phase of immune response.

The earliest evidence of the autologous mixed lymphocyte reaction (AMLR) was reported by Fridman and Kourilsky (1969). These investigators showed that peripheral blood lymphocytes could be stimulated in one-way mixed lymphocyte cultures by autologous leukemic lymphocytes. However, it was not clear whether the stimulating antigen was a "self" antigen or a tumor-associated antigen. Steel and Hardy (1970) and Junge *et al.* (1970) observed increased DNA synthesis by peripheral blood leukocytes on stimulation with autologous lymphoid cell lines established during acute infectious mononucleosis. Green and Sell (1970), Knight *et al.* (1971), and Birnbaum *et al.* (1972) reported

---

Sudhir Gupta • Department of Medicine, Division of Basic and Clinical Immunology, University of California, Irvine, California 92717.

lymphocyte proliferation on stimulation with noninfected autologous lymphoblastoid cells from healthy donors. Opelz *et al.* (1975), using fractionated T and non-T cells from normal donors, observed an increased proliferative response of T cells upon stimulation with autologous non-T cells.

Recently, there has been concern among investigators about the true existence of the AMLR. Huber *et al.* (1982) reported data to suggest that the proliferative responses of T cells in the AMLR are not caused by self antigens but rather by xenoantigens [sheep red blood cells (SRBC) or fetal calf serum] used in the culture medium or during the separation procedure for T and non-T cells. However, under experimental conditions in which no xenoantigens were used, it was clearly shown that both the syngeneic mixed lymphocyte reaction (SMLR) in mice and the AMLR in man were largely caused by stimulation by self antigens (Moody *et al.*, 1983; Laffon *et al.*, 1983; Thorbecke *et al.*, 1983). The true existence of the AMLR is further supported by the establishment of T-cell clones and T-cell hybrids in man and experimental animals that recognize self antigen and not the xenoantigens (Richardson and Stobo, 1983; Glimcher and Shevach, 1982).

Although the true significance of the AMLR is presently unclear, it is considered an immune response in which immunoregulatory and effector T-cell functions are generated and perhaps are essential for maintaining normal immunostasis. Furthermore, the author believes that the AMLR provides perhaps the best model to study various interactions in cellular and cytokine cascades that might take place *in vivo*. The AMLR and SMLR have recently been reviewed (Weksler *et al.*, 1981; Battisto and Ponzio, 1981; Gupta, 1983). In this chapter, a detailed review of the AMLR, with regard to cell types responding to and stimulating it, production and influence of cytokines, generation of immunoregulatory and cytotoxic effector functions, and the surface molecules involved in the self-recognition, is presented. The cellular and molecular bases of abnormal AMLR in rheumatic disorders are discussed in detail. Recently, it has become apparent that the AMLR is not only between T and non-T cells but also between T and T cells.

II. T–NON-T INTERACTIONS IN THE AMLR

A. Cell Types Responding in T–Non-T AMLR

There is a general agreement among investigators that in the AMLR, the major responding population is T lymphocytes; however, the nature of the major stimulating population remains somewhat controversial (discussed below). Opelz *et al.* (1975), using a purified population of T and non-T cells, found that T lymphocytes were the responding cells in the AMLR and that increasing or decreasing the number of stimulator non-T cells could increase or decrease the AMLR response. Kuntz *et al.* (1976), using macrophages, B cells, or third-population lymphoid cells as stimulators against autologous responder T cells, demonstrated that T cells proliferate in the AMLR. Smith and Knowlton (1981), using a percoll gradient to isolate T-cell subsets, observed that the low-density T cells were most responsive to autologous non-T cells and to the lectin concanavalin A (Con A). In contrast, both high- and low-density T cells responded in the allogeneic MLR.

Stobo and Loehnen (1978) fractionated purified T cells into five fractions using a discontinuous bovine serum albumin (BSA) density gradient. The maximum autologous reactivity was observed in fraction II, whereas allogeneic reactivity was maximum in fraction III. Using BuDR and light to deplete alloreactive or autoreactive T cells, these investigators found that the depletion of autoreactive T cells resulted in complete abrogation of response of residual T cells to autologous non-T cells in the secondary stimulus, and the response to allogeneic non-T cells was only slightly reduced. These observations suggest that autoreactive T cells are distinct from those responding to allogeneic non-T cells. More recently, Smith (1983) examined the precursor frequency of autoreactive T cells in man: AMLR-responding cells were found to have a precursor frequency of 1/7500 to 1/44,000 T cells. T cells responding to TNP-modified self-antigen were twice, and those responding to alloantigens ten times more frequent than AMLR-reactive T-cell precursors. Kozak *et al.* (1982) found the precursor frequency of AMLR-reactive T cells to be 1/2200 to 1/5000.

To define which subpopulation(s) of T cells respond in the AMLR, various methods were used to separate T-lymphocyte subpopulations and examine their response to autologous non-T cells. These included T-cell subsets defined with receptors for immunoglobulin isotypes (Gupta, 1978; Gupta and Good, 1979), sensitivity or resistance to the inhibitory effect of theophylline on T cells to form rosettes with SRBC (Shore *et al.*, 1978), rosette formation between T cells and autologous human RBC (Baxley *et al.*, 1973; Santilands *et al.*, 1974), and the presence of differentiation antigens defined with monoclonal antibodies (Reinherz and Schlossman, 1980). Sakane *et al.* (1978) demonstrated that both Tγ cells and non-Tγ cells were capable of responding in the AMLR. Wolos and Davey (1979) observed that the depletion of Tγ cells from a T-cell-enriched fraction did not reduce the capacity of the remaining T cells ($T\gamma^-$) to proliferate in the AMLR. This would indicate that Tγ cells did not respond in the AMLR. Since IgG Fc receptors on Tγ cells are modulated after interacting with immune complexes, the discrepancy in the results of these two investigators could be explained by the different techniques used in their experiments. Sakane *et al.* (1978) used positively selected Tγ cells to study their function, whereas Wolos and Davey (1979) depleted Tγ cells from the responding T cells and thereby examined the function of Tγ cells in the AMLR indirectly.

Damle and Gupta (1982a) and Gupta and Damle (1981a,b) separated human T cells into theophylline-resistant (TR) and theophylline-sensitive (TS) subsets and examined their proliferative response against autologous and allogeneic non-T cells. The TR are enriched for helper functions, whereas the TS cells express suppressor functions (Shore *et al.*, 1978). The TR cells responded vigorously in the AMLR, but TS cells failed to respond in the AMLR and allogeneic MLR. Furthermore, TR cells enhanced the AMLR and MLR between fresh T and non-T cells; in contrast, TS cells suppressed both responses (Gupta and Damle, 1981a,b,c).

Several investigators have shown that a small population of peripheral blood T cells and thymocytes form spontaneous rosettes with autologous RBC (Baxley *et al.*, 1973; Kaplan, 1975; Santilands *et al.*, 1974). These have been designated autologous rosette-forming cells (ARFC or Tar). Conflicting data have accumulated regarding the response of ARFC in the AMLR and their relationship with suppressor functions. Kumagai *et al.* (1981) demonstrated that approximately 5–9% of human peripheral blood T cells are

ARFC. They observed that ARFC-negative T cells were the major responders in both AMLR and MLR and also to TNP-modified self antigens. They found no difference in the distribution of $OKT4^+$ and $OKT8^+$ T cells in ARFC and non-ARFC T cells. However, when ARFC and non-ARFC T cells were analyzed after 7 days of stimulation with autologous non-T cells, an increase in $OKT8^+$ cells was observed only in the ARFC fraction. These observations contradict the data that show that the major subpopulation of T cells responding in T–non-T AMLR is $OKT4^+$ (discussed later in this chapter).

Smolen *et al.* (1981c) have also found no differential distribution of $OKT4^+$ or $OKT8^+$ T cells among ARFC prior to activation. Sakane *et al.* (1981) observed only 1–3% ARFC; however, a marked increase in the proportion of ARFC was observed following treatment of T cells with neuraminidase. Using this approach, they separated ARFC and non-ARFC T cells and examined their proliferative response to mitogens, autologous non-T cells, and Con-A-inducible suppressor cell activity. The ARFC expressed suppressor activity, whereas non-ARFC showed no suppressor activity but responded vigorously to mitogen and in the AMLR. No differential distribution of $OKT4^+$ and $OKT8^+$ T cells was observed in ARFC and non-ARFC T cells. Sakane *et al.* (1981), by activating T cells with Con A (which increases ARFC) and separating ARFC and non-ARFC T cells, demonstrated that ARFC cells contain suppressor activity and non-ARFC T cells contain helper activity.

In contrast, several investigators have reported that ARFC are the major responders in the AMLR (Palacios *et al.*, 1980; Fournier and Charriere, 1981; Rucheton *et al.*, 1981; Uchida and Micksche, 1981). The percentage of ARFC reported by these investigators varied over a wide range. Palacios *et al.* (1980) found $T\mu$ and $T\gamma$ cells lacking from ARFC; whereas Rucheton *et al.* (1981) observed marked enrichment of $T\mu$ cells in ARFC. Uchida and Micksche (1981) also reported that the ARFC responded in the AMLR and expressed Con-A-inducible suppressor cell activity. It is apparent that there are conflicting data regarding phenotypically defined T-cell subsets and functions in the ARFC. It is very likely that these differences arise from different proportions of ARFC (3–50%) observed in these studies. These appear to be caused by technical variations and the very fragile nature of these rosettes. Therefore, data on ARFC in health and disease states should be critically evaluated.

The development of monoclonal antibodies to define differentiation antigens on functionally distinct subpopulations of T cells has facilitated the study of distinct subsets in various immune responses including the AMLR. Damle *et al.* (1981) were first to report the study of monoclonal antibody-defined T-cell subset response in the AMLR. They utilized various monoclonal antibodies, including 9.6, defining all T cells (Kamoun *et al.*, 1981), 9.3 and OKT4 (helper/inducer), and OKT8 (suppressor/cytotoxic) monoclonal antibodies. *In vitro* addition of 9.6, 9.3, or OKT4 monoclonal antibodies to the cultures of T and non-T cells in the absence of complement markedly inhibited the AMLR; in contrast, addition of OKT8 antibody to the culture had no significant effect on the AMLR (Damle *et al.*, 1981; Gupta and Damle, 1982a,c; Gupta *et al.*, 1981). This suggested to us that in the AMLR, T cells with helper/inducer phenotype are the major responders, and the molecule defined with 9.3 and OKT4 monoclonal antibodies could be the recognition unit for stimulating antigen.

We then examined the response of OKT4-enriched and OKT8-enriched T-cell subsets (prepared by complement-dependent cytotoxicity) in the AMLR. $OKT4^+$ T cells proliferated vigorously in the AMLR, whereas $OKT8^+$ T cells failed to respond to autologous non-T cells (Damle *et al.*, 1981; Gupta and Damle, 1981b 1982c). Since then, a number of investigators have also found that helper/inducer phenotype T cells respond in the AMLR (Van Wauwe and Goosens, 1981; Kozak *et al.*, 1982; Engleman *et al.*, 1981; Ellis and Mohanakumar, 1983). Ellis and Mohanakumar (1983) utilized a monoclonal antibody KT69-7 that recognizes the same epitope that is recognized by OKT4, T4, or Leu 3 monoclonal antibodies.

Reinherz *et al.* (1982) have utilized a monoclonal antibody anti-TQ1 to further subdivide $OKT4^+$ cells. This antibody reacts with approximately 70 to 85% of $T4^+$ cells. $T4^+TQ1^+$ cells responded vigorously in the AMLR, whereas $T4^+TQ1^-$ T cells are helpers for immunoglobulin synthesis. $TQ1^+T4^+$ cells also react with JRA sera. Romain *et al.* (1982a) have also shown that the interactions involving non-T-cell determinants and the T3-Ti T-cell antigen–receptor complex are important in autologous reactivity. Hausman *et al.* (1980) reported that two distinct subpopulations of T cells respond to two distinct autologous stimuli. Using a monoclonal antibody (Mac-120) against a subpopulation of peripheral blood monocytes and a monoclonal antibody (T-29) that defines approximately 10% of T cells, they showed that $T\text{-}29^+$ T cells respond to Mac 120^+ monocytes whereas $T\text{-}29^-$ T cells respond to B lymphocytes (monocyte-depleted non-T cells) in the AMLR.

Experiments with BuDR and light further confirmed that the T cells responding to B cells are distinct from those responding to monocytes. Smolen *et al.* (1981a) reported that $OKT8^+$ cells will respond to autologous non-T cells if exogenous IL-2 is added to the cultures. Romain *et al.* (1984b) and our group (Gupta *et al.*, 1985) have also observed similar results. The failure of $T8^+$ cells to respond to autologous non-T cells in absence of exogenous IL-2 could be for the following reasons: (1) $T8^+$ cells on stimulation with non-T cells in the AMLR do not produce IL-2 (cf. $T4^+$ cells); (2) fewer IL-2 receptors are expressed on $T8^+$ cells in $T8^+$–non-T AMLR; (3) or the low affinity of IL-2 receptors on activated $OKT8^+$ cells. We found no difference in Tac antigen (IL-2 receptor) expression on $OKT8^+$ T cells activated in T–non-T AMLR when compared to Tac^+OKT4^+ T cells (Gupta *et al.*, 1985). Therefore, it is likely that the lack of IL-2 production by $T8^+$ cells in the AMLR could be responsible for the failure of their proliferation, although these cells are activated in response to autologous non-T cells as evident from the expression of Tac antigen, HLA-DR antigens, and their capacity to stimulate in the T–T AMLR (Gupta *et al.*, 1985).

B. Cell Types Stimulating in T–Non-T AMLR

In contrast to the general agreement about responder T cells in the AMLR, the nature of the predominant stimulating cell type remains controversial. Kuntz *et al.* (1976) observed some enhancement of the AMLR when the stimulating cells were depleted of phagocytic and adherent cells, suggesting either that cells of monocyte–macrophage lineage are not stimulatory (therefore their depletion resulted in enrichment of stimulator non-T cells) or else that they are suppressive in the AMLR. The latter evidence is presented by several investigators (Tomonari and Aizawa 1979; Katz and Fauci, 1979; Smolen *et al.*, 1981b, 1982).

In contrast, other investigators have presented direct evidence that monocytes stimulate in the AMLR (Beale *et al.*, 1980; Dock and Davey, 1980; Gupta and Damle, 1981b,

1982a,c; MacDermott and Stacey, 1981; Hausman *et al.*, 1980; Huber *et al.*, 1981). Kuntz-Crow and Kunkel (1982) reported that the dendritic cells were the major stimulators in the AMLR compared to B lymphocytes. Lattime *et al.* (1980) demonstrated that in murine SMLR, the responder T cells are Ly1$^+$, 2 3$^-$, Qa 1$^-$ and the stimulator cells are Ia-bearing macrophagelike cells. Lederman *et al.* (1983) reported that monocytes cultured for 3 days at 37°C display fewer HLA-DR antigens and are less potent stimulators in the AMLR than fresh macrophages. Kuntz *et al.* (1976), by further fractionation of non-T cells into mouse red blood cell rosette-forming B cells (a subset of relatively immature B cells) and Ripley rosette-forming (third-population) cells, demonstrated that the third-population lymphoid cells were the major stimulators in the AMLR. Sakane *et al.* (1978), by depleting the third-population lymphoid cells, demonstrated that residual non-T cells (B cells) were the major stimulators in the AMLR. Gottlieb *et al.* (1979) also provided evidence to support the view that surface IgM$^+$ B lymphocytes provided more stimulation than IgM$^-$ B lymphocytes in the AMLR. The discrepancies in these observations appear to arise from a difference in technique used to isolate a particular stimulator cell type, which could be modified by different separation procedures. Palacios (1982) reported that Epstein–Barr virus (EBV)-infected stimulator cells are stronger stimulators in the AMLR that noninfected non-T cells.

C. Nature of Stimulating Antigen(s)

Although the nature of stimulating cell type is controversial, there is general agreement that the major (may not be exclusive) stimulating antigen in the AMLR is HLA-DR or Ia antigen. The AMLR has been shown to be inhibited by the addition of anti-HLA-DR heteroantisera to the cultures or by pretreatment of the stimulator non-T cells with anti-DR antisera (Bergholtz *et al.*, 1977; Gottlieb *et al.*, 1979; Huber *et al.*, 1981). Mingari and Moretta (1982) and Damle *et al.* (1981) used anti-HLA-DR framework-specific monoclonal antibodies and demonstrated that the addition of anti-DR monoclonal antibody in the absence of complement to the cultures of T–non-T cells or pretreatment of non-T cells with anti-HLA-DR antibody abrogated the AMLR; however, the treatment of responder T cells with anti-DR antibody had no affect on the AMLR (Damle *et al.*, 1981; Gupta *et al.*, 1981; Gupta and Damle, 1981b).

Gupta and Damle (1981a,b,c) used an anti-DR monoclonal antibody (17.15) with a restricted specificity against HLA-DR 4 and 5 and demonstrated that this antibody inhibited the stimulatory capacity of the macrophages and non-T cells (B cells plus third-population cells) from an individual with HLA-DR 4 only. Dock and Davey (1980) failed to find a correlation between the degree of proliferation in the AMLR and the expression of HLA-DR on the stimulating non-T cells. Smith (1978), using sera from multiparous women, observed that some sera will inhibit AMLR and not allogeneic MLR and vice versa, suggesting that distinct serologic determinants might stimulate in the AMLR and allogeneic MLR. Although both Mac 120$^+$ and Mac 120$^-$ macrophages express HLA-DR antigens, Mac 120$^+$ cells stimulate in the AMLR (Hausman *et al.*, 1980), whereas Mac 120$^-$ macrophages stimulate in allogenic MLR (J. D. Stobo, personal communication), suggesting that distinct antigens (could be a subtype of DR antigens) stimulate in the AMLR and allogeneic MLR. Lederman *et al.* (1983) also reported a correlation between the density of HLA-DR on macrophages and their capacity to stimulate in the

AMLR. Recently, we observed that *in vitro* treatment of human monocytes with recombinant interferon increases the fluorescence intensity of HLA-DR expression with a concomitant increase in their capacity to stimulate in the AMLR (unpublished report).

III. T–T INTERACTIONS IN THE AMLR

There is a general agreement that DR antigens are lacking from the majority of resting T cells; however, upon activation with mitogens, soluble antigens, alloantigens, and autoantigens, T cells express HLA-DR antigens (Charron *et al.*, 1980; Damle and Gupta, 1982a; Gupta and Damle, 1982a,b,c; Gupta, 1983a,b,c; Indiveri *et al.*, 1980; Ko *et al.*, 1979; Reinherz *et al.*, 1981; Yu *et al.*, 1980a,b; Engleman *et al.*, 1980; Russo *et al.*, 1981). Indiveri *et al.* (1980) and Russo *et al.* (1981) observed that phytohemagglutinin (PHA-activated T cells express surface HLA-DR antigens and can induce proliferation of autologous T cells (T–TPHA AMLR). Engleman *et al.* (1980) and Charron *et al.* (1980) also found that allogeneic MLR-activated T cells were capable of stimulating autologous responder T cells.

We extended the studies of T–TPHA AMLR to monoclonal-antibody-defined T-cell subsets (Damle and Gupta, 1982a; Gupta and Damle, 1982a–c). OKT4$^+$ and OKT8$^+$ were separated by complement-mediated cytotoxicity. Unseparated T cells (55–75%) following activation with PHA express HLA-DR antigen as defined with monoclonal antibody 7.2 and FACS. Pretreatment of PHA-activated T cells with 7.2 monoclonal antibody completely abrogated their capacity to stimulate in the T–TPHA AMLR. Using BuDR and light to deplete autoreactive or alloreactive T cells in T–TPHA AMLR or allogeneic MLR and then examining the response of the residual T cells to PHA-activated autologous or allogeneic T cells, we observed that T cells responding in T–TPHA AMLR were distinct from those responding in T–TA allogeneic MLR. These observations also suggest that DR antigens expressed on PHA-activated autologous T cells might be different from those present on activated allogeneic T cells. Furthermore, with a similar approach, we also demonstrated that T cells responding in T–non-T AMLR and T–TPHA AMLR were distinct. When OKT4$^+$ and OKT8$^+$ T cells were used as responder, it was shown that in T–TPHA AMLR, OKT8$^+$ T cells were the major responders. Therefore, distinct subsets of T cells appear to respond in T–non-T (OKT4$^+$) and T–TPHA (OKT8$^+$) AMLR. Using Ia antibodies with different specificities, Indiveri *et al.* (1983) observed that the Ia antigens stimulating in T–non-T and T–TPHA AMLR are distinct.

In order to simulate AMLR *in vivo,* we investigated the interaction between T cells activated in T–non-T AMLR (TA) and fresh autologous responder T cells (T–TA AMLR). We proposed that *in vivo,* initially, T–non-T AMLR occurs and results in activation of T cells that express HLA-DR antigen and in turn stimulate other resting T cells (T–TA AMLR). First, we observed that T cells activated in T–non-T AMLR for 4 days provided maximum stimulation in the T–TA AMLR. The TA cells were irradiated and used as stimulators against fresh autologous T cells and OKT4$^+$ and OKT8$^+$ T cells (Gupta, 1983a,b,c; Gupta *et al.*, 1985). The TA cells stimulated unseparated T cells and OKT4$^+$ cells but not OKT8$^+$ cells. This was in contrast to OKT8$^+$ cells responding in T–TPHA AMLR (Damle and Gupta, 1982b). However, the addition of IL-2 to the cultures resulted in the proliferation of OKT8$^+$ cells. We observed that both OKT4$^+$ and OKT8$^+$ T cells after activation with TA express Tac antigen but only OKT4$^+$ cells responded. This could be because of lack of IL-2 production in TA–T8$^+$ AMLR, whereas in TA–T4$^+$ AMLR, IL-2 is produced and used by OKT4$^+$ cells to proliferate. We also examined the stimulatory capacity of activated OKT4$^+$ and OKT8$^+$ T cells (activated in T–non-T AMLR) in T–TA AMLR. Both activated OKT4$^+$ and OKT8$^+$ T cells stimulated proliferation of unseparted T cells and OKT4$^+$ cells; however, both subsets failed to stimulate OKT8$^+$ T cells in T–TA AMLR. Therefore, in T–non-T and T–TA AMLR, phenotypically similar (OKT4$^+$) T-cell subsets respond but express distinct immunoregulatory functions (discussed later in this chapter).

IV. IMMUNOLOGIC MEMORY AND SPECIFICITY OF T–NON-T AND T–T AMLR

Immunologic memory and specificity are considered two cardinal features of an immune response. Both T–non-T (Weksler and Kozak, 1977) and T–T (Damle and Gupta, 1982b) AMLR demonstrate immunologic memory and specificity. Weksler and Kozak (1977) showed that the peak proliferative response in T–non-T AMLR was on day 7. At day 9, when the AMLR had subsided, T cells were washed and rechallenged with fresh autologous non-T cells (that were used in primary cultures). In this secondary AMLR, the peak proliferative response was observed on day 3, thus demonstrating immunologic memory. The specificity of the AMLR was demonstrated by the fact that the rechallenge of T cells activated in primary AMLR with allogeneic non-T cells gave the primary immune response, whereas with autologous non-T cells a secondary response was observed. In T–TPHA AMLR we also demonstrated immunologic memory and specificity (Damle and Gupta, 1982b). T cells activated in primary T–TPHA AMLR, when rechallenged with activated PHA autologous and allogeneic T cells (stimulators), proliferated more vigorously to autologous activated T cells than to allogeneic activated T cells. When BuDR and light experiments were performed to deplete auto- or alloreactive T cells from primary T–TPHA AMLR and secondary cultures were done using activated autologous or allogeneic T cells as stimulators against the remaining T cells from primary cultures, evidence of immunologic specificity was obtained. Therefore both T–non-T and T–T AMLR represent true immune responses.

V. IMMUNOREGULATORY AND CYTOTOXIC FUNCTIONS IN THE AMLR

A. Generation of Helper Function

Induction of immunoglobulin secretion in the AMLR has been reported by several investigators (Shin *et al.*, 1981; Gatenby *et al.*, 1982; Romain and Lipsky, 1983). Shin *et al.* (1981) demonstrated that autologous reactive T cells are triggered to proliferate by HLA-DR antigens on PWM-pulsed non-T cells, and a subpopulation of these proliferating cells in turn help PWM-primed B cells to differentiate into immunoglobulin-secreting cells. These helper T cells displayed a proliferative kinetics different from that of other autologous reactive T cells in peaking on the second day of culture and were relatively resistant to irradiation or treatment with mitomycin C. Chiorrazzi *et al.* (1979) reported that supernatants from the AMLR cultures contain factor(s) that help immunoglobulin synthesis and secretion from autologous B lymphocytes or tonsil B cells. Yu *et al.* (1980) observed that the AMLR culture supernatants induced the generation of antibody-producing cells from monocyte-depleted peripheral blood lymphocytes in the absence of antigen. These factors are not removed by anti-HLA-DR or anti-Ig columns and also help in the differentiation of cytotoxic effector functions.

It remains to be determined whether B-cell growth factor or B-cell differentiation factor is produced in the AMLR. We examined the function of $OKT4^+$ T cells activated in T–non-T AMLR on the proliferative response of fresh autologous responder T cells to PHA and alloantigens (Damle and Gupta, 1982b). Activated $OKT4^+$ T cells enhanced the proliferative responses. This enhancing influence of $OKT4^+$ was independent of HLA-DR antigen expression. Recently, we found an enhancing factor produced by $OKT4^+$ T cells activated in T–non-T AMLR (unpublished observations). The enhancing influence of this factor(s) is not MHC restricted.

B. Generation of Suppressor Functions in the AMLR

A number of investigators have reported generation of suppressor functions in T–non-T (Smith and Knowlton, 1979; Gatenby *et al.*, 1982; Sakane and Green, 1979; Fitzharris and Knight, 1981) and T–T AMLR (Damle and Gupta, 1982b; Gupta and Damle, 1982c; Gupta *et al.*, 1985). Fitzharris and Knight (1981) reported that autoactivated T cells suppressed PWM-induced and Hong Kong B virus-induced antibody production; AMLR-activated T cells also suppressed the proliferative response of fresh autologous T cells in the AMLR and allogeneic MLR. Suppressor activity was resistant to mitomycin treatment. Innes *et al.* (1979) found suppressor activity in AMLR-activated T cells against staphylococci-induced immunoglobulin-producing cells. This suppressor influence was radiation sensitive. Smith and Knowlton (1979) observed that T cells activated in T–non-T AMLR suppressed the proliferative and cytotoxic responses of fresh, unstimulated autologous T cells to allogeneic cells in MLR. The suppressive influence was sensitive to mitomycin C treatment.

These experiments did not distinguish whether the suppression of cytotoxic response was at the afferent or efferent limb. Palacios (1981) also reported the generation of suppressor activity in autoreactive T cells against the proliferative response of responder T cells to PHA and alloantigens. The suppressor influence was resistant to mitomycin C treatment but was abrogated by cyclosporin A. Stephen *et al.* (1981) also demonstrated that T cells activated with non-T cells, B cells, or macrophages suppressed immunoglobulin synthesis in a PWM-driven system. The suppressor function was sensitive to hydrocortisone and irradiation. Gatenby *et al.* (1982) showed that activated Leu 2^+, DR^+ T cells but neither Leu 2^+, DR^- nor Leu 3^+ T cells from primary AMLR cultures suppressed immunoglobulin synthesis in the second AMLR. The suppressor amplifier activity was radiation resistant. The activation of Leu 2^+ DR^+ suppressor T cells requires Leu 3^+ cells in the primary culture. Furthermore, in the absence of fresh Leu 2^+ cells in second culture, little or no suppression was observed. This suggests that for the optimum suppression at least two distinct subpopulations of Leu 2^+ cells are required.

We examined the generation of suppression in T–T AMLR. Damle and Gupta (1982b) and Gupta and Damle (1982c) demonstrated that $OKT8^+$ cells activated in T–TPHA AMLR would suppress the proliferative response of fresh autologous T cells to PHA and alloantigens. This suppression is not mediated by HLA-DR antigens on the activated regulator cells and is resistant to mitomycin C. In the T–TA AMLR, activated $OKT4^+$ cells suppressed the proliferative response of fresh autologous T cells (Gupta *et al.*, 1985). Control $OKT4^+$ had no influence. In contrast, control and activated $OKT8^+$ cells expressed similar suppressor activity. The suppressor activity was resistant to mitomycin treatment. We have also observed production of a suppressor factor in the supernatants of T4–TA AMLR that can suppress the proliferation of autologous T cells (unpublished observations). This suppressive influence was MHC restricted. The characteristics of this factor remain to be determined.

Sakane and Green (1979) and Smith and Knowlton (1981) examined the relationship between autoreactive T cells and suppressor function. Using the BuDR and light technique to delete the autoreactive T cells, Sakane and Green (1979) observed a concomitant loss of Con-A-inducible suppressor cell activity, suggesting that autoreactive T cells contain precursors of Con-A-inducible suppressors. Smith and Knowlton (1981) also reached the same conclusion. They exposed Con-A-responding T cells to BuDR and light and found loss of AMLR, but response to PHA and alloantigens were preserved. However, a recent study of AMLR in polymyositis/dermatomyositis suggests that autoreactive T cells are distinct from Con-A-induced suppressors (Ransohoff and Dastom, 1983). These investigators found deficient AMLR but normal Con-A-induced suppressor activity.

C. Generation of Cytotoxic Functions in the AMLR

In the conventional T–non-T AMLR, specific cytolytic T lymphocytes (CTL) are not generated (Katz *et al.*, 1978). Zarling *et al.* (1976) also failed to generate CTL when remission lymphocytes were cultured with irradiated autologous leukemic cells. However, by using the "three-cell" approach in which remission lymphocytes, irradiated leukemia cells, and irradiated allogeneic stimulating cells were cocultured, they were able to generate CTL for autologous leukemia cells. Lee and Oliver (1978) were also able to generate cytotoxic T lymphocytes against autologous leukemia cells in acute myelogenous leukemia by using coculture of autologous leukemic blast cells, remission lymphocytes, and allogeneic lymphocytes. Van de Stouwe *et al.* (1977) were unable to generate CTL in the AMLR between peripheral blood T cells and autologous B lymphocytes and autologous B lymphoid cell lines against peripheral blood lymphocytes as targets. A low cytotoxicity was, however, detected when lymphoid cell lines were used both as stimulator and targets. However, this cytotoxicity was nonspecific and was always greater for heterologous lines than for the stimulator line.

Weksler *et al.* (1980) were also unable to generate CTL in the AMLR. No specific cytotoxic T lymphocytes were generated in cultures containing T cells and irradiated autologous, allogeneic, or hapten-modified autologous T lymphocytes. However, when allogeneic T lymphocytes or hapten-modified autologous T lymphocytes were added to an AMLR, specific CTL were generated. These investigators also demonstrated that supernatants from the AMLR facilitated the generation of specific CTL in T-cell cultures to which allogeneic T cells or hapten-modified autologous T cells were added. Miller and Kaplan (1978) reported cytotoxic activity in autoactivated T cells against lipopolysaccharide-induced autologous B lymphoblasts, but autologous T or non-T cells or the histocytic lymphoma cell lines could not be killed. Sumiya *et al.* (1980) demonstrated generation of specific CTL in the AMLR against lymphoblastoid cell line (stimulator) as targets.

It appears that target antigens are expressed on activated or dividing autologous cells in such a manner that they render the target cells more susceptible to lysis by autoactivated T cells. Tomonari (1980) and Tomonari *et al.* (1980) were able to generate nonspecific cytotoxic T-lymphocytes that will lyse a variety of malignant and nonmalignant targets, but normal autologous or allogeneic non-T cells are less susceptible to cytotoxic functions. Zagury *et al.* (1983) produced T-cell clones in the presence of IL-2 following stimulation with autologous EBV-induced B lymphocytes or with autologous Burkitt's lymphoma and examined their cytotoxic functions. The cytotoxicity was MHC restricted, since cloned CTL sensitized against autologous EBV-induced B cells lysed their autologous targets but not allogeneic B cell targets or K-562, and cloned CTL sensitized against autologous Burkitt's lymphoma cells lysed their corresponding lymphoma targets or autologous EBV-induced B cells but did not lyse allogeneic EBV-induced B cells. The cloned CTL were homogeneous and expressed T8 antigen but lacked T4, T10, or M1 antigens.

Strassmann *et al.* (1983) demonstrated the generation of NK and cytotoxic T cells without NK activity in the AMLR between peripheral blood mononuclear cells and autologous lymphoblastoid cell lines. The NK cells generated in the AMLR expressed OKM1 or B73.1 antigens. Depletion of OKM1$^+$ or B73.1$^+$ cells from mononuclear cells resulted in the loss of generation of NK activity without loss of CTL activity. More recently, Goto and Zvaifler (1983) also examined the conditions for the production of cytotoxic T cells in the AMLR and attempted to define the surface phenotype of the responsible cells using monoclonal antibodies and distinguishing them from other cytotoxic effector cells such as NK and CTL. Cytotoxic activity was developed in the AMLR between normal T and non-T cells in the presence of fresh autologous serum or plasma. The maximal cytotoxic activity was developed between 7 and 9 days. Cytotoxic cells were IgG Fc negative and killed autologous T and B lymphoblastoid cell lines. K-562 cells were the most sensitive targets, whereas Raji cells were least sensitive. No attempt was made to demonstrate the presence or absence of cytotoxicity against autologous normal stimulator cells. The AMLR-generated killer cells were 9.6$^+$ (monoclonal antibody that defines SRBC receptor on T cells) and Ia$^+$, 4F2$^+$ (activated cell markers) but lacked OKM1, Leu 7, T8, and 9.3 antigens. Therefore, these killers were different from classical NK and CTL cells. The AMLR killing was proportional to the percentage of 4F2$^+$ cells but unrelated to the expression Ia antigens.

In summary, in the AMLR, cytotoxic T cells are generated, and autologous serum and plasma appear to be better than pooled human serum or fetal calf serum. No specific CTL activity could be generated in the AMLR between normal T and non-T cells against autologous normal stimulator or responder cells. However, when lymphoblastoid cell lines are used as stimulators, killer activity could be generated against autologous stimulator lymphoblastoid cell lines. Cytotoxic cells are distinct from specific CTL cells and differ somewhat from classical NK cells (with regard to phenotype). Specific CTL activity in the AMLR can be generated against stimulator lymphoblastoid or leukemic cells only in a "three-cell" system in which irradiated allogeneic T cells are added to the autologous cultures.

VI. GENERATION OF CYTOKINES IN THE AMLR

A number of soluble factors are produced in the AMLR and are discussed here in brief. These include helper factor, suppressor factor, interleukin 2, and γ-interferon. The author believes that other lymphokines are also produced in the AMLR; e.g., lymphotoxins. One of the lymphotoxins has a property analogous to the cytotoxic target cell specificity of the AMLR killer cells. Arvilommi and Rasanen (1980) reported lack of leukocyte migration inhibition factor (LIF) production in the AMLR between T cells and B lymphocytes. Experiments using subsets of T cells remain to be done to determine whether in the AMLR, T cells indeed do not produce LIF. Occasionally, inhibitors of biologically active molecules are produced concomitantly by the cell type that produces the active molecule. This can be best exemplified by the production of IL-1 and its inhibitor by activated macrophages. Therefore, in the study of LIF, supernatants should be used in various dilutions, which would result in dilution of the inhibitor (if it is produced in the AMLR), and LIF activity will become apparent.

Chiorazzi *et al.* (1979) reported that the supernatants from T–non-T AMLR help in the production of immunoglobulins by autologous peripheral blood lymphocytes and tonsilar lymphocytes. Yu *et al.* (1980) showed that AMLR supernatants would induce the generation of antibody-producing cells from monocyte-depleted peripheral blood lymphocytes. This helper factor could be generated in the absence of antigen or third-party T lymphocytes. The helper factor also induced the differentiation of precytotoxic cells to effector cytotoxic T cells. This helper activity was not removed by anti-DR or anti-Ig columns.

Recently, we have analyzed supernatants from the AMLR of $T4^+$–non-T and $T8^+$–non-T cocultures. Helper activity was observed in the supernatants of $T4^+$–non-T AMLR but not by $T8^+$–non-T AMLR (unpublished observation). The helper activity was MHC nonrestricted. In the AMLR using a three-cell system in which irradiated allogeneic T cells or TNP-modified self antigen was added to autologous mixture of T and non-T cells, after 48 hr supernatants contained factor that differentiated pre-CTL to CTL. In the T–TA AMLR, using $T4^+$ and $T8^+$ cells as responders, we observed the production of suppressor factor by T–TA or T4–TA AMLR. The suppressor activity was MHC restricted (unpublished observation). Palacios and Moller (1981) reported production of IL-2 by $OKT4^+$ in T–non-T AMLR. The production of IL-2 in the AMLR was enhanced by IL-1, which sensitized $T4^+$ cells to stimulation by non-T cells. Both $T4^+$ and $T8^+$ cells appear to respond to IL-2. Although Manger *et al.* (1980) failed to demonstrate the production of γ-interferon (γ-INF) in the AMLR; Hasler *et al.* (1983a) have shown production of γ-INF in both AMLR and allogeneic MLR. Furthermore, they demonstrated deficient production of γ-INF in AMLR but normal γ-INF production in allogeneic MLR in patients with rheumatoid arthritis.

VII. FACTORS REGULATING THE AMLR

As indicated before, T-cell subsets responding in the T–non-T and T–T4 AMLR express helper and suppressor activities that regulate by feedback the T–non-T AMLR (Gupta, 1983b). In addition, the AMLR is extremely sensitive to the affect of corticosteroids. Ilfeld *et al.* (1977) examined the inhibitory effects of thymic factor, fresh autologous plasma, hepatoma-derived α-fetoprotein, and hydrocortisone on the AMLR and allogeneic MLR. Hydrocotisone but not the other agents in physiological concentrations markedly inhibited AMLR but had no effect on the allogeneic MLR. Katz and Fauci (1979) examined *in vitro* and *in vivo* effects of hydrocortisone on the AMLR and allogeneic MLR. *In vitro* hydrocortisone suppressed the AMLR to a much greater extent than the allogeneic MLR. *In vivo* administration of hydrocortisone to normal volunteers suppressed the AMLR 4 hr after injection. The T cells after 4 hr of I.V. hydrocortisone responded poorly to both autologous and allogeneic non-T cells. Non-T cells obtained after 4 hr of hydrocortisone treatment had greater stimulatory capacity for autologous or allogeneic T cells than those non-T cells obtained before injection. This indicates that the inhibitory effect of hydrocortisone is at the T-cell level.

We also examined the AMLR after I.V. administration of hydrocortisone (single dose) in normal volunteers (Gupta and Damle, 1981c). At 4 hr after injection, both AMLR and allogeneic MLR were depressed. The responses returned to normal levels 24 hr after injection of hydrocortisone. The peak proliferative response was observed on day 6 in samples drawn before or 24 hr following injection. The peak proliferative response of T cells at 4 hr was on day 7. Analysis of T-cell subsets revealed a decrease in Tμ cells and an increase in Tγ cells at 4 hr after injection. At 24 hr, values of T-cell subsets returned to preinjection levels. Yu *et al.* (1978) reported that methylprednisone *in vitro* inhibits the stimulatory capacity of non-T cells and not the responding capacity of T cells. MacDermott and Stacey (1981) also observed that hydrocortisone inhibits the stimulatory capacity of macrophages in the AMLR.

More recently, Palacios and Sugawara (1982) examined the cellular and molecular basis of hydrocortisone-induced inhibition of the AMLR. They demonstrated that hydrocortisone *in vitro* inhibits the T-cell proliferation in the AMLR by causing the IL-2 producer T cells to become unresponsive to IL-1 and unable to synthesize IL-2. It is evident that there are certain discrepancies between *in vitro* and *in vivo* effects of hydrocortisone on the AMLR. The depression appears to be caused by redistribution of responding and IL-2 producer T cells as well as by inhibition of the response to IL-1 of IL-2 producer T cells. *In vivo* influence on stimulator cells needs further investigation.

Histamine also regulates the AMLR. Histamine in a dose-dependent manner appears to inhibit the AMLR (Damle and Gupta, 1981). The targets of inhibition are responder T cells and not the stimulator non-T cells. The inhibitory influence could be stimulated by H_2 agonists but not by H_1 agonists. Similarly, histamine-induced inhibition of the AMLR could be reversed by H_2 blockers but not by H_1 blockers. Studies of histamine-treated $OKT4^+$ and $OKT8^+$ T cells demonstrated that histamine-induced inhibition of the AMLR is mediated by activation of $OKT8^+$ suppressor cell function (Damle and Gupta, 1981). The histamine-induced inhibition of the AMLR was mediated by a suppressor factor. The production of such a factor could be evoked by an H_2 agonist, and histamine-induced suppressor factor production could be inhibited by H_2 antagonists.

VIII. CONCLUSION

In summary, in the AMLR various functionally and phenotypically distinct subsets respond by proliferation and production of a variety of biologically active molecules. In the AMLR, suppressor, helper, and cytotoxic functions are generated. Therefore, the AMLR represents perhaps the best *in vivo* equivalent model for the study of cellular and molecular interactions in health and their perturbations in disease states (Fig. 1). Perhaps it is via the AMLR that immune hemostasis is maintained by the generation of immunoregulatory and effector functions.

IX. THE AUTOLOGOUS MIXED LYMPHOCYTE REACTION IN RHEUMATIC DISEASES

Among the rheumatic diseases, the AMLR is best studied in systemic lupus erythematosus (SLE).

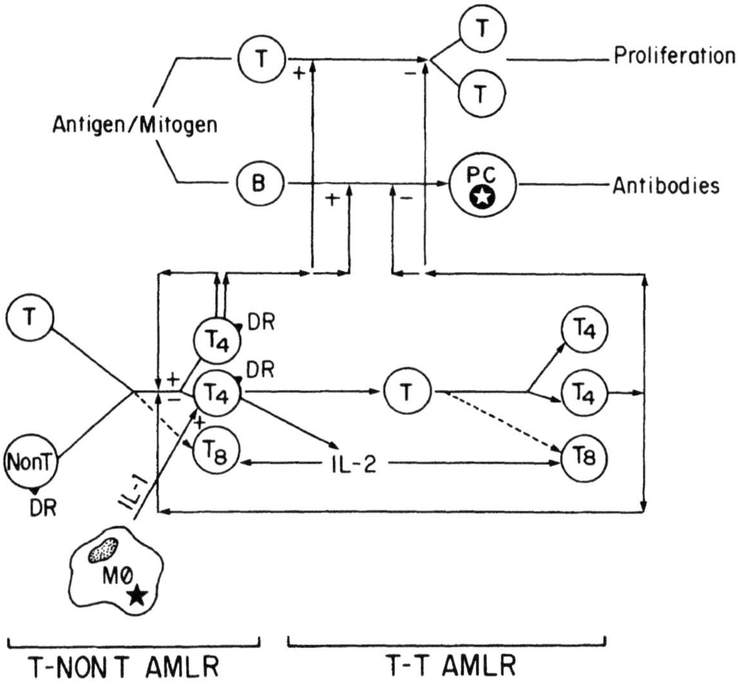

Figure 1. A model of T–non-T and T–T AMLR with cellular and cytokine cascade. MØ = macrophage, IL-1 = Interleukin 1, IL-2 = Interleukin 2, PC = Plasma cell.

A. Systemic Lupus Erythematosus

Lupus is a prototype of autoimmune disorders and is characterized by multisystem involvement, polyclonal hyperimmunoglobulinemia, and a variety of autoantibodies. A deficiency of suppressor T cells has been implicated in polyclonal B-cell activation and autoantibody production in SLE. Several investigators have reported impairment of the AMLR in patients with SLE. Sakane *et al.* (1978) observed a lack of AMLR in patients with active SLE (who were not receiving any immunosuppressive treatment or prednisone more than 10 mg/day) and decreased AMLR in some patients with inactive SLE. The allogeneic MLR was normal in both the groups. In active SLE, unfractionated T cells as well as Tγ and non-Tγ cells failed to respond to autologous or allogeneic non-T cells. In patients with inactive SLE, only the Tγ cells failed to respond; the non-Tγ and unfractionated T cells responded normally in the AMLR. These observations suggested that the defect was in the responder T cells rather than of the stimulatory T cells. Sakane *et al.* (1980) reported that in active SLE both Con-A-induced suppressor function and the AMLR were deficient but returned to normal levels during inactive stages of disease. This suggests that the T-cell defect in SLE is not simply genetically determined.

Palacios and Alarcon-Segovia (1981) also demonstrated decreased AMLR in both unfractionated T and Tar cells in SLE. However, this defect was corrected by incubating with thymic factor. This further suggests that the SLE defect in the AMLR is at the T-cell level. Kuntz et al (1979) also reported impaired AMLR but intact allogeneic MLR in SLE. The non-T cells from patients did not stimulate allogeneic T-cells normally. The cellular basis of impaired AMLR was studied using nontwin siblings who were matched at HLA-A and B; MLR identity was used as the sole criterion of HLA-D locus identity. Their study showed that the decreased AMLR was caused by a decreased capacity of the non-T cells to stimulate in the AMLR.

Sakane *et al.* (1979) studied the cellular basis of deficient AMLR in two sets of twins. In the first set of twins, the disease was inactive, and her identical twin sister was normal. The patient demonstrated decreased AMLR in the Tγ cell fraction only; unseparated T cells and non-Tγ cells responded normally to autologous non-T cells. Reciprocal mixing experiments among T, Tγ, and non-T cells from the patient and her healthy identical twin revealed that the defect in the patient with inactive SLE was at the level of responder Tγ cells. The stimulatory capacity of non-T cells was normal. In the second set, the patient had active SLE and was receiving 100 mg/day prednisone. Her twin sister had mild clinical and serologic abnormalities of SLE (inactive SLE). The identical sister with inactive SLE showed decreased AMLR only in Tγ cells. In contrast, the patient with active SLE (her sister) had diminished AMLR in unfractionated T, Tγ, and non-Tγ fractions. In a mixing experiment, T cells from the active SLE sister did not respond to non-T cells from the sister with inactive SLE, whereas those non-T cells could stimulate autologous T cells. Non-T cells from the patient also failed to stimulate T cells or non-Tγ cells of the sister despite their normal response to the sister's non-T cells. This suggests that in this set of twins the defect was both at the responder T- and stimulator non-T-cell level. A note of caution: this patient was on high-dose prednisone at the time of study, and, therefore, the defect in the stimulator cells could have been caused by the prednisone (Yu *et al.*, 1978; McDermott and Stacy, 1981).

More recently Sakane *et al.* (1983) examined the proliferative response of $OKT4^+$ cells in the AMLR and immunoregulatory properties in patients with SLE. Lupus $OKT4^+$ proliferated poorly in the MLR, expressed normal helper activity, but lacked suppressor function. The $OKT4^+$ cell abnormality was independent of disease activity and occurred in the absence of autoantibodies, including anti-T antibodies. Instead, anti-T-cell antibodies could preferentially eliminate $OKT8^+$ suppressor cells and normal T cells. Sakane *et al.* suggested that the defect in the $OKT4^+$ T-cell suppressor activity is intrinsic to SLE and that the $OKT8^+$ suppressor T-cell defect is caused by anti-T-cell antibodies.

Hahn *et al.* (1982) examined the influence of sera from 15 patients with active SLE and seven with inactive SLE. Twelve of 22 sera reduced the AMLR, which correlated with the defective AMLR in fresh lymphocytes from those patients. When normal T and non-T cells were preincubated with suppressive sera and then added to AMLR cultures containing normal serum, AMLR was reduced. The suppressive serum factors were directed against various T responders and stimulators, monocytes, and B cells plus null cells. Monocyte–T-cell AMLR was suppressed most frequently. The serum inhibitors were not removed by high-speed centrifugation or by depletion of antibodies to DNA, and no correlation was observed with antilymphocytotoxic antibodies. Frajman *et al.* (1983) reported normalization of both AMLR and suppressor cell activity during pregnancy in patients with SLE. These investigators suggested that the reconstitution of these functions may explain in part the remission of lupus during pregnancy.

B. Rheumatoid Arthritis

Recently, several investigators have reported deficient AMLR in the peripheral blood from RA. Beck *et al.* (1981) and Kaldan *et al.* (1983) reported deficient AMLR in the peripheral blood of RA that was independent of disease activity, clinical course, or treatment schedule. Kalden *et al.* (1983) found no difference in suppressor factor production in the AMLR between RA and controls. These investigators also failed to demonstrate γ-INF production in the AMLR from RA and controls. This is in contrast to the observations by Hasler *et al.* (1983a), who demonstrated production of a γ-INF-like substance in the supernatants of AMLR from normal controls and in the allogeneic MLR of RA but found deficient γ-INF production in the AMLR from RA. Surprisingly, they did not find any deficiency of proliferative response in the AMLR from RA. They also observed that adherent-cell depletion of RA non-T cells led to a marked increased γ-INF production, whereas the proliferative response fell sharply.

Hasler *et al.* (1983b) showed that defective γ-INF production in RA AMLR is at least in part caused by enhanced sensitivity of the RA lymphocytes to adherent-cell-produced prostaglandin. Smith and DeHoratius (1982) also reported low AMLR in seven of 12 patients with RA. Six of seven had active disease; in contrast, only one of five with normal AMLR had active disease. Forre *et al.* (1982, 1983) also examined the AMLR in 51 patients with juvenile rheumatoid arthritis (JRA) and 11 with RA. Reduced AMLR was observed in the peripheral blood of RA and JRA. In contrast, the AMLR in synovial tissue and synovial fluid lymphocytes was normal. Furthermore, they observed that the synovial fluid T cells were able to stimulate autologous peripheral blood T cells (T–T AMLR). The non-T cells from the synovial fluid of RA are more stimulatory than their peripheral blood non-T cells; however, the T cells from synovial fluid and synovial tissue were less responsive to peripheral blood non-T cells (Forre *et al.*, 1982, 1983; Beck *et al.*, 1981; Silver *et al.*, 1983). Forre *et al.* (1983) also reported that a rabbit antiserum produced against a fragment comprising the variable heavy (V_H) chain region of an IgG3 human myeloma protein reacted with peripheral blood T cells and inhibited the AMLR. Thus, V_H antigens appear to be integral parts of the T-cell receptor for autologous DR antigens. The role of circulating and joint fluid immune complexes in abnormal AMLR remains to be determined.

C. Progressive Systemic Sclerosis

The pathogenesis of progressive systemic sclerosis (PSS) is unknown, but a number of immunologic defects have been described. Morse and Bodi (1982) studied the AMLR and allogeneic MLR in 20 patients with PSS. The AMLR was examined between T cells and non-T cells (macrophages, B cells, and third-population cells). The responses were measured on day 6. The AMLR in PSS were comparable to age- and sex-matched healthy controls. In the allogeneic MLR, non-T cells from PSS appear to be poor stimulators. More recently, Alcocer-Varela *et al.* (1984) examined the AMLR between T and non-T cells (B cells and third-population cells) in 20 patients with PSS. The AMLR at day 7 was diminished in PSS compared to the control group. In the time kinetic studies, the AMLR at 7 days decline after an early proliferative response occuring on day 4. The allogeneic MLR was comparable to controls. These data suggest that either autoreactivity between T and non-T cells might have occurred *in vivo* in PSS and is recalled in *in vitro* AMLR or that alterations of immunoregulatory cells permit this earlier activation in the system.

D. Sjogren's Syndrome

A combination of genetic, immunologic, and environmental factors appears to play a role in the pathogenesis of Sjogren's Syndrome (SS), which is characterized by lymphocytic infiltration of exocrine glands, hyperimmunoglobulinemia, and presence of autoantibodies. Miyasaka *et al.* (1980) studied the AMLR in 25 patients with SS. The AMLR was decreased in 15 of 25 patients compared with controls. Increasing the number of stimulator cells had no influence on the deficient AMLR. Eight of 15 patients with deficient AMLR had only glandular disease. Patients with SS and associated pseudolymphoma, SLE, RA, or primary biliary cirrhosis had lower AMLR than patients with SS alone. No correlation was observed among the levels of serum immunoglobulin, response to PHA, and titers of antilymphocyte antibodies; however, a direct correlation was observed between the AMLR and deficient Con-A-induced suppressor activity. In the AMLR, monocytes from patients with SS were poorer stimulators than monocytes from healthy controls. In the allogeneic MLR, non-T cells from patients were poor stimulators, but their monocyte stimulatory capacity was comparable to controls. Studies are required using T-cell subsets on production and influence of IL-2 in HLA-matched siblings to understand the cellular and molecular basis of deficient AMLR in SS.

E. Polymyositis/Dermatomyositis and Mixed Connective Tissue Disease

Polymyositis (PM)/dermatomyositis (DM) is a disease of unknown etiology, but cell-mediated immunity appears to play an important role in its pathogenesis. Ransohoff and Dastom (1983) studied the AMLR and Con-A-induced suppressor cell activity in adults with PM/DM. Patients with associated malignancy, overlap syndrome, and childhood DM were excluded. No patient was on cytotoxic or immunosuppressive drugs. Patients on antimalarial or antiinflammatory medications were studied at least 24 hr after the last dose of medication. The AMLR was deficient in six of nine patients with PM/DM. No correlation was found between disease activity and deficient AMLR. The AMLR could not be enhanced by increasing the numbers of non-T stimulator cells in culture or by varying the day on which cultures were harvested. Monocytes in the stimulator cells were comparable in the two groups. Allogeneic MLR was studied in two patients and found to be normal. Concanavalin-A-induced suppressor activity was normal in all four patients studied; one of these patients had normal AMLR, in one AMLR was deficient, and in the remaining two, the AMLR was not studied. The claim by the authors that there is a dissociation between AMLR and Con-A-induced suppressor activity in PM/DM appears to be an overstatement; more patients have to be examined in whom both of these functions should be simultaneously assessed.

Palacios and Alarcon-Segovia (1981) found lower AMLR in unfractionated T and Tar cells in mixed connective tissue disease (MCTD); however, addition of thymic factor to the cultures did not enhance the AMLR. This is in contrast to SLE, in which AMLR was enhanced by thymic hormone.

X. CONCLUSION

In various rheumatic disorders, the abnormalities of AMLR have been described. Systemic lupus erythematosus is the only disorder in which the cellular basis of deficient AMLR has been characterized. Study of identical or matched siblings is needed to understand the cellular and molecular basis of deficient AMLR in rheumatic diseases. Studies of production of IL-2, helper, suppressor, and cytotoxic factors and response of IL-1 and IL-2 on the AMLR in rheumatic diseases are required. Since in T–T AMLR suppressor function is generated that feedback inhibits T–non-T AMLR, T–T AMLR in rheumatic disease should also be studied to understand the mechanism of feedback regulation to explain deficient T–non-T AMLR.

ACKNOWLEDGMENTS. Part of the work cited here was supported by grants from the U.S. Public Health Service: AG-04361, AI-20717, and AI-21808.

REFERENCES

Alcocer-Varela, J., Laffon, A., Alarcon-Segovia, D., and Ibanez de Kasep, G., 1984, Early proliferative response in the human autologous mixed lymphocyte reaction in scleroderma, *J. Rheumatol.* **11**:48–52.

Arvilommi, H., and Rasanen, L., 1980, Cellular interactions in spontaneous or autologous cell-induced proliferative and lymphokine responses of human lymphocytes, *Immunology* **40**:695–700.

Battisto, J. R., and Ponzio, N. M., 1981, Autologous and syngeneic mixed lymphocyte reactions and their immunological significance, *Prog. Allergy* **28**:160–192.

Baxley, G., Bishop, G. B., Cooper, A. G., and Wortis, H. H., 1973, Rosetting of human red blood cells to thymocytes and thymus-derived cells, *Clin. Exp. Immunol.* **15**:385–392.

Beale, M. G., MacDermott, R. P., Stacey, M. C., Nash, G. S., Hahn, B. H., Seiden, M. V., Burkholder-Jacobs, S. L., and Loewenstein, L. S. P., 1980, Stimulating cell types in the autologous mixed leukocyte reaction in man, *J. Immunol.* **124**:227–232.

Beck, P., Burmester, G. R., Ledwoch, A., Urban, C., and Kalden, J. R., 1981, Autologous and allogeneic MLC reactivity in patients with rheumatoid arthritis, *J. Clin. Lab. Immunol.* **6**:27–33.

Bergholtz, B., Albrechtsen, D., and Thorsby, E., 1977, Stimulation of T lymphocytes by autologous non-T lymphoid cells, Participation of HLA-DR, *Tissue Antigens*, **10**:27–38.

Birnbaum, G., Siskind, G., and Weksler, M. E., 1972, Autologous and allogeneic stimulation of peripheral human leukocytes, *Cell Immunol.* **3**:44–52.

Burnet, F. M., 1959, *The Clonal Selection Theory of Acquired Immunity*, Cambridge University Press, Cambridge.

Charron, D. J., Engleman, E. G., Benike, C. J., and McDevitt, H. O., 1980, Ia antigens on alloreactive T cells in man detected by monoclonal antibodies. Evidence for synthesis of HLA/D/DR molecules of the responder type, *J. Exp. Med.* **152**:127–136.

Chiorazzi, N., Fu, S. M., and Kunkel, H. G., 1979, Induction of polyclonal antibody synthesis by human allogeneic and autologous helper factors, *J. Exp. Med.* **149**:1543–1548.

Damle, N., and Gupta, S., 1981, $OKT8^+$ T cells mediate histamine-induced suppressor T cell function, *ICRS Med. Sci.* **9**:912–919.

Damle, N. K., and Gupta, S., 1982a, Heterogeneity of concanavalin A-induced suppressor T cells in man defined with monoclonal antibodies, *Clin. Exp. Immunol.* **40**:581–588.

Damle, N. K., and Gupta, S., 1982b, Autologous mixed lymphocyte reaction in man. V. Functionally and phenotypically distinct human T cell subpopulations respond to non-T and activated T cells in AMLR, *Scand. J. Immunol.* **16**:59–68.

Damle, N. K., and Gupta, S., 1982c, Autologous mixed lymphocyte reaction in man. III. Regulation of autologous MLR by theophylline-resistant and sensitive T lymphocyte subpopulations, *Scand. J. Immunol.* **15**:493–500.

Damle, N. K., Hansen, J. A., Good, R. A., and Gupta, S., 1981, Monoclonal antibody analysis of human T lymphocyte subpopulations exhibiting autologous mixed lymphocyte reaction, *Proc. Natl. Acad. Sci. U.S.A.* **78**:5096–5098.

Dock, N. L., and Davey, F. R., 1980, Peripheral blood monocytes in autologous mixed lymphocyte reaction, *Clin. Immunol. Immunopathol.* **17**:123–131.

Ehrlich, P., 1957, Uber den jetzigen Stand der Karzinomforschung: In Himmelweit, in: *The Collected Papers of Paul Ehrlich*, Vol. II, Pergamon Press, Oxford, pp. 550–562.

Ellis, T. M., and Mohanakumar, T., 1983, Dissociation of autologous and allogeneic mixed lymphocyte reactivity by using a monoclonal antibody specific for human T helper cells, *J. Immunol.* **131**:2323–2327.

Engleman, E. G., Benike, C. J., and Charron, D. J., 1980, Ia antigens on peripheral blood leukocytes in man. Functional studies of HLA-DR positive T cell activated in MLR, *J. Exp. Med.* **152**:114–126.

Engleman, E. G., Benike, C. J., Grumet, F. C., and Evans, R. L., 1981, Activation of human T lymphocyte subsets: Helper and suppressor/cytotoxic T cells recognize and respond to distinct histocompatibility antigens, *J. Immunol.* **127**:2124–2129.

Fitzharris, P., and Knight, R. A., 1981, Generation of suppressor cells in the autologous mixed lymphocyte reaction, *Clin. Exp. Immunol.* **46**:185–195.

Forre, O., Egeland, T., Doblough, J. H., Krien, T. K., and Natvig, J. B., 1982, Autologous mixed lymphocyte reaction in patients with rheumatoid arthritis and juvenile rheumatoid arthritis: Both non T cells and *in vivo* activated T cells can act as stimulator cells, *Scand. J. Immunol.* **16**:173–179.

Forre, O., Thoen, J., Waalen, K., and Natvig, B., 1983, Autologous mixed lymphocyte reaction in rheumatoid arthritis. Characterization of stimulator cells and the recognition unit for autoantigens on responder cells, *Behring Inst. Mitt.* **72**:188–192.

Fournier, C., and Charriere, J., 1981, Autologous mixed lymphocyte reaction in man. I. Relationship with age and sex, *Cell. Immunol.* **60**:212–219.

Frajman, M., Diaz-Jouanen, E., Alcocer-Varela, J., Fishbein, E., Guevara, M., and Alarcon-Segovia, D.,

1983, Effect of pregnancy on functions of circulating T cells from patients with systemic lupus erythematosus: Correction of T-cell suppression and autologous mixed lymphocyte responses, *Clin. Immunol. Immunopathol.* **29**:94–102.

Fridman, W. H., and Kourilsky, F. J., 1969, Stimulation of lymphocytes by autologous leukemic cells in acute leukemia, *Nature* **224**:277–279.

Gatenby, P. A., Kotzin, B. L., Kansas, G. S., and Engleman, E. G., 1982, Immunoglobulin secretion in the human autologous mixed leukocyte reaction: Definition of a suppressor-amplifier circuit using monoclonal antibodies, *J. Exp. Med.* **156**:55–67.

Glimcher, L. H., and Shevach, E. M., 1982, Production of autoreactive I region-restricted T cell hybridoma, *J. Exp. Med.* **156**:640–645.

Goto, M., and Zvaifler, N. J., 1983, Characterization of the killer cells generated in the autologous mixed lymphocyte reaction, *J. Exp. Med.* **157**:1309–1399.

Gottlieb, A. B., Fu, S. M., Yu, D. T. Y., Wang, C. Y., Halper, J. P., and Kunkel, H. G., 1979, The nature of the stimulatory cell in human allogeneic and autologous MLC reactions; role of isolated IgM-bearing B cells, *J. Immunol.* **123**:1497–1503.

Green, S., and Sell, K. W., 1970, Mixed leukocyte stimulation of normal peripheral blood leukocytes by autologous lymphoblastoid cells, *Science* **170**:989–990.

Gupta, S., 1978, Functionally distinct subpopulations of human T lymphocytes. A review, *Clin. Bull.* **8**:100–107.

Gupta, S., 1983a, Autologous mixed lymphocyte reaction in health and disease states in man, *Vox Sang.* **44**:265–268.

Gupta, S., 1983b, Cellular interactions in the human T–T autologous mixed lymphocyte reaction, *Behring Inst. Mitt.* **72**:101–106.

Gupta, S., 1983c, In T–T AMLR, distinct T cell subsets respond to mitogen- or AMLR-activated stimulator T cells, *Fed. Proc.* **42**:719 (Abstract).

Gupta, S., and Damle, N., 1981a, Regulation of autologous and allogeneic MLR in man, *Fed. Proc.* **40**:977 (Abstract).

Gupta, S., and Damle, N., 1981b, Autologous mixed lymphocyte culture response in man, in: *Fundamental Mechanisms in Human Cancer Immunology,* (J. P. Saunders, J. C. Daniels, B. Serrou, C. Rosenfield, C. B. Denney eds.), Elsevier, New York, pp. 375–383.

Gupta, S., and Damle, N., 1981c, Autologous mixed lymphocyte culture response in man. I. Effect of intravenous hydrocortisone *in vivo, Hum. Lymph. Diff.* **1**:77–82.

Gupta, S., and Damle, N. K., 1982a, Regulation of autologous mixed culture response in man, in: *Symposium on Cellular and Humoral Mechanisms of Immune Regulation* (G. Phonake, ed.), Government of India Press, Bombay, pp. 83–98.

Gupta, S., and Damle, N. K., 1982b, Monoclonal antibody-defined T cell subsets responding in T–T AMLR, *Fed. Proc.* **41**:800 (Abstract).

Gupta, S., and Damle, N. K., 1982c, Monoclonal antibody-defined T cell subsets responding in T–T and T–non-T autologous mixed lymphocyte reaction. Generation of immunoregulatory functions, in: *Current Concepts in Human Immunology and Cancer Immunomodulation* (B. Serrou, ed.), North Holland, Amsterdam, pp. 183–188.

Gupta, S., and Good, R. A., 1979, T cell subpopulations as defined by Fc receptors, *Thymus* **1**:139–149.

Gupta, S., Damle, N. K., Platsoucas, C. D., and Hansen, J. A., 1981, Complement-independent inhibition of autologous mixed lymphocyte response by monoclonal antibodies, *Clin. Res.* **29**:368 (Abstract).

Gupta, S., Chandy, K. G., Thornton, M., and Goldberg, M., 1985, Autologous mixed lymphocyte reaction in man. XIII. Characterization of T–T autologous mixed lymphocyte reaction, *J. Clin. Immunol.* **5**:187–194.

Hahn, B. M., Pletscher, S., Mumiain, M., and MacDermott, R. P., 1982, Suppression of the normal autologous mixed leukocyte reaction by sera from patients with systemic lupus erythematosus, *Arthritis Rheum.* **25**:381–389.

Hasler, F., Bluestein, H. G., Zvaifler, N. J., and Epstein, L. B., 1983a, Analysis of the defects responsible for the impaired regulation of Epstein–Barr virus-induced B cell proliferation by rheumatoid arthritis lymphocytes. I. Diminished gamma interferon production in response to autologous stimulation, *J. Exp. Med.* **157**:173–188.

Hasler, F., Bluestein, H. G., Zvaifler, N. N., and Epstein, L. B., 1983b, Analysis of the defects responsible for the impaired regulation of EBV-induced B cell proliferation by rheumatoid arthritis lymphocytes. II. Role of monocytes and increased sensitivity of rheumatoid arthritis lymphocytes to prostaglandin E, *J. Immunol.* **131**:768–772.

Hausman, P. B., Raff, H. V., Gilbert, R. C., Picker, J. J., and Stobo, J. D., 1980, T cells and macrophages involved in the autologous mixed lymphocyte reaction are required for the response to conventional antigen, *J. Immunol.* **125:**1374–1379.

Huber, C., Fink, U., Liebold, W., Schmalzl, F., Peterson, P. A., Klareskog, L., and Braunsteiner, H., 1981, The role of adherent HLA-DR$^+$ mononuclear cells in autologous and allogeneic MLR, *J. Immunol.* **127:**72–73.

Huber, C., Merkenschlager, M., Gattringer, C., Royston, L., Fink, U., and Braunsteiner, H., 1982, Human autologous mixed lymphocyte reactivity is primarily specific for xenoprotein determinants absorbed to antigen-presenting cells during rosette formation with SRBC, *J. Exp. Med.* **155:**1222–1227.

Ilfeld, D., Krakauer, R. S., and Blaese, R. M., 1977, Expression of the human autologous mixed lymphocyte reaction by physiologic concentration of hydrocortisone, *J. Immunol.* **119:**428–434.

Indiveri, F., Wilson, B. S., Russo, C., Quaranta, V., Pellegrino, M. A., and Ferrone, F., 1980, Ia-like antigens on human T lymphocytes relationship to other marker role in MLR and structural profile, *J. Immunol.* **125:**2673–2678.

Indiveri, F., Scudeletti, M., Bende, D., Barabino, A., Russo, C., Pellegrino, M. A., and Ferrone, S., 1983, Role of distinct domain of Ia antigens in autologous and allogeneic mixed lymphocyte reaction, *Behring Inst. Mitt.* **72:**95–100.

Innes, J. B., Kuntz, M. M., Kim, Y. T., and Weksler, M. E., 1979, Induction of suppressor activity in the autologous mixed lymphocyte reaction and in cultures with concanavalin A, *J. Clin. Invest.* **64:**1608–1613.

Junge, U., Hoekstra, J., and Deinhardt, F., 1970, Altered antigenicity of cultural mononucleosis lymphocytes, *Lancet* **2:**217.

Kalden, J. R., Leitner, O., Klockel, O., Kirchner, H., Manger, B., and Koch, B., 1983, The autologous mixed lymphocyte reaction in patients with rheumatoid arthritis, *Behring Inst. Mitt.* **72:**193–202.

Kamoun, M., Martin, P. J., Hansen, J. A., Brown, A. W., Siadak, A. W., and Nowinski, R. C., 1981, Identification of a human T lymphocyte surface protein associated with E-rosette receptor, *J. Exp. Med.* **153:**207–214.

Kaplan, J., 1975, Human T lymphocytes form rosettes with autologous and allogeneic human red blood cells, *Clin. Immunol. Immunopathol.* **3:**471–475.

Katz, P., and Fauci, A. S., 1979, Autologous and allogeneic intracellular interactions: Modulation by adherent cells, irradiation, and *in vitro* and *in vivo* corticosteroids, *J. Immunol.* **123:**2270–2277.

Katz, P., Haynes, B. F., and Fauci, A. S., 1978, Lack of generation of killer cells in the mixed lymphocyte reaction between mitogen stimulated and unstimulated autologous lymphocytes, *J. Immunol.* **121:**1998–2001.

Knight, S. C., Moore, G. E., and Clarkson, B. D., 1971, Stimulation of autocthonous lymphocytes by cells from normal and leukemic lines, *Nature* **229:**185–187.

Ko, H. S., Fu, S. M., Winchester, R. J., Yu, D. T. Y., and Kunkel, H. G., 1979, Ia determinants on stimulated human T lymphocytes. Occurrence on mitogen and antigen-activated T cells, *J. Exp. Med.* **150:**246–255.

Kozak, R. W., Moody, C. E., Staiano-Coico, L., and Weksler, M. E., 1982, Lymphocyte transformation induced by autologous cells. XII. Quantitative and qualitative differences between human autologous and allogeneic reactive T lymphocytes, *J. Immunol.* **128:**1723–1727.

Kumagai, S., Scher, I., and Green, I., 1981, Autologous rosette-forming T cells regulate responses of T cells. Phenotypic and functional analysis of suppressor cells generated from autologous rosette-forming T cells after autologous mixed lymphocyte reaction, *J. Clin. Invest.* **68:**356–364.

Kuntz, M. M., Innes, J. B., and Weksler, M. E., 1976, Lymphocyte transformation induced by autologous cells. IV. Human T-lymphocyte proliferation induced by autologous or allogeneic non-T lymphocytes, *J. Exp. Med.* **143:**1049–1054.

Kuntz, M. M., Innes, J. B., and Weksler, M. E., 1979, The cellular basis of the impaired autologous mixed lymphocyte reaction in patients with systemic lupus erythematosus, *J. Clin. Invest.* **63:**151–153.

Kuntz-Crow, M., and Kunkel, H. G., 1982, Human dendritic cells: Major stimulators of the autologous and allogeneic mixed lymphocyte reaction, *Clin. Exp. Immunol.* **49:**338–346.

Laffon, A., Alcocer-Varela, J., and Alarcon-Segovia, D., 1983, The autologous mixed lymphocyte reaction is not primarily due to xenoantigenic stimulation, *Clin. Immunol. Immunopathol.* **28:**304–308.

Lattime, E., Golub, S. H., and Stutman, O., 1980, Lyt 1$^+$ cells respond to Ia-bearing macrophages in the murine syngeneic mixed lymphocyte reaction, *Eur. J. Immunol.* **10:**723–726.

Lederman, M. M., Liebman, M. L., Hassid, A. I., and Berk, G. I., 1983, Preincubation of human monocytes results in loss of effector activity and diminished stimulation of the autologous mixed lymphocyte reaction, *Clin. Exp. Immunol.* **53:**482–490.

Lee, S. K., and Oliver, R. T. D., 1978, Autologous leukemia specific T cell-mediated lymphocytotoxicity in patients with acute myelogenous leukemia, *J. Exp. Med.* **147**:912–922.

Manger, B., Zawatzky, R., Kirschner, H., and Kalden, J. R., 1980, Interferon production in human allogeneic mixed lymphocyte cultures (MLC), in: *Fourth International Congress of Immunology,* (J. L. Preud'Homone and V. A. L. Hawken eds.), p. 11.7 (Abstract).

MacDermott, R. P., and Stacey, M. C., 1981, Further characterization of the human autologous mixed leukocyte reaction (MLR), *J. Immunol.* **126**:729–734.

Miller, R. A., and Kaplan, H. S., 1978, Generation of cytotoxic lymphocytes in the autologous mixed lymphocyte culture, *J. Immunol.* **121**:2165–2167.

Mingari, M. C., and Moretta, L., 1982, Role of Ia antigens in the human autologous mixed lymphocyte reaction, *Eur. J. Immunol.* **12**:98–100.

Miyasaka, N., Sauvezie, B., Pierce, D. A., Daniels, T. E., and Talal, N., 1980, Decreased autologous mixed lymphocyte reaction in Sjögren's syndrome, *J. Clin. Invest.* **66**:928–933.

Moody, C. E., Gupta, S., and Weksler, M. E., 1983, Lymphocyte transformation induced by autologous cells. XV. Xenoantigens are not required for the proliferative response observed in the autologous mixed lymphocyte reaction, *J. Clin. Immunol.* **3**:100–102.

Morse, J. H., and Bodi, B. S., 1982, Autologous and allogeneic mixed lymphocyte reactions in progressive systemic sclerosis, *Arthritis Rheum.* **25**:390–395.

Opelz, G., Kuchi, M., Takasugi, M., and Terasaki, P. I., 1975, Autologous stimulation of human lymphocyte subpopulations, *J. Exp. Med.* **142**:1327–1333.

Palacios, R., 1981, Cyclosporin A inhibits the proliferative response and the generation of helper, suppressor and cytotoxic T cell functions in the autologous mixed lymphocyte reaction, *Cell. Immunol.* **61**:453–462.

Palacios, R., 1982, Epstein–Barr virus increases the proliferative response and the generation of suppressor and cytotoxic T cells functions in autologous mixed lymphocyte reaction, *Scand. J. Immunol.* **15**:17–24.

Palacios, R., and Alarcon-Segovia, D., 1981, Human postthymic precursor cells in health and disease. VI. Effect of serum thymic factor on the response of cells from patients with systemic lupus erythematosus or mixed connective tissue disease in autologous mixed lymphocyte reaction, *Clin. Immunol. Immunopathol.* **18**:362–367.

Palacios, R., and Sugawara, I., 1982, Hydrocortisone abrogates proliferation of T cells in autologous mixed lymphocyte reaction by rendering the interleukin-2 producer T cells unresponsive to interleukin I and unable to synthesize the T-cell growth factor, *Scand. J. Immunol.* **15**:25–31.

Palacios, R. and Moller, G., 1981, HLA-DR rendering resting T cells to interleukin 2 and induced production of the growth factor in the autogons mixed lymphocyte reaction, *Cell Immunol.* **63**:143–153.

Palacios, R., Llorente, L., Alarco-Segovia, D., Ruiz-Arguelles, D., and Diaz-Jouanen, E., 1980, Autologous rosette-forming T cells as the responding cells in human autologous mixed lymphocyte reaction, *J. Clin. Invest.* **65**:1527–1530.

Ransohoff, R. M., and Dastom, M. M., 1983, Impaired autologous mixed lymphocyte reaction with normal concanavalin A-induced suppression in adult polymyositis/dermatomyositis, *Clin. Exp. Immunol.* **53**:67–75.

Reinherz, E. L., and Schlossman, S. F., 1980, The differentiation and function of human T lymphocytes, *Cell* **19**:821–826.

Reinherz, E. L., Morimoto, C., Penta, A C., and Schlossman, S. F., 1981, Subpopulations of $T4^+$ inducer T cell subset in man: Evidence of an amplifier population preferentially expressing Ia antigens upon activation, *J. Immunol.* **126**:67–70.

Reinherz, E. L., Morimoto, C., Fitzgerald, K. A., Huzzey, R. E., Daley, J. F., and Schlossman, S. F., 1982, Heterogeneity of human T4 inducer T cells defined by a monoclonal antibody that delineates two distinct functional subpopulations, *J. Immunol.* **128**:463–468.

Richardson, B., and Stobo, J. D., 1983, Autologous reactive T cell clones and T–T hybrids, *Behring Inst. Mitt.* **72**:87–88.

Romain, P. L., and Lipsky, P., 1983, Immunoglobulin secretion during the autologous mixed lymphocyte reaction in man, *J. Immunol.* **130**:1146–1151.

Romain, P. L., Schlossman, S. F., and Reinherz, E. L., 1984a, Surface molecules involved in self-recognition and T cell activation in the autologous mixed lymphocyte reaction, *J. Immunol.* **133**:1093–1100.

Romain, P. L., Morimoto, C., Daley, J. F., Palley, L. S., Reinherz, E. L., and Schlossman, S. F., 1984b, Reactivity of inducer cell subsets and T8-cell activation during the human autologous mixed lymphocyte reaction, *Clin. Immunol. Immunopathol.* **30**:117–128.

Rucheton, M., Caraux, J., Rey, A., Thierry, C., Esteve, C., Valles, H., Duffer, J., Desplaces, A., Zaguri, D., and Serrou, B., 1981, Human autologous rosettes. II. Further characterization: Markers and functions, *Cell. Immunol.* **64**:312–323.

Russo, C., Indiveri, F., Quaranta, V., Molanario, G. A., Pellegrino, M. A., and Ferrone, S., 1981, Stimulation of human T lymphocytes by PHA-activated autologous T lymphocytes: An analysis of the role of Ia-like antigens with monoclonal antibodies, *Immunogenetics* **12**:267–274.

Sakane, T., and Green, I., 1979, Specificity and suppressor function of human T cells responsive to autologous non-T cells, *J. Immunol.* **123**:584–589.

Sakane, T., Steinberg, A. D., and Green, I., 1978, Failure of autologous mixed lymphocyte reaction between T and non-T cells in patients with systemic lupus erythematosus, *Proc. Natl. Acad. Sci. U.S.A.* **75**: 3464–3468.

Sakane, T., Steinberg, A. D., Arnett, F. C., Reinertsen, J. L., and Green, I., 1979, Studies of immune functions of patients with systemic lupus erythematosus. III. Characterization of lymphocyte subpopulations responsible for defective autologous lymphocyte reaction, *Arthritis Rheum.* **22**:770–776.

Sakane, T., Steinberg, A. D., and Green, I., 1980, Studies of immune functions of patients with systemic lupus erythematosus. V. T cells suppressor function and autologous mixed lymphocyte reaction during active and inactive phase of disease, *Arthritis Rheum.* **23**:225–231.

Sakane, T., Honda, M., Taniguchi, Y., and Kotani, H., 1981, Separation of concanavalin A-induced human helper and suppressor T cells by the autologous erythrocyte rosette technique, *J. Clin. Invest.* **68**:447–453.

Sakane, T., Kotani, H., Takada, S., Murakawa, Y., and Ueda, Y., 1983, A defect in the suppressor circuit among $OKT4^+$ cell populations in patients with systemic lupus erythematosus occurs independently of a defect in the $OKT8^+$ suppressor T cell function, *J. Immunol.* **131**:758–761.

Santilands, G. P., Gray, K. G., Cooney, A. E., Browning, J. D., and Anderson, J. R., 1974, Autorosette formation by human thymocytes and lymphocytes, *Lancet* **1**:27–28.

Shin, H. S., Wang, C. Y., and Choi, Y. S., 1981, Activation of autologous reactive helper T lymphocytes for differentiation of human B lymphocytes, *J. Immunol.* **126**:2485–2489.

Shore, A., Dosch, H. M., and Gelfand, E. W., 1978, Induction and separation of antigen-dependent T helper and T suppressor cells in man, *Nature* **274**:586–588.

Silver, R. M., Redelman, D., and Zvaifler, N. J., 1983, Studies of rheumatoid synovial fluid lymphocytes. II. A comparison of their behavior with blood mononuclear cells in the autologous mixed lymphocyte reaction and response to TCGF, *Clin. Immunol. Immunopathol.* **27**:15–27.

Smith, J. B., 1978, Stimulation of autologous and allogeneic human T cells by B cells occurs through separate B cell antigen systems, *Cell. Immunol.* **36**:203–209.

Smith, J. B., 1983, Frequency in human peripheral blood of T cells which respond to self, modified self and alloantigens, *Immunology* **50**:181–187.

Smith, J. B., and DeHoratius, R. J., 1982, Different autologous mixed lymphocyte reactions correlate with disease activity in systemic lupus erythematosus and rheumatoid arthritis, *Clin. Exp. Immunol.* **48**:155–162.

Smith, J. B., and Knowlton, R. P., 1979, Activation of suppressor T cells in human autologous mixed lymphocyte culture, *J. Immunol.* **123**:419–422.

Smith, J. B., and Knowlton, R. P., 1981, Autologous mixed lymphocyte culture responder T cells are in the concanavalin A reactive subpopulation and separate from alloreactive cells, *Clin. Immunol. Immunopathol.* **20**:31–38.

Smolen, J. S., Luger, T. A., Chused, T. M., and Steinberg, A. D., 1981a, Responder cells in the human autologous mixed lymphocyte reaction, *J. Clin. Invest.* **68**:1601–1604.

Smolen, J. S., Sharrow, S. O., Reeves, J. P., Boegel, W. A., and Steinberg, A. D., 1981b, The human autologous mixed lymphocyte reaction. Suppression by macrophages and T cells, *J. Immunol.* **127**:1987–1993.

Smolen, J. S., Sharrow, S. O., and Steinberg, A. F., 1981c, Characterization of autologous rosette-forming cells. A non-restricted phenomenon, *J. Immunol.* **127**:737–741.

Smolen, J. S., Raveche, E. S., Steinberg, R. T., Sharrow, S. O., Fauci, A. S., and Steinberg, A. D., 1982, The human autologous mixed lymphocyte reaction. II. Analysis of activation and proliferation, *J. Clin. Lab. Immunol.* **9**:185–192.

Steel, C. M., and Hardy, D. A., 1970, Evidence of altered antigenicity in cultured lymphoid cells from patients with infectious mononucleosis, *Lancet* **1**:1322.

Stephen, J. P., Yenokida, G. G., Graeff, A. S., Elson, C. O., and Strober, W., 1981, Immunoregulatory function of T cells activated in the autologous mixed lymphocyte reaction, *J. Immunol.* **127**:2605–2609.

Stobo, J. D., and Loehnen, C. P., 1978, Proliferative reactivity of T cells to autologous cell-associated antigens, *Arthritis Rheum.* **21**(Suppl):210–214.

Strassmann, G., Bach, F. H., and Zarling, J. M., 1983, Depletion of human NK cells with monoclonal antibodies allows the generation of cytotoxic T lymphocytes without NK-like cells in mixed cultures, *J. Immunol.* **130**:1556–1560.

Sumiya, M., Kano, S., Gonda, N., Oshimi, K., and Takaku, F., 1980, Generation of autoreactive established autologous lymphoblastoid cell line, *J. Immunol.* **125**:1625–1629.

Thorbecke, G. J., Chapman-Alexander, J., Katz, I. R., Bienenstock, A., and Asofsky, R., 1983, Role of B cels in the stimulation of syngeneic mixed lymphocyte response, *Behring Inst. Mitt.* **72**:107–116.

Tomonari, K., 1980, Cytotoxic T cells generated in the autologous mixed lymphocyte reaction. I. Primary autologous mixed lymphocyte reaction, *J. Immunol.* **124**:1111–1121.

Tomonari, K., and Aizawa, M., 1979, Induction of autoreactive cells by the preculture of human peripheral blood mononuclear cells with the fresh autologous plasma, *J. Immunol.* **122**:2478–2483.

Tomonari, K., Wakisaka, A., and Aizawa, M., 1980, Self recognition by autologous mixed lymphocyte reaction primed cells, *J. Immunol.* **125**:1596–1600.

Uchida, A., and Micksche, M., 1981, Reactivity to autologous non-T cells and suppressor function of human autologous rosettes, *Immunol. Lett.* **3**:145–149.

Van de Stouwe, R. A., Kunkel, H. G., Halper, J. P., and Weksler, M. E., 1977, Autologous mixed lymphocyte culture reactions and generation of cytotoxic cells, *J. Exp. Med.* **146**:1809–1814.

Van Wauwe, J., and Goosens, J., 1981, Monoclonal anti-human T lymphocyte antibodies. Enumeration and characterization of T cell subsets, *Immunology* **42**:157–164.

Weksler, M. E., and Kozak, R. W., 1977, Lymphocyte transformation induced by autologous cells. V. Generation of immunologic memory and specificity during the autologous mixed lymphocyte reaction, *J. Exp. Med.* **146**:1833–1838.

Weksler, M. E., Moody, C. E., Ostry, R. F., Casazza, B. A., 1980, Lymphocyte transformation induced by autologous cells. X. Soluble factors that generate cytotoxic T lymphocytes, *J. Exp. Med.* **152**(Suppl.):284–291.

Weksler, M. E., Moody, C. E., and Kazak, R. W., 1981, The autologous mixed lymphocyte reaction, *Adv. Immunol.* **31**:271–312.

Wolos, J. A., and Davey, F. R., 1979, T cell subpopulations in autologous and allogeneic mixed lymphocyte reaction, *Cell Immunol.* **48**:415–419.

Yu, D. T. Y., Ramer, S. J., Clement, P. J., 1978, Effect of methyl prednisone on autologous mixed lymphocyte cultures, *Transplantation* **25**:163–165.

Yu, D. T. Y., McCune, J. M., Fu, S. M., Winchester, R. J., and Kunkel, H. G., 1980a, Two types of Ia-positive T cells. Synthesis and exchange of Ia antigens, *J. Exp. Med.* **152**(Suppl.):89–98.

Yu, D. T. Y., Chiorazzi, N., and Kunkel, H. G., 1980b, Helper factors derived from autologous mixed lymphocyte cultures, *Cell. Immunol.* **50**:305–313.

Zagury, D., Morgan, D., Lenoir, G., Fouchard, M., and Feldman, M., 1983, Human normal CTL clones: Generation and properties, *Int. J. Cancer* **31**:427–432.

Zarling, J. M., Raich, P. C., McKeough, M., and Bach, F. H., 1976, Generation of cytotoxic lymphocytes *in vitro* against autologous human leukemia cells, *Nature* **262**:691–693.

4

Interleukins

Molecular and Biological Characteristics

Sudhir Gupta

I. INTRODUCTION

Lymphocyte reactions are complex and involve interactions between lymphocyte subsets and accessory cells and a number of soluble molecules that they produce. A major contribution to the study of T-cell biology was provided by the observations of Morgan *et al.* (1976) that a cytokine, then designated as T-cell growth factor (TCGF), released into conditioned media of lectin-stimulated mononuclear cells could support the long-term growth of T cells in a culture system. This has led to the development of homogeneous clones of various T-cell subsets that permitted functional studies of T-cell subsets, their capacity to produce various effector and immunoregulatory molecules, mechanisms of interactions with various growth and inhibitory factors, and requirement for various molecules for their own growth.

Since then, a number of mitogenic factors have been produced in human and experimental animals. In 1979, at the International Lymphokine Workshop, a common nomenclature was proposed. The name interleukin 1 (IL-1) was given to factors that do not support continuous proliferation of T lymphocytes and are products of activated cells of monocyte–macrophage lineage. Interleukin 2 (IL-2) was the name given to factors derived from mitogen-stimulated mononuclear cell supernatants that could support long-term proliferation of T lymphocytes. Interleukin 2 includes previously designated molecules such as TCGF, thymocyte-stimulating factor, cytotoxic T-cell-inducing factor, and killer cell helper factor. In this chapter, attempts have been made to discuss the molecular and biological features of IL-1 and IL-2 and their alterations in various rheumatic disorders.

Sudhir Gupta • Department of Medicine, Division of Basic and Clinical Immunology, University of California, Irvine, California 92717.

II. INTERLEUKIN 2

Interleukin 2 is a single polypeptide that is released from antigen- or mitogen-triggered lymphocytes within hours of activation and that functions to switch T cells from G_1 phase to S, G_2, and M phases. Interleukin 2 also directly or indirectly plays a role in the proliferation and maturation of other cell types. It is released by T cells in response to two signals provided by antigen-pulsed accessory cells. The first signal is antigen, presented in the context of DR (Ia) antigen, and the second signal is IL-1. Certain lectins can substitute for antigen in the accessory-cell signal. The subject of IL-2 has recently been reviewed (Smith, 1984; Robb, 1984; Sarin and Gallo, 1983).

A. Production of IL-2

Fresh lymphocytes do not contain intracellular IL-2 or release IL-2 spontaneously. However, when stimulated with mitogens (PHA, Con A, or PWM) or antigens (alloantigens, autoantigens, tumor antigens, soluble proteins), they release IL-2 into the culture medium. Among the lectins, PHA has been used most extensively. Concanavalin A has not been used extensively to produce human IL-2 because it either does not cause any release of IL-2 or very low levels of IL-2. It is possible that Con-A-induced suppressor cells could be responsible for the termination of IL-2 production. The factors that are considered to be crucial or important for optimal IL-2 production include binding of antigen/mitogen to the cell surface of producer cell, interaction with Ir gene product (Ia or DR), and IL-1 produced by macrophages (Smith *et al.*, 1979; Schreier *et al.*, 1980; Larsson and Contimiho, 1979). Neefe *et al.* (1981) demonstrated that PHA-induced IL-2 production has an absolute requirement for adherent cells; exhaustive removal of adherent cells by nylon wool column resulted in a lack of IL-2 production that was restored by the addition of adherent cells to T lymphocytes. Macphail and Stutman (1984) demonstrated that the treatment of stimulator cells in the mixed lymphocyte reaction (MLR) with anti-Ia antibody inhibited IL-2 production. Exogenous IL-2 failed to reconstitute T-cell proliferation. Reconstitution experiments carried out with an exogenous source of IL-1 showed that the inhibition of IL-2 production was not, solely at least, caused by inhibition of IL-1 production.

The culture medium commonly used for IL-2 production contains fetal calf serum. Although a specific need for serum protein in the production of IL-2 has been claimed, IL-2 has been produced in serum-free condition (Mier and Gallo, 1980). Studies on activation of both murine (Wagner and Rollinghoff, 1978) and human (Ruscetti *et al.*, 1980) T cells suggest that transcription and translation precede the appearance of IL-2 in the culture medium, and the kinetics indicate that IL-2 appears in measurable quantities within 4 to 6 hr after stimulation, and peak levels are attained after 12 to 24 hr.

As mentioned earlier, macrophages (1–5%) are required for optimum IL-2 production; however, excessive numbers of the adherent cells suppress IL-2 production. This inhibition might be caused by production of prostaglandin by adherent cells, since the addition of the prostaglandin synthetase inhibitor indomethacin augments IL-2 production (Baker *et al.*, 1981). Addition of Epstein–Barr virus-transformed lymphoblastoid cells or phorbol myristic acetate (PMA) to T cells or γ irradiation of peripheral blood lymphocytes results in enhanced IL-2 production (Bonnard *et al.*, 1980; Inouye *et al.*, 1980;

Ruscetti *et al.*, 1980). Interleukin 2 is probably produced in the G_1 phase of the cell cycle (Stadler *et al.*, 1981). Increased IL-2 production by irradiated peripheral blood lymphocytes appears to be related to an accumulation of lymphocytes in the G_1 phase. Inhibitors of DNA synthesis (colchicine or cytosine arabinoside) do not influence IL-2 release, whereas IL-2 production is inhibited by the protein synthesis inhibitor puromycin (Ruscetti *et al.*, 1980). Phorbol myristic acetate increases the level of IL-2 mRNA in the mitogen-stimulated T cells (Hirano *et al.*, 1984).

Recently, we have demonstrated the role of functional K^+ channels in T-cell activation (DeCoursey *et al.*, 1984; Chandy *et al.*, 1985a,b). 4-Aminopyridine (4-AP), a specific K^+ channel blocker that inhibits DNA synthesis and protein synthesis, also inhibited IL-2 production in response to PHA (Chandy *et al.*, 1984; Gupta *et al.*, 1985). Gillis *et al.* (1979a) reported that the corticosteroid-induced immunosuppression of T cells was caused by its inhibitory effect on IL-2 production, because addition of IL-2 to cultures stimulated with PHA in the presence of dexamethasone completely abolished the glucocorticoid-induced suppression.

The cell origin of IL-2 has been extensively studied. In the murine system, lectin-stimulated lymphocytes release very little IL-2 as compared to splenocytes and cortisol-resistance thymocytes; the lymphoid cells from athymic nude mice do not produce detectable IL-2 (Gillis *et al.*, 1978, 1979b). This suggests that mature T cells are the source of IL-2. More recently, Ortaldo and Herberman (1984) have shown a clone of large granular lymphocytes (LGL) having natural killer activity that, on stimulation with PHA and cells of K-562 cell line, will produce IL-2. The phenotype of this clone was B73.1$^+$, OKT11$^+$, OKMI$^-$, and DR . Since the cellular lineage of the LGL is unclear and could be heterogeneous, it is possible that this particular clone is of T-cell lineage. Cells and cell lines with B-cell or macrophage characteristics do not produce any IL-2, whereas cell lines and lymphomas and leukemias of T cells do produce IL-2 (Gillis *et al.*, 1980; Gootenberg *et al.*, 1981; Harwell *et al.*, 1980; Schrader and Clark-Lewis, (1981).

Meuer *et al.* (1982) examined the monoclonal-antibody-defined T cell subsets as sources of IL-2 production on stimulation with lectin or in the allogeneic MLR: PHA/PMA and Con A/PMA triggered equivalent amounts of IL-2 production from both T4$^+$ and T8$^+$ activated T cells; however, the majority of IL-2 activity after allogeneic MLR was restricted to T4$^+$ cells. Palacios and Moller (1981) demonstrated the production of IL-2 by OKT4$^+$ cells in the autologous mixed lymphocyte reaction (AMLR). Therefore, it appears that both major subsets of T cells are capable of producing IL-2 (depending on the stimulus); however, OKT4$^+$ cells appear to be the predominant source of IL-2. In the murine studies, it was found that when stimulator–responder major histocompatability complex (MHC) antigens differed at only the I region, Lyt 1$^+$ T cells and not Lyt 2$^+$ T cells produced IL-2. In contrast, when the MLR combination differed singularly at the K/D region of MHC, the Lyt 2$^+$ and not the Lyt 1$^+$ cells were responsible for IL-2 production (Kern *et al.*, 1981; Okada and Henney, 1980; Okada *et al.*, 1979).

These studies emphasize the importance of stimulus in the activation of individual T-cell subpopulations. Using a limiting-dilution culture system, Pfizenmaier *et al.* (1984) have shown that on stimulation with Con A, 90% of Lyt 2$^-$ T cells were capable of producing IL-2 activity. In addition, IL-2 activity is produced by 8–10% of Lyt 2$^+$ T cells. At the clonal level, the average of IL-2 activity produced by Lyt 2$^+$ T cells is about eightfold less than that produced by Lyt 2$^-$ cells. In a number of clones analyzed, it was observed that the capacity to produce IL-2 activity and the capacity to express cytotoxic activity were mutually exclusive. A minority of clones (<3%) were found to simultaneously produce IL-2 activity and express cytotoxicity.

B. Molecular Characteristics of IL-2

During the past 5 years a number of approaches have been employed to purify IL-2 to homogeneity. These included dye-affinity chromatography, immunoaffinity chromatography, and reverse-phase high-pressure liquid chromatography (HPLC). A number of structural and functional similarities suggest that the IL-2 from human, rat, murine, and ape lymphocytes are analogues of one another. Human, rat, and ape IL-2 are secreted as single polypeptide chains with approximate molecular weights of 19–22,000 on gel-permeation chromatography and 15–17,000 on SDS-PAGE gel (Schreier *et al.*, 1980; Henderson *et al.*, 1983; Robb and Smith, 1981). Murine IL-2 behaves on gel filtration as a noncovalent dimer (30–40,000 molecular weight) of a 15- to 17,000-molecular-weight subunit. Purified IL-2 from each species exhibits nearly equivalent specific activity.

Several investigators have isolated the messenger RNA (mRNA) from human and gibbon IL-2-producing cells and transplanted them in *Xenopus laevis* to produce biologically active IL-2 (Lin *et al.*, 1982; Erfat *et al.*, 1982; Sarin and Gallo, 1983). When analyzed on a sucrose density gradient under denaturing conditions, the poly-A-selected mRNA from human tonsil lymphocytes has been shown to be around 10 S (Erfat *et al.*, 1982), whereas under nondenaturing conditions, the size of mRNA from a gibbon ape lymphoma cell line has been shown to be 14 to 15 S (Lin *et al.*, 1982). A minor (13 to 13.5 S) species of mRNA has been detected in human cells that can be translated to produce biologically active IL-2 (Erfat *et al.*, 1982). The mRNA species of 10 S corresponds to an RNA of 650 bases. Assuming 200 nucleotides for the 5′ leader and 3′ untranslated region, the remaining portion of the IL-2 mRNA can code for 130 to 160 amino acids corresponding to a protein of 14,000–18,000 daltons, which is in agreement with the reported molecular weight of IL-2.

Taniguchi *et al.* (1983) prepared a cDNA library from the fractionated poly(A) mRNA that sedimented at around 11.5 S and showed the highest IL-2 mRNA activity. From this library, a hybrid plasmid, P3-16, containing the cDNA copy of the human IL-2 was identified by an IL-2 mRNA hybridization translation assay. Subsequent screening of the cDNA library indicated that the frequency of IL-2-specific clones was 1 : 2000. This would translate the frequency of the IL-2-specific mRNA in poly(A) mRNA fraction to be approximately 1 : 20,000 because tenfold enrichment of the IL-2 mRNA is achieved by the sucrose density gradient fractionation. Therefore, the screening of an unselected cDNA library would be exceedingly time-consuming.

The structure of human IL-2 is fully characterized with respect to its amino acid sequence and posttranslational modification. Human IL-2 consists of a 133-amino-acid single polypeptide containing a single intramolecular disulfide bridge between two cysteines in positions 58 and 105. This bond plays an important role in maintaining an active conformation of the molecule since reduction under denaturing conditions caused a loss of biological activity (Robb, 1984). The nucleotide sequence was derived from cDNA prepared from transformed and nontransformed T cells (Taniguchi *et al.*, 1983; Devos *et al.*, 1983).

In both cases, the cDNA coded for a molecule of 153 amino acids containing an amino-terminal signal sequence of 20 amino acids. The sequence analysis of mature protein showed that those 20-amino-terminal residues are removed prior to secretion (Robb and Smith, 1981). Similar analysis of tryptic fragments from throughout the molecule confirmed the order of the remaining residues predicted by the cDNA data (Robb, 1984). Amino-terminal sequence analysis of human IL-2 indicates that the amino acid in position 3 of the polypeptide chain is modified. Examination of the N-terminal octapeptide with an amino acid analyzer and mass spectrometry demonstrated that position 3 is a threonine that is linked to N-acetyl-D-galactosamine.

These data identify one site of posttranslational modification of human IL-2 and emphasize the importance of complementing sequence analysis at the cDNA level with similar data at the protein level. The posttranslational addition of carbohydrate has no effect on *in vitro* bioactivity, although it may yet play a role in *in vivo* clearance of the molecule and appears to prolong its half-life. The carbohydrate attached to Thr3 provides an explanation for the charge and size heterogeneity of human IL-2. Since there is a single copy of the gene for the IL-2 (Seigal *et al.*, 1984; Fujita *et al.*, 1984), apart from possible allelic differences, all heterogeneity of human IL-2 arises from posttranslational modification (Robb *et al.*, 1983). Since neither IL-2 activity nor IL-2-specific mRNA is produced by producer cells without induction by lectins or antigens and the levels of IL-2 secretion correlate well with the level of mRNA in the cells, it suggests that IL-2 production is controlled at the mRNA transcription level.

The gene for IL-2 has recently been shown to be located on human chromosome 4q (Seigal *et al.*, 1984). Sequence analysis of genomic DNA indicated that the IL-2 gene contains three introns, and the exon sequences can be aligned with the previously reported cDNA sequence except for a few nucleotides in the 3′ nontranslated region (Fujita *et al.*, 1983). The promotor region contains a prototype "TATA" sequence as well as a notable palindromic sequence. There are sequences in this region that are homologous to the promotor region of the human γ-interferon gene. In the second intron, a sequence closely resembling the core sequence for the viral enhancer element has been found. Such sequences may play a role in the expression of the interleukin 2 gene in lectin- or antigen-stimulated T lymphocytes.

C. Interleukin 2 Receptor

Similar to any other peptide hormone or growth factor, IL-2 requires binding to its specific membrane receptor to perform its biological activities. The IL-2 receptor has been purified (Leonard *et al.*, 1983) and more recently cloned (Leonard *et al.*, 1984; Nikaido *et al.*, 1984). Originally, the IL-2 receptor was described only on activated T cells, but recently the IL-2 receptor has also been shown on activated B lymphocytes, B-cell lines, certain B-cell leukemias and lymphomas, and natural killer cells (Uchiama *et al.*, 1981a,b; Tsudo *et al.*, 1984; Waldmann *et al.*, 1984; Robb *et al.*, 1984; Leonard *et al.*, 1982, 1983; Depper *et al.*, 1984a; Reske-Kunz *et al.*, 1984; Robb and Green, 1983; Korsmeyer *et al.*, 1983). The definition of IL-2 receptor or IL-2 binding site on the surface membrane has been made possible by the purification of IL-2 to homogeneity or recombinant IL-2 and the development of monoclonal antibodies against IL-2 and IL-2 receptors in both human and animal systems (Ortega *et al.*, 1984; Malek *et al.*, 1983, 1984; Osawa and

Diamantstein, 1983, 1984; Uchiama *et al.*, 198la,b; Mier and Gallo, 1980, 1982; Welte *et al.*, 1982; Smith *et al.*, 1983).

The mechanism of action of IL-2 involves binding to high-affinity receptor on the surface of responsive cells (Robb *et al.*, 1984). The anti-Tac (IL-2 receptor antibody) antibody is capable of blocking high-affinity IL-2 binding to activated T cells (Leonard *et al.*, 1982; Robb and Green, 1983) and all the T-cell responses attributed to such interaction with IL-2. Analyses of the molecules recognized by the anti-IL-2-receptor antibodies on human, rat and murine cells have shown concordant results. In each case, a glycoprotein molecule of 50–55,000 molecular weight (p50) was found (Robb and Green, 1983; Osawa and Diamantstein, 1983; Malek *et al.*, 1983; Leonard *et al.*, 1983). Leonard *et al.* (1983) demonstrated that both anti-Tac monoclonal antibody and anti-IL-2 antibody immunoprecipitated a protein band that appears to represent IL-2 cross linked to its receptor on HUT-102 B2 cells. In HUT-102 B2 cells, the IL-2 receptor is a p50 glycoprotein with internal disulfide bond(s) and a pI of 5.5–6.0, and it represents 0.05% of total cellular *de novo* protein synthesis. It contains a peptide of p33 that is processed to a mature form that includes N-linked and O-linked sugars and sialic acid. Furthermore, affinity supports coupled with the antibody and with IL-2 bound the same 50- to 55,000-molecular-weight glycoprotein from a mixture of detergent-solubilized cellular molecules (Robb and Green, 1983).

Because the antibody-coupled support removed all cellular proteins reactive with the IL-2-coupled support, and the IL-2-coupled support was capable of removing all antibody-reactive molecules, it is apparent that the number of IL-2 receptors is equal to the number of Tac protein molecules. However, quantitative binding assays with radiolabeled IL-2 and anti-Tac indicate that activated T cells have 10–20 times more binding sites for the antibody than high-affinity sites of IL-2 (Green and Robb, 1984).

One of the possible explanations for the quantitative difference between the two binding assays is that a large portion of the Tac protein possess a low affinity for IL-2. In fact, more recently, Robb *et al.* (1984) have demonstrated the existence of a class (or classes) of low-affinity binding sites. They demonstrated that anti-Tac antibody could substantially or totally block the entire spectrum of IL-2 binding and that IL-2 could block all radiolabeled anti-Tac binding. This suggests that low-affinity binding sites were present on lectin-activated T cells, several human and murine T cell lines, and selected Tac-positive B-cell lines.

The proportion of high- and low-affinity binding sites on the different cell types varies. The low affinity binding sites are found on 9-day-old PHA-induced T cell blasts, PMA-induced HSB2 cells, and B cells in hairy-cell leukemia. The ratio of low- to high-affinity binding for the murine CTL and HT-2 lines is higher than that for the CTLL-2 line. Therefore, display of the protein recognized by anti-Tac or 7D4 monoclonal antibodies (murine IL-2 receptor antibody) is not necessarily a quantitative measure of the capacity of the cells for high-affinity interaction with IL-2. It seems unlikely that the low-affinity binding sites for IL-2 participate in normal physiological responses to IL-2, since at concentrations that might occur *in vivo* (<200 pM), only less than 1% of such sites would be occupied. It remains to be determined whether the low-affinity sites act as a pool for the generation of high-affinity receptors.

Receptors for IL-2 have been found on human activated B cells and various B-cell lines from various lymphomas and leukemias (Waldmann *et al.*, 1984; Tsudo *et al.*,

1984; Zubler *et al.*, 1984). Interleukin 2 induces proliferation and immunoglobulin synthesis/secretion in normal activated B cells and various B-cell lines; both of these effects of IL-2 are blocked by anti-Tac monoclonal antibody. The IL-2 receptor on cloned normal B cell is of similar molecular weight (53–57,000) to that present on PHA-activated T cell blasts (Waldmann *et al.*, 1984). The level of Tac antigen expression on two activated Tac-positive B-cell lines was only 4500 and 7500 Tac receptors, respectively, whereas PHA-activated T cells express 30–60,000 receptors per cell, and an HTLV-positive adult T-cell leukemia cell line (HUT 102) expresses 150–600,000 Tac receptors per cell.

Recently, IL-2 receptor from human T cells has been purified to apparent homogeneity using anti-Tac monoclonal antibody immunoaffinity chromatography and cloned, and its N-terminal amino acids have been sequenced (Nikaido *et al.*, 1984; Leonard *et al.*, 1984.) A single gene encodes the IL-2 receptor; however, the possibility of a recently duplicated gene cannot be completely excluded. The amino acid sequence of the IL-2 receptor does not have any significant homology with any known eukaryotic or oncogenes.

Based on clones of cDNA and sequencing, a primary structure of the IL-2 receptor precursor with 272 amino acids was deduced (Nikaido *et al.*, 1984). The receptor is separated into domains by a putative 19-residue transmembrane region. Two mRNAs (1.5 and 3.5 kilobases), which differ in their polyadenylation signals, that are capable of encoding functions for IL-2 receptor have been identified. Leonard *et al.* (1984) have isolated an additional cDNA that may correspond to an alternatively spliced mRNA that lacks a 216-base segment and appears to encode an altered membrane protein that does not bind IL-2. The data from the studies of Leonard *et al.* (1984) also suggest that IL-2 receptor expression may be regulated at the level of transcription as well as through posttranscriptional changes in mRNA processing.

The entire protein sequence of the human IL-2 receptor consists of the carboxy terminus of the protein encoded by these mRNAs with a stretch of positively charged basic amino acids (six of the terminal 13 amino acids are arginines or lysines). These could be intracytoplasmic. This region contains one serine and one threonine, which may serve as potential phosphorylation sites. This region is preceded by a 19-amino-acid hydrophobic region, which could readily form a transmembrane region. There is a second hydrophobic region, which is included in the splicable region; this could represent a fold in the protein or a loop into but not through the membrane, or it may be important in binding IL-2, which also has hydrophobic regions. In addition, there are numerous serines and threonines immediately extracytoplasmic to the transmembrane region, which may serve as the potential O-linked glycosylation sites. Because of a very short cytoplasmic tail (13 amino acids), too short to mediate enzymatic activity, the mechanisms of signal transduction by this receptor remain unclear. It remains to be investigated whether the ligand itself communicates the signal to the cell or else whether other proteins serve as subunits in a receptor complex.

The interaction of IL-2 with its surface receptor is characterized by a particular high-affinity (K_d 3.5 $\times$ 10^{-12} M for human T cells). Followng T- or B-cell activation, receptors for IL-2 are expressed that parallel transformation of the cell from an IL-2-unresponsive to an IL-2-responsive state. Following binding with its receptor sites, IL-2 rapidly ($t_{1/2}$ = 20–30 min) enters a pH-4-resistant state, presumably through internalization of the IL-2–receptor complex. Thereafter, the factor undergoes lysosomal-dependent degradation ($t_{1/2}$ = 70–80 min). Preliminary studies suggest that this putative IL-2–receptor complex may be phosphorylated (Robb, 1984) and may be involved in signal transmission to the cell nucleus. Interleukin 2 binding causes cells to progress from the late G_1 phase into the S phase of the cell cycle (Bettens *et al.*, 1984). The sigmoidal dose–response curve for binding of radiolabeled IL-2 to the receptor and parallel dose–response curve to DNA synthesis, blocking of the cellular proliferation by anti-IL-2 and anti-IL-2 receptor antibodies, and time course of receptor expression clearly demonstrate that the high-affinity IL-2 receptor mediates the physiological role of IL-2 on T-cell functions.

Following activation, T cells express Tac antigen within 6 hr, and the peak level of the Tac expression is observed between 48 and 72 hr. Thereafter, IL-2 receptors decline, and by day 13 T cells resemble resting T cells and are unresponsive to IL-2. This loss of IL-2 responsiveness is restored by restimulation with antigen or lectin and is concomitant with the reexpression of IL-2 receptors (Kaplan *et al.*, 1984; Andrew *et al.*, 1984). This observation clearly demonstrates that induction and down-regulation of IL-2 receptor play a crucial role in controlling the extent of cellular response.

A number of factors regulate the expression of IL-2 receptor. Malek and Shevach (1984) have shown that IL-2 receptor expression on normal Lyt^- T cells is accessory-cell dependent. Kay *et al.* (1984) also reported the requirement of IL-1 in the induction of IL-2 receptor on a cloned murine helper T-cell line. Recently, Welte *et al.* (1984) and Reem and Yeh (1984) have shown that IL-2 up-regulates the expression of IL-2 receptor on activated T cells. Waldmann *et al.* (1984) have also shown that IL-2 increases the expression of Tac antigen on a B-cell line (5B5) from 520 to 4500 Tac antigens per cell. This suggests that IL-2 also influences the number of IL-2 receptors expressed on B cells.

The requirement for RNA transcription and protein synthesis suggests that *de novo* receptor synthesis is occurring rather than the unmasking of cryptic receptors. Phorbol myristic acetate (PMA) also induces IL-2 receptor expression on both Tac-negative leukemic T-cell lines (Greene *et al.*, 1984) and normal human T cells (Depper *et al.*, 1984b). Greene *et al.* (1984), using JURKAT and HSB-2 cell lines, showed that the signals required for IL-2 synthesis and IL-2 receptor expression are not identical and that induction of Tac antigen and IL-2 production are not obligately linked in these cells. The expression of Tac antigen is inhibited by actinomycin D and cycloheximide but not by mitomycin C (Depper *et al.*, 1984a) or γ radiation (Waldmann *et al.*, 1984), demonstrating the requirement of *de novo* RNA and protein synthesis but not DNA synthesis. Phospholipase C has also been shown to augment the expression of IL-2 receptors (Depper *et al.*, 1984a).

The fact that both PMA and phospholipase C activate protein kinase C suggests that activation of protein kinase C may induce IL-2 receptor expression. Miyawaki *et al.* (1983) showed that cyclosporin A, although it inhibits the DNA synthesis, did not inhibit IL-2 receptor expression on lectin-stimulated T cells. Similar findings were found with potassium-channel blockers that blocked DNA synthesis but had no significant influence on Tac expression on PHA-activated human T cells (Chandy *et al.*, 1984; Gupta *et al.*, 1984, 1985). Both cyclosporin A and potassium-channel blockers inhibit the production of IL-2. In collaboration with W. C. Greene, we have observed that potassium-channel blockers inhibit 80% of the Tac message. Therefore, it would appear that 20% of the Tac message could be independent of K^+ channel and might explain the lack of response of K^+ channel blockers on Tac expression. Kronker *et al.* (1984) have shown that cyclosporin A inhibits IL-2 gene expression at the level of mRNA transcription.

D. Biological Effects of Interleukin 2

Interleukin 2 has been useful in generating long-term clones of helper, suppressor, and cytotoxic T cells that have facilitated their functional studies in terms of immunoregulatory and effector functions as well as their capacity to produce a variety of other soluble mediators capable of influencing the functions of other cell types.

1. Cytotoxic T Cells

Activation and proliferation of cytotoxic T lymphocytes (CTL) appear to require specific antigen and IL-2. After interaction with specific antigen, precursors of CTL (P-CTL) express receptors for IL-2; the binding of IL-2 to IL-2 receptors results in the differentiation and proliferation of P-CTL into effector cytotoxic T cells (Pactkau *et al.*, 1976; Wagner and Rollinghoff, 1978; Lalande *et al.*, 1980; Symington and Teh, 1980; Teh and Teh, 1980). It is possible that more than one factor is required for the proliferation and differentiation of P-CTL into CTL effectors (Raulet and Bevan, 1982; Wagner *et al.*, 1982). It has been possible, however, to establish long-term CTL lines or helper T-cell lines by IL-2-containing culture medium (Schreier *et al.*, 1980; Gillis and Smith, 1977; Nabholz *et al.*, 1978; Von Boehmer *et al.*, 1979). The addition of IL-2 and specific allogeneic stimulator cells has resulted in antigen-specific P-CTL differentiation to antigen-specific effector CTL (Teh and Teh, 1980; Symington and Teh, 1980; MacDonald *et al.*, 1980). This approach has been used in determining the frequencies of allospecific P-CTL and fine specificity of CTL clones, analysis of the CTL repertoire, and for the limiting-dilution analyses of primary CTL responses to nonalloantigens, e.g., viral antigens (Symington and Teh, 1980; MacDonald *et al.*, 1980; Wagner *et al.*, 1981). Schreier *et al.* (1980) demonstrated that both CTL and helper T-cell clones require IL-2 absolutely for their growth and survival; however, only helpers and not CTL clones are able to interact with accessory cells to initiate the mechanisms leading to IL-2 release in culture.

Recent studies have shown that nonspecific CTL can be induced by IL-2-containing supernatants (Teh *et al.*, 1981). These nonspecific CTL are a potential source of interference in the analysis of the specificities and frequency of antigen-specific CTL clones in limiting-dilution assays for P-CTL. More recently, Teh and Yu (1983) described some of the parameters for the induction of nonspecific CTL by IL-2-containing supernatants in the absence of antigenic stimulation. These investigators were able to generate nonspecific killer cells by culturing C57BL/6 lymph node or spleen cells with IL-2-containing supernatants obtained from PMA-stimulated EL4 T-cell lymphoma or Con-A-stimulated rat spleen cells. The induction of cytotoxic cells by IL-2 was sensitive to γ radiation. The majority of P-CTL and effector CTL bear Thy-1 alloantigens and therefore are T cells. These nonspecific killer cells have cytotoxicity against a broad spectrum of target cells. The frequency of nonspecific P-CTL in C57BL/6 lymph node and spleen cells is 1/7000 and 1/12,000 respectively. The induction of nonspecific killer cells by IL-2-containing supernatants is partially dependent on nylon-wool-adherent cells. Since these nonspecific CTL can kill syngeneic splenic blasts efficiently, they are unlikely to be natural killer (NK) cells.

Interleukin 2 has been used to grow cytotoxic T cells capable of killing autologous or syngeneic leukemic cells. Murine spleen cells primed against friend leukemia cells have been sustained in IL-2-containing medium (Gillis and Smith, 1977). These T cells retain specific cytolytic activity against leukemic cells. Similarly, lymphocytes from leukemic patients in remission have been cultured with irradiated autologous blasts and IL-2-containing medium (Zarling and Bach, 1979).

Although evidence supports IL-2 modulation of *in vitro* immune responses, only a few studies have reported *in vivo* effects of IL-2. Wagner *et al.* (1981) reported induction of CTL activity in nude mice after *in vivo* treatment with IL-2-containing supernatants; however, purified IL-2 was not used. Gillis (1983) examined *in vivo* influence of purified IL-2 on the generation of CTL effector function in BALB/c mice immunized with EL-4 tumor cells intraperitoneally. An augmentation of CTL activity was observed. Since cytotoxic activity was specific for the appropriate H-2 haplotype, it appeared that the augmented cytolytic activity seen following IL-2 administration was T-cell mediated. Further characterization of effector cells confirmed T-cell lineage.

It remains to be determined whether specific CTL could be used for adoptive immunotherapy for solid tumors; the potentials are real.

2. *Natural Killer Cells*

It has recently been shown that human NK cells express IL-2 receptors, and NK clones have been propagated in IL-2-containing medium (Abo *et al.*, 1983; Ortaldo and Herberman, 1984). Trinchiari *et al.* (1984) reported IL-2-mediated enhancement of NK activity. Henney *et al.* (1981) and Minato *et al.* (1981) have shown *in vitro* enhancement of NK activity in murine spleen cells incubated with purified IL-2. Abo *et al.* (1983) demonstrated the presence of Tac antigen on a subset of HNK-1$^+$ large granular cells that carry T-cell markers (Leu 4 antigen or receptors for sheep erythrocytes). These cells require polyclonal mitogen or allogeneic stimulation to express IL-2 receptor and will undergo proliferation in the presence of IL-2. Interleukin-2-containing Con-A-activated murine spleen cell supernatants have been used to sustain NK cells in suspension and to clone murine NK cells (Dennert *et al.*, 1981). These cells have no antibody-dependent cellular cytotoxicity (ADCC) but were able to kill all NK targets used in routine assays. In addition, cloned cell lines mediating both NK and ADCC have been described, suggesting a single cell type mediating both functions (Nabel *et al.*, 1981).

The stimulation of NK by IL-2 is more pronounced than that of interferon and synergistic to the stimulatory effect of interferon (Ortaldo *et al.*, 1984). It is likely that the potentiating effect of IL-2 on NK activity is in part related to its capacity to induce production of γ-interferon. Gillis (1983) investigated whether the IL-2 could enhance NK-cell response *in vivo*. A significant augmentation of cytolytic activity of splenic cells from CBA/J mice against a YAC-1 target was observed 48 hr following *in vivo* administration of IL-2. They further demonstrated that the augmentation of cytotoxic activity was against NK-susceptible targets that could be killed by appropriately sensitized CTL. These data suggest that the augmentation of splenic cytolytic activity observed after 48 hr of *in vivo* IL-2 administration was mediated by NK cells.

3. Helper T Cells

Antigen-specific helper T-cell clones have been developed in the presence of exogenous IL-2 (Schreier *et al.*, 1980). These clones will support an antibody response to the antigen in T-cell-depleted cultures of spleen cells. The frequency of specific helper T cells in antigen-stimulated spleen cells may be as high as one in 1000 depending on the priming schedule. Restimulation with antigen and accessory cells is not a prerequisite for maintenance of specific helper function. Cloned helper T cells release humoral factors that influence the growth of T cells, B cells, macrophages, and myeloid and erythroid progenitor cells. These factors include macrophage colony-stimulating factor (Stanley *et al.*, 1976), granulocyte colony-stimulating factor(s) (Williams *et al.*, 1978), erythroid and mixed myeloid and erythroid burst-promoting activity (Johnson and Metcalf, 1977; Iscove, 1978), and IL-2 and B-cell growth-factor activity.

4. Suppressor T Cells

The generation of a SRBC-specific suppressor T-cell line has been reported (Fresno *et al.*, 1981a,b). Antigen-activated Lyt $1^{-}2^{+}3^{+}$ cells were sorted and then grown in the presence of IL-2. The resultant cell line exerted antigen-specific suppression of the generation of antibody-forming cells. This cell line released a 70,000-dalton polypeptide, which dissociated into two 45,000- and 24,000-dalton polypeptides. The 70,000-dalton polypeptide specifically bound to SRBC glycophorin and suppressed the effect of antigen-specific helper T cells added to the cultures. This suggests that suppressor T cells are also capable of growing in the presence of IL-2 and maintaining their suppressor function. Recently, a soluble suppressor for B-cell immunoglobulin synthesis has been identified in a human suppressor T-cell line (Fleisher *et al.*, 1981).

Analysis of suppressor T-cell clones suggests that they share several properties with antibody-forming B cells (Cantor, 1981). Both have receptors that bind antigens in the absence of MHC products and are regulated by soluble factors from helper T cells (Fresno *et al.*, 1981a,b). Ting *et al.* (1984) also reported induction of suppressor T cells by interleukin 2. In *nu*/*nu* spleen cells, higher concentrations of IL-2 support the T-cell growth, whereas lower concentrations are needed to generate alloreactive CTL. It has also been shown that the addition of a high concentration of IL-2 suppressed the generation of alloreactive CTL in a conventional mixed lymphocyte culture (MLC) reaction. A high concentration of IL-2 induced the generation of antigen-nonspecific suppressor T cells in normal spleen cell cultures and augmented the antigen-specific suppressor T cells in MLC. These suppressor cells could be induced by rat, murine, and human IL-2 preparations and suppressed the generation of CTL in fresh MLC and in polyclonal CTL cultures.

The ability to induce suppressor cells correlated with the activity of IL-2 present in these preparations and was independent of their ability to induce cytotoxic effectors. These data suggest a dual role of IL-2 in the regulation of CTL responses. It appears that during antigen sensitization, the initial endogenous production of lower levels of IL-2 provides the second signal for the differentiation and proliferation of CTL; when higher levels of IL-2 are produced later, the suppressor T-cell precursors are activated and differentiated into suppressor effectors that regulate the CTL response.

5. Lymphokine Production

Interleukin 2 has been shown to induce secretion of γ-interferon by T cells (Farrar *et al.*, 1981). This is one of the mechanisms by which IL-2 augments natural killer activity. γ-Interferon also affects generation of CTL, macrophage activation, and MHC antigen expression, and therefore IL-2 could play (indirectly) an important role in several immune responses.

Recently, Howard *et al.* (1983) reported induction with highly purified IL-2 of T-cell lines that secrete B-cell growth factor I (BCGF-I). Supernatants from these antigen-stimulated T-cell lines are not directly mitogenic for resting B cells but synergize in an H_2-unrestricted manner with anti-Ig-activated B cells to produce polyclonal proliferation but not antibody-forming-cell development. Analysis of the mechanism of BCGF-I production by antigen-stimulated T cells showed that optimum amounts of BCGF-I were obtained as quickly as 24 hr post-stimulation and that the factor-producing cells in the T-cell line bore the Lyt 1^+2^- phenotype. The activation of normal T-cell lines to produce BCGF-I requires either antigen presented in the context of syngeneic antigen-presenting cells of IL-2.

6. B Lymphocytes

Recent evidence suggests that activated B lymphocytes express receptors of IL-2 (Waldmann *et al.*, 1984); therefore, IL-2 appears to have direct effects on certain B-cell functions. These investigators showed inhibition by anti-Tac antibody of induced immunoglobulin synthesis by rigorously T-cell-depleted B cells. Robb *et al.* (1984) and Tsudo *et al.* (1984) have reported a direct effect of IL-2 on anti-Ig-induced B-cell proliferation. Waldmann *et al.* (1984) reported producing two- to fourfold increases in immunoglobulin production in the absence of a concomitant increase in cell number by a cloned B-cell line (5B4) from a normal individual by addition of purified IL-2. This increase in immunoglobulin synthesis was blocked completely by the addition of anti-Tac antibody. Augmentation of immunoglobulin synthesis in conjunction with the observation that neither IL-2 nor anti-Tac affected DNA replication by these B cells suggests that IL-2 can facilitate the terminal differentiation by B cells.

E. CONCLUSIONS

It has been apparent from the foregoing description that IL-2 is not merely a T-cell growth factor but also regulates the differentiation and proliferation of immunoregulatory and cytotoxic precursor T cells, induces production of various lymphokines, augments the NK function, and induces proliferation and differentiation of B cells to immunoglobulin-synthesizing and -secreting cells.

III. INTERLEUKIN 1

The antigen-specific activation of T cells is dependent on two distinct interdependent macrophage signals. The initial signal is to present antigen in conjunction with Ia antigen, and the second signal is provided by a low-molecular-weight antigen-nonspecific peptide, interleukin 1 (IL-1), by inducing synthesis and secretion of IL-2. Therefore, the link between IL-1 and IL-2 involves the conversion of a macrophage-derived maturational signal to a secondary T-cell-derived proliferative response that in turn determines the tempo of immune response. It appears that IL-1 may permit the macrophage to regulate *in vivo* behavior of a variety of cell types that are involved in immunologic and inflammatory reactions.

Interleukin 1 is the term used for previously described factors that were given names according to their biological effects; these included endogenous pyrogen, lymphocyte-activating factor, leukocyte endogenous mediator, B-cell-activating factor, thymocyte proliferating factor, helper peak-1, mononuclear cell factor, mitogenic proteins, and T-cell-replacing factor III. The subject of IL-1 has recently been reviewed (Dinarello, 1984a,b; Oppenheim *et al.*, 1982; Mizel, 1982), and therefore only salient features are discussed here.

A. Production of IL-1

The production of IL-1 has been demonstrated by the use of the endogenous pyrogen (EP) assay in rabbits, by the lymphocyte-activating factor (LAF) assay, by the capacity to proliferate murine thymocytes to submitogenic doses of mitogen, and by the leukocyte endogenous mediator (LEM) assay for the induction of acute-phase responses (c-reactive protein, decrease in serum iron and zinc, and increase in fibrinogen and neutrophil counts). The LAF or thymocyte proliferation is the most commonly used assay to measure IL-1 activity. It is based on the principle that IL-1 in the presence of lectin induces thymocytes to produce IL-2, which results in [^{3}H]thymidine incorporation by thymocytes. By these assays, IL-1 has been shown to be produced by almost all the cells of monocyte–macrophage lineage.

A list of the cell sources for IL-1 is given in Table 1. The majority of these cells have now been shown to possess the property of antigen presentation as well. Recently, Sauder (1984) has shown that both Langerhans cells and keratinocytes of the skin produce a factor similar to IL-1, termed epidermal cell thymocyte-activating factor (ETAF). It is also a 15,000-molecular-weight factor that enhances thymocyte proliferation, stimulates cells in the hypothalamus to mediate fever, stimulates leukocyte chemotaxis and hepatic synthesis of acute-phase proteins, induces muscle proteolysis, and augments IL-2 production and autocrine growth stimulation. Mayernik *et al.* (1984) demonstrated that fresh monocytes secrete IL-1 readily in response to lipopolysaccharide (LPS) and latex particles. Macrophages cultured for 2 or more days *in vitro* failed to produce significant IL-1 activity. This failure of monocytes does not appear to be caused by the presence of an inhibitor. Stimulated T cells, when cultured with macrophages, do not correct this defect. Both murine and human placental mononuclear phagocytic cells are rich sources of IL-1 (Flynn *et al.*, 1982).

It is unclear at this writing whether the resting monocytes produce IL-1 spontaneously, although such claims have been made, but in these circumstances, "spontaneous" IL-1 production was caused by contaminating traces of endotoxin in the culture medium. A large number of agents that stimulate monocyte–macrophage cells, induce IL-1 production. A list of IL-1 inducers is given in Table 2. Antigen–antibody complexes in antigen excess or Fc fragments trigger IL-1 production, presumably via the surface Fc

Table 1. Interleukin-1-Producing Cells[a]

Peripheral blood monocytes
Synovial membrane macrophages
Pulmonary alveolar macrophages
Splenic macrophages
Peritoneal macrophages
Kupffer's cells of liver
Placental macrophages
Bone marrow adherent cells
Monocytic and myelomonocytic leukemia cells and cell lines
Hodgkin's lymphoma cell line
Astrocytes
Keratinocytes and Langerhans cells of skin
Corneal epithelial cells
Renal mesangial cells
Vascular endothelial cells
Renal cell carcinoma

[a] Modified from Dinarello, 1984.

receptors of the macrophage (Blyden and Handschumacher, 1977; Dayer *et al.*, 1980). Lectin-induced IL-1 production appears to be indirectly mediated via the production of lymphokines. γ-Interferon appears to increase IL-1 production by activated macrophages by suppressing PGE_2 production by macrophages (Boraschi *et al.*, 1984).

Not all stimulators of phagocytic cells result in IL-1 production. This could be because of increased PGE_2 synthesis by these agents, because PGE_2 will inhibit IL-1 production. Tuftsin, N-formyl-Met-Leu-Phe, levamisole, and $NaIO_2$ activate macrophages but do not stimulate IL-1 production. Phagocytosis of a microorganism is not a necessary event for IL-1 induction, although adherence of spirochetes to monocytes results in IL-1 production. Similarly, silica and urate crystals induce IL-1 production but do not require their phagocytosis. Therefore, it is evident that the activation of mononuclear phagocytic cell surface is critical for the induction of IL-1.

The process of membrane activation leading to IL-1 production involves products of lipoxygenation. Interleukin 1 is an inducible protein requiring new RNA and protein synthesis. Activation of mononuclear phagocytes to produce IL-1 requires contact with inducing agents for less than 1 hr. There is little evidence to suggest that IL-1 is preformed or stored. Once induced, IL-1 is detectable intracellularly, and most of it is secreted into the medium within 3–12 hr. There are, however, certain murine and human cell lines that spontaneously secrete IL-1.

Recently, it has been shown that macrophages have receptors for C5a, and purified C5a will induce IL-1 production (Goodman *et al.*, 1982). Ia or DR expression on the surface of mononuclear phagocytic cells is important for IL-1 production. It is not clear whether Ia antigen is required for the activation, synthesis, or secretion steps involved in IL-1 production. The role of Ia in IL-1 production is of particular interest because γ-interferon increases IL-1 production and also increased expression of Ia on murine macrophages. Phorbol myristic acetate is a low-molecular-weight tumor promoter and an agonist of IL-1: PMA is known to activate directly protein kinase C, which, when bound to free intracellular Ca^{2+}, will lead to cellular activation. Recently, Fontana *et al.* (1984)

Table 2. Inducers/Enhancers of Interleukin 1 Production[a]

Mitogens
Phytohemagglutinin
Concanavalin A
Antigens
Alloantigens
Microbial antigens
Nonmicrobial antigens
Lymphokines
Colony-stimulating factor
γ-Interferon
Macrophage-activating factor
Microorganisms
Viruses
Bacteria
Spirochetes
Microbial products
E. coli lipopolysaccharide
Endotoxin from gram-negative bacteria
Peptidoglycans
Some exotoxins
Tumor promoters
TPA (12-O-tetradecanoylphorbol-13-acetate)
PMA (Phorbol myristate acetate)
Others
Polysaccharide from plant *Echinacea purpurea*
Bile acids
C5a
Immune complexes
Bleomycin
Silica and urate crystals
Latex particles
Butyrates

[a]Modified from Dinarello, 1984.

have shown the production of IL-1-like substance from a glioblastoma cell line. In addition, this cell line also produces an inhibitor of IL-2 mediated effects.

A number of agents are known to regulate IL-1 production by macrophages or macrophage cell lines. Addition of indomethacin enhances IL-1 production, suggesting that PGE_2 inhibits IL-1 production. This is supported by the fact that γ-interferon increases IL-1 production by inhibiting PGE_2 release (Boraschi *et al.*, 1984). Corticosteroids and cyclosporin A have also been shown to inhibit IL-1 production. We have recently shown that K^+ channel blockers will inhibit IL-1 production by the $P388D_1$ cell line and human macrophages (Vayuvegula *et al.*, 1985). Actinomycin, cycloheximide, and puromycin also block IL-1 production.

B. Physical, Chemical, and Molecular Characterization of IL-1

Experiments using inhibitors of mRNA and protein synthesis have established that new mRNA synthesis and its translation into new protein are required for the production of biologically active IL-1. Evidence that IL-1 is newly synthesized protein has been obtained by translation of mRNA in frog oocytes and assay of biological activity of IL-1 in culture supernatants. Interleukin 1 activity is destroyed by proteases such as pronase or proteinase K. Mizel (1982) reported that murine IL-1 is resistant to treatment with several endopeptidases including trypsin, chymotrypsin, and papain as well as several exopeptidases, including lucine aminopeptidase and carboxypeptidase A. It is sensitive to papain in 8 M urea. Oppenheim *et al.* (1982) have reported that human IL-1 is sensitive to chymotrypsin and urea but resistant to trypsin and papain. Interleukin 1 is also resistant to neuraminidase, ribonuclease, and serine esterase inhibitors (Dinarello, 1984a). The relative insensitivity of IL-1 to proteolytic attack may have physiological significance in inflammatory processes.

In the murine system, the P388D$_1$ cell line has been a good source of IL-1, although three other cell lines also actively produce IL-1. Mizel (1982) reported that IL-1 is an approximately 15,000-dalton protein. The results of gel filtration studies with biological activities for IL-1 derived from several species have demonstrated a molecular weight of 14,000–17,000 on Sephadex and Biogel. Higher molecular weights have also been reported (35,000–60,000). It has also been observed that in addition to the 15,000-dalton species in serum-free medium a 35,000- to 40,000-molecular-weight protein is also secreted. It is possible that the higher-molecular-weight species is a precursor of the 15,000-dalton species.

Auron *et al.* (1984) have recently isolated human IL-1 cDNA that encodes a precursor polypeptide of 269 amino acids (30,747 molecular weight). Messenger RNA isolated by hybridization to this cDNA, on translation in a reticulocyte cell-free system, yielded immunoprecipitable IL-1. This hybridized mRNA, when injected into *Xenopus laevis* oocytes, secreted biologically active IL-1. The cDNA nucleotide sequence suggests that IL-1 is initially translated as a large-molecular-weight precursor molecule that is subsequently cleaved into an approximately 15,000-dalton species with biological activities of IL-1. Recently, Dinarello *et al.* (1984) have purified a 4.2-kd peptide from the plasma of febrile humans. This small-molecular-weight peptide will induce muscle proteolysis *in vitro* and is active in the thymocyte proliferation assay. The 4.2-kd peptide appears to be a cleavage product of the 15,000-dalton IL-1 that can mediate several IL-1 functions. It is also suggested that *in vivo* IL-1 may circulate in this small-molecular-weight cleavage form.

C. Biological Effects of IL-1

Interleukin 1 has several effects on the immune system as well as on cells outside the immune system. Therefore, the biological effects of IL-1 are discussed under two separate headings, namely, effects on the immune system and on nonimmune systems.

1. Immunologic Effects of Interleukin 1

a. Cells of T-Cell Lineage. The role of IL-1 in T-cell proliferation and generation of helper T cells and cytotoxic T cells is well established. More recently, IL-1 has been shown to support the expansion of suppressor T cells as well. All of these effects of IL-1 have a common pathway, that is, the induction of IL-2. The stimulation of IL-2 synthesis by IL-1 is dependent on the presence of another activating signal, either a specific antigen or a polyclonal mitogen (Con A or PHA). In the lectin system, the requirement for a macrophage can be completely replaced by TPA or PMA; however, in antigen-specific T-cell proliferation, TPA or PMA cannot replace the macrophage requirement because the macrophages are essential for processing and presentation of antigen.

The nature of the interplay between the IL-1 and antigen signal is not well understood. One possibility is that IL-1 may convert target cells to a primed state during which they develop the capacity to bind specific antigen. This IL-1-mediated activation step may involve the induction of the synthesis of cell surface receptors on T cells for antigens. Interleukin 1 increases the frequency of T-cell binding of synthetic antigen (Puri *et al.* 1980). Kaye *et al.* (1984) have shown evidence that IL-1 is required for the expression of IL-2 receptors on a cloned helper T-cell line. Therefore, IL-1 is required for the induction of IL-2 production and for the expression of IL-2 receptors on T cells. Phenotypic characterization of the thymocytes that produce IL-2 in the presence of IL-1 plus PHA or Con A revealed them to be $Ly2^-$, PNA^- (helper/inducer phenotype) T cells. Interleukin 1 has also been shown to enhance the generation of stable binding between sheep erythrocytes and human T cells. This occurs through the induction of new receptors on T cells. It is interesting in this context that stable rosette-forming T cells are increased in rheumatoid arthritis (Galili *et al.*, 1979). Interleukin 1 could also regulate the cell surface phenotype of immature thymocytes: IL-1-treated cortical thymocytes exhibit a marked decrease in Thy 1 and Ly 2 surface markers, the phenotype changes that are characteristic of thymocyte maturation. Interleukin 1 is also chemotactic for T lymphocytes (Sauder, 1984) and could be responsible for T-cell infiltration at the local inflammatory site.

b. Cells of B-Cell Lineage. Antigen-induced antibody synthesis is dependent on the presence of macrophages and helper T cells. It is likely that IL-1 acts by enhancing the production of IL-2 and increasing the number of helper T cells. Hoffman (1980) has presented evidence that IL-1 can enhance the expression of surface Ig, complement receptors, and Ia antigens on murine B cells and increase the frequency of reactive B cells. Recent evidence has supported the view that IL-1 acts directly on cells of B-cell lineage. Giri *et al.* (1984) demonstrated that IL-1 can enhance *in vitro* functional maturation of surface-immunoglobulin-negative pre-B cells from normal bone marrow and in a pre-B-cell line. The IL-1-mediated enhancement of surface Ig expression was associated with stimulation of κ light chain synthesis. Booth and Watson (1984) demonstrated that a B-cell growth and differentiation factor that copurified with IL-1 (BGDF/IL-1) induced proliferation of two distinct murine B cells activated with IgM or dextran sulfate. Lipsky *et al.* (1983) showed evidence that IL-1 acts directly on B cells, perhaps to prepare them to receive appropriate T-cell signals. Their results support the conclusion that IL-1 plays an important role in B-cell proliferation and in the generation of immunoglobulin-secreting cells. Falkoff *et al.* (1984) demonstrated that highly purified IL-1 failed to induce Ig secretion by purified human B cells on activation with *Staphylococcus aureus* Cowan I. However, IL-1 consistently synergized with B-cell differentiation factor produced by a T–T hybrid clone. It remains to be determined whether IL-1, like IL-2, also induces the production of T-cell-derived B-cell proliferative and differentiation factors.

c. Natural Killer Cells. Dempsey *et al.* (1982) reported that IL-1 synergizes with other lymphokines to enhance NK activity against a variety of tumor targets. Interleukin 1 synergizes the effects of IL-2 and γ-interferon in enhancing NK-cell activity against both NK-sensitive and NK-resistant targets. Interleukin 1 has little or no direct effect on NK cells. This role of IL-1 supports the observed beneficial effect of the use of microbial toxins in the treatment of malignant tumors at the turn of this century.

2. Nonimmunologic Effects of Interleukin 1

a. Interleukin 1 and Fibroblasts. Several chronic inflammatory disorders are characterized by extensive granulomatous and fibrotic reactions. Fibroblast proliferation and stimulation of fibroblast secretory products are features of wound healing, granuloma formation, and the generalized process of fibrosis. Studies of *in vitro* fibroblast cultures in such disease processes have demonstrated that several mononuclear-cell-derived soluble factors stimulate fibroblast proliferation and production of collagen factor. One such factor is IL-1 (Schmidt *et al.*, 1982). Wharton *et al.* (1982) and Wharton (1983) described a macrophage-derived growth factor that caused quiescent fibroblasts to become competent to progress from G_0 phase to S and M phases of the cell cycle. Their preliminary data suggested that macrophage-derived growth factor (MDGF) was distinct from IL-1. Schmidt *et al.* (1982), however, reported that IL-1 has mitogenic activity for fibroblasts. In contrast, Bitterman *et al.* (1982) demonstrated that a human alveolar macrophage-derived factor that did not have IL-1 activity had "progressive activity" for fibroblasts. Estes *et al.* (1984) demonstrated that MDGF is biochemically and functionally distinct from IL-1; MDGF and IL-1 activities produced by $P388D_1$ cell line can be separated by gel-filtration chromatography, and MDGF has a molecular weight of approximately 56,000, whereas IL-1 has a molecular weight of 14–16,000.

The elaboration of MDGF and IL-1 activities is differentially modulated by classical macrophage activators. The RAW 264.1 cell line spontaneously produces MDGF but not IL-1. However, when the cell line is first stimulated by lymphokine-rich supernatants and then triggered by LPS, increased IL-1 production is observed, but MDGF production is completely inhibited. Antibody-purified IL-1 had no or little growth-stimulating activity for quiescent fibroblasts; however, it could do so in the presence of platelet-derived growth factor (PDGF). This could explain the observation of IL-1-induced fibroblast proliferation in serum-supplemented culture medium, which could contain minute amounts of PDGF. The mechanism of MDGF action is presently unknown. Partially purified MDGF does not have proteolytic activity.

Postlethwaite *et al.* (1983) reported that human IL-1 stimulates collagenase production by fibroblasts in a dose-dependent manner. Analysis of highly purified IL-1 revealed that thymocyte proliferation and fibroblast collagenase-stimulating activity are nondissociable. Interleukin 1 from $P388D_1$ cells has been shown to be capable of stimulating collagenase production by adherent rheumatoid synovial cells. A human mononuclear cell factor having similar effect on synovial cells has been found to have some properties common with IL-1 obtained from the $P388D_1$ cell line (Mizel *et al.*, 1980; Krane, 1975; Dayer *et al.*, 1976, 1979). Interleukin 1 may play an important role in regulating collagenase production by fibroblasts and thereby influence the remodeling of collagen at sites of inflammation *in vivo*.

b. Interleukin 1 and Acute-Phase Response. Fever is a prominent sign of the acute-phase response and is the result of an effect of IL-1 on the thermoregulatory center in the anterior hypothalamus. Interleukin 1 abruptly increases the synthesis of PGE_2 in the anterior hypothalamus, which raises the thermostatic set point and drives the mechanisms of heat conservation and heat production until blood and core temperature are elevated to match the hypothalamic set point (Dinarello and Wolff, 1982). Antipyretics reduce fever by inhibiting the cyclooxygenase pathway of arachidonic acid metabolism. Interluekin 1 may act by inducing phospholipases, which then release arachidonic acid from membrane phospholipids.

The acute response to most infectious agents is manifested by neutrophilia. Interleukin 1 increases the number and immaturity of circulating neutrophils. The release of neutrophils is apparently evoked by a direct action of IL-1 on bone marrow. Interleukin-1 is also chemotactic for neutrophils, and the local concentrations of IL-1 in inflammatory site could determine the intensity of cellular infiltration (Lugler *et al.*, 1983).

Interleukin 1 induces the synthesis of a number of acute-phase proteins by hepatocytes; however, albumin synthesis is reduced. It increases hepatic synthesis of haptoglobin, α_1-antichymotrypsin, α_1-acid glycoprotein, α_1-macroglobulin, hemopexin, ceruloplasmin, complement components, fibrinogen, c-reactive protein, and serum amyloid A protein. The increased production of plasma protein could (at least in rat hepatocytes) be mediated by an elevated level of functional mRNA.

Chronic inflammatory disorders are characterized by decreased levels of iron and zinc. Zinc is incorporated into several proteases and certain nucleic acid polymerases and transcriptases. It is also a normal component of microbial membranes and ribosomes. Therefore, both iron and zinc are essential for rapid microbial growth. The mechanism of anemia associated with infections and inflammatory diseases includes the sequestration of iron–lactoferrin complexes (Van Snick *et al.*, 1974). Interleukin 1 has also been shown to activate lactoferrin release from neutrophils (Klempner *et al.*, 1978). Therefore in anemia of chronic disease, bone marrow stores of iron are normal or even increased.

Interleukin 1 has also been shown to induce slow-wave sleep (Kreuger *et al.*, 1985). Interleukin 1 may mediate factor-5-induced sleep in the brain, possibly by its release from astrocytes. The increased sleep that accompanies many infectious diseases probably provides the host with reduced energy demands and contributes to overall efficiency of the host defense mechanism.

Muscle wasting, weakness, and atrophy are observed in chronic infections. Interleukin 1 takes part in the protein degradation process. Purified IL-1 increases urinary excretion of 3-methylhistidine when infused in guinea pigs. Interleukin 1 has also been shown to produce skeletal muscle proteolysis. It appears to induce PGE_2 synthesis either directly from muscle cells or from associated cells in the muscle strips, and PGE_2 increases lysosomal protease activity, leading to proteolysis. The effect is blocked by indomethacin as well as by removal of Ca^{2+} from the muscle. Increase in muscle fiber Ca^{2+} leads to proteolysis and increased PGE_2 production.

In summary, IL-1 has numerous immunologic and nonimmunologic biological activities. Immunologic influences require interactions with other cells (along with an antigen or mitogen), resulting in induction of lymphokine production that induces the proliferation and differentiation of suppressor, helper, and cytotoxic T cells, B-cell proliferation and differentiation, and enhanced NK activity (Fig. 1).

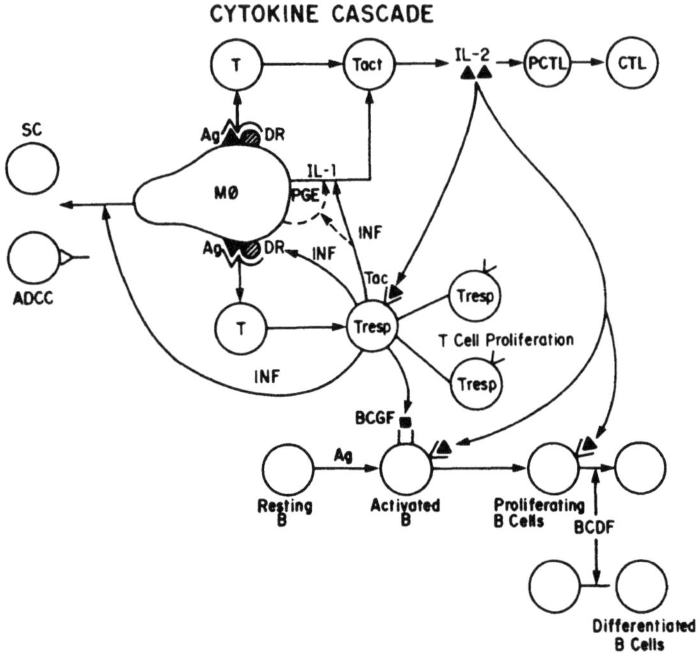

Figure 1. Cellular and cytokine interactions and their regulation. Tact, activated T cells; Tac, IL-2 receptor; IL-2, interleukin 2; Ag, antigen; IL-1, interleukin 1; pCTL, precursor cytotoxic T lymphocyte; CTL, effector cytotoxic T lymphocyte; INF, γ interferon; MØ, monocyte–macrophage; Tresp, responder T cell; BCGF, B-cell growth factor; BCDF, B-cell differentiation factor; PGE, prostaglandin E_2.

IV. INTERLEUKINS IN RHEUMATIC DISEASES

Autoimmune diseases, disorders of immunoregulation, have been studied using several animal models systems, including MRL/MP 1pr-1pr (MRL-1pr), C57BL/6-1pr, NZB/NZW F_1, and C3H-1pr/1pr mice. Animals with 1pr gene manifest an age-related autoimmune disorder that has characteristics of human SLE manifested by development of antibodies to nucleic acids, immune-complex glomerulonephritis, enhanced T-helper-cell activity, and in addition have lymphoproliferation of Lyt $1^+2^-3^-$, $Lyb5^+$ T cells. Mitogen-induced IL-2 reduction and response of T cells to exogenous IL-2 have been shown to be deficient in these animals (Dauphinee *et al.*, 1981a,b; Wofsy *et al.*, 1981; Altman *et al.*, 1981; Santoro *et al.*, 1983a,b; Talal *et al.*, 1982).

Talal *et al.* (1982) have shown that the androgen-mediated amelioration of autoimmune disease in NZB/NZW F_1 mice is associated with IL-2 activity. This led several investigators to suggest that deficiency of IL-2 production and effect is involved in the development of autoimmune disease. Davidson *et al.* (1984) reported that IL-2 production by C3H-1pr spleen and lymph node cells was normal up to 6 weeks of age and was impaired thereafter, with lymph nodes more severely affected than spleen. The IL-2 defect could be significantly repaired by the addition of PMA to the cultures. In spite of impaired

IL-2 production, Davidson *et al.* (1984) observed normal CTL responses to alloantigens. Although C3H-1pr mice share many of the lymphoid abnormalities observed in MRL-1pr mice, they do not develop the severe early-onset SLE-like disease characteristic of MRL-1pr. This suggests that a factor other than defective IL-2 is required for the development of fulminant automimmune disease. Hefeneider *et al.* (1984), using a limiting-dilution assay, demonstrated normal frequencies of IL-2 and colony-stimulating factor (CSF) in autoimmune MRL-1pr mice. This also argues against the hypothesis that deficient IL-2 production may be involved in the etiopathogenesis of autoimmune disease. This is further supported by the fact that addition of PMA to the cultures will correct the defective IL-2 production in MRL 1-1pr mice (Santoro *et al.*, 1983b).

A. Systemic Lupus Erythematosus

In patients with SLE, depressed T-cell proliferation, reduced natural killer (NK) function, and decreased γ-interferon (discussed in Chapter 5) have been described. All the above functions are regulated by IL-2, which in turn is dependent on the presence of IL-1. Findings with respect to IL-2 production and response to IL-2 in SLE have been conflicting. Alcocer-Varela *et al.* (1984), Alcocer-Varela and Alarcon-Segovia (1982), Linker-Israeli *et al.* (1983), and Miyasaka *et al.* (1984) have reported deficient production of IL-2 when T cells were stimulated with PHA, in the AMLR, or by phorbol myristate acetate (PMA).

In general, no correlation was observed between deficient IL-2 production and clinical or serologic disease activity, proportion of $OKT4^{+}$ cells, or antilymphocyte antibodies. Linker-Israeli *et al.* (1983) demonstrated that addition of purified IL-1 to lymphocyte culture of untreated SLE patients did not normalize the IL-2 production. The response of activated T cells to purified IL-2 in SLE has been reported to be deficient (Alcocer-Varela *et al.*, 1984; Alcocer-Varela and Alarcon-Segovia, 1982) or normal (Miyasaka *et al.*, 1984). Sibbitt *et al.* (1984) found normal IL-2 production in patients with SLE in response to Con A and PWM. They also demonstrated a lack of IL-2 response in the deficient NK functions in SLE (Sibbitt *et al.*, 1983). Absorption studies of purified IL-2 with activated T cells from SLE demonstrate decreased numbers of IL-2-receptor-bearing T cells or decreased numbers of IL-2 receptors per T cell in SLE (Miyasaka *et al.*, 1984, and Alcocer-Varela and Alarcon-Segovia, 1982). However, no studies have been reported for IL-2 receptor expression using anti-Tac or other IL-2 receptor monoclonal antibodies. It is also likely that decreased IL-2 response could be caused by anti-IL-2-receptor antibodies in SLE.

Interleukin 1 purification by monocytes from SLE has also been investigated. Lipopolysaccharide- or PMA-stimulated macrophages from SLE produce reduced amounts of IL-1 (Linker-Israeli *et al.*, 1983; Alcocer-Varela *et al.*, 1983). Both groups of investigators observed a decreased response of T cells to purified IL-1. The mechanism(s) for decreased IL-1 production in SLE has not been investigated. It could be related to decreased γ-interferon (which is known to increase IL-1 production by inhibiting prostaglandin E synthesis by monocytes), increased PGE production, or an intrinsic defect of monocytes. It is likely that an abnormal interleukin production or response to them could be responsible for abnormal immunoregulatory and effector functions in SLE.

B. Rheumatoid Arthritis

Dingle (1984) and Rafter (1982) proposed the hypothesis that synovial macrophages in rheumatoid arthritis patients continue to produce interleukin-1 (IL-1), which perpetuates the inflammation so characteristic of the disease. Rafter (1982) proposed that a microbe, or some part of it, enters into a joint space (subclinical stage), which initiates an inflammatory reaction with the release of IL-1 by synovial macrophages. Interleukin 1 in the joint space elicits fibroblast proliferation, enhanced collagenase and prostaglandin synthesis (Dayer *et al.*, 1981), and alteration in serum copper levels. The disturbed serum copper levels lead to altered macrophage glutathione metabolism, which promotes the disease by causing synovial macrophages to release IL-1 and by interfering with normal catabolism of IgG. The latter results in RF and immune complex formation and these are ingested by macrophages, causing release of mediators.

The role of IL-1 in RA joint pathology is further supported by some beneficial effects of chloroquin, which is known to interfere with IL-1 secretion (Salmeron and Lipsky, 1983). As a matter of fact, Bodel and Hollingsworth (1968) were first to report the presence of a pyrogen resembling endogenous pyrogen in RA joint fluid. Since endogenous or leukocyte pyrogen is indistinguishable from IL-1, their results would be consistent with the results of more recent studies. Nouri *et al.* (1984a) reported IL-1-like activity in two of 13 sera of RA patients but in 13 of 13 synovial fluids in RA. Fontana *et al.* (1982) and Ise *et al.* (1982) have also reported IL-1-like activity in synovial fluid from RA. Wood *et al.* (1983) showed the presence of an IL-1-like factor from synovial fluid of RA patients. This factor has molecular similarities to IL-1, could be elicited from an IL-1 affinity column, and exhibited lymphocyte-activating factor activity. The amount of IL-1 did not correlate with the number of macrophages, suggesting that IL-1 may be produced by both free macrophages and macrophages in the pannus, or it may be produced by synoviocytes themselves. In RA, a defect in antigen-specific suppressor T (T_s)-cell function has been reported. Keystone *et al.* (1983) examined the possibilities of whether diminished Ts activity was caused by interleukin-dependent clonal expansion of Ts cells or by prior *in vivo* activation. Patients with recent onset of RA or disease flare exhibited enhanced IL generation (IL-1 and/or IL-2). This suggests that the deficient Ts activity in RA is not a result of deficient interleukin generation. Nouri *et al.* (1984a) and Wilkins *et al.* (1983) recently reported the presence of IL-2 in the synovial fluid from patients with rheumatoid arthritis. Emery *et al.* (1984) reported IL-2-induced reconstitution of deficient cell-mediated immunity in RA.

C. Interleukins in Other Rheumatic Diseases

Alcocer-Varela *et al.* (1984) examined the production of IL-2 in 83 untreated patients with six connective tissue diseases. Interleukin 2 production in AMLR and in response to PHA was measured. Patients with mixed connective tissue disease had decreased PHA-induced IL-2 production but normal IL-2 production in AMLR. The response to IL-2 was moderately diminished. In contrast, patients with dermatopolymyositis showed decreased AMLR-induced IL-2 production but normal PHA-induced IL-2 production as well as normal response to IL-2. Patients with scleroderma had normal IL-2 production in AMLR and in response to PHA and responded normally to exogenous IL-2. Patients with Sjogren's syndrome had decreased production and decreased response to IL-2, a defect similar to that in SLE but less severe. Miyasaka *et al.* (1984) reported widely varied production and response to IL-2 in patients with Sjogren's syndrome. The differences between these two studies could reflect different patient populations and different inducing agents. Gonzalez-Amaro *et al.* (1984) reported a decreased IL-2 response on NK function in mixed connective tissue disease (MCTD) patients. In two patients, no response to IL-2 was observed. Further studies showed the presence of IgM inhibitory factor acting on the IL-2 receptor (possibly IL-2 receptor antibody). Nouri *et al.* (1984a) reported the presence of IL-1 in the synovial fluid from patients with ankylosing spondylitis, psoriatic arthritis, osteoarthritis, and rubella arthritis. This suggests that IL-1 is an important mediator in the inflammatory pathway of different types of joint diseases. More recently, Nouri *et al.* (1984b) have demonstrated varying amounts of IL-2 in synovial fluids from patients with ankylosing spondylitis, osteoarthritis, and psoriatic arthritis.

V. SUMMARY

In this chapter the physical, chemical, molecular, and biological properties of interleukin 1 and interleukin 2 are reviewed. Their role in rheumatic disease is discussed in detail.

ACKNOWLEDGMENTS. Part of work cited here was supported by grants from the U.S. Public Health Service: AG-04361, AI-20717 and AI-21808.

REFERENCES

Abo, T., Miller, C. A., Balch, C. M., and Cooper, M. D., 1983, Interleukin-2 receptor expression by activated HNK 1^+ granular lymphocytes. A requirement for their proliferation, *J. Immunol.* **131:**1822–1826.

Alcocer-Varela, J., and Alarcon-Segovia, D., 1982, Decreased production and response to interleukin-2 by cultured lymphocytes from patients with systemic lupus erythematosus, *J. Clin. Invest.* **69:**1388–1392.

Alcocer-Varela, J., Laffon, A., and Alarcon-Segovia, D., 1983, Specific monocyte production of, and T lymphocyte response to, interleukin-1 in the peripheral blood of patients with systemic lupus erythematosus, *Clin. Exp. Imunol.* **54:**125–132.

Alcocer-Varela, J., Laffon, A., and Alarcon-Segovia, D., 1984, Differences in the production of and/or the response to interleukin-2 by T lymphocytes from patients with the various connective tissue diseases, *Rheumatol. Int.* **4:**39–44.

Altman, A., Theofilopoulos, A. N., Weiner, R., Katz, K. M., and Dixon, F. J., 1981, Analysis of T cell function in autoimmune murine strain. Defects in production of and responsiveness to interleukin-2, *J. Exp. Med.* **154:**791–808.

Andrew, M. E., Braciale, V. L., and Braciale, T. J., 1984, Regulation of interleukin 2 receptor expression on murine cytotoxic T lymphocyte clones, *J. Immunol.* **132:**839–844.

Auron, P. E., Webb, A. C., Rossenwasser, L. J., Mucci, S. F., Rich, A., Wolff, S. M., and Dinarello, C. A., 1984, Nucleotide sequence of human monocyte interleukin-1 precursor DNA, *Proc. Natl. Acad. Sci. U.S.A.* **81:**7907–7911.

Baker, P. E., Fahey, J., and Munck, A., 1981, Prostaglandin inhibition of T-cell proliferation is mediated at low levels, *Cell Immunol.* **61:**52–61.

Bettens, F., Kristensen, F., Walker, C., Bonnard, G. D., and DeWeck, A. L., 1984, Lymphokine regulation of human lymphocyte proliferation: Formation of resting G_0 cells by removal of interleukin-2 in cultures of proliferating T lymphocytes, *Cell. Immunol.* **86:**337–346.

Bitterman, P. B., Rennard, S. I., Hunninghake, G. W., and Crystal, R. G., 1982, Human alviolar macrophage growth factor for fibroblasts. Regulation and partial characterization, *J. Clin. Invest.* **70**:806.

Blyden, G., and Handschumacher, R. E., 1977, Purification and properties of human lymphocyte activating factor (LAF), *J. Immunol.* **118**:1631–1638.

Bodel, P. T., and Hollingsworth, J. W., 1968, Pyrogen release from human synovial exudate cells, *Br. J. Exp. Pathol.* **49**:11–19.

Bonnard, G. D., Yasaka, K., and Maca, R. D., 1980, Continuous growth of functional human T Lymphocytes: Production of human T cell growth factor, *Cell. Immunol.* **51**:390–401.

Booth, R. J., and Watson, J. D., 1984, Interleukin-1 induces proliferation in two distinct B cell subpopulations responsive to two different murine B cell growth factors, *J. Immunol.* **133**:1346–1349.

Boraschi, D., Censini, S., and Tagliabue, A., 1984, Interferon-2 reduces macrophage-suppressive activity by inhibiting prostaglandin E_2 release and inducing interleukin-1 production, *J. Immunol.* **133**:764–768.

Cantor, H., 1981, Regulation of immune responses: Analysis with lymphocyte clones, *Cell* **25**:7–8.

Chandy, K. G., DeCoursey, T. E., Cahalan, M. D., McLanghlin, C., and Gupta, S., 1984, Voltage-gated potassium channels are required for human T lymphocyte activation, *J. Exp. Med.* **160**:369–385.

Chandy, K. G., DeCoursey, T. E., Cahalan, M. D., and Gupta, S., 1985a, Electroimmunity: The physiological role of ion channels in the immune system, *J. Immunol.* (in press).

Chandy, K. G., DeCoursey, T. E., Cahalan, M. D., and Gupta, S., 1985b, Ion channels in T lymphocytes, *J. Clin. Immunol.* **5**:1–7.

Dauphinee, M. J., Kipper, S. B., Wofsy, D., and Talal, N., 1981a, Interleukin-2 deficiency is a common feature of autoimmune mice, *J. Immunol.* **127**:2483–2487.

Dauphinee, M. J., Kipper, S., Roskos, K., Wofsy, D., and Talal, N., 1981b, Deficient interleukin-2 activity in MRL/MP and C57B1/6J mice bearing Lpr gene, *J. Exp. Med.* **154**:1671–1680.

Davidson, W. F., Roths, J. B., Holmes, K. L., Rudikoft, E., and Morse III, H. C., 1984, Dissociation of severe lupus-like disease from polyclonal B cell activation and IL-2 Deficiency in C3H-1pr/lpR mice, *J. Immunol.* **133**:1048–1056.

Dayer, J. M., Krane, S. M., Russel, R. G. G., and Robinson, D. R., 1976, Production of collagenase and prostaglandin by isolated adherent rheumatoid synovial cells, *Proc. Natl. Acad. Sci. U.S.A.* **73**:945–949.

Dayer, J. M., Breard, J., Chess, L., and Krane, S. M., 1979, Participation of monocyte–macrophage and lymphocytes in the production of a factor that stimulates collagenase and prostaglandin released by rheumatoid synovial cells, *J. Clin. Invest.* **64**:1384–1392.

Dayer, J. M., Passwell, J. H., Schneeberger, E. F., and Krane, S. M., 1980, Interactions among rheumatoid synovial cells and monocyte-macrophages: 1. Description and partial biochemical analysis, *J. Exp. Med.* **142**:151–160.

Dayer, J. M., Stephenson, M. L., Schmidt, E., Karge, W., and Krane, S. M., 1981, Purification of a factor from human blood monocytes macrophages which stimulates the production of collagenase and prostaglandin E2 by cells cultured from rheumatoid synovial tissue, *FEBS Lett.* **124**:253–256.

DeCoursey, T. E., Chandy, K. G., Gupta, S., and Cahalan, M. D., 1984, Voltage gated K^+ channel in human T lymphocytes: A role in mitogenesis? *Nature* **307**:465–468.

Dempsey, R. A., Dinarello, C. A., Mier, J. W., Rosenwasser, L. J., Allegrelta, M., Brown T. E., and Parkinson, D. R., 1982, The differentiation effects of human leukocytic pyrogen/lymphocyte human activating factor, T cell growth factor and interferon on human natural killer activity, *J. Immunol.* **129**:2504–2510.

Dennert, G., Yogeeswaran, G., and Yamagata, S., 1981, Cloned cell lines with natural killer activity: Specificity, function and cell surface markers, *J. Exp. Med.* **153**:545–556.

Depper, J. M., Leonard, W. J., Kronke, M., Waldmann, T. A., and Greene, W. C., 1984a, Augmentated T cell growth factor receptor expression in HTLV 1-infected human leukemic T cells, *J. Immunol.* **133**:1691–1695.

Depper, J. M., Leonard, W. J., Kronke, M., Noguchi, P. D., Cunningham, R. E., Waldmann, T. A., and Greene, W. C., 1984, Regulation of interleukin-2 receptor expression: Effect of phorbol diester, phospholipase C and reexposure to lectin or antigen, *J. Immunol.* **133**:3054–3061.

Devos, R., Plaetinck, G., Cheronte, H., Simons, G., Degrave, W., Traverniere, J., Remout, E., and Fiers, W., 1983, Molecular cloning of human interleukin-2 cDNA and its expression in *E. coli*, *Nucleic Acid Res.* **11**:4307–4323.

Dinarello, C. A., 1984a, Interleukin 1, *Rev. Infect. Dis.* **6**:51–95.

Dinarello, C. A., 1984b, Interleukin 1 and the pathogenesis of the acute phase response, *N. Engl. J. Med.* **311**:1413–1418.

Dinarello, C. A., and Wolff, S. M., 1982, Molecular basis of fever in humans, *Am. J. Med.* **72**:799–819.

Dinarello, C. A., Clowes, Jr., G. H. A., Gordon, H., Saraves, C. A., and Wolff, S. M., 1984, Cleavage of human interleukin 1: Isolation of a peptide fragment from plasma of febrile humans and activated monocytes, *J. Immunol.* **133**:1332–1338.

Dingle, J. T., 1984, The role of cellular interactions in joint erosions, *Clin. Orthoped.* **182**:24–30.

Emery, P., Panayi, G. S., and Nouri, A. E. E., 1984, Interleukin-2 reverses deficient cell mediated immune responses in rheumatoid arthritis, *Clin. Exp. Immunol.* **57**:123–129.

Erfat, S., Pilo, S., and Kaempfer, R., 1982, Kinetics of induction and molecular size of mRNAs encoding human interleukin-2 and gamma interferon, *Nature* **297**:236–239.

Estes, J. E., Pledger, W. J., and Gillespie, G. Y., 1984, Macrophage-derived growth factor for fibroblasts and interleukin-1 are distinct entities, *J. Leuko. Biol.* **35**:115–129.

Falkoff, R. J. M., Butler, J. L., Dinarello, C. A., and Fauci, A. S., 1984, Direct effects of a monoclonal B cell differentiation factor and of purified interleukin-1 on B cell differentiation, *J. Immunol.* **133**:692–696.

Farrar, W. L., Johnson, H. M., and Farrar, J. J., 1981, Regulation of the production of immune interferon and cytotoxic T lymphocytes by interleukin 2, *J. Immunol.* **126**:1120.

Fleisher, T. A., Greene, W. C., Uchiama, T., Goldman, C. K., Nelson, D. L., Blaese, R. M., and Waldmann, T. A., 1981, Characterization of a soluble suppressor of human B cell immunoglobulin biosynthesis produced by a continuous human suppressor T cell line, *J. Exp. Med.* **154**:156–167.

Flynn, A., Finke, J. H., and Hilfiker, M. L., 1982, Placental mononuclear phagocytes as a source of interleukin-1, *Science* **218**:475–477.

Fontana, A., Hengartner, H., Weber, E., Fehr, K., Grob, P. J., and Cohen, G., 1982, Interleukin-1 activity in synovial fluid of patients with rheumatoid arthritis, *Rheumatol. Int.* **2**:49–53.

Fontana, A., Hengartner, H., DeTribolet, N., and Weber, E., 1984, Glioblastoma cells release interleukin-1 and factors inhibiting interleukin-2-mediated effects, *J. Immunol.* **132**:1837–1844.

Fresno, M., Nabel, G., McVay-Boudreau, L., Furthmayer, H., and Cantor, H., 1981a, Antigen-specific T lymphocyte clones. I. Characterization of a T cell clone expressing antigen-specific suppressive activity, *J. Exp. Med.* **153**:1245–1259.

Fresno, M., McVay-Boudreau, L., Nabel, G., and Cantor, H., 1981b, Antigen-specific T lymphocyte clones. II. Purification and biological characterization of an antigen-specific suppressive protein synthesized by cloned T cells, *J. Exp. Med.* **153**:1260–1274.

Fujita, T., Takaoka, C., Matsui, H., and Taniguchi, T., 1983, Structure of the human interleukin-2 gene, *Proc. Natl. Acad. Sci. U.S.A.* **80**:7437–7441.

Galili, U., Rosenthal, L., Galili, N., and Klein, E., 1979, Activated T cells in the synovial fluid of arthritis patients: Characterization and comparison with *in vitro* activated human and murine T cells in cooperation with monocytes in cytotoxicity, *J. Immunol.* **122**:878–883.

Gillis, S., 1983, Interleukin-2: Biology and biochemistry, *J. Clin. Immunol.* **3**:1–13.

Gillis, S., and Smith, K. A., 1977, Long-term culture of tumor specific cytotoxic T cells, *Nature* **268**:154.

Gillis, S., Ferm, M. M., Ou, W., and Smith, K. A., 1978, T cell growth factor: Parameters for production and a quantitative microassay for activity, *J. Immunol.* **120**:2027–2032.

Gillis, S., Crabtree, G. R., and Smith, K. A., 1979, Glucocorticoid-induced inhibition of T cell growth factor production. I. The effect on mitogen-induced lymphocyte transformation, *J. Immunol.* **123**:1624–1631.

Gillis, S., Baker, P. E., Union, N. A., and Smith, K. A., 1979b, The *in vitro* generation and sustained culture of nude mouse cytolytic T-lymphocytes, *J. Exp. Med.* **149**:1460–1476.

Gillis, S., Scheid, M., and Watson, J., 1980, The isolation and characterization of interleukin-2 producing T cell lymphoma, *J. Immunol.* **125**:2570–2578.

Giri, J. G., Kincade, P. W., and Mizel, S. B., 1984, Interleukin-1 mediated induction of K-light-chain synthesis and surface immunoglobulin expression on pre-B cells, *J. Immunol.* **132**:223–228.

Gonzalez-Amaro, R., Alcocer-Varela, J., Martinez-Cordero, E., and Alarcon-Segovia, D., 1984, Natural killer cell-mediated activity in mixed connective tissue disease and its response to induction by interleukin-2, *J. Clin. Immunol.* **4**:273–279.

Goodman, M. G., Chenoweth, D. E., and Weigle, W. O., 1982, Induction of interleukin-1 secretion and enhancement of humoral immunity by binding of human C5a to macrophage surface C5a receptor, *J. Exp. Med.* **156**:912–917.

Gootenberg, J. E., Ruscetti, F. W., Mier, J. W., Gazdar, A., and Gallo, R. C., 1981, Human cutaneous T cell lymphoma and leukemic cell lines produce and respond to T cell growth factor, *J. Exp. Med.* **154:**1403–1418.

Greene, W. C., and Robb, R. J., 1984, Receptors for T cell growth factor: Structure, function, and expression on normal and neoplastic cells, *Contemp. Top. Mol. Immunol.* **10:**1–34.

Greene, W. C., Robb, R. J., Depper, J. M., Leonard, W. J., Drogula, C., Svetlik, P. B., Wong-Staal, F., Gallo, R. C., and Waldmann, T. A., 1984, Phorbol diester induces expression of Tac antigen on human acute T lymphocytic leukemic cells, *J. Immunol.* **133:**1042–1047.

Gupta, S., Chandy, K. G., DeCoursey, T. E., and Cahalan, M. D., 1984, Role of potassium channels in interleukin 2 synthesis and interleukin 2 receptor expression, *Lymphokine Res.* **3:**246.

Gupta, S., Chandy, K. G., Vayuvegula, B., Rhulig, L., DeCoursey, T. E., and Cahalan, M. D., 1985, Role of potassium channels in interleukin 1 and interleukin 2. Synthesis and interleukin 2 receptor expression, in: *Cellular and Molecular Biology of Lymphokines* (C. Sorg and A. Schnimpl, eds.), Academic Press, New York (in press).

Harwell, L. B., Skidmore, B., Marrack, P., and Kappler, J. W., 1980, Concanavalin A inducible interleukin-2 producing T-cell hybridoma, *J. Exp. Med.* **152:**893–904.

Hefeneider, S. M., Conlon, P. F., Dower, S. K., Henney, C. S., and Gillis, S., 1984, Limiting dilution analysis of interleukin-2 and colony-stimulating factor producer cells in normal and autoimmune mice, *J. Immunol.* **132:**1863–1868.

Henderson, L. E., Hewetson, J. F., Hopkins, R. F. III, Sowder, R. C., Neubauer, R. H., and Rabin, H., 1983, A rapid, large scale purification procedure for gibbon interleukin-2, *J. Immunol.* **131:**810–815.

Henney, C. S., Kuribaysashi, K., Kern, D. E., and Gillis, S., 1981, Interleukin-2 augments natural killer cell activity, *Nature* **291:**335–338.

Hirano, T., Fujimoto, K., Teranishi, T., Nishino, N., Onoue, K., Maeda, S., and Shimada, K., 1984, Phorbol ester increases the level of interleukin-2 mRNA in mitogen-stimulated human lymphocytes, *J. Immunol.* **312:**2165–2167.

Hoffman, M., 1980, Macrophages and T cells control distinct phases of B cell differentiation in the humoral immune responses *in vitro*, *J. Immunol.* **125:**2076–2081.

Howard, M., Matis, L., Malek, T. R., Sevach, E., Kell, W., Cohen, D., Nakanishi, K., and Paul, W. E., 1983, Interleukin-2 induces antigen-reactive T cell lines to secrete BCGF-1, *J. Exp. Med.* **158:**2024–2039.

Iscove, N. N., 1978, Erythropoietin-independent stimulation of early erythropoiesis in adult bone marrow cultures by condition media from lectin-stimulated mouse spleen cells, in: *Hematopoietic Cell Differentiation* (D. Golde, M. J. Cline, D. Metcalf, and C. Fox, eds.), Academic Press, New York, pp. 37–52.

Ise, K., Nakamura, S., Ohkamura, S., and Yoshinaga, M., 1982, DNA synthesis-potentiating activity on mouse thymocytes of synovial fluid of rheumatoid arthritis patients, *Acta Pathol. Jpn.* **32:**49–503.

Johnson, G. R., and Metcalf, D., 1977, Pure and mixed erythroid colony formation *in vitro* stimulated by spleen conditioned medium with no detectable erythropoietin, *Proc. Natl. Acad. Sci. U.S.A.* **74:**3879–3882.

Kaplan, D. R., Braciale, V. L., and Braciale, T. J., 1984, Antigen-dependent regulation of interleukin-2 receptor expression on cloned human cytotoxic T lymphocytes, *J. Immunol.* **133:**1966–1969.

Kaye, J., Gillis, S., Mizel, S. B., Shevach, E. M., Malek, T. R., Dinarello, C. A., Lachman, L. B., and Janeway, C. A., 1984, Growth of a cloned helper T cell line induced by a monoclonal antibody specific for the antigen receptor: Interleukin-1 is required for the expression of receptors for interleukin-2, *J. Immunol.* **133:**1339–1345.

Kern, E. E., Gillis, S., Okada, M., and Henney, C. S., 1981, The role of interleukin-2 (IL-2) in the differentiation of cytotoxic T cells: The effect of monoclonal anti-IL-2 antibody and absorption with IL-2 dependent T cell lines, *J. Immunol.* **127:**1323–1328.

Keystone, E. C., Shore, A., Miller, R. G., Tan, P., Poplouski, L., Leary, P., and Albert, S., 1983, Evidence for activated peripheral blood T cells in rheumatoid arthritis, *J. Rheumatol.* **11**(Suppl.)**:**85–92.

Klempner, M. S., Dinarello, C. A., and Gallin, J. L., 1978, Human leukocyte pyrogen induces release of specific granule contents from human neutrophils, *J. Clin. Invest.* **61:**1330–1336.

Korsmeyer, S., Greene, W. C., Cossman, J., Hsu, S. M., Jensen, J. P., Neckers, L. M., Marshall, S. L., Bakshi, A., Depper, J. M., Leonard, W. J., Jaffe, E. S., and Waldmann, T. A., 1983, Rearrangement and expression of immunoglobulin genes and expression of Tac antigen in hairy cell leukemia, *Proc. Natl. Acad. Sci. U.S.A.* **80:**4522–4526.

Krane, S. M., 1975, Collagenase production by human synovial tissue, *Ann. N. Y. Acad. Sci.* **256:**289–303.

Kreuger, J. M., Walter, J., Dinarello, C. A., Wolff, S. M., and Chedid, L., 1985, Sleep promoting effects of endogenous pyrogen (interleukin-1), *Am. J. Physiol.* (in press).

Kronker, M., Depper, J. M., Leonard, W. J., Wong-Staal, F., Gallo, R. C., Waldmann, T. A., and Greene, W. C., 1984, Cyclosporin A inhibits interleukin-2 gene expression at the level of MRNA transcription, *Lymphokine Res.* **3:**(abstract)253.

Lalande, M. E., McCutcheon, M. J., and Miller, R. G., 1980, Quantitative studies on the precursor of cytotoxic lymphocytes. VI. Second signal requirements of specifically activated precursors isolated 12 hr after stimulation, *J. Exp. Med.* **151:**12.

Larsson, E. L., and Contimiho, A., 1979, The role of mitogenic lectins in T-cell triggering, *Nature* **280:** 239–241.

Leonard, W. J., Depper, J. M., Uchiama, T., Smith, K. A., Waldmann, T. A., and Greene, W. C., 1982, A monoclonal antibody that appears to recognize the receptor for human T cell growth factor. Partial characterization of receptor, *Nature* **300:**267–269.

Leonard, W. J., Depper, J. M., Robb, R. J., Waldmann, T. A., and Greene, W. C., 1983, Characterization of the human receptor for T cell growth factor, *Proc. Natl. Acad. Sci. U.S.A.* **80:**6957–6961.

Leonard, W. J., Depper, J. M., Crabtree, G. R., Rudukoff, S., Pumphery, J., Robb, R. J., Kronke, M., Setlik, P. B., Pegger, N. J., Waldmann, T. A., and Green, W. C., 1984, Molecular cloning and expression of cDNAs for the human interleukin-2 receptor, *Nature* **311:**626–631.

Lin, Y., Stadler, B. M., and Rabin, H., 1982, Synthesis of biologically active interleukin-2 by xenopus oocytes in response to poly A-RNA from a gibbon T cell line, *J. Biol. Chem.* **257:**1587–1590.

Linker-Israeli, M., Bakke, A. C., Kitridon, R. C., Gendler, S., Gillis, S., and Horowitz, D. A., 1983, Defective production of interleukin-1 and interleukin-2 in patients wih systemic lupus erythematosus, *J. Immunol.* **130:**2651–2655.

Lipsky, P. E., Thompson, P. A., Rossenwasser, L. J., and Dinarello, C. A., 1983, The role of interleukin-1 in human B cell activation: Inhibition of B cell proliferation and the generation of immunoglobulin-secreting cells by an antibody against human leukicytic pyrogen, *J. Immunol.* **130:**2708–2714.

Lugler, T. A., Charon, J. A., Colot, M., Micksche, M., and Oppenheim, J. J., 1983, Chemotactic properties of partially purified human epidermal cell-derived thymocyte activating factor (ETAF) for polymorphonuclear and mononuclear cells, *J. Immunol.* **131:**816–820.

MacDonald, H. R., Cerottini, J.-C., and Ryser, J. E., 1980, Quantitation and cloning of cytotoxic T lymphocytes and their precursors, *Immunol. Rev.* **51:**93–123.

Macphail, S., and Stutman, O., 1984, Independent inhibition of IL-2 synthesis and cell proliferation by anti-Ia antibodies in mixed lymphocyte response to MLs, *Eur. J. Immunol.* **14:**318–324.

Malek, T. R., and Shevach, E. M., 1984, Cellular and humoral requirements for the induction of IL-2 receptor expression on T cell subpopulations, *Leukemia Res.* **3:**257.

Malek, T. R., Robb, R. J., and Shevach, E. M., 1983, Identification and initial characterization of a rat monoclonal antibody reactive with the murine interleukin-2 receptor–ligard complex, *Proc. Natl. Acad. Sci. U.S.A.* **80:**5694–5698.

Malek, T. R., Ortega, G., Jakway, J. P., Chan, C., and Shevach, E. M., 1984, The murine IL-2 receptor. II. Monoclonal anti-IL-2 receptor antibodies as specific inhibitors of T cell function *in vitro, J. Immunol.* **133:**1976–1982.

Mayernik, D. G., Hag, A., and Rinehart, J. J., 1984, Interleukin-1 secretion by human monocytes and macrophages, *J. Leukocyte Biol.* **36:**551–557.

Meuer, S. C., Hussey, R. E., Penta, A. C., Fitzgerald, K. A., Stadler, B. M., Schlossman, S. F., and Reinherz, E. L., 1982, Cellular origin of interleukin-2 (IL-2) in man: Evidence for stimulus-restricted IL-2 production by $T4^+$ and $T8^+$ T lymphocytes, *J. Immunol.* **129:**1076–1079.

Mier, J. W., and Gallo, R. C., 1980, Purification and some properties of human T-cell growth factor from phytohemagglutinin-stimulated lymphocyte conditioned media, *Proc. Natl. Acad. Sci. U.S.A.* **77:**6134–6138.

Mier, J. W., and Gallo, R. C., 1982, The purification and properties of human T cell growth factor, *J. Immunol.* **128:**1122–1127.

Minato, N., Reid, L., and Blood, B. R., 1981, On the heterogeneity of murine natural killer cells, *J. Exp. Med.* **154:**750–762.

Miyasaka, N., Nakamura, T., Russell, I. J., and Talal, N., 1984, Interleukin-2 deficiencies in rheumatoid arthritis and systemic lupus erythematosus, *Clin. Immunol. Immunopathol.* **31**:109–117.

Miyawaki, T., Yachie, A., Ohzeki, S., Nagaoki, T., and Taniguchi, N., 1983, Cyclosporin A does not prevent expression of Tac antigen, a possible TCGF receptor molecule, on mitogen-stimulated human T cells, *J. Immunol.* **130**:2727–2742.

Mizel, S. B., 1982, Interleukin-1 and T cell activation, *Immunol. Rev.* **63**:51–72.

Mizel, S. B., Dayer, J. M., Krane, S. M., and Mergenhagen, S. E., 1980, Stimulation of rheumatoid synovial cell collagenase and prostaglandin production by partially purified lymphocyte-activating factor (interleukin-1), *Proc. Natl. Acad. Sci. U.S.A.* **78**:2474–2477.

Morgan, D. A., Ruscetti, F. W., and Gallo, R. C., 1976, Selective *in vitro* growth of T lymphocytes from normal human bone marrow, *Science* **193**:1007–1009.

Nabel, G., Bucalo, L. R., Allard, J., Wigzell, H., and Cantor, H., 1981, Multiple activities of a clone cell line mediating natural killer cell function, *J. Exp. Med.* **153**:1582–1591.

Nabholz, M., Engers, M. D., Collavo, D., and North, M., 1978, Cloned T cell lines with specific cytotoxic activity, *Curr. Top. Microbiol. Immunol.* **81**:176–187.

Neefe, J. R., Curl, R., and Woody, J. N., 1981, Absolute requirement for adherent cells in the production of human interleukin-2 (IL-2) cell, *Immunology* **67**:71–80.

Nikaido, T., Shimizu, A., Ishida, N., Sabe, H., Teshigawara, K., Maeda, M., Uchiama, T., Yodoi, J., and Honjo, T., 1984, Molecular cloning of cDNA encoding human IL-2 receptor, *Nature* **311**:631–635.

Nouri, A. M. E., Panayi, G. S., and Goodman, S. M., 1984a, Cytokines and chronic inflammation of rheumatic disease. I. The presence of interleukin-1 in synovial fluid, *Clin. Exp. Immunol.* **55**:295–302.

Nouri, A. M. E., Panayi, G. S., and Goodman, S. M., 1984b, Cytokines and the chronic inflammation of rheumatic disease. II. The presence of interleukin-2 in synovial fluids, *Clin. Exp. Immunol.* **58**:402–409.

Okada, M., and Henney, C. S., 1980, The differentiation of cytotoxic T cells in vitro. II. Amplifying factor(s) produced in primary mixed lymphocyte cultures against K/D stimuli require the presence of $Ly2^+$ cells but not $Lyt1^+$ cells, *J. Immunol.* **125**:300–307.

Okada, M., Klimpel, G. R., Kupper, R. C., and Henney, C. S., 1979, The differentiation of cytotoxic T cells *in vitro*. I. Amplifying factor(s) in the primary response is $Lyt\ 1^+$ cell dependent, *J. Immunol.* **122**:2527–2533.

Oppenheim, J. J., Stadler, B M., Siraganian, R. P., Mage, M., and Mathieson, B., 1982, Lymphokines: Their role in lymphocyte response. Properties of interleukin-1, *Fed. Proc.* **41**:257–262.

Ortaldo, J. R., and Herberman, R. B., 1984, Heterogeneity of natural killer cells, *Annu. Rev. Immunol.* **2**:359–394.

Ortaldo, J. R., Mason, A. T., Gerard, J. P., Henderson, L. E., Farrar, W., Hopkins, R. F. III, Herberman, R. B., and Rabin, H., 1984, Effects of natural and recombinant IL-2 on regulation of IFNY production and natural killer activity: Lack of involvement of the Tac antigen for these immunoregulatory effects, *J. Immunol.* **133**:779–783.

Ortega, G., Robb, R. J., Shevach, E. M., and Malek, T. R., 1984, The murine IL-2 receptor. I. Monoclonal antibodies that define distinct functional epitopes on activated T cells and react with activated B cells, *J. Immunol.* **133**:1970–1975.

Osawa, H., and Diamantstein, T., 1983, Studies on T lymphocyte activation: II. Monoclonal antibody inhibiting the capacity of rat T lymphoblasts to absorb and to respond to IL-2, an anti-IL-2 receptor antibody, *Immunology* **48**:617–621.

Osawa, H., and Diamantstein, T., 1984, A rat monoclonal antibody that binds specifically to mouse T lymphoblasts and inhibits IL-2 receptor function: A putative anti-IL-2 receptor antibody, *J. Immunol.* **132**:2445–2450.

Paetkaun, V., Mills, G., Gerhart, S., and Monnticone, V., 1976, Proliferation of murine thymic lymphocytes *in vitro* is mediated by the Con A induced release of a lymphokine (co-stimulator), *J. Immunol.* **117**:1320–1324.

Palacios, R., and Moller, G., 1981, HLA-DR antigens render resting T cells sensitive to interleukin-2 and induce production of the growth factor in the autologous mixed lymphocyte reaction, *Cell Immunol.* **63**:143–153.

Pfizenmaier, K., Schewich, P., Danbener, W., Kronke, M., Rollinghoff, M., and Wagner, H., 1984, Quantitative representation of all T cell committed to develop into cytotoxic effector cells and/or interleukin-2 activity-producing helper cells within murine T lymphocyte subsets, *Eur. J. Immunol.* **14**:33–39.

Postlethwaite, A. E., Lachman, L. B., Mainardi, C. L., and Kang, A. H., 1983, Interleukin-1 stimulation of collagenase production by cultured fibroblasts, *J. Exp. Med.* **157**:801–806.

Puri, J., Shinitzky, M., and Conai, P., 1980, Concomitant increase in antigen binding and in T cell membranes lipid viscosity induced by the lymphocyte activating factor (LAF), *J. Immunol.* **124**:1937–1942.

Rafter, G. W., 1982, Etiology of rheumatoid arthritis, *Med. Hypotheses* **9**:437–443.

Raulet, D. M., and Bevan, M. J., 1982, A differentiation factor required for the expression of cytotoxic T cell function, *Nature* **269**:754–757.

Reem, G., and Yeh, N. H., 1984, Interleukin-2 regulates expression of its receptor and synthesis of gamma interferon by human T lymphocytes, *Science* **225**:429–430.

Reske-Kunz, A. B., Von Steldren, D., Rude, E., Osawa, H., and Diamentstein, T., 1984, Interleukin-2 receptors on an insulin-specific T cell clone: Dynamic of receptor expression, *J. Immunol.* **133**:1356–1361.

Robb, R. J., 1984, Interleukin-2: The molecule and its function, *Immunol. Today* **5**:203–209.

Robb, R. J., and Greene, W. C., 1983, Direct demonstration of the identity of T cell growth factor binding proterri and the Tac Antigen, *J. Exp. Med.* **158**:1332–1337.

Robb, R. J., and Smith, K. A., 1981, Human T-cell growth factor is glycosylated, *Mol. Immunol.* **18**:1087–1094.

Robb, R. J., Kutney, R. M., Panico, M., Morris, H., DeGrado, W. F., and Chowdlvey, V., 1983, Posttranslational modification of human-T cell growth factor, *Biochem. Biophys. Res. Commun.* **116**:1049–1055.

Robb, R. J., Greene, W. C., and Rusk, C. M., 1984, Low and high affinity cellular receptors for interleukin-2. Implications for the level of Tac antigen, *J. Exp. Med.* **160**:1126–1146.

Ruscetti, F. W., Mier, J. W., and Gallo, R. C., 1980, Human T cell growth factor: Parameters for production, *J. Supramol. Struct.* **13**:229–241.

Salmeron, G., and Lipsky, P. E., 1983, Immunosuppressive potentials of antimalarials, *Am. J. Med.* **75**:19–24.

Santoro, T. J., Benjamin, W. R., Oppenheim, J. J., and Steinberg, A. D., 1983a, The cellular basis for immune interferon production in autoimmune MRL-lpr/lpr mice, *J. Immunol.* **131**:265–268.

Santoro, T. J., Luger, T. A., Ravache, E. S., Smolen, J. S., Oppenheim, J. J., and Steinberg, A. D., 1983b, *In vitro* correction of the interleukin-2 defect of autoimmune mice, *Eur. J. Immunol.* **13**:601 –604.

Sarin, P. S., and Gallo, R. C., 1983, Human T-cell growth factor, *CRC Crit. Rev. Immunol.* **4**:279–305.

Sauder, D. H., 1984, Epidermal cytokines: Properties of epidermal cell thymocyte-activating factor (ETAF), *Lymph Res.* **4**:145–152.

Schmidt, J. A., Mizel, S. B., Cohen, D., and Green, I., 1982, Interleukin-1, a potent regulator of fibroblast-proliferation, *J. Immunol.* **128**:2177–2182.

Schrader, J. W., and Clark-Lewis, I., 1981, T-cell hybridoma derived regulatory factor. I. Production of T cell growth factor following stimulation by concanavalin A, *J. Immunol.* **126**:1101–1105.

Schreier, M. H., Iscove, N. N., Tees, R., Aarden, L., and VonBoehmer, H., 1980, Clones of killer and helper T cells: Growth requirements, specificity and retention of function in long term culture, *Immunol. Rev.* **51**:315–336.

Seigal, L. J., Harper, M. E., Wong-Staal, F., Gallo, R. C., Nash, W. G., and O'Brien, S. J., 1984, Gene for T cell growth factor: Location on human chromozone 4q and feline chromosome B1, *Science* **223**:175–178.

Sibbitt, W. L., Jr., Likar, L., Spellman, C. W., and Bankhurst, A. D., 1983, Impaired natural killer cell function in systemic lupus erythematosus. Relationship to interleukin-2 production, *Arthritis Rheum.* **26**:1316–1320.

Sibbit, W. L., Kenny, C., Spellman, C. W., Ley, K. D., and Bankhurst, A. D., 1984, Lymphokines in autoimmunity: relationship between interleukin-2 and interferon-γ production in systemic lupus erythematosus, *Clin. Immunol. Immunopathol.* **32**:166–173.

Smith, K. A., 1984, Interleukin-2, *Annu. Rev. Immunol.* **2**:319–333.

Smith, K. A., Gillis, S., Baker, P. E., McKenzie, D., and Ruscetti, F. W., 1979, T-cell growth factor mediated T cell proliferation, *Ann. N. Y. Acad. Sci.* **332**:423–432.

Stadler, B. M., Dougherty, S. F., Farrar, J. J., and Oppenheim, J. J., 1981, Relationship of cell cycle to recovery of IL-2 activity from human mononuclear cells, human and mouse T cell lines, *J. Immunol.* **127**:1936–1940.

Stanley, E. R., Cifone, M., Heard, P. M., and Defendi, V., 1976, Factors regulating macrophage production and growth: Identity of colony-stimulating factor and macrophage growth factor, *J. Exp. Med.* **143**:631–647.

Symington, F. W., and Teh, H. S., 1980, A two signal mechanism for the induction of cytotoxic T lymphocytes, *Scand. J. Immunol.* **12**:1–12.

Talal, N., Dauphinee, M. J., and Wofsy, D., 1982, Interleukin-2 deficiency, genes, and systemic lupus erythematosus, *Arthritis Rheum.* **25**:838–842.

Taniguchi, T., Matsui, H., Fujita, T., Takaota, C., Hashima, N., Yoshimoto, R., and Hamuro, J., 1983, Structure and expression of a cloned cDNA for human interleukin-2, *Nature* **302**:305–309.

Teh, M. S., and Teh, S. J., 1980, Direct evidence for a two-signal mechanism of cytotoxic T cell activation, *Nature* **285**:163–165.

Teh, H. S., and Yu, M., 1983, Activation of nonspecific killer cells by interleukin-2-containing supernatants, *J. Immunol.* **131**:1827–1833.

Teh, M. S., Kwong, L., Yu, M., and Kilburn, D. G., 1981, A simple method for the quantitation of specific cytotoxic precursors to syngeneic tumors, *J. Immunol. Methods* **46**:97–111.

Ting, C. C., Yang, S. S., and Hargrove, M. E., 1984, Induction of suppressor T cells by interleukin-2, *J. Immunol.* **133**:261–266.

Trinchiari, G., Matsumoto-Kobayashi, M., Clark, S. C., Seehra, J., London, L., and Perussia, B., 1984, Response of resting human peripheral blood natural killer cells to interleukin-2, *J. Exp. Med.* **160**:1147–1169.

Tsudo, M., Uchiama, T., and Uchino, H., 1984, Expression of Tac antigen on activated normal human B cells, *J. Exp. Med.* **160**:612–617.

Uchiama, T., Broder, S., and Waldmann, T. A., 1981a, A monoclonal antibody (anti-Tac) reactive with activated and functionally mature human T cells. I. Production of anti-Tac monoclonal antibody and distribution of Tac(+) cells, *J. Immunol.* **126**:1393–1397.

Uchiama, T., Nelson, D. L., Fleisher, T. A., and Waldmann, T. A., 1981b, A monoclonal antibody (anti-Tac) reactive with activated and functionally mature human T cells. II. Expression of Tac antigen on activated cytotoxic killer T cells, Suppressor cells and on one of two types of helper cells, *J. Immunol.* **126**:1398–1403.

Van Snick, J. L., Masson, P. L., and Heremans, J. F., 1974, The involvement of lactoferrin in the hyposideremia of acute inflammation, *J. Exp. Med.* **140**:1068–1084.

Vayuvegula, B., Butler, G., Chandy, K. G., Ruhling, M. L., and Gupta, S., 1985, Requirement of functional K+ channel for interleukin-1 production, *Fed. Proc.* **44**:1864 (Abstract).

Von Boehmer, H. S., Mengartner, H., Nabholz, M., Lenhardt, W., Schreier, M., and Haas, W., 1979, Fine specificity of a continuously growing killer cell clone specific for M-Y antigen, *Eur. J. Immunol.* **9**:592–597.

Waldmann, T. A., Goldman, C., Robb, R. J., Depper, J. M., Leonard, W. J., Sharrow, S. O., Bongiovanni, K. F., Korsmeyer, S. J., and Greene, W. C., 1984, Expression of interleukin-2 receptors on activated B cells, *J. Exp. Med.* **160**:1450–1466.

Wagner, H., and Rollinghoff, M., 1978, T cell interactions during *in vitro* cytotoxic allograft responses, *J. Exp. Med.* **148**:1523–1538.

Wagner, H. C., Herdt, C., Stockinger, M., Pfizenmaier, K., Bartlett, R., and Rollinghoff, M., 1981, Impact of the thymus on the generation of immunocompetence and diversity of antigen-specific MHC-restricted cytotoxic T lymphocyte precursors, *Immunol. Rev.* **58**:95–129.

Wagner, H. C., Hardt, C., Rouse, B. T., Rollinghoff, M., Schewrich, P., and Pfzenmaier, K., 1982, Dissection of the proliferative and differentiation signals controlling murine cytotoxic T lymphocyte response, *J. Exp. Med.* **155**:1876–1881.

Welte, K., Wang, C. Y., Mertelsmann, R., Venuta, S., Feldman, S. P., and Moore, M. A., 1982, Purification of human interleukin-2 to apparent homogeneity and its molecular heterogeneity, *J. Exp. Med.* **156**:454–464.

Welte, K., Andreeff, M., Platzer, E., Holloway, K., Rubin, B. Y., Moore, M. A. S., and Merkelsmann, R., 1984, Interleukin-2 regulates the expression of Tac antigen on peripheral blood T lymphocytes, *J. Exp. Med.* **160**:1390–1403.

Wharton, W., 1983, Human macrophage-like cell line U937-1 elaborates mitogenic activity for fibroblasts, *J. Reticuloendothel. Soc.* **33**:151–156.

Wharton, W., Gillespie, G. Y., Russel, S. W., and Pledger, W. J., 1982, Mitogenic activity elaborated by macrophage-like cell lines acts as competence factor(s) for BALB/c 3T3 cells, *J. Cell. Physiol.* **110**:93–100.

Wilkins, J. A., Warrington, R. J., Sigurdson, S. L., and Rutherford, W. J., 1983, The demonstration of an interleukin-2 like activity in the synovial fluids of rheumatoid arthritis patients, *J. Rheumatol.* **10**:109–113.

Williams, N., Eger, R. R., Moore, M. A. S., and Mendelsohn, N., 1978, Differentiation of mouse bone marrow precursor cells into neutrophil granulocytes by an activity separated from WEH1-3 cell conditioned medium, *Differentiation* **11**:59–63.

Wofsy, D., Murphy, E. D., Roth, J. B., Dauphinee, M. J., Kipper, S. B., and Talal, N., 1981, Deficient interleukin-2 activity in MRL/MP and C57B1/6J mice bearing lpr gene, *J. Exp. Med.* **154**:1671–1680.

Wood, D. D., Ihrie, E. J., Dinarello, C. A., and Cohen, P. L., 1983, Isolation of an interleukin-1-like factor from human joint effusions, *Arthritis Rheumat.* **26**:975–983.

Zarling, J. M., and Bach, F. H., 1979, Continuous culture of T cells cytotoxic for autologous human leukemic cells, *Nature* **280**:685–687.

Zubler, R. H., Lowenthal, J. W., Erard, F., Hashimoto, N., Devos, R., and MacDonald, H. R., 1984, Activated B cells express receptors for, and proliferate in response to interleukin-2, *J. Exp. Med.* **160**:1170–1183.

5

Interferon and Natural Killer Cells in Rheumatic Diseases

Norman Talal

I. INTRODUCTION

The interferons, a family of protein and glycoprotein molecules secreted by a variety of animal cells, are known for their antiviral, antiproliferative, and immunoregulatory properties (Preble *et al.*, 1983; Ho, 1982; Pestka *et al.*, 1981; Stewart, 1981). Interferon was first characterized as an antiviral protein by Isaacs and Lindenmann in 1957 (Isaacs and Lindenmann, 1957). Today we classify human interferons into three distinct groups on the basis of their antigenic, biological, and chemical properties (Table 1). These are called α-interferon, which is produced by leukocytes, β-interferon, which is produced by fibroblasts and epithelial cells, and γ-interferon, which is a lymphokine secreted by lymphocytes. The longstanding clinical interest in the interferons comes from their known antiviral and antiproliferative activities and their current usage in clinical trials to treat a variety of malignancies as well as the acquired immunodeficiency syndrome (AIDS). The ability to clone interferon has contributed greatly to the supply of interferon as well as to our knowledge of its molecular structure and biological properties (Pestka *et al.*, 1981). Interferons act on the virus-infected cell rather than on the virus itself, although the exact mechanism of action is still uncertain. Their ability to inhibit cell multiplication and interfere with tumor growth is thought to be independent of their antiviral activity.

The effect of interferon on immunity has been somewhat confusing. Both positive and negative influences have been observed, depending to some extent on dosage and timing. Low doses of interferon enhance the antibody response to sheep red blood cells

Norman Talal • Clinical Immunology Section, Audie L. Murphy Memorial Veterans Administration Hospital, and Department of Medicine, The University of Texas Health Science Center at San Antonio, San Antonio, Texas 78284.

Table 1. Types of Human Interferon[a]

Type	Made by	Characteristics
α	Leukocytes	19 to 24,000 daltons, pH 2 stable, several subtypes, less species specific, not glycoprotein
β	Fibroblasts	19 to 24,000 daltons, pH 2 stable, more species specific, glycoprotein
γ	T lymphocytes stimulated with antigens or mitogens	pH 2 labile, 50,000 daltons (native), species specific, glycoprotein

[a]From Preble and Friedman (1983).

in mice, whereas high doses are inhibitory. Interferon administered 24 hr before antigen inhibits delayed hypersensitivity, whereas an enhanced delayed hypersensitivity response occurs when interferon is given a few hours after antigen. Interferon can inhibit cell-mediated immune responses to antigens or mitogens, inhibit the mixed lymphocyte reaction, augment immune and nonimmune macrophage phagocytosis, and increase IgE-mediated histamine release. The discovery that interferon and interferon inducers can augment natural killer cell activity has attracted great attention in recent years (Herberman *et al.*, 1981–1982; Huddlestone *et al.*, 1979; Minato *et al.*, 1980; Targan and Stebbing, 1982).

Natural killer (NK) cells are a subpopulation of lymphoid cells that are spontaneously cytotoxic for a variety of viral infected or malignantly transformed target cells (Herberman, 1982). The NK function is independent of prior recognition and sensitization of target cells, is not mediated by clonally distributed receptor molecules, and is not restricted by the major histocompatibility locus. Recent studies of NK cells have investigated their lineage and heterogeneity and have emphasized their role as mediators of immunologic surveillance, particularly with regard to prevention of metastases (Herberman, 1982; Hoffman, 1983). Morphologically, these cells appear as large granular lymphocytes (LGLs) characterized by azurophilic, electron-dense, intracytoplasmic granules normally containing acid hydrolases. The NK cells share certain characteristics in common with T cells such as the ability to form E-rosettes and to grow in response to interleukin 2 (IL-2) or T-cell growth factor. However, they also have some characteristics of macrophages such as the presence of Fc receptors. Additionally, they have unique phenotypic cell surface markers, which can be detected with monoclonal antibodies to Leu-7 and Leu-11.

The NK cell may have emerged early in phylogeny and may possess a broad regulatory role in controlling the proliferation and differentiation of many other types of cells, particularly those involved in hematopoiesis and granulopoiesis (Hoffman and Ferranrini, 1983; Kiessling *et al.*, 1983). The interaction of the NK cell with bone marrow stem cells may represent a primitive cell/cell recognition mechanism.

Decreased NK function is often present in patients with various malignancies, AIDS, serious infections, various autoimmune and rheumatic disorders, and the Chediak–Higashi syndrome.

The ability of interferon to enhance NK activity plays a role in potentiating defense against viral infections and neoplasms. However, the precise relationship between interferon and NK cells is complicated by the fact that the natural killer effector cell can itself produce a variety of cytokines (Herberman *et al.*, 1984). Curiously, there is no correlation between therapeutic efficacy of interferon and the level of NK cell activity in a given individual. Indeed, patients treated over long periods of time with interferon may show depressed NK-cell activity. Because of the general complexities of the immune system and the specific uncertainties concerning interferon and natural killing, it is difficult to construct a simple model that will adequately express all possible interrelationships. Nevertheless, it is necessary to attempt such a model to serve as a basis for understanding the possible role of both interferon and NK cells in rheumatic diseases (Fig. 1).

There is increasing evidence that interferon is necessary for the adequate maintenance and function of NK cells, whose activity is greatly diminished under circumstances in which interferon is deleted. Poly-I:C, a potent interferon inducer, is also an inducer of NK-cell activity (Herberman, 1982; Miyasaka *et al.*, 1984a). In both animal and human studies, antiinterferon antibodies eliminate the booster effect of interferon itself or of poly-I:C (Herberman *et al.*, 1981–1982). Repeated administration of antiinterferon to normal mice diminishes NK cell activity. Pathogen-free rodents have very low NK activity until they are exposed to a conventional environment. Thus, environmental factors may be responsible for the induction of interferon and the consequent appearance and maintenance of NK activity. The ability of interferon to augment NK cells does not require accessory cells and probably represents a direct effect of the mediator on the NK effector cell itself. The LGLs appear to bind interferon within a few minutes, and detectable augmentation of activity can be measured within the first hour. Augmentation by interferon of either mouse or human NK activity is dependent on both RNA and protein synthesis. Interferon appears to mediate these effects through several mechanisms, including binding of NK cells to the target as well as increased ability to recycle and interact with multiple target cells.

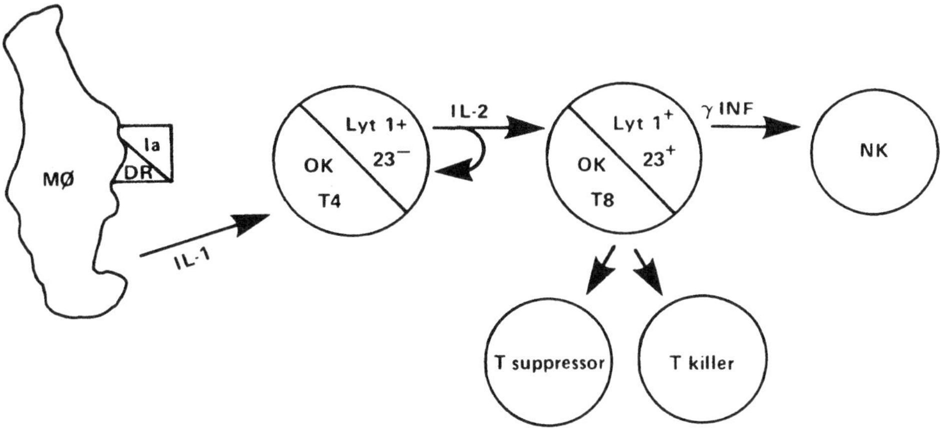

Figure 1. Schematic representation of the immunoregulatory network illustrating how the critical interaction of class II molecules on antigen-presenting cells (e.g., macrophage) triggers OKT4 cells (Lyt-1^+23^- in the mouse) to produce IL-2, which then binds to specific receptors on both OKT4 and OKT8 cells (Lyt-1^+23^+ in the mouse), favoring the generation of T suppressor and T killer cells and the production of γ-interferon (γ INF), a stimulator of NK cells. This model is a generalization based on the best available evidence and is not intended to explain all the facts available.

II. BIOLOGICAL EFFECTS OF INTERFERON

Human and mouse interferons have generally been classified into three antigenically distinct groups by use of specific antisera (Table 1). α-Interferons are produced by leukocytes primarily and, to a lesser extent, by fibroblasts. β-Interferon is the major interferon produced by fibroblastlike cells. Mixtures of α- and β-interferons studied in early experiments on virus-induced interferon are often called type I or "classical" interferon. These interferons are generally stable at pH 2 except for the unusual acid-labile interferon often seen in immunoregulatory diseases (discussed in Section IV). γ- or type II interferon is a lymphokine produced by activated T lymphocytes that is sometimes referred to as "immune" interferon. This interferon is destroyed at acid pH.

Genes for over 13 distinct subtypes of human α-interferon have recently been cloned using recombinant DNA techniques (Preble and Friedman, 1983). The reason for the existence of so many forms of α-interferon is unknown. Different subtypes of α-interferon may vary in molecular weight and in other biological properties. Human leukocyte interferon contains various proportions of each subtype. Only one gene has been cloned for human β-interferon, and only one gene is known for human γ-interferon. The β-interferon gene has 40% homology with the α-interferons, which themselves show 70% homology. γ-Interferon shares only 11% of its structure with the α species.

The various α-interferon subtypes show remarkable differences in view of their structural similarity. Differences in pharmacological properties may arise from structural alterations of only three amino acid residues. Monoclonal antibodies to both human and mouse interferons are currently available. Radioimmunoassays and possible other biological assays for interferon are under development.

Viruses were the first recognized but are not the only inducers of interferon. Many natural and synthetic nonviral substances can induce α- and/or β-interferons in animals or in cell cultures. These inducers include double-stranded RNAs such as poly-I:C, intracellular microorganisms including bacteria, rickettsia, mycoplasma, and chlamydia, lipopolysaccharides, pyran copolymers, polyvinyl sulfate, cycloheximide, and tilorone. T lymphocytes produce γ-interferon after exposure to mitogens or specific antigens in the presence of macrophages. Interleukin 2 is a potent stimulator of γ-interferon (Kawase *et al.*, 1983).

Many cell types including fibroblasts, epithelial cells, lymphocytes, macrophages, and NK cells can be stimulated to produce interferon given an appropriate inducer. Leukocytes produce α-interferons, whereas fibroblasts or epithelial cells produce primarily β-interferon under similar conditions. Lymphoblastoid cell lines produce a mixture of α- and β-interferons, with α-interferon predominating.

The exact mechanism whereby interferon exerts its antiviral activity is not totally understood (Fig. 2). Interferon appears to bind to specific cell surface receptors composed of gangliosides and/or glycoprotein. Repetitive binding studies suggest that α- and γ-interferons share one class of receptors, whereas β- and γ-interferons bind to other receptors. Some of the interferon appears to be internalized via receptor-mediated endocytosis. After binding to the cell surface, interferon induces the synthesis of new cellular messenger RNA and protein, which are the mediators of the antiviral state. Thus, inhibitors of RNA and protein synthesis can block the antiviral effects of interferon.

Several proteins appear to be associated with the antiviral state. One is a protein

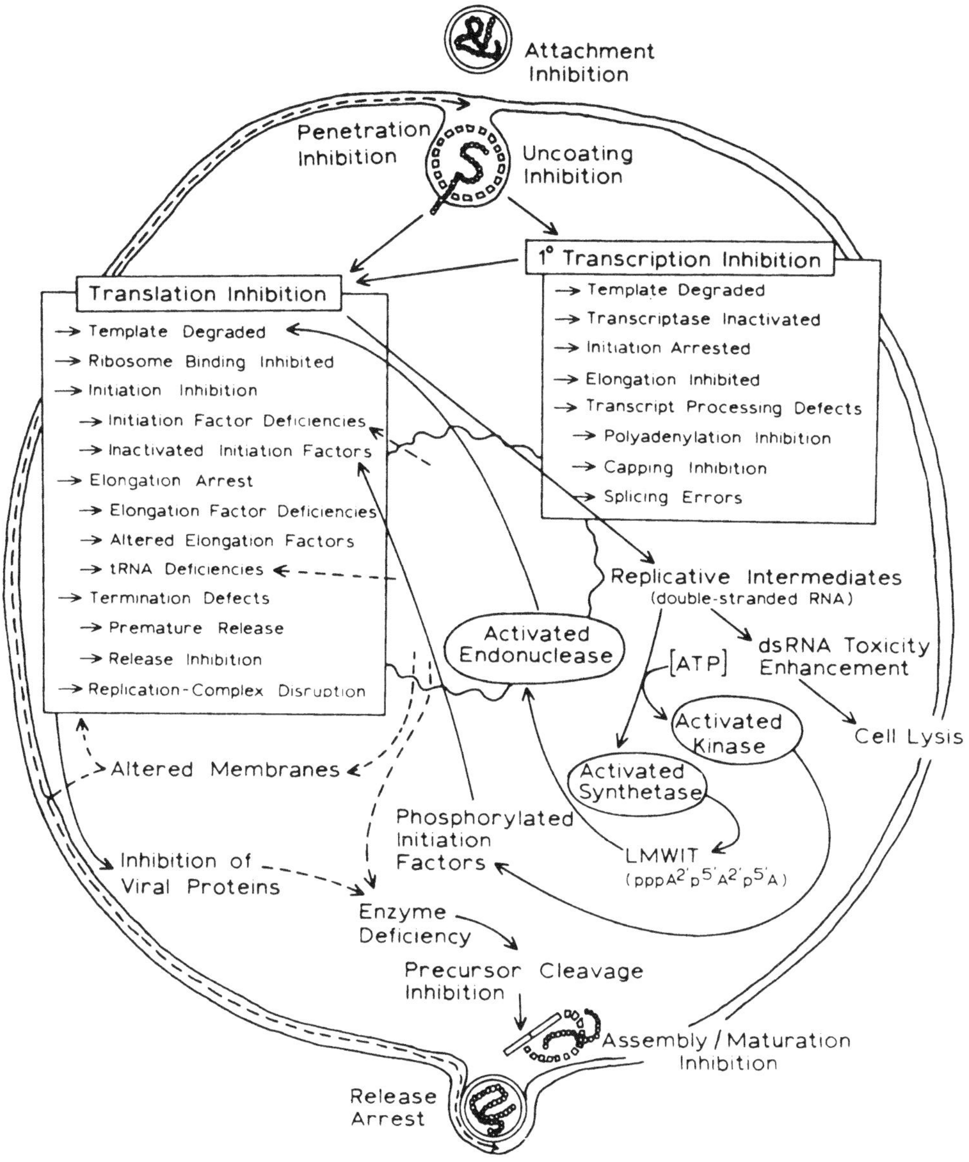

Figure 2. A simplistic view of the antiviral action of interferon. (From Stewart, 1981, page 222.)

kinase found in interferon-treated cells, 2–5 A synthetase, which synthesizes 2′,5′-oligoadenylate (2–5 A). The level of this enzyme in cells has been used clinically to monitor the effects of interferon. The 2–5 A synthetase is activated by all three types of interferon as well as by double-stranded RNA, which itself is a component of or is produced during replication of different viruses. Several postulated mechanisms leading to the inhibition of virus-specific protein synthesis and degradation of viral messenger RNA are shown in Fig. 2. Interferon may also affect other steps in the virus infection cycle, and the efficacy of the antiviral state depends very much on the particular virus strain and host cell under investigation.

Antibody to interferon significantly influences the course of viral infection in mice, resulting in enhanced viral replication, shorter latent period, and more severe systemic disease with higher mortality. Local interferon production may be more important than high levels of circulating interferon in mediating the antiviral state. For example, the early presence of significant numbers of interferon-producing white cells in virus-infected lungs possibly contributes to host defense against influenza. The rapid clearance of circulating interferon from the blood makes it difficult to measure in patients. Therefore, quantitation of the enzyme 2–5 A synthetase in blood cells has proved useful in evaluating the role of interferon in recovery from viral infection. In general, this enzyme seems to reflect the course of clinical disease.

Interferon has several important effects on cell growth and proliferation in addition to its antiviral properties (Table 2). Abnormal organization and rigidity of the cell cytoskeleton may be related to the anticellular proliferative effects of interferon, which account for its use in clinical trials as an anticancer agent. β-Interferon decreases membrane fluidity and induces rigidity, resulting in cell enlargement and decreased cell locomotion. Persistent membrane changes occur in mouse cells treated with mouse β-interferon, including an increase in the ratio of saturated : unsaturated fatty acids in the lipid bilayer. Increased rigidity results in a decreased ability to redistribute cell surface receptors for concanavalin A (Con A). Interferon treatment of mouse or human cells causes actin-containing microfilaments to organize into a dense fibrous submembranous meshwork. These changes in microfilament structure probably explain the abnormalities in cell shape, mitosis, and cell surface mobility of Con A receptors. The increased rigidity of the plasma membrane and cytoskeleton also explains the inhibition of virus uptake by receptor-mediated endocytosis that may occur in interferon-treated cells. There are also changes in microtubules of mouse macrophages accompanied by increases in the rate of phagocytosis.

There is no general agreement as to exactly how interferon mediates its antineoplastic effects. Indeed, many of the side effects observed in clinical trials of interferon therapy such as leukopenia, thrombocytopenia, and hair loss may reflect the anticellular proliferative effects of the modulator. Interferon appears to act independent of stage in the cell cycle, but new protein synthesis may be required for its action. For example, mitogenic induction of orthnithine decarboxylase and S-adenosyl-L-methionine decarboxylase activities are inhibited by inteferon. However, although Daudi human lymphoblastoid cell lines are extremely sensitive to the antiproliferative effects of human interferon, there is no evidence to implicate the enzyme 2–5 A in this activity. As with its antiviral effect, the local concentration of interferon creating enriched microenvironments may be more important for its anticancer effect than the serum concentration.

Table 2. Biological Effects of Interferon

1. Antiviral.
2. Antiproliferative; effect on tumors.
3. Modulation of humoral and cellular immunity (antibody synthesis and delayed hypersensitivity).
4. Increased expression of cell surface antigens, particularly class II phenotypic proteins of the major histocompatibility complex.
5. Activation of macrophages with enhanced antimicrobial effects.
6. Enhancement of natural killer (NK) cells.

III. EFFECT OF INTERFERON ON THE IMMUNE SYSTEM

All three classes of interferon have potent immunoregulatory properties influencing both humoral and cellular immunity (Preble and Friedman, 1983; Sonnenfeld and Pick, 1980; Vilesk *et al.*, 1980). Both human and mouse interferon can increase the expression of IgG Fc receptors on macrophages (Guyre *et al.*, 1983) and suppress the lymphocyte proliferative response to mitogens and antigens. In experiments performed over 10 years ago, low doses of mouse α/β-interferon were able to augment antibody responses, whereas high doses were inhibitory. Pretreatment of sensitized B cells reduced antigen-driven proliferation. The response to T-cell-dependent antigens was more sensitive to inhibition by interferon than were T-cell-independent responses. Interferon is less effective as a suppressor of pokeweed-mitogen-driven B-cell proliferation. It is interesting that the level of 2–5 A synthetase is higher in mature Balb/c splenic immunocompetent T cells than in immature thymic T cells.

It is likely that the inhibitory effects of interferon on humoral immunity are mediated through actions on immunoregulatory cells, possibly T and/or NK cells, rather than being direct effects on B cells themselves. γ-Interferon, itself the product of T cells, is the most potent immunoregulator of the three different classes. Mouse γ-interferon is 20 to 250 times more immunosuppressive of primary antibody responses *in vitro* than is α or β interferon. In one study, α-interferon enhanced *in vitro* production of pokeweed-mitogen-driven IgG and IgM including IgM rheumatoid factor (Rodriquez *et al.*, 1983).

One of the most interesting aspects of interferon as an immunoregulator is its ability to induce changes in membrane-associated antigens and receptors. γ-Interferon increases the expression of class II major histocompatibility antigens, both Ia in the mouse and DR in man, in a highly preferential and selective manner (Steeg *et al.*, 1982; Basham and Merigam, 1983; Wallach *et al.*, 1982; Virelizier *et al.*, 1984). This is accomplished with doses of γ-interferon as low as 2 units, orders of magnitude less than that required for induction of 2–5 A and an antiviral effect. New messenger RNA is required for this Ia expression, which occurs on macrophages, melanoma cells, myelomonocytic cell lines, B-cell lines, and even vascular endothelium (Pober *et al.*, 1983; de Waal *et al.*, 1983). Class I MHC antigens and B_2-microglobulin can also be induced by α- and γ-interferon, but at much higher concentrations. The expression of class I and class II MHC antigens appears to be independently regulated by α-interferon (Wong *et al.*, 1984). Recent evidence suggests that interferon does not exert this effect directly but requires a second family of Ia-inducing factors, which are the products of activated macrophages (Walker *et al.*, 1985). Moreover, the continued presence of interferon may be necessary for maintenance of the Ia-positive state.

Macrophages exposed to interferon *in vivo* or *in vitro* become activated, Ia-positive, produce hydrogen peroxide, become more antimicrobial, and mediate nonspecific tumor cell killing (Unanue *et al.*, 1984; Nathan *et al.*, 1983). γ-Interferon-treated macrophages demonstrate an increase in messenger RNA coding for I-region cell surface molecules and have an immunoenhancing capability on antibody formation (Nakamura *et al.*, 1984). There is good evidence that the macrophage-activating factor (MAF) and perhaps the macrophage-Ia-recruiting factor (MIRF) are identical with γ-interferon (Schultz and Kleinschmidt, 1983; Sverdersky *et al.*, 1984). Macrophage expression of Ia is inhibited by E-class prostaglandins and by α-fetoprotein (Unanue *et al.*, 1984).

Ia expression represents an inducible cell phenotype rather than a marker of fixed cell lineage. Lipopolysaccharide (LPS) through the production of prostaglandins, is a down-regulator of murine macrophage Ia expression. Nevertheless, LPS is a potent stimulator of macrophage IL-1 production, suggesting that macrophage Ia expression and IL-1 production can be dissociated and may be regulated independently. Incubation of adherent and nonadherent cells with antibody to interferon leads to a dose-dependent decrease in adherent cell DR expression, suggesting that low levels of interferon constitutively produced by resting peripheral lymphocytes are sufficient to maintain DR expression (Sztein *et al.*, 1984). Thus, there are bidirectional interactions between macrophages and lymphocytes that are important in immunoregulation.

DR antigen can be expressed on numerous cell types including follicular thyroid cells (Pujol-Borrell *et al.*, 1983), raising the possibility that these could even present antigen and contribute thereby to autoimmune reactions. Induction of Ia by viruses or interferon has been proposed as a mechanism contribution to target-organ-specific autoimmune disorders (Bottazzo *et al.*, 1983).

One of the most exciting aspects of cellular immunology today is the discovery of the important immunoregulatory role of interleukin 2 (IL-2), also called T-cell growth factor (S. Gupta, Chapter 4, this volume). Interleukin 2 is produced by Lyt-1^+2^- T helper/inducer cells and acts on many different cells that express IL-2 receptors (Fig. 1). Among its many biological effects, IL-2 induces the production of γ-interferon by Lyt-2^+ cells, which is the population that also expresses suppressor/cytotoxic activity (Torres *et al.*, 1982). Aberrant production of γ-interferon can be induced in autoimmune-susceptible MRL/lpr mice by exposure to mitogen and phorbol esters (Santoro *et al.*, 1983). Both IL-2 (Henney *et al.*, 1981; Handra *et al.*, 1983; Domzig *et al.*, 1983) and γ-interferon (Huddlestone *et al.*, 1979; Minato *et al.*, 1980; Targan and Stebbing, 1982) stimulate NK cells.

IV. INTERFERON AND AUTOIMMUNE DISORDERS

Fifty-one percent of SLE patients have an unusual acid-labile form of human α-interferon present in the serum (Table 3; Hooks *et al.*, 1979; Preble *et al.*, 1982). Since this interferon is inactivated at pH 2, a property of γ- but not classical α-interferon, it was not immediately identified as belonging to the α class. However, it was shown to be α-interferon by neutralization with specific antibody and by its antiviral activity on bovine cells (Preble *et al.*, 1982). Since natural human α-interferon produced by virus-stimulated leukocytes *in vitro* is a mixture of at least 13 subtypes of α-interferon, it is likely that this autoimmune-associated acid-labile interferon represents a subtype of normal human α-interferon. Indeed, a normal human interferon with antigenic properties of α and physiochemical acid-labile properties of γ is produced by normal peripheral blood mononuclear cells during an immune response (Balkwill *et al.*, 1983). An acid-labile interferon also occurs in rheumatoid arthritis, scleroderma, Sjogren's syndrome, and autoimmune vasculitis but not in drug-induced lupus. There is disagreement as to a correlation between acid-labile interferon and SLE activity (Hooks *et al.*, 1979; Preble *et al.*, 1982). Leukocytes from SLE but not RA patients have a diminished capacity to produce interferon in response to several inducers (Neighbour and Grayzel, 1981). A similar abnormality occurs in

Table 3. Interferon in Sera of Patients with Autoimmune Disease[a]

Serum source	Interferon: No. positive/ no. tested	Interferon: Percent positive
Systemic lupus erythematosus	25/49	51
Rheumatoid arthritis	6/11	55
Scleroderma	6/10	60
Sjogren's syndrome	4/15	27
Vasculitis	7/12	33
Behcet's disease	30/58	51
Aphthous stomatitis	0/13	0
Normal	1/34	3

[a] Modified from Moutsopoulos and Hooks (1983).

lepromatous leprosy, where it may be related to deficient IL-2 production since it is correctable by IL-2 and *M. leprae* antigen (Nogueira *et al.*, 1983). Mononuclear cells from both interferon-positive and -negative SLE patients contain elevated levels of the enzyme 2–5 A synthetase, suggesting that these patients respond to their own endogenously produced acid-labile α-interferon (Preble *et al.*, 1983).

Interferons including the acid-labile interferon are inducers of tubuloreticular inclusions (TRI) often present in the endoplasmic reticulum of vascular endothelial cells and in lymphocytes of lupus patients (Preble and Friedman, 1983). When originally described, these structures were first mistakenly thought to be viral particles but are now generally considered nonspecific markers of cellular injury. Interferon may induce TRI in a long-lived lymphocyte subpopulation that can persist in the circulation even after the interferon serum concentration disappears. High local concentrations of interferon in lymphoid organs might also contribute to the production of cells containing TRI. These inclusions have also been observed in lymphocytes and monocytes from patients receiving long-term interferon therapy in clinical trials.

There are only rare reports of antibodies to interferon in SLE patients (Panem *et al.*, 1982; Moutsopoulos and Hooks, 1983). Interferon is a poor immunogen and does not appear to circulate as an immune complex in SLE.

The exact biological significance of the acid-labile interferon is currently being studied in several laboratories. Although administration of interferon can accelerate the onset and severity of autoimmune disease in NZB mice (Engleman *et al.*, 1981), there is no evidence to implicate interferon directly in the pathogenesis of autoimmunity. Nevertheless, the potent immunoregulatory effects of interferon might very well come into play and contribute to creating the state of disordered immunoregulation that is thought to underlie generalized autoimmune diseases such as SLE.

Further reason to implicate interferon in pathogenesis comes from recent observations in homosexual and hemophiliac patients with AIDS, whose serum often contains acid-lable α-interferon (Preble *et al.*, 1985; Eyster *et al.*, 1983; DeStefano *et al.*, 1982). Approximately 12% of patients with generalized lymphoadenopathy and 71% of patients with Kaposi's sarcoma and/or opportunistic infection had elevated serum interferon titers. Acid-labile α-interferon was also present in 10% of asymptomatic homosexual men, where it may precede the development of frank immunologic disease and possibly have predictive value. A similar suggestion has been proposed for the elevated levels of serum β_2-microglobulin in AIDS patients (Zolla-Pazner *et al.*, 1984), which also occurs in patients with autoimmune disorders (Talal *et al.*, 1975). Furthermore, lymphocytes from AIDS patients had elevated levels of 2–5 A synthetase as well as characteristic TRI, suggesting that AIDS patients, like those with lupus, respond to their own endogenously produced interferon (Preble and Friedman, 1983).

V. NATURAL KILLER CELLS

Natural killer cells were first discovered as "background" cytotoxicity among lymphocytes from normal, nonimmune donors. They are defined operationally by the ability of non-primed lymphocytes from healthy donors to kill diverse tumors or virally infected targets in short-term cytotoxicity assays. Natural killing is independent of the thymus and can easily be demonstrated in athymic nude mice. The NK effector cells lack classical markers for T and B cells, are radioresistant, nonphagocytic, nonadherent, show no immunologic memory, and can be activated nonspecifically and rapidly by interferon and agents that induce interferon (Herberman *et al.*, 1981–1982; Huddlestone *et al.*, 1979; Minato *et al.*, 1980; Targan and Stebbing, 1982). They have the appearance of LGLs and react with certain monoclonal antibodies, particularly anti-Leu 11, OKM1, and Leu-7 (HNK1). Various target cells differ in their susceptibility to natural killing. The target structure recognized is as yet unknown. Cells with spontaneous cytotoxic activity occur early in the human fetus, in mouse yolk sac cells, and in lower life forms such as earthworms (Herberman, 1985), suggesting that the NK system may constitute a primitive defense mechanism.

Natural killer cells function in tumor surveillance and are responsible for the rapid elimination of intravenously inoculated tumor cells. Suppression or augmentation of NK activity in mice is associated with parallel alterations in susceptibility or resistance to artificial metastases produced by intravenous inoculation of tumor cells. Cells recoverable from metastatic lung nodules from a transplantable tumor in mice are more resistant to NK activity than locally growing tumor cells. Injection of a cloned NK line into NK-deficient mice confers resistance against metastatic spread and against primary radiation-induced leukemia. Although the mouse mutant beige has impaired NK function and rejects tumor transplants poorly, there is still no conclusive information to suggest that NK cells protect against spontaneous tumor appearance. Humans with the Chediak–Higashi syndrome, thought to be a human correlate of the beige mouse, have impaired NK function and an 85% incidence of spontaneous lymphoproliferative disorders (Roder *et al.*, 1980).

Many diverse types of tumors are susceptible to NK killing, which is not dependent on a requirement for MHC products and thus not subject to syngeneic restriction. Virus-infected cells, normal hematopoietic and lymphoid cells, and some microbial agents are targets. Many laboratories are currently studying how NK cells actually kill and whether soluble factors are involved. Both the binding of NK cells to their targets and postbinding events are involved in cytotoxicity and influenced in interferon-mediated augmentation of killing. In general, NK-sensitive tumors show a higher frequency of binding cells than do resistant tumors even when cloned NK lines are usual. Primitive normal hematopoietic cells are also recognized and lysed by NK cells *in vitro*. Thymocytes and bone marrow cells from man and mouse are unusually sensitive. The NK sensitive thymocytes are a subpopulation of immature, cortisone-sensitive, large, rapidly dividing cells. Similarities between this thymocyte target and the proposed target for the murine leukemia virus-transformed cell have led to speculation that the NK cell normally regulates immature T cells. As for the bone marrow, the target appears to be a true stem cell, suggesting that NK cells play a role in controlling hematopoiesis. Indeed, NK cells may be the most important factor in rejection of allogeneic and parenteral bone marrow transplants. *In vivo* treatment with antiserum directed to the NK cell suppresses resistance to such bone marrow transplants.

The characteristics of NK cells include some features shared with classical T cells (e.g., ability to produce and respond to IL-2) and others shared with classical macrophages (e.g., presence of OKM1 and Fc receptors). To add to the confusion, NK cells have recently been found to produce a great array of factors including interleukins 1 and 2 as well as α- and γ-interferon (Table 4). This has created considerable doubt as to the true nature of the NK cell and has left unresolved two major and conflicting possibilities. On the one hand, there may be a true heterogeneity such that cells belonging to both the T and macrophage lineage can mediate natural cytotoxicity (Hercend *et al.*, 1983a,b; Fitzgerald *et al.*, 1983). Supporters of the alternative position propose a true NK lineage constituting a unique type of cell that has overlap features of the two other populations. Analysis at the clonal level has not resolved this issue. Clones derived from purified LGLs expanded in IL-2 demonstrated a heterogenous pattern of reactivity against various tumor targets (Allavena and Ortaldo, 1984). Clones expressed both T-cell antigens (OKT3, OTK4, OKT8) and LGL antigens (OKM1, OKT10, B73.1). There was no correlation between surface phenotype and cytotoxic activity. Mixtures of clones could explain the heterogeneity of the entire NK population. Curiously and totally unrelated to NK cells, there exists evidence for another kind of overlap cell that has features of both B and T cells and occurs in autoimmune NZB mice (Hayakawa *et al.*, 1983; Manohar *et al.*, 1982).

Maintenance of NK-cell activity is dependent on interferon (Fig. 3) and probably

Table 4. Cytokines Produced by Human LGL[a]

γ-Interferon
α-Interferon
Interleukin 2 (IL-2)
Interleukin 1 (IL-1)
B-cell growth factor (BCGF)
Colony-stimulating factor (CSF)
Lymphotoxin
NK cytotoxic factor (NKCF)

[a]From Herberman (1985).

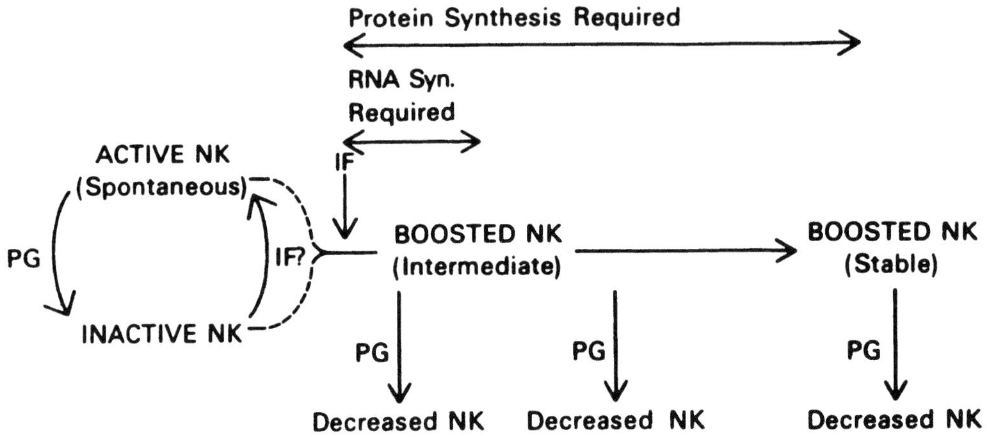

Figure 3. Model for regulation of mouse NK activity. Interferon (IF) appears to be responsible for augmentation of spontaneous NK activity to the "boosted NK" state. It remains unclear, as indicated in the left side of the model, whether IF acts on inactive precursors of NK cells or whether it augments the reactivity of already spontaneously activated NK cells. During the early period of boosting, RNA and protein synthesis is required, as indicated by the ability of the appropriate inhibitors to block or reverse augmentation. After 4–6 hr for RNA synthesis, and approximately 18 hr for protein synthesis, the boosted NK state becomes stable and is no longer affected by the metabolic inhibitors. Prostaglandins E_1 or E_2 (PG) have been found to inhibit both spontaneous and boosted NK activity and may be important negative regulatory factors. (From Herberman *et al.*, 1980.)

IL-2, just as Ia positivity also is interferon dependent. As already discussed, this interferon induction may take place locally in microenviromental sites of relatively high lymphokine concentration. It is certainly conceivable that the growth inhibitory properties of the NK cell on bone marrow and other targets might be mediated via interferon. The recent evidence from Herberman (Herberman, 1985) that NK cells produce a wide variety of cytokines (Table 4) opens the door for possible self-regulation of natural killing. For example, LGLs exposed to appropriate targets might initially secrete interferon and IL-2, which in turn could further drive the cells for cytotoxic activity (Herberman, 1985).

Kiessling feels that NK-cell–target recognition represents some primitive cell/cell recognition phenomenon by which immature malignant and normal cells can be distinguished from more mature counterparts and eliminated from the organism (Kiessling *et al.*, 1983). Natural killer cells may thus have a basic regulatory function on stem cells. Very recent experiments suggest that NK cells may also down-regulate the antibody response by acting on accessory cells that have interacted with antigen (Abruzzo and Rowley, 1983). The authors suggest that these antigen-exposed accessory cells become targets for NK killing and that loss of this function in NK-deficient states (e.g., aging) may lead to dysregulation and elevated IgM. These observations suggest a model (Fig. 4) in which IL-2 and interferon, by acting on the NK cell, can inhibit human polyclonal immunoglobulin synthesis through mechanisms that are independent and perhaps more important than suppressor T cells (Fleisher *et al.*, 1982). Large granular lymphocytes also inhibit antibody production by autologous human lymphoblastoid B cells, which appear in the circulation 5–7 days after *in vivo* immunization (Brieva *et al.*, 1984). This inhibition is enhanced by interferon and blocked by anti-Leu 7 plus complement.

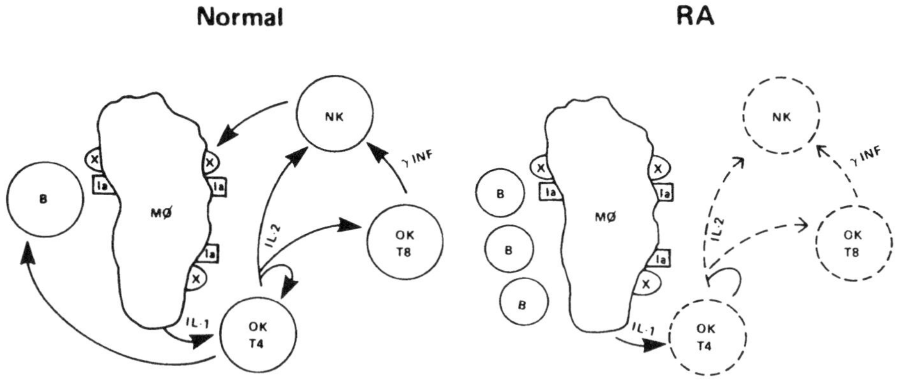

Figure 4. A model showing IL-2 and interferon acting on the NK cell and causing the inhibition of human polyclonal immunoglobulin synthesis through mechanisms that are independent of suppressor T cells.

VI. NATURAL KILLER CELLS AND AUTOIMMUNE DISORDERS

Numerous laboratories have reported significantly diminished NK-cell activity in SLE patients using a standard K562 cell line as a target (Silverman and Cathcart, 1980; Goto *et al.*, 1980; Neighbour, 1982; Katz *et al.*, 1982; Sibbit *et al.*, 1983a) as well as lymphoblastoid and myeloid cell lines (Hoffman, 1980) and a mammary epithelial cell line (Fitzharris *et al.*, 1982). Cytotoxicity was lower in patients with active or untreated disease (Silverman and Cathcart, 1980; Neighbour 1981; Katz *et al.*, 1982; Sibbit *et al.*, 1983a), although not all laboratories agreed (Goto *et al.*, 1980). There was also disagreement as to the presence of serum inhibitory factors and the effect of overnight incubation. Cytotoxicity increased following overnight incubation in one study (Silverman and Cathcart, 1980), suggesting the presence of membrane-bound inhibitory factors. These investigators also found that SLE serum could markedly inhibit natural killing by peripheral blood lymphocytes of normal subjects. This is not surprising in view of the fact that antibody-dependent cellular cytotoxicity (ADCC) is decreased in lupus, and this activity is known to be blocked by circulating immune complexes. Furthermore, there is some evidence to suggest that both NK and ADCC activities are overlapping functions possibly mediated by similar if not at times identical cell populations. By contrast, other workers found that NK function in SLE remained low even after prolonged *in vitro* incubation at 37°C or protease treatment (Sibbit *et al.*, 1983a; Hoffman, 1980). There was no evidence for a cell-mediated supressive mechanism, and indomethacin was without effect.

The normal ability of interferon to augment NK is also impaired in SLE (Neighbour *et al.*, 1982; Fitzharris *et al.*, 1982; Sibbit *et al.*, 1983a,b,c). Fewer than 50% of SLE patients showed any increase in NK after treatment with interferon or Newcastle disease virus; the level of cytotoxicity was minimally increased above endogenous NK levels (Neighbour *et al.*, 1982). Indeed, SLE sera were found to inhibit the inteferon-mediated augmentation of natural killing found with normal peripheral blood mononuclear cells (Sibbit *et al.*, 1983c). There was no significant correlation between interferon production and endogenous NK activity either in normals or in SLE patients (Neighbour *et al.*, 1982). Similarly, incubation of lymphocytes from SLE patients with exogenous interleukin 2 failed to restore NK activity to normal levels (Sibbit *et al.*, 1983b).

In studies designed to further elucidate the mechanisms responsible for impaired natural killing in SLE, one laboratory (Katz *et al.*, 1982) found evidence for an abnormality in the lytic event itself rather than a deficiency of NK cells, an abnormality in target binding, or an inability of NK cells to lyse multiple targets. Serum factors did not appear to play a major etiologic role in the abnormal killing, although this is contradicted by another study (Sibbit *et al.*, 1983b). The presence of specific antibody to NK cells in lupus sera has also been suggested (Goto *et al.*, 1980).

Natural killing is also decreased in patients with Sjogren's syndrome (Goto *et al.*, 1981; Miyasaka *et al.*, 1983). More than one mechanism may be involved. There is evidence for both inhibitory serum factors, which do not correlate with levels of immune complexes or with antilymphocyte antibodies, and for inhibitory adherent cells (Miyasaka *et al.*, 1983). Addition of indomethacin or catalase partially restored NK activity in some patients, indicating that both prostaglandins and hydrogen peroxide may play a pathogenetic role in reducing natural killing. This impaired NK-cell activity could play a pathogenetic role in the development of lymphoma and pseudolymphoma, which are well-recognized complications of Sjogren's syndrome (Strand and Talal, 1980).

There is more uncertainty and disagreement about the status of natural killing in patients with rheumatoid arthritis. In part, this uncertainty relates to differences in technique but might also reflect the extent of disease activity in the particular patient population studied.

Natural killer activity was depressed in RA patients but could be augmented by interferon (Itoh *et al.*, 1981). One laboratory (Karsh *et al.*, 1981) found it significantly decreased only in patients with active disease, whereas another found it low in seropositive but not seronegative RA (McDaniel *et al.*, 1983). Surprisingly, still another laboratory reported NK activity increased in females but not males with RA, especially those being treated with gold (Goto, 1981). Other studies found NK activity to be similar in RA and controls (Dobloug *et al.*, 1982; Silver *et al.*, 1982). When a human melanoma cell line was used as the target, NK activity of rheumatoid patients was not different from controls except at very high effector-to-target ratios (Burmester *et al.*, 1978).

We find that NK-cell activity in RA peripheral blood is diminished, but this is best documented in patients with active disease. We performed two separate studies using our own San Antonio clinic population. In the first study, employing unselected seropositive patients, there was a modest impairment in peripheral blood NK-cell activity, but this did not achieve statistical significance (Lynn *et al.*, 1983). The second study utilized RA patients with joint effusions who had more active disease than those in the first study. There we found a significant impairment in peripheral blood NK activity ($P < 0.001$) that correlated inversely with the erythrocyte sedimentation rate (Combe *et al.*, 1985a). Natural killing using RA blood cells can be augmented normally by the interferon inducer poly-I:C, by interleukin 2, and especially by the two modulators acting together (Combe *et al.*, 1985b). Indomethacin augments peripheral blood NK activity in RA just as it does in normal individuals. In RA synovial fluid, NK is decreased compared to blood and appears to be mediated by a cell lacking Fc receptors but having broad target specificity (Silver *et al.*, 1982).

Table 5. Induction of IL-2 by PHA in Normal Controls and Patients with Rheumatoid Arthritis

Subjects	IL-2 (units/ml)
Normal PB (n = 15)	28.0 ± 17.4[a]
RA PB (n = 13)	10.2 ± 11.9[b]
SF (n = 13)	14.8 ± 26.3[c]
ST (n = 4)	2.6 ± 3.4
Gout SF (n = 4)	61.5 ± 32.8

[a] Mean ± S.D.
[b] Significantly reduced compared to normal PB ($P < 0.001$).
[c] Significantly reduced compared to normal PB ($P < 0.02$).

We have also studied NK activity in the rheumatoid synovium and find it markedly diminished compared even to RA peripheral blood. Like blood NK, synovial fluid NK is very responsive to the immunomodulators poly-I:C and interleukin 2. This sensitivity to exogenous immunopotentiation probably reflects the fact that the synovial environment is relatively devoid of inherent capacity to produce interferon and IL-2. For example, matched blood (PB) and synovial fluid lymphocytes from 13 RA patients showed markedly impaired IL-2 production following PHA stimulation (Table 5). Lymphocytes recovered from RA synovial tissue specimens produced almost no IL-2 in response to PHA (Combe *et al.*, 1985a). Lymphocytes from the synovial fluid of control patients with gout produced abundant quantities of IL-2 following PHA stimulation, indicating that the low IL-2 seen in RA is not merely a general characteristic of inflammation. Interleukin 2 production by RA blood or synovial fluid did not correlate with therapeutic regimen or clinical activity.

Rheumatoid arthritis synovial lymphocytes also showed a diminished ability to respond to IL-2 ($P < 0.001$) (Table 6). Indeed, the proliferative response of synovial lymphoid cells to added IL-2 was even more impaired than that of blood ($P < 0.05$).

Interleukin 2 has diverse effects on the immune response including the ability to induce lymphocytes to produce γ-interferon (IFN). Since the proliferative response of RA blood and synovial lymphocytes to IL-2 is diminished, we studied whether the IFN response to IL-2 would also be decreased (Combe *et al.*, 1985). The IFN activity released spontaneously by either RA or normal unstimulated cells was negligible. Following

Table 6. Response to Exogenous IL-2 by Lymphocyte Blasts from Patients with RA and Normal Controls

	Lymphocyte proliferation	
	No IL-2 (cpm)	Plus IL-2 (cpm)
Normal PB (n = 10)	681 ± 547[a]	39,685 ± 13,759
RA PB (n = 6)	604 ± 600	27,466 ± 6,447
RA SF (n = 8)	561 ± 373	17,408 ± 6,700[b]

[a] Mean ± S.D.
[b] Significantly different from both normal PB ($P < 0.001$) and RA PB ($P < 0.05$).

Table 7. Induction of Interferon by Incubation of Mononuclear Cells with IL-2

	Interferon (units/ml)	
	No IL-2	+IL-2
Normal PB (n = 8)	1.3 ± 1.2[a]	62.5 ± 12.5
RA PB (n = 8)	2.5 ± 2.5	16.1 ± 7.6[b]
RA SF (n = 8)	2.5 ± 4.6	29.6 ± 11.5[c]

[a] Interferon concentration is presented as mean ± S.E.
[b] Decreased compared to normal PB ($P < 0.001$).
[c] Decreased compared to normal PB ($P < 0.02$).

exposure to IL-2, both blood ($P < 0.001$) and synovial ($P < 0.02$) lymphocytes produced significantly less IFN than did normal PB lymphocytes (Table 7). The IFN produced was primarily of the γ class, since incubation at pH 3.0 and treatment with an antibody specific for γ-IFN either abolished or greatly reduced the IFN activity compared to the pretreatment values.

As already mentioned, NK cell activity in synovial fluid is very responsive to augmentation by IL-2 (Table 8). All increases were significant compared to base line ($P < 0.005$). Interleukin 2 enhanced NK activity of RA synovial lymphocytes to a greater degree than that seen with normal or rheumatoid ($P < 0.02$) peripheral blood. The NK activity of rheumatoid synovial fluid was enhanced to a level comparable to that seen in normal peripheral blood even though the base-line values tended to be lower in the synovial fluid.

Despite the defective induction of IFN by IL-2, IL-2 increased the *in vitro* activity of RA blood and synovial lymphoid cells to a degree comparable to normals (Tables 7, 8). Thus, there was a discordance between the poor ability of IL-2 to stimulate IFN production and its excellent ability to augment NK activity in RA. Removal of adherent cells did not restore but further decreased the IFN induced by IL-2 from 34.7 ± 10.1 units/ml (mean ± S.E.) to 3.3 ± 3.3 units/ml. Therefore, synovial adherent cells, which have been shown in numerous studies to produce abundant quantities of suppressing prostaglandins, failed to suppress the IL-2 induction of interferon. In fact, adherent cells

Table 8. Effect of IL-2 on NK Activity in Rheumatoid Arthritis and Normal Controls

	Mean percentage cytotoxicity		
	No IL-2	+IL-2	Percent increase
Normal PB (n = 16)	47.1 ± 4.8[a]	64.0 ± 3.6	36[b]
RA PB (n = 9)	29.0 ± 4.6	42.3 ± 6.3	46
RA SF (n = 9)	37.9 ± 5.6	60.1 ± 4.3	59

[a] Whole mononuclear cells were employed at an E : T ratio of 20 : 1 to measure NK activity (as percent of maximal ^{51}Cr release from K562).
[b] Percent increase over base line by addition of IL-2.

Table 9. Reduced NK Activity in Aged C57BL/1pr Mice

Strain	Age (months)	Percent NK Killing at effector : target cell ratio		
		200 : 1	100 : 1	50 : 1
C57	3	25.7	23.9	10.9
	9	31.5	9.3	0.0
C57-1pr	3	20.5	34.9	36.1
	9	0.0	3.9	6.7

may promote this effect of IL-2, since we have found that synovial macrophages regulate NK cell activity differently than do peripheral blood macrophages (Combe *et al.*, 1985a). Rheumatoid arthritis synovial macrophages augment NK activity, and this effect is independent of indomethacin, whereas RA blood macrophages, like normal blood macrophages, down-regulate blood NK cells through an indomethacin-sensitive mechanism.

One laboratory found that natural cytotoxicity of spleen cells from autoimmune NZB mice was within the same range as several normal strains when tested with various cultured cell lines (Croker *et al.*, 1979). By contrast, we found high levels of natural killing against the YAC target (Seaman *et al.*, 1978). Similar technical variations, particularly the nature of the target cells, may account for different findings in autoimmune MRL/1pr mice. Both elevated (Clark *et al.*, 1981) and reduced (Tai and Warner, 1980) NK-cell activity have been observed. Interestingly, mesenteric lymph node cells from older MRL/1pr mice were more active than MRL/n cells against WEHI-22. We find that many autoimmune-susceptible strains of mice show an age-dependent decline in NK cell activity measured against the conventional YAC-1 target cell line (Table 9).

VII. CONCLUDING COMMENTS

Our current understanding of how autoimmune and malignant disease may develop out of a background of disordered immunoregulation is shown schematically in Fig. 5. This concept of pathogenesis is very similar to one proposed 15 years ago (Talal, 1970) and discussed more recently in relation to the impaired autologous mixed lymphocyte response that often accompanies these diseases (Smith and Talal, 1982).

The immune response gene predisposition is probably related to common structural products of DR and DS loci such as those recently found for HLA-DR4 in RA patients (Nepom *et al.*, 1984). Whether transposable genetic elements or structures similar to oncogenes (?autogenes) are also involved is a matter for speculation. Less speculative is the immunologic imbalance characteristic not only of autoimmunity but also seen in patients with AIDS (Talal, 1983) and those immunosuppressed with cyclosporin A (Touraine *et al.*, 1983). The crux of this imbalance is a depressed cellular immunity accompanied by IL-2 deficiency and a polyclonal B-cell activation with augmented and often inappropriate antibody responses. Several factors may account for this heightened humoral immunity, including intrinsic mechanisms related to EB or other viruses (Vaughan *et al.*, 1983; Depper and Zvaifler, 1981), T-cell-derived B-cell growth and differentiation factors

Immune response gene (? Autogene)

↓

Immunologic imbalance

↓ ↓

Cellular immunity depressed	Antibody responses augmented
(↓ Interleukin 2)	(Polyclonal B-cell activation)
↓	↓
Impaired immune surveillance	Immunization with viral
(↓ NK Cells)	antigens and nucleic acids
↓	↓
Malignancy	"Autoantibodies"
	↓
	Immune complex nephritis

Figure 5. A scheme showing the development of autoimmune and malignant disease out of a background of disordered immunoregulation.

(Prud'homme *et al.*, 1983), or the recently described down-regulation of B cells by NK cells (Abruzzo and Rowley, 1983). Probably as a consequence of several mechanisms, "autoantibodies" are produced that may be induced by viral antigens and/or nucleic acids and not be truly anti-self in that sense. Indeed, such reactivity might even derive from a physiological basis as previously hypothesized (Talal, 1978).

My own laboratory's interest in NK cells grew out of our finding that IL-2 production and response are diminished in autoimmune mice (Wofsy *et al.*, 1981; Dauphinee *et al.*, 1981). We find that RA and SLE patients similarly manifest IL-2 abnormalities (Miyasaka *et al.*, 1984), and we have recently focused on the rheumatoid joint, which is a site of intense B-cell hyperactivity. Synovial lymphocytes from RA patients produce little IL-2 in response to mitogenic stimulation and respond poorly to exogenous IL-2 as measured by proliferation and interferon production. Systemic as well as local production of interferon would be extremely important both for the maintenance of NK cell activity and for more direct antiviral defense.

We looked directly at NK cell activity in RA and found that it, like IL-2, is also diminished both in blood and even more in the synovium. Several mechanisms in the RA synovium are present to bolster what little residual NK activity remains. For example, activated macrophages in the RA synovium are augmenters of NK, whereas RA blood macrophages suppress NK, as do normal peripheral blood macrophages. Interleukin 2, although it is a poor inducer of interferon in RA, is a good activator of NK both in RA blood and particularly in the synovium.

We are intrigued by the possibility that NK cells play a role in down-regulating B cells and that the failure of this mechanism contributes to the persistent immunoglobulin, autoantibody, and rheumatoid factor production seen in RA (Fig. 4B).

One model (Abruzzo and Rowley, 1983) suggests that the antigen-activated macrophage is a target for NK and that this mechanism normally operates to shut off immunoglobulin production, particulary of IgM. Failure of this mechanism would leave unchecked the activated macrophage and thereby account for the macrophage abnormalities and excessive monokines and IL-1 characteristic of RA (Pope and Talal, 1985).

The requirement for IL-2 and interferon to maintain NK activity is impressive. The actual number of NK cells in RA is probably not diminished, although their activity is markedly reduced by virtue of their living in a milieu deficient in precisely those immunoregulatory factors necessary for maintenance of function. This additional role for IL-2 as a sustainer of NK adds yet another important function to the many already described for this extraordinary molecule. Interleukin 2 deficiency may be a final common pathway through which multiple immunoregulatory mechanisms become enfeebled, thereby creating a subsoil out of which autoimmune diseases may more easily emerge.

ACKNOWLEDGMENT. These studies were supported in part by the General Medical Research Service of the Veterans Administration.

REFERENCES

Abruzzo, L. V., and Rowley, D. A., 1983, Homeostasis of the antibody response: Immunoregulation by NK cells, *Science* **222**:581–585.

Allavena, P., and Ortaldo, J. R., 1984, Characteristics of human NK clones: Target specificity and phenotype, *J. Immunol.* **132**(5):1–7.

Balkwill, F. R., Griffin, D. B., Band, H. A., and Beverley, P. C. L., 1983, Immune human lymphocytes produce an acid-labile α-interferon, *J. Exp. Med.* **157**:1059–1063.

Basham, T. Y., and Merigan, T. C., 1983, Recombinant interferon-γ increases HLA-DR synthesis and expression, *J. Immunol.* **130**:1492–1494.

Bottazzo, G. F., Pujol-Borrell, R., Hanafusa, T., and Feldmann, M., 1983, *Lancet* **2**:1115–1119.

Brieva, J. A., Targan, S., and Stevens, R. H., 1984, NK and T cell subsets regulate antibody production by human *in vivo* antigen-induced lymphoblastoid B cells, *J. Immunol.* **132**:611–615.

Burmester, G. R., Kalden, J. R., Peter, H. H., Schedel, I., Beck, P., and Wittenborg, A., 1978, Immunological and functional characteristics of peripheral blood and synovial fluid lymphocytes from patients with rheumatoid arthritis, *Scand. J. Immunol.* **7**:405–417.

Clark, E. D., Shultz, L. D., and Pollack, S. B., 1981, Mutations in mice that influence natural killer (NK) cell activity, *Immunogenetics* **12**:601–613.

Combe, B., Pope, R., Darnell, B., and Talal, N., 1984, Modulation of natural killer cell activity in the rheumatoid joint and peripheral blood, *Scand. J. Immunol.* **20**:551–558.

Combe, B., Pope, R. M., Fischbach, M., Darnell, B., Baron, S., and Talal, N., 1985, Interleukin-2 in rheumatoid arthritis: Production of and response to interleukin-2 in rheumatoid synovial fluid, synovial tissue and peripheral blood, *Clin. Exp. Immunol.* **59**:520–528.

Croker, B. P., Zinkernagel, R. M., and Dixon, F. J., 1979, Natural cytotoxic cells in NZB mice: Spontaneous *in vivo* and *in vitro* primed activity and structural characteristics, *Clin. Immunol. Immunopathol.* **12**:410–424.

Dauphinee, M. J., Kipper, S. B., Wofsy, D., and Talal, N., 1981, Interleukin-2 deficiency is a common feature of autoimmune mice, *J. Immunol.* **127**(6):2483.

Depper, J. M., and Zvaifler, N. J., 1981, Epstein–Barr virus. Its relationship to the pathogenesis of rheumatoid arthritis, *Arthritis Rheum.* **24**:755.

DeStefano, E., Friedman, R. M., Friedman-Kien, A. E., Goedert, J. J., Henriksen, D., Preble, O. T., Sonnabend, J. A., and Vilcek, J., 1982, Acid-labile human leukocyte interferon in homosexual men with Kaposi's sarcoma and lymphadenopathy, *J. Infec. Dis.* **146**:451–455.
de Waal, R. M. W., Bogman, M. J. J., Maass, C. N., Cornelissen, L. M. H., Tax, W. J. M., and Koene, R. A. P., 1983, Variable expression of Ia antigens on the vascular endothelium of mouse skin allografts, *Nature* **303**:426–429.
Dobloug, J. H., Forre, O., Kvien, T. K., Egeland, T., and Degre, M., 1982, Natural killer (NK) cell activity of peripheral blood, synovial fluid and synovial tissue lymphocytes from patients with rheumatoid arthritis and juvenile rheumatoid arthritis, *Ann. Rheum. Dis.* **41**:490–494.
Domzig, W., Stadler, B. M., and Herberman, R. B., 1983, Interleukin 2 dependence of human natural killer (NK) cell activity, *J. Immunol.* **130**:1970–1973.
Engleman, E. G., Sonnenfeld, G., Dauphinee, M., Greenspan, J. S., and Talal, N., 1981, Treatment of NZB/NZW F_1 hybrid mice with *Mycobacterium bovis* strain BCG or type II interferon preparations accelerates autoimmune disease, *Arthritis Rheum.* **24**:(11):1396–1402.
Eyster, M. E., Goeder, J. J., Poon, M. C., and Preble, O. T., 1983, Acid-labile alpha interferon. A possible preclinical marker for the acquired immunodeficiency syndrome in hemophilia, *N. Engl. J. Med.* **309**:583–586.
Fitzgerald, P. A., Evans, R., Kirkpatrick, D., and Lopez, D., 1983, Heterogeneity of human NK cells: Comparison of effectors that lyse HSV-1-infected fibroblasts and K562 erythroleukemia targets, *J. Immunol.* **130**:1663–1667.
Fitzharris, P., Alcocer, J., Stephens, H. A. F., Knight, R. A., and Snaith, M. L., 1982, Insensitivity to interferon of NK cells from patients with systemic lupus erythematosus, *Clin. Exp. Immunol.* **47**:110–118.
Fleisher, T. A., Attallah, A. M., Tosato, G., Blaese, R. M., and Greene, W. C., 1982, Interferon-mediated inhibition of human polyclonal immunoglobulin synthesis, *J. Immunol.* **129**:1099–1103.
Goto, M., Tanimoto, K., and Horiuchi, Y., 1980, Natural cell mediated cytotoxicity in systemic lupus erythematosus: Suppression by antilymphocyte antibody, *Arthritis Rheum.* **23**(11):1274–1281.
Goto, M., Tanimoto, K., Chihara, T., and Horiuchi, Y., 1981, Natural cell-mediated cytotoxicity in Sjogren's syndrome and rheumatoid arthritis, *Arthritis Rheum.* **24**(11):1377–1383.
Guyre, P. M., Morganelli, P. M., and Miller, R., 1983, Recombinant immune interferon increases immunoglobulin G Fc receptors on cultured human mononuclear phagocytes, *J. Clin. Invest.* **72**:393–397.
Handra, K., Suzuki, R., Matsui, H., Shimizu, Y., and Kumagai, K., 1983, Natural killer (NK) cells as a responder to interleukin-2 (IL 2). II. IL 2-induced interferon γ production, *J. Immunol.* **130**:988–992.
Hayakawa, K., Hardy, R. R., Parko, D. R., and Herzenberg, L. A., 1983, The "Ly-1 B" cell subpopulation in normal, immunodefective, and autoimmune mice, *J. Exp. Med.* **157**:202.
Henney, C. S., Kuribayashi, K., Kern, D. E., and Gillis, S., 1981, Interleukin-2 augments natural killer cell activity, *Nature* **291**:335–338.
Herberman, R. (ed.), 1982, *NK Cells and Other Natural Effector Cells,* Academic Press, New York.
Herberman, R. B., 1985, Multiple functions of natural killer (NK) cells, including immunoregulation as well as resistance to tumor growth, in: *Progress in Immunopathology,* Vol. I, S. Karger, Basel (in press).
Herberman, R. B., Ortaldo, J. R., Djeu, J. Y., Holden, H. T., Jett, J., Lang, N. P., Rubinstein, M., Pestka, S., 1980, Role of interferon in regulation of cytotoxicity by natural killer cells and macrophages, *Ann. N. Y. Acad. Sci.* **350**:63–71.
Herberman, R. B., Ortaldo, J. R., Timonen, T., Reynolds, C. W., Djeu, J. Y., Pestka, S., and Stanton, J., 1981–1982, Interferon and natural killer (NK) cells, *Texas Rep. Biol. Med.* **41**:590–595.
Herberman, R. B., Allavena, P., Scala, G., Djeu, J., Kasahara, T., Domzig, W., Procopio, A., Blanca, I., Ortaldo, J., and Oppenheim, J. J., 1984, Cytokine production by human large granular lymphocytes (LGL), in: *Natural Killer Activity and Its Regulation* (T. Hoshino, H. S. E. Korin, and A. Uchida, eds.), Tokyo Exerpta Medica Limited, Tokyo, pp. 409–413.
Hercend, T., Meuer, S., Brennan, A., Edson, M. A., Acuto, O., Reinherz, E. L., Schlossman, S. F., and Ritz, J., 1983a, Identification of a clonally restricted 90 dK heterodimer on two human cloned natural killer cell lines, *J. Exp. Med.* **158**:1547–1560.
Hercend, T., Reinherz, E. L., Meuer, S., Schlossman, S. F., and Ritz, J., 1983b, Phenotypic and functional heterogeneity of human cloned natural killer cell lines, *Nature* **301**:158–160.
Ho, M., 1982, Recent advances in the study of interferon, *Pharmacol. Rev.* **34**:119–129.
Hoffman, T., 1980, Natural killer function in systemic lupus erythematosus, *Arthritis Rheum.* **23**:(1):30–35.

Hoffman, T., and Ferranrini, M., 1983, Analytical review. A role for natural killer cells in survival: Functions of large granular lymphocytes, including regulation of cell proliferation, *Clin. Immunol. Immunopathol.* **29**:323–332.

Hooks, J. J., Moutsopoulos, H. M., Geis, S. A., Stahl, N. I., Decker, J. L., and Notkins, A. L., 1979, Immune interferon in the circulation of patients with autoimmune disease, *N. Engl. J. Med.* **301**:5–8.

Huddlestone, J. R., Merigan, T. C., Jr., and Oldstone, M. B. A., 1979, Induction of kinetics of natural killer cells in humans following interferon therapy, *Nature* **282**:417–419.

Isaaca, A., and Lindenmann, J., 1957, Virus interference. I. The interferon, *Proc. R. Soc. Lon. (Biol.)* **147**:258–267.

Itoh, K., Saitoh, F., Kumagai, K., and Kosaka, S., 1981, Depressed natural killer activity in rheumatoid arthritis and its *in vitro* augmentation with interferon and N-2-carboxyphenol-4 chloranthranilic acid disodium salt (CCA), an anti-arthritis agent, *Ryumachi* **21**:69–74.

Karsh, J., Dorval, G., and Osterland, C. K., 1981, Natural cytotoxicity in rheumatoid arthritis and systemic lupus erythematosus, *Clin. Immunol. Immunopathol.* **19**:437–446.

Katz, P., Zaytoun, A. M., Lee, J. H., Jr., Panush, R. S., and Longley, S., 1982, Abnormal natural killer cell activity in systemic lupus erythematosus: An intrinsic defect in the lytic event, *J. Immunol.* **129**(5):1966–1971.

Kawase, I., Brooks, C. G., Kuribayashi, K., Olabuenaga, S., Newman, W., Gillis, S., and Henney, C. S., 1983, Interleukin-2 induces γ-interferon production: Participation of macrophages and NK-like cells, *J. Immunol.* **131**:288–290.

Kiessling, R., Hansson, M., and Gronberg, A., 1983, Natural killer cells as regulators of malignant and normal cell growth, in: *Progress in Immunology V. Fifth International Congress of Immunology* (Y. Yamamura and T. Tada, eds.), Academic Press, New York, pp. 1181–1194.

Lynn, J., Darnell, B., and Talal, N., 1983, The enhancement of natural killer cell activity in rheumatoid arthritis by interleukin-2 and poly I : C, *Arthritis Rheum.* (Abstract).

Manohar, V., Brown, E., Leverson, W. M., and Chused, T. M., 1982, Expression of Lyt-1 by a subset of B lymphocytes, *J. Immunol.* **129**:532–538.

McDaniel, D. O., Barger, B. O., Alarcon, G. S., and Acton, R. T., 1983, NK activity in rheumatoid arthritis and its association with HLA-DR antigen, *Clin. Res.* **31**:652A.

Minato, N., Reid, L., Cantor, H., Lengyel, P., and Bloom, B. R., 1980, Mode of regulation of natural killer cell activity by interferon, *J. Exp. Med.* **152**:124–137.

Miyasaka, N., Seaman, W., Bakshi, A., Sauvezie, B., Strand, V., Pope, R., and Talal, N., 1983, Natural killing activity in Sjogren's syndrome, *Arthritis Rheum.* **26**(8):954–960.

Miyasaka, N., Darnell, B., Baron, S., and Talal, N., 1984a, Interleukin 2 enhances natural killing of normal lymphocytes, *Cell. Immunol.* **84**:154–162.

Miyasaka, N., Nakamura, T., Russell, I. J., and Talal, N., 1984b, Interleukin 2 deficiencies in rheumatoid arthritis and systemic lupus erythematosus, *Clin. Immunol. Immunopathol.* **31**:109–117.

Moutsopoulos, H. M., and Hooks, J. J., 1983, Interferon and autoimmunity, *Clin. Exp. Rheumatol.* **1**:81–84.

Nakamura, M., Manser, T., Pearson, G. D. N., Daley, M. J., and Gefter, M. L., 1984, Effect of IFN-γ on the immune response *in vivo* and on gene expression *in vitro, Nature* **307**:381–382.

Nathan, C. F., Murray, H. W., Wiebe, M. E., and Rubin, B. Y., 1983, Identification of interferon-γ as the lymphokine that activates human macrophage oxidative metabolism and antimicrobial activity, *J. Exp. Med.* **158**:670–689.

Neighbour, P. A., Grauzel, A. I., Miller, A. E., 1982, Endogenous and interferon-augmented natural killer cell activity of human peripheral blood mononuclear cell *in vitro*. Studies of patients with multiple sclerosis, systemic lupus erythematosus or rheumatoid arthritis, *Clin. Exp. Immunol.* **49**:11–21.

Neighbour, P. A., and Grayzel, A. I., 1981, Interferon production *in vitro* by leucocytes from patients with systemic lupus erythematosus and rheumatoid arthritis, *Clin. Exp. Immunol.* **45**:576–582.

Nepom, B. S., Nepom, G. T., Mickelson, E., Schaller, J. G., Antonelli, P., and Hansen, J. A., 1984, Specific HLA-DR4-associated histocompatibility molecules characterize patients with seropositive juvenile rheumatoid arthritis, *J. Clin. Invest.* **74**:287–291.

Nogueira, N., Kaplan, G., Levy, E., Sarno, E. R., Kushner, P., Granelli-Piperno, A., Vieira, L., Gould, V. C., Levis, W., Steinman, R., Yip, Y. K., and Cohn, Z. A., 1983, Defective γ interferon production in leprosy, *J. Exp. Med.* **158**:2165–2170.

Panem, S., Check, I. J., Henriksen, D., and Vilcek, J., 1982, Antibodies to alpha interferon in a patient with systemic lupus erythematosus, *J. Immunol.* **129**(1):1–3.

Pestka, S., Maeda, S., Hobbs, D. S., Levy, W. P., McCandliss, R., Stein, S., Moshera, J. A., and Staehelin, T., 1981, The human interferons, in: *Cellular Responses To Molecular Modulators* (L. W. Mozes, ed.), Academic Press, New York, pp. 455–489.

Pober, J. S., Gimbrone, M. A., Cotran, R. S., Reiss, C. S., Burakoff, S. J., Fiers, W., and Ault, K. A., 1983, Ia expression by vascular endothelium is inducible by activated T cells and by human γ interferon, *J. Exp. Med.* **157**:1339–1353.

Pope, R., and Talal, N., 1985, Autoimmunity in rheumatoid arthritis, in: *Concepts in Immunopathology,* Vol. 1 (J. Cruse, ed.), S. Karger, Basel, New York, pp. 219–250.

Preble, O. T., and Friedman, R. M., 1983, Biology of disease. Interferon-induced alterations in cells: Relevance to viral and nonviral diseases, *Lab. Invest.* **49**:4–18.

Preble, O. T., Black, R. J., Friedman, R. M., Klippel, J. H., and Vilcek, J., 1982, Systemic lupus erythematosus: Presence in human serum of an unusual acid-labile leukocyte interferon, *Science* **216**:429–431.

Preble, O. T., Rothko, K., Klippel, J. H., Friedman, R. M., and Johnston, M. I., 1983, Interferon-induced 2′-5′ adenylate synthetase *in vivo* and interferon production *in vitro* by lymphocytes from systemic lupus erythematosus patients with and without circulating interferon, *J. Exp. Med.* **157**:2140–2146.

Preble, O. T., Rook, A. H., Quinnan, G. V., Vilcek, J., Friedman, R. M., Steis, R., Gelmann, E. P., and Sonnabend, J. A., 1985, Role of interferon in AIDS, *Ann. N.Y. Acad. Sci.* (in press).

Prud'homme, G. L., Park, C. L., Fieser, T. M., Kofler, R., Dixon, F. J., and Theofilopoulos, A. N., 1983, Identification of a B cell differentiation factor spontaneously produced by proliferating T cells in murine lupus strains of the *lpr/lpr* genotype, *J. Exp. Med.* **157**:730.

Pujol-Borrell, R., Hanafusa, T., Chiovato, L., and Bottazzo, G. F., 1983, Lectin-induced expression of DR antigen on human cultured follicular thyroid cells, *Nature* **303**:71–73.

Roder, J. C., Haliotis, T., Klein, M., Korec, S., Jett, J. R., Ortaldo, J., Heberman, R. B., Katz, P., and Fauci, A. S., 1980, A new immunodeficiency disorder in humans involving NK cells, *Nature* **284**:553–555.

Rodriquez, M. A., Prinz, W. A., Sibbitt, W. L., Bankhurst, A. D., and Williams, R. C., Jr., 1983, Human alpha-interferon enhances *in vitro* IgM rheumatoid factor synthesis by lymphocytes from normal subjects and rheumatoid arthritis patients, *Arthritis Rheum.* **26**:1091–1097.

Santoro, T. J., Benjamin, W. R., Oppenheim, J. J., and Steinberg, A. D., 1983, The cellular basis for immune interferon production in autoimmune MRL-1pr/1pr mice, *J. Immunol.* **131**(1):265–268.

Schultz, R. M., and Kleinschmidt, W. J., 1983, Functional identity between murine γ interferon and macrophage activating factor, *Nature* **305**:239–243.

Seaman, W. E., Blackman, M. A., Gindhart, T. D., Roubinian, J. R., Loeb, J. M., and Talal, N., 1978, β-Estradiol reduces natural killer cells in mice, *J. Immunol.* **121**:2193–2198.

Sibbitt, W. L., Jr., Mathews, P. M., and Bankhurst, A. D., 1983a, Natural killer cell in systemic lupus erythematosus, *J. Clin. Invest.* **71**:1230–1239.

Sibbitt, W. L., Jr., Froelich, C. J., and Bankhurst, A. D., 1983b, Abnormal interferon modulation of natural cytotoxicity in systemic lupus erythematosus: Relation to suppressive serum factors, *Arthritis Rheum.* **26**(12):1452–1459.

Sibbitt, W. L., Jr., Likar, L., Spellman, C. W., and Bankhurst, A. D., 1983c, Impaired natural killer cell function in systemic lupus erythematosus: Relationship to interleukin-2 production, *Arthritis Rheum.* **26**(11):1316–1320.

Silver, R. M., Redelman, D., Zvaifler, N. J., and Naides, S., 1982, Studies of rheumatoid synovial fluid lymphocytes. I. Evidence for activated natural killer-(NK) like cells, *J. Immunol.* **128**:1758–1763.

Silverman, S. L., and Cathcart, E. S., 1980, Natural killing in systemic lupus erythematosus: Inhibitory effects of serum, *Clin. Immunol. Immunopathol.* **17**:219–226.

Smith, J. B., and Talal, N., 1982, Significance of self-recognition and interleukin-2 for immunoregulation, autoimmunity and cancer, *Scand. J. Immunol.* **16**:269–278.

Sonnenfeld, G., and Pick, E., (eds.), 1980, *Lymphokines I,* Academic Press, New York, p. 113.

Steeg, P. S., Moore, R. N., Johnson, H. W., and Oppenheim, J. J., 1982, Regulation of murine macrophage Ia antigen expression by a lymphokine with immune interferon activity, *J. Exp. Med.* **156**:1780–1793.

Stewart, W. E. II, 1981, *The Interferon System,* 2nd ed., Springer-Verlag, New York.

Strand, V., and Talal, N., 1980, Advances in the diagnosis and concept of Sjogren's syndrome (autoimmune exocrinopathy), *Bull. Rheum. Dis.* **30**:1046–1052.

Svedersky, L. P., Benton, C. V., Berger, W. H., Rinderknecht, E., Harkins, R. N., and Palladino, M. A., 1984, Biological and antigenic similarities of murine interferon-γ and macrophage-activating factor, *J. Exp. Med.* **159**:812–827.

Sztein, M. B., Steeg, P. S., Johnson, H. M., and Oppenheim, J. J., 1984, Regulation of human peripheral blood monocyte DR antigen expression *in vitro* by lymphokines and recombinant interferons, *J. Clin. Invest.* **73**:556–565.

Tai, A., and Warner, N. L., 1980, Analysis of recognition patterns of NK cells through use of varying combinations of mouse strains and tumor targets, in: *Natural Cell-Mediated Immunity Against Tumors*, (R. B. Herberman, ed.), Academic Press, New York, pp. 257–264.

Talal, N., 1970, Immunologic and viral factors inthe pathogenesis of systemic lupus erythematosus, *Arthritis Rheum.* **13**:887–894.

Talal, N., 1978, Autoimmunity and the immunologic network, *Arthritis Rheum.* **21**(7):853–861.

Talal, N., 1983, A clinician and a scientist look at acquired immune-deficiency syndrome (AIDS). A validation of immunology's theoretical foundation, *Immunol. Today* **4**(7):180–183.

Talal, N., Grey, H. M., Zvaifler, N., Michalski, J. P., and Daniels, T. E., 1975, Elevated salivary and synovial fluid β_2-microglobulin in Sjogren's syndrome and rheumatoid arthritis, *Science* **187**:1196–1198.

Targan, S., and Stebbing, N., 1982, *In vitro* interactions of purified cloned human interferons on NK cells: enhanced activation, *J. Immunol.* **129**:934–935.

Torres, B. A., Farrar, W. L., and Johnson, H. M., 1982, Interleukin 2 regulates immune interferon (IFNγ) production by normal and suppressor cell cultures, *J. Immunol.* **128**:2217–2219.

Touraine, J. L., Elyafi, S. E., Dosi, E., Chapuis-Cellier, C., Ritter, C., Blanc, N., DuBernard, J., Pouteil-Noble, C., Chevalier, M., Creyssel, R., and Traeger, J., 1983, Immunoglobulin abnormalities and infectious lymphoproliferative syndrome in cyclosporine treated transplant patients, *Transplant Proc.* **15**:2798.

Unanue, E. R., Beller, D. I., Lu, C. Y., and Allen, P. M., 1984, Antigen presentation: Comments on its regulation and mechanism, *J. Immunol.* **132**(1):1–5.

Vaughan, J., Carson, D., and Fox, R., 1983, The Epstein–Barr virus and rheumatoid arthritis, *Clin. Exp. Rheumatol.* **1**:165.

Vilesk, J., Gresser, I., and Merigan, T. C., (eds.), 1980, *Regulatory Functions of Interferon*, New York Academy of Sciences, New York.

Virelizier, J. L., Perez, N., Arenzana-Seisdedos, F., and Devos, R., 1984, Pure interferon gamma enhances class II HLA antigens on human monocyte cell lines, *Eur. J. Immunol.* **14**:106–108.

Walker, E. B., Maino, V., Sanchez-Lanier, M., Warner, N., and Stewart, C., 1985, Murine gamma interferon activates the release of a macrophage-derived Ia-inducing factor which transfers Ia inductive capacity, *J. Exp. Med.* (in press).

Wallach, D., Fellous, M., and Revel, M., 1982, Preferential effect of γ interferon on the synthesis of HLA antigens and their mRNAs in human cells, *Nature* **299**:833–836.

Wofsy, D., Roths, J. B., Murphy, E. D., Dauphinee, M. J., Kipper, S. B., and Talal, N., 1981, Deficient interleukin-2 activity in MRL/Mp and C57B1/6J mice bearing the lpr gene, *J. Exp. Med.* **154**:1671.

Wong, G. H. W., Clark-Lewis, I., Harris, A. W., and Schrader, J. W., 1984, Effect of cloned interferon-γ on expression of H-2 and Ia antigens on cell lines of hemopoietic, lymphoid, epithelial, fibroblastic and neuronal origin, *Eur. J. Immunol.* **14**:52–56.

Zolla-Pazner, S., William, D., El-Sadr, W., Marmor, M., and Stahl, R., 1984, Quantitation of beta-2 microglobulin and other immune parameters in a prospective study of men at risk for AIDS, *J.A.M.A.* **251**:2951–2955.

II

Autoimmunity

6

Rheumatoid Factor

Sherman Fong, Dennis A. Carson, and
John H. Vaughan

1. RHEUMATOID FACTOR

A. Introduction

Rheumatoid factors (RF) are a group of autoantibodies with anti-IgG reactivity. Because they were first discovered in patients with rheumatoid arthritis (RA), in whom they are present in large amounts and persistently over time, they were designated as rheumatoid factors. They occur, however, in a wide variety of illnesses and can be provoked in almost all normal individuals by appropriate stimuli. In this chapter, we review what is known about the structure, binding characteristics, and genetics of RF, emphasizing developments in our knowledge during the last few years. We also discuss the prevalence of RF in rheumatoid arthritis and other conditions and possible reasons for this. Finally, we outline possible roles of RF in normal physiological as well as pathological processes.

B. Historical Considerations

Rheumatoid factor activity was first recognized by the peculiar ability of the sera of patients with RA to agglutinate erythrocytes coated with small amounts of IgG antibody, a reagent commonly employed to detect complement-fixing antibodies to microbial antigens (Waaler, 1940; Rose *et al.*, 1948). The antiantibody nature of RF was subsequently shown (*vide infra*). It was thought that the high activity of antistreptococcal agglutinations that had previously been recognized in RA patients indicated a streptococcal etiology

Sherman Fong, Dennis A. Carson, and John H. Vaughan • Department of Basic and Clinical Research, Scripps Clinic and Research Foundation, La Jolla, California 92037.

(Dawson *et al.*, 1932). In fact, the high agglutination was caused by RF interacting with normal amounts of antibody to streptococci (Lamont Havers, 1952). Quantitative techniques were first brought to the study of RF by the demonstration that RF could be absorbed from serum by immune complexes with a measurable increment of protein to the complexes (Vaughan, 1956) or by precipitation with soluble IgG aggregates (Epstein *et al.*, 1956). Ultracentrifugal techniques demonstrated that most of the RF was IgM protein and that RF circulated as an IgG–IgM complex (Franklin *et al.*, 1957).

The antibody nature of RF was delineated in a series of careful studies (reviewed in Vaughan, 1972). Rheumatoid factors were shown to be contained in multiple immunoglobulin classes. They cross reacted with various animal IgG as one would predict for any heterologous antihuman IgG. The binding to IgG was through the Fab regions of the RF molecules to sites on the Fc portion of IgG molecules. They were produced in experimental animals by immunization with bacteria or with heat-aggregated IgG, and in each case, autoreactive anti-IgG molecules having the characteristics of RF were produced. In humans, RF were recognized to accompany a number of infectious diseases, including subacute bacterial endocarditis, and to disappear with cure of the disease. The development of RF was therefore theorized to be by autoimmunization by circulating immune complexes.

C. Methods of Detection

In the classic Rose–Waaler reaction, RF were detected by agglutination of sheep red blood cells coated with nonagglutinating concentrations of rabbit IgG anti-red-cell antibodies (Waaler, 1940; Rose *et al.*, 1948). Agglutination of the sheep cells by normal heterophile anti-red cell-antibody was avoided by preabsorption of the sera to be tested, or else the test was read as a differential agglutinating titer between that of the heterophile antibody with the uncoated sheep cells and that of the RF with the coated sheep cells. Nonagglutinating or incomplete IgG anti-Rh antibodies coating human red cells have been used, which avoids the problem of heterophile antibody (Waller and Vaughan, 1956; Grubb and Laurell, 1956; Natvig and Kunkel, 1967; Steinberg and Wilson, 1963). Nonerythrocyte particulate systems were also developed (Heller *et al.*, 1954; Boyden, 1951; Singer and Plotz, 1956; Greenbury, 1960), with human IgG–latex agglutination (or flocculation) becoming the standard in most clinical laboratores. However, the Rose–Waaler test is more specific for the RF associated with RA than is the latex test since (1) the latex test uses a human IgG-coated particle and therefore can detect non-RF antibodies such as antiallotype IgG resulting from transplacental immunization or blood transfusion (Steinberg and Wilson, 1963); and (2) the RF in RA almost always cross reacts with rabbit IgG, whereas the RF occurring in other disorders frequently does not. Nephelometric measurements (Finley *et al.*, 1979) have recently been advocated for increasing the sensitivity of flocculation tests to small changes in the amount of RF.

Recently, solid-phase radioimmunoassays (RIA) and enzyme-linked immunosorbent assays (ELISA) have been extensively used to detect IgM, IgG, and IgA RF in a very sensitive and reproducible manner (Carson *et al.*, 1977; Pope and McDuffy, 1981; Gripenberg *et al.*, 1979; Koopman and Schrohenloher, 1980a; Koopman *et al.*, 1982). The amount of RF is estimated by determining the quantity of patients' serum Ig that binds to human or rabbit IgG attached to the plate, using iodinated or enzyme-linked antibodies to human Ig as the detector. Appropriate absorptions or fractionations can insure that the tagged antibody detector does not react with the IgG originally attached to the plate.

Since RF activity is directed against the Fc region of IgG, the RF exists in serum complexed to IgG. For the most part, this complex is highly dissociable, and the RF is therefore easy to demonstrate. However, some RF apparently binds autologous IgG much more avidly and therefore is "hidden" in the usual assays for it. Such "hidden RF" can be detected following use of acid or another dissociating agent. "Hidden RF" with specificity for native human IgG have been reported in the sera of adults with RA by Allen and Kunkel (1966). Subsequent investigators, using a variety of options (Bluestone *et al.*, 1969; Cracchiolo *et al.*, 1970; Hansson and Winblad, 1970; Uesson and Hansson, 1981), have come to similar conclusions in adults, and Moore *et al.* (1974, 1978, 1980, 1983) have noted "hidden IgM-RF" in children with RA. Robbins *et al.* (1978) noted that peripheral blood lymphocytes produced *in vitro* RF that could not be detected in the simultaneously obtained serum and, more recently (Robbins and Wistar, 1984), that synovial fluid leukocytes exhibit an anti-IgG_3 RF specificity not seen in the serum.

Techniques to detect cell-associated RF began with immunofluorescence. Plasma cells producing RF were first stained by Mellors *et al.* (1959) with fluorescent-labeled aggregated IgG, which was subsequently also done by Mellors *et al.* (1961), Munthe and Natvig (1972), McCormick (1963), and Bonomo *et al.* (1968). The detection of the active secretion of RF by lymphoid cells was reported by Vaughan *et al.* (1976) using a direct plaque-forming cell assay with sheep red blood cells coated with reduced and alkylated rabbit IgG. The assay was further developed by Egeland *et al.* (1982) and Petersen *et al.* (1983), to distinguish IgG RF from IgM RF. Both workers found more IgG RF- than IgM RF-secreting cells in RA joints. Attempts at detecting B lymphocytes carrying RF as membrane immunoglobulin have included mixed agglutination in fixed tissues (Milde and Tonder, 1968) and rosetting of IgG-coated erythrocytes with lymphocytes (Bach *et al.*, 1970; Durance *et al.*, 1974). These approaches are confused, however, by Fc receptors on cell surfaces, which give similar binding with IgG-coated erythrocytes. More promising is the use of antiidiotype sera to stain the cell surfaces (Carson *et al.*, 1981; Bonagura *et al.*, 1982).

II. IMMUNOCHEMICAL PROPERTIES

A. The IgG Antigens with Which RF React

Seven different sites on the Fc portions of human IgG molecules have been described at which RF react (Natvig *et al.*, 1972) (Table 1). These are localized in both the $C\gamma 2$ and $C\gamma 3$ domains. They include cross-reactive antigens shared by IgG molecules of both human and lower animal species as well as isotypic and allotypic (Gm) antigens found in humans and some primates (Grubb, 1970; Gaarder and Natvig, 1974) but not in lower animal species. The Gm alloantigens are present on only single human IgG subclasses. An important distinction exists between the anti-Gm antibodies that may develop in normal persons as a result of transfusion or pregnancy (Steinberg and Wilson, 1963) and those

Table 1. Antigenic Determinants on the Fc Fragment of IgG with which Rheumatoid Factors React[a]

	Portion of the Fc fragment involved			
	C γ 2		C γ 3	
Subclass	Original	Proposed	Original	Proposed
IgG_1	Ga	Ga	Gm (a)	G1m (a)
			Gm (x)	G1m (x)
			"Non-a"	nG1m (a)
IgG_2	Ga	Ga	"Non-a"	nG1m (a)
IgG_3	Gm (g)	G3m (g)	"Non-a"	nG1m (a)
	Gm (b1)	G3m (b1)		
IgG_4	Ga	Ga	'γ 4 non-a'	nG4m (a)

[a] Human rheumatoid factors recognize both the subclass antigen Ga and the allotypic Gm antigens. The original designations are t hose used by Natvig *et al.* (1972). The proposed notation is drawn from the review of notation for allotypic and related markers of human immunoglobulins by World Health Organization (1976).

that develop in patients with rheumatoid arthritis as a part of the RF. The former show strict allospecific reactivity, not recognizing the individual's own Gm antigens, whereas the latter are autospecific; i.e., true anti-Gm autoantibodies.

The cross reactions of RF with IgG of lower species were examined early by quantitative immunochemical techniques. Rheumatoid factors were found to be composed of a heterogeneous population of molecules, some of which reacted with human as well as with rabbit, bovine, or equine IgG, and others of which reacted with human IgG alone (Butler and Vaughan, 1964, 1965). Studies on the effects of chemical modification and enzymatic digestion of human and rabbit IgG molecules have led to the suggestion that the major cross-reactive autoantigenic determinant of human IgG may be conformationally dependent and structurally distinct from the Gm determinants (Hunneyball and Stanworth, 1976a). It was concluded that a tyrosine but not a lysine residue is involved in the human (but not the rabbit) cross-ractive determinant. By thermolysin digestion, the human determinant was localized on the COOH-terminal end of the Cγ2 domain (Hunneyball and Stanworth, 1976a). In studies with Facb and pFc′ fragments of rabbit IgG produced by plasmin cleavage, which contain the Cγ2 and Cγ3 domains, respectively, neither fragment alone could inhibit RF, but recombined they did (Stewart *et al.*, 1973; Gaarder and Michaelson, 1974; Hunneyball and Stanworth, 1976b). Therefore, the antigen in the rabbit IgG may require the presence of both the Cγ2 and Cγ3 domains. Alternatively, there may be two antibody populations, each reacting with a separate domain. Since rabbit IgG inhibits the anti-Ga activity of RF and also can be used to immunopurify it, Ga is closely associated with, if not identical with, the cross-reactive determinant.

Whether or not human RF recognize neoantigenic determinants generated in immune complexes is controversial. It has been shown that RF from RA sera react better with aggregated IgG than with native IgG in both precipitation and agglutination systems (Edelman *et al.*, 1958; Oreskes *et al.*, 1963). However, it has also been shown that the binding affinity of each IgM-RF for monomeric IgG is the same as for aggregated IgG

(Normansell, 1970; Normansell and Stanworth, 1966). Although RF reactivity can be inhibited with either native or aggregated IgG, both forms of IgG have closely parallel inhibition curves, suggesting that no new antigenic determinant is created by aggregated IgG (Gaarder and Natvig, 1974). Thus, the greater reactivity of RF with aggregated IgG has been attributed to the increased valency of the aggregated IgG, enabling it more readily to form aggregates with IgM RF, with subsequent precipitation or agglutination (Normansell, 1971; Eisenberg, 1976).

Some evidence nevertheless supports the possible importance of neoantigens in IgG in promoting RF production. Neoantigenic determinants may be created within IgG in immune complexes, and similar changes may occur in stored IgG in the absence of antigen (Henney *et al.*, 1965). Circular dichroism spectral analyses have shown that IgG in patients with RA may differ in conformation from normal IgG (Alkner *et al.*, 1982). The IgG from RA patients yields abnormal fragments on papain digestion (Watkins *et al.*, 1970), and autologous IgG in RA is more readily catabolized in RA patients than is normal IgG (Catalano *et al.*, 1977). Antibodies to altered IgG have been reported in RA (Johnson *et al.*, 1976), and a population of RF has been described that reacts preferentially with mildly reduced and alkylated IgG (Brown and Brown, 1981). Rheumatoid factor has been reported to react preferentially with autologous IgG (Bandilla and McDuffie, 1969).

Antibodies can be found in both normal and pathological sera that are directed against various enzymatic cleavage products of human IgG. Included among these are the "pepsin agglutinators," which are antibodies that react with antigenic determinants exposed on the $F(ab')_2$ fragment but not on the native intact IgG (Osterland *et al.*, 1963). Whether these should be considered as part of the RF group of molecules can be debated.

Recent studies of RF in murine strains with different genetic backgrounds have prompted investigations on the genetics, fine specificities, and biological role of RF. A comparative study of the three normal murine strains (129/SV, CBA/Ht, and C57BL/6) with two autoimmune lupus-prone strains (MRL/1 and NZB) showed that the spontaneous RF consisted of distinct non-cross-reactive antibody subpopulations, each specific for one murine IgG subclass (Van Snick *et al.*, 1983). The sera of normal strains contained IgG_1- and IgG_{2a}-specific RF, whereas the autoimmune strain contained additionally IgG_{2b}-specific RF. Lipopolysaccharide-stimulated normal mouse spleen cells secreted distinct subpopulations for IgG_1 or IgG_{2a}. Similarly, normal A/J mice secreted IgG_1-specific RF following secondary immunization with a number of protein antigens (Nemazee and Sato, 1983). Hybridomas from MRL/1 mouse spleen fusions were found to secrete IgM RF specific for murine IgG_{2a} or IgG_{2b} with no cross reaction with heterologous IgG (Theofilopoulos *et al.*, 1983).

The determinants recognized by murine rheumatoid factors have been localized in one study (Stassin *et al.*, 1983). In a panel of mouse myeloma variants with abnormalities in the heavy chains, both allotypic and isotypic determinants were recognized by mouse RF. The determinants were localized to the COOH-terminal regions of IgG_1, IgG_{2a}, and IgG_{2b}. It was found that both polyclonal RF derived from autoimmune mouse strains (MRL/MPJ-1pr and NZB/Bin J) and most monoclonal RF derived from normal strains (BALB/c, C57BL/6, and 129/SV) recognized end eight-amino-acid residues of the COOH-terminal end of the $C\gamma2$ domain and the complete $C\gamma3$ domain.

B. Affinity

The affinity with which IgM RF reacts with IgG has been determined by analytical ultracentrifugation and by equilibrium molecular sieving. The association constant of IgM RF with monomer IgG is generally low, ranging from 10^4 to 10^5 liters/mol (Stone and Metzger, 1968; Normansell, 1970, 1971; Stewart *et al.*, 1973; Lyet and Normansell, 1974; Eisenberg, 1976; Wager and Teppo, 1978). This is much lower than the association constants of common heteroantibodies with their antigens. Despite the intrinsically low association constant of IgM RF, this molecule can produce stable complexes with aggregated IgG. An IgM RF with higher affinity has been implied in studies with acid-dissociated IgM fractions of serum (Allen and Kunkel, 1966) and with a plaque-forming cell assay (Robbins *et al.*, 1978). Such RF may be so firmly complexed with autologous IgG that it cannot be demonstrated in whole serum or, when made extravascularly, may complex so firmly with local IgG that it never reaches the peripheral blood. The IgG RF, when serving both as antigen and antibody in self-association complexes, can have association constants as high as 10^{10} liters/mol (Pope *et al.*, 1974).

C. IgG, IgA, and IgE RF

Although RF was originally recognized in the IgM class of proteins as a molecule forming 22 S complexes with IgG (Franklin *et al.*, 1957), "intermediate complexes" sedimenting between 7 S and 19 S were subsequently seen in RA patients and were shown to contain IgG RF (Kunkel *et al.*, 1961). Such IgG RF immune complexes have subsequently been detected by others not only in the serum (Chodirker and Tomasi, 1963; Schrohenloher, 1966; Pope *et al.*, 1974, 1975) but also in the synovium (Munthe and Natvig, 1971, 1972) and synovial fluids (Hannestad, 1968; Winchester *et al.*, 1970; Winchester, 1975).

Pope *et al.* (1975) showed that the isolated IgG from those complexes bore either κ or λ light chains, but the IgG RF itself exhibited predominantly κ light chains similar to IgM RF. This has proved true not only in patients with RA but also in patients with subacute bacterial endocarditis (Carson and Lawrence, 1978). The IgG RF form self-associating complexes when they are molecularly autospecific (Pope *et al.*, 1974). In these cases, monomeric normal human IgG did not successfully compete with the IgG RF molecules themselves for reassociation. When the complexes are dissociated and reformed in the presence of excess normal IgG, the normal IgG do not successfully compete with the IgG RF molecules in the reassociation (Pope *et al.*, 1975). The antigenic determinants responsible for the self-association are probably in the $C\gamma2$ domain (Nardella *et al.*, 1981) and may require intactness of both the $C\gamma2$ and $C\gamma3$ regions for expression. The complexes are most stable in dimers, tetramers, and octamers. In other patients, IgG RF apparently can exist in complex with non-RF IgG. This depends on the IgG RF being directed against a different subclass of IgG than its own; e.g., IgG_1 RF versus IgG_3 molecules. A physicochemical analysis based on viscosity and light-scattering measurements showed that at physiological pH these complexes probably consist of cyclic tetramers with two antigen and two antibody molecules (Gabriel and Hadler, 1981).

Immunoglobulin A RF have been demonstrated in both sera and synovial fluids of patients with rheumatoid arthritis (Heimer and Levin, 1966; Torrigiani and Roitt, 1967; Panush *et al.*, 1971; Stankaitiene *et al.*, 1978; Dunne *et al.*, 1979; Koopman *et al.*,

1982). Especially high levels may be seen in Sjogren's syndrome, in which they exist as polymers (Elkon *et al.*, 1981, 1982). The predominance of the polymer form suggests a mucosal origin. The IgA RF of the saliva is complexed with the secretory component, as is classically the case with other IgA mucosal antibodies.

Measurable levels of IgG and IgA RF are extremely uncommon in normal persons. They are also much less common among the RF that may occur in systemic lupus erythematosus and other connective tissue diseases than they are in RA (Pope *et al.*, 1981; Quisimorio *et al.*, 1983).

The existence of IgE RF was first suggested by a reduction in the quantity of IgE present in the sera of patients with severe seropositive RA and vasculitis after *in vitro* absorption with IgG (Mizushima *et al.*, 1981). Subsequently, Zuraw *et al.* (1981) and Meretey *et al.* (1982) also reported IgE RF. All of these reports are subject to technical criticism that makes their interpretation somewhat uncertain. Nevertheless, the existence of IgE RF would explain nicely the abilities of some RA sera to cause the release of histamine from isolated perfused guinea pig lung (Broder *et al.*, 1969).

D. Idiotypic Characteristics of RF

A considerable interest has recently developed in the idiotypic characteristics of RF. Antibody molecules of a given specificity in a given class or subclass of immunoglobulins differ structurally from the other antibodies of that class or subclass only in the regions where they bind to antigen. Therefore, when a monoclonal RF (mRF) is injected into another species and the resultant antiserum is absorbed extensively with normal human immunoglobulin, there may be left a small amount of antibody that reacts exclusively with the original immunizing mRF at or near its antigen-binding site. This is antiidiotypic antibody. It may be a "private" antiidiotype, in which case it reacts exclusively with the immunizing mRF, or it may be cross-reactive idiotype (CRI), in which case it reacts not only with the particular immunizing mRF but also with other mRF. Kunkel *et al.* (1973) first showed that in a large collection of mIgM RF paraproteins 60% could be classified into one CRI, which they designated Wa after the prototype mRF of the group. Twenty percent could be classified into another CRI, which they designated Po. Sixty percent of all mRF belong to a minor κ-IIIb subgroup of the light chain variable region subgroup (Kunkel *et al.*, 1974), and all of the Wa^+ CRI are in that subgroup. In a second series, mRF from mixed cryoglobulinemia were examined; all the mRF proteins were IgM κ, and the majority belong to the Wa (Powell and Agnello, 1983). A third cross-reactive idiotype, Bla, has been described for polyclonal and monoclonal RF that have dual reactivity for IgG and DNA-histone (Agnello *et al.*, 1980).

Whether idiotypic specificities involve structural features in the antigen-binding site itself or structures distant from but related to it has remained unclear. Many antiidiotypic antibodies have appeared to be directed to conformations formed by H–L chain interactions. An opening approach at better understanding this area in respect to RF was an examination of the primary amino acid sequences of a series of mRF (Capra and Kehoe, 1974; Andres and Capra, 1981a,b,c). The complete and partial variable regions of the heavy and light chains of 12 monoclonal mIgM RF paraproteins are shown in Fig. 1.

The two Wa^+ proteins, Sie and Wol, differ almost completely in the complementarity-determining regions (CDR) of their heavy chains and less so in two of the three

```
LIGHT CHAINS
                         CDR1                                       CDR2                          CDR3
      ______________________________________________   ___________________________   ___________________________

      24  25  26  27  27A 28  29  30  31  32  33  34    50  51  52  53  54  55  56    89  90  91  92  93  94  95

Sie^a Arg Ala Ser Gln Ser Val Ser Asn Ser Tyr Leu Ala   Gly Ala Ser Ser Arg Ala Thr   Gln Gln Tyr Gly Ser Ser Pro
Glo^a --------------------------- Ser ---------------
Wol^a --------------------------- Ser Gly ------- Gly   ---------------------------   ------------------- Leu Gly
Pom^b ------------------- Ile --- Asn ---------------   ----------- Thr -----------   ----------- Asn Asn Trp ---
Lay^b Gln ----------- ( ) Asn Val Asn Ala ------- Asn   ----------- Thr --- Glu Ala   ----------- Asn Asn Trp ---
Gar^c --------------------------- Ser ---------------   ---------------------------
Neu^c --------------------------- Ser Arg -----------   ---------------------------
Got^c ----------------------- Arg Ser ---------------   ---------------------------
Pay^c ------------------- Lys --- Ser ---------------   ---------------------------
Flo^c ------------------- Lys --- Ser ---------------
Cur^c -------
Cla^c -----------

HEAVY CHAINS

             CDR1                              CDR2                                                CDR3
      _________________________   _______________________________________________________   ____________________________________________________

      30  31  32  33  34  35      50  51  52  53  54  55  56  57  58  59  60  61  62  63    99  100 101 102 103 104 105 106 107 108 109 110 111

Sie^a Ser Gly Tyr Thr Ile Ser     Ser Pro Ala Lys Trp Thr Asp Pro Phe Gln Gly Val Tyr Ile   Glu Trp Lys Gly Gln Val Asn Val Asn Pro Phe Asp Tyr
Wol^a Val Asp --- Lys Gly Leu     Gln Ile Pro Leu Arg Phe Asn Gly Glu Val Lys Asn Pro Gly   --- Tyr Gly Phe Asp Thr Ser Asp Tyr Tyr Tyr Try ---
Pom^b --- Ser Ser Ala Met ---     Trp Lys Tyr Asn Gly Asn --- Lys His Tyr Ala Asp Ser Val   Asp Ala Gly Pro Tyr --- Ser Pro Thr Phe Phe Ala His
Lay^b --- Ala Ser Ala Met ---     Trp Lys Tyr Asn Gly Asn --- Lys His Tyr Ala Asp Ser Val   Asp Ala Gly Pro Tyr --- Ser Pro Thr Phe Phe Ala His
```

Figure 1. The complete and partial amino acid sequences of the light and heavy chain complementarity-determining regions (CDR) of human monoclonal IgM rheumatoid factor paraproteins (Capra and Kehoe, 1974; Andrews and Capra, 1981a,b; Ledford *et al.*, 1983). The dashed lines indicate identity of amino acids with those in the Sie mRF; a, Wa idiotype positive; b, Po idiotype positive; c, yet unclassified idiotypes.

CDR in their light chains, but they are identical in the CDR-2 of their light chains. This sequence is similar to that of four other idiotypically unclassified RF proteins, Gar, Neu, Got, and Pay (Ledford *et al.*, 1983). In the framework regions, Sie and Wol are almost identical, which is consistent with both proteins being of the VkIIIb light chain subclass. Since the CDR, but not the framework regions, are involved directly in antigen binding (Cebra *et al.*, 1974), the identity between the two mRF in the CDR-2 suggested that this could be a basis for CRI between these proteins. Synthetic peptides corresponding to the CDR-3 of the heavy chain and to the CDR-2 of the light chain were therefore prepared and injected into rabbits (Chen *et al.*, 1984a,b). The rabbit antiserum to the CDR-3 peptide behaved like a private idiotype, reacting with Sie but with no other mRF (Fig. 2). The antiserum to the CDR-2 of the light chain behaved like a CRI antibody, reacting with three Wa mRF, Sie, Glo, and Teh, but only weakly with Pom (which differs from Sie in the CDR-2 by one amino acid) and not with Wa$^-$ mRF (Lay). Therefore, the antipeptide antibody identifies a public idiotype on human IgM RF that is largely dependent on the primary sequence of the second CDR of the light chain.

A third type of antiidiotype can be generated in some cases. This is an antiidiotype that bears the "internal image" of the antigen and mimics the antigen in its interaction with antibody (Fong *et al.*, 1983b, 1984). These antiidiotypes are highly cross reactive, do not conform to the Wa, Po, or Bla CRI, and are specific for conformational features of the RF rather than amino acid sequences.

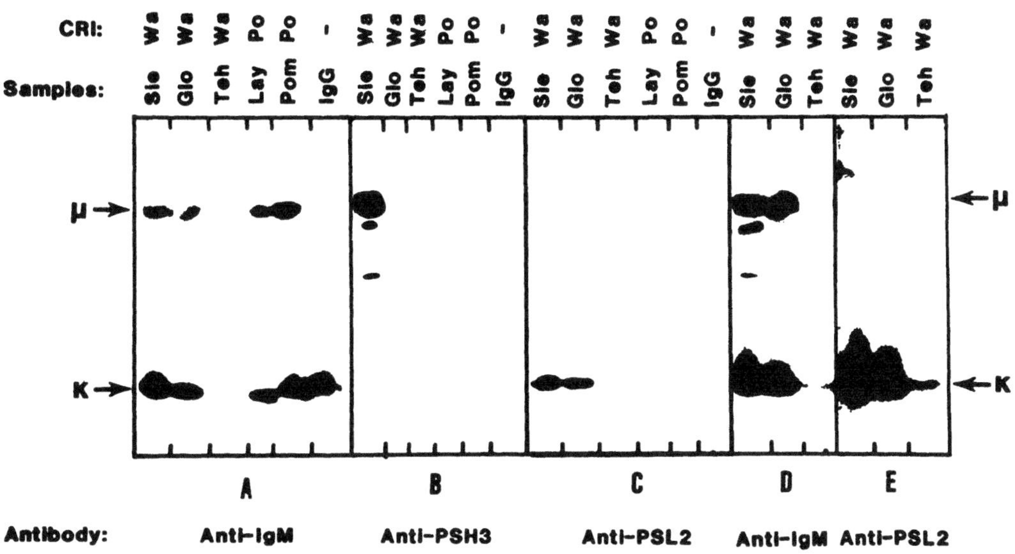

Figure 2. Detection of private and cross-reactive idiotypes of IgM rheumatoid factors with rabbit antisera against IgM or against synthetic peptides representing the third complementarity-determining regions of the heavy chain (PSH3) or the second of the light chain (PSL2). The individual mRF were run from top to bottom in a reducing gel, electrotransferred to nitrocellulose, and probed with the above sera. The light and heavy chains (μ and κ) are shown by the anti-IgM probe (panel A). The private idiotype of Sie is recognized by anti-PSH3, which sees the Sie heavy chain but none of the other heavy chains (panel B). The cross-reactive idiotype (CRI) is recognized on Sie, Glo, and Teh by anti-PSL2 (panels B and C). Panels D and E show longer exposures to bring out the Teh reaction, which was weak because only a very small amount of this mRF was available. (From Chen *et al.*, 1985).

The basis for the CRI in the Po group is not known. Two of the three CDR in the variable region of the heavy chains and one of the three CDR in the light chains of Pom and Lay are identical (Fig. 1) (Capra and Kehoe, 1974; Klapper and Capra, 1976). They differ substantially in the framework regions of their light chains; Pom is VkIII, and Lay is VkI. No synthetic peptide studies have yet been done with these proteins.

The use of murine monoclonal antiidiotypic antibody reagents for subdividing the human RF molecules into distinct idiotypic groups has recently been reported (Pasquali *et al.*, 1983; Carson and Fong, 1983). These homogeneous reagents will provide further improvement in the antiidiotype approach and will facilitate the systematic classification of human RF.

The idiotypes of antibodies may be genetically determined, as implied by the presence of idiotypic and cross-reactive idiotypic molecules in pre-B cells (Eichmann and Kindt, 1971; Pawlak *et al.*, 1973; Eichmann and Berek, 1973; Kubagawa *et al.*, 1979). A genetic basis for an idiotypic determinant in RF was first shown by Pasquali *et al.* (1980) with an antiidiotype prepared against the RF of a RA patient who had multiple relatives with RA. This antiidiotype had "private" characteristics in that it failed to react with 11 of 12 monoclonal and polyclonal RF from unrelated individuals and was only poorly reactive with the 12th (a monoclonal RF). This antiidiotype reacted well, however, with the RF present in multiple members of the family spanning three generations (Fig. 3).

Antiidiotypic antisera have also been used to demonstrate cross-idiotypic specificities within polyclonal IgM RF paraproteins isolated from RA patients. Shared idiotypic antigens were found between some monoclonal and polyclonal RF as well as between IgM and IgG RF (Forre *et al.*, 1979; Pasquali *et al.*, 1983).

III. INDUCTION AND CONTROL

A. Induction of RF

Three basic types of stimuli have been considered to trigger the production of RF. These are (1) stimulation by aggregated IgG, normally in the form of immune complexes, (2) induction by exogenous antigens bearing cross-reactive determinants to human IgG, and (3) stimulation by polyclonal B-cell activators. Prolonged immunization of rabbits with immune complexes containing autologous IgG can induce the formation of RF (Williams and Kunkel, 1963; McClusky *et al.*, 1962; Bokisch *et al.*, 1973). Chronic immunization with bacterial antigens also can induce RF in rabbits (Christian, 1963; Bokisch *et al.*, 1973) and in patients with subacute bacterial endocarditis (Williams and Kunkel, 1962; Sheagren *et al.*, 1976; Carson *et al.*, 1978). Sustained RF production depended on the continued presence of the immunologic stimulation, and elimination of the immunizing bacteria in subacute bacterial endocarditis by antibiotics led to a decline of the RF titer (Williams and Kunkel, 1962; Carson *et al.*, 1978). Vaccination of normal persons with tetanus toxoid induced increased numbers of precursors of RF-secreting cells in the peripheral blood (Welch *et al.*, 1983) (Fig. 4), and heat-aggregated human IgG induced normal human peripheral blood mononuclear cells to secrete RF *in vitro* (Pisko *et al.*, 1982). The basis for thinking that RF can be induced by immune complexes is thus substantial.

Evidence for participation of autologous IgG in the induction of mouse RF has been presented by Van Snick *et al.* (1984). By analysis of allotypic specificity of anti-IgG_{2a}

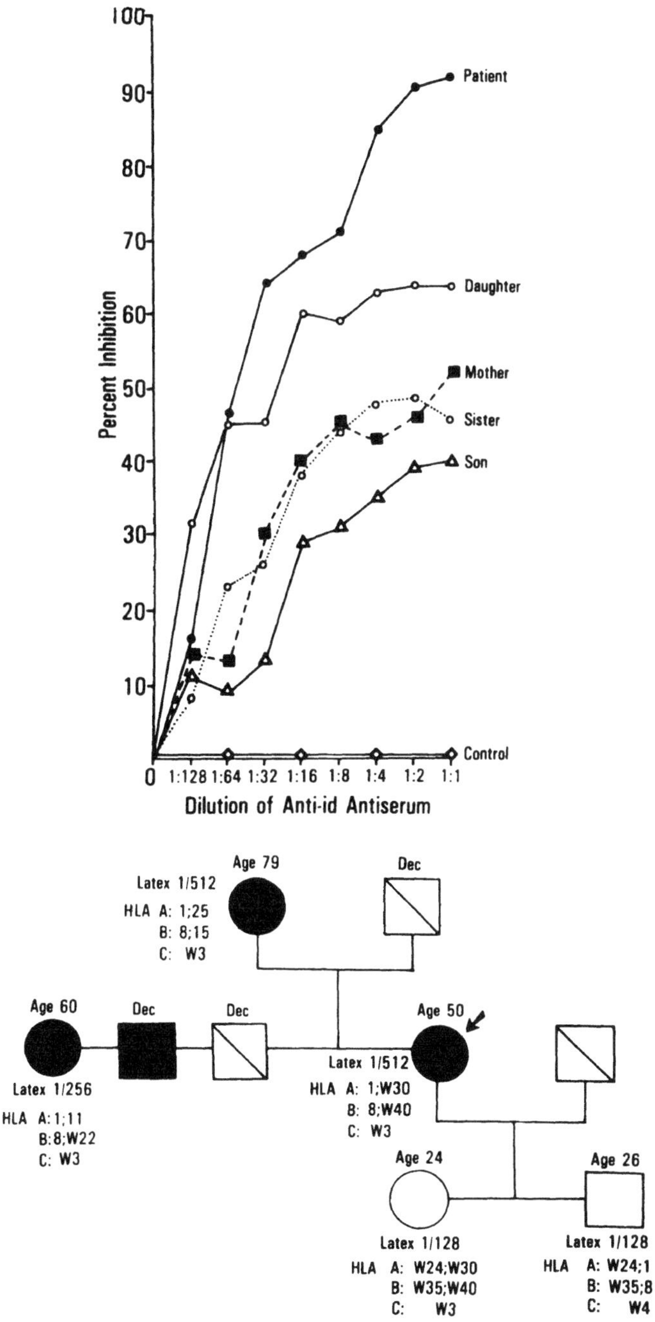

Figure 3. Inheritance of IgM rheumatoid factor idiotypes in a family spanning three generations. The patient and four first-degree relatives, mother, sister, daughter, and son, are shown in the family tree. The closed circles (female) and squares (males) indicate subjects with definite rheumatoid arthritis. The arrow indicates the proband. The expression of the idiotype is shown by the relative ability of the antiidiotype to interfere with the binding of the individual RF to IgG. The patients RF was inhibited by >90%. The four first-degree relatives were inhibited by 40–60%. (From Pasquall *et al.*, 1980.)

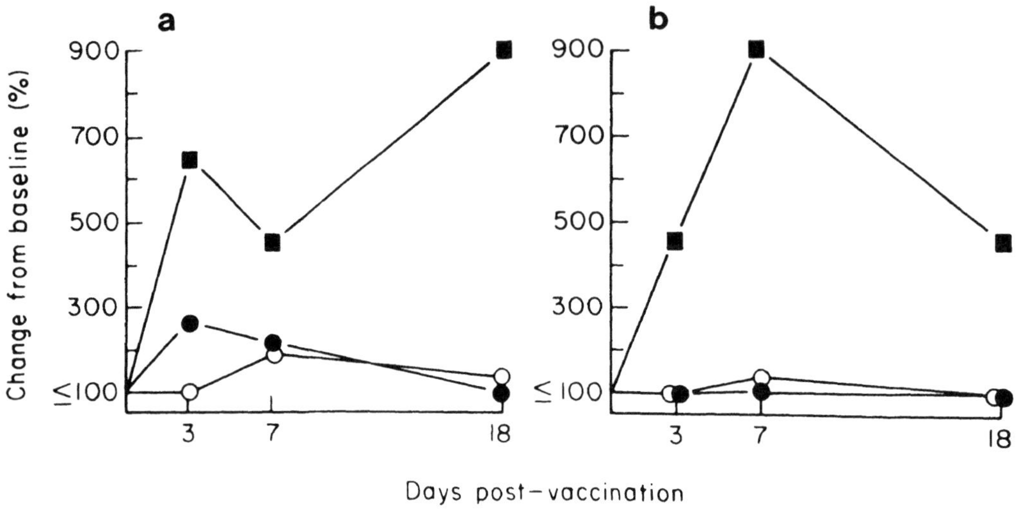

Figure 4. Increase in the IgM RF B-cell frequency and plasma IgM RF after tetanus toxoid vaccination in the two individuals, a and b. (■) IgM RF B-cell frequency; (○) IgM RF in plasma; (●) total IgM. (From Welch *et al.*, 1983.)

RF in recombinant inbred strains of 129/SV (IgH-1^a) and C57BL/6 (IgH-1^b) mice, it was observed that RF specific for a given allotype was only found in the presence of that allotype. The data thus suggested that autologous IgG must play a role in the induction of mouse RF in these mice.

The thought that RF may arise as an immune response against cross-reactive antigens arose from the fact that a portion of RF molecules may react not only with human IgG but also with other antigens. Reactivity of RF with nuclear antigen (McCormick and Day, 1963; Hannestad and Johannessen, 1976), dinitrophenylhapten (Hannestad, 1969), and bromelain-treated erythrocytes (Cunliffe and Cox, 1980) have been described. Both anti-IgG and antinuclear specificities of mRF were shown to reside on the Fab pieces of the RF molecule (Hannestad and Stollar, 1978; Johnson, 1979a,b), and the antinuclear reactivity could be masked by excess serum IgG (Johnson, 1979a). The antinuclear activity had an anti-DNA/histone specificity, and it bore a distinct cross-reactive idiotype (Agnello *et al.*, 1980). A majority of seropositive RA patients possessed similar dually reactive RF within a subset of their polyclonal RF (Hannestad and Johannessen, 1976; Johnson, 1979a). The fact that the dual reactivities existed on only a minority of RF molecules makes it less likely that these antigens are the primary stimuli to RF production.

A wide variety of microbial and plant products can act as polyclonal B-cell activators (PBA). Murine lymphocytes can be induced to secrete RF after stimulation with bacterial lipopolysaccharide (Dresser, 1978; Izui *et al.*, 1979). Pokeweed mitogen (a T-cell-dependent PBA) (Keightley *et al.*, 1976), and Epstein–Barr virus (EBV) (A T-cell-independent PBA) (Bird and Britton, 1979) have been extensively studied. Both have been shown to induce the production of RF from normal human PBL (Koopman and Schrohenloher, 1980b; Fong *et al.*, 1981) and from RA PBL (Slaughter *et al.*, 1978; Tsoukas *et al.*, 1980; Koopman and Schrohenloher, 1980c; Fong *et al.*, 1982a; Olsen *et al.*, 1982). Both PWM- and EBV-stimulated peripheral blood lymphocytes secreted RF that carried idiotypic markers shared by serum IgM RF (Pasquali *et al.*, 1981). However, the EBV-stimulated cells synthesized RF with idiotypes present on only a portion of the RF in the serum or in the supernatants from PWM-stimulated cells, thus suggesting that different B-cell subsets were involved in the production. In fact, EBV-induced IgM RF in elderly humans without RA is preferentially derived from early B cells, which form rosettes with mouse erythrocytes (Lucivero *et al.*, 1981; Fong *et al.*, 1983a). Pokeweed-mitogen-induced IgM RF preferentially arises from T-cell-dependent, more mature B cells, which lack the mouse erythrocyte receptor. The RF of RA patients are probably derived from both of these cell types. Whether the rosette-forming B cells are progenitors of the more mature, nonrosetting B cells as depicted in Fig. 5, or an independent subset is not known.

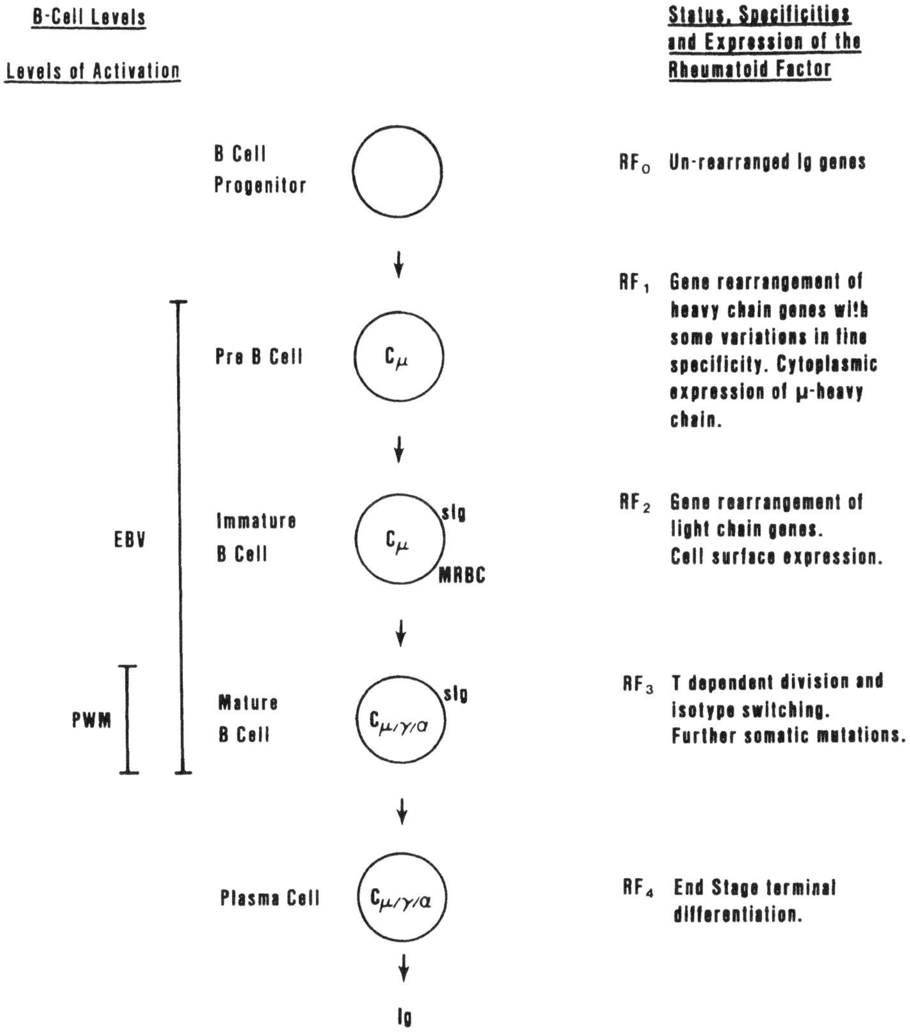

Figure 5. A scheme of RF production. Information coding for primordial RF is present in the germ line V_L and V_H gene segments. Pre-B cells express cytoplasmic μ chains of RF. With further rearrangement of L-chain genes, the B cell expresses cell surface RF receptors. These early B cells bear the mouse erythrocyte (MRBC) receptor. On activation, these cells secrete IgM RF. Mature memory B cells bearing cell surface Ig respond to pokeweed mitogen (PWM) and secrete IgM RF by a T-dependent process. The terminally differentiated plasma cells similarly secrete both IgM RF and other isotypes of RF. The levels at which EBV and PWM, two polyclonal B-cell activators, induce RF are indicated at the left.

However, the mouse erythrocyte receptor is lost following B-cell activation (Forbes *et al.*, 1981; McGraw *et al.*, 1982), thus suggesting the former hypothesis. A hypothetical schemetic of RF-secreting cells during B-cell differentiation is shown in Fig. 5.

It has been proposed that RF may constitute a family of closely related antibody molecules derived by mutational events from germ-line gene segments that specify an original RF important to the species (Carson *et al.*, 1981). Consistent with this hypothesis are a number of observations. Up to 10% of IgM paraproteins, which arise from neoplastic proliferation of immature lymphocytes, are comprised of IgM RF (Preud'homme and Segligmann, 1972). Also, IgM RF precursor B cells are also present in human umbilical cord blood (Fong *et al.*, 1981) (Fig. 6) and are prevalent in normal adult bone marrow, a site for generation of new B cells (Fong *et al.*, 1982b). The qualitative difference in the RF that the earlier cells produce can be interpreted to imply that their RF is closer to the RF of the germ-line genes than it is to the RF produced by the more mature B cells. As shown by the similarity of the idiotypes of the serum and to those of the PWM-induced RF, it is the RF of the more mature B cells that dominates the peripheral blood in RA patients.

If PBA is an important basis for RF production in RA, there must be an independent control mechanism in RA to explain the fact that PBA are unselective in respect to the specific autoantibodies they induce, whereas RA exhibits high selectivity for RF. Ab-

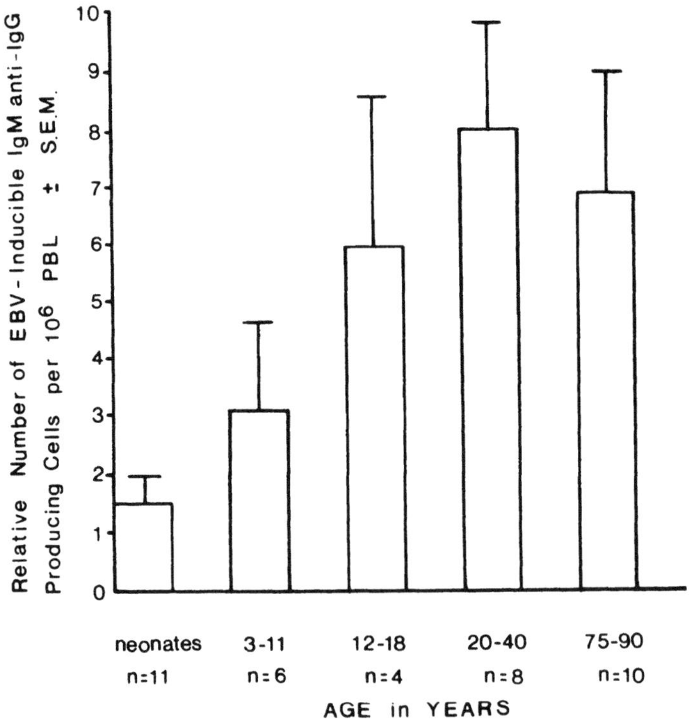

Figure 6. Relative frequencies of EBV-inducible IgM RF autoantibody-secreting lymphocytes as a function of age. (From Fong *et al.*, 1981, 1982a.)

normalities in T-cell control could conceivably contribute this mechanism, but definitive information is not yet available on this point.

B. Control of RF Production

In both normal and RA PBL, PWM can stimulate *in vitro* production of RF, and in both cases this depends on T-cell help. Addition of Tγ (suppressor) cells to mixed populations of B and T helper cells results in decreased secretion of IgM RF, but the RF was not reduced differentially from other IgM molecules (Tsoukas *et al.*, 1980) (Fig. 7). T cells capable of suppressing RF producton are also present in normal persons (Koopman, 1981). Thus, RF secretion *in vitro* is subject to classical regulation by helper and suppressor T cells, but there is no demonstrated selectivity or abnormality of this suppression of RF in RA. Spontaneous production of RF by the PBL occurs in about half the patients with RA but not at all in normal persons (Vaughan *et al.*, 1976; Tsoukas *et al.*, 1980; Koopman and Schrohenloher, 1980a,b). A similar spontaneous production of antitetanus antibody occurs in the PBL 5–7 days after booster immunizations of normal persons (Stevens *et al.*, 1979). Therefore, we take the spontaneous production of RF to signal an active immunizing process in these patients. It is of note that those patients with spontaneous producton exhibit more severe disease than do the others (Vaughan *et al.*, 1976).

It has been hypothesized by Jerne (1974) that antibody production is controlled through a network of idiotypic and antiidiotypic antibodies. In humans, the capacity of heterologously derived antiidiotypic antibodies to suppress the corresponding idiotype expression has been demonstrated both *in vitro* (Bona and Fauci, 1980; Mudawwar *et al.*, 1980) and *in vivo* (Miller *et al.*, 1982). In respect to whether RF production is subject to antiidiotype control, one study of PWM-stimulated PBL reported inhibition by a rabbit anti-Wa idiotype of the appearance of plasma cells bearing the Wa idiotype (Bonagura *et al.*, 1982). A rabbit antiidiotype to the IgM RF of a patient with a B-cell lymphoma

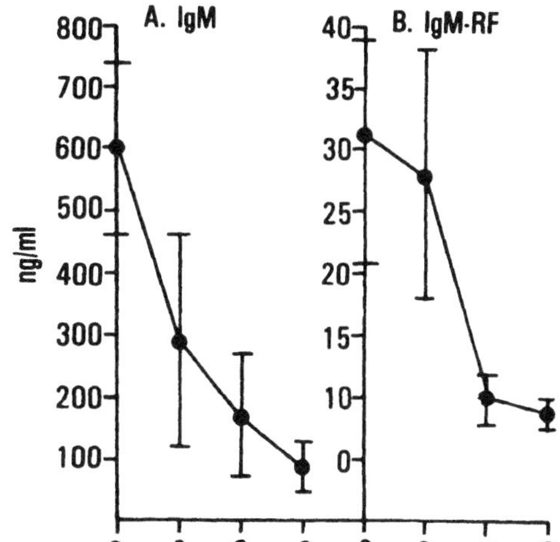

Figure 7. B cells of patients with rheumatoid arthritis are responsive to pokeweed-mitogen-generated "suppressor" signals. The patient's B cells were mixed with an equal number of enriched T γ-negative (helper) cells. Addition of T γ-positive (suppressor) cells reduced in a dose-dependent parallel manner the amount of secreted IgM RF and IgM. (From Tsoukas *et al.*, 1980.)

was capable of suppressing *in vitro* B-cell synthesis of the idiotype (Koopman *et al.*, 1983). The suppression was T-cell independent. Intact $F(ab')_2$ fragments, but not Fab, of the antiidiotype were also effective in mediating the suppression, although less well than the intact molecule. Rabbit antiidiotypic antibodies bearing the "internal image" of IgG Fc fragments have similarly been able to modulate *in vitro* the human RF response (Fong *et al.*, 1983b, 1984) (Fig. 8). The mechanisms mediating these antiidiotype suppressions of RF production are uncertain. Prior animal studies indicated that antiidiotype may modulate idiotypic expression either through activation of specific suppressor T cells or directly on the B cells (Rajewsky and Takemori, 1983). In humans, the evidence suggests that antiidiotypic antibodies can directly inhibit B-cell release as well as synthesis of antibody (Bona and Fauci, 1980; Mudawwar *et al.*, 1980), including RF (Koopman *et al.*, 1983).

Whether autoantiidiotypic antibodies capable of these types of suppression actually exist in RA and function in control of RF production is not yet certain. Several laboratories have reported the existence of anti-Fab antibodies, especially in rheumatoid arthritis, that have variable degrees of reactivities with Fab of different individual origins (Nasu *et al.*, 1980; Heimer *et al.*, 1982; Birdsall *et al.*, 1983). The suggestion that this variation may reflect idiotypic specificity has generally failed to rule out allotypic specificity; i.e., that the variation is not related to immunoglobulin class or subclass differences rather than differences at the antigen binding sites of the RF molecules. No studies were carried out in any of those reports to determine whether any of the anti-Fab were capable of suppressing RF activity. In a study of mixed cryoglobulinemia with associated hepatitis B virus (HBV) infection, it was shown that a significant proportion of the Fab–autoanti-

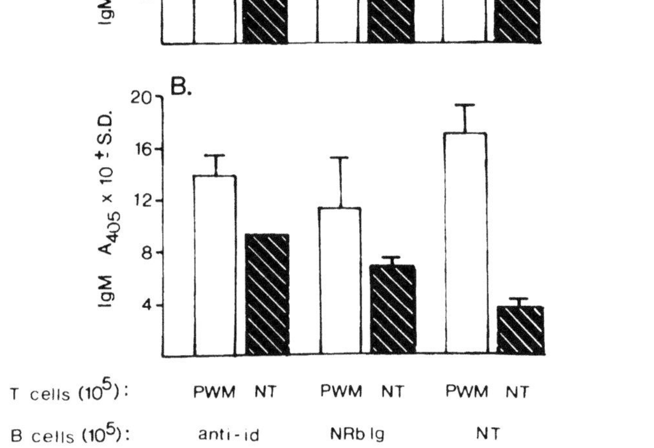

Figure 8. Preincubation of purified B cells with antiidiotype bearing the internal image of IgG Fc fragments inhibited the IgM RF-secreting response but not the total of IgM response. B cells were preincubated with either antiidiotype or normal Ig for 48 hr. Peripheral T cells were preincubated with or without PWM for a similar period of time. The B and T cells were then mixed at a ratio of 1 : 1, and the level of IgM RF and IgM was analyzed by ELISA after 9 days of culture. The presence of the anti-id resulted in a marked reduction in the amount of PWM-stimulated RF production (panel A) without affecting total IgM production (panel B). NT, not treated with PWM; NRb Ig, normal rabbit immunoglobulin; Id, idiotype. (From Fong *et al.*, 1984.)

Fab reaction seen in that condition was inhibited by HBV particles (Geltner *et al.*, 1980). This, however, suggests an antiidiotype related to the HBV rather than the RF.

C. Relation to HLA-D and to Ig Genetic Markers

Although the frequency of HLA-DRW4 was increased in seropositive patients (Dobloug *et al.*, 1980; Stastny, 1978), there is no tendency for the RF to be higher in the $DR4^+$ RF^+ patients than in the $DR4^-$ RF^+ patients (Alarcon *et al.*, 1982). Moreover, RF are found in normal $DR4^+$ persons no more frequently than in normal $DR4^-$ persons (Engleman *et al.*, 1978), and *in vitro* and on stimulation of normal PBL by PWM, $DR4^+$ and $DR4^-$ donors yielded the same quantities of RF (Rodriquez *et al.*, 1983). An association between Gm allotypes and RF production was reported in coal workers with pneumoconiosis (Mentnech *et al.*, 1980). A possible genetic linkage between RF production in mice and the IgG_{2b} heavy chain locus (Igh-1) has also been reported (Van Snick, 1981).

IV. PHYSIOLOGICAL AND PATHOLOGICAL ROLE

A. Complement Activation by RF

Rheumatoid factor autoantibodies occur in several chronic disease states. They may potentiate the inflammatory response by activation of complement following antigen–antibody complex formation. It has been shown that complexing between RF and reduced and alkylated IgG can result in the activation of complement (Zvaifler and Schur, 1968). Similarly, RF bound to reduced and alkylated IgG anti-sheep-red-blood-cells on sheep erythrocytes activated the classical pathway of complement (Tanimoto *et al.*, 1975; Taylor-Upsahl *et al.*, 1977). The degree of complement activation is highly dependent on the amount of IgG coupled to the red cells. When a large amount of IgG was used to coat the cells, the condition was optimal for direct complement lysis of the cells, and the presence of IgM RF reduced the lysis (Schmid *et al.*, 1970). In contast, at suboptimal concentrations of IgG on the cells, direct lysis by complement did not occur or was weak, and RF initiated it or enhanced it. These results were interpreted as showing a weak complement-fixing capability of IgM RF compared to IgG antibodies.

One study comparing IgM RF and IgG RF and their reactivities with aggregated reduced and alkylated IgG reported that they activated complement to similar extents (Bianco *et al.*, 1974). However, when IgM and IgG RF were studied for their complement-activating abilities on surfaces, IgM RF was 100- to 1000-fold more active than IgG RF on a weight basis (500- to 5000-fold on a molar basis) and ten- to 100-fold more active than a rabbit IgG antibody to human IgG (Sabharwal *et al.*, 1982) (Fig. 9). These results are consistent with previous ones showing the generally greater ability of IgM antibodies than IgG antibodies to activate the classical complement pathway (Borsos and Rapp, 1965). The relative inability of the IgG RF to activate complement could be caused by preferential self-association of IgG RF molecules, sterically hindering the complement binding site (Pope *et al.*, 1975). Also, soluble immune complexes with fewer than three IgG molecules have been reported to be incapable of fixing complement and to bind

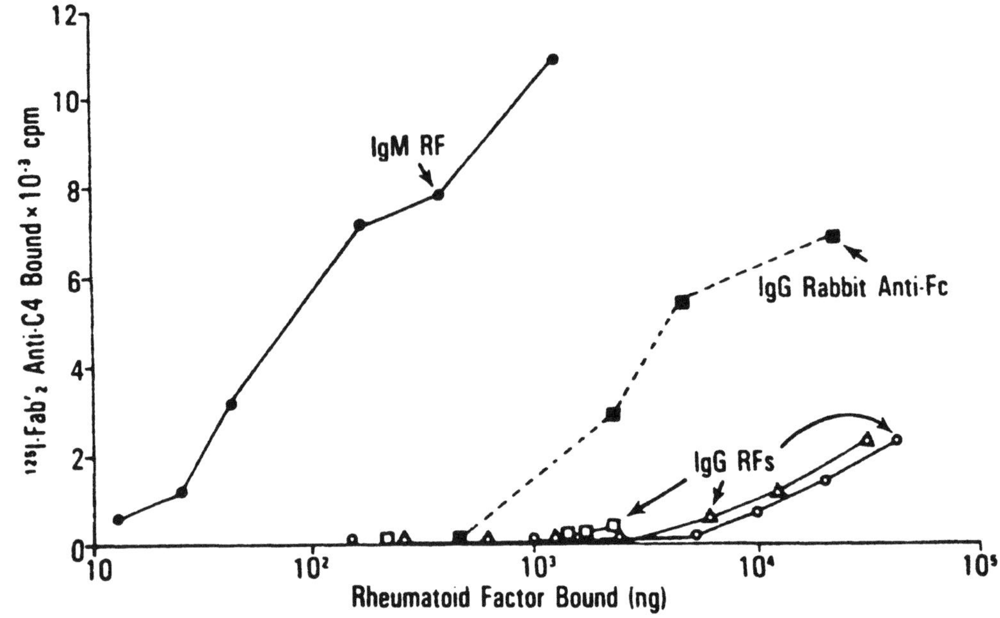

Figure 9. Comparative complement-activating ability of IgM RF and IgG RF. Activation of C4 by RF was measured in an ELISA assay. The IgG RF is 100- to 1000-fold less active, and rabbit IgG anti-FC 10- to 100-fold less active than IgM RF. Three separate IgG RF preparations were examined. (From Sabharwal *et al.*, 1982.)

relatively poorly to IgM RF (Hyslop *et al.*, 1970). Large IgG complexes in rheumatoid synovium do fix complement and bind IgM RF and therefore are probably important in potentiating inflammation.

B. Rheumatoid Factor in Rheumatoid Arthritis

Rheumatoid factors are found in the sera of 70–90% of patients with rheumatoid arthritis (reviewed in Vaughan, 1972). Often they are present at the earliest recognition of the disease, but they may appear only after the disease has been manifest for up to a year or two. Once present in high titer, RF tend to persist at that titer indefinitely, although they may diminish along with other evidences of the disease following treatment with immunosuppressive agents.

Extensive studies of synovial tissues and fluids of patients with rheumatoid arthritis have revealed that the joints are a major source of production of RF. Using fluorescein-tagged preparations of aggregated IgG to stain for cells containing IgG, Munthe and Natvig (1972) showed that up to 50% of plasma cells in rheumatoid synovial tissues may be producing RF. In further studies (Egeland *et al.*, 1982; Petersen *et al.*, 1983), it was demonstrated that the majority of these plasma cells stain for IgG RF. With a hemolytic plaque-forming cell assay for enumeration of Igm RF-producing lymphocytes, Vaughan *et al.* (1976) demonstrated that both the synovial fluid and bone marrow were relatively rich sources of these cells. The numbers in the blood were more scanty, and their presence was limited to patients with more severe disease. Other workers have extended these observations to show that the synovial tissues yield even larger numbers of RF-producing cells and that IgG RF-producing cells outnumber IgM RF-producing cells (Egeland *et al.*, 1982; Petersen *et al.*, 1983).

Examination of the immune complexes of the synovial fluids of RA patients (Winchester *et al.*, 1970) has emphasized the presence of IgG–IgG complexes and shown that lowered levels of intraarticular hemolytic complement levels correlated best with the IgG–IgG complexes, suggesting that IgG RF plays a major pathogenetic role in the joint disease. In studies of complexes isolated on a sucrose–polyethylene glycol gradient, Male *et al.* (1980) noted that IgG and IgM were the predominant molecular species and that moderate amounts of IgA and lesser amounts of the complement components C1q, C4, and C3 were present. Albumin, fibrinogen, and α_2-macroglobulin were also present in small amounts, apparently as entrapped serum proteins. Ninety-six percent of the protein in the complexes was thereby accounted for. The cumulative data thus suggest that the immune complexes in the joint fluids of patients with rheumatoid arthritis are locally generated, are composed of relatively more IgG RF than IgM RF, activate the complement system, and thereby are locally pathogenic. Although bacterial, viral, or other exogenous antigen may be present in the complexes, this could be only in very small quantities.

Patients with rheumatoid arthritis and RF have more aggressive joint disease than those without RF, and those with highest titers of RF are also more likely to exhibit extraarticular, vasculitic disease (Mongan *et al.*, 1969). These latter patients also were found to have slightly depressed titers of hemolytic complement when compared to patients without vasculitic disease, which suggested that circulating RF complexes in these patients can activate complement extraarticularly. Studies of the turnover of IgG (Catalano *et al.*, 1977) and C4 (Kaplan *et al.*, 1980) in RA patients showed both values to be high, that the enhanced turnover was occurring in extravascular as well as in intravascular compartments of the body, and that the enhanced C4 turnover was more closely correlated with RF titers than with other antibodies or with the Raji cell or C1q binding assays for immune complexes (Fig. 10).

Direct *in vivo* binding of C3 to RF in patients with severe disease has been shown in an enzyme-linked immunosorbent assay (Elson *et al.*, 1983). Extraarticular generation of RF has been illustrated by Halla *et al.* (1983), who demonstated IgM RF production from pleural explants in two of three patients with rheumatoid pleuritis with effusion. Some patients with rheumatoid arthritis do not exhibit elevated RF titers, and some rheumatoid synovial tissues may be almost devoid of B cells and plasma cells. Thus, other mechanisms of pathogenesis than RF may be operative, and the finding in some patients' synovial fluids of T-cell lymphokines indicates a T-cell role in the arthritic manifestation of the disease. Extraarticular vasculitic disease, however, is essentially confined to those who have circulating RF complexes.

Thus, it seems likely that RF and their complexes are the basis of extraarticular vasculitic disease but are only one component of the inflammatory process in the synovial disease itself. A high association of IgG RF in the serum of patients with systemic vasculitis (Quismorio *et al.*, 1983; Pope *et al.*, 1981) emphasizes the possible importance of this particular RF in extraarticular disease. Indeed, IgG RF might be expected to serve admirably to form a nidus of complexed IgG on which all other RF can react to build the aggregates required for the most potent complement activation and thus the most pathogenetic complex.

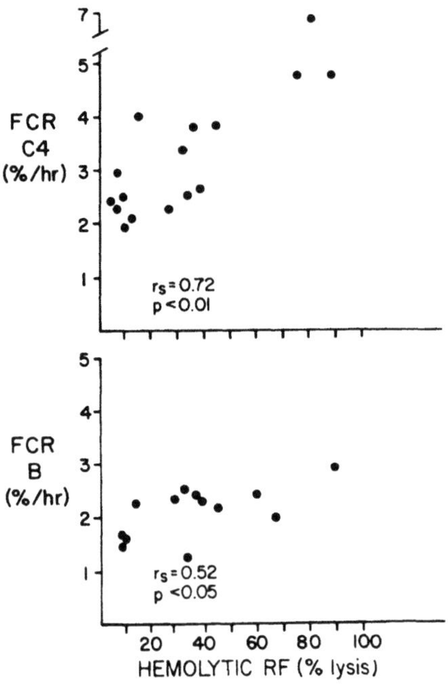

Figure 10. Correlation of C4 turnover with titer of hemolytic RF. Enhanced C4 turnover (FCR C4) is more closely correlated with the RF titer than is FCR Factor B of the alternative complement pathway; FCR C4 also correlates better with RF than with other antibodies or with assays of immune complexes (data not shown). (From Kaplan *et al.*, 1980.)

C. Occurrence in Other Diseases

Since RF are produced in response to immunization by IgG complexes as well as in response to polyclonal B-cell stimulation by a number of bacterial products (see above), it is not surprising that RF appear in a wide variety of infectious diseases, particularly chronic infectious diseases. Among these have been endocarditis, tuberculosis, leprosy, schistosomiasis, leishmaniasis, kala azar, chronic hepatitis, and complicated typhoid fever. In instances in which these diseases are curable, the RF disappeared as the infection was eliminated. Additionally, rheumatoid factors are seen in a variety of inflammatory diseases of undetermined etiology. They occur in 20% of patients with systemic lupus erythematosus and in essentially all patients with Sjogren's syndrome. They occur in a proportion of patients with polyarteritis nodosa and in most patients with the so-called "mixed connective tissue disease" syndrome (MCTD). In many of these non-RA disorders, the RF differs in having less cross reactivity with animal IgG and in having less RF in the immunoglobulin classes other than IgM (Pope *et al.*, 1981). The principal exception to this is the RF in Sjogren's syndrome, which may be rich in IgA RF, consistent with the mucosal nature of that disease (Dunne *et al.*, 1979; Elkon *et al.*, 1982). In respect to systemic lupus, it is interesting that the IgM-to-IgG shift, which is so prominent in the anti-DNA in that disease, is much less prominent for RF (Pope *et al.*, 1981). The opposite is true for rheumatoid arthritis, in which the IgM-to-IgG shift is very significant for rheumatoid factor and more poorly expressed for anti-DNA antibodies (Pope *et al.*, 1981; Karsh *et al.*, 1982).

The demonstrated efficacy of standard immunization procedures in humans to increase the numbers of precursors of circulating RF-producing cells (Welch *et al.*, 1983) and to yield increased titers of RF in the serum (Aho *et al.*, 1962) emphasizes that RF production is a normal immune response for humans. The RF production in rheumatoid arthritis, however, is quantitatively much greater, and the RF are qualitatively different both in distribution among the immunoglobulin classes and in the breadth of their reactivities with IgG. In these ways, the RF in rheumatoid arthritis are in a significantly different category from the RF in other states, and the basis for this difference needs better understanding.

D. Physiological Significance of RF

If RF specificities are represented in the germ-line genes, then RF, or at least the more "primordial" RF generated by very early B cells, must have some survival value for the species. The finding that IgM RF is an effective complement-fixing antibody capable of lysing and killing cells that are coated with otherwise ineffective quantities of IgG antibodies provides a very good rationale for their existence (Tesar and Schmid, 1973; Tanimoto *et al.*, 1975). This capability of IgM RF was initially shown with erythrocytes coated with small quantities of IgG antierythrocyte antibodies, which do not lyse the cells unless RF is present to augment the reactants on the cell surface. The possible survival value of this has been shown with murine trypanosomal organisms, which were not eliminated when coated with IgG antibodies alone but were in the presence of RF (Clarkson and Mellow, 1981).

Another means by which RF may protect animals is against circulating immune complexes in chronic infections. By providing a means by which the aggregate size of complexes can be increased and thereby quickly cleared into the reticuloendothelial system, animals may be protected from the development of immune complex vasculitic disease (Van Snick *et al.*, 1978). A variant on this is that since RF bind IgG molecules in the hinge region very close to where the first component of complement also binds IgG, RF may reduce the total complement binding to immune complexes and thereby reduce the attachment of the complexes to C3 receptors in the renal glomerulus, preventing glomerulonephritis (Bolton *et al.*, 1982).

Of more general biological significance, however, is the possibility that RF could clear the tissues of idiotype–antiidiotype immune complexes, thereby qualifying RF as a regulatory component in the control of the immune response (Morgan *et al.*, 1979). Studies with mice have been instructive, suggesting that RF may be a component of the normal immune response in this species, too. Mice produce RF in response to secondary immunization, whereas no RF response is detected following a primary immunization (Nemazee and Sato, 1982, 1983; Van Snick and Coulie, 1983; Coulie and Van Snick, 1983). These results suggest that RF-like autoantibodies are produced *in vivo* in response to immune complexes and that RF occurrence is a physiological phenomenon.

E. Pathogenetic Potentials

Whatever survival value there may be for RF, they clearly have pathogenetic potential. When they combine with IgG on surfaces, IgM RF are potent activators of the complement system of proteins. They activate complement poorly when they react with IgG in solution (Tanimoto *et al.*, 1975), but to the extent that soluble IgG complexes achieve sufficient size in the circulation to consititute a "surface," IgM RF may presumably fix complement here too (Zvaifler and Schur, 1968). As with other antibodies, IgM RF is a much more effective complement activator than IgG RF (Sabharwal *et al.*, 1982). Early data (Tanimoto *et al.*, 1975) suggested that there may be a heterogeneity in the ability of IgM RF to activate the complement, some but not all being capable of this. Our later data, however, have indicated a good complement-activating capability for some of the same monoclonal RF that failed in the earlier systems. The difference may have been related to whether the IgG used as antigen was presented in univalent or polyvalent form.

That RF can augment vasculitic disease caused by immune complexes has been shown in studies of mesenteric vasculitis (Baum *et al.*, 1964), nephrotoxic nephritis (McCormick *et al.*, 1969), and vasculitic lung disease (De Horatius and Williams, 1972). In all of these instances, immune complexes injected intravascularly produced mild disease but in the company of RF produced significantly enhanced disease. Rheumatoid factors and RF-like proteins have been recovered from the glomeruli of patients with glomerulonephritis (Rossen *et al.*, 1975). However, some authors have reported that the glomerulonephritis experienced with SLE is no more severe in those having circulating RF than in those without them (Estes and Christian, 1971). In patients with leprosy, tuberculosis, and subacute bacterial endocarditis, those patients exhibiting high titers of RF in the serum had significantly more activation of complement and more severe disease than did those lacking RF (Reyes *et al.*, 1983).

REFERENCES

Abruzzo, J. L., and Christian, C. L., 1961, The induction of a rheumatoid factor-like substance in rabbits, *J. Exp. Med.* **114**:791–806.

Agnello, V., Arbetter, A., de Kasep, G. I., Powell, R., Tan, E. M., and Joslin, F., 1980, Evidence for a subset of rheumatoid factors that cross-react with DNA-histone and have a distinct cross-idiotype, *J. Exp. Med.* **151**:1514–1527.

Aho, K., Konttinen, A., Rajasalmi, M., and Wager, O., 1962, Transient appearance of the rheumatoid factor in connection with prophylactic vaccinations, *Acta Pathol. Microbiol. Scand.* **56**:478–479.

Alarcon, G. S., Koopman, W. J., and Schroenloher, R. E., 1982, Differential patterns of *in vitro* IgM rheumatoid factor synthesis in seronegative and seropositive rheumatoid arthritis, *Arthritis Rheum.* **25**:150–155.

Alkner, U., Uesson, M., Hansson, U. B., and Glans, J., 1982, Circular dichroism of immune complexes with rheumatoid factor activity, *Mol. Immunol.* **19**:21–25.

Allen, J. C., and Kunkel, H. G., 1966, Hidden rheumatoid factors with specificity for native globulins, *Arthritis Rheum.* **9**:758–768.

Andrews, D. W., and Capra, J. D., 1981a, Complete amino acid sequences of variable domains from two monoclonal human anti-gammaglobulins of the Wa cross-idiotypic group: Suggestions that the J segments are involved in the structural correlates of the idiotype, *Proc. Natl. Acad. Sci. U.S.A.* **78**:3799–3803.

Andrews, D. W., and Capra, J. D., 1981b, Amino acid sequences of the variable regions of light chains from two idiotypically cross-reactive human IgM anti-γ-globulins of the Wa group, *Biochemistry* **20**:5816–5822.

Andrews, D. W., and Capra, J. D., 1981c, Amino acid sequence of the variable regions of heavy chains from two idiotypically cross-reactive human IgM anti-γ-globulins of the Wa group, *Biochemistry* **20**:5822–5830.

Bach, J.-F., Delrieu, F., and Delbarre, F., 1970, The rheumatoid rosette. A diagnostic test unifying seropositive and seronegative rheumatoid arthritis, *Am. J. Med.* **49**:213–222.

Bandilla, K. K., and McDuffie, F. C., 1969, Reactivity of rheumatoid factor with autologous IgG antibodies, *Arthritis Rheum.* **12**:74–81.

Baum, J., Stastny, P., and Ziff, M., 1964, Effects of the rheumatoid factor and antigen–antibody complexes on the vessels of the rat mesentery, *J. Immunol.* **93**:985–992.

Bianco, N. E., Dobkin, L. W., and Schur, P. H., 1974, Immunological properties of isolated IgG and IgM anti-gamma-globulins (rheumatoid factor), *Clin. Exp. Immunol.* **17**:91–101.

Bird, A. G., and Britton, S., 1979, A new approach to the study of human B lymphocyte function using an indirect plaque assay and a direct B cell activator, *Immunol. Rev.* **45**:41–67.

Birdsall, H. H., Lidsky, M. D., and Rossen, R. D., 1983, Anti-Fab′ antibodies in rheumatoid arthritis. Measurement of the relative quantities incorporated in soluble immune complexes in sera and supernatants from cultured peripheral blood lymphocytes, *Arthritis Rheum.* **26**:1481–1492.

Bluestone, R., Goldberg, L. S., and Cracchiolo, A., 1969, Hidden rheumatoid factors in seronegative nodular rheumatoid arthritis, *Lancet* **2**:878–879.

Bokisch, V. A., Chiao, J. W., Bernstein, D., and Krause, R. M., 1973, Homogeneous rabbit 7s anti-IgG with antibody specificity for peptidoglycans, *J. Exp. Med.* **138**:1184–1193.

Bolton, W. K., Schrock, J. H., and Davis, J. S., IV, 1982, Rheumatoid factor inhibition of *in vitro* binding of IgG complexes in the human glomerulus, *Arthritis Rheum.* **25**:297–303.

Bona, C. A., and Fauci, A. S., 1980, *In vitro* idiotypic suppression of chronic lymphocytic leukemia lymphocytes secreting monoclonal immunoglobulin M anti-sheep erythrocyte antibody, *J. Clin. Invest.* **69**:1356–1365.

Bonagura, V. R., Kunkel, H. G., and Pernis, B., 1982, Cellular localization of rheumatoid factor idiotypes, *J. Clin. Invest.* **69**:1356–1365.

Bonomo, L., Tursi, A., and Gillardi, U., 1968, Distribution of the anti-gamma globulin factors in the synovial membrane and other tissues in various diseases, *Ann. Rheum. Dis.* **27**:122–129.

Borsos, T., and Rapp, H. J., 1965, Hemolysin titration based on fixation of the activated first component of complement: Evidence that one molecule of hemolysin suffices to sensitise an erythrocyte, *J. Immunol.* **95**:559–566.

Boyden, V. S., 1951, The absorption of protein on erythrocytes treated with tannic acid and subsequent hemagglutination by anti-protein sera, *J. Exp. Med.* **93**:107–128.

Broder, I., Baumal, R., Gordon, D., and Bell, D., 1969, Histamine-releasing activity of rheumatoid and non-rheumatoid serum and synovial fluid, *Ann. N.Y. Acad. Sci.* **168**:126–139.

Brown, C. S., and Brown, J. C., 1981, Preferential reactivity of certain human and rabbit IgM and IgG rheumatoid factors with mildly reduced and amidomethylated IgG, *J. Immunol.* **126**:2373–2377.

Butler, V. P., and Vaughan, J. H., 1964, Hemmagglutination by rheumatoid factor of cells coated with animal gamma globulin, *Proc. Soc. Exp. Biol. Med.* **116**:585–593.

Butler, V. P., and Vaughan, J. H., 1965, The reaction of rheumatoid factor with animal gamma-globulins: Quantitative considerations, *Immunology* **8**:144–159.

Capra, J. D., and Kehoe, J. M., 1974, Structure of antibodies with shared idiotype: The complete sequence of the heavy chain variable region of two immunoglobulin M anti-gamma globulins, *Proc. Natl. Acad. Sci. U.S.A.* **71**:4032–4036.

Carson, D. A., and Fong, S., 1983, A common idiotype on human rheumatoid factors identified by a hybridoma antibody, *Mol. Immunol.* **20**:1081–1087.

Carson, D. A., and Lawrance, S., 1978, Light chain heterogeneity of 19s and 7s anti-γ-globulins in rheumatoid arthritis and subacute bacterial endocarditis, *Arthritis Rheum.* **21**:438–440.

Carson, D. A., Lawrance, S., Catalano, M. A., Vaughan, J. H., and Abraham, G., 1977, Radioimmunoassay of IgG and IgM rheumatoid factors reacting with human IgG, *J. Immunol.* **119**:295–300.

Carson, D. A., Bayer, A. S., Eisenberg, R. A., Lawrance, S., and Theofilopoulos, A., 1978, IgG rheumatoid factor in subacute bacterial endocarditis: Relationship to IgM rheumatoid factor and circulating immune complexes, *Clin. Exp. Immunol.* **31**:100–103.

Carson, D. A., Pasquali, J.-L., Tsoukas, C. D., Fong, S., Slovin, S. F., Lawrance, S. K., Slaughter, L., and Vaughan, J. H., 1981, Physiology and pathology of rheumatoid factors, *Springer Semin. Immunopathol.* **4**:161–179.

Catalano, M. A., Krick, E. H., De Heer, D. H., Nakamura, R. M., Theofilopoulos, A. N., and Vaughan, J. H., 1977, Metabolism of autologous and homologous IgG in rheumatoid arthritis, *J. Clin. Invest.* **60**:313–322.

Cebra, J. J., Koo, P. H., and Ray, A., 1974, Specificity of antibodies: Primary structural basis of antibody binding, *Science* **186**:263–264.

Chen, P. P., Houghten, R. A., Fong, S., Rhodes, G. A., Gilbertson, T. A., Vaughan, J. H., Lerner, R. A., and Carson, D. A., 1984a, Anti-hypervariable region antibody induced by a defined peptide. A new approach for studying the structural correlates of idiotypes, *Proc. Natl. Acad. Sci. U.S.A.* **81**:1784–1788.

Chen, P. P., Fong, S., Normansell, D., Karras, J. G., Vaughan, J. H., and Carson, D. A., 1984b, Delineation of a cross-reactive idiotype of human autoantibodies with antibody against a synthetic peptide, *J. Exp. Med.* **159**:1502–1511.

Chen, P. P., Goni, F., Fong, S., Jirik, F., Vaughan, J. H., Frangione, B., and Carson, D. A., 1985, The majority of human monoclonal IgM rheumatoid factors express a primary structure-dependent cross-reactive idiotype, *J. Immunology* **134:**3281–3285.

Chodirker, W. B., and Tomasi, T. B., Jr., 1963, Low molecular-weight rheumatoid factor, *J. Clin. Invest.* **42:**876–884.

Christian, C. L., 1963, Rheumatoid factor properties of hyperimmune rabbit sera, *J. Exp. Med.* **118:**827–844.

Clarkson, A. B., and Mellow, G. H., 1981, Rheumatoid factor-like immunoglobulin M protects previously uninfected rat pups and dams from *Trypanosoma lewisi, Science* **214:**186–188.

Coulie, P., and Van Snick, J., 1983, Rheumatoid factors and secondary immune responses in the mouse. II. Incidence, kinetics and induction mechanisms, *Eur. J. Immunol.* **13:**895–899.

Cracchiolo, A., Bluestone, R., and Goldberg, L. S., 1970, Hidden antiglobulins in rheumatoid disorders, *Clin. Exp. Immunol.* **7:**651–656.

Cunliffe, D. A., and Cox, K. O., 1980, IgM-autoantibodies against isologous erythrocytes also react with isologous IgG (Fc), *Nature* **26:**720–722.

Dawson, M. H., Olmstead, M., and Boots, R. H., 1932, Agglutination reactions in rheumatoid arthritis: Agglutination reactions with *Streptococcus hemolyticus, J. Immunol.* **23:**187–204.

De Horatius, R. J., and Williams, R. C., 1972, Rheumatoid factor accentuation of pulmonary lesions associated with experimental diffuse proliferative lung disease, *Arthritis Rheum.* **15:**293–301.

Dobloug, J. H., Førro, Ø., Kass, E., and Thorsby, E., 1980, HLA antigens and rheumatoid arthritis, *Arthritis Rheum.* **23:**309–313.

Dresser, D. W., 1978, Most IgM-producing cells in the mouse secrete autoantibodies (rheumatoid factor), *Nature* **274:**480–482.

Dunne, J. V., Carson, D. A., Speigelberg, H. L., Aspaugh, M. D., and Vaughan, J. H., 1979, IgA rheumatoid factor in the sera and saliva of patients with rheumatoid arthritis and Sjogren's syndrome, *Ann. Rheum. Dis.* **38:**161–170.

Durance, R. A., Micheli, A., and Fallet, F. H., 1974, Rosette formation in rheumatoid and non-rheumatoid states, *Ann. Rheum. Dis.* **33:**216–220.

Edelman, G. M., Kunkel, H. G., and Franklin, E. C., 1958, Interaction of the rheumatoid factor with antigen–antibody complexes and aggregated gamma globulin, *J. Exp. Med.* **108:**105–120.

Egeland, T., Lea, T., Saari, G., Mellbye, O. J., and Natvig, J. B., 1982, Quantitation of cells secreting rheumatoid factor of IgG, IgA, and IgM class after elution from rheumatoid synovial tissue, *Arthritis Rheum.* **25:**1445–1450.

Eichmann, K., and Berek, C., 1973, Mendelian segregation of a mouse antibody idiotype, *Eur. J. Immunol.* **3:**599–601.

Eichmann, K., and Kindt, T. J., 1971, The inheritance of individual antigenic specificities of rabbit antibodies to streptococcal carbohydrates, *J. Exp. Med.* **134:**532–552.

Eisenberg, R., 1976, The specificity and polyvalency of binding of a monoclonal rheumatoid factor, *Immunochemistry* **13:**355–359.

Elkon, K. B., Caeiro, F., Gharavi, A. E., Patel, B. M., Ferjencik, P. P., and Hughes, G. R. V., 1981, Radioimunoassay profile of anti-globulins in the connective tissue disorders: Elevated levels of IgA antiglobulin in systemic sicca syndrome, *Clin. Exp. Immunol.* **46:**547–552.

Elkon, K. B., Delacroix, D. L., Gharavi, A. E., Vaerman, J. P., and Hughes, G. R. V., 1982, Immunoglobulin A and polymeric IgA rheumatoid factors in systemic sicca syndrome: Partial characterization, *J. Immunol.* **129:**576–581.

Elson, C. J., Scott, D. G. I., Blake, D. R., Bacon, P. A., and Holt, P. D. J., 1983, Complement activating rheumatoid-factor-containing complexes in patients with rheumatoid vasculitis, *Ann. Rheum. Dis.* **42:**147–150.

Engleman, E. G., Sponzilli, E. E., Batey, M. E., Ramcharan, S., and McDevitt, H. O., 1978, Mixed lymphocyte reaction with healthy women with rheumatoid factor, *Arthritis Rheum.* **21:**690–693.

Epstein, W., Johnson, A. M., and Ragan, C., 1956, Observations on a precipitin reaction between serum of patients with rheumatoid arthritis and a preparation (Cohn fraction II) of human gamma globulin, *Proc. Soc. Exp. Biol. Med.* **91:**235–237.

Estes, D., and Christian, C. L., 1971, The natural history of systemic lupus erythematosus by prospective analysis, *Medicine* **50:**85–95.

Finley, P. R., Hicks, M. J., Williams, R. J., Hinlicky, J., and Lichti, D. A., 1979, Rate of nephelometric measurement of rheumatoid factor in serum, *Clin. Chem.* **25:**1909–1914.

Fong, S., Tsoukas, C. D., Frincke, L. A., Lawrance, S. K., Holbrook, T. L., Vaughan, J. H., and Carson, D. A., 1981, Age-associated changes in Epstein–Barr virus-induced human lymphocyte autoantibody responses, *J. Immunol.* **126:**910–914.

Fong, S., Miller, J. J. III, Moore, T. L., Tsoukas, C. D., Vaughan, J. H., and Carson, D. A., 1982a, Frequencies of Epstein–Barr virus-inducible IgM anti-IgG B lymphocytes in normal children with children with juvenile rheumatoid arthritis, *Arthritis Rheum.* **25:**959–965.

Fong, S., Vaughan, J. H., Tsoukas, C. D., and Carson, D. A., 1982b, Selective induction of autoantibody secretion in human bone marrow by Epstein–Barr virus, *J. Immunol.* **129:**1941–1945.

Fong, S., Vaughan, J. H., and Carson, D. A., 1983a, Two different rheumatoid factor-producing cell populations distinguished by the mouse erythrocyte receptor and responsiveness to polyclonal B cell activators, *J. Immunol.* **130:**162–164.

Fong, S., Gilbertson, T. A., and Carson, D. A., 1983b, The internal image of IgG in cross-reactive anti-idiotypic antibodies against human rheumatoid factors, *J. Immunol.* **131:**719–724.

Fong, S., Gilbertson, T. A., Chen, P. P., Vaughan, J. H., and Carson, D. A., 1984, Modulation of human rheumatoid factor specific lymphocyte responses with a cross-reactive anti-idiotype bearing the internal image of antigen, *J. Immunol.* **132:**1183–1189.

Forbes, I. J., Zalewski, P. D., Valente, L., and Murray, A. W., 1981, Loss of receptor activity for mouse erythrocytes precedes tumour promotor-induced maturation of chronic lymphocytic leukemia cells, *Cancer Lett.* **14:**187–192.

Forre, O., Dobloug, J. H., Michaelson, T. E., and Natvig, J. B., 1979, Evidence of similar idiotypic determinates on different rheumatoid factor populations, *Scand. J. Immunol.* **9:**281–289.

Franklin, E. C., Holman, H. R., Muller-Eberhard, H. J., and Kunkel, H. G., 1957, An unusual protein component of high molecular weight in the serum of certain patients with rheumatoid arthritis, *J. Exp. Med.* **105:**425–438.

Gaarder, P. I., and Michaelsen, T. E., 1974, Specificity of rheumatoid factors cross-reacting with human and rabbit IgG, *Acta Pathol. Microbiol. Scand. (B)* **82:**733–741.

Gaarder, P. I., and Natvig, J. B., 1974, The reaction of rheumatoid anti-Gm antibodies with native and aggregated Gm-negative IgG, *Scand. J. Immunol.* **3:**559–571.

Gabriel, D. A., and Hadler, N. M., 1981, The physical characterization of an aggregating IgG heteropolymer containing rheumatoid factor, *J. Biol. Chem.* **256:**3240–3244.

Geltner, D., Franklin, E. C., and Frangione, B., 1980, Anti-idiotypic activity in the IgM fraction of mixed cryoglobulins, *J. Immunol.* **125:**1530–1535.

Greenbury, C. L., 1960, A comparison of the Rose–Waaler latex fixation "RA-Test," and bentonite flocculation tests, *J. Clin. Pathol.* **13:**325–330.

Gripenberg, M., Wafin, F., Isomaki, H., and Linder, E., 1979, A simple enzyme immunoassay for the demonstration of rheumatoid factor, *J. Immunol. Methods* **31:**109–118.

Grubb, R., 1970, *The Genetic Markers of Human Immunoglobulins,* Springer-Verlag, Berlin, Heidelberg, New York.

Grubb, R., and Laurell, A. B., 1956, Hereditary serological human serum groups, *Acta. Pathol. Microbial. Scand.* **39:**390–398.

Halla, J. T., Koopman, W. J., Schrohenloher, R. E., Darby, W. L., and Heck, L. W., 1983, Local synthesis of IgM and IgM rheumatoid factor in rheumatoid pleuritis, *J. Rheumatol.* **10:**204–209.

Hannestad, K., 1968, Rheumatoid factor reacting with autologous native γG-globulin and joint fluid γG aggregates, *Clin. Exp. Immunol.* **3:**671–690.

Hannestad, K., 1969, M rheumatoid factors reacting with nitrophenyl groups and denatured deoxyribonucleic acid, *Ann. N.Y. Acad. Sci.* **168:**63–75.

Hannestad, K., and Johannessen, A., 1976, Polyclonal human antibodies to IgG (rheumatoid factors) which cross-react with cell nuclei, *Scand. J. Immunol.* **5:**541–547.

Hannestad, K., and Stollar, B. D., 1978, Certain rheumatoid factors react with nucleosomes, *Nature* **275:**671–673.

Hansson, U.-B., and Winblad, S., 1970, A simple routine method for detecting hidden rheumatoid factors, *J. Immunol. Methods* **22:**155–164.

Heimer, R., and Levin, F. M., 1966, On the distribution of rheumatoid factors among the immunoglobulins, *Immunochemistry* **3:**1–10.

Heimer, R., Wolfe, L. D., and Abruzzo, J. L., 1982, IgM and IgG anti-F(ab')$_2$ antibodies in rheumatoid arthritis and systemic lupus erythematosus, *Arthritis Rheum.* **25:**1298–1306.

Heller, G., Jacobson, A. S., Kolodny, M. H., and Kammerer, W. H., 1954, The hemagglutination test for rheumatoid arthritis. II. The influence of human plasma fraction II (gamma globulin) on the reaction, *J. Immunol.* **72**:66–78.

Henney, C. S., Stanworth, D. R., and Gell, P. G. H., 1965, Exposure of new antigenic determinants following antigen–antibody combination, *Nature* **205**:1079–1081.

Hunneyball, I. M., and Stanworth, D. R., 1976a, Subfragmentation of the Fc fragment of human IgG-1 myeloma protein by thermolysin, *Immunology* **30**:579–586.

Hunneyball, I. M., and Stanworth, D. R., 1976b, The effects of chemical modification on the antigencity of human and rabbit immunoglobulin G, *Immunology* **30**:881–894.

Hyslop, N. E., Jr., Dourmashkin, R. R., Green, N. M., and Porter, R. R., 1970, The fixation of complement and the activated first component (C1) of complement by complexes formed between antibody and divalent hapten, *J. Exp. Med.* **131**:783–802.

Izui, S., Eisenberg, R. A., and Dixon, F. J., 1979, IgM rheumatoid factors in mice injected with bacterial lipopolysaccharides, *J. Immunol.* **125**:2096–2102.

Jerne, N. K., 1974, Towards a network theory of the immune system, *Ann. Immunol. Inst. Pasteur (Paris)* **125c**:373–389.

Johnson, P. M., 1979a, IgM rheumatoid factors cross-reactive with IgG and a cell nuclear antigen: Apparent 'masking' in original serum, *Scand. J. Immunol.* **9**:461–466.

Johnson, P. M., 1979b, Stimuli for anti-IgG antibody production in rheumatoid arthritis, in: *Immunopathogenesis of Rheumatoid Arthritis,* (G. S. Panayi and P. M. Johnson, eds.), Reedbrooke, London, pp. 45–50.

Johnson, P. M., Watkins, J., and Holborow, E. J., 1975, Anti-globulin production to altered IgG in rheumatoid arthritis, *Lancet* **1**:611–613.

Kaplan, R. A., Curd, J. G., DeHeer, D. H., Carson, D. A., Pangburn, M. K., Muller-Eberhard, H. J., and Vaughan, J. H., 1980, Metabolism of C4 and factor B in rheumatoid arthritis. Relation to rheumatoid factor, *Arthritis Rheum.* **23**:911–920.

Karsh, J., Haibert, S. P., Anken, M., Klima, E., and Steinberg, A. D., 1982, Anti-DNA, anti-deoxyribonucleoprotein and rheumatoid factor measured by ELISA in patients with systemic lupus erythematosus, Sjogren's syndrome and rheumatoid arthritis, *Int. Arch. Allergy Appl. Immunol.* **68**:60–69.

Keightley, R. G., Cooper, M. D., and Lawton, A. R., 1976, The T cell dependence of B cell differentiation induced by pokeweed mitogen, *J. Immunol.* **117**:1538–1544.

Klapper, D. G., and Capra, J. D., 1976, The amino acid sequence of the variable regions of the light chains from two idiotypically cross-reactive IgM anti-gammaglobulins, *Ann. Immunol. Inst. Pasteur (Paris)* **127c**:261–271.

Koopman, W. J., 1981, Suppressor T cells prevent *in vitro* expression of IgM rheumatoid factor in some healthy adults, *Proc. Soc. Exp. Biol. Med.* **168**:344–349.

Koopman, W. J., and Schrohenloher, R. E., 1980a, Sensitive radioimunoassay for quantification of IgM rheumatoid factor, *Arthritis Rheum.* **23**:302–308.

Koopman, W. J., and Schrohenloher, R. E., 1980b, *In vitro* synthesis of IgM rheumatoid factor by lymphocytes from healthy adults, *J. Immunol.* **125**:934–939.

Koopman, W. J., and Schrohenloher, R. E., 1980c, Enhanced *in vitro* synthesis of IgM rheumatoid factor in rheumatoid arthritis, *Arthritis Rheum.* **23**:985–992.

Koopman, W. J., Shcrohenloher, R. E., and Solomon, A., 1982, A quantitative assay for IgA rheumatoid factor, *J. Immunol. Methods* **50**:89–96.

Koopman, W. J., Schrohenloher, R. E., Barton, J. C., and Greenleaf, E. C., 1983, Suppression of *in vitro* monoclonal human rheumatoid factor synthesis by anti-idiotypic antibody, *J. Clin. Invest.* **72**:1410–1419.

Kubagawa, H., Vogler, L. B., Capra, J. D., Conrad, M. E., Lawton, A. R., and Cooper, M. D., 1979, Studies on the clonal origin of multiple myeloma. Use of individually specific (idiotype) antibodies to trace the oncogenic events to its earliest point of expression in B-cell differentiation, *J. Exp. Med.* **159**:792–807.

Kunkel, H. G., Muller-Eberhard, H. J., Fudenberg, H. H., and Tomasi, T. B., 1961, Gamma globulin complexes in rheumatoid arthritis and certain other conditions, *J. Clin. Invest.* **40**:117–129.

Kunkel, H. G., Agnello, V., Joslin, F. G., Winchester, R. J., and Capra, J. D., 1973, Cross-idiotypic specificity among monoclonal IgM proteins with anti-γ-globulin activity, *J. Exp. Med.* **137**:331–342.

Kunkel, H. G., Winchester, R. J., Joslin, F. G., and Capra, J. D., 1974, Similarities in the light chains of anti-γ-globulins showing cross-idiotypic specificities, *J. Exp. Med.* **139**:128–136.

Lamont-Havers, R. W., 1952, Nature of serum factors causing agglutination of sensitized sheep cells and group A hemolytic streptococci, *Proc. Soc. Exp. Biol. Med.* **88:**35–38.

Ledford, D. K., Goni, F., Pizzolato, M., Franklin, E. C., Solomon, A., and Frangione, B., 1983, Preferential association of kIIIb light chains with monoclonal human IgM k autoantibodies, *J. Immunol.* **131:**1322–1325.

Lucivero, G., Lawton, A. R., and Cooper, M. D., 1981, Rosette formation with mouse erythrocytes defines a population of human B lymphocytes unresponsive to pokeweed mitogen, *Clin. Exp. Immunol.* **45:**185–190.

Lyet, J. P., and Normansell, D. E., 1974, Low molecular weight rheumatoid factors in rheumatoid arthritis sera, *Immunochemistry* **11:**417–421.

Male, D., Roitt, I. M., and Hay, F. C., 1980, Analysis of immune complexes in synovial effusions of patients with rheumatoid arthritis, *Clin. Immunol.* **39:**297–306.

McCluskey, R. T., Miller, F., and Benacerraf, B., 1962, Sensitization to denatured autologous gamma globulins, *J. Exp. Med.* **115:**253–273.

McCormick, J. N., 1963, An immunofluorescence study of rheumatoid factor, *Ann. Rheum. Dis.* **22:**1–10.

McCormick, J. N., and Day, J., 1963, The association of rheumatoid factor with anti-nuclear factor activity, *Lancet* **2:**554–557.

McCormick, J. N., Day, T., Morris, C. J., and Hill, A. G. S., 1969, The potentiating effect of rheumatoid arthritis serum in the immediate phase of nephrotoxic nephritis, *Clin. Exp. Immunol.* **4:**17–28.

McGraw, D. J., Kurec, A. S., and Davey, F. R., 1982, Mouse erythrocyte formation. A marker for resting B lymphocytes, *Am. J. Clin. Pathol.* **77:**177–183.

Mellors, R. C., Heimer, R., Corcos, J., and Korngold, L., 1959, Cellular origin of rheumatoid factor, *J. Exp. Med.* **110:**875–886, Plates 92–96.

Mellors, R. C., Nowoslawski, A., Korngold, L., and Sengson, L., 1961, Rheumatoid factor and the pathogenesis of rheumatoid arthritis, *J. Exp. Med.* **113:**475–484, Plates 49–54.

Mentnech, M. S., Pearson, D. J., Elliott, J. A., Taylor, G., and Major, P. C., 1980, Correlation of Gm allotypes with the incidence of anti-IgG antibody in coal workers' pneumoconiosis, *Clin. Immunol. Immunopathol.* **17:**274–279.

Meretey, K., Falus, A., Erhardt, C. C., and Maini, R. N., 1982, IgE and IgE-rheumatoid factors in circulating immune complexes in rheumatoid arthritis, *Ann. Rheum. Dis.* **41:**405–408.

Milde, E.-J., and Tonder, O., 1968, Demonstration of rheumatoid factor in tissue by mixed agglutination with tissue sections, *Arthritis Rheum.* **11:**537–545.

Miller, R. A., Maloney, D. G., Warnke, R., and Levy, R., 1982, Treatment of B cell lymphoma with monoclonal anti-idiotype antibody, *N. Engl. J. Med.* **306:**517–522.

Mizushima, Y., Hoshi, K., Shoji, Y., and Ogita, T., 1981, IgE rheumatoid factor, *Experientia* **37:**200–201.

Mongan, E. S., Cass, R. M., Jacox, R. F., and Vaughan, J. H., 1969, A study of the relation of seronegative and seropositive rheumatoid arthritis to each other and to necrotizing vasculitis, *Am. J. Med.* **47:**23–35.

Moore, T. L., Dorner, R. W., and Zuckner, J., 1974, Hidden rheumatoid factor in seronegative juvenile rheumatoid arthritis, *Ann. Rheum. Dis.* **33:**255–257.

Moore, T. L., Zuckner, J., Baldassore, A. R., Weiss, T. D., and Dorner, R. W., 1978, Complement-fixing hidden rheumatoid factor in juvenile rheumatoid arthritis, *Arthritis Rheum.* **21:**930–934.

Moore, T. L., Dorner, R. W., Weiss, T. D., Baldassore, A. R., and Zuckner, J., 1980, 19S IgM hidden rheumatoid factor in juvenile rheumatoid arthritis, *Pediatr. Res.* **14:**1135–1138.

Moore, T. L., Sheridan, P. W., Zuckner, J., and Dorner, R. W., 1983, Separation and characterization of immune complexes containing 19S IgM rheumatoid factor IgG in juvenile arthritis, *Arthritis Rheum.* **26:**165–169.

Morgan, A. C., Jr., Rossen, R. D., and Twomey, J. J., 1979, Naturally occurring circulating immune complexes: Normal human serum contains idiotype–antiidiotype complexes dissociable by certain IgG antiglobulins, *J. Immunol.* **122:**1672–1680.

Mudawwar, F., Awdeh, Z., Ault, K., and Geha, R. S., 1980, Regulation of monoclonal immunoglobulin G synthesis by anti-idiotypic antibody in a patient with hypogammaglobulinemia, *J. Clin. Invest.* **65:**1202–1209.

Munthe, E., and Natvig, J. B., 1971, Characterization of IgG complexes in elutes from rheumatoid tissue, *Clin. Exp. Immunol.* **8:**249–262.

Munthe, E., and Natvig, J. B., 1972, Complement fixing intracellular complexes of IgG rheumatoid factor in rheumatoid plasma cells, *Scand. J. Immunol.* **1:**217–229.

Nardella, F. A., Teller, D. C., and Mannik, M., 1981, Studies on the antigenic determinants in the self-association of IgG rheumatoid factor, *J. Exp. Med.* **154:**112–125.

Nasu, H., Chia, D. S., Knutson, D. W., and Barnett, E. V., 1980, Naturally occurring human antibodies to the $F(ab')_2$ portion of IgG, *Clin. Exp. Immunol.* **42:**378–386.

Natvig, J. B., and Kunkel, H. G., 1967, Detection of genetic antigens utilizing gamma globulins coupled to red blood cells, *Nature* **215:**68–69.

Natvig, J. B., Gaarder, P. I., and Turner, M. W., 1972, IgG antigens of the Cγ2 and Cγ3 homology regions interacting with rheumatoid factors, *Clin. Exp. Immunol.* **12:**177–183.

Nemazee, D. A., and Sato, V. L., 1982, Enhancing antibody: A novel component of the immune response, *Proc. Natl. Acad. Sci. U.S.A.* **79:**3828–3832.

Nemazee, D. A., and Sato, V. L., 1983, Induction of rheumatoid antibodies in the mouse, regulated production of autoantibody in the secondary humoral response, *J. Exp. Med.* **158:**529–545.

Normansell, D. E., 1970, Anti-γ-globulin in rheumatoid arthritis sera. I. Studies on the 22S complexes, *Immunochemistry* **7:**787–797.

Normansell, D. E., 1971, Anti-γ-globulin in rheumatoid arthritis sera. II. The reactivity of anti-γ-globulin rheumatoid factors with altered γ-G-globulin, *Immunochemistry* **8:**593–602.

Normansell, D. E., and Stanworth, D. R., 1966, Ultracentrifugal studies of the reactions of rheumatoid factor with native human γ-G-globulins, *Immunology* **10:**527–533.

Olsen, N., Ziff, M., and Jasin, H. E., 1982, *In vitro* synthesis of immunoglobulins and IgM-rheumatoid factor by blood mononuclear cells of patients with rheumatoid arthritis, *Rheumatol. Int.* **2:**59–66.

Oreskes, I., Singer, J. M., and Plotz, C. M., 1963, Reactivity of rheumatoid arthritis sera with altered and aggregated human γ-globulins, *J. Immunol.* **90:**107–115.

Osterland, C. K., Harboe, M., and Kunkel, H. G., 1963, Anti-γ-globulin factors in human sera revealed by enzymatic splitting of anti-Rh antibodies, *Vox Sang.* **8:**133–152.

Panush, R. S., Bianco, N. E., and Schur, P. H., 1971, Serum and synovial fluid IgG, IgA and IgM antigammaglobulins in rheumatoid arthritis, *Arthritis Rheum.* **14:**737–747.

Pasquali, J.-L., Fong, S., Tsoukas, C., Vaughan, J. H., and Carson, D. A., 1980, Inheritance of immunoglobulin M rheumatoid-factor idiotypes, *J. Clin. Invest.* **66:**863–866.

Pasquali, J.-L., Fong, S., Tsoukas, C. D., Slovin, S. F., Vaughan, J. H., and Carson, D. A., 1981, Different populations of rheumatoid factor idiotypes induced by two polyclonal B cell activators, pokeweed mitogen and Epstein–Barr virus, *Clin. Immunol. Immunopathol.* **21:**184–189.

Pasquali, J.-L., Urlacher, A., and Storck, D., 1983, A highly conserved determinant on human rheumatoid factor idiotypes defined by a mouse monoclonal antibody, *Eur. J. Immunol.* **13:**197–201.

Pawlak, L. L., Mushinski, E. B., Nisonoff, A., and Potter, M., 1973, Evidence for the linkage of the IgC_H locus to a gene controlling the idiotypic specificity of anti-*p*-azophenylarsonate antibodies in strain A mice, *J. Exp. Med.* **137:**22–31.

Petersen, J., Heilmann, C., Bjerrum, O. J., Ingemann-Hansen, T., and Halkjaer-Kristensen, J., 1983, IgG rheumatoid factor-secreting lymphocytes in rheumatoid arthritis: Evaluation of a haemolytic plaque-forming cell technique, *Scand. J. Immunol.* **17:**471–478.

Pisko, E. J., Turner, R. A., and Foster, S. L., 1982, Induction of human rheumatoid factor producing cells by aggregated IgG, *Arthritis Rheum.* **25:**1108–1116.

Pope, R. M., and McDuffy, S. J., 1981, IgG rheumatoid factor: Analysis of various species of IgG for detection by radioimmunoassay, *J. Lab. Clin. Med.* **97:**842–853.

Pope, R. M., Teller, D. C., and Mannik, M., 1974, The molecular basis of self-association of antibodies to IgG (rheumatoid factors) in rheumatoid arthritis, *Proc. Natl. Acad. Sci. U.S.A.* **71:**517–521.

Pope, R. M., Teller, D. C., and Mannik, M., 1975, The molecular basis of self-association of IgG rheumatoid factors, *J. Immunol.* **115:**365–373.

Pope, R. M., Yoshinoya, S., and McDuffy, S. J., 1981, Detection of immune complexes and their relationship to rheumatoid factor in a variety of autoimmune disorders, *Clin. Exp. Immunol.* **46:**259–267.

Powell, R., and Agnello, V., 1983, Characterization of complement-fixing activity and cross-idiotypes of rheumatoid factors in idiopathic mixed cryoglobulinemia, *Clin. Immunol. Immunopathol.* **29:**146–151.

Preud'homme, J. L., and Seligmann, 1972, Anti-human immunoglobulin G activity of membrane-bound monoclonal immunoglobulin M in lymphoproliferative disorders, *Proc. Natl. Acad. Sci. U.S.A.* **69:** 2132–2135.

Quismorio, F. P., Beardmore, T., Kaufman, R. L., and Mongan, E. S., 1983, IgG rheumatoid factors and anti-nuclear antibodies in rheumatoid arthritis, *Clin. Exp. Immunol.* **52:**333–340.

Rajewsky, K., and Takemori, T., 1983, Genetics, expression and functions of idiotypes, *Annu. Rev. Immunol.* **1:**569–607.

Reyes, P. A., Maluf, J. G., Curd, J. G., and Vaughan, J. H., 1983, Association of rheumatoid factor with complement activation in rheumatoid arthritis and other diseases, *Clin. Exp. Immunol.* **53**:391–396.

Robbins, D. L., and Wistar, R. J., 1985, Comparative specificities of serum and synovial cell 19S IgM rheumatoid factors in rheumatoid arthritis, *J. Rheumatol.* (in press).

Robbins, D. L., Moore, T. L., Carson, D. A., and Vaughan, J., 1978, Relative reactivities of rheumatoid factors in serum and cells. Evidence for a selective deficiency in serum and cells, *Arthritis Rheum.* **21**:820–826.

Rodriquez, M. A., Bankhurst, A. D., Williams, R. C., Jr., Troup, G. M., and Stastny, P., 1983, Studies on the relationship between HLA DR4 and *in vitro* IgM rheumatoid factor production, *Clin. Immunol. Immunopathol.* **27**:96–109.

Rose, H. M., Ragan, C., Pearce, E., and Lipman, M. O., 1948, Differential agglutination of normal and sensitized sheep erythrocytes by sera of patients with rheumatoid arthritis, *Proc. Soc. Exp. Biol. Med.* **68**:1–6.

Rossen, R. D., Reisberg, M. A., Sharp, J. T., Suki, W. N., Schloeder, F. X., Hill, L. L., and Eknoyan, G., 1975, Antiglobulins and glomerulonephritis: Classification of patients by the reactivity of their sera and renal tissue with aggregated and native human IgG. *J. Clin. Invest.* **56**:427–437.

Sabharwal, U. K., Vaughan, J. H., Fong, S., Bennett, P. H., Carson, D. A., and Curd, J. G., 1982, Activation of the classical pathway of complement by rheumatoid factors. Assessment by radioimmunoassay for C4, *Arthritis Rheum.* **25**:161–167.

Schmid, F. R., Roitt, I. M., and Rocha, M. J., 1970, Complement fixation by a two component antibody system, immunoglobulin G and immunoglobulin M anti-globulin (rheumatoid factor): Paradoxical effect related to immunoglobulin G concentration, *J. Exp. Med.* **132**:673–693.

Schrohenloher, R. D., 1966, Characterization of the γ-globulin complexes present in certain sera having high titers of anti-γ-globulin activity, *J. Clin. Invest.* **115**:501–512.

Sheagren, J. H., Tuazon, C. V., Griffin, C., and Padman, N., 1976, Rheumatoid factor in acute bacterial endocarditis, *Arthritis Rheum.* **19**:887–890.

Singer, J. M., and Plotz, C. M., 1956, The latex fixation test. I. Application to the serologic diagnosis of rheumatoid arthritis, *Am. J. Med.* **21**:888–892.

Slaughter, L., Carson, D. A., Jensen, F. C., Holbrook, T. L., and Vaughan, J. H., 1978, *In vitro* effects of Epstein–Barr virus on peripheral blood mononuclear cells from patients with rheumatoid arthritis and normal subjects, *J. Exp. Med.* **148**:1429–1434.

Stankaitiene, D. J., Matulis, A. A., Guabyr, H., and Jusenaite, J. P., 1978, Serum anti-immunoglobulins reactive with human and rabbit IgG in rheumatoid arthritis and other conditions, *Arthritis Rheum.* **61**:120–128.

Stassin, V., Coulie, P. G., Birshtein, B. K., Secher, D. S., and Van Snick, J., 1983, Determinants recognized by murine rheumatoid factors: Molecular localization using a panel of mouse myeloma variant immunoglobulins, *J. Exp. Med.* **158**:1763–1768.

Stastny, P., 1978, Association of the B-cell alloantigen DRW4 with rheumatoid arthritis, *N. Engl. J. Med.* **29**:869–871.

Steinberg, A. C., and Wilson, J. A., 1963, Hereditary globulin factors and immune tolerance in man, *Science* **140**:303–304.

Stevens, R. H., Macy, E., Morrow, C., and Saxon, A., 1979, Characterization of a circulating subpopulation of spontaneous antitetanus toxoid antibody producing B cells following *in vivo* booster immunization, *J. Immunol.* **122**:2498–2504.

Stewart, G. A., Smith, A. K., and Stanworth, D. R., 1973, Biological activities associated with the Facb fragment of rabbit IgG, *Immunochemistry* **10**:755–760.

Stone, M. J., and Metzger, H., 1968, Binding properties of a Waldenstrom macroglobulin antibody, *J. Biol. Chem.* **243**:5977–5984.

Tanimoto, K., Cooper, N. R., Johnson, J. S., and Vaughan, J. H., 1975, Complement fixation by rheumatoid factor, *J. Clin. Invest.* **55**:437–445.

Taylor-Upsahl, M. M., Johnson, P. M., Mellbye, O. J., and Natvig, J. B., 1977, A study of complement fixation by complement rheumatoid factor using a hemolytic assay system, *Clin. Exp. Immunol.* **28**:204–211.

Tesar, J. T., and Schmid, F. R., 1973, Heterogeneity among rheumatoid factors for complement fixation, *J. Immunol.* **110**:993–1002.

Theofilopoulos, A. N., Balderas, R. S., Hang, L., and Dixon, F. J., 1983, Monoclonal IgM rheumatoid factors derived from arthritis MRL/MP-1pr/1pr mice, *J. Exp. Med.* **158**:901–919.

Torrigiani, G., and Roitt, I. M., 1967, Antiglobulin factors in sera from patients with rheumatoid arthritis and normal subjects. Quantitative estimation in different immunoglobulin classes, *Ann. Rheum. Dis.* **26**:334–340.

Tsoukas, C. D., Carson, D. A., Fong, S., Pasquali, J.-L., and Vaughan, J. H., 1980, Cellular requirements for pokeweed mitogen induced autoantibody production in rheumatoid arthritis, *J. Immunol.* **125**:1125–1129.

Uesson, M., and Hansson, U.-B., 1981, Quantitative precipitin analysis of free and hidden RF IgM, *Scand. J. Immunol.* **14**:61–69.

Van Snick, J. L., 1981, A gene linked to the Igh-C locus controls the production of rheumatoid factor in the mouse, *J. Exp. Med.* **153**:738–742.

Van Snick, J., and Coulie, P., 1983, Rheumatoid factors and secondary immune responses in the mouse. I. Frequent occurrence of hybridomas secreting IgM anti-IgG, autoantibodies after immunization with protein antigen, *Eur. J. Immunol.* **13**:890–894.

Van Snick, L., Van Roost, E., Markowetz, B., Cambiaso, C. L., and Masson, P. L., 1978, Enhancement of IgM rheumatoid factor of *in vitro* ingestion by macrophages and *in vivo* clearance of aggregated IgG or antigen–antibody complexes, *Eur. J. Immunol.* **8**:279–285.

Van Snick, J. L., Stassin, V., and De Lestre, B., 1983, Isotypic and allotypic specificity of mouse rheumatoid factors, *J. Exp. Med.* **157**:1006–1019.

Van Snick, J., Coutelier, J.-P., Van Roost, E., and Guenet, J.-L., 1984, Rheumatoid factors in 129XB recombinant inbred strains. Igh-1-linked control of allotypic and isotypic specificies, *J. Exp. Med.* **159**:355–364.

Vaughan, J. H., 1956, Behavior of the rheumatoid arthritis agglutinating factor with immune precipitates, *J. Immunol.* **77**:181–188.

Vaughan, J. H., 1972, Infectious and immunological considerations in rheumatic diseases, in: *Arthritis and Allied Conditions,* ed. 8 (J. L. Hollander, ed.), Lea & Febiger, Philadelphia, p. 153.

Vaughan, J. H., Chihara, T., Moore, T. L., Robbins, D. L., Tanimoto, K., Johnson, J., and McMillan, R., 1976, Rheumatoid factor-producing cells detected by direct hemolytic plaque assay, *J. Clin. Invest.* **58**:933–941.

Waaler, E., 1940, On the occurrence of a factor in human serum activating the specific agglutination of sheep blood corpuscles, *Acta. Pathol. Microbiol. Scand.* **17**:172–188.

Wagar, O., and Teppo, A.-M., 1978, Binding affinity of human autoantibodies: Studies of cryoglobulin IgM rheumatoid factors and IgG autoantibodies to albumin, *Scan. J. Immunol.* **7**:503–509.

Waller, M. V., and Vaughan, J. H., 1956, Use of anti-Rh sera for demonstrating agglutinating activating factors in rheumatoid arthritis, *Proc. Soc. Exp. Biol. Med.* **92**:198–200.

Watkins, J., Unger, A., and Mahon, N., 1970, Differences between the papain hydrolysis patterns of the serum G immunoglobulins of healthy individuals and of rheumatoid patients, *Clin. Sci.* **38**:15P.

Welch, M. J., Fong, S., Vaughan, J., and Carson, D., 1983, Increased frequency of rheumatoid factor precursor B lymphocytes after immunization of normal adults with tetanus toxoid, *Clin. Exp. Immunol.* **51**:299–304.

Williams, R. C., and Kunkel, H. G., 1962, Rheumatoid factor, complement, and conglutinin aberrations in patients with subacute bacterial endocarditis, *J. Clin. Invest.* **41**:666–675.

Williams, R. C., and Kunkel, H. G., 1963, Antibodies to rabbit-γ-globulins after immunizing with various preparations of autologous-γ-globulins, *Proc. Soc. Exp. Biol. Med.* **112**:554–561.

Winchester, R. J., 1975, Characterization of IgG complexes in patients with rheumatoid arthritis, *Ann. N.Y. Acad. Sci.* **256**:73–81.

Winchester, R. J., Agnello, V., and Kunkel, H. G., 1970, Gamma globulin complexes in synovial fluids of patients with rheumatoid arthritis: Partial characterization and relationship to lowered complement levels, *Clin. Exp. Immunol.* **6**:689–706.

World Health Organization, 1976, Review of the notation for the allotypic and related markers of human immunoglobulins, *Eur. J. Immunol.* **6**:599–601.

Zuraw, B. L., O'Hair, C. H., Vaughan, J. H., Mathison, D. A., Curd, J. G., and Katz, D. H., 1981, Immunoglobulin E-rheumatoid factor in the serum of patients with rheumatoid arthritis, asthma and other diseases, *J. Clin. Invest.* **68**:1610–1613.

Zvaifler, N. J., and Schur, P. H., 1968, Reactions of aggregated merceptoethanol treated gamma globulin with rheumatoid factor-precipitation and complement fixation studies, *Arthritis Rheum.* **11**:523–536.

7

Autoantibodies to Nonhistone Nuclear Antigens
Their Immunobiology and Clinical Relevance

Gordon C. Sharp and Margaret A. Alspaugh

I. INTRODUCTION

In the absence of precise etiologic and pathogenetic information, the diagnosis of the rheumatic diseases is based on a combination of clinical, laboratory, and pathological features. Serologic findings have assumed increasing diagnostic importance since the discovery by Hargraves *et al.* (1948) of the LE cell, the forerunner of the antinuclear antibodies. Subsequent studies by Holman and Kunkel (1957) showed that the LE cell phenomenon was caused by a circulating autoantibody reacting with autologous nuclear material (DNA–histone). More recently, the widely used indirect immunofluorescent test has served as a sensitive screening test and has revealed the presence of circulating autoantibodies to nuclear antigens (ANA) in systemic rheumatic diseases such as systemic lupus erythematosus (SLE), progressive systemic sclerosis or scleroderma (PSS), mixed connective tissue disease (MCTD), Sjogren's syndrome, and poly/dermatomyositis.

During the past 30 years a variety of immunologic techniques (e.g., immunoprecipitation, complement fixation, hemagglutination) have been used to identify antibodies to specific nuclear constituents. Testing of patient sera by the immunofluorescent method (fluorescent ANA), typically using sections of cryopreserved tissues as substrates, has revealed a wide spectrum of patterns. Certain fluorescent ANA patterns were shown to

---

Gordon C. Sharp and Margaret A. Alspaugh • Department of Medicine and Pathology, University of Missouri-Columbia, School of Medicine and Cancer Research Center, Columbia, Missouri 65201.

correlate with the presence of specific antinuclear antibodies defined by other immunologic tests (e.g., the rim fluorescent ANA pattern correlated with antibody to DNA). However, a complex array of speckled ANA patterns with variations in size and density of speckles is produced by sera containing antibodies to many different nonhistone nuclear antigens (Nakamura and Tan, 1977). The more recent use of tissue culture cell lines, which have larger nuclei and nucleoli than those in tissue sections, has improved the sensitivity and differentiation of patterns and has facilitated the detection of distinct new ANAs such as anticentromere (Tan *et al.*, 1980) and anti-mitotic-spindle-apparatus (McCarty *et al.*, 1981).

Of all the systemic rheumatic diseases, SLE is the one in which the greatest abundance of autoantibodies have been described. Initially it was not known which of these autoantibodies might have the most clinical significance. However, numerous published reports document the special relationship between antibody to native DNA and SLE and the role of DNA–anti-DNA complexes in SLE nephritis (Tan *et al.*, 1966; Koffler *et al.*, 1967; Bruneau and Benveniste, 1979). Antibodies to single-strand DNA lack the same specificity for SLE since they are found in numerous diseases (Koffler *et al.*, 1971), but they may also be involved in pathological changes in lupus kidneys (Koffler *et al.*, 1974). Antibodies to histones have also been detected in SLE, have a particularly strong relationship with drug-induced LE, and have also been detected in rheumatoid arthritis (Tan, 1982). These important autoantibodies are discussed in detail elsewhere in this book. The remainder of this chapter focuses on another group of autoantibodies reactive with various nonhistone antigens that have become of increasing biological and clinical interest during the past two decades.

The list of autoantibodies to nonhistone antigens is long and no doubt will increase steadily as ANAs presently under investigation prove to have biological and/or clinical significance. Shown in Fig. 1 are nuclear antigens (excluding DNA and histone) that have proven or potential clinical relevance and the rheumatic diseases with which their atuoantibodies are associated. Some of these autoantibodies are restricted to certain diseases or subsets and therefore can serve as disease markers, whereas others occur in combination or are more widely distributed. High titers of antibody to nuclear ribonucleoprotein (RNP) in the absence of other ANAs constitute a serologic pattern that is especially related to MCTD. Antibodies to Sm and native DNA are markers for SLE. Other antibodies that appear useful as markers include anticentromere in the CREST subset of PSS, anti-Scl-70 in PSS, and antibodies to Ku, PM-1, and Jo-1, which are closely linked with polymyositis (PM) or PM–PSS overlap syndrome. Although antibodies to Me, Su, and MA are still in a preliminary phase of investigation and their true clinical significance remains uncertain, these systems are discussed since the work has been pursued in the authors' laboratory, and this permits inclusion of new information that has not been widely disseminated.

Other systems that are of considerable biological interest but whose clinical diagnostic and prognostic roles have not been fully elucidated [e.g., rheumatoid arthritis nuclear antigen (RANA), Alspaugh *et al.*, 1976; proliferating cell nuclear antigen (PCNA), Miyachi *et al.*, 1978; mitotic spindle apparatus (MSA), McCarty *et al.*, 1981; and SL antigen, Harmon *et al.*, 1981] are not discussed in this chapter. Particular emphasis is given to the elucidation of nuclear RNP and Sm antigens and to the new clinical, immunopathological, and molecular biological information that has been generated as a result of scientific investigation of these systems.

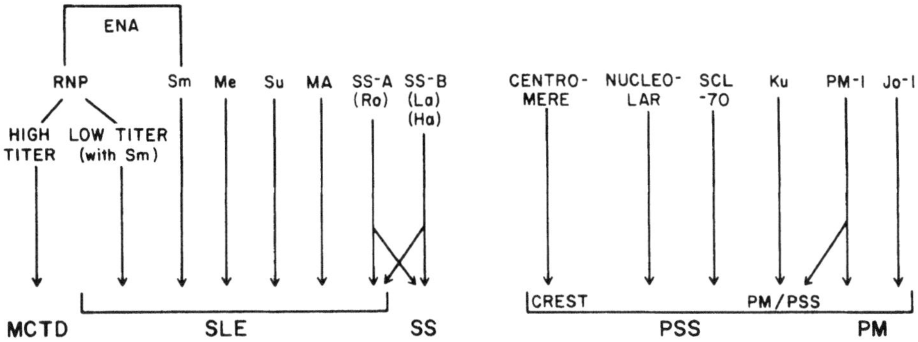

Figure 1. Various nuclear nonhistone antigens to which circulating autoantibodies are found in the rheumatic diseases are listed at the top of the figure. Arrows are drawn from each antigen to the disease listed below in which the system is most frequently observed. ENA, extractable nuclear antigen consisting of ribonucleoprotein (RNP) and Sm components. Sm, Me, Su, MA, Ro, La, Ha, Ku, and Jo-1 are antigen designates by various authors, taken from the names of the prototype patients. SS-A and SS-B are systems associated with Sjogren's syndrome (SS). Scl-70 and PM-1 designations refer to their association with scleroderma (PSS) and polymyositis (PM). The PM-1 and Ku systems are most closely related to polymyositis–scleroderma overlap syndrome (PM/PSS). Ro and La were originally reported as cytoplasmic systems but are immunologically identical to the nuclear SS systems. Antibodies to the centromere and nucleolar antigens are identified by the fluorescent ANA method and are associated with the CREST variant of PSS and systemic sclerosis, respectively. MCTD, mixed connective tissue disease; SLE, systemic lupus erythematosus.

II. NUCLEAR RIBONUCLEOPROTEIN AND SM ANTIGENS

A. Early Studies

In the early and mid-1960s at Stanford University, some interesting patients were observed who had overlapping clinical features of systemic lupus erythematosus, progressive systemic sclerosis, and polymyositis and hence were referred to as having mixed connective tissue disease (MCTD)(Sharp *et al.*, 1972b). Their characteristic serologic finding was that they has persistent high titers of antibody to whole calf thymus nuclei by complement fixation both during active disease and in remission. This was in contrast to typical SLE patients, whose antibody titer would diminish as the disease became inactive. The nature of the circulating antinuclear antibody in these MCTD patients was subsequently clarified by Sharp *et al.* (1972b) through the development of a very sensitive passive hemagglutination test in which various nuclear antigens were adsorbed on to tannic-acid-treated sheep erythrocytes. In these studies, all the MCTD patients had very high hemagglutination titers (1:1000 to 1:10,000,000) of antibodies directed against a partially purified extractable nuclear antigen (ENA) that had been described earlier by Holman (1965). In contrast, ENA antibodies were usually present at lower levels in about 50% of patients with typical SLE and were rarely found in other rheumatic diseases.

It was postulated that this partially purified ENA might contain more than a single antigenic specificity. In order to investigate the possibility that ENA antibodies occurring in MCTD might be different from those detected in SLE, enzyme digestion studies were performed in which ENA-coated erythrocytes treated with ribonuclease (RNase), trypsin, or deoxyribonuclease were reacted with MCTD and SLE sera. Digestion with RNase and trypsin eliminated or greatly reduced the hemagglutination reaction to ENA in all cases of MCTD but had little effect on ENA antibody titers in SLE (Sharp *et al.*, 1972b). When Tan performed fluorescent antinuclear antibody analyses on these MCTD sera, he found that they produced speckled reactions in high titer and that RNase treatment of the tissue sections eliminated the speckled reactions of MCTD sera (Sharp *et al.*, 1972b). These findings suggested that the circulating antibody in MCTD has a specificity for a nuclear ribonucleoprotein (RNP) antigen.

B. Distinct Immunologic Specificities

Immunodiffusion analyses in the early 1970s further elucidated the fact that ENA contains at least two immunologically distinct antigenic components, the RNase- and trypsin-sensitive RNP antigen and the RNase- and trypsin-resistant Sm antigen (Sharp *et al.*, 1972a; Northway and Tan, 1972; Reichlin and Mattioli, 1972; Parker, 1973). The Sm antigen has previously been described by Tan and Kunkel (1966). Although the immunodiffusion test provides a more definitive identification of RNP and Sm antibodies, the hemagglutination test with titers before and after RNase is also very useful since it is much more sensitive and quantitative. This was substantiated by studies that demonstrated that RNP antibody is rarely detectable by immunodiffusion when the hemagglutination titer is <1 : 1000. The hemagglutination test for RNP antibody is also 100 to 1000-fold more sensitve than the fluorescent ANA test in the detection of RNP antibodies. (Table 1; Sharp *et al.*, 1972a). In some cases, counterimmunoelectrophoresis will demonstrate RNP or Sm antibodies that have not been detected by other techniques (Kurata and Tan, 1976; Bresnihan *et al.*, 1977). This sensitivity is important in early diagnosis, as RNP antibody is not detected in normal individuals.

C. Clinical Correlates of RNP and Sm Antibodies

The serologic pattern of very high titers of RNP antibodies and no Sm antibodies occurs in 95–100% of patients with MCTD, is infrequent in SLE and PSS, and occurs rarely if

Table 1. Serologic Studies on MCTD and SLE Sera[a]

		Immunodiffusion			Hemagglutination titer	
		RNP Ab titer	Sm Ab	ANA[d] Titer	ENA Ab	ENA Ab after RNase
MCTD[b]	−1	1 : 128	0	1 : 4096	1 : 8,000,000	0
	−2	1 : 64	0	1 : 2048	1 : 8,000,000	0
	−3	1 : 32	0	1 : 2048	1 : 32,000,000	0
	−4	1 : 32	0	1 : 2048	1 : 32,000,000	0
	−5	1 : 32	0	1 : 1024	1 : 8,000,000	0
SLE[c]	−1	0	+	1 : 256	1 : 1000	1 : 1000
	−2	0	+	1 : 64	1 : 2000	1 : 2000
	−3	0	+	1 : 64	1 : 2000	1 : 1000
	−4	0	+	1 : 64	1 : 4000	1 : 4000

[a]Sharp *et al.* (1972).
[b]Patient with MCTD, analysis of five different serum specimens.
[c]Patient with SLE, analysis of four different serum specimens.
[d]Indirect immunofluorescent test; all gave speckled ANA patterns.

at all in other rheumatic diseases (Sharp *et al.*, 1972b, 1976; Northway and Tan, 1972; Parker, 1973; Notman *et al.*, 1975; Farber and Bole, 1976; Singsen *et al.*, 1977; Tan *et al.*, 1980; Sharp, 1982). Recent reports of long-term studies (Grant *et al.*, 1981; Sullivan *et al.*, 1984) indicate that the clinical manifestations of MCTD may not all be present at the time of disease onset, and the disease undergoes transitions in its clinical features with increasing overlap over time. In our prospective, longitudinal study of MCTD at the University of Missouri (Table 2), 60% of the patients initially had more limited clinical involvement and were thought to have SLE, PSS, polymyositis, rheumatoid arthritis, or an undifferentiated connective tissue disease. By the time of their most recent medical evaluation, 91% had developed typical overlapping features consistent with a diagnosis of MCTD, and only 9% persisted with a mild, undifferentiated syndrome.

This experience (Sullivan *et al.*, 1984) illustrates the problem inherent in drawing diagnostic and prognostic conclusions from short-term studies of connective tissue diseases and is a further indication that the serologic pattern of high titers of RNP antibody may have a high specificity for MCTD. The typical serologic findings in MCTD are a high-titer speckled fluorescent ANA (often > 1 : 1000), very high titers (frequently 1 : 1,000,000) of antibody to RNase-sensitive ENA by hemagglutination, and RNP antibody by immunodiffusion. Antibodies to native DNA and Sm antibodies are infrequent in MCTD, and their appearance usually is associated with a severe flare of SLE-like disease (Grant *et al.*, 1981; Frank *et al.*, 1983; Sullivan *et al.*, 1984). The serologic pattern of Sm antibodies, usually in association with lower titers of RNP antibodies, is found in 25–30% of lupus patients and has a high specificity for SLE (Notman *et al.*, 1975; Sharp *et al.*, 1976).

Patients with clinical features of MCTD will rarely be negative for RNP antibody (Sharp *et al.*, 1976), and occasionally they may transiently have negative fluorescent ANA and RNP antibody tests early in their course. Subsequently these tesets will become positive, usually following corticosteroid therapy (Sharp *et al.*, 1972b; Alarcon-Segovia, 1979; Grant *et al.*, 1981). Once present, high titers of circulating RNP antibody usually persist during periods of both active and inactive disease, but a long-term study has disclosed that in some patients after 5–11 years RNP antibody levels may fall or become undetectable (Sullivan *et al.*, 1984). This phenomenon is more often seen in patients in prolonged remission and less frequently in association with active disease, where it may relate to the presence of circulating immune complexes, which have been described in active MCTD (Halla *et al.*, 1978; Frank *et al.*, 1983). Other recent reports also emphasize

Table 2. Transitions in Disease over Longitudinal Study of 34 Patients[a]

Disease classification	Number classified at initial evaluation	Number classified at latest evaluation
Mixed connective tissue disease	14	31
Undifferentiated connective tissue disease	7	3
Systemic lupus erythematosus	6	0
Rheumatoid arthritis or JRA	4	0
Progressive systemic sclerosis	2	0
Polymyositis	1	0

[a]Sullivan *et al.* (1984).

that ENA antibody titers and fluorescent ANA patterns, as well as other serologic tests, may change with time in MCTD (Nimelstein *et al.*, 1980; Grant *et al.*, 1981).

The initial description of typical clinical characteristics in MCTD included Raynaud's phenomenon, polyarthralgia or arthritis, swollen hands with a sausage appearance of the fingers, esophageal hypomotility, inflammatory myopathy, lupuslike skin rashes, serositis, leukopenia, and anemia. Infrequent renal disease, responsiveness to corticosteroids, and a relatively good prognosis were suggested by that first report (Sharp *et al.*, 1972b). Over the past decade it has been recognized that renal disease may occur (though progressive renal failure is rare), and, of particular note, pulmonary disease is very common (Table 3; Sullivan *et al.*, 1984). Pulmonary hypertension associated with proliferative vascular lesions is a serious complication in some patients, and the prognosis, therefore, is not always favorable (Nimelstein *et al.*, 1980; Singsen *et al.*, 1980a; Grant *et al.*, 1981; Sharp, 1981; Sullivan *et al.*, 1984).

D. Immunopathological Abnormalities in MCTD

1. General Comments

The etiology and pathogenesis of mixed connective tissue disease are unknown. The frequency of disseminated infection as a cause of death (Singsen *et al.*, 1980a) suggests that normal immune and other host defense systems might be impaired, although drugs used in treatment could contribute to such impairment. In fact, there are many immunologic abnormalities that have been reported in MCTD patients, further supporting the possibility that immune injury plays a role in the pathogenesis of the disease (Table 4).

Table 3. Clinical Characteristics of 34 MCTD Patients[a]

Characteristic	Number	Percent
Raynaud's phenomenon	31	91
Swollen hands/sclerodactyly	29	85
Polyarthritis	29	85
Pulmonary involvement	29	85
Inflammatory myopathy	27	79
Esophageal dysfunction	25	74
Lymphadenopathy	17	50
Alopecia	13	41
Pleuritis	12	35
Malar rash	10	29
Pulmonary hypertension	10	29
Cardiac abnormalities	9	26
Renal disease	9[b]	26[b]
Anemia	8	24
Leukopenia	7	21
Diffuse scleroderma	7	21
Sjogren's syndrome	4	12

[a]Sullivan *et al.* (1984).
[b]Only six patients (18%) had clinical evidence of renal disease.

Table 4. Immunologic Abnormalities in Mixed Connective Tissue Disease

Persistence over years of extremely high antibody titers to nuclear ribonucleoprotein
Marked polyclonal hypergammaglobulinemia
Hypocomplementemia in 25–30% of cases
Circulating immune complexes
Deposition of immunoglobulins G and M and complement along sarcolemmal basement membrane, in vascular walls, and along glomerular basement membrane
Widespread lymphocytic and plasma cell infiltration of numerous tissues
Immunoregulatory T-cell defects
Penetration of living mononuclear cells by nuclear ribonucleoprotein antibody

2. Evidence of B Cell Hyperactivity

The persistence, in some cases for many years, of extraordinarily high titers of antibody to nuclear RNP (Sullivan *et al.*, 1984) and polyclonal hypergammaglobulinemia frequently in the range of 2–8 g/dl (Sharp *et al.*, 1972b) suggest a continuing B-cell response and a loss of normal regulatory mechanisms. A direct measurement of the actual amount of circulating RNP antibody in MCTD, compared to the amount of circulating antinuclear antibodies in other rheumatic diseases, has not been reported. However, the available evidence indicates that the level of RNP antibody in many MCTD patients is higher than the level of antinuclear antibodies in other diseases. Levels of hemagglutinating RNP antibody in the 1–100 million range are common, and speckled fluorescent ANA titers exceeding 1 : 1000 and sometimes 1 : 10,000 are much more frequent than in the case of other antinuclear antibodies. Maddison and Reichlin (1977) estimated that RNP antibody constituted 33% of the total immunoglobulin in one case.

3. Circulating Immune Complexes and Deposition of IgG, IgM, and Complement in Tissues

Circulating immune complexes have been detected by Raji cell Clq binding techniques during active disease in MCTD (Halla *et al.*, 1978; Frank *et al.*, 1983). In only one study has the presence of circulating RNP antigen and antibody been described (Fishbein *et al.*, 1977). Deposition of IgG, IgM, and complement have been observed in vascular walls, within muscle fibers, in the sarcolemmal–basement membrane region in muscle, and along the glomerular basement membrane in MCTD (Oxenhandler *et al.*, 1977; Singsen *et al.*, 1978).

4. Reticuloendothelial System Clearance of Immune Complexes

In a recent study of 18 patients with MCTD (most of whom had active disease), only four patients had defective reticuloendothelial system (RES) Fc-specific immune clearance as measured by clearance of IgG-sensitized erythrocytes even though 17 had circulating immune complexes by Raji cell and Clq binding assays (Frank *et al.*, 1983). The four patients with defective clearance had an illness that more resembled typical SLE with antibodies to Sm and/or DNA, higher levels of immune complexes, glomerulonephritis, and severe skin lesions. Since renal disease was absent in the 14 patients with normal

RES clearance, possibly the maintenance of normal RES function enabled these patients to clear immune complexes efficiently, precluding serious renal damage.

5. Mononuclear Cell Infiltration of Tissues

In addition to the abnormalities already described, there is widespread pathological evidence of lymphocytic and plasma cell infiltration of numerous human tissues in MCTD (Singsen *et al.*, 1980a). Lymph nodes are often enlarged, sometimes to enormous proportions, and muscle, spleen, salivary glands, and synovium are particularly affected.

6. Abnormalities in Immune Regulation

Alarcon-Segovia and colleagues have studied the numbers and functions of postthymic precursor T cells, helper T cells (T_H), and suppressor T cells (T_S) in various rheumatic diseases (Alarcon-Segovia *et al.*, 1981; Alarcon-Segovia, 1981; Alarcon-Segovia and Palacios, 1981; Palacios *et al.*, 1981). Their findings in MCTD suggest adequacy of postthymic precursor cells and serum thymic factor but a defect at the level of the T_H either in their signaling to precursor cells for feedback inhibition or in the reception of suppressor signals from T_S (Alarcon-Segovia and Palacios, 1981) (Fig. 2). There is a

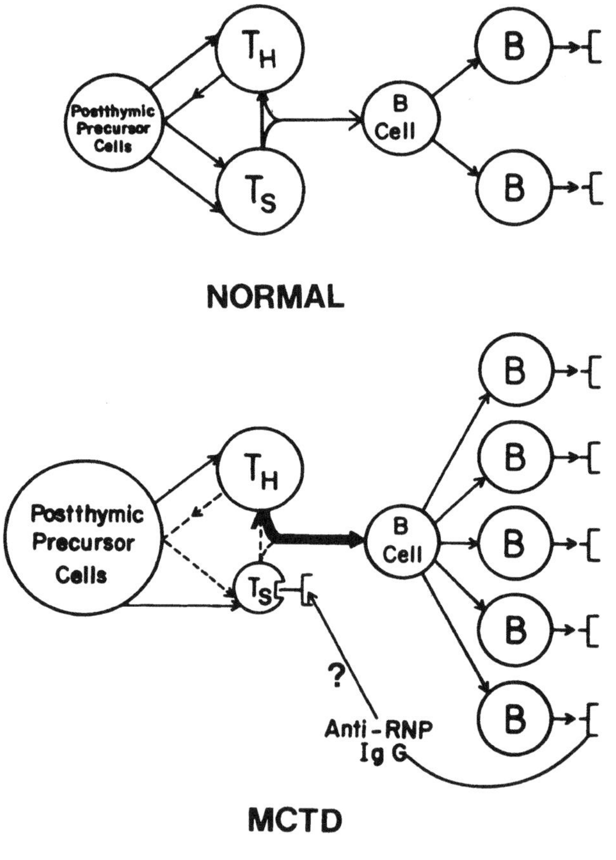

Figure 2. Schematic representation of immunoregulation in normal subjects and patients with MCTD, showing the immunoregulatory imbalance in MCTD. Normal postthymic precursor T cells generate T_H and T_S cells, which are in equilibrium, providing a balanced helper and suppressor function and a normal B-cell response in the healthy subject. T_H cells normally produce a feedback inhibition signal, which acts on the postthymic precursor T cells. This leads to suppressor signals from T_S cells, which helps to maintain normal regulation. In the MCTD patient, the pool of postthymic precursor T cells is increased; these cells are qualitatively normal and generate adequate numbers of T_H cells. Although numerically adequate, the T_H cells are functionally defective either in their signaling to precursor T cells or in the reception of suppressor signals from the T_S cells. Decreased generation of T_S cells, and the consequent loss of suppression, causes increased B-cell activation by uncontrolled T_H cells. This results in production of high levels of IgG autoantibodies to RNP. Penetration of RNP antibodies into T_S cells through their Fc receptors may further accentuate the loss of T_S cells and abrogate their suppressor function, thus leading to an autoperpetuating phenomenon. (Modified from Alarcon-Segovia and Palacios, 1981.)

defect in the T_S that could be caused by a decreased stimulus from feedback inhibition or be a result of the effect of antibodies to RNP, which apparently can penetrate living mononuclear cells through Fc receptors (Alarcon-Segovia *et al.*, 1978, 1979). These abnormalities of immunoregulatory T-cell circuits in MCTD are different from those found in PSS, SLE, Sjogren's syndrome, and rheumatoid arthritis (Alarcon-Segovia, 1981), supporting the concept that MCTD is a distinct entity.

Alarcon-Segovia's report of RNP antibody penetrating living mononuclear cells is of considerable interest since there have been few instances in which antibodies have been shown to penetrate living cells. Possibly, there is something unique about RNP antibodies, perhaps their sheer quantity compared to other antibodies, that would permit this to occur. In this regard, it is pertinent that over the past few years there have been several reports of direct speckled nuclear fluorescence noted in tissues from MCTD patients when they were incubated with fluoresceinated anti-human γ-globulin (Alarcon-Segovia *et al.*, 1979; Gilliam and Prystowsky, 1977; Mundy *et al.*, 1981). There has been controversy as to whether these findings are the result of *in vivo* penetration of cells by RNP antibody or whether the observations are caused by an artifact in which high levels of circulating RNP antibodies enter the cells during the processing of nonviable tissue.

E. Purification and Biochemical Characterization of RNP and Sm Antigens

Studies of the biological role of RNP and Sm antigens might result in a better understanding of the pathogenesis of the rheumatic diseases with which they are associated. In order to perform such studies, it is first necessary to purify and characterize these antigens. In earlier studies, Northway and Tan (1972) had emphasized the immunologic distinctness of the RNP and Sm antigens, whereas Mattioli and Reichlin (1973) had shown their close molecular relationship. The recent observations of Takano *et al.*, (1981), consistent with both of these concepts, indicate that RNP and Sm are distinct antigenic sites on the same macromolecular complex. Purification of RNP and Sm from calf thymus nuclei with preservation of their antigenic activities was achieved by affinity chromatography of the antigens on column resins covalently bound to purified human antibodies specific for RNP and Sm (Takano *et al.*, 1980, 1981). Purified RNP and Sm had molecular weights of 160,000 and 70,000, respectively. Purification and biochemical analyses of immunologically active RNP from many different preparations of calf thymus extract have revealed that the majority of antibodies from MCTD patient sera recognize an antigen composed of the 165-nucleotide RNA, U1 RNA, and five peptides (Takano *et al.*, 1981; Agris *et al.*, 1984). Polypeptides of about 65,000 and 30,000 molecular weight were found to be associated with the RNP antigenic determinant, whereas the Sm antigenic determinant was associated with 12,000–13,000 molecular weight polypeptides. Studies from other laboratories show some variability in the molecular weight of the Sm polypeptides (Lerner and Steitz, 1979; White *et al.*, 1981; Dang *et al.*, 1983). These differences could arise from limited proteolysis during isolation (Dang *et al.*, 1983).

Studies of RNP, Sm, and other nuclear antigens may also contribute to our understanding of basic cell biology, since Lerner, Steitz, and colleagues have recently reported that small nuclear RNPs may have an important role in the processing of hnRNA to mature mRNA (Lerner *et al.*, 1980; Yang *et al.*, 1981). If RNP antibodies are able to penetrate living cells, this could result in inhibition of one or more of the specific steps in the RNA-processing pathway. Further definition of the structure of the RNP/Sm complex has resulted from more recent investigations. Nucleotide sequence studies (Agris *et al.*, 1984; Fig. 3) showed that calf thymus U1 RNA was identical in sequence to that of man and that the minimal RNase-sensitive RNP antigen recognized by the majority of RNP antibodies from MCTD sera is composed of a 55-nucleotide sequence (numbers 37–92) within U1aRNA in association with the largest two of the five polypeptides of the RNA–protein complex. In other studies (Liautard *et al.*, 1983), the lower-molecular-weight peptides associated with Sm antigenic activity were found to protect the uridine-rich nucleotides at the 3′ end of U1a RNA. Protein protection of the middle and 3′ terminus of the RNA leaves the 5′ end open for the hypothesized functions of RNP in the processing of messenger RNA (Lerner *et al.*, 1980; Rogers and Wall, 1980).

F. RNP and Sm Antibodies in MRL Mice

The autoimmune disease in MRL/Mp–1pr/1pr (MRL/1) mice is characterized by massive lymphoproliferation, arthritis, arteritis, and the presence of circulating immune complexes

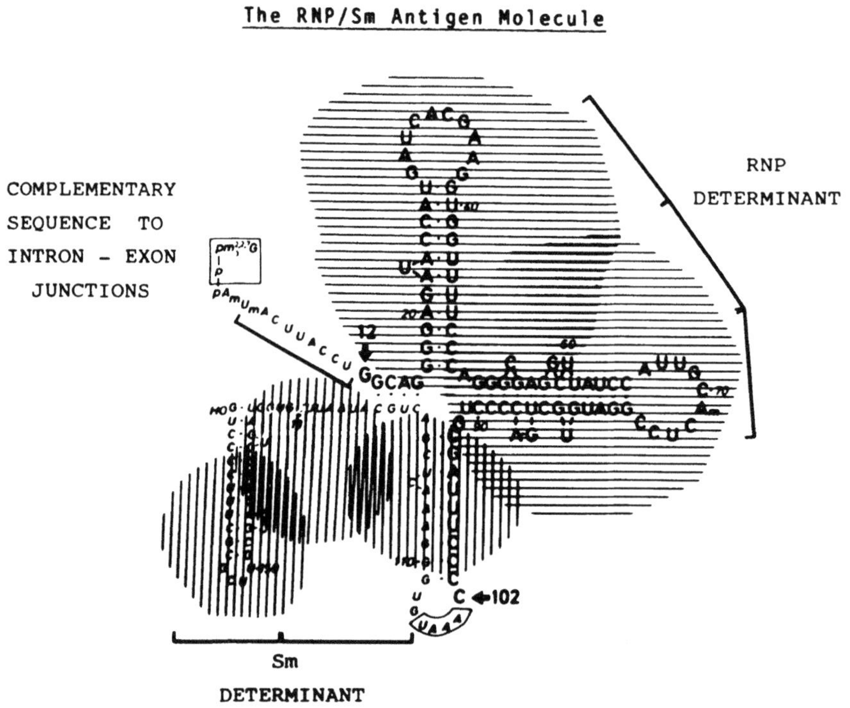

Figure 3. Diagrammatic representation of U1RNP and the autoimmune antigenic peptides for RNP and Sm sera. The predominant small nuclear ribonucleoprotein complex is composed of U1RNA and between five and seven peptides. The figure shows the U1RNA sequence displayed in its secondary structure and covered with peptides. The RNP antigenic determinant is composed of two peptides of larger molecular weights (30K and 65K, approximately) located on the RNA between nucleosides 40 and 90. The Sm antigenic determinant is on the smaller peptides (12–15K) that reside near the 3′-terminal sequence of the U1RNA, as depicted. The nucleotide sequence at the 5′ terminus is free of protein and hypothesized to be an aid in splicing of hnRNA by its complementariness to intron–exon junctions.

and antibodies to DNA, RNP, and Sm (Eisenberg *et al.*, 1978; Singsen *et al.*, 1980b; Pisetsky *et al.*, 1980; Billings *et al.*, 1982). Since these mice produce RNP and Sm antibodies, they are being used to construct hybridomas for the production of monoclonal antibodies to these antigens (Lerner *et al.*, 1981b; Billings *et al.*, 1982; Wise *et al.*, 1982).

III. Me, Su, AND MA ANTIGENS

A. Me Antigen

In the process of analyzing rheumatic disease sera for the presence of RNP and Sm antibodies, several new RNase-resistant antigens were identified that are immunologically distinct from systems previously described. The Me antigen (named after the initial prototype patient and formerly referred to as "system C") appears to have a close molecular association with the RNP/Sm complex, particularly with the Sm antigen (Boak *et al.*, 1984). The physiochemical properties (thermal, pH, and enzyme sensitivity) of Me and Sm are very similar even though they are immunologically distinct. Prototype Me serum (which did not contain detectable Sm antibody), when incubated with the purified RNP/Sm complex, was able to remove Sm but not RNP antigenic activity. The competition between the Me and Sm systems was very specific because incubation of the RNP/Sm complex with other unrelated antinuclear antibodies had no effect. Western blot analyses showed that both anti-Me and anti-Sm sera reacted with peptides of approximately 22,000 and 12–14,000 Daltons.

Clinical diagnoses of ten patients positive for Me antibodies include undifferentiated connective tissue disease in six, SLE in three, and MCTD in one. Thus, some patients with various rheumatic diseases previously reported to have Sm antibodies might actually have circulating Me antibodies.

B. Su Antigen

Another RNase-resistant nonhistone nuclear antigen recently described by Treadwell and associates (1984a) has been designated Su (after the patient in whom this antinuclear antibody was first identified). The Su antibody was detected by immunodiffusion and is immunologically distinct from previously described nuclear antigens and from bovine IgG. The latter exclusion is an important one since the antigen is present in greatest amounts in calf thymus extract, and a serologic reaction with bovine IgG has recently been described in rheumatic diseases (Targoff *et al.*, 1983). Physiochemical analysis showed that the Su antigen was sensitive to trypsin, weakly acidic, and had a molecular weight of approximately 150,000.

Although the Su antibody was detected in only about 4% of unselected SLE patients, it may be of some diagnostic use since 27 of 37 patients in whom this system has been detected had SLE (alone or in overlap), and six had an undifferentiated connective tissue disease (Treadwell *et al.*, 1984a). The fact that antibodies to native DNA, Sm, and RNP were not detected in 37% of the Su-positive SLE patients further suggests its potential clinical importance as a new serologic marker for lupus. Lupus patients with Su antibodies had lower frequencies of malar rash, alopecia, and arthritis and a higher frequency of Raynaud's phenomenon when compared to previously published series.

C. MA Antigen

Another immunologically distinct nuclear nonhistone antigen, designated MA, was reported by Winn and associates in 1979. Antibodies to MA are seen in fewer than 5% of SLE patients and have not been identified in other rheumatic diseases. The MA system may be of some clinical importance since it has only been identified in patients with very severe SLE. The MA system produces a unique fluorescent ANA pattern in which there is a ring of speckles around the periphery of the nucleus. The finding by Winn *et al.* (1979) of the alternating presence of circulating MA antigen and MA antibody in association with flares of lupus nephritis suggests that this system, like DNA–anti-DNA, may be capable of participating in an immune complex nephritis.

IV. SS-A (Ro) AND SS-B (La) (Ha) ANTIGENS

A. Clinical Associations of SS-A (Ro) and SS-B (La) (Ha) Antibodies

Using an extract of a human lymphocyte cell line (WI-L2), Alspaugh and Tan (1975) defined the SS-A and SS-B precipitating antigen–antibody systems in the sera of patients with Sjogren's syndrome. Anti-SS-A and anti-SS-B occurred more commonly in the sera of patients with the sicca syndrome (70% and 48%, respectively) than in the sera of patients with Sjogren's syndrome and accompanying rheumatoid arthritis (9% and 3%, respectively) (Alspaugh *et al.*, 1976). Anti-SS-B gave a speckled pattern of nuclear fluorescence on all substrates. On WI-L2 cells as substrate, anti-SS-A produced a powdery, homogeneous stain of both the nucleus and cytoplasm. Anti-Ro and anti-La were reported as precipitating systems occurring in SLE (Mattioli, and Reichlin, 1974) and were thought to be reactive with cytoplasmic antigens. Later studies by Alspaugh and Maddison (1979) showed immunologic identity of anti-SS-A with anti-Ro and anti-SS-B with anti-La. Further studies in 1980 by Scopelitis *et al.* demonstrated that 33% of SLE patients had anti-SS-A, which was in agreement with the frequency of anti-Ro in SLE. Recent studies (Harmon *et al.*, 1984) suggest that SS-A antigen is in the nucleus of HEp-2 cells, but certain questions remain on the location of SS-A (Ro) in various cells.

In 1977, the Ha system was described in Sjogren's syndrome, but this antigen was later shown to be immunologically identical with SS-B (Akizuki *et al.*, 1977). By the passive hemagglutination technique, anti-Ha (SS-B) is not associated with specific clinical features, but antibody titers increased with the onset of vasculitis and decreased with drug-induced remission.

The diagnostic value of anti-SS-A and anti-SS-B antibodies has been emphasized in the past and in several more recent studies (Alspaugh *et al.*, 1978; Martinez-Lavin *et al.*, 1979; Moutsopoulous *et al.*, 1980; Forstot *et al.*, 1981; Isenberg *et al.*, 1982). Table 5 shows the frequency of these antibodies based on initial studies as well as recent studies. Two recent studies particularly stressed their aid in early diagnosis (Forstot *et al.*, 1981; Isenberg *et al.*, 1982). Serial stuides showing changes in anti-SS-A levels have been

Table 5. Frequency of Precipitins to SS-A and SS-B in Connective Tissue Diseases

Disease	Percent positive	
	Anti-SS-A	Anti-SS-B
Keratoconjunctivitis sicca (alone)	28	22
SS–sicca complex	50–88	23–71
SS–RA	9–39	3–6
SLE	24–33	0–5
SLE–SS	58	17
Discoid lupus erythematosus	0	0
PSS	0	1
PSS–SS	20	0
RA (seropositive)	3	0
RA (seronegative)	0	0
Normal healthy subjects	0	0
Geriatric sera	2	0

performed in SLE patients (Scopelitis *et al.*, 1980). Anti-SS-A antibody levels were generally more stable in well-controlled patients. Titers increased and decreased with exacerbation and remission of disease, particularly with pleural effusions but not with kidney disease. Although titers tended to fluctuate in these cases, SS-A antibody, unlike DNA antibody, seldom disappeared with corticosteroid therapy. Thus, SS-A antibody may be an important diagnostic marker in a patient with nephritis who has already received treatment.

B. Other Specific Clinical Problems Associated with Anti-SSA/Ro

1. Congenital Complete Heart Block

The evidence is accumulating that pregnant women (usually clinically healthy) with circulating anti-SS-A/Ro presumably pass these IgG antibodies to the fetus in the second or third trimesters, resulting in congenital complete heart block (CCHB) and/or neonatal LE. In 1981, Franco *et al.* reported an association between the neonatal LE syndrome and maternal antibodies to SS-A/Ro, with two infants continuing to demonstrate heart block 2–3 years later. Kephart and associates (1981) also described an SS-A/Ro-positive infant with neonatal LE and CCHB. Weston *et al.* (1982) subsequently reported that seven of eight infants with neonatal LE had SS-A/Ro antibodies; four of eight had CCHB. The mothers were all SS-A/Ro positive, but only two had overt rheumatic disorders. Scott *et al.*, in 1983, reported on 45 cases of CCHB in which sera were available from 41 mothers, 24 of whom were healthy and 17 of whom had some rheumatic disorder. Eighty-three percent of the mothers had antibodies to SS-A/Ro, as did seven of eight infants less than 3 months old. Two infants with isolated CCHB, one of whom was detected intrauterine at 24 weeks' gestation, have been reported from the University of Missouri (Singsen *et al.*, 1985); in both cases, the mothers were clinically well and had only SS-A/Ro antibodies.

Congenital complete heart block is a significant clinical problem, as the current mortality rate approximates 25%. The clue of SS-A/Ro antibodies and possibility of detecting CCHB *in utero* by ultrasonography many weeks prior to the expected date of delivery afford the opportunity for clinical intervention with elective cesarean section and immediate availability of cardiac pacing, which may reduce this mortality. Studies are in progress to try to gain a better understanding of the timing of damage to the cardiac conduction system and to determine if maternal SS-A/Ro antibodies are the mediator of fetal conduction tissue damage as opposed to being only an epiphenomenon. If it can be proven, this would be one of the few instances of direct antibody-mediated cell damage resulting in circumscribed organ-specific consequences.

2. Subacute Cutaneous Lupus Erythematosus

Subacute cutaneous lupus erythematosus is a clinically and histologically distinct subset of lupus that occurs in patients who share similar autoimmune and genetic features (Sontheimer *et al.*, 1979, 1981, 1982; Bangert *et al.*, 1981). These patients have predominantly skin and joint involvement and only rarely have significant CNS, renal, or serosal disease. Antibodies to SS-A/Ro (sometimes associated with anti-SS-B/La) were present in 63% of a series of these patients (Sontheimer *et al.*, 1982) which is significantly higher than for an unselected population with SLE (Maddison *et al.*, 1979). Patients with annular skin lesions in particular showed a strong concordance of anti-SS-A/Ro antibodies and the HLA-DR3 phenotype. Similar annular skin eruptions have been noted in neonates with placental transfer of anti-SSA/Ro antibodies (Miyagawa *et al.*, 1981; Kephart *et al.*, 1981). Patients reported as having "ANA-negative" SLE because they have no detectable serum antibodies that bind to mouse liver cell nuclei appear to have a similar if not identical form of cutaneous lupus erythematosus with a low incidence of significant nephritis or CNS disease (Maddison *et al.*, 1981; Sontheimer *et al.*, 1982). These "ANA-negative" lupus patients also had a high frequency (62%) of antibodies to SS-A/Ro, and two-thirds were found to have a positive fluorescent ANA when their sera were tested with human KB cells instead of mouse tissue sections (Maddison *et al.*, 1981). It has become clear that murine cell nuclei lack certain antigens (such as SS-A/Ro) that are present in human nuclei (Harmon *et al.*, 1984).

3. Other Clinical Subsets

In contrast to the relatively mild subacute cutaneous LE syndrome, SLE patients with antibodies to SS-A/Ro in combination with DNA antibodies have been reported to have a much greater frequency of serious renal disease than SLE patients with both SS-A/Ro and SS-B/La antibodies (Wasicek and Reichlin, 1982). Antibodies to SS-A/Ro have also been reported in 86% of patients with Sjogren's syndrome who have vasculitis (Alexander *et al.*, 1982).

C. Purification and Biochemical Characterization of SS-A/Ro and SS-B/La/Ha Antigens

Recent studies have added greatly to our knowledge of the possible nature of SS-A/Ro and SS-B/La antigens. Lerner and associates (1981a) showed that SS-A/Ro may be a protein determinant of a small cytoplasmic RNA–protein. However, studies by Harmon and associates (1984) indicate that SS-A/Ro is predominantly a nuclear antigen with a highly variable species distribution, significant quantities being detected in human, monkey, dog, and guinea pig tissues, and low quantities being detected in the mouse, rat, rabbit, hamster, and chicken. These investigators suggest that the reported differences in the intracellular location of the SS-A and Ro antigens may be related to quantitative differences in the SS-A antigen from species to species and the coexistence of antibodies other than anti-SS-A/Ro in the sera tested.

SS-B/La sera from patients with autoimmune disorders precipitate a set of nuclear and cytoplasmic small RNA–protein complexes. Analyses in several laboratories have shown that the SS-B/La antigen is associated with RNAs transcribed by RNA polymerase III, including precursors of tRNA and 5 S ribosomal RNA (Hendrick *et al.*, 1981), and with ribonucleoprotein particles containing small nuclear U1 RNA, which is transcribed by RNA polymerase II (Madore *et al.*, 1984). In purified preparations of SS-B, immunoreactive peptides of 29,000, 40,000, and 67,000 molecular weight have been reported (Venables *et al.*, 1983; Teppo *et al.*, 1982). Although initial studies suggested that SS-A antigen might be a fairly large protein, recent studies by Tsu-San Lieu and associates (1983) suggest that it may have a molecular weight of 48,000.

V. CENTROMERE, NUCLEOLAR, AND Scl-70 ANTIGENS

A diverse group of antinuclear antibodies can be identified in the sera of patients with PSS. With the use of tissue culture cell lines as substrate for the fluorescent ANA test, almost all PSS sera are positive (Bernstein *et al.*, 1982). In particular, anticentromere antibodies were not detected initially when mouse kidney sections were used as substrate but were first observed when HEp-2 cells were used. The anticentromere pattern is produced by autoantibody to the centromere kinetochore (Moroi *et al.*, 1980) and has been reported to be present in 49–96% of patients with the limited CREST form of scleroderma (Tan *et al.*, 1980; Fritzler *et al.*, 1980; McCarty *et al.*, 1983; Tramposch *et al.*, 1984; Steen *et al.*, 1984). This autoantibody has been detected much less frequently in patients with Raynaud's phenomenon or with the diffuse scleroderma form of PSS and very rarely in other rheumatic diseases (Tan *et al.*, 1980; Fritzler *et al.*, 1980; McCarty *et al.*, 1983; Tramposch *et al.*, 1984; Steen *et al.*, 1984). Often this is the only autoantibody specificity present in the sera of CREST patients. The fact that some patients with anticentromere antibodies initially presenting only with Raynaud's phenomenon subsequently developed findings consistent with the CREST syndrome (Fritzler *et al.*, 1980; Tramposch *et al.*, 1984; Steen *et al.*, 1984) is a further indication of the high specificity of this serologic pattern for the CREST form of PSS.

Patients with PSS may also exhibit diffuse fine speckled or nucleolar fluorescent ANA patterns. The fine speckled pattern is produced by antibody to the Scl-70 antigen, a basic nonhistone nuclear protein with a molecular weight of 70,000 (Douvas *et al.*, 1979). The nucleolar immunofluorescent pattern may be associated with multiple antigens, one being a 4–6 S nucleolus-specific RNA (Tan *et al.*, 1980). Antibody to Scl-70 is found with a relatively low frequency (approximating 18%) in PSS but may represent a marker antibody for the disease since it is found very infrequently in other rheumatic diseases (Tan *et al.*, 1980). In the study by McCarty and associates (1983), compared with patients who exhibitied speckled or nucleolar ANA patterns, those with anticentromere antibody has significantly less renal, cardiac, pulmonary, and lower gastrointestinal tract disease. Fritzler *et al.* (1980) have also pointed out the decreased frequency of cardiac and renal involvement in patients with anticentromere antibodies.

VI. Mi-1, PM-1, Jo-1, AND Ku ANTIGENS

Immunodiffusion studies employing extracts of whole calf thymus or thymus nuclei have revealed a spectrum of precipitating antibodies in plymyositis (PM) and dermatomyositis (DM). In 1976, Reichlin and Mattioli reported the Mi system, which was initially detected by an indirect complement fixation method. They also demonstrated a precipitating antibody, anti-Mi-1, which was distinct from the Mi antibody detected by complement fixation. A more recent study (Targoff *et al.*, 1983) revealed that anti-Mi-1 is a form of antibovine IgG but is not a classical rheumatoid factor because the reactivity is directed against Fab as well as Fc fragments. The low frequency in both DM and SLE and lack of specificity indicate that anti-Mi-a will not be a clinically useful diagnostic test (Targoff *et al.*, 1983).

In 1977, Wolfe *et al.* reported that 64% (9/14) of patients with PM and 87% (7/8) of PM–PSS overlap patients had precipitaitng antibody to an immunologically distinct antigen designated PM-1. Because of the weak precipitation reaction in immunodiffusion, it is possible that some of these reactions originally reported could have been of a different specificity. Recent technical improvements employing partially purified PM-1 antigen and polyethylene glycol added to the gel have considerably enhanced the clarity of the PM-1 precipitation reaction. This has facilitated a more recent investigation by Treadwell *et al.* (1984b) of the immunologic, physiochemical, and biochemical properties of the PM-1 antigen and of the clinical characteristics of patients with PM-1 antibodies. The PM-1 antigen was noted to be sensitive to heat and trypsin, to have a modecular weight approximating 150,000, and to be present in higher concentrations in calf thymus nuclear extract than in other sources. Another recent study of this antigen by Reichlin and associates (1984) indicates that it is probably nucleolar, since sera precipitating the antigen stained the nucleoli of HEp-2 cells by indirect immunofluorescence.

Treadwell *et al.*(1984b) found positive reactions for PM-1 antibody in PM–PSS overlap (12%, 9/77), PM (9%, 2/22), and PSS (8%, 2/32), whereas patients with SLE, rheumatoid arthritis, and other rheumatic diseases and normals were negative. The diagnoses and clinical characteristics of 18 patients positive for PM-1 antibody (Table 6) provide a further indication of the high specificity of this system for PM–PSS, PM, and DM. The predominant clnical feature was inflammatory myositis, and extensive sclerodermatous skin changes and severe internal organ involvement were rare. An interlaboratory collaborative study confirmed that this antinuclear antibody is associated with PM, DM, and PM–PSS (Reichlin *et al.*, 1984). The circulating antinuclear antibody profile was examined in 77 patients with PM–PSS overlap (Treadwell *et al.*, (1984b; Table 7). It is of note that, when present, PM-1 was usually the only detectable antibody (78%). Thus, PM-1 antibody appears to be a useful serolgic marker for PM/DM and in particular to distinguish a possible subset of patients with clinical features of PM–PSS overlap disease. Although detailed long-term studies have not been performed, in several patients in the series of Treadwell *et al.* (1984b), PM-1 antibodies persisted following treatment with corticosteroids.

Nishikai and Reichlin (1980a,b) characterized another nuclear antigen designated

Table 6. Diagnoses and Clinical Characteristics in 18 Patients with PM-1 Antibody[a]

Diagnosis	Percent	Clinical characteristics	Percent
PM–PSS	50	Positive muscle biopsy	92[b]
DM–PSS	17	Proximal muscle weakness	83
PM	11	Sclerodactyly	78
PSS	11	Raynaud's phenomenon	72
DM	6	Elevated serum CPK	61
Pronestyl LE	6	Pulmonary disease	50
(possible PM)		Dysphagia	44
		Arthritis	44

[a]Treadwell *et al.* (1984b).
[b]Positive in 11/12 who had biopsies.

Jo-1, which appears to be protein in nature and of approximately 150,000 molecular weight. Although the Jo-1 and PM-1 antigens have similar physiochemical properties, they are immunologically distinct on immunodiffusion analysis (Treadwell *et al.*, 1984). Antibodies to Jo-1 have a strong association with polymyositis, being detected in 18–31% of patients with PM, rarely in DM, and not detected in SLE, PSS, or other diseases (Nishikai and Reichlin, 1980a,b; Reichlin *et al.*, 1984).

Molecular biological investigations with the Jo-1 system have also yielded important new information. Jo-1 antibodies from PM patients have been shown to immunoprecipitate a subunit of histidyl-tRNA synthetase (Mathews and Bernstein, 1983). Thus, the addition of such antisera to a protein-synthesizing system may affect translation by inhibiting aminoacylation. Utilizing a rabbit reticulocyte *in vitro* translation system, Reedy *et al.* (1984) have examined the effect of sera of different antinuclear antibody specificities on protein synthesis. The translation system employed efficiently translated exogeneously supplied rabbit globin mRNA in a dose–response manner. Jo-1 antibody from a PM patient, but not other antibodies, inhibited globin mRNA translation by as much as 40%. Polyacrylamide gel electrophoresis was employed to examine the translation product. Autoradiography of the gel showed a decrease in the synthesis of globin peptides that was proportional to the amount of antibody added to the translation system. Thus, this

Table 7. Frequency of Specific Antinuclear Autoantibodies in 77 Patients with PM–PSS Overlap Syndrome[a]

Autoantibodies to	Percent positive
PM–1	12
RNP	29
Sm	10[b]
SS–A	14
SS–B	5
Scl–70	10
Native DNA	6
None of these antibodies	39

[a]Treadwell *et al.* (1984b).
[b]PM–PSS overlap patients with Sm antibodies also had features of SLE.

is another example in which the use of sera from rheumatic disease patients with elucidation of antigenic specificities and molecular biological methodologies can provide new insights into cellular biological function in health and disease.

The Ku antigen reported by Mimori *et al.* (1981) is a RNase-resistant, trypsin-sensitive nuclear acidic protein with an estimated molecular weight of 300,000. The most frequent clinical features in patients positive for Ku antibodies are characteristic of PM–PSS overlap syndrome, which appears to be very similar to the clinical picture most frequently associated with the PM-1 system. However, the PM-1 and Ku systems were found to be distinct by immunodiffusion, physiochemical properties, estimated molecular weight, and in their localization in various tissues (Mimori *et al.*, 1981; Treadwell *et al.*, 1984b).

VII. CONCLUSION

As a result of increasing scientific investigation and, in particular, with the application of very sensitive molecular biological methodologies (e.g., radioimmunoassays, enzyme-linked immunoadsorbent assays, Western blots, hybridomas generating monclonal antibodies), antibodies to nuclear antigens have been detected in increasing frequency in certain systemic rheumatic diseases including SLE, PSS, MCTD, DM/PM, Sjogren's syndrome,and rheumatoid arthritis. Autoantibodies to some of the nonhistone nuclear antigens have proven to be useful in establishing a diagnosis and projecting the prognosis in some of these diseases. The correlation of certain of these autoantibodies with particular patterns of organ system involvement (e.g., anti-RNP with pulmonary, esophageal, and muscle disease, and anti-SS-A/Ro with congenital complete heart block) has led to the earlier identification of these clinical complications. Thus, these serologic markers have provided us with a greater appreciation of possible disease subsets, and this affords the opportunity for new clinical investigation that may ultimately result in more selective and effective therapeutic or preventive measures.

In addition to their diagnostic and prognostic use, some of the nonhistone nuclear antigens and autoantibodies may have a biological role in the pathogenesis of certain rheumatic diseases. The identification of some of these autoantibodies in murine models of autoimmune disease has provided an opportunity for more incisive genetic, immunologic, and hormonal investigations related to immune regulation, RES clearance of immune complexes, and immunopathological mechanisms of tissue injury. This has also provided a means of generating monoclonal antibodies that can be employed as molecular biological probes and for the development of more sensitive and specific laboratory tests. Finally, a remarkable consequence of the molecular biological investigations facilitated by the availability of purified nuclear antigens and antibodies is the elucidation of a possible role for some of these RNA–protein complexes in basic cell biology.

REFERENCES

Agris, P. F., KiKuchi, Y., Gross, H.J., Takano, M., and Sharp, G. C., 1984, Characterization of the autoimmune antigenic determinant for ribonucleoprotein (RNP) antibody, *Immunol. Commun.* **13**(2): 137–149.

Akizuki, M., Powers, R., Jr., and Holman, H. R., 1977, A soluble acidic protein of the cell nucleus which reacts with serum from patients with systemic lupus erythematosus and Sjogren's syndrome, *J. Clin. Invest.* **59**:264–272.

Alarcon-Segovia, D., 1979, Mixed connective tissue disease: Appearance of antibodies to ribonucleoprotein following corticosteroid treatment, *J. Rheumatol.* **6**:694–699.

Alarcon-Segovia, D., 1981, Mixed connective tissue disease—a decade of growing pains, *J. Rheumatol.* **8**:535–540.

Alarcon-Segovia, D., and Palacios, R., 1981, Human postthymic precursor cells in health and disease. IV. Abnormalities in immunoregulatory T cell circuits in mixed connective tissue disease, *Arthritis Rheum.* **24**:1486–1494.

Alarcon-Segovia, D., Ruiz-Arguelles, A., and Fishbein, E., 1978, Antibody to nuclear ribonucleoprotein penetrates live human mononuclear cells through Fc receptors, *Nature* **271**:67–69.

Alarcon-Segovia, D., Ruiz-Arguelles, A., and Fishbein, E., 1979, Antibody penetration into living cells. I. Intranuclear immunoglobulin in peripheral blood mononuclear cells in mixed connective tissue disease and systemic lupus erythematosus, *Clin. Exp. Immunol.* **35**:364–375.

Alarcon-Segovia, D., Palacios, R., and Ibanez de Kasep, G., 1981, Human postthymic precursor cells in health and disease. VII. Immunoregulatory circuits of the peripheral blood mononuclear cells from patients with progressive systemic sclerosis, *J. Clin. Lab. Imunol.* **5**:143–148.

Alexander, E. L., Provost, T. T., Stevens, M. B., and Alexander, G. E., 1982, Neurologic complications of primary Sjogrens syndrome, *Medicine (Baltimore)* **61**:247–257.

Alspaugh, M. A., and Maddison, P. J., 1979, Resolution of the identity of certain antigen–antibody systems in systemic lupus erythematosus and Sjogren's syndrome, *Arthritis Rheum.* **22**:796–798.

Alspaugh, M. A., and Tan, E. M., 1975, Antibodies to cellular antigens in Sjogren's syndrome, *J. Clin. Invest.* **55**:1067–1073.

Alspaugh, M. A., Talal, N., and Tan, E. M., 1976, Differentation and characterization of autoantibodies and their antigens in Sjogren's syndrome, *Arthritis Rheum.* **19**:216–222.

Alspaugh, M. A., Buchanan, W. W., and Whaley, K., 1978, Precipitating antibodies to cellular antigens in Sjogren's syndrome, rheumatoid arthritis, and other organ and nonorgan specific autoimmune diseases, *Ann. Rheum. Dis.* **37**:244 –246.

Bangert, J., Freeman, R. G., Sontheimer, R. D., and Gilliam, J. N., 1981, Comparative analysis of the histopathology of subacute cutaneous lupus erythematosus and discoid lupus erythematosus, *Clin. Res.* **29**:587A.

Bernstein, R. M., Steigerwald, J. C., and Tan, E. M., 1982, Association of antinuclear and antinucleolar antibodies in progressive systemic sclerosis, *Clin. Exp. Immunol.* **48**:43–51.

Billings, P. B., Allen, R. W., Jensen, F. C., and Hoch, S. O., 1982, Anti-RNP monoclonal antibodies derived from a mouse strain with lupus-like autoimmunity, *J. Immunol.* **128**:1176–1180.

Boak, A. M., Treadwell, E. L., Searing , B., and Agris, P. F., 1984, The autoimmune antigen system C is a component of the snRNP/Sm complex, *Fed. Proc.* **43**:1839.

Bresnihan, B., Bunn, C., Snaith, M. L., and Hughes, G. R. V., 1977, Antiribonucleoprotein antibodies in connective tissue diseases: Estimation by counterimmunoelectrophoresis, *Br. Med. J.* **1**:610–611.

Bruneau, C., and Benveniste, J., 1979, Circulating DNA : anti-DNA complexes in systemic lupus erythematosus, *J. Clin. Invest.* **64**:191–198.

Dang, H., Fischbach, M., Lerner, E., and Talal, N., 1983, Molecular and antigenic nature of isolated Sm, *J. Immunol.* **130**:2782–2785.

Douvas, A. S., Achten, M., and Tan, E. M., 1979, Identification of a nuclear protein (Scl-70) as a unique target of human antinuclear antibodies in scleroderma, *J. Biol. Chem.* **254**:10514–10522.

Eisenberg, R. A., Tan, E. M., and Dixon, F. J., 1978, Presence of anti-Sm reactivity in autoimmune mouse strains, *J. Exp. Med.* **147**:582–587.

Farber, S. J., and Bole, G. G., 1976, Antibodies to components of extractable nuclear antigen, *Arch. Intern. Med.* **136**:425–431.

Fishbein, E., Alarcon-Segovia, D., and Ramos-Niembro, F., 1977, Free serum ribonucleoprotein (RNP) in mixed connective tissue disease (MCTD), in: *Proceedings XIV International Congress Rheumatology*, American Rheumatism Association, San Francisco, p. 14.

Forstot, S. L., Forstot, J. Z., Peebles, C. L., and Tan, E. M., 1981, Serologic studies in patients with keratoconjunctivitis sicca, *Arch. Ophthalmol.* **99**:888–890.

Franco, H. L., Weston, W. L., Peebles, C., Forstot, S. L., and Phanuphak, P., 1981, Autoantibodies directed against sicca syndrome antigens in the neonatal lupus syndrome, *J. Am. Acad. Dermatol.* **4**:67–72.

Frank, M. M., Lawley, T. J., Hamburger, M. I., and Brown, E. J., 1983, Immunoglobulin G Fc receptor-mediated clearance in autoimmune disease, *Ann. Intern. Med.* **98**:206–218.
Fritzler, M. J., Kinsella, T. D., and Garbutt, E., 1980, The CREST syndrome—a distinct serologic entity with anticentromere antibodies, *Am. J. Med.* **69**:520–526.
Gilliam, J. N., and Prystowsky, S. D., 1977, Mixed connective tissue disease syndrome: The cutaneous manifestations of patients with epidermal nuclear staining and high titer antibody to RNAse sensitive extractable nuclear antigen (ENA), *Arch. Dermatol.* **113**:583–587.
Grant, K. D., Adams, L. E., and Hess, E. V., 1981, Mixed connective tissue disease—a subset with sequential clinical and laboratory features, *J. Rheumatol.* **8**:587–598.
Halla, J. T., Schrohenloher, R. E., Hardin, J. G., and Volanakis, J. E., 1978, Circulating immune complexes in mixed connective tissue disease (MCTD), *Arthritis Rheum.* **21**:562–563.
Hargraves, M. M., Richmond, H., and Morton, R., 1948, Presentation of two bone marrow elements: The "tart" cell and "L.E." cell, *Proc. Staff Meet. Mayo Clin.* **23**:25–28.
Harmon, C., Peebles, C., and Tan, E. M. 1981, SL—a new precipitating system, *Arthritis Rheum.* **24**:S122.
Harmon, C. E., Deng, J., Peebles, C. L., and Tan, E. M., 1984, The importance of tissue substrate in the SS-A/Ro antigen–antibody system, *Arthritis Rheum.* **27**:166–173.
Hendrick, J. P., Wolin, S. L., Rinke, J., Lerner, M. R., and Steitz, J. A., 1981, Ro small cytoplasmic ribonucleoproteins are a subclass of La ribonucleoproteins: Further characterization of the Ro and La small ribonucleoproteins from uninfected mammalian cells, *Mol. Cell Biol.* **1**:1138–1149.
Holman, H. R., 1965, Partial purification and characterization of an extractable nuclear antigen which reacts with SLE sera, *Ann. N.Y. Acad. Sci.* **124**:800–806.
Holman, H. R., and Kunkel, H. G., 1957, Affinity between the lupus erythematosus serum factor and cell nuclei and nucleoprotein, *Science* **126**:162–163.
Isenberg, D. A., Hammond, L., Fisher, C., Griffiths, M., Stewart, J., and Bottazzo, G. F., 1982, Predictive value of SS-B precipitating antibodies in Sjogren's syndrome, *Br. Med. J.* **284**:1738–1740.
Kephart, D. C., Hood, A. F., and Provost, T. T., 1981, Neonatal lupus erythematosus: New serologic findings, *J. Invest. Dermatol.* **77**:331–333.
Koffler, D., Schur, P. H., and Kunkel, H. G., 1967, Immunological studies concerning the nephritis of systemic lupus erythematosus, *J. Exp. Med.* **126**:607–624.
Koffler, D., Agnello, V., Thoburn, R., and Kunkel, H. G., 1971, Systemic lupus erythematosus: Prototype of immune complex nephritis in man, *J. Exp. Med.* **134**:169s–179s.
Koffler, D., Agnello, V., and Kunkel, H. G., 1974, Polynucleotide immune complexes in serum and glomeruli of patients with systemic lupus erythematosus, *Am. J. Pathol.* **74**:109–122.
Kurata, N., and Tan, E. M., 1976, Identification of antibodies to nuclear acidic antigens by counterimmunoelectrophoresis (CIE), *Arthritis Rheum.* **19**:574–580.
Lerner, M. R., and Steitz, J. A., 1979, Antibodies to small nuclear RNA's complexed with protein are produced by patients with systemic lupus erythematosus, *Proc. Natl. Acad. Sci. U.S.A.* **76**:5495–5499.
Lerner, M. R., Boyle, J. A., Mount, S. M., Wolin, S. L., and Steitz, J. A., 1980, Are snRNP's involved in splicing? *Nature* **283**:220–224.
Lerner, M. R., Boyle, J. A., Hardin, J. A., and Steitz, J. A., 1981a, Two novel classes of small ribonucleoproteins detected by antibodies associated with lupus erythematosus, *Science* **211**:400–402.
Lerner, E. A., Lerner, M. R., Janeway, C. A., and Steitz, J. A., 1981b, Monoclonal antibodies to nucleic acid-containing cellular constituents: Problems for molecular biology and autoimmune disease, *Proc. Natl. Acad. Sci. U.S.A.* **78**:2737–2741.
Liautard, J. P., Sri-Widada, J., Brunel, C., and Jeanteur, P., 1982, Structural organization of ribonucleoproteins containing small nuclear RNAs (SnRNPs) from Hela cells. Proteins interact closely with a similar structural domain of U_1, U_2, U_4 and U_5 snRNAs, *J. Mol. Biol.* **162**:623–643.
Lieu, T. S., Steigerwald, J. C., and Tan, E. M., 1983, Purification and identification of SSA antigen (Ro) reacting with sera of patients with Sjogren's syndrome, *Arthritis Rheum.* **26**:S64.
Maddison, P. J., and Reichlin, M., 1977, Quantitation of precipitating antibodies to certain soluble nuclear antigens in SLE: Their contributions to hypergammaglobulinemia, *Arthritis Rheum.* **20**:819–824.
Maddison, P., Mogavero, H., Provost, T. T., and Reichlin, M., 1979, The clinical significance of autoantibodies to a soluble cytoplasmic antigen in systemic lupus erythematosus and other connective tissue disease, *J. Rheumatol.* **6**:189–195.
Maddison, P. J., Provost, T. T., and Reichlin, M., 1981, Serological findings in patients with "ANA-negative" systemic lupus erythematosus, *Medicine (Baltimore)* **60**:87–94.

Madore, S. J., Wieben, E. D., and Pederson, T., 1984, Eukaryotic small ribonucleoproteins, anti-La human autoantibodies react with U1 RNA–protein complexes, *J. Biol. Chem.* **259:**1929–1933.

Martinez-Lavin, M., Vaughan, J. H., and Tan, E. M., 1979, Autoantibodies and the spectrum of Sjogrens syndrome, *Ann. Intern. Med.* **91:**185–190.

Mathews, M. B., and Bernstein, R. M., 1983, Myositis autoantibody inhibits histidyl-tRNA synthetase. A model for autoimmunity, *Nature* **304:**177–179.

Mattioli, M., and Reichlin, M., 1973, Physical association of two nuclear antigens and mutual occurrence of their antibodies: The relationship of the Sm and RNA protein (Mo) systems in SLE sera, *J. Immunol.* **110:**1318–1324.

Mattioli, M., and Reichlin, M., 1974, Heterogeneity of RNA protein antigens reactive with sera of patients with systemic lupus erythematosus: Description of a cytoplasmic nonribosomal antigen, *Arthritis Rheum.* **17:**421–429.

McCarty, G. A., Barada, F. A., Snyderman, R., and Fritzler, M. J., 1981, A new autoantibody staining pattern, the mitotic spindle apparatus: Immunologic characteristics, clinical occurrence, and cytoskeletal studies, *Arthritis Rheum.* **24:**S109.

McCarty, G. A., Rice, J. R., Bembe, M. L., and Barada, R. A., Jr., 1983, Anticentromere antibody: Clinical correlations and association with favorable prognosis in patients with scleroderma variants, *Arthritis Rheum.* **26:**1–7.

Mimori, T., Akizuki, M., Yamagata, H., Inada, S., Yoshida, S., and Homma, M., 1981, Characterization of a high molecular weight acidic nuclear protein recognized by autoantibodies in sera from patients with polymyositis–sclerderma overlap, *J. Clin. Invest.* **68:**611–620.

Miyachi, K., Fritzler, M. J., and Tan, E. M., 1978, Autoantibody to a nuclear antigen in proliferating cells, *J. Immunol.* **121:**2228–2234.

Miyagawa, S., Kitamura, W., Yoshioka, J., and Sakamoto, K., 1981, Placental transfer of anticytoplasmic antibodies in annular erythema of newborns, *Arch. Dermatol.* **117:**569–572.

Moroi, Y., Peebles, C., Fritzler, M. H., Steigerwald, J., and Tan, E. M., 1980, Autoantibody to centromere (kinetochore) in scleroderma sera, *Proc. Natl. Acad. Sci. U.S.A.* **7:**1627–1631.

Moutsopoulous, H. M., Klippel, J. H., Pavlidis, N., Wolf, R. O., Sweet, J. B., Steinberg, A. D., Chu, F. C.,and Tarpley, T. M., 1980, Correlative histologic and serologic findings of sicca syndrome in patients with systemic lupus erythematosus, *Arthritis Rheum.* **23:**36–40.

Mundy, T. M., Landing, B. H., Hanson, V., Bernstein, B., and King, K., 1981, Direct immunofluorescence in patients with high titer antibodies to extractable nuclear antigen (ENA), *Arthritis Rheum.* **24:**S101.

Nakamura, R. M., and Tan, E. M., 1977, Recent progress in the study of autoantibodies to nuclear antigens, *Hum. Pathol.* **9:**85.

Nimelstein, S. H., Brody, S., McShane, D., and Holman, H. R., 1980, Mixed connective tissue disease: A subsequent evaluation of the original 25 patients, *Medicine (Baltimore)* **59:**239–248.

Nishikai, M., and Reichlin, M., 1980a, Heterogeneity of precipitating antibodies in polymyositis and dermatomyositis, *Arthritis Rheum.* **23:**881–888.

Nishikai, M., and Reichlin, M., 1980b, Purification and characterization of a nuclear non-histone basic protein (Mi-1) which reacts with anti-immunoglobulin sera and the sera of patients with dermatomyositis, *Mol. Immunol.* **17:**1129–1141.

Northway, J. D., and Tan, E. M., 1972, Differentiations of antinuclear antibodies giving speckled staining patterns in immunofluorescence, *Clin. Immunol. Immunopathol.* **1:**140–154.

Notman, D. D., Kurata, N., and Tan, E. M., 1975, Profiles of antinuclear antibodies in systemic rheumatic diseases, *Ann. Intern. Med.* **83:**464–469.

Oxenhandler, R., Hart, M., Corman, L., Sharp, G., and Adelstein, E., 1977, Pathology of skeletal muscle in mixed connective tissue disease, *Arthritis Rheum.* **20:**985–988.

Palacios, R., Alarcon-Segovia, D., Llorente, L., Ruiz-Arguelles, A., and Fishbein, E., 1981, Human postthymic precursor cells in health and disease. II. Their loss and dysfuntion in systemic lupus erythematosus and their partial correction with serum thymic factor, *J. Clin. Lab. Immunol.* **5:**71–80.

Parker, M. D., 1973, Ribonucleoprotein antibodies: Frequencies and clinical significance in systemic lupus erythematosus, scleroderma and mixed connective tissue disease, *J. Lab. Clin. Med.* **82:**769–775.

Pisetsky, D. S., McCarty, G. A.., and Peters, D. V., 1980, Mechanisms of autoantibody production in autoimmune MRL mice *J. Exp. Med.* **151:**1302–1310.

Reedy, D. B., Boak, A. M., Zwillich, S. H., and Agris, P. F., 1984, Evaluation of specific autoimmune antibodies utilizing *in vitro* translation, *Fed. Proc.* **43:**1717.

Reichlin, M., and Mattioli, M., 1972, Correlation of a precipitin reaction to an Rnaprotein antigen and low prevalence of nephritis in patients with systemic lupus erythematosus, *N. Engl. J. Med.* **286**:908–911.

Reichlin, M., and Mattioli, M., 1976, Description of a serological reaction characteristic of polymyositis, *Clin. Immunol. Immunopathol.* **51**:12–20.

Reichlin, M., Maddison, P. J., Targoff, I., Bunch, T., Arnett, F., Sharp, G., Treadwell, E., and Tan, E. M., 1984, Antibodies to an nuclear/nucleolar antigen in patients with polymyositis-overlap syndromes, *J. Clin. Immunol.* **4**:40–44.

Rogers, J., and Wall, R., 1980, A mechanism for RNA splicing, *Proc. Natl. Acad. Sci. U.S.A.* **77**:1877–1879.

Scopelitis, E., Biundo, J. J., Jr., and Alspaugh, M. A., 1980, Anti-SS-A antibody and other antinuclear antibodies in systemic lupus erythematosus, *Arthritis Rheum.* **23**:287–293.

Scott, J. S., Maddison, P. J., Taylor, P. V., Esscher, E., Scott, O., and Skinner, R. P., 1983, Connective tissue disease, antibodies to ribonucleoprotein, and congenital heart block, *N. Engl. J. Med.* **309**:209–212.

Sharp, G. C., 1981, Mixed connective tissue disease and overlap syndromes, in: *Textbook of Rheumatology*, Vol. II (W. N. Kelley, E. D. Harris, Jr., S. Ruddy, and C. B. Sledge, eds.) W. B. Saunders, Philadelphia, pp. 1151–1161.

Sharp, G. C., 1982, Subsets of SLE and mixed connective tissue disease, *Am. J. Kidney Dis.* **2**(Suppl. 1):201–205.

Sharp, G. C., Irvin, W. S., Northway, J. D., and Tan, E. M., 1972a, Specificity of antibodies to extractable nuclear antigens (ENA) in mixed connective tissue disease (MCTD) and systemic lupus erythematosus (SLE), *Arthritis Rheum.* **15**:125.

Sharp, G. C., Irvin, W. S., Tan, E. M., Gould, R. G., and Holamn, H. R., 1972b, Mixed connective tissue disease. An apparently distinct rheumatic disease syndrome associated with a specific antibody to an extractable nuclear antigen (ENA), *Am. J. Med.* **52**:148–159.

Sharp, G. C., Irvin, W. S., May, C. M., Holman, H. R., McDuffie, F. C., Hess, E. V., and Schmid, F. R., 1976, Association of antibodies to ribonucleoprotein and Sm antigens with mixed connective tissue disease, systemic lupus erythematosus and other rheumatic diseases, *N. Engl. J. Med.* **295**:1149–1154.

Singsen, B. H., 1981, Mixed connective tissue disease, scleroderma and morphea in childhood, in: *Brennemans Practice of Pediatrics* (R. Wedgewood, ed.), Harper & Row, Philadephia, pp. 1–17.

Singsen, B. H., Bernstein, B. H., Kornreich, H. K., King, K. K., and Hanson, V., 1977, Mixed connective tissue disease in childhood. A clinical and serologic survey, *J. Pediatr.* **90**:893–900.

Singsen, B. H., Landing, B., Wolfe, J. F., Bernstein, B., Oxenhandler, R. W., Sharp, G. C., and Hanson, V., 1978, Histologic evaluation of mixed connective tissue disease in children and adults, *Arthritis Rheum.* **21**:593.

Singsen, B. H., Swanson, V. L., Bernstein, B. H., Heuser, E. T., Hanson, V., and Landing, B. H., 1980a, A histologic evaluation of mixed connective tissue disease in childhood, *Am. J. Med.* **68**:710–717.

Singsen, B. H., Olive, P. M., Luger, A. M., Benage, D. D., Takano, M., Walker, S. E., and Sharp, G. C., 1980b, Identification of nuclear ribonucleoprotein antibodies in MRL mice, *Arthritis Rheum.* **23**:747.

Singsen, B. H., Akhter, J. E., Weinstein, M. M., and Sharp, G. C., 1985, Congenital complete heart block and SSA antibodies: Obstetric implications *Am. J. Obst. Gynecol.* (in press)

Sontheimer, R. D., Thomas, J. R., and Gilliam, J. N., 1979, Subacute cutaneous lupus erythematosus: A cutaneous marker for a distinct lupus erythematosus subset, *Arch. Dermatol.* **115**:1409–1415.

Sontheimer, R. D., Stastny, P., and Gilliam, J. N., 1981, Human histocompatibility antigen associations in subacute cutaneous lupus erythematosus, *J. Clin. Invest.* **67**:312–316.

Sontheimer, R. D., Maddison, P. J., Reichlin, M., Jordon, R. E., Stastny, P., and Gilliam, J. N., 1982, Serologic and HLA associations in subacute cutaneous lupus erythematosus, a clinical subset of lupus erythematosus, *Ann. Intern. Med.* **97**:664–671.

Steen, V. D., Ziegler, G. L., Rodnan, G. P., and Medsger, T. A., Jr., 1984, Clinical and laboratory associations of anticentromere antibody in patients with progressive systemic sclerosis, *Arthritis Rheum.* **27**:125–131.

Sullivan, W. D., Hurst, D. J., Harmon, C. E., Esther, J. H., Agia, G. A., Maltby, J. D., Lillard, S. B., Held, C. N., Wolfe, J. F., Sunderrajan, E. V., Miricq, H. R., and Sharp, G. C., 1984, A prospective evaluation emphasizing pulmonary involvement in patients with mixed connective tissue disease, *Medicine (Baltimore)* **63**:92–106.

Takano, M., Agris, P. F., and Sharp, G. C., 1980, Purification and biochemical characterization of nuclear ribonucleoprotein antigen using purified antibody from serum of a patient with mixed connective tissue disease, *J. Clin. Invest.* **65**:1449–1456.

Takano, M., Golden, S. S., Sharp, G. C., and Agris, P. F., 1981, Molecular relationships between two nuclear antigens, ribonucleoprotein and Sm: Purification of active antigens and their biochemical characterization, *Biochemistry* **21**:5929–5935.

Tan, E. M., 1982, Autoantibodies to nuclear antigens (ANA): Their immunobiology and medicine, *Adv. Immunol.* **33**:167–240.

Tan, E. M., and Kunkel, H. G., 1966, Characterisitics of a soluble nuclear antigen precipitating with sera of patients with systemic lupus erythematosus, *J. Immunol.* **96**:464–471.

Tan, E. M., Schur, P. H., Carr, R. I., and Kunkel, H. G., 1966, Deoxyribonucleic acid (DNA) and antibodies to DNA in the serum of patients with systemic lupus erythematosus, *J. Clin. Invest.* **45**:1732–1740.

Tan, E. M., Rodnan, G. P., Garcia, I., Moroi, Y., Fritzler, M. J., and Peebles, C., 1980, Diversity of antinuclear antibodies in progressive systemic sclerosis, *Arthritis Rheum.* **23**:617–625.

Targoff, I. N., Raghu, G., and Reichlin, M., 1983, Antibodies to Mi-1 in SLE: Relationship to other precipitins and reaction with bovine immunoglobulin, *Clin. Exp. Immunol.* **53**:76–82.

Teppo, A. M., Gripenberg, M., Kuki, P., Baklien, K., Helve, T., and Wegelius, O, 1982, Purification and characterisation of a nuclear SS-B antigen, *Scand. J. Immunol.* **15**:1–7.

Tramposch, H. D., Smith, C. D., Senecal, J., and Rothfield, N., 1984, A long-term longitudinal study of anticentromere antibodies, *Arthritis Rheum.* **27**:121–124.

Treadwell, E. L., Alspaugh, M. A., and Sharp, G. C., 1984a, Characterization of a new antigen-antibody system (Su) in patients with systemic lupus erythematosus, *Arthritis Rheum.* **27**:1263–1271.

Treadwell, E. L., Alspaugh, M. A., Wolfe, J. F., and Sharp., G. C., 1984b, Clinical relevance of PM-1 antibody and physiochemical characterization of PM-1 antigen, *J. Rheumatol.* **11**:658–662.

Venables, P. J. W., Charles, P. J., Buchanan, R. R. C., Yi, T., Mumford, P. A., Schrieber, L., Room, G. R. W., and Maini, R. N., 1983, Quantitation and detection of isotypes of anti-SS-B antibodies by ELISA and Farr assays using affinity purified antigens, *Arthritis Rheum.* **26**:146–155.

Wasicek, C. A., and Reichlin, M., 1982, Clinical and serological differences between systemic lupus erythematosus patients with antibodies to Ro versus patients with antibodies to Ro and La, *J. Clin. Invest.* **69**:835–843.

Weston, W. L., Harmon, C., Peebles, C., Manchester, D., Franco, H. L., Huff, J. C., and Norris, D. A., 1982, A serological marker for neonatal lupus erythematosus, *Br. J. Dermatol.* **107**:377–382.

White, P. J., Gardner, W. D., and Hoch, S. O., 1981, Identification of the immunologically active components of the Sm and RNP antigens, *Proc. Natl. Acad. Sci. U.S.A.* **78**:626–630.

Winn, D. M., Wolfe, J. F., Harmon, D., and Sharp, G. C., 1979, Characterization of a distinct nuclear acidic protein antigen (MA) and clinical findings in systemic lupus erythematosus patients with MA antibodies, *J. Clin. Invest.* **64**:820–823.

Wise, K. S., Takano, M., and Sharp. G. C., 1982, Polypeptide of ribonucleoprotein complex recognized by murine monoclonal autoantibody, *Arthritis Rheum.* **25**:S16.

Wolfe, J. F., Adelstein, E., and Sharp, G. C., 1977, Antinuclear antibody with distinct specificity for polymyositis, *J. Clin. Invest.* **59**:176–178.

Yang, V. W., Lerner, M. R., Steitz, J. A., and Flint, S. J., 1981, A small nuclear ribonucleoprotein is required for splicing of adenoviral early RNA sequences, *Proc. Natl. Acad. Sci. U.S.A.* **78**:1371–1375.

8

Antibodies to DNA Epiphenomena or Pathogens?

Bevra H. Hahn

I. HISTORY

The study of antibodies directed against DNA began in the 1950s with the discovery of the L.E. cell by Hargraves. Several investigators found that the L.E. cell phenomenon resulted from ingestion of altered nuclear material by circulating phagocytic cells. Close examination of that material showed that it consisted of DNA–protein (predominantly DNA–histone) and IgG. Thus, the existence of antibodies to the supposedly "forbidden" constituents of the human nucleus was recognized.

Over the next decades it became clear that patients with systemic lupus erythematosus (SLE) had circulating antibodies to multiple nuclear constituents in addition to DNA–histone; that group of antibodies became known as antinuclear antibodies (ANA). Furthermore, the ability to produce ANA was not confined to patients with SLE but also occurred in many other chronic rheumatic diseases, chronic inflammatory states, and even after acute viral infections in otherwise healthy individuals. As ANA tests became more sensitive, low titers of the antibodies were found in normal persons, with an increased incidence in the aged.

The first reports that the family of ANA included immunoglobulins that reacted with DNA alone appeared in 1957 (Ceppellini *et al.*, 1957; Robbins *et al.*, 1957; Seligmann, 1957). At the same time, investigators in three laboratories discovered not only that antibodies to DNA existed but also that they had significant associations with SLE.

Since that time, numerous investigators have studied antibodies to DNA. It is agreed that antibodies reactive with the double-stranded or native molecule of DNA (dsDNA) are indeed relatively disease-specific for SLE, whereas antibodies to denatured, single-

Bevra H. Hahn • Department of Medicine, Division of Rheumatology, University of California, Los Angeles, California 90024.

stranded DNA (ssDNA) are not, that rising titers of either anti-dsDNA or anti-ssDNA often herald a disease flare, that SLE patients with high titers of anti-DNA are at increased risk for nephritis (Fig. 1), and that manipulation of antibodies to DNA can profoundly alter disease in the murine models of SLE.

Specifically, ssDNA inoculated into NZB/NZW mice in immunogenic form (on methylated BSA) can significantly accelerate anti-DNA antibody formation and nephritis (Lambert and Dixon, 1968), whereas ssDNA inoculated into newborn mice of the same strain in tolerogenic form (on poly-D-lysine) can protect mice from development of anti-DNA and renal disease (Parker *et al.*, 1974). Nucleoside bases are also effective tolerogens if presented on appropriate carriers—dGL or isologous IgG (Eschav *et al.*, 1975; Borel *et al.*, 1978).

However, as evidence for anti-DNA playing a pathogenic role in disease was being accumulated, it was also learned that healthy mice and humans have the capacity to make antibodies to DNA in their immunoglobulin repertoires and that, in fact, polyclonal activators of B-cell secretion frequently cause appearance of anti-ssDNA and even of anti-dsDNA with no obvious adverse sequelae. Thus, the argument was joined: Are antibodies to DNA one more epiphenomenon resulting from any conditions that activate B cells? Or are they actually pathogenic in some situations (especially SLE)? In this chapter, we discuss current information about DNA antibodies that relate to their epitope specificity, the importance of their immunoglobulin class and subclass, the characteristics of those that appear after polyclonal activation and those that deposit in target tissues (including idiotype and charge characteristics), and the multiple factors that control production and destruction of those antibodies. We attempt to convince the reader that two populations of anti-DNA exist, the nonpathogenic and the pathogenic, and that the former may represent an epiphenomenon, whereas the latter should be targeted for specific suppression as new methods to treat SLE nephritis are developed.

II. EPITOPE SPECIFICITY

The anti-DNA response in most individuals, human and murine, consists of multiple different immunoglobulin subpopulations. In a single individual, one can find antibodies to DNA of IgM and IgG classes, of all IgG subclasses, with complement-fixing and non-complement-fixing capabilities, and with specificities for different regions, or epitopes, of the DNA molecule. Before monoclonal antibody technology became available, attempts

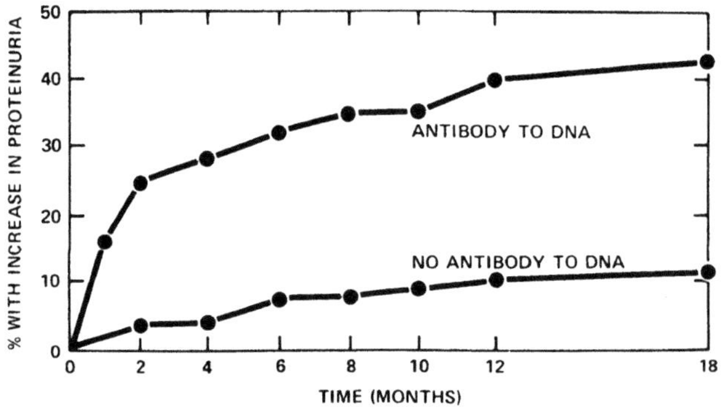

Figure 1. Lupus patients with antibodies to DNA in their serum were more likely to develop proteinuria over an 18-month period of follow-up than SLE patients without anti-DNA. (Reprinted from Fries and Holman, 1975, with permission of the publisher.)

to separate antibodies of different epitope specificities were hampered by interference of other specificities in the polyclonal, heterogeneous sera studied and by different avidities and physical properties of various antibody subpopulations. Nevertheless, early studies (Arana and Seligmann, 1967; Koffler *et al.*, 1971) showed that SLE sera contain three general families of anti-DNA antibodies: (1) those that react with both ds- and ssDNA substrates (the majority); (2) those that react exclusively with ssDNA; and (3) those that react exclusively with dsDNA substrates (usually a small proportion). The advent of monoclonal antibody technology, in addition to available better-defined, more stable ssDNA and dsDNA substrates (such as fdDNA for ss and the kinetoplast of *Crithidia luciliae* for dsDNA), has allowed further classification of epitope specificity. Sketches of the structure of DNA are shown in Fig. 2, and the four general groups of epitope specificities are listed in Table 1.

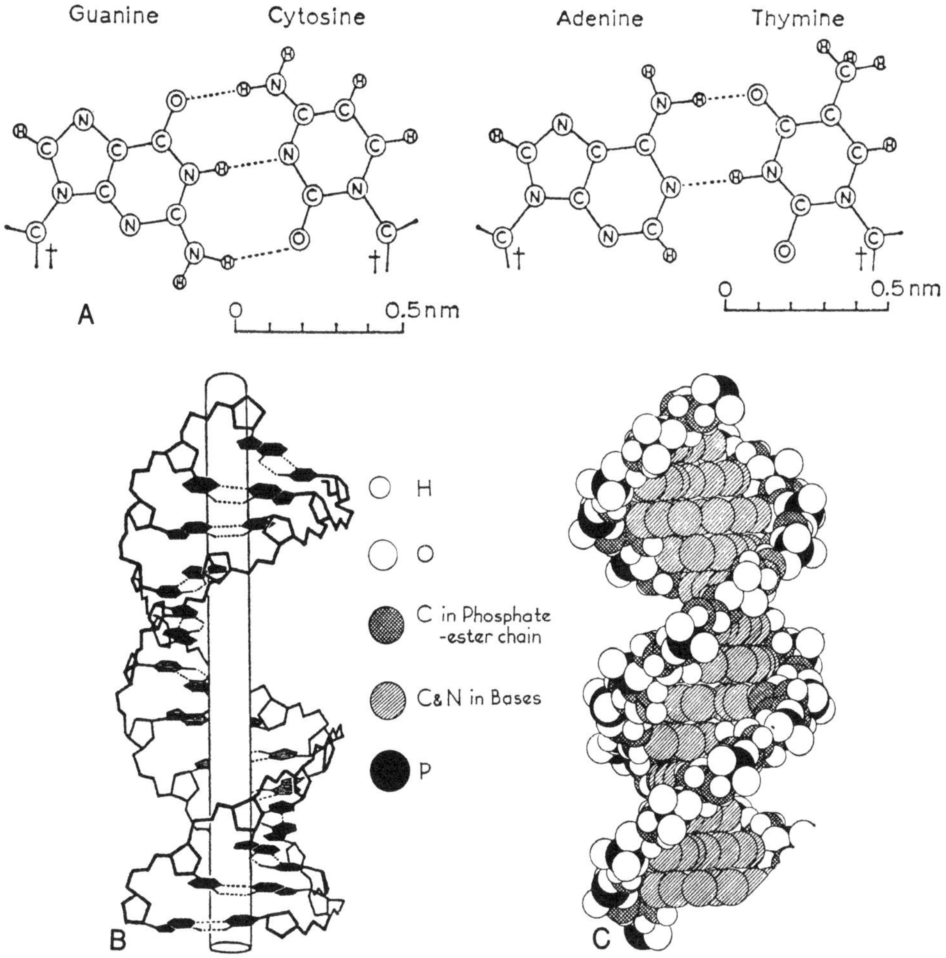

Figure 2. Structure of DNA. A: Base pairs in DNA: adenine–thymine and guanine–cytosine. B: Sketch of base pairs in B helix with ribose–phosphate backbone. C: Sketch of B helix of DNA showing positions of carbon and phosphate groups in the backbone. (Reprinted from Adams *et al.*, 1976, with permission of the publisher.)

Table 1. Epitope Specificities of Antibodies to DNA

Specificity	Antibody
Individual nucleoside bases	Anti-ssDNA
Base sequences	Either anti-ssDNA or anti-dsDNA depending on sequence
Sugar–phosphate backbone	Either anti-ssDNA or anti-dsDNA
Secondary structures	Anti-Z-DNA

It is likely that each individual antibody to DNA reacts with one of four structures on the DNA molecule: (1) individual nucleoside bases; (2) base sequences; (3) the ribose–phosphate backbone; or (4) secondary structures. The first can be typified by a monoclonal anti-DNA IgG derived from an MRL/lpr mouse and studied by Munns *et al.* (1982), which is specific for guanosine. Obviously, that immunoglobulin can react with either ssDNA, in which multiple guanosine residues are exposed, or with ssRNA, where the same is true. Andrzejewski *et al.* (1980) also found reactivity with individual bases in monoclonal antibodies derived from MRL/lpr mice, although reactivity with the ribose phosphate backbone was more frequent. An example of the second type of reactivity, with base sequences, was found in the studies of a monoclonal anti-DNA derived from an NZB/NZW F_1 female mouse studied by our group (Hahn and Ebling, 1984) and found to recognize guanosine–cytosine presented in the B helix of DNA. Since the specificity was G–C, the antibody could only be anti-dsDNA; if the specificity were, for example, G–T or G–T–C–G, the antibody would be an anti-ssDNA. In contrast, Lafer *et al.* (1983) have shown that many anti-DNA antibodies from patients with SLE react preferentially with the Z conformations of DNA. In Z-DNA, there is a left-hand twist at guanosine residues rather than the right-hand twists characteristic of the B conformation of the helix, so that secondary structure is different, and guanosine and neighboring bases are presented at a different angle from the B helix. Of the three specificities, base sequence has been the most difficult to demonstrate.

Interesting recent examples of specificity for the ribose–phosphate backbone of DNA were reported by Andrzejewski *et al.* (1980), who described several monoclonal antibodies to DNA from MRL/lpr mice and later from humans with SLE (Lafer *et al.*, 1981; Schoenfeld *et al.*, 1983) that reacted with cardiolipin as well as with DNA. One antibody with that reactivity also acted as a circulating anticoagulant. They suggested that many "DNA antibodies" react with the 2-carbon-3-phosphate structure contained in the backbone of DNA (see Fig. 2B,C), in cardiolipin, in the platelet lipid associated with prothrombin-activating factor, and possibly with the same structure contained in the phospholipid of cell membranes. For example, one of the human monoclonal antibodies to DNA cloned in their laboratory reacted with ssDNA and with platelets. If this concept is correct, then one antibody can actually have several activities, including anti-DNA, anti-cell-membrane (e.g., antilymphocyte), and anticoagulant. In fact, Schwartz and colleagues (Lafer *et al.*, 1981; Schoenfeld *et al.*, 1983) have suggested that DNA is simply a convenient antigen to detect "lupus antibodies" that react with ribose–phosphate and phospholipid. They have subsequently suggested that this subgroup of cardiolipin-reactive antibodies to DNA are induced by immunizations with intestinal bacteria. In contrast, other investigators (Jarros *et al.*, 1983) have reported that most antibodies to cardiolipin do not cross react with DNA and that anti-CL may be associated with arterial clotting in patients with SLE. In addition, some investigators have reported that incubation with cardiolipin does not remove antibodies to DNA from most human SLE sera.

lipid–phosphate structures is one of the most interesting current directions in SLE research. It is the opinion of the author that such cross reactivity characterizes one subpopulation of antibodies to DNA (but probably not a majority), that such antibodies may arise from bacterial immunization or polyclonal B-cell activation, and that they may indeed exhibit multiple antigenic specificities including pathogenic interactions that alter clotting.

Recent studies of Weisbart and Munns (Weisbart *et al.*, 1983; Munns *et al.*, 1984) have shown that at least some of these three epitope specificities can be found in polyclonal human and murine SLE sera. Guanosine is the single base with which the largest number of sera react most frequently, but quite different patterns occur in individual sera, sometimes with equivalent reactivity with two or three bases, suggesting sequence specificity, and sometimes with very little reactivity with individual bases, suggesting that the bulk of antibody activity in that serum may be directed against the backbone structure or base sequences.

Now that the four general classes of epitope specificity of antibodies to DNA have been defined, the question remains, are they of any consequence? Does it matter clinically if an antibody reacts with ssDNA, with dsDNA, or with a shared structure in DNA, RNA, clotting factors, etc? Probably it does, but we are no closer to that answer than we were a decade ago. For practical purposes, laboratories should still offer tests that detect anti-dsDNA whether the substrate be *Crithidiae*, endonuclease-treated mammalian or bacterial DNA, or bacteriophage DNA such as PM-2 because the group of antibodies that react with dsDNA is still more specific for SLE than the group that reacts exclusively with ssDNA. Patients with circulating antibodies to dsDNA almost always have antibodies to ssDNA as well. A rise in the titer of either group of antibodies is often, although not always, associated with a disease flare. Therefore, once it is established that a patient has anti-dsDNA, follow-up tests with either ssDNA or dsDNA substrates may be equally useful. However, for practical purposes, one laboratory test of anti-DNA antibodies will suffice, and anti-dsDNA is therefore the best choice.

III. IMMUNOGLOBULIN CLASS, SUBCLASS, AND PHYSICAL PROPERTIES OF ANTIBODIES TO DNA

Circulating antibodies to DNA can be found in both IgM and IgG classes. In general, IgG antibodies are more likely to be associated with clinically active SLE and with nephritis than are IgM antibodies (Rothfield and Stollar, 1967; Sonteheimer and Gilliam, 1978). This is dramatically illustrated in the NZB/NZW F_1 mouse models of SLE, as described by Talal (1980). Early in life, males and females develop circulating IgM antibodies to DNA. Several weeks later, a switch to IgG occurs in the females, followed shortly by proteinuria and eventually by death from nephritis. In contrast, males do not experience the class switch and do not develop clinical nephritis until much later.

In humans with SLE, there are also statistically significant correlations among IgG antibodies to DNA, active SLE, and nephritis (Rothfield and Stollar, 1967; Sonteheimer and Gilliam, 1978). These correlations are also true for antibodies to DNA of the subclasses of IgG that fix complement (IgG_{2a}, IgG_{2b}, and IgG_3 in the mouse; IgG_1 and IgG_3 in the human). For example, immunoglobulin eluted from glomeruli of mice with spontaneous SLE contain predominantly IgG_{2a} or IgG_{2b} antibodies to DNA (Ebling and Hahn, 1980), although large quantities of eluate contain small amounts of IgM, IgG_1 and IgG_3 (Slack *et al.*, 1984). In humans with severe nephritis, IgG_1 and IgG_3 usually predominate in sera (Sonteheimer and Gilliam, 1978).

In addition to the importance of immunoglobulin class and subclass, the physical properties of antibodies to DNA are also important in determining pathogenicity. Some investigators have reported that precipitating antibodies to DNA have a significantly higher association with nephritis than nonprecipitating antibodies (Gershwin and Steinberg, 1974); one group reported opposite findings (Johnson *et al.*, 1973). There has been disagreement regarding the importance of antibody avidity. Perhaps the best study is one in which the avidities of antibodies to DNA in sera and in matching glomerular eluates were compared (Winfield *et al.*, 1977); the sera from patients with nephritis contained predominantly low-avidity antibodies, whereas the eluates contained high-avidity anti-DNA. Those findings illustrate the hazards of assuming that circulating antibodies contain all of the antibody subpopulations that are deposited in target tissues. Taylor and his colleagues have reported that antibodies to DNA that dissociate slowly from antigen are more pathogenic than rapidly dissociating populations (Taylor *et al.*, 1979); Pearson and Lightfoot have shown that disease activity in SLE correlates with rapidly associating antibodies to DNA (Pearson and Lightfoot, 1981).

One of the most interesting recent concepts regarding the factors that make an antibody pathogenic for glomeruli is the importance of charge. Glomerular basement membrane contains multiple polyanionic sites. It is possible that antigens, antibodies, or immune complexes with a net cationic charge fix preferentially to those structures. For example, cationized albumin injected into rabbits fixed to glomeruli and persisted for days; neutral and anionic forms did not (Border *et al.*, 1982). Cationic immune complexes injected into mice caused chronic nephritis; complexes with other charges did not (Gallo *et al.*, 1981). In mice with SLE, antibodies to DNA eluted from glomeruli are a restricted subpopulation with a highly cationic charge (pI 8.0–9.0), as shown in Fig. 3 (Ebling and Hahn, 1980).

Furthermore, in experiments in which serum antibodies to DNA from NZB/NZW F_1 mice were incubated with glomeruli from 36-week-old syngeneic mice, only the cationic populations (pI 7.0–9.0) adhered to glomeruli (Dang and Harbeck, 1984). However, this adherence was prevented by pretreatment of the glomeruli with DNase, and glomeruli from younger mice did not fix any anti-DNA, suggesting that more is involved than a simple charge interaction between cationic antibodies and polyanionic sites in glomerular basement membrane (GBM). It is possible that DNA fixes to basement membrane structures, perhaps to collagen, as suggested by Izui *et al.* (1976), and then cationic anti-DNA fixes to DNA and/or neighboring anionic basement membrane determinants. This concept is different from the model of passive entrapment of circulating, complement-fixing complexes of DNA–anti-DNA in GBM; it is possible that both mechanisms occur in SLE.

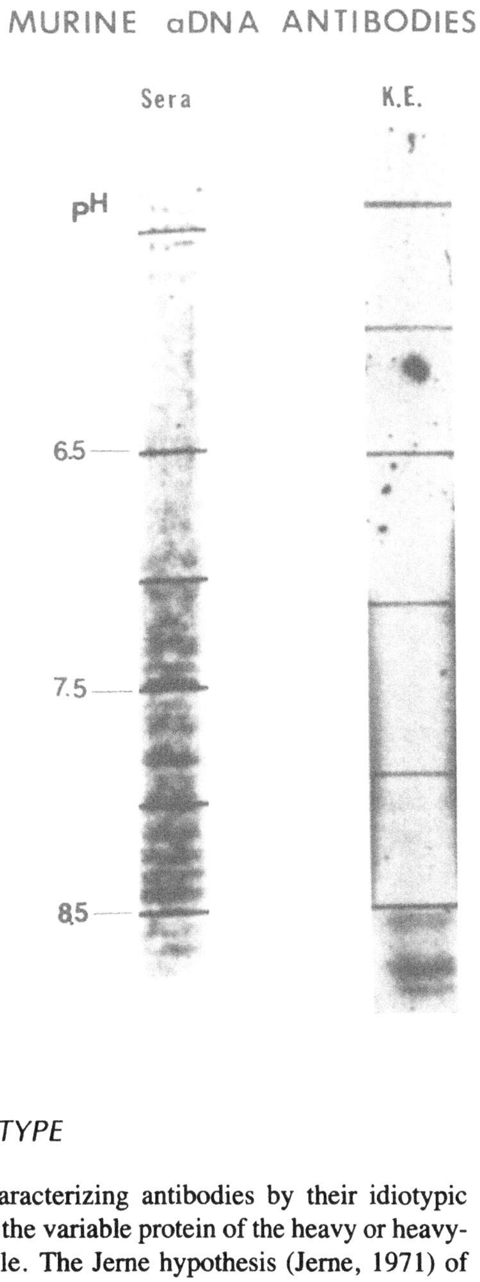

Figure 3. Restriction of antibodies to DNA in glomerular eluates of NZB/NZW F_1 female mice. The IgG antibodies from serum (on the left) and glomeruli (on the right) were focused at their isoelectric points in a vertical gel and overlaid with [^{125}I]dsDNA. Each black band is an antibody to DNA (or a group of lines representing a single clone). Antibodies in glomeruli were restricted to three cationic bands (pI 8.0–9.0).

IV. IDIOTYPE

Recently, there has been great interest in characterizing antibodies by their idiotypic structures. Idiotype is an antigenic sequence on the variable protein of the heavy or heavy-plus-light chain of an immunoglobulin molecule. The Jerne hypothesis (Jerne, 1971) of a network of antigen–antibody–antiidiotype control of the immune response is correct for at least some humoral immune responses. This author's concept of the network is illustrated in Fig. 4. Antigen (e.g., DNA) calls forth several different antibodies to various epitopes on that antigen. The sequence on Ab_1 that confers exact epitope specificity is a unique, private idiotype (Id) confined to one subpopulation of identical immunoglobulin (Ig) molecules. Some immunoglobulins contain an additional Id sequence that is shared by other Ig molecules with different epitope specificities, the "public" or "cross-reactive" or "framework" Id. Since all Id regions are antigenic, Ab_1 calls forth another immune

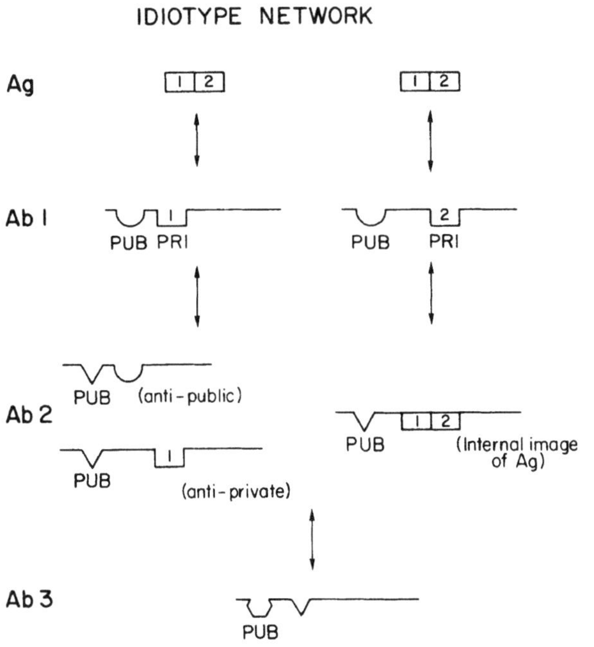

Figure 4. The idiotype–antiantibody network of control of the humoral immune response. Ag, antigen; Ab_1, antibody (idiotype); Ab_2, antiidiotype; Ab_3, antianti-idiotype; PUB, public; PRI, private. See text for detailed explanation.

response, Ab_2, or anti-Id. Anti-Ids may be directed against the private or public Ids on Ab_1. Some anti-Ids contain structures that are similar to the immunizing antigen; these are called "internal image" anti-Ids. Internal image anti-Ids are common in the repertoire of anti-Ids to rheumatoid factors (Fong *et al.*, 1983). Another example of an internal image Id is found in the immune response to antiinsulin antibodies; some Ab_2 anti-Ids have insulinlike activity (Schecter *et al.*, 1982). Ab_2 elicits an Ab_3 (antianti-Id) response, and the network continues. Under some conditions, each Ab down-regulates the preceding Ag or Ab; in other conditions, up-regulating occurs.

Studies of antibodies to DNA in patients with SLE and in mouse models of that disease have shown that a large proportion of antibodies to DNA are constructed from cross-reactive public Ids. Solomon *et al.* (1983) found a public Id on DNA antibodies from eight of nine patients with SLE. Almost all NZB/NZW F_1 females and MRL/lpr males and females construct some of their anti-DNA repertoire from public Ids (Hahn and Ebling, 1984; Marion *et al.*, 1982; Rauch *et al.*, 1982). Furthermore, similar cross-reactive Ids can be found on antibodies to DNA from NZB/NZW F_1, MRL/lpr/lpr, and BXSB mice (Hahn and Ebling, 1984), suggesting that V region genes are highly conserved or produce closely related sequences on antibodies to DNA. Most data suggest that public Ids on anti-DNA are not confined to those antibodies or to autoimmune strains of mice. Normal mice can be induced to assemble public-Id-positive antibodies in response to polyclonal B-cell activation (Datta *et al.*, 1983).

The public Id described in our laboratory, which is present on anti-DNA in multiple lupus mouse strains, is largely confined to IgG with a pI of >7.0, which may make it a useful marker for potentially nephritogenic antibodies regardless of their epitope specificity. The description of idiotypic characteristics of antibodies may provide clues to genetic control of the immune response and to structures that determine pathogenicity

Table 2. Characteristics of Pathogenic Antibodies to DNA IgG Class

Complement-fixing subclasses of IgG
High avidity for DNA
Cationic charge

for various target tissues and may serve to target undesirable antibodies for specific suppression, perhaps by anti-Id reagents. See Section V for a discussion of the mechanisms by which the anti-DNA response is controlled.

To summarize, the characteristics of antibodies to DNA that probably render them pathogenic, especially for glomeruli, are listed in Table 2.

V. MECHANISMS CONTROLLING PRODUCTION AND PERSISTENCE OF ANTIBODIES TO DNA

As discussed more fully in other chapters of this text, multiple factors govern the ability of a human or mouse to make antibodies to DNA of both pathogenic and nonpathogenic types and the ability of the organism to dispose of these antibodies. A list of these factors is presented in Table 3.

The genetic control of the ability to make antibodies to DNA is probably quite complex in humans. Although most individuals, man and mouse, can make antibodies to ssDNA (and even low quantities of anti-dsDNA) in response to multiple B-cell activation (Izui *et al.*, 1977), very few develop any adverse clinical effects. Therefore, individuals with SLE must have some differences in antibody subpopulations or in target tissue susceptibility or in catabolism of DNA and/or anti-DNA that result in disease, and that predisposition must be partially under genetic control. Clearly, several HLA-linked genes contribute to the expression of SLE in man (especially DR3, MB1, and MT1), but the disease can exist in patients lacking those markers. Family studies have suggested the presence of at least one Mendelian dominant non-HLA-linked gene, which has not been identified (Arnett, 1983). Patients with high titers of anti-DNA and with nephritis have a significantly increased incidence of DR2 and MT1 markers.

Table 3. Factors Influencing the Production and Persistence of Antibodies to DNA

Genetic control of the immune response
Environmental stimuli: viruses, bacteria, drugs, ultraviolet light
Sex hormone status of the host
Idiotype–antiidiotype networks
T–B–macrophage-cell interactions
Clearance of immune complexes by the reticuloendothelial system
Availability of DNA antigen

The three major murine models of SLE—NZB (or NZB/NZW F_1), MRL/lpr, and BXSB—have different H_2 loci as well as different Ig allotypes and lymphocyte surface alloantigens. Anti-DNA formation and immune nephritis are controlled by at least four genes in the NZ strains. However, in the BXSB mouse, the ability to make a pathogenic anti-DNA response may be controlled by a single gene or set of genes on the Y chromosome; that chromosome accelerates SLE in mice with a genetic predisposition but cannot induce severe SLE when passed into normal strains (Dixon, 1982). The lpr gene of MRL/lpr mice also serves as an accelerating factor influencing production of anti-DNA-associated nephritis as well as massive lymphoproliferation of an unusual early T cell but is not the sole gene governing the anti-DNA response. In mouse as in man, there is evidence that production of different autoantibodies (e.g., anti-Sm, antierythrocyte, anti-DNA) is controlled by different genes (Arnett, 1982; Raveche *et al.*, 1983; Dixon, 1982; Roths, 1979).

Certain environmental triggers may produce not only polyclonal B-cell activation but pathogenic anti-DNA in susceptible hosts. For example, there has been great interest in the possibility that viral infections cause SLE, possibly by altering DNA enough to render it "foreign" instead of "self." All of the murine SLE strains have deposits of retrovirus gp-70–anti-gp-70 as well as DNA–anti-DNA in their glomeruli (Dixon, 1982). We have already discussed the hypothesis that enteric bacteria evoke antibodies to DNA by virtue of cross-reacting 2-carbon-3-phosphate structures (Lafer *et al.*, 1981). A noninfectious environmental accelerator of SLE in man, and possibly in mice, is ultraviolet light. This acceleration may be mediated through anti-DNA, since exposure of DNA to UV light renders it more immunogenic (Tan, 1976).

In humans, certain drugs can promote the development of circulating antibodies to DNA (usually anti-ssDNA) and, in some cases, disease resembling SLE. The two most important drugs in this category are hydralazine and procainamide; isoniazid, hydantoin, chlorpromazine, and β blockers are also suspect (Blomgren *et al.*, 1972; Hahn *et al.*, 1972; Alarcon-Segovia, 1975). All of these drugs have in common the ability to interact physically or chemically with DNA and, in some cases, to render it more immunogenic (Alarcon-Segovia, 1975).

Another important environmental factor influencing the ability of an organism to produce IgG antibodies to DNA is the sex hormone status of the host. Lupus is predominantly a disease of females of the childbearing age in humans and in the NZ strains of mice. Women and men with SLE have increased α-hydroxylation of estrone to metabolites with estrogenic properties; women have accelerated breakdown of testosterone to inactive products (Lahita *et al.*, 1981). In general, androgenic hormones are protective in NZB/NZW and MRL/lpr mouse models of SLE; estrogens are permissive and modulate the switch from IgM to IgG antibodies to DNA, thus permitting the emergence of nephritis. Castrated male NZB/NZW mice develop severe SLE with the female pattern of IgG antibodies to DNA; castrated females or those treated with androgens or antiestrogens are protected from their disease (Roubinian *et al.*, 1978, 1979). An interesting example of the interplay between sex hormone status and genetic predisposition to SLE was shown in experiments of Laskin *et al.* (1981) in which resistance to tolerance could be transferred to (NZB × DBA/2) F_1 hybrids via NZB thymus cells only if testosterone was absent (i.e., in females or castrated males).

The control of the immune response by Id–anti-Id networks may also be defective in SLE. Patients develop anti-Ids directed against their autologous antibodies to DNA (Abdou *et al.*, 1981; Nasa *et al.*, 1982). Abdou and colleagues (1981) have demonstrated that anti-Id is detectable in sera during periods of disease remission but not during exacerbations. The author and her colleagues have been successful in suppressing IgG bearing a public Id on anti-DNA antibodies in NZB/NZW mice by administering exogenous Id (which induces anti-Id) or anti-Id (Hahn and Ebling, 1984; Hahn and Ebling, 1983). Suppression of Id was associated with suppression of total antibodies to DNA and a temporary but significant delay in nephritis. In contrast, in other experiments, administration of anti-public-Id to very young MRL/lpr mice increased the quantity of Id-positive Ig without altering the level of antibodies to DNA (Teitelbaum *et al.*, 1984). Studies of autoregulation and therapeutic regulation of the anti-DNA response by manipulation of Id and anti-Id are an exciting area of current research.

Genetic, environmental, sex hormone, and immune network control mechanisms all impact at the level of cell–cell interactions. Exactly which cells behave abnormally in patients and mice with SLE is a point of controversy. Most authorities agree that an unusually large number of mature B cells secreting Ig are present (Steinberg *et al.*, 1982; Theofilopoulus *et al.*, 1980). Whether their presence reflects genetic control, polyclonal B-cell activation, overactive helper T-cell function, defective suppressor T-cell control, or combinations of these is currently being debated. There is evidence for and against each of these hypotheses. The reader is referred to some excellent discussions of this topic (Steinberg *et al.*, 1982; Talal *et al.*, 1982; Creighton *et al.*, 1979; Williams, 1979).

We must not confine our thinking to factors that influence the production of antibodies to DNA without considering the factors that determine the rate at which antibodies and immune complexes are cleared from tissues and from the circulation. There is good evidence that the capacity of the reticuloendothelial system (RES) to remove immune complexes can be saturated (Haakenstad and Mannik, 1974). Patients with clinically active SLE have defective clearances, probably because of such saturation (Frank *et al.*, 1979). The problem may be compounded by the genetically controlled reduced numbers of CR-1 receptors characteristic of some SLE patients (Wilson *et al.*, 1982), which result in a reduced capacity to transport and clear complexes that have activated complement. NZB/NZW F_1 and MRL/lpr mice also have a decreased number of binding sites available for immune complex removal, possibly because of saturation or a defect in Fc receptor expression (Magilavy *et al.*, 1983).

Finally, a discussion of antibodies to DNA is not complete without mention of the availability of the antigen and its various epitopes. The presence of free DNA in the circulation of patients with SLE was initially reported in 1966 (Tan *et al.*, 1966). Levels are usually high in patients with clinically active disease, and the DNA is of a relatively uniform small size (molecular weight $0.2–0.45 \times 10^6$), suggesting some protection from the activity of DNase, possibly afforded by anti-DNA antibodies (Raptis and Menard, 1980). These data are compatible with an earlier report that antibodies to dsDNA from patients with active SLE bind a dsDNA fragment of 20–1200 base pairs (Fig. 5; Papalian *et al.*, 1980). Spleen cells from mice with SLE release larger quantities of DNA then do normal mouse cells (Golan and Borel, 1983). Similarly, stimulated human SLE lymphocytes release large quantities of DNA rich in a low-molecular-weight fragment that has a high content of guanosine–cytosine, a specificity with which some antibodies to dsDNA react (Sano *et al.*, 1983). Patients with active SLE have the capacity to bind

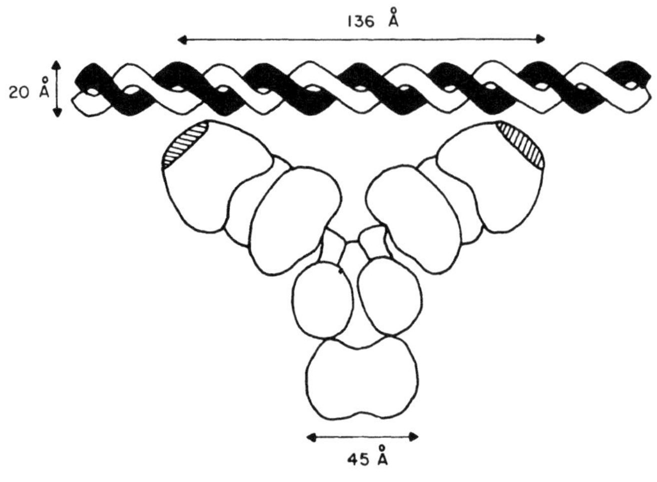

Figure 5. The prevalent DNA–anti-DNA complex present in sera of patients with SLE. A single IgG molecule binds bivalently to a dsDNA fragment of 20–1200 base pairs. Stability of this complex and protection of DNA fragments of this size from degradation may promote persistence of complexes and active disease. (Reprinted from Stollar, 1980, with permission of the publisher.)

increased amounts of DNA on the surfaces of both B and T lymphocytes (Bankhurst and Williams, 1975). Therefore, DNA antigens are quantitatively increased in SLE, and configurations that can stimulate and/or react with antibodies to DNA are widely available.

VI. SUMMARY

In summary, one mechanism by which antibodies to DNA are produced is in response to polyclonal B-cell activation. However, abundant DNA antigen is available in patients and mice with SLE to stimulate a specific antigen-induced antibody response in which macrophages, T cells, and B cells all participate. Fischbach and colleagues (Fischbach *et al.*, 1981) have reported that the spectrotypes of antibodies to DNA do not differ in spontaneous antibodies to DNA and those induced by administration of drugs, LPS, or DNA antigens. However, data from several laboratories have suggested that in certain situations, probably influenced by multiple genetic and environmental stimuli, subpopulations of anti-DNA emerge that are pathogenic and cause the target organ damage that results in clinical SLE. Further attempts to define those subpopulations and to control their expression is a major focus of current research efforts.

REFERENCES

Abdou, N. I., Wall, H., Lindsley, H. B., Halsey, J. F., and Suzuki, T., 1981, Network theory in autoimmunity. *In vitro* suppression of serum anti-DNA antibody binding to DNA by anti-idiotypic antibody in SLE, *J. Clin. Invest.* **67:**1297–1304.

Adams, R. L. P. (ed.), 1976, *Davidson's The Biochemistry of the Nucleic Acids,* Academic Press, New York.

Alarcon-Segovia, D., 1975, Drug induced systemic lupus erythematosus and related syndromes, *Clin. Rheum. Dis.* **1:**573–592.

Andrezejewski, C., Jr., Stollar, B. D., Lalor, T. M., and Schwartz, R. S., 1980, Hybridoma auto-antibodies to DNA, *J. Immunol.* **124:**1499–1503.

Arana, R., and Seligmann, M., 1967, Antibodies to native and denatured deoxyribonucleic acid in SLE, *J. Clin. Invest.* **46:**1867–1882.

Arnett, F. C., Jr., 1983, Systemic lupus erythematosus: Current state of the genetic hypothesis, in: *Current Topics in Rheumatology* (B. H. Hahn, F. C. Arnett, T. M. Zizic, and M. C. Hochberg, eds.), The Upjohn Co., Kalamazoo, MI, pp. 1–160.

Bankhurst, A. D., Williams, R. D., Jr., 1975, Identification of DNA-binding lymphocytes in patients with SLE, *J. Clin. Invest.* **56:**1378–1385.

Blomgren, S. E., Condemi, J. J., and Vaughan, J. H., 1972, Procainamide induced lupus. Clinical and laboratory manifestations, *Am. J. Med.* **52:**338–348.

Border, W. A., Ward, H. J., Kamil, E. S., and Cohen, A. H., 1982, Induction of membranous nephropathy in rabbits by administration of cationic antigen, *J. Clin. Invest.* **69:**451–456.

Borel, Y., Lewis, R. M., Andre-Schwartz, J., Stollar, B. D., and Deinen, L., 1978, Treatment of lupus nephritis in adult (NZB × NZW) F_1 mice by cortisone-facilitated tolerance to nucleic acid antigens, *J. Clin. Invest.* **61:**276–286.

Ceppellini, R., Polli, E., and Celada, F., 1957, A DNA reacting factor in serum of a patient with lupus erythematosus diffusus, *Proc. Soc. Exp. Biol. Med.* **96:**572–575.

Creighton, W. D., Katz, D. H., and Dixon, F. J., 1979, Antigen-specific immunocompetency, B cell function, and regulatory helper and suppressor T cell activities in spontaneously autoimmune mice, *J. Immunol.* **123:**2627–2636.

Dang, H., and Harbeck, R. J., 1984, The *in vivo* and *in vitro* glomerular deposition of isolated anti-double-stranded-DNA antibodies in NZB/W mice, *Clin. Immunol. Immunopathol.* **30:**265–270.

Datta, S. K., Stollar, B. D., and Schwartz, R. S., 1983, Normal mice express idiotypes related to autoantibody idiotypes of lupus mice, *Proc. Natl. Acad. Sci. U.S.A.* **80:**2723–2727.

Dixon, F. J., 1982, Murine lupus—an overview, *Arthritis Rheum.* **25:**721–725.

Ebling, F. M., and Hahn, B. H., 1980, Restricted subpopulations of DNA antibodies in kidneys of mice with SLE, *Arthritis Rheum.* **23:**392–403.

Eschar, Z., Benecerraf, B., and Katz, D. H., 1975, Induction of tolerance to nucleic acid determinants by administration of a complex of nucleoside D-glutamic acid and D-lysine (D-GL), *J. Immunol.* **114:**872–876.

Fischbach, M., Rabbie, J., and Talal, N., 1981, Comparison of different antinucleic acid antibody spectrotypes in spontaneous, induced and murine lupus, *J. Clin. Invest.* **68:**1036–1043.

Fong, S., Gilbertson, T. A., and Carson, D. A., 1983, The internal image of IgG in cross-reactive anti-idiotype antibodies against human rheumatoid factors, *J. Immunol.* **131:**719–724.

Frank, M. M., Hamburger, M. I., Lawley, T. J., Kimberly, R. P., and Plotz, P. H., 1979, Defective reticuloendothelial system Fc-receptor function in SLE, *N. Engl. J. Med.* **300:**518–523.

Fries, J. F., and Holman, H. R., 1975, *Systemic Lupus Erythematosus: A Clinical Analysis*, W. B. Saunders, Philadelphia.

Gallo, G. R., Caulin-Glaser, T., and Lamm, M. E., 1981, Charge of circulating immune complexes as a factor in glomerular basement membrane localization in mice, *J. Clin. Invest.* **67:**1305–1313.

Gershwin, E. M., and Steinberg, A. D., 1974, Qualitative characteristics of anti-DNA antibodies in lupus nephritis, *Arthritis Rheum.* **17:**947–954.

Golan, D. T., and Borel, Y., 1983, Spontaneous increase of DNA turnover in murine SLE, *Eur. J. Immunol.* **13:**430–433.

Haakenstad, A. O., and Mannik, M., 1974, Saturation of the reticuloendothelial system with soluble immune complexes, *J. Immunol.* **112:**1939–1948.

Hahn, B. H., and Ebling, F. M., 1983, Suppression of NZB/NZW murine nephritis by administration of syngeneic monoclonal antibody to DNA. Possible role of anti-idiotypic antibodies, *J. Clin. Invest.* **71:**1728–1736.

Hahn, B. H., and Ebling, F. M., 1984, Suppression of murine lupus nephritis by administration of an anti-idiotypic antibody to anti-DNA, *J. Immunol.* **132:**187–190.

Hahn, B. H., and Ebling, F. M., 1984, Similar public idiotype determinants are present on cationic IgG antibodies to DNA in mice of unrelated lupus-prone strains, *J. Immunol.* **133:**3015–3019.

Hahn, B. H., Sharp, G. C., Irvin, W. S., Kantor, O. S., Gardner, C. A., Bagby, M., Perry, H. M., Jr., and Osterland, C. K., 1972, Immune responses to hydralazine and nuclear antigens in hydralazine-induced lupus erythematosus, *Am. J. Med.* **76:**365–374.

Izui, J., Lambert, P.-H., and Miescher, P. A., 1976, *In vitro* demonstration of a particular affinity of glomerular basement membrane and collagen for DNA, *J. Exp. Med.* **144**:428–443.

Izui, S., Zaldivar, N., Scher, I., and Lambert, P. H., 1977, Mechanisms for induction of anti-DNA antibodies by bacterial lipopolysaccharide in mice, *J. Immunol.* **119**:2151–2154.

Jarros, E. M., Gjaravo, N. E., and Hughes, G. R. V., 1983, Cardiolipin antibodies: Detection by radioimmunoassay and association with thrombosis in SLE, *Lancet* **2**:1211–1214.

Jerne, N. K., 1971, Towards a network theory of the immune system, *Ann. Immunol.* **125C**:373–377.

Johnson, G. E., Edmonds, J. P., and Holborow, E. J., 1973, Precipitating antibodies to DNA detected by two-stage electroimmunodiffusion: Studies in SLE and in RA, *Lancet* **2**:883–885.

Koffler, D., Carr, R., Agnello, V., Thoburn, R., and Kunkel, H. G., 1971, Antibodies to polynucleotides in human sera: Antigenic specificity and relation to disease, *J. Exp. Med.* **134**:294–312.

Lafer, E. M., Rauch, J., Andrezejewski, C., Jr., Mudd, D., Furic, B., Schwartz, R. S., and Stollar, B. D., 1981, Polyspecific monoclonal lupus antibodies reactive with both polynucleotides and phospholipids, *J. Exp. Med.* **153**:897–909.

Lafer, E. M., Valle, R. P. C., Moller, A., Nordheim, A., Schur, P. H., Rich, A., and Stollar, B. D., 1983, Z-DNA-specific antibodies in human SLE, *J. Clin. Invest.* **71**:314–320.

Lahita, R. G., Bradlow, H. L., Kunkel, H. G., and Fishman, J., 1981, Increased 16-hydroxylation of estradiol in SLE, *J. Clin. Endocrinol. Metab.* **53**:174–178.

Lambert, P. H., and Dixon, F. J., 1968, Pathogenesis of glomerulonephritis of NZB/W mice, *J. Exp. Med.* **127**:507–522.

Laskin, C. A., Taurog, J. D., Smathers, P. A., and Steinberg, A. D., 1981, Studies of defective tolerance in murine lupus, *J. Immunol.* **127**:1743–1747.

Magilavy, D. B., Hundley, T. R., Steinberg, A. D., and Finbloom, D. S., 1983, Abnormal binding of soluble IgG immune complexes to hepatic nonparenchymal cells of autoimmune mice, *J. Immunol.* **131**:2784–2788.

Marion, T. N., Lawton, A. R. III, Kearney, J. F., and Briles, D. E., 1982, Anti-DNA autoantibody in (NZB × ZW) F_1, mice are clonally heterogeneous, but the majority share a common idiotype, *J. Immunol.* **128**:668–671.

Munns, T. W., Liszewski, M. K., Tellam, J. T., Ebling, F. M., and Hahn, B. H., 1982, Antibody mucleic acid complexes. Indentification of the antigenic determinant of a murine monoclonal antibody specific for single-stranded nucleic acids, *Biochemistry* **21**:2929–2939.

Munns, T. W., Liszewski, M. K., and Hahn, B. H., 1984, Antibody nucleic acid complexes. Conformational and base specificities associated with spontaneously-occurring poly-acid monoclonal anti-DNA antibodies from autoimmune mice, *Biochemistry* **23**:2964–2970.

Nasa, H., Chia, D. S., Taniguchi, O., and Barnett, E. V., 1982, Characterization of antiF(ab')2 antibodies in SLE patients, *Clin. Immunol. Immunopathol.* **25**:80–84.

Papalian, M., Lafer, E., Wong, R., and Stollar, B. D., 1980, Reaction of SLE anti-native DNA antibodies with native DNA fragments from 20 to 1200 base pairs, *J. Clin. Invest.* **65**:469–477.

Parker, L. P., Hahn, B. H., and Osterland, C. K., 1974, Modification of NZB/NZW F_1 autoimmune disease by development of tolerance to DNA, *J. Immunol.* **113**:292–312.

Pearson, L., and Lightfoot, R. W., Jr., 1981, Correlation of DNA–anti-DNA association rates with clinical activity in SLE, *J. Immunol.* **126**:16–19.

Raptis, L., and Menard, H. A., 1980, Quantitation and characterization of plasma DNA in normals and patients with SLE, *J. Clin. Invest.* **66**:1391–1399.

Rauch, J., Murphy, E., Roths, J. B., Stollar, B. D., and Schwartz, R. S., 1982, A high frequency idiotypic marker of anti-DNA antibodies in MRL/lpr/lpr mice, *J. Immunol.* **129**:236–241.

Raveche, E. S., Novotny, E. A., Hansen, C. T., Tjio, J. H., and Steinberg, A. D., 1983, Genetic studies in NZB mice. V. Recombinant inbred lines demonstrate that separate genes control autoimmune phenomena, *J. Exp. Med.* **153**:1187–1197.

Robbins, W. C., Holman, J. R., Diecher, H., and Kunkel, H. G., 1957, Complement fixation with cell nuclei and DNA in lupus erythematosus, *Proc. Soc. Exp. Biol. Med.* **96**:575–579.

Rothfield, N. F., and Stollar, B. D., 1967, The relation of immunoglobulin class, pattern of antinuclear antibody, and complement-fixing antibodies to DNA in sera from patients with SLE, *J. Clin. Invest.* **46**:1785–1794.

Roths, J. B., 1979, in: *Genetic Control of Autoimmune Disease* (N. R. Rose, P. E. Bigazzi, and N. L. Warner, eds.), Elsevier/North-Holland, New York, pp. 207–217.

Roubinian, J. R., Talal, N., Greenspan, J. S., Goodman, J. R., and Siiteri, P. K., 1978, Effect of castration and sex hormone treatment on survival, anti-nucleic-acid antibodies and glomerulonephritis in NZB/NZW F_1 mice, *J. Exp. Med.* **147**:1568–1583.

Roubinian, J. R., Talal, N., Greenspan, J. S., Goodman, J. R., and Siiteri, P. K., 1979, Delayed androgen treatment prolongs survival in murine lupus, *J. Clin. Invest.* **63**:902–911.

Sano, H., Imokawa, M., Steinberg, A. D., and Morimoto, C., 1983, Accumulation of guanosine–cytosine enriched low MW DNA fragments in lymphocytes of patients with SLE, *J. Immunol.* **130**:187–190.

Schecter, Y., Maron, R., Elias, D., and Cohen, I. R., 1982, Autoantibodies to insulin receptor spontaneously develop as anti-idiotypes in mice immunized with insulin, *Science* **216**:452–454.

Schoenfeld, Y., Rauch, J., Massicotte, H., Datta, S. K., Andre-Schwartz, J., Stollar, B. D., and Schwartz, R. S., 1983, Polyspecificity of monoclonal lupus antibodies produced by human-human hybridomas, *N. Engl. J. Med.* **308**:414–418.

Seligmann, M., 1957, Mise en evidence dans le serum de malades atteints de lupus erythemateux dissemine d'une substance determinant une reaction de precipitation avec l'acide desoxyribonucleique, *C. R. Acad. Sci. (D) (Paris)* **245**:243–247.

Slack, J. H., Hang, L., Barkley, J., Fulton, R. J., D'Hoostelaere, L., Robinson, A., and Dixon, F. J., 1984, Isotypes of spontaneous and mitogen-induced autoantibodies in SLE-prone mice, *J. Immunol.* **132**:1271–1275.

Solomon, G., Schiffenbauer, J., Keiser, H. D., and Diamond, B., 1983, Use of monoclonal antibodies to identify shared idiotypes on human antibodies to DNA from patients with SLE, *Proc. Natl. Acad. Sci. U.S.A.* **80**:850–853.

Sonteheimer, R. D., and Gilliam, J. N., 1978, DNA antibody class, subclass, and complement fixation in SLE with and without nephritis, *Clin. Immunol. Immunopathol.* **10**:459–467.

Steinberg, A. D., Raveche, E. S., Laskin, C. A., Miller, M. L., and Steinberg, R. T., 1982, Genetic, environmental, and cellular factors in the pathogenesis of SLE, *Arthritis Rheum.* **25**:734–743.

Stollar, B. D., 1980, Reaction of systemic lupus erythematosus antinative DNA antibodies with native DNA fragments from 20 to 1200 base pairs, *J. Clin. Invest.* **65**:469–477.

Talal, N., 1980, Tolerance and autoimmunity, in: *Clinical Immunology* (C. P. Parker, ed.), W. B. Saunders, Philadelphia, pp. 105–109.

Talal, N., Dauphinee, M. J., and Wofsy, D., 1982, Interleukin-2 deficiency, genes, and SLE, *Arthritis Rheum.* **25**:838–842.

Tan, E. M., 1976, Sunlight as a potential aetiological factor in systemic lupus erythematosus, in: *Modern Topics in Rheumatology* (G. R. Hughes, ed.), Year Book Publishers, Chicago, pp. 99–106.

Tan, E. M., Schur, P. H., Carr, R. H., and Kunkel, H. G. 1966, DNA and antibodies to DNA in the serum of patients with SLE, *J. Clin. Invest.* **45**:1732–1740.

Taylor, R. P., Weber, D., Broccoli, A. V., and Winfield, J. R., 1979, Stability of DNA/anti-DNA complexes, *J. Immunol.* **122**:115–120.

Teitelbaum, D., Rauch, J., Stollar, B. D., and Schwartz, R. J. 1984, *In vivo* effects of antibodies against a high frequency idiotype of anti-DNA antibodies in MRL mice, *J. Immunol.* **132**:1282–1285.

Theofilopoulus, A. N., Shawler, D. L., Eisenberg, R. A., and Dixon, F. J., 1980, Splenic immunoglobulin secreting cells and their regulation in autoimmune mice, *J. Exp. Med.* **151**:446–466.

Weisbart, R. H., Garrett, R. A., Leibling, M. R., Barnett, E. V., Paulus, H. E., and Katz, D. H., 1983, Specificity of anti-nucleoside antibodies in SLE, *Clin. Immunol. Immunopathol.* **27**:403–411.

Williams, R. C., Jr., 1982, Cellular mechanism of tissue injury and immune derangement in SLE, *Arthritis Rheum.* **25**:810–813.

Wilson, J. G., Wong, W. W., Schur, P. H., and Fearon, D. T., 1982, Mode of inheritance of decreased C3b Receptors on erythrocytes of patients with systemic lupus erythematosus, *N. Engl. J. Med.* **307**:981–985.

Winfield, J. B., Faiferman, J., and Koffler, D., 1977, Avidity of anti-DNA antibodies in serum and IgG glomerular eluates from patients with SLE. Association of high avidity anti-native DNA antibody with glomerulonephritis, *J. Clin. Invest.* **59**:90–96.

9

Neuron-Reactive Antibodies in Systemic Lupus Erythematosus

Ken D. Pischel and Harry G. Bluestein

I. INTRODUCTION

Neuropsychiatric involvement is a frequent clinical problem in systemic lupus erythematosus (SLE), occuring in 25–60% of cases at some time during the course of the illness. As is true of the effects of SLE elsewhere, there are protean manifestations of central nervous system (CNS) dysfunction, but most commonly it presents as seizures or organic brain syndrome with psychosis and/or impaired mentation. Despite advances in understanding some of the mechanisms of tissue damage that affect other organs, the pathogenesis of the diffuse CNS involvement in SLE remains uncertain. Inflammatory destruction of small blood vessels, the major pathogenic mechanism affecting other organs, does not appear to play an important role in the CNS (Ellis and Verity, 1979; Johnson and Richardson, 1968). However, accumulating evidence suggests that autoantibodies reacting with cell surface molecules, the immune-mediated mechanism responsible for some of the hematological problems in SLE, is also a major contributor to the pathogenesis of much of lupus CNS disease.

II. AUTOANTIBODY HYPOTHESIS OF LUPUS NEUROPSYCHIATRIC DISEASE

Autoantibodies are a hallmark of SLE. Those that react with cell membrane structures, particularly on platelets, erythrocytes, and lymphocytes, have been intensively studied because of their pathogenic potential. The levels of those antibodies in serum of SLE

Ken. D. Pischel and Harry G. Bluestein • Division of Rheumatology, Department of Medicine, University of California Medical Center, San Diego, California 92103.

patients correlate with cytopenias and functional defects in the target cell type. It has been proposed that the pathogenesis of SLE CNS disease involves a similar sequence of events. However, it is not sufficient to have antibodies directed against neuronal tissue in the serum. One must also postulate an alteration of the blood–brain barrier that allows those antibodies to enter the CNS. Then the antineuronal antibodies may bind to neuronal membranes and interfere with their function (Bluestein and Zvaifler, 1983; Zvaifler and Bluestein, 1982).

A. Antineuronal Antibodies in SLE Sera

Antineuronal antibodies are frequently present in SLE patients' sera (Bluestein and Zvaifler, 1976). They have been detected by several different assay systems and shown to react with human brain tissue and cultured human neuronal cells (Bluestein and Zvaifler, 1976; Bluestein, 1978, 1979; Bresnihan *et al.*, 1979; H. A. Wilson *et al.*, 1979). Antineuronal activity has been quantitated using a human neuroblastoma cell line SK-N-SH (Biedler *et al.*, 1973). This cell line retains many neuronal features, including an electrically excitable membrane and normal brain surface antigens (West *et al.*, 1977) as shown by rabbit antisera raised against normal human brain tissue reacting with SK-N-SH cells and antisera to SK-N-SH cells binding to normal human brain tissue. This cell line has provided a reproducible substrate to evaluate the presence of antineuronal antibodies in SLE. By use of this cell line, neurocytotoxic antibodies have been demonstrated in the sera of 75% of SLE patients (Bresnihan *et al.*, 1979). These cytotoxic antibodies are reactive with cell surface antigens and may be removed by absorption with normal human brain or various cultured neuronal cell lines.

B. Heterogeneity and Cross Reactivities of Antineuronal Antibodies

The antineuronal antibodies, like others present in lupus sera, are heterogeneous and have complex cross-reactive patterns. Absorption studies have shown that most of the reactive sera also react with other neuronal-derived cell lines (LA-N-1 and IMR-32) as well as two glial cell lines (A-172 and U-118MG) (Bluestein, 1979). Forty percent of sera react with each cell line, 25% react with both neuronal and glial cells, 15% with neuronal but not glial cells, and none with just glial cells. Absorption studies of sera cytotoxic to all five cell lines provided further information about the target antigens. At least six antibody specificities were shown by this means (Bluestein, 1979).

Lymphocytes and neuronal cells express common antigens, as previously shown by cross absorption of antineuronal and antilymphocyte antibodies (Bluestein and Zvaifler, 1976). When lupus sera were absorbed with lymphocytes and neuronal cell lines, three distinct patterns were observed: (1) shared activity toward antigens present on both lymphoid and neuronal cells, usually seen for the majority of IgG activity but uncommonly with IgM; (2) neuron-reactive but lymphocyte-nonreactive antibodies, typically seen with IgM but rarely with IgG; and (3) lymphocyte-antigen-specific, neuronal-nonreactive antibodies, which were detected in a very small number of cases.

The finding that antineuronal antibodies are frequently present in SLE sera satisfies one requirement of the autoantibody model for the pathogenesis of CNS lupus, but the serum antineuronal levels from patients with active CNS lupus do not differ significantly from those of nonaffected SLE patients when a sensitive radioimmunoassay is used (Bluestein *et al.*, 1981). This may be because the antibodies' access to the CNS is normally limited by the blood–brain barrier. However, the lack of clinical correlation with serum antineuronal antibodies has not been a universal observation. Other studies that employed immunofluorenscence assays have reported an association between serum antineuronal levels and CNS disease activity (Brensnihan *et al.*, 1979; H. A. Wilson *et al.*, 1979). The reason for this difference is not clear but may relate to differences in assays. Bresnihan *et al.* (1979) measured an erythrocyte cross-reactive antigen, which probably represents a fraction of the antineuronal activity. The explanation for differences with H. A. Wilson *et. al.* (1979) is uncertain, as the target cell line (SK-N-SH) is the same, and may relate to differences in sensitivity between the indirect immunofluorescence and radioimmunobinding assays. The radioimmunoassay is the most all-encompassing, and, when applied to SLE sera, it fails to distinguish between those with and without CNS disease.

C. Elevated Cerebrospinal Fluid Antineuronal Antibodies with Active Disease

In order to test the second requirement of the autoantibody model (i.e., that entry of antineuronal antibody into the CNS is necessary to produce the clinical manifestations of diffuse CNS disease) a sensitive radioimmunoassay was developed to measure antibody in cerebrospinal fluid. It quantitatively measures IgG and IgM antibody binding to the SK-N-SH neuroblastoma cell line with either a direct or two-stage radioiodinated protein A binding assay (Bluestein *et al.*, 1981). Cerebrospinal fluid (CSF) provided an accessible intra-CNS source to test for antineuronal antibody. Lupus patients with active CNS disease had markedly elevated IgG antineuronal levels in their CSF compared to those individuals without neuropsychiatric manifestations and to appropriate controls (Bluestein, 1984; Bluestein *et al.*, 1981; Bluestein and Woods, 1982; Bluestein and Zvaifler, 1983). There was a small incidence of elevated IgG antineuronal binding in CSF from SLE patients without active CNS involvement, but it was at a low level (Fig. 1). Mean IgM antineuronal levels were elevated in all groups of SLE patients with or without active CNS manifes-

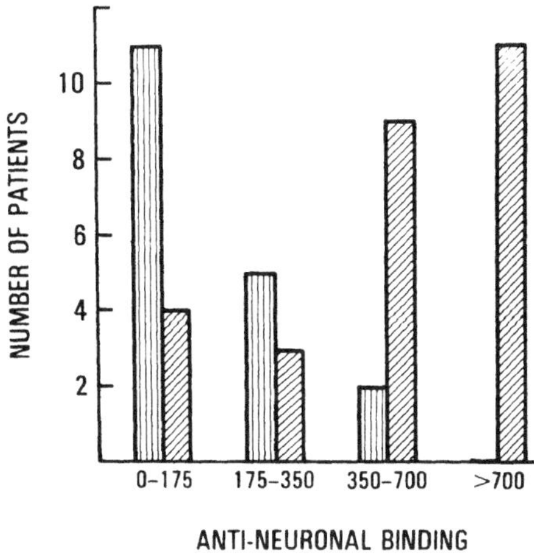

Figure 1. The frequency distribution of antineuronal activity in cerebrospinal fluid of SLE patients with (▨) or without (▥) active nervous system disease. The upper limit of normal for antineuronal binding in CSF is 350. (Reproduced with permission from Bluestein and Woods, 1982.)

tations, and although its levels were higher in patients with active CNS disease, IgM antineuronal titer was a poor discriminator of disease activity (Bluestein *et al.*, 1981). The IgG antineuronal activity was most elevated in patients with psychosis, organic brain syndrome, or generalized seizures, and it was a good indicator of neuropsychiatric involvement. These findings are consistent with the second premise of the autoantibody model, that antineuronal antibodies are present within the nervous system during exacerbations of CNS lupus.

D. Antineuronal Antibodies and Neuronal Dysfunction

The third tenet of the proposed autoantibody model, (i.e., that the interactions of antibodies with neuronal membrane antigens cause the CNS dysfunction) has not been demonstrated directly. However, it has been shown in animals that introducing antineuronal antibodies into the CSF may perturb neuronal function. The introduction of antibodies reactive with brain constituents causes convulsions, meningitis, impaired memory, and motor dysfunction (Kobiler *et al.*, 1976; Lassmann *et al.*, 1983; Rappaport *et al.*, 1978; Simon and Simon, 1975). In addition to their direct effects on neuronal function, those antibodies potentially could impair neurotransmitter function via antireceptor activities in an analogous fashion to the neuromuscular block of myasthenia gravis (reviewed by Biesecker and Koffler, 1983), and they could inhibit essential interactions between neurons and glia (Grumet *et al.*, 1983).

E. Antineuronal Levels in Subsets of CNS Lupus

Despite the supporting findings for the autoantibody model, it has been suggested that antineuronal antibodies are elevated in active CNS disease as a secondary phenomenon. According to that alternative explanation, vascular damage itself causes the dysfunction and only incidentally allows antineuronal antibodies to enter the CNS. Evidence against this possibility is the observation that the lupus patients with focal neurological deficits secondary to vascular damage are less likely than those with more common global syndromes to have elevated IgG antineuronal activity in the CSF. Patients with the more diffuse neuropsychiatric manifestations such as psychosis, generalized seizures, or organic brain syndrome generally do not have vasculitis on pathological examination, but most have elevated IgG antineuronal levels (75–90% of cases), whereas those with localized lesions such as hemiparesis caused by arterial disease have a much lower incidence (10–25%). Thus, the high levels of antineuronal antibodies in the CNS do not appear to be secondary to those vascular events that are known to be involved in the pathogenesis of lupus neurological disease.

Cerebrospinal fluid antineuronal antibodies were not elevated in one subset of CNS lupus patients, those with the involuntary movement disorders chorea and hemiballismus. Initially, that was surprising, since serum antibodies to neurons in the basal ganglia had been previously demonstrated in studies of Sydenham's chorea and Huntington's disease (Husby *et al.*, 1976, 1977). However, in those diseases, the antibody reactivity is restricted to differentiation antigens unique to the subthalamic and caudate nuclei. It is possible that similar antibodies exist in the CSF of SLE patients with chorea but were not detected because the target antigens are not expressed on SK-N-SH cells. The recent finding of system-specific antigens on limbic system neurons (Levitt, 1984) further reinforces the importance of developing assays capable of detecting antibodies to neuronal differentiation antigens.

The strong correlation of elevated antineuronal antibodies in CSF with clinically active CNS lupus has made the antineuronal radioimmunoassay the most useful clinical laboratory test for diagnosing active SLE neuropsychiatric disease. Elevated levels are detected in 90% of lupus patients with diffuse CNS disease but in fewer than 5% of SLE patients with neurological problems from causes other than lupus. Often, CNS disease coincides with flares of other aspects of lupus; thus, it is not surprising that hypocomplementemia and high titers of antibody to DNA correlate with SLE CNS disease (Sergent *et al.*, 1975; Feinglass *et al.*, 1976). However, those tests are not reliable for diagnosis in those patients whose neuropsychiatric disorder is their sole lupus manifestation. The classic lupus serologies, complement, and DNA antibodies are rarely abnormal in those situations (Winfield *et al.*, 1978).

III. FACTORS REGULATING CSF ANTINEURONAL LEVELS

Little is known about the critical factors regulating the level of antineuronal antibodies in the CSF. Even the source of the antibodies, whether they originate from the circulation or are synthesized locally, is controversial. Normally, serum proteins have limited access to the CSF, being blocked at both the choroid plexus and the cerebral capillaries.

A. Choroid Plexus Transfer of Proteins

In the choroid plexus, the access of proteins to the CSF is normally restricted by the tight junctions between cells adjoining the epithelial basement membrane (Brightman and Reese, 1969) and not by the capillary endothelium, which is fenestrated. Access of antibodies to the CSF is further restricted by interstitial cells having Fc receptors (Husby *et al.*, 1979). Nevertheless, the choroid plexus has been considered a possible alternative route by which proteins from the circulation could gain access to the CSF. Immunofluorescense and electron microscopy have shown immune complexes deposited in the choroid plexus walls (Atkins *et al.*, 1972; Boyer *et al.*, 1980; Gershwin *et al.*, 1975; Davis *et al.*, 1978; Sher and Pertschuk, 1974). Deposition of immune complexes and complement components could damage these tight junctions. In a rabbit model, circulating immune complexes of BSA–anti-BSA antibodies were found to deposit in the choroid plexus (Harbeck *et el.*, 1979), followed by proportional rises in CSF albumin and IgG levels, suggesting a breakdown of the blood–CSF barrier. Immune reactants have been detected in the choroid plexus of SLE patients, but they are found in material from patients with or without a history of CNS disease. In fact, the rich capillary bed of the choroid seems to act as a nonspecific trap for immune complexes; thus, the presence of deposits is of uncertain importance.

B. Transendothelial Transfer of Proteins

An alternative site for immunoglobulin to enter the CSF is via the cerebral capillaries. Proteins are selectively transported across capillary endothelial cells by microcytosis, after which they appear to percolate through the tissue and enter the CSF (Broadwell *et al.*, 1983). The rate of this transport process may be accelerated by various factors, including ischemic injury, increased vascular pressure, or infusion of hypertonic solutions of 5-hydroxytryptamine (serotonin) (Westergaard, 1977). In SLE, vascular injury from immune complexes or thrombosis could lead to accelerated IgG influx. Although pathological examination so far has shown little frank vasculitis, there is evidence of vascular damage. Microinfarcts occur in brain tissue, and proliferative changes similar to those associated with hypertensive encephalopathy and thrombotic thrombocytopenic purpura have been seen in small vessels (Ellis and Verity, 1979; Johnson and Richardson, 1968). These changes resemble those seen in the coronary arteries of autoimmune strains of mice, many of which develop coronary thrombosis (Accinni and Dixon, 1979; Dixon, 1983). These vascular changes may allow the leak of serum proteins into the nervous system. The empirical observation that CNS disease is associated with dermal vasculitis and arteritis (Feinglass *et al.*, 1976) supports the concept of vascular damage contributing to CNS disease. Why the complexes, if they are, in fact, present in the small vessels of the brain, do not result in an inflammatory response is not understood, but it could reflect inhibitory effects of glial cells on the inflammatory response (Dick *et al.*, 1983) or differences in the type of immune complexes that lodge in the cerebral vessels. For example, it has been suggested that CNS disease is associated with small aggregates and renal disease with large ones (Tung *et al.*, 1981).

C. Local Synthesis of Antineuronal Antibodies

Another mechanism to account for the presence of antineuronal antibodies, besides entry from the circulation, is local synthesis within the CNS, such as has been described in multiple sclerosis and subacute sclerosing panencephalitis (Ewan and Lachmann, 1979; Tourtellotte, 1970). In those conditions, IgG levels in the CSF are elevated disproportionately in comparison with albumin and other plasma proteins (Tibbling *et al.*, 1977). This selective IgG elevation is also found in the CSF from SLE patients. The IgG index, which computes the relative IgG (albumin ratios in CSF and serum), has been used in multiple sclerosis to quantitatively express the disproportionate elevation of CSF IgG. In one study of CSF from 19 patients with CNS lupus, the IgG index was reportedly elevated in 25%, and all of those with high indices also had oligoclonal IgG bands on isoelectric focusing of the CSF (Winfield *et al.*, 1983).

The combination of restricted heterogeneity of the CSF IgG and the selective increase in IgG concentration was interpreted as evidence for antibody production within the nervous system in a subset of patients with neuropsychiatric manifestations of SLE. However, some caution may be appropriate in interpreting those findings. In our experience, the IgG index is frequently elevated in SLE regardless of the presence of clinically apparent CNS disease (Table 1). This index elevation may be seen with normal CSF IgG levels because of low albumin levels, which underscores the fallibility of relying stringently on the IgG index to determine CSF synthesis. Furthermore, oligoclonal bands have been detected in a variety of nonimmunologic neurological conditions, including acute infarctions (Lin and Kostulas, 1983; Hershey and Trotter, 1980). An influential argument against local synthesis in lupus is that, in contrast to multiple sclerosis, immunoglobulin-secreting lymphocytes or plasma cells have not been seen in the CNS of affected SLE patients.

It is not necessary to invoke intrathecal IgG synthesis to account for its disproportionate elevation in some lupus CSF. Possible explanations include: (1) selective entry of IgG as compared to albumin into the CSF, perhaps enhanced by the Fc-receptor-bearing cells in the choroid plexus; (2) more rapid clearance of albumin as compared to IgG from the CSF; and (3) disproportionate retention of IgG complexed with antigen. Immune complexes have been found in CSF from SLE patients in association with active CNS disease by some investigators (Keeffe *et al.*, 1974; Sebold *et al.*, 1982) but not by others (Winfield *et al.*, 1983). In many of the reported cases, immune complexes were detected in CSF but not in the patient's serum. That suggested that the complexes had formed within the CNS, although the antibody may have come from the circulation. Since a significant portion of the CSF IgG is antineuronal antibody, it seems reasonable to assume that after leaking across the blood–brain barrier, those antibodies bind to and subsequently are shed from neuronal membranes. That could cause a relative increase in CSF IgG as compared to albumin and account for the increased specific activity of antineuronal activity in CSF as compared to serum (Bluestein *et al.*, 1981). The similarity in binding specificity of the antineuronal antibodies in CSF and serum lends further support to the serum origin of CSF IgG antineuronal antibody.

IV. ANTIGENIC TARGETS OF ANTINEURONAL ANTIBODIES

Just as the site of antineuronal antibody production and the regulators of CSF antineuronal antibody levels are of great interest, so too is the identification of the specific antigens inducing and reacting with the antineuronal antibodies. Although absorptions using neuronal cell lines suggest that several antigens are involved (Bluestein, 1979), an attractive possibility is that much of the antigenic complexity may be explained by cross reactivity of similar molecules containing related structures, such as those that occur between phospholipids and polynucleotides with SLE antibodies (Lafer *et al.*, 1981).

The stimulating antigens for these antibodies have not been identified, and it may be difficult to do so given the complexity of their cross reactivities. The inducing antigens for antineuronal antibodies might be neuronal in origin and somehow be released into the circulation, perhaps by damage to neuronal tissue, invasion by immune cells, transfer by infectious particles, or transport into the blood across cerebral endothelium (Broadwell *et al.*, 1983; Van Deurs, 1977; Wagner *et al.*, 1974). Alternatively, the stimulating

Table 1. Cerebrospinal Fluid IgG Index in SLE

CNS disease[a]	Number tested	Number elevated[b]	IgG index[c] (mean ± S.E.M)
+	31	18	0.70 ± 0.06
−	20	14	0.86 ± 0.1

[a] +, clinically apparent neuropsychiatric manifestations of SLE; −, no evidence of CNS lupus.
[b] IgG index > 0.6.
[c] IgG index = $(IgG_{CSF} \times Albumin_{serum})/(IgG_{serum} \times Albumin_{CSF})$.

antigens may exist outside the nervous system and share immunoreactive determinants with identical or similar molecules residing on neuronal cells. An example of such an antigen is asialo-GM_1, a neutral glycolipid present on lymphoid cells (Nakahara *et al.*, 1980; Young *et al.*, 1980) and in the brain. Some SLE patients with neurological disease form antibody to that molecule (Hirano *et al.*, 1980). Many potentially cross-reactive antigens exist on both hemopoietic cells and neuroectoderm-derived cells, including HNK-1 (Lipinski *et al.*, 1983), HLA-DR (Carrel *et al.*, 1982), BA2 (Kemshed *et al.*, 1982), Leu-4 (Garson *et al.*, 1982), GM_2 (Tai *et al.*, 1983), and spectrin (Lazarides and Nelson, 1983) (see Table 2). Further intriguing possibilities include phospholipid structures present in the membranes that may cross react with DNA and phospholipid molecules (Lafer *et al.*, 1981).

Studies using antigenic material from serum cryoprecipitates reinforce the idea that antigens in the circulation may stimulate antineuronal antibodies. The cryoglobulins from SLE patients contain proportionally elevated amounts of antilymphocyte antibody (Winfield *et al.*, 1975; Zvaifler and Bluestein, 1976), postulated to be complexed with antigens. Rabbit sera raised against these cryoglobulins frequently reacted with antigens on lymphocytes (Klippel *et al.*, 1979), and many of the reactive sera also contained antibodies to neuronal cells (Bluestein *et al.*, 1978). Thus, the lupus cryoglobulins contain molecules that share antigenic determinants with human neurons. The neuron-reactive antibodies in SLE sera and in anticryoglobulin sera have a similar pattern of cross reactivity to several neural and glial cell lines (Bluestein and Woods, 1982). Furthermore, in both cases, brain is able to remove the antineuronal and antilymphocyte reactivity, whereas lymphocytes only partially deplete antineuronal activity (Bluestein, 1983; Bluestein and Woods, 1982; Bluestein and Zvaifler, 1983). This suggests that the natural immunogens for the antineuronal reactivities are not all represented on the surface of lymphocytes. Additionally, the immunogen does not appear to be from normal human serum proteins, platelets, or human erythrocytes (Bluestein, 1984). Nevertheless, molecules sharing antigenic determinants with neurons are present in the circulation, and the SLE antineuronal antibodies could result from an immune response to them. Further work is needed to delineate the stimulatory molecules and those of neuronal cells with which they react. Once the target antigens are identified, a proper test of the capacity of antibodies that bind to them to interfere with neuronal function can be constructed.

V. CONCLUSION

The evidence to support an autoantibody-mediated pathogenesis for the major CNS manifestations of SLE has been reviewed. The autoantibody hypothesis has three requirements: (1) antibodies reactive with neuronal cells are present; (2) these antibodies need to gain access to the nervous system; and (3) once within the CNS, the antibodies react with their target antigens, resulting in neuronal dysfunction (Bluestein, 1984; Bluestein and Zvaifler, 1983). It has been shown that antineuronal antibodies are present in SLE, and they probably originate from the circulation, although intrathecal synthesis is possible. Implied in the model is the need for concomitant vasculopathy. Whether the blood–brain barrier is disrupted at the capillary level, at the choroid plexus, or both is not known. Immune complexes probably contribute to the disruption of the blood–brain barrier at

Table 2. Common Neuronal–Lymhocyte Surface Antigens

Antigen	Neuronal cell type	Lymphocyte cell type
Acetylcholine receptor	Neurons (Rotter *et al.*, 1979)	Lymphocytes (Fuchs *et al.*, 1980)
Asialo-GM_1	Brain (Svennerholm, 1963)	Lymphocytes (Nakahara *et al.*, 1980; Young *et al.*, 1980)
BA2	Neuroblastomas (Kemshead *et al.*, 1982)	Leukemia and progenitor cells (Kersey *et al.*, 1981)
CALLA	Glioma (Carrel *et al.*, 1982)	Lymphoblastoid leukemia (Ritz *et al.*, 1980)
Fc Receptor	Oligodendrocytes (Ma *et al.*, 1981)	T lymphocytes (Yoshida and Anderson, 1972)
		B lymphocytes (Basten *et al.*, 1972)
F10-44-2	Brain (Dalchau *et al.*, 1980)	T lymphocytes (Dalchau *et al.*, 1980)
HNK-1	Neuroectoderm (Lipinski *et al.*, 1983)	NK lymphocytes (Abo and Balch, 1981)
HLA-DR	Melanomas (Winchester *et al.*, 1978)	B lymphocytes (Winchester *et al.*, 1975)
	Neuroectoderm (B. S. Wilson *et al.*, 1979)	T lymphocytes (Fu *et al.*, 1978)
IL-2 Receptor	Oligodendrocytes (Merrill *et al.*, 1984)	T lymphocytes (Leonard *et al.*, 1982)
Leu-4	Purkinje cells (Garson *et al.*, 1982)	T lymphocytes (Kaneoka *et al.*, 1983)
OKT9	Neuroblastoma (Kemshead *et al.*, 1982)	Immature thymocytes (Kung *et al.*, 1979)
OKT8	Oligodendrocytes (Oger *et al.*, 1982)	Suppressor T lymphocytes (Reinherz *et al.*, 1980)
Opiate Receptors	Brain (Hiller *et al.*, 1973)	Lymphocytes (Wybran *et al.*, 1979)
PC.1	Brain (Takahashi *et al.*, 1970)	B lymphocytes (Takahashi, 1970)
T, Tn	Nerve tissue (trace) (Springer *et al.*, 1979)	T lymphomas (Springer, 1984)
		Thymomas (Springer, 1984)
Thy 1	Neurons (Reif and Allen, 1964)	Lymphocytes (Golub, 1971; Ritter *et al.*, 1983)
Thy 2	Brain tissue (Siadak and Nowinski, 1981)	Thymocytes (Siadak and Nowinski, 1981)

either site, explaining why CNS disease may correlate with indices of systemic disease activity, but interestingly, the complexes typically do not induce an associated inflammatory cell response. Unique properties of the cerebral vasculature may inhibit the usual pattern of inflammation. Once antibodies enter the CNS, they may interact with neuronal and glial membranes, and they may interfere with those cells' functions in a reversible manner. Although not directly shown with patients' sera, experimental models demonstrate such effects. Correction of the perturbations may lead to a rapid recovery. Current studies of the vascular lesions and antineuronal specificities are examining the important details of antigenic cross reaction and factors modulating CFS antineuronal IgG levels and are thereby continuing to test the antineuronal antibody hypothesis for the pathogenesis of CNS lupus.

REFERENCES

Abo, T., and Balch, C. M., 1981, A differentiation antigen of human NK and K Cells identified by a monoclonal antibody (HNK-1), *J. Immunol.* **127**:1024–1029.

Accinni, L., and Dixon, F. J., 1979, Degenerative vascular disease and myocardial infarction in mice with lupus-like syndrome, *Am. J. Pathol.* **96**:447–492.

Atkins, C. J., Kondon, J., Quismorio, F. P., and Friou, G., 1972, The choroid plexus in systemic lupus erythematosus, *Ann. Intern. Med.* **76**:65–72.

Basten, A., Miller, J. F. A. P., Sprent, M. J., and Pye, J., 1972, A receptor for antibody on B lymphocytes, *J. Exp. Med.* **135**:610–626.

Biedler, J. L., Helson, L., and Spengler, B. A, 1973, Morphology and growth, tumorigenicity, and cytogenetics of human neuroblastoma cells in continuous culture, *Cancer Res.* **33**:2643–2652.

Biesecker, G., and Koffler, D., 1983, Immunology of myasthenia gravis, *Hum. Pathol.* **14**:419–423.

Bluestein, H. G., 1978, Neurocytotoxic antibodies in serum of patients with systemic lupus erythematosus *Proc. Natl. Acad. Sci. U.S.A.* **75**:3965–3969.

Bluestein, H. G., 1979, Heterogeneous neurocytotoxic antibodies in systemic lupus erythematosus, *Clin. Exp. Immunol.* **35**:210–217.

Bluestein, H. G., 1984, Antineuronal antibodies in the pathogenesis of neuropsychiatric manifestations of systemic lupus erythematosus, in: *Neuroimmunology* (P. O. Behan and F. Spreafico, eds.), Raven Press, New York, pp. 157–165.

Bluestein, H. G., and Woods, V. L., Jr., 1982, Antineuronal antibodies in systemic lupus erythematosus, *Arthritis Rheum.* **25**:773–778.

Bluestein, H. G., and Zvaifler, N. J., 1976, Brain-reactive lymphoctotoxic antibodies in the serum of patients with systemic lupus erythematosus, *J. Clin. Invest.* **57**:509–516.

Bluestein, H. G., and Zvaifler, N. J., 1983, Antibodies reactive with central nervous system antigens, *Human Pathol.* **14**:424–428.

Bluestein, H. G., Klippel, J. H., and Zvaifler, N. J. 1978, Antibodies to neuronal cells in antisera to SLE cryoproteins, *Arthritis Rheum.* **21**:546.

Bluestein, H. G., Williams, G. W., and Steinberg, A. D., 1981, Cerebrospinal fluid antibodies to neuronal cells: Association with neuropsychiatric manifestations of systemic lumps erythematosus, *Am. J. Med.* **70**:241–246.

Boyer, R. S., Sun, N. C., Verity, M. A., Nies, K. M., and Louie, J. S., 1980, Immunoperoxidase staining of the choroid plexus in systemic lupus erythematosus, *J. Rheumatol.* **7**:645–650.

Bresnihan, B., Oliver, M., Williams, B., and Hughes, G. R. V., 1979, An antineuronal antibody cross-reactivity with erythrocytes and lymphocytes in systemic lupus erythematosus, *Arthritis Rheum.* **22**:313–320.

Brightman, M. W., and Reese, T. S., 1969, Junctions between intimately opposed cell membranes in the vertebrate brain, *J. Cell. Biol.* **40**:648–677.

Broadwell, R. D., Balin, B. J., Salcman, M., and Kaplan, R. S., 1983, Brain–blood barrier? Yes and no, *Proc. Natl. Acad. Sci. U.S.A.* **80**:7352–7356

Carrel, S., de Tribolet, N., and Gross, N., 1982, Expression of HLA-DR and common acute lymphoblastic leukemia antigens on glioma cells, *Eur. J. Immunol.* **12:**12:354–357.

Dalchau, R., Kirkley, J., and Fabre, J. W., 1980, Monoclonal antibody to a human brain-granulocyte T lymphocyte antigen probably homologous to the W 3/13 antigen of the rat, *Eur. J. Immunol.* **10:**745–749.

Davis, J. A., Weisman, M. H., and Dail, D. H., 1978, Vascular disease in infective endocarditis, *Arch. Intern. Med.* **138:**480–483.

Dick, S. J., Macchi, B., Papazoglou, S., Oldfield, E. H., Kornblith, P. L., Smith, B. H., and Gately, M. K., 1983, Lymphoid cell–glioma cell interaction enhances cell coat production by human gliomas: Novel suppressor mechanism, *Science* **220:**739–742.

Dixon, F. J., 1982, Murine SLE—an overview, *Arthritis Rheum.* **25:**721–725.

Ellis, S. G., and Verity, M. A.. 1979, Central nervous system involvement in systemic lupus erythematosus: A review of neuropathologic findings in 57 cases, 1955–1977, *Semin. Arthritis Rheum.* **8:***212–221.*

Ewan, P. W., and Lachmann, P. J., 1979, IgG synthesis within the brain in multiple sclerosis and subacute sclerosing panencephalitis, *Clin. Exp. Immunol.* **35:**227–235.

Feinglass, E. J., Arnett, F. C., Dorsch, C. A., Zizac, T. M., and Stevens, M. B., 1976, Neuropsychiatric manifestations of systemic lupus erythematosus: Diagnosis, clinical spectrum, and relationship to other features of the disease, *Medicine* **55:**323–339.

Fu, S. M., Chiorazzi, N., Wang, C. Y., Montazeri, G., Kunkel, H. G., Ko, H. S., and Gottlieb, A. B., 1979, Ia-bearing T lymphocytes in man, *J. Exp. Med.* **148:**1423–1428.

Fuchs, S., Schmidt-Hopfeld, I., Tridente, G., and Tarrab-Hazdai, R., 1980, Thymic lymphocytes bear a surface antigen which cross-reacts with acetylocholine receptor, *Nature* **287:**162–164.

Garson, J. A., Beverley, P. C. L., Coakham, H. B., and Harper, E. I., 1982, Monoclonal antibodies against human T lymphocytes label Purkinje neurones of many species, *Nature* **298:**375–377.

Gershwin, M. E., Hyman, L. R., Steinberg, A. D., 1975, The choroid plexus in CNS involvement of systemic lupus erythematosus, *J. Pediat.* **87:**588–590.

Golub, E. S., 1971, Brain-associated θ antigen: Reactivity of rabbit anti-mouse brain with mouse lymphoid cells, *Cell. Immunol.* **2:**353–361.

Grumet, M., Rutishauser, U., and Edelman, G. M., 1983, Neuron–glia adhesion is inhibited by antibodies to neural determinants, *Science* **222:**60–62.

Harbeck, R. J., Hoffman, A. A., Hoffman, S. A., and Shucard, D. W., 1979, Cerebrospinal fluid and the choroid plexus during acute immune complex disease, *Clin. Immunol. Immunopathol.* **13:**413–425.

Hershey, L. A., and Trotter, J. L., 1980, The use and abuse of the cerebrospinal fluid profile in the adult: A practical evaluation, *Ann. Intern. Med.* **80:**426–434.

Hiller, J. M., Pearson, J., and Simon, E. J., 1973, Distribution of stereospecific binding of the potent narcotic analgesic etorphine in the human brain: Predominance in the limbic system, *Res. Commun. Chem. Pathol. Pharmacol.* **6:**1052–1062.

Hirano, T., Hashimoto, H., and Shiokawa, Y., 1980, Antiglycolipid autoantibody detected in the sera from systemic lupus erythematosus patients, *J. Clin. Invest.* **66:**1437–1440.

Husby, G., van de Rijn, I., Zabriskie, J. B., Abdin, Z. H., and Williams, R. C., Jr., 1976, Antibodies reacting with cytoplasm of subthalamic and caudate nuclei neurons in chorea and acute rheumatic fever, *J. Exp. Med.* **144:**1094–1110.

Husby, G., Li, L., Davis, L. E., Wedge, E., Kokmen, E., and Williams, R. C., Jr., 1977, Antibodies to human caudate nucleus neurons in Huntington's chorea, *J. Clin. Invest.* **59:**922–932.

Husby, G., Williams, R. C., Jr., and Wedege, E., 1979, Huntington's disease, antineuronal antibodies, brain antigens, and receptors of IgG in human choroid plexus, *Adv. Neurol.* **23:**435–442.

Johnson, R. T., and Richardson, E. P., 1968, The neurological manifestations of systemic lupus erythematosus: A clinical–pathological study of 24 cases and review of the literature, *Medicine* **47:**337–369.

Kaneoka, H., Perez-Rojas, G., Sasasuki, T., Benike, C. J., and Engleman, E. G., 1983, Human T lymphocyte proliferation induced by a pan-T monoclonal antibody (anti-leu 4): Heterogeneity of response is a function of monocytes, *J. Immunol.* **131:**158–164.

Keeffe, E. B., Bardana, E. J., Harbeck, R. J., Pirofsky, B., and Carr, R. I., 1974, Lupus meningitis: Antibody to deoxyribonucleic acid (DNA) and DNA : anti-DNA complexes in cerebrospinal fluid, *Ann. Intern. Med.* **80:**58–60.

Kemshead, J. T., Fristchy, J., Asser, U., Sutherland, R., and Greaves, M. F., 1982, Monoclonal antibodies defining markers with apparent selectivity for particular haemopoietic cell types may also detect antigens on cells of neural crest origin, *Hybridoma* **1:**109–123.

Kersey, J. H., Lebien, T. W. Abramson, C. S., Newman, R. A., Sutherland, R., and Greaves, M. F., 1981, A human leukemia-associated and lymphohemopoietic progenitor cell surface structure identified with monoclonal antibody, *J. Exp. Med.* **153**:726–731.

Klippel, J. H., Bluestein, H. G., and Zvaifler, N. J., 1979, Lymphocyte reactivity of antisera to cryoproteins in systemic lupus erythematosus, *Clin. Immunol. Immunopathol.* **12**:52–61.

Kobiler, D., Fuchs, S., and Samuel, D., 1976, The effect of antisynaptosomal plasma membrane antibodies on memory, *Brain Res.* **115**:129–138.

Kung, P. C., Goldstein, G., Rheinherz, E. L., and Schlossman, S. F., 1979, Monoclonal antibodies defining distinctive human T-cell surface antigens, *Science* **206**:347–349.

Lafer, E. M., Rauch, J., Andrzejewski, C., Jr., Mudd, D., Furie, B., Furie, B., Schwartz, R. S., and Stollar, B. D., 1981, Polyspecific monoclonal lupus autoantibodies reactive with both polynucleotides and phospholipids, *J. Exp. Med.* **153**:897–909.

Lassmann, H., Stemberger, H., Kitz, K., and Wisniewski, H. M., 1983, *In vivo* demyelinating activity of sera from animals with chronic experimental allergic encephalomyelitis. Antibody nature of the demyelinating factor and the role of complement, *J. Neurol. Sci.* **59**:123–137.

Lazarides, E., and Nelson, W. J., 1983, Erythrocyte and brain forms of spectrin in cerebellum: Distinct membrane–cytoskeletal domains in neurons, *Science* **220**:1295–1296.

Leonard, W. J., Depper, J. M., Uchiyama, T., Smith, K. A., Waldman, T. A., and Greene, W. C., 1982, A monoclonal antibody that appears to recognize the receptor for human T-cell growth factor, partial characterization of the receptor, *Nature* **300**:267–269.

Levitt, P., 1984, A monoclonal antibody to limbic system neurons, *Science* **223**:299–301.

Link, H., and Kostulas, V., 1983, Utility of isoelectric focusing of cerebrospinal fluid and serum on agarose evaluated for neurological patients, *Clin. Chem.* **29**:810–815.

Lipinski, M., Braham, K., Caillaud, J., Carlu, C., and Tursz, T., 1983, HNK-1 antibody detects an antigen expressed on neuroectodermal cells, *J. Exp. Med.* **158**:1775–1780.

Ma, B. I., Joseph, B. S., Walsh, M. J., Potvin, A. R., and Tourtellotte, W. W., 1981, Multiple sclerosis serum and cerebrospinal fluid immunoglobulin binding to Fc receptors of oligodendrocytes, *Ann. Neurol.* **9**:371–377.

Merrill, J. E., Kutsunai, S., Mohlstrom, C., Hofman, F., Groopman, J., and Golde, D. W., 1984, Proliferation of astroglia and oligodendroglia in response to human T cell-derived factors, *Science* **224**:1428–1430.

Nakahara, K., Ohashi, T., Oda, T., Hirano, T., Kasai, M., Okumura, K., and Tada, T., 1980, Asialo GM_1 as a cell surface marker detected in acute lymphoblastic leukemia, *N. Engl. J. Med.* **302**:674–677.

Oger, J., Szuchet, S., Antel, J., and Arnason, B. G. W., 1982, A monoclonal antibody against human T suppressor lymphocytes binds specifically to the surface of cultured oligodendrocytes, *Nature* **295**:66–68.

Rappaport, M. M., Karpiak, S. E., and Mahadik, S. P., 1978, Biological activities of antibodies injected into the brain, *Fed. Proc.* **38**:2391–2396.

Reif, A. E., and Allen, J. M., 1964, The AKR thymic antigen and its distbribution in leukemias and nervous tissues, *J. Exp. Med.* **120**:413–433.

Reinherz, E. L., Kung, P. C., Goldstein, G., Levey, R. H., and Schlossman, S. F., 1980, Discrete stages of human intrathymic differentiation: Analysis of normal thymocytes and leukemic lymphoblasts of T-cell lineage, *Proc. Natl. Acad. Sci. U.S.A.* **77**:1588–1592.

Ritter, M. A., Sauvage, C. A., and Delia, D., 1983, Human thy-1 antigen: Cell surface expression on early T and B lymphocytes, *Immunology* **49**:555–564.

Ritz, J., Pesando, J. M., Notis-McConarty, J., Lazarus, H., and Schlossman, S. F., 1980, A monoclonal antibody to human acute lymphoblastic leukemia antigen, *Nature* **283**:583–585.

Rotter, A., Birdsall, N. J. M., Burgen, A. S. V., Field, P. M., Hulme, E. C., and Raisman, G., 1979, Muscarinic receptors in the central nervous system of the rat, *Brain Res. Rev.* **1**:141–165.

Seibold, J. R., Buckingham, R. B., Medsger, T. A., Jr., and Kelly, R. H., 1982, Cerebrospinal fluid immune complexes in systemic lupus erythematosus involving the central nervous system, *Semin. Arthritis Rheum.* **12**:68–76.

Sergent, J. S., Lockshin, M. D., Klempner, M. S., and Lipsky, B. A., 1975, Central nervous system disease in systemic lupus erythematosus—therapy and prognosis, *Am. J. Med.* **58**:644–654.

Sher, J. H., and Pertschuk, L. P., 1974, Immunoglobulin G deposits in the choroid plexus of a child with systemic lupus erythematosus, *Pediatrics* **85**:385–387.

Siadak, A. W., and Nowinski, R. C., 1981, Thy-2: A murine thymocyte–brain alloantigen controlled by a

Simon, J., and Simon, O., 1975, Effects of passive transfer of antibrain antibodies to a normal recipient, *Exp. Neurol.* **47**:523–534.

Springer, G. F., 1984, T and Tn, general carcinoma antigens, *Science* **244**:1198–1206.

Springer, G. F., Desai, P. R., Murthy, M. S., Tegtmeyer, H., and Scanlon, E. F., 1979, Human carcinoma-associated precursor antigens of the blood group MN system and the host's immune response to them, *Prog. Allergy* **26**:42–96.

Svennerholm, L., 1963, Chromatographic separation of human brain gangliosides, *J. Neurochem* **10**:613–623.

Tai, T. T., Paulson, J. C., Cahan, L. D., and Irie, R. F., 1983, Ganglioside GM_2 as a human tumor antigen (OFA-I-1), *Proc. Natl. Acad. Sci. U.S.A.* **80**:5392–5396.

Takahashi, T., Old, L. J., and Boyse, E. A., 1970, Surface alloantigens of plasma cells, *J. Exp. Med.* **131**:1325–1341.

Tibbling, G., Link, U. H., and Ohman, S., 1977, Principles of albumin and IgG analysis in neurologic disorders. I. Establishment of reference values, *Scand. J. Clin. Lab Invest.* **37**:385–390.

Tourtellotte, W. W., 1970, On cerebrospinal fluid IgG quoitients in multiple sclerosis and other diseases, *J. Neurol. Sci.* **10**:279–304.

Tung, K. S., DeHoratius, R. J., and Williams, R. C., Jr., 1981, Studies of circulating immune complex size in systemic lupus erythematosus, *Clin. Exp. Immunol.* **43**:615–625.

Van Deurs, B., 1977, Vesicular transport of horseradish peroxidase from brain to blood in segments of the cerebral microvasculature in adult mice, *Brain Res.* **124**:1–8.

Wagner, H. J., Pilgrim, C., and Brandl, J., 1974, Penetration and removal of horseradish peroxidase injected into the cerebrospinal fluid. Role of cerebral perivascular spaces, endothelium, and microglia, *Acta Neuropathol.* **27**:299–315.

West, G. J., Uki, J., Herschman, H. R., and Seeger, R. C., 1977, Andrenergic, cholinergic and inactive human neuroblastoma cell lines with the action potential Na^+ ionophore, *Cancer Res.* **37**:1372–1376.

Westergaard, E., 1977, The blood–brain barrier to horseradish peroxidase under normal and experimental conditions, *Acta Neuropathol.* **39**:181–187.

Wilson, B. S., Indiveri, F., Pellegrino, M. A., and Ferrone, S., 1979, DR (Ia-like) antigens on human melanoma cells, *J. Exp. Med.* **149**:658–668.

Wilson, H. A., Winfield, J. B., Lahita, R. G., and Koffler, D., 1979, Association of IgG antibrain antibodies with central nervous system dysfunction in systemic lupus erythematosus, *Arthritis Rheum.* **22**:458–462.

Winchester, R. J., Fu, S. M., Wernet, P., Kunkel, H. G., Dupont, B., and Jersild, C., 1975, Recognition by pregnancy serums of non-HLA alloantigens selectively expressed on B lymphocytes, *J. Exp. Med.* **141**:924–928.

Winchester, R. J., Wang, C., Gibofsky, A., Kunkel, H. G., Lloyd, K. O., and Old, L. J., 1978, Expression of Ia-like antigens on cultured human malignant melanoma cell lines, *Proc. Natl. Acad. Sci. U.S.A.* **75**:6235–6239.

Winfield, J. B., Winchester, R. J., Wernet, P., and Kunkel, J. G., 1975, Specific concentration of antilymphocyte antibodies in the serum cryoprecipitates of patients with systemic lupus erythematosus, *Clin. Exp. Immunol.* **19**:399–406.

Winfield, J. B., Brunner, C. M., and Koffler, D., 1978, Serologic studies in patients with systemic lupus erythematosus and central nervous system dysfunction, *Arthritis Rheum.* **21**:289–294.

Winfield, J. B., Shaw, M., Silverman, L. M., Eisenberg, R. A., Wilson, H. A., and Koffler, D., 1983, Intrathecal IgG synthesis and blood–brain barrier impairment in patients with systemic lupus erythematosus and central nervous system dysfunction. *Am. J. Med.* **774**:837–844.

Wybran, J., Appleboom, T., Famaey, J., and Govaerts, A., 1979, Suggestive evidence for receptors for morphine and methionine-enkephalin on normal human blood T lymphocytes, *J. Immunol.* **123**:1068–1070.

Yoshida, T. O., and Anderson, B., 1972, Evidence for a receptor recognizing antigen complexed immunoglobulin on the surface of activated mouse thymus lymphocytes, *Scand. J. Immunol.* **1**:401–408.

Young, W. W., Jr., Hakomori, S., Durdik, J. M., and Henney, C. S., 1980, Identification of ganglio-N-tetrasylceramide as a new cell surface marker for murine natural killer (NK) cells, *J. Immunol.* **124**:199–201.

Zvaifler, N. J., and Bluestein, H. G., 1976, Lymphocytotoxic antibody activity in the cryoprecipitates from serum of patients with SLE, *Arthritis Rheum.* **19**:844–850.

Zvaifler, N. J., and Bluestein, H. G., 1982, The pathogenesis of central nervous system manifestations of systemic lupus erythematosus, *Arthritis Rheum.* **25**:862–866.

10

Antiphospholipid Antibodies

G. R. V. Hughes, E. N. Harris, and A. E. Gharavi

I. INTRODUCTION

Of the several types of antibodies described in autoimmune disorders, the antiphospholipid antibodies have received relatively little attention. There are two well-described groups of antiphospholipid antibodies, anticardiolipin antibodies (Pangborn, 1941; De Bruijn, 1966; Inoue and Nojima, 1969; Harris *et al.*, 1983, 1985c) and the lupus anticoagulant (Conley and Hartmann, 1952; Margolius *et al.*, 1961; Feinstein and Rapaport, 1972; Veltkamp *et al.*, 1974; Byron, 1982; Shapiro and Thiagarajan, 1982). Based on the demonstration of cross reactivity of some monoclonal DNA antibodies with cardiolipin and other phospholipids (Lafer *et al.*, 1981; Schoenfeld *et al.*, 1983; Koike *et al.*, 1984a,b), it is believed by some investigators that a subgroup of anti-DNA antibodies may bind to the repeating phosphodiester groups on the polynucleotide backbone of DNA and that these antibodies, too, may be antiphospholipid antibodies.

Anticardiolipin antibodies, traditionally detected by the various standard test for syphilis (STS), first became important in diagnosing syphilis. However, with mass serologic screening of patients during the Second World War and with the development of the treponemal immobilization test (TPI) in the late 1940s, it became evident that several people had a persistently positive test for syphilis without any clinical evidence of syphilis (Moore and Mohr, 1952). Further, this false-positive test for syphilis was found to occur in a number of patients with SLE and could even precede the onset of SLE by several years (Haserick and Long, 1951; Moore and Lutz, 1955).

At about the time when the biological false-positive reactors were first being described, there were reports of a "circulating anticoagulant," detected in the blood of some SLE patients, which prolonged blood clotting and prothrombin time *in vitro* (Conley and Hartmann, 1952; Lee and Sanders, 1955; Laurell and Nilsson, 1957; Medal and Lisker,

---

G. R. V. Hughes, E. N. Harris, and A. E. Gharavi • Rheumatology Unit, Royal Postgraduate Medical School, The Hammersmith Hospital, London W12 0HS, England.

1959; Margolius *et al.*, 1961). This circulating anticoagulant was subsequently termed the "lupus anticoagulant" because it was detected primarily in patients with SLE. It should be emphasized, however, that the lupus anticoagulant has been described in patients with autoimmune disorders other than SLE (Margolius *et al.*, 1961; Schleider *et al.*, 1976; Mueh, *et al.*, 1980; Carreras and Vermelyn, 1982) and in infectious, malignant (Schleider *et al.*, 1976; Mueh *et al.*, 1980), and drug-induced disorders (Canoso and Sise, 1982). Several investigators noted the frequency with which a false-positive test for syphilis occurred in patients with the lupus anticoagulant (Laurell and Nilsson, 1957; Margolius *et al.*, 1961; Lechner, 1974; Lee and Miotti, 1975; Johansson and Lassus, 1974; Boey *et al.*, 1983). The relationship between the lupus anticoagulant and a false positive test for syphilis was further established by Laurell and Nilsson, who demonstrated that the lupus anticoagulant activity could be absorbed out with cardiolipin (Laurell and Nilsson, 1957).

Interest in the lupus anticoagulant was initially aroused because it was described in SLE patients with hemorrhage (Conley and Hartmann, 1952; Laurell and Nilsson, 1957). However, it soon became evident that hemorrhage was infrequent in patients with this anticoagulant (Medal and Lisker, 1959; Margolius *et al.*, 1961; Schleider *et al.*, 1976). Then the lupus anticoagulant was treated as merely "another antibody in SLE," of no apparent significance. The false-positive test for syphilis was treated too as merely one of the several "markers" for SLE and other autoimmune disorders.

Recently, there has been a resurgence of interest in these antibodies. Several investigators have found that these antibodies are not "benign" but may be associated with recurrent venous and/or arterial thrombosis (Bowie *et al.*, 1963; Johansson and Lassus, 1974; Lechner, 1974; Angeles-Cano *et al.*, 1979; Mueh *et al.*, 1980; Carreras and Vermelyn, 1982; Boey *et al.*, 1983; Elias and Eldor, 1984), thrombocytopenia (Lechner, 1974; Lee and Miotti, 1975; Boey *et al.*, 1983; Harris *et al.*, 1983, 1985b), recurrent intrauterine death (Nilsson *et al.*, 1975; Firkin *et al.*, 1980; Carreras and Vermelyn, 1982; Valesini *et al.*, 1982; Hull *et al.*, 1983), and possibly transverse myelopathy (Hughes, 1983) in patients with SLE and other autoimmune disorders. Reports of the cross reactivity of anti-DNA antibodies with cardiolipin has also been the subject of much interest among immunologists. It is likely that a more commplete understanding of antiphospholipid antibodies will be of considerable importance to both clinicians and immunologists.

II. ANTICARDIOLIPIN ANTIBODIES

A. Historical Background

It is possible that anticardiolipin antibodies were first reported in 1906, when Wasserman described a complement-fixation test to detect "reagin" in the sera of syphilitic patients, which reacted with a saline extract of livers from fetuses with congenital syphilis. Over the next three decades, alcoholic extracts of a variety of normal tissues were found to be suitable sources of antigenic material, and several complement-fixation tests (Wasserman, Kahn) and flocculation tests (Price, Hinton, Venereal Disease Reference Laboratory) were developed to detect reagin (Catterall, 1973; Harvey and Shulman, 1974).

In 1941, Pangborn showed that the antigen isolated from alcoholic extracts of ox heart muscle was an acid phospholipid, and this compound was subsequently named cardiolipin (Pangborn, 1941). Cardiolipin was shown to be a diphosphatidylglycerol structure with a free median β-hydroxyl group and the phosphatidyl groups in the γ-positions (Fig. 1) (MacFarlane and Gray, 1957; Gray and MacFarlane, 1958). The position of the fatty acids was determined by identification of the fragments obtained on hydrolysis of cardiolipin with hot acetic acid (MacFarlane and Wheeldon, 1958). Pure cardiolipin, mixed with carefully adjusted quantities of lecithin and cholesterol as sensitizing agents, is presently used for the complement-fixation and flocculation tests to detect reagin (Catterall, 1973).

As a result of widespread screening of military and nonmilitary personnel during the Second World War, it became evident that a number of people had a positive standard test for syphilis without clinical evidence of the disease (Moore and Mohr, 1952). Development of the treponemal immobilization test (TPI) in 1949 allowed better distinction between patients with "true-positive" and "false-positive" tests for syphilis (Nelson and

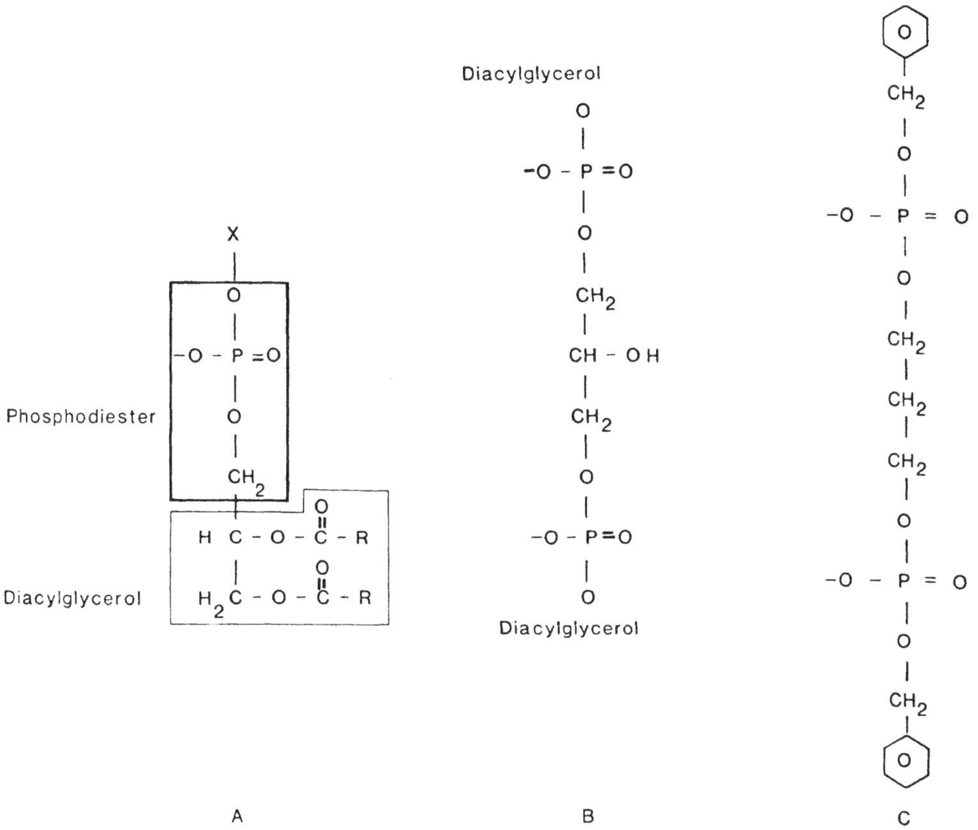

Figure 1. A: Basic structure of a phospholipid, consisting of a diacylglycerol group, a phosphodiester group, and (X) a substituted group characteristic of the specific phospholipid. B: Structure of a cardiolipin. The polar region of the molecule, consisting of two phosphodiester groups and a γ-hydroxyl, is the presumed epitope of the molecule. C: Portion of a single strand of DNA showing the similarity between the polar antigenic region of cardiolipin and the backbone of DNA. Some studies suggest that although the glyceride portions of cardiolipin may not be part of the epitope, they are nevertheless essential for its antigenicity. Thus, a molecule with phosphodiester groups attached to structures other than a glyceride (e.g., DNA) may not bind antiphospholipid antibodies as effectively as a phospholipid molecule.

Mayer, 1949; Nelson *et al.*, 1950). Moore and Mohr found that there were two groups of "false-positive reactors," those who had transient false-positive tests (usually as a result of intercurrent infection) and a second group whose tests remained persistently positive (Moore and Mohr, 1952). This latter group was identified as chronic "biologic false–positive" (BFP) reactors, defined as individuals without clinical or epidemiologic evidence of syphilis who had repeatedly positive standard serologic syphilis tests (STS) and repeatedly negative TPI determinations for 6 months or longer.

In 1955, Moore and Lutz showed that patients with the BFP STS reaction had a high incidence of autoimmune diseases, in particular, systemic lupus erythematosus, Sjogren's disease, autoimmune hemolytic anemia, Hashimoto's thyroiditis, and rheumatoid arthritis (Moore and Lutz, 1955). Several large prospective series since then have shown that a chronic BFP STS can precede certain autoimmune disorders, in particular SLE, by several years (Harvey and Shulman, 1966; Berglund and Carlsson, 1966; Weupper *et al.*, 1966; Putkonen *et al.*, 1967; Tuffanelli, 1968; Catterall, 1973). Further, abnormal autoimmune serologic tests were frequent among this group of patients, antinuclear antibodies (ANA) in particular being noted in about 50% of patients studied (Catterall, 1973; Harvey and Shulman, 1974). It is difficult to predict which patients with the BFP STS will develop SLE, but Harvey and Shulman (1974) suggest that young females are most at risk. In a series of studies by Johansson and collegues, they suggested that BFP STS patients most likely to develop SLE were young females who also had a positive ANA, the lupus anticoagulant, and immunoglobulins bound to the dermoepidermal junction on skin biopsy (Johansson *et al.*, 1972; Johansson and Lassus, 1974).

B. Immunology

Immunologic and physicochemical studies have shown that reagin is an antibody of either the IgG or IgM immunoglobulin class (Fowler and Allen, 1962; Inoue and Nojima, 1967a,b; Aho, 1968). Using a solid-phase radioimmunoassay to detect anticardiolipin antibodies, Harris *et al.* were able to detect IgA anticardiolipin antibodies in 13 SLE patients (Harris *et al.*, 1983). Anticardiolipin antibodies raised in animal systems or derived from the sera of patients with syphilis exhibit a great deal of cross reactivity with synthetic cardiolipin analogues and a variety of other phospholipids (Inoue and Nojima, 1967a,b, 1969; Tamamura *et al.*, 1971; Wicken *et al.*, 1972; De Siervo, 1974; Guarnieri, 1974a; Cooper *et al.*, 1974). Because of the considerable cross reactivity of anticardiolipin antibodies, there are still questions about the specificity or specificities of the antibodies (Alving, 1977). Early studies used antisera to cardiolipin or phospholipids raised in animal systems or confined themselves to sera of patients with syphilis. Cardiolipin and other phospholipid antigens used were mixed with varying concentrations of lecithin and cholesterol to enable detection of the antibodies by flocculation or complement-fixation tests. Therefore, results of these studies must be interpreted with caution, and, for reasons discussed below, anticardiolipin antibodies in syphilitic patients probably differ from the antibodies in biological false-positive reactors (Alving, 1977).

Two groups of workers have shown that anticardiolipin antibodies raised in animal systems or derived from patients with syphilis react best with the intact cardiolipin molecule (Faure and Coulon-Morelec, 1963; Inoue and Nojima, 1969). There was decreased reactivity of the anticardiolipin antibodies tested following the removal of a phosphatidic acid from the cardiolipin molecule or removal of the central hydroxyl group, or shortening or lengthening the distance between the posphodiester groups (Fig. 1). Cardiolipin lost its antigenicity if the glyceride portions of the molecule were replaced by benzyl groups (Inoue and Nojima, 1969) or if more than two fatty acids were removed from the molecule (Faure and Coulon-Morelec, 1963). These authors concluded that the antibodies bind one or both phosphodiester groups of the cardiolipin molecule, but the glyceride portions of the molecule were essential for its reactivity. De Siervo, in a subsequent study, suggested that immunization with cardiolipin may result in a mixture of antibodies reacting either with the whole cardiolipin molecule or with different sites on the molecule (De Siervo, 1974).

Most intriguing of all was the work of Guarnieri and Eisner (1974), who demonstrated that anticardiolipin and antiphosphatidylinositol sera raised in rabbits cross reacted with DNA and to a small extent with RNA but that such cross reactivity only occurred when the DNA or RNA was mixed with auxiliary lipids; i.e., lecithin and cholesterol. These workers explained this cross reactivity on the basis of the similarity between the antigenic polar region of cardiolipin and the phosphodiester-linked backbone of DNA. Recently, monoclonal anti-DNA antibodies raised in mouse–mouse hybridomas (Lafer *et al.*, 1981; Koike *et al.*, 1984b) and in human–human hybridomas (Shoenfeld *et al.*, 1983) have been shown to cross react with cardiolipin. Monoclonal anticardiolipin antibodies raised in lupus-prone mice have also been shown to cross react with DNA (Rauch *et al.*, 1984). This work was extended by Koike and his colleagues, who reported with anti-ssDNA and, to a lesser extent, anti-dsDNA from patients with SLE cross reacted with cardiolipin (Koike *et al.*, 1982). In a follow-up study, they reported cross reactivity of anticardiolipin antibodies in SLE patients with ssDNA and dsDNA (Koike *et al.*, 1984a). Tincani and colleagues have also reported a strong statistical correlation between anticardiolipin antibody and anti-ssDNA antibody positivity but no correlation between anticardiolipin antibody and anti-dsDNA antibody positivity (Tincani *et al.*, 1984).

Some groups, however, have not confirmed the above findings. Morgan and colleagues reported that monoclonal anti-dsDNA and anti-ssDNA hybridomas were not inhibited by cardiolipin or other phospholipids (Morgan *et al.*, 1983). Harris and coworkers did not find a correlation between anticardiolipin antibody levels and anti-dsDNA antibody levels by regression analysis (Harris *et al.*, 1983). In a study of ten SLE patients with high anticardiolipin antibody levels, we found that cardiolipin and other negatively charged phospholipids inhibited anticardiolipin antibody activity, but there was no significant inhibition of anticardiolipin antibody activity by ssDNA or dsDNA. Further, we found that cardiolipin did not inhibit anti-dsDNA or anti-ssDNA antibody-binding activity in another ten SLE patients studied (Harris *et al.*, 1985c). There have been several instances, too, in which we have found patients who are ANA negative but have high anticardiolipin antibody levels and lupus anticoagulant activity. It is likely that a small population of anticardiolipin antibodies cross react with DNA. However, several studies in our laboratory suggest that the anticardiolipin antibodies cross react primarily with negatively charged phospholipids such as phosphatidylserine, phosphatidic acid, and phosphatidylinositol. We have found little cross reactivity with the zwitterionic phospholipids such as phosphatidylethanolamine and sphingomyelin (Harris *et al.*, 1985c).

It appears likely too that the antibodies responsible for the BFP STS differ from those in syphilis patients. Some support for this suggestion is that the biological false-positive test is usually positive at low titers, unlike the high-titer positivity of untreated syphilis sera (Fiumara, 1963). On the other hand, preliminary findings using solid-phase radioimmunoassay to detect anticardiolipin antibodies show that syphilis sera give low positive or negative results but that biological false-positive reactors and some patients with negative VDRLs give very high anticardiolipin antibody levels (Harris *et al.*, 1985c). On the basis of these results, it is probable that the epitope of the cardiolipin molecule, when mixed with lecithin and cholesterol in standard tests for syphilis, differs from that of cardiolipin adsorbed to a plastic surface in the solid-phase radioimmunoassay. Cardiolipin is located on the inner membrane of mitochondria, and Wright and colleages showed that syphilis sera gave a pattern of antimitochondrial immunofluorescence different from that of primary biliary cirrhosis (Wright *et al.*, 1970). Subsequent studies have shown that anticardiolipin antibodies in patients with collagen vascular disorders, some of whom had the lupus anticoagulant, gave yet another pattern of immunofluorescence (the "M5" pattern) different from that of patients with syphilis (the "M1" pattern) (Labro *et al.*, 1978). The detection of lupus anticoagulant activity in biological false-positive but not in syphilis sera also suggests differences between these groups of anticardiolipin antibodies (Johansson and Lassus, 1974). There are possibly also variations in specificities of anticardiolipin antibodies even in the group of biological false-positive reactors (Alving, 1977).

III. THE LUPUS ANTICOAGULANT

A. Detection, Mechanism of Action, and Immunology

The first description of the lupus anticoagulant is usually attributed to Conley and Hartmann (1952), who described two SLE patients, both of whom had a biological false-positive test for syphilis, with a hemorrhagic disorder and prolonged prothrombin and whole-blood clotting times. It is possible, however, that the lupus anticoagulant may have been first described by Aggeler *et al.* (1946) in a patient with SLE.

B. Mechanism of Action

The lupus anticoagulant acts at the level of the prothrombin converter complex of the clotting cascade (Fig. 2) as evidenced by its effects on routine coagulation tests (Yin and Gaston, 1965; Gonyea *et al.*, 1968; Lechner, 1969). The lupus anticoagulant is usually detected by prolongation of the activated partial thromboplastin time or, less frequently, prolongation of the prothrombin time (Feinstein and Rapaport, 1972). In the presence of dilute thromboplastin, there is disproportionate prolongation of the prothrombin time in lupus-anticoagulant-positive plasma compared to normal control plasma (Lee and Sanders, 1955; Frick, 1955; Laurell and Nilsson, 1957). The thrombin time is usually normal. This particular group of tests suggests that the lupus anticoagulant has no effect on the intrinsic or extrinsic pathway up to the activation of factor X. A normal thrombin time suggests that the anticoagulant does not act in the late stages of clotting. The abnormal partial thromboplastin time is not corrected by mixing with an equal volume of normal platelet-poor plasma, as would be expected with a normal clotting factor deficiency. In the mixing test, the inhibition is immediate and does not increase progressively with time, unlike anticoagulants that inhibit specific clotting factors; e.g., the factor VIII anticoagulant (Lee and Miotti, 1975; Editorial, 1984).

Evidence that the lupus anticoagulant acts against the phospholipid component of the prothrombin activator complex is largely indirect but persuasive (Feinstein and Rapoport, 1972; Veltkamp *et al.*, 1974). The only direct evidence that the lupus anticoagulant binds specifically to phospholipids is obtained from the work of Thiagarajan and collegues, who showed that a monoclonal IgM antibody from a patient with Waldenstrom's macroglobulinemia had lupus anticoagulant activity and cross reacted with negatively charged phospholipids by an Ouchterlony technique (Thiagarajan *et al.*, 1980). Of relevance is the demonstration in our laboratory of cross reactivity of IgG anticardiolipin antibodies primarily with negatively charged phospholipids, which, taken with Thiagarajan work on the lupus anticoagulant, reinforces suggestions that the two antibodies are related. Recently, we have affinity purified anticardiolipin antibodies using cardiolipin liposomes and have shown them to have lupus anticoagulant activity (unpublished). These affinity-purified antibodies cross react with negatively charged phospholipids.

The enhanced effect of the lupus anticoagulant on prothrombin time when thromboplastin, a phospholipid extract, is diluted is also indirect evidence suggesting antiphospholipid activity (Lee and Sanders, 1955; Frick, 1955; Laurell and Nilsson, 1957). Several workers have shown that increasing phospholipid concentration can partially correct the effects of the lupus anticoagulant (Veltkamp *et al.*, 1974; Exner *et al.*, 1975; Coots *et al.*, 1981). Further, studies by Firkin and other workers have shown that normal platelets, activated platelets, or lysed platelets could correct the effects of the lupus anticoagulant, suggesting that the phospholipid(s) that the lupus anticoagulant binds are present in the platelet membrane (Exner *et al.*, 1978; Firkin *et al.*, 1978; Howard and Firkin, 1983). The strong correlation between presence of the lupus anticoagulant and the anticardiolipin antibody, determined either by standard tests for syphilis (Margolius

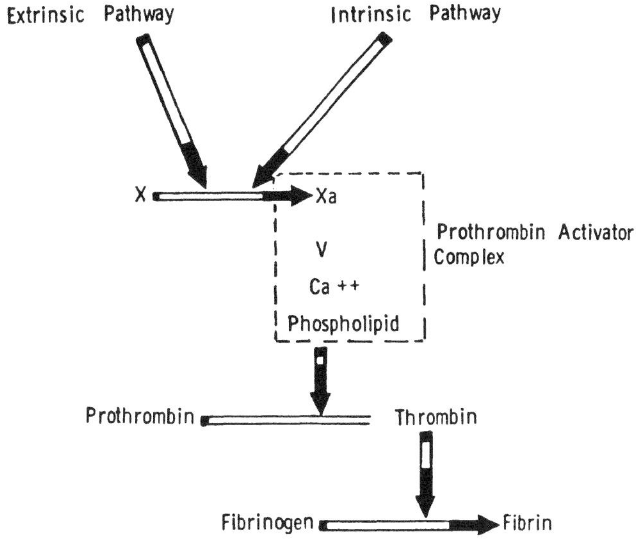

Figure 2. Blood coagulation scheme. The lupus anticoagulant acts at the level of the prothrombin activator complex. It may bind a platelet phospholipid, thereby disturbing the interaction of factors Xa, V, and prothrombin on the platelet surface, and delay the conversion of prothrombin to thrombin.

et al., 1961; Johansson and Lassus, 1974; Lee and Miotti, 1975; Boey *et al.*, 1983) or solid-phase radioimmunoassay (Harris, 1983), suggests that these are cross-reacting antiphospholipid antibodies. Significantly, Laurell and Nilsson (1957) found that cardiolipin and thromboplastin could absorb out lupus anticoagulant activity. The particular phospholipid with which the lupus anticoagulant binds is unknown. Thiagarajan's work and our own, mentioned previously, tend to suggest that the lupus anticoagulant binds a negatively charged phospholipid, and recent studies by Howard and Firkin suggest that this phospholipid is probably located in the platelet membrane.

C. Characterization of the Lupus Anticoagulant

Several studies have demonstrated that the lupus anticoagulant is an antibody. Perhaps the first suggestion that the lupus anticoagulant was an antibody was contained in a unique case report by Frick in 1955. He described a woman with clinical features of SLE and circulating anticoagulant as well as a BFP STS. Both antibodies were detected in the sera of the baby, and the circulating anticoagulant persisted for 3 months, whereas the BFP STS remained positive for 6 months.

Over the succeeding decade there was increasing evidence that the lupus anticoagulant was an antibody (Laurell and Nilsson, 1957; Medal and Lisker, 1959; Margolius *et al.*, 1961), but it was Yin and Gaston (1965) who first isolated an IgG protein fraction with anticoagulant activity using Sephadex G-200 gel filtration with subsequent purification on DEAE-cellulose. Lechner, using similar methods, found anticoagulant activity either solely in the IgM fraction (Lechner, 1969) or in both IgG and IgM fractions. A monoclonal IgM antibody with lupus anticoagulant activity has been described in a patient with Waldenstrom's macroglobulinemia (Thiagarajan *et al.*, 1980). Of particular interest recently was the description by Lafer and coworkers (1981) of a mouse monoclonal anti-DNA antibody with lupus anticoagulant activity that cross reacted with other phospholipids, giving rise to the hypothesis, mentioned previously, that subpopulations of anti-DNA antibodies may bind to phospholipids.

IV. CLINICAL FEATURES OF ANTIPHOSPHOLIPID ANTIBODIES

A. Frequency of Occurrence

Most studies quote the frequency of the lupus anticoagulant to be 6–10% in patients with SLE (Frick, 1955; Margolius *et al.*, 1961; Schleider *et al.*, 1976; Mueh *et al.*, 1980; Lee and Miotti, 1975; Byron, 1982). Our experience suggests that this antibody occurs more frequently. Thus, in an unpublished survey of 167 patients with SLE and other autoimmune disorders, the lupus anticoagulant was detected in 56 patients, 40 of whom had SLE. Variations in sensitivities of tests to detect the lupus anticoagulant and variations in activity of the lupus anticoagulant with treatment make its frequency of occurrence difficult to estimate. It should be reemphasized, too, that the lupus anticoagulant is not exclusive to SLE and has been described in other autoimmune, drug-induced, malignant, and infectious disorders (Frick, 1955; Margolius *et al.*, 1961; Schleider *et al.*, 1976; Mueh *et al.*, 1980; Carreras and Vermelyn, 1982; Canoso and Sise, 1982).

Similarly, estimates of the frequency of anticardiolipin antibody in SLE patients, detected by standard tests for syphilis, vary considerably. Harvey and Shulman suggest a frequency of 10% in adult SLE patients (Harvey, 1974). However, using a solid-phase radioimmunoassay to detect anticardiolipin antibodies, we found elevated IgG anticardiolipin antibody levels in 82 (42%) of 197 SLE patients and elevated IgM anticardiolipin antibody levels in 48 (25%) of 189 SLE patients. Elevated anticardiolipin antibody levels have also been detected in patients with other autoimmune disorders such as primary Sjogren's syndrome, mixed connective tissue disease, rheumatoid arthritis, idiopathic thrombocytopenic purpura, Behcet's disease, myasthenia gravis, and other undefined autoimmune disorders (Fig. 3). Elevated antibody levels have also been noted in pregnancy and occasionally in patients without autoimmune disorders.

B. Antiphospholipid Antibodies and Thrombosis

Early studies of the lupus anticoagulant emphasized hemorrhagic disorders in patients with this antibody (Conley and Hartmann, 1952; Lee and Sanders, 1955; Frick, 1955; Laurell and Nilsson, 1957). It soon became evident that there was no increased risk of bleeding in patients with the lupus anticoagulant even when they underwent surgery (Medal and Lisker, 1959; Margolius *et al.*, 1961; Schleider *et al.*, 1976; Boxer *et al.*, 1976; Elias and Eldor, 1984). When bleeding did occur, it usually could be attributed to

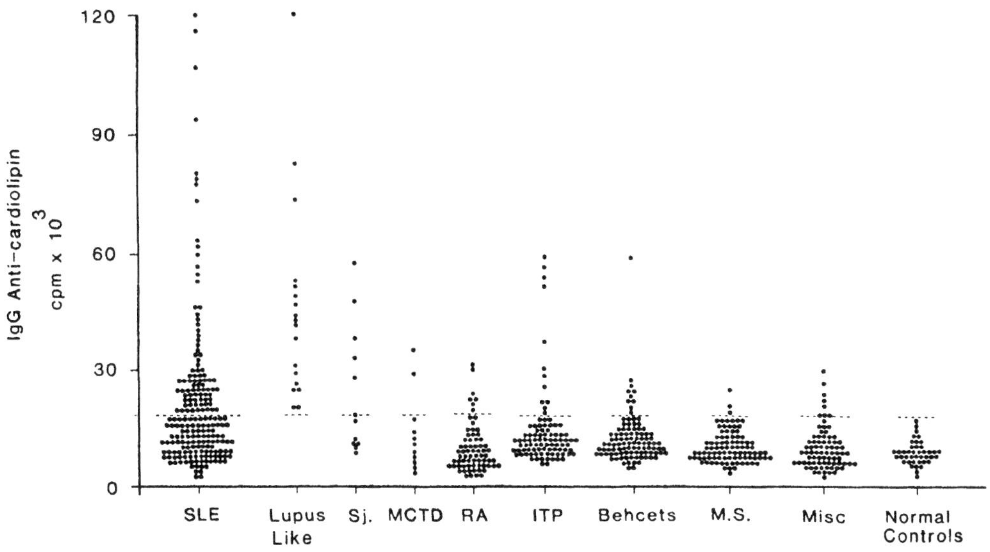

Figure 3. Anticardiolipin IgG antibody levels measured by solid-phase radioimmunoassay in various disorders, including systemic lupus erythematosus (SLE), "lupuslike" disorders, primary Sjogren's syndrome (Sj), mixed connective tissue disease (MCTD), rheumatoid arthritis (RA), idiopathic thrombocytopenic purpura (ITP), Behcet's disease, multiple sclerosis (MS), a miscellaneous group (including dermatomyositis, scleroderma, osteoarthritis and other disorders), and normal controls. Patients with "lupuslike" disorders had thrombosis and/or thrombocytopenia and/or recurrent abortion with some clinical features of SLE. None of these patients had ever had elevated DNA binding. The interrupted line is the upper limit of normal, taken as 2.25 standard deviations above the mean normal control level.

an associated thrombocytopenia (Margolius *et al.*, 1961; Schleider *et al.*, 1976; Lechner, 1974; Elias and Eldor, 1984) or clotting factor deficiency, most frequently hypoprothrombinemia (Loeliger, 1959; Margolius *et al.*, 1961; Gonyea *et al.*, 1968; Lee and Miotti, 1975). Paradoxically, the lupus anticoagulant, although associated with prolongation of the partial thromboplastin time *in vitro,* appears to be associated with recurrent venous or arterial thrombosis *in vivo*. This association between the lupus anticoagulant and thrombosis has been reported by several investigators (Bowie *et al.*, 1963; Johansson and Lassus, 1974; Lechner, 1974; Angeles-Cano *et al.*, 1979; Mueh *et al.*, 1980; Williams *et al.*, 1980, Carreras and Vermelyn, 1982; Boey *et al.*, 1983; Elias and Eldor, 1984). Boey and co-workers (1983) reported a history of venous or arterial thrombosis in 18 of 31 patients with the lupus anticoagulant, and Elias and Eldor (1984) reported venous or arterial thrombosis in 19 of 35 patients with the lupus anticoagulant.

An association of the BFP STS, circulating anticoagulant, and thrombosis was reported by Johansson and Lassus (1974), who studied 96 patients with a chronic BFP STS. Thirty-five had the circulating anticoagulant, and eight of these patients had recurrent thromboses. These authors in a subsequent report described eight patients, three women and five men, with chronic BFP STS and circulating anticoagulants who had recurrent deep vein thrombosis of the extremities, necrotizing purpura with painful starlike ulcers around the ankle, and proliferation of dermal capillaries without significant inflammation on skin biopsy (Johansson *et al.*, 1977). Using the solid-phase radioimmunoassay to detect anticardiolipin antibodies in a series of 65 patients with SLE and other autoimmune disorders, anticardiolipin antibodies were elevated in 15 of 18 patients with a history of venous or arterial thrombosis, and there was a statistical correlation between elevated anticardiolipin antibody levels and thrombosis (Harris *et al.*, 1983). Sixteen of the 18 patients with thrombosis also had the lupus anticoagulant. In a follow-up study of 15 patients with autoimmune disorders and cerebral infarction, 13 had elevated IgG anticardiolipin antibody levels (Harris *et al.*, 1984). Of interest too is that in reviewing results of anticardiolipin antibody levels in 800 sera tested, we have found that of the 50 patients with the highest IgG anticardiolipin antibody levels, 19 had a history of venous and/or arterial thrombosis.

It is still uncertain whether antiphospholipid antibodies play a pathogenetic role in thrombosis or are merely "markers" for thrombotic disease. The work of Carreras and his colleagues (1981) suggest that these antibodies may play a causative role in thrombosis. These workers first studied a woman with the lupus anticoagulant who had a history of recurrent arterial thrombosis and recurrent abortion. They found that an IgG fraction of the patient's serum with lupus anticoagulant activity blocked the production of prostacyclin from the endothelium of rat aorta rings, but this inhibitory effect could be abolished by addition of arachidonic acid. In a follow-up study of 14 patients with the lupus anticoagulant, they found that plasma from eight of these patients inhibited prostacyclin production from vascular tissue, and six of the eight patients had a history of thrombosis (Carreras and Vermelyn, 1982). On the basis of these studies, they have proposed that the lupus anticoagulant can cross react with phospholipids in the membrane of an endothelial cell, thereby blocking arachidonic acid release and resulting in decreased prostacyclin production. Decreased prostacyclin levels would result in enhanced platelet aggregation and thrombosis. An alternative mechanism is proposed on the basis of a study by Angeles-Cano and colleagues. They showed decreased plasminogen activator release after venous occlusion in a group of SLE patients, many of whom had the lupus anticoagulant (Angeles-Cano, 1979). It is conceivable that antiphospholipid antibodies can damage endothelial cells, resulting in decreased plasminogen activator release and an increased tendency to thrombosis.

C. Thrombocytopenia

There have been several reports of an association between the lupus anticoagulant and thrombocytopenia (Lechner, 1974; Lee and Miotti, 1975; Boxer, 1976; Boey *et al.*, 1983), and recent studies suggest that anticardiolipin antibodies are also associated with thrombocytopenia (Harris *et al.*, 1983, 1985a). In a study of 116 patients with SLE and other autoimmune disorders, IgG anticardiolipin antibody levels were elevated in 30 of 43 patients with thrombocytopenia (Harris *et al.*, 1985a). There was a strong statistical correlation between elevated IgG anticardiolipin antibody levels and thrombocytopenia ($P < 0.001$), and of the 20 patients with the highest IgG anticardiolipin antibody levels, 16 had thrombocytopenia (Fig. 4). In a survey of sera from 96 patients with idiopathic thrombocytopenia purpura, elevated anticardiolipin antibody levels of IgG and/or IgM immunoglobulin classes were found in 30 (Harris *et al.*, 1985b).

On the basis of these observations, it seems reasonable to suggest that antiphospholipid antibodies may bind phospholipids in platelet membrane, resulting in enhanced platelet uptake and destruction by the reticuloendothelial system. Some support for this hypothesis comes from unpublished studies in our laboratory that show that platelets

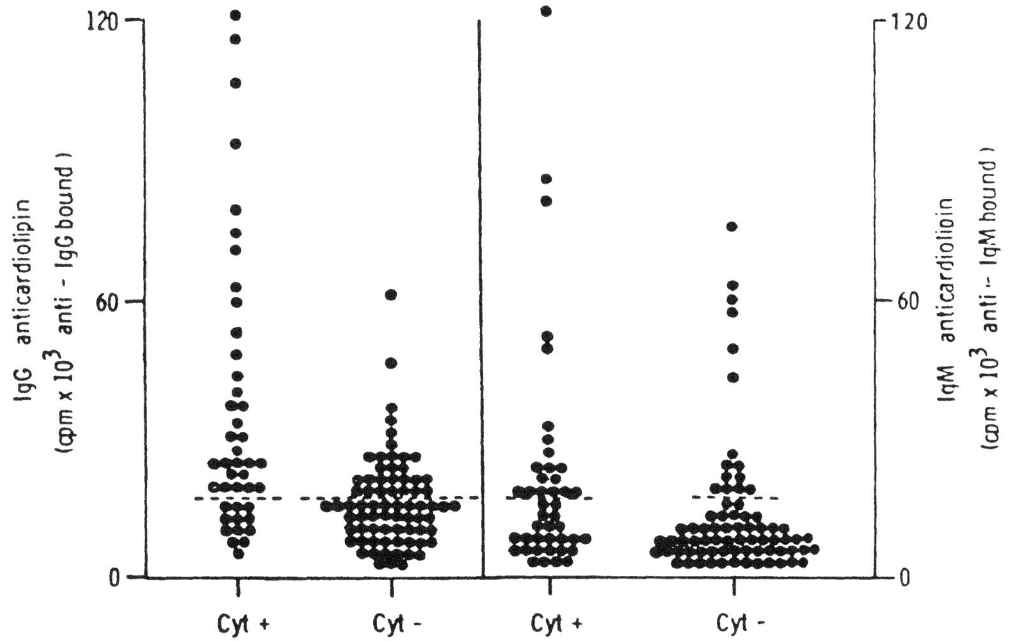

Figure 4. Comparison of IgG and IgM anticardiolipin antibody levels in SLE patients with (Cyt +) and without (Cyt −) a history of thrombocytopenia. Thrombocytopenia was defined as a platelet count less than 100,000/ml. The interrupted line is the upper limit of normal.

disrupted by sonication can inhibit anticardiolipin antibody-binding activity. Analysis of the phospholipids in the platelet membrane suggests that the negatively charged phospholipids are primarily located on the inner (endoplasmic) portion of the bimolecular lipid membrane (Alving, 1977). We have already cited our own and other studies suggesting that both the lupus anticoagulant and anticardiolipin antibodies react best with negatively charged phospholipids. Hence, disruption of platelet membrane by sonication may result in exposure of negatively charged phospholipids and thus would explain inhibition of anticardiolipin-binding activity. It is possible that activation of platelets may somehow "expose" negatively charged phospholipids in their membrane and result in enhanced binding of antiphospholipid antibodies to the platelet. The requirement for activation of platelets prior to antiphospholipid binding may help to explain why all patients with antiphospholipid antibodies do not develop thrombocytopenia.

D. Recurrent Intrauterine Death

Antiphospholipid antibodies also appear to be associated with recurrent intrauterine death (Nilsson *et al.*, 1975; Firkin *et al.*, 1980; Soulier and Boffa, 1980; Valesini *et al.*, 1982; Lubbe *et al.*, 1983; Ros *et al.*, 1983; Hull *et al.*, 1983). We have recently studied 21 patients with recurrent intrauterine deaths and found that 16 had the lupus anticoagulant and/or elevated anticardiolipin antibody levels. Our own and other studies (Firkin *et al.*, 1980; Lubbe *et al.*, 1983) suggest that intrauterine deaths usually occur in the second or third trimester of pregnancy. Many of these patients do not have SLE, often presenting only with recurrent intrauterine death and few other features of an autoimmune disorder (Firkin *et al.*, 1980; Lubbe *et al.*, 1983; Prentice *et al.*, 1984). An unpublished survey of women with recurrent intrauterine deaths in the third trimester of pregnancy showed many patients with the lupus anticoagulant (G. Gregorini, personal communication).

Carreras and colleagues have reported that the lupus anticoagulant inhibits prostacyclin production by pregnant human myometrium (Carreras *et al.*, 1981; Carreras and Vermelyn, 1982). They postulate that prostacyclin may play an important role in the regulation of fetal circulation; hence, a deficiency of prostacyclin production by placental vessels could result in reduced blood flow, placental infarction, and fetal distress. We have reviewed the pathology reports of placentas from aborted fetuses of SLE patients with the lupus anticoagulant and elevated anticardiolipin antibody levels and have found a few instances in which multiple placental infarcts have been present.

E. Nonlupus Disorders

The association of antiphospholipid antibodies with thrombosis, thrombocytopenia, and recurrent abortion is not limited only to patients with SLE. Since starting our work with antiphospholipid antibodies, we have collected several patients who have been referred because of unexplained recurrent venous or arterial thrombosis, thrombocytopenia, and/or recurrent abortion. Some of these patients have had some features of an autoimmune disorder, but many have been ANA negative, and none have had elevated DNA binding by Farr assay. Many were found to have very elevated anticardiolipin antibody levels (Fig. 3), and the lupus anticoagulant was usually detected. We have also found that two patients with Behcet's disease and two other patients with primary Sjogren's syndrome who had elevated anticardiolipin antibody levels, cerebral infarction, and/or recurrent thrombosis. Hence, antiphospholipid antibodies and their association with thrombosis, thrombocytopenia, and recurrent abortion, although manifest mainly in SLE patients, do occur in patients with other autoimmune disorders.

F. Cerebral Disease

It is also possible that antiphospholipid antibodies may bind directly to brain tissue and so account for some of the neurological disorders of SLE and other autoimmune disorders. In a prospective study of patients with a BFP STS, Catterall found six women who developed transverse myelopathy similar to multiple sclerosis. Because these patients had some features of systemic lupus, Catterall called this syndrome "lupoid sclerosis." In a subsequent study of these six women, Fulford and colleagues (1972) suggested that lupoid sclerosis might be a variant of SLE characterized by chronic neurological symptoms and signs suggesting multiple sclerosis and laboratory abnormalities that included elevated ESR, a weakly positive ANA, scanty LE cells, and a chronic BFP STS. This syndrome resembles, in some respects, another disorder described in Jamaica and the Caribbean, termed the Jamaican neuropathy, features of which include transverse myelopathy, posterior column defects, optic atrophy, and eighth nerve deafness (Wilson and Hughes, 1975). Several patients with the Jamaican neuropathy have a false-positive test for syphilis. We have recently found a patient with transverse myelopathy who was ANA positive and DNA-binding normal with elevated IgM anticardiolipin antibody levels. Although it would be tempting to suggest that antiphospholipid antibodies may play a role in multiple sclerosis, Catterall failed to find a positive Wasserman test on screening 69 unselected patients with multiple sclerosis, and our own studies have not located significantly elevated anticardiolipin antibody levels in sera from 94 patients with multiple sclerosis. Further, any proposed role for antiphospholipid antibodies in causing neurological damage will require screening of CSF from these patients, a study that we are in the process of completing.

Several studies have demonstrated antibodies that react with brain tissue in patients with CNS lupus (Bluestein and Zvaifler, 1976; Bresnihan *et al.*, 1977, 1979; Bluestein, 1978; Wilson *et al.*, 1979; Zvaifler and Bluestein, 1982). Some of these antibodies are lymphocytotoxic, presumably because of cross reaction with antigen determinants present in both lymphocyte membranes and brain tissue. Cross-reacting antiglycolipid antibodies reacting with T-cell membrane and brain tissue have been demonstrated in patients with CNS lupus (Hirano *et al.*, 1980). Phospholipids are also found both in lymphocyte membranes and brain tissue. Two studies have shown that antiphospholipid antibodies raised in animals can bind to neural membrane structures (Guarnieri, 1975; Teitelbaum *et al.*, 1973). Hence, it is conceivable that a subpopulation of cross-reacting lymphocytotoxic antibodies may be antiphospholipid antibodies.

V. TREATMENT

Several investigators have noted decreased lupus anticoagulant activity with steroid and/or immunosuppressive therapy (Medal and Lisker, 1959; Margolius *et al.*, 1961; Schleider *et al.*, 1976; Williams *et al.*, 1980; Landi *et al.*, 1983; Gladman *et al.*, 1983; Elias and Eldor, 1984). Preliminary work in our laboratory also suggests that plasmapheresis and prednisolone and/or other immunosuppressive therapy can lower both lupus anticoagulant activity and anticardiolipin antibody levels. Of particular importance is a study by Lubbe and colleagues (1983) who reported six women with SLE and recurrent abortion, all of whom had the lupus anticoagulant. Treatment of these women with prednisolone, 50 mg daily, and aspirin resulted in disappearance of lupus anticoagulant activity and successful pregnancies. An SLE patient similarly treated in Italy (G. Gregorini, personal communication) also had a successful outcome of her pregnancy after several previous recurrent intrauterine deaths.

Treatment of patients with antiphospholipid antibodies is based on the premise that they play a causative role in thrombosis, thrombocytopenia, or recurrent abortion. Not all patients with elevated antiphospholipid antibodies have these complications. Hence, we believe that treatment of patients with antiphospholipid antibodies but without clinically active disease is probably not justified at this time. There appear to be sufficient grounds to justify treatment of women with recurrent intrauterine deaths who have the lupus anticoagulant. Similarly, given the morbidity and potential mortality of recurrent cerebral vascular accident or of venous thrombosis and pulmonary embolism in otherwise healthy young people with antiphospholipid antibodies, an effort to remove these antibodies in patients with these complications would seem to be justified.

The role of antiplatelet agents or oral anticoagulants in preventing recurrent thrombosis in patients with antiphospholipid antibodies is uncertain (Schleider *et al.*, 1976; Mueh *et al.*, 1980; Williams *et al.*, 1980). Our own experience and that of other workers have suggested that some patients continue to have recurrent thrombosis despite apparently adequate anticoagulant therapy. Until further evidence becomes available, we recommend that either anticoagulants or antiplatelet agents be used in addition to immunosuppressive therapy in patients with a history of thrombosis and demonstrable antiphospholipid antibodies.

VI. OUTSTANDING QUESTIONS

There are several questions that must arise about this group of antibodies. Given the considerable cross reactivity of these antibodies, the question arises whether the lupus anticoagulant and anticardiolipin antibodies are the same or cross-reacting antibodies. We have found a few patients with detectable lupus anticoagulant without elevated anticardiolipin antibodies and several instances in which very elevated anticardiolipin antibodies have been found without detectable lupus anticoagulant activity. The phospholipid against which the lupus anticoagulant acts is still unknown. Of further interest is whether the anticardiolipin antibodies are one population of antibodies with one specificity or several populations of antibodies with varying specificities. Differences between the antibody found in syphilis and that responsible for the biological false-positive test for syphilis suggest that more than one population exists. Work in experimental animals also suggests more than one population (Alving, 1977). Of considerable importance to many investigators is whether anti-DNA antibodies include a subpopulation of antiphospholipid antibodies, a question that we believe will require further investigation.

Of clinical relevance is whether these antibodies play a pathogenic role in thrombosis, thrombocytopenia, and/or recurrent abortion. If this is true, one must ask why all patients with these antibodies do not have some or all of these complications. It is conceivable that given subpopulations of these antibodies with given specificities for specific phospholipids may be responsible for specific complications such as thrombocytopenia. Alternatively, other factors that operate *in vivo,* such as platelet activation, may also be operative in enabling these antibodies to bind to target membranes. It would also be interesting to determine whether these antibodies can play a role in CNS disease, since there is certainly a theoretical possibility that they can bind phospholipids in lymphocyte membranes ("?"lymphocytotoxic antibodies) and in neural membranes (antibrain or antineuronal antibodies).

The roles of immunosuppressive therapy and of anticoagulant or antiplatelet agents in preventing recurrent thrombosis or recurrent abortion in patients with antiphospholipid antibodies remain to be determined.

Finally, as with all autoantibodies, one must ask what the stimulus is for production of antiphospholipid antibodies. Phospholipids are ubiquitous in nature. Antiphosphatidylglycerol and anticardiolipin antisera have been prepared in rabbits by using phospholipids purified from bacteria (De Siervo, 1974). Hence, several infectious organisms either by virtue of phospholipids in their cell membranes or because of tissue destruction after infection can potentially induce antiphospholipid antibody production. The role of genetic predisposition to antiphospholipid antibody production is also uncertain. There have been isolated reports of the lupus anticoagulant occurring in more than one family member (Exner, *et al.*, 1980). Similar isolated reports have been made of more than one family member with a BFP STS (Konstant, 1972) or, more frequently, of family members with serologic abnormalities other than the BFP STS (Tuffanelli, 1968). Our own studies have not shown a correlation between elevated anticardiolipin antibody levels and any HLA phenotype. We are in the process of conducting family studies to ascertain whether there might be an increased familial frequency of antiphospholipid antibodies.

It is clear that antiphospholipid antibodies are of considerable interest both for immunologic and clinical reasons, and, doubtless, much more will be learned about these interesting antibodies in the near future.

REFERENCES

Aggeler, P. M., Lindsay, S., and Lucia, S. P., 1946, Studies on the coagulation defect in a case of thrombocytopenic purpura complicated by thrombosis, *Am. J. Pathol.* **22:**1181–1203.

Aho, K., 1968, Studies of syphilitic antibodies, *Br. J. Vener. Dis.* **44:**283–286.

Alving, C., 1977, Immune reactions of lipids and lipid model membranes, in: *The Antigens,* Vol. 4 (M. Sela, ed.), Academic Press, New York, pp. 1–56.

Angeles-Cano, E., Sultan, Y., and Clauvel, J. P., 1979, Predisposing factors to thrombosis in systemic lupus erythematosus: Possible relation to endothelial cell damage, *J. Lab. Clin. Med.* **94:**315–323.

Berglund, S., and Carlsson, M., 1966, Clinical significance of chronic biologic false postive Wasserman reaction and "antinuclear factors," *Acta. Med. Scand.* **180:**407–412.

Bluestein, H. G., 1978, Neurocytotoxic antibodies in serum of patients with systemic lupus erythematosus, *Proc. Natl. Acad. Sci. U.S.A.* **75:**3965–3969.

Bluestein, H. G., and Zvaifler, N. J., 1976, Brain reactive lymphocytoxic antibodies in the serum of patients with systemic lupus erythematosus. *J. Clin Invest.* **57:**509–516.

Boey, M. L., Colaco, C. B., Gharavi, A. E., Elkon, K. B., Loizou, S., and Hughes, G. R. V., 1983, Thrombosis in SLE: Striking association with the presence of circulating "lupus anticoagulant," *Br. Med. J.* **287**:1021–1023.

Bowie, W. E. J., Thompson, J. H., Pascuzzi, C. A., and Owen, C. A., 1963, Thrombosis in systemic lupus erythematosus despite circulating anticoagulants, *J. Clin. Invest.* **62**:416–430.

Boxer, M., Ellman, L., and Carvalho, A., 1976, The lupus anticoagulant, *Arthritis Rheum.* **19**:1244–1248.

Bresnihan, B., Oliver, M., Grigor, G., and Hughes, G. R. V., 1977, Brain reactivity of lymphocytotoxic antibodies in systemic lupus erythematosus with and without cerebral involvement, *Clin. Exp. Immunol.* **30**:333–337.

Bresnihan, B., Oliver, M., Williams, B., and Hughes, G. R. V., 1979, An antineuronal antibody cross-reactive with erythrocytes and lymphocytes in systemic lupus erythematosus, *Arthritis Rheum.* **22**:313–320.

Byron, M. A., 1982, The clotting defect in SLE, *Clin. Rheum. Dis.* **8**:137–151.

Canoso, R. T., and Sise, H. S., 1982, Chlorpromazine-induced lupus anticoagulant and associated immunologic abnormalities, *Am. J. Hematol.* **13**:121–129.

Carreras, L. O., and Vermelyn, J. G., 1982, "Lupus" anticoagulant and thrombosis—possible role of inhibition of prostacyclin formation, *Thromb. Haemostas. (Stuttgart)* **48**:38–40.

Carreras, L. O., Defreyn, G., and Machin, S. J., 1981, Arterial thrombosis, intrauterine death and lupus anticoagulant: Detection of immunoglobulin interfering with prostacyclin formation, *Lancet* **1**:244–246.

Catterall, R. D., 1973, Biological false positive reactions and systemic disease, in: *Ninth Symposium on Advanced Medicine* (G. Walker, ed.), Pitman Medical, London, pp. 97–111.

Conley, C. L., and Hartmann, R. C., 1952, A hemorrhagic disorder caused by circulating anticoagulant in patients with disseminated lupus erythematosus, *J. Clin. Invest.* **31**:621–622.

Cooper, M. R., Cohen, H. J., Huntley, C. C., Waite, B. M., Spees, L., and Spurr, L., 1974, A monoclonal IgM with antibodylike specificity for phospholipids in a patient with lymphoma, *Blood* **43**:493–504.

Coots, M. C., Miller, M. A., and Glueck, H. I., 1981, The lupus inhibitor. A study of its heterogeneity, *Thromb. Haemostas.* **46**:734–739.

De Bruijn, J. H., 1966, Chemical structure and serological activity of natural and synthetic cardiolipin and related compounds, *Br. J. Vener. Dis.* **42**:125–128.

De Siervo, A. J., 1974, Anti-cardiolipin and anti-phosphatidylglycerol antibodies prepared against bacterial phospholipids, *Infect. Immun.* **9**:835–838.

Editorial, 1984, Lupus anticoagulant, *Lancet* **1**:1157–1158.

Elias, M., and Eldor, A., 1984, Thromboembolism in patients with the 'lupus'-like circulating anticoagulant, *Arch. Intern. Med.* **144**:510–515.

Exner, T., Rickard, K. A., and Kronenberg, H., 1975, Studies on phospholipids in the action of a lupus coagulation inhibitor, *Pathology* **7**:319–328.

Exner, T., Rickard, K. A., and Kronenberg, H., 1978, A sensitive test demonstrating lupus anticoagulant and its behavioural patterns, *Br. J. Haematol.* **40**:143–151.

Exner, T., Barber, S., Kronenberg, H., and Rickard, K., 1980, Familial association of the lupus anticoagulant, *Br. J. Haematol.* **45**:89–96.

Faure, M., and Coulon-Morelec, M., 1963, Entre la structure chimique du cardiolipide et son activite serologique. Conservation du cardiolipide, *Ann. Inst. Pasteur (Paris)* **104**:246–263.

Feinstein, D. I., and Rapaport, S. I., 1972, Acquired inhibitors of blood coagulation, in: *Progress in Hemostasis and Thrombosis*, Vol. 1 (T. N. Spaet, ed.), Grune & Stratton, New York, pp. 79–95.

Firkin, B. G., Booth, P., Hendrix, L., and Howard, M. A., 1978, Demonstration of a platelet by-pass mechanism in the clotting system using an acquired anticoagulant, *Am. J. Hematol.* **5**:81–92.

Firkin, B. G., Howard, M. A., and Radford, N., 1980, Possible relationship between lupus inhibitor and recurrent abortion in young women, *Lancet* **2**:366.

Fiumara, N. S., 1963, Biologic false-positive reaction for syphilis, *N. Engl. J. Med.* **268**:402–405.

Fowler, E., and Allen, R. H., 1962, Studies on the production of Wasserman reagin, *J. Immunol.* **88**:591–594.

Frick, P. G., 1955, Acquired circulating anticoagulants in systemic "collagen disease": Autoimmune thromboplastin deficiency, *Blood* **10**:691–706.

Fulford, K. W., Catterall, R. D., Delhanty, J. J., Donjach, V., and Kremer, M., 1972, A collagen disorder of the nervous system presenting as multiple sclerosis, *Brain* **95**:373–386.

Gladman, D. D., Urowitz, M. B., Tozman, E. C., and Glynn, M. X., 1983, Haemostatic abnormalities in systemic lupus erythematosus, *Q. J. Med.* **207**:424–433.

Gonyea, L., Herdman, R., and Bridges, R. A., 1968, The coagulation abnormalities in systemic lupus erythematosus, *Thromb. Diathes. Haemorrh.* **20**:457–464.

Gray, G. M., and MacFarlane, M. G., 1958, Separation and composition of the phospholipids of ox heart, *Biochem. J.* **70**:409–433.

Guarnieri, M., 1974, Reaction of cardiolipin and phosphatidylinositol antisera with phospholipids antigens, *Lipids* **9**:692–695.

Guarnieri, M., 1975, Reaction of anti-phosphatidyl inositol antisera with neural membrane, *Lipids* **10**:294–298.

Guarneiri, M., and Eisner, D., 1974, A DNA antigen that reacts with antisera to cardiolipin, *Biochem. Biophys. Res. Commun.* **58**:347–353.

Harris, E. N., Gharavi, A. E., Boey, M. L., Patel, B. M., Mackworth-Young, C. G., Loizou, S., and Hughes, G. R. V., 1983, Anticardiolipin antibodies: Detection by radioimmunoassay and association with thrombosis in systemic lupus erythematosus, *Lancet* **2**:1211–1214.

Harris, E. N., Gharavi, A. E., Asherson, R. A., Boey, M. L., and Hughes, G. R. V., 1984, Cerebral infarction in systemic lupus: Association with anticardiolipin antibodies, *Clin. Exp. Rheum.* **1**:47–51.

Harris, E. N., Asherson, R. A., Gharavi, A. E., Morgan, S. H., Derue, G., and Hughes, G. R. V., 1985a, Thrombocytopenia in SLE and related autoimmune disorders: Association with anticardiolipin antibody, *Br. J. Haematol.* **59**:227–230.

Harris, E. N., Gharavi, A. E., Hegde, V., Morgan, S. H., Derue, G., Englert, H., Chan, J. K. H., Asherson, R. A., and Hughes, G. R. V., 1985b, Anticardiolipin antibodies in autoimmune thrombocytopenic purpura, *Br. J. Haematol.* **59**:1–6.

Harris, E. N., Gharavi, A. E., Loizou, S., Derue, G., Chan, J. K., Patel, B. M., Mackworth-Young, C. G., Bunn, C. C., and Hughes, G. R. V., 1985c, Crossreactivity of antiphospholipid antibodies, *J. Clin. Lab. Immunol.* **16**:1–6.

Harvey, A. M., and Shulman, L. E., 1966, Connective tissue disease and chronic biologic false-positive test for syphilis (BFP reaction), *Med. Clin. North Am.* **50**:1271–1279.

Harvey, A. M., and Shulman, L. E., 1974, Systemic lupus erythematosus and the chronic biologic false-positive test for syphilis, in: *Lupus Erythematosus,* 2nd edition (E. I. Dubois, ed.), University of California Press, Los Angeles, pp. 196–209.

Haserick, J. R., and Long, R., 1951, Systemic lupus erythematosus preceded by false-positive tests for syphilis: Presentation of five cases, *Ann. Int. Med.* **37**:559–565.

Hirano, T., Hashimoto, H., Shiokawa, Y., Iwamora, M., Nagai, Y., Kasai, M., and Ochiai, K., 1980, Antiglycolipid autoantibody detected in the sera from systemic lupus erythematosus patients, *J. Clin. Invest.* **66**:1437–1440.

Howard, M. A., and Firkin, B. G., 1983, Investigations of the lupus-like inhibitor bypassing activity of platelets, *Thromb. Haemostas. (Stuttgart)* **50**:775–779.

Hughes, G. R. V., 1983, Thrombosis, abortion, cerebral disease and the lupus anticoagulant, *Br. Med. J.* **287**:1088–1089.

Hull, R. G., Harris, E. N., Morgan, S. H., and Hughes, G. R. V., 1983, Anti-Ro antibodies and abortions in women with SLE, *Lancet* **2**:1138.

Inoue, K., and Nojima, S., 1967a, Immunochemical studies of phospholipids. I. Reactivity of various synthetic cardiolipin derivatives with Wasserman antibody, *Chem. Phys. Lipids* **1**:360–367.

Inoue, K., and Nojima, S., 1967b, Immunochemical studies of phospholipids II. Production of antibody to cardiolipin, *Biochim. Biophys. Acta* **144**:409–414.

Inoue, K., and Nojima, S., 1969, Immunochemical studies of phospholipids. IV: The reactivities of antisera against natural cardiolipin and synthetic cardiolipin analogues-containing antigens, *Chem. Phys. Lipids* **3**:70–77.

Johansson, E. A., and Lassus, A., 1974, The occurrence of circulating anticoagulants in patients with syphilitic and biologically false positive antilipoidal antibodies, *Ann. Clin. Res.* **6**:105–108.

Johansson, E. A., Lassus, A., and Salo, O. P., 1972, Occurrence of antinuclear factors with immunoglobulins bound to the dermo–epidermal junction in patients with chronic biological false positive (CBFP) reactions for syphilis, *Acta Derm. Vener. (Stockholm)* **52**:196–200.

Johansson, E. A., Niemi, K. M., and Mustakallio, K. K., 1977, A peripheral vascular syndrome overlapping with systemic lupus erythematosus: Recurrent venous thrombosis and hemorrhagic capillary proliferation with circulating anticoagulants and false-positive seroreactions for syphilis, *Dermatologica* **155**:257–267.

Koike, T., Tomioka, H., and Kumagai, A., 1982, Antibodies cross-reactive with DNA and cardiolipin in patients with systemic lupus erythematosus, *Clin. Exp. Immunol.* **50**:298–302.

Koike, T., Seuishi, M., Funaki, H., Tomioka, H., and Yoshida, S., 1984a, Antiphospholipid antibodies and biological false positive serological test for syphilis in patients with systemic lupus erythematosus, *Clin. Exp. Immunol.* **56**:193–199.

Koike, T., Maruyama, N., Funaki, H., Tomioka, H., and Yoshida, S., 1984b, Specificity of mouse hybridoma antibodies to DNA II. Phospholipid reactivity and biological false positive serological test for syphilis, *Clin. Exp. Immunol.* **57**:345–350.

Konstant, H., 1972, Familial chronic biologic false-positive seroreactions for syphilis: Report of two families, one with three generations affected, *JAMA* **219**:45–48.

Labro, M. T., Andrieu, M., Weber, M., and Homberg, J. C., 1978, A new pattern of non-organ and non-species-specific anti-organelle antibody detected by immunofluorescence: The mitochondrial antibody number 5, *Clin. Exp. Immunol.* **31**:357–366.

Lafer, E. M., Rauch, J., Andrzejewski, C., Mudd, D., Furie, B., Schwarz, R. S., and Stollar, B. D., 1981, Polyspecific monoclonal lupus autoantibodies reactive with both polynucleotides and phospholipids, *J. Exp. Med.* **153**:897–909.

Landi, G., Calloni, M. V., and Sabbadini, M. G., 1983, Recurrent ischemic attacks in young adults with lupus anticoagulant, *Stroke* **14**:377–379.

Laurell, A. B., and Nilsson, I. M., 1957, Hypergammaglobulinemia, circulating anticoagulant, and biologic false positive Wasserman reaction: A study of two cases, *J. Lab. Clin. Med.* **49**:694–707.

Lechner, K., 1969, A new type of coagulation inhibitor, *Thromb. Diathes. Haemorrh.* **21**:482–499.

Lechner, K., 1971, Acquired inhibitors in auto- and isoimmune disease, *Thromb. Diathes. Haemorrh.* (*Suppl.*) **45**:227–241.

Lechner, K., 1974, Acquired inhibitors in nonhemophilic patients, *Haemostasis* **3**:65–93.

Lee, S. L., and Miotti, A. B., 1975, Disorders of hemostatic function in patients with systemic lupus erythematosus, *Semin. Arthritis Rheum.* **4**:241–252.

Lee, S. L., and Sanders, M., 1955, A disorder of blood coagulation in systemic lupus erythematosus, *J. Clin. Invest.* **34**:1814–1822.

Loeliger, A., 1959, Prothrombin as cofactor of the circulating anticoagulant in systemic lupus erythematosus, *Thromb. Diathes. Haemorrh.* **3**:237–256.

Lubbe, W. F., Palmer, S. J., Butler, W. S., and Laggins, G. C., 1983, Fetal survival after prednisone suppression of maternal lupus anticoagulant, *Lancet* **1**:1361–1363.

MacFarlane, M. G., and Gray, G. M., 1957, Composition of cardiolipin, *Biochem. J.* **67**:25.

MacFarlane, M. G., and Wheeldon, L. W., 1958, Position of the fatty acids in cardiolipin, *Nature* **183**:1808.

Margolius, A., Jackson, D. P., and Ratnoff, O. D., 1961, Circulating anticoagulants: A study of 40 cases and a review of the literature, *Medicine* (*Baltimore*) **40**:145–202.

Medal, L. S., and Lisker, R., 1959, Circulating anticoagulants in disseminated lupus erythematosus, *Br. J. Haematol.* **5**:284–293.

Moore, J. E., and Lutz, W. B., 1955, The natural history of systemic lupus erythematosus: An approach to its study through chronic biologic false positive reactors, *J Chron. Dis.* **1**:297–316.

Moore, J. E., and Mohr, C. F., 1952, Biologically false positive serologic tests for syphilis: Type, incidence, and cause, *JAMA* **150**:467–473.

Morgan, A., Thompson, S., Rogers, L. A., and Staines, N. A., 1983, Specificity of murine monoclonal anti-DNA autoantibodies: Reactivity with nucleotides, nucleosides and phospholipids, British Society of Immunology Meeting, Spring 1983.

Mueh, J. R., Herbst, K. D., and Rapaport, S. I., 1980, Thrombosis in patients with the lupus anticoagulant, *Ann. Intern. Med.* **92**:156–159.

Nelson, R. A., and Mayer, M. M., 1949, Immobilization of treponema pallidum *in vitro* by antibody produced in syphilitic infection, *J. Exp. Med.* **89**:369.

Nelson, R. A., Zhuetlin, H. E. C., Diesendrick, J., and Austin, P. A., 1950, Studies on treponemal immobilizing antibodies in syphilis, *Ann. J. Syph. Gonorr. Vener. Dis.* **34**:101.

Nilsson, I. M., Astedt, B., Hedner, U., and Berezin, D., 1975, Intrauterine death and circulating anticoagulant ("antithromboplastin"), *Acta. Med. Scand.* **197**:159.

Pangborn, M. C., 1941, A new serologically active phospholipid from beef heart, *Proc. Soc. Exp. Biol.* **48**:484–486.

Prentice, R. L., Gatenby, P. A., Loblay, R. H., Shearman, R. P., Kronenberg, H., and Basten, A., 1984, Lupus anticoagulant in pregnancy, *Lancet* **1**:464.

Putkonen, T., Jokinen, E. J., and Mustakallio, K. K., 1967, Chronic biologic false positive seroreactions for syphilis as a harbinger of systemic lupus erythematosus, *Arch Derm. Vener.* **47**:83–88.

Rauch, J., Tannenbaum, H., Stollar, B. D., and Schwarz, R. S., 1984, Monoclonal anticardiolipin antibodies bind DNA, *Eur. J. Immunol.* **14**:529–534.

Ros, J. O., Tarres, M. V., Baucells, M. V., Maired, J. V., and Solano, J. T., 1983, Prednisone and maternal lupus anticoagulant, *Lancet* **2**:576.

Schleider, M. A., Nachman, R. L., Jaffe, E. A., and Coleman, M., 1976, A clinical study of the lupus anticoagulant, *Blood* **48**:499–509.

Shapiro, S. S., and Thiagarajan, P., 1982, Lupus anticoagulants, *Prog. Hemostasis Thromb.* **6**:263–285.

Shoenfeld, Y., Rauch, J., Massicotte, H., Datta, S. K., Andre-Schwarz, J., Stollar, B. D., and Schwarz, R. S., 1983, Polyspecificity of monoclonal lupus autoantibodies produced by human–human hybridomas, *N. Engl. J. Med.* **308**:414–420.

Soulier, R. P., and Boffa, M. C., 1980, Avortements a repetition, thromboses et anticoagulant circulant antithromboplastine, *Nouv. Presse Med.* **9**:859–864.

Tamamura, S., Hashimoto, T., and Hara, I., 1971, The immunological relations between acidic phospholipids and their antibodies, *Jpn. J. Exp. Med.* **41**:31–38.

Teitelbaum, D., Arnon, R., Sela, M., Rabinsohn, Y., and Shapiro, D., 1973, Sphingomyelin specific antibodies elicited by synthetic conjugates, *Immunochemistry* **10**:736–743.

Thiagarajan, P., Shapiro, S. S., and De Marco, L., 1980, Monoclonal immunoglobulin M coagulation inhibitor with phospholipid specificity—mechanism of a lupus anticoagulant, *J. Clin. Invest.* **66**:397–405.

Tincani, A., Meroni, P. L., Mantelli, P. G., and Balestrieri, G., 1984, Anti-phospholipid antibodies: Their relationship with anti-DNA and anti-mitochondrial activity, ANA symposium, Leuven, Belgium.

Tuffanelli, D. L., 1968, False positive reactions for syphilis: Serological abnormalities in relatives of chronic reactors, *Arch Dermatol.* **98**:606–611.

Valesini, G., Carsetti, R., Patricelli, S., Conti, L., Grandolfo, G. M., and Nicotra, M., 1982, Autoimmunity and abortion, in: *Serono Symposium No. 45. Immunological Factors in Human Reproduction* (S. Shulman, F. Dondero, and M. Nicotra, eds.), Academic Press, London, New York.

Veltkamp, J. J., Kerkhoven, P., and Loeliger, E. A., 1974, Circulating anticoagulant in disseminated lupus erythematosus: Proposed mode of action, *Haemostasis* **2**:253–259.

Weupper, K. D., Bodily, H. L., and Tuffanelli, D. L., 1966, Serologic tests for syphilis and the false-positive reactor, *Arch. Dermatol.* **94**:152–155.

Wicken, A. J., Gibbens, J. W., and Knox, K. W., 1972, Anti-techoic acid antibodies and non-treponemal serological tests for syphilis, *Infect. Immun.* **5**:982–984.

Williams, H., Laurent, R., and Gibson, T., 1980, The lupus coagulation inhibitor and venous thrombosis: A report of four cases, *Clin. Lab. Haematol.* **2**:139–144.

Wilson, H. A., Winfield, J. B., Lahita, R. G., and Koffler, D., 1979, The association of IgG anti-brain antibodies with central nervous system dysfunction and systemic lupus erythematosus, *Arthritis Rheum.* **12**:458–462.

Wilson, W. A., and Hughes, G. R. V., 1975, Aetiology of Jamaican neuropathy, *Lancet* **1**:240.

Wright, D. J. M., Doniach, D., Lessof, M. H., Turk, J. L., Grimble, A. S., and Catterall, R. D., 1970, New antibody in early syphilis, *Lancet* **1**:740–743.

Yin, E. T., and Gaston, L. W., 1965, Purification and kinetic studies on a circulating anticoagulant in a suspected case of lupus erythematosus, *Thromb. Diathes. Haemostas.* **14**:88–115.

Zvaifler, N. J., and Bluestein, H. G., 1982, The pathogenesis of central nervous system manifestations of systemic lupus erythematosus, *Arthritis Rheum.* **25**:862–866.

11

The Heterogeneity of Autoimmune Responses

Marc Feldmann, Deborah Doniach, and Gian Franco Bottazzo

I. INTRODUCTION

The contrasts between organ-specific endocrine autoimmunity (AI) and the more widespread "collagen disorders" such as SLE and RA have been insufficiently emphasized. In this context, it is now also important to separate the receptor diseases characterized by hormone overproduction, hyperplasia, or hypertrophy of the glands from destructive autoimmunity, exemplified by classical thyroiditis, gastritis, adrenalitis, etc. Hypertrophic receptor diseases are still relatively unexplored, except for Graves' thyrotoxicosis, because of the difficulties in demonstrating receptor antibodies or disturbed receptor function generally, but great progress may be expected in the near future.

Destructive autoimmunity, on the other hand, has been analyzed in great detail with animal models, and in human disease, the previously "idiopathic" atrophies of practically all endocrine glands have been demonstrated to be caused by autoimmunity (Doniach and Bottazzo, 1983). These studies are now extended to the paracrine system of the gastrointestinal tract (Mirakian *et al.*, 1981) and the hypothalamus (Scherbaum *et al.*, 1984). Both cellular and humoral immune mechanisms are involved in these contrasting disorders, although lymphoid cells are more conspicuous in the destructive lesions. It is a remarkable fact that the entire structure of a lymph node including germinal centers, paracortical areas with their typical interdigitating cells, and the "high endothelium" venules that separate cortex from paracortex in normal lymph nodes may develop in the

Marc Feldmann • ICRF Tumour Immunology Unit, Department of Zoology, University College London, London WC1E 6BT, England. *Deborah Doniach and Gian Franco Bottazzo* • Department of Immunology, Middlesex Hospital Medical School, London W1P 9PG, England.

thyroid gland in lymphoid thyroiditis and at certain stages in the development of similar lesions in the other endocrine glands.

The genetic predisposition and environmental contributions are different in "hypertrophic" and "atrophic" types of autoimmunity despite their conspicuous overlap. Similarly, these two basic types of AI affecting the endocrine system differ fundamentally from what is known to occur in the connective tissue disorders described in detail in this book.

The degree of initial environmental contribution and genetic predisposition and the sequence of events leading to the expression of different forms of autoimmune attack are not yet clear. In this context, remarkable facts must be considered; i.e., that the majority of patients with Graves' disease have evidence of focal lymphocytic thyroiditis, however mild, and that different types of thyroid disorders can all occur in the same patient at different times in life as well as in different members of their families despite the apparently opposite natures of the autoimmune phenomena in the effector phase. Furthermore, autoimmunity in different glands is inextricably mixed from a familial point of view as well as in individual cases. So-called polyendocrine autoimmunity may be rare in clinical practice, but it is now realized that serologically polyendocrine cases are far from rare even though many of the organs affected have lesions that may remain subclinical for the duration of the patient's life (Bottazzo and Doniach, 1985).

There is also a substantial degree of overlap between the organ- and non-organ-specific ends of the AI spectrum. This is particularly notable in receptor disease such as myasthenia gravis and "insulin-resistance with acanthosis." In myasthenia, about 50% of the cases have antinuclear antibodies, and in the AI insulin-receptor disease, practically all the patients have ribonucleoprotein antibodies as seen in mixed connective tissue disease, and half the patients suffer from a clinical Sjogren's syndrome (Kahn *et al.*, 1982). The overlap also varies with the age of onset. For instance, 30% of children with thyroiditis have ANA, and a small proportion actually develop clinical SLE (2/64 in our series; Doniach *et al.*, 1965).

The other remarkable overlapping area is observed in the autoimmune liver diseases. In primary biliary cirrhosis in which the intrahepatic bile ducts are selectively destroyed (International Pathology Group, 1983), primary atrophic and goitrous AI thyroiditis are present in up to 20% of the cases, and there is a substantial overlap with the CREST syndrome (calcinosis, Raynaud's phenomenon, esophagopathy, sclerodactyly telangiectasia). In lupoid hepatitis, the prevalence of thyroid antibodies is about two to three times higher than would be expected by chance (Doniach *et al.*, 1966). Interestingly, the chronic hepatitis associated with the so-called liver and kidney microsomal antibodies (LKM) shows a high prevalence of organ-specific reactions (Rizzetto *et al.*, 1973). This is of special interest in view of the "semi-organ-specific" nature of the endoplasmic reticulum LKM antigen and the fact that this variety of autoimmunity can be induced temporarily in predisposed individuals by drugs such as halothane (Walton *et al.*, 1976).

In view of the extraordinary complexity of interweaving relationships and our relative ignorance of the layers of regulatory "fail-safe" mechanisms that must break down before an actual autoimmune process can develop as a clinical disease manifestation, this chapter describes our own experience and working hypotheses about one aspect of endocrine destructive autoimmunity; i.e., the means by which endocrine cells become induced to act as self-antigen presenters (Fig. 1). We then discuss other prevalent ideologies such as the "H-gene" theory of autoimmunity put forward by Adams *et al.* (1984) and the "idiotype–antiidiotype" theories (Roitt, 1984) recently emerging in several areas of experimental and clinical autoimmunity (Cooke *et al.*, 1983; Plotz, 1983).

II. OUR WORKING HYPOTHESIS

Of the several stages in the generation of an autoimmune response, the first is initiation: the development of autoantibody or of autoreactive cells. The second is the development of tissue damage as a result of these immune reactions. It is known that autoantibodies

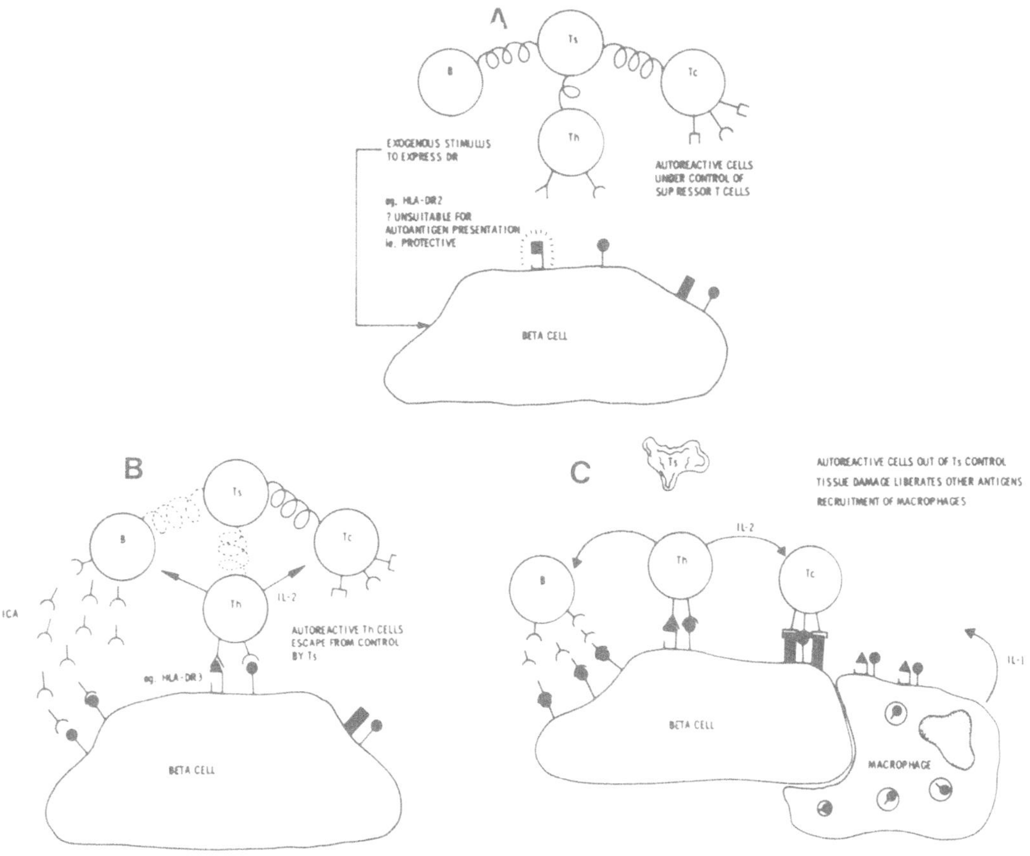

Figure 1. Three stages in induction of autoimmune disease using the β-cell as an example. (A) In genetically nonsusceptible individuals and in the absence of environmental stimuli, there is a lack of HLA-DR expression and consequently no autoimmunity. Environmental agents may induce DR (▮) as illustrated, but the molecule (e.g., DR-2) has a particular shape that is not ideal for presenting surface autoantigens efficiently (⚲); e.g., DR-2 suppressor T cells (Ts) maintain other lymphocytes under control (ᘓᘓ). (B) In genetically predisposed individuals, environmental agents induce DR expression. The configuration of DR (e.g., DR-3) is of importance and permits the correct presentation of autoantigens to T-helper cells (T_H). The T_H induce B lymphocytes to generate autoantibodies (Y). During the long latency period that precedes the onset of clinical symptoms, there is mild but continuous damage. (c) With abnormality of T-suppressor-cell function (specific to β-cells in the case of diabetes), organ damage becomes clinically manifest. With infiltration of cytotoxic T cells (Tc) and macrophages, Tc have a preferential receptor for class I (HLA-A,B,C ▮) molecules. Their expression is increased in affected organs. This ultimate attack leads to the release of many autoantigens and to the generation of other autoantibodies, which perpetuate the disease.

to endocrine organs may exist for many years without the appearance of overt clinical disease (reviewed by Doniach and Bottazzo, 1983), so it is necessary to consider the two stages separately. Unfortunately, relatively little is known of the initiating and precipitating causes of autoimmune disease after the onset of autoantibody production.

A. Mechanism of Induction of Immune Responses

Both cell-mediated (delayed hypersensitivity or cytotoxic T-cell) and long-term humoral responses involve T cells that recognize antigenic determinants associated with class II major histocompatibility, HLA-DR antigens (Ia in animals) (reviewed by Bodmer, 1981). Unlike MHC class I (HLA-A,B,C), MHC class II DR molecules are of restricted tissue distribution. They are normally present on cells of the immune system such as B and activated T lymphocytes, antigen-presenting cells (APC) such as Langerhans cells, dendritic cells, and macrophages and also vascular endothelial cells but not on connective tissue or endocrine cells (Barclay and Mason, 1983). As the recognition of DR antigen is critical for the induction of immune responses, only cells expressing DR are able to induce T cells to respond.

T-cell recognition of DR molecules and extrinsic antigen, in an appropriate form in the presence of IL-1, leads to cell division and the induction of receptors for T-cell growth factor (IL-2). The lymphocyte-activating factor IL-1 is required unless the T cells are already inactivated, and IL-2 is mainly produced by activated T helper cells. Interleukin 2 amplifies the growth of the relevant T-cell clones and of nearby clones with receptors for IL-2, and in this way relevant autoreactive clonal progeny develop either to act as effector cells or to induce effector B or T cells (Singer and Hodes, 1983).

T-cell recognition of DR* molecules and antigen also leads to the release of a variety of lymphokines such as IL-2, B-cell growth and differentiating factors, macrophage-activating factor, and interferon γ (INF_{γ}). Interferons, especially INF_{γ}, have been shown to be potent inducers of DR expression (Steeg *et al.*, 1982; Rhodes and Stokes, 1982).

In order to activate T cells, antigen has to be processed into an appropriate form. Both cellular (e.g., bacteria or viruses) and protein antigens need to be broken down to polypeptides of various sizes. This is mediated by enzymes either in or on the antigen-presenting cells and may be stimulated experimentally by enzymes, e.g., trypsin or elastase. These polypeptides are recognized by T cells in association with MHC class II (DR) antigens. It is still unclear whether DR molecules bind antigen selectively. The evidence to support this idea is not conclusive as yet (Werdelin, 1982; Rock and Benacerraf, 1983). T cell receptors, by possessing binding sites for both DR and antigen, could bring the two sufficiently close to permit T-cell triggering. Recent evidence suggests the need for an optimum quantity of DR and antigen for effective presentation, and, when an excess is present, diminished responses occur (Matis *et al.*, 1983).

* We will use HLA-DR abbreviated to DR to encompass all subtypes of human MHC Class II antigens at the D locus (HLA-DR, HLA-DC and HLA-SB), or in the new WHO nomenclature, HLA-DR, HLA-DQ and HLA-DP).

B. Expression of DR/Ia Molecules on Other Cells

Aberrant expression of DR or Ia has been noted in endothelium and in a variety of epithelia—gut, skin, kidney, bronchi, and mammary glands, in conditions, such as graft-versus-host (GVH) disease and dermatoses, parasitic infestation, and lactation (reviewed by Barclay and Mason, 1983; Steeg *et al.*, 1982). It is pertinent that GVH disease, with widespread aberrant DR expression, has features in common with some autoimmune disorders (Epstein *et al.*, 1980; Gleichmann *et al.*, 1978). It is not yet known whether all cells may express these antigens under appropriate stimulus, nor is it known whether the mechanism of DR regulation is the same in all cells. Preliminary evidence suggests that there is a heterogeneity of signals inducing DR; e.g., B cells respond to BCGF and other stimuli.

Culturing normal human thyroid epithelial cells with mitogenic lectins demonstrated that these cells may be induced to express DR antigens, as detected by a panel of monoclonal antibodies (Pujol-Borrell *et al.*, 1983). Most important, sections of thyroid glands or cultures of freshly dispersed thyroid follicles from patients with Graves' disease showed a spontaneous, patchy distribution of DR molecules on thyrocytes (Fig. 2), positively identified in monolayers by their reaction with antimicrosomal/microvillar an-

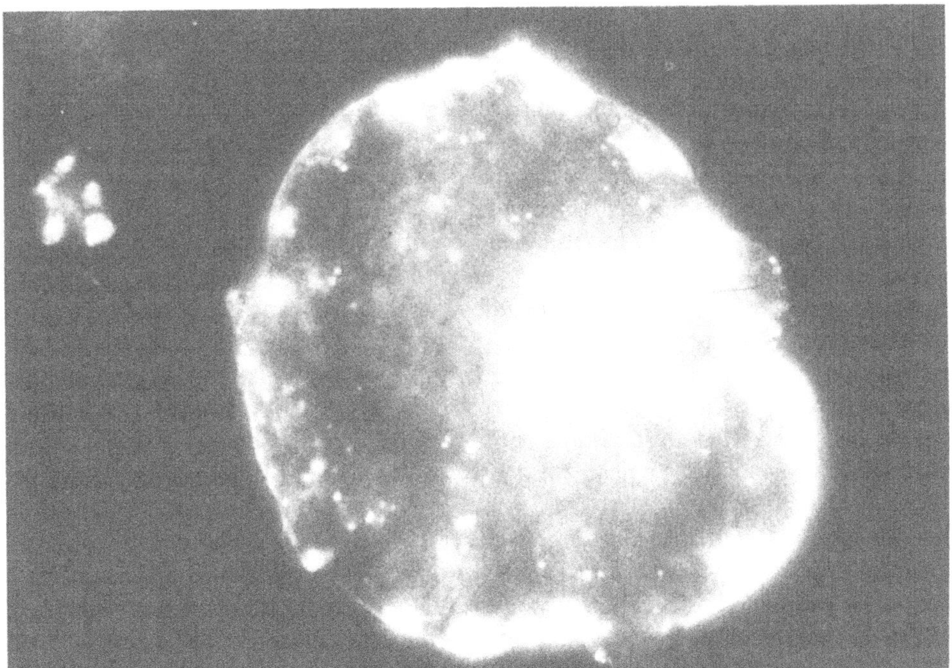

Figure 2. Photomicrograph of a freshly dispersed intact thyroid follicle from a gland removed at thyroidectomy for Graves' thyrotoxicosis and stained by indirect immunofluorescence for HLA-DR antigen. The outer surface of the follicle was DR^+, suggesting *in vivo* spontaneous synthesis of the glycoproteins in some of the thyrocytes. The larger white blobs represent pink autofluorescence from lipofuscin, easy to distinguish from the green DR^+ staining (×472). (Reproduced from Hanafusa *et al.*, 1983.)

tibodies spontaneously present in the sera of patients with Hashimoto's disease (Hanafusa *et al.*, 1983). An expansion of this work has proved that this phenomenon is by no means restricted to thyroid cells. Inappropriate DR expression has recently been observed on β-islet cells (Fig. 3) in a newly diagnosed diabetic pancreas obtained soon after death (Bottazzo *et al.*, 1985) in bile ducts of liver biopsies (Fig. 4) taken from stage I primary biliary cirrhosis cases (Ballardini *et al.*, 1984), and in a variety of intestinal disorders including Crohn's and celiac diseases (Selby *et al.*, 1983) as well as on biopsies from children with intractable diarrhea caused by autoimmune enteritis (Fig. 5) (R. Mirakian, A. C. Richardson, P. Milla, J. Unsworth, J. Walker-Smith, M. O. Savage and G. F. Bottazzo unpublishd data). In all of these conditions, the DR expression appeared as an early marker of the disease before the appearance of an active lymphocytic invasion of the organ. In BB rats, DR expression on pancreatic β-cells was seen mainly before the animals became diabetic, always associated with a lymphocyte infiltrate (Dean *et al.*, 1984).

C. Induction of Responses to Autoantigens

Organ-specific autoantigens are generally present in very low concentration in the circulation (Hijmans *et al.*, 1961) and consequently are probably unable to cause T-cell tolerance or suppression. Conversely, from what is known, those antigens present at high concentrations and involved in the collagen diseases should by right cause T-cell tolerance and maintain it. Receptors for hormones such as TSH or insulin or surface autoantigens on rare cells (e.g., pancreatic islet cells) would be expressed at concentrations too low to induce tolerance, and so if these antigens were presented by DR molecules synthesized by the corresponding endocrine cells, autoimmunity could result, assuming other requirements for T-cell stimulation were fulfilled. It is known that autoantigens can be presented by autologous antigen-presenting cells (Winchester *et al.*, 1984).

Usually one requirement for effective T-cell stimulation is the presence of IL-1, but since keratinocytes can secrete IL-1 (Oppenheim and Gery, 1982), other epithelial cells could also produce it. Furthermore, certain T-cell clones can be stimulated by DR^+ B lymphocytes in the absence of IL-1 (Kappler *et al.*, 1982). Thus, aberrant DR expression on epithelial endocrine cells could be sufficient to activate T cells. We have recently tested this possibility using DR^+ thyrocytes from thyrotoxic patients and cloned human T cells recognizing influenza A hemagglutinin or synthetic peptide corresponding to amino acids 306–329 of the HA-1 sequence (Londei *et al.*, 1984). It was found that the thyrocytes presented the peptide effectively, and the response was blocked by appropriate anti-MHC Class II antibody (Fig. 6). The problem was to verify that presentation was by the thyrocytes and not by contaminating macrophages or dendritic or B cells. This was resolved by cell purification but most convincingly by the fact that the thyrocytes, unlike blood cells, presented peptide antigen but not the intact virus. Thus, they were able to present but not to process antigen. This would of course permit the presentation of autoantigens already on the cell membrane.

Provided that there are enough autoreactive precursors present, which is likely for antigens too rare to induce tolerance or suppressor T cells, then autoimmune reactions could be initiated. The consequences depend on the types of cells activated, whether tissue damage takes place, and whether various immunoregulatory mechanisms can efficiently stop this response.

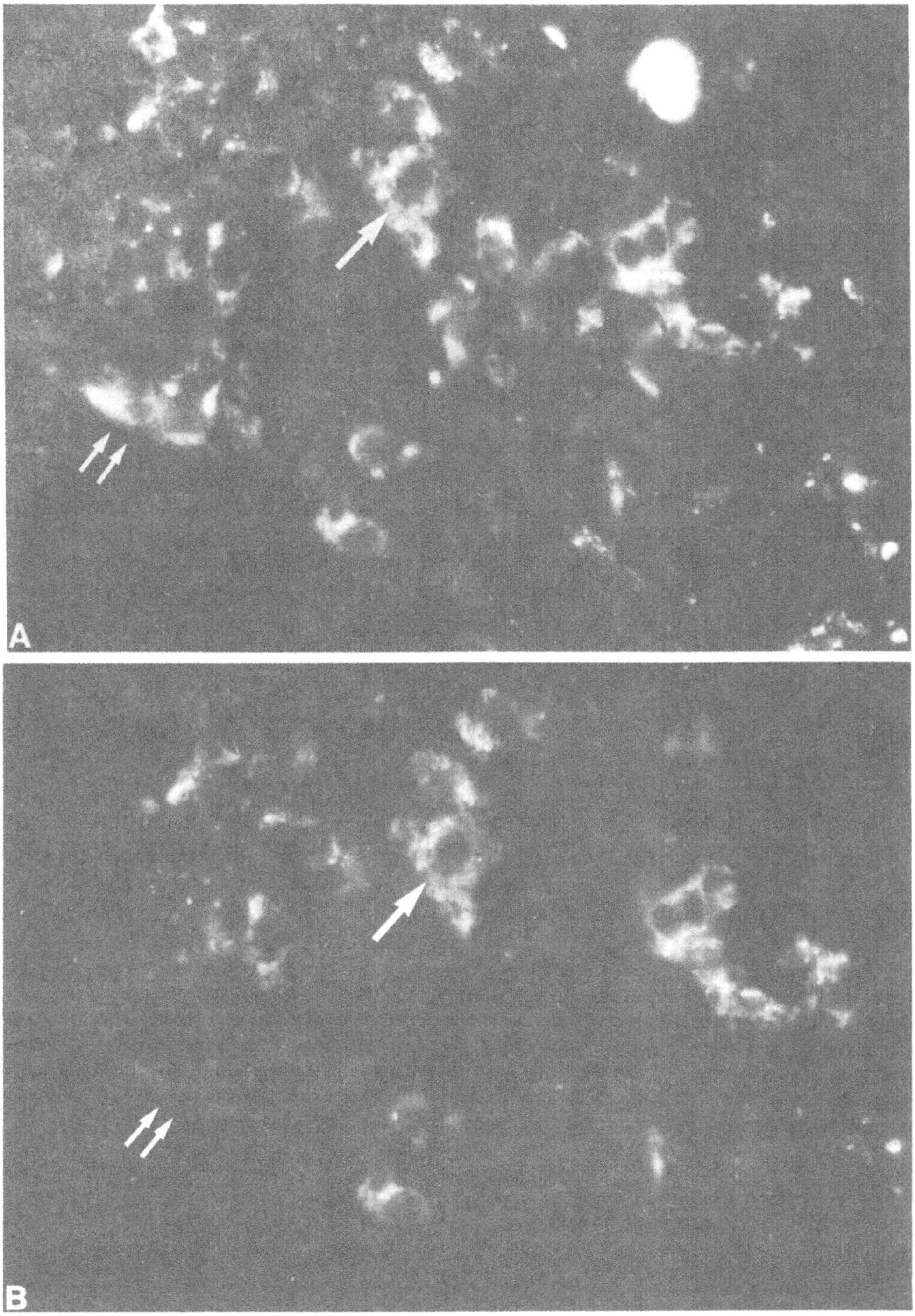

Figure 3. Cryostat section of a diseased islet from the postmorten pancreas of a diabetic child with insulitis stained by double fluorochrome immunofluorescence for (A) human insulin (green) or (B) HLA-DR antigen (red). The same field was photographed with red or green filters. Some large β-cells (one arrow) producing insulin also stained DR$^+$, a feature not seen in normal islet cells. Other insulin-producing cells at edge of islet (two arrows) were DR$^-$. The white blob in A is an artifact (×480). (By courtesy of Dr. B. M. Dean.)

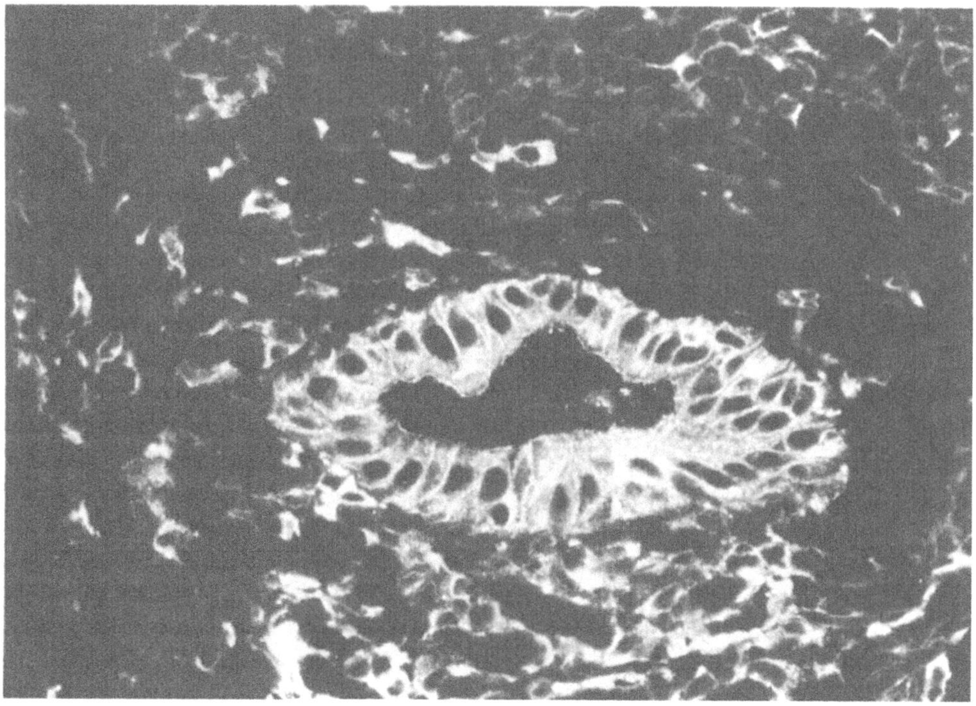

Figure 4. Unfixed cryostat section of liver biopsy from a symptomless patient with stage 1 primary biliary cirrhosis, stained by immunofluorescence for HLA-DR glycoproteins, showing a septal bile duct with strongly positive biliary epithelium. Adjacent sections stained by conventional H and E also showed features of early PBC including irregular nuclei, cell reduplication, and lymphoid invasion. The needle biopsy contained four portal tracts, three of which showed DR^+ bile ducts, whereas one duct was negative. Sections taken at five levels in the biopsy clearly illustrated the focal nature of the duct lesions. The degree of periductular cell infiltration varied with the intensity of DR staining on the bile duct cells ($\times 450$).

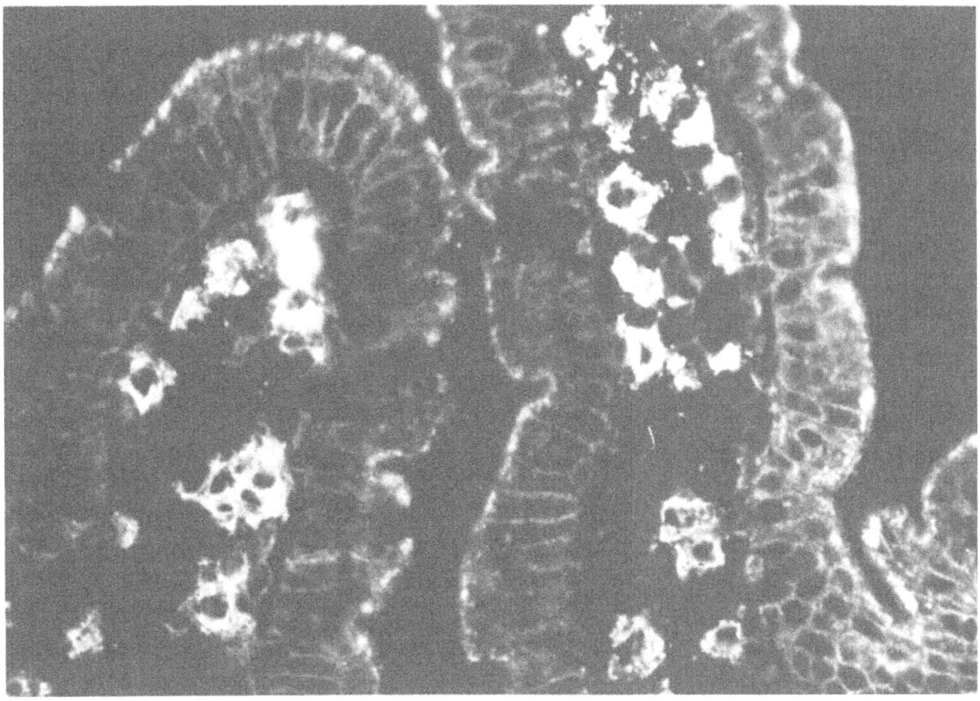

Figure 5. Jejunal biopsy from a child with circulating antibodies to enterocytes (ECA) and diarrhea, stained by immunofluorescence for HLA-DR antigens, showing increased expression both in the epitheliuim and in the cells of the lamina propria as compared with normal small intestine. In the enterocytes, the strongest DR$^+$ reactivity was on the microvillar border. The DR$^+$ lamina propria cells included macrophages, dendritic APCs, and mast cells (×480). (Courtesy of Dr. R. Mirakian.)

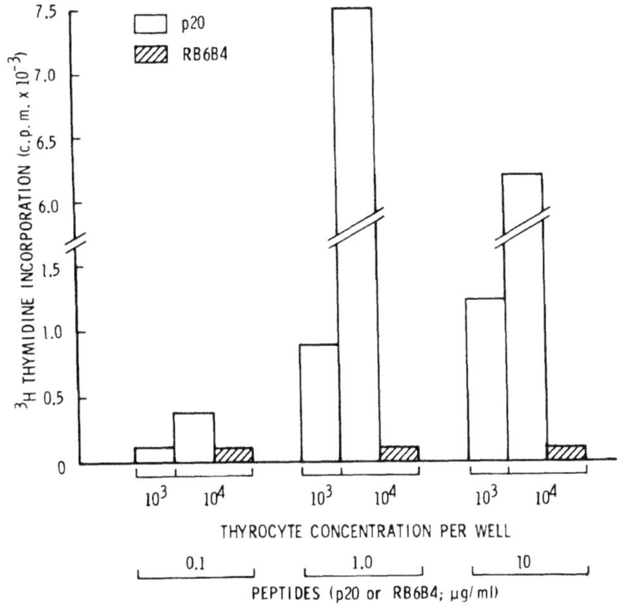

Figure 6. This experiment demonstrated that the proliferation of the flu-specific T-helper clone was not caused by the release of growth factors from the HLA-DR$^+$ thyrocytes acting as APCs and was dose related for the relevant viral peptide (p20). No proliferation was observed when another flu peptide was added (RB6B4). (From Londei *et al.*, 1984.)

The recent development of methods for cloning T cells using interleukin-2 has made it possible to attempt to analyze the T cells that are present in an autoimmune organ. We have now cloned out intrathyroid already activated T cells from two patients with Graves' disease (Fig. 7). A number of specific clones of helper phenotype (T4) were identified in each. They were of two specificities: one set recognized autologous thyrocytes only, and the other recognized autologous thyrocytes and blood cells but not histoincompatible thyroid or blood. The cloned cells that recognize autologous thyrocytes adhere and grow on their surface, proving that the thyrocytes can act as antigen-presenting cells. Further analysis of these clones should yield insights into the mechanisms of autoimmune thyroidities (Londei *et al.*, 1985).

D. Viruses and Autoimmunity

There are some suggestions that endocrine autoimmune diseases, especially diabetes, have followed viral infections (Oldstone *et al.*, 1984); however, the search for specific viruses has rarely been successful. Viruses could be involved in the induction of autoimmunity by providing an antigen recognized by T cells that would induce responses to the virus-infected cells (Allison, 1977). The HLA-DR linkage of endocrine autoimmune responses (reviewed by Bodmer, 1981; Doniach *et al.*, 1982a) could thus reflect a genetic predisposition to respond effectively or not respond to that virus. However, this Ir gene concept does not explain why viral infections usually do not lead to persistent autoimmunity.

Although it is certainly possible that viruses may act as helper determinants (Bromberg *et al.*, 1982) that T cells recognize and then stimulate autoreactive B cells, there is no evidence to support this concept. We wish to propose that failure to detect specific

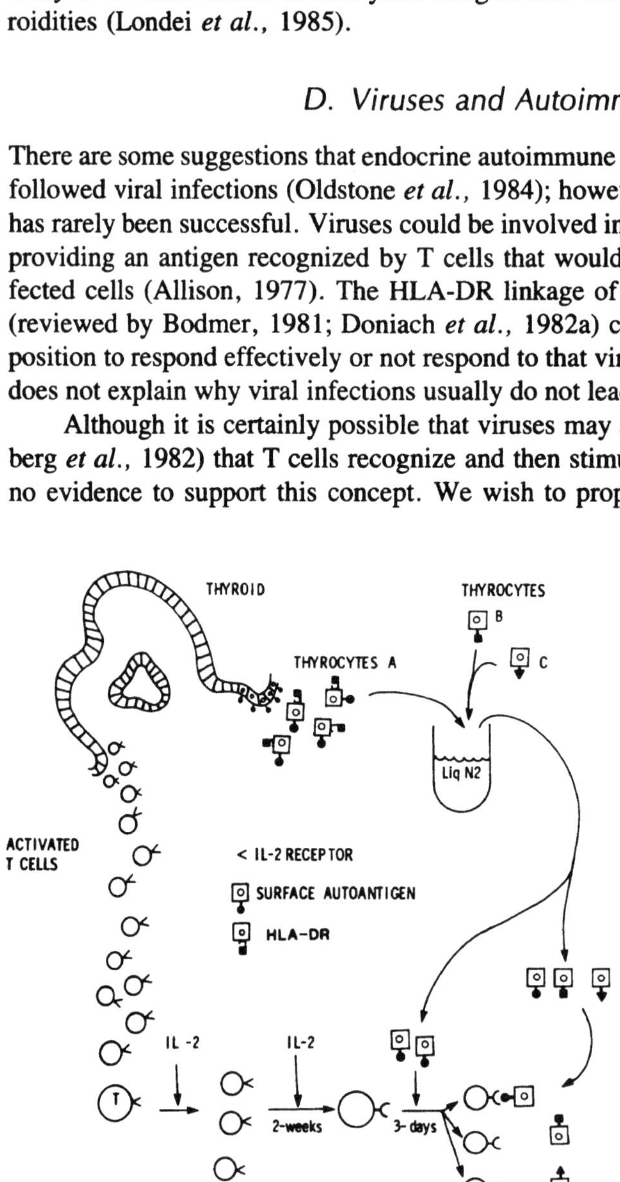

Figure 7. Diagram of method used to establish self-reactive T-cell clones from thyroidectomy glands of patients with Graves' disease. *In vivo* "activated" lymphoid cells were teased out of the thyroid and cultured in mitogen-free interleukin-2-enriched medium for up to 2 weeks. The thyrocytes were obtained by collagenase digestion and stored in liquid nitrogen until required. Growing T-cell clones were challenged with the patient's own viable thyrocytes. This approach demonstrated that some "sensitized" T cells are able to proliferate when in contact with autologous thyroid cells but not with HLA-DR-mismatched glands (see Londei *et al.*, 1985).

causal viruses in the pathogenesis of these autoimmune conditions is because, as for the common cold, there is no single specific virus. As already mentioned, organ-specific autoantibodies may be demonstrable years before the clinical expression of the corresponding endocrine disease. This suggests that DR antigen expression and the subsequent slow autoimmune damage has begun much earlier than previously anticipated. This is well documented in juvenile diabetes (Bottazzo, 1984). Prospective studies have also indicated that there need not be an irrevocable course towards clinical manifestations (Spencer *et al.*, 1984).

E. Interferon and Autoimmunity

Antecedent viral infections or other environmental factors could induce interferon α or β release and would also activate T cells, with the subsequent release of interferon γ, all of which could cause enhanced expression of DR antigens on antigen-presenting macrophages and endothelial cells and could also induce and maintain aberrant DR expression on neighboring epithelial cells in genetically predisposed individuals. It is known that IFN_γ induces DR on APC and endothelial cells (Steeg *et al.*, 1982; Pober *et al.*, 1983), and there is some evidence that IFN_α and IFN_β can act on APC (Rhodes and Stokes, 1982).

Once the initial activation of T helper cells has taken place as a result of the aberrant DR expression, effector mechanisms may be initiated. Activated T cells will help the induction of B lymphocytes and of cytotoxic or delayed-hypersensitivity T cells. Since B-cell tolerance has higher thresholds, and since autoreactive B cells can readily be demonstrated by antigen binding (Bankhurst *et al.*, 1973) or mitogens, antibody responses will follow once sufficient helper T cells are induced.

Since we demonstrated that IFN_γ induces HLA-DR expression in normal thyroid cells from laryngectomy patients (Fig. 8), it was of interest that supernatants of T cells also induced DR expression, which was blocked by anti-IFN_γ antiserum (Todd *et al.*, 1984). These results are in keeping with those of other groups who have shown that IFN_γ induced HLA-DR expression in endothelial cells, myeloid cells, and macrophages. In the tissues in which it has been tested, Ia or DR molecules have been associated with antigen-presenting capacity whether the antigen was present normally or abnormally; e.g., L cells (fibroblasts) transfected with I-A_α and I-A_β chains can present antigen to T-cell hybrids (Malissen *et al.*, 1984). Thus, there was every reason to suspect that thyroid epithelial cells expressing DR antigens should be able to present antigen. This was recently tested and shown to be correct (Londei *et al.*, 1984). DR^+ thyroid cells were capable of presenting peptides, and thus the consequence of IFN_γ-induced DR expression is the capacity of cells that normally could not to activate T cells and initiate the chain of events leading to an immune response: if T cells capable of recognizing autoantigens are present, then autoimmunity would result.

Interferon abnormalities have been described in systemic autoimmune disease. It has been found that patients with active SLE and some other autoimmune diseases (e.g., RA, psoriasis) have higher serum IFN titers than patients with inactive disease. It is possible that IFN production, in response to whatever stimulus, by increasing DR expression, could explain the generalized autoimmune status observed in these conditions. There has

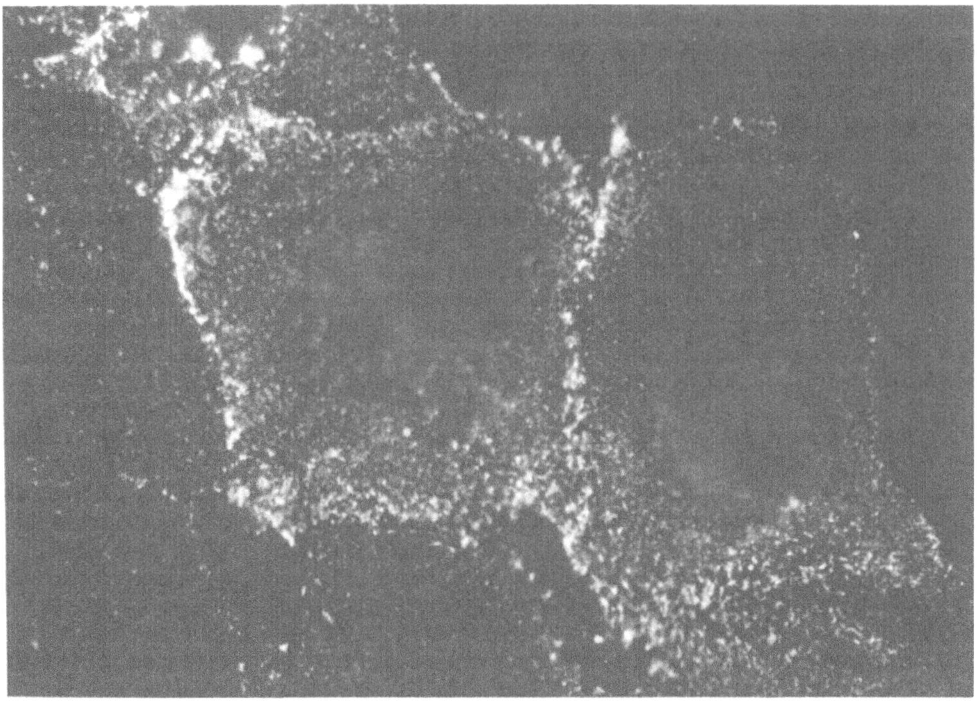

Figure 8. Induction of HLA-DR by γ-interferon (100 U/ml) in human thyrocytes. This monolayer was stained on day 7 by indirect immunofluorescence with a monoclonal antibody (MID-3) to the nonpolymorphic region of the glycoprotein. The two living thyrocytes in the center of the photo show intense DR^+ dots on their plasma membrane. (×450). (Reproduced from Todd *et al.*, 1984.)

been speculation that the autologous MLR may be involved in the autoimmune process (Talal and Smith, 1982), with T cells releasing IFN in an uncontrolled manner (Rosenberg *et al.*, 1984).

In SLE, RA, and a few other conditions, including AIDS, the interferon in the circulation is not one of the well-studied IFN species (α, β, γ). It has properties of both α and γ, being acid labile like IFN_γ and reacting with anti IFN_α antisera (Prebble *et al.*, 1982). The properties of this interferon are not yet well understood, but since α, β, and γ all share functional properties but at different efficiencies, it seems likely that this type of IFN may also be capable of inducing DR. As there is a correlation between titers of circulating IFN and disease activity, this seems to be a strong argument for the involvement of IFN in the pathogenesis of systemic autoimmunity.

F. HLA-A,B,C, Behavior in Autoimmune Lesions

Class I MHC antigens are normally present on all tissue cells, but in tissues taken from autoimmune patients their expression is greatly increased both on vascular endothelium and on endocrine cells. This was seen in sections of thyroiditis specimens (Hanafusa *et al.*, 1983), in liver biopsies from autoimmune hepatitis cases (Ballardini *et al.*, 1984), and in the diabetic pancreas (Fig. 9). More recently, we have shown that interferon α,

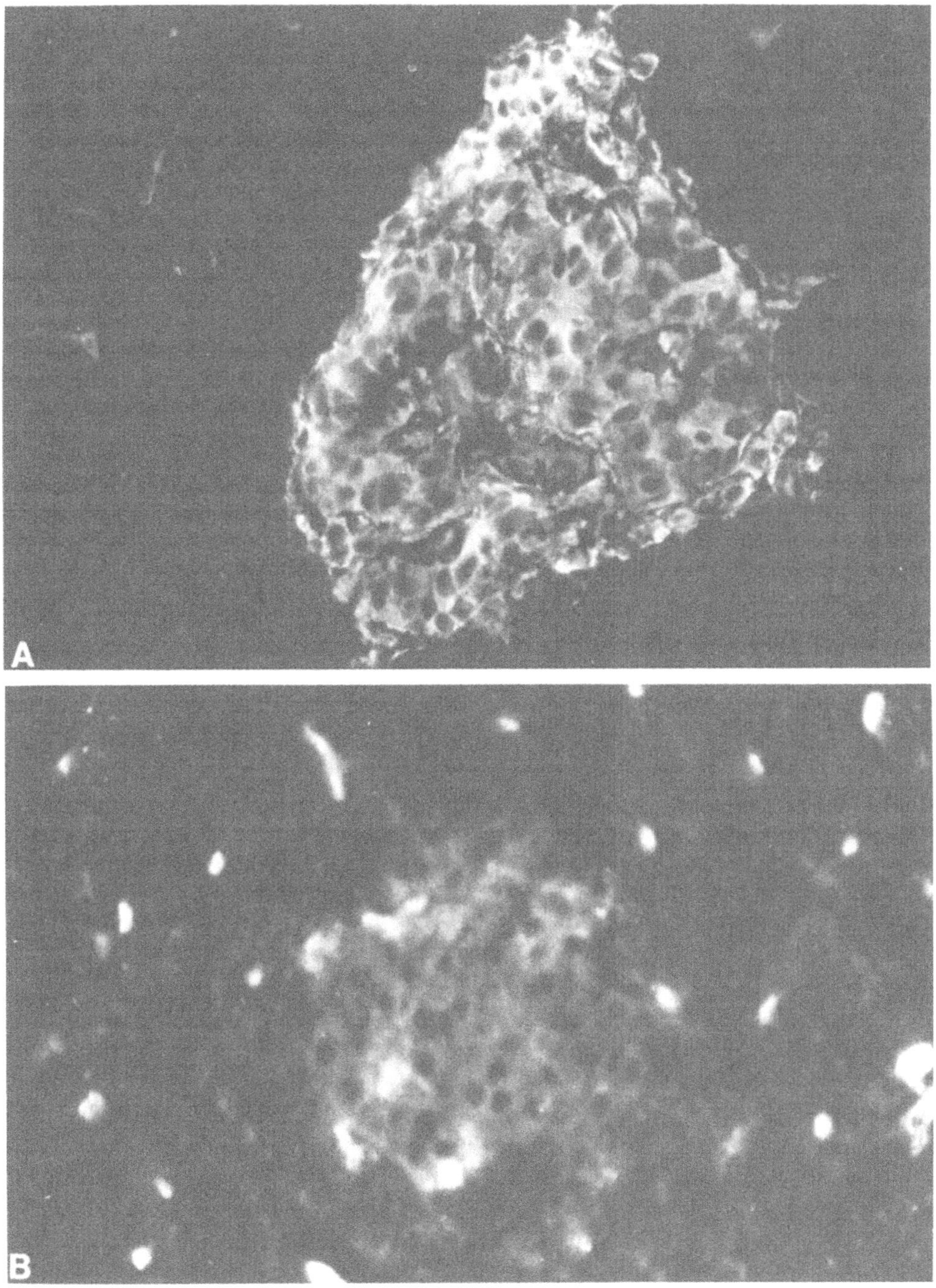

Figure 9. Cryostat section of a diseased pancreatic islet taken at postmortem from a newly diagnosed type-1 diabetic child, stained by immunofluorescence for MHC class I HLA-A,B,C antigens. The expression of these glycoproteins was greatly increased in the diabetic pancreas (A) as compared with islets in a non-diabetic postmortem control pancreas stained with the same reagents (B) (×338).

β, and γ, but not IL-2, all have a potent enhancing effect on the expression of HLA-A,B,C when incubated with monolayer cultures of normal thyrocytes (Todd *et al.*, 1984). Immunostaining studies to identify T-lymphocyte subsets in autoimmune thyroiditis (Jansson *et al.*, 1984) and insulitis (Bottazzo *et al.*, 1985) constantly show a predominance of suppressor cytotoxic phenotype ($T8^+$) cells in early lesions where damage to endocrine cells is occurring. The magnified expression of class I MHC molecules would be compatible with and would facilitate cellular damage via cytotoxic T lymphocytes but may merely be a consequence of augmented IFN levels.

G. Relationship of Autoimmune Response and Disease

Whether the initial induction of an autoimmune response via the sequence described above results in an autoimmune disease depends on a variety of factors. The incidence of autoantibodies increases in middle age, especially in females, suggesting that their induction in the absence of overt disease is not a rare event. Disease may depend on the rate of regeneration of tissues or on abnormalities, either temporary or inborn and more permanent (Arulanantham *et al.*, 1979), of the suppressor T-cell pathways. If an episode of autoimmune T-cell generation is associated with a concomitant or subsequent depression of the suppressor-cell pathway, then sufficient tissue damage could take place to activate many T-cell clones, with the release or exposure of large quantities of autoantigen, which could then generate a progressive autoimmune response.

Experimental maneuvers that deplete suppressor cells (e.g., irradiation or cyclophosphamide) permit autoimmunity (e.g., Tarsic and Naor, 1982), and T cells of suppressor ($T8^+$) phenotypes are reduced in a variety of human endocrine autoimmune diseases during their active phases (Starkosch *et al.*, 1982; Buschard *et al.*, 1982). In our scheme, diminution of suppressor function, either congenital or acquired, is a later event. The autoreactivity in the organ-specific syndromes indicates that depressed non-antigen-specific suppressor function occurs only rarely and cannot explain the relative reproducibility and specificity of each autoimmune syndrome.

H. Mechanisms of Self-Nonreactivity

A multitude of explanations have been offered to account for the usual state of self-nonreactivity. Initially, immunologic tolerance, conceived by Burnet (1959) as the deletion of self-reactive clones, was the preferred hypothesis. Subsequently, when suppressor cells were discovered, their role was emphasized (Gershon, 1978). The hypothesis of the idiotype network of lymphocyte receptor interactions as an important form of immune regulation has led to speculation that it may prevent harmful autoreactivity.

Current concepts of self-nonreactivity do not usually envisage a single mechanism to account for a wide variety of self antigens. It is also now evident that self-reactivity is a normal component of T-cell physiology: most T cells need to recognize MHC components that they have learned to recognize as self during lymphopoiesis in the thymus (Schoenfeld and Schwartz, 1984).

Immunologic tolerance may be induced experimentally with either high concentrations of antigen or prolonged low concentrations (Mitchison, 1964). Tolerance is easier to induce in T cells than B cells, which fits in well with much evidence that there is no self-tolerance to a variety of self antigens. Thus, there are antigen-binding B cells for thyroglobulin and for myelin basic protein in normal subjects, and autoimmunity may be induced by the administration of hapten-modified antigens that helper T cells can recognize (reviewed by Weigle, 1977). Tolerance to the liver autoantigen F is at the level of T cells. With this autoantigen, there is no evidence for suppressor cells in mice spontaneously tolerant, and there is evidence for induction of self-tolerance (Nardi, 1985).

The role of antigen-specific suppression in self-tolerance is by no means clear. Volpé and his school studied this subject extensively by means of direct leucocyte migration inhibition (LMI). They were able to demonstrate that patients with autoimmune thyroid disease have a T-cell suppressor defect for thyroid homogenate, whereas type I diabetics have a similar defect regarding islet cell homogenate. In both instances, addition of a small proportion of normal T cells can correct the increased LMI. The tests are based on an 18-hr incubation with or without antigen using 95% pure E-rosetting lymphocytes, and the normalization of LMI can be abolished if the control T cells are pretreated with mitomycin, X rays, or cimetidine (Topliss *et al.*, 1983). These authors also showed that the excessive LMI seen in newly diagnosed diabetics with islet antigens can be corrected with T cells from Graves' patients, and, *vice versa*, diabetic T lymphocytes are able to normalize the LMI to thyroid in Graves' disease. Some unaffected predisposed relatives of thyroid or diabetic patients show the same organ-specific suppressor defects.

More recently, Vento *et al.* (1984), using the indirect LMI test, demonstrated the same phenomenon in autoimmune and virally induced chronic liver disorders in relation to the liver-specific lipoprotein (LSP). They also presented evidence that the correction of LMI is mediated by soluble suppressor factor. Full characterization of this factor is required to confirm the organ-specific nature of these reactions. However, the exact physiological relevance of the LMI assay is not fully understood, and it would be useful to have other assays of suppressor function.

The role of the idiotype network in self-tolerance remains to be clarified, as does its role in many other aspects of immune regulation. It is conceivable that antiidiotypic antibody may inhibit autoreactive T cells, but there is no evidence for it that we know of. There are certain reasons to suspect that antiidiotypic antibody would not be effective at suppressing T-cell responses to the level required as a sole mechanism of self-tolerance. One reason is that a separate antibody would be needed for virtually every T-cell clone (e.g., Meuer *et al.* 1983): Haskins *et al.* (1983) have demonstrated exquisite specificity of anticlonotypic antibodies. Secondly, some clonotypic antibodies inhibit responses only at high concentrations, whereas others do not inhibit but stimulate the cells, presumably by mimicking antigen (Kaye *et al.*, 1983). Even inhibitory antibodies may stimulate when presented on the surface of beads, which could mirror the *in vivo* effect of APCs (Meuer *et al.*, 1983).

A more likely role for idiotype regulation would involve T cells, whose normal function is immune regulation. Suppressor T cells recognizing helper T cells have been described (Lamb and Feldmann, 1982), and these cells may be of importance in preventing excess clonal proliferation *in vivo*. Clearly, much more information is necessary before we understand the role of various possible mechanisms in self-nonreactivity.

I. Hidden Determinants: A Role in Self-Unresponsiveness?

Accessibility of the relevant autoantigens to immune-reactive lymphocytes is also of crucial importance, especially with respect to the nervous system. In the thyroid, microvillar surface antigens are normally localized on the apical pole of thyroid follicles. Thus, various mechanisms have to be invoked to explain the finding of *in vivo* intrafollicular deposition of immunoglobulins (Khoury *et al.*, 1984) (Fig. 10A,B). At the apical pole, there is no access to lymphocytes, and thus reversal of polarity is needed to render these antigens accessible *in vivo*. Human thyroid cells in culture can be easily induced to reverse their polarity (Hanafusa *et al.*, 1984). This would enable membrane DR molecules to present the relevant autoantigen to helper T cells. In support of this notion, we have recently demonstrated that the partially disrupted follicles from thyrotoxic patients show spontaneous expression of HLA-DR on the external vascular follicular wall as illustrated in Fig. 11 (Hanafusa *et al.*, 1984).

We believe that inaccessibility of certain autoantigens to the T-cell system is an important component of self-nonreactivity. This is because there are many rare specialized cells (e.g., most of the endocrine cells) that have specific surface antigens (e.g., their receptors for hormones) which are expressed in the body in very low amounts. It seems

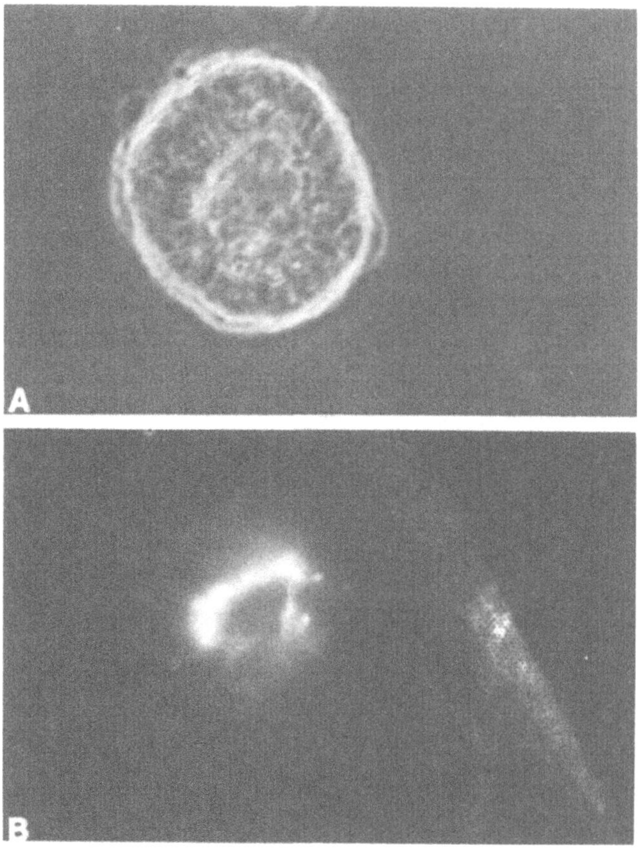

Figure 10. Partially disrupted follicle from a thyrotoxic gland. (A) Phase contrast showing the three-dimensional structure ("half-melon"); focus is on the row of follicular cells in the plane of rupture. (B) Direct immunofluorescence staining with anti-Fab reveals Ig deposits restricted to the inner apical surface (×650). (Reproduced from Khoury *et al.*, 1984.)

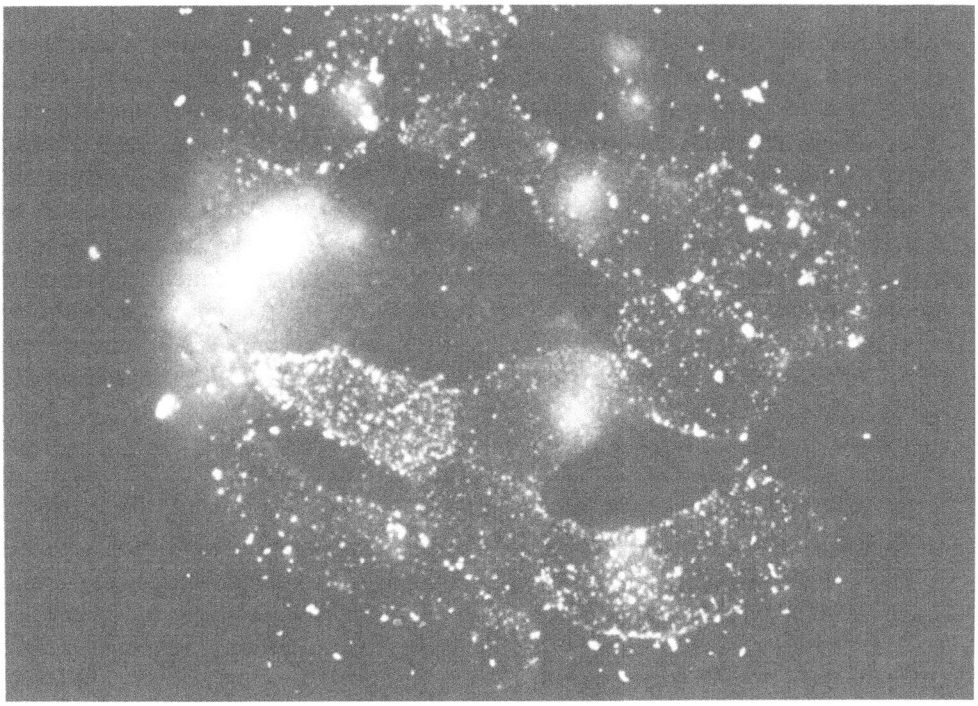

Figure 11. Photomicrograph of a reconstituted human thyroid follicle cultured with 10% fetal calf serum for 8 days and stained by indirect immunofluorescence with a patient's serum containing thyroid microsomal antibodies. The "microvillar" cell-surface-reactive antigen is normally confined to the inner border of thyrocytes near the colloid edge, but under these culture conditions up to 70% of the thyrocytes reverse their polarity and express the antigen on their outside surface, thus making it accessible to damage by complement-fixing antibodies or to indirect cytotoxicity by K cells coated with antigen–antibody complexes (ADCC) (×488). (Reproduced from Hanafusa *et al.*, 1984.)

highly unlikely that they are sufficiently accessible on cell membranes to tolerize maturing T cells migrating past their surfaces (especially at distal poles of cells) that potentially reactive clones would be tolerized. It seems equally inconceivable that sufficient antigen would be released into the circulation to induce tolerance in other remote lymphoid tissue compartments.

Recent observations that the injection of purified rat glomerular basement membrane (GBM) protein into brown Norway rats in the absence of adjuvants or polyclonal activators induces anti-GBM antibody (C. M. Lockwood, personal communication) lend support to the notion that there may not be tolerance to certain antigens (or in this instance, significant suppression). Lack of response to their own autologous GBM could be because it is insoluble and not associated with Ia antigens and thus is not presented effectively.

J. The Concept of Organ Specificity

One of the dogmas of endocrine autoimmunity has been the absolute organ specificity of the antibodies. There is no correlation between reactions to one organ and those to any other in individual sera, and it has been demonstrated with thyroid, gastric, and adrenal cells that each of the antibodies can be selectively absorbed out with one organ extract, leaving the titers of the other reactions unchanged. Nevertheless, the remarkable overlap that exists among the AI endocrinopathies is not explained, and neither was our total inability to separate the genetic predisposition to gastric and thyroid autoimmunty in family studies of pernicious anemia and Hashimoto patients, respectively (Roitt and Doniach, 1967).

Recent work from Notkins' group (Satoh *et al.*, 1983) is a further challenge to long-held notions. These authors prepared mixed hybridomas from diabetic blood lymphocytes, and some of the resulting monoclonal antibodies reacted by immunofluorescence with more than one endocrine gland and produced staining patterns on thyroid, stomach, pancreatic islets, and pituitary almost identical to those seen with sera of polyendocrine patients. Admittedly, some of these monoclonal antibodies reacted with growth hormone, whereas in human patients the organ-specific microsomal antigens are invariably membrane-bound receptor proteins, and the antibodies cannot be absorbed with an excess of the relevant hormones. Nevertheless, specific organs share many antigens.

We also have the example of "semi-organ-specific" antibodies such as LKM already mentioned and the shared islet-cell antigen present on all four types of endocrine pancreas cells (Bottazzo and Doniach, 1978). Certain diabetic sera react with several types of pituitary cells, and that could be another example of the same phenomenon (Mirakian *et al.*, 1982). This contrasts with lymphocytic hypophysitis, in which reactions are against prolactin cells or growth hormone cells, respectively (Bottazzo *et al.*, 1980b). Looking at it another way, the B lymphocytes in the circulation can be pictured as potentially able to produce a myriad of "monoclonal" antibodies. In real patients, however, physiologically useful (Grabar, 1983) and some "dangerous" potential clones are amplified to the degree necessary to express a disease state, and they appear to be strictly organ specific. Even on known autoantigens, i.e., thyroglobulin, selected epitopes appear to be involved in thyrotoxicosis (Ruf *et al.*, 1985) as compared with the large number stimulated in immunized animals.

It remains unclear why antibody responses in autoimmune disease vary from completely polyclonal (Hay and Torrigiani, 1973) to a highly restricted clonality (Dean *et al.*, 1983; Zakarija *et al.*, 1983).

In mild cases we can envisage that few clones are activated. In more severe instances of each of the endocrine diseases, the derepression of particular clones is so uncontrolled that somatic mutations play a part in the great proliferation of antibodies directed at very closely related epitopes. A good example is Graves' disease, where antibodies to the TSH receptors may become so varied that they pick out selected parts of the molecules involved in message transmission. The challenge now is to work out the mechanisms by which these autoimmune clones become derepressed at the immunoglobulin gene level and what causes them to expand.

K. Asymptomatic Autoimmunity

The demonstration of autoantibodies in clinically healthy individuals needs to be explained. Above, we discussed a lack of self-tolerance.

From a variety of approaches, it has become evident that the reaction of an antibody with its antigenic determinant *in vivo* does not necessarily lead to the destruction of that cell. Immunoglobulin-coated cells may look perfectly healthy. Experimental therapeutic injection of large quantities of anti-T-cell antibodies may cause cytolysis and opsonization of cells; but in other circumstances merely modulation of the cell surface antigen, leaving the cell functionally intact (Miller *et al.*, 1982; Linch *et al.*, 1983). The outcome depends on many factors: the antibody (quantity, affinity, Ig class), antigen (density, ease of modulation, role in cell physiology), macrophage Fc receptor and phagocytosis function, rate of repair/regeneration of cells under the influence of growth factors, complement activity, which is influenced by the patient's complotype, and function of other cells (macrophages, NK, K). It seems likely that many autoantibodies could exist in conditions where gross cell damage would be unlikely to result, and thus be asymptomatic. The presence of asymptomatic autoantibodies would reflect past episodes of induction of autoantibodies at levels that were controllable by the host.

L. Autoimmunity and the Idiotype Network

A variety of workers have studied the role of idiotype interactions in autoimmunity. An important finding is that both in human diseases and in animal models there are cross-reactive idiotypes. Examples in humans are those anti-Id connected with DNA antibodies in SLE (Isenberg *et al.*, 1984), IgG rheumatoid factors in RA, acetylcholine receptor antibodies in myasthenia gravis (Dwyer *et al.*, 1983), and antithyroglobulin in Hashimoto's disease (Matsuyama *et al.*, 1983). Cross-reactive idiotypes to the same set of antigens have also been demonstrated in the corresponding animal models of these diseases.

Do these observations have any implications for etiology, pathogenesis, or therapy? It seems unlikely that idiotype network abnormalities can be the *sole* cause of autoimmunity, as discussed elsewhere (Bottazzo *et al.*, 1985; Roitt, 1984), as T cells recognizing and regulating idiotypic interactions are not MHC restricted (Bottomley and Mosier, 1981; Singhai *et al.*, 1984). Idiotypic dysregulation by itself does not explain the HLA-DR associations (e.g., Svejgaard *et al.*, 1983), which indicate a role for cells of the T helper lineage. Nor does it easily explain the striking interferon abnormalities.

1. A Role for Cross-Reactive Idiotypes?

It was recently suggested (Cooke *et al.*, 1983) that if an environmental agent, virus bacteria, or parasite, triggered an antibody response with a cross-reactive idiotype (CRI) that was shared with an autoantibody set, then T helper cells with specificity for the CRI could augment the autoantibody response. This concept is based on the regulation of antibody responses by idiotype-recognizing T cells. However, it is by no means clear that these cells are routinely involved apart from the regulation of dominant idiotypes, as there are a number of studies showing that antigen-specific helper clones are sufficient to induce responses (e.g., Hodes *et al.*, 1981; Lamb and Feldmann, 1982), and thus, idiotype-specific T cells are not an absolute requirement.

2. Are Autoantibodies Antiidiotype Antibodies to Viral Antibodies?

Plotz (1983) suggested that certain viral antibodies directed at the viral structures that react with the cell surface may elicit antiidiotype antibodies with a complementary configuration to the viral cell binding site and thus would react with the cell surface receptor for the virus. Arguments in favor of this concept include the fact that antihormone antiidiotype antibodies mimic hormone; e.g., antiinsulin antiidiotype shows insulinlike activity (reviewed Strosberg *et al.*, 1983). Antibodies to acetylcholine analogues can elicit antiidiotype antibodies that induce a myasthenia-gravis-like illness.

A prediction of this hypothesis is that in sera after viral infection there should be antibodies against the viral receptors; i.e., autoantibodies should be common in antiviral antisera and should react with non-virally-infected tissues. However that is not the usual observation; viral antisera usually do not stain uninfected tissues, suggesting that these antiidiotypic antibodies are not a common occurrence. However, titers may be low, and more critical tests are needed (e.g., autoantibodies should block antiviral antibodies) autoantibodies should block viral binding to tissues. This has been tried on endocrine pancreas, and Coxsackie antibodies did not cross react with islets (King *et al.*, 1983). Until there is evidence that this occurs, then the importance of this mechanism in autoimmunity remains unproven.

M. Genetic Contributions to the Etiology of Diabetes Mellitus

Type I insulin-dependent diabetes is caused by a selective destruction of the insulin-secreting β-cells of the pancreatic islets (Bottazzo, 1984). In about 2% of cases, the initial injury can be attributed to specific causes: rat poison, known viruses (e.g., mumps, rubella, Coxsackie, and others) but practically always there is a superimposed autoimmune insulitis that can be identified by the islet-cell antibodies in the patient's serum (Papadopulos and Lernmark, 1983) and/or cell-mediated immunity to islet-cell constituents (Pozzili and DiMario, 1984). Another 10% of type I diabetics belong to the subgroup of older females with polyendocrine autoimmunity (Bottazzo *et al.*, 1978). This still leaves the great majority of cases with an unknown initiating external agent.

The total genetic contribution does not exceed 50% since this is the maximum estimate of concordance rate in identical twins. At least four different haplotypes in the major histocompatibility complex (MHC) are now implicated, involving HLA-DR3, DR4, and several "complotypes"; i.e., allotypes of the complement components C2, C4, and Bf (Alper *et al.*, 1984). In addition, it is suspected that differences in the DQ portion of the D region may also be found in type I diabetics. This entire set of genes on chromosome 6 has been calculated by Rimoin and Rotter (1984) to account for between 60 and 70% of the genetic susceptibility. This leaves another 30–40% that must be accounted for by genes on other chromosomes. The present candidates include chromosome 11, where DNA sequences flanking the insulin gene probably contribute to susceptibility (Bell *et al.*, 1984; Hitman *et al.*, 1985), and chromosome 14, where the immunoglobulin heavy-chain genes are situated. There is controversy about whether or not Ig heavy-chain genes contribute to type I diabetes, but there is some evidence that they are involved in susceptibility to Graves' disease (Bothwell, 1983). Last but not least is chromosome 2, which contains the κ light-chain immunoglobulin genes and the blood groups Lewis and Kidd (Hodge *et al.*, 1981). At the moment there are only three known human allotypes, Km1, Km1,2, and Km3, in the constant region of the κ light chains. T-cell receptor polymorphism may also be of importance. Duncan Adams (1983) has tried for some years to put forward a hypothesis of autoimmunity based on Burnet's (1959) forbidden clone theory, on Adams' own extensive understanding of the human thyroid-stimulating antibody field, which he initiated, and on more recent studies in mice (Knight and Adams, 1981).

A version of this "H-gene theory of autoimmunity" (H, histocompatibility) implicates IgV genes in addition to H genes in predisposition to autoimmunity (Adams *et al.*, 1984). Essentially, they obtained evidence based on highly selected multiplex families of diabetic children or thyrotoxics that the Ig kappa light chain allotype Km1 was overrepresented in affected versus nonaffected sibs. Although these observations were of potential interest, the same authors and other laboratories could not confirm these preliminary results.

The "H gene" model depends on the clonal deletion of B lymphocytes recognizing the patient's own major and minor histocompatibility antigens. Such deletions would influence, either directly or via modification of regulatory idiotype networks (Jerne *et al.*, 1982), the appearance by somatic mutation of autoreactive forbidden clones from "pre-forbidden" clones. The effect could be to diminish or enhance the risk of autoimmunity depending on which H antigen alleles the patient possessed. For example, recognition of HLA-DR2 might protect from diabetes, as it is known to do in half of the DR2-positive cases by causing tolerization of clones that, following somatic mutation of their V regions, could have reacted with islet-cell autoantigens. By contrast, HLA-DR3 might delete antiidiotype clones and liberate from suppression preforbidden idiotypes, which might go on to recognize islet cells following appropriate somatic mutation. In the thyroid stimulating antibodies of thyrotoxicosis there is restricted clonality with excess of lambda light chains and this is attributed to somatic mutations of derepressed "forbidden clones" (Knight *et al.*, 1984).

The importance of somatic mutation in this model may help to explain the abrupt onset of diabetes in some susceptible individuals who have had anti-islet-cell antibodies for months or years without clinical symptoms (Gorsuch *et al.*, 1981). Perhaps "mutating antibodies" particularly harmful to islet cells appear in patients predestined to become diabetic. Such antibodies could have increased affinity for particular β-cell antigens, facilitating the fixation of complement components, which in turn are influenced by the patient's particular "complotype." All of these events might act in synergy with a mutated T-cell idiotype repertoire.

It must be stressed that the H-gene theory, our own hypothesis involving DR-mediated self-antigen presentation by endocrine cells, and other idiotypic hypotheses that depend on cross reactions between unknown infective agents (see also Ebringer and Shipley, 1983) and surface antigens are not mutually exclusive. Adams' theory deals with the generation of effector mechanisms and the genetic background necessary for the development of an autoimmune response. We postulated that the local expression of DR on endocrine cells induced by an environmental factor will initiate or perpetuate antigen presentation and maintain the autoimmune response in patients with the right HLA constitution (Bottazzo *et al.*, 1983).

N. Antihormones and Antireceptor Diseases

Pituitary TSH stimulates thyroid growth and hormone synthesis in equal measure, whereas pathological immunoglobulins in Graves' disease or sporadic "simple" goiters may act selectively on growth (Drexhage *et al.*, 1980; Doniach *et al.*, 1982b). A similar separation has been achieved with hybridomas produced by fusing lymphocytes from Graves' patients with mouse myeloma cells (Valente *et al.*, 1982). These artificial "immortalized" cells may secrete monoclonal antibodies that selectively affect either thyrocyte growth or hormone output. Growth-promoting antibodies have now been demonstrated by four different methods in several laboratories (Drexhage *et al.*, 1982; Chiovato *et al.*, 1983; Schatz *et al.*, 1983; McMullan and Smyth, 1984). The titers are ten times higher in goitrous Graves' than in euthyroid goiters. Now that iodine deficiency is no longer responsible for these cases in some Western countries, the growth antibodies could be the principal cause in some 70% of sporadic goiters (Van der Gaag *et al.*, 1985a).

It is of interest that TSH-receptor-blocking antibodies have also proved to be of at least two kinds, and they block growth or hormone synthesis separately. In primary myxedema, growth blockers prevent the regrowth of thyrocytes despite increased pituitary TSH secretion (Drexhage *et al.*, 1981). In neonatal athyreotic cretinism, thyroid growth-blocking antibodies were detected in about half the mothers of such babies (Van der Gaag *et al.*, 1985b). Hormone synthesis-blocking antibodies are known to exist in thyrotoxic sera (Zakarija *et al.*, 1983; Steel *et al.*, 1984) as well as in babies showing transient hypothyroidism (Matsuura *et al.*, 1980).

It is likely that other growth-stimulating autoantibodies will be discovered in the future. For instance, microprolactinomas behave in many ways like hyperplastic thyroid nodules rather than true tumors.

An exciting and important new possibility is that some peptic ulcers may be caused by autoantibodies that stimulate the histamine receptors on gastric parietal cells. Dobi and Lenkey (1982) demonstrated increased gastric acid secretion *in vivo* after injecting rats with Ig prepared from duodenal ulcer patients. We have recently obtained more direct evidence for stimulating anti-H_2-receptor antibodies in these patients using cultured gastric parietal cells isolated from guinea pig stomach and measuring the cAMP response. Interestingly, the majority of patients with these long-acting-thyroid-stimulator-like gastric antibodies were resistent to cimetidine (DeLazzari *et al.*, 1984). The notable hypertrophy of parietal cells seen in some of these cases suggests that a "growth" variant of these antibodies may also exist. Blocking of the gastrin receptors on parietal cells by parietal-cell antibodies was demonstrated by Loveridge *et al.* (1980).

In other rare families, a hypertrophy of the gastrin (G) cells in the stomach antrum could similarly result from an Ig with trophic effects, and it is interesting to note that in some families the duodenal ulcer patients had sibs suffering from Graves' disease (Taylor *et al.*, 1981).

Autoantibodies to TSH interfere with the RIA methods but do not influence clinical symptoms. Two types were detected in patients with thyroiditis or with Graves' disease who had never received TSH injections for diagnostic purposes. Some TSH antibodies react better with beef TSH (Kajita *et al.*, 1983). This is reminiscent of the rheumatoid factors that react preferentially with rabbit IgG. In other studies, the human anti-TSH reacted better with the human hormone (Beall and Kruger, 1983; Lazarus *et al.*, 1983). The main interest is that the TSH antibodies may be the initial reaction, which is then followed by idiotypic responses that lead to internal image antiidiotypes, which can mimic TSH. This could explain the genesis of some forms of thyroid-stimulating antibodies and possibly account for some cases of intermittent hyperthyroidism.

In the context of pancreatic autoimmunity, the spontaneous development of insulin autoantibodies is gaining prominence at the present time. The full insulin autoimmune syndrome (IAIS) was seen mainly in Japan (Hirata, 1983) but exists in other countries to a lesser extent (Burden and Rosenthal, 1983). The patients have attacks of hypoglycemia that can last for months but show a tendency to spontaneous remission. Recently, insulin antibodies have also been described in newly diagnosed patients with type 1 diabetes (Palmer *et al.*, 1983) and in some polyendocrine nondiabetic cases (Wilkin and Nicholson, 1984). As in thyroiditis, the question arises of whether the insulin autoantibodies are the precursors of insulin receptor antiidiotypes that mimic insulin actions. Such a network reactivity has been well documented in mice injected with insulin (Schechter *et al.*, 1982). These antiidiotypes were able to stimulate adipocyte metabolism. When Maron *et al.* (1983) tried the same tests in untreated children with IDDM included as negative controls for a prospective study on insulin-treated diabetics, they found antiinsulin receptor antibodies in about half the sera. These antibodies were all of the IgM class and were able to displace radioactive insulin from its receptors and also to stimulate adipocyte metabolism.

Until now IgG anti-insulin-receptor antibodies were associated with a rare form of diabetes characterized by extreme insulin resistance and associated with acanthosis nigricans as mentioned above (Kahn *et al.*, 1982).

Although this work needs confirmation in view of the known effects of normal Fc on adipocyte function (Khoker and Dandona, 1983), one wonders whether these receptor antibodies are secondary to the spontaneous insulin autoimmunization. Recent evidence in genetically predisposed relatives in juvenile diabetic families suggests that spontaneous insulin-antibodies appear in the serum several years before clinical onset of diabetes, when measured by a sensitive micro-ELISA assay (Dean *et al.*, 1985). The possibility of idiotype network control in some forms of IDDM is of great theoretical interest since it is obvious that we are not separating all the possible forms of IDDM, and there is still great heterogeneity, which masks the basic pathogenetic mechanisms.

Insulin may act as a powerful immunogen, especially if inappropriate secretion of immature molecules occurs during the slow process of autoimmune β-cell damage (Rotter and Rimoin, 1983). The demonstration that insulin is an integral surface protein expressed on the plasma membrane of dispersed rat islet cells reinforces this possibility (Kaplan *et al.*, 1983). T cells could then "see" insulin molecules in conjunction with major histocompatibility products, and this mechanism could form another arm of the autoimmune process directed against β-cells (Kaplan, 1984). HLA-DR7- and HLA-DR4-positive individuals are more liable to produce insulin antibodies to both animal and human preparations (Reeves *et al.*, 1984; Schernthaner *et al.*, 1983), and these patients may be the best candidates for spontaneous autoimmunization to their own insulin or proinsulin.

Alternatively T-cell participation in insulin-receptor autoimmunization cannot be entirely excluded, especially in view of the finding that MHC class I molecules are closely associated to insulin receptors on the plasma membrane, possibly sharing common determinants (Brossette *et al.*, 1984).

Another organ also appears to be involved with reactions to a hormone and resulting antiidiotypic networks. In some cases of renal failure, the patients appear to develop antibodies to the parathyroid hormone (PTH) receptors on renal tubules (Jüppner *et al.*, 1978). In one of these cases, antibodies to a segment of the PTH molecule have now been identified (Jüppner *et al.*, 1984), and it is just possible that such antihormones would be found more often after acid dissociation of circulating complexes involving antiidiotypic reactions.

There are also interesting reports that autoantibodies to the gonadotrophin receptors on ovarian cells account for some cases of ovarian atrophy in patients with coexisting myasthenia gravis, giving rise to gonadotrophin-resistant hypogonadism (Escobar *et al.*, 1982).

Despite these new data covering autoimmunity in different endocrine systems, the question of which is the "chicken" and which is the "egg" is paramount. We believe that primary receptor antibodies are more important in the causation of severe and persistent Graves' disease or of insulin-resistant diabetes with acanthosis (Flier *et al.*, 1979). The great variety of different thyroid-stimulating antibodies, many of them reacting better with TSH-sensitive receptors on adipocytes or retroorbital tissues (Kodama *et al.*, 1982; Kendall-Taylor *et al.*, 1984), must in part be the effect of somatic mutations occurring as a result of the enormous expansion of B cell clones making TSH-receptor antibodies, as previously discussed.

III. DO ANIMAL MODELS ACCURATELY REFLECT CLINICAL DISEASE ENTITIES?

Experimental autoimmunity has much to tell us concerning mechanisms of immune regulation and induction and yields clues about the human autoimmune diseases. There was a lot to be said for a meticulous investigation of animal models in the past, when methods of studying human tissues were not as well developed as those available now.

What of the present? It is evident that the techniques available to evaluate human responses *in vitro* have progressed dramatically in recent years, and almost every response can be assayed, T cells and NK cells can be cloned in IL-2, and B cells can be cloned, though with greater difficulty, by fusion. It seems appropriate now to make the complete description of the existing human diseases a higher priority rather than to meticulously analyze animal models, which are of unknown relevance to the clinical entities.

Although it should be stressed that there are many useful models about which much needs to be learned, it is in areas of immune physiology *in vivo* that the models can teach us things that cannot be investigated in humans.

ACKNOWLEDGMENTS. We thank our numerous colleagues for their contribution to generating the results and contributing to the ideas put forward here and Philippa Wells for her considerable efforts on this manuscript.

REFERENCES

Adams, D. D., 1983, Autoimmune mechanisms, in: *Autoimmune Endocrine Disease* (T. F. Davies, ed.), John Wiley & Sons, New York, pp. 1–39.

Adams, D. D., 1984, V genes and autoimmune disease, *Lancet* **2**:463–464.

Adams, D. D., Adams, Y. J., Knight, J. G., McCall, J., White, P., Horrocks, R., and van Loghem, E., 1984, A solution to the genetic and environmental puzzles of insulin-dependent diabetes mellitus, *Lancet* **1**:420–424.

Allison, A. C., 1977, Autoimmune diseases: Concepts of pathogenesis and control, in: *Autoimmunity: Genetic, Immunologic, Virologic and Clinical Aspects* (N. Talal, ed.), Academic Press, New York, pp. 91–139.

Alper, C. A., Awdeh, Z. L., Raum, D. D., Fleischnick, E., and Yunis, E. J., 1984, Complement genes of human majority histocompatibility complex: Implications for linkage disequilibrium and disease associations, in: *Clinical Immunology,* Vol. 1, *Immunogenetics* (G. S. Panayi and C. Davids, eds.), Butterworth, London, pp. 50–91.

Arulanantham, K., Dwyer, J. M., and Genel, M., 1979, Evidence for defective immunoregulation in the syndrome of familial candidiasis endocrinopathy, *N. Engl. J. Med.* **300:**164–168.

Ballardini, G., Bianchi, F., Mirakian, R., Pisi, E., Doniach, D., and Bottazzo, G. F., 1984, Aberrant expression of HLA-DR antigens on bile duct epithelium in primary biliary cirrhosis: Relevance to pathogenesis, *Lancet* **2:**1009–1015.

Bankhurst, A. D., Torrigiani, G., and Allison, A. C., 1973, Lymphocytes binding human thyroglobulin in healthy people and its relevance for tolerance to autoantigens, *Lancet* **1:**226–230.

Barclay, A. N., and Mason, D. W., 1983, Graft rejection and Ia antigens—paradox resolved? *Nature* **303:**382–383.

Beall, G. N., and Kruger, S. R., 1983, Binding of ^{125}I-human TSH by gamma globulins of sera containing thyroid-stimulating immunoglobulin (TSI), *Life Sci.* **32:**77–83.

Bell, G. I., Horita, S., and Karam, J. H., 1984, A polymorphic locus near the human insulin gene is associated with insulin-dependent diabetes mellitus, *Diabetes* **33:**176–183.

Bodmer, W. F., 1981, MHC gene clusters of man and mouse, in: *Mammalian Genetics and Cancer, Jackson Laboratory 50th Anniversary Symposium* (E. Russell, ed.), Alan R. Liss, New York, pp. 213–240.

Bothwell, A., 1983, Enhancement, translocation and the behaviour of V genes, *Immunol. Today* **4:**315–316.

Bottazzo, G. F., 1984, Beta-cell damage in diabetic insulitis: Are we approaching the solution? *Diabetologia* **26:**241–250.

Bottazzo, G. F., and Doniach, D., 1978, Islet-cell antibodies in diabetes mellitus. Evidence of an autoantigen common to all cells in the islet of Langerhans, *Ric. Clin. Lab.* **8:**29–38.

Bottazzo, G. F., and Doniach, D., 1985, Polyendocrine autoimmunity: An extended concept, in: *Endocrine Autoimmunity* (R. Volpe, ed.), Marcel Dekker, New York (in press).

Bottazzo, G. F., Cudworth, A. G., Moul, D. J., and Doniach, D., 1978, Evidence for a primary autoimmune type of diabetes mellitus, *Br. Med. J.* **2:**1253–1255.

Bottazzo, G. F., Vandelli, G., and Mirakian, R., 1980, The detection of autoantibodies to discrete endocrine cells in complex endocrine organs, in: *Autoimmune Aspects of Endocrine Disorders* (A. Pinchera, D. Doniach, G. F. Fenzi, and L. Baschieri, eds.), Academic Press, London, pp. 367–377.

Bottazzo, G. F., Dean, B. M., McNally, J. M., and McKay, E. H., 1983a, Direct evidence of various immunological phenomena associated with the 'insulitis' process, *Diabetologia* **25:**142–143.

Bottazzo, G. F., Pujol-Borrell, R., Hanafusa, T., and Feldmann, M., 1983b, Role of aberrant HLA-DR expression and antigen presentation in induction of endocrine autoimmunity, *Lancet* **2:**1115–1119.

Bottazzo, G. F., Pozzilli, P., Mirakian, R., Dean, B. M., and Doniach, D., 1984, Early immunological events in diabetes, in: *Immunology of Diabetes* (D. Adreani, K. F. Federlin, L. G. Heding, and U. Di Mario, eds.), Kimpton Medical Publications, Edinburgh, London, pp. 95–104.

Bottazzo, G. F., Dean, B. M., McNally, J. M., McKay, E. H., Swift, P. G. F., Gamble, D. R., 1985, Spotlight on diabetic insulitis: *In situ* characterization of autoimmune phenomena and demonstration of increased and aberrant expression of HLA molecules, *N. Engl. J. Med.* (in press).

Bottomly, K., and Mosier, D. E., 1981, Antigen specific helper T cells required for idiotype expression are not H-2 restricted, *J. Exp. Med.* **154:**411–421.

Bromberg, T. J., Lake, P., and Brunswick, M., 1982, Viral antigens act as helper determinants to cell surface antigens, *J. Immunol.* **129:**683–688.

Brossette, N., Van Obberghen, E., and Fehlmann, M., 1984, Interaction between insulin-receptors and major histocompatibility complex antigens in mouse liver membranes, *Diabetologia* **27:**74–76.

Burden, A. C., and Rosenthal, F. D., 1983, Methimazole and insulin autoimmune syndrome, *Lancet* **2:**1311.

Burnet, F. M., 1959, *The Clonal Selection Theory of Acquired Immunity,* Cambridge University Press, Cambridge.

Buschard, K., Madsbad, S., Krarup, T., and Rygaard, J., 1982, Glycaemic control and suppressor cell activity in patients with insulin-dependent diabetes mellitus, *Clin. Exp. Immunol.* **48:**189–195.

Chiovato, L., Hammond, L. J., Hanafusa, T., Pujol-Borrell, R., Doniach, D., and Bottazzo, G. F., 1983, Detection of thyroid growth immunoglobulins (TGI) by (^{3}H)-thymidine incorporation in cultured rat thyroid follicles, *Clin. Endocrinol.* **19:**581–590.

Cooke, A., Lydyard, P. M., and Roitt, I. M., 1983, Mechanisms of autoimmunity: A role for cross-reactive idiotypes, *Immunol. Today* **4**:170–175.

Dean, B. M., Bottazzo, G. F., and Cudworth, A. G., 1983, IgG subclass distribution in organ-specific autoantibodies. The relationship to complement-fixing ability, *Clin. Exp. Immunol.* **52**:61–66.

Dean, B. M., Walker, R., Bone, A. J., Cooke, A., Bottazzo, G. F., and Baird, J. D., 1984, Development of diabetes in the BB/E rat (II): Expression of class II molecules (Ia) in islet-cells, *Diabetologia* **27**:269 A.

Dean, B. M., Becker, F., Tarn, A. C., Schwarz, G. L., Gale, E. A. M., Bottazzo, G. F., 1985, Class and species specificity of insulin antibodies in members of the Barts-Windsor-Middlesex family study. Pre- and post-insulin therapy, *Diabetes* (in press).

DeLazzari, F., Hammond, L. J., Mirakian, R., Venturi-Pasini, C., Naccarato, R., Doniach, D., and Bottazzo, G. F., 1985, Gastric parietal-cell stimulating antibodies (PCSAb): Evidence for an autoimmune variant of duodenal ulcer disease, *Ital. J. Gastroenterol.* (in press).

Dobi, S., and Lenkey, B., 1982, Role of a secretagogue immunoglobulin in gastric acid secretion, *Acta Physiol. Acad. Sci. Hung.* **60**:9–25.

Doniach, D., and Bottazzo, G. F., 1983, Early detection of autoimmune endocrine disorders, *Hosp. Up-date* **9**:1145–1159.

Doniach, D., Nilsson, L. R., and Roitt, I. M., 1965, Autoimmune thyroiditis in children and adolescents. II. Immunological correlation and parent study, *Acta. Paediatr. (Stockholm)* **54**:260–274.

Doniach, D., Roitt, I. M., Walker, J. G., and Sherlock, S., 1966, Tissue antibodies in primary biliary cirrhosis, active chronic (lupoid) hepatitis, cryptogengic cirrhosis and other live diseases and their clinical implications, *Clin. Exp. Immunol.* **31**:237–250.

Doniach, D., Cudworth, A. G., Khoury, E. L., and Bottazzo, G. F., 1982a, Autoimmunity and HLA-system in endocrine diseases, in: *Recent Progress in Endocrinology II* (J. L. H. O'Riordan, ed.), Churchill, Livingston Edinburgh, pp. 99–132.

Doniach, D., Chiovato, L., Hanafusa, T., and Bottazzo, G. F., 1982b, The implication of 'thyroid-growth-immunoglobulins' (TGI) for the understanding of sporadic non-toxic-nodular goitre, *Springer Semin. Immunopathol.* **5**:433–446.

Drexhage, H. A., Bottazzo, G. F., Doniach, D., Bitensky, L., and Chayen, J., 1980, Evidence for thyroid-growth-stimulating immunoglobulins in some goitrous thyroid diseases, *Lancet* **2**:287–292.

Drexhage, H. A., Bottazzo, G. F., Bitensky, L., Chayen, J., and Doniach, D., 1981, Thyroid growth blocking antibodies in primary myxedema, *Nature* **289**:594–596.

Drexhage, H. A., Bitensky, L., Chayen, J., Bottazzo, G. F., and Doniach, D., 1982, The involvement of the pentose shunt in thyroid metabolism after stimulation with TSH or with immunoglobulins from patients with thyroid disease. I. The generation of NADPH in relation to stimulation of thyroid growth, *Clin. Endocrinol.* **16**:49–56.

Dwyer, D. S., Bradley, R. J., Urquhar, C. K., and Kearney, J. F., 1983, Naturally occurring anti-idiotype antibodies in myasthenia gravis patients, *Nature* **301**:611–614.

Ebringer, A., and Shipley, M., (eds.), 1983, Pathogenesis of HLA-27 associated diseases, *Br. J. Rheumatol. (Suppl.)* **2**:1–186.

Epstein, O., Thomas, H. C., and Sherlock, S., 1980, Hypothesis: Primary biliary cirrhosis is a dry gland syndrome with features of chronic graft-versus-host disease, *Lancet* **1**:1166–1168.

Escobar, M. E., Cigorrage, S. B., Chiauzzi, V. A., Charreau, E. H., and Rivarola, M. A., 1982, Development of the gonadotrophin resistant ovary syndrome in myasthenia gravis: Suggestions of similar autoimmune mechanisms, *Acta Endocrinol. (Kbh.)* **99**:431–436.

Field, L. L., Anderson, C. E., and Rimoin, D. L., 1984, Inheritance of immunoglobulin light chain genes in pairs of siblings with insulin-dependent diabetes mellitus, *Lancet* **1**:1132.

Flier, J. S., Kahn, C. R., and Roth, J. C., 1979, Receptors, antireceptor antibodies and mechanisms of insulin resistance, *N. Engl. J. Med.* **300**:413–419.

Gershon, R. K., 1978, Suppressor T cells, *Contemp. Top. Immunobiol.* **3**:1–37.

Gleichmann, E., Issa, P., Van Elven, E. H., and Lamers, M. C., 1978, The chronic graft-versus-host reaction: A lupus erythematosus like syndrome caused by abnormal T–B interactions, *Clin. Rheum. Dis.* **4**:587–602.

Gorsuch, A. N., Spencer, K. M., Lister, J., Bottazzo, G. F., and Cudworth, A. G., 1981, Evidence for a long prediabetic period in type I (insulin-dependent) diabetes mellitus, *Lancet* **2**:1363–1365.

Grabar, P., 1983, Autoantibodies and the physiological role of immunoglobulins, *Immunol. Today* **4**:337–340.

Hanafusa, T., Pujol-Borrell, R., Chiovato, L., Russell, R. C. G., Doniach, D., and Bottazzo, G. F., 1983, Aberrant expression of HLA-DR antigen on thyrocytes in Graves' disease: Relevance for autoimmunity, *Lancet* **2**:1111–1115.

Hanafusa, T., Pujol-Borrell, R., Chiovato, L., Doniach, D., and Bottazzo, G. F., 1984, *In vitro* and *in vivo* reversal of thyroid epithelial polarity: Its relevance for autoimmune thyroid disease, *Clin. Exp. Immunol.* **57**:639–646.

Haskins, K., Kubo, R., White, J., Pigeon, M., Kappler, J., and Marrack, R., 1983, The major histocompatibility complex restricted antigen receptor on T cells. I. Isolation with a monoclonal antibody, *J. Exp. Med.* **157**:1149–1169.

Hay, F. C., and Torrigiani, G., 1973, The distribution of anti-thyroglobulin antibodies in the immunoglobulin G subclass, *Clin. Exp. Immunol.* **15**:517–521.

Hijmans, W., Doniach, D., Roitt, I. M., and Holborow, E. J., 1961, Serological overlap between lupus erythematosus, rheumatoid arthritis and thyroid auto-immune disease, *Br. Med. J.* **2**:909–914.

Hirata, Y., 1983, Methimazole and insulin autoimmune syndrome with hypoglycaemia, *Lancet* **2**:1037–1038.

Hitman, G. A., Tarn, A. C., Drummond, V., Williamson, L. G., Jowett, N. I., Bottazzo, G. F., and Galton, D. J., 1985, An association of insulin-dependent diabetes with a highly variable locus close to the insulin gene on chromosome II. *Diabetologia* (in press).

Hodes, R. J., Kimoto, M., Hathcock, K. S., Fathman, C. G., and Singer, A., 1981, Functional helper activity of monoclonal T cell populations. Antigen specific and H-2 restricted cloned T cell populations help for *in vitro* antibody responses to TNP(T,G)A—L, *Proc. Natl. Acad. Sci. U.S.A.* **78**:6431–6435.

Hodge, S. E., Anderson, C. E., Weiswanger, K., Field, L. L., Spence, M. A., Sparks, R. S., Sparks, M. C., Crist, M., Terasaki, P. I., Rimoin, D. L., and Rotter, G. I., 1981, A second genetic locus for insulin dependent diabetes mellitus, evidence for close linkage between IDDM and Kidd blood group, *Lancet* **2**:893–895.

International Pathology Group, 1983, Histopathology of the intrahepatic biliary tree, *Liver* **3**:161–175.

Isenberg, D. A., Schoenfeld, Y., Madaio, M. P., Rauch, J., Reichlin, M., Stollar, B. D., and Schwartz, R. S., 1984, Anti-DNA antibody idiotypes in systemic lupus erythematosus, *Lancet* **2**:417–422.

Jansson, R., Karlsson, A., and Forsum, U., 1984, Intrathyroidal HLA-DR expression and T lymphocyte phenotypes in Graves' thyrotoxicosis, Hashimoto's goitre and non-toxic nodular goitre, *Clin. Exp. Immunol.* **58**:264–272.

Jerne, N. K., Roland, G., and Cazenave, P. A., 1982, Recurrent idiotypes and internal images, *EMBO J.* **1**:234–242.

Jüppner, H., Bialasiewicz, A. A., and Hesch, R. D., 1978, Autoantibodies to parathyroid hormone receptor, *Lancet* **2**:1222–1223.

Jüppner, H., Atkinson, M. J., Baethke, R., and Hesch, R. D., 1984, Autoantibodies to mid-C-regional PTH in a patient with terminal renal insufficiency, *Lancet* **1**:1379–1381.

Kahn, C. R., Kasuga, M., King, G. S., and Grunfeld, C., 1982, Autoantibodies to insulin receptors in man: Immunological determinants and mechanism of action, in: *Receptor, Antibodies and Disease, CIBA Symposium 90* (D. Evered, ed.), Pitman, London, pp. 91–105.

Kajita, Y., Nakajima, Y., Ishida, M., Ochi, Y., Miyazaki, T., Hachiya, T., and Ijichi, H., 1983, Characteristics of autoantibodies to bovine TSH in the serum of two patients with Graves' disease, *Acta Endocrinol. (Kbh.)* **104**:423–430.

Kaplan, D. R., 1984, Possible target antigens in autoimmune endocrine disease, *Immunol. Today* **5**:130–131.

Kaplan, D. R., Colca, J. R., and McDaniel, M. L., 1983, Insulin as a surface marker on isolated cells from the rat pancreatic islets, *J. Cell. Biol.* **97**:433–437.

Kappler, J., White, J., Wegmann, D., Mustain, E., and Marrack, P., 1982, Antigen presentation by Ia^+ B cell hybridomas to H-2 restricted T cell hybridomas, *Proc. Natl. Acad. Sci. U.S.A.* **79**:3604–3607.

Kaye, J., Purcell, S., Tite, J., Jones, B., and Janeway, C. A., 1983, Both a monoclonal antibody and antisera specific for determinants unique to individual cloned helper T cell lines can substitute for antigen and antigen-presenting cells in activation of T cells, *J. Exp. Med.* **158**:836–856.

Kendall-Taylor, P., Atkinson, S., and Holcome, M., 1984, A specific IgG in Graves' ophthalmopathy and its relation to retro-orbital and thyroid autoimmunity, *Br. Med. J.* **288**:1183–1186.

Khoker, M. A., and Dandona, P., 1983, Insulin-like stimulatory effect of Fc fragments of human immunoglobulin G on rat adipocyte lipogenesis: Indirect evidence for Fc receptor on adipocytes, *J. Clin. Endocrinol. Metab.* **56**:393–396.

Khoury, E. L., Bottazzo, G. F., and Roitt, I. M., 1984, The thyroid 'microsomal' antibody revisited: Its paradoxical binding *in vivo* to the apical surface of the follicular epithelium, *J. Exp. Med.* **195**:577–591.

King, M., Chaikh, A., Bidwell, D., Voller, A., and Banatvala, J. E., 1983, Coxsackie B virus specific IgM responses in children with insulin-dependent (juvenile onset; type I) diabetes mellitus, *Lancet* **1**:1397–1398.

Knight, J. G., and Adams, D. D., 1981, Genes determining autoimmune disease in New Zealand mice, *J. Clin. Lab. Immunol.* **5**:156–170.

Kodama, L., Sikorska, H., Bandy-Dafoe, P., Bayly, R., and Wall, J. R., 1982, Demonstration of a circulating antibody against a soluble eye-muscle antigen in Graves' ophthalmopathy, *Lancet* **2**:1355–1356.

Lamb, J. R., and Feldmann, M., 1982, A human suppressor T cell clone which recognizes an autologous helper T cell clone, *Nature* **300**:456–458.

Lazarus, J. H., John, R., Ginsberg, J., Hughes, I. A., Shewring, G., Rees Smith, B., Woodhead, J. S., and Hall, R., 1983, Transient neonatal hyperthyrotrophiaemia: A serum abnormality due to transplacentally acquired antibody to thyroid stimulating hormone, *Br. Med. J.* **286**:592–594.

Linch, D. C., Beverley, P. C. L., Newland, A., and Twinhill, A., 1983, Treatment of a low grade T cell proliferation with monoclonal antibody, *Clin. Exp. Immunol.* **51**:133–140.

Londei, M., Lamb, J. R., Bottazzo, G. F., and Feldmann, M., 1984, Epithelial cells expressing aberrant MHC Class II determinants can present antigen to cloned human T lymphocytes, *Nature* **312**:639–641.

Londei, M., Bottazzo, G. F., and Feldmann, M., 1985, T cell clones recognizing autologous thyroid cells from Graves' disease patients, *Science* **288**:85–88.

Loveridge, N., Bitensky, L., Chayen, J., Hausamen, T. U., Fisher, J. M., Taylor, K. B., Gardner, J. D., Bottazzo, G. F., and Doniach, D., 1980, Inhibition of parietal cell function by human gammaglobulin containing gastric parietal cell antibodies, *Clin. Exp. Immunol.* **41**:264–270.

Malissen, B., Price, M. P., Gaverman, J. M., McMillan, M. M., White, J., Kappler, J., Marrack, P., Pierres, A., Pierres, M., and Hood, L., 1984, Gene transfer of H-2 Class II genes: Antigen presentation by mouse fibroblast and hamster B cell lines, *Cell* **36**:319–327.

Maron, R., Elias, D., Jongh, B. M., Bruining, G. J., Van Rood, J. J., Schechter, Y., and Cohen, I. R., 1983, Autoantibodies to the insulin receptor in juvenile onset insulin-dependent diabetes, *Nature* **303**:817–818.

Matis, L., Glimcher, L., Lindgren, A., Longo, D. L., and Schwartz, R. H., 1983, Effect of normal antigen and Ia concentration on the magnitude of the proliferative response of T cell clones, in: *Ir Genes, Past, Present and Future* (C. W. Pierce, S. E. Cullen, J. A. Kapp, B. D. Schwartz, and D. C. Schreffler, eds.), Humana Press, New Jersey, pp. 439–444.

Matsuura, N., Yamada, Y., Nohara, Y., Konishi, J., Kasagi, K., Endo, K., Kogima, H., and Wataya, K., 1980, Familial neonatal transient hypothyroidism due to maternal TSH-binding inhibitor immunoglobulins, *N. Engl. J. Med.* **303**:738–741.

Maysuyama, T., Fukumori, H., and Tanaka, H., 1983, Evidence of unique idiotypic determinant and similar idiotypic determinant on human anti-thyroglobulin antibodies, *Clin. Exp. Immunol.* **51**:318–386.

McMullan, N. M., and Smyth, P. P. A., 1984, *In vitro* generation of NADPH as a index of thyroid stimulating immunoglobulins (TGI) in goitrous disease, *Clin. Endocrinol.* **20**:269–280.

Meuer, S. C., Fitzgerald, K. A., Hussey, R. E., Hodgdon, J. C., Schlossman, S. F., and Reinherz, E. L., 1983, Clonotypic structures involved in antigen-specific human T cell function. Relationship to T3 molecular complex, *J. Exp. Med.* **157**:705–719.

Miller, R. A., Maloney, D. G., Warnke, R., and Levy, R., 1982, Treatment of a B cell lymphoma with monoclonal antiidiotype antibody, *N. Engl. J. Med.* **306**:517–522.

Mirakian, R., Richardson, C. A., Bottazzo, G. G., and Doniach, D., 1981, Humoral autoimmunity to gut-related endocrine cells, *Clin. Immunol. Newslett.* **2**:161–167.

Mirakian, R., Cudworth, A. G., Bottazzo, G. F., Richardson, C. A., and Doniach, D., 1982, Autoimmunity to anterior pituitary cells and the pathogenesis of type I (insulin-dependent) diabetes mellitus, *Lancet* **1**:755–759.

Mitchison, N. A., 1964, Induction of immunological paralysis in 2 zones of dosage, *Proc. R. Soc. (London) (Biol.)* **161**:275–292.

Nardi, N., 1985, Absence of suppression in natural and induced tolerance to F antigen, *Immunogenetics* **20**:387–395.

Oldstone, M. B. A., Southern, P., Rodriguez, M., and Lampert, P., 1984, Virus persists in beta cells of islets of Langerhans and is associated with chemical manifestation of diabetes, *Science* **224**:1440–1443.

Oppenheim, J. J., and Gery, I., 1982, Interleukin 1 is more than an interleukin, *Immunol. Today* **3**:113–119.

Palmer, J. P., Asplin, C. M., Clemons, P., Lyen, K., Tatpati, O., Raghu, P. K., and Paquette, T. L., 1983, Insulin antibodies in insulin-dependent diabetics before insulin treatment, *Science* **222:**1337–1339.

Papadopoulos, G. K., and Lernmark, A., 1983, The spectrum of islet cell antibodies, in: *Autoimmune Endocrine Disease* (T. F. Davies, ed.), John Wiley & Sons, New York, pp. 167–180.

Plotz, P. H., 1983, Autoantibodies are anti-idiotype antibodies to antiviral antibodies, *Lancet* **2:**824–826.

Pober, J., Gimbrane, M. A., Cotran, R. S., Reiss, C. S., Burakoft, S. J., Fiers, W., and Alt, K., 1983, Ia expression by vascular endothelium is inducible by activated T cell and by human γ interferon, *J. Exp. Med.* **157:**1339–1359.

Pozzilli, P., and DiMario, U., 1984, Lymphocyte subpopulations and circulating immune complexes: Their relationship in the pathogenesis of Type I (insulin-dependent) diabetes, in: *Immunology in Diabetes* (D. Andreani, U. DiMario, K. F. Federlin, and L. G. Heding, eds.), Kimpton Medical Publications, London, pp. 133–142.

Prebble, O. T., Black, R. J., Friedman, R. M., Klippel, J., and Vilcek, J., 1982, Systemic lupus erythematosus: Presence in human serum of an unusual acid-labile leukocyte interferon, *Science* **216:**429–431.

Pujol-Borrell, R., Hanafusa, T., Chiovato, L., and Bottazzo, G. F., 1983, Lectin-induced expression of DR antigens on human cultured follicular thyroid cells, *Nature* **303:**71–73.

Reeves, W. G., Barr, D., Douglas, C. A., Gelsthorpe, K., Kanning, I., Skene, A., Wells, L., Wilson, R. M., and Tattersall, R. B., 1984, Factors governing the human immune response to injected insulin, *Diabetologia* **26:**266–271.

Rhodes, J. M., and Stokes, P., 1982, Interferon induced changes in the monocyte membrane: Inhibition by retinol and retinoic acid, *Immunology* **45:**531–536.

Rimoin, D. L., and Rotter, J. I., 1984, The genetics of diabetes mellitus, in: *Immunology in Diabetes* (D. Andreani, U. Di Mario, K. F. Federlin, and L. G. Heding, eds.), Kimpton Medical Publications, London, pp. 45–62.

Rizzetto, M., Swana, G., and Doniach, D., 1973, Microsomal antibodies in active chronic hepatitis and other disorders, *Clin. Exp. Immunol.* **15:**331–344.

Rock, K. L., and Benacerraf, B., 1983, Inhibition of antigen specific T lymphocyte activation by structurally related Ir gene-controlled polymers evidence of specific competition for accessory cell antigen presentation, *J. Exp. Med.* **157:**1618–1634.

Roitt, I. M., 1984, Prevailing theories in autoimmune disorders, *Triangle* **23:**67–76.

Roitt, I. M., and Doniach, D., 1967, A reassessment of studies on the aggregation of thyroid autoimmunity in families of thyroiditis patients, *Clin. Exp. Immunol.* **2:**727–736.

Rosenberg, Y., Steinberg, A. D., and Santoro, T. J., 1984, The basis of autoreactivity in MRL-lpr/lpr mice: A role for self Ia reactive T cells, *Immunol. Today* **5:**64–66.

Rotter, J. I., and Rimoin, D. L., 1983, Genetics of Type-I diabetes, *Acta Endocrinol. (Kbh.)* **103**(Suppl. 256):26A.

Ruf, J., Carayon, P., and Lissitzky, S., 1985, Various expressions of a unique anti-human thyroglobulin antibody repertoire in normal state and autoimmune disease, *Eur. J. Immunol.* **15:**268–272.

Satoh, J., Prabhakar, B. S., Haspel, M. V., Ginsberg-Fellner, F., and Notkins, A. L., 1983, Human monoclonal autoantibodies that react with multiple endocrine organs, *N. Engl. J. Med.* **309:**217–220.

Schatz, H, Beckmann, F. H., and Floren, M., 1983, Radioassay for thyroid growth stimulating immunoglobulins (TGI) with cultivated porcine thyroid follicles, *Horm. Metab. Res.* **15:**627–628.

Schechter, Y., Maron, R., Elias, D., and Cohen, I. R., 1982, Autoantibodies to insulin receptor spontaneously develop as anti-idiotypes in mice immunized with insulin, *Science* **216:**542–544.

Scherbaum, W. A., Bottazzo, G. F., Czernichow, A. P., Wass, J. A. H., and Doniach, D., 1984, Role of autoimmunity in the pathogenesis of central diabetes insipidus P_2JC, in: *International Symposium on Diabetes Insipidus* (A. P. Czernichow, ed.), S. Karger, Basel, pp. 232–239.

Schernthaner, G., Borkenstein, M., Fink, M., Mayr, W. R., Menzel, J., and Schuber, E., 1983, Immunogeneity of human insulin (Novo) or pork component insulin in HLA-DR typed insulin-dependent diabetic individuals, *Diabetes Care* **6**(Suppl. 1):43–48.

Selby, W. S., Janossy, G., Mason, D. Y., and Jewell, D. P., 1983, Expression of HLA-DR antigens by colonic epithelium in inflammatory bowel disease, *Clin. Exp. Immunol.* **53:**614–618.

Shoenfeld, Y., and Schwartz, R. S., 1984, Immunologic and genetic factors in autoimmune diseases. *N. Engl. J. Med.* **311:**1019–1029.

Singer, A., and Hodes, R. J., 1983, Mechanisms of T cell–B cell interactions, *Annu. Rev. Immunol.* **1:**211–242.

Singhai, R., Weaver, M., Sikora, L., and Levi, J. G., 1984, Evidence for the presence of idiotype-bearing regulatory T-cells in which idiotype expression is not linked to either Igh or MHC. *Immunology* **51**:743–754.

Spencer, K. M., Tarn, A. C., Dean, B. M., Lister, J., and Bottazzo, G. F., 1984, Family studies in type 1 (insulin dependent) diabetes: Evidence of fluctuating islet cell autoimmunity in unaffected relatives, *Lancet* **1**:764–766.

Steeg, P., Moore, R. N., Johnson, H. M., and Oppenheim, J. J., 1982, Regulation of murine macrophage Ia antigen expression by a lymphokine with immune interferon activity, *J. Exp. Med.* **156**:1780–1793.

Steel, N. R., Weightman, D. R., Taylor, J. J. and Kendall-Taylor, P., 1984, Blocking activity to action of thyroid stimulating hormone in serum from patients with primary hypothyroidism, *Br. Med. J.* **288**:1556–1562.

Strakosch, C. R., Wenzel, B. E., Row, V. V., and Volpe, R., 1982, Immunology of autoimmune thyroid diseases, *N. Engl. J. Med.* **307**:1499–1507.

Strosberg, A. D., 1983, Anti-idiotype and anti-hormone receptor antibodies, *Springer Semin. Immunopathol.* **6**:67–78.

Svejgaard, A., Platz, P., and Ryder, L. P., 1983, HLA and disease—1982. A survey, *Immunol. Rev.* **70**:193–218.

Talal, N., and Ŝmith, J. B., 1982, Significance of self-recognition and interleukin-2 for immunoregulation, autoimmunity and cancer, *Scand. J. Immunol.* **16**:269–273.

Tarcic, N., and Naor, D., 1982, Delayed-type hypersensitivity induced in immunodeficient mice with syngeneic modified self antigens: A suggestive model of autoimmune response, *Eur. J. Immunol.* **12**:961–966.

Taylor, I. L., Calam, J., Rotter, J. I., Vaillant, C., Samloff, I. M., Cook, A., Simkin, E., and Dockray, G. J., 1981, Family studies of hypergastrinemic, hyperpepsinogenemic I duodenal ulcer, *Ann. Intern. Med.* **95**:421–425.

Todd, I., Pujol-Borrell, R., Hammond, L. J., Bottazzo, G. F., and Feldmann, M., 1985, Inferferon-gamma induces HLA-DR expression by thyroid epithelium *Clin. Exp. Immunol.* **61**:265–273.

Topliss, D., How, J., Lewis, M., Row, V., and Volpe, R., 1983, Evidence for cell-mediated immunity and specific suppressor T-lymphocyte dysfunction in Graves' disease and diabetes mellitus, *J. Clin. Endocrinol. Metab.* **57**:700–705.

Valente, W. A., Vitti, P., Yavin, Z., Yavin, E., Rotella, M. C., Grossman, E. F., Toccafondi, R. S., and Khon, L. D., 1982, Monoclonal antibodies to the thyrotropin receptor: Stimulating and blocking antibodies derived from the lymphocytes of patients with Graves' disease, *Proc. Natl. Acad. Sci. U.S.A.* **79**:6680–6684.

Van der Gaag, R. D., Drexhage, H. A., and Dussault, J. H., 1985a, Role of maternal immunoglobulins blocking TSH-induced thyroid growth in sporadic forms of congenital hyperthyroidism. *Lancet* **1**:246–250.

Van der Gaag, R. D., Drexhage, H. A., Wiersinga, W. M., Bottazzo, G. F., and Doniach, D., 1985b, Further studies on thyroid growth stimulating immunoglobulins (TG1) in euthyroid nonendemic goitre, *J. Clin. Endocrinol. Metab.* (in press).

Vento, S., Hegarty, J. E., Bottazzo, G. F., Macchia, E., Williams, R., and Eddleston, A. L. W. F., 1984, Antigen specific suppressor cell function in autoimmune chronic active hepatitis, *Lancet* **1**:1200–1204.

Walton, B., Simpson, B. R., Strunin, L., Doniach, D., Perrin, J., and Appleyard, A. J., 1976, Unexplained hepatitis following halothane, *Br. Med. J.* **1**:1171–1176.

Weigle, W. O., 1977, Cellular events in experimental autoimmune thyroiditis allergic encephalomyelitis and tolerance to self, in: *Autoimmunity: Genetic, Immunologic, Virologic and Clinical Aspects* (N. Talal, ed.), Academic Press, New York, pp. 141–170.

Werdelin, O., 1982, Chemically related antigens compete for presentation by accessory cells to T cells, *J. Immunol.* **129**:1883–1891.

Wilkin, T. J., and Nicholson, S., 1984, Autoantibodies against human insulin, *Br. Med. J.* **288**:349–352.

Winchester, G., Sunshine, G. H., Nardi, N., and Mitchison, N. A., 1984, Antigen-presenting cells do not discriminate between self and non-self *Immunogenetics*, **19**:487–491.

Zakarija, M., McKenzie, J. M., and Munro, D., 1983, IgG TSI blockers, *J. Clin. Invest.* **72**:1344–1357.

12

Immune Response to Collagen

David E. Trentham

I. INTRODUCTION

This chapter briefly analyzes current concepts regarding the immunologic properties of collagen with major emphasis devoted to the hypothesis that antiself reactivity specific for the cartilage type (native type II) of collagen is an effector mechanism in the connective tissue diseases, rheumatoid arthritis, and relapsing polychondritis. The intent is to update earlier reviews of immunity to collagen (Furthmayr and Timpl, 1976; Beard *et al.*, 1977; Trentham, 1981, 1982a, 1983, 1985a; Stuart *et al.*, 1982a).

II. THE NORMAL AND ABNORMAL SYNOVIUM

Histology studies of the human synovium in various diseases suggest that this membrane has a limited capacity to react to immunologic, viral, bacterial, physical, or metabolic insults. There are two basic kinds of immunologically mediated synovitis in humans. The first type consists of pannus formation and mononuclear inflammatory cell infiltration and culminates in articular cartilage and bone destruction. This situation is typified by the disease rheumatoid arthritis. The second type is comprised, predominantly, of polymorphonuclear leukocyte infiltration and subsynovial neovascularization in the absence of pannus formation and connective tissue destruction. The diarthrodial joint lesion in systemic lupus erythematosus is representative of this process. Proliferative synovitis is the focus of this review (Fig. 1).

The morphological studies of the human synovium have been extended by recent ultrastructural investigations of the synovium of the knee in healthy young adult rats (Caulfield *et al.*, 1982; Graabaek, 1982; DeSimone *et al.*, 1983). These analyses have

David E. Trentham • Department of Medicine, Harvard Medical School, and Department of Rheumatology and Immunology, The Brigham and Women's Hospital, Boston, Massachusetts 02115.

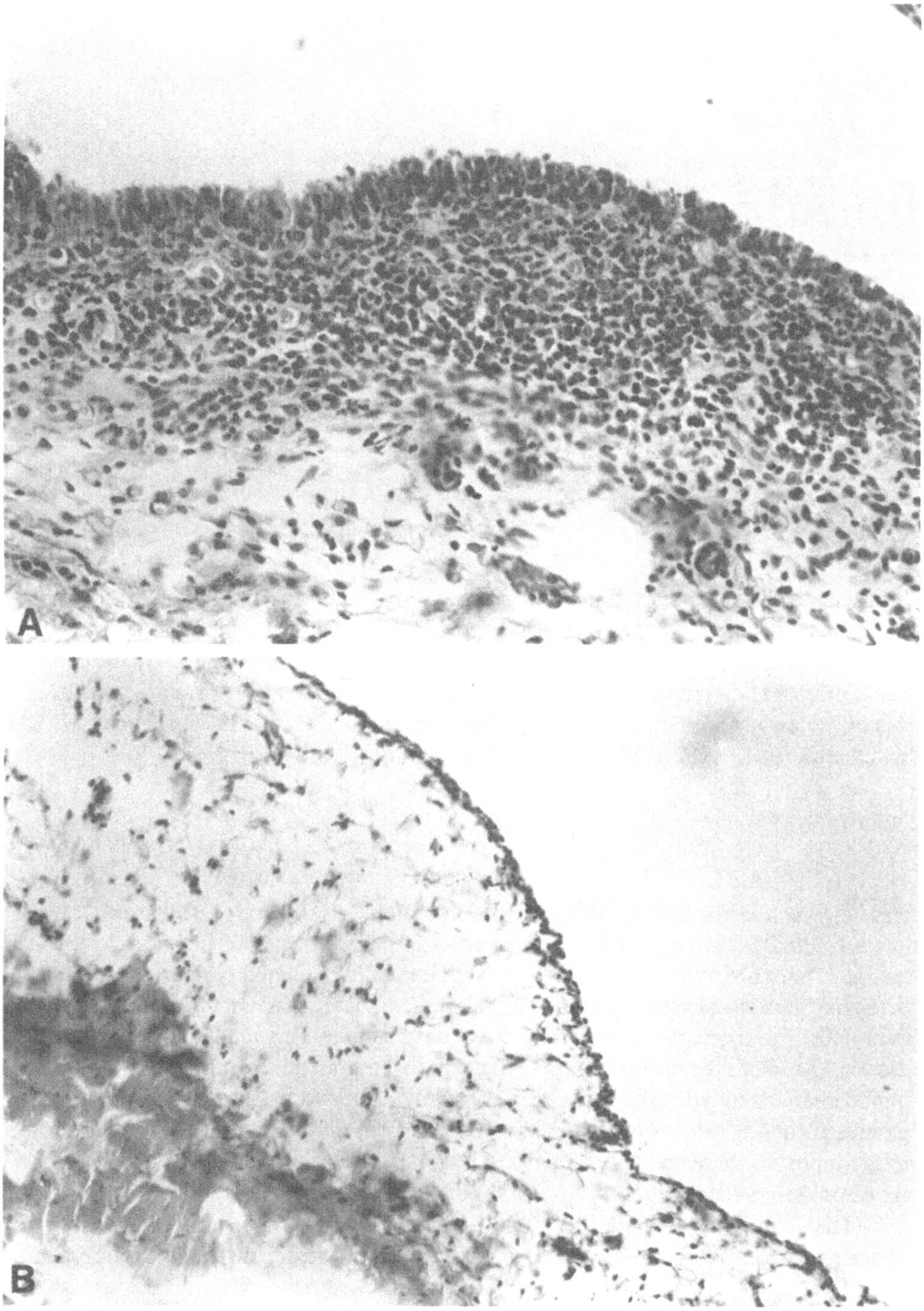

Figure 1. A mildly hyperplastic rat synovial membrane with subsynovial mononuclear-cell infiltration and neovascularization (A), the common appearance of proliferative synovitis regardless of its etiology, versus (B) a normal synovium (×341).

reaffirmed the existence of the dichotomous synovial cell types proposed by Barland *et al.* (1962); i.e., the type A phagocytic-appearing cells and the type B synoviocyte, the principal function of which is apparently the secretion of joint lubricants.

These rodent studies have also shown that the normal synovium is not universally a one- to two-cell-layer-thick lining. Areas in the rat knee contiguous to cartilage can attain a thickness of five to eight cell layers in the absence of inflammatory cell infiltrates (Caulfield *et al.*, 1982). Whether this occurrence is a premorbid event, is indicative of microtrauma-induced injury, or merely delimits areas providing the bulk of hyaluronate synthesis is unknown. It is equally uncertain whether there is a counterpart of this regional synovial thickening in human diarthrodial joints.

Another insight afforded by electron microscopic studies of the normal rat synovium is the frequent occurrence of pentalaminar inclusions resembling viral particles within the lysosomes of synoviocytes (Caulfield *et al.*, 1982). The existence of inclusion bodies has been reported in human synoviocytes as well (Zvaifler, 1973). The potential physiological or pathological role of these inclusion bodies is conjectural.

III. CONCEPTS REGARDING THE PATHOGENESIS OF RHEUMATOID ARTHRITIS

Although an exogenous-agent etiology for rheumatoid arthritis continues to be an attractive theory (Person and Sharp, 1976), no direct evidence of viral involvement in this disease exists. Rheumatoid arthritis was first perceived as an expression of autoimmunity with the recognition of rheumatoid factor. In the past decade, rheumatoid arthritis has begun to be further appreciated as an immunologically mediated disease.

Initial work suggested that rheumatoid arthritis represented an intraarticular immune-complex-induced process (Zvaifler, 1973). The profound decreases in complement in the synovial fluid of patients with this disease (Pekin and Zvaifler, 1964; Marcus and Townes, 1971; Zubler *et al.*, 1976) provided evidence for this theory. But the majority of the findings since that time have been consistent with the possibility that the articular manifestations of rheumatoid arthritis are propagated, at least in part, by cellular hypersensitivity (Trentham, 1985b). Early evidence for this concept was afforded by the recognition that immunocompetent cells could passively transfer disease in the model of inflammatory synovitis induced in rats with complete Freund's adjuvant, adjuvant arthritis (Waksman and Wennersten, 1963; Pearson and Wood, 1964). The theory that rheumatoid arthritis is a T-cell-influenced disorder was fostered by the abrupt amelioration of joint inflammation in rheumatoid arthritis patients during thoracic-duct drainage (Paulus *et al.*, 1977), the recognition that the majority of lymphocytes within the rheumatoid synovium are T cells (Van Boxel and Paget, 1975; Abrahamsen *et al.*, 1975), the identification of lymphokinelike substances in the synovial fluid of patients with rheumatoid arthritis (Stasny *et al.*, 1975), and the data from uncontrolled studies that total lymphoid irradiation can selectively suppress T-cell but not B-cell processes in concert with disease improvement (Kotzin *et al.*, 1981; Trentham *et al.*, 1981; Field *et al.*, 1983; Brahn *et al.*, 1984). Immunohistochemical techniques have hinted recently that the rheumatoid synovium is the site of antigen-presenting macrophages contiguous to activated T cells (Klareskog *et al.*, 1982), the lesion in its entirety resembling a delayed-type hypersensitivity response to relevant-antigen challenge.

Although the intraarticular events of rheumatoid arthritis could prove to be subserved partially by T cells and their soluble mediators, it is equally probable that at least some of the extraarticular manifestations of RA, such as vasculitis, are B-cell and complement provoked. This global envisioning of the pathogenesis of rheumatoid arthritis would integrate the immunologically mediated features of the disease. Regardless of the precise mechanisms involved, if rheumatoid arthritis is propagated by immune mechanisms, the search for autoantigens participating in the disease becomes a paramount issue.

IV. COLLAGEN AS AN AUTOANTIGEN IN RHEUMATOID ARTHRITIS

The hypothesis that collagen functions as an autoantigen in rheumatoid arthritis was partially formulated before the era of rheumatoid factor (Jarco, 1936; Klemperer *et al.*, 1942; Waksman and Mason, 1949; Glynn, 1969; Steffen, 1970). Initial studies of the immunologic properties of collagen used type I and found that it possessed antigenicity (Waksman and Mason, 1949; Steffen and Timpl, 1963; Schmitt *et al.*, 1964; Steffen *et al.*, 1968, 1971, 1972, 1973, 1974, 1975, 1977; Steffen, 1969; Michaeli *et al.*, 1969, 1972; Steffen and Wick, 1971; Lindsley *et al.*, 1971; Beil *et al.*, 1973; Hahn and Timpl, 1973; Michaeli and Fudenberg, 1974a,b; Cracchiolo *et al.*, 1975; Adelmann *et al.*, 1972; Adelmann, 1972; Adelmann and Kirrane, 1973; Senyk and Michaeli, 1973; Gentner and Adelmann, 1976a,b; Stuart *et al.*, 1976; Kravis *et al.*, 1976; McAdam *et al.*, 1978). The isolation of type II collagen from cartilage (Miller and Matukas, 1969; Trelstad *et al.*, 1970; Miller, 1971a,b) and the eye and type III collagen from several human tissues, including blood vessels (Chung and Miller, 1974; Trelstad, 1974; Weiss *et al.*, 1975; Seyer *et al.*, 1976, 1977a,b), demonstrated that these three interstitial collagens comprised a family of biochemically distinct macromolecules providing support for different tissues (Traub and Piez, 1971; Gallop *et al.*, 1972; Nimni, 1974; LeRoy, 1974; Seraffini-Fracassini and Smith, 1974; Miller, 1973, 1976; Lane and Weiss, 1975; Fietzek and Kühn, 1976; Prockop *et al.*, 1979). This discovery prompted additional interest in the possible role of these collagens as type-specific autoantigens in rheumatoid arthritis (Nowack *et al.*, 1974; Hahn *et al.*, 1974, 1975; Beard *et al.*, 1978). While raising reference antisera, we found that native type II collagen is arthritogenic in the rat (Trentham *et al.*, 1977). Type II collagen-induced arthritis can also occur in mice (Courtenay *et al.*, 1980).

V. THE MORPHOLOGY OF EXPERIMENTALLY INDUCED SYNOVITIS IN THE RAT

Morphological studies of the peripheral joint lesion in collagen (Caulfield *et al.*, 1982) and adjuvant (Pearson and Wood, 1963; Burstein and Waksman, 1964; Mohr *et al.*, 1975; Trentham *et al.*, 1980) arthritis of rats have shown shared features. In both diseases, the initial lesion that can be discerned histologically occurs intrasynovially and consists of two events: (1) synoviocyte disruption and a change from a flattened appearance to a vertical cellular polarity; and (2) intrasynovial edema and fibrin deposition within and on the surface of the synovium and the joint-space margin of the articular cartilage (Caulfield *et al.*, 1982). Within a day or two, synovial hyperplasia, intra- and subsynovial neovascularization, and pannus extending over the surface of the cartilage are apparent. Mitotic events in cells that appear to have originated within the synovium are occasionally seen (the possibility has not been completely excluded that the dividing cells are macrophagelike elements carried to the synovium in the blood). Pannus formation continues for several days in the absence of inflammatory-cell infiltration, but by the time debris fills the lysosomes of synoviocytes, polymorphonuclear leukocytes and mononuclear inflammatory cells enter this granulation tissue. Coincident with the ingress of these inflammatory cells is the inception of cartilage and bone destruction. Microabscesslike areas comprised of either polymorphonuclear leukocytes or mononuclear inflammatory cells are often juxtaposed with the erosive lesions in these models.

A final inflammatory stage of experimentally induced synovitis in the rat is a persistent, hyperplastic synovium packed with dense infiltrates of mononuclear cells and granulomatous areas (Caulfield *et al.*, 1982). Aspects of this stage can last for at least 90 days post-immunization. Immunofluorescence techniques show a paucity of immunoglobulin and complement deposited in the arthritic synovium (Caulfield *et al.*, 1982). Although immunoglobulin deposits on the surface of the articular cartilage have been reported in collagen arthritis (Stuart *et al.*, 1983a; Kerwar *et al.*, 1983a), the concurrent dense fibrin precipitates at this site make the exact specificity of this immunofluoresence finding somewhat uncertain. As in the rheumatoid synovium (Van Boxel and Paget, 1975; Abrahamsen *et al.*, 1975; Klareskog *et al.*, 1982), T cells predominate in collagen arthritis (Klareskog *et al.*, 1983). Thus, there is a close histological resemblance in the experimental models to the biopsy picture of rheumatoid arthritis (Schumacher and Kitridou, 1972; Lindblad *et al.*, 1983).

VI. IMMUNOLOGIC ASPECTS OF EXPERIMENTAL ARTHRITIS

Humoral and cellular responses to collagen develop around the inception of collagen arthritis in rats (Trentham *et al.*, 1978a, 1980; Stuart *et al.*, 1979a,b; McCune *et al.*, 1980; Morgan *et al.*, 1980; Clague *et al.*, 1980a; Dynesius-Trentham *et al.*, 1981; Sloboda *et al.*, 1981; Kerwar *et al.*, 1981; McCune *et al.*, 1982b; Stuart *et al.*, 1982b; Ofosu-Appiah *et al.*, 1983). Paralleling the exceptional arthritogenicity of this protein, sensitization to type II collagen in both rats (Hahn *et al.*, 1974; Trentham *et al.*, 1978a; Clague *et al.*, 1980a,b) and mice (Nowack *et al.*, 1974; Stuart *et al.*, 1982c) is antigen specific. In one study, an antibody-mediated pathogenesis of collagen arthritis in mice was suggested by a peaking of antibody titers to collagen coincident with the onset of arthritis in immunized mice (Stuart *et al.*, 1981). Thymidine-incorporation assays indicated that there was a transient cellular sensitization to type II collagen that occurred prior to the beginning of arthritis (Stuart *et al.*, 1982c), further implying that antibodies rather than T-cell immunity to collagen were critical to the inception of this disease. However, murine experiments in the reviewer's laboratory, using a radiometric ear assay to measure delayed-type hypersensitivity to collagen, have shown that *in vivo* evidence of cellular sensitivity to collagen develops later, around the time that arthritis emerges. This situation differs from the rapid onset of delayed-type hypersensitivity to ovalbumin in immunized mice of this DBA-1 strain. Thus, it is impossible to conclude at present from studies of afferent sensitization to collagen whether antibody or cellular mechanisms play a role in the pathogenesis of collagen arthritis in either rats or mice.

Investigations using cobra-venom factor to induce transient complement depletion (Morgan *et al.*, 1981; Kerwar *et al.*, 1982) or induce delayed-type hypersensitivity in the absence of arthritis and antibody responses to collagen (Schoen *et al.*, 1981) have also suggested that antibody responses to collagen are involved in the induction of collagen arthritis in rats. However, nonspecific effects of cobra venom (Salant *et al.*, 1980) and the theoretical possibility that suppressor lymphocytes or macrophages influencing arthritis were primed by the antigen-presentation protocol (Greene and Benacerraf, 1980) mandate caution in the interpretation of these data. Environmental manipulation can affect the morphological manifestations of collagen arthritis (Rogers *et al.*, 1980, 1983) and could have affected the results obtained in these studies.

Moreover, evidence suggesting that collagen arthritis in rats is more complex than simply an antibody-mediated disease has been obtained in studies using psychological stress (Rogers *et al.*, 1980, 1983), passive transfer of the phenomenon of collagen-specific suppression of disease (Brahn and Trentham, 1984a), and administration of eicosapentaenoic acid (Prickett *et al.*, 1984), dimethyl sulfoxide (Trentham and Rowland, 1983), and analogues of retinoic acid (Trentham and Brinckerhoff, 1982). The observation that T-cell-deficient (nude) rats are refractory to the induction of collagen arthritis (Klareskog *et al.*, 1983) suggests a T-cell dependence for this disease, as do studies with an anti-T-cell serum in our laboratory (Brahn and Trentham, 1984b). Nonetheless, it is possible that the resistance found in the nude rat strain is conferred by non-T-cell-mediated genetic mechanisms, and the precise specificities of polyclonal antisera are always a concern. Thus, these studies have not provided definitive evidence regarding the role of B and T cells in the primary pathogenesis of collagen arthritis.

The possible role of collagen immunity in adjuvant arthritis is controversial. Cellular sensitivity to collagen in this model has been found in some (Steffen and Wick, 1971; Trentham *et al.*, 1980; Holoshitz *et al.*, 1983) but not all (Trentham and Dynesius-Trentham, 1983) studies. Serum antibodies to collagen occur only in low titer and either late in the disease (Trentham *et al.*, 1980) or not at all (Trentham and Dynesius-Trentham, 1983; Cremer *et al.*, 1983). Only extremely preliminary indications exist that collagen immunity is involved in any aspect of the primary pathogenesis of this disease (Welles and Battisto, 1981; Holoshitz *et al.*, 1983; Trentham and Dynesius-Trentham, 1983), and evidence to the contrary has also been reported (Cremer *et al.*, 1980, 1983; Iizuka and Chang, 1982).

VII. THE PATHOGENESIS OF EXPERIMENTAL ARTHRITIS

More substantive data regarding the pathogenesis of collagen arthritis and adjuvant arthritis have been provided by passive transfer experiments (Trentham *et al.*, 1978b; Stuart *et al.*, 1982d, 1983a; Stuart and Dixon, 1983; Taurog *et al.*, 1983; Kerwar *et al.*, 1983a,b). Although these studies have implied that collagen and adjuvant arthritis are immunologically mediated, transfer experiments in neither model have shown the relative roles of T- and/or B-cell pathways in the primary disease.

Collagen arthritis has been transferred by intravenously injected spleen and lymph node cells from syngeneic rats immunized with type II collagen (Trentham *et al.*, 1978b). Subsequent work has demonstrated that synovitis can be induced in rats (Stuart *et al.*, 1982d, 1983a; Kerwar *et al.*, 1983a,b) or mice (Stuart and Dixon, 1983) by intravenous injection of IgG antibodies specific for native type II collagen. Unanswered questions exist regarding the results of all of these experiments.

Cell transfer produced a lesion that resembled a milder form of the primary disease; i.e., substantial pannus formation, cartilage and bone erosion, and mononuclear inflammatory cell infiltration. The disease persisted until the latest time of evaluation, 24 days after cell transfer. No antibodies to collagen were detected in the sera of the arthritic recipients (Trentham *et al.*, 1978b), suggesting that antibody production by the recipient did not explain the induction of synovitis in these experiments. However, collagen arthritis has not been passively transferred by T cells. For this reason, cell transfer of collagen arthritis fails to provide conclusive evidence of T-cell involvement in collagen arthritis.

Serum transfer experiments have not furnished irrefutable evidence that collagen arthritis is a B-cell-mediated disease. Negative results were obtained with several serum-transfer protocols (Trentham *et al.*, 1978b; Schoen *et al.*, 1981). Subsequent work showed that synovitis can be induced by this system, but disease in the recipient occurred only when large amounts of immunoglobulin-containing material was injected (Stuart *et al.*, 1982d; Stuart and Dixon, 1983; Kerwar *et al.*, 1983b). The lesion induced by antibody is transient, resolving in a week or 10 days (Stuart *et al.*, 1982d; Stuart and Dixon, 1983; Kerwar *et al.*, 1983b). Although cartilage damage can occur, other morphological aspects of the synovitis induced by antibody may differ from the primary disease. One group reported some pannus formation in rats (Stuart *et al.*, 1982d) and mice (Stuart and Dixon, 1983), but another laboratory has concluded that intravenous injection of affinity-purified IgG antibody to type II collagen induces polymorphonuclear leukocyte infiltration but not pannus in rats (Kerwar *et al.*, 1983b). An articular disease characterized by scant synovial hyperplasia and polymorphonuclear leukocyte dominance would not recapitulate the chronic proliferative synovitis observed after cell transfer (Trentham *et al.*, 1978b), in collagen arthritis induced by primary immunization (Caulfield *et al.*, 1982), or in rheumatoid arthritis. It would more closely simulate the picture in systemic lupus erythematosus.

In conclusion, the present importance of cell and serum transfer of collagen arthritis is in showing that products of B cells, and perhaps T cells, reactive to heterologous type II collagen can induce synovitis. The exact relationship of these data to collagen arthritis is unknown.

Although there is no passive transfer evidence that T-cell sensitization to collagen can induce arthritis, indications do exist that T cells can incite a proliferative synovitis in rats. Syngeneic T cells from rats with adjuvant arthritis stimulated with concanavalin A *in vitro* can induce synovitis following intravenous injection (Taurog *et al.*, 1983). However, it has not been demonstrated that the transferred disease represents the complete counterpart of adjuvant arthritis, since T cells not exposed to concanavalin A are ineffectual in disease transfer (Taurog *et al.*, 1983). *In vitro* propagated T cells from rats with adjuvant arthritis, reactive to both mycobacterial and homologous type II collagen (Holoshitz *et al.*, 1983) or exclusively to mycobacterial (Holoshitz *et al.*, 1984) antigenic stimulation, are also capable of inducing proliferative synovitis in irradiated recipients. These data provide further evidence that T cells can incite experimental synovitis. However, erosive arthritis can develop spontaneously on rare occasions in rats, and total lymphoid irradiation is capable of inducing an inflammatory synovitis in this species as well (Trentham *et al.*, 1984). For these reasons, the possibility exists that the irradiation regimen was involved in the induction of arthritis in these propagated T cell transfers.

Until recently, the only immunologic product that was clearly capable of inducing joint inflammation was IgG antibody to native type II collagen. Work by Helfgott *et al.*, (1984) has delineated a mechanism whereby T cells could function in the pathogenesis of collagen arthritis and, conceivably, other arthritic diseases. Sensitized rat T cells generate *in vitro* a type II collagen-specific lymphokine with an apparent molecular weight of approximately 60,000 to 70,000 that induces a persistent erosive proliferative synovitis when instilled into the knee joints of immunologically naive syngeneic recipients. The arthritogenicity of this lymphokine is independent of the complement pathway. It is unknown whether collagen-induced arthritogenic factor is present in other diseases such as adjuvant arthritis, but the identification of arthritogenic factor in collagen arthritis and the presence of cellular sensitivity to collagen in patients with rheumatoid arthritis (Trentham *et al.*, 1978c, 1981a,b; Endler *et al.*, 1978; Smolen *et al.*, 1980; Stuart *et al.*, 1980; Dayer *et al.*, 1982; Klareskog *et al.*, 1982; Solinger *et al.*, 1981; Solinger and Stobo, 1982; Golds *et al.*, 1983; Kammer and Trentham, 1984) are consistent with the proposal that production of arthritogenic factor is a T-cell-mediated effector mechanism in rheumatoid arthritis. Further studies of this new lymphokine have the potential to afford critical insights into the pathogenesis of chronic synovitis in humans.

The arthritic lesions induced by type II collagen-specific IgG antibody and the T-cell factor in the rat have additional implications. The results of passive transfer studies in experimental allergic orchitis in guinea pigs (Tung *et al.*, 1971a,b) may be instructive in this regard. In the orchitis model, intravenously injected antibodies to sperm induced a transient acute inflammatory response in the testes consisting of polymorphonuclear leukocyte infiltration and deposition of immunoglobulin and complement (Tung *et al.*, 1971b), whereas intravenous injection of sensitized lymph node cells produced mild orchitic lesions in an inconsistent fashion. However, local injection of cells into the interstitium of the testes initiated a severe prolonged lesion that recapitulated the disease observed after primary immunization, characterized by mononuclear inflammatory cells (Tung *et al.*, 1971a). Striking similarities with passive transfer studies in collagen arthritis exist. In the reviewer's experience, intraarticular instillation of anticollagen antibodies induces only a mild synovitis of the rat knee joint. In contrast, the histological features of collagen arthritis induced by primary immunization develop after intraarticular injection of arthritogenic-factor-enriched material. These observations suggest that collagen arthritis in the rat is primarily a T-cell-mediated disease.

In the rat model, Brahn and Trentham (1984b) have shown that T cells subserve a critical function in the induction of collagen arthritis during the first 5 days after immunization with collagen using a polyclonal T-cell-specific heterologous antiserum. This finding is similar to the observations of Kaibara *et al.* (1983) using cyclosporin A in the model. The nature of this cellular mechanism is unknown, but it is possible that it involves production of arthritogenic factor as well as providing T-cell help for collagen antibody production by B cells.

Another aspect of collagen arthritis may afford insights into the pathogenesis of this model. To induce disease, it is obligatory to use native (helical) collagen for immunization (Trentham *et al.*, 1977). This requisite has been interpreted as evidence that collagen arthritis is an antibody-mediated disease, since T cells traditionally are considered to react to sequential antigenic determinants on proteins, whereas antibodies frequently are conformationally dependent. However, recent findings in mice have identified conformationally dependent T-cell reactivities to the multideterminant protein insulin (Glimcher *et al.*, 1983). It is possible that clones of T cells exist in rodents that recognize quarternary epitopes on native type II collagen. Indirect evidence in rats consistent with this proposal has been obtained by thymidine-incorporation assays (Trentham *et al.*, 1978a) and antigen-presentation experiments (Schoen *et al.*, 1981). However, the cellular response to type II collagen in mice has been reported to lack helical specificity (Stuart *et al.*, 1982c). This is another important area for further investigation.

VIII. SENSITIVITY TO COLLAGEN IN RHEUMATOID ARTHRITIS

Some patients with rheumatoid arthritis have antibodies to the interstitial collagens in their sera (Steffen and Timpl, 1963; Michaeli and Fudenberg, 1974b; Cracchiolo *et al.*, 1975; Andriopoulos *et al.*, 1976a,b; Menzel *et al.*, 1978; Trentham *et al.*, 1978c, 1981a,b; Foidart *et al.*, 1978; Clague *et al.*, 1980b; Beard *et al.*, 1980; Meghlaoui *et al.*, 1981; Dyer *et al.*, 1982; Stuart *et al.*, 1983b; Kammer and Trentham, 1984), and a proportion exhibit cellular sensitivity to collagen (Trentham *et al.*, 1978c, 1981a,b; Endler *et al.*, 1978; Smolen *et al.*, 1980; Stuart *et al.*, 1980; Dayer *et al.*, 1982; Klareskog *et al.*, 1982; Solinger *et al.*, 1981; Solinger and Stobo, 1982; Golds *et al.*, 1983; Kammer and Trentham, 1984). Antibodies to collagen are also reported to be present in the synovial fluid of some patients with this disease (Cracchiolo *et al.*, 1975; Menzel *et al.*, 1978; Andriopoulos *et al.*, 1976b). These humoral (Andriopoulos *et al.*, 1976b; Trentham *et al.*, 1978c; Stuart *et al.*, 1983b) and cellular (Trentham *et al.*, 1978c; Klareskog *et al.*, 1982) reactivities appear to be specific for collagenous determinants. However, the titers of serum antibodies to collagen are low, and they have not correlated with signs or symptoms of this disease (Andriopoulos *et al.*, 1976a; Trentham *et al.*, 1978c; Dyer *et al.*, 1982; Stuart *et al.*, 1983b). Moreover, collagen reactivity is not restricted to rheumatoid arthritis; it is present in a variety of diseases characterized by inflammation of connective tissue (Michaeli and Fudenberg, 1974a; Stuart *et al.*, 1976, 1980, 1983b; Kravis *et al.*, 1976; McAdam *et al.*, 1978; Cracchiolo *et al.*, 1975; Foidart *et al.*, 1978; Suou and Hirayama, 1980; Trentham *et al.*, 1981b; Meghlaoui *et al.*, 1981; Ebringer *et al.*, 1981; Mackel *et al.*, 1982; Yoo *et al.*, 1982; Adar *et al.*, 1983; Golds *et al.*, 1983) and even in normal subjects (Solinger *et al.*, 1981; Kammer and Trentham, 1984). These data tell us little concerning possible collagen-induced efferent pathways in rheumatoid arthritis.

IX. EVIDENCE THAT AUTOIMMUNITY TO TYPE II COLLAGEN IS INVOLVED IN THE PRIMARY PATHOGENESIS OF RELAPSING POLYCHONDRITIS

Perhaps the most persuasive evidence that autoimmunity to type II collagen is involved in the pathogenesis of any human disease is found in relapsing polychondritis. Antibodies to type II collagen have been detected in some patients with relapsing polychondritis, and their presence appears to correlate with periods of active extraarticular inflammation (Foidart *et al.*, 1978; Ebringer *et al.*, 1981). These findings have been confirmed in our laboratory. One of four patients with active relapsing polychondritis had high serum titers of IgG antibodies specific for native type II collagen by an ELISA. Although the incidence of antibodies to type II collagen may appear to be low in these surveys, it is possible that antibody production is a localized or evanescent phenomenon in polychondritis. This proposal would be consistent with the relapsing nature of the disorder.

Further evience of a role for immunologic responses to type II collagen in the pathogenesis of inflammatory chondritis was provided by the finding that auricular lesions histologically resembling relapsing polychondritis develop on occasion in rats immunized with type II collagen (Griffiths *et al.*, 1981; Cremer *et al.*, 1981; McCune *et al.*, 1982a). The identification of complement and immunoglobulin, as well as fibrin, in these chondritic lesions (McCune *et al.*, 1982a) suggests that the inflammation in this model is antibody induced. Total lymphoid irradiation, a technique that produces complex immunoregulatory changes in rodents (Strober *et al.*, 1979), can also induce experimental polychondritis in the rat (Trentham *et al.*, 1984). This irradiation-induced lesion may indicate that the immune system can be manipulated to permit clones of effector lymphocytes for this chondritic process to expand. Further studies could ascertain whether this proposed relation of autoimmunity to type II collagen in human and experimental polychondritis is valid (Trentham, 1982b).

If autoimmunity to type II collagen functions in the primary pathogenesis of rheumatoid arthritis as well as in relapsing polychondritis or even inner ear disease (Yoo *et al.*, 1982, 1983a,b), the question arises as to how these phenotypically different diseases could be sequelae of one antigenic response. Several explanations can be offered, but all lack supporting data. Different contributions of B and T cells in each disorder might produce disparate pathological processes; i.e., polychondritis could be an antibody-induced lesion, whereas the joint inflammation in rheumatoid arthritis might be primarily T cell mediated. Immunologic responses directed to separate epitopes on native type II collagen could be involved in the two diseases and explain their clinical differences. Alternatively, different efferent pathways in the two diseases could be primed by similar afferent sensitivity responses to collagen. For example, many patients administered procainamide or hydralazine develop antibodies to DNA; however, only a minority of cases eventuate in clinical manifestations of drug-induced lupus triggered by as yet unidentified efferent processes (Schoen and Trentham, 1981). Efforts to identify effector mechanisms involved in autoimmune diseases will undoubtedly receive greater attention in the future.

X. IMMUNOGENETIC REGULATION OF COLLAGEN IMMUNITY IN RODENTS

The immune response to collagen in rats (Griffiths *et al.*, 1981; Griffiths and Dewitt, 1981) and mice (Rosenwasser *et al.*, 1980; Wooley *et al.*, 1981) is, like most protein immunogens (Rosenwasser *et al.*, 1980), regulated by immune-response (Ir) genes. Susceptibility to collagen arthritis in rats (Griffiths *et al.*, 1981; Griffiths and Dewitt, 1981) and mice (Wooley *et al.*, 1981, 1983) and adjuvant-arthritis susceptibility (Battisto *et al.*, 1982) are also influenced by genetic mechanisms. But immunogenetic pathways that control collagen reactivity in humans have not been clearly identified. Preliminary indications that HLA-DR4 governs one's ability to respond cellularly to collagen (Solinger *et al.*, 1981; Solinger and Stobo, 1982) have failed to receive support from the findings in other studies (Smolen *et al.*, 1980; Kammer and Trentham, 1984). However, familial clustering of subjects with autoantibodies to type II collagen has been found (Kammer and Trentham, 1984). This observation necessitates additional work to elucidate collagen-specific Ir genes in humans.

XI. HOW MIGHT AUTOIMMUNITY TO COLLAGEN ARISE?

Sufficient data exist to permit a brief hypothetical discussion of ways in which autoimmunity to collagen might emerge. Since the evidence is derived solely from rodent experiments, its relevance for human disease is conjectural.

Murine immunity is subserved by a phenotypic and functional network that, under normal conditions, is precisely regulated. The critical role of distinct populations of self-regulatory lymphocytes in initiating, controlling the amplitude and epitope specificities, and terminating specific responses to protein immunogens is beyond dispute. What is uncertain is the degree to which idiotypic mechanisms and antigen-specific helper and suppressor factors participate in regulating the immune system. This fine orchestration of immunity incorporates the potential for pertubations to offset its balance. Such dysregulation could be the pivotal mechanism by which clones of anti-self-reacting lymphocytes emerge and eventuate in autoimmune disease. Rather than being primary aberrations *per se,* autoimmune diseases could represent a phenomenon in which these clones are byproducts of an imbalanced helper–suppressor T-cell milieu.

Autoimmunity in rodents is achieved in a reproducible fashion by injecting a host protein that is normally sequestered from the immune system in concert with an adjuvant preparation. Traditionally, adjuvants were considered to be potent activators of cellular immunity; i.e., they were thought to act simply as an immunostimulant. Today, their functions appear to be more complex; the available evidence suggests that the essential action of adjuvants is to realign immunologic homeostasis. In most situations, this adjuvant-induced reregulation favors augmenting activities, and neosensitizations are accomplished. But in other instances, adjuvant-triggered mechanisms can preferentially activate suppressor pathways. In addition to adjuvants, the capacity of antigen-coupled cells and low doses of irradiation, hydrocortisone, and cyclophosphamide (Schoen *et al.*, 1981) to alter the outcome of immunization protocols further demonstrates that the rodent immune system is a complex repertoire of amplifying and dampening influences.

Autoimmunity in rodents must, in general, be experimentally induced. In contrast, autoimmune disease in humans is perceived to have a spontaneous inception unrelated to environmental factors. This conclusion would be premature if underlying endogenous or exogenous mechanisms responsible for the emergence of autoimmunity in humans exist. This possibility can be illustrated by studies with type II collagen.

To function effectively as autoimmunogens, host proteins must be injected in complete Freund's adjuvant (Trentham, 1981). Native type II collagen appears to violate this rule in the rat, since equivalent degrees of arthritogenicity and immunogenicity are observed when either complete or incomplete Freund's adjuvant is used (Trentham *et al.*, 1977). The explanation for this phenomenon remains unclear. Although it appears that type II collagen cannot substitute for mycobacteria in providing a universal adjuvant effect for other protein immunogens (Cremer *et al.*, 1980), it is possible that conventionally purified type II collagen possesses contaminating material, such as proteoglycans, that provides a "self-adjuvanticity." Alternatively, portions of the native molecule could provide a unique autoadjuvanticity. Type II collagen can act as a ligand to stimulate human monocytes to produce interleukin-1 (Dayer *et al.*, 1982). This activity or other ligand-induced effects by type II collagen on immunoinducing cells could function in afferent pathways culminating in sensitization to this protein.

Type II collagen can function in a unique manner in antigen-presentation protocols to produce selective responses by the immune system without adjuvant oil. For example, subcutaneous injection of type II collagen-coupled syngeneic spleen cells induces delayed-type hypersentivity but no antibody responses in rats, whereas use of allogeneic-carrier cells triggers both T- and B-cell autosensitization to collagen. B cells can also be stimulated to produce antibodies by subcutaneous injection of syngeneic collagen-coupled cells into cyclophosphamide-pretreated rats. These responses are antigen specific and can be achieved with the use of homologous type II collagen (Schoen *et al.*, 1981). The data from these experiments illustrate the complexity of the immune system in generating reactivity to this host constituent and suggest that antigen presentation of released type II collagen by endogenous macrophage monocytes may be one mechanism whereby autoimmunity to this protein develops in rheumatic disease. For example, cartilage collagen breakdown during inflammatory arthritis in humans could lead to antigen processing by synovial macrophages or other Ia (immune associated)-bearing antigen-presenting cells and explain the development of collagen reactivity in rheumatoid arthritis, psoriatic arthritis, and even crystal-induced arthropathy (Trentham *et al.*, 1981b; Stuart *et al.*, 1983b).

Other mechanisms can give rise to autoimmunity to collagen. Cellular sensitivity to collagen can be evoked by injecting rats with complete Freund's adjuvant (Steffen and Wick, 1971; Trentham *et al.*, 1980; Holoshitz *et al.*, 1983) or by inducing pulmonary inflammation with bleomycin (Schrier *et al.*, 1982). Preliminary evidence suggests that the intravenous injection of cell-membrane-associated heterologous or homologous native proteins, such as type II collagen, type I collagen, or ovalbumin, combined with the intradermal injection of the synthetic alkyldiamine adjuvant CP-20961 induces cellular reactivity to type II collagen (Trentham and Dynesius-Trentham, 1983). Although the mechanism(s) accounting for this surprising result are unknown, the phenomenon further illustrates the fact that immunomodulatory protocols not involving the injection of type II collagen can eventuate in afferent sensitivity to this cartilage constituent. This finding argues against the theory that all situations involving autoimmunity to collagen in human disease merely reflect a secondary epiphenomenon attributable to cartilage breakdown at sites of joint inflammation.

Other information concerning the possible role of immunologic dysregulation in the pathogenesis of connective tissue diseases has been derived from studies showing that a low percentage (5–10%) of young-adult Sprague–Dawley rats injected with ketamine anesthesia and receiving 3400 rad of fractionated total lymphoid irradiation (TLI) develop a severe polyarthritis during the 2-week period following the end of the irradiation protocol. The disease is a persistent severe peripheral polyarthritis with pannus formation, mononuclear cell infiltration, and cartilage and bone erosion (Trentham *et al.*, 1984). The lesion includes deposits of fibrin within and on the surface of the inflamed synovium. On rare occasions, unmanipulated rats develop this syndrome. The morphological picture of the spontaneous or post-TLI arthritis resembles collagen and adjuvant disease. An auricular chondritis that is histologically identical to that observed after type II collagen immunization has also been observed in the post-TLI period (Trentham *et al.*, 1984). These connective tissue lesions do not resemble those induced by infection, and there are no cultural or serologic indications that the involved rats have become colonized with *Mycoplasma arthritidis*. Evidence favoring an immunologically mediated pathogenesis is afforded by the recognized ability of TLI to produce complex modulatory changes in the immune system (Strober *et al.*, 1979) as well as by the finding of immunoglobulin and complement deposited within the arthritic synovium (Fig. 2). Antibodies to collagen have not been detected in the sera of these arthritic rats. However, a small percentage of involved rats have exhibited evidence of delayed-type hypersensitivity to type II collagen. These findings are preliminary, and it is unknown whether the spontaneous and post-TLI diseases are the same. Nonetheless, this new model furnishes the opportunity of providing additional information regarding the pathogenesis of connective tissue disease.

The finding that inflammatory arthritis can be induced in the rat by the injection of collagen or adjuvant preparations and the use of TLI suggests that different external factors can affect the immune system and lead to connective tissue disease in the rat. The appreciation that inflammatory arthritis can also develop spontaneously in an experimental strain further argues that animal models can furnish insights into human disease. The morphological features of these inflammatory arthritides in the rat are similar, and indirect evidence of immunologic involvement in the pathogenesis of all of these models exists. What remains to be identified is whether common pathogenetic processes, such as autoimmune reactions to type II collagen, operate or whether widely divergent immune mechanisms incite the inflammation in these diseases. If the former possibility is shown to be true in the future, it would become more likely that these experimental models of autoimmune arthritis are relevant for human disease.

XII. COLLAGEN IMMUNITY AND THE PATHOGENESIS OF RHEUMATOID ARTHRITIS: A HYPOTHESIS

Based on the available evidence, a theory regarding the possible role of collagen immunity in the pathogenesis of rheumatoid arthritis can be offered. This speculation relates to epitope-specific collagen reactivities being critical to the pathogenesis of rodent and human disease. Findings in human lupus and myasthenia gravis illustrate this potential. Autoimmune diseases represent states in which a panoply of autoantibodies and sensitized lymphocytes exist (Schoen and Trentham, 1981). Autoantibodies against denatured DNA are found in many diseases, but increasing evidence suggests that exquisitely specific anti-native-DNA responses are a major effector mechanism in lupus (Schoen and Trentham, 1981). In myasthenia gravis, a number of antiself reactivities are also present, but it now appears that anti-acetylcholine-receptor reactivities are the process intimately involved in the primary pathogenesis of the disease (Drachman *et al.*, 1982). A few patients with

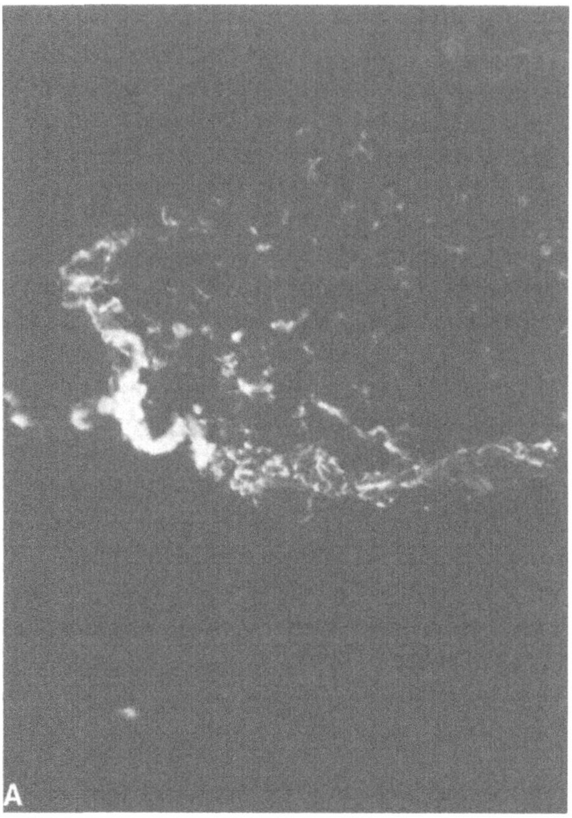

Figure 2. Direct immunofluorescence staining revealing (A) immunoglobulin, (B) complement C3, and (C) fibrin deposited in a histological section from the synovium overlying the infrapatellar fat pat of three different rats with post-TLI arthritis. Arthritis began 11 days after completion of TLI in all three rats, and the tissue was obtained 8 days later (× 134 for A, B, and C).

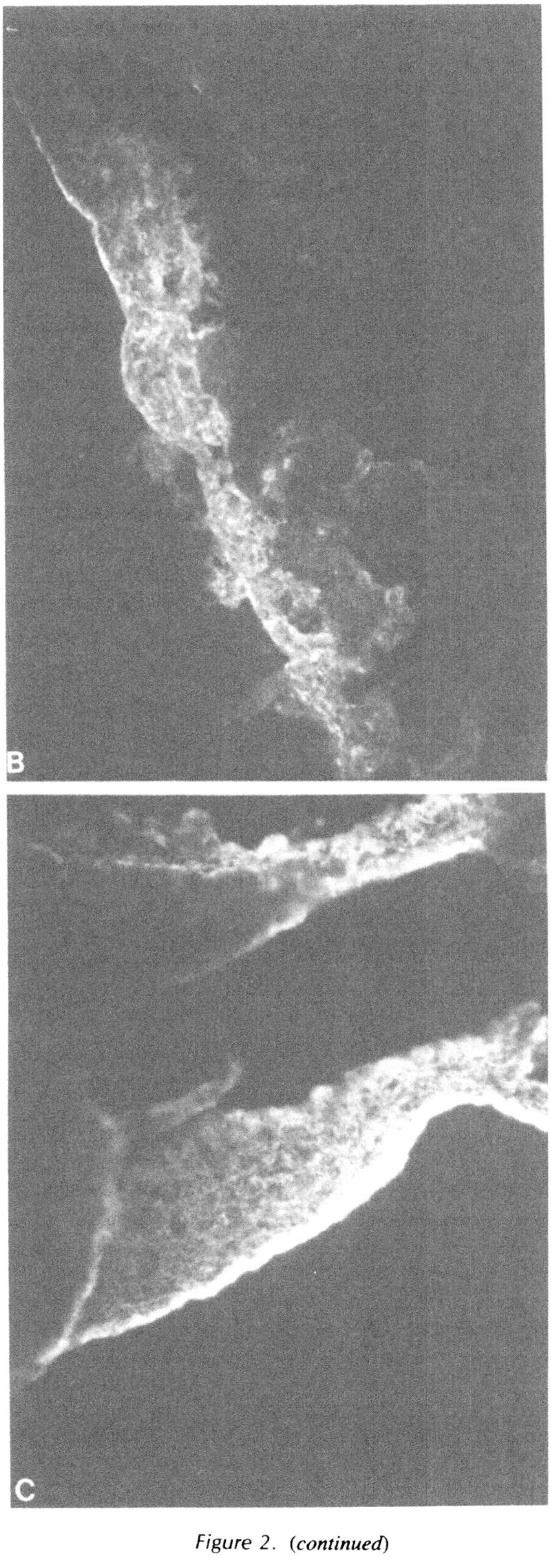

Figure 2. (*continued*)

rheumatoid arthritis who possess high titers of antibodies specific for native type II collagen have been identified (Stuart *et al.*, 1983b). All of these data are consistent with the possibility that critical epitopes on type II collagen, a probably complex multideterminant protein antigen (Trentham, 1981), may function in the primary pathogenesis of rheumatoid arthritis. Alternatively, preliminary evidence from a leukapheresis trial suggests that rheumatoid arthritis is a heterogeneous disorder (Wahl *et al.*, 1983). Should this conclusion be correct, then a subset of patients with rheumatoid arthritis in which anticollagen reactivity is a fundamental pathogenetic mechanism may exist. If rheumatoid arthritis is a T-cell-mediated disease, and should autoimmunity to collagen be involved, then a unifying pathway would be provided by a type II collagen-specific arthritogenic lymphokine functioning in the human disease.

The rigorous test of whether collagen immunity participates in the pathogenesis of rheumatoid arthritis must await trials involving antigen-specific immunosuppression (Trentham, 1981, 1982a). Protocols capable of achieving antigen-specific attenuation of experimental arthritis in the rat (Staines *et al.*, 1981; Schoen *et al.*, 1982; Holoshitz *et al.*, 1983; Cremer *et al.*, 1983; Brahn and Trentham, 1984a) have been identified. Adaptations of these techniques may someday be evaluated in human disease.

XIII. CONCLUSION

Studies of the immunologic properties of native type II collagen in the past decade have delineated a new field in connective tissue disease. They have suggested that the emergence of synovial hyperplasia could, in some way, be related to cartilage. The recent advances in the field of collagen immunology have provided data, the significance of which is only partially evident at present. In the near future, additional work may answer the question of whether autoimmunity to collagen is an effector mechanism in human disease.

ACKNOWLEDGMENT. This work was supported in part by U.S. Public Health Service grant AM-21490.

REFERENCES

Abrahamsen, T. G., Froland, S. S., Natvig, J. B., and Pahle, J., 1975, Elution and characterization of lymphocytes from rheumatoid inflammatory tissue, *Scand. J. Immunol.* **4**:823–830.

Adar, R., Papa, M. Z., Halpern, Z., Mozes, M., Shoshan, S., Sofer, B., Zinger, H., Dayan, M., and Mozes, E., 1983, Cellular sensitivity to collagen in thromboangiitis obliterans, *N. Engl. J. Med.* **308**:1113–1116.

Adelmann, B. C., 1972, The structural basis of cell-mediated immunological reactions of collagen: Reactivity of separated α chains of calf and rat collagen in cutaneous delayed hypersensitivity reactions, *Immunology* **23**:739–748.

Adelmann, B. C., and Kirrane, J., 1973, The structural basis of cell-mediated immunological reactions of collagen: The species specificity of the cutaneous delayed hypersensitivity reaction, *Immunology* **25**:123–130.

Adelmann, B. C., Kirrane, J. A., and Glynn, L. E., 1972, The structural basis of cell-mediated immunological reactions of collagen: Characteristics of cutaneous delayed hypersensitivity reactions in specifically sensitized guinea pigs, *Immunology* **23**:723–738.

Andriopoulos, N. A., Mestecky, J., Miller, E. J., and Bradley, E. L., 1976a, Antibodies to native and denatured collagens in sera of patients with rheumatoid arthritis, *Arthritis Rheum.* **19**:613–617.

Andriopoulos, N. A., Mestecky, J., Wright, G. P., and Miller, E. J., 1976b, Characterization of antibodies to the native human collagens and to their component α chains in the sera and the joint fluid of patients with rheumatoid arthritis, *Immunochemistry* **13:**709–712.

Barland, P., Novikoff, A. B., and Hammerman, D., 1962, Electron microscopy of the human synovial membrane, *J. Cell Biol.* **14:**207–220.

Battisto, J. R., Smith, R. N., Beckman, K., Sternlicht, M., and Welles, W. L., 1982, Susceptibility to adjuvant arthritis in DA and F_{344} rats: A dominant trait controlled by an autosomal gene locus linked to the major histocompatibility complex, *Arthritis Rheum.* **25:**1194–1200.

Beard, H. K., Faulk, W. P., Conochie, L. B., and Glynn, L. E., 1977, Some immunological aspects of collagen, *Prog. Allergy* **22:**45–106.

Beard, H. K., Ueda, M., Faulk, W. P., and Glynn, L. E., 1978, Cell-mediated and humoral immunity to chick type II collagen and its cyanogen bromide peptides in guinea pigs, *Immunology* **34:**323–335.

Beard, H. K., Ryvar, R., Skingle, J., and Greenbury, C. L., 1980, Anticollagen antibodies in sera from rheumatoid arthritis patients, *J. Clin. Pathol.* **33:**1077–1081.

Beil, W., Timpl, R., and Furthmayr, H., 1973, Conformation dependence of antigenic determinants on the collagen molecule, *Immunology* **24:**13–24.

Brahn, E., and Trentham, D. E., 1984a, Antigen-specific suppression of collagen arthritis by adoptive transfer of spleen cells, *Clin. Immunol. Immunopathol.* **31:**124–131.

Brahn, E., and Trentham, D. E., 1984b, Effect of anti-T cell serum on collagen arthritis in rats: Evidence that T cells are involved in its pathogenesis, *Cell Immunol.* **86:**421–428.

Brahn, E., Helfgott, S. M., Belli, J. A., Anderson, R. J., Reinherz, E. L., Schlossman, S. F., Austen, K. F., and Trentham, D. E., 1984, Total lymphoid irradiation therapy of refractory rheumatoid arthritis: Fifteen- to forty-month followup, *Arthritis Rheum.* **27:**481–488.

Burstein, N. A., and Waksman, B. H., 1964, The pathogenesis of adjuvant disease in the rat. I. A histologic study of early lesions in the joints and skin, *Yale J. Biol. Med.* **37:**177–194.

Caulfield, J. P., Hein, A., Dynesius-Trentham, R., and Trentham, D. E., 1982, Morphologic demonstration of two stages in the development of type II collagen-induced arthritis, *Lab. Invest.* **46:**321–343.

Chung, E., and Miller, E. J., 1974, Collagen polymorphism: Characterization of molecules with the chain composition $[\alpha 1(III)]_3$ in human tissues, *Science* **183:**1200–1201.

Clague, R. B., Morgan, K., Shaw, M. J., and Holt, P. J. L., 1980a, Native type II collagen-induced arthritis in the rat. II. Relationship between the humoral immune response to native type II collagen and arthritis, *J. Rheumatol.* **7:**775–782.

Clague, R. B., Shaw, M. J., and Lennox Holt, P. J., 1980b, Incidence of serum antibodies to native type I and type II collagens in patients with inflammatory arthritis, *Ann. Rheum. Dis.* **39:**201–206.

Courtenay, J. S., Dallman, M. J., Dayan, A. D., Martin, A., and Mosedale, B., 1980, Immunisation against heterologous type II collagen induces arthritis in mice, *Nature* **283:**666–668.

Cracchiolo, A., Michaeli, D., Goldberg, L. S., and Fudenberg, H. H., 1975, The occurrence of antibodies to collagen in synovial fluids, *Clin. Immunol. Immunopathol.* **3:**567–574.

Cremer, M. A., Stuart, J. M., Townes, A. S., and Kang, A. H., 1980, Collagen-induced polyarthritis in rats: A study of native type II collagen for adjuvant activity, *J. Immunol.* **124:**2912–2918.

Cremer, M. A., Pitcock, J. A., Stuart, J. M., Kang, A. H., and Townes, A. S., 1981, Auricular chondritis in rats: An experimental model of relapsing polychondritis induced with type II collagen, *J. Exp. Med.* **154:**535–540.

Cremer, M. A., Hernandez, A. D., Townes, A. S., Stuart, J. M., and Kang, A. H., 1983, Collagen-induced arthritis in rats: Antigen-specific suppression of arthritis and immunity by intravenously injected native type II collagen, *J. Immunol.* **131:**2995–3000.

Dayer, J.-M., Trentham, D. E., and Krane, S. M., 1982, Collagens act as ligands to stimulate human monocytes to produce mononuclear cell factor (MCF) and prostaglandins (PGE_2), *Collagen Rel. Res.* **2:**523–540.

DeSimone, D. P., Parsons, D. B., Johnson, K. E., and Jacobs, R. P., 1983, Type II collagen-induced arthritis: A morphologic and biochemical study of articular cartilage, *Arthritis Rheum.* **26:**1245–1258.

Drachman, D. B., Adams, R. N., Josifek, L. F., and Self, S. G., 1982, Functional activities of autoantibodies to acetylcholine receptors and the clinical severity of myasthenia gravis, *N. Engl. J. Med.* **307:**769–775.

Dyer, P. A., Clague, R. B., Klouda, P. T., Firth, S., Harris, R., and Holt, P. J. L., 1982, HLA antigens in patients with rheumatoid arthritis and antibodies to native type II collagen, *Tissue Antigens* **20:**394–396.

Dynesius-Trentham, R. A., Rowland, D., LaRoche, E., and Trentham, D. E., 1981, Rat leukocyte inhibitory factor (LIF): Similarities to human LIF and generation by cells from rats with collagen-induced arthritis, *Cell. Immunol.* **63**:362–373.

Ebringer, R., Rook, G., Swana, G. T., Bottazzo, G. F., and Doniach, D., 1981, Autoantibodies to cartilage and type II collagen in relapsing polychondritis and other rheumatic diseases, *Ann. Rheum. Dis.* **40**:473–479.

Endler, A. T., Zielinski, C., Menzel, E. J., Smolen, J. S., Schwägerl, W., Endler, M., Eberl, R., Frank, O., and Steffen, C., 1978, Leukocyte migration inhibition with collagen type I and collagen type III in rheumatoid arthritis and degenerative joint diseases, *Z. Rheumatol.* **37**:87–92.

Field, E. H., Strober, S., Hoppe, R. T., Calin, A., Engleman, E. G., Kotzin, B. L., Tanay, A. S., Calin, H. J., Terrell, C. P., and Kaplan, H. S., 1983, Sustained improvement of intractable rheumatoid arthritis after total lymphoid irradiation, *Arthritis Rheum.* **26**:937–946.

Fietzek, P. P., and Kühn, K., 1976, The primary structure of collagen, *Int. Rev. Connect. Tissue Res.* **7**:1–60.

Foidart, J.-M., Abe, S., Martin, G. R., Zizic, T. M., Barnett, E. V., Lawley, T. J., and Katz, S. I., 1978, Antibodies to type II collagen in relapsing polychondritis, *N. Engl. J. Med.* **299**:1203–1207.

Furthmayr, H., and Timpl, R., 1976, Immunochemistry of collagens and procollagens, *Int. Rev. Connect. Tissue Res.* **7**:61–99.

Gallop, P. M., Blumenfeld, O. O., and Seifter, S., 1972, Structure and metabolism of connective tissue proteins, *Annu. Rev. Biochem.* **41**:617–672.

Gentner, G. J., and Adelmann, B. C., 1976a, Specific suppression of delayed hypersensitivity skin reactions to collagen in guinea pigs after immunization with collagen and Freund's incomplete adjuvant, *Immunology* **31**:87–94.

Gentner, G. J., and Adelmann, B. C., 1976b, The relation between the cell-mediated immunological response and the induction of circulating antibodies to collagen in guinea pigs: Investigation of cell functions, *Immunology* **31**:95–100.

Glimcher, L. H., Schroer, J. A., Chan, C., and Shevach, E. M., 1983, Fine specificity of cloned insulin-specific T cell hybridomas: Evidence supporting a role for tertiary conformation, *J. Immunol.* **131**:2868–2874.

Glynn, L. E., 1969, Aetiology of rheumatoid arthritis with regard to its chronicity, *Ann. Rheum. Dis.* **28**(Suppl.):3–4.

Golds, E. E., Stephen, I. B. M., Esdaile, J. M., Strawczynski, H., and Poole, A. R., 1983, Lymphocyte transformation to connective tissue antigens in adult and juvenile rheumatoid arthritis, osteoarthritis, ankylosing spondylitis, systemic lupus erythematosus, and a nonarthritic control population, *Cell. Immunol.* **82**:196–209.

Graabaek, P. M., 1982, Ultrastructural evidence for two distinct types of synoviocytes in rat synovial membrane, *J. Ultrastruct. Res.* **78**:321–339.

Greene, M. I., and Benacerraf, B., 1980, Studies on hapten specific T cell immunity and suppression, *Immunol. Rev.* **50**:163–186.

Griffiths, M. M., and Dewitt, C. W., 1981, Immunogenetic control of experimental collagen-induced arthritis in rats. II. ECIA susceptibility and immune response to type II collagen (calf) are linked to RTI, *J. Immunogenet.* **8**:463–470.

Griffiths, M. M., Eichwald, E. J., Martin, J. H., Smith, C. B., and Dewitt, C. W., 1981, Immunogenetic control of experimental type II collagen-induced arthritis. I. Susceptibility and resistance among inbred strains of rats, *Arthritis Rheum.* **24**:781–789.

Hahn, E., and Timpl, R., 1973, Involvement of more than a single polypeptide chain in the helical antigenic determinants of collagen, *Eur. J. Immunol.* **3**:442–446.

Hahn, E., Timpl, R., and Miller, E. J., 1974, The production of specific antibodies to native collagens with the chain compositions, $[\alpha 1(I)]_3$, $[\alpha 1(II)]_3$ and $[\alpha 1(I)]_2\ \alpha 2$, *J. Immunol.* **13**:421–423.

Hahn, E., Nowack, D., Götze, D., and Timpl, R., 1975, H-2-linked genetic control of antibody response to soluble calf skin collagen in mice, *Eur. J. Immunol.* **5**:288–291.

Helfgott, S. M., Dynesius-Trentham, R., and Trentham, D. E., 1984, Type II Collagen induced arthritogenic factor in the rat, *Clin. Res.* **32**:348.

Holoshitz, J., Naparstek, Y., Ben-Nun, A., and Cohen, I. R., 1983, Lines of T lymphocytes induce or vaccinate against autoimmune arthritis, *Science* **219**:56–58.

Holoshitz, J., Matitiau, A., and Cohen, I. R., 1984, Arthritis induced in rats by cloned T lymphocytes responsive to mycobacteria but not to collagen type II, *J. Clin. Invest.* **73**:211–215.

Iizuka, Y., and Chang, Y.-H., 1982, Adjuvant polyarthritis. VII. The role of type II collagen in pathogenesis, *Arthritis Rheum.* **25**:1325–1332.

Jarcho, S., 1936, Lupus erythematosus associated with visceral vascular lesions: A series of autopsied cases, *Bull. Johns Hopkins Hosp.* **59:**262–273.

Kaibara, N., Hotokebuchi, T., Takagishi, K., and Katsuki, I., 1983, Paradoxical effects of cyclosporin A on collagen arthritis in rats, *J. Exp. Med.* **158:**2007–2015.

Kammer, G. M., and Trentham, D. E., 1984, HLA-DR4 is not a requisite for autoimmunity to collagen in rheumatoid arthritis, *Arthritis Rheum.* **27:**489–494.

Kerwar, S. S., Sloboda, A. E., Birnbaum, J. E., and Oronsky, A. L., 1981, Studies on the effect of D-penicillamine on type II collagen-induced polyarthritis, *J. Rheumatol.* **8:**84–88.

Kerwar, S. S., Bauman, N., Oronsky, A. L., and Sloboda, A. E., 1982, Studies on type II collagen-induced polyarthritis: Effect of complement depletion, *J. Immunopharmacol.* **3:**323–338.

Kerwar, S. S., Gordon, S., McReynolds, R. A., and Oronsky, A. L., 1983a, Localization of ^{125}I-labeled anticollagen immunoglobulin in passive transfer of arthritis, *Clin. Immunol. Immunopathol.* **29:**318–321.

Kerwar, S. S., Englert, M. E., McReynolds, R. A., Landes, M. J., Lloyd, J. M., Oronsky, A. L., and Wilson, F. J., 1983b, Type II collagen-induced arthritis: Studies with purified anticollagen immunoglobulin, *Arthritis Rheum.* **26:**1120–1131.

Klareskog, L., Forsum, U., Scheynius, A., Kabelitz, D., and Wigzell, H., 1982, Evidence in support of a self-perpetuating HLA-DR-dependent delayed-type cell reaction in rheumatoid arthritis, *Proc. Natl. Acad. Sci. U.S.A.* **79:**3632–3636.

Klareskog, L., Holmdahl, R., Larsson, E., and Wigzel, H., 1983, Role of T lymphocytes in collagen II induced arthritis in rats, *Clin. Exp. Immunol.* **51:**117–125.

Klemperer, P., Pollack, A. D., and Baehr, G., 1942, Diffuse collagen disease: Acute disseminated lupus erythematosus and diffuse scleroderma, *JAMA* **119:**331–332.

Kotzin, B. L., Strober, S., Engleman, E. G., Calin, A., Hoppe, R. T., Kansas, G. S., Terrell, C. P., and Kaplan, H. S., 1981, Treatment of intractable rheumatoid arthritis with total lymphoid irradiation, *N. Engl. J. Med.* **305:**969–975.

Kravis, T. C., Ahmed, A., Brown, T. E., Fulmer, J. D., and Crystal, R. G., 1976, Pathogenic mechanisms in pulmonary fibrosis: Collagen-induced migration inhibition factor production and cytotoxicity mediated by lymphocytes, *J. Clin. Invest.* **58:**1223–1232.

Lane, J. M., and Weiss, C., 1975, Review of articular cartilage collagen research, *Arthritis Rheum.* **18:**553–562.

LeRoy, E. C., 1974, Collagens and human disease, *Bull. Rheum. Dis.* **25:**778–784.

Lindblad, S., Klareskog, L., Hedfors, E., Forsum, U., and Sundström, C., 1983, Phenotypic characterization of synovial tissue cells *in situ* in different types of synovitis, *Arthritis Rheum.* **26:**1321–1332.

Lindsley, H., Mannik, M., and Bornstein, P., 1971, The distribution of antigenic determinants in rat skin collagen, *J. Exp. Med.* **133:**1309–1324.

Mackel, A. M., Delustro, F., Harper, F. E., and LeRoy, E. C., 1982, Antibodies to collagen in scleroderma, *Arthritis Rheum.* **25:**522–531.

Marcus, R. L., and Townes, A. S., 1971, The occurrence of cryoproteins in synovial fluid; the association of a complement-fixing activity in rheumatoid synovial fluid with cold-precipitable protein, *J. Clin. Invest.* **50:**282–293.

McAdam, K. P. W. J., Fudenberg, H. H., and Michaeli, D., 1978, Antibodies to collagen in patients with leprosy, *Clin. Immunol. Immunopathol.* **9:**16–21.

McCune, W. J., Trentham, D. E., and David, J. R., 1980, Gold does not alter the arthritic, humoral or cellular responses in rats with type II collagen-induced arthritis, *Arthritis Rheum.* **23:**932–936.

McCune, W. J., Schiller, A. L., Dynesius-Trentham, R. A., and Trentham, D. E., 1982a, Type II collagen-induced auricular chondritis, *Arthritis Rheum.* **25:**266–273.

McCune, W. J., Buckley, J. A., Belli, J. A., and Trentham, D. E., 1982b, Immunosuppression by fractionated total lymphoid irradiation in collagen arthritis, *Arthritis Rheum.* **25:**532–539.

Meghlaoui, A., Herbage, D., Huc, A., and Monier, J.C., 1981, Mise au point d'une technique immunoenzymatique (ELISA) pour la détection des anticorps anti-collagène de type I et II: Recherche de ces anticorps au cours de la polyarthrite rhumatoïde du lupus érythémateux disséminé et de la lèpre, *Ann. Immunol.* **132:**287–305.

Menzel, J., Steffen, C., Kolarz, G., Kojer, M., and Smolen, J., 1978, Demonstration of anticollagen antibodies in rheumatoid arthritis synovial fluids by ^{14}C-radioimmunoassay, *Arthritis Rheum.* **21:**243–248.

Michaeli, D., and Fudenberg, H. H., 1974a, Antibodies to collagen in patients with emphysema, *Clin. Immunol. Immunopathol.* **3:**187–192.

Michaeli, D., and Fudenberg, H. H., 1974b, The incidence and antigenic specificity of antibodies against denatured human collagen in rheumatoid arthritis, *Clin. Immunol. Immunopathol.* **2:**153–159.
Michaeli, D., Martin, G. R., Kettman, J., Benjamini, E., Leung, D. V. K., and Blatt, B. A., 1969, Localization of antigenic determinants in the polypeptide chains of collagen, *Science* **166:**1522–1524.
Michaeli, D., Senyk, G., Maoz, A., and Fuchs, S., 1972, Ascaris cuticle collagen and mammalian collagens: Cell mediated and humoral immunity relationships, *J. Immunol.* **109:**103–109.
Miller, E. J., 1971a, Isolation and characterization of a collagen from chick cartilage containing 3 identical α chains, *Biochemistry* **10:**1652–1659.
Miller, E. J., 1971b, Isolation and characterization of the CNBr-peptides from α1(II) chains of chick cartilage collagen, *Biochemistry* **10:**3030–3035.
Miller, E. J., 1973, A review of biochemical studies on the genetically distinct collagens of the skeletal system, *Clin. Orthop.* **92:**260–280.
Miller, E. J., 1976, Biochemical characteristics and biological significance of the genetically-distinct collagens, *Mol. Cell. Biochem.* **13:**165–192.
Miller, E. J., and Matukas, V. J., 1969, Chick cartilage collagen: A new type of α1 chain not present in bone or skin of the species, *Proc. Natl. Acad. Sci. U.S.A.* **64:**1264–1268.
Mohr, W., Wild, A., and Paulini, K., 1975, Proliferation of synovial tissue cells in rats with adjuvant disease, *Pathol. Microbiol. (Basel)* **43:**1–9.
Morgan, K., Clague, R. B., Shaw, M. J., and Holt, P. J. L., 1980, Native type II collagen-induced arthritis in the rat: I. Incidence and humoral response to collagen, *Ann. Rheum. Dis.* **39:**285–290.
Morgan, K., Clague, R. B., Shaw, M.J., Firth, S. A., Twose, T. M., and Lennox Holt, P. J., 1981, Native type II collagen-induced arthritis in the rat: The effect of complement depletion by cobra venom factor, *Arthritis Rheum.* **24:**1356–1362.
Nimni, M. E., 1974, Collagen: Its structure and function in normal and pathological connective tissues, *Semin. Arthritis Rheum.* **4:**95–150.
Nowack, H., Hahn, E., and Timpl, R., 1974, Specificity of the antibody response in inbred mice to bovine type I and type II collagen, *Immunology* **29:**621–628.
Ofosu-Appiah, W. A., Morgan, K., and Lennox Holt, P. J., 1983, Native type II collagen-induced arthritis in the rat. III. Relationship between the cellular immune response to native type II collagen and arthritis, *Ann. Rheum. Dis.* **42:**331–337.
Paulus, H. E., Machleder, H. I., Levine, S., Yu, D. T. Y., and MacDonald, N. S., 1977, Lymphocyte involvement in rheumatoid arthritis: Studies during thoracic duct drainage, *Arthritis Rheum.* **20:**1249–1262.
Pearson, C. M., and Wood, F. D., 1963, Studies of arthritis and other lesions induced in rats by the injection of mycobacterial adjuvant. VII. Pathologic details of the arthritis and spondylitis, *Am. J. Pathol.* **42:**73–86.
Pearson, C. M., and Wood, F. D., 1964, Passive transfer of adjuvant arthritis by lymph node or spleen cells, *J. Exp. Med.* **120:**547–560.
Pekin, Jr., T. J., and Zvaifler, N. J., 1964, Hemolytic complement in synovial fluid, *J. Clin. Invest.* **43:**1372–1382.
Person, D. A., and Sharp, J. T., 1976, The etiology of rheumatoid arthritis, *Bull. Rheum. Dis.* **27:**888–893.
Prickett, J. D., Trentham, D. E., and Robinson, D. R., 1984, Dietary fish oil augments the induction of arthritis in rats immunized with type II collagen, *J. Immunol.* **132:**725–729.
Prockop, D. J., Kivirikko, K. I., Tuderman, L., and Guzman, N. A., 1979, The biosynthesis of collagen and its disorders, *N. Engl. J. Med.* **301:**13–23, 77–85.
Rogers, M. P., Trentham, D. E., McCune, W. J., Ginsberg, B. I., Rennke, H. G., Reich, P., and David, J. R., 1980, Effect of psychological stress on the induction of arthritis in rats, *Arthritis Rheum.* **23:**1337–1342.
Rogers, M. P., Trentham, D. E., Dynesius-Trentham, R., Daffner, K., and Reich, P., 1983, Exacerbation of collagen arthritis by noise stress, *J. Rheumatol.* **10:**651–654.
Rosenwasser, L. J., Bhatnagar, R. S., and Stobo, J. D., 1980, Genetic control of the murine T lymphocyte proliferative response to collagen: Analysis of the molecular and cellular contributions to immunogenicity, *J. Immunol.* **124:**2854–2859.
Salant, D. J., Belok, S., Madaio, M. P., and Couser, W. G., 1980, A new role for complement in experimental membranous nephropathy in rats, *J. Clin. Invest.* **66:**1339–1350.
Schmitt, F. O., Levine, L., Drake, M. P., Rubin, A. L., Pfahl, D., and Davidson, P. F., 1964, The antigenicity of tropocollagen, *Proc. Natl. Acad. Sci. U.S.A.* **51:**493–497.
Schoen, R. T., and Trentham, D. E., 1981, Drug-induced lupus: An adjuvant disease? *Am. J. Med.* **71:**5–8.
Schoen, R. T., Mehlman, H., Trentham, D. E., Perry, L., Greene, M. I., and David, J. R., 1981, Autoimmunity induced by type II collagen-coupled spleen cells, *J. Immunol.* **127:**2275–2279.

Schoen, R. T., Greene, M. I., and Trentham, D. E., 1982, Antigen-specific suppression of type II collagen-induced arthritis by collagen-coupled spleen cells, *J. Immunol.* **128:**717–719.

Schrier, D. J., Phan, S. H., and Ward, P. A., 1982, Cellular sensitivity to collagen in bleomycin-treated rats, *J. Immunol.* **129:**2156–2159.

Schumacher, H. R., and Kitridou, R. C., 1972, Synovitis of recent onset: A clinicopathologic study during the first month of disease, *Arthritis Rheum.* **15:**465–485.

Senyk, G., and Michaeli, D., 1973, Induction of cell-mediated immunity and tolerance to homologous collagen in guinea pigs: Demonstration of antigen-reactive cells for a self-antigen, *J. Immunol.* **111:**1381–1388.

Seraffini-Fracassini, A., and Smith, J. W. (eds), 1974, Collagen, in: *The Structure and Biochemistry of Cartilage,* Churchill, Livingston, Edinburgh, pp. 29–63.

Seyer, J. M., Hutcheson, E. T., and Kang, A. H., 1976, Collagen polymorphism in idiopathic chronic pulmonary fibrosis, *J. Clin. Invest.* **57:**1498–1507.

Seyer, J. M., Kang, A. H., and Whitaker, J. N., 1977a, The characterization of type I and type III collagens from human peripheral nerve, *Biochim. Biophys. Acta* **492:**415–425.

Seyer, J. M., Hutcheson, E. T., and Kang, A. H., 1977b, Collagen polymorphism in normal and cirrhotic human liver, *J. Clin. Invest.* **59:**241–248.

Sloboda, A. E., Birnbaum, J. E., Oronsky, A. L., and Kerwar, S. S., 1981, Studies on type II collagen-induced polyarthritis in rats: Effect of antiinflammatory and antirheumatic agents, *Arthritis Rheum.* **24:**616–624.

Smolen, J. S., Menzel, E. J., Scherak, O., Kojer, M., Kolarz, G., Steffen, C., and Mayr, W. R., 1980, Lymphocyte transformation to denatured type I collagen and B lymphocyte alloantigens in rheumatoid arthritis, *Arthritis Rheum.* **23:**424–432.

Solinger, A. M., and Stobo, J. D., 1982, Immune response gene control of collagen reactivity in man: Collagen unresponsiveness in HLA-DR4 negative nonresponders is due to the presence of T-dependent suppressive influences, *J. Immunmol.* **129:**1916–1920.

Solinger, A. M., Bhatnagar, R., and Stobo, J. D., 1981, Cellular, molecular, and genetic characteristics of T cell reactivity to collagen in man, *Proc. Natl. Acad. Sci. U.S.A.* **78:**3877–3881.

Staines, N. A., Hardingham, T., Smith, M., and Henderson, B., 1981, Collagen-induced arthritis in the rat: Modification of immune and arthritic responses by free collagen and immune anti-collagen antiserum, *Immunology* **44:**737–744.

Stasny, P., Rosenthal, M., Andreis, M., Cooke, D., and Ziff, M., 1975, Lymphokines in rheumatoid synovitis, *Ann. N.Y. Acad. Sci.* **256:**117–131.

Steffen, C., 1969, Tissue antibodies in rheumatoid arthritis and other connective tissue diseases, *Ann. Immunol.* **1:**47–58.

Steffen, C., 1970, Consideration of the pathogenesis of rheumatoid arthritis as collagen autoimmunity, *Z. Immunitätsforsch.* **139:**219–227.

Steffen, C., and Timpl, R., 1963, Antigenicity of collagen and its application in the serologic investigation of rheumatoid arthritis sera, *Int. Arch. Allergy Appl. Immunol.* **22:**333–349.

Steffen, C., and Wick, G., 1971, Delayed hypersensitivity reactions to collagen in rats with adjuvant-induced arthritis, *Z. Immunitätsforsch.* **141:**169–180.

Steffen, C., Schuster, F., Tausch, G., Timpl, R., and Pecker, I., 1968, Weitere Untersuchungen über Kollagenantikörper bei Patienten mit primär chronischer Polyarthritis, *Klin. Wochenschr.* **46:**976–981.

Steffen, C., Carmann, H., Tausch, G., Bosch, J., and Freilinger, G., 1971, Untersuchungen uber die Autoantikorpereigenschaft von Kollagen-Antikörpern und ihre Patienten mit rheumatoider Arthritis, *Z. Rheumaforsch.* **30:**92–97.

Steffen, C., Knapp, W., Thumb, N., Schuster, F., Bosch, J., Brunner, H., and Eibl, M., 1972, Demonstration of collagen in synovial fluid cells of rheumatoid arthritis by immunofluorescence, *Z. Immunitätsforsch.* **143:**252–263.

Steffen, C., Ludwig, H., Thumb, N., Frank, O., Ebert, R., and Tausch, G., 1973, Demonstration of antibodies with different specificity for collagen in rheumatoid arthritis and comparison of human and calf collagen as test antigen, *Klin. Wochenschr.* **51:**222–229.

Steffen, C., Ludwig, H., and Knapp, W., 1974, Collagen-anticollagn immune complexes in rheumatoid arthritis synovial fluid cells, *Z. Immunitätsforsch.* **147:**229–235.

Steffen, C., Ludwig, H., Kovac, W., and Menzel, J., 1975, Collagen-induced acute synovitis in collagen-immunized rabbits, *Z. Immunitätsforsch.* **150:**432–446.

Steffen, C., Kovac, W., Endler, T. A., Menzel, J., and Smolen, J., 1977, Induction of acute and chronic arthritis by intraarticular injection of preformed collagen-anticollagen complexes, *Immunology* **32:**161–170.

Strober, S., Slavin, S., and Gottlieb, M., 1979, Allograft tolerance after total lymphoid irradiation (TLI), *Immunol. Rev.* **46**:87–112.

Stuart, J. M., and Dixon, F. J., 1983, Serum transfer of collagen-induced arthritis in mice, *J. Exp. Med.* **158**:378–392.

Stuart, J. M., Postlethwaite, A. E., and Kang, A. H., 1976, Evidence for cell-mediated immunity to collagen in progressive systemic sclerosis, *J. Lab. Clin. Med.* **88**:601–607.

Stuart, J. M., Cremer, M. A., Dixit, S. N., Kang, A. H., and Townes, A. S., 1979a, Collagen-induced arthritis in rats: Comparison of vitreous and cartilage derived collagens, *Arthritis Rheum.* **22**:347–352.

Stuart, J. M., Cremer, M. A., Kang, A. H., and Townes, A. S., 1979b, Collagen-induced arthritis in rats: Evaluation of early immunologic events, *Arthritis Rheum.* **22**:1344–1351.

Stuart, J. M., Postlethwaite, A. E., Kang, A. H., and Townes, A. S., 1980, Cell-mediated immunity to collagen in rheumatoid arthritis and other rheumatic diseases, *Am. J. Med.* **69**:13–18.

Stuart, J. M., Myers, L. K., Townes, A. S., and Kang, A. H., 1981, Effect of cyclophosphamide, hydrocortisone, and levamisole on collagen-induced arthritis in rats, *Arthritis Rheum.* **24**:790–794.

Stuart, J. M., Townes, A. S., and Kang, A. H., 1982a, The role of collagen autoimmunity in animal models and human diseases, *J. Invest. Dermatol.* **79**(Suppl):121S–127S.

Stuart, J. M., Bandy, P. R., Townes, A. S., and Pinals, R. S., 1982b, Failure of calcitonin to inhibit collagen-induced arthritis in rats, *Agents Actions* **12**:671–673.

Stuart, J. M., Townes, A. S., and Kang, A. H., 1982c, Nature and specificity of the immune response to collagen in type II collagen-induced arthritis in mice, *J. Clin. Invest.* **69**:673–683.

Stuart, J. M., Cremer, M. A., Townes, A. S., and Kang, A. H., 1982d, Type II collagen-induced arthritis in rats: Passive transfer with serum and evidence that IgG anticollagen antibodies can cause arthritis, *J. Exp. Med.* **155**:1–16.

Stuart, J. M., Tomoda, K., Yoo, T. J., Townes, A. S., and Kang, A. H., 1983a, Serum transfer of collagen-induced arthritis. II. Identification and localization of autoantibody to type II collagen in donor and recipient rats, *Arthritis Rheum.* **26**:1237–1244.

Stuart, J. M., Huffstutter, E. H., Townes, A. S., and Kang, A. H., 1983b, Incidence and specificity of antibodies to types I, II, IV and V collagen in rheumatoid arthritis and other rheumatic diseases as measured by ^{125}I-radioimmunoassay, *Arthritis Rheum.* **26**:832–840.

Suou, T., and Hirayama, C., 1980, Antibodies to denatured bovine collagens in sera of patients with liver disease, *Clin. Exp. Immunol.* **39**:119–124.

Taurog, J. D., Sandberg, G. P., and Mahowald, M.L., 1983, The cellular basis of adjuvant arthritis. II. Characterization of the cells mediating passive transfer, *Cell. Immunol.* **80**:198–204.

Traub, W., and Piez, K. A., 1971, The chemistry and structure of collagen, *Adv. Protein Chem.* **25**:243–352.

Trelstad, R. L., 1974, Human aorta collagens: Evidence for three distinct species, *Biochem. Biophys. Res. Commun.* **57**:717–725.

Trelstad, R. L., Kang, A. H., Igarashi, S., and Gross, J., 1970, Isolation of two distinct collagens from chick cartilage, *Biochemistry* **9**:4993–4998.

Trentham, D. E., 1981, Autoimmunity to collagen as a disease mechanism, in: *Advances in Inflammation Research,* Vol. II (G. Weissmann, ed.), Raven Press, New York, pp. 149–164.

Trentham, D. E., 1982a, Collagen arthritis as a relevant model for rheumatoid arthritis: Evidence pro and con, *Arthritis Rheum.* **25**:911–916.

Trentham, D. E., 1982b, Case records of the Massachusetts General Hospital, *N. Engl. J. Med.* **307**:1631–1639.

Trentham, D. E., 1983, Immunity to collagen in rheumatoid and experimental arthritis, in: *Clinical Immunology Update* (E. C. Franklin, ed.), North-Holland/American Elsevier, New York, pp. 37–55.

Trentham, D. E., 1984a, Immunity to type II collagen in rheumatoid arthritis: A current appraisal, *Proc. Soc. Exp. Biol. Med.* **176**:95–104.

Trentham, D. E., 1984b, Strategies for medical treatment based on current understanding of the pathogenesis of rheumatoid arthritis, *Clin. Orthop.* **182**:31–36.

Trentham, D. E., and Brinckerhoff, C. E., 1982, Augmentation of collagen arthritis by synthetic analogues of retinoic acid, *J. Immunol.* **129**:2668–2672.

Trentham, D. E., and Dynesius-Trentham, R. A., 1983, Attenuation of an adjuvant arthritis by type II collagen, *J. Immunol.* **130**:2689–2692.

Trentham, D. E., and Rowland, D., 1983, Dimethyl sulfoxide does not suppress the clinical manifestations of collagen arthritis, *J. Rheumatol.* **10**:114–116.

Trentham, D. E., Townes, A. S., and Kang, A. H., 1977, Autoimmunity to type II collagen: An experimental model of arthritis, *J. Exp. Med.* **146**:857–868.

Trentham, D. E., Townes, A. S., Kang, A. H., and David, J. R., 1978a, Humoral and cellular sensitivity to collagen in type II collagen-induced arthritis in rats, *J. Clin. Invest.* **61**:89–96.

Trentham, D. E., Dynesius, R. A., and David, J. R., 1978b, Passive transfer by cells of type II collagen-induced arthritis in rats, *J. Clin. Invest.* **62**:359–366.

Trentham, D. E., Dynesius, R. A., Rocklin, R. E., and David, J. R., 1978c, Cellular sensitivity to collagen in rheumatoid arthritis, *N. Engl. J. Med.* **299**:327–332.

Trentham, D. E., McCune, W.J., Susman, P., and David, J. R., 1980, Autoimmunity to collagen in adjuvant arthritis of rats, *J. Clin. Invest.* **66**:1109–1117.

Trentham, D. E., Belli, J. A., Anderson, R. J., Buckley, J. A., Goetzl, E. J., David, J. R., and Austen, K. F., 1981a, Clinical and immunologic effects of fractionated total lymphoid irradiation in refractory rheumatoid arthritis, *N. Engl. J. Med.* **305**:976–982.

Trentham, D. E., Kammer, G. M., McCune, W. J., and David, J. R., 1981b, Autoimmunity to collagen: A shared feature of psoriatic and rheumatoid arthritis, *Arthritis Rheum.* **24**:1363–1369.

Trentham, D. E., Brahn, E., Williams, W., McCune, W. J., and Belli, J. A., 1984, Connective tissue disease can develop in rats either spontaneously or after total lymphoid irradiation, *J. Rheumatol.* **11**:410–412.

Tung, K. S. K., Unanue, E. R., and Dixon, F. J., 1971a, Pathogenesis of experimental allergic orchitis. I. Transfer with immune lymph node cells, *J. Immunol.* **106**:1453–1462.

Tung, K. S. K., Unanue, E. R., and Dixon, F. J., 1971b, Pathogenesis of experimental allergic orchitis. II. The role of antibody, *J. Immunol.* **106**:1463–1472.

Van Boxel, J. A., and Paget, S. A., 1975, Predominantly T-cell infiltrate in rheumatoid synovial membranes, *N. Engl. J. Med.* **293**:517–520.

Wahl, S. M., Wilder, R. L., Katona, I. M., Wahl, L. M., Allen, J. B., Scher, I., and Decker, J. L., 1983, Leukapheresis in rheumatoid arthritis: Association of clinical improvement with reversal of anergy, *Arthritis Rheum.* **26**:1076–1084.

Waksman, B. H., and Mason, H. L., 1949, The antigenicity of collagen, *J. Immunol.* **63**:427–433.

Waksman, B. H., and Wennersten, C., 1963, Passive transfer of adjuvant arthritis in rats with living lymphoid cells of sensitized donors, *Int. Arch. Allergy Appl. Immunol.* **23**:129–139.

Weiss, J. B., Shuttleworth, C. A., and Brown, R., 1975, Occurrence of type III collagen in inflammed synovial membrane. A comparison between nonrheumatoid, rheumatoid and normal synovial collagens, *Biochem. Biophys. Res. Commun.* **65**:907–912.

Welles, W. L., and Battisto, J. R., 1981, Suppression of adjuvant arthritis by antibodies specific for collagen type II, *Immunol. Commun.* **10**:673–685.

Wooley, P. H., Luthra, H. S., Stuart, J. M., and David, C. S., 1981, Type II collagen-induced arthritis in mice. I. Major histocompatibility complex (I region) linkage and antibody correlates, *J. Exp. Med.* **154**:688–700.

Wooley, P. H., Dillon, A. M., Luthra, H. S., Stuart, J. M., and David, C. S., 1983, Genetic control of type II collagen-induced arthritis in mice: Factors influencing disease susceptibility and evidence for multiple MHC-associated gene control, *Transplant. Proc.* **15**:180–186.

Yoo, T. J., Stuart, J. M., Kang, A. H., Townes, A. S., Tomoda, K., and Dixit, S. N., 1982, Collagen autoimmunity in otosclerosis and Meniere's disease, *Science* **217**:1153–1155.

Yoo, T. J., Tomoda, K., Stuart, J. M., Kang, A. H., and Townes, A. S., 1983a, Type II collagen-induced autoimmune otospongiosis, *Ann. Otol. Rhinol. Laryngol.* **92**:103–108.

Yoo, T. J., Yazawa, Y., Tomoda, K., and Floyd, R., 1983b, Type II collagen-induced autoimmune endolymphatic hydrops in guinea pig, *Science* **222**:65–67.

Zubler, R. H., Nydegger, U., Perrin, L. H., Fehr, K., McCormick, J., Lambert, P. H., and Miescher, P. A., 1976, Circulating and intraarticular immune complexes in patients with rheumatoid arthritis, *J. Clin. Invest.* **57**:1308–1319.

Zvaifler, N. J., 1973, The immunopathology of joint inflammation in rheumatoid arthritis, *Adv. Immunol.* **16**:265–336.

III

Classical Concepts of Rheumatic Diseases

13

Immune Response to Streptococcal Antigens in Rheumatic Fever

Ralph C. Williams, Jr.

I. INTRODUCTION

Acute rheumatic fever still represents the one only of the connective tissue disorders in which a basic causative agent has been clearly identified. We know that rheumatoid arthritis is commonly associated with the production of rheumatoid factors and a positive latex fixation test and that systemic lupus erythematosus represents a generalized often severe disease of connective tissues associated with anti-DNA antibodies, but in neither of the two latter disorders has the original inciting agent been defined. By contrast, it has been firmly established that acute rheumatic fever results from prior pharyngeal infection by β-hemolytic group A streptococci and that each subsequent attack is set off by throat reinfection with group A streptococci (Anderson *et al.*, 1948; Wannamaker, 1959).

II. CLINICAL PICTURE

The classic story involves initial streptococcal throat infection followed 2 to 3 weeks later by a true migratory arthritis, fever, acute illness, and chest pain or rapidly progressive dyspnea associated with generalized myocarditis and heart failure. Besides this typical story there are numerous other possible variations in the clinical picture of an acute

---

Ralph C. Williams, Jr. • Department of Medicine, University of New Mexico School of Medicine, Albuquerque, New Mexico 87131.

rheumatic attack. In some instances the initial throat infection may go unrecognized, and the child may appear to his parents to be suffering from rapid onset of coughing and progressive shortness of breath presumed to be a bad cold and possibly pneumonia, but which in fact represents rapidly progressive left ventricular failure associated with a pancarditis usually including mitral and/or aortic valve involvement and dysfunction. An example of massive cardiomegaly in such a patient who presented to the hospital with a 4- to 5-day history of progressive dyspnea is shown in Fig. 1.

In some patients, the only clinical manifestation of rheumatic activity is Sydenham's chorea or St. Vitus dance. This curious disturbance represents a dramatic involuntary movement disorder usually occurring in children or young adults, ages 4–12 years, and considerably more common in females than in males (Lessof, 1958). Chorea as a manifestation of acute rheumatic fever is very uncommon after the age of 20, and, in fact, when chorea occurs in an adult, completely different diagnoses must be considered, including systemic lupus, thyrotoxicosis, or Huntington's disease. Chorea as a clinical manifestation of rheumatic activity may be transient, lasting only a few days or several weeks. On the other hand, severe rheumatic chorea may persist for months and can be extremely disabling for the affected individual, inducing weight loss, irritability, and emotional listlessness or withdrawal along with inability to function at home or in a school situation. It is fair to say that the clinical description of chorea has been very little improved on, if at all, since its initial, very accurate analysis by Sydenham over 200 years ago (Sydenham, 1740). In many instances personally observed by us, a child

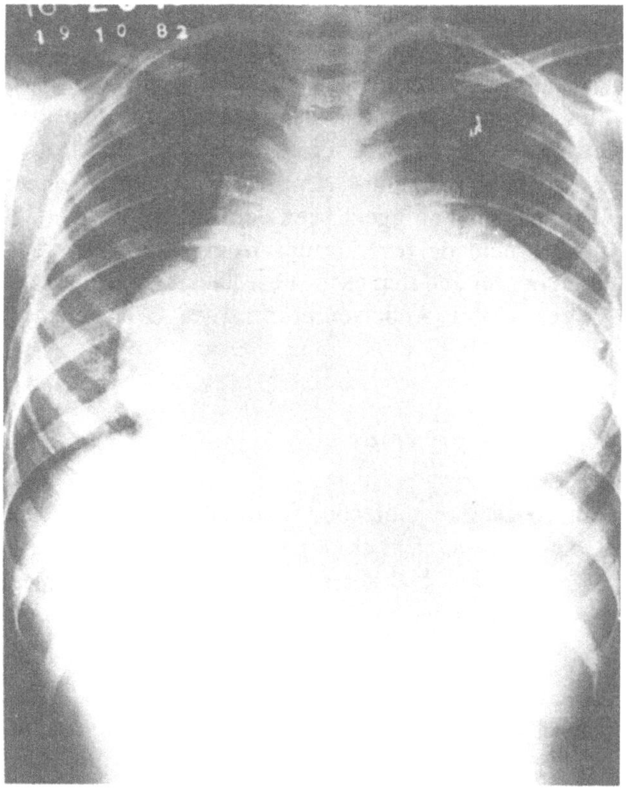

Figure 1. Massive cardiomegaly in a 9-year-old child presenting with a brief history of sore throat followed by fatigue and progressive dyspnea. Clinical signs of left ventricular failure were flagrantly present in this patient with acute rheumatic carditis.

showing severe or repeated bouts of chorea will also manifest soft but definite mitral presystolic or systolic murmurs indicating concurrent rheumatic cardiac activity despite no clinical symptomatic evidence of cardiac involvement. It is interesting to note that chorea rarely occurs in the presence of arthritis in rheumatic fever.

Attacks of acute rheumatic fever in some individuals may appear as mild transitory episodes of polyarthritis or merely arthralgia associated with malaise, low-grade fever, and elevation of erythrocyte sedimentation rate and acute phase reactants such as C-reactive protein (CRP). Again, during these episodes the patient may experience no direct symptoms of cardiac involvement such as chest pain, dyspnea, pleurisy, or shortness of breath on exertion. However, clearly, at the same time there may be very strong clinical evidence for cardiac involvement such as soft mitral diastolic murmurs, minimal cardiac enlargement by fluoroscopy or echocardiographic analysis, soft pericardial friction rubs, or progressive elevations of CRP, with antistreptolysin O/streptokinase or anti-DNase B as evidence of recent group A β-hemolytic streptococcal infection. A number of other variations of this general theme may be encountered as definite clinical presentations of acute rheumatic fever; however, there is one point that for us has proven to be of great clinical usefulness, and that is the general uniformity in pattern of recurrent rheumatic attacks within the same individual patient. Thus, if rheumatic fever occurs in a child of 5 in association with severe or moderate Sydenham's chorea and little else, then it is very likely that all subsequent rheumatic activity will also be associated with chorea. In another individual, if chest pain secondary to acute pericarditis or pancarditis with associated pericarditis is the major initial presenting symptom during a first episode, it is highly likely that this general clinical pattern will run true and will be repeated each time that particular individual suffers a recurrent rheumatic fever attack.

The great variability of the actual presenting clinical picture of acute rheumatic fever has prompted clinicians to adopt the so-called Jones criteria, which are now referred to as the revised Jones criteria (American Heart Association Committee Report, 1965). These general parameters by which the diagnosis of acute rheumatic fever can be substantiated are shown in Table 1. Although the specific items listed often prove extremely useful in assessing the individual patient being considered by the clinician, it is important to point out that the revised Jones criteria represent only a rough, still imperfect guide in establishing a firm diagnosis. For instance, in individual circumstances a child or young adult with systemic lupus, infective endocarditis, or even mixed connective tissue disease

Table 1. Revised Jones Criteria for Diagnosis of Acute Rheumatic Fever[a]

Major manifestations	Minor manifestations
Carditis	Fever
Polyarthritis	Arthralgias
Chorea	Previous rheumatic fever or rheumatic heart disease
Erythema marginatum	Elevated erythrocyte sedimentation rate (ESR) or positive C-reactive protein (CRP)
Subcutaneous nodules	Prolonged PR interval

[a] Plus supporting evidence of preceding streptococcal infection; history of recent scarlet fever; positive throat culture for group A streptococcus; increased ASO titer or other streptococcal antibodies. From Stollerman *et al.* (1965).

may fulfill enough of the Jones criteria to fit a diagnosis of acute rheumatic fever, but, indeed, such a designation may be entirely inappropriate. For this reason, great care must be exercised in application and interpretation of the Jones criteria in individual patients. We have found these criteria most deficient in evaluating patients with low-grade recurrences of acute rheumatic activity. Considerably more effort and reappraisal are now needed to strengthen these criteria and help clinicians with their practical application. This particular problem becomes even more difficult when patients experience recurrences of previous rheumatic activity during the course of subacute or occasionally extended courses of immunosuppressive therapy with corticosteroids.

III. PREVALENCE OF RHEUMATIC FEVER

At the present time it is the general consensus that the incidence of acute rheumatic fever has declined substantially within the populations of North America (Canada and the United States) as well as Europe, particularly during the last three or four decades (DiSciascio and Taranta, 1980; Strasser, 1978; Rosenstein, 1973; Hassell and Stuart, 1974). The decline in prevalence has been attributed to a more widespread, even sometimes indiscriminate use of antibiotics, better sanitary and housing conditions for relatively large segments of the population, or possibly to changes in the relative rheumatogenicity or rheumatic-fever-inducing potential of various strains of group A streptococci within various populations. Of interest, however, is the actual fact that sequential studies of the prevalence of acute rheumatic fever in the United States have indicated that the actual decline in new cases had started to occur before widescale introduction of antibiotics, so that more ready availability of antimicrobials seems an unlikely explanation for the distinct decline in incidence and prevalence of new cases of rheumatic fever seen in countries such as the United States or Canada.

There are at present no reproducible test systems or criteria by which various strain isolates of group A streptococci can be clearly identified as those prone to be associated with subsequent development of acute rheumatic fever as poststreptococcal sequelae. There are some indications, however, that M types 5, 18, 19, and 24 may frequently be isolated from individual patients with acute rheumatic activity. This stands in contrast to the situation regarding acute poststreptococcal glomerulonephritis, where certain repeatedly isolated strains such as type 6 or type 12 appear to have relatively strong nephritogenic potential. Studies by Villarreal *et al.* (1980) have actually identified an immunochemical marker that may be directly related to the nephritogenic potential of various group A streptococcal isolates. No such identifiable marker for rheumatic-fever-inducing potential is yet available for group A typing, and all discussion of relative rheumatogenicity among various group A isolates is merely speculation, though certainly the M types mentioned above (5, 18, 19, and 24) are frequently isolated in individual instances.

In contrast to the apparent decline in prevalence of new cases of acute rheumatic fever in North America, Europe, and Japan (Lue *et al.*, 1975, 1979; Kawakita *et al.*, 1976), the disorder still represents a serious health problem in many parts of the world, particularly in so-called Third-World countries such as Egypt, other parts of the Middle East, India, Southeast Asia, the Philippines, parts of Central and South America, as well as many populations living on islands in the Caribbean (Strasser, 1978; Shaper, 1972;

Shrestha and Padmavati, 1979; Abdin and Eissa, 1965; Berry, 1972; Potter *et al.*, 1978; Dharmasakti and Hanafiah, 1979). In India alone, it is estimated that there are six to eight million children during any one year who either experience an acute rheumatic fever attack or who already have established rheumatic heart disease. At the present time there is very little clear understanding of why underdeveloped areas of the world, particularly many that have high average ambient temperatures, still represent high prevalance areas for acute rheumatic fever activity. From a logistic standpoint, the human disability and long-term morbidity of rheumatic fever and subsequent chronic, progressive rheumatic heart disease still constitute a major health problem for many underdeveloped countries and, consequently, a large proportion of the world population.

IV. THE PROCESS OF STREPTOCOCCAL SENSITIZATION AND SUBSEQUENT ACUTE RHEUMATIC FEVER ITSELF

If one focuses on the actual process that eventually generates an attack of acute rheumatic fever, one must start in the pharynx of the affected child (Catanzaro *et al.*, 1958; Wannamaker, 1976). In most countries or well-delimited populations where prevalence has been carefully and reliably documented, the peak age at which the very first or primary attack of acute rheumatic fever occurs appears to be between ages 4 and 6. One of the striking findings, particularly when prevalence studies are conducted in underdeveloped countries, is the young age at which some children are affected. The syndrome of juvenile mitral stenosis is still frequently seen in India, Thailand, and areas such as Khartoum or Pakistan (Ayuthya *et al.*, 1976; D'Arbela *et al.*, 1976). The disorder is slightly more common in female children, particularly if rheumatic chorea is present as a major presenting manifestation of the acute attack (Taranta and Stollerman, 1956; Lessof, 1958).

A great deal of study has been directed at what actually happens in the pharynx and tonsils that allows active, invasive streptococcal infection and not merely colonization (E. L. Kaplan *et al.*, 1971; Tompkins *et al.*, 1977). The subsequent acute rheumatic fever attack clearly has to proceed after some sort of sensitizing immunologic process that begins in the pharynx. Many children with acute rheumatic fever can be shown to have concurrent streptococcal pyoderma, but streptococcal skin infection alone virtually never induces subsequent acute rheumatic fever (Potter *et al.*, 1972). Indeed, streptococcal pyoderma is often associated in a direct causal way with subsequent acute poststreptococcal glomerulonephritis (Potter *et al.*, 1972; Stollerman, 1971; Poon-King *et al.*, 1973). Also of interest is the clinical fact that a given initial group A streptococcal infection rarely if ever produces both acute rheumatic fever and poststreptococcal acute glomerulonephritis in the same patient at the same time (Bisno *et al.*, 1970). These two well-known poststreptococcal sequelae therefore appear to be mutualy exclusive. Whether this curious exclusion is somehow related to genetic factors operating in the susceptible host or to something about the sensitizing bacteria is not yet understood.

Since acute rheumatic fever follows pharyngeal group A streptococcal infection, there have been a number of studies that have attempted to examine what role, if any, the oral or pharyngeal secretions have in allowing the whole process to become activated (Wannamaker, 1973). If secretory IgA or other specific components of the secretory immunoglobulin system were somehow defective or overly permissive of group A β-hemolytic streptococcal infection, it would perhaps afford an excellent explanation or hypothesis as to precisely how the whole process is initiated. Thur far, studies of specific or generalized secretory IgA responses in both pharyngeal and serum samples obtained from children and young adults have not supported any well-documented secretory IgA defect (Svartman *et al.*, 1975a). This particular line of investigation, however, needs to be considerably extended.

During the last decade a number of salient observations have been made that relate specific adherence properties of various bacteria to their pathogenic potential. In particular, this has proven to be directly correlated in infective endocarditis, where the relative adherence of various bacterial strains isolated from blood cultures appears to be highly correlated with ability to infect heart valves or other endocardial surfaces (Gibbons and van Houte, 1971; Sheld *et al.*, 1978).

Our own studies of the potential importance of bacterial adherence to the initial pharyngeal colonization and subsequent infection with respect to group A streptococci and rheumatic heart disease (Selinger *et al.*, 1978; Reed *et al.*, 1980) have shown an interesting and as yet unexplained predilection for much higher adherence of group A strains isolated from subjects during acute rheumatic episodes to pharyngeal cells actually obtained from rheumatic patients as compared to normal, nonrheumatic controls.

An example of this interesting difference in adherence or actual stickiness between the bacterial surface and the pharyngeal epithelial cell surfaces is shown in Fig. 2. No clear understanding of these interesting preliminary observations has yet been found, but this particular area of work has great potential importance in explaining how the initial pharyngeal implantation may occur. From a clinical standpoint, the difference between mere colonization and actual significant infection of the pharynx in an individual subject appears to be whether or not a significant protective immune response occurs within the affected individual. This response is usually measured in terms of titers of antibodies to streptococcal products such as streptolysin O or DNase B. The response to these two latter streptococcal products appears to be the most relable one for clinical assessment; these serologic procedures have been standardized through WHO reference laboratories throughout the world and are available in many underdeveloped countries where streptococcal infection and sequelae still represent a serious health problem.

The general area of host–organism interaction has been repeatedly examined in currently ongoing and extensive previous epidemiologic studies of the rate of carriage and frequency of isolates of group A streptococci (Stollerman, 1960; Gordis *et al.*, 1969). If substantial numbers of individuals at risk, for instance, within a certain segment of school children, are repeatedly sampled on a monthly basis by routine throat culture, it is surprising that 4–5% of several thousand such children in parts of the world endemic for acute rheumatic fever such as Cairo or New Delhi show pharyngeal presence of group A streptococci, often without obvious clinical signs of sore throat, fever, or grossly purulent exudate (Stollerman, *et al.*, 1955; Wood *et al.*, 1964; Padmavati, 1978). Among many such populations studied, the prevalence of positive throat cultures clearly varies to some extent with the season and in general appears to be somewhat higher (6–7%) during the winter or rainy portions of the year.

Since 4–7% of routinely sampled school children presumably at risk show positive throat culture isolates for group A streptococci but only a small fraction (estimated at 0.1–0.2%) of these same children actually go on to develop serious poststreptococcal

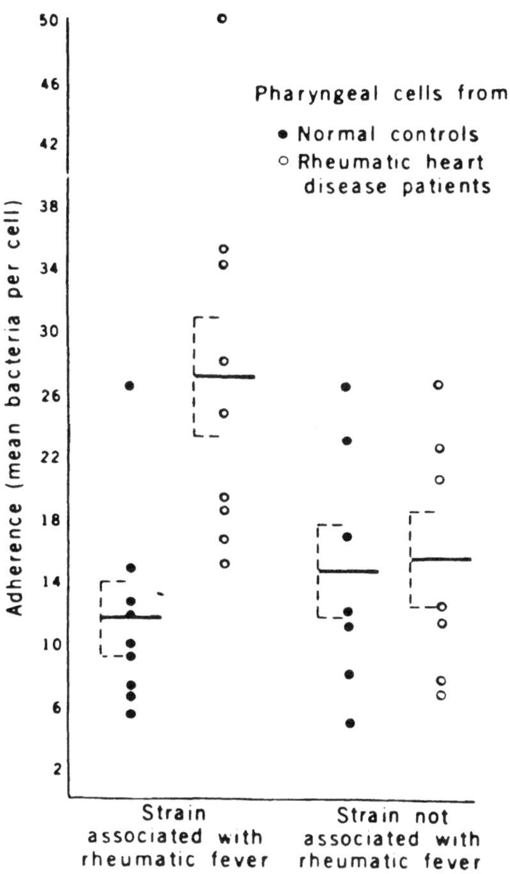

Figure 2. Comparison of adherence of pharyngeal cells taken from rheumatic heart disease (RHD) patients and age- and sex-matched controls. There is increased adherence of pharyngeal cells from RHD patients when a rheumatic-fever-associated strain of streptococcus is used, but no difference in adherence when a control streptococcal strain is used. Horizontal bars indicate means. Standard error of the mean is indicated by dashed lines. (Reproduced with permission from Selinger *et al.*, 1978.)

sequelae such as acute rheumatic fever, it is obvious that there must be important features of the host–bacterium interface that select or somehow predispose certain individuals to develop an abnormal or exaggerated response, in this case, rheumatic fever. Whether the selective predisposing factors are genetic, possibly related to the phenomenon of bacterial stickiness/adherence, to various properties of the secretory IgA and pharyngeal salivary secretions, or to other as yet poorly defined variables, has not yet been determined. In addition, attention has also been directed at the characteristics of streptococcal infections that fail to cause recurrences of rheumatic fever, particularly in carefully studied U.S. populations (Bisno *et al.*, 1977). In these recent surveys, decreases in virulent organisms as measured by opacity factor production and a higher proportion of so-called skin serotypes were recorded.

Perhaps the most compelling single piece of evidence that the complex clinical picture that we see as an attack of acute rheumatic fever represents some sort of immunologic response to streptococcal infection lies in the so-called latent interval. In clinical experience, there is virtually no exception to the rule— patients show a relatively clinically silent period of between 14 and 21 days after throat infection before clinical symptomatology begins. At times in the case of recurrences of rheumatic fever, the interval between pharyngeal infection and manifestations of rheumatic activity may occasionally be shorter

(7–10 days), again suggesting the type of hastened activation of the immune system that might be expected in an anamnestic response. Clinical and serologic studies of patients suffering from bouts of rheumatic chorea suggest that the interval of time between streptococcal exposure and initial onset of the movement disorder may be considerably longer (4–6 weeks) (Taranta and Stollerman, 1956), for reasons that are not yet clearly understood.

In many early studies that focused primarily on the height and intensity of various phases of the humoral immune response, it was repeatedly demonstrated that patients with acute rheumatic fever developed much higher antibody levels to various streptococcal antigens than did those of controls (Stollerman *et al.*, 1956). Because of this rather consistent finding, rising or high titers of antistreptococcal antibodies (such as antistreptolysin O or anti-DNase B) are actually used as a reliable parameter in the diagnosis as, for instance, in the application of the modified Jones criteria.

V. PATHOLOGICAL CHANGES NOTED IN ASSOCIATION WITH RHEUMATIC FEVER

Patients with acute rheumatic fever show many florid signs of a generalized inflammatory process involving widely distributed areas of the connective tissue. The acute synovitis associated with transient, usually truly migratory arthritis may produce considerable swelling and volume of detectable synovial fluid. There are very few detailed descriptions of actual inflammatory histological alterations in the locally inflamed rheumatic synovium; however, studies of synovial fluid obtained during acute inflammatory episodes show individual complement component profiles compatible with local *in vivo* immune complex activation and subsequent potentiation of the inflammatory process (Svartman *et al.*, 1975b).

Cardiac involvement in general takes the form of a pancarditis with pericardium, myocardium, and endocardial surfaces sharing equal uniform inflammatory foci. Pericardial involvement may be extensive and is often associated clinically with prolonged or intermittent chest pain and pericardial effusions. Studies of the immunopathology of rheumatic pericarditis by Persellin *et al.* (1982), showed extensive deposition of IgG, IgM, and C3 on the pericardial surface and within the walls of pericardial blood vessels. Examples of these findings are shown in Fig. 3. Pericarditis is one of the major manifestations of acute rheumatic fever, and its presence is nearly universally seen at autopsy in cases of fatal rheumatic carditis (Friedberg and Gross, 1936). Rheumatic pericarditis is usually associated with myocarditis and bears a worse prognosis when associated with pericardial effusion (Ash, 1942; Thomas *et al.*, 1956).

The hallmark of acute rheumatic fever, of course, is the myocarditis and generalized myocardial involvement. Scattered focal areas of mononuclear cellular infiltration, often in close association with arterioles, are noted throughout the ventricular myocardium. An example of typical myocardial involvement is shown in Fig. 4. These areas often progress to show so-called Aschoff bodies or local collections of lymphocytes, monocytes, and macrophagelike cells, which are associated with a characteristic histological picture (Fig. 5). The precise relationship of Aschoff bodies to the acute rheumatic process has been the subject of considerable debate.

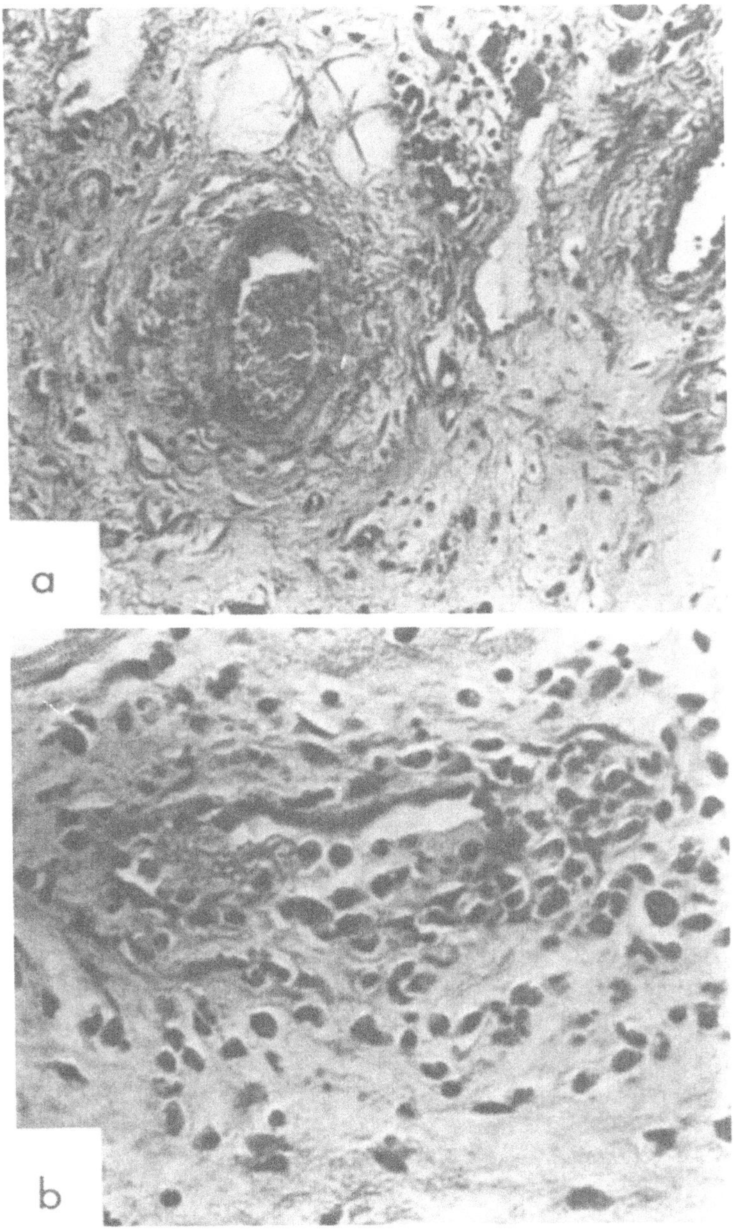

Figure 3. Histological picture of acute rheumatic pericarditis showing (a) blood vessel almost completely occluded with a thrombus in the wall of the pericardium. The interstitial tissues are edematous and scantily infiltrated by inflammatory cells (× 750). b shows blood vessel with focal wall destruction and infiltration with neutrophils, plasma cells, and monocytes, (× 750). c shows strong diffuse reaction with antifibrinogen antibody of inflamed pericardial tissues (× 750). d illustrates deposition of C3 in coarse granular form in the wall of a blood vessel (× 750). (Reproduced with permission from Persellin *et al.*, 1982.)

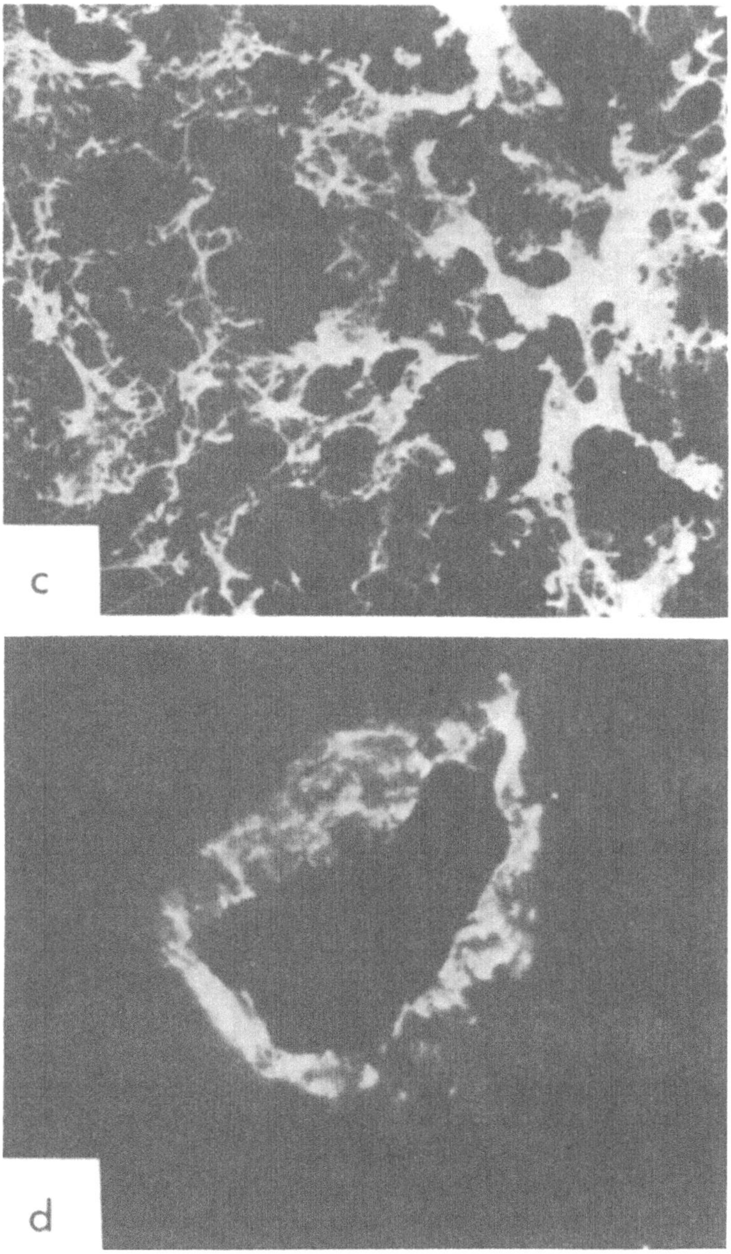

Figure 3. (*continued*)

Certainly, these pathological changes appear to be unique to rheumatic fever and are not seen during the course of viral myocarditis or Chagas' disease. Several decades ago, during the early days of modern cardiac surgery, atrial appendages removed incidental to closed valvulotomy or valvuloplasty often showed numerous Aschoff bodies in the absence of concurrent clinical acute rheumatic activity. The precise relationship between

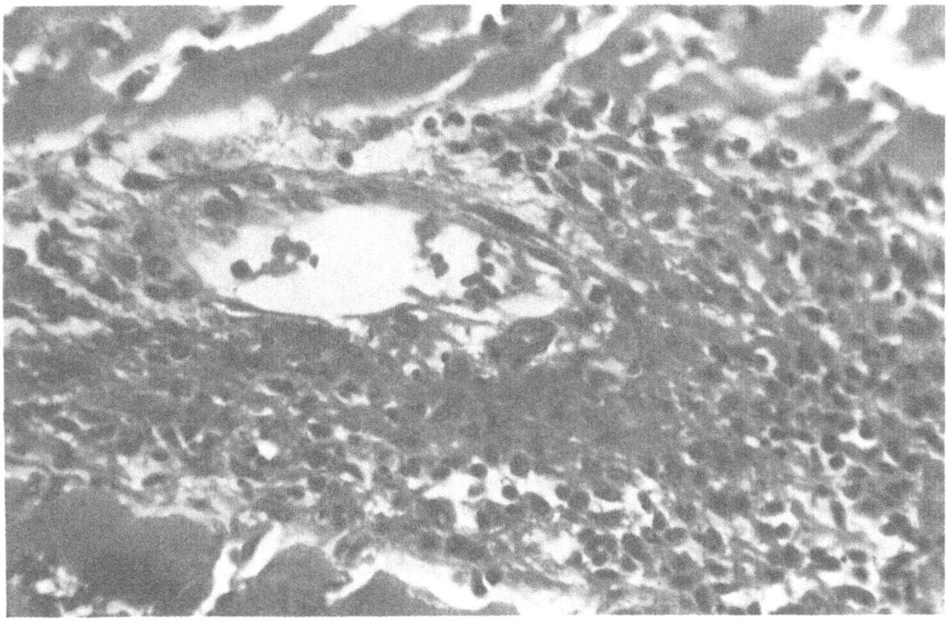

Figure 4. Typical mononuclear cell infiltrates present in the perivascular distribution of heart from child who died of acute rheumatic carditis (×493).

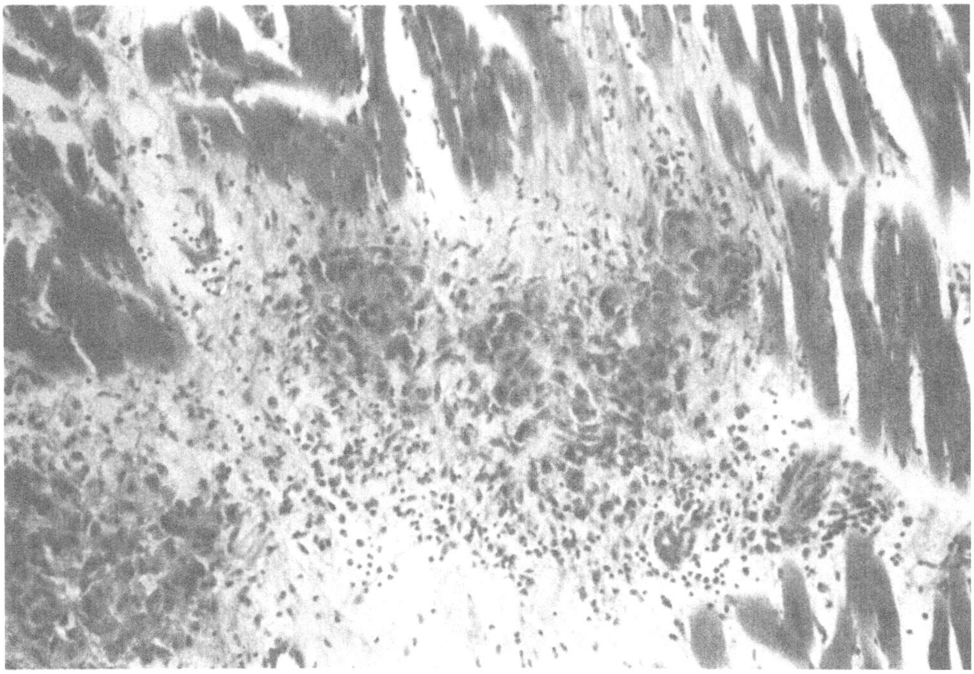

Figure 5. Histological appearance of typical Aschoff lesion present in myocardium from a 10-year-old boy who died during the course of acute rheumatic myocarditis (×300).

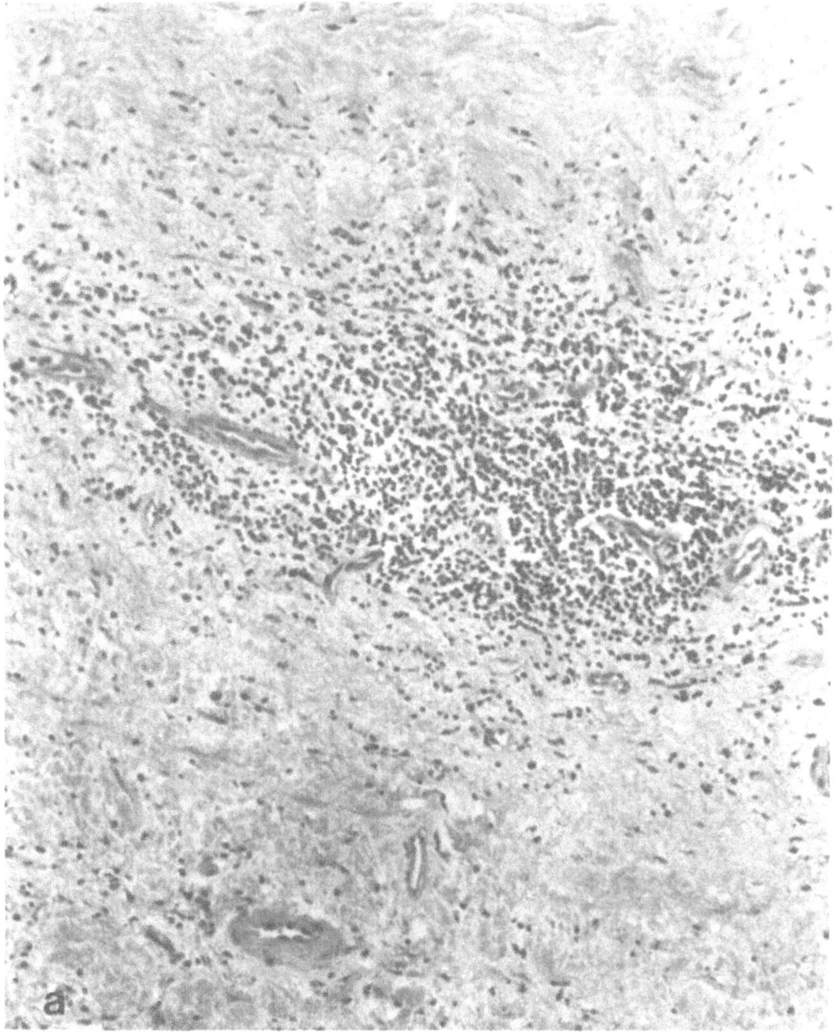

Figure 6. (a) Typical mononuclear cell infiltrates present within mitral valve from patient with rheumatic heart disease in which valve was excised 20 years after the first attack of rheumatic fever (×250). (b) Higher-power view of cells comprising mitral valve infiltrate showing activated lymphocytes and histiocytes (×750).

the presence of Aschoff bodies and clear-cut acute rheumatic activity still remains uncertain. This is illustrated in a study by Virmani and Roberts (1977) in which 21% of 191 operatively removed left atrial appendages showed Aschoff bodies in a retrospective study of patients undergoing mitral valve surgery for rheumatic mitral disease. Parallel examination of the same group of patients showed very little in the way of clinical or laboratory signs of what would be considered clear-cut rheumatic activity or acute rheumatic fever.

Cardiac valvular tissues as well as endocardium are also involved in a generalized

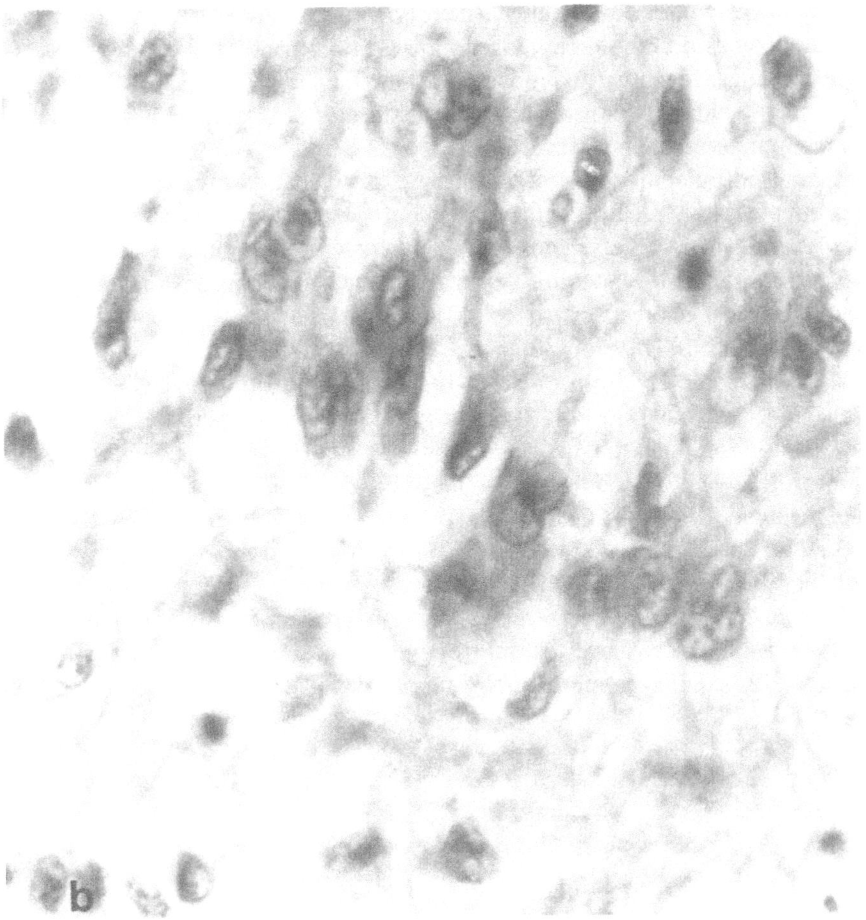

Figure 6. (*continued*)

inflammatory process. Examination of mitral and aortic valves removed during the course of cardiovascular surgery in India has recently shown a surprisingly high incidence of focal intense collections of lymphocytes and plasma cells (Raizada *et al.*, 1983). An example of such mononuclear-cell intravalvular infiltrates is shown in Fig. 6. In the case of this remarkable clinical material, many patients operated on were much younger than comparable mitral or aortic valve patients currently being operated on for rheumatic heart disease in the United States. Thus, the Indian material examined sometimes showed chronic changes with rheumatic valves only several years after the original series of episodes of acute rheumatic carditis. By contrast, although similar mitral valve material from American patients also showed focal mononuclear-cell infiltrates, the inflammatory foci were not as extensive or intense as in the younger Indian patients studied, possibly because many of the U.S. patients were operated on three to four decades after the last of their clinically perceived rheumatic attacks. However, regardless of these differences, the presence of striking focal collections of apparently immunological activated cells within rheumatic valvular tissues many years following the acute rheumatic episode clearly implicates some sort of chronic ongoing immunologic process in the pathogenesis of the pathological changes eventually produced within the heart valves themselves. In our studies, no direct evidence for retained residual streptococcal antigen was obtained using indirect immunofluorescence (Raizada *et al.*, 1983).

A generalized inflammatory process such as is present during acute rheumatic fever also often involves the pleura, with consequent pleuritis and occasional vasculitis of pulmonary vessels or so-called rheumatic pneumonia. From a clinical standpoint, this is frequently very difficult to distinguish from pulmonary embolic phenomena.

One of the most interesting aspects of acute rheumatic fever relates to its frequent association with successive crops of subcutaneous nodules. These nodules cannot be distinguished histologically from those of rheumatoid arthritis. A characteristic microscopic appearance is shown in Fig. 7. Severity of nodules and persistence with multiple new crops of such nodules have been strongly related to ongoing relative severity of rheumatic carditis. The olecranon area is the most commonly involved site; in patients with acute rheumatic fever, artificial repeated trauma is capable of inducing the formation of nodules at the site of trauma (Massel *et al.*, 1937). As noted above, the histopathological picture of the affected myocardium, subcutaneous nodules, and many other tissues including the endocardium and heart valves suggests primary involvement of the cellular immune system. Precisely how the initial streptococcal stimulus is translated into a longstanding cell-mediated immune autoreactivity is still not certain.

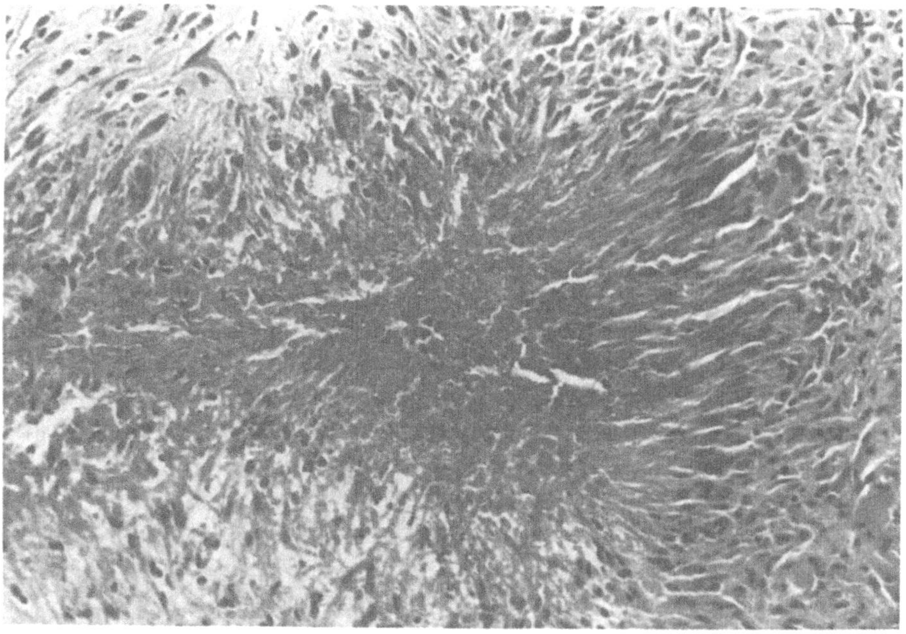

Figure 7. Typical histological appearance of a rheumatic nodule showing granuloma with central disorganization and necrosis, surrounded by pallisading mononuclear cells and lymphocytes (×280).

VI. MOLECULAR MIMICRY

A. Molecular Mimicry and Acute Rheumatic Fever

How the group A streptococcus actually induces acute rheumatic fever in the host is still not settled; however, the concept of molecular mimicry has achieved a leading role as a reasonable theoretical explanation for the entire process. Molecular mimicry essentially refers to the fact that there appear to be a number of antigenic components residing in the streptococcus that share very close antigenic similarity with similar substances present within human tissues. A partial tabulation of these cross reactions between streptococcal components and various human tissues is presented in Table 2; the diversity and extent of this cross reactivity are indeed impressive.

The earliest work documenting antigenic cross reactivity between components of streptococci and human heart tissues were observations by Kaplan *et al.* (Kaplan, 1962, 1963; Kaplan and Meyerserian, 1962) and concurrently by Zabriskie and Freimer (1966). Clear-cut cross reactivity between streptococcal antigens and human myocardium was demonstrated by Kaplan and coworkers; in parallel studies, Zabriskie and Freimer (1966) showed that a cross reaction was present between antigenic determinants in group A streptococcal membranes and human myocardial sarcolemmal membrane. The cross reactivity could best be demonstrated using serum antibody from patients with accute rheumatic fever. Such sera often contained so-called heart-reactive antibodies, which stained sar-

Table 2. A Comparative List of Streptococcal Antigens that have been Reported to Show Cross Reaction with Various Human Tissues

Streptococcal antigen	Human cross reactive material	Reference
Group A cell wall extracts (? copurify with acid extracts of M protein)	Human myocardium	Kaplan (1962) Kaplan and Meyeserian (1962) Lyampert *et al.* (1966) Nakhla and Glynn (1967)
Group A membranes	Human myocardial sarcolemmal membranes	Zabriskie and Freimer (1966) van de Rijn *et al.* (1977)
Group A polysaccharide and glycoproteins	Human heart valve glycoproteins	Goldstein *et al.* (1968)
M-protein components (specific polypeptide)	Human sarcolemmal membranes	Dale and Beachey (1982)
Group A streptococcal antigens	Human brain antigens	Kingston and Glynn (1976)
Group A streptococcal membranes	Neuronal cytoplasmic antigens in human caudate and subthalamic nuclei	Husby *et al.* (1976)
Group A streptococcal antigens	Human cardiac conduction system	Kasp-Groschowska and Kingston (1977)
Group A polysaccharide	Epithelial cells of thymus and skin	Lyampert *et al.* (1976)

colemmal membranes in frozen sections of human heart (Zabriskie *et al.*, 1970; Kaplan and Svec, 1964). An example of a heart-reactive antibody is shown in Fig. 8. Such strongly positive immunofluorescence could be completely removed by immunoadsorption with purified membranes obtained from group A streptococci (Zabriskie and Friemer, 1966; van de Rijn *et al.*, 1977). Serial studies of heart-reactive antibodies in patients with acute rheumatic fever showed high titers initially during the acute phases of carditis with subsequent fall in heart-reactive antibody activity as clinical disease parameters subsided (Zabriskie *et al.*, 1970). The immunochemical specificity of this reaction was later extended by van de Rijn *et al.* (1977), with cross reactivity again being most obviously demonstrable using serum antibody obtained from human subjects with acute rheumatic fever.

These latter studies also indicated that group A streptococcal membranes were composed of a host of protein or glycoprotein components and also that rabbit antisera prepared against group A streptococcal membranes recognized different antigenic components from those reacting with human antibodies present in sera from rheumatic fever subjects. The cross reactivity between antigenic components of group A streptococci and constituents of human heart muscle has also been recognized independently by other workers (Lyampert *et al.*, 1966; Danilova, 1966; Nakhla and Glynn, 1967).

Characterization of this well-defined cross reactivity between group A streptococcal materials and human myocardium presents an important central problem for investigators attempting to develop protective vaccines against strains of streptococci capable of ini-

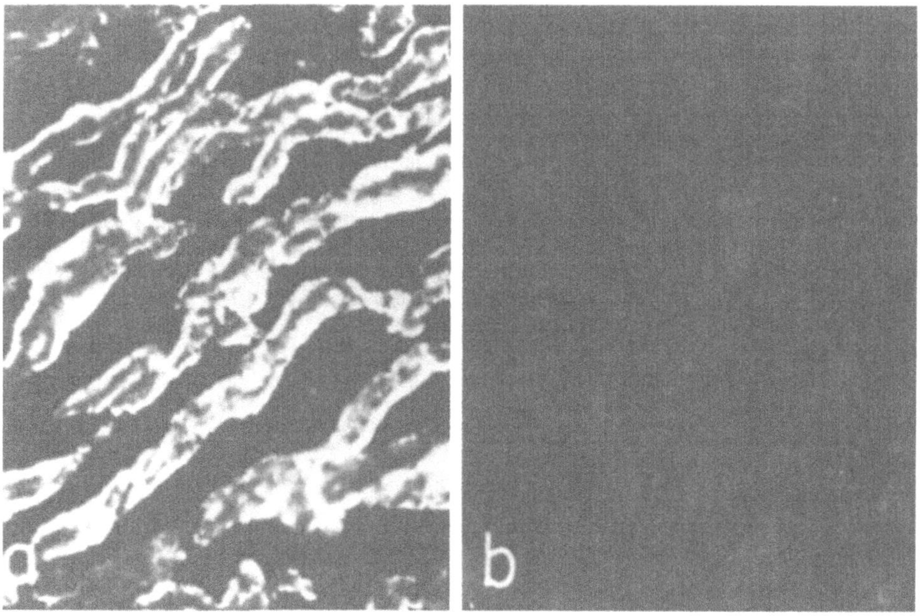

Figure 8. Immunofluorescence appearance of typical pattern of heart-reactive antibody. (a) The antibody bound to the sarcolemma of cardiac myofibers. (b) Absence of staining pattern when heart-reactive antibody was absorbed with purified cross-reactive antigens derived from streptococcal membrane. (Reproduced with permission from van de Rijn *et al.*, 1977.)

tiating acute rheumatic fever (Beachey *et al.*, 1977, 1980). Most of the cross-reactive antigens appear to be associated with material derived from the bacterial cell wall or cell membrane but not with the surface M protein, which confers type-specific immunity and enhanced opsonization for the infected or immunized host. In the original studies by Kaplan (Kaplan, 1962, 1963), the heart cross-reactive antigen appeared to be restricted to cell wall materials and also restricted to types 5 and 19. Also, in Kaplan's initial work (Kaplan, 1962, 1963), heart cross-reactive antigens copurified with acid extracts of M protein from streptococcal serotypes 5 and 19. Similar findings were also recorded independently by Lyampert and coworkers (Lyampert *et al.*, 1966).

This particular point has become more and more relevant to the idea of a possible protective antistreptococcal vaccine. Recent work by Dale and Beachey (1982) has indeed provided direct evidence of heart cross-reactive materials within highly purified polypeptide fragments of type 5 M protein. Antibodies made against this polypeptide M protein fragment cross reacted with human heart sarcolemmal membranes, and after elution and dissociation from human sarcolemmal membranes, the same cross-reactive antibody opsonized both types 5 and 19 M-protein-bearing streptococci. Subsequent reports from this same group have indicated that the cardiac cross-reactive material contained within the M protein polypeptide can be eliminated by pepsin digestion (Dale *et al.*, 1983). This latter finding now paves the way for a rational approach toward developing a potentially protective vaccine against pathogenic streptococci. Development of this approach is now anticipated with much interest and expectation.

The pattern of immunofluorescence distribution of heart-reactive antibody among patients with acute rheumatic carditis suggests a cardiac-membrane-related phenomenon. It seems possible, therefore, that heart-reactive antibody, occurring as it does in direct parallel with rheumatic carditis, may be capable of playing a direct pathophysiological role in myocardial muscle dysfunction since important cardioreceptors such as myocardian α- and β-adrenergic receptors are concentrated in this particular anatomic site. Studies are currently under way in our laboratory to examine this possibility. Similar studies of the possible pathophysiological capacity of heart-reactive antibodies have already been performed by investigators interested in the functional cardiac disturbances associated with Chagas' disease. These studies have shown clear-cut physiological effects of chagasic heart-reactive antibodies examined in an *in vitro* system (Gimeno *et al.*, 1979; Sterin-Borda *et al.*, 1976). In this context, it is important to point out that heart-reactive antibodies as a general class of immunoglobulin reactivity are not solely limited to acute rheumatic fever but are also present in heart transplant patients, in individuals with the so-called postpericardiotomy syndrome, in patients with Dressler's syndrome, as well as in patients with Chagas' disease and consequent chronic chagasic cardiomyopathy (Zabriskie *et al.*, 1971; McCabe *et al.*, 1973; Engle *et al.*, 1974; Santos-Buch and Teixeira, 1974; Kennedy and Das, 1976).

The second major type of molecular mimicry between group A streptococci and mammalian tissues involves cross reactions between streptococcal antigens and human cardiac valvular glycoproteins. This cross reactivity was demonstrated using valvular glycoprotein components carefully isolated by chromatographic techniques (Goldstein *et al.*, 1967, 1968). Rabbit antisera prepared against either glycoproteins extracted from human cardiac valves or against polysaccharide from group A streptococci showed high degrees of cross reactivity as demonstrated by mutual cross-absorption experiments. The apparent cross reaction between group A polysaccharide and heart valve glycoprotein is of considerable interest in view of subsequent work by Dudding and Ayoub (1968), who demonstrated persistence of anti-group-A-polysaccharide antibodies in the serum of rheumatic heart disease patients many years after any clinical evidence of acute rheumatic activity. Subsequent studies from this group have shown that these same anti-group-A-polysaccharide antibody elevations decrease in rheumatic patients undergoing valve resection and replacement with prosthetic valves (Ayoub *et al.*, 1974).

Several reports have documented cross reactions between streptococcal antigens and components of the nervous system. Kingston and Glynn (1976) showed apparent cross-reacting antigens present within group A streptococcal bacteria and nervous tissue, although in this latter study no controls were included to rule out possible nonspecific interactions between the immunoglobulins used and possible tissue-fixed Fc receptors. More convincing were reports by Husby *et al.* (1976) of antineuronal antibody in serum samples from children and young adults with Sydenham's chorea (Husby *et al.*, 1976). This antibody reacted with cytoplasmic antigens apparently clearly concentrated or relatively localized in caudate and subthalamic nuclei of normal human brain. The cytoplasmic neuronal staining could be completely abolished by absorption of positively reacting serum samples using relatively purified preparations of membranes from group A but not from control group D streptococci (Table 3). An example of a strongly positive reaction demonstrating antineuronal antibody from a child with active Sydenham's chorea is shown in Fig. 9. Clinical correlations between the presence of antineuronal antibody and actual chorea showed a distinct relationship between perceived severity of the choreiform attacks and relative serum titer of the antineuronal antibody. A typical chart of serial studies of two patients with repeated chorea attacks is shown in Fig. 10. Moreover, although the antibody was sometimes detected in children with primarily carditis and arthritis, it usually was found principally in patients with active chorea.

There has been considerable practical difficulty in understanding how serum antibody to cytoplasmic neuronal antigenic constituents might conceivably be involved in the genesis of chorea itself, since there is a theoretical problem with potential access of the antibody to central nervous system neurons because of the blood–brain barrier (Williams *et al.*, 1980a,b). At present, this problem has not been solved, since there are no differential direct observations on rheumatic chorea patients in whom titer and immunochemical specificity of antineuronal antibody have been measured simultaneously in both serum and cerebrospinal fluid (CSF). Thus far, our own attempts at passive transfer of chorea to animals (mice and rats) with serum have not proven successful. Since the few pathological or postmortem studies available on patients who have died during acute Sydenham's chorea episodes have shown little more than minimal changes or minuscule interstitital round cell infiltrates within the brain itself (Lessof, 1958), it seems possible that chorea may be a neurofunctional rather than a tissue-altering disorder. It is also possible, but by no means proven, that the movement disorder itself represents a humoral immune response to important cross-reacting neuroreceptors that share antigenic determinants with conformations on group A streptococcal membranes. This is clearly an exciting area that needs additional investigation.

Cross reactions between streptococcal antigens and the cardiac conduction system have been described (Kasp-Grochowska and Kingston, 1977). In these reports, no extensive characterization of the exact streptococcal cross-reacting determinants was given.

Table 3. Results of Absorption of Serum Showing Positive Immunofluorescent Reactions with Neuronal Cytoplasm in Caudate Nuclei Using Streptococcal Antigens, Tissue Homogenates, and Cohn Fraction IV[a]

	Reaction tested	Group A unabsorbed	Group A T6 membrane (D471)	Group A T6 cell wall (D471)	Group D T6 carbohydrate (D471)	Group D membrane (A932)	Cell wall (A932)	Isol. neurons, caudate nucleus	Lyophil. cerebral cortex	Lyophil. mouse liver	Cohn fraction IV
Serum 298 (chorea) undiluted	Caudate nucleus neuron staining	+	0	±	+	+	+	0	+	+	+
Serum W.W. (SLE) 1/50	Antinuclear antibody	++	++	++	++	++	++	+	+	+	++

[a] Reproduced with permission from Husby *et al.* (1976).

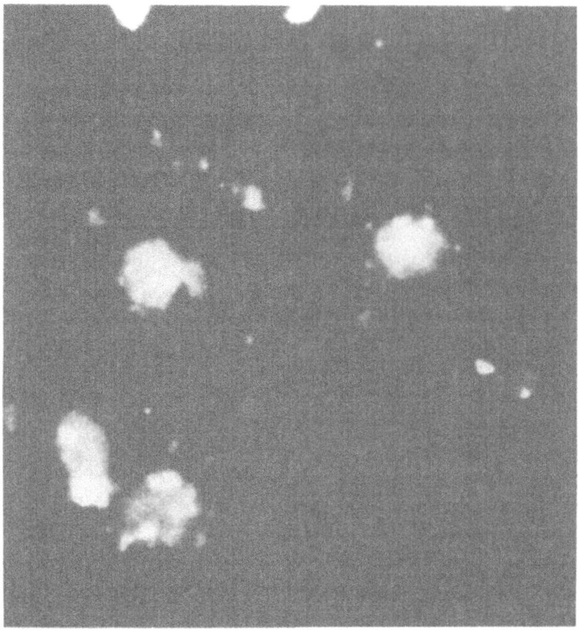

Figure 9. Immunofluorescence appearance of antineuronal antibody staining of frozen sections of normal human caudate nucleus using serum sample from a child with Sydenham's chorea. Positive fluorescence staining of neuronal cytoplasm was completely removed by absorption with membranes from group A streptococci.

The potential importance of this finding lies in the fact that prolongation of the PR interval occurs in 40% of patients with acute rheumatic fever, and an antibody cross reacting with streptococcal membranes being a potential mediator of this phenomenon remains an attractive possibility.

In addition, there have also been reports of cross reactivity between streptococcal polysaccharides and antigens present in thymic materials (Lyampert *et al.*, 1976; Zabriskie, 1967). The studies of Lyampert *et al.* were performed largely using immunofluorescence, and the precise identity of the thymic antigens involved has never subsequently been defined using, for instance, any of the current OKT3, T4, or T8 monoclonal reagents. Cross-reacting determinants reacted within epithelial cells of mammalian thymus as well as skin. Further work on this particular problem is clearly indicated, since if significant or extensive cross reactions occurred between various T cell determinants and streptococci, it might well represent an additional important potential mechanism whereby the initial inciting group A streptococcal infection with subsequent immune response could profoundly alter the intrinsic immune reactivity of the host.

If one accepts the idea of molecular mimicry as being a leading contender, the general theoretical scheme is that group A streptococci infecting the host induce immune responses to a number of their own antigenic determinants, which in turn cross react with autologous tissues of the host and produce the clinical signs and tissue lesions of acute rheumatic fever. Whether the actual clinical manifestations of the disorder itself are caused principally by humoral, antibody-mediated mechanisms or, alternatively, by cell-mediated immunity has not been established.

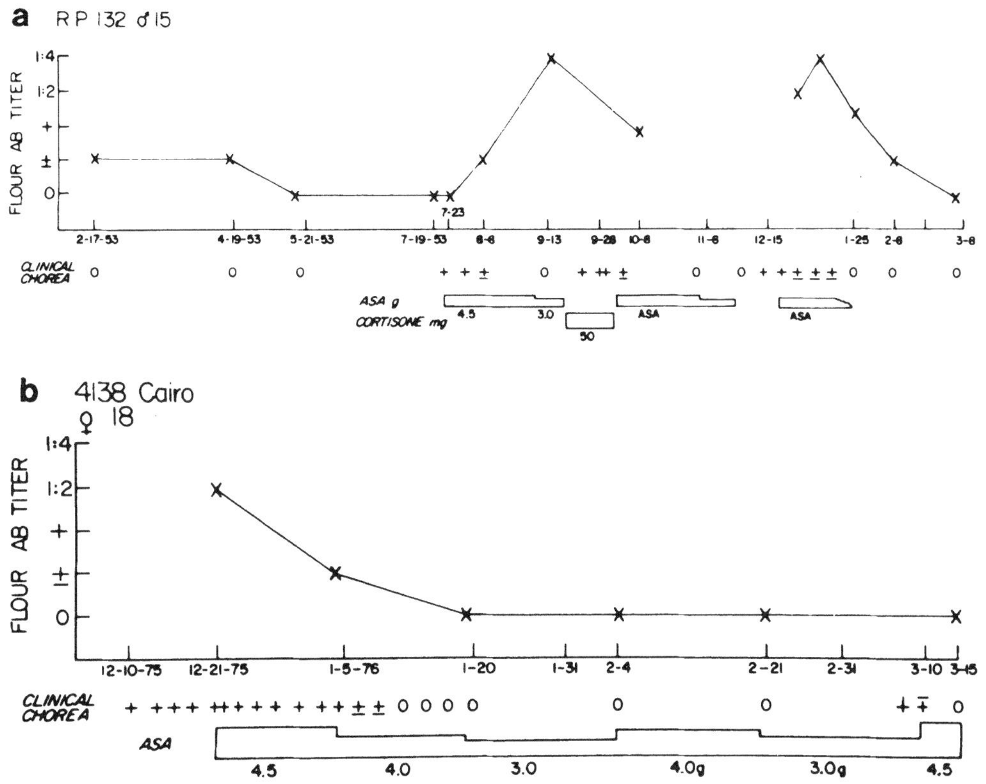

Figure 10. (a) Serial studies of serum samples of a Rockefeller University patient before and after several clinical episodes of chorea. It can be seen that although weak antineuronal immunofluorescence was present without clinically manifest chorea on 2-17-53 and 4-19-53, the subsequent clinical episodes of chorea were associated with a rise in titer of antineuronal antibody staining. Antibody was no longer evident 7 weeks after subsidence of clinical chorea. (b) Serial studies of Cairo patient 4138 show presence of antineuronal antibody detected on admission, 12-21-75, coincident with moderately severe chorea. Besides aspirin therapy, the patient also received phenobarbital and reserpine. Subsequent subsidence of clinical chorea was associated with disappearance of detectable serum antineuronal antibody. A transient mild recurrence of chorea on 3-8-75 was not accompanied by the presence of detectable serum antineuronal antibody. (Reproduced with permission from Husby *et al.*, 1976).

B. Molecular Mimicry in Other Disorders

The general concept of molecular mimicry being of potential central importance in the pathogenesis of other poorly understood human disease states has recently been dramatically emphasized by work related to Chagas' disese. This latter disorder, caused by *Trypanosoma cruzi,* affects an estimated 12 million people in Central and South America. Major clinical manifestations include neuronal and ganglia involvement of both parasympathetic and sympathetic nervous systems and in some patients a chronic progressive severe myocarditis (Koberle, 1974). Of particular interest with respect to rheumatic fever is the fact that when patients die of chagasic myocarditis, often no trace of the original infecting *T. cruzi* can be found. Particularly interesting in this regard were reports by

Wood *et al.* (1982) that a monoclonal antibody raised against rat dorsal root ganglion showed cross reactivity with both human myocardium and determinants on the surface of *T. cruzi* organisms. The case for molecular mimicry in this particular instance is especially striking since the trypanosome, human myocardium, and autonomic nervous system neuronal elements all share involvement in the direct pathogenesis of the disease picture. Subsequent work from this same group has shown cross reactions by two additional murine mmonoclonal antibodies raised against *T. cruzi* antigens and antigens shared by both brain and spinal cord extracts (Snary *et al.*, 1983).

A large body of evidence has begun to develop concerning antigenic similarities among diverse components present in nature. Much of this sort of observation has received particular impetus with the widespread application of monoclonal antibodies. That such uniform, identical immunoglobulins may show combining sites with conformations or three-dimensional shapes that are similar or identical but that nonetheless are present on materials with no apparent natural relationship to each other might be expected *a priori*. Recent examples of this phenomenon now include apparent cross reactions between antigens defining Thy-1 on murine lymphocites and vimentin (Dulbecco, *et al.*, 1981), a fibrillar cellular skeletal protein. Similar cross reactivity has also been shown for vimentin and a cell surface phosphoprotein associated with measles virus infection of cells (Fujinami *et al.*, 1983).

Additional fascinating examples of extensive molecular mimicry have recently been reported in the description of insulinlike molecules in unicellular parasites or bacteria (Roth *et al.*, 1982; Le Roith *et al.*, 1980). In addition, platelet growth factor has, by sequence analysis, a strong homology for products that have been previously identified with the simian sarcoma *onc* gene v-sis (Doolittle *et al.*, 1983). Finally, more in line with the situation encountered in acute rheumatic fever, certain strains of bacteria notorious for their capacity to induce meningitis in children show strong or partial antigenic cross reactivity with components of nervous tissue (Finne *et al.*, 1983), the very target organ for the infections they are most likely to cause in human subjects. The list of other possible or less well-defined examples of molecular mimicry is long indeed, and it will remain for the future to explore in greater detail whether such natural similarities are in any way related either to disease susceptibility or to actual favored autoimmune responsiveness.

VII. STUDIES OF HUMORAL AND CELLULAR PHENOMENA IN ASSOCIATION WITH ACUTE RHEUMATIC FEVER

Perhaps the first work to link the general process of rheumatic fever with humoral evidence of inflammation was the discovery by Tillet and Francis (1930) of pronounced elevation of C-reactive protein (CRP) in association with pneumonia. Later elevations of CRP were also recorded in other inflammatory states and in rheumatic fever (MacLeod and Avery, 1980; Anderson and McCarty, 1950). Much of the early and subsequent work linking CRP to rheumatic activity dealt with the specificity and sensitivity of the reaction and later with the sites for production of CRP within hepatocytes (Kushner, 1982; Kushner and Kaplan, 1961). Currently, the concept of CRP as an acute-phase reactant and possibly as a primordial antibodylike molecule at least in an evolutionary sense has become more firmly established (Gewurz *et al.*, 1982).

Early epidemiologic and clinical studies established that the first symptoms of an acute rheumatic fever attack were also accompanied by heightened serologic evidence of recent group A streptococcal infection. A number of streptococcal components and extracellular products were studied, and the general consensus has been that antistreptolyin O and possibly also anti-DNase B were most frequently reliably elevated. Elevations of such antibodies are generally higher among patients with acute rheumatic fever than in parallel normal controls; however, there are occasional exceptions to this general rule. Antistreptococcal antibody responses are generally lower among patients with Sydenham's chorea than in patients with arthritis, carditis, and the full-blown rheumatic fever syndrome.

Serial studies of heart-reactive antibody can be correlated with changes in clinical acute rheumatic activity (Zabriskie *et al.*, 1970). An example of such sequential change is shown in Fig. 11. However, detectable heart-reactive antibody is not found in all patients with rheumatic fever, although this may merely represent the practical thresholds for detection with present techniques.

Several studies have documented moderate or marked elevations of circulating immune complexes during acute rheumatic fever episodes (Yoshinoya and Pope, 1980; van de Rijn *et al.*, 1978; Williams *et al.*, 1976). Although a possible relationship between immune complex elevations and HLA-B5 was noted in one study (Yoshinoya and Pope, 1980), the usefulness of elevated serum immune complexes in general does not seem to be great, particularly in terms of either differential diagnosis or immediate prognosis. In our own studies, relative quantitative amounts of complexes as well as molecular weight distributions were similar when patients with chorea alone were compared to those with carditis, arthritis, and generalized systemic involvement (Williams *et al.*, 1976). The presence of circulating immune complexes in the serum of patients with acute rheumatic fever probably fits with the initial manifestations of some sort of intensely activated immune process. In addition, circulating complexes could be directly responsible for

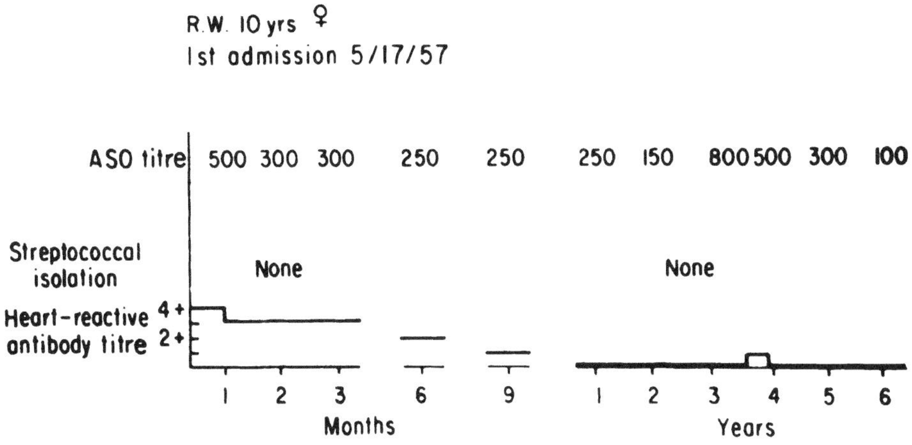

Figure 11. Heart-reactive antibody titers in patient R.W. following a single episode of rheumatic fever. Heart-reactive antibody titers were negative by the fourth year following the initial episode and have remained negative for over 6 years. (Reproduced with permission from Zabriskie *et al.*, 1970.)

various features of the acute clinical profile such as transient arthritis or arthralgia or even the strange skin lesions of erythema multiforme, which sometimes accompany the acute episode. Direct confirmation of the importance of immune complexes in erythema multiforme will require careful immunofluorescence study of serial skin biopsies among individual patients.

A. Changes in Peripheral Blood Lymphocytic Profile

Studies of the lymphocyte or general mononuclear-cell changes that may be present during acute carditis, arthritis, or even chorea have now extended in our hands over a period of several years (Lueker *et al.*, 1975; Williams *et al.*, 1977, 1982). Most of the clinical material was derived from Trinidad in the West Indies, the population of children hospitalized at the Free Rheumatic Heart Centre in Cairo, and most recently from several large clinical centers in New Delhi and at the Postgraduate Institute of Medical Research at Chandigarh in Northern India (Williams *et al.*, 1982). All patients studied were seen and personally examined to substantiate a clear-cut clinical diagnosis of rheumatic fever at the time of each set of studies undertaken.

Initial studies of peripheral blood T- and B-cell changes during acute rheumatic fever showed an early T-cell depression of both absolute numbers and proportion of T lymphocytes determined by E-rosetting or with heterologous anti-T-cell antibody using indirect immunofluorescence (Lueker *et al.*, 1975). As rheumatic episodes progressed, T-cell numbers and proportions gradually rose to normal. Initial depression of T cells within peripheral blood was subsequently confirmed independently by another group working in Northern India at Chandigarh (Ganguly *et al.*, 1982). Later studies appeared to indicate a relative increment in T cells with IgG Fc receptors or Tγ cells coincident with bouts of clear-cut clinical rheumatic activity (Williams *et al.*, 1978). This apparent increase in the putative Tγ suppressor/cytotoxic cell subset during rheumatic attacks may represent cell subpopulations involved in direct toxic injury to cardiac muscle. More recently, using mouse monoclonal anti-T-cell-subset reagents, we have shown that patients with acute rheumatic fever and active carditis may show a relative decrease in peripheral blood T suppressor phenotype subsets as identified with the OKT8 reagent (Williams *et al.*, 1982).

An attempt was also made to examine alteration in B cells and, in particular, antigen-binding cells detectable in assay systems employing rosette formation with autologous patient's erythrocytes coated with sonicated preparations of group A streptococcal membranes (Williams *et al.*, 1978). This particular technique was therefore directed at detecting B cells present in peripheral blood that were capable of binding to antigenic determinants present on sonicated group A streptococcal membranes, some of which have been presumed to be closely related to the spectrum of inciting antigens in acute rheumatic fever. Considerable elevation of these putative antigen-binding cells was recorded in acute rheumatics studied both in Trinidad and in Egypt. Examples of these findings are shown in Fig. 12. It is important to point out that the actual numbers of cells thought to be antigen binding using this technique were found to be several orders of magnitude higher than levels of antigen-binding cells calculated from experimental animal model systems (Cudkowicz *et al.*, 1978; Shearer *et al.*, 1968). The pronounced increment of streptococcal membrane antigen-binding cells in the patients with acute rheumatic fever suggests an intense immune B-cell activation during early phases of the disease. These findings were

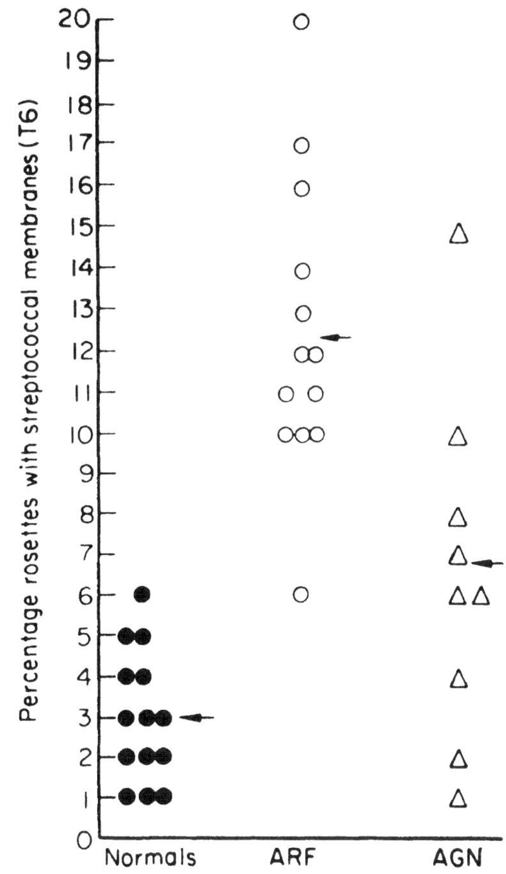

Figure 12. Percentage of peripheral blood lymphocytes showing rosette formation with autologous erythrocytes coated with group A streptococcal membranes (type 6). Values are shown for normal children as controls, acute rheumatic fever (ARF), and acute glomerulonephritis (AGN), with mean values indicated by arrows. Differences between mean of normals and those of rheumatic fever or acute glomerulonephritis were significant ($P < 0.01$) by χ^2 analysis. (Reproduced with permission from Williams *et al.*, 1977.)

reminiscent of the previously well-documented marked elevations of antibodies to various streptococcal antigens during acute rheumatic episodes. The relatively large proportions of putative antigen-binding cells detected by the autologous rosetting technique may reflect a marked heterogenicity among streptococcal membrane antigens.

As has been noted above, marked elevations of plasma or serum CRP had long been associated with acute rheumatic activity. For this reason, we examined peripheral blood mononuclear cells during acute rheumatic episodes for possible *in vivo* CRP binding. Marked elevations of CRP-binding cells were noted during acute rheumatic fever episodes. Examples of these data are shown in Table 4. The CRP binding appeared to be quite tight and relatively nonreversible when peripheral blood mononuclear cells from rheumatic subjects were studied before and after incubation in 37°C, 5% CO_2–oxygen conditions for periods of 12–20 hr. The CRP binding to peripheral blood lymphocytes in acute rheumatic fever was approximately equally distributed between T and B cells and also appeared to show some predilection for cell populations bearing Fc receptors.

A series of experiments conducted both in Egypt and in Trinidad was directed at the question of whether CRP bound to the surface of immunologically competent cells was in effect playing some protective or possibly self-modulating role during the course of acute rheumatic attacks. This hypothesis was proposed on the basis of a large body

Table 4. Lymphocytes Binding CRP in Normal Controls and Children with Rheumatic Fever[a]

	CRP-binding lymphocytes (%)	Total no. of CRP (lymphocytes/mm^3)
Acute rheumatic fever (30)	16.3 ± 8.3	821.8 ± 509.6
Normal children controls (30)	3.3 ± 2.9	137.6 ± 61.5
Significance of difference	$P < 0.0001$	$P < 0.0001$

[a] Reproduced with permission from Williams *et al.* (1978).

of concurrent work on possible physiological functions of CRP that had indicated potential modulatory or protective features for CRP in regard to complement activation as well as in platelet release of various important mediator molecules (Fiedel and Gewurz, 1976; Kaplan and Volanakis, 1974; Siegel *et al.*, 1975; Volanakis and Narkates, 1981). A series of studies using double-color immunofluorescence (simultaneous rhodamine/fluorescein staining) and sequential addition *in vitro* of preparations of sonicated group A streptococcal membranes to peripheral blood lymphocytes of patients with active rheumatic fever indicated that *in vivo* CRP binding to B cells had appeared to diminish the ability of this cell population to adhere to or react with group A streptococcal membranes (Williams *et al.*, 1980a,b). Representative data from this series of experiments are shown in Table 5. These observations suggested, therefore, that at least one of the possible consequences of *in vivo* CRP binding to lymphocyte membranes during the course of acute rheumatic fever might be to down-modulate the autoimmune process by blocking or defusing antigen-binding B cells from being restimulated or activated through potentially harmful antigens present in streptococcal membranes. If such a hypothesis eventually proves correct, the strong host response by way of rapid induction of hepatic CRP synthesis during acute rheumatic fever might be explained as an important early protective reaction aimed mainly at controlling a potentially harmful self-injurious immune stimulus for the host.

B. Group A Polysaccharide

A curious feature that has been reported about rheumtic fever and chronic rheumatic heart disease relates to the apparent long-term persistance of antibody to group A polysaccharide in the serum of rheumatic subjects (Dudding and Ayoub, 1968). This initial observation has now been confirmed by several other groups. Moreover, it has been noted that the persistent elevation of anti-group-A-carbohydrate antibody in patients with rheumatic heart disease often abruptly falls when they undergo mitral valve resection and prosthetic valve placement (Ayoub *et al.*, 1974).

A number of possibilities originally reviewed by Dudding and Ayoub (1968) exist to explain these observations. First, the serologic, immunochemical, and cross-absorption data of Goldstein *et al.* (1967, 1968) indicating extensive immunologic cross reactivity between group A polysaccharides and cardiac valvular glycoproteins or polysaccharides

Table 5. Double-Cell Surface Marker Analysis of Non-T-Rosetting Cells for Streptococcal Membrane Binding CRP and Ia Antigen in Patients with ARF[a]

Patient	Percent cells in whole non-T-rosetting fraction binding T_{12} *Strep.* membranes	Percent cells binding to T_{12} *Strep.* membranes also positive for CRP	Percent cells with Ia antigen in whole nonrosetting population	Percent cells with T_6 *Strep.* membrane binding in whole nonrosetting fraction	Percent cells binding to T_6 *Strep.* membrane with detectable Ia
3	19	10			
4	18	15			
23	28	12			
22	20	8			
5105	16	10			
Mean	20.2	11.0			
26			66	4	38
316			68	39	49
9			55	33	48
31			69	34	50
4			54	15	83
T3			52	8	65
Mean				22.2	55.5

Relative Streptococcal Membrane-Binding Capacities of Neuraminidase T-Rosetting and Nonrosetting Cells in Children with ARF

Patient	Percent cells binding *Strep.* membrane in T-rosetting population	Percent cells binding *Strep.* membrane in nonrosetting population
3	10	19
4	9	18
23	10	38
22	11	20
5105	9	16
26	5	4
316	8	39
9	8	33
31	2	34
T-3	2	8
T-4	2	13
Mean	6.9	21.1
Mean of normal control children (13)	0.9 ± 0.06	2.5 ± 1.3

[a] Reproduced with permission from Williams *et al.* (1980b).

might suggest that the latter are somehow altered during the chronic inflammatory process that affects rheumatic valves and that this in turn induces an extended immune response stretching over a number of years in the host. Secondly, it could be postulated that there is something about the chronic rheumatic process that turns off normal immunomodulatory forces that ordinarily would gradually shut down or turn off a strong immune response to group A polysaccharide. In such an instance, a selective defect in suppressor cells or suppressor activity for group A polysaccharide humoral immune reactivity would have to be postulated. At present, to our knowledge, there seems to be very little in the way of positive data or clear experimental support for this explanation. A considerable literature has, however, developed relative to immunoregulatory and, in particular, suppressor-cell influence on immune responsiveness to other bacterial polysaccharide products; e.g., in pneumococcal infection or to several of the pneumococcal type-specific polysaccharides (Wright, 1927; Brown *et al.*, 1981; Baker *et al.*, 1970). Nevertheless, the persistence of relatively high titers of anti-group-A-carbohydrate antibody among many patients with rheumatic heart disease remains a curious and thus far unexplained finding.

C. Cell-Mediated Immune Studies

When one examines the basic lesions of acute rheumatic fever, particularly the myocarditis, valvular and subvalvular connective tissue inflammation, subsequent slow evolution of chronic inflammation, and, finally, extensive scarring within heart valves and endocardium, much of the histological picture in both acute and chronic rheumatic heart disease suggests prominent involvement of cell-mediated immunity in the basic rheumatic progress. The types of cells that are seen in Aschoff bodies or focal areas of subacute or chronic myocarditis are mainly lymphocytes, histiocytes, and occasional plasma cells. The precise origin of the Anitschkow myocyte—whether a transformed cardiac muscle cell, an activated macrophagelike cell, or even an unusual dendritic cell—has never been clearly defined. Immunohistological studies of Aschoff bodies by Becker and Murphy (1969) showed that cells and cell fragments in Aschoff lesions contained actomyosin similar to that of normal cardiac and striated muscle cells. By contrast, cells characteristic of endocardial Aschoff lesions were demonstrated by immunofluorescence techniques to contain actomyosin similar antigenically to uterine smooth muscle. Nevertheless, the basic histological appearance of the myocardial lesions as well as many of the mononuclear cell infiltrates within epicardial, subvalvular, and valvular tissues in rheumatic fever/rheumatic heart disease clearly is very reminiscent of a cell-mediated immune process.

Several clinical studies support the potential importance of cell-mediated immunity in the rheumatic process (Read *et al.*, 1974; Gowrishankar and Agarwal, 1980). The report by Read *et al.* (1974) provides clear evidence of positive assays for increased cell-directed immune responsiveness in rheumatic fever patients or even those with subsequent low-grade rheumatic activity. In these latter studies, strongly positive responses in lymphocyte transformation or leukocyte migration inhibition were most often seen when particulate streptococcal membrane antigenic material was used. Studies by Sapru *et al.* (1977), which included patients with established rheumatic heart disease as well as those with acute rheumatic fever, indicated an increase in thymidine incorporation when peripheral blood lymphocytes from established rheumatics as well as those with acute rheumatic activity were exposed to group A streptococcal membrane preparations. In this latter study, phytohemagglutinin stimulation indices were reduced among rheumatic patients compared with controls, but no other base-line control antigen stimulation, for instance, with group D or group C streptococcal membranes, was recorded.

Similar positive evidence for delayed-type hypersensitivity reactions to various streptococcal products has been reported by Gowrishankar and Agarwal (1980) in studies of patients both with established rheumatic heart disease and a separate group with active rheumatic carditis. Of great interest in this report were positive tests for cell-mediated immunity, including leukocyte migration inhibition, noted in these patients using streptococcal RNA preparations as antigens. In addition, positive reactions were also noted using human heart valve glycoprotein preparations as stimulating antigens. Healthy normal volunteers and subjects with poststreptococcal glomerulonephritis did not show any increased *in vitro* results for cell-mediated immunity. These latter findings suggest that the pertinent or significant streptococcal antigenic message might indeed be contained within RNA sequences rather than as original antigenic pieces of degraded steptococci, as had previously been suggested by results obtained with several animal models (Cromartie and Craddock, 1966; Cromartie *et al.*, 1977).

In the study by Gowrishankar and Agarwal (1980), essentially no difference in leukocyte migration inhibition was recorded in nine patients with acute rheumatic carditis from results obtained in 15 patients with established rheumatic heart disease not manifesting flagrant disease activity. Control observations included test systems employing group C streptococcal antigens; these latter showed no difference in leukocyte migration between rheumatics and controls. Additional studies of cell-mediated immune functions have recently been recorded by Anand *et al.* (1983a). In this report, leukocyte migration inhibition was studied using human heart muscle antigens as well as streptoccal membranes. Patients with acute rheumatic fever as well as chronic rheumatic heart disease were compared to normal controls and to patients with recent myocardial infarction. Positive assays against streptococcal membrane antigens were again noted in both acute and chronic rheumatics. Cardiac muscle antigens produced positive leukocyte migration inhibitory results in rheumatic patients as well as in those with acute myocardial infarction. No parallel control observations using other non-group-A streptococcal-related antigens were provided as base-line controls in this study.

The exact role of cell-mediated immune reactions in the pathogenesis of the valvular lesions in rheumatic heart disease is perhaps of most importance in attempts to understand the actual pathogenesis of the basic disease process. Our studies of the distribution of various lymphocytic phenotypes within the mononuclear collections of cells noted in rheumatic mitral valves (Raizada *et al.*, 1983) indicated that most of the lymphocytes in these lesions were T cells. In addition, the vast majority of these same T cells were found to be of the OKT4 or helper/inducer phenotype, with only a minority of the cells identified as being of the OKT8 or cytotoxic/suppressor variety. In many instances, clusters of OKT4 T cells were noted in close apposition to tissue fibroblasts, which appeared to be laying down collagen. These findings suggest that one of the final common pathways involved with valvular scarring and eventual rheumatic cardiac dysfunction may be related to clusters of chronically activated T cells of helper/inducer phenotype that secrete lymphokines or messenger molecules capable of inducing fibroblast stimulation and collagenous scarring of the involved valves and endocardium. At present, such a hypothesis remains mostly conjecture and will require direct experimental testing before any valid conclusion can be reached. Precise knowledge about the exact mechanisms involved in valvular and other types of tissue damage and scarring that occur during the course of chronic rheumatic heart disease may help us eventually to design effective treatment or intervention even after the basic underlying process has been initiated.

One other experimental model that has been utilized to examine the potential role of direct lymphocyte-mediated damage to cardiac muscle cells in acute rheumatic fever was described by Yang *et al.*, (1977). In this model, the authors utilized target cells constituted as a syncitium of beating fetal heart cells. Animals sensitized previously by parenteral immunization with streptococcal antigens produced lymphocytes that were capable of directly killing or damaging the syncitium of beating heart cells. These observations provided substantial evidence for the potential role of cell-mediated immunity in the overall pathogenesis of acute rheumatic fever. Thus far, there do not appear to be similar direct cell-killing data on beating heart cell cultures and primed acute rheumatic fever lymphocyte donors indicating a possible likely parallel situation within humans. One of the major problems in adapting such an assay for human myocardial cell syncitia as targets and peripheral blood lymphocytes as the source of potential killer cells would be in establishing a nonallogeneic system. With the inbred stains of mice or guinea pigs that were used by Yang *et al.* (1977), no cross-histocompatability problems were encountered; however, if such a system were employed in a human model, virtually all cell-mixture experiments would of necessity have to be isologous or allogeneic. Despite these potential drawbacks, it would seem that similar assays might provide results of great interest if adapted to comparable human systems.

D. Genetic Influence and Possible Contribution of Immune Response Genes

One of the most interesting fundamental problems related to rheumatic fever is to define the exact features that allow an initial pharyngeal infection to proceed on to acute carditis and/or chorea in only approximately 0.1–0.2% of the individuals in a given population at risk or actually harboring group A streptococci in their throats. Recent observations by Patarroyo *et al.* (1979) may eventually provide a clearer insight into this basic problem of host/bacterium interface. These studies showed a distinct association between B-cell alloantigen defined by an alloantiserum called 883 and the occurrence of rheumatic fever or rheumatic heart disease within two different populations studied in New York City and Bogota, Colombia. Representative data from this study are shown in Table 6. No

Table 6. Typing of B-Cell Alloantigens in Patients with Rheumatic Fever

	New York group %		Bogota group %		
DR specificity	Normal subjects (52)	RF (21)	Normal subjects (60)	RF (41)	Combined series relative risk
Undefined (883)	17	71	16	75	12.94
1	31	20	24	20	0.686
2	28	33	20	30	1.463
3	24	25	20	15	0.68
4 × 10	26	25	20	30	1.26
4 × 7 × 10	28	35	32	40	1.54
5	12	0	10	15	1.21

Table 7. A Comparison of the Frequency of Reactivity with Monoclonal Antibody 83S19.23 in Rheumatic and Nonrheumatic Individuals from Various Geographical Areas

Subjects	No. pts. pos./total	Frequency (%)
Rheumatics		
New Delhi and Chandigarh	13/22	59.1
New Mexico	30.39	76.9
New York	17/23	74.0
Nonrheumatics		
New Delhi and Chandigarh	3/18	16.6
New Mexico	5/30	16.6
New York	3/15	20.0

clear relationship to any of the known B-cell DR or DR-like antigens was apparent. Subsequently, studies by our group have shown that a similar segregation for alloantigen 883 exists for rheumatic heart disease within a comparable population in New Mexico. Comparative data showing the relative population 883 typing results for New York, Bogota, Colombia, and New Mexico are shown in Table 7. These data appear to indicate a high correlation or relative segregation for acute rheumatic fever and presence of B-cell alloantigen 883.

Subsequent to this initial work recorded by Patarroyo *et al.* (1979), several mouse monoclonal reagents have been developed that appear to have specifities identical to that of the original human alloantiserum 883 (Yeadon *et al.*, 1983). These mouse monoclonal reagents were developed using B cells from known positive and negative 883-typed rheumatic patients with subsequent cell fusion and generation of multiple clones of antibody-secreting cells. Of great interest during these experiments was the production of a second monoclonal antibody (256), which appeared to show high specificity for a second B-cell alloantigen that is also related to rheumatic heart disease. Many rheumatic heart disease patients who were negative for 883 appeared to be positive for 256. With B-cell typing using both 883 and 256 mouse monoclonals, 90–95% of patients with rheumatic heart disease were typed as positive. There appeared to be no overlap in the same individual for either alloantigen, and no subjects in either normal controls or rheumatic heart disease groups were positive for both 883 and 256 B-cell alloantigens. Representative data using both 883 and 256 monoclonal reagents are shown in Table 8. Considerably more work needs to be done using these reagents in attempts to define whether or not a clear DR-like specificity is being detected and, secondly, whether the 883 and 256 specificities can be shown to be have clear genetically understandable distributions in family studies. These studies of kindreds are now under way.

The finding of a clear association between 883 and 256 typing and the occurrence of rheumatic heart disease stands in sharp contrast to the negative or discrepant studies previously published that attempted to ascertain whether in fact there was any clear correlation between genetic of family studies, HLA or HLB typing, and rheumatic in-

Table 8. A Comparison of the Original 883⁺ Rheumatics with Hybridoma Clones 83S19.23 and 256S10

Subjects	883[a]	83S19.23[b]	256S10[c]
883^+ rheumatics (10)	10/10[d]	9/10	0/10
Normals	1/10	1/10	2/10

[a] Original multiparous 883^+ serum used by Patarroyo.
[b] Hybridoma clone isolated from animals immunized with B cells from 883^+ rheumatics.
[c] Hybridoma clone isolated from animals immunized with B cells from 883^- rheumatics.
[d] Assay by both immunofluorescence and cytotoxicity assays.

volvement (Wilson and Schweiter, 1954; Ward *et al.*, 1976; Falk *et al.*, 1973; Read *et al.*, 1977). Very little if any uniform agreement was recorded by a series of workers who had previously examined this question. Moreover, previous studies of identical twins had also failed to record a clearly defined genetic predisposition towards development of rheumatic heart disease (Taranta *et al.*, 1961). In view of the recent findings concerning 883 and 256 typing, the studies of additional twins need to be extended and examined independently.

Considerably more work is now needed to define the relationship between 883/256 B-cell alloantigens and the host reponse to streptococcal disease, in particular to development of rheumatic fever and various patterns of disease expression of rheumatic heart disease throughout the world.

VII. EXPERIMENTAL MODELS OF ACUTE RHEUMATIC FEVER AND RHEUMATIC HEART DISEASE

Much of the early work related to attempts to understand the pathogenesis of acute rheumatic fever was carried out by Murphy (1964) using rabbits as the main experimental animal (Murphy and Swift, 1950). Repeated injection along with infection of animals with group A streptococci appeared to induce rheumaticlike lesions in both rabbits and mice (Murphy, 1964). No extensive attempts to repeat or confirm this work were then carried out. In 1966, Cromartie and Craddock (1966) reported that pathological lesions involving the heart, joints, and other connective tissue structures could be induced using a single intraperitoneal injection of streptococcal mucopeptide in mice. The cardiac pathology of this particular murine model was extremely similar to that observed in human rheumatic diseases. Extension of work using this mouse model indicated that the inflammatory changes induced in connective structures might be directly related to lack of ready biodegradability of much of the original group A streptococcal antigen injected (Cromartie *et al.*, 1977; Schwab, 1965; Ohanian *et al.*, 1969).

Recently, experimental results reported by Dos Reis and coworkers (Dos Reis and Barcinski, 1980; Dos Reis *et al.*, 1982), again using parenteral sensitization with various streptococcal antigens, have clearly defined what appears to be a critical role for macrophages and presumably the Ia antigens expressed on these antigen-processing cells in the generation of initial antistreptococcal immune responsiveness and subsequent direct cell-mediated cytotoxic or T-cell-mediated immunity capable of inducing lesions within the myocardium and other cardiac structures. Cells obtained from mice injected with extracts of group A streptococci were capable of inducing heart lesions when transferred to syngeneic recipients. In addition, streptococcal-antigen-pulsed macrophages were also able to induce heart lesions when injected into syngeneic recipients. Peritoneal macrophages pulsed with streptococcal extract were able to induce specific immune responsiveness to cardiac tissue antigen extracts. Control observations indicated no similar findings if macrophages were pulsed with group G streptococcal extracts.

The findings using this latest mouse model and various inbred, clearly defined mouse strains indicate the central importance of macrophage antigen processing and subsequent antigenic presentation to the development of T-cell immune reactivity showing cross reactivity with cardiac tissues. In this respect, our recent findings related to 883/256 B-cell allospecifities and the rheumatic process take on additional interest. It would therefore appear to be of particular importance to study macrophage functions and Ia or DR-like expression of potential antigen-processing cells within the human pharynx or in human tonsillar tissues. The potential importance of the small population of dendritic antigen-processing cells in this anatomic location also would be important to define. Studies in animals have already established that cardiac tissues, for reasons that are not at all clear from a teleological standpoint, are relatively enriched in the so-called dendritic-cell population (Hart and Fabre, 1981).

An experimental model that also appears to provide some promise in deciphering some of the sequence of events occurring in rheumatic fever has been described by Anand and coworkers using repeated and sometimes prolonged immunizations of rhesus monkeys with group A streptococcal membranes (Anand *et al.*, 1983b). Studies using this interesting primate model have indicated that animals repeatedly sensitized with group A streptococcal membranes rapidly develop cross-reacting heart-reactive antibody that stains marginal sarcolemmal membranes of both monkey and human hearts. Somewhat disappointing in this primate model are the relative rarity of distinct cardiac or myocardial granulomata after the long course of parenteral group A membrane sensitization and the apparent absence of well-defined or progressive valvular lesions and valvular deformities. Concurrent sensitization of monkeys with group A polysaccharides or with other glycoprotein fractions might possibly extend the spectrum of primate lesions observed after streptococcal product immunization. At the present time, we are examining this monkey model in collaboration with Dr. Ganguly and the group at Chandigarh in India using antihuman 883/256 B-cell monoclonal typing alloantisera, which appear to cross react with rhesus monkey B-cell antigens. Thus far, induction of gross granulomatous lesions in these rhesus animals has been disappointingly slight. The eventual production of chronic myocarditis or valvular deformities using this primate model may require long-term or intermittent sensitization as well as pharyngeal infection as an entry point for the streptococcal antigens.

Final understanding of the ways in which group A streptococcal throat infection induces acute rheumatic fever in the affected human host still awaits further analysis. There are many fascinating, potentially critical areas of interaction between the group A streptococcus and the patient that may indeed play a key role in deciding whether an ordinary pharyngeal infection with β-hemolytic streptococcus will eventually induce acute rheumatic fever. Some of the most important possibilities at the present time include: (1) Specific antigenic or surface-modulating characteristics that are unique for their ability to induce the rheumatic syndrome; (2) Specific adherence qualities or relative stickiness between selected strains of streptococci and either pharyngeal epithelial cells or macrophage/dendritic cells; (3) Genetically determined factors that govern basic human responses to critical cross-reactive antigens within infecting streptococci; and (4) Other factors including extracellular streptococcal products or even streptococcal-associated phage material that could profoundly influence the immune response or the host tissue reaction to injury. Which of these particular features will prove to be the most important in determining the actual clinical course or expression of rheumatic fever and eventual rheumatic heart disease remains for future work to determine. Certainly, the study of the streptococcus and its intimate, longstanding relationship with mankind provides a stimulating area for future work.

REFERENCES

Abdin, Z. H., and Eissa, A., 1965, Rheumatic fever and rheumatic heart disease in children below the age of 5 years in the tropics, *Ann. Rheum. Dis.* **24**:389–391.

American Heart Association Committee Report, 1965, Jones criteria (revised) for guidance in the diagnosis of rheumatic fever, *Circulation* **32**:664–680.

Anand, I. S., Ganguly, N. K., Khanna, A. K., Rissam, H. S., and Wahi, P. L., 1983a, Specificity of cellular reactivity to streptococcal membrane antigen in rheumatic heart disease, *Indian J. Med. Res.* **77**:213–218.

Anand, I. S., Ganguly, N. K., Khanna, A. K., Chakravarti, R. N., and Wahi, P. L., 1983b, Pathogenesis of immune-mediated carditis in monkeys, in: *Advances in Myocardiology*, Vol. 4 (E. Chazov, V. Saks, and G. Rona, eds.), Plenum Press, New York, pp. 215–226.

Anderson, H. C., and McCarty, M., 1950, Determination of C-reactive protein in the blood as a measure of the activity of the disease process in acute rheumatic fever, *Am. J. Med.* **8**:445–455.

Anderson, H. C., Kunkel, H. G., and McCarty, M., 1948, Quantitative antistreptokinase studies in patients infected with group A hemolytic streptococci: A comparison with serum antistreptolysin and gamma globulin levels with special reference to the occurrence of rheumatic fever, *J. Clin. Invest.* **27**:425–434.

Ash, R., 1942, Cardiac signs of rheumatic infection of childhood, *Am. J. Dis. Child.* **63**:1–14.

Ayoub, E. M., Taranta, A., and Bartley, T. D., 1974, Effect of valvular surgery on antibody to the group A streptococcal carbohydrate, *Circulation* **50**:144–150.

Ayuthya, P. S. N., Ratanabanagkoon, K., and Pongpanich, B., 1976, Juvenile rheumatic fever and rheumatic heart disease at Rhamathibodi Hospital, Thailand, *Southeast Asian J. Trop. Med. Public Health* **7**:77–80.

Baker, P. J., Stashak, P. N., Amsbaugh, D. F., Prescott, B., and Barth, R. F., 1970, Evidence for the existence of two functionally distinct types of cells which regulate the antibody response to type III pneumococcal polysaccharide, *J. Immunol.* **105**:1581–1583.

Beachey, E. H., Chiang, E. T., Seyer, J. M., Kang, A. H., Chiang, T. M., and Stollerman, G. H., 1977, Separation of type specific M protein from toxic cross-reactive antigens of group A streptococci, *Trans. Assoc. Am. Physicians* **90**:390–400.

Beachey, E. H., Seyer, J. M., and Kang, A. H., 1980, Primary structure of protective antigens of type 24 streptococcal M protein, *J. Biol. Chem.* **255**:6284–6289.

Becker, C. G., and Murphy, G. E., 1969, Demonstration of contractile protein in endothelium and cells of the heart valves, endocardium, intima, arteriosclerotic plaques, and Aschoff bodies of rheumatic heart disease, *Am. J. Pathol.* **55**:1–37.

Berry, J. N., 1972, Prevalence survey for chronic rheumatic heart disease and rheumatic fever in Northern India, *Br. Heart J.* **34**:143–149.

Bisno, A. L., Pearce, I. A., Wall, H. P., Moody, M. D., and Stollerman, G. H., 1970, Contrasting epidemiology of acute rheumatic fever and acute glomerulonephritis. Nature of the antecedent streptococcal infection, *N. Engl. J. Med.* **283**:561–565.

Bisno, A. L., Pearce, I. A., and Stollerman, G. H., 1977, Streptococcal infections that fail to cause recurrences of rheumatic fever, *J. Infect. Dis.* **156**:278–285.

Brown, E. J., Hosea, S. W., and Frank, M. M., 1981, The role of the spleen in experimental pneumococcal bacteremia, *J. Clin. Invest.* **67**:975–982.

Catanzaro, F. J., Rammelkamp, C. H., Jr., and Chamovitz, R., 1958, Prevention of rheumatic fever by treatment of streptococcal infections. II. Factors responsible for failures, *N. Engl. J. Med.* **259**:51–62.

Cromartie, W. J., and Craddock, J. G., 1966, Rheumatic-like cardiac lesions in mice, *Science* **154**:285–287.

Cromartie, W. J., Craddock, J. G., Schwab, J. H., Anderle, S. K., and Yang, C., 1977, Arthritis in rats after systemic injection of streptococcal cells or cell walls. *J. Exp. Med.* **146**:1585–1602.

Cudkowicz, G., Shearer, G. M., and Ito, T., 1978, Cellular differentiation of the immune system of mice. VI. Strain differences in class differentiation and other properties of marrow cells, *J. Exp. Med.* **148**:466–483.

Dale, J. B., and Beachey, E. H., 1982, Protective antigenic determinant of streptococcal M protein shared with sarcolemmal membrane protein of human heart, *J. Exp. Med.* **156**:1165–1176.

Dale, J. B., Seyer, J. M., and Beachey, E. H., 1983, Type-specific immunogenicity of a chemically synthesized peptide fragment of type 5 streptococcal M protein, *J. Exp. Med.* **158**:1727–1732.

Danilova, T. A., 1966, An immunofluorescent study of the antigens of group A streptococcus and heart tissue from humans and experimental animals, *Fed. Proc.* **25**:1099–1102.

D'Arbela, P. G., Patel, A. K., and Somers, K., 1976, Juvenile rheumatic fever and rheumatic heart disease at Mulago Hospital, Kampala, Uganda: Some aspects of the pattern of the disease, *E. Afr. Med. J.* **51**:710–718.

DiSciascio, H., and Taranta, A., 1980, Rheumatic fever in children, *Am. Heart J.* **99**:635–658.

Doolittle, R. F., Hunkapiller, M. W., Hood, L. E., Devare, S. G., Robbins, K. C., Aaronson, S. A., and Antoniades, H. N., 1983, Simian sarcoma virus *onc* gene, v-sis, is derived from the gene (or genes) encoding a platelet-derived growth factor, *Science* **221**:275–276.

Dos Reis, G. A., and Barcinski, M. A., 1980, Role of macrophage-dependent determinant selection in induction phase of streptococcal carditis, *Lancet* **2**:777–779.

Dos Reis, G. A., Gaspar, M. I. G., and Barcinski, M. A., 1982, Immune recognition in the streptococcal carditis of mice: The role of macrophages in the generation of heart-reactive lymphocytes, *J. Immunol.* **128**:1514–1521.

Dudding, B. A., and Ayoub, E. M., 1968, Persistence of streptococcal group A antibody in patients with rheumatic valvular disease, *J. Exp. Med.* **128**:1081–1098.

Dulbecco, R., Unger, M., Bologna, M., Bettifora, H., Syka, P., and Okada, S., 1981, Cross-reactivity between Thy-1 and a component of intermediate filaments demonstrated using a monoclonal antibody, *Nature* **292**:772–774.

Engle, M. A., McCabe, J. C., Ebert, P. A., and Zabriskie, J. B., 1974, The postpericardiotomy syndrome and anti-heart antibodies, *Circulation* **49**:401–406.

Falk, J. Z., Fleischman, J. L., Zabriskie, J. B., and Falk, R. E., 1973, A study of HLA antigen phenotype in rheumatic fever and rheumatic heart disease patients, *Tissue Antigens* **3**:173–178.

Fiedel, B. A., and Gerwurz, H., 1976, Effects of C-reactive protein on platelet function. I. Inhibition of platelet aggregation and release reactions, *J. Immunol.* **116**:1289–1294.

Finne, J., Leinonen, M., and Makela, P. H., 1983, Antigenic similarities between brain components and bacteria causing meningitis. Implications for vaccine development and pathogenesis, *Lancet* **2**:355–357.

Friedberg, C. K., and Gross, L., 1936, Pericardial lesions in rheumatic fever, *Pathology* **12**:183–203.

Fujinami, R. S., Oldstone, M. B. A., Wroblewska, Z., Frankel, M. E., and Korpowski, H., 1983, Molecular mimicry in virus infection: Cross-reaction of measles virus phosphoprotein or of herpes simplex virus protein with human intermediate filaments, *Proc. Natl. Acad. Sci. U.S.A.* **80**:2346–2350.

Ganguly, N. K., Anand, I. S., Khanna, A. K., Kohli, R. S., and Wahi, P. L., 1982, T cells and T cell subsets in rheumatic heart disease, *Indian J. Med. Res.* **76**:854–858.

Gerwurz, H., Mold, C., Siegel, J., and Fiedel, B., 1982, C-reactive protein and the acute-phase response, *Adv. Intern. Med.* **27**:343–371.

Gibbons, R. J., and van Houte, J., 1971, Selective bacterial adherence to oral epithelial surfaces and its role as an ecological determinant, *Infect. Immun.* **3**:567–573.

Gimeno, A. L., Gimeno, M. F., Sterin-Borda, L., Cossio, D. M., Sterin-Speziale, N., Diez, C., Seara, S. M., and Arana, R. M., 1979, Altered inotropic and chronotropic effects of nor-adrenaline on isolated rat atria exposed to chagasic sera. Influences of cocaine, normetanephrine and U-0521 (3'-4'-dihydroxy-2-methyl propiophenome), *Cardiovasc. Res.* **13**:723–731.

Goldstein, I., Halpern, B., and Robert, L., 1967, Immunological relationship between steptococcus A polysaccharide and the structural glycoproteins of heart valve, *Nature* **213:**44–47.

Goldstein, I., Rebeyrotte, P., Parlebas, J., and Halpern, B., 1968, Isolation from heart valves of glycopeptides which share immunological properties with *Streptococcus haemolyticus* group A polysaccharides, *Nature* **219:**866–868.

Gordis, L., Lilenfeld, A., and Rodriguez, R., 1969, Studies in the epidemiology and preventability of rheumatic fever. I. Demographic factors and the incidence of acute attacks, *J. Chron. Dis.* **21:**665–666.

Gowrishankar, R., and Agarwal, S. C., 1980, Leucocyte migration inhibition with human heart valve glycoproteins and group A streptococcal ribonucleic acid proteins in rheumatic heart disease and post streptococcal glomerulonephritis, *Clin. Exp. Immunol.* **39:**519–525.

Hart, D. N. J., and Fabre, J. W., 1981, Demonstration and characterization of Ia-positive dendritic cells in the interstitial connective tissues of rat heart and other tissues, but not brain, *J. Exp. Med.* **153:**347–361.

Hassell, T. A., and Stuart, K. I., 1974, Rheumatic fever, a three-year study, *Br. Med. J.* **2:**39–40.

Husby, G., van de Rijn, I., Zabriskie, J. B., Abdin, Z. H., and Williams, R. C., Jr., 1976, Antibodies reacting with cytoplasma of subthalamic and caudate nuclei neurons on chorea and acute rheumatic fever, *J. Exp. Med.* **144:**1094–1110.

Kaplan, E. L., Dudding, B. A., Top, R. H., and Wannamaker, L. W., 1971, Diagnosis of streptococcal pharyngitis: Differentiation of active infection from the carrier state in the symptomatic child, *J. Infect. Dis.* **123:**490–501.

Kaplan, M. H., 1962, An immunological cross-reaction between group A streptococcal cells and human heart tissue, *Lancet* **1:**706–710.

Kaplan, M. H., 1963, Immunologic relation of streptococcal tissue and antigens. I. Properties of an antigen in certain strains of group A streptococci exhibiting an immunologic cross-reaction with human heart tissue, *J. Immunol.* **90:**595–606.

Kaplan, M. H., and Meyerserian, M., 1962, Immunologic studies of heart tissue. V. Antigens related to heart tissue revealed by cross-reaction of rabbit antisera to heterologous heart, *J. Immunol.* **88:**450–461.

Kaplan, M. H., and Svec, K. H., 1964, Immunologic relation of streptococcal and tissue antigens. III. Presence in human sera of streptococcal antibody cross-reactive with heart tissue, *J. Exp. Med.* **119:**651–666.

Kaplan, M. H., and Volanakis, J. E., 1974, Interaction of C-reactive protein complexes with the complement system. I. Consumption of human complement associated with the reaction of C-reactive protein with pneumococcal C-polysaccharide and the choline phosphatides lecithin and sphingomyelin, *J. Immunol.* **112:**2135–2147.

Kasp-Grochowska, E., and Kingston, D., 1977, Streptococcal cross-reacting antigen and the bundle of His, *Clin. Exp. Immunol.* **27:**63–65.

Kawakita, S., Takeuchi, T., Uemura, Y., Onishi, T., Saito, K., Nagami, H., Watanabe, T., and Watanabe, T., 1976, Group A streptococcal infections as related to rheumatic fever, *Jpn. Heart J.* **17:**592–598.

Kennedy, H. L., and Das, S. K., 1976, Postmyocardial infarction (Dressler's) syndrome: Report of a case with immunological and viral studies, *Am. Heart J.* **91:**233–239.

Kingston, D., and Glynn, L. E., 1976, Antistreptococcal antibodies reacting with brain tissue. I. Immunofluorescent studies, *Br. J. Exp. Pathol.* **57:**114–128.

Koberle, F., 1974, Pathogenesis of Chagas' disease, *Ciba Found. Symp.* **20:**137–197.

Kushner, I., 1982, The phenomenon of the acute phase response, *Ann. N.Y. Acad. Sci.* **389:**39–48.

Kushner, I., and Kaplan, M. H., 1961, Studies of acute phase protein. I. An immunohistochemical method for the localization of C-reactive protein in rabbits. Association with necrosis in local inflammatory lesions, *J. Exp. Med.* **114:**961–974.

Le Roith, D., Shiloach, J., Roth, J., and Lesniak, M. A., 1980, Evolutionary origins of vertebrate hormones: Substances similar to mammalian insulins are native to unicellular eukaryotes, *Proc. Natl. Acad. Sci. U.S.A.* **77:**6184–6186.

Lessof, M., 1958, Sydenham's chorea, *Guy's Hosp. Rep.* **107:**185–206.

Lue, H.-C., Chen, C. M., Hsu, J. Y., Chen, C. I., and Wei, H. Y., 1975, Prevalence of rheumatic heart disease in the young in Northern Taiwan, *Jpn. Circ. J.* **39:**188.

Lue, H.-C., Chen, C.-L., Wei, H., Okuni, M., Mabilangan, L. M., Dharmasakti, D., and Hanafiah, A., 1979, The natural history of rheumatic fever and rheumatic heart disease in the orient, *Jpn. Heart J.* **20:**237–252.

Lueker, R. D., Abdin, Z. H., and Williams, R. C., Jr., 1975, Peripheral blood T and B lymphocytes during acute rheumatic fever, *J. Clin. Invest.* **55:**975–985.

Lyampert, I. M., Vedenskaya, O. L., and Danilova, T. A., 1966, Study on streptococcus group A antigens common with heart-tissue elements, *Immunology* **11**:313–320.

Lyampert, I. M., Beletskaya, L. V., Borodiyuk, N. A., Gnezditskaya, E. V., and Rassokhina, I. I., 1976, Autoantibodies against the common antigenic determinant of group A streptococcal polysaccharide and epithelial cells of mammalian thymus and skin, *Bull. Exp. Biol. Med.* **81**:712–715.

MacLeod, C. M., and Avery, O. T., 1982, The occurrence during acute infections of a protein not normally present in the blood. II. Isolation and properties of the reactive protein, *J. Exp. Med.* **73**:183–190.

McCabe, J. C., Ebert, P. S., Engle, M. A., and Zabriskie, J. B., 1973, Circulating heart-reactive antibodies in the postpericardiotomy syndrome, *J. Surg. Res.* **14**:158–168.

Massel, B. F., Mote, J. R., and Jones, T. D., 1937, The artificial induction of subcutaneous nodules in patients with rheumatic fever, *J. Clin. Invest.* **16**:125–128.

Murphy, G. E., 1964, Experimental and histological investigation of the nature of rheumatic heart disease, in: *The Streptococcus, Rheumatic Fever and Glomerulonephritis* (J. Uhr, ed.), Williams & Wilkins, Baltimore, pp. 209–237.

Murphy, G. E., and Swift, H. F., 1950, The induction of rheumatic-like cardiac lesions in rabbits by repeated focal infections with group A streptococci; comparison with the cardiac lesions of serum disease, *J. Exp. Med.* **91**:485–498.

Nakhla, L. S., and Glynn, L. E., 1967, Studies on the antigen in β-hemolytic streptococci that cross-reacts with an antigen in human myocardium, *Immunology* **13**:209–218.

Ohanian, S. H., Schwab, J. H., and Cromartie, W. J., 1969, Relation of rheumatic-like lesions of the mouse to localization of group A streptococcal cell walls, *J. Exp. Med.* **129**:37–49.

Padmavati, S., 1978, Rheumatic fever and rheumatic heart disease in developing countries, *Bull. WHO* **56**:543–550.

Patarroyo, M. E., Winchester, R. J., Vejerano, A., Gibofsky, A., Chalem, F., Zabriskie, J. B., and Kunkel, H. G., 1979, Association of a B-cell alloantigen with susceptibility to rheumatic fever, *Nature* **278**:173–174.

Persellin, S. T., Ramirez, G., and Moatamed, F., 1982, Immunopathology of rheumatic pericarditis, *Arthritis Rheum.* **25**:1054–1058.

Poon-King, T., Potter, E. V., Svartman, M., and Mohammed, I., 1973, Epidemic acute nephritis with reappearance of M-type 55 streptococci in Trinidad, *Lancet* **1**:475–479.

Potter, E. V., Svartman, M., Burt, E. G., Finklea, J. F., Poon-King, T., and Earle, D. P., 1972, Relationship between acute rheumatic fever to acute glomerulonephritis in Trinidad, *J. Infect. Dis.* **125**:619–625.

Potter, E. V., Svartman, M., Mohammed, I., Cox, R., Poon-King, T., and Earle, D. P., 1978, Tropical acute rheumatic fever and associated streptococcal infections compared with concurrent endemic and early epidemic acute glomerulonephritis, *J. Pediatr.* **92**:325–333.

Raizada, V., Williams, R. C., Jr., Chopra, P., Gopinath, N., Prakash, K., Sharma, K. B., Cherian, K. M., Panday, S., Arora, R., Nigam, M., Zabriskie, J. B., and Husby, G., 1983, Tissue distribution of lymphocytes in rheumatic heart valves as defined by monoclonal and anti-T cell antibodies, *Am. J. Med.* **74**:90–96.

Read, S. E., Fischetti, V. A., Utermohlen, V., Falk, R. E., and Zabriskie, J. B., 1974, Cellular activity studies to streptococcal infections and rheumatic fever, *J. Clin. Invest.* **54**:439–450.

Read, S. E., Reid, H., Poon-King, T., Fischetti, V. A., Zabriskie, J. B., and Rapaport, F. T., 1977, HLA and predisposition to the nonsuppurative sequelae of group A streptococcal infections, *Transplant. Proc.* **9**:543–546.

Reed, W. P., Selinger, D. S., Albright, E. L., Abdin, Z. H., and Williams, R. C., Jr., 1980, Streptococcal adherence to pharyngeal cells of Egyptian children with acute rheumatic fever, *J. Infect. Dis.* **142**:803–810.

Rosenstein, B., 1973, Streptococcal infections and their control in the inner city: The Sinai–Druid, Baltimore experience, *Connecticut Med.* **37**:8–10.

Roth, J., Le Roith, D., Shiloach, J., Rosenzweig, J. L., Lesniak, M. A., and Havrankova, J., 1982, The evolutionary origins of hormones, neurotransmitters, and other extracellular chemical messengers: Implications for mammalian biology, *N. Engl. J. Med.* **306**:523–527.

Santos-Buch, C. A., and Teixeira, A. R. L., 1974, The immunology of experimental Chagas' disease. III. Rejection of allogeneic heart cells *in vitro*, *J. Exp. Med.* **140**:38–53.

Sapru, R. P., Ganguly, N. K., Sharma, S., Chandani, R. E., and Gupta, A. K., 1977, Cellular reaction to group A beta-haemolytic streptococcal membrane antigen and its relation to complement levels in patients with rheumatic heart disease, *Br. Med. J.* **2**:422–424.

Schwab, J. H., 1965, Biological properties of streptococcal cell-wall particles. I. Determinants of the chronic nodular lesions of connective tissue, *J. Bacteriol.* **90**:1405–1411.

Selinger, D. S., Julie, N., Reed, W. P., and Williams, R. C., Jr., 1978, Adherence of group A streptococci to pharyngeal cells: A role in the pathogenesis of rheumatic fever, *Science* **201**:455–457.

Shaper, A. G., 1972, Cardiovascular disease in the tropics. I. Rheumatic heart, *Br. Med. J.* **3**:683–686.

Shearer, G. M., Cudkowicz, G., Connell, M. S. J., and Priore, R. L., 1968, Cellular differentiation of the immune system of mice. I. Separate splenic antigen-sensitive units for different types of anti-sheep antibody-forming cells, *J. Exp. Med.* **128**:437–457.

Sheld, W. M., Valone, J. A., and Sande, M. A., 1978, Bacterial adherence in the pathogenesis of endocarditis. Interaction of bacterial dextran, platelets, and fibrin, *J. Clin. Invest.* **61**:1394–1404.

Shrestha, N. K., and Padmavati, S., 1979, Prevalence of rheumatic heart disease in Delhi school children, *Indian J. Med. Res.* **69**:821–833.

Siegel, J., Osmand, A. P., Wilson, M. F., and Gewurz, H., 1975, Interactions of C-reactive protein with the complement system. II. C-reactive protein-mediated consumption of complement by poly-L-lysine polymers and other polycations, *J. Exp. Med.* **142**:709–721.

Snary, D., Flint, J., Wood, J. N., Scott, M. T., Chapman, M. D., Dodd, J., Jessell, T. M., and Miles, M. A., 1983, A monoclonal antibody with specificity for *Trypanosoma cruzi,* central and peripheral neurones and glia, *Clin. Exp. Immunol.* **54**:617–624.

Sterin-Borda, L., Cossio, D. M., Gimeno, A. L., Diez, C., Laguens, R. P., Meckert, P. C., and Arana, R. M., 1976, Effect of chagasic sera in rat isolated atrial preparations: Immunological, morphological and functional aspects, *Cardiovasc. Res.* **10**:613–622.

Stollerman, G., 1960, Factors that predispose to rheumatic fever, *Med. Clin. North Am.*, **44**:17–28.

Stollerman, G. H., 1971, Rheumatogenic and nephritogenic streptococci, *Circulation* **43**:915–921.

Stollerman, G. H., Rusoff, J. H., and Hirschfeld, I., 1955, Prophylaxis against group A steptococci in rheumatic fever. The use of single monthly injections of benzathine penicillin G, *N. Engl. J. Med.* **252**:787–792.

Stollerman, G. H., Lewis, A. J., Schultz, I., and Taranta, A., 1956, Relationship of immune response to group A streptococci to the course of acute, chronic and recurrent rheumatic fever, *Am. J. Med.* **20**:163–169.

Stollerman, G. H., Markowitz, M., Taranta, A., Wannamaker, L. W., and Whittermore, R., 1965, Jones criteria (revised) for guidance in the diagnosis of rheumatic fever, *Circulation* **32**:664–668.

Strasser, T., 1978, Rheumatic fever and rheumatic heart disease in the 1970s, *WHO Chron.* **32**:18–25.

Svartman, M., Potter, E. V., Poon-King, T., and Earle, D. P., 1975a, Salivary immunoglobulins and streptococcal antibodies in patients with acute rheumatic fever, *J. Lab. Clin. Med.* **85**:1013–1021.

Svartman, M., Potter, E. V., Poon-King, T., and Mohammed, I., 1975b, Immunoglobulin and complement components in synovial fluid of patients with acute rheumatic fever, *J. Clin. Invest.* **56**:111–117.

Sydenham, T., 1740, *Schedula Monitoria de Novae Febris,* reprinted 1805, Opera Universa, London, Heppin-Stall, p. 495, (trans. J. Pechey), pp. 417–419, 11th ed., R. Ware, London.

Taranta, A., and Stollerman, G. H., 1956, The relationship of Sydenham's chorea to infection with group A streptococci, *Am. J. Med.* **20**:170–175.

Taranta, A., Torosday, S., Metrakos, J., Jegier, W., and Uchida, I., 1961, Rheumatic fever in monozygotic and dizygotic twins, in: *Proceedings of the Tenth International Congress of Rheumatology,* Minerva Medica, Turin, pp. 96–98.

Thomas, G. T., Besterman, E. M. M., and Holman, A., 1956, Rheumatic pericarditis, *Am. Heart J.* **52**:29–36.

Tillet, W. S., and Francis, T., Jr., 1930, Serological reactions in pneumonia with a non-protein fraction from pheumococcus, *J. Exp. Med.* **52**:561–571.

Tompkins, R. K., Burnes, D. C., and Cable, W. E., 1977, An analysis of the cost-effectiveness of pharyngitis management and acute rheumatic fever prevention, *Ann. Intern. Med.* **86**:481–492.

van de Rijn, I., Zabriskie, J. B., and McCarty, M., 1977, Group A streptococcal antigens cross-reactive with myocardium. Purification of heart-reactive antibody and isolation and characterization of the streptococcal antigen, *J. Exp. Med.* **146**:579–599.

van de Rijn, I., Fillit, H., Brandeis, W. E., Reid, H., Poon-King, T., McCarty, M., Day, N. K., and Zabriskie, J. B., 1978, Serial studies on circulating immune complexes in post-streptococcal sequelae, *Clin. Exp. Immunol.* **34**:318–325.

Villarreal, H., Jr., Fischetti, V. A., van de Rijn, I., and Zabriskie, J. B., 1980, Observations on an extracellular protein unique to nephritogenic streptococci, in: *Streptococcal Diseases and the Immune Response* (S. E. Read and J. B. Zabriskie, eds.), Academic Press, New York, pp. 181–198.

Virmani, R., and Roberts, W. C., 1977, Aschoff bodies in operatively excised atrial appendages and in papillary muscles. Frequency and clinical significance, *Circulation* **55**:559–563.

Volanakis, J. E., and Narkates, A. J., 1981, Interaction of C-reactive protein with artificial phosphatidylcholine bilayers and complement, *J. Immunol.* **126**:1820–1825.

Wannamaker, L. W., 1959, The paradox of antibody response to streptodornase. The usefulness of antidesoxyribonuclease B as an indication of streptococcal infection in patients with acute rheumatic fever, *Am. J. Med.* **27**:567–574.

Wannamaker, L. W., 1973, The chain that links the heart to the throat, *Circulation* **48**:9–18.

Wannamaker, L. W., 1976, A penicillin shot without culturing the child's throat, *JAMA* **235**:913–914.

Ward, C., Gelsthorpe, K., Doughty, R. W., and Hardisty, C. A., 1976, HLA antigens and acquired valvular heart disease, *Tissue Antigens* **7**:227–231.

Williams, R. C., Jr., Walker, L. C., Kassaby, M., Mahros, R., Hassaballa, F., Abdin, Z. H., and Tung, K. S. K., 1976, Circulating immune complexes in acute rheumatic fever, *J. Lab. Clin. Immunol.* **2**:185–190.

Williams, R. C., Jr., Zabriskie, J. B., Mahros, F., Hassaballa, F., and Abdin, Z. H., 1977, Lymphocyte surface markers in acute rheumatic fever and post streptococcal glomerulonephritis, *Clin. Exp. Immunol.* **27**:135–142.

Williams, R. C., Jr., Kilpatrick, K. A., Kassaby, M., and Abdin, Z. H., 1978, Lymphocytes binding C-reactive protein during acute rheumatic fever, *J. Clin. Invest.* **61**:1384–1393.

Williams, R. C., Jr., Husby, G., Wedege, E., Walker, L. C., and Tung, K. S. K., 1980a, Antigen-binding cells, C-reactive protein, antineuronal antibodies and immunocomplexes in acute rheumatic fever, in: *Streptococcal Diseases and Their Immune Response* (J. B. Zabriskie and S. E. Read, eds.), Academic Press, New York, pp. 695–714.

Williams, R. C., Jr., van de Rijn, I., Mahros, F., Abdin, Z. H., Reid, H., and Poon-King, T., 1980b, Lymphocytes binding C-reactive protein and streptococcal membranes in acute rheumatic fever, *J. Lab. Clin. Med.* **96**:803–814.

Williams, R. C., Jr., Raizada, V., Prakash, K., van de Rijn, I., Zabriskie, J. B., Stobo, J. D., and Sharma, K. B., 1982, Changes in T-lymphocyte subsets during acute rheumatic fever, *J. Clin. Immunol.* **2**:166–172.

Wilson, M. G., and Schweitzer, M., 1954, Pattern of hereditary susceptibility in rheumatic fever, *Circulation* **10**:699–704.

Wood, H. F., Feinstein, A. R., Taranta, A., and Piersson, J. E., 1964, Rheumatic fever in children and adolescents: A long-term epidemiologic study of subsequent prophylaxis, streptococcal infections, and clinical sequelae: III. Comparative effectiveness of three prophalaxis regimens in preventing streptococcal infections and rheumatic recurrences, *Ann. Inter. Med.* **60**(Suppl. 5):31–46.

Wood, J. N., Hudson, L., Jessell, T. M., and Yamamoto, M., 1982, A monoclonal antibody defining antigenic determinants on subpopulations of mammalian neurones and *Trypanosoma cruzi* parasites, *Nature* **296**:34–38.

Wright, H. D., 1927, Experimental pneumococcal septicemia and antipneumococcal immunity, *J. Pathol. Bacteriol.* **30**:185–252.

Yang, L. C., Soprey, P. R., Wittner, M. K., and Fox, E. N., 1977, Streptococcal-induced cell-mediated immune destruction of cardiac myofibers *in vitro, J. Exp. Med.* **146**:344–360.

Yeadon, C., Buskirk, D., Lavanchy, D., Braun, D., Fotino, M., and Zabriskie, J. B., 1983, The B cell annoantigen 883. A marker for rheumatic fever (RF) susceptibility gene? Characterization by a monoclonal antibody, *Arthritis Rheum.* **26**:165.

Yoshinoya, S., and Pope, R. M., 1980, Detection of immune complexes in acute rheumatic fever and their relationship to HLA-B5, *J. Clin. Invest.* **65**:136–145.

Zabriskie, J. B., and Freimer, E. H., 1966, An immunological relationship between the group A streptococcus and mammalian muscle, *J. Exp. Med.* **124**:661–678.

Zabriskie, J. B., 1967, Mimetic relationships between group A streptococci and mammalian tissues, *Adv. Immunol.* **7**:147–188.

Zabriskie, J. B., Hsu, K. C., and Seegal, B. C., 1970, Heart-reactive antibody associated with rheumatic fever: characterization and diagnostic significance, *Clin. Exp. Immunol.* **7**:147–193.

Zabriskie, J. B., Read, S. E., and Ellis, R. J., 1971, Cellular and humoral studies in diseases with heart-reactive antibodies in: *Progress of Immunology* (A. Bernard, ed.), Academic Press, New York, pp. 213–229.

14

Infectious Agents in Rheumatic Diseases

Frank R. Schmid

I. INTRODUCTION

In contrast to our incomplete understanding of many of the rheumatic diseases, information is more abundant about the pathogenesis of those caused by recognized infectious agents. Yet even here, great gaps exist in our ability to identify the presence of these agents promptly and to cope with their virulence. More striking is our ignorance of the complex immune apparatus that the host invokes to counter their attack.

Nevertheless, considerable theoretical insight has been gained from our current knowledge of the means by which the infectious agent gains a foothold at a primary site of infection, enters the bloodstream, and finally colonizes a given bone, joint, or other connective tissue. The damage that is produced is the direct result of toxic factors released by the microorganism at the site of inflammation and to varying degrees is also the consequence of an accompanying immune response mounted by the host. Treatment is directed, therefore, toward microbial killing as well as toward removal of any antigenic material that persists. Once this is accomplished, the inflammatory process subsides, and further tissue damage is averted (Table 1).

Another type of joint inflammation occurs as a result of entrance into the host of the infectious agent at the primary site of infection but absence of at least viable forms of the agent in the joint, a so-called reactive arthritis. In this case, it is thought that the entire inflammatory process is caused by the host's response to a component of the microorganism. Treatment, of course, is directed toward eradication of the primary infection and, equally if not more vigorously, toward control of inflammation in the joint.

Frank R. Schmid • Department of Medicine, Section of Arthritis-Connective Tissue Diseases, Northwestern University Medical School, Chicago, Illinois 60611.

Table 1. Infectious Agents in Rheumatic Diseases

Disease state	Microorganism at primary site of infection	Microorganism in bone/joint or vessel	Pathogenesis of inflammation
Infectious arthritis Osteomyelitis	Yes	Viable microorganism Nonviable components of microorganism	Toxic products of microorganism Immune response to microorganism
Reactive arthritis	Yes	Not found[a]	Immune response to microorganism
Rheumatoid arthritis Lupus erythematosus Vasculitis	No	Not found[a]	Immune response to unknown stimulus (e.g., infectious agent)

[a] Nonviable microbial components detected in some animal models that mimic reactive form or rheumatoid arthritis. Hepatitis B components noted in some vasculitic lesions.

When one looks at the role of infectious agents in rheumatic disease in this way, several well characterized clinical entities can be viewed as special examples of reactive arthritis, particularly Reiter's syndrome, some of the spondyloarthropathies, and rheumatic fever. In some cases of infectious arthritis, particularly when all viable agents have been killed, the process in the joint resembles that seen in reactive arthritis, although the immune mechanisms may be different.

Finally, infectious agents, particularly viruses, continue to be sought in the chronic inflammatory syndromes of rheumatoid arthritis (Simpson *et al.*, 1984; Aho and Raunio, 1982), systemic lupus erythematosus, and vasculitis (Duffy *et al.*, 1976). Such an agent, were it to be found, could easily account for the major portion of the pathology so characteristic of these conditions.

In this chapter the pathogenesis and some relevant clinical applications are provided first about those rheumatic diseases in which infectious agents are the proven cause of the inflammatory reaction in the joint or bone. Then, except for rheumatic fever, which is covered elsewhere in this volume, a similar presentation is given for reactive arthritis. Bridging these two is a discussion of the contribution that nonviable antigenic fragments of microorganisms make toward inflammation, particularly where this has been worked out in selected animal models.

II. RHEUMATIC DISEASES CAUSED BY VIABLE MICROORGANISMS

A. Overview

Infection of the bone or joint begins in the metaphysis or synovium. Here bacteria and other microorganisms lodge, having traveled in the bloodstream from a distant primary site of infection. Their proliferation creates a small abscess that extends into the medullary canal of the bone to cause osteomyelitis or into the joint space from the bony cortex or synovium to cause septic arthritis (Schmid, 1985; Waldvogel *et al.*, 1970). Other modes of entry into the bone or joint are much less common. Direct penetration may occur from an injury, from contamination of an operative wound (Inman *et al.*, 1984), or from intraarticular injection.

In light of the many steps that are involved, it is indeed remarkable that successful hematogenous infection of the bone or joint occurs at all. Different components of the host's defense system must have had to be overcome and/or the virulence of the infecting agent must have been so great in order to permit microbial metastasis and propagation at a skeletal site far removed from the initial portal of entry. For example, gram-negative bacilli, which are frequent causes of bacteremia, are not usually associated with septic arthritis unless the patient has evidence of a major local or systemic flaw in his ability to fight infection (Goldenberg *et al.*, 1974).

Inflammation in septic arthritis or osteomyelitis results from the combined effects of toxic factors elaborated by viable microorganisms and of mediators generated by the immune response of the host. In the interval of days or weeks after the infection has developed at the primary site but before the bone or synovium is colonized, the normal host will have mounted an immune response that, although unable to control the spread of the infection, can still contribute to the inflammatory response (Manicourt and Orloff, 1982; Walker *et al.*, 1978). This response will include a variety of cellular and humoral mechanisms, among which are the production of antibody, complement activation, and phagocytic cell stimulation. Although geared toward the killing and removal of the infecting agent and its breakdown products, these also contribute to pain, swelling, and erythema within the bone and joint and later to tissue destruction and repair.

B. The Initial Extraarticular Microbial Infection

Most commonly, a site remote from the bone or joint becomes infected before the bone or joint itself. A contiguous infectious lesion can occasionally penetrate an adjacent synovial or osseous structure as, for example, when a peritoneal abscess extends into the hip joint or a diabetic foot ulcer into the metatarsal bone, but usually the microbes disseminate widely in the bloodstream to any part of the musculoskeletal system as well as to other tissues.

The primary site of infection, therefore, is usually found in the skin or mucous membranes—structures at the interface of the host with the environment. Frequent examples are the proliferation of staphylococci in skin abscesses; spirochetes of *Borrelia burgdorferi* in the lesion of erythema chronicum migrans or of *T. pallidum* in the genital chancre; gram-negative bacilli in a septic gallbladder or urinary bladder; gonococci in urethritis, cervicitis, proctitis, or pharyngitis; or opportunistic agents in the infected shunt of a patient on dialysis. Recognition of such a process either in the immediate past or currently active in a patient with bone or joint pathology is of cardinal importance to reinforce the suspicion of sepsis. Unfortunately, however, many patients lack a positive history or have no clinical evidence of a lesion; this is particularly the case in those in whom staphylococci or streptococci are the offending agents (Goldenberg and Cohen, 1976).

Latent infections, too, may be the source of seeding the bloodstream. These may have lain dormant for prolonged periods of time, as in some gonococcal infections in both male and female patients. When local factors such as menstruation intervene, then bacteremia follows (Eisenstein and Masi, 1981).

C. Bloodstream Invasion

Entry into the bloodstream by microbes from a primary site of infection is common; most are overcome by an effective reticuloendothelial system in the liver, spleen, and lung that traps and kills these pathogens. However, when the microbial bolus has favorable characteristics such as size or membrane constituents or when the host's defenses fail because of a genetic defect or are overwhelmed by sheer numbers of the invading microorganisms, then conditions develop in which sufficient numbers of pathogens can be present in the circulation of sufficiently long periods of time to allow microbial attachment to an endothelial surface and subsequent colonization.

It is unlikely that most microorganisms are controlled or killed within the bloodstream itself. What is required is sticking to and subsequent phagocytosis by endothelial or other lining cells such as macrophages to prevent lodgment, survival, and growth of microbes in the interstitial tissues beneath the endothelium in the synovium or Haversian canals.

D. Bone and Joint Colonization

Microbes that bind to endothelial or to basement membrane components of vessels may propagate and spread to initiate a synovial or bone infection. Factors that favor such colonization are not clear but must be related to local phenomena in a particular bone or joint since symptoms develop in only one or two locations (Argen *et al.*, 1966). In some cases, however, polyarthralgia of a migratory nature is noted instead of or preceding the more persistent involvement of one or a few joints (Brandt *et al.*, 1974). This clinical observation suggests that various types of colonization occur, most of which become contained or are aborted, but a few of which progress to a full-blown infection (Wehrbein, 1929).

In bone, the infection starts in the metaphyseal sinusoidal veins. This site is favored because the afferent limb of the metaphyseal capillary lacks phagocytic lining cells; the efferent limb frequently has multiple channels with a broad diameter so that blood flow becomes slow and more turbulent; and, furthermore, the capillary loops adjacent to the epiphyseal growth plate are nonanastomotic so that necrosis can more easily follow vascular thrombosis. In children, the metaphyseal infection does not cross the epiphyseal growth plate but spreads laterally, perforating the cortex to cause a subperiosteal abscess. In some joints such as the hip and shoulder, the synovial reflection reaches beyond this region so that infection penetrates directly into the joint from such an abscess. In the infant below age 1 and in the adult (Atcheson and Ward, 1978), capillaries perforate the region of the growth plate so that infection can spread through epiphysis into the joint.

Although any microbe that causes human disease can cause a bone and joint infection, a small number account for most of the cases: staphylococci in patients of all ages for both bone and joint infections, gonococci for joint infections, especially in the younger population, and, to a lesser extent, streptococci, *Hemophilus influenzae* in children below the age of 2, and gram-negative bacilli in debilitated hosts. Other agents such as *M. tuberculosus* and fungi are infrequent (Schmid, 1985).

Staphylococci and gonococci, which most commonly affect bone and synovium, are not the most common causes of clinical septicemia. Gram-negative bacilli are (Newman,

1976), but these do not invade osseous or synovial tissue as often and then usually only when these sites have been previously damaged or when the host has become immunocompromised. These observations suggest that some microorganisms enjoy a special affinity for skeletal structures.

Prior damage predisposes to successful invasion of a particular bone or joint. The rheumatoid joint (Kellgren *et al.*, 1958) or the joint in tophaceous gout is more readily infected. Gross trauma may create a hematoma or a structurally altered environment in which seeded microbes can propagate. The knee, which is the most common joint involved in sepsis, is also the most easily traumatized. Even microtrauma may be a factor, as in the occasional case in which an intraarticular needle injection is performed during a period of septicemia.

Gross contamination of a bone or joint by injury leads to direct infection. More subtle examples of direct rather than hematogenous colonization, however, occasionally occur and can be overlooked. Penetration by a foreign body such as a thorn or a nail may be forgotten and yet have been the means for introduction of sepsis. Therapeutic arthrocentesis, despite the frequency with which this procedure is done, is not a common cause of sepsis, and even such major procedures as total joint replacement by a prosthesis are responsible for infection in fewer than 1% of cases in centers in which the volume of this operation is large (Inman *et al.*, 1984).

Nevertheless, most cases of infectious arthritis or osteomyelitis are not associated with an obvious local predisposing factor. In these cases, one is forced to postulate an altered microvasculature and/or perivascular environment that favors the selection of a particular joint or bone over many other potential ones for the successful establishment of the infection.

E. Response of the Host's Defense Mechanisms

The normal host is well provided with mechanisms to recognize the presence of foreign agents as microbes, to distinguish them from indigenous tissue, and to destroy them. This represents a major mission of the multiple components of the immune system and its related effector cells and molecules.

The introduction of a new antigen into the host may activate the alternative complement pathway directly without the interposition of antibody (Greenblatt *et al.*, 1978), an effect that can destroy bacteria before the immune response begins or signs of inflammation have appeared. Without this activity, as in those individuals born without C3b inactivator and therefore with little usable C3, multiple pyogenic infections occur (Reed *et al.*, 1976). The same antigen can also be readily recognized by the macrophage–T-cell system, which then begins to trigger the chain of events that stimulates the host's normal immune response. In this response, additional lymphocytes modulate the degree to which clones of committed T and B cells proliferate and ultimately form specific antibodies. Humans undoubtedly differ one from another for this genetically regulated event, a feature that has been well established in animal models. Some animals react vigorously to specific microbes, others tardily or weakly. It is just such genetic programming that accounts in an as yet unexplained way for the development of a sterile reactive arthritis in patients exposed to gram-negative bacilli such as *Shigella* and *Yersinia* if they possess the B27 antigen. Whether some qualitative difference in the immune-response gene segment also predisposes one person to direct microbial invasion and makes another resistant has not been determined.

The consequences of this clonal expansion of committed lymphocytes are twofold: one, the production of such products as lymphokines from lymphocytes that cause fever and stimulate macrophages, fibroblasts, and other lymphocytes; and two, the production by 5–10 days of antibody that more effectively activates the complement–polymorphonuclear-cell system. Antimicrobial antibody, therefore, will have been stimulated in most cases by the time or even before the bone or joint has become seeded by the infecting agent. Antibody and complement proteins individually and together draw phagocytic cells toward the nidus of infection (chemotaxis), dilate blood vessels (anaphylotactic action), bind microbes to phagocytic cell membranes (opsonization), and stimulate intracellular phagocytosis and killing.

Defects in either the presence of specific antibody or of a complement protein are associated with a greater risk of infection (Hughes, 1977; Reed *et al.*, 1976). As an example, children below the age of 2 who have little or no specific antibody for *H. influenzae* are especially vulnerable to this agent. Others with a more general reduction of immunoglobulin, as in the agammaglobulinemic syndromes, are prone to various bacterial infections including infectious arthritis (Oxelius, 1984). Genetic deficiencies of complement proteins such as C3 predispose to a variety of bacterial infections, whereas deficiency of the terminal pathway components, C5 through C8, produces a unique susceptibility to hematogenous neisserial infections (Peterson *et al.*, 1979). Defects in phagocytic cell function, as in the chronic granulomatous disease of children, to name but one, render the child unable to resist various bacterial infections.

Other mediator systems contribute to the host's response toward the infection, including the prostaglandin, the kinin, and the clotting systems. Specific failure of any of these has not been established, although it is clear that each is activated in and about sites of infection.

F. The Inflammatory Process

As microorganisms penetrate the joint cavity, a rapid series of events occurs. The synovial microvasculature dilates, subsynovial tissue becomes edematous, and the volume of synovial fluid increases dramatically with a rise in intraarticular pressure (Phemister, 1924). Concentrations of macromolecules such as immunoglobulins and complement proteins in joint fluid approach those in plasma (Kushner and Somerville, 1971). Since hematogenous dissemination usually occurs at least several days after the infection has become established at a primary site, lymphocyte activation and antibody production against the microorganism ordinarily will have begun. Thus, immune complexes can form between antibody and the microorganism or its antigenic fragments, and these can induce such complement-mediated events in the joint as histamine release, chemotaxis, and phagocytosis. Bacterial products alone, even in the absence of antibody, can trigger complement activation through the alternate pathway (Greenblatt *et al.*, 1978).

Other synovial tissues, such as bursae and tendon sheaths, share the same pathogenetic mechanism for infection as described for the joint synovium except for the suggestion that direct penetration of microorganisms from the overlying skin rather than hematogenous spread might be the means by which superficial bursae such as the olecranon and prepatellar bursae become infected (Canoso and Sheckman, 1979).

1. Microbial Identification

Specific identification of the infecting agent in the bone or joint is critical. For the joint, careful examination of synovial fluid must be performed rapidly. Delays in obtaining synovial fluid and examining it properly are associated with inadequate restoration of joint function. Thus, the diagnostic approach to septic arthritis must be viewed as a medical emergency. For the bone, aspiration or biopsy is usually done, although in some circumstances (see below) diagnosis of the infecting agent is inferred from the clinical presentation or culture from the blood or other tissue.

Synovial fluid in septic arthritis is usually turbid and contains large numbers of polymorphonuclear leukocytes. The glucose content is reduced compared to that in a simultaneously obtained serum specimen. Synovial fluid lactic acid levels do not discriminate between septic and nonseptic arthritis (Arthur *et al.*, 1983). On Gram's stain of synovial fluid, organisms are seen in only half or three-quarters of cases. The purulent character of synovial fluid can be less striking in some instances. Lesser numbers of white cells and higher values for glucose, too, are noted in these patients, particularly those with gonococcal arthritis.

Appropriate culture media must be inoculated whenever sepsis is suspected regardless of the quality of the synovial fluid. The specimen obtained from the infected joint should be taken immediately to the microbiology laboratory for study. Based on the impression gained from clinical evaluation, the physician should direct the laboratory's attention to the more probable suspected infectious agents so that special media can be used.

Agents responsible for the majority of cases of septic arthritis and osteomyelitis are the cocci, especially the staphylococci and gonococci, and, to a lesser extent, gram-negative bacilli (Newman, 1976). Each of these agents is considered in more detail in the following sections.

2. Gram-Positive Coccal Infections

Staphylococci are the most common invaders of the joint in all age groups save for the gonococci in young adults. Frequency of infection is as high as 40% or more, whereas with streptococci it is only about a third as frequent. The pathogenesis of the disease is marked by two special features: one, the primary site can be missed in many patients compared to those with gram-negative bacilli (Goldenberg and Cohen, 1976), and two, staphylococci and other gram-positive cocci, as noted above, appear to have a special affinity for bone and joint structures (Newman, 1976).

Characteristically, the involved joint is warm, swollen, and painful. Intrasynovial fluid pressure can be markedly increased. The knee and the hip are most often involved, in that order, but with a tendency for hip involvement to be seen more frequently in children. The shoulder, elbow, wrist, and ankle account for most of the remaining joints. Vertebrae and the sacroiliac joints are infected in fewer than 5% of patients.

Hip joint involvement by staphylococci carries an unusually bad prognosis, especially in children (Nelson, 1972). The main reason for this is delay in diagnosis and treatment of infection in this deep-seated joint.

Identification of gram-positive cocci in a smear of joint fluid and of the specific species by culture is achieved in over two-thirds of patients in whom infection is thought to have occurred. Negative cultures in the face of convincing clinical evidence of infection may result from prior abortive treatment with antibiotics or from the presence of too few viable microorganisms in synovial fluid compared to the larger number contributing to the inflammation in the synovium. On the other hand, the lack of bacteria may simply indicate the absence of sepsis even in the face of convincing signs and symptoms including values of synovial fluid white blood cell counts greater than 50,000 or even 100,000/mm^3, predominantly polymorphonuclear cells, and a low-grade fever. These findings may sometimes occur, albeit rarely, in noninfectious inflammatory arthritides such as chondrocalcinosis, gout, and rheumatoid arthritis. In all instances, however, careful bacteriological studies need to be completed before the possibility of infection is finally excluded. While these are in progress, antibiotic treatment should be initiated and maintained.

Osteomyelitis that results from hematogenous spread presents the same general features of infection as pyogenic arthritis. Local findings include bone pain and tenderness with overlying skin and subcutaneous redness if a peripheral long bone is involved. Vertebral or other deep-seated bone involvement will not usually be detected on clinical examination. A scan by radioactive technetium polyphosphonate or gallium is needed to determine localization in these areas. Bacterial identification may not need to be proven by biopsy of bone but can be inferred from the clinical presentation and recovery of bacteria on blood culture. The teichoic-acid–antibody assay may be useful in ruling out such serious disseminated infections as deep-seated osteomyelitis (Sheagren, 1984). In recurrent or protracted disease, however, bone biopsy or tissue obtained at debridement should be submitted for culture (Waldvogel *et al.*, 1970).

In the elderly or debilitated patient, the intensity of the inflammatory response in the bone or joint may be muted and thus easy to overlook. To compound this dilemma, these patients and others under treatment with drugs that reduce host defense mechanisms are more vulnerable to septic arthritis (Willkens *et al.*, 1960).

Although joints that were not previously injured can be readily infected by staphylococci, prior joint damage or impairment of host defenses will enhance the likelihood of septic involvement. A striking example of such a superimposed infection occurs in patients with rheumatoid arthritis (Kellgren *et al.*, 1958). In these patients, staphylococci are by far the most common infecting agent. The resulting illness is severe, with death or poor restoration of joint function in over a third. Often several joints are infected simultaneously. In some, the clinical signs of sepsis in the infected joint are diminished so that infection is not suspected. Helpful diagnostic clues are the presence of a primary site of infection such as an open leg ulcer caused by vasculitis or, perhaps, a draining subcutaneous nodule, the development of fever and sometimes a chill, or the appearance of one or a few even mildly swollen or painful joints in a patient in whom evidence elsewhere of a flare of the rheumatoid process is lacking.

Septic arthritis and osteomyelitis may also occur in habitual users of intravenous drugs as heroin addicts. Although gram-negative bacilli, particularly *Pseudomonas* and *Serratia,* are closely associated with this type of infection, staphylococci still constitute an equally common threat (Ross *et al.*, 1975).

Within the past decade, infection at the site of implantation of a joint prosthesis has emerged as a serious problem. *Staphylococcus epidermidis* and *aureus* are recovered most often during the early postoperative period, the result of contamination of the surgical wound. A lesser number of late cases are recognized, some occurring even several years after surgery. In these, it is thought that the prior operative site has been seeded during a recent bacteremic episode (Inman *et al.*, 1984).

Infections of such superficial bursae as olecranon bursae are almost always caused by staphylococci (Canoso and Sheckman, 1979).

Group B streptococci have become a common cause of neonatal infections and account for a large fraction of septic arthritis and osteomyelitis in the very young. Symptoms usually occur several weeks after birth (Baker, 1977). Adults also have had more joint infections caused by this agent (Small *et al.*, 1984). Much less commonly, groups A, C, F, G, and D are responsible for infections of the musculoskeletal system. *Streptococcus viridans* and strictly anaerobic streptococci lack group-specific carbohydrates in their cell walls and are usually not typable.

The diagnosis of streptococcal infection is made by demonstration of gram-positive cocci on the stained smear and by culture of synovial fluid, bone, or blood. Group identification is made by appropriate antisera.

Patients with a staphylococcal infection have a high probability that the disease has been caused by penicillin-resistant strains, particularly in hospital-acquired infections (Sheagren, 1984). For this reason, a β-lactamase-resistant antibiotic should be used initially, preferably nafcillin, 100–150 mg/kg per day in four divided dosages given intravenously into a running infusion. Alternative drugs include cephalothin, 100 mg/kg per day, and vancomycin, 30 mg/kg per day. Another antibiotic can be chosen, if necessary, after the identity and sensitivity of the microorganism becomes known. If the microorganism proves to be sensitive to penicillin, penicillin G can be substituted, 20 million units daily, intravenously, in four divided doses. Antibiotics other than penicillin are usually reserved for patients infected with staphylococci resistant to penicillin analogues or for those with a known allergy to penicillin.

The expected duration of antibiotic therapy is 2 to 4 weeks, at first intravenously and later orally, but no exact timetable can be given. Rather, the response to therapy is assessed on a daily basis. At the end of the first week, signs of joint inflammation should have lessened. If joint swelling persists unabated and purulent synovial fluid continues to accumulate despite regular, even daily, needle aspiration (see below), then a comprehensive review of the patient's illness should be done to determine if the appropriate antibiotic is being used based on the microbial sensitivity to the drug. Changes in the antibiotic can be made if indicated.

In hematogenous osteomyelitis of long bones or vertebrae caused by staphylococci, antibiotic therapy is maintained, sometimes for several months. As with septic arthritis, oral administration of the drug can be substituted for intravenous use after improvement has begun to occur. Much of this later phase of treatment can be attempted outside the hospital. In the majority of patients a cure will be achieved. In vertebral disease, spontaneous fusion may occur.

Most streptococci, particularly those of groups A and B, are penicillin sensitive. However, enterococci such as *Streptococcus faecalis* and *Streptococcus fecium* are resistant to a variety of antibiotics. These relatively resistant microorganisms may require the intravenous use of ampicillin, 12 g daily in divided doses, or the intravenous use of penicillin G, 20 million units daily in divided doses, plus either streptomycin, 0.5 g every

12 hr, or gentamicin, 80 mg every 8 hr, intramuscularly or intravenously. Vancomycin may be given 1.0 g every 12 hr as an alternative medication. Antibiotic treatment may be required for from 2 to 4 weeks, but, as with other infecting microorganisms, the exact time depends on the host response.

3. Gonococcal Arthritis

This infectious agent is the most common cause of infectious arthritis in young adults, producing disease in up to 50% of such patients. In contrast to cases of the disease seen in the preantibiotic era, most cases now respond readily to treatment. Nevertheless, this expectation is not always realized. An occasional patient may still develop a destructive arthritis. Thus, management of a patient with gonococcal arthritis should assume the same urgency and the same full medical program that is used for infectious arthritis from other microbial agents (O'Brien *et al.*, 1983).

The primary site of infection is the mucosa of the urethra, vagina, rectum, or pharynx. From these sites, the infection becomes blood-borne and seeds readily to the joint tissue. In fact, gonococci appear to have the same preferential affinity for infection of synovial tissues of the joint, tendon, or bursa as gram-positive cocci. Along with synovial involvement, many patients develop a vasculitis with erythema and microinfarction of the skin. These relatively painless and scattered lesions appear as small papules or vesicles on an erythematous base with an area of central necrosis or pustule. Gonococci can sometimes be recovered on culture from them.

The hematogenous phase of the illness is associated with a migratory polyarthritis or polyarthralgia as well as with a monarthritis. When the polyarthritis is striking, the differential diagnosis includes not only arthritis caused by this and other infectious agents but also noninfectious inflammatory arthritides such as systemic lupus erythematosus, rheumatoid arthritis, and the spondyloarthropathies such as Reiter's syndrome. After several days, the more disseminated process may settle into one or two joints or tendons. In this second phase of the illness, the inflammation tends to persist, and, in contrast to the lesser chance for recovery of microorganisms from joints during the migratory phase, microorganisms may now be recovered more easily but still perhaps in only half or fewer of cases (Brandt *et al.*, 1974).

Strains of gonococci responsible for the disseminated form of the infection tend to be penicillin sensitive. In contrast, those strains that remain at the primary site of infection can sometimes be penicillin resistant (Crider *et al.*, 1984). These distinctions, however, are not absolute. Therefore, one must still attempt to test the sensitivity of the infecting strain to antibiotics.

Gonococci are released from the primary site of infection of an active, recently acquired infection and also from a latent focus in both the male and female. In the latter instance, microorganisms that may have remained quiescent in the mucosal tissues for prolonged periods of time may, under favorable circumstances such as during menstruation, break out into the bloodstream (Eisenstein and Masi, 1981). Two clinical applications follow from these observations: first, the absence of a reliable history of recent sexual activity does not exclude the diagnosis of gonococcal arthritis, and secondly, specimens for culture should be taken from multiple mucosal areas even if the patient is asymptomatic.

Disseminated gonococcal infections are associated in a small fraction of cases with a well-characterized defect in the host's complement system. Individuals with the rare genetic deficiency of either C5, C6, C7, or C8 are unduly predisposed to one or more systemic episodes of neisserial infections, either gonococcal or meningococcal. This vulnerability reveals the striking dependency of the host's immune system on the complement-dependent lytic mechanism mediated by these complement proteins in order to control these bacteria (Peterson *et al.*, 1979). In the absence of this mechanism, these microorganisms can successfully invade the bloodstream and colonize synovial and dermal tissues despite the presence of other host defense mechanisms that remain intact including the potent opsonic action of antigonococcal antibody and C3b complement.

Gonococcal arthritis is best diagnosed by demonstration of microorganisms in the synovial fluid. Special media and reduced oxygen tension are required for their successful growth in culture. When the synovial fluid culture is negative, unfortunately all too often, the diagnosis can be strongly suspected if a positive culture is obtained from the blood or primary site of infection in the patient whose clinical presentation suggests an infectious etiology for the arthritis.

Gonococcal arthritis is best treated by penicillin G, 10 million units intravenously in divided doses two or three times a day. If the organism is resistant to the penicillin, other agents may be used including erythromycin, 2.0 g/day intravenously in four doses, or cefoxitin, 100 mg/kg per day in four doses.

Most patients respond quickly and completely to antibiotic therapy, with resolution of the arthritic inflammation within a week or two.

Despite this optimistic outlook, however, the same principles of management apply as with septic arthritis caused by other bacteria. Treatment should not be offered on an outpatient basis since the exact bacterial diagnosis can at best be only suspected at the outset and an occasional gonococcal strain may be resistant to the initial antibiotic drug. Also, in a small number of patients, destructive changes may occur. For these reasons, all patients should be hospitalized until the diagnosis has been established and parenteral therapy shown to be efficacious. Afterwards, the antibiotic can be given orally and the outcome observed outside the hospital.

4. Gram-Negative Bacillary Infections

Gram-negative bacilli encompass a large number of bacteria that share a common morphology and pose similar problems in diagnosis, treatment, and prognosis whenever they cause arthritis or osteomyelitis (Goldenberg *et al.*, 1974; Bayer *et al.*, 1977). Although many facets of the bone and joint disease caused by this group can be discussed in common, differences among them make it necessary to know their individual characteristics. For instance, *Hemophilus influenzae* arthritis is rarely seen except in children below the age of 2, and *Salmonella* arthritis or osteomyelitis has a strong association with patients with sickle cell disease. Prevention of *H. influenzae*, at least in children over 18 months of age, may be possible by prophylactic immunization using a type b capsular polysaccharide vaccine (Peltola *et al.*, 1984).

Primary sites of infection or colonization are the bowel and the urinary tract and gallbladder. Instrumentation, catheterization, and surgery are some of the means that lead to dissemination from these sites. As medical intervention for major medical problems has increased, so also has the risk for joint infection by these agents. Many individuals in whom bacteremia develops have a compromised immune system as a result of a serious illness such as lymphoma, diabetes, or renal failure or of treatment by corticosteroid or cytotoxic drugs (Bayer *et al.*, 1977).

Septic arthritis caused by these bacilli characteristically presents as a monarticular or occasionally oligoarticular disease. The onset is acute, with obvious signs of swelling, redness, and pain. Bacteremia is manifested by chills in some and fever in most patients. Because of the presence of endotoxin in gram-negative bacterial cell walls, shock may develop.

The joint fluid typically is purulent with markedly elevated white blood cell counts, mainly polymorphonuclear cells, and a low synovial fluid glucose level. Gram-negative rod or coccobacillary microorganisms may be seen on a stained specimen of joint fluid. Further identification can be achieved by observation of growth characteristics on selective media and typing with antisera.

Among the wide spectrum of gram-negative bacilli that cause septic arthritis, the more common ones are *E. Coli, Klebsiella pneumoniae,* Enterobacteriaceae, *Pseudomonas, Serratia marcessans, Proteus, Hemophilus influenzae,* and *Salmonella.* Their exact identification is critical because the initial choice of antibiotic therapy is based on this knowledge and further refined after sensitivities to various antibiotics become known. Drug resistance is common and must be carefully evaluated.

Antibiotic therapy should be initiated promptly based on evidence obtained from the clinical presentation and results of the Gram stain of synovial fluid. If a gram-negative bacillary infection is suspected, an aminoglycoside such as gentamicin, 5 mg/kg per day in three divided doses, should be given intravenously. Carbenicillin, 400 mg/kg per day, can be added if a *Pseudomonas aeruginosa* infection is considered. For *H. influenzae* infections, ampicillin, 150–200 mg/kg per day in six equal portions, is used, but since strains resistant to this drug have been reported, antibiotic susceptibility testing is essential. In that event, chloramphenicol, 30–50 mg/kg per day in four equal portions, can be substituted.

Careful monitoring of the joint response will indicate the efficacy of the treatment plan. Because these patients often have a major underlying systemic illness, treatment must be precise, vigorous, and prolonged. On average, drugs probably will be needed for at least 4 to 6 weeks before the joint is restored to normal. In addition, needle aspiration of purulent joint contents should be performed repeatedly, and, if this procedure proves inadequate, arthroscopy or arthrotomy carried out (see below).

5. *Antiinflammatory Drug Treatment*

Inflammation in septic arthritis is not only the result of toxic factors produced by viable microorganisms but also the result of the host's response to microbial antigens. Bacterial killing by antibiotics achieves the major goal of treatment, but it does not affect removal of already formed microbial fragments. Such material may lodge in the joint for varying periods of time either in loculated areas of necrotic debris or embedded in articular cartilage. Release from these sites over a further period of time, therefore, contributes to persistence of the inflammatory response even though all infecting agents may have been killed.

The clinical picture posed by postinfectious synovitis mimics that caused by the infection itself. Because viable microorganisms may still be present in joint tissues even after the synovial fluid culture has become sterile, antibiotics are usually not discontinued. Instead, a nonsteroidal antiinflammatory drug is added, but only after a week or more of antibiotic treatment during which the infectious process has begun to be controlled. The combination of antibiotic and antiinflammatory therapy usually reduces the inflammatory process. Both drugs can continue to be used until all signs of active disease have disappeared. Corticosteroid drugs are rarely indicated, and their intraarticular use is contraindicated.

G. Bone and Joint Destruction

A major difference between a closed-space infection, such as septic arthritis, and one dispersed throughout the fibrillar scaffolding of the connective tissue, such as cellulitis, is the slower rate of exchange of its contents with the surrounding vascular and lymphatic spaces. Solutes and particulate matter in synovial fluid must diffuse across the synovial cavity, often held at increased pressure, to reach distant subsynovial vessels in contrast to the easy access of materials in interstitial tissues to nearby capillary networks. But diffusion of solutes between joint and blood vessels, although slowed in the joint, does reach equilibrium within several hours. Thus, the diminished effectiveness of antibiotics against bacteria in a closed-space infection is not caused by suboptimal local concentrations of the drug (Parker and Schmid, 1971). Rather, the slowed diffusion into and egress from the joint of metabolic byproducts of the infection retard bacterial cell growth (Eagle, 1952). Bacteria remain dormant under these conditions and are able to survive in the presence of otherwise bactericidal drug concentrations. For this reason, the time-honored principle of drainage of pus and its replacement by more normal body fluids is a critical component of an effective therapeutic program.

Structures at risk for injury by the infectious process are those that lie within the confines of the synovial-lined capsule or sheath, although surrounding soft tissues outside this space are sometimes breached in the rare instance of rupture or sinus formation. Damage to the synovium and capsule of a bursa is reversible, but tendons within synovial sheaths are vulnerable to the effects of the inflammatory process with significant loss of function. Even more vulnerable is articular cartilage. Chondrolysis is readily demonstrated in the presence of pus, and destroyed hyaline cartilage cannot be replaced. These anatomic considerations influence the need for drainage, which is obviously more critical for joints and tendons than for bursae.

In bone, edema, cellular infiltration, and accumulation of products of inflammation develop in much the same manner as has been noted for septic arthritis and contribute to the necrotic breakdown of bone trabeculae and loss of matrix and mineral. Even greater in bone, however, is the part played by vascular obstruction. Large segments of bone devoid of blood supply can separate to form sequestrae. In cross section, the infected bone shows a core of necrosis with fibrin deposits and massive polymorphonuclear-cell infiltration surrounded by an area with granulation tissue containing lymphocytes and plasma cells and, finally, an outer layer of fibrous tissue in which new bone is being formed. When the infection ruptures beneath the periosteum, which is more common in children than adults, the periosteum overgrows to form an involucrum. Cortical destruction can predispose to fractures (Waldvogel *et al.*, 1970).

Loss of cartilage, large-bone erosion, and rupture or weakening of capsular and intrasynovial structures such as ligaments and tendons cannot be restored by natural means even though the infection has been successfully eradicated. Instead, fibrosis occurs with varying degrees of restriction and painful motion and subluxation.

1. Drainage of Synovial Fluid by Needle Aspiration

Except for infants with septic arthritis of the hip, who require open surgical drainage as soon as the diagnosis is made, initial drainage can be accomplished by needle aspiration in almost all cases of infectious arthritis (Goldenberg *et al.*, 1975). All possible fluid is removed on a daily or less frequent basis. Initially, the joint cavity can be lavaged with sterile physiological saline or Ringer's solution. At each aspiration, the volume, cell count, and, less often, the fasting glucose level, are determined.

In the deep-seated joint of the older child or adult, the question of whether open surgical drainage should be chosen initially in preference to needle drainage poses a problem because of the difficulty associated with repeated aspiration. If sepsis is recognized early, and if the organism recovered from the joint is sensitive to antibiotics, particularly if it is a gonococcus or another nonstaphylococcal coccus, then needle drainage is still preferred, since this technique prevents conversion of a closed-space infection into an open wound. If recognition of sepsis is delayed, or if sepsis is caused by a "difficult" organism such as some staphylococcus or a gram-negative bacillus, or if the infected joint is the result of extension of infection from a periarticular site such as a contiguous bone or soft tissue, arthroscopy (Jarret *et al.*, 1981) or open drainage should be carried out.

2. Surgical Drainage and Debridement

At regular intervals the response of the joint infection to the treatment program is assessed according to changes in tenderness, heat, swelling, and range of motion of the joint. The frequency of joint aspiration is reduced as the volume and the inflammatory character of the fluid revert toward normal. If doubt exists that effective bactericidal levels are being achieved because a change was made in the type, dose, or route of administration of an antibiotic drug, a tube-dilution assay of serum and synovial fluid can be performed. When joint fluid is no longer obtainable, assay of antibiotic concentrations of blood alone provides a reasonably close approximation of drug concentration in the joint. The results of this continuous monitoring should be charted chronologically, so that effectiveness of the treatment program can be quickly and accurately determined. Consultation from the outset with those expert in infectious diseases and with the orthopedic surgeon is invaluable in planning a coordinated approach.

Any septic joint untreated or inadequately treated for more than 1 or 2 weeks may have developed some of the pathological changes of a chronic infection. These include damage to cartilage and bone, increased fibrosis, and, ultimately, destruction of the normal joint mechanism. Fortunately, the number of such cases has decreased since the introduction of antibiotic therapy.

If joint damage has developed, reconstructive procedures may be considered, but the operation should be deferred until all evidence of infection has been absent for several months. Arthroplasty or fusion of a joint may be indicated in certain cases. Prosthetic replacement to restore normal joint function is now widely accepted (Jupiter *et al.*, 1981).

The possibility of reexacerbating a dormant infection, however, must always be considered, particularly with tuberculosis. Nevertheless, prosthetic replacement of a damaged hip, knee, and other joints has been undertaken with beneficial results.

More necessary than in the patient with infectious arthritis is the need to monitor the therapeutic program for the patient with osteomyelitis. Clinical findings at the site of the bone infection and radiological and scintiphotographic examinations are used to determine whether the infection has been eradicated. In hematogenous osteomyelitis of a long bone or vertebra, antibiotics are given orally for several weeks after intravenous use; in chronic osteomyelitis, most often when secondary to contiguous infection, long-term oral therapy for months has proven successful.

III. POSTINFECTIOUS INFLAMMATION IN RHEUMATIC DISEASES

During the initial stage of bone or joint infection, the inflammatory stimulus is mainly triggered by toxic factors released from proliferating microorganisms. Even at this point, however, mediators of inflammation produced by the immune response of the host play a role, having been activated by the offending agent days or weeks earlier, at the time of its initiation of the primary site of infection or during dissemination in the bloodstream. As the inflammation continues to persist, these antibody- or lymphokine-mediated reactions become increasingly important. Only when effective antibiotic treatment has eradicated all viable agents or, occasionally, when the host may have accomplished the same goal without treatment, a likely possibility for those joints that become inflamed but spontaneously subside during the polyarthritic phase of some infections (Wehrbein, 1929), can the remaining inflammatory response be assigned entirely to the host's immune system, a response that continues to be fueled by residual antigenic fragments present in synovial fluid, synovial membrane, cartilage, or bone (Goldenberg, 1983).

In clinical situations, therefore, it is usually not possible to independently measure the phlogistic contributions of the microorganism or of the host within the inflamed tissues. Viable microorganisms are found together with immune complexes containing antigen in the patient's serum or synovial fluid during the height of the illness (Manicourt and Orloff, 1982; Walker *et al.*, 1978). A residual tissue focus of infection can persist but remain undetected at a time when cultures of synovial fluid are sterile because only the synovial fluid is usually available for testing. Only in well-controlled experimental circumstances as in animal models can the various components of the inflammatory process be dissected apart from one another and analyzed.

A. Experimental Infectious Arthritis

A variety of infectious agents have been used to produce an infectious arthritis in animals. Generally, the microorganisms must be injected intraarticularly in order to create the counterpart of the natural infection. Rarely has it been possible to use a hematogenous route because the resulting septicemia overwhelms and kills the animal or produces unwanted metastatic disease in organs other than the bone or joint. An interesting exception was noted when blood-borne bacteria did colonize the inflamed joint of a rabbit in which a sterile immune synovitis had already been induced. No infection became implanted in the contralateral normal joint (Lofgren *et al.*, 1982). This experiment emphasizes the requirement for prior alteration within a given joint to enhance its susceptibility to infection.

Intraarticular injections of *Staphylococcus aureus, Escherichia coli,* group A streptococci, or *Neisseria gonorrhoeae* into rabbits produce an acute and sometimes rapidly destructive arthritis in the involved joint. The acute phase peaks in a few days, lasts up to 7 or more days, and is marked by a polymorphonuclear cellular infiltration in synovium and synovial fluid with abscess formation and necrosis. By the second week, the pathology changes to a chronic synovitis in which lining cell hyperplasia and mononuclear cell infiltration in the synovium occurs. Although most types of bacteria could be grown for prolonged periods of time from the inflamed synovial tissue, *N. gonorrhoeae* could not (Goldenberg *et al.*, 1983). Within 24 hr or even after 2 hr (Goldenberg *et al.*, 1984), cultures for this agent were sterile, yet the inflammation persisted in much the same fashion as that caused by the other agents that continued to grow on culture. When killed *N. gonorrhoeae* or its lipopolysaccharide fraction was injected, results were similar to those caused by the injection of viable organisms, that is, an acute synovitis early followed by a chronic synovitis later (Goldenberg *et al.*, 1984).

These findings mimic the course of the natural disease in man. Infectious arthritis caused by gonococci more often than the arthritis caused by gram-positive cocci or gram-negative bacilli is diagnosed without the benefit of a positive synovial fluid culture yet responds dramatically to antibiotic therapy. The most reasonable explanation based on the animal model for the ultimate control of gonococcal inflammation in man is the early death of viable microbes, either naturally or hastened by drug treatment, followed by elimination of those microbial fragments that continue to induce immune response.

B. Experimental Postinfectious Arthritis

When cellular components such as cell walls are used to mimic the nonviable or immunologic phase of the inflammatory process, the requirement for an intraarticular route of injection in order to localize disease within the joint need not be met. Systemic as well as intraarticular administration can be effective. The type of arthritis that is produced, however, resembles the late, chronic phase of monarticular septic arthritis if the material is injected locally but resembles more nearly a reactive arthritis or even rheumatoid arthritis if it is injected systematically.

When given intraarticularly, cell wall materials such as lipopolysaccharide from *N. gonorrhoeae* and *E. coli* (Braude *et al.*, 1963; Goldenberg, 1984; Hollingsworth and Atkins, 1965; Schurman *et al.*, 1977), streptococcal cell walls (Schwab *et al.*, 1967), and mycoplasma antigens (Washburn *et al.*, 1982) create a monarticular inflammatory arthritis. A single intraperitoneal injection into experimental rats of cell wall fragments from group A streptococci, on the other hand, induces a symmetrical polyarthritis that involves peripheral and not axial joints and is characterized by extensive synovial proliferation and marginal joint erosions—features similar to those seen in rheumatoid arthritis (Clark *et al.*, 1979; Cromartie *et al.*, 1977; Wilder *et al.*, 1982, 1983). The systemic administration of an aqueous suspension of purified bacterial cell wall peptidoglycans and the synthetic peptidoglycan fragment muramyl dipeptide has but transient biological effects (Dziarski, 1982; Parant *et al.*, 1979) and does not produce arthritis (Fox *et al.*,

1982), possibly because of the rapid *in vivo* degradation of the purified material, which is not protected by its natural linkage to complex polysaccharide heteropolymers (Cromartie *et al.*, 1977; Gallis *et al.*, 1966; Smialowicz and Schwab, 1977). The complexity of the experimental model is further illustrated by the ability of systemic infection by *Mycoplasma pulmonis* to ameliorate, not accentuate, the severity of adjuvant- or collagen-induced arthritis in LEW/N rats (Taurog *et al.*, 1984).

The inflammation in the laboratory rats, whether injected locally or systemically, is biphasic: an acute phase with a peak at day 3 marked by an intense fibrous exudate and polymorphonuclear-cell infiltration in the synovial membrane, particularly around blood vessels, and a chronic phase marked by extensive synovial hyperplasia, especially of lining cells, and variable but often intense mononuclear-cell infiltration, marginal erosions, and cartilage destruction. These two phases may overlap. The acute phase is thymus independent and may reflect the toxic effect of cell wall components on synovial tissue. The chronic exacerbation is thymus dependent since it does not occur in athymic littermates and may represent a cell-mediated immunologic reaction driven by the cell wall material, which can be demonstrated in the synovium (Wilder and Allen, 1984).

An entirely comparable series of events is produced in laboratory rats using cell wall material from *Lactobacillus casei*, a gram-positive, facultative, aerobic bacterium commonly found in the oral, vaginal, and gastrointestinal flora of rats and humans (London, 1976). A simple injection of an aqueous suspension of *L. casei* cell walls induces a chronic inflammatory polyarthritis in the distal joints of the rat (Lehman *et al.*, 1983).

Host factors play a significant role in the development of the experimental synovitis caused by the streptococcal or *L. casei* cell wall materials. Susceptibility in laboratory rats is strongly dependent on the strain chosen (LEW/N are susceptible; F344/N are resistant) and on hormonally mediated sex-linked effects (LEW/N females develop severe arthritis; F344/N females do not) (Allen *et al.*, 1983; Lehman *et al.*, 1984; Wilder *et al.*, 1983). These differences are not so much related to the amount and the persistence of antigen in the inflamed synovium tissues or in other sites such as the liver and spleen but rather to the relatively greater ability of the resistant animal to more effectively neutralize the toxic actions of the cell wall components.

In summary, data from these animal models permit a more detailed analysis of events that in all likelihood occur in the natural disease. Viable microbes or nonviable intact microbes or cell wall components reach selected target joint(s), directly if inoculated locally and indirectly via the bloodstream if injected intraperitoneally or intravascularly. In both cases, an acute fibrous polymorphonuclear response ensues, mainly in response to toxic effects of microbial components, followed later in some hosts or with certain microbes by a chronic mononuclear destructive arthropathy caused mainly by the host's immunologic response. The animal models suggest that the chronic phase develops in the susceptible animal because it is unable to eliminate the offending antigen as completely or rapidly as does the resistant animal.

In human disease, infectious arthritis most nearly corresponds to the acute-phase reaction in which toxic microbial products attack joint tissues to cause the major symptoms and findings; the host's immunologically mediated effects are evident to a much lesser degree, especially if a curative antibiotic drug is given early. Yet, with more virulent microbes and in impaired hosts, the chronic phase in which immune-directed events occur begins to dominate the clinical and pathological picture but still locally, within the one or a few joints that were originally infected. Undoubtedly, in humans, as in the resistant animal models, there are many cases of natural resistance to the development of synovial inflammation because only a relatively small number of patients develop infected joints out of the much larger number that experience episodes of septicemia.

Reactive forms of arthritis (see below) and even possibly such other inflammatory arthritides as rheumatoid arthritis most closely resemble the more chronic polyarthritis induced by systemic administration of selected bacteria. In these cases, as in the animal model, the genetic makeup of the patient is critical. A patient who is B27 positive is at much higher risk to develop a reactive arthritis just as the LEW/N laboratory animal is to develop a chronic polyarthritis. The animal data further suggest that vulnerability to chronic arthritis is more closely linked to the host's inability to readily remove the offending antigen before it can induce damage, although if such is indeed the case in humans with reactive arthritis, toxic microbial materials have yet to be demonstrated in articular tissues.

IV. REACTIVE ARTHRITIS

Reactive arthritis results from the interaction of an exogenous infectious agent, which may be innocuous or nonarthrogenic for most individuals, and an immunogenetically predisposed host. The prototypic illnesses in man of this type of arthritis are those grouped under the heading of spondyloarthropathies, particularly Reiter's syndrome. In these, the portal of entry of the microorganism is often the gastrointestinal or the urogenital tract. Subsequently, surface antigens of the infective agent react with cell membrane markers on macrophages and/or lymphocytes of the host that are coded by genes within the histocompatibility gene segment, particularly those coding for HLA-B27. Thereafter, by largely unknown mechanisms, inflammation is induced at selected locations: the enthesis (the site of insertion of ligament or tendon into bone), synovium, uveal tract, and the elastic layer of the aorta.

In patients who have rheumatic fever, a similar but less-well-defined interaction occurs between the group A *Streptococcus* and a non-HLA-B27 immune response of the host that involves the endocardium, synovium, skin, and central nervous system (see Chapter 13). An aseptic form of arthritis sometimes develops after infections caused by brucellosis (Alarcon *et al.*, 1981) and tuberculosis (Poncet's disease) (Summers and Jayson, 1980), in meningococcemic patients (Herrick and Parkhurst, 1919), and possibly in patients with an arthritis during the prodromal phase of hepatitis B infection (Duffy *et al.*, 1976). Grouped under the same heading of postinfectious diseases are a number of incomplete syndromes in which an exposure to a suitable infectious agent such as a gram-negative bacillus is followed by an inflammatory arthritis but without any other symptoms (Arnett, 1979).

A. Genetic Factors

The HLA system in man is comprised of a series of closely spaced genes on the short arm of the human chromosome 6. Four of the loci, HLA-A, B, C, and D/DR, encode polypeptide chains that in three, HLA-A, B, and C, form dimers with β_2,-microglobulin (encoded by a gene on chromosome 15) and in one, HLA-D/DR, dimerizes with another polypeptide that may or may not be coded for on chromosome 6. These dimeric proteins are integrated into the membrane of nucleated cells. Each locus is highly polymorphic, and antibodies are readily produced by alloimmunization. It is not yet clear whether the gene product of HLA-D is identical to that of HLA-DR (McMichael and McDevitt, 1977).

Although knowledge of the functions of the HLA system in man is limited, it has been shown that HLA-D is intimately involved in antigen presentation by macrophages to T cells (Rodey *et al.*, 1979), that HLA genes are linked to specific immune responses to synthetic polypeptides (Hsu *et al.*, 1981), and that specific immune suppressor genes are present within the histocompatibility gene segment (Sasazuki *et al.*, 1980). In addition, the structural genes for complement proteins, C4, C2, and factor B, which also are polymorphic, map between HLA-B and D (Rittner and Bertrams, 1981).

HLA-B27 is strongly associated with spondylitis in almost all racial groups in which its frequency has been studied (Woodrow, 1977). Caucasians and some North American Indians have a greater than 90% association; American blacks only about a 50% association. However, other antigens are found with increased frequency in many of the B27-negative patients, including Bw16 (Khan *et al.*, 1980; Van den Berg-Loonen *et al.*, 1977), which has been split into Bw38 and Bw39 and is associated with psoriasis and psoriatic arthritis and spondylitis (Espinoza *et al.*, 1978), and B7, Bw22, or B40. These latter three HLA antigens belong to a cross-reactive group (acronym CREG) called B7-CREG, which also includes Bw42 (Arnett *et al.*, 1977; Joysey and Wolf, 1978). CREG antigens cross react with B27. The basis for this cross reactivity is a common public antigenic determinant located on the heavy chain of HLA-B7, B27, Bw22, and B40 molecules distinct from the private antigenic determinants, which are not shared among the CREG members and which therefore allow these molecules to be distinguished one from the other (Schwartz *et al.*, 1979).

Monoclonal antibodies have been prepared against the HLA-B27 antigen. Of two that have been characterized, one reacts almost entirely with a B27 epitope, and the other mainly with a B27 epitope but also to a lesser degree with an epitope on the B7 molecule. Cross reactivity with B7 is attributed to a B27-like epitope on B7 distinct from the B7-specific epitope itself (Grumet, 1983).

The risk of developing ankylosing spondylitis among HLA-B27-positive individuals drawn from the community at large or from family members of asymptomatic HLA-B27-positive subjects is less than that of B27-positive relatives of spondylitic patients. Among family members 45 years or older, 21% of HLA-B27-positive relatives of HLA-B27-positive spondylitic patients have spondylitis as compared to only 1.3% of HLA-B27-positive individuals in the population at large, a 16-fold greater risk for spondylitis among HLA-B27-positive relatives of patients (van der Linden *et al.*, 1984). In another study, the risk of having spondyloarthropathy was 5.6-fold greater for the B27-positive relatives of B27-positive patients compared with relatives of B27-positive healthy subjects (Calin *et al.*, 1983). Still other studies indicate that ankylosing spondylitis is found more frequently in some B27-positive families and not at all in other families of spondylitic patients (Hochberg *et al.*, 1978; LeClerq and Russell, 1984). Although genetic factors cannot be excluded, these differences imply that nongenetic, probably environmental factors influence expression of disease.

The striking association of B27 and spondylitis suggests that the arthritis is initiated either as a direct result of the action of the histocompatibility gene product or as an indirect result of linkage disequilibrium between the B27 gene and a second gene or group of genes. Most favor a direct role for B27 itself or a possible subset epitope of B27 in disease development (Ebringer, 1983).

If the HLA-B27 antigen alone is responsible for the increased incidence of disease, it may be triggered either by a cross reactivity or similarity between B27 and a foreign antigen found in the bacterial cell wall or by the function of the HLA-B27 molecule to act as a receptor for microbial antigens. In the first or cross-tolerance hypothesis, an inflammatory spondylitis would be produced by microorganisms such as *Klebsiella, Yersinia,* or other gram-negative microorganisms, which partially resemble or cross react with HLA-B27. Such microorganisms evoke the formation of antibacterial antibodies, which then bind to the partially cross-reacting B27 and cause an immune-complex-mediated disease (Damian, 1964; Ebringer, 1979). In the second or receptor hypothesis, HLA-B27 itself or an HLA-B27-associated structure acts as a receptor for a gram-negative microorganism, an association that facilitates or enhances the potential of the bacteria to produce disease (Seager *et al.*, 1979). The cross-tolerance and receptor theories, which are by definition mutually exclusive remain to be proven.

B. Pathology

Unfortunately, information is sparse concerning the pathology of the early lesion of the enthesopathy seen in the spondyloarthropathies. Biopsies are rarely performed at articular sites, particularly at the onset of the illness. In nonarticular sites such as the iliac crest, the enthesopathy consists of a nonspecific nongranulomatous inflammatory lesion that characteristically leads to destruction at the attachment site of the ligament to the bone. The resulting bony erosion is then repaired by deposition of reactive bone, which may combine with the eroded end of the ligament to form a new enthesis. In the vertebral body, the enthesopathy occurs at the attachment of the outer fibers of the annulus to the vertebral plate, especially anteriorly and anterolaterally. Repair of the erosive lesion in this site results in a syndesmophyte composed of reactive bone that undergoes remodeling and replacement via lamellar bone. Similarly, lesions at the capsular attachment of the facet joints can lead to capsular ossification and ankylosis, leaving most of the intraarticular cartilage intact. A similar sequence is thought to occur in the sacroiliac joints (Ball, 1983).

Lymphocytic clusters occur in the fibrous and fibroadipose tissues near ligamentous attachments. They may either be part of the inflammatory process at this site or only a reflection of nonspecific increased cellular traffic through the tissue. Focal edema with a few polymorphonuclear leukocytes and lymphocytes may be seen. In more severe lesions, lymphocytes and polymorphonuclear leukocytes occur in variable numbers, and polymorphonuclear leukocytes may be numerous. Plasma cells tend to be present in the adjacent marrow spaces, but they are not conspicuous. There is no associated necrotizing arteritis. Bound deposits of immunoglobulins or complement have not been detected in the few instances in which this was studied (Ball, 1983).

Thus, the manner by which bacterial antigens may exert their phlogistic effects in patients who are B27 positive remains elusive. Available studies are incomplete and somewhat contradictory. Efforts to determine whether, among other mechanisms, bacterial adherence to gut or mucosal membranes is altered, whether macrophages have an impaired function in antigen presentation or as effector cells, or whether polymorphonuclear cells are limited in their ability to undergo chemotaxis or other functions have yet to be clarified.

C. Clinical Syndromes

Infections caused by gram-negative bacteria, chlamydia, and other agents have been associated with the development of arthritis in individuals who are B27 positive. In some cases, these patients develop the typical features of a well-recognized illness such as Reiter's syndrome; in others, the clinical presentation may be incomplete, so that a specific diagnosis cannot be made. In order to encompass the wide number of possible presentations of patients who may have a reactive or postinfectious arthritis, these conditions are discussed from different viewpoints even though some overlap may occur. Data from patients in whom a causal relationship to an infectious agent is obvious are presented first; then additional data are presented on patients in whom the diagnosis of Reiter's disease, or of an enteric disease and arthritis, or of ankylosing spondylitis is clear-cut but in whom the relationship to a prior infection is less certain.

1. Reactive Arthritis Caused by Specific Gram-Negative Bacilli

a. Shigella Postinfectious Reactive Arthritis. A reactive arthritis has been reported in 0–12% of cases of bacillary dysentery caused by *Shigella flexneri*. Most of the outbreaks occurred in conjunction with military field operations. In a large Finnish outbreak, only three out of 555 patients experienced the typical Reiter's triad of arthritis, urethritis, and conjunctivitis, but 20% had conjunctivitis and 17% urethritis or dysuria. No well-documented case of reactive arthritis has been reported following *Shigella sonnei* dysentery despite the higher proportion of bowel infections with that species that occur in the United States and other developed nations (Calin *et al.*, 1979; Kaslow *et al.*, 1979).

b. Salmonella Postinfectious Reactive Arthritis. Salmonellosis has been associated at times with reactive arthritis, although the evidence is not as compelling as with some species of *Shigella* or *Yersinia*. Although it is more common than shigellosis in developed nations, many outbreaks of salmonellosis caused by a great variety of *Salmonella* species have been carefully investigated without mention of reactive arthritis. Nevertheless, the features in several small series of cases and in four outbreaks in which the rheumatic complications were recorded support the belief that certain species of group B (*S. typhimurium* and *S. heidelberg*) and group D (*S. enteritidis*) do induce a reactive arthritis (Kaslow, 1984).

In an epidemic of *Salmonella typhimurium* in Scotland in 1981, approximately 700 patients, mostly youngsters, out of a general practice of 7000 individuals developed gastroenteritis. Four hundred eighteen were bacteriologically proven. Among these, eight cases were identified in whom a reactive arthritis or erythema nodosum occurred, and among these eight individuals, B27 was present in three, Bw22 in one, and B7 in three others (Eastmond, 1983).

c. Yersinia Postinfectious Reactive Arthritis. The genus *Yersinia* comprises the species *Y. pestis, Y. enterocolitica,* and *Y. pseudotuberculosis*. The last two are intestinal pathogens causing acute enteritis and mesenteric lymphadenitis. The intestinal infection can be complicated by erythema nodosum and a reactive arthritis. A definitive diagnosis of a recent *Yersinia* infection can be made only by isolation of the microbe from the patient together with a demonstration of a rising antibody level. Most cases of *Yersinia* infection of the bowel are mild, and patients may not seek medical care for the infection. Patients seeking treatment for intestinal *Yersinia* infection only seldom develop arthritis, implying a rate of arthritis that is clearly low and not much different from those of other gram-negative bacteria (Aho, 1983).

Yersinia arthritis typically occurs in young adults, although the disease is also recognized in children and elderly people. Males and females are affected to about the same degree. Arthritis is characteristically oligoarticular. The joints most frequently affected are those of lower extremities and the hands. The acute phase itself is self-limited and usually lasts from a few weeks to several months. Monoarthritis, which typically affects the knee joints, is probably more frequent than is apparent from patient series collected from specialized clinics. In some patients the disease runs a prolonged course with a relapsing periarticular swelling and even effusions (Aho, 1983).

A variety of immune changes have been reported in patients with this infection. These include increased polyclonal immunoglobulin levels, increased circulating immune complexes (a similar rise also occurs in patients without arthritis who have *Yersinia* infection), and T-cell abnormalities (Aho, 1983). T lymphocytes from patients with the spontaneous onset of Reiter's syndrome are capable of recognizing and proliferating on exposure to determinants on formalin-killed strains of *Y. enterocolitica,* serum type 3. A similar response did not occur for serum type 8, which, unlike 3, is not associated with reactive arthritis (Brenner *et al.,* 1984).

d. Postinfectious Reactive Arthritis Caused by Other Bacilli. Other gram-negative bacilli that have been linked to reactive arthritis include *Campylobacter fetus* and *Campylobacter jejuni*. In the latter case, this infection preceded initial rheumatic symptoms in patients with an associated B27 antigen (Kasunen *et al.,* 1980; Urman *et al.,* 1977).

2. Reiter's Syndrome

In 1916 Reiter described the case of a young soldier with an acute febrile illness that included conjunctivitis, urethritis, and severe polyarthritis after an episode of bloody diarrhea, although cases of the syndrome to which Reiter's name has become attached had long been described in the literature. Over 40 years ago, Bauer and Engleman organized the clinical findings of these patients about the triad of polyarthritis or monoarthritis, nongonococcal urethritis, and inflammation of the eye (Bauer and Engleman, 1942). The additional presence of mucocutaneous lesions on the skin of the extremities and on the oral and genital mucosa firmly established the complete syndrome. Nevertheless, the number of individuals with the complete triad or tetrad represents a minority; most patients acutally present with an incomplete form of this syndrome, usually only arthritis following a dysenteric episode or urethritis.

Reiter's syndrome is classified within the family of spondyloarthropathies because approximately one-fourth of patients develop radiologic sacroiliitis or spondylitis, rheumatoid factor is typically absent, and almost three-quarters are B27 positive. The disease generally affects several peripheral joints, particularly those of the lower extremities. Sites of attachment of tendons or fascia to bone (enthesis) are characteristic locations of this disease; however, peripheral joint synovitis also occurs.

The inflammatory lesions of Reiter's syndrome are sometimes a consequence of infection within the genitourinary or gastrointestinal tract, although the skeletal lesions themselves are always sterile. When an infectious focus cannot be demonstrated, its presence in the pathogenesis is assumed, thus making the definition of this syndrome virtually identical to that of reactive arthritis (Keat, 1983).

The frequency of the different features of the triad varies from study to study. Arthritis develops in approximately 1% of men presenting with nongonococcal urethritis at hospital clinics. It occurs in approximately 2 to 3% of all patients with *Shigella, Salmonella,* and *Campylobacter* infections but in a much higher proportion of those infected with *Yersinia*. The male/female ratio is roughly equal for Reiter's syndrome following enteric infections, whereas a very high male predominance is associated with genital infections. The interval between the onset of infection and the rheumatic symptoms is usually less than 30 days. The first episode often resolves completely within a number of months, but a majority of patients experience recurrences, more commonly after genital infections. Some patients develop a chronic progressive arthritis. Whether recurrences are associated with reexposure to the inciting agent is not usually known. Since *Chlamydia* and possibly other pathogens can remain dormant in the host, they may be the source of a recurrence. In epidemics, most cases occur among B27-positive patients who are not related to each other.

The involved synovium shows an increased vascular permeability and infiltration by inflammatory cells, particularly polymorphonuclear leukocytes. Similarly, the predominant cell type in the synovial fluid is the polymorphonuclear leukocyte. Little or no synovial lining cell hyperplasia occurs (Norton *et al.*, 1966). During the acute stage, intracellular inclusions including ingested erthrocytes and nucleated cells within synovial fluid cells have occasionally been noted. Later, the pathological changes more closely resemble the chronic inflammation of rheumatoid arthritis. Inflammatory lesions at the entheses are characteristic, notably at tendon and fascial attachments. Ocular lesions occur with a varying degree of frequency. Conjunctivitis is the most common. Asynchronous anterior uveitis is associated with severe or recurring arthritis, particularly with sacroiliitis (Keat, 1983).

3. Inflammatory Bowel Diseases and Arthritis

Ulcerative colitis and Crohn's disease are associated with an inflammatory arthritis and spondylitis. Both a nondeforming large-joint arthritis and sacroiliitis can occur, the peripheral arthritis being found in about 20% of patients and back involvement in about 10%. The degree of peripheral arthritis often runs parallel with the intensity of the bowel inflammation; back involvement, on the other hand, is more chronic and independent of the bowel disease. No infectious agent has as yet been implicated as a cause for either the bowel or the joint lesions of this disease, although it is considered possible that intestinal organisms may sensitize the host, perhaps in a manner similar to that induced by injection of *L. casei,* a gut microorganism, into laboratory rats (Lehman *et al.*, 1984). A strong association exists between B27 and spondylitis but not peripheral joint involvement (Ansell and Wigley, 1964; Wright and Watkinson, 1966).

A second enteric condition associated with arthritis is so-called bypass arthritis. In some patients in whom an anastomosis has been carried out between the small and large intestine to control morbid obesity, arthritis develops (Shagrin *et al.*, 1971). Small papules and pustules may appear on the extremities and the upper part of the trunk along with an erythema-nodosum-like panniculitis and disappear after several weeks (Dicken and Seehafer, 1979). Immune complexes have been detected in the serum of bypass patients, both in those in whom arthritis developed and in others in whom no arthritis has occurred. Bacterial residues have been identified within the immune complex. It has been suggested that these may deposit within joint tissue to create the arthritic syndrome. Factors that support this theory are the presence of large numbers of microorganisms in the blind loop, detection of circulating immune complexes during active arthritis, identification of cryoprecipitates that contain complement and antibodies to *E. coli, B. fragilis,* and streptococci, a favorable response to antibiotics in some patients, and, finally, the resolution of the syndrome when the bypass is taken down (Utsinger, 1980; Wands *et al.*, 1976).

A third condition is Whipple's disease, a rare condition in which the presenting features are protean but the most common symptoms are abdominal discomfort and diarrhea (Maizel *et al.*, 1970). Most patients are young and middle-aged males. Arthritis occurs in the majority of the patients, sometimes years before the bowel complaints are evident (Kelly and Weisiger, 1963). Bacterial remnants—cell wall material—have been found in the synovium, but no viable agents have been recovered from these tissues (Hawkins *et al.*, 1976).

4. Ankylosing Spondylitis

Ankylosing spondylitis is the prototypic disease for the family of related disorders grouped under the heading of spondyloarthropathies. Until recently, its relationship to an infectious agent was unknown, although concern for prostatic infection as a possible inciting factor in the sacroiliitis had been considered in the past. Now, interesting data suggest a relationship to an increased fecal carriage of and an immune hypersensitivity to *Klebsiella* species.

This disorder is characterized by inflammation of the spine and sacroiliac joints. Distal joint involvement is unusual except in teenage boys. Women are much less commonly and less severely affected than men, although they have a high frequency of HLA-B27—90% or greater. Acute uveitis may be the presenting symptom and occur episodically during the course of chronic back disease. A small number of patients develop aortic insufficiency as a result of necrosis of elastic fibers in the aortic root (Calabro, 1980).

A cross reactivity exists between *Klebsiella aerogenes* and the HLA-B27 antigen, a finding that would support the notion of cross reactivity or molecular mimicry between a host component and an infectious agent (Avakian *et al.*, 1980; Welsh *et al.*, 1980). Some studies also have noted a relationship between recovery of *Klebsiella* from the feces and the presence of increased activity of the spondylitis as measured either clinically or by tests of acute-phase reactants (Cowling *et al.*, 1980; Eastmond *et al.*, 1980; Ebringer,

1978). Others have failed to establish such a relationship (Warren and Brewerton, 1980). These provocative findings need further study, however, before a convincing case can be established for an etiologic role for gram-negative bacilli such as *Klebsiella* in ankylosing spondylitis.

V. SUMMARY

The greater the degree to which information about the pathogenesis of straightforward infectious arthritis or osteomyelitis is gathered, the more it will be possible to diagnose and treat these conditions. Possibly of greater interest is the likelihood that knowledge of this process will have relevance for less-well-understood conditions such as the reactive arthritides and even for inflammatory diseases of unknown cause such as rheumatoid arthritis and systemic lupus erythematosus, for which infectious agents have been postulated with unfailing regularity but not yet detected. Thus, a view of some of the inflammatory rheumatic diseases as a continuum could yield dividends for those at one end of the spectrum, in which the virulence of the microorganisms rapidly overpowers a normally constituted host, to those at the other end, in which an effete or almost symbiotic agent cannot be entirely eradicated by a host either not programmed adequately or flawed in some of the components needed to eliminate the offending agent.

REFERENCES

Aho, K., 1983, *Yersinia* reactive arthritis, *Br. J. Rheumatol.* **22**(Suppl. 2):41–45.

Aho, K., and Raunio, V., 1982, EB-virus and rheumatoid arthritis: New insights into their interrelation, *Med. Biol.* **60**:49–52.

Alarcon, G. S., Bocanegra, T. S., Gotuzzo, E., Hinostroza, S., Carrillo, C., Vasey, F. B., Germain, B. F., and Espinoza, L. R., 1981, Reactive arthritis associated with brucellosis: HLA studies, *J. Rheumatol.* **8**:621–625.

Allen, J. B., Blatter, D., Calandra, G. B., and Wilder, R. L., 1983, Sex hormonal effects on the severity of streptococcal cell wall-induced polyarthritis in the rat, *Arthritis Rheum.* **26**:560–563.

Ansell, B. M., and Wigley, R. A. D., 1964, Arthritic manifestations in regional enteritis, *Ann. Rheum. Dis.* **23**:64–72.

Argen, R. J., Wilson, C. H., and Wood, P., 1966, Suppurative arthritis: Clinical features of 42 cases, *Arch. Intern. Med.* **117**:661–671.

Arnett, F. C., 1979, Incomplete Reiter's syndrome: Clinical comparisons with classical triad, *Ann. Rheum. Dis.* **38**(Suppl. 1):73–78.

Arnett, F. C., Jr., Hochberg, M. C., and Bias, W. B., 1977, Cross-reactive HLA antigens in B27-negative Reiter's syndrome and sacroiliitis, *Johns Hopkins Med. J.* **141**:193–197.

Arthur, R. E., Stern, M., Galeazzi, M., Basdassare, A. R., Weiss, T. D., Rogers, J. R., and Zuckner, J., 1983, Synovial fluid lactic acid in septic and nonseptic arthritis, *Arthritis Rheum.* **26**:1499–1505.

Atcheson, S. G., and Ward, J. R., 1978, Acute hematogenous osteomyelitis progressing to septic synovitis and eventual pyrarthrosis: The vascular pathway, *Arthritis Rheum.* **21**:968–971.

Avakian, H., Welsh, J., Ebringer, A., and Entwistle, C. C., 1980, Ankylosing spondylitis, HLA-B27 and *Klebsiella*. II. Cross-reactivity studies with human tissue typing sera, *Br. J. Exp. Pathol.* **61**:92–96.

Bauer, W., and Engleman, E. P., 1942, A syndrome of unknown etiology characterized by urethritis, conjunctivitis and arthritis (so-called Reiter's disease), *Trans. Assoc. Am. Physicians* **57**:307–313.

Bayer, A. S., Chow, A. W., Louie, J. S., Nies, K. M., and Guze, L. B., 1977, Gram-negative bacillary septic arthritis: Clinical, radiographic, therapeutic and prognostic features, *Semin. Arthritis Rheum.* **17**:503–510.

Brandt, K. D., Cathcart, E. S., and Cohen, A. S., 1974, Gonococcal arthritis: Clinical features correlated with blood, synovial fluid and genitourinary cultures, *Arthritis Rheum.* **17**:503–510.

Braude, A. I., Jones, J. L., and Douglas, H., 1963, The behavior of *Escherichia coli* endotoxin (somatic antigen) during infectious arthritis, *J. Immunol.* **90**:297–311.

Brenner, M. B., Kobayashi, S., Weisenhutter, C. W., Huberman, A. K., Bales, P., and Yu, D. T. Y., 1984, *In vitro* T lymphocyte proliferative response to *Yersinia enterocolitica* in Reiter's syndrome: Lack of response in other HLA-B27 positive individuals, *Arthritis Rheum.* **27**:250–257.

Calabro, J. J., 1980, The spondyloarthropathies: An overview, *Scand. J. Rheumatol.* **9**(Suppl. 32):21–24.

Calin, A., Kaslow, R. A., Simon, D., Ryder, R. P., Kaye, R., and Dritz, S., 1979, Reiter's syndrome and the seroepidemiology of *Shigella, Ann. Rheum. Dis.* **38**:190.

Calin, A., Marder, A., Becks, E., and Burns, T., 1983, Genetic differences between B27 positive patients with ankylosing spondylitis and B27 positive healthy controls, *Arthritis Rheum.* **26**:1460–1464.

Canoso, J. J., and Sheckman, P. R., 1979, Septic subcutaneous bursitis: Report of sixteen cases, *J. Rheumatol.* **6**:96–102.

Clark, R. L., Cuttino, J. T., Anderle, S. K., Cromartie, W. J., and Schwab, J. H., 1979, Radiologic analysis of arthritis in rats after systemic injection of streptococcal cell walls, *Arthritis Rheum.* **22**:25–35.

Cowling, P., Ebringer, R., Cawdell, D., Ishii, M., and Ebringer, A., 1980, C-reactive protein, ESR and *Klebsiella* in ankylosing spondylitis, *Ann. Rheum. Dis.* **39**:45–49.

Crider, S. R., Colby, S. D., Miller, L. K., Harrison, W. O., Kerbs, S. B. J., and Berg, S. W., 1984, Treatment of penicillin-resistant *Neisseria gonorrhoeae* with oral norfloxacin, *N. Engl. J. Med.* **311**:137–140.

Cromartie, W. J., Craddock, J. G., Schwab, J. H., Anderle, S. K., and Yang, C. H., 1977, Arthritis in rats after systemic injection of streptococcal cells or cell walls, *J. Exp. Med.* **146**:1585–1602.

Damian, R. T., 1964, Molecular mimicry: Antigen sharing by parasite and host and its consequences, *Am. Nat.* **98**:129–149.

Dicken, C. H., and Seehafer, J. R., 1979, Bowel bypass syndrome, *Arch. Dermatol.* **115**:837–839.

Duffy, P., Lidsky, M. D., Sharp, J. T., Davis, J. S., Person, D. A., Hollinger, F. B., and Min, K.-W., 1976, Polyarthritis, polyarteritis and Hepatitis B., *Medicine (Baltimore)* **55**:19–37.

Dziarski, R., 1982, Preferential induction of autoantibody secretion in polyclonal activation by petidoglycan and lipopolysaccharide: II. *In vivo* studies, *J. Immunol.* **128**:1026–1030.

Eagle, H., 1952, Experimental approach to the problem of treatment failure with penicillin: I. Group A streptococcal infection in mice, *Am. J. Med.* **13**:389–399.

Eastmond, J. C., 1983, Gram-negative bacteria and B27 disease, *Br. J. Rheumatol.* **22**(Suppl. 2):67–74.

Eastmond, C. J., Wilshaw, H. E., Burgess, S. E., Shinebaum, R., Cooke, E. M., and Wright, V., 1980, The frequency of faecal *Klebsiella aerogenes* in patients with ankylosing spondylitis and controls with respect to individual features of the disease, *Ann. Rheum. Dis.* **39**:118–123.

Ebringer, A., 1978, The link between genes and disease, *New Sci.* **79**:865–867.

Ebringer, A., 1979, Ankylosing spondylitis, immune response genes and molecular mimicry, *Lancet* **1**:1186.

Ebringer, A., 1983, The cross-tolerance hypothesis, HLA-B27 and ankylosing spondylitis, *Br. J. Rheumatol.* **22**(Suppl. 2):53–66.

Eisenstein, B. I., and Masi, A. T., 1981, Disseminated gonococcal infection (DGI) and gonococcal arthritis (GCA): I. Bacteriology, epidemiology, host factors, pathogen factors, and pathology, *Semin. Arthritis Rheum.* **10**:155–172.

Espinoza, L. R., Vasey, F. B., Oh, J. H., Wilkinson, R., and Osterland, C. K., 1978, Association between HLA-Bw38 and peripheral psoriatic arthritis, *Arthritis Rheum.* **21**:72–75.

Fox, A., Brown, R. G., Anderle, S. K., Chetty, C., Cromartie, W. J., Gooder, H., and Schwab, J. H., 1982, Arthropathic properties related to the molecular weight of peptidoglycan–polysaccharide polymers of streptococcal cell wall, *Infect. Immun.* **35**:1003–1010.

Gallis, H. A., Miller, S. E., and Wheat, R. W., 1966, Degradation of 14-C labelled streptococcal cell walls by egg white lysozyme and lysosomal enzymes, *Infect. Immun.* **13**:1459–1466.

Goldenberg, D. L., 1983, Post-infectious arthritis: A new look at an old concept with particular attention to disseminated gonococcal infection (DGI), *Am. J. Med.* **74**:925–928.

Goldenberg, D. L., and Cohen, A. S., 1976, Acute infectious arthritis: A review of patients with nongonococcal joint infections (with emphasis on therapy and prognosis), *Am. J. Med.* **60**:369–377.

Goldenberg, D. L., Brandt, K. D., Cathcart, E. S., and Cohen, A. S., 1974, Acute arthritis caused by gram negative bacilli: A clinical characterization, *Medicine (Baltimore)* **53**:197–208.

Goldenberg, D. L., Brandt, K. D., Cohen, A. S., and Cathcart, E. S., 1975, Treatment of septic arthritis: Comparison of needle aspiration and surgery as initial modes of joint drainage, *Arthritis Rheum.* **18:**83–90.

Goldenberg, D. L., Chisholm, P. L., and Rice, P. A., 1983, Experimental model of bacterial arthritis: A microbiologic and histopathologic characterization of the arthritis after the intraarticular injection of *Neisseria gonorrhoeae, Staphylococcus aureus,* group A streptococci and *Escherichia coli, J. Rheumatol.* **10:**5–11.

Goldenberg, D. L., Reed, J. I., and Rice, P. A., 1984, Arthritis in rabbits induced by killed *Neisseria gonorrhoeae* and gonococcal lipopolysaccharide, *J. Rheumatol.* **11:**3–8.

Greenblatt, J., Boackle, R. J., and Schwab, J. H., 1978, Activation of the alternate complement pathway by peptidoglycan from streptococcal cell wall, *Infect. Immun.* **19:**296–303.

Grumet, F. C., 1983, Monoclonal antibodies to HLA-B27, *Br. J. Rheumatol.* **22**(Suppl. 2):110–118.

Hawkins, C. F., Farr, M., Morris, C. J., Hoare, A. M., and Williamson, N., 1976, Detection of electron microscopy of rod-shaped organisms in synovial membrane from a patient with the arthritis of Whipple's disease, *Ann. Rheum. Dis.* **35:**502–509.

Herrick, W. W., and Parkhurst, G. M., 1919, Meningococcus arthritis, *Am. J. Med. Sci.* **158:**473–481.

Hochberg, M. C., Bias, B., and Arnett, F. C., Jr., 1978, Family studies in HLA-B27 associated arthritis, *Medicine (Baltimore)* **57:**463–475.

0ecHollingsworth, J. W., and Atkins, E., 1965, Synovial inflammatory response to bacterial endotoxin, *Yale J. Biol. Med.* **38:**241–256.

Hsu, S. H., Chan, M. M., and Bias, W. B., 1981, Genetic control of major histocompatibility complex-linked immune responses to synthetic polypeptides in man, *Proc. Natl. Acad. Sci. U.S.A.* **78:**440–444.

Hughes, W. T., 1977, Infections in the compromised host, *Adv. Intern. Med.* **22:**73–81.

Inman, R. D., Gallegos, K. V., Brause, B. D., Redecha, P. B., and Christian, C. L., 1984, Clinical and microbial features of prosthetic joint infection, *Am. J. Med.* **77:**47–53.

Jarrett, M. P., Grossman, L., Sadler, A. H., and Grayzel, A. I., 1981, The role of arthroscopy in the treatment of septic arthritis, *Arthritis Rheum.* **24:**737–739.

Joysey, V. C., and Wolf, E., 1978, HLA-A, -B, and -C antigens, their serology and cross reaction, *Br. Med. Bull.* **34:**217–222.

Jupiter, J. B., Karchmer, A. W., Lowell, J. D., and Harris, W. H., 1981, Total hip arthroplasty in the treatment of adult hips with current or quiescent sepsis, *J. Bone Joint Surg.* **63A:**194–200.

Kaslow, R. A., 1984, The epidemiology of *Yersinia* and other reactive arthropathies, in: *Epidemiology of the Rheumatic Diseases* (R. C. Lawrence and L. E. Shulman, eds.), Gower Medical, New York, London, pp. 89–100.

Kaslow, R. A., Ryder, R. P., and Calin, A., 1979, Search for Reiter's syndrome after an outbreak of *Shigella sonnei* dysentery, *J. Rheumatol.* **6:**562–566.

Kasunen, T. U., Kaurenen, O., Martio, J., Pitkänen, J., Pönkä, A., Hortling, L., Aittoniemi, S., Mutru, O., Penttila, O., and Koskimies, S., 1980, Reactive arthritis after *Campylobacter jejuni* enteritis in patients with HLA-B27, *Lancet* **1:**1312–1313.

Keat, A., 1983, Reiter's syndrome and reactive arthritis in perspective, *N. Engl. J. Med.* **309:**1606–1615.

Kellgren, J. H., Ball, J., Fairbrother, R. W., and Barnes, K. L., 1958, Suppurative arthritis complicating rheumatoid arthritis, *Br. Med. J.* **1:**1193–1200.

Kelly, J. J., and Weisiger, B. B., 1963, The arthritis of Whipple's disease, *Arthritis Rheum.* **6:**615–632.

Khan, M. A., Kushner, I., and Braun, W. E., 1980, Genetic heterogeneity in primary ankylosing spondylitis, *J. Rheumatol.* **7:**383–386.

LeClerq, S. A., and Russell, A. S., 1984, The risk of sacroiliitis in B27 positive persons: A reappraisal, *J. Rheumatol.* **11:**327–329.

Lehman, T. J. A., Allen, J. B., Plotz, P. H., and Wilder, R. L., 1983, Polyarthritis in rats following the systemic injection of *Lactobacillus casei* cell walls in aqueous suspension, *Arthritis Rheum.* **26:**1259–1265.

Lehman, T. J. A., Allen, J. B., Plotz, P. H., and Wilder, R. L., 1984, *Lactobacillus casei* cell wall-induced arthritis in rats: Cell wall fragment distribution and persistence in chronic arthritis-susceptible LEW/N and -resistant F344/N rats, *Arthritis Rheum.* **27:**939–942.

Lofgren, R. P., Mahowald, M. L., Peterson, L. R., Jagiella, W. M., Raddatz, D. A., Raskind, J. R., Shafer, R. B., and Gereing, D. N., 1982, Staphylococcal bacteremia in rabbits with antigen induced arthritis, *Arthritis Rheum.* **25:**S83.

London, J. C., 1976, The ecology and taxonomic status of the lactobacilli, *Annu. Rev. Microbiol.* **30:**279–301.

Maizel, H., Rufin, J. M., and Dobbins, W. O., 1970, Whipple's disease: A review of 19 patients from one hospital and a review of the literature since 1950, *Medicine (Baltimore)* **49:**175–205.

Manicourt, D. H., and Orloff, S., 1982, Gonococcal arthritis–dermatitis syndrome: Study of serum and synovial fluid immune complex levels, *Arthritis Rheum.* **25:**574–578.

McMichael, A., and McDevitt, H. O., 1977, The association between the HLA system and disease, *Prog. Med. Genet.* **2:**39–95.

Nelson, J. D., 1972, The bacterial etiology and antibiotic management of septic arthritis in infants and children, *Pediatrics* **50:**437–440.

Newman, J. H., 1976, Review of septic arthritis throughout the antibiotic era, *Ann. Rheum. Dis.* **35:**198–205.

Norton, W. L., Lewis, D., and Ziff, M., 1966, Light and electron microscopic observations in the synovitis of Reiter's disease, *Arthritis Rheum.* **9:**747–757.

O'Brien, J. P., Goldenberg, D. L., and Rice, P. A., 1983, Disseminated gonococcal infection: A prospective analysis of 49 patients and a review of pathophysiology and immune mechanism, *Medicine (Baltimore)* **62:**395–406.

Oxelius, J.-A., 1984, Immunoglobulin G (IgG) subclasses and human disease, *Am. J. Med.* **76**(3A):7–18.

Parant, M., Parant, F., Chedid, L., Yapa, A., Petit, J. F., and Lederer, D., 1979, Fate of the synthetic immunoadjuvant, muramyl dipeptide (14-C-labelled) in the mouse, *Int. J. Immunopharmacol.* **1:**35–41.

Parker, R. H., and Schmid, F. R., 1971, Antibacterial activity of synovial fluid during therapy of septic arthritis, *Arthritis Rheum.* **14:**96–104.

Peltola, H., Käyaty, H., Virtanen, M., Mäkelä, P. H., 1984, Prevention of *Hemophilus influenzae* type b bacteremic infections with the capsular polysaccharide vaccine, *N. Engl. J. Med.* **310:**1561–1566.

Peterson, B. H., Lee, T. J., Snyderman, R., and Brooks, G. F., 1979, *Neisseria meningitidis* and *Neisseria gonorrhoeae* bacteremia associated with C6, C7 or C8 deficiency, *Ann. Intern. Med.* **90:**917–920.

Phemister, D. B., 1924, The effect of pressure on articular surfaces in pyogenic and tuberculous arthritides and its bearing on treatment, *Ann. Surg.* **80:**481–500.

Reed, W. P., Davidson, M. S., and Williams, R. C., Jr., 1976, Complement system in pneumococcal infection, *Infect. Immun.* **13:**1120–1128.

Rittner, C., and Bertrams, J., 1981, On the significance of C2, C4 and factor B polymorphisms in disease, *Human Genet.* **56:**235–247.

Rodey, G. E., Luehrman, L. K., and Thomas, D. W., 1979, *In vitro* primary immunization of human peripheral blood lymphocytes to KLH: Evidence for HLA-D region restriction, *J. Immunol.* **123:**2250–2253.

Ross, G. N., Baroff, L. J., and Quismorio, F. P., 1975, *Serratia* arthritis in heroin users, *J. Bone Joint Surg.* **57A:**1158–1160.

Sasazuki, T., Kaneoka, H., Nishimura, Y., Kaneoka, R., Hayama, M., and Ohkuni, H., 1980, An HLA-linked immune suppression gene in man, *J. Exp. Med.* **152:**297s–313s.

Schmid, F. R., 1985, Principles of diagnosis and treatment of bone and joint infections, in: *Arthritis and Allied Conditions* (D. J. McCarty, ed.), Lea & Febiger, Philadelphia, pp. 1627–1650.

Schurman, D. L., Mirra, J., Ding, A., and Nagel, D. A., 1977, Experimental *E. coli* arthritis in rabbits. A model of infectious and post-infectious inflammatory synovitis, *J. Rheumatol.* **4:**118–127.

Schwab, J. H., Cromartie, W. J., Ohanian, S. H., and Craddock, J. G., 1967, Association of experimental chronic arthritis with the persistence of group A streptococcal cell walls in the articular tissue, *J. Bacteriol.* **94:**1728–1735.

Schwartz, B. D., Luehrman, L. K., and Rodey, G. E., 1979, Public antigenic determinant on a family of HLA-B molecules, *J. Clin. Invest.* **64:**938–994.

Seager, K., Bashir, H. V., Gelzy, A. F., Edmonds, J., and Tyndall, A., 1979, Evidence for a specific B27 associated cell surface marker on lymphocytes of patients with ankylosing spondylitis, *Nature* **277:**68–70.

Shagrin, J. W., Frame, B., and Duncan, H., 1971, Polyarthritis in obese patients with intestinal bypass, *Ann. Intern. Med.* **75:**377–380.

Sheagren, J. N., 1984, *Staphylococcus areus:* The persistent pathogen, *N. Engl. J. Med.* **310:**1368–1373,1437–1442.

Simpson, R. W., Smith, C., and Godzeski, C., 1984, Association of parvoviruses with rheumatoid arthritis of humans, *Science* **223:**1425.

Small, C. B., Slater, L. N., Lowy, F. D., Small, R. D., Salvati, E. A., and Casey, J. I., 1984, Group B streptococcal arthritis in adults, *Am. J. Med.* **76:**367–375.

Smialowicz, R. J., and Schwab, J. H., 1977, Processing of streptococcal cell walls by rat macrophages and human monocytes *in vitro, Infect. Immun.* **17:**591–598.

Summers, G. D., and Jayson, M. I. V., 1980, Does Poncet's disease exist? *Rheumatol. Rehabil.* **19:**149–150.

Taurog, J. D., Leary, S. L., Cremer, M. A., Mahowald, M. L., Sandberg, G. P., and Manning, P. J., 1984, Infection with *Mycoplasma pulmonis* modulated adjuvant- and collagen-induced arthritis in Lewis rats, *Arthritis Rheum.* **27:**943–946.

Urman, J. D., Zurier, R. B., and Rothfield, N. F., 1977, Reiter's syndrome associated with *Campylobacter* infection, *Ann. Intern. Med.* **86:**444–446.

Utsinger, P. D., 1980, Bypass disease: A bacterial antigen–antibody systemic immune complex disease, *Arthritis Rheum.* **23:**758.

Van den Berg-Loonen, E. M., Dekker-Saeys, B. J., Meuwissen, S. G. M., Nijenhuis, L. E., and Engelfriet, C. R., 1977, Histocompatibility antigens and other genetic markers in ankylosing spondylitis and inflammatory bowel diseases, *J. Immunogenet.* **4:**167–175.

van der Linden, S. M., Valkenburg, H. A., de Jongh, B. M., and Cats, A., 1984, The risk of developing ankylosing spondylitis in HLA-B27 positive individuals: A comparison of relatives of spondylitis patients with the general population, *Arthritis Rheum.* **27:**241–249.

Waldvogel, F. A., Medoff, G., and Schwartz, M. N., 1970, Osteomyelitis: A review of clinical features, therapeutic considerations and unusual aspects, *N. Engl. J. Med.* **282:**198–206,260–266,316–322.

Walker, L. C., Ahlin, T. D., Tung, K. S., and Williams, R. C., Jr., 1978, Circulating immune complexes in disseminated gonorrheal infection, *Ann. Intern. Med.* **89:**28–33.

Wands, J. R., LaMont, J. T., Mann, E., and Isselbacher, K. J., 1976, Arthritis associated with intestinal bypass procedure for morbid obesity: Complement activation and characterization of circulating cryoproteins, *N. Engl. J. Med.* **294:**121–124.

Warren, R. E., and Brewerton, D. A., 1980, Faecal carriage of *Klebsiella* by patients with ankylosing spondylitis and rheumatoid arthritis, *Ann. Rheum. Dis.* **39:**37–44.

Washburn, L. R., Cole, B. C., and Ward, J. R., 1982, Chronic arthritis of rabbits induced by mycoplasmas: III. Induction with non-viable *Mycoplasma arthritidis* antigens, *Arthritis Rheum.* **25:**937–946.

Wehrbein, H. L., 1929, Gonococcus arthritis: A study of six hundred and ten cases, *Surg. Gynecol. Obstet.* **49:**105–113.

Welsh, J., Avakian, H., Cowling, P., Ebringer, A., Wooley, P., Panayi, G., and Ebringer, R., 1980, Ankylosing spondylitis, HLA-B27 and *Klebsiella*. I. Cross-reactivity studies with rabbit antisera, *Br. J. Exp. Pathol.* **61:**85–91.

Wilder, R. L., and Allen, J. B., 1984, The role of thymus-dependent lymphocytes in the pathogenesis of group A streptococcal cell wall-induced arthritis (SCWIA) in rats, *Arthritis Rheum.* **37:**S36.

Wilder, R. L., Calandra, G. B., Garvin, A. J., Wright, K. D., and Hansen, C. T., 1982, Strain and sex variation in the susceptibility to streptococcal cell wall-induced polyarthritis in the rat, *Arthritis Rheum.* **25:**1064–1072.

Wilder, R. L., Allen, J. B., Wahl, L. M., Calandra, G. B., and Wahl, S. M., 1983, The pathogenesis of group A streptococcal cell wall-induced polyarthritis in the rat, *Arthritis Rheum.* **26:**1442–1451.

Willkens, R. F., Healey, L. A., and Decker, J. L., 1960, Acute infectious arthritis in the aged and chronically ill, *Arch. Intern. Med.* **106:**334–364.

Woodrow, J. C., 1977, Histocompatibility antigens and rheumatic diseases, *Semin. Arthritis Rheum.* **6:**257–276.

Wright, V., and Watkinson, G., 1966, Articular complications of ulcerative colitis, *Am. J. Proctol.* **17:**107–115.

15

Scleroderma as a Fibrotic Disorder

J. Eugene Huffstutter and E. Carwile LeRoy

I. INTRODUCTION

Scleroderma (SD) is a multisystem disease of unknown etiology. Its study has involved collaboration between clinicians and basic scientists. Clinical studies have helped to define the natural variation of disease manifestations (subsets) and to gain empirical insight into pathogenic mechanisms; such careful categorization of patients is also important in experiments involving patients' cells or body fluids to understand potential differences in results.

The unique feature of scleroderma, diffuse fibrosis, has been a focal point in the investigation of its cellular mechanisms. New cell-culture techniques and better understanding of cellular responses have enhanced our knowledge of fibrotic processes. Investigation of animal models such as the tight-skin mouse may explain some aspects of the hidebound skin of SD. Also, the further characterization of some recently described human diseases (e.g., chronic graft-versus-host disease, toxic-oil syndrome) that share characteristics of SD may define common cellular responses to different stimuli.

This chapter gives a broad overview of the study of SD, attempting to consolidate diverse areas of investigation with an emphasis on interrelationships between immune responses and fibrosis.

II. CLINICAL ASPECTS

A detailed review of recent clinical and therapeutic observations is beyond the scope of this chapter. Recent developments that have enlarged our understanding of disease man-

---

J. Eugene Huffstutter and E. Carwile LeRoy • Department of Medicine, Division of Rheumatology and Immunology, Medical University of South Carolina, Charleston, South Carolina 29425.

ifestations and may be key to learning the mechanism(s) involved in pathogenesis are briefly discussed.

A. Renal

Perhaps the greatest single achievement in SD therapy has been the current treatment for hypertension/renal crisis. Since the initial case reports by Mitnick and Feig (1978) and by Wasner *et al.* (1978), aggressive medical management without nephrectomy has become the standard of care. With the development of captopril, control of hypertension is improved, as is our understanding of its mechanisms (Lopez-Ovejero *et al.*, 1979). The initial enthusiasm regarding the reversibility of renal failure has been tempered by reports of progressive kidney failure despite optimal blood pressure control (Brown *et al.*, 1983). One reason for this variable response concerns the clinical status of the patient when therapy is initiated (Whitman *et al.*, 1982). It is possible for the SD kidney to evolve through several phases before "permanent" failure ensues. Basal and stimulated plasma renin levels have been correlated with renal histology (Kovalchik *et al.*, 1978), but the mechanisms involved in the pathogenesis of these lesions are unknown. Further study is needed to clarify the sequence of events responsible for renal disease in SD.

B. Pulmonary

With improved therapy for SD renal disease, the focus has shifted to the lungs as a major cause of morbidity and mortality. The advent of reproducible spirometry and diffusion capacities has allowed lung function to be evaluated noninvasively over time (Schneider *et al.*, 1982). Newer scanning techniques have demonstrated inflammatory infiltrates (Baron *et al.*, 1983) and abnormalities in vascular dynamics (Furst *et al.*, 1981); correlation of these findings with disease pathogenesis is needed. Prospective analysis of patients may elucidate disease mechanisms. Although other organ involvement may correlate with pulmonary function abnormalities (Denis *et al.*, 1981), the nature of these associations is still under investigation.

The use of bronchoalveolar lavage in the investigation of idiopathic pulmonary fibrosis has proven valuable. From study of cells and cell products in lavage fluid, mechanisms of lung fibrosis may be clarified (Reynolds *et al.*, 1977; Martin *et al.*, 1983). Since this technique is relatively safe and reproducible, patients may be followed longitudinally, correlating lavage data with clinical parameters. Silver and colleagues (1984) have demonstrated that bronchoalveolar lavage can be applied safely to SD patients. New information regarding mechanisms of inflammation and fibrosis should be forthcoming.

C. Cardiac

Primary heart involvement in SD, although easy to detect histologically, may be difficult to identify clinically. Advances in echocardiography and scanning techniques facilitate diagnosis of clinically silent lesions so that the natural history and therapeutic interventions can be monitored (Gottdiener *et al.*, 1979; Botstein and LeRoy, 1981). A correlation of heart involvement with severity of skin involvement has been established (Follansbee *et al.*, 1984) and may reflect widespread small-vessel disease (LeRoy, 1984).

One new technique that may be useful in the evaluation of SD heart disease is nuclear magnetic resonance imaging (James *et al.*, 1982). This modality will allow better resolution of structures in addition to metabolic information.

In summary, clinical studies are a useful guide to understanding SD. Correlation of specific disease features and longitudinal evaluation of patients to detect early disease (Harper *et al.*, 1982) are critical in these studies.

III. MODELS OF SCLERODERMA

Since the description by Stastny *et al.* in 1963 of homologous disease in the rat, the search for an adequate animal model for SD continues. Although several exist, none completely demonstrates the lesions of SD. Investigation of these models may give clues to pathogenic mechanisms applicable to SD. There are other human diseases that share clinical characteristics with SD. Animal models of some of these diseases have been developed; also, animal models to study wound healing may reveal mechanisms of fibroblast regulation.

A. Tight-Skin Mouse

A spontaneous disease in mice resembling SD, first reported by Green *et al.* in 1976, is the tight-skin (TSK) mouse. Skin manifestations closely resemble changes noted in SD but lack inflammatory components. Analysis of the skin reveals an increase in collagen and glycosaminoglycans analogous to SD (Osborn *et al.*, 1983). In culture, TSK mouse fibroblasts produce increased amounts of collagen (Jimenez *et al.*, 1984). Variations of internal organ involvement in the TSK mouse are the major differences between this model and SD (Russell, 1983). Table 1 lists some of the major characteristics of the TSK mouse and SD. Further experiments are needed to understand alterations in fibroblast regulation that lead to thickened skin.

B. Sclerosing Disease of White Leghorn Chickens

An inherited, fibrosing disease occurring in White Leghorn chickens has many features analogous to human SD (Gershwin *et al.*, 1981). Abnormalities seen in both diseases include arthritis, esophageal fibrosis, skin thickening, and peripheral necrosis as well as antibodies to antinuclear antigens. However, these diseases demonstrate different dermal, vascular, and renal histology. Antibodies against type II collagen have been noted in the chicken but not in SD. Although this model may be useful in understanding certain aspects of fibrosis, it may not help in SD because of these histopathological differences.

C. Skin Sclerosis Induced by Glycosaminoglycan Injection

The induction of sclerodermatous changes in mice by injection of glycosaminoglycans (GAG) was first described in 1975 by Ishikawa *et al.* Morphological comparison of the skin in SD and in mice with experimentally induced fibrosis revealed striking similarities with only a few differences involving the vascular appearance and elastic fibers (Ishikawa

Table 1. Comparison of the Tight-Skin Mouse (TSK) and Scleroderma (SD)

	TSK	SD
Skin		
Clinical thickening	+	+
Increased collagen	+	+
Ratio of type I/III collagen	?	Normal
Increased GAG	+	+
Increased fibronectin	?	+
Inflammatory infiltrate	—	+
Skin appendages	Well preserved	Lost
Fibroblasts *in vitro*		
Synthesize increased collagen	+	+
Synthesize increased GAG	?	+
Internal organs		
Lung	Emphysema	Fibrosis
Heart	Enlargement	Pericarditis, myofibrosis
Vascular system	Intimal thinning	Intimal proliferation
Bone	Hypertrophy	Erosion and resorption
Gastrointestinal tract	Normal	Esophageal motility problems, wide-mouth colonic diverticuli, intestinal statis
Renal	Normal	Multiple abnormalities

et al., 1978). The observation that involved skin from the mice demonstrated decreased collagen content (Ishikawa *et al.*, 1980), coupled with a failure to reproduce fibrotic changes using similar techniques (Fox *et al.*, 1982), raises doubt as to the validity of this model for SD. Future studies may identify mechanisms that contribute to disease production after GAG injection.

D. Bleomycin-Induced Fibrosis

Bleomycin, a glycopeptide antibiotic with potent activity against a variety of cancers, is used in conjunction with a variety of antitumor agents because of its lack of bone marrow toxicity. It is concentrated in the lungs and skin, where its major toxicity occurs (Kiely, 1981). Pulmonary fibrosis is seen at cumulative doses greater than 400 mg; lower doses have been associated with skin changes which include hyperpigmentation, erythema, alopecia, ulceration, and infiltrative plaques suggestive of SD. Two patients have been described with bleomycin-induced SD, characterized by proximal hidebound skin without Raynaud's phenomenena or internal organ involvement (Finch *et al.*, 1980); fibroblasts from one patient demonstrated increased collagen and GAG synthesis. Peripheral blood mononuclear cells from this patient were stimulated to proliferate by low concentrations of bleomycin. The patient's skin disease resolved slowly with no specific therapy other than withholding further bleomycin. As his skin disease improved, collagen and GAG synthesis normalized, and his peripheral blood mononuclear cells lost reactivity to bleomycin. This report certainly warrants further investigation into the relationship between bleomycin and fibrosis, including animal models of bleomycin-induced injury (Tom and Montgomery, 1980).

In the lung, bleomycin produces endothelial injury followed by epithelial cell damage, edema, macrophage migration, and epithelial cell hyperplasia. Fibroblasts appear, and fibrosis ensues (Fasske and Morgenroth, 1983). One possible mechanism of bleomycin injury is its effects on DNA. Bleomycin produces breaks in both single- and double-stranded DNA (Haidle, 1971; Lloyd *et al.*, 1979; Love *et al.*, 1981). Bleomycin induces DNA breaks in human fibroblasts *in vitro,* which are rapidly corrected when the drug is removed (Hurt *et al.*, 1983). Effects of DNA breakage on fibroblast proliferation and matrix synthesis are under investigation. It is tempting to postulate an analogy between bleomycin-induced DNA breakage and the chromosome breakage factor described in SD (Emerit, 1979; Sherer *et al.*, 1981). More study is needed to determine the role of DNA breakage in human fibrosis.

E. Serotonin and Fibrosis

The observation that rats injected with serotonin develop thickened skin (MacDonald *et al.*, 1958) prompted speculation about its involvement in the pathogenesis of SD. However, this rat model lacks visceral organ involvement, demonstrates no inflammatory reaction, and has normal skin away from the injection site. Fibroblasts *in vitro* are stimulated by serotonin to replicate (Boucek and Alvarez, 1970). However, they do not produce increased amounts of collagen independent of general protein synthesis (Boucek *et al.*, 1972), a characteristic of SD fibroblasts. Descriptions of SD-like lesions associated with carcinoid tumors (Fries *et al.*, 1973) and therapy with 5-hydroxytryptophan and carbidopa (Sternberg *et al.*, 1980) have intensified recent speculation concerning the role of serotonin in SD. However, these patients lack Raynaud's phenomenon and visceral organ involvement. Proponents of a serotonin mechanism emphasize the vascular effects of serotonin, its location in platelet granules, and interactions of platelet secretion with the immune system (Meuer *et al.*, 1981) as evidence that tryptophan metabolism is important in SD expression. Preliminary trials of ketanserin, a selective antagonist of the serotonin-2 receptor, demonstrate subjective and objective improvement in SD patients with Raynaud's phenomenon (Seibold and Jageneau, 1984). Further work may clarify the role of serotonin in SD. Long-term experiments involving blockade of serotonin receptors may not only confirm possible involvement of this substance in pathogenesis but also demonstrate the efficacy of therapeutic intervention.

F. Wound Healing

Analysis of normal and hypertrophic scars in animal models and human skin should increase our knowledge of connective tissue metabolism and fibroblast regulation. Normal wound healing involves an orderly sequence of events resulting in collagen deposition and maturation (Bailey *et al.*, 1975). Hypertrophic scars demonstrate several abnormalities, which include excess collagen, absence of macrophages with increased numbers of mast cells, decreased elastic fibers, increased GAG, decreased fibrin clearance, and occlusion of microvessels by cellular proliferation (Kurkinen *et al.*, 1980; Kischer *et al.*,

1982). The mechanism(s) responsible for these alterations may be important in the connective tissue abnormalities of SD. Analysis of the sequential events that occur in wound healing may increase understanding of stimulatory and inhibitory factors of fibroblasts. Macrophages are important in promoting wound healing (Thakral *et al.*, 1979; Leibovich and Danon, 1980). The absence of macrophages in hypertrophic scars also implicates their importance in down-regulation. Several factors that stimulate collagen production and disappear when healing is complete have been isolated from early wounds (O'Hare *et al.*, 1983). The cellular source of these factors and the stimulus that induces their production are under active investigation.

One potential stimulus is the low oxygen tension that occurs in wounds as a result of interruption of the blood supply. Rats exposed to hypoxia demonstrated increased collagen deposition in experimental granulation tissue (Chvapil *et al.*, 1970). Capillary growth is also influenced by low oxygen tension (Chvapil, 1974). Using a rabbit model of wound repair, Hunt *et al.* (1978) demonstrated increased lactate, decreased oxygen tension, and increased carbon dioxide at sites of repair. The role these factors play in the regulation of connective tissue metabolism is speculative. However, this does provoke an interesting argument that local hypoxia occurring in poorly perfused tissues of SD patients may be a stimulus for continued collagen synthesis. This model provides a method to investigate the contribution of anaerobic metabolism to wound healing. Certainly other factors are involved, such as platelets and inflammatory cells; their role in fibroblast regulation is reviewed later.

G. Chronic Graft-versus-Host Disease

Reports of SD-like skin changes occurring after bone marrow transplantation (Masters *et al.*, 1975; Spielvogel *et al.*, 1977), coupled with the immunologic abnormalities known to occur in SD, prompted several investigators to propose chronic graft-versus-host disease (GVHD) as a model for SD (Furst *et al.*, 1979; Jaffee and Claman, 1983). The skin disease is similar, with inflammatory infiltrates and increased collagen content. The clinical course may be similar with appearance of esophageal dysfunction, pulmonary fibrosis, cardiac abnormalities, and myositis (Shulman *et al.*, 1980). However, there are important differences, which include the presence of eosinophilia in GVHD and variations in hepatic, intestinal, and renal manifestations. Investigations of the pathogenesis of GVHD have demonstrated effector cells with two characteristics essential for disease expression: proliferation and protracted activation in response to host antigens (Wick *et al.*, 1983). Immunocompetent donor cells that react to minor histocompatibility determinants on host cells have been cultured from skin biopsies (Reinsmoen and Bach, 1983). The prolonged activation of donor cells (by continued stimulation and/or absence of suppression) may be important in fibroblast regulation (*vide infra*). Preliminary studies indicate that suppressor T cells are lacking in acute GVHD, and their reappearance heralds the cessation of disease activity. Studies of T cells in chronic GVHD demonstrate heterogeneity regarding helper/suppressor T-cell ratios and are inconclusive (Reinherz *et al.*, 1979). The sequence of events involved in the pathogenesis of chronic GVHD is still under investigation. Elucidation of the immunologic alterations that result in fibrosis may have application to mechanisms important in SD.

H. Toxin-Induced Sclerosis

Various chemicals have been implicated in the induction of a SD-like illness. In addition to serotonin (previously described), the offending agents include a wide range of aromatic and chlorinated solvents and epoxy resins (Yamakage *et al.*, 1980; Walder, 1983). Exposed subjects present with skin sclerosis and Raynaud's phenomenon, usually without the visceral organ involvement of SD. The disease may be self-limiting. Although not an adequate model for SD, they may serve as a model for the development of skin sclerosis.

Probably the most recognized form of this model is vinyl-chloride-induced disease. All cases have been described in people who clean the polymerizers in vinyl chloride production (Dinman *et al.*, 1971). Although these patients developed Raynaud's phenomenon and internal organ involvement (e.g., hepatic fibrosis, linear pulmonary fibrosis) (Suciu *et al.*, 1975; Dodson *et al.*, 1971), it is not the internal organ involvement characteristic of SD (Maricq *et al.*, 1976).

A SD-like illness occurring after cosmetic surgery with silicone or paraffin injections has recently been reviewed (Kumagai *et al.*, 1984). These patients demonstrate skin changes that range from morphea to sclerodactyly to diffuse SD. Other manifestations include myositis, pulmonary fibrosis, digital ulcers, and Sjogren's syndrome. Immunologic responses to the injected material are considered causal. Further work is needed to define the immune alterations and how they result in fibrosis.

Spanish toxic-oil syndrome (TOS) is a multisystem disease caused by the ingestion of adulterated rapeseed oil. The disease has two phases. The acute phase is characterized by fever, headaches, exanthems, pulmonary disease, and eosinophilia. Several patients died of respiratory failure or thromboembolic complications from a nonnecrotizing vasculitis. Later, a chronic phase develops with neuromuscular problems, sclerodermiform skin lesions, and weight loss (Martinez-Tello *et al.*, 1982). Other similarities to SD include the presence of myositis and renal disease. In one case, a renal biopsy was reported to have changes similar to those in SD (Gutierrez-Millet *et al.*, 1982). The vascular lesions of TOS include endothelial swelling, vacuolization, and necrosis (Toxic Epidemic Syndrome Study Group, 1982). This is followed by infiltration of the vessel wall by eosinophils, plasma cells, and lymphocytes. Finally, there is obliterative fibrosis of the intima. There are other differences in addition to the vascular lesions. Autopsies on 20 patients with TOS failed to reveal kidney lesions similar to those of SD but instead found interstitial inflammatory infiltrates and vascular lesions previously described. Toxic-oil syndrome is also characterized by a pulmonary lesion with no fibrosis, inflammatory liver infiltrates, a lack of immune complexes in the serum, and eosinophilia. Thus, despite similarities, there are important differences. It is interesting to speculate that the skin fibrosis may be the result of endothelial damage. Since the lung is the major initial site of endothelial injury, the absence of interstitial lung disease thus far is enigmatic. Future work may identify the causal agent of the disease and clarify the mechanism(s) of pathogenesis.

I. Miscellaneous Sclerodermalike Diseases

A number of other illnesses have SD-like features. These include scleredema, scleromyxoedema, porphyria cutanea tarda, eosinophilic fasciitis, and SD-like changes in insulin-dependent diabetes (Fleischmajer and Pollock, 1979; Kent *et al.*, 1981). The etiologies of these disorders are diverse, and further research into their pathogenesis may not be applicable to SD. However, certain similarities to SD do exist. Sclerodactyly occurs commonly in juvenile diabetes and may be associated with the extent of vascular disease (Seibold, 1982). Fibroblasts from these patients exhibit increased collagen synthesis *in vitro* (Kohn and Hensse, 1977). Decreases in lung compliance have been noted and attributed to glycosolation of collagen, resulting in thickened fibrils, decreased breakdown, and increased cross linkage (Garza-Elizondo *et al.*, 1983). Thus, further investigation of this illness may reveal mechanisms of connective tissue interaction and fibroblast regulation.

IV. GENETICS

Several diseases that exhibit autoimmune phenomena are associated with certain HLA tissue types. Reports of familial SD (Gray and Altman, 1977; Sheldon *et al.*, 1981) implicated an inherited mechanism of disease expression. Preliminary studies suggested that SD may also have one or more HLA associations (Freudenberg *et al.*, 1978; Di-Bartolomeo *et al.*, 1981; Ercilla *et al.*, 1981; Germain *et al.*, 1981; Gladman *et al.*, 1981). However, typing of 237 SD patients noted only a very small increase in HLA-Bw35 (0.30 vs. 0.17 in normals). There was an association of the DR-3 antigen with pulmonary fibrosis (0.42 vs. 0.20) and of the DR-1 antigen with the presence of anticentromere antibody (0.46 vs. 0.17; $P < 0.05$), but the significance of these observations is unknown (Lynch *et al.*, 1982).

HLA-D associations may be important in pathogenesis since these antigens resemble rodent immune response antigens in structure and tissue distribution (Stobo, 1982). The recent demonstration of human antigens that resemble HLA-DR antigens but are immunologically distinct implies that other immune response genes exist (Lampson and Levy, 1980; Goyert *et al.*, 1982). Further work is needed to characterize these antigens and define their role in immune response and disease pathogenesis.

V. IMMUNOLOGIC ASPECTS

A. Humoral Immunity

Although immunologic mechanisms have long been thought to be involved in the pathogenesis of SD, attempts at elucidating disease-specific immune mechanisms have been largely unsuccessful. As new techniques are developed, immune mechanisms are partially clarified, and new questions raised. An example involves the use of actively dividing human cells (HEp2) in assays for antinuclear antibodies (ANA). By utilizing cultured cell lines, one can reduce preparation artifacts. A positive ANA can be detected in a higher percentage of scleroderma patients with this system than with older methods utilizing fixed rodent tissue sections (Tan, 1981).

At least four different ANA staining patterns exist; some describe nine separate, definable patterns (Bernstein *et al.*, 1982). The most common pattern seen consists of fine speckles. A second ANA pattern is centromeric, indicating the presence of anticentromere antibodies (ACA). This antibody pattern seems to be correlated with the limited cutaneous (CREST) variant of generalized SD and Raynaud's phenomenon (Tan *et al.*, 1980; Fritzler and Kinsella, 1980; Moroi *et al.*, 1980; McCarty *et al.*, 1983). The antigen appears to be a protein or polypeptide tightly bound to centromeric DNA (kinetochore). Longitudinal studies indicate the antibodies to be IgG at a fairly constant titer (Tramposch *et al.*, 1984). Other clinical correlates include telangiectasias of the digits, calcinosis, and an inverse association with pulmonary involvement; the presence of ACA in these patients does not predict survival (Steen *et al.*, 1984). A third ANA pattern described in SD patients consists of diffuse, fine speckles indicative of antibodies to an extractable nucleoprotein termed Scl-70. This antigen is a nonhistone, chromosome-associated protein with an approximate molecular weight of 70,000 (Douvas *et al.*, 1979). It is present in about 20% of all SD patients but has a higher prevalence in patients with diffuse disease and correlates with lung involvement (Catoggio *et al.*, 1983). It is rarely found in other diseases. Patterns of discrete, course speckles, nucleolar dots, and homogeneous staining have also been noted, but the nature of the antigens remains unknown. Three different nucleolar patterns occur and probably reflect multiple antigens.

Immune complexes detected in the serum of SD patients seem to correlate with the presence of pulmonary involvement (Seibold *et al.*, 1982; Siminovitch *et al.*, 1982). The nature of the antigen(s) involved is unknown; antibodies to types I and IV collagen have been detected in scleroderma sera. These antibody levels also correlate with lung involvement (Mackel *et al.*, 1982a).

With regard to further research in the area of humoral immunity in SD, the nature of the centromeric antigen and Scl-70 will be further defined. It is likely that the specific antigens resulting in the other patterns will also be identified. Correlations between serologic and clinical parameters may give clues to mechanisms involved both in antibody induction and in propagation of disease.

Localization of immune complexes to particular tissues may indicate their role in disease expression. Techniques exist for separating immune complexes into component antibodies and antigens. Antigen identification may define the immune alteration(s) resulting in specific antibody production.

B. Cellular Immunity

Histological examination of newly diagnosed SD patients provides a morphological argument that cellular immunity is involved in the pathogenesis of SD. During the earliest identifiable clinical phase, mononuclear cells are noted in both involved and uninvolved skin (Fleischmajer *et al.*, 1977a,b; Rodnan *et al.*, 1979). This infiltrate, consisting of lymphocytes, plasma cells, and macrophages, usually precedes fibrosis. The quantity of dermal lymphocytes in skin biopsies seems to correlate not only with the degree of thickened skin but also with the progression of skin disease (Roumm *et al.*, 1983). T lymphocytes are present in these infiltrates in the normal helper-to-suppressor ratio. However, lymphocyte characterization from peripheral blood of SD patients demonstrates an increased helper-to-suppressor ratio (Alarcon-Segovia *et al.*, 1981; Krakauer *et al.*, 1981; Claudy *et al.*, 1982; Morse and Bodi, 1982; Whiteside *et al.*, 1983); this finding is not universal (Keystone *et al.*, 1982). Some experiments have demonstrated increased suppressor cell activity in peripheral blood (Keystone *et al.*, 1981; Krawitt *et al.*, 1982). Suppressor monocytes have been postulated as a mechanism to explain decreased *in vitro* antibody responses (Segond *et al.*, 1982); increased suppressor function could explain the decreased reactivity to mitogens such as phytohemagglutinin observed in SD patients (Lockshin *et al.*, 1983). However, several experiments document normal responses to mitogens (Baron *et al.*, 1981; Winkelstein *et al.*, 1982).

Thus, experiments to elucidate abnormalities in immune cell function have yielded conflicting results (Jimenez, 1983). Alterations observed in these experiments may reflect variations in cell number. A decrease in T cells has been documented with normal numbers of circulating B cells (Wright *et al.*, 1979; Baron *et al.*, 1981). Scleroderma sera have been observed to be cytotoxic to lymphocytes (Pruzanski *et al.*, 1983); this cytotoxicity has not been shown to be consistently T-cell selective and may not explain the observed T-cell paucity. Lymphocytes of SD patients have demonstrated cytotoxicity against various target cells (Currie *et al.*, 1970; Wright *et al.*, 1982b); this has not been a consistent finding (Cooper and Friou, 1979; Wright *et al.*, 1982a).

A potential reason for such differing results involves the phase of disease. As patients evolve in their disease, their immune system may also change. It is possible that a single patient may demonstrate an altered helper/suppressor T-cell ratio or a defect in mitogen responsiveness at a particular phase of SD. The stage of disease is the key to interpreting these studies; carefully documented longitudinal evaluation of patients with and without these immunologic abnormalities is needed to study these questions.

Experiments to determine mechanisms responsible for alterations in cellular immunity have been inconclusive, although several potential self-antigens have been identified. Lymphocyte transformation to cellular components (Hughes *et al.*, 1974) and to collagen has been demonstrated (Currie *et al.*, 1970; Stuart *et al.*, 1976). Lymphokine production in response to crude skin homogenates (Kondo *et al.*, 1976, 1979) and purified collagens has been observed. It is not known what role these alterations play in pathogenesis, but they do provide a mechanism by which lymphocytes may become activated at potential sites of fibrosis. These activated cells could recruit monocytes and plasma cells, producing the inflammatory skin infiltrates noted in SD. Products of these inflammatory cells secreted in close proximity to fibroblasts may induce activation and/or proliferation (Mackel *et al.*, 1982b). Although cell-mediated immunity to collagen is not disease specific (Trentham *et al.*, 1978; Adar *et al.*, 1983), future experiments may clarify the antigens involved and mechanisms resulting in this autoimmunity. The possibility that collagen type-specific immune responses result in different clinical patterns deserves further study.

VI. CONNECTIVE TISSUE

One method of investigating the fibrosis of SD concerns the biochemical analysis of connective tissue components. Although some reports describe a decrease in both thickness and collagen content of clinically involved skin (Fleischmajer, 1964; Black *et al.*, 1970), most studies demonstrate skin thickening histologically and by weight that closely correlates with clinical estimates (Rodnan *et al.*, 1979). Characterization of scleroderma skin collagens reveals types I and III in similar proportions to those found in normal adult dermis (Lovell *et al.*, 1979; Nimni, 1983). Investigation of other organs involved in fibrosis reveals collagen deposition in increased amounts but similar proportions of types I and III collagens (Russell *et al.*, 1982; Black *et al.*, 1983). The mechanisms involved in collagen synthesis, deposition, and maturation in SD are unclear (LeRoy, 1981; Uitto and Bauer, 1982). Increases in procollagen (Fleischmajer *et al.*, 1980a) and type III collagen (Fleischmajer *et al.*, 1980b) have been identified around capillaries, implicating small vessels as sites for initial fibrosis. Serum factors released into the interstitium after vascular injury would be at higher concentrations around vessels. Further work is needed to clarify the vascular interactions with connective tissue.

Analysis of other connective tissue components reveals increases in glycosaminoglycans (Fleischmajer and Perlish, 1972; Ishikawa and Horiuchi, 1975) and fibronectin (Cooper *et al.*, 1979). The distribution of fibronectin seems to parallel the location of collagen. It may function as a site for fibroblast migration and attachment (Pearlstein, 1976) and therefore act as an important component of the extracellular matrix involved in maintaining cell location. The interaction of fibronectin with fibrin and inflammatory cells are being actively investigated (Bianco, 1983; Colvin, 1983). Elucidation of these complex interactions may be important in understanding links between vascular and inflammatory aspects of SD. Further analysis of tissues involved in SD may reveal the factors resulting in the hidebound quality of skin, whether it be alterations in collagen linkage or interaction with glycosaminoglycans or fibronectin or other substances not yet identified.

VII. FIBROBLAST METABOLISM

Although the nature of the fibrosis and the cells involved in SD are still being investigated, it is felt that fibroblasts play a key pathogenetic role. To understand fibroblast alterations in disease, their function in health must be better understood. It is evident that fibroblasts are metabolically active in normals, being responsible for the production and maintenance of the connective tissue matrix. They also play a major role in tissue repair after injury. Increased numbers of dermal fibroblasts have been noted in SD and may be responsible for the resulting fibrosis (Fleischmajer *et al.*, 1983). This increased population could result from migration from surrounding tissues or local proliferation or both. Alternative explanations for the apparent increase in fibroblast numbers involve problems in methods of analysis and interpretation of cell morphology. *In situ* measurements of cell number are difficult and may be inaccurate when dependent on only two-dimensional observations. Morphological changes may reflect enhanced metabolic activity with no change in absolute numbers (Fleischmajer *et al.*, 1977a). *In vitro,* these cells produce increased quantities of collagen (LeRoy, 1972, 1974). Thus, three aspects of fibroblast regulation may be important in SD disease expression: migration, proliferation, and activation.

This section reviews experiments regarding these three aspects of fibroblast regulation and their potential role in SD.

A. Chemotactic Factors

Fibroblast migration has been documented both *in vitro* and *in vivo* (Abercrombie *et al.*, 1971; Baum, 1971). Several chemoattractants have been identified. They include components of connective tissue such as collagen (Postlethwaite *et al.*, 1978), elastin (Senior *et al.*, 1982), and fibronectin (Seppa *et al.*, 1981). Peripheral blood mononuclear cells and cells from granulomas also produce factors that attract fibroblasts (Postlethwaite *et al.*, 1976; Wyler and Postlethwaite, 1983). Platelet products such as platelet factor four, platelet-derived growth factor, and β-thromboglobulin have all been shown to be fibroblast chemoattractants (Senior *et al.*, 1983) in addition to activated complement (C5a) components (Postlethwaite *et al.*, 1979). Thus, multiple mechanisms can result in fibroblast migration; however, the sequence of events involved in fibroblast migration in normal and disease processes is still incompletely understood.

B. Proliferation

It is probable that under certain conditions, fibroblasts migrate, whereas other stimuli result in cellular proliferation to increase numbers. This proliferation is controlled by several mechanisms. Insulin, neuraminidase, thrombin, platelet-derived growth factor, and trypsin all demonstrate a direct stimulatory effect on fibroblasts. Addition of these substances to density-inhibited cultures results in cell proliferation (Vaheri *et al.*, 1973). The effects of inflammatory cells on fibroblast metabolism are more complex. Peripheral blood mononuclear cells, when stimulated specifically (by antigen) and nonspecifically (by mitogen), release substances into the media that result in fibroblast proliferation (Wahl *et al.*, 1978; DeLustro *et al.*, 1980; Schmidt *et al.*, 1982; Postlethwaite and Kang, 1983). Mononuclear cells also produce factors that inhibit fibroblast growth (Korn *et al.*, 1980; Elias *et al.*, 1982). It appears that these experiments are in direct contradiction, but analysis of the methods utilized reveals potential reasons for the differences. Table 2 lists some of the differences in the methods of two of these studies showing different results.

Table 2. Differences in Methods of Two Studies of Effects of PBM-Derived Supernatants on Cultured Fibroblasts[a]

	DeLustro *et al.* (1980)	Korn *et al.* (1980)
PBM culture		
Serum	10% fetal calf	20% human AB
Time	48 hr	72 hr
Container	Culture dishes (anchorage dependent)	Polypropylene tubes (suspension culture)
Factor first noted	2 hr	6 hr
Cell concentration	2.5×10^5/cc	5×10^5/cc
Fibroblast culture		
Serum	5% fetal calf	10% fetal calf
Subculture passage	4–10	8–30
Time	48–96 hr	48 hr
Cell concentration	2.5×10^4/cc	5×10^4/cc
Supernatants added	24 hr after fibroblasts plated	At same time fibroblasts plated

[a] Differences in methods of two studies demonstrating opposite effects of peripheral blood mononuclear (PBM) derived supernatants on cultured fibroblasts are listed. The DeLustro *et al.* study reported fibroblast stimulation while the article by Korn *et al.* observed suppression. The explanation for these "contradictory" results may well be methodologic.

Although all of the factors listed may be important, certain aspects seem to have greater potential for producing different results. These include the use of suspension cultures versus an anchorage-dependent system, variations in the concentration and type of sera, and different times for harvesting supernatants and addition to the fibroblasts. Therefore, fibroblasts may be controlled by both stimulatory and inhibitory factors produced by mononuclear cells.

The number of mitogens and chemoattractants identified is further evidence that fibroblast regulation must occur at several levels. This regulation may occur through the presence or absence of soluble mediators (Wharton, 1983) or by a differential response to varying concentrations of the same mediator. For example, prostaglandin E_2 is stimulatory at low concentrations and inhibitory at high concentrations (Castor and Fremuth, 1982). Another difference in these regulators is the observation that some act at a specific phase of the cycle of cell division whereas others are not cell-cycle specific (Bitterman *et al.*, 1982). The duration of effects that these factors have on fibroblasts may not depend on length of exposure or the half-life of the factor *in vitro*. Expression of an abnormal phenotype, which may continue for several generations, can be induced by brief exposures of fibroblasts to cell supernatants (Korn, 1983). Thus, biological assays that measure a summation of multiple activities may not reflect the variety of substances contained in the sample (DeLustro *et al.*, 1983). More work is needed to define the time course involved in production of the factors. Purification and characterization will facilitate the search for the source of these substances and permit a study of their mechanisms in the complex process of fibroblast proliferation.

C. Matrix Synthesis

In addition to proliferation, a number of factors have been identified that influence protein and proteoglycan synthesis by fibroblasts. Several different products from mononuclear cells cultured with and without nonspecific and specific mitogens have been identified that stimulate fibroblast collagen synthesis (Johnson and Ziff, 1976; Spielvogel *et al.*, 1978; Postlethwaite *et al.*, 1981; Jalkanen and Penttinen, 1982). Coculture of mononuclear cells with fibroblasts also results in enhanced collagen secretion into the medium (Hibbs *et al.*, 1983). The synthesis of other components can be altered by addition of these lymphokines and monokines as well as certain platelet-derived products (Castor *et al.*, 1977; Jaffe *et al.*, 1983; Postlethwaite *et al.*, 1983a,b). Mononuclear cells also produce factors that inhibit collagen synthesis (Jimenez *et al.*, 1979; McArthur *et al.*, 1982; Rosenbloom *et al.*, 1983; Hart *et al.*, 1983).

As is the case with proliferation, fibroblast synthesis of matrix is a complex process involving stimulatory and inhibitory components. Subtle differences in culture conditions, incubation times, and methods of analysis may produce striking changes in results (Horlein *et al.*, 1981). For example, the measurement of free collagen in the medium is reflective of net secretion and does not measure the collagen synthesized but not secreted (Bienkowski *et al.*, 1978) or that degraded before assembly (Vaheri *et al.*, 1978; Dayer *et al.*, 1982; Laub *et al.*, 1982; Postlethwaite *et al.*, 1983a; Welgus and Stricklin, 1983). Another example of variations in methods as a potential factor in differing results involves the low cleavage rate of procollagen peptides in rapidly dividing cells. Assay systems that detect only fully processed mature collagens would measure this protein as low under conditions of rapid cell division and high as cells reached confluence. Assays that include procollagens in the measurement of total collagens would give different results (Aumailley *et al.*, 1982).

It is also apparent that cell interactions with the extracellular matrix are important aspects to consider in interpreting cell culture experiments (Keski-oja *et al.*, 1981; Ehrlich and Wyler, 1983). Future work may elucidate the factors involved in these varied responses and determine where each fits in the complex process of fibroblast metabolism (Duksin *et al.*, 1983; Harris *et al.*, 1972). Analysis of cell behavior in a matrix that simulates the *in vivo* environment may produce results that more closely approximate their natural behavior.

VIII. SCLERODERMA FIBROBLASTS

Since we do not fully understand normal fibroblast metabolism, analysis and comparison of these cells in SD patients is difficult. Fibroblasts derived from skin biopsies of SD patients demonstrate enhanced collagen synthesis *in vitro* with a normal ratio of type I/III collagens (LeRoy, 1974; Uitto *et al.*, 1979). However, some studies fail to demonstrate increased collagen synthesis (Perlish *et al.*, 1976; Kjellstrom *et al.*, 1981). Reasons for these discrepant results include the study of patients in different phases of disease (Krieg *et al.*, 1981), culture of fibroblasts from different layers of the dermis (Buckingham *et al.*, 1978; Uitto *et al.*, 1979), and other alterations in methodology. Most investigators agree that SD fibroblasts produce more collagen and that this abnormal production continues for several cell cycles. Fibroblasts derived from three patients who demonstrated a marked reduction in skin thickening clinically continued to demonstrate elevated collagen synthesis (Shapiro *et al.*, 1983). This continuation of abnormal collagen synthesis in patients who are clinically improving indicates involvement of other factors in disease expression. Sera from SD patients contain a factor(s) that stimulates fibroblast collagen synthesis (Tan *et al.*, 1981) and proliferation (LeRoy *et al.*, 1983; Potter *et al.*, 1984). The origin of these factors is unknown; peripheral blood mononuclear cells of scleroderma patients secrete a substance(s) that activate fibroblasts (Cathcart and Krakauer, 1981; Tamura and Ishikawa, 1983). Responses to these factors may also be altered in SD fibroblasts compared with normals (LeRoy *et al.*, 1982).

Abnormalities in production of other connective tissue components occur in SD and are also being actively investigated. Although some experiments document normal synthesis of glycosaminoglycans (Bashey *et al.*, 1977), other work demonstrates increases of up to fivefold (Buckingham *et al.*, 1983; Cabral and Castor, 1983). The last study indicates a marked degree of heterogeneity observed in the cultured fibroblasts. The nonuniform responses of SD fibroblasts (Potter *et al.*, 1981; Fleischmajer *et al.*, 1981) raise the possibility that SD represents a process of fibroblast selection. The demonstration of subpopulations of normal human fibroblasts that have different receptors, protein synthesis, and growth characteristics may be the first step in understanding this phenomenon (Botstein *et al.*, 1982; Korn *et al.*, 1984; Bordin *et al.*, 1984). Future experiments are needed to define how SD fibroblasts differ from normals and the factors responsible for these differences.

IX. VASCULAR ASPECTS

Vascular abnormalities observed in SD include Raynaud's phenomena, telangiectasias, and diffuse small-vessel disease characterized by intimal proliferation and obliteration of the vessel lumen (Norton and Nardo, 1970). The role these vascular lesions play in pathogenesis is controversial (Campbell and LeRoy, 1975; Kahaleh and LeRoy, 1979; Jayson, 1983; Whicher *et al.*, 1984). This section reviews work in this area with particular reference to new investigations.

A. Microvasculature

Although small-vessel involvement has been described for many years, it is only recently that these abnormalities have been systematically analyzed (Maricq and LeRoy, 1979; Rodnan *et al.*, 1980; Russell and Hanna, 1983). One of the easiest methods for observing these vessels is direct *in vivo* capillary microscopy of the nailfold. This technique correlates very well with histology (Thompson *et al.*, 1984). It has been used to predict patients at high risk for subsequent development of SD (Maricq *et al.*, 1982) and may prove to be a valuable tool in the diagnosis of early disease. Large, longitudinal trials classifying patients with various capillary patterns may determine which abnormalities signify disease progression. Serial determinations of parameters of endothelial cell injury and platelet activation (*vide infra*) coupled with capillary microscopy findings may explain why some patients progress to clinical disease.

B. Endothelial Cells

The observation that SD sera contain a factor that is cytotoxic for human endothelial cells may be an important key to understanding the vascular changes of this disease (Kahaleh *et al.*, 1979). Although its disease (Shanahan and Korn, 1982; Bocanegra *et al.*, 1981) and cellular (Cohen *et al.*, 1983) specificities have been questioned, its presence can explain many aspects of SD. Subtle differences in methodology may explain the discrepant sensitivities and specificities, especially when dealing with endothelial cell culture techniques (Balconi *et al.*, 1983; Rogers and Kalnins, 1983). Partial purification of this factor reveals that it is a heat stable, nondialyzable protease (Kahaleh and LeRoy, 1983). Further studies may define the disease(s) associated with this factor and the cells that produce it. Identification of the stimulus that induces synthesis of this factor may be a key to understanding early events in the pathogenesis of SD.

The interactions of endothelial cells and the immune system may be critical to learning the etiology of SD. Mononuclear cells secrete product(s) that increase endothelial cell growth, but the cell(s) responsible are still under investigation (Wall *et al.*, 1978; Ooi *et al.*, 1983). Sublethal injury to endothelial cells changes their surface characteristics, unmasking previously hidden receptors (Ryan *et al.*, 1981). The observation that endothelial cells may actually function as antigen-presenting cells for T lymphocytes stresses the potential interactions of these cells (Pober *et al.*, 1983; Ashida *et al.*, 1981; Nunez *et al.*, 1983; Pober and Gimbrone, 1982). Although the precise role endothelial cells play in the immune response is debated (Roska *et al.*, 1984), further work in the area should define this interaction and determine how it may be important in diseases with prominent vascular and immune abnormalities (Maynard *et al.*, 1977; Sage *et al.*, 1982).

Platelets are known to have several properties that may be important in SD pathogenesis. Increased platelet activation has been documented in SD (Kahaleh *et al.*, 1982; Kallenberg *et al.*, 1982). Platelet aggregates and adherence to vessel walls denuded of endothelial cells have been observed (Brown and McClusky, 1978; Amenta and Katz, 1983). This activation and adherence would result in release of platelet granules that contain a number of vasoactive and growth factors. Growth factors contained in platelets have been isolated that stimulate endothelial cells (King and Buchwald, 1984), smooth muscle cells (Ross *et al.*, 1974), and fibroblasts (Antoniades *et al.*, 1979; Heldin *et al.*, 1979). These factors may be important in intimal proliferation.

Evidence implicating coagulation factors in the vascular events of SD center around fibrinogen and factor VIII. Increases in the euglobulin clot lysis time and fibrinogen turnover have been noted (Gratwick *et al.*, 1978; Holland and Jayson, 1981). This may reflect the fibrin deposition characteristic of SD (Kincaid-Smith, 1975). Increases in factor VIII activity and antigen have been observed in SD and Raynaud's phenomena (Kahaleh *et al.*, 1981). This factor mediates adherence of platelets to deendothelialized vessel walls (Green, 1979).

Thus, a series of events that can result in the vascular alterations observed in SD has been outlined in Fig. 1. The microcirculation is most severely affected perhaps because the low, nonpulsatile flow, impeded by platelet aggregates, makes it most susceptible to substances affecting endothelial cells (Dawson *et al.*, 1983; Ryan and Ryan, 1983). Further

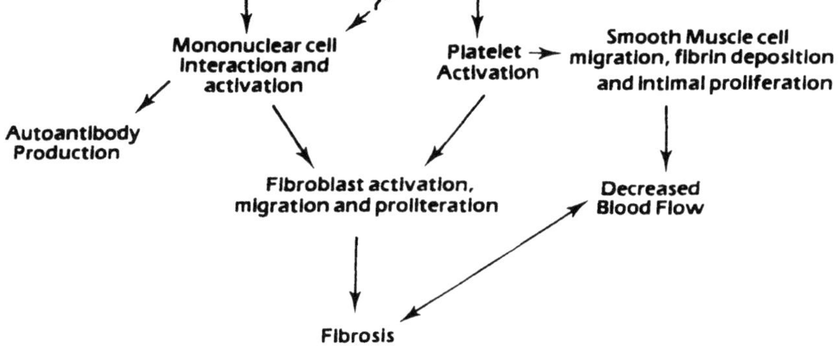

Figure 1. The stimulus for endothelial cell cytotoxic factor production, immune system activation, and the interaction between the immune system and endothelial cells are poorly understood. Clarification of these aspects may be critical to understanding the etiology of SD.

work is needed to identify the initiating process(es) and establish the link(s) between the vascular aspects of SD and fibrosis.

X. SUMMARY

The achievements of immunology and connective tissue research are many. This chapter has dealt with some of the experiments dealing with SD and fibroblast metabolism in light of possible future work. Certainly, the unknown factors involved in the etiology and pathogenesis of SD may frustrate physicians who lack effective therapy for this disabling and fatal disease (Gershwin, 1982). However, because of new techniques and knowledge gained regarding possible mechanisms of disease expression, we feel more optimistic toward future SD research: ". . . while mindful of the vastness of our ignorance and of the severe limitations in our ability to assist the victims of the many rheumatic diseases, I believe that we can be rightly proud of the achievements. . ." (Rodnan, 1977).

REFERENCES

Abercrombie, M., Heaysman, J. E. M., and Pegrum, S. M., 1971, The locomotion of fibroblasts in culture IV: Electron microscopy of the leading lamella, *Exp. Cell Res.* **67**:359–367.

Adar, R., Papa, M. Z., Halpern, Z., Mozes, M., Shoshan, S., Sofer, B., Zinger, H., Dayan, M., and Mozes, E., 1983, Cellular sensitivity to collagen in thromboangiitis obliterans, *N. Engl. J. Med.* **308**:1113–1116.

Alarcon-Segovia, D., Palacios, R., and de Kasep, G. I., 1981, Human postthymic precursor cells in health and disease VII. Immunoregulatory circuits of the peripheral blood mononuclear cells from patients with progressive systemic sclerosis, *J. Clin. Lab. Immunol.* **5**:143–148.

Allan, D. A., Bashey, R. I., Conway, P. A., and Jimenez, S. A., 1981, Effects of homologous and heterologous sera on proliferation of normal and scleroderma skin fibroblasts, *Arthritis Rheum.* **24**:S60.

Amenta, P. S., and Katz, S. M., 1983, Platelets in renal scleroderma, *Arch. Pathol. Lab. Med.* **107**:439–440.

Antoniades, H. N., Scher, C. D., and Stiles, C. D., 1979, Purification of human platelet-derived growth factor, *Proc. Natl. Acad. Sci. U.S.A.* **76**:1809–1813.

Ashida, E. R., Johnson, A. R., and Lipsky, P. E., 1981, Human endothelial cell-lymphocyte interaction: Endothelial cells function as accessory cells necessary for mitogen-induced T lymphocyte activation *in vitro*, *J. Clin. Invest.* **67**:1490–1499.

Aumailley, M., Krieg, T., Razaka, G., Muller, P. K., and Bricaud, H., 1982, Influence of cell density on collagen biosynthesis in fibroblast cultures, *Biochem. J.* **206**:505–510.

Bailey, A. J., Bazin, S., Sims, T. J., LeLous, M., Nicoletis, C., and Delaunay, A., 1975, Characterization of the collagen of human hypertrophic and normal scars, *Biochim. Biophys. Acta* **405**:412–421.

Balconi, G., Pietra, A., Busacca, M., DeGaetano, G., and DeJana, E., 1983, Success rate of primary human endothelial cell culture from umbilical cords is influenced by maternal and fetal factors and interval from delivery, *In Vitro* **19**:807–810.

Baron, M., Keystone, E. C., Gladman, D. D., Lee, P., and Poplonski, L., 1981, Lymphocyte subpopulations and reactivity to mitogens in patients with scleroderma, *Clin. Exp. Immunol.* **46**:70–76.

Baron, M., Feiglin, D., Hyland, R., Urowitz, M. B., and Shiff, B., 1983, 67-Gallium lung scans in progressive system sclerosis, *Arthritis Rheum.* **26**:969–974.

Bashey, R. I., Perlish, J. S., Nochumson, S., Stephens, R. E., and Fleischmajer, R., 1977, Connective tissue synthesis by cultured scleroderma fibroblasts. II. Incorporation of ^{3}H-glucosamine and synthesis of glycosaminoglycans, *Arthritis Rheum.* **20**:879–885.

Baum, J. L., 1971, Source of the fibroblast in central corneal wound healing, *Arch. Ophthalmol.* **85**:473–477.

Bernstein, R. M., Steigerwald, J. C., and Tan, E. M., 1982, Association of antinuclear and antinucleolar antibodies in progressive systemic sclerosis, *Clin. Exp. Immunol.* **48**:43–51.

Bianco, C., 1983, Fibrin, fibronectin, and macrophages, *Ann. N.Y. Acad. Sci.* **408**:602–609.

Bienkowski, R. S., Baum, B. J., and Crystal, R. G., 1978, Fibroblasts degrade newly synthesized collagen within the cell before secretion, *Nature* **276**:413–416.
Bitterman, P. B., Rennard, S. I., Hunninghake, G. W., and Crystal, R. G., 1982, Human alveolar macrophage growth factor for fibroblasts, *J. Clin. Invest.* **70**:806–822.
Black, C. M., Duance, V. C., Sims, T. J., and Light, N. D., 1983, An investigation of the biochemical and histological changes in the collagen of the kidney and skeletal muscle in systemic sclerosis, *Collagen Rel. Res.* **3**:231–244.
Black, M. M., Bottoms, E., and Shuster, S., 1970, Skin collagen content and thickness in systemic sclerosis, *Br. J. Dermatol.* **83**:552–555.
Bocanegra, T. S., Germain, B. F., Saba, H. I., Bridgeford, P. H., Saba, S. R., Vasey, F. B., and Espinoza, L. R., 1981, Cytotoxicity of sera from patients with polymyalgia rheumatica giant cell arteritis for human endothelial cells, *Arthritis Rheum.* **24**:S89.
Bordin, S., Page, R. C., and Narayanan, A. S., 1984, Heterogeneity of normal human diploid fibroblasts: Isolation and characterization of one phenotype, *Science* **223**:171–173.
Botstein, G. R., and LeRoy, E. C., 1981, Primary heart disease in systemic sclerosis (scleroderma): Advances in clinical and pathologic features, pathogenesis, and new therapeutic approaches, *Am. Heart J.* **102**:913–919.
Botstein, G. R., Sherer, G. K., and LeRoy, E. C., 1982, Fibroblast selection in scleroderma—an alternative model of fibrosis, *Arthritis Rheum.* **25**:189–195.
Boucek, R. J., and Alvarez, T. R., 1970, 5-Hydroxytryptamine: A cytospecific growth stimulator of cultured fibroblasts, *Science* **167**:898–899.
Boucek, R. J., Speropoulos, A. J., and Noble, N. L., 1972, Serotonin and ribonucleic acid and collagen metabolism of fibroblasts *in vitro*, *Proc. Soc. Exp. Biol. Med.* **140**:599–603.
Brown, E. A., MacGregor, G. A., and Maini, R. N., 1983, Failure of captopril to reverse the renal crisis of scleroderma, *Ann. Rheum. Dis.* **42**:52–53.
Brown, R. S., and McCluskey, R. T., 1978, Case records of the Massachusetts General Hospital: Weekly clinico-pathological exercises, Case 34–1978, *N. Engl. J. Med.* **299**:466–474.
Buckingham, R. B., Prince, R. K., Rodnan, G. P., and Taylor, F., 1978, Increased collagen accumulation in dermal fibroblast cultures from patients with progressive systemic sclerosis (scleroderma), *J. Lab. Clin. Med.* **92**:5–21.
Buckingham, R. B., Prince, R. K., and Rodnan, G. P., 1983, Progressive systemic sclerosis (PSS, scleroderma) dermal fibroblasts synthesize increased amounts of glycosaminoglycan, *J. Lab. Clin. Med.* **101**:659–669.
Cabral, A., and Castor, C. W., 1983, Connective tissue activation. XXVII. The behavior of skin fibroblasts from patients with scleroderma, *Arthritis Rheum.* **26**:1362–1369.
Campbell, P. M., and LeRoy, E. C., 1975, Pathogenesis of systemic sclerosis: A vascular hypothesis, *Semin. Arthritis Rheum.* **4**:351–368.
Castor, C. W., and Fremuth, T. D., 1982, Factors modifying DNA synthesis by lung fibroblasts *in vitro*, *Proc. Soc. Exp. Biol. Med.* **171**:109–113.
Castor, C. W., Wright, D., and Buckingham, R. B., 1968, Effects of rheumatoid sera on fibroblast proliferation and hyaluronic acid synthesis, *Arthritis Rheum.* **11**:652–659.
Castor, C. W., Ritchie, J. C., Scott, M. E., and Whitney, S. L., 1977, Connective tissue activation. XI. stimulation of glycosaminoglycan and DNA formation by a platelet factor, *Arthritis Rheum.* **20**:859–868.
Cathcart, M. K., and Krakauer, R. S., 1981, Immunologic enhancement of collagen accumulation in progressive systemic sclerosis (PSS), *Clin. Immunol. Immunopathol.* **21**:128–133.
Catoggio, L. J., Bernstein, R. M., Black, C. M., Hughes, G. R. V., and Maddison, P. J., 1983, Serological markers in progressive systemic sclerosis: Clinical correlations, *Ann. Rheum. Dis.* **42**:23–27.
Chvapil, M., 1974, Pharmacology of fibrosis and tissue injury, *Environ. Health Perspect.* **9**:283–294.
Chvapil, M., Hurych, J., and Mirejovska, E., 1970, Effect of long-term hypoxia on protein synthesis in granuloma and in some organs in rats, *Proc. Soc. Exp. Biol. Med.* **135**:613–617.
Claudy, A. L., Le Petit, J. C., Barthelemy, H., and Garcier, F., 1982, T-cell imbalance in progressive systemic sclerosis defined by monoclonal antibodies, *Arch. Dermatol. Res.* **274**:189–192.
Cohen, S., Johnson, A. R., and Hurd, E., 1983, Cytotoxicity of sera from patients with scleroderma, *Arthritis Rheum.* **26**:170–178.
Colvin, R. B., 1983, Fibrinogen–fibrin interactions with fibroblasts and macrophages, *Ann. N.Y. Acad. Sci.* **408**:621–633.

Cooper, S. M., and Friou, G. J., 1979, Cytotoxicity in progressive systemic sclerosis: No evidence for increased cytotoxicity against fibroblasts of different origin, *J. Rheumatol.* **6**:25–29.

Cooper, S. M., Keyser, A. J., Beaulieu, A. D., Ruoslahti, E., Nimni, M. E., and Quismorio, F. P., 1979, Increase in fibronectin in the deep dermis of involved skin in progressive systemic sclerosis, *Arthritis Rheum.* **22**:983–987.

Currie, S., Saunders, M., and Knowles, M., 1970, Immunological aspects of systemic sclerosis: *In vitro* activity of lymphocytes from patients with the disorder, *Br. J. Dermatol.* **84**:400–409.

Dawson, C. A., Bronikowski, T. A., Linehan, J. H., and Hakim, T. S., 1983, Influence of pulmonary vasoconstriction on lung water and perfusion heterogeneity, *J. Appl. Physiol.* **54**:654–660.

Dayer, J. M., Trentham, D. E., and Krane, S. M., 1982, Collagens act as ligands to stimulate human monocytes to produce mononuclear cell factor (MCF) and prostaglandins (PGE_2), *Collagen Rel. Res.* **2**:523–540.

DeLustro, F., Sherer, G. K., and LeRoy, E. C., 1980, Human monocyte stimulation of fibroblast growth by a soluble mediator(s), *J. Reticuloendothel. Soc.* **28**:519–532.

DeLustro, F., Mackel, A. M., DeLustro, B., and LeRoy, E. C., 1983, Human monocyte regulation of connective tissue growth, *Am. Zool.* **23**:213–220.

Denis, P., Ducrotte, P., Pasquis, P., and Lefrancois, R., 1981, Esophageal motility and pulmonary function in progressive systemic sclerosis, *Respiration* **42**:21–24.

DiBartolomeo, A. G., Rabin, B. S., and Rodman, G. P., 1981, HLA-D antigens in progressive systemic sclerosis (scleroderma), *Immunol. Commun.* **10**:733–740.

Dinman, B. D., Cook, W. A., Whitehouse, W. M., Magnuson, H. J., and Ditcheck, T., 1971, Occupational acroosteolysis. I. An epidemiological study, *Arch. Environ. Health* **22**:61–73.

Dodson, V. N., Dinman, B. D., Whitehouse, W. M., Nasr, A. N. M., and Magnuson, H. J., 1971, Occupational acroosteolysis. III. A clinical study, *Arch. Environ. Health* **22**:83–91.

Douvas, A. S., Achten, M., and Tan, E. M., 1979, Identification of a nuclear protein (Scl-70) as a unique target of human antinuclear antibodies in scleroderma, *J. Biol. Chem.* **254**:10514–10522.

Duksin, D., Gal, A., and Goodman, R. M., 1983, Altered protein glycosylation and procollagen to collagen conversion in human fibroblasts, *Lab. Invest.* **49**:346–352.

Ehrlich, H. P., and Wyler, D. J., 1983, Fibroblast contraction of collagen lattices *in vitro:* Inhibition by chronic inflammatory cell mediators, *J. Cell. Physiol.* **116**:345–351.

Elias, J. A., Rossman, M. D., and Daniele, R. P., 1982, Inhibition of human lung fibroblast growth by mononuclear cells, *Am. Rev. Respir. Dis.* **125**:701–705.

Emerit, I., 1979, Chromosomal abnormalities in progressive systemic sclerosis, *Clin. Rheum. Dis.* **5**:201–214.

Ercilla, M. G., Arriaga, F., Gratacos, M. R., Coll, J., Lecha, V., Vives, J., and Castillo, R., 1981, HLA antigens and scleroderma, *Arch. Dermatol. Res.* **271**:381–385.

Fasske, E., and Morgenroth, K., 1983, Experimental bleomycin lung in mice: A contribution to the pathogenesis of pulmonary fibrosis, *Lung* **161**:133–146.

Finch, W. R., Rodnan, G. P., Buckingham, R. B., Prince, R. K., and Winkelstein, A., 1980, Bleomycin-induced scleroderma, *J. Rheumatol.* **7**:651–659.

Fleischmajer, R., 1964, The collagen in scleroderma, *Arch. Dermatol.* **89**:437–441.

Fleischmajer, R., and Perlish, J. S., 1972, Glycosaminoglycans in scleroderma and scleredema, *J. Invest. Dermatol.* **58**:129–132.

Fleischmajer, R., and Pollock, J. L., 1979, Progressive systemic sclerosis: Pseudoscleroderma, *Clin. Rheum. Dis.* **5**:243–261.

Fleischmajer, R., Perlish, J. S., and West, W. P., 1977a, Ultrastructure of cutaneous cellular infiltrates in scleroderma, *Arch. Dermatol.* **113**:1661–1666.

Fleischmajer, R., Perlish, J. S., and Reeves, J. R. T., 1977b, Cellular infiltrates in scleroderma skin, *Arthritis Rheum.* **20**:975–984.

Fleischmajer, R., Dessau, W., Timpl, R., Krieg, T., Luderschmidt, C., and Wiestner, M., 1980a, Immunofluorescence analysis of collagen, fibronectin, and basement membrane protein in scleroderma skin, *J. Invest. Dermatol.* **75**:270–274.

Fleischmajer, R., Gay, S., Perlish, J. S., and Cesarini, J. P., 1980b, Immunoelectron microscopy of type III collagen in normal and scleroderma skin, *J. Invest. Dermatol.* **75**:189–191.

Fleischmajer, R., Perlish, J. S., Krieg, T., and Timpl, R., 1981, Variability in collagen and fibronectin synthesis by scleroderma fibroblasts in primary culture, *J. Invest. Dermatol.* **76**:400–403.

Fleischmajer, R., Perlish, J. S., and Duncan, M., 1983, Scleroderma: A model for fibrosis, *Arch. Dermatol.* **119**:957–962.

Follansbee, W. P., Curtiss, E. I., Medsger, T. A., Steen, V. D., Uretsky, B. F., Owens, G. R., and Rodnan, G. P., 1984, Physiologic abnormalities of cardiac function in progressive systemic sclerosis with diffuse scleroderma, *N. Engl. J. Med.* **310**:142–148.

Fox, P. K., White, D. D., Cavanagh, M., Davies, M. G., and Wusterman, F., 1982, Failure to demonstrate fibrotic changes in the skin of mice injected with glycosaminoglycan fractions from the urine of scleroderma patients, *Dermatology* **164**:90–94.

Freudenberg, J., Holzmann, H., Schneider, S., and Korting, G. W., 1978, HLA-Antigenfrequenzen bei Patienten mit progressiver Sklerodermie und Morphaea, *Arch. Dermatol. Res.* **263**:197–205.

Fries, J. F., Lindgren, J. A., and Bull, J. M., 1973, Scleroderma-like lesions and the carcinoid syndrome, *Arch. Intern. Med.* **131**:550–553.

Fritzler, M. J., and Kinsella, T. D., 1980, The CREST syndrome: A distinct serologic entity with anticentromere antibodies, *Am. J. Med.* **69**:520–526.

Furst, D. E., Clements, P. J., Graze, P., Gale, R., and Roberts, N., 1979, A syndrome resembling progressive systemic sclerosis after bone marrow transplantation—a model for scleroderma? *Arthritis Rheum.* **22**:904–910.

Furst, D. E., Davis, J. A., Clements, P. J., Chopra, S. K., Theofilopoulos, A. N., and Chia, D., 1981, Abnormalities of pulmonary vascular dynamics and inflammation in early progressive systemic sclerosis, *Arthritis Rheum.* **24**:1403–1408.

Garza-Elizondo, M. A., Diaz-Jouanen, E., Franco-Casique, J. J., and Alarcon-Segovia, D., 1983, Joint contractures and scleroderma-like skin changes in the hands of insulin-dependent juvenile diabetics, *J. Rheumatol.* **10**:797–800.

Germain, B. F., Espinoza, L. R., Bergen, L. L., Vagesh, M., and Vasey, F. B., 1981, Increased prevalence of DRw3 in the CREST syndrome, *Arthritis Rheum.* **24**:857–859.

Gershwin, M. E., 1982, Slow progress with scleroderma, *Ann. Intern. Med.* **97**:776–778.

Gershwin, M. E., Abplanalp, H., Castles, J. J., Ikeda, R. M., van de Water, J., Eklund, J., and Haynes, D., 1981, Characterization of a spontaneous disease of white leghorn chickens resembling progressive systemic sclerosis (scleroderma), *J. Exp. Med.* **153**:1640–1659.

Gladman, D. D., Keystone, E. C., Baron, M., Lee, P., Cane, D., and Mervert, H., 1981, Increased frequency of HLA-DR5 in scleroderma, *Arthritis Rheum.* **24**:854–856.

Gottdiener, J. S., Moutsopoulos, H. M., and Decker, J. L., 1979, Echocardiographic identification of cardiac abnormality in scleroderma and related disorders, *Am. J. Med.* **66**:391–398.

Goyert, S. M., Shively, J. E., and Silver, J., 1982, Biochemical characterization of a second family of human Ia molecules, HLA-DS, equivalent to murine I-A subregion molecules, *J. Exp. Med.* **156**:550–566.

Gratwick, G. M., Klein, R., Sergent, J. S., and Christian, C. L., 1978, Fibrinogen turnover in progressive systemic sclerosis, *Arthritis Rheum.* **21**:343–347.

Gray, R. G., and Altman, R. D., 1977, Progressive systemic sclerosis in a family, *Arthritis Rheum.* **20**:35–41.

Green, D., 1979, Role of the von Willebrand factor in atherogenesis, *Artery* **5**:262–272.

Green, M. C., Sweet, H. O., and Bunker, L. E., 1976, Tight-skin, a new mutation of the mouse causing excessive growth of connective tissue and skeleton, *Am. J. Pathol.* **82**:493–507.

Gutierrez-Millet, V., Navas-Palacios, J., Gomez-Reino, J., and Fernandez–Epifanio, J. L., 1982, Renal involvement in toxic oil syndrome, *Lancet* **1**:1120.

Haidle, C. W., 1971, Fragmentation of deoxyribonucleic acid by bleomycin, *Mol. Pharmacol.* **7**:645–652.

Harper, F. E., Maricq, H. R., Turner, R. E., Lidman, R. W., and LeRoy, E. C., 1982, A prospective study of Raynaud phenomenon and early connective tissue disease: A five-year report, *Am. J. Med.* **72**:883–888.

Harris, A., and Dunn, G., 1972, Centripetal transport of attached particles on both surfaces of moving fibroblasts, *Exp. Cell. Res.* **73**:519–523.

Hart, P. H., Powell, L. W., Cooksley, W. G. E., and Halliday, J. W., 1983a, Mononuclear cell factors that inhibit fibroblast collagen synthesis. I. *In vitro* conditions determining their production and expression, *Scand. J. Immunol.* **18**:41–49.

Hart, P. H., Powell, L. W., Cooksley, W. G. E., and Halliday, J. W., 1983b, Mononuclear cell factors that inhibit fibroblast collagen synthesis. II. Properties of the factors, *Scand. J. Immunol.* **18**:51–58.

Heldin, C. H., Westermark, B., and Wasteson, A., 1979, Platelet-derived growth factor: Purification and partial characterization, *Proc. Natl. Acad. Sci. U.S.A.* **76**:3722–3726.

Hibbs, M. S., Postlethwaite, A. E., Mainardi, C. L., Seyer, J. M., and Kang, A. H., 1983, Alterations in collagen production in mixed mononuclear leukocyte–fibroblast cultures, *J. Exp. Med.* **157**:47–59.

Holland, C. D., and Jayson, M. I. V., 1981, Venous blood fibrinolysis and fibrinolytic potential in Raynaud's phenomena (RP) and systemic sclerosis (SS), *Ann. Rheum. Dis.* **40**:518–519.

Horlein, D., McPherson, J., Goh, S. H., and Bornstein, P., 1981, Regulation of protein synthesis: Translational control by procollagen-derived fragments, *Proc. Natl. Acad. Sci. U.S.A.* **78**:6163–6167.

Hormia, M., Lehto, V. P., and Virtanen, I., 1983, Factor VIII-related antigen: A pericellular matrix component of cultured human endothelial cells, *Exp. Cell. Res.* **149**:483–497.

Hughes, P., Holt, S., and Rowell, N. R., 1974, Leukocyte migration inhibition in progressive systemic sclerosis, *Br. J. Dermatol.* **91**:1–6.

Hunt, T. K., Conolly, W. B., Aronson, S. B., and Goldstein, P., 1978, Anaerobic metabolism and wound healing: An hypothesis for the initiation and cessation of collagen synthesis in wounds, *Am. J. Surg.* **135**:328–332.

Hurt, M. M., Beaudet, A. L., and Moses, R. E., 1983, Repair response of human fibroblasts to bleomycin damage, *Mutation Res.* **112**:181–189.

Ishikawa, H., and Horiuchi, R., 1975, Initial change of glycosaminoglycans in systemic scleroderma, *Dermatologica* **150**:334–345.

Ishikawa, H., Suzuki, S., Horiuchi, R., and Sato, H., 1975, An approach to experimental scleroderma, using urinary glycosaminoglycans from patients with systemic scleroderma, *Acta. Derm. Vener.* **55**:97–107.

Ishikawa, H., Saito, Y., Yamakage, A., and Kitabatake, M., 1978, Scleroderma-inducing glycosaminoglycan in the urine of patients with systemic scleroderma, *Dermatologica* **156**:193–204.

Ishikawa, H., Yamakage, A., Kitabatake, M., Katayama, H., and Saito, Y., 1980, Detection of sclerosis-inducing glycosaminoglycan in the skin of an amine-induced experimental skin sclerosis, 1980, *Dermatologica* **161**:145–151.

Jaffe, B. D., and Claman, H. N., 1983, Chronic graft-versus-host disease (GVHD) as a model for scleroderma. I. Description of model systems, *Cell. Immunol.* **77**:1–12.

Jaffee, E. A., Ruggiero, J. T., Leung, L. L. K., Doyle, M. J., McKeown-Longo, P. J., and Mosher, D. F., 1983, Cultured human fibroblasts synthesize and secrete thrombospondin and incorporate it into extracellular matrix, *Proc. Natl. Acad. Sci. U.S.A.* **80**:998–1002.

Jalkanen, M., and Penttinen, R., 1982, Enhanced fibroblast collagen production by a macrophage-derived factor (CEMF), *Biochem. Biophys. Res. Commun.* **108**:447–453.

James, A. E., Price, R. R., Rollo, F. D., Patton, J. A., Erickson, J. J., Coulam, C. M., and Partain, C. L., 1982, Nuclear magnetic resonance imaging—a promising technique, *JAMA* **247**:1331–1334.

Jayson, M. I. V., 1983, Systemic sclerosis—a microvascular disorder? *J. R. Soc. Med. (London)* **76**:635–642.

Jimenez, S. A., 1983, Cellular immune dysfunction and the pathogenesis of scleroderma, *Semin. Arthritis Rheum.* (Suppl. 1)**13**:104–113.

Jimenez, S. A., McArthur, W., and Rosenbloom, J., 1979, Inhibition of collagen synthesis by mononuclear cell supernates, *J. Exp. Med.* **150**:1421–1431.

Jimenez, S. A., Millan, A., and Bashey, R. I., 1984, Scleroderma-like alterations in collagen metabolism occurring in the TSK (tight skin) mouse, *Arthritis Rheum.* **27**:180–185.

Johnson, R. L., and Ziff, M., 1976, Lymphokine stimulation of collagen accumulation, *J. Clin. Invest.* **58**:240–252.

Kahaleh, M. B., and LeRoy, E. C., 1979, Progressive systemic sclerosis: Kidney involvement, *Clin. Rheum. Dis.* **5**:167–184.

Kahaleh, M. B., and LeRoy, E. C., 1983, Endothelial injury in scleroderma: A protease mechanism, *J. Lab. Clin. Med.* **101**:553–560.

Kahaleh, M. B., Sherer, G. K., and LeRoy, E. C., 1979, Endothelial injury in scleroderma, *J. Exp. Med.* **149**:1326–1335.

Kahaleh, M. B., Osborn, I., and LeRoy, E. C., 1981, Increased factor VIII/von Willebrand factor antigen and von Willebrand factor activity in scleroderma and in Raynaud's phenomenon, *Ann. Intern. Med.* **94**:482–484.

Kahaleh, M. B., Osborn, I., and LeRoy, E. C., 1982, Elevated levels of circulating platelet aggregates and beta-thromboglobulin in scleroderma, *Ann. Intern. Med.* **96**:610–613.

Kallenberg, C. G. M., Vellenga, E., Wouda, A. A., and The, T. H., 1982, Platelet activation, fibrinolytic activity and circulating immune complexes in Raynaud's phenomenon, *J. Rheumatol.* **9**:878–884.

Kent, L. T., Cramer, S. F., and Moskowitz, R. W., 1981, Eosinophilic fasciitis—clinical, laboratory, and microscopic considerations, *Arthritis Rheum.* **24**:677–683.

Keski-oja, J., Tadaro G. J., and Vaheri, A., 1981, Thrombin affects fibronectin and procollagen in the pericellular matrix of cultured human fibroblasts, *Biochim. Biophys. Acta* **673**:323–331.

Keystone, E. C., Gladman, D. D., Baron, M., Cane, D., and Poplonski, L., 1981, Antigen-specific suppressor cell activity in patients with scleroderma, *J. Rheumatol.* **8**:747–751.

Keystone, E. C., Lau, C., Gladman, D. D., Wilkinson, S., Lee, P., and Shore, A., 1982, Immunoregulatory T-cell subpopulations in patients with scleroderma using monoclonal antibodies, *Clin. Exp. Immunol.* **48**:443–448.

Kiely, J. M., 1981, Series on pharmacology in practice. 12. Antineoplastic agents, *Mayo Clin. Proc.* **56**:384–392.

Kincaid-Smith, P., 1975, Participation of intravascular coagulation in the pathogenesis of glomerular and vascular lesions, *Kidney Int.* **7**:242–253.

King, G. L., and Buchwald, S., 1984, Characterization and partial purification of an endothelial cell growth factor from human platelets, *J. Clin. Invest.* **73**:392–396.

Kischer, C. W., Shetlar, M. R., and Chvapil, M., 1982, Hypertrophic scars and keloids: A review and new concept concerning their origin, *Scan. Electron Microsc.* **4**:1699–1713.

Kjellstrom, T., Malmquist, J., and Persson, B., 1981, Synthesis of collagen and sulfated glycosaminoglycans by normal and scleroderma fibroblasts in culture, with and without addition of cyclofenil, *Acta Med. Scand.* **210**:125–128.

Kohn, R. R., and Hensse, S., 1977, Abnormal collagen in cultures of fibroblasts from human beings with diabetes mellitus, *Biochem. Biophys. Res. Commun.* **76**:765–771.

Kondo, H., Rabin, B. S., and Rodnan, G. P., 1976, Cutaneous antigen-stimulating lymphokine production by lymphocytes of patients with progressive systemic sclerosis (scleroderma), *J. Clin. Invest.* **58**:1388–1394.

Kondo, H., Rabin, B. S., and Rodnan, G. P., 1979, Stimulation of lymphocyte reactivity by a low molecular weight cutaneous antigen, *J. Rheumatol.* **6**:30–37.

Korn, J. H., 1983, Fibroblast prostaglandin E_2 synthesis: Persistence of an abnormal phenotype after short-term exposure to mononuclear cell products, *J. Clin. Invest.* **71**:1240–1246.

Korn, J. H., Halushka, P. V., and LeRoy, E. C., 1980, Mononuclear cell modulation of connective tissue function, *J. Clin. Invest.* **65**:543–554.

Korn, J. H., Torres, D., and Downie, E., 1984, Clonal heterogeneity in the fibroblast response to mononuclear cell derived mediators, *Arthritis Rheum.* **27**:174–179.

Kovalchik, M. T., Guggenheim, S. J., Silverman, M. H., Robertson, J. S., and Steigerwald, J. C., 1978, The kidney in progressive systemic sclerosis: A prospective study, *Ann. Intern. Med.* **89**:881–887.

Krakauer, R. S., Sundeen, J., Sauder, D. N., and Scherbel, A., 1981, Abnormalities in immunoregulation in progressive systemic sclerosis, *Arch. Dermatol.* **117**:80–82.

Krawitt, E. L., Holdstock, G., Bland, J. H., Chastenay, B. F., and Albertini, R. J., 1982, Suppressor cell activity in progressive systemic sclerosis, *J. Rheumatol.* **9**:263–267.

Krieg, T., Luderschmidt, C., Weber, L., Muller, P. K., and Braun-Falco, O., 1981, Scleroderma fibroblasts: Some aspects of *in vitro* assessment of collagen synthesis, *Arch. Dermatol. Res.* **270**:263–272.

Kumagai, Y., Shiokawa, Y., Medsger, T. A., Jr., and Rodnan, G. P., 1984, Clinical spectrum of connective tissue disease after cosmetic surgery: Observations on eighteen patients and a review of the Japanese literature, *Arthritis Rheum.* **27**:1–12.

Kurkinen, M., Vaheri, A., Roberts, P. J., and Stenman, S., 1980, Sequential appearance of fibronectin and collagen in experimental granulation tissue, *Lab. Invest.* **43**:47–51.

Lampson, L. A., and Levy, R., 1980, Two populations of Ia-like molecules on a human B cell line, *J. Immunol.* **125**:293–299.

Laub, R., Huybrechts-Godin, G., Peeters-Joris, C., and Vaes, G., 1982, Degradation of collagen and proteoglycan by macrophages and fibroblasts—individual potentialities of each cell type and cooperative effects through the activation of fibroblasts by macrophages, *Biochim. Biophys. Acta* **721**:425–433.

Leibovich, S. J., and Danon, D., 1980, Promotion of wound repair in mice by application of glucan, *J. Reticuloendothel. Soc.* **27**:1–11.

LeRoy, E. C., 1972, Connective tissue synthesis by scleroderma skin fibroblasts in cell culture, *J. Exp. Med.* **135**:1351–1362.

LeRoy, E. C., 1974, Increased collagen synthesis by scleroderma skin fibroblasts *in vitro*, *J. Clin. Invest.* **54**:880–889.

LeRoy, E. C., 1981, The connective tissue in scleroderma, *Collagen Rel. Res.* **1**:301–308.

LeRoy, E. C., 1984, The heart in systemic sclerosis, *N. Engl. J. Med.* **310**:188–190.

LeRoy, E. C., Mercurio, S., and Sherer, G. K., 1982, Replication and phenotypic expression of control and scleroderma human fibroblasts: Responses to growth factors, *Proc. Natl. Acad. Sci. U.S.A.* **79**:1286–1290.

LeRoy, E. C., Kahaleh, M. B., and Mercurio, S., 1983, A fibroblast mitogen present in scleroderma but not control sera: Inhibition by proteinase inhibitors, *Rheumatol. Int.* **3**:35–38.

Lloyd, R. S., Haidle, C. W., and Robberson, D. L., 1979, Bleomycin fragmentation of duplex DNA occurs as staggered single-strand scissions, *Gene* **7**:303–316.

Lockshin, M. D., Markenson, J. A., Fuzesi, L., Kazanjian-Aram, S., Joachim, C., and Ordene, M., 1983, Monocyte-induced inhibition of lymphocyte response to phytohaemagglutinin in progressive systemic sclerosis, *Ann. Rheum. Dis.* **42**:40–44.

Lopez-Ovejero, J. A., Saal, S. D., D'Angelo, W. A., Cheigh, J. S., Stenzel, K. H., and Laragh, J. H., 1979, Reversal of vascular and renal crises of scleroderma by oral angiotensin-converting-enzyme blockage, *N. Engl. J. Med.* **300**:1417–1419.

Love, J. D., Liarakos, C. D., and Moses, R. E., 1981, Nonspecific cleavage of ϕ174 XRFI deoxyribonucleic acid by bleomycin, *Biochemistry* **20**:5331–5336.

Lovell, C. R., Nicholls, A. C., Duance, V. C., and Bailey, A. J., 1979, Characterization of dermal collagen in systemic sclerosis, *Br. J. Dermatol.* **100**:359–369.

Lynch, C. J., Singh, G., Whiteside, T. L., Rodnan, G. P., Medsger, T. A., and Rabin, S. B., 1982, Histocompatibility antigens in progressive systemic sclerosis (PSS; scleroderma), *J. Clin. Immunol.* **2**: 314–318.

MacDonald, R. A., Robbins, S. L., and Mallory, G. K., 1958, Dermal fibrosis following subcutaneous injections of serotonin creatinine sulfate, *Proc. Soc. Exp. Biol. Med.* **97**:334–337.

Mackel, A. M., DeLustro, F., Harper, F. E., and LeRoy, E. C., 1982a, Antibodies to collagen in scleroderma, *Arthritis Rheum.* **25**:522–531.

Mackel, A. M., DeLustro, F., DeLustro, B., Fudenberg, H. H., and LeRoy, E. C., 1982b, Immune response to connective tissue components of the basement membrane, *Connect. Tissue Res.* **10**:333–343.

Maricq, H. R., and LeRoy, E. C., 1979, Progressive systemic sclerosis: Disorders of the microcirculation, *Clin. Rheum. Dis.* **5**:81–101.

Maricq, H. R., Johnson, M. N., Whetstone, C. L., and LeRoy, E. C., 1976, Capillary abnormalities in polyvinyl chloride production workers: Examination by *in vivo* microscopy, *JAMA* **236**:1368–1371.

Maricq, H. R., Weinberger, A. B., and LeRoy, E. C., 1982, Early detection of scleroderma-spectrum disorders by *in vivo* capillary microscopy: A prospective study of patients with Raynaud's phenomenon, *J. Rheumatol.* **9**:289–291.

Martin, W. J. II, Williams, D. E., Dines, D. E., and Sanderson, D. R., 1983, Interstitial lung disease—assessment by bronchoalveolar lavage, *Mayo Clin. Proc.* **58**:751–757.

Martinez-Tello, F. J., Navas-Palacios, J. J., Ricoy, J. R., Gil-Martin, R., Conde-Zurita, J. M., Delgado, F. C. R., Tellez, I., Cabello, A., and Madero-Garcia, S., 1982, Pathology of a new toxic syndrome caused by ingestion of adulterated oil in Spain, *Virchows Arch. Pathol. Anat.* **397**:261–285.

Masters, R., Hood, A. F., and Cosini, A. B., 1975, Chronic cutaneous graft-vs-host reaction following bone marrow transplantation, *Arch. Dermatol.* **111**:1526.

Maynard, J. R., Dreyer, B. E., Stemerman, M. B., and Pitlick, F. A., 1977, Tissue-factor coagulant activity of cultured human endothelial and smooth muscle cells and fibroblasts, *Blood* **50**:387–396.

McArthur, W., Derr, K., Dixon, M., Jimenez, S. A., and Rosenbloom, J., 1982, Immune modulation of connective tissue functions: Studies on the production of collagen synthesis inhibitory factor by populations of human peripheral blood mononuclear cells, *Cell. Immunol.* **74**:126–139.

McCarty, G. A., Rice, J. R., Bembe, M. L., and Barada, F. A., Jr., 1983, Anticentromere antibody. Clinical correlations and association with favorable prognosis in patients with scleroderma variants, *Arthritis Rheum.* **26**:1–7.

Meuer, S., Hugli, T. E., Andreatta, R. H., Hadding, U., and Bitter-Suermann, D., 1981, Comparative study on biological activities of various anaphylatoxins (C4a, C3a, C5a): Investigations on their ability to induce platelet secretion, *Inflammation* **5**:263–273.

Mitnick, P. D., and Feig, P. U., 1978, Control of hypertension and reversal of renal failure in scleroderma, *N. Engl. J. Med.* **299**:871–872.

Moroi, Y., Peebles, C., Fritzler, M. J., Steigerwald, J. D., and Tan, E. M., 1980, Autoantibody to centromere (kinetochore) in scleroderma sera, *Proc. Natl. Acad. Sci. U.S.A.* **77**:1627–1631.

Morse, J. H., and Bodi, B. S., 1982, Autologous and allogeneic mixed lymphocyte reactions in progressive systemic sclerosis, *Arthritis Rheum.* **25**:390–395.

Nimni, M. E., 1983, Collagen: Structure, function and metabolism in normal and fibrotic tissues, *Semin. Arthritis Rheum.* **13**:1–86.

Norton, W. L., and Nardo, J. M., 1970, Vascular disease in progressive systemic sclerosis (scleroderma), *Ann. Intern. Med.* **73**:317–324.

Nunez, G., Ball, E. J., and Stastny, P., 1983, Accessory cell function of human endothelial cells. I. A subpopulation of Ia positive cells is required for antigen presentation, *J. Immunol.* **131**:666–673.

O'Hare, R. P., Fallon, A., Bradley, J. F., Burns, J., and McGee, J. O'D., 1983, Isolation of collagen stimulating factors from healing wounds, *J. Clin. Pathol.* **36**:707–711.

Ooi, B. S., MacCarthy, E. P., Hsu, A., and Ooi, Y. M., 1983, Human mononuclear cell modulation of endothelial cell proliferation, *J. Lab. Clin. Med.* **102**:428–433.

Osborn, T. G., Bauer, N. E., Ross, S. C., Moore, T. L., and Zuckner, J., 1983, The tight-skin mouse: Physical and biochemical properties of the skin, *J. Rheumatol.* **10**:793–796.

Pearlstein, E., 1976, Plasma membrane glycoprotein which mediates adhesion of fibroblasts to collagen, *Nature* **262**;497–500.

Perlish, J. S., Bashey, R. I., Stephens, R. E., and Fleischmajer, R., 1976, Connective tissue synthesis by cultured scleroderma fibroblasts. I. *In vitro* collagen synthesis by normal and scleroderma dermal fibroblasts, *Arthritis Rheum.* **19**:891–901.

Pober, J. S., and Gimbrone, M. A., Jr., 1982, Expression of Ia-like antigens by human vascular endothelial cells is inducible *in vitro:* Demonstration by monoclonal antibody binding and immunoprecipitation, *Proc. Natl. Acad. Sci. U.S.A.* **79**:6641–6645.

Pober, J. S., Gimbrone, M. A., Jr., Cotran, R. S., Reiss, C. S., Burakoff, S. J., Fiers, W., and Ault, K. A., 1983, Ia expression by vascular endothelium is inducible by activated T cells and by human gamma interferon, *J. Exp. Med.* **157**:1339–1353.

Postlethwaite, A. E., and Kang, A. H., 1983, Induction of fibroblast proliferation by human mononuclear leukocyte-derived proteins, *Arthritis Rheum.* **26**:22–27.

Postlethwaite, A. E., Snyderman, R., and Kang, A. H., 1976, The chemotactic attraction of human fibroblasts to a lymphocyte-derived factor, *J. Exp. Med.* **144**:1188–1203.

Postlethwaite, A. E., Seyer, J. M., and Kang, A. H., 1978, Chemotactic attraction of human fibroblasts to types I, II, and III collagens and collagen-derived peptides, *Proc. Natl. Acad. Sci. U.S.A.* **75**:871–875.

Postlethwaite, A. E., Snyderman, R., and Kang, A. H., 1979, Generation of a fibroblast chemotactic factor in serum by activation of complement, *J. Clin. Invest.* **64**:1379–1385.

Postlethwaite, A. E., Smith, G. N., Mainardi, C. L., Seyer, J. M., and Kang, A. H., 1981, Characterization of a human lymphokine that stimulates fibroblasts to produce collagen, *Arthritis Rheum.* **24**:S61.

Postlethwaite, A. E., Lachman, L. B., Mainardi, C. L., and Kang, A. H., 1983a, Interleukin 1 stimulation of collagenase production by cultured fibroblasts, *J. Exp. Med.* **157**:801–806.

Postlethwaite, A. E., Lachman, L. B., and Kang, A. H., 1983b, Stimulation of fibroblast hyaluronic acid production by human interleukin I, *Arthritis Rheum.* **26**:S59.

Potter, S. R., Bienenstock, J., Buchanan, W. W., and Goldstein, S., 1981, Fibroblast stimulation factor(s) in sera from patients with progressive systemic sclerosis (PSS), *Arthritis Rheum.* **24**:S61.

Potter, S. R., Bienenstock, J., Lee, P., Wilkinson, S., and Buchanan, W. W., 1984, Clinical associations of fibroblast growth promoting factor in scleroderma, *J. Rheumatol.* **11**:43–47.

Pruzanski, W., Lee, P., Willshire, A., Gladman, D., and Keystone, E. C., 1983, Lymphocytotoxic and phagocytotoxic activity in progressive systemic sclerosis, *J. Rheumatol.* **10**:55–60.

Reinherz, E. L., Parkman, R., Rappeport, J., Rose, F. S., and Schlossman, S. F., 1979, Aberrations of suppressor T cells in human graft-versus-host disease, *N. Engl. J. Med.* **300**:1061–1068.

Reinsmoen, N. L., and Bach, F. H., 1983, Detection of HLA restricted anti-minor histocompatibility antigen(s) reactive cells from skin GVHD lesions, *Hum. Immunol.* **8**:300.

Reynolds, H. Y., Fulmer, J. D., Kazmierowski, J. A., Roberts, W. C., Frank, M. M., and Crystal, R. G., 1977, Analysis of cellular and protein content of broncho-alveolar lavage fluid from patients with idiopathic pulmonary fibrosis and chronic hypersensitivity pneumonitis, *J. Clin. Invest.* **59**:165–175.

Rodnan, G. P., 1977, Growth and development of rheumatology in the United States—a bicentennial report. Presidential address to the American Rheumatism Association, *Arthritis Rheum.* **20:**1149–1168.

Rodnan, G. P., Lipinski, E., and Luksick, J., 1979, Skin thickness and collagen content in progressive systemic sclerosis and localized scleroderma, *Arthritis Rheum.* **22:**130–140.

Rodnan, G. P., Myerowitz, R. L., and Justh, G. O., 1980, Morphologic changes in the digital arteries of patients with progressive systemic sclerosis (scleroderma) and Raynaud phenomenon, *Medicine (Baltimore)* **59:**393–408.

Rogers, K. A., and Kalnins, V. I., 1983, Comparison of the cytoskeleton in aortic endothelial cells *in situ* and *in vitro, Lab. Invest.* **49:**650–654.

Rosenbloom, J., McArthur, W., Malamud, D., and Jimenez, S., 1983, Characterization of a lymphokine produced by human T cells which inhibits collagen synthesis, *Cell. Immunol.* **81:**192–198.

Roska, A. K., Johnson, A. R., and Lipsky, P. S., 1984, Immunologic function of endothelial cells: Guinea pig aortic endothelial cells support mitogen-induced T lymphocyte activation, but do not function as antigen-presenting cells, *J. Immunol.* **132:**136–145.

Ross, R., Glomset, J., Kariya, B., and Harker, L., 1974, A platelet-dependent serum factor that stimulates the proliferation of arterial smooth muscle cells *in vitro, Proc. Natl. Acad. Sci. U.S.A.* **71:**1207–1210.

Roumm, A. D., Whiteside, T. L., Medsger, T. A., Jr., and Rodnan, G. P., 1983, Quantitation and subtyping of lymphocytes in skin and peripheral blood (PB) of patients with progressive systemic sclerosis (PSS), *Arthritis Rheum.* **26:**S61.

Russell, M. L., 1983, The tight-skin mouse: Is it a model for scleroderma? *J. Rheumatol.* **10:**679–681.

Russell, M. L., and Hanna, W. M., 1983, Ultrastructure of muscle microvasculature in progressive systemic sclerosis: Relation to clinical weakness, *J. Rheumatol.* **10:**741–747.

Russell, M. L., Friesen, D., Henderson, R. D., and Hanna, W. M., 1982, Ultrastructure of the esophagus in scleroderma, *Arthritis Rheum.* **25:**1117–1123.

Ryan, U. S., and Ryan, J. W., 1983, Endothelial cells and inflammation, *Clin. Lab. Med.* **3:**577–599.

Ryan, U. S., Schultz, D. R., and Ryan, J. W., 1981, Fc and C3b receptors on pulmonary endothelial cells: Induction by injury, *Science* **214:**557–558.

Sage, H., Pritzl, P., and Bornstein, P., 1982, Endothelial cells secrete a novel collagen type *in vitro* independently of prolyl hydroxylation, *Collagen Rel. Res.* **2:**465–479.

Schmidt, J. A., Mizel, S. B., Cohen, D., and Green, I., 1982, Interleukin I, a potential regulator of fibroblast proliferation, *J. Immunol.* **128:**2177–2182.

Schneider, P. D., Wise, R. A., Hochberg, M. C., and Wigley, F. M., 1982, Serial pulmonary function in systemic sclerosis, *Am. J. Med.* **73:**385–394.

Segond, P., Salliere, D., Galanaud, P., Desmottes, R. M., Massias, P., and Fiessinger, J. N., 1982, Impaired primary *in vitro* antibody response in progressive systemic sclerosis patients: Role of suppressor monocytes, *Clin. Exp. Immunol.* **47:**147–154.

Seibold, J. R., 1982, Digital sclerosis in children with insulin-dependent diabetes mellitus, *Arthritis Rheum.* **25:**357–361.

Seibold, J. R., and Jageneau, A. H. M., 1984, Treatment of Raynaud's phenomenon with ketanserin, a selective antagonist of the serotonin$_2$ (5-HT$_2$) receptor, *Arthritis Rheum.* **27:**139–146.

Seibold, J. R., Medsger, T. A., Jr., Winkelstein, A., Kelly, R. H., and Rodnan, G. P., 1982, Immune complexes in progressive systemic sclerosis (scleroderma), *Arthritis Rheum.* **25:**1167–1173.

Senior, R. M., Griffin, G. L., and Mecham, R. P., 1982, Chemotactic responses of fibroblasts to tropoelastin and elastin derived peptides, *J. Clin. Invest.* **70:**614–618.

Senior, R. M., Griffin, G. L., Huang, J. S., Walz, D. A., and Deuel, T. F., 1983, Chemotactic activity of platelet alpha granule proteins for fibroblasts, *J. Cell Biol.* **96:**382–385.

Seppa, H. E. J., Yamada, K. M., Seppa, S. T., Silver, M. H., Kleinman, H. K., and Schiffmann, N. E., 1981, The cell binding fragment of fibronectin is chemotactic for fibroblasts, *Cell. Biol. Int. Rep.* **5:** 813–819.

Shanahan, W. R., Jr., and Korn, J. H., 1982, Cytotoxic activity of sera from scleroderma and other connective tissue diseases, *Arthritis Rheum.* **25:**1391–1395.

Shapiro, L. S., Prince, R. K., Buckingham, R. B., and Rodnan, G. P., 1983, D-Penicillamine treatment of progressive systemic sclerosis (scleroderma): A comparison of clinical and *in vitro* effects, *J. Rheumatol.* **10:**316–318.

Sheldon, W. B., Lurie, D. P., Maricq, H. R., Kahaleh, M. B., DeLustro, F. A., Gibofsky, A., and LeRoy, E. C., 1981, Three siblings with scleroderma (systemic sclerosis) and two with Raynaud's phenomenon from a single kindred, *Arthritis Rheum.* **24**:668–676.

Sherer, G. D., Jackson, B. B., and LeRoy, E. C., 1981, Chromosome breakage and sister chromatid exchange frequencies in scleroderma, *Arthritis Rheum.* **24**:1409–1413.

Sherman, L. A., 1983, Binding of soluble fibrin to macrophages, *Ann. N.Y. Acad. Sci.* **408**:610–620.

Shulman, H. M., Sullivan, K. M., Weiden, P. L., McDonald, G. B., Striker, G. E., Sale, G. E., Hackman, R., Tsoi, M. S., Storb, R., and Thomas, E. D., 1980, Chronic graft-versus-host syndrome in man, *Am. J. Med.* **69**:204–217.

Silver, R. M., Metcalf, J. F., Stanley, J. H., and LeRoy, E. C., 1984, Bronchoalveolar lavage (BAL) analysis of scleroderma lung disease, *Arthritis Rheum.* **27**:S19.

Siminovitch, K., Klein, M., Pruzanski, W., Wilkinson, S., Lee, P., Yoon, S. J., and Keystone, E., 1982, Circulating immune complexes in patients with progressive systemic sclerosis, *Arthritis Rheum.* **25**:1174–1179.

Spielvogel, R. L., Goltz, R. W., and Kersey, J. H., 1977, Scleroderma-like changes in chronic graft vs host disease, *Arch. Dermatol.* **113**:1424–1428.

Spielvogel, R. L., Kersey, J. H., and Goltz, R. W., 1978, Mononuclear cell stimulation of fibroblast collagen synthesis, *Clin. Exp. Dermatol.* **3**:25–30.

Stastny, P., Stembridge, V. A., and Ziff, M., 1963, Homologous disease in the adult rat, a model for the autoimmune disease. I. General features and cutaneous lesions, *J. Exp. Med.* **118**:635–648.

Steen, V. D., Ziegler, G. L., Rodnan, G. P., and Medsger, T. A., 1984, Clinical and laboratory associations of anticentromere antibody in patients with progressive systemic sclerosis, *Arthritis Rheum.* **27**:125–131.

Sternberg, E. M., Van Woert, M. H., Young, S. N., Magnussen, I., Baker, H., Gauthier, S., and Osterland, C. K., 1980, Development of a scleroderma-like illness during therapy with L-5-hydroxytryptophan and carbidopa, *N. Engl. J. Med.* **303**:782–787.

Stobo, S. D., 1982, The influence of immune response genes on the expression of disease, *J. Lab. Clin. Med.* **100**:822–828.

Stuart, J. M., Postlethwaite, A. E., and Kang, A. H., 1976, Evidence for cell-mediated immunity to collagen in progressive systemic sclerosis, *J. Lab. Clin. Med.* **88**:601–607.

Suciu, I., Prodan, L., Ilea, E., Puaduraru, A., and Pascu, L., 1975, Clinical manifestations of vinyl chloride poisoning, *Ann. N.Y. Acad. Sci.* **246**:53–69.

Tamura, T., and Ishikawa, H., 1983, Activation of fibroblasts induced by mononuclear cells from patients with systemic sclerosis and inactivation by mitogen stimulation, *Dermatologica* **166**:10–14.

Tan, E. M., 1981, Antinuclear antibodies in scleroderma, *Int. J. Dermatol.* **20**:569–573.

Tan, E. M., Rodnan, G. P., Garcia, I., Moroi, Y., Fritzler, M. J., and Peebles, C., 1980, Diversity of antinuclear antibodies in progressive systemic sclerosis, *Arthritis Rheum.* **23**:617–625.

Tan, E. M. L., Uitto, J., Bauer, E., and Eisen, A. Z., 1981, Human skin fibroblasts in culture: Procollagen synthesis in the presence of sera from normal human subjects and from patients with dermal fibroses, *J. Invest. Dermatol.* **76**:462–467.

Thakral, K. K., Goodson, W. H., and Hunt, T. K., 1979, Stimulation of wound blood vessel growth by wound macrophages, *J. Surg. Res.* **26**:430–436.

Thompson, R. P., Harper, F. E., Maize, J. C., Ainsworth, S. K., LeRoy, E. C., and Maricq, H. R., 1984, Nailfold biopsy in scleroderma and related disorders: Correlation of histologic, capillaroscopic, and clinical data, *Arthritis Rheum.* **27**:97–103.

Tom, W. M., and Montgomery, M. R., 1980, Biochemical and morphological assessments of bleomycin pulmonary toxicity in rats, *Toxicol. Appl. Pharmacol.* **53**:64–74.

Toxic Epidemic Syndrome Study Group, 1982, Toxic epidemic syndrome, Spain, 1981, *Lancet* **2**:697–702.

Tramposch, H. D., Smith, C. D., Senecal, J. L., and Rothfield, N., 1984, A long-term longitudinal study of anticentromere antibodies, *Arthritis Rheum.* **27**:121–124.

Trentham, D. E., Dynesius, R. A., Rocklin, R. E., and David, J. R., 1978, Cellular sensitivity to collagen in rheumatoid arthritis, *N. Engl. J. Med.* **299**:327–332.

Uitto, J., and Bauer, E. A., 1982, Diseases associated with collagen abnormalities, in: *Collagen in Health and Disease* (J. B. Weiss and M. I. V. Jayson, eds.), Churchill Livingston, New York, pp. 289–312.

Uitto, J., Bauer, E. A., and Eisen, A. Z., 1979, Scleroderma: Increased biosynthesis of triple-helical type I and III procollagens associated with unaltered expression of collagenase by skin fibroblasts in culture, *J. Clin. Invest.* **64**:921–930.

Vaheri, A., Ruoslahti, E., Sarvas, M., and Nurminen, M., 1973, Mitogenic effect by lipopolysaccharide and pokeweed lectin on density-inhibited chick embryo fibroblasts, *J. Exp. Med.* **138:**1356–1364.

Vaheri, A., Kurkinen, M., Lehto, V. P., Linder, E., and Timpl, R., 1978, Codistribution of pericellular matrix proteins in cultured fibroblasts and loss in transformation: Fibronectin and procollagen, *Proc. Natl. Acad. Sci. U.S.A.* **75:**4944–4948.

Wahl, S. M., Wahl, L. M., and McCarthy, J. B., 1978, Lymphocyte-mediated activation of fibroblast proliferation and collagen production, *J. Immunol.* **121:**942–946.

Walder, B. K., 1983, Do solvents cause scleroderma? *Int. J. Dermatol.* **22:**157–158.

Wall, R. T., Harker, L. A., Quadracci, L. J., and Striker, G. E., 1978, Factors influencing endothelial cell proliferation *in vitro, J. Cell. Physiol.* **96:**203–214.

Wasner, C., Cooke, C. R., and Fries, J. F., 1978, Successful medical treatment of scleroderma renal crisis, *N. Engl. J. Med.* **299:**873–875.

Welgus, H. G., and Stricklin, G. P., 1983, Human skin fibroblast collagenase inhibitor: Comparative studies in human connective tissues, serum, and amniotic fluid, *J. Biol. Chem.* **258:**12259–12264.

Wharton, W., 1983, Human macrophage-like cell line U937-1 elaborates mitogenic activity for fibroblasts, *J. Reticuloendothel. Soc.* **33:**151–156.

Whicher, J. T., Bell, A. M., Martin, M. F. R., Marshall, L. A., and Dieppe, P. A., 1984, Prostaglandins cause an increase in serum acute-phase proteins in man, which is diminished in systemic sclerosis, *Clin. Sci.* **66:**165–171.

Whiteside, T. L., Kumagai, Y., Roumm, A. D., Almendinger, R., and Rodnan, G. P., 1983, Suppressor cell function and T lymphocyte subpopulations in peripheral blood of patients with progressive systemic sclerosis, *Arthritis Rheum.* **26:**841–847.

Whitman, H. H. III, Case, D. B., Laragh, J. H., Christian, C. L., Botstein, G., Maricq, H., and LeRoy, E. C., 1982, Variable response to oral angiotensin-converting-enzyme blockade in hypertensive scleroderma patients, *Arthritis Rheum.* **25:**241–248.

Wick, M. R., Moore, S. B., Gastineau, D. A., and Hoagland, H. C., 1983, Immunologic, clinical, and pathologic aspects of human graft-versus-host disease, *Mayo Clin. Proc.* **58:**603–612.

Winkelstein, A., Bernstein, M. L., Stevens, M. A., Rodnan, G. P., Medsger, T. A., Jr., and Dobson, S. A., 1982, Reduced T lymphoid colony growth in patients with progressive systemic sclerosis and rheumatoid arthritis, *J. Lab. Clin. Med.* **100:**240–247.

Wright, J. K., Hughes, P., Rowell, N. R., and Sneddon, I. B., 1979, Antibody-dependent and phytohaemagglutinin-induced lymphocyte cytotoxicity in systemic sclerosis, *Clin. Exp. Immunol.* **36:**175–182.

Wright, J. K., Hughes, P., and Rowell, N. R., 1982a, Spontaneous lymphocyte-mediated (NK cell) cytotoxicity in systemic sclerosis: A comparison with antibody-dependent lymphocyte (K cell) cytotoxicity, *Ann. Rheum. Dis.* **41:**409–413.

Wright, J. K., Hughes, P., and Rowell, N. R., 1982b, Lymphocyte cytotoxicity in systemic sclerosis: No increase on short-term culture with established human cell lines, *Ann. Rheum. Dis.* **41:**414–416.

Wyler, D. J., and Postlethwaite, A. E., 1983, Fibroblast stimulation in schistosomiasis. IV. Isolated egg granulomas elaborate a fibroblast chemoattractant *in vitro, J. Immunol.* **130:**1371–1375.

Yamakage, A., Ishikawa, H., Saito, Y., and Hattori, A., 1980, Occupational scleroderma-like disorder occurring in men engaged in the polymerization of epoxy resins, *Dermatologica* **161:**33–44.

16

Gout

Daniel J. McCarty

I. INTRODUCTION

Gout is defined by the presence of tissue deposits of microcrystalline monosodium urate monohydrate (MSU). The MSU crystals are almost always found in synovial fluid aspirated from patients affected by attacks of gouty arthritis (Fig. 1). When aggregates of MSU crystals achieve sufficient mass, they can produce destruction of hard tissues about joints. This is called tophaceous gout. It is likely that MSU crystals often exist in lanthanic (asymptomatic) form without producing either acute or chronic arthritis. Hyperuricemia is not gout but is an antecedent factor in most gouty patients related to the deposition and growth of MSU crystals. Gout as a consequence of primary hyperuricemia is referred to as primary gout, whereas that associated with secondary hyperuricemia is called secondary gout.

Acute gouty arthritis and chronic tophaceous gout are usually easy to recognize clinically and often afflict the rich and powerful, who are in a position to be bibulous, gluttonous, and successfully lecherous. There are, therefore, many reports of gout afflicting both historically and contemporaneously important persons, providing material for some excellent reviews (Rodnan, 1961; Hartung, 1957; Bywaters, 1962). Uric acid was first identified by Scheele as urolithic acid (Scheele, 1776), and the first demonstration of crystals in gout was provided by the inventor of the optical microscope, the Dutch upholsterer Antoni van Leeuwenhoek, who examined the contents of a draining tophus from one of his relatives in 1679 (McCarty, 1970). The MSU crystals were first specifically identified in joint fluid in 1961 (McCarty and Holander, 1961). Calcium pyrophosphate dihydrate (CPPD) crystals were discovered as a byproduct of this work, leading to the concept of the crystal deposition diseases (McCarty, *et al.*, 1965) and crystal-induced inflammation (McCarty, 1963). This MSU crystal deposition disease is, therefore, a

Daniel J. McCarty • Department of Medicine, Medical College of Wisconsin, Milwaukee, Wisconsin 53226.

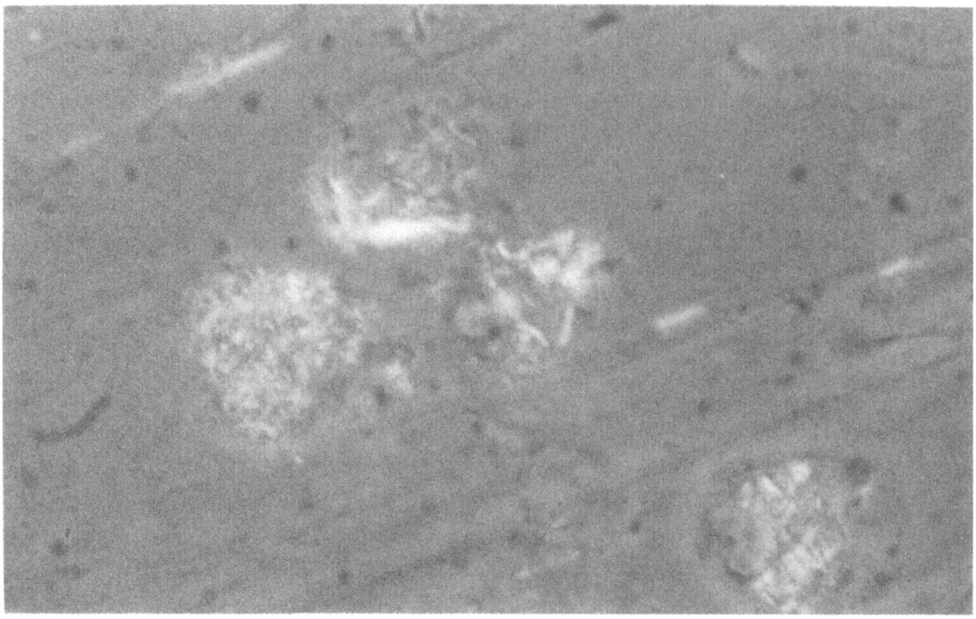

Figure 1. Four neutrophilic leukocytes engorged with MSU crystals in a drop of fluid from an acute gouty joint (polarized light, ×938).

specific example of a generic class of diseases associated with joint inflammation and/or destructive arthropathy. Colchicine, an alkaloid obtained from the autumn crocus that is effective in the treatment of gouty inflammation, has a long and interesting history of its own (Wallace, 1973). The introduction of probenecid (Gutman and Yu, 1951) and allopurinol (Rundles *et al.*, 1966) were breakthroughs in the effective treatment of hyperuricemia and of tophaceous gouty arthritis.

II. HYPERURICEMIA

Hyperuricemia has been defined physicochemically and also on the basis of epidemiologic studies. Sodium urate in serum is saturated at about 6.4 mg/dl. About 0.3 to 0.4 mg/dl is precipitated with plasma proteins, so that plasma is saturated at approximately 6.8 mg/dl.

The epidemiologic definition of hyperuricemia is based on the means + 2 S.D. with a given analytic method applied to randomly chosen sample populations. With colorimetric or specific uricase enzymatic spectrophotometric (Mikkelsen *et al.*, 1965) methods, the upper limits of normal are about 7.0 mg/dl in men and 6 mg/dl in premenopausal women. Automated colorimetric methods given values about 0.4 to 1.0 mg/dl higher than do the specific methods (Crowley and Alton, 1968). This difference reflects the measurement of chromagens other than uric acid. Colorimetric methods lend themselves to automation and mass testing and in a normal population are highly correlated with the results obtained with specific methods. In uremic subjects or in urine, however, the colorimetric methods often give much higher levels because of the inclusion of much nonurate chromagen. The physicochemical definition is preferable because the distribution of plasma urate values from population studies is not symmetric about the mean but is skewed so that the majority of values outside the 2-S.D. range are high. Values of serum urate in children are lower but rise with puberty in boys. Serum urate values in postmenopausal women approach or equal those of men.

III. CLINICAL COURSE

The natural history of gout is divided into three stages, namely, acute gouty arthritis, intercritical (between attacks) gout, and chronic tophaceous gout.

A. Acute Gout

Acute attacks are usually monoarticular and associated with little constitutional symptoms; giving way eventually to polyarticular bouts. The attacks last from 3 days to many weeks in untreated patients. They typically recur at progressively shorter intervals and eventually resolve incompletely, leaving a chronic inflammation that slowly progresses to crippling. Acute exacerbations are superimposed, usually with decreasing frequency and severity. The peak age of onset of acute gouty arthritis occurred in the fourth (Delbarre *et al.*, 1967), fifth (Brochner-Mortensen, 1941; Graham and Scott, 1970), or sixth (Harth and Robinson, 1962) decades in various reported studies.

The first metatarsal phalangeal joint is involved in about 50% of first attacks and constitutes classical podagra. Only 3% of initial attacks were polyarticular in 143 men, but 26% were polyarticular in 40 women in one report (Delbarre *et al.*, 1967). But 14.5% of first attacks in another series of 76 patients (71% men) involved multiple joints (Salzman *et al.*, 1965). Fully 90% of gouty patients experience acute attacks in the great toe at some time during the course of their disease. Other common sites initially involved include the insteps, ankles, heels, knees, wrists, fingers, and elbows. Acute gout is predominantly a disease of the lower extremity, but any joint of any extremity may be involved. Acute attacks may rarely affect the shoulders, hips, spine, sacroiliac, sternoclavicular, and temporomandibular joints, but these are almost preceded by typical attacks in the usual distal appendicular joints. The more distal the site of the involvement, the more typical is the attack.

Some patients report numerous short twinges of pain in the great toe, sometimes years before the first full-blown dramatic episode. Such twinges are also described by gouty subjects as preceding an acute attack. These "petite attacks" most often pass away in a few hours. Subpainful atacks of MSU-crystal-proven gout definitely do occur. In most patients, however, the initial attacks of gout occur with explosive suddenness, without warning. Attacks most commonly begin at night, with symptoms often first noted only as the foot is placed on the floor on arising, although the pain may awaken the victim even from deep sleep. The skin over the affected joint soon becomes reddened and warm, and the joint and periarticular tissues become extremely tender (Fig. 2). Leukocytosis, fever, and, after 48 hr, elevation of the erythrocyte sedimentation rate often occur. Even the slightest pressure from bedsheets may produce exquisite pain.

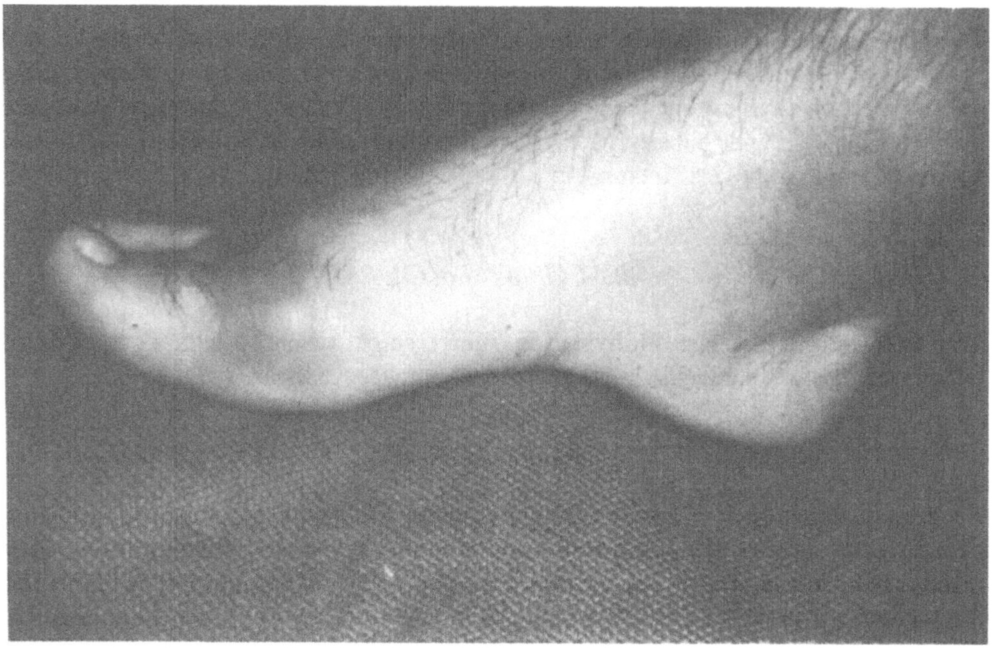

Figure 2. Acute gouty arthritis in both the ankle and the first metatarsophalangeal joint of the right foot of a 52-year-old man.

Subcutaneous attacks, which are not particularly painful, may occur in patients who have had untreated gout for many years.

The course of untreated attacks is highly variable. Mild attacks may subside within several hours or persist for only a day or two and never reach full intensity. Severe attacks may last several weeks or even months. The skin over the joint may desquamate as the attack subsides. Resolution is usually complete, and the patient is again well. This freedom from symptoms between attacks is an important diagnostic point.

1. Provocative Features

Acute gout is often triggered by trauma, alcohol ingestion, exercise, certain drugs, and by either surgery or acute medical illness. The first metatarsal–phalangeal joint is exposed to the greatest pressure (force per unit area) of any joint in the body. Attacks may follow exercise. Occupational trauma may predispose. But the inflammation in gout is out of proportion to the severity of injury, an important point of differentiation from traumatic arthritis. Alcohol both predisposes to hyperuricemia and provokes acute attacks. The mechanisms by which ethanol contributes to hyperuricemia are discussed below. Gouty attacks may be precipitated by drugs as an idiosyncrasy. Other drugs may alter urate homeostasis, producing hyperuricemia, such as attacks following administration of vitamin B_{12} to patients with pernicious anemia or of thiazides in the treatment of hypertension or hypouricemia. A sudden fall in serum urate levels (e.g., in patients soon after treatment with probenecid or allopurinol) often precipitates attacks. Rapid lowering of the serum urate concentration following a temporary elevation, such as that seen during overindulgence of food and alcohol, may release MSU microcrystals from preexisting intraarticular deposits, leading to the development of acute gouty arthritis (Rodnan, 1980). Thus, a sudden change in serum urate concentration in either direction may lead to an acute attack of gout in a predisposed individual.

Attacks of gout may develop in association with the stress of an acute medical illness or postoperatively. In patients with known gout, the risk of a postoperative attack is extremely high in the absence of preventive therapy. Acute gout occurred in 86% of 22 gouty patients subjected to surgery without prophylactic colchicine therapy (Linton and Talbott, 1943). Acute arthritis tended to occur between the third and fifth postoperative day, less commonly as late as the tenth day. Acute pseudogout is also often precipitated by surgery or acute medical illness (Wallace *et al.*, 1977); postsurgical attacks in this condition are most common on the first or second postoperative day. Attacks of gout in predisposed hyperuricemic subjects are also common during acute medical illnesses. Factors leading to attacks of gout in these settings are still not identified.

2. Recurrent Attacks

Some patients never have a second attack, but most have second attacks within 6 months to 2 years. In one large series, 62% had recurrences within the first year, 16% in 1 to 2 years, 11% in 2 to 5 years, 4% in 5 to 10 years, and 7% not for 10 or more years (Gutman, 1958). The frequency of attacks usually increases with time in an untreated patient. Later attacks are often polyarticular, more severe, last longer, and are more likely to be accompanied by fever. Erosive bony changes may develop, and the attacks may abate more gradually than before, but the affected joints usually recover completely.

In one series of patients with late polyarticular attacks, one-third reported that their initial attack was also polyarticular (Hadler *et al.*, 1974). Various joints may be involved in sequence in a migratory attack, which may include bursae, tendons, or other extraarticular sites. As in pseudogout, a number of neighboring joints may become involved, the "cluster attack" (McCarty, 1963).

Eventually, the patient may enter a phase of chronic polyarticular gout, which is often confused with rheumatoid arthritis. But unlike rheumatoid arthritis in which joint inflammation is "in phase," inflamed gouty joints are out of phase, and a flare in one joint often coincides with subsidence in another. Some patients progress directly from the initial acute attack into chronic arthritis with no remissions, and early development of tophi and incapacity. The clinical course of gout may mimic that of rheumatoid arthritis with synovial thickening and flexion deformities; tophi may be mistaken for rheumatoid nodules. This is especially true of patients treated with systemic corticosteroids. The articular and subcutaneous nodules seen in patients with rheumatoid nodulosis are easily confused with tophi (Ginsberg *et al.*, 1975). Positive tests for rheumatoid factor in the patient with rheumatoid nodules is helpful diagnostically, although 10% of gouty patients also have positive tests for rheumatoid factor (Wallace *et al.*, 1977), and fully one-third of patients with tophaceous gout are positive, although the titers are generally lower than in RA (Kozin and McCarty, 1977a). A similar prevalence of low-titer rheumatoid factor in another study of gouty patients correlated with the presence of liver disease with seropositivity (Reynolds *et al.*, 1983).

B. Chronic Tophaceous Gout

The beginning of chronic symptoms or visible tophaceous involvement is highly variable, ranging in one series from 3 to 42 years after the first acute attack, with an average of 11.6 years (Hench, 1936). A retrospective analysis of 1165 patients with primary gout who had not received therapy for hyperuricemia showed that 1 to 5 years after the first attack of arthritis, 70% were free of demonstrable tophi, and of the remainder, few had more than minimal deposits (Gutman, 1973). Ten years after the first acute attack, about half of the patients were still free of tophi, and most of the remainder still had only small deposits. Thereafter, the proportion of nontophaceous cases slowly declined to 28% after 20 years. Severe crippling disease reached appreciable proportions (24%) only 20 years after the initial attack. Tophaceous gout is often associated with early age of onset, long duration of disease, long period of active but untreated gout, frequent attacks, high serum urate values, and increased tendency toward upper extremity and polyarticular episodes (Nakayama *et al.*, 1984).

The rate of MSU crystal deposition in the joint tissues correlated directly with the degree and duration of an elevated serum level. The mean serum urate concentration was 9.1 mg/dl (uricase method) in nontophaceous patients, 10 to 11 mg/dl in patients with minimal to moderate tophaceous deposits, and greater than 11.0 mg/dl in patients with extensive tophaceous involvement in one series (Gutman, 1952).

Occasionally, tophi may already be present at the time of the first acute attack. This is rare in primary gout but was recorded in nearly 0.5% of subjects with gout secondary to myeloproliferative disease (Yu, 1965) and may also occur in juvenile gout; e.g., that complicating glycogen storage disease (Smythe and Huffman, 1955) or the Lesch–Nyhan syndrome (Wood *et al.*, 1972). Tophi rarely if ever develop in gout secondary to primary renal disease.

A classic location of tophi is the helix of the ear. Tophaceous deposits may produce irregular asymmetric lumps in the fingers (Fig. 3), feet, or other joints. The classic "gouty" shoe is one cut to accommodate such enlarged joints. Tophi commonly form along the ulnar surface of the forearm or in the olecranon bursae or Achilles tendon. They may develop subcutaneously along the tibial surface or in the distal interphalangeal joints, especially in Heberden's nodes. The predilection for developing tophi in the distal part of the extremities and in the ear may be related to their coolness relative to the central part of the body and the decreasing solubility of urate at lower temperatures (Loeb, 1972).

As tophi and renal disease advance, acute attacks recur less frequently and are milder; late in the illness they may disappear altogether. But they may be superimposed on a chronically inflamed joint or may involve previously uninvolved sites.

Tophi grow slowly, and there is often progressive stiffness and persistent aching in the involved joints. Extensive destruction of joints and large subcutaneous tophi may lead to grotesque deformities, particularly of hands and feet, and to progressive crippling (Fig. 3). The thin skin overlying a tophus may ulcerate and exude white chalky material. Rarely, ulcerted tophi may become secondarily infected. The axial skeleton does not escape urate crystal deposition, but acute gouty spondylitis is unusual. Tophaceous involvement of the sacroiliac joint and aseptic necrosis of the hip have been reported as manifestations of gout (McCallum *et al.*, 1970): MSU crystals were identified in one

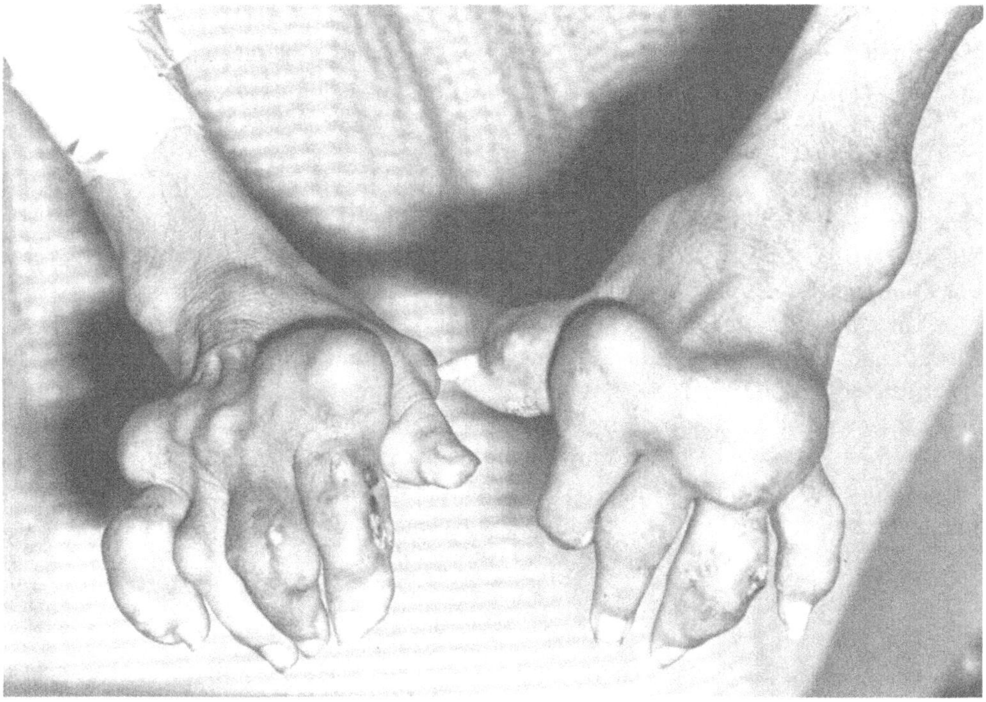

Figure 3. Chronic tophaceous gouty arthritis affecting the hands.

case in the avascular bone (Hunder *et al.*, 1968). But no cases of avascular necrosis of the femoral head were found in a systematic study of 138 gouty patients (Stockman *et al.*, 1980). The cases of avascular necrosis of the femoral head that I have seen in gouty patients were attributable to alcoholism, which is a known predisposing factor; i.e. both for gout and for avascular necrosis.

Before the availability of uricosuric drugs, 50 to 70% of gouty patients developed visible tophi, permanent joint changes, or chronicity of symptoms (Bartels and Matossian, 1959; Bauer and Klemperer, 1947). The incidence of tophi has dropped to less than 35% since hyperuricemia became treatable (Yu, 1974). A further drop since 1968 is probably attributable to the use of allopurinol. At the Mayo Clinic, the incidence of tophi decreased from 11 to 3% between 1959 and 1972 without an appreciable change in the overall prevalence of acute gout (O'Duffy *et al.*, 1975). Future incidence figures should be lower still.

IV. PREVALENCE AND INCIDENCE

The prevalence of gout varies widely in different populations worldwide but is similar in Europe and North America (0.3 vs. 0.27%) (Lawrence, 1960; Wyngaarden, 1960). A prevalence of 0.2% was found in a population of 5127 subjects studied in Framingham, Massachusetts (2293 men and 2844 women) aged 30 to 59 years (mean age 44) (Hall *et al.*, 1967). Fourteen years later (mean age 58), the prevalence had risen to 1.5%, 2.8% in men and 0.4% in women. In the Maori of New Zealand, the mean serum urate is 7.1 mg/dl in men, and the prevalence of gout is 10% (Lennane *et al.*, 1960; MacLachlan and Rodnan, 1967). Prevalence of gout is related to the serum urate level (Hall *et al.*, 1967).

Primary gout is predominantly a disease of men. In most large series, only 3 to 7% of cases occurred in women, most of whom were postmenopausal (Bartels, 1957; Gutman and Yu, 1961; Hoffman, 1959). Higher percentages of women have been recorded in series that include cases of secondary gout.

Primary gout is uncommon before the third decade, and its incidence peaks in the fourth to sixth decades (Harth and Robinson, 1962; Turner *et al.*, 1960). In general, the higher the serum urate level, the earlier is the onset of gouty arthritis. In the Framingham study, the cumulative incidence of gouty arthritis in men appeared to plateau at mean age 58 years, although only one-third of the men with urate levels of 8 mg/dl or more had developed gout (Hall *et al.*, 1967). Some patients with persistently normal serum urate levels developed clinical gout, although this was not proven by crystal identification.

V. DIAGNOSIS

Diagnosis should be established on firm criteria to insure that expensive, lifelong, and potentially toxic medications are not prescribed needlessly. I diagnose gout only after finding sodium urate monohydrate crystals in synovial fluid or in a tophus. In a multicenter study conducted by an American Rheumatism Association Subcommittee on Diagnostic and Therapeutic Criteria, approximately 85% of patients with gouty arthritis had demonstrable intracellular crystals of sodium urate monohydrate in acutely inflamed joints, a finding absolutely specific for gout (Wallace *et al.*, 1977). Extracellular urate crystals have been described in synovial fluid from approximately 70% of patients with gout when these individuals are asymptomatic (Rouault *et al.*, 1982). Only one of 19 asymptomatic hyperuricemic controls had synovial fluid urate crystals, whereas two of nine patients with renal failure and no history of synovitis had extracellular urate crystals in synovial fluid.

In the absence of specific crystal identification, the following combination of findings is useful in diagnosing gout (Wallace *et al.*, 1977): (1) a classical history of monoarticular arthritis followed by an intercritical period free of symptoms; (2) rapid resolution of synovitis after colchicine therapy; and (3) hyperuricemia. Criteria for improvement as a result of colchicine therapy have been established, namely: (1) Major subsidence of objective joint inflammatory changes within 48 hr of colchicine therapy; and (2) No recrudescence of inflammatory joint manifestations within 7 days (Wallace *et al.*, 1967). Arthralgia or synovitis alone in a hyperuricemic patient is not sufficient to establish the diagnosis. Pseudogout (CPPD) or basic calcium phosphate (BCP) crystal-induced inflammation are the most difficult diseases to differentiate, and acute attacks caused by these crystals may also respond to colchicine therapy, especially if it is given intravenously (Spilberg *et al.*, 1980; Thompson *et al.*, 1968).

VI. ROENTGENOGRAPHIC FINDINGS

The major value of radiographic examination is to exclude other types of arthritis and to detect bony tophi in patients with established gout.

Sharply "punched-out" defects in bone near joints suggest gout. Such lesions occur most often in subchondral bone in the bases of heads of phalanges. They may be seen about joints that have never been inflamed clinically. The most typical location is the medial aspect of the head of the first metatarsophalangeal joint (Fig. 4). Bony tophaceous lesions almost always antedate subcutaneous tophi (Nakayama *et al.*, 1984).

About 40% of 78 gouty patients with erosions exhibited a "thin shell-like configuration continuous with adjacent bone contour"—the "overhanging margin" (Martel, 1968). This sign correlated with the concomitant presence of the ankylosing hyperostosis syndrome of Rotes-Querol and Forestier (DISH) (Littlejohn and Hall, 1982). Although bony erosions often occur in other diseases that affect joints, the "overhanging margin" is highly characteristic of gout. Bony erosions usually occur relatively late in the disease. Many patients with repeated attacks of gout show neither bony nor soft-tissue lesions.

Bony erosions are caused by deposits of MSU crystals (tophi) and are directly related to the severity and the duration of the disease. Bony erosive changes occurred in a significant percentage of gouty patients before subcutaneous tophi developed (Nakayama *et al.*, 1984). Joint destruction may become extensive; bony ankylosis or pathological fractures occur rarely. Substantial repair of the bony lesions often follows control of serum urate levels, which allows slow resorption of the crystal deposits. Soft-tissue swelling is often seen, as tophi have the same density as other soft tissues. The lesions are usually asymmetric, and the swelling is often accompanied by the typical erosions in adjacent bone, helping to distinguish tophi from the symmetrical swelling associated with other types of arthritis. Rheumatoid "nodulosis" may appear superficially similar by X-ray examination, but "overhanging bony margins" are never seen (Ginsberg *et al.*, 1975).

One series showed that one-third of patients with gout had meniscal calcifications of the type usually associated with CPPD crystal deposits (Dodds and Steinbach, 1966), but another study found calcification of one or more menisci in only two of 43 patients with gout, roughly the incidence of chondrocalcinosis observed in elderly populations (5%) (Good and Rapp, 1967). Because of the high incidence of gout in patients with pseudogout (5%) and vice versa, the presence of such calcification in the patient with gout should suggest the possibility that CPPD crystal deposition and pseudogout may also be present. Tophi may also calcify as an extension of the overhanging margin, and calcification may occur in tophaceous masses.

Periarticular osteopenia may occur, although this is much less common than in rheumatoid arthritis. The demonstration that MSU crystals stimulate synovial cells to secrete prostaglandin E_2 (Hasselbacher *et al.*, 1981), which in turn can stimulate calcium mobilization from bone (Robinson *et al.*, 1975), suggests that subchondral osteopenia in gout may be related to active synovitis. Destruction of articular cartilage may lead to progressive narrowing of joint space. Collagenase, as well as PGE_2, is secreted by synovial cells exposed to MSU crystals, and this may contribute to bony erosion and joint destruction in chronic gouty arthritis. Ankylosis, bony or fibrous, may occur (Hughes *et al.*, 1968). Bone infarcts may also occur in gouty patients.

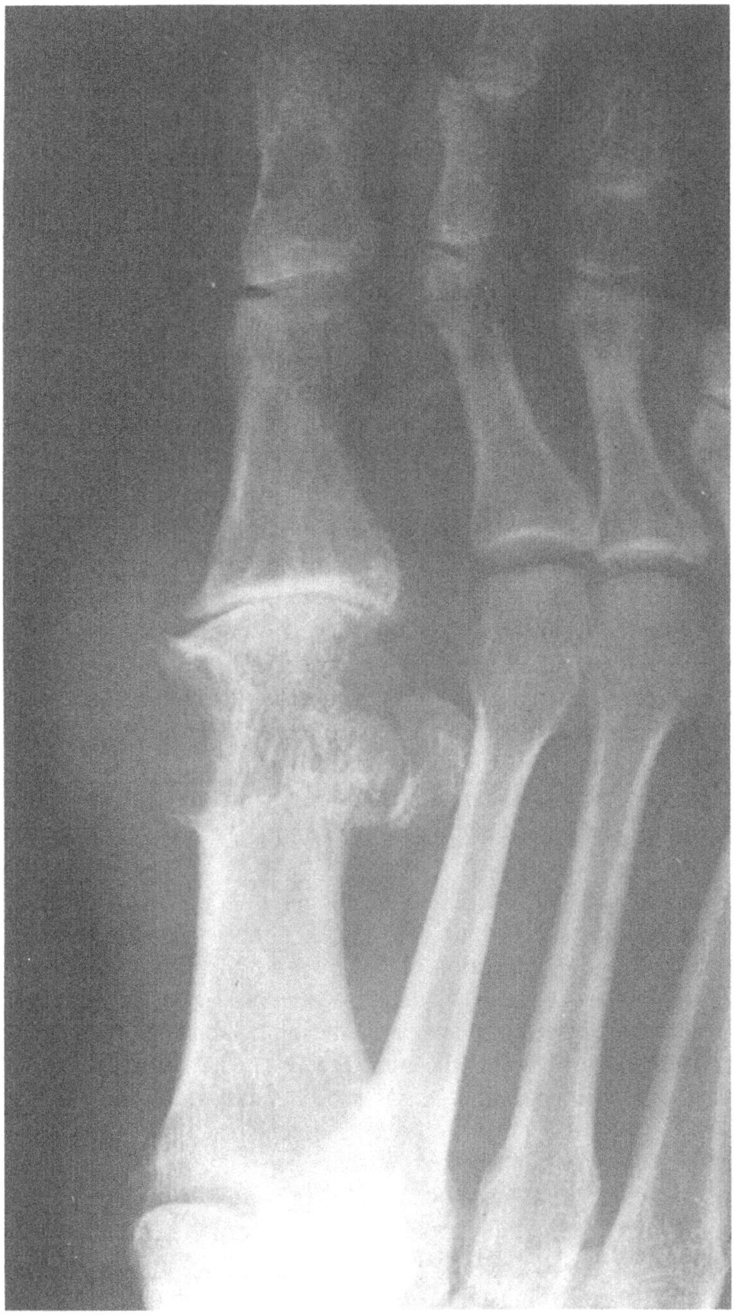

Figure 4. Typical gouty erosion in the medial side of the first metatarsal.

Uric acid renal stones are radiolucent and appear radiographically as a "filling defect." Cystine, xanthine, and 2,8-dihydroxyadenine stones are also radiolucent, but most radiolucent stones are composed of uric acid. Uric acid and stones or gravel may be white or pink ("brick dust") as a result of absorption of a pigment, which has not been identified. Some patients with "brick-dust urine" may present with what they believe is hematuria.

Radiopaque stone also occur in gouty subjects and are composed largely of calcium oxalate. These often contain a small amout of uric acid, which possibly serves as a nidus for the deposition of calcium oxalate by epitaxial overgrowth (*vide infra*).

VII. HEREDITY

The familial tendency of gout has long been recognized. A familial incidence of gout was found in 38 to 80% of English cases (Cohen, 1955) and in 6 to 22% of American gouty patients (Neel, 1947). Evidence for heredity of hyperuricemia was found in studies of families of gouty patients and in certain populations. A study of Blackfeet and Pima Indians showed strong hereditary determinants of serum urate levels, which appeared to be polygenic. Transmission patterns suggested that some of the genes were autosomal dominant, and others possibly X-linked (O'Brien *et al.*, 1966). Other studies (Mikkelsen *et al.*, 1965; Hall *et al.*, 1967) also favored multifactorial inheritance. The frequency histograms were skewed toward high values without evidence of biomodality. But other studies of more restricted populations showed bimodal distributions of serum urate values, suggesting the effect of a single dominant gene (Lawrence, 1960; Cobb, 1963; Decker *et al.*, 1962; Burch *et al.*, 1966).

VIII. PATHOLOGY

Monosodium urate (MSU) crystals deposit in cartilage, epiphyseal bone, periarticular structures, and kidneys. Urate deposits produce local necrosis and, unless the tissue is avascular, an ensuing foreign body reaction with proliferation of fibrous tissue. The characteristic tophaceous nodule consists of a multicentric deposit of urate crystals and intercrystalline matrix together with a foreign body reaction. The needle-shaped MSU crystals are arranged radially in small clusters. Tophi commonly occur in the ear, in bursae, in various tendons, in skin of finger tips, palms, or soles, in the tarsal plates of the eyelids, in nasal cartilages, and in the ocular cornea or sclera. Affected joints may develop cartilaginous degeneration, synovial proliferation (even pannus), destruction of subchondral bone, proliferation of marginal bone, and (rarely) fibrous or bony ankylosis (Ludwig *et al.*, 1938). No joint is exempt, although those of the lower extremity are most commonly involved. Tophaceous involvement of the sacroiliac joint can occur (Malawista *et al.*, 1965). Urates tend to deposit in relatively cool avascular tissues, especially those rich in proteoglycans (Hartung, 1957).

IX. RENAL DISEASE

Renal disease is the most frequent extraarticular complication of gout (Barlow and Beilin, 1968; Talbott and Terplan, 1960; Wyngaarden, 1958). Crystals of MSU depositing in the renal interstitium give rise to urate nephropathy. Uric acid crystals may precipitate in the collecting tubules, and this is called uric acid nephropathy. Uric acid may form stones or act as a nidus allowing epitaxial overgrowth of calcium oxalate. Distinction between these two entities is often unclear, and the term "gouty kidney" has been used for both. Uric acid nephropathy is uncommon in the absence of marked overproduction and overexcretion of uric acid as a result of lymphoreticular malignancy or gross enzymatic defects, whereas urate nephropathy is most common in patients with gout not associated with marked overproduction of uric acid. Hypertension and lead nephropathy are also prevalent in gouty patients.

Urate nephropathy usually progresses so slowly that it does not materially reduce life expectancy (Talbott and Lilienfeld, 1959). The incidence of proteinuria and of hypertension in gouty patients varies from 20 to 40%. It is unclear whether hypertension is the result of hyperuricemia and urate nephropathy or whether it is the cause of renal dysfunction (Messerli *et al.*, 1980). Uncontrolled hypertension is probably responsible for most of the renal dysfunction observed in gouty patients (Berger and Yu, 1965; Fessel, 1979; Messerli *et al.*, 1980).

The only distinctive histological feature of urate nephropathy is the presence of MSU crystals and the surrounding giant cell reaction, but these may be associated with interstitial and/or vascular changes (Talbott and Terplan, 1960). Some of the former may be related to hypertension. The changes labeled as chronic pyelonephritis may not be of infectious origin but rather a sterile manifestation of MSU-crystal-induced inflammation (Gonick *et al.*, 1965). A few patients with severe tophaceous gout have minimal clinical evidence of renal insufficiency, whereas others with severe renal disease have suffered only minimal joint disease. The extreme degree of this latter phenomenon may be represented by the rare reports of "gouty nephrosis" occurring without clinical evidence of articular gout (Brown and Mallory, 1950; Ebstine, 1906; Talbott, 1964).

Other causes, such as lead toxicity, may contribute to renal dysfunction in gouty patients. Study of one large series of gouty patients showed that hypertension correlated with a reduced glomerular filtration rate (Berger and Yu, 1975). Excessive lead stores associated with decreased creatinine clearance was found in another series of gouty patients, suggesting that lead nephropathy may be a common cause of renal dysfunction (Batuman *et al.*, 1981). Only half of the subjects with excessive lead stores had a history of drinking moonshine whiskey.

Renal failure was the eventual cause of death in about one-fourth of gouty subjects (Mayne, 1956; Lawrence, 1960), emphasizing the need for aggressive treatment of commonly associated and preventable causes of renal damage such as hypertension.

X. PATHOGENESIS OF HYPERURICEMIA

Hyperuricemia can result from increased intake of precursor purines, increased *de novo* production of uric acid, decreased excretion, or from a combination of these factors.

Uricolysis in man can be accounted for almost entirely by the action of colonic bacteria on uric acid entering the gastrointestinal tract in various secretions (Sorensen, 1959; Wyngaarden and Stetten, 1953). Gastrointestinal excretion is increased from the normal one-third of excreted urate to about one-half in nearly all hyperuricemic subjects and may constitute the chief route of urate disposal in patients with reduced renal function. Both increased production of uric acid and reduced renal clearance of uric acid play important roles in the pathogenesis of hyperuricemia.

The rate of purine synthesis theoretically may be assessed by measurement of the difference between purine excretion and intake in the steady state, but as urinary excretion of uric acid represents a variable fraction of total purine excretion, only gross estimates of purine production are achieved by urinary measurements. Purine intake may be reduced to as low as 3 mg of purine nitrogen per day by dietary restriction, and urinary uric acid then becomes a minimal estimate of purine production. Values in normal men eating a purine-restricted diet ranged from 264 to 588 mg per day (mean 426 $\pm$ 81 mg) (Seegmiller *et al.*, 1961).

Daily urinary uric acid excretion in men with gout ranged from values of less than 150 mg to more than 1500 mg. Lower values were found in patients with overt renal damage. In some series, 21 to 28% of patients excreted quantities of urate exceeding the mean + 2 S.D. (Hauge and Harvald, 1955; Seegmiller *et al.*, 1961), but in the general population of gouty patients, this percentage is probably less than 10–15%. Decreased extrarenal disposal of urate has been excluded as a cause of uric acid overexcretion by normal urinary recoveries of injected isotopically labeled uric acid (Seegmiller *et al.*, 1961). Overexcretion of uric acid is good evidence for excessive synthesis of purines *de novo,* but normal urinary excretion does not exclude overproduction because in hyperuricemic patients with reduced renal urate clearance, the gastrointestinal loss of urate is often increased as discussed above.

Isotopic uric acid has been given intravenously, and its concentration in urinary uric acid used to estimate the size and turnover rate of the "miscible uric acid pool." In 25 normal men, the pool averaged 1200 mg (range 866 to 1587 mg), and its turnover averaged 695 mg per day (range 513 to 1108 mg per day) (Scott *et al.*, 1969; Seegmiller *et al.*, 1961; Wyngaarden, 1965). In most gouty subjects the pool was enlarged to 2000 to 4000 mg in patients without tophi and to 18,000 to 31,000 mg in patients with severe tophaceous gout (Benedict, 1950). The miscible pool often represents only a small fraction of the total body urate in gouty subjects, as only the outer layers of tophi are readily exchangeable with urate in solution in body fluids.

Purines are synthesized *de novo* in the body from various low-molecular-weight precursors such as glycine, CO_2, aspartic acid, formate, and glutamine. The rate of urate production can be estimated by measurement of the rate of incorporation of isotopically labeled precursors into urinary uric acid. When [^{15}N]- or [^{14}C]glycine was fed to normal men, the isotopic enrichment of urinary uric acid reached a maximum on the second or third day and thereafter decline (Benedict *et al.*, 1952; Wyngaarden, 1957a,b). The pattern of incorporation was abnormal in gouty patients (Benedict *et al.*, 1952, 1953; Seegmiller *et al.*, 1961; Wyngaarden, 1958). Particularly in overexcretors, the peak enrichment values were higher, occurred earlier, and were followed by a more rapid decline because of increased urate synthesis. Marked overincorporation of precursor glycine into urinary uric acid occurred in all overexcretor subjects, and significant overincorporation was found in many patients with normal excretion. Glycine incorporation in subjects with primary gout showed urate production rates ranging from normal to four- or fivefold higher. Correction for large tophaceous deposits and for poor renal function was accomplished by injecting urate labeled with a different isotope intravenously and determining the fraction that failed to appear in the urine (Seegmiller *et al.*, 1961). Two of five gouty subjects whose uncorrected [^{14}C]glycine incorporation values were normal then showed excessive incorporation.

A. De Novo Purine Biosynthesis

Phosphoribosylpyrophosphate (PRPP) and purine ribonucleotides are important in the control of purine biosynthesis *de novo* (Fig. 5). Both PRPP and purine ribonucleotides may exert their role in the regulation of purine biosynthesis at the first and rate-limiting step of the synthetic pathway, a reaction catalyzed by the enzyme amidophosphoribosyltransferase: PRPP is a substrate for this enzyme, and the purine ribonucleotides (IMP, AMP, and GMP) lead to its allosteric inhibition. The rate of purine biosynthesis *de novo* is therefore regulated by the availability of substrate, especially PRPP, and by the concentration of these inhibitors.

The apparent K_m of human amidophosphoribosyltransferase for PRPP is greater than the intracellular PRPP concentration (Holmes *et al.*, 1973; Wood and Seegmiller, 1973). Increased PRPP levels therefore lead to an increased rate of purine biosynthesis *de novo*.

The molecular mechanism of the inhibitory action of purine ribonucleotides is known (Holmes *et al.*, 1973; Itakura *et al.*, 1981; Wood and Seegmiller, 1973). Amidophos-

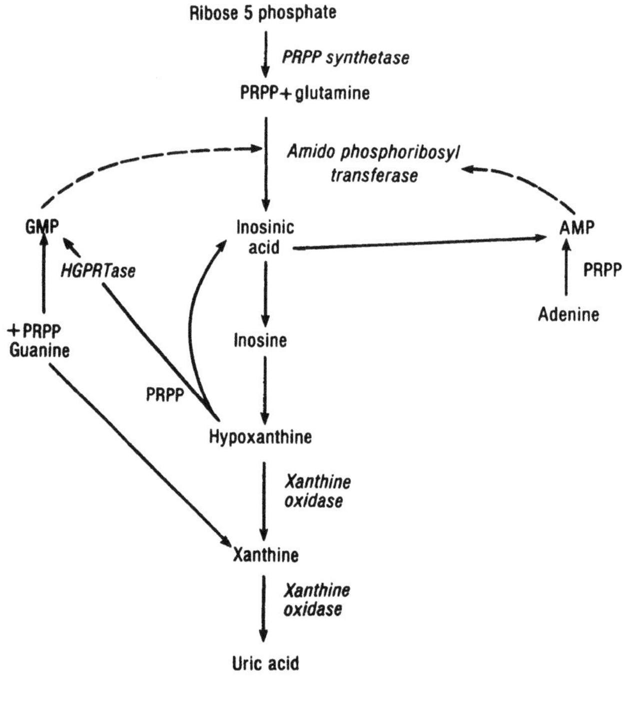

Figure 5. Simplified scheme of purine biosynthesis *de novo*. Inosinic acid (IMP), guanylic acid (GMP), and adenylic acid (AMP) are feedback inhibitors of the first and rate-limiting step in the synthesis of inosinic acid, the parent purine. Hypoxanthine is salvaged to GMP by hypoxanthine–guanine phosphoribosyltransferase (HGPRTase). *De novo* synthesis is driven chiefly by the concentration of intracellular PRPP. Xanthine oxidase is found chiefly in the liver, which is the organ directly responsible for uric acid synthesis. Clearly, most xanthine derives from guanine, not hypoxanthine, because in xanthine oxidase deficiency, xanthine, not hypoxanthine, is the main compound excreted in the urine.

phoribosyltransferase exists in a small active form of 133,000 daltons and a large inactive form of 270,000 daltons. Its catalytic activity is directly proportional to the amount of enzyme present in the active form. The small form was converted to the large form by the purine ribonucleotides; conversely, the large form was converted to the small form by PRPP.

Only a small minority of patients with primary gout show an increased rate of purine biosynthesis *de novo*. The florid overproducer of uric acid can be easily detected by measuring the 24-hr urinary urate excretion. More than 600 mg of uric acid on a low-purine diet or more than 800 mg on an average unrestricted diet suggests an augmented rate of purine synthesis (Gutman and Yu, 1957a,b; Seegmiller *et al.*, 1961). However, more sensitive tests such as isotopic precursor incorporation techniques with correction for excessive pool size and/or poor renal function as outlined above are required to detect individuals with less pronounced urate overproduction. Specific enzymatic defects have been identified in a few of the patients who overproduce uric acid. Some of these lead to an increase in the concentration of PRPP, whereas others lead to a decreased intracellular purine ribonucleotide pool.

Although it has been proposed that the concentration or availability of PRPP is increased in a number of conditions, this has been established only in the case of the hypoxanthine–guanine phosphoribosyltransferase (HGPRTase) and PRPP synthetase mutants. Enzymatic abnormalities can lead to increased synthesis or a decrease in utilization of PRPP in the "salvage" pathway, thus increasing its availability for *de novo* purine synthesis. Glucose-6-phosphatase deficiency, increased activity of glutathione reductase, and increased activity of PRPP synthetase all increase the PRPP pool. Glucose-6-phosphatase deficiency may lead to increased PRPP production by increasing substrate availability for the pentose phosphate pathway. Increased activity of glutathione reductase may lead to an increase in PRPP production as a consequence of an increased NADP/NADPH ratio. Two gouty patients had increased concentrations of ribose-5-phosphate and PRPP in their cultured skin fibroblasts (Becker, 1976). They had both increased rates of purine biosynthesis *de novo* and hyperuricemia, suggesting that increased availabilty of ribose-5-phosphate increases the rate of purine biosynethesis. Increased activity of PRPP synthetase obviously leads to an increased production of PRPP.

Deficiency of HGPRTase is one of a group of abnormalities leading to an accumulation of PRPP because less PRPP is consumed in the salvage pathway. The reaction catalyzed by this enzyme is depicted in Fig. 5. Its substrates are PRPP and hypoxanthine (or guanine), and the products are IMP and inorganic pyrophosphate (PPi). Marked deficiency of this enzyme results in a decreased consumption of both substrates, PRPP and hypoxanthine; PRPP accumulation leads to increased purine biosynthesis for the reasons already cited, and the unsalvaged hypoxanthine is oxidized by xanthine oxidase to uric acid.

The deficiencies of HGPRTase and glucose-6-phosphatase and increased activity of PRPP synthetase are the best-characterized enzymatic abnormalities leading to purine overproduction. The deficiency of HGPRTase catalytic activity, an X-linked disorder, has been ascribed to several enzymatic abnormalities. In extracts from cells of most patients, there is no demonstrable immunologically cross-reactive protein (Kelley and Wyngaarden, 1983), but in others a decreased substrate affinity or increased sensitivity to inhibition by reaction products accounted for the reduced catalytic activity. Specific amino acid substitutions have been identified in some of these mutations (Wilson and Kelley, 1983a,b). HGPRTase deficiency presents as one of two clinical phenotypes (Kelley *et al.*, 1969; Kelley and Wyngaarden, 1983). The Lesch–Nyhan syndrome occurs in boys with nearly complete deficiency of enzyme catalytic activity. In addition to hyperuricemia, hyperuricaciduria, and a tendency to form uric acid calculi, a severe neurological disorder characterized by compulsive self-mutilation develops. In patients with a partial deficiency of HGPRTase activity, the neurological manifestations are minimal or absent, but serum urate concentrations are often greater than 10 mg/dl, with urinary uric acid excretion often exceeding that of creatinine. Gouty arthritis often begins in the second or third decade, and renal calculi are common.

Patients with glucose-6-phosphatase deficiency (glycogen storage disease type I) have hyperuricemia from infancy (Howell and Williams, 1983). Gouty arthritis develops early in life; chronic tophaceous gout and/or gouty nephropathy may develop later.

Increased PRPP synthetase activity also shows genetic heterogeneity (Becker, 1978; Becker and Seegmiller, 1974). This complex enzyme is subject to several different types of regulation. The availability of its substrate, ribose-5-phosphate, may be important in determining the rate of synthesis of PRPP, and it is inhibited by a number of different compounds. Increased enzyme activity was the result of decreased sensitivity to inhibition by the purine ribonucleotides ADP and GDP in one family, and in another increased PRPP synthetase activity was caused by increased catalytic activity per enzyme molecule; in a third family, increased synthetase activity resulted from an increased affinity for its substrate ribose-5-phosphate. The genes for PRPP synthetase and HGPRTase are both located on the X chromosome (Sperling *et al.*, 1977). Affected individuals have shown marked overproduction of purines, hyperuricemia, and hyperuricaciduria, with gouty arthritis and/or renal calculi occurring at an early age.

B. Decrease in Purine Ribonucleotides

The hepatic content of purine ribonucleotides in patients with glucose-6-phosphatase deficiency falls after fasting or glucagon administration. Fructose administration to normal subjects caused similar hepatic purine nucleotide depletion. Reduction in hepatic cell purine nucleotide levels causes hyperuricemia as a result initially of increased catabolism of endogenous purine ribonucleotides and subsequently an increased rate of purine biosynthesis *de novo* (Ravio *et al.*, 1975). Both decreased hepatic content of purine nucleotides and the increased purine biosynthesis induced by fructose are associated with a shift of amidophosphoribosyltransferase, the rate-limiting enzyme in the purine biosynthetic pathway, to the active form (Itakura *et al.*, 1981).

C. Excretion

Approximately two-thirds of the urate produced daily is normally excreted by the kidney, and one-third is eliminated thorough the gastrointestinal tract (Buzard *et al.*, 1955; Sorensen, 1959; Wyngaarden and Stetten, 1953). Decreased renal clearance commonly leads to hyperuricemia despite increased gastrointestinal urate excretion (Pollycove *et al.*, 1957; Skupp and Ayvazian, 1969; Sorensen, 1959).

Uric acid excretion is thought to be regulated by a three-component system composed of glomerular filtration, tubular reabsorption, and tubular secretion of uric acid (Gutman and Yu, 1961). It is often assumed that urate is freely filterable at the glomerulus, but the reported studies are conflicting with regard to urate binding to human serum proteins. One *in vitro* study suggested that as much as 30% of urate may be bound to serum protein (Champion *et al.*, 1973), but others have failed to show significant binding of urate to human serum proteins at 37° (Farrell *et al.*, 1971; Kovarsky *et al.*, 1979; Sheikh and Moller, 1968). The few *in vivo* studies that have been performed did not show that a significant amount of urate is bound to albumin (Holmes and Blondet, 1979) or to other plasma proteins (Kelton *et al.*, 1978a,b). Urate is clearly reabsorbed by the human nephron since on the average cnly 7.6 ± 2.4% of the filtered load of urate appears in urine (Gutman and Yu, 1957a,b). Clearance studies in man suggest reabsorptive sites for urate in the collecting ducts (Diamond and Meisel, 1975). Tubular secretion of uric acid was first demonstrated in a patient known as the "human dalmation" who had a serum urate concentration of less than 0.6 mg/dl and in whom urate clearance exceeded that of inulin (Praetorius and Kirk, 1950). Uric acid secretion was shown to occur in normal subjects after urate loading, mannitol diuresis, and large doses of probenecid (Gutman *et al.*, 1959). Urate secretion in man is probably mediated by pathways common to other organic acids, since pyrazinoic acid, lactate, β-hydroxybutyrate, acetoacetate, salicylate, and other organic acids all decrease excretion (Weiner and Mudge, 1964).

A "postsecretory reabsorptive" model proposing two sites for uric acid reabsorption in the proximal nephron, separated by a uric acid secretory site, is the best attempt thus far to accommodate all of the observations on the renal handling of uric acid inman (Fig. 6).

A reduction in urate clearance contributes to hyperuricemia in most patients with primary gout. A comparison of urate excretion rates and plasma urate concentrations in gouty patients and in controls showed that excretion increased as plasma urate concentration increased in both groups, but a higher plasma urate concentration was required for the gouty subjects to achieve equivalent rates of excretion (Wyngaarden, 1965; Simkin, 1977). Nongouty subjects with primary hyperuricemia also showed a greater increment

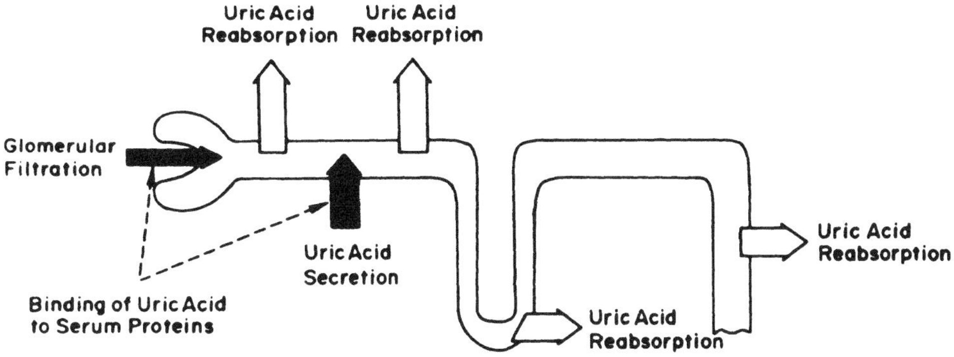

Figure 6. Scheme of urate renal excretion. Reproduced with permission from Lea & Febiger.)

in plasma urate in response to the oral ingestion of purines than did normouricemic controls (Zollner and Griebsch, 1974).

The filtered load of urate is influenced by the glomerular filtration rate and by the extent to which urate is bound to plasma proteins. As some dyes known to bind to plasma proteins are completely filtered at the glomerulus, it is very unlikely that urate protein binding is a limiting factor at the glomerular level.

Many gouty subjects exhibit both increased urate production and decreased renal clearance. Patients with glucose-6-phosphatase deficiency show both increased purine biosynthesis *de novo* and decreased uric acid clearance. The former is caused by increased availability of PRPP and/or decreased intracellular concentrations of purine ribonucleotides, and the latter is a result of hyperlactacidemia and decreased urate secretion. The simultaneous occurrence of both pathogenetic mechanisms leading to hyperuricemia also occurs in patients with idiopathic gout.

XI. SECONDARY HYPERURICEMIA AND SECONDARY GOUT

A. Hematologic Disorders

Hyperuricemia and secondary gout occur in lymphoproliferative and myeloproliferative disorders, multiple myeloma, secondary polycythemia, certain hemoglobinopathies, thalassemia, and pernicous anemia, all associated with chronically increased bone marrow activity (Talbott, 1959).

Mean urinary urate excretion was 634 mg per 24 hr in a series of patients with gout secondary to hematologic disorders versus a mean of 497 mg per 24 hr in normal controls (Gutman and Yu, 1962). Urate excretion was either normal or increased in the gouty subjects, and the incorporation of labeled precursors into urinary purine bases and uric acid revealed striking labeling of the bases during the first day followed by secondary labeling of both bases and uric acid between 7 and 12 days. Cumulative incorporation of isotope into uric acid was normal during the first few days but greatly exceded normal after 1 or 2 weeks as a result of an increased turnover of nucleic acid purine (Wyngaarden *et al.*, 1959).

B. Drugs and Other Agents

A study of hyperuricemic hospitalized men implicated diuretics in 20% (Paulus *et al.*, 1970), and half of the new cases of gout in the Framingham study occurred in persons taking thiazides or ethacrynic acid. A prerequisite for diuretic-induced hyperuricemia is volume contraction (Suki *et al.*, 1967; Steele, 1969; Steele and Oppenheimer, 1969). Diuretics both increase the tubular reabsorption of filtered urate and inhibit tubular secretion. Neither of these effects represents a direct action of the drug on tubular transport, as urate excretion returns to near control values when volume depletion is prevented by intravenous saline. Furosemide induces hyperlactacidemia, which further suppresses secretion of urate.

There is a strong correlation between serum urate levels and alcohol intake (Evans *et al.*, 1968; Saker *et al.*, 1967). Infusion of ethanol results in hyperuricemia. Gouty patients are often bibulous and consume more alcohol than the nongouty population (Evans *et al.*, 1968; MacLachlan and Rodnan, 1967; Reynolds *et al.*, 1983; Saker *et al.*, 1967). Both of the mechanisms leading to hyperuricemia follow alcohol ingestion: NAD is reduced as ethanol is metabolized by alcohol dehydrogenase; hyperlactacidemia achieved in some patients consuming ethanol suppresses renal urate excretion sufficiently to induce hyperuricemia. The hyperuricemia and hyperuricosuria associated with habitual alcohol consumption may disappear after periods of abstinence and intake of a normal diet (Delbarre *et al.*, 1967a,b). Increased catabolism of liver purine nucleotides occurs after ethanol intake (Faller and Fox, 1982; Grunst *et al.*, 1977). It is likely that liver purine biosynthesis is increased by ethanol.

A number of other drugs produce hyperuricemia, which may lead to confusion in the evaluation of patients with acute arthritis. Low doses of salicylates (plasma concentration of less than 5 mg/dl) (Yu and Gutman, 1959), pyrazinamide (Weiner and Tinker, 1972), ethambutol (Postlethwaite *et al.*, 1972), nicotinic acid (Gershon and Fox, 1974), fructose (Ravio *et al.*, 1975), methoxyflurane (Hamilton and Robertson, 1974), and levodopa (Honda and Gindin, 1972) all lead to hyperuricemia. And low-dose salicylates, pyrazinamide, and ethambutol decrease urate renal clearance. Nicotinic acid both decreases urate clearance and stimulates purine biosynthesis *de novo*.

C. Other Factors

A strong positive correlation exists between body weight and serum urate concentration, but the relationship is probably multifactorial (Brauer and Prior, 1978; Fessel and Barr, 1977; Fessel *et al.*, 1973; Glynn *et al.*, 1983; Scott, 1977; Sturge *et al.*, 1977). Hyperuricemia, obesity, hypertension, and diabetes are often associated (Fessel *et al.*, 1973; Reynolds *et al.*, 1983). Obesity has a number of effects of urate metabolism including decreased clearance and increased production (Emmerson, 1968, 1973). Factors such as muscle mass also play a role in producing hyperuricemia (Brauer and Prior, 1978; Fessel and Barr, 1977), and nonadipose body weight was best correlated with serum urate concentration (Fessel and Barr, 1977). Weight reduction was followed by a modest lowering of serum urate concentrations in one series (Scott, 1977).

About 80% of patients with hypertriglyceridemia also have hyperuricemia, and 50–75% of patients with gout have hypertriglyceridemia (Barlow, 1968; Berkowitz, 1964; Scott, 1977). No correlation was found between hyperuricemia and isolated hypercholesterolemia, but the latter is often associated with hypertriglyceridema in patients with gout (Rondier *et al.*, 1977; Scott, 1977).

In untreated hypertensive patients with normal renal function, the incidence of hyperuricemia ranged form 22 to 27% (Breckenridge, 1966; Cannon *et al.*, 1966). When therapy and renal disease were included, the incidence increased even further (Dollery *et al.*, 1960; Itskovitz and Sellers, 1963; Kinsey, 1963). The overall incidence of gout in hypertensive patients is 2 to 12% (Breckenridge, 1966; Cannon *et al.*, 1966). Conversely, the incidence of hypertension in gouty populations varies from 30 to 52% (Rapado, 1974). In most hypertensive patients, hyperuricemia appears to be related to reduced urate clearance (Simon *et al.*, 1969). Although the mechanism(s) relating gout and hypertension are unclear, the association is important clinically since uncontrolled hypertension is the chief cause of renal dysfunction in gouty patients as discussed above.

Despite high serum urate concentrations in many uremic patients, gouty arthritis is rare. Only six of 496 chronically uremic patients had gout (Sarre, 1964). The rarity of gout associated with uremia has been attributed to a shortened life-span and a decreased ability to respond to an inflammatory stimulus (Buchanan *et al.*, 1965). Tophi in gouty patients with primary renal disease are very rare.

Recurrent attacks of acute arthritis of periarthritis initially thought to represent gout may occur in patients with chronic renal failure treated with periodic hemodialysis (Caner and Decker, 1964). But examination of the involved tissues has shown calcium phosphate (apatite) crystals in addition to MSU crystals (McCarty, 1965). Crystals in muscles of renal failure patients have been identified as calcium phosphate (apatite and possibly dicalcium phosphate), not urate (Moskowitz *et al.*, 1969).

Reduced urate clearance is the primary mechanism leading to hyperuricemia in patients with saturnine gout (Ball and Sorensen, 1969). The primary source of lead exposure in the United States is illicit or "moonshine" alcohol. Lead intoxication is probably a fairly common cause of renal dysfunction and of gout in the United States (Batuman *et al.*, 1981). A history of lead exposure and excretion of more than 1000 μg of lead after calcium EDTA administration has been documented in the absence of any measureable reduction in creatinine or urate clearance in gouty subjects (Reynolds *et al.*, 1983). Lead may nucleate MSU crystals (Tak *et al.*, 1981).

Total caloric restriction results in extreme degrees of hyperuricemia as a consequence of both reduced renal urate clearance and urate overproduction (Cristofori and Duncan, 1964; Drenick *et al.*, 1964). Urate retention correlated best with ketosis, especially with the serum concentration of β-hydroxybutyrate (Goldfinger *et al.*, 1965; Healey, 1964; Shapiro *et al.*, 1963). Carbohydrate refeeding resulted in correction of ketosis, temporarily excessive excretion, and reduced serum urate levels. Attacks of gouty arthritis may occur during periods of starvation but are unusual except in patients with a prior history of gout (MacLachlan and Rodnan, 1967). They often occurred in morbidly obsese hospitalized patients who were starved for several weeks (Duncan diet).

There is a high incidence of hyperuricemia in hyperparathyroidism (Scott *et al.*, 1964). Hyperuricemia was found in 11 of 12 patients in one series, and five of these gave a history suggestive of gout. Synovial fluid examination is essential to differentiate MSU crystals from the CPPD crystals of pseudogout, which is found in 20 to 50% of patients with hyperparathyroidism. The relationship between hyperuricemia and psoriasis is not clear; 21 to 50% of psoriatic patients had hyperuricemia in some series, but in others the incidence of hyperuricemia was no greater than that in the general population (Eisen and Seegmiller, 1961; Lambert and Wright, 1977). A high percentage of patients with sarcoidosis were hyperuricemic (Bunim *et al.*, 1962; Zimmer and Demis, 1966). Half of a small series of patients with Bartter's syndrome were found to be hyperuricemic, and 20% had episodes of acute gout (Meyer *et al.*, 1975). All patients showed reduced urate clearance; CPPD crystal deposits have also been associated with Bartter's syndrome.

XII. UROLITHIASIS

The incidence of renal calculi was 22% in patients with primary gout and 42% in patients with secondary gout. This is about three orders of magnitude greater than that in the general population (Yu and Gutman, 1967). In 40% of cases of primary gout, renal stones preceded gouty arthritis by up to 20 years. About one-third of nongouty patients who develop uric acid and stones have a family history of gout. Over 80% of calculi in gouty subjects were composed of uric acid (Yu and Gutman, 1967). The other stones had only a central nidus of uric acid or contained only calcium oxalate or calcium phosphate. Hyperuricosuric subjects are predisposed to develop calcium oxalate stones (Coe, 1980). Reduction in urinary urate excretion by allopurinol decreased calcium oxalate stone formation in hyperuricosuric subjects. Factors predisposing to uric acid nephrolithiasis in gout include undue acidity of the urine, increased urinary excretion of uric acid, and increased urinary concentration or abnormalities of urinary constituents affecting uric acid solubility (Atsmon *et al.*, 1963).

Gouty patients often excrete an unusually acid urine and show a decreased rise of urinary pH in response to oral alkali (Yu and Gutman, 1967). Urine pH correlated with a low NH_4^+/titratable acid ratio, which has been attributed to a subnormal ammonium excretion at a given acid load (Gutman and Yu, 1965; Henneman *et al.*, 1962; Plante *et al.*, 1968) or to higher values of titratable acidity (Barzel *et al.*, 1964). In the three-fourths of gouty subjects whose urinary uric acid excretion is normal, the high incidence of renal stones may be related to their low urinary pH. The pK_{a1} and pK_{a2} values of uric acid are 5.75 and 10.3. At urinary pH values of 4.5 to 5, the predominant form should be uric acid, not sodium urate. This has been shown by X-ray diffraction studies (Howell *et al.*, 1963; Prien and Prien, 1968). The prevalence of renal stones rises with increasing plasma urate levels and was nearly 50% when serum urate levels exceed 12 mg/dl (Yu and Gutman, 1967). The prevalence of urolithiasis increased from 11% in patients with excretion values under 300 mg per day to 50% in patients with values over 1100 mg per day.

Only about 20% of patients without clinical gout who form uric acid stones are hyperuricemic (Talbott, 1957), but this group includes patients with a tendency toward a low urine pH.

XIII. TREATMENT

Progress in the understanding of purine metabolism, knowledge of its potential adverse consequences, and the availability of effective drugs have led to the rational management of hyperuricemia.

Hyperuricemia *per se* is neither a disease nor an indication for therapy, but it should prompt a study of its etiology. A decision to treat is based on the possible consequences of the hyperuricemia in each patient. Treatment should not be based solely on the result of one assay. Serum urate concentrations vary with age and sex, fluctuate throughout the day in some individuals, and may be subject to seasonal variation. Recent weight loss, heavy physical exertion, renal function impairment, ingestion of substances such as alcohol, and drugs may all result in hyperuricemia, as discussed above. The cause can be easily determined in 70% of cases by history and physical examination alone (Paulus *et al.*, 1970).

A 24-hr urinary uric acid measurement should be obtained to determine grossly whether hyperuricemia is the consequence of overproduction or decreased excretion. Hyperuricemic individuals excreting more than 600 mg of uric acid per day on a purine-free diet are hyperuricemic because of purine overproduction, and those excreting less than 600 mg are most often hyperuricemic because of an inadequate excretion. If the urine is collected when the patient is consuming a regular diet, which is the most practical approach in clinical practice, then a value of 800 mg per 24 hr can be used (see above). The values given above were determined in subjects with noraml renal function. Since impaired renal function decreases the amount of urate filtered in the glomeruli, less uric acid appears in the urine. Consequently, normal 24-hr urinary uric acid values do not necessarily rule out urate overproduction in a patient with renal dysfunction. Similarly, the increased extrarenal excretion of urate that occurs in hyperuricemic subjects might mask modest degrees of urate overproduction as already discussed.

The normal values given above were obtained using the specific uricase method. Colorimetric methods are even less specific in urine than they are in serum because drugs and nonurate chromogens found in urine often cause spuriously 9 high values, and these normal chromagens are increased in renal failure as already discussed. Intake of corticosteroids, ascorbic acid, phenylbutazone, or salicylates confuse the interpretation of 24-hr urinary urate excretion values.

Exactly when hyperuricemia should be treated is still debated. In patients with frequent attacks of acute gouty arthritis or with tophi, therapy is clearly indicated. But treatment of individuals with asymptomatic hyperuricemia, either idiopathic or secondary to antihypertensive drug therapy, or with only one acute episode and a serum urate of less than 9.0 mg/dl, remains controversial. Treatment is lifelong, costly, and potentially toxic. The decision to treat should be based on the needs of each patient. A mistake made in the treatment of a chronic disease is a chronic mistake.

A. Asymptomatic Hyperuricemia

Little data exist concerning the benefits of treatment of asymptomatic hyperuricemia. The chance of complications if therapy is withheld must be estimated.

The risk of gouty arthritis rises with both the degree of hyperuricemia and age (Hall *et al.*, 1967; Meyers *et al.*, 1968). It seems unwise to treat asymptomatic hyperuricemia simply to prevent the first attack of acute gout. There is no evidence to show that structural kidney damage will occur first (Emmerson, 1968; Klinenberg *et al.*, 1975), and tophi are rarely present prior to the first gouty attack. Antihyperuricemic therapy should be withheld until arthritis occurs and the diagnosis is confirmed by crystal identification.

Renal disease is an important potential consequence of hyperuricemia. Progressive renal failure is a major cause of death in patients with gout, as already discussed. Urate nephropathy leading to irreversible chronic renal failure is rare. Urate nephropathy is a late event in the natural history of gout and only rarely is reported in the absence of gouty arthritis (*vide supra*). The risk of renal failure from hyperuricemia *per se* is extremely low. One study of 113 patients with asymptomatic hyperuricemia and 193 normouricemic controls followed for 8 years found that azotemia, defined as a serum creatinine greater than 1.6 mg in men and 1.3 mg in women, occurred in 1.8 and 2.1%, respectively (Fessel, 1979). No statistically significant differences in renal function were found between hyperuricemic patients treated with allopurinol versus placebo for at least 2.5 years (Rosenfeld, 1974). Even in patients with known gout, hyperuricemia *per se* is rarely damaging to renal function (Berger and Yu, 1975). Long-term follow-up of renal clearance in 149 gouty patients suggested that coexisting diseases, especially hypertension, have the most effect on renal function, with age *per se* a second important factor (Yu *et al.*, 1979). Studies of renal hemodynamics in 624 gouty patients showed that hyperuricemia alone did not adversely affect renal function, but associated cardiovascular disease, hypertension, nonrelated intrinsic renal disease, and age did correlate with decreased renal function (Yu and Berger, 1982).

In gouty patients, the risk of nephrolithiasis was related to the magnitude of the urinary uric acid excretion and serum urate elevation (Yu and Gutman, 1967). The rate of stone formation was 2.8 times higher in asymptomatic hyperuricemic individuals than in normouricemic controls (Fessel, 1979). This risk is sufficiently low to justify withholding therapy until the occurrence of the first stone.

Acute uric acid nephropathy is rare, occurring almost exclusively in patients receiving chemotherapy for hematologic malignancies. It is of little or no concern in the context of aysmptomatic hyperuricemia.

Whether hyperuricemia is a independent risk factor for atherosclerotic cardiovascular disease is unknown. Hyperuricemic individuals with or without gout have a high incidence of hypertension and coronary artery disease. One analysis of a large series of hyperuricemic patients correlated cardiovascular mortality with serum uric acid levels independent of obesity (Fessel, 1980). Hyperuricemia was thought to be an "associated" rather than a "risk" factor for vascular disease. In patients with essential hypertension, hyperuricemia most likely reflects early renal vascular involvement; i.e., nephrosclerosis, and if it persists following myocardial infarction, it is a sign of a poor prognosis (Woolliscroft *et al.*, 1982). There is no evidence that lowering the serum urate concentration in either an asymptomatic hyperuricemic or a gouty patient prevents heart disease.

There is probably no indication to screen for hyperuricemia in asymptomatic individuals, but if found, its cause should be determined.

B. Symptomatic Hyperuricemia

1. Gout

The most common indication for lowering the serum urate concentration is articular gout. The differential diagnosis of acute monoarticular arthritis is extensive, and accurate diagnosis must precede therapy, as already discussed.

It is generally agreed that hyperuricemia should be treated in patients with frequent recurrent attacks of gout, tophi, classic radiographic (bone tophi) changes, or uric acid stones. Some believe that the first attack of acute gout is indication for therapy; others hold that first attacks are easily, inexpensively, and effectively treated and postpone urate-lowering therapy. Some patients experience only one attack and may not have another for many years. In the Framingham study, one-fourth of the patients with acute gouty arthritis had only one attack in the 12 years of observation (Hall *et al.*, 1967).

A gouty patient should be educated about the disease and the goals and potential side effects of therapy. Weight control is important, and meticulous attention should be given to blood pressure control. A 24-hr urinary uric acid measurement as outlined above helps determine the etiology of the hyperuricemia, aids in selecting the most appropriate hypouricemic agent, and also influences the decision of whether or not to start hypouricemic therapy after a first attack, because, as mentioned already, the formation of stones correlates with urinary uric acid excretion.

If hypouricemia therapy is withheld from a patient with gout, there is a definite risk of tophaceous destruction of bone and cartilage. In one series of gouty patients, 42% without tophi on physical examination had radiographic changes characteristic of bony tophi (Nakayama *et al.*, 1984). The frequency of acute attacks, history of therapy, and serum urate levels at the time of evaluation failed to predict which patients would show bony changes. Radiographic study is useful in defining the severity of the disease and provides useful information concerning the treatment decision (Barthelemy *et al.*, 1984).

Before one gives hypouricemic agents: (1) All signs of acute inflammation should be absent; (2) The patient should be advised regarding factors capable of precipitating an acute attack; and (3) Prophylactic treatment with colchicine, 0.5 to 1.5 mg daily, or a nonsteroidal antiinflammatory drug should be started. Because any sudden decrease in the serum urate concentration can trigger an acute attack, urate-lowering drugs should not be given until joint inflammation is controlled. Colchicine is extremely successful in preventing gout (Cohen, 1936; Yu, 1982). It is most effective if started at least 1 week before the hypouricemic agent is given, and it should be continued until the serum urate has been well controlled and the patient has been free of acute attacks for at least one year. Drug dosage is titrated to maintain a serum urate concentration below 5.0 mg/dl.

2. *Nephrolithiasis*

Medical prophylaxis of either uric acid or calcium stones in hyperuricemic patients is highly effective (Coe, 1977; Pak *et al.*, 1981). Both types of stones occur in association with hyperuricosuria. The chemical composition of the stone should be identified whenever possible, but regardless of the nature of the calculi, maintenance of a daily urine volume greater than 2 liters is recommended. Alkalinization of the urine with sodium bicarbonate or acetazolamide (Diamox®) maybe useful for patients with uric acid stones, but care must be taken not to raise urinary pH above 7.0, as this will favor the formation of calcium-containing stones. At pH 5.0, urine is saturated at a uric acid concentration of 15 mg/dl; at pH 7.0, saturation occurs with 200 mg/dl (Klinenberg *et al.*, 1975). Specific treatment of hyperuricosuria is achieved with allopurinol.

3. *Uric Acid Nephropathy*

This rare reversible form of acute renal failure develops most often in patients experiencing an aggressive or "blastic" phase of leukemia or lymphoma prior to or during cytotoxic therapy (Gelbart *et al.*, 1977; Rieselbach *et al.*, 1964) but has also been observed with disseminated adenocarcinoma (Crittenden and Ackerman, 1977), after vigorous exercise with heat stress (Knochel *et al.*, 1974), and following epileptic seizures (Warren *et al.*, 1975). Intraluminal uric acid precipitates are accompanied by dilated proximal tubules and normal glomeruli (Seegmiller and Frazier, 1966). This syndrome is often preventable. Appropriate therapy has reduced the associated mortality from 47% to nearly zero (Rieselbach *et al.*, 1964). Marked hyperuricemia (range 12 to 80 mg/dl), oliguria, and a urinary uric-acid-to-creatinine ratio greater than 1.0 are the hallmarks of this condition (Steele and Rieselbach, 1967; Kelton *et al.*, 1978). Intravenous fluids and furosemide are given to develop a flow of 100 ml per hr or more. Acetazolamide, 250 to 500 mg every 6 to 8 hr, and sodium bicarbonate, 90 meq/liter given intravenously, usually achieve an alkaline urine (Kelley *et al.*, 1966). The urine pH should be measured periodically, and circulatory overload must be avoided. Allopurinol, 8 mg/kg, is given as a single dose to inhibit uric acid production and thereby decrease the concentration of urinary uric acid. If renal insufficiency persists, the daily dose should be reduced to 100 to 200 mg. Hemodialysis may be needed if these measures fail (Kjellstrand *et al.*, 1974).

C. Hypouricemic Therapy

Diet now plays a minor role (Talbott, 1981). A very-low-purine diet reduces mean serum urate concentration by only 1.0 mg/dl and urinary uric acid excretion by only 200 to 400 mg per day (Gutman and Yu, 1952). But dietary counseling regarding alcohol and associated problems such as obesity, hyperlipidemia, diabetes, or hypertension is still important.

1. Uricosuric Drugs

Criteria for uricosuric drug use are listed in Table 1. These agents enhance the excretion of uric acid by inhibition of proximal tubular reabsorption of urate from the luminal side of the renal tubule (Levinson and Sorensen, 1979; Meisel and Diamond, 1977; Steele and Boner, 1973). If the serum urate concentration can be maintained at 5.0 mg per 100 ml or less, tophi may shrink or even disappear (Gutman and Yu, 1957a,b).

Urinary uric acid excretion is elevated above pretreatment levels during the initial phase of therapy with a risk of renal stones as great at 9%. Once the excess urate has been excreted, urinary uric acid values return essentially to their original levels but are maintained with a lower serum urate concentration (Gutman and Yu, 1951). Uricosuric agents are effective in 70 to 80% of gouty patients. Salicylates block the uricosuric effects of these agents, possibly by inhibition of urate secretion (Hansten, 1979). They lose effectiveness as the creatinine clearance falls, becoming completely impotent at 30 ml/min (Wyngaarden, 1957a,b; Yu, 1974).

a. Probenecid. Probenecid is readily absorbed from the gastrointestinal tract. Its half-life ranges from 6 to 12 hr, is dose dependent (Dayton *et al.*, 1963), and is prolonged by allopurinol (Tjandramaga *et al.*, 1972). The drug is extensively bound to plasma proteins, largely confined to extracellular fluid, and rapidly metabolized (Dayton *et al.*, 1973; Gutman and Yu, 1957a,b; Tjandramage *et al.*, 1972). Therapy is begun at 250 mg twice a day and increased as necessary up to 3.0 g/day. One gram per day is effective

Table 1. Criteria for Use of Uricosuric Drugs

1. Hyperuricemia attributable to decreased uric acid excretion (less than 800 mg of uric acid in a 24-hr urine specimen collected on a regular diet or less than 600 mg on a purine-restricted diet).
2. Under 60 years old.
3. Good renal function (a creatinine clearance greater than 80 ml/min is ideal, but it should be at least 50 ml/min; except for benzbromarone—see text).
4. No history of nephrolithiasis.

in about 50% of gouty patients (Gutman and Yu, 1957a,b; Yu, 1974). Because the half-life is 6 to 12 hr, it should be taken in two to three evenly spaced doses. Complications most likely to occur soon after its use include acute gouty arthritis and nephrolithiasis. The former is avoided by the use of prophylactic colchicine, the latter by starting therapy at low doses and increasing at a rate of 0.5 g every 1 to 2 weeks and by maintenance of a high urine volume. Acetazolamide, 500 mg taken at night, helps alkalinize the concentrated morning urine. Hypersensitivity, skin rash, and gastrointestinal complaints are the major side effects. Serious toxicity is exceedingly rare, but hepatic necrosis (Reynolds *et al.*, 1957) and nephrotic syndrome (Ferris *et al.*, 1957; Hertz *et al.*, 1972) have been reported.

b. Sulfinpyrazone. This analogue of phenylbutazone is well absorbed from the gastrointestinal tract with peak serum levels observed within 1 hr. The half-life is 1 to 3 hr (Burns *et al.*, 1957; Dayton *et al.*, 1961). Sulfinpyrazone is 98% bound to plasma proteins and is distributed in extracellular fluids. About 20 to 45% of the drug is excreted unchanged in the urine, and the rest is excreted as the parahydroxyl metabolite, which is also uricosuric. Sulfinpyrazone also has antiplatelet activity through its inhibition of thromboxane synthesis (Ali and McDonald, 1977). Therapy with sulfinpyrazone is initiated at a dose of 50 mg twice a day. The usual maintenance level is 300 to 400 mg a day in three to four divided doses, but up to 800 mg a day can be used. Sulfinpyrazone has side effects similar to those for probenecid. Bone marrow suppression occurs rarely (Emmerson, 1963; Persellin and Schmid, 1961).

c. Benzbromarone. This drug is not available in the United States. It is debrominated in the liver and excreted free or in the conjugated form primarily in the bile. Although a weak inhibitor of xanthine oxidase activity *in vitro* the drug acts *in vivo* by inhibiting the tubular reabsorption of uric acid (DeGery *et al.*, 1974; Jain *et al.*, 1974; Sinclair and Fox, 1975).

Benzbromarone is well tolerated at doses of 25 to 120 mg per day. It is effective even in patients with serum creatinine concentrations greater than 2.0 mg/dl and therefore may be used in patients with renal insufficiency (Zollner *et al.*, 1970).

2. Inhibitors of Uric Acid Synthesis

Allopurinol is the most widely used compound. Its major metabolite, oxipurinol, available in other countries, is useful in some but not all patients who are sensitive to allopurinol (Lockard *et al.*, 1976; Rundles, 1966).

Allopurinol, a hypoxanthine analogue, was originally synthesized to potentiate antitumor agents such as 6-mercaptopurine and is both a competitive inhibitor of and a substrate for xanthine oxidase (Feigelson *et al.*, 1957). It is completely absorbed and has a half-life of about 3 hr. Most of the oxipurinol formed as its major metabolite is excreted unchanged in the urine. Oxipurinol has a half-life of 14 to 28 hr; its excretion is enhanced by uricosuric agents and reduced by renal insufficiency (Elion *et al.*, 1968).

These compounds partially block the conversion of hypoxanthine to xanthine and xanthine to uric acid. Administration of allopurinol leads to a sharp decrease in both serum urate concentration and urinary uric acid excretion within 24 hr. Maximum effects occur within 4 days to 2 weeks (Rundles *et al.*, 1966a,b; Wyngaarden *et al.*, 1965). This is accompanied by increased excretion of the so-called "oxypurines" (hypoxanthine and xanthine) in serum and urine. Uric acid itself is the most "oxy" purine, but the term is usually meant to include only its less "oxy" precursors. Total purine excretion falls 10 to 60% of pretreatment levels (Delbarre *et al.*, 1966; Klinenberg *et al.*, 1965; Rundles *et al.*, 1966a,b) as a result of salvage of hypoxanthine and because of a reduction in the rate of *de novo* purine biosynthesis secondary to depletion of PRPP as allopurinol is metabolized to its ribonucleotide (Fox *et al.*, 1970).

Criteria for use of metabolic inhibitors are given in Table 2. The dose is titrated for each patient dependent on the severity of the tophaceous disease and on renal function. The average effective dose for most individuals is one 300-mg tablet a day (Yu, 1965a,b). Failure of 600 mg a day to control serum urate level is rare. Dosage should be reduced in the presence of a reduced glomerular filtration rate because of the long half-life of oxipurinol. Allopurinol need be taken only once a day because of the long half-life of its active major metabolite (Brewis *et al.*, 1975).

Gradual resolution of tophi generally occurs, the frequency of gouty attacks is reduced, and the patient's functional status usually improves if the serum urate concentration has been controlled effectively for 6 to 12 months. Attacks of gouty arthritis are infrequent in patients discontinuing allopurinol after 2 years of therapy, but it is advisable to prescribe the drug indefinitely (Loebl and Scott, 1974).

Side effects are surprisingly few. Colchicine is about 85% effective in preventing acute attacks caused by the sudden fall in serum urate (Yu, 1982). Because of the increased concentations of urinary oxypurines, xanthine stones can develop, but this is rare (Greene *et al.*, 1969; Sorensen and Seegmiller, 1968; Band *et al.*, 1970; Albin *et al.*, 1972). The much more soluble hypoxanthine poses no threat of stone. The overall incidence of side effects is 5 to 20%, but only about half of them are severe enough to require stopping therapy. Skin rash, gastrointestinal distress, diarrhea, and headache are most frequent (Rundles *et al.*, 1966a,b; Yu and Gutman, 1964). A maculopapular erythema is usual, although exfoliative dermatitis and toxic epidermal necrolysis have been reported (Lang, 1979; Steele and Rieselbach, 1967). A mild rash does not contraindicate further therapy. Desensitization may be helpful in some patients (Fam *et al.*, 1980).

Table 2. Criteria for Use of Metabolic Inhibitors

I. Patients with gout who have/are:
   a. urate overexcretion (24-hr urinary uric acid greater than 800 mg on ordinary diet or 600 mg on a purine-restricted diet)
   b. nephrolithiasis
   c. renal insufficiency (creatinine clearance less than 80 mg/min)
   d. tophaceous deposits
   e. more than 60 years old
   f. unable to take uricosuric agents because of ineffectiveness or intolerance
II. Patients with nephrolithiasis caused by uric acid or calcium oxalate and hyperuricosuria (>600 mg per 24 hr)
III. Patients with 2,8-dihydroxyadenine renal stones
IV. Patients at risk for or with uric acid nephropathy

Alopecia, fever, lymphadenopathy, bone marrow suppression, hepatic toxicity, interstitial nephritis, renal failure, hypersensitivity vasculitis and death have all been reported (Lupton and Odon, 1979; Young *et al.*, 1974). The drug may cause or enhance cataracts (Fraunfelder *et al.*, 1982; Lerman *et al.*, 1982). Such toxicity occurs most often in patients with renal insufficiency or who are also receiving diuretics.

Drug–drug interactions must be considered. Because 6-mercaptopurine and azathioprine are metabolized by xanthine oxidase, allopurinol prolongs the half-life of these agents and potentiates their effects (Elion *et al.*, 1963). Cyclophosphamide effects may be enhanced (Boston Collaborative Drug Surveillance Program, 1974), and the incidence of ampicillin- and amoxicillin-related skin rashes increases about threefold (Jick and Porter, 1981).

Allopurinol and a uricosuric agent have been used together in a few patients where serum urate could not be controlled by either used alone (Kelley, 1975). Uricosurics increased the urinary excretion of oxipurinol, but allopurinol increases the half-life of probenecid by inhibition of microsomal enzymes, and the drugs can be used in combination without change in the usual dose of either. Combined therapy usually results in increased urinary uric acid excretion and a further lowering of the serum urate concentration (Rundles *et al.*, 1966a,b).

a. Pathogenesis and Treatment of Acute Gouty Attacks Monosodium urate (MSU) crystals are nearly always found in exudate aspirated from the affected joints (McCarty and Hollander, 1961). Many MSU crystals are located within the neutrophilic leukocytes and to a lesser extent within monocytes (McCarty, 1962). As gouty attacks correlated with a rapid fall in serum urate levels (Rodnan, 1980), it is likely that the slight increase in crystal solubility caused them to shed into the joint space from preexisting asymptomatic deposits in joint tissues. Once in the joint fluid, adsorption of various polypeptides probably determines their biological actions.

Immunoglobulin G is adsorbed strongly as a monomolecular layer (Kozin and McCarty, 1977b). The Fc portion of the adsorbed molecules is completely available, suggesting that the more electronegative Fab part of the molecule is adsorbed more strongly to the crystal surface (Kozin and McCarty, 1980). Elution studies followed by two dimensional (O'Farrell) gel analysis has disclosed that many other molecules are adsorbed preferentially to the crystals (Terkeltaub *et al.*, 1983). C_{1q} is adsorbed and activated as is kallekrein. Complement activation occurs also via the adsorbed IgG (Doherty *et al.*, 1983; Hasselbacher, 1979). Hagemen factor is both absorbed and activated (Kellermeyer and Breckenridge, 1965; Ginsberg *et al.*, 1980). Fibronectin and IgG are opsonins promoting crystal phagocytosis, while lipoprotein adsorption interferes with neutrophil uptake (Terkeltaub *et al.*, 1984).

Crystal uptake leads to the generation of prostaglandin E_2 (Hasselbacher *et al.*, 1981; McMillan *et al.*, 1981) leukotrienes, including the powerful chemoattractant (LTB_4) (Rae *et al.*, 1982), and release of collagenase (Hasselbacher, 1982), neutral proteases including elastin, lysosomal hydrolases (Andrews and Phelps, 1971; Cheung *et al.*, 1983). MSU crystals specifically induce messenger RNA for collagenase. A potent chemotactic glycopeptide (cell derived chemotactic factor—CCF) is also synthesized and released (Spilberg *et al.*, 1976). Reactive oxygen species are released and may contribute to tissue damage (Abramson *et al.*, 1982; Simchowitz *et al.*, 1982). Endogenous pyrogen (IL-1) release from monocytes has been documented and may account for the fever of gout (Duff *et al.*, 1983). After ingestion, adsorbed proteins are digested and the naked crystals exert a lytic effect on the phagolysosomal membrane, resulting in "perforation from within" and death of the leukocyte (Hoffstein and Weissmann, 1975; Mandel, 1976; Schumacher and Phelps, 1971; Sirahama and Cohen, 1974). These mechanisms have been reviewed recently in detail (McCarty, 1985).

Colchicine blocks release both CCF (10^{-6}M) (Andrews and Phelps, 1971; Phelps, 1970) and LTB_4 (10^{-5}M) (Serhan *et al.*, 1983). These drug concentrations are those expected inside neutrophils, whose labile pool of microtubules bind colchicine; 1 molecule of drug binds to a specific receptor site on 1 dimer of microtubule protein (tubulin). Neutrophil motility, chemotaxis, phagolysosome formation degranulation, adhesiveness, and phagocytic ability are all decreased by colchicine, but these effects require higher drug concentrations than are likely to be achieved by the usual intravenous (1 mg) or oral (0.5 mg per hour) doses given to patients.

Nonsteroidal agents such as indomethacin, phenylbutazone, sulindac, ibuprofen, etc, are also quite effective in suppressing MSU crystal–induced inflammation; although their mechanism of action is still unclear and the doses required are usually large.

Colchicine or nonsteroidal antiinflammatory drugs are also effective in preventing acute attacks when taken in low daily doses. The mechanism of prevention is unclear, although colchicine in prophylactic doses (0.5 to 1.5 mg daily) has been said to normalize the elevated serum hexosamine levels found in gouty subjects (Katz, 1975).

XIV. NEW DIRECTIONS

As is evident from this discussion, gouty arthritis is a solved problem. Enough has been learned about the disease to allow its precise and specific diagnosis and to permit evaluation of the etiology of the attendant hyperuricemia so that the most appropriate treatment can be selected. Practically speaking, the only patients suffering from gout now are those with inadequate physicians or who are noncompliant with regard to taking their medications as directed.

But much remains to be learned about this ancient disease. The relationship of serum urate level to occlusive vascular disease, to hypertension, to hypertriglyceridemia, and to renal dysfunction remains unclear. The potent action of uric acid as a free-oxygen-radical scavenger has been postulated to protect humans against aging and cancer (Ames *et al.*, 1981). Perhaps the mutation resulting in loss of uricase had a distinct survival value in our species.

Similarly, the apparent strong negative association between gout and rheumatoid arthritis has defied explanation. I have never seen a single case after 25 years of searching. The frequent coexistence of MSU crystals with CPPD crystals also needs explanation. The local mechanism(s) responsible for nucleation and growth of either crystal remains a mystery. The reasons for spontanteous subsidence of acute gouty arthritis are still unclear, although studies showing adsorption of proinflammatory substances such as IgG, C1q, and fibronectin and of antiphlogistic molecules such as lipoproteins are beginning to shed some light on this question.

Perhaps more important than MSU crystal disease (gout) are the more recently recognized arthritides associated with calcium-containing crystals such as calcium pyrophosphate dihydrate (CPPD) and the basic calcium phosphate (BCP) (carbonate-substituted hydroxyapatite, octacalcium phosphate, tricalcium phosphate) (Ryan and McCarty, 1984; McCarty and Halverson, 1984). Incidence of both BCP and CPPD crystal deposition appears to rise sharply with age. As the mean are of the populations of the industrialized countries is rapidly rising, these conditions must, of necessity, become an increasing health problem. As in gout, CPPD or BCP crystals may be associated with an acute inflammatory response and, even more commonly, with a chronic destructive arthropathy that appears to differ in some respects from primary osteoarthritis. The biological effects of these crystals are just beginning to be unraveled. Whether enough of the pathogenetic mechanism can be understood to permit effective treatment or prophylaxis of these types of arthritis remains a moot question.

REFERENCES

Albin, A., Stephens, B. F., Hirata, T., Wilson, K., Williams, H. E., 1972, Nephropathy, xanthinuric and oratic aciduria complicating Burkitt's lymphoma treated with chemotherapy and allopurinol, *Metabolism* **21**:771–778.

Ali, M., and McDonald, W. D., 1977, Effects of sulfinpyrazone on platelet prostaglandin synthesis and platelet release of serotonin, *J. Lab. Clin. Med.* **89**:868–875.

Abramson S., Hoffstein S. T., Weissmann G., 1982, Superoxide anion generation by human neutrophils exposed to monosodium urate: Effect of protein adsorption and complement activation. *Arthritis. Rheum.* **25**:174–180.

Andrews, R., and Phelps, P., 1971, Release of lysosomal enzymes from polymorphonuclear leukocytes (PMN) after phagocytosis of monosodium urate (MSU) and calcium pyrophosphate dihydrate (CPPD) crystals: Effects of colchicine and indomethacin. *Arthritis Rheum.* **14**:368 (abstract).

Ames, B. M., Cathcart, R., Schweirs, E., Hochstein, P., 1981, Uric acid provides an anti-oxidant defense in humans against oxidant- and radical-caused aging and cancer: A hypothesis, *Proc. Natl. Acad. Sci. U.S.A.* 78:6858–6862.

Atsmon, A., DeVries, A., and Frank, M., 1963, *Uric Acid Lithiasis*, Elsevier, Amsterdam.

Ball, G. V., and Sorensen, L. B., 1969, Pathogenesis of hyperuricemia in saturnine gout, *N. Engl. J. Med.* **280**:1199–1202.

Band, P. R., Silverberg, D. S., and Henderson, J. F., 1970, Xanthine nephropathy in a patient with lymphosarcoma treated with allopurinol, *N. Engl. J. Med.* **283**:354–357.

Barlow, K. A., 1968, Hyperlipidemia in primary gout, *Metabolism* **17**:289–299.

Barlow, K. A., and Beilen, L. J., 1968, Renal disease in primary gout, *Q. J. Med.* **37**:79–96.

Bartels, E. C., 1957, Gout as a complication of surgery, *Surg. Clin. North Am.* **38**:845–848.

Bartels, E. C., Matossian, G. S., 1959, Gout: Six year follow up on probenecid (Benemid) therapy. *Arthritis Rheum.* **2**:193–202.

Barthelemy, C. R., 1984, Gouty arthritis. A prospective radiographic evaluation of sixty patients, *Skel. Radiol.* (in press).

Barzel, U. S., Sperling, O., Frank, M., and de Vries, A., 1964, Renal ammonium excretion and urinary pH in an idiopathic uric acid lithiasis, *J. Urol.* **92**:1–5.

Batuman, V., Maesaka, J. M., Haddad, B., Tepper E., Landy, E., Wedeen, R. P., 1981, The role of lead in gout nephropathy. *N. Engl. J. Med.* **304**:520–23.

Bauer, W., and Klemperer, F., 1947, Gout, In: *Disease of Metabolism*, ed. 2, (G. Duncan, ed.), W. B. Saunders, Philadelphia, p. 611.

Becker, M. A. 1976, Patterns of phosphoribosylpyrophosphate and ribose-5-phosphate concentration and generation in fibroblasts from patients with gout and purine overproduction, *J. Clin. Invest.* **57**:308–313.

Becker, M. A., 1978, Abnormalities PRPP metabolism leading to an overproduction of uric acid, in: *Handbook of Experimental Pharmacology*, Vol. 51, *Uric Acid* (W. N. Kelley and I. M. Weiner, eds.), Springer-Verlag, New York, pp. 155–183.

Becker, M. A., and Seegmiller, J. E., 1974, Genetic aspects of gout, *Annu. Rev. Med.* **25**:15–28.
Benedict, J. D., 1950. The effect of salicylates and adrenocorticotropin hormone upon the miscible pool of uric acid in gout. *J. Clin. Invest.* **29**:1104–1111.
Benedict, J. D., Roche, M., Yu, T.-F., Bien, E. J., 1952, Incorporation of glycine nitrogen into uric acid in normal and gouty man, *Metabolism* **1**:3–12.
Benedict, J. C., Yu, T.-F., Bien, E. J., Gutman, A. B., 1953, A further study of the utilization of dietary glycine nitrogen for uric acid synthesis in gout, *J. Clin Invest.* **32**:775–777.
Berger, L., and Yu, T.-F., 1975, Renal function in gout: IV. An analysis of 524 gouty subjects including long-term follow-up studies, *Am. J. Med.* **59**:605–613.
Berkowitz, D., 1964, Blood lipid and uric acid inter-relationships, *JAMA* **190**:856–858.
Boston Collaborative Drug Surveillance Program, 1974, Allopurinol and cytotoxic drugs. Interactions in relation to bone marrow depression, *JAMA* **227**:1036–1040.
Brauer, G. W., and Prior, I. A. M., 1978, A prospective study of gout in New Zealand Maoris, *Ann. Rheum. Dis.* **37**:466–472.
Breckenridge, A., 1966, Hypertension and hyperuricemia, *Lancet* **1**:15–18.
Brewis, I., Ellis, R. M., and Scott, J. T., 1975, Single daily dose of allopurinol. *Ann. Rheum. Dis.* **34**:256–259.
Brochner-Mortensen, K., 1941, 100 gouty patients, *Acta Med. Scand.* **106**:81–107.
Brown, J., and Mallory, G. K., 1950, Renal changes in gout, *N. Engl. J. Med.* **243**:325–329.
Buchanan, W. W., Klinenberg, J. R., and Seegmiller, J. E., 1965, The inflammatory response to injected microcrystalline monosodium urate in normal hyperuricemic, gouty and uremic subjects, *Arthritis Rheum.* **8**:361–367.
Bunim, J. J., Kimberg, D. V., Thomas, L. B. Scott, J., 1962, The syndrome of sarcoidosis, psoriasis and gout, *Ann. Intern. Med.* **57**:1018–1040.
Burch, T. A., O'Brien, W. M., Need, R., and Kurland, L. T., 1966, Hyperuricemia and gout in the Mariana Islands, *Ann. Rheum. Dis.* **215**:114–119.
Burns, J. J., 1957, A potent new uricosuric agent, the sulfoxide metabolite of the phenylbutazone analogue, G-25671, *J. Pharmacol. Exp. Ther.* **119**:418–426.
Buzard, J, Bishop, C., and Talbott, J. H., 1955, The fate of uric acid in the normal and gouty human being, *J. Chron. Dis.* **2**:42–49.
Bywaters, E. G. L., 1962, Gout in the time and person of George IV: A case history, *Ann. Rheum. Dis.* **21**:325–338.
Caner, J. E. Z., and Decker, J. L., 1964, Recurrent acute (?gouty) arthritis in chronic renal failure treated with periodic hemodialysis, *Am. J. Med.* **36**:571–582.
Cannon, P. J., Stason, W. B., Demartini, F. E., Sommers, S. C., 1966, Hyperuricemia in primary and renal hypertension, *N. Eng. J. Med.* **275**:457–464.
Champion, D. W., Bluestone, R., and Klinenberg, J. R., 1973, Uric acid: Characterization of its interaction with human serum albumin, *J. Clin. Invest.* **52**:2383–2387.
Cheung, H. S., Bohan, S., and, Kozin, F., 1983, Kinetics of collagenase and neutral protease release by neutrophils exposed to microcrystalline sodium urate, *Connect. Tissue Res.* **11**:78–85.
Cobb, S., 1963, Hyperuricemia in executives, in: *The Epidemiology of Chronic Rheumatism,* Vol. 1 (J. H. Killgren, M. R. Jeffrey, and J. Ball (eds.), F. A. Davis, Philadelphia, pp. 182–186.
Coe, F. L., 1977, Treated and untreated recurrent calcium nephrolithiasis in patients with idiopathic hypercalcuria, hyperuricosuria or no metabolic disorder, *Ann. Intern. Med.* **87**:404–410.
Coe, F. L., 1980, Hyperuricosuric calcium oxalate nephrolithiasis, *Contemp. Issues Nephrol.* **5**:116–135.
Cohen, A., 1936, Gout, *Am. J. Med. Sci.***192**:448–493.
Cohen, H., 1955, Gout and other metabolic disorders producing joint disease, in: *Textbook of the Rheumatic Disease* (W. S. C. Copeman ed.), Livingstone, Edinburgh, p. 361.
Cristofori, F. C., and Duncan, G. G., 1964, Uric acid excretion in obese subjects during period of total fasting, *Metabolism* **13**:303–311.
Crittenden, D. R., and Ackerman, G. I., 1977, Hyperuricemic acute renal failure in disseminated carcinoma, *Arch. Intern. Med.* **137**:97–99.
Dayton, P. G., Sicam, L. E., Landrau, M., and Burns, J. J., 1961, Metabolism of sulfinpyrazone (Anturane) and other thio analogues of phenylbutazone in man, *J. Pharmacol. Exp. Ther.* **132**:287–290.
Dayton, P. G., 1963, The physiological disposition of probenecid including renal clearance in man studied by an improved method for its estimation in biological material, *J. Pharmacol. Exp. Ther.* **140**:278–286.

Dayton, P. G., 1973, Studies of the fate of metabolites and analogs of probenecid. The significance of metabolic sites, especially lack of ring hydroxylation, *Drug Metab. Dispos.* **1**:742–751.
Decker, J. L., Lane, J. J., Jr., and Reynolds, W. E., 1962, Hyperuricemia in a male Filipino population, *Arthritis Rheum.* **5**:144–155.
deGery, A., Auscher, C., Saporta, L., and Delbarre, F., 1974, Treatment of gout and hyperuricemia by benzbromarone, ethyl-2(dibromo-3,5,-hydrox-4-benzoyl)-3 benzofuran, *Adv. Exp. Med. Biol.* **41B**:683–689.
Delbarre, F., Amor, B., Auscher, C., and deGery, A., 1966, Treatment of gout with allopurinol: A study of 106 cases, *Ann. Rheum. Dis.* **25**:627–633.
Delbarre, F., Auscher, C., Brouilhet, H., and deGery, A., 1967a, Action de l'ethanol dans la goutte et sur le metabolisme de l'acide urique, *Semin. Hop. Paris* **43**:659–664.
Delbarre, F., Braun, S., and St. George-Chaumet, F., 1967b, La goutte, Problèmes clinques, biologiques et therapeutiques, *Semin. Hop. Paris* **43**:623–633.
Diamond, H. S., and Meisel, A. D., 1975, Collecting duct urate reabsorption in man, *Clin. Res.* **23**:360A.
Dodds, W. J., and Steinback, H. L., 1966, Gout associated with calcification of cartilage, *N. Engl. J. Med.* **275**:745–749.
Doherty, M., Whicker, J. T., and Dieppe, P. A., 1983, Activation of the alternative pathway of complement by monosodium urate monohydrate crystals and other inflammatory particles. *Ann. Rheum. Dis.* **42**:285–291.
Dollery, C. T., Duncan, H., and Schumer, B., 1960, Hyperuricemia related to treatment of hypertension, *Br. Med. J.* **2**:832–835.
Drenick, E. J., Swendseid, M. E., Blahd, W. H., and Tuttle, S. G., 1964, Prolonged starvation as treatment for severe obesity, *JAMA* **187**:100–105.
Duff, G. W., Atkins, E., and Malawista, S. E., 1983, The fever of gout. *Clin. Res.* **31**:361A.
Ebstein, W., 1906, *Die Natur und Behandlung der Gicht,* Bergmann, Wiesbaden.
Eisen, A. Z., and Seegmiller, J. E., 1961, Uric acid metabolism in psoriasis, *J. Clin. Invest.* **40**:1486–1494.
Elion, G. B., 1963, Potentiation by inhibition of drug degradation 6-substituted purines and xanthine oxidase, *Biochem. Pharmacol.* **12**:85–93.
Elion, G. B., Yu, T.-F., Gutman, A. B., and Hitchings, G. H., 1968, Renal clearance of oxypurinol, the chief metabolite of allopurinol, *Am. J. Med.* **45**:69–77.
Emmerson, B. T., 1963, A comparison of uricosuric agents in gout, with special reference to sulfinpyrazone, *Med. J. Aust.* **1**:839–844.
Emmerson, B. T., 1968, The clinical differentiation of lead gout from primary gout, *Arthritis Rheum* **11**:623–634.
Emmerson, B. T., 1973, Alteration of urate metabolism by weight reduction, *Aust. N. Z. J. Med.* **3**:410–412.
Evans, J. G., Prior, I. A. M., and Harvey, H. P. B., 1968, Relation to serum uric acid to body bulk, hemoglobin and alcohol intake in two South Pacific Polynesian populations, *Ann. Rheum. Dis.* **27**:319–324.
Faller, J., and Fox, I. H., 1982, Ethanol-induced hyperuricemia: Evidence of increased urate production by activation of adenine nucleotide turnover, *N. Engl. J. Med.* **307**:1598–1602.
Fam, A. G., Paton, T. W., and Chaiton, A., 1980, Reinstitution of allopurinol therapy for gouty arthritis after cutaneous reactions, *Can. Med. Assoc. J.* **123**:128–129.
Farrell, P. C., Popovich, R. P., and Babb, A. L., 1971, Binding levels of urate ions in human serum albumin and plasma, *Biochim. Biophys. Acta* **243**:49–52.
Feigelson, P., Davidson, J. K., and Robins, P. K., 1957, Pyrazolopyrimidines as inhibitors and substrates of xanthine oxidase, *J. Biol. Chem.* **726**:993–1000.
Ferris, T. F., Morgan, W. S., and Leviten, H., 1957, Nephrotic syndrome caused by probenecid, *N. Engl. J. Med.* **256**:592–596.
Fessel, W. J., 1979, Renal outcomes of gout and hyperuricemia, *Am. J. Med.* **67**:74–82.
Fessel, W. J., 1980, High uric acid as an indicator of cardiovascular disease—independence from obesity, *Am. J. Med.* **68**:401–404.
Fessel, W. J., and Barr, G. D., 1977, Uric acid, lead body weight and creatinine interactions: Results from regression analysis of 78 variables, *Semin. Arthritis. Rheum* **7**:115–121.
Fessel, W. J., Siegelaub, A. B., and Johnson, E. S., 1973, Correlates and consequences of asymptomatic hyperuricemia, *Arch. Intern. Med.* **132**:44–54.
Fox, I. H., Wyngaarden, J. B., and Kelley, W. N., 1970, Depletion of erythrocyte phosphoribosylpyrophosphate in man. A newly observed effect of allopurinol, *N. Engl. J. Med.* **283**:1177–1182.
Fraunfelder, F. T., Hanna, C., Dreis, M. W., and Cosgrove, K. W., 1982, Cataracts associated with allopurinol therapy, *Am. J. Ophthalmol.* **94**:137–140.

Gelbart, D. J., Weinstein, A. B., and Fajardo, 1977, Allopurinol-induced interstitial nephritis, *Ann. Intern. Med.* **86**:196–198.

Gershon, S.I., and Fox, I.H., 1974, Pharmacologic effects of nicotinic acid on human purine metabolism, *J. Lab. Clin. Med.* **84**:179–186.

Ginsberg, J. H., Genant, H. K. Yu, T.-F., and McCarty, D. J., 1975, Rheumatoid nodulosis. An unusual variant of rheumatoid disease, *Arthritis Rheum.* **18**:49–58.

Ginsberg, M. H., Jaques, B., Cochrane, C. G., and Griffin, J. H., 1980, Urate crystal-dependent cleavage of Hageman factor in human plasma and synovial fluid, *J. Lab. Clin. Med.* **95**:497–506.

Glynn, R. J., Champion, E. W., and Silbert, J. E., 1983, Trends in serum uric acid levels 1961–1980, *Arthritis Rheum* **26**:87–93.

Goldfinger, S., Klinenberg, J. R., and Seegmiller, J. E., 1965, Renal retention of uric acid induced by infusion of beta-hydroxybutyrate and acetoacetate, *N. Engl. J. Med.* **272**:351–355.

Gonick, H. C., Rubini, M. E., Gleason, I. O., and Sommers, S. C., 1965, The renal lesion in gout, *Ann. Intern. Med.* **62**:667–674.

Good, A. E., and Rapp, R., 1967, Chondrocalcinosis of the knee with gout and rheumatoid arthritis, *N. Engl. J. Med.* **277**:286–290.

Graham, R., and Scott, J. T., 1970, Clinical survey of 354 patients with gout, *Ann. Rheum. Dis.* **29**:461–468.

Greene, M. L., Fujimoto, W. Y., and Seegmiller, J. E., 1969, Urinary xanthine stones—a rare complication of allopurinol therapy, *N. Engl. J. Med.* **280**:426–427.

Grunst, J., Dietze, G., and Wicklmayr, M., 1977, Effect of ethanol on uric acid production of human liver, *Nutr. Metab.* **21**:138–141.

Gutman, A. B., 1958, Gout and gouty arthritis, in: *Textbook of Medicine* (P. B. Beeson and W. McDermott, eds.), W. B. Saunders, Philadelphia, p. 595.

Gutman, A. B., 1973, The past four decades of progress in the knowledge of gout, with an assessment of the present status, *Arthritis Rheum* **16**:431–445.

Gutman, A. B., and Yu, T.-F., 1951, Benemid (*p*[di-*n*-prophysulfamyl]benzoic acid) as uricosuric agent in chronic gouty arthritis, *Trans. Assoc. Am. Physicians* **64**:279–287.

Gutman, A. B., and Yu, T.-F., 1952, Gout, a derangement of purine metabolism, *Adv. Intern Med.* **5**:227–302.

Gutman, A. B., and Yu, T.-F, 1957a, Renal function in gout: With a commentary on the renal regulation of urate excretion and the role of the kidney in the pathogenesis of gout, *Am. J. Med.* **23**:600–622.

Gutman, A. B., and Yu, T.-F., 1957b, Protracted uricosuric therapy in tophaceous gout, *Lancet* **2**:1258–1260.

Gutman, A. B., and Yu, T.-F, 1961, A three-component system for regulation of renal excretion of uric acid in man, *Trans. Assoc. Am. Physicians* **74**:353–365.

Gutman, A. B., and Yu, T.-F., 1962, Secondary gout, *Ann. Intern. Med.* **56**:675.

Gutman, A. B., and Yu, T.-F., 1965, Urinary ammonium excretion in primary gout, *J. Clin, Invest.* **44**:1474–1481.

Gutman, A. B., Yu, T.-F., and Berger, L., 1959, Tubular secretion of urate in man, *J. Clin. Invest.* **38**:1778–1781.

Hadler, H. M., Franck, W. A., Bress, N. M., and Robinson, D. R., 1974, Acute polyarticular gout, *Am. J. Med.* **56**:715–719.

Hall, A. P., Barry, P. E., Dawber, T. R., 1967, Epidemiology of gout and hyperuricemia: A long term population study, *Am. J. Med.* **42**:27–37.

Hamilton, W. F. D., and Robertson, G. S., 1974, Changes in serum uric acid related to the dose of methoxyflurone, *Br. J. Anaesth* **46**:54–58.

Hansten, P. D., 1979, *Drug Interactions,* ed. 4, Lea & Febiger, Philadelphia, p. 255.

Harth, M. and Robinson, C. E. G., 1962, Gouty arthritis in a D.V.A. hospital: A retrospective study, *Med. Serv. J. Canada* **18**:671–674.

Hartung, E. F., 1957, Symposium on gout: Historical considerations, *Metabolism* **6**:196–208.

Hasselbacher P., 1979, C3 activation by monosodium urate monohydrate and other crystalline material, *Arthritis Rheum.* **22**:571–578.

Hasselbacher, P., 1982, Stimulation of synovial fibroblasts by calcium oxalate and monosodium urate monohydrate: A mechanism of connective tissue degradation in oxalosis and gout, *J. Lab. Clin. Med.* **100**:977–985.

Hasselbacher, P., McMillan, R. M., Vater, C. A., Hahn, J., 1981, Monosodium urate monohydrate crystals stimulate secretion of collagenase and PGE_2 by synovial fibroblasts: A model of joint destruction in chronic gouty arthritis, *Arthritis Rheum.* **24**:577–583.

Hauge, M., and Harvald, B., 1955, Heredity in gout and hyperuricemia, *Acta Med. Scand.* **152**:247–257.

Healey, L. A., 1964, The effect of fasting and kitosis on uric acid excretion, *Arthritis Rheum* **7**:313.

Hench, P. S., 1936, Diagnosis of gout and gouty arthritis, *J. Lab. Clin. Med.* **22**:48–55.

Henneman, P. H., Wallach, S., and Dempsey, E. F., 1962, The metabolic defect responsible for uric acid stone formation, *J. Clin. Invest.* **41**:537–542.

Hertz, P., Yager, H., and Richardson, J. A., 1972, Probenecid induced nephrotic syndrome, *Arch. Pathol.* **94**:241–243.

Hoffman, W. S., 1959, Some unsolved problems of gout, *Med. Clin. North Am.* **43**:595–606.

Hoffstein, S., and Weissmann, G., 1975, Mechanisms of lysosomal enzyme release from leukocytes. *Arthritis Rheum.* **18**:153–165.

Holmes, E. W., and Blondet, P., 1979, Urate binding to serum albumin: Lack of influence on renal clearance of uric acid, *Arthritis Rheum.* **22**:737–739.

Holmes, E. W., Wyngaarden, J. B., and Kelley, W. N., 1973, Human glutamine phosphoribosylpyrophosphate amidotransferase. Two molecular forms interconvertible by purine ribonucleotides and phosphoribosylpyrophosphate, *J. Biol. Chem.* **248**:6035–6040.

Honda, H., and Gindin, R. A., 1972, Gout while receiving levodopa for parkinsonism, *JAMA* **219**:55–57.

Howell, R. R., and Williams, J. C., 1983, the glycogen storage disease, in: *The Metabolic Basis of Inherited Disease,* ed. 5 (J. B. Stanbury, J. B. Wyngaarden, D. S. Frederickson, J. L. Goldstein, M. S. Brown eds.), McGraw-Hill, New York, pp. 141–166.

Howell, R. R., Eanes, E. D., and Seegmiller, J. E., 1963, X-ray diffraction studies of the tophaceous deposits in gout, *Arthritis Rheum.* **41**:537–542.

Hughes, G. R., Barnes, C. G., and Mason, R. M., 1968, Bony ankylosis in gout, *Ann. Rheum. Dis.* **27**:67–70.

Hunder, G. G., Worthington, J. W., and Bickel, W. H., 1968, Avascular necrosis of the femoral head in a patient with gout, *JAMA* **203**:47–49.

Itakura, M., Sabina, R. L., Heald, P. W., and Holmes, E. W., 1981, Basis for the control of purine biosynthesis by purine ribonucleotides, *J. Clin. Invest.* **67**:994–1002.

Itskovitz, H. D., and Sellers, A. M., 1963, Gout and hyperuricemia after adrenalectomy for hypertension, *N. Engl J. Med.* **268**:1105–1108.

Jain, A. K., Ryan, J. R., McMahon, F. G., and Novick, R. J., 1974, Effect of single oral doses of benzbromarone on serum and urinary uric acid, *Arthritis Rheum* **17**:149–157.

Jick, H., and Porter, J. B., 1981, Potentiation of ampicillin skin reactions by allopurinol or hyperuricemia, *J. Clin. Pharmacol.* **21**:456–458.

Katz, W. A., 1975, Deposition of urate crystals in gout, *Arthritis Rheum.* **18**:751–756.

Kellermeyer, R. W., and Breckenridge, R. T., 1965, The inflammatory process in acute gouty arthritis. I. Activation of Hageman factor by sodium urate crystals, *J. Lab. Clin. Med.* **65**:307–315.

Kelley, W. N., 1975, Pharmacologic approach to the maintenance of urate homeostasis, *Nephron* **14**:99–115.

Kelley, W. N., and Wyngaarden, J. B., 1983, Clinical syndromes associated with hypoxanthine–guanine phosphoribosyltransferase deficiency, in: *Metabolic Basis of Inherited Diseases,* ed. 5, J. B. Stanburg, J. B. Wyngaarden, D. S. Frederickson, J. L. Goldstein, and M. S. Brown, eds.), McGraw-Hill, New York, pp. 115–1143.

Kelley, W. N., Richardson, A. P., Mason, M. F., and Rector, F. C., 1966, Acetazolamide in phenobarbital intoxication, *Arch. Intern. Med.* **117**:64–69.

Kelley, W. N., Greene, M. L., Rosenbloom, F. M., and Henderson, F. G., 1969, Hypoxanthine guanine phosphoribosyltransferase deficiency in gout, *Ann. Intern. Med.* **70**:155–206.

Kelton, J., Kelley, W. N., and Holmes, E. W., 1978a, A rapid method for the diagnosis of actue uric acid nephropathy, *Arch. Intern. Med.* **138**:612–615.

Kelton, J. G., Ulan, R., Steller, C., and Holmes, E., 1978b, A method for monitoring dialysis patients and a tool for assessing binding to serum proteins, *in vivo, Ann. Intern. Med.* **89**:67–70.

Kinsey, D., 1963, Gout and hyperuricemia in hypertensive patients 15–25 years following lumbo–dorsal splanchnicectomy, *Arthritis Rheum.* **6**:778–779.

Kjellstrand, C. M., Campbell, D. C., von Hartitzsch, B., and Buselmeier, T. J., 1974, Hyperuricemic acute renal failure, *Arch Intern. Med.* **133**:349–359.

Klinenberg, J. R., Goldfinger, S. E., and Seegmiller, J. E., 1965, The effectiveness of the xanthine oxidase inhibitor allopurinol in the treatment of gout, *Ann. Intern. Med.* **62**:639–647.

Klinenberg, J. R., Gonick, H. C., and Dornfield, L., 1975, Renal function abnormalities in patients with asymptomatic hyperuricemia, *Arthritis Rheum.* **18**:725–730.

Knochel, J. P., Doten, L. N., and Hamburger, R. J., 1974, Heat, stress, exercise and muscle injury: Effects on urate metabolism and renal function, *Ann. Intern. Med.* **81**:321–328.

Kovarsky, J., Holmes, E. W., and Kelley, W. N., 1979, Absence of significant urate binding to human serum proteins, *J. Lab. Clin. Med.* **93**:85–91.

Kozin, F., and McCarty, D. J., 1977a, Rheumatoid factors in the serum of gouty patients, *Arthritis Rheum.* **20**:1559.

Kozin, F., McCarty, D. J., 1977b, Protein binding to monosodium urate monohydrate calcium pyrophosphate and silicon dioxide crystals. I. Physical characteristics, *J. Lab. Clin. Med.* **89**:1314–1425.

Kozin, F., McCarty, D. J., 1980, Molecular orientation of immunoglobulin G adsorption to microcrystalline monosodium urate monohydrate, *J. Lab. Clin. Med.* **95**:49–58.

Lambert, J. R., and Wright, V., 1977, Serum uric acid levels in psoriatic arthritis, *Ann. Rheum. Dis.* **36**:264–267.

Lang, P. G., 1979, Severe hypersensitivity reactions to allopurinol, *South Med. J.* **72**:1361–1368.

Lawrence, J. S., 1960, Heritable disorders of connective tissue, *Proc. R. Soc. Med.* **53**:522–526.

Lennane, G. A. Q., Rose, B. S., and Isdale, I. C., 1960, Gout in the Maori, *Ann. Rheum. Dis.* **19**:120–125.

Lerman, S., Megau, J. W., and Gardner, K., 1982, Allopurinol therapy and cataractogenesis in humans, *Am. J. Ophthalmol.* **94**:141–146.

Levinson, D. J., and Sorensen, L. B., 1979, Renal handling of uric acid in normal gouty subjects: Evidence for a 4-component system, *Ann. Rheum. Dis.* **39**:173–179.

Linton, R. R., and Talbott, J. H., 1943, The surgical treatment of tophaceous gout, *Ann. Surg.* **117**:161–182.

Littlejohn, G. O., and Hall, S., 1982, Diffuse idiopathic skeletal hyperostosis and new bone formation in male gouty subjects. A radiologic study, *Rheum. Int.* **2**:83–86.

Lockard, O., Jr., Harmon, C., Nolph, K., and Irvin, W., 1976, Allergic reaction to allopurinol with cross-reactivity to oxypurinol, *Ann. Intern. Med.* **85**:333–335.

Loeb, J. N., 1972, The influence of temperature on the solubility of uric acid and monosodium urate, *Arthritis Rheum.* **15**:189–192.

Loebl, W. Y., and Scott, J. T., 1974, Withdrawal of allopurinol in patients with gout, *Ann. Rheum. Dis.* **33**:304–307.

Ludwig, A. P., Bennett, G. A., and Bauer, W., 1938, A rare manifestation of gout: Widespread ankylosis simulating rheumatoid arthritis, *Ann. Intern. Med.* **11**:1248–1276.

Lupton, G. P., and Odon, R. B., 1979, The allopurinol hypersensitivity syndrome, *J. Am. Acad. Dermatol.* **1**:365–379.

MacLachlan, M. J., and Rodnan, G. P., 1967, Effects of food, fast and alcohol on serum uric acid and acute attacks of gout, *Am. J. Med.* **42**:38–57.

Malawista, S. E., Seegmiller, J. E., Hathaway, E., and Sokoloff, L., 1965, Sacroiliac gout, *JAMA* **194**:954–956.

Mandel, N. S., 1976, The structural basis of crystal-induced membranolysis, *Arthritis Rheum.* **19**:439–445.

Martel, W., 1968, The overhanging margin of bone: A roentgenologic manifestation of gout, *Radiology* **91**:755–756.

Mayne, J. G., 1956, Pathological study of the renal lesions found in 27 patients with gout, *Ann. Rheum. Dis.* **15**:61–62.

McCallum, D. E., Mathews, R. S., and O'Neil, M. T., 1970, Aseptic necrosis of the femoral head: Associated diseases and evaluation of treatment, *South Med. J.* **63**:241–253.

McCarty, D. J., 1962, Phagocytosis of urate crystals in gouty synovial fluid, *Am J. Med. Sci.* **243**:288–295.

McCarty, D. J., 1963, Crystal-induced inflammation; syndromes of gout and pseudogout, *Geriatrics* **18**:467–478.

McCarty, D. J., 1965, The inflammatory reaction to microcrystalline sodium urate, *Arthritis Rheum.* **8**:726–735.

McCarty, D. J., 1970, A historical note: Leeuwenhoek's description of crystals from a gouty tophus, *Arthritis Rheum.* **13**:414–418.

McCarty, D. J., and Halverson, P. B., 1984, Arthritis associated with apatite and other calcium phosphate crystals, in: *Arthritis and Allied Conditions*, ed. 10, (D. J. McCarty, ed.), Lea & Febiger, Philadelphia pp. 1547–1564.

McCarty, D. J., and Hollander, J. L., 1961, Identification of urate crystals in gouty synovial fluid, *Ann. Intern. Med.* **54**:452–460.

McCarty, D. J., Gatter, R. A., Brill, J. M., and Hogan, J. M., 1965, Crystal deposition diseases. Sodium urate (gout) and calcium pyrophosphate (chondrocalcinosis, pseudogout), *JAMA* **193**:129–132.

McMillan, R. M., Hasselbacher, P., Hahn, J. L., Harris, E. D., 1981, Interactions of murine macrophages with monosodium urate crystals: Stimulation of lysosomal enzyme release and prostaglandin synthesis, *J. Rheumatol.* **8**:555–562.

Meisel, A. D., and Diamond, H. S., 1977, Inhibition of probenecid uricosuria by pyrazinamide and para-aminohippurate, *Am. J. Physiol.* **232**:222–226.

Messerli, F. H., Frohlich, E. D., Dreslinski, G. R., Suarez, D. H., and Aristimuno, G., 1980, Serum uric acid and essential hypertension: An indicator of renal vascular involvement, *Ann. Intern. Med.* **93**:817–821.

Meyer, W. J., III, Gill, J. R., Jr., and Bartter, F. C., 1975, Gout as a complication of Barrter's syndrome: A possible role for alkalosis in the decreased clearance of uric acid, *Ann. Intern. Med.* **83**:56–59.

Meyers, A. R., Epstein, F., H. Dodge, H. J., and Mikkelsen, W. M., 1968, The relationship of serum uric acid to risk factors in coronary heart disease, *Am. J. Med.* **45**:520–528.

Mikkelsen, W. M., Dodge, H. J., and Valkenburg, H., 1965, The distribution of serum uric acid values in a population unselected as to gout or hyperuricemia—Tecumseh, Michigan 1959–1960, *Am. J. Med.* **39**:242–251.

Moskowitz, R. W., Vertes, V., Schwartz, A., Marshall, G., 1969, Crystal-induced inflammation associated with chronic renal failure treated with periodic hemodialysis, *Am. J. Med.* **47**:450–460.

Nakayama, D. A., Barthelemy, C., Carrera, G., Lightfoot, R. W., Wortmann, R., 1984, Tophaceous gout: A clinical assessment, *Arthritis Rheum.* **27**:468–471.

Neel, J. V., 1947, The clinical detection of the genetic carriers of inherited disease, *Medicine* **26**:115–153.

O'Brien, W. M., Burch, T. A., and Bunim, J. J., 1966, Genetics of hyperuricemia in Blackfeet and Pima Indians, *Ann. Rheum. Dis.* **25**:117–119.

O'Duffy, J. D., Hunder, G. G., and Kelly, P. J., 1975, Decreasing prevalence of tophaceous gout, *Mayo Clin. Proc.* **50**:227–228.

Pak, C. Y. C., Peters, P., Hurt G., Kodesky, M., Fine, M., Reisman, D., Splann, F., Caramela, C., Freeman, A., Britton, F., Sakhau, K., Breslau, N. A., 1981, Is selective therapy of recurrent nephrolithiasis possible? *Am. J. Med.* **71**:615–622.

Paulus, H. E., 1970, Clinical significance of hyperuricemia in routinely screened hospitalized men, *JAMA* **211**:277–281.

Persellin, R. H., and Schmid, F. R., 1961, The use of sulfinpyrazone in the treatment of gout reduces serum uric acid levels and diminishes severity of arthritis attacks with freedom from significant toxicity, *JAMA* **175**:971–975.

Phelps, P., 1970, Polymorphonuclear leukocyte motility *in vitro*. IV. Colchicine inhibition of chemotactic activity formation after phagocytosis of urate crystals. *Arthritis Rheum.* **131**:1–9.

Plante, G. E., Durivage, J., and Lemieux, G., 1968, Renal excretion of hydrogen in primary gout, *Metabolism* **17**:377–385.

Pollycove, M., Tolbert, B. M., Lawrence, J. H., and Harman, D., 1957, Uric acid metabolism: The oxidation of uric acid in normal subjects and patients with gout, polycythemia and leukemia, *Clin. Res.* **5**:38.

Postlethwaite, A. E., Bartel, A. G., and Kelley, W. N., 1972, Hyperuricemia due to ethambutol, *N. Engl. J. Med.* **286**:761–763.

Praetorius, E., and Kirk, J. E., 1950, Hypouricemia with evidence for tubular elimination of uric acid, *J. Lab. Clin. Med.* **35**:865–868.

Prien, E. L., and Prien, E. L., 1968, Composition and structure of urinary stone, *Am. J. Med.* **45**:654–672.

Rae, S. E., Davidson, E. M., and Smith, M. J. H., 1982, Leukotriene B_4 an inflammatory mediator in gout. *Lancet* **2**:1122–1138.

Rapado, A., 1974, Relationship between gout and arterial hypertension, *Adv. Exp. Med. Biol.* **41B**:451–459.

Ravio, K. O., Becker, M. A., Meyer, L. J., Greene, M. L., Wuki, G., Seegmiller, J. E., 1975, Stimulation of human purine synthesis *de novo* by fructose infusion. *Metabolism* **24**:861–869.

Reynolds, E. S., Schlant, R. C., Goneck, H. C., and Dammin, G. J., 1957, Fatal massive necrosis of the liver as a manifestation of hypersensitivity to probenecid, *N. Eng. J. Med.* **256**:592–596.

Reynolds, P. P., Knapp, M. J., Baraf, H. S. B., and Holmes, E. W., 1983, Moonshine and lead: Relationship to the pathogenesis of hyperuricemia in gout, *Arthritis Rheum.* **26**:59–67.

Rieselback, R. E., 1964, Uric acid excretion and renal function in the acute hyperuricemia of leukemia, *Am. J. Med.* **37**:872–904.

Robinson, D. R., Tashjian, A. H., and Levin, L., 1975, Prostaglandin induced bone resorption by rheumatoid synovia, *Clin. Res.* **23**:443A.

Rodnan, G. P., 1961, A gallery of gout: Being a miscellany of prints and caricatures from the 16th century to the present day, *Arthritis Rheum.* **4**:27–46.
Rodnan, G. P., 1980, The pathogenesis of aldermanic gout: Procatarctic role of fluctuation in serum urate concentrations in gouty arthritis provoked by feast and alcohol, *Clin. Res.* **28**:359A.
Rondier, J., Truffert, J., le Go, A., Cayla, J., 1977, Gout and hyperlipidemia effect of overweight on the levels of circulating lipids, *Ann. Clin. Res.* **9**:239.
Rosenfeld, J. B., 1974, Effect of long-term allopurinol administration of GFR in normotensive and hypertensive subjects, *Adv. Exp. Biol. Med.* **41B**:581–596.
Rouault, T., Caldwell, D. S., and Holmes, E. W. 1982, Aspiration of the asymptomatic metatarsophalangeal joint in gout patients and hyperuricemia controls, *Arthritis Rheum.* **25**:209–212.
Rundles, R. W., 1966, Metabolic effects of allopurinol and alloxanthine, *Ann. Rheum. Dis.* **25**:615–620.
Rundles, R. W., Elion, G. B., and Hitchings, G. H., 1966A, Allopurinol in the treatment of gout and secondary hyperuricemia, *Bull. Rheum. Dis.* **16**:400–403.
Rundles, R. W., Metz, E. N., and Silberman, H. R., 1966b, Allopurinol in the treatment of gout, *Ann. Intern. Med.* **64**:229–258.
Ryan, L. M., and McCarty, D. J, 1984, Calcium pyrophosphate crystal deposition disease, in: *Arthritis and Allied Conditions,* ed. 10 (D. J. McCarty, ed.), Lea & Febiger, Philadelphia pp. 1515–1546.
Saker, B. M., Tofler, O. B., Burvill, M. J., and Reilly, K. A., 1967, Alcohol consumption and gout, *Med. J. Aust.* **1**:1213–1216.
Salzman, R. T., Howell, D. S., and Ricca, L. R., 1965, Aberrancy in clinical hallmarks of gouty arthritis: Brief clinical report, *Arthritis Rheum.* **8**:998–1001.
Sarre, H., 1964, *Congres International de al Goutte et de la Lithiase Urique,* Evian, France.
Scheele, K. W., 1776, Examen chemicum calculi urinarii, *Opuscula* **2**:73.
Schumacher, H. R., and Phelps, P. 1971, Sequential changes in human polymorphonuclear leukocytes after urate crystal phagocytosis. *Arthritis Rheum.* **14**:513–526.
Scott, J. T., 1977, Obesity and hyperuricaemia, *Clin, Rheum. Dis.* **3**:25–35.
Scott, J. T., Dixon, A., and Bywaters, E. G. L., 1964, Association of hyperuricemia and gout with hyperparathyroidism, *Br. Med. J.* **1**:1070–1073.
Scott, J. T., Holloway, V. P., Glass, H. H., and Arnot, R. N., 1969, Studies of uric acid pool size and turnover rate, *Ann. Rheum. Dis.* **28**:366–373.
Seegmiller, J. E., and Frazier, P. D., 1966, Biochemical considerations of the renal damage of gout, *Ann. Rheum. Dis* **25**:668–672.
Seegmiller, J. F., Grayzel, A. I., Laster, L., and Little, L., 1961, Uric acid production in gout, *J. Clin. Invest.* **40**:1304–1314.
Serhan, C. N., Lundberg, U., Weissmann, G., Samuelsson, B., 1983, Formation of leukotrienes and hydroxy acids by human neutrophils and platelets exposed to monosodium urate, *Clin. Res.* **31**:521A.
Shapiro, J. R., Klinenberg, J. R., Peck, W., Goldfinger, S. E., and Seegmiller, J. E., 1963, Hyperuricemia associated with obesity and intensified by caloric restriction, *Arthritis Rheum.* **7**:343 (abstract).
Sheikh, M. I., and Moller, J. R., 1968, Binding of urate to proteins of human and rabbit plasma, *Biochim. Biophys Acta* **158**:456–458.
Simchowitz, L., Atkinson, J. P., and Spilberg, I., 1982, Stimulation of the respiratory burst in human neutrophils by crystal phagocytosis. *Arthritis Rheum.* **25**:181–188.
Simkin, P. A., 1977, Urate excretion in normal and gouty men, *Adv. Exp. Med. Biol.* **76B**:41–45.
Simon, N. M., Smucker, J. E., O'Connor, J., and Del Greco, F., 1969, Differential uric acid excretion in essential and renal hypertension, *Circulation* **39**:121–125.
Sinclair, D. S., and Fox, I. H., 1975, The pharmacology of hypouricemic effect of benzbromarone, *J. Rheumatol.* **2**:437–445.
Skupp, S., and Ayvazian, J. H., 1969, Oxidation of 7-methylguanine by human xanthine oxidase, *J. Lab. Clin. Med.* **73**:909–916.
Smythe, C. M., and Huffman. E. R., 1955, Gouty arthritis: Diagnosis and treatment, *Rocky Mountain Med. J.* **52**:513–518.
Sirahama, T., and Cohen, A., 1974, Ultrastructural evidence for leakage of lysosomal contents after phagocytosis of monosodium urate crystals. *Am. J. Pathol.* **76**:500–511.
Skupp, S., and Ayvazian, J. H., 1969, Oxidation of 7-methylguanine by human xanthine oxidase. *J. Lab. Clin. Med.* **73**:909–916.

Sorensen, L. B., 1959, Degradation of uric acid in man, *Metabolism* **8**:687–703.

Sorensen, L., and Seegmiller, J. E., 1968, Seminars on the Lesch–Nyham syndrome: Management and treatment, discussion, *Fed. Proc.* **27**:1097–1104.

Sperling, O., Boer, P., Brosch, S., Zoref, E., 1977, Superactivity of phosphoribosylpyrophosphate synthetase, due to feedback resistance causing purine overproduction and gout, *Ciba Found. Symp.* **48**:143–164.

Spilberg, I., 1980, Colchicine and pseudogout, *Arthritis Rheum.* **23**:1062–1063.

Spilberg, I., Gallagher, A., Mehta, J., Mandell, B., 1976, Urate crystal-induced chemotactic factor isolation and partial characterization. *J. Clin. Invest.*, **58**:815–819.

Spilberg, I., McLain, D., Simchowitz, L., Bemy S., 1980, Colchicine and pseudogout, *Arthritis Rheum.* **23**:1062–1063.

Steele, T. H., 1969, Evidence for altered renal urate reabsorption during changes in volume of the extracellular fluid, *J. Lab. Clin. Med.* **74**:288–299.

Steele, T. H., and Boner, G., 1973, Origins of the uricosuric response, *J. Clin. Invest.* **52**:1368–1375.

Steele, T. H., and Oppenheimer, S., 1969, Factors affecting urate excretion following diuretic administration in man, *Am. J. Med.* **47**:564–574.

Steele, T. H., and Rieselbach, R. E., 1967, The contribution of residual nephrons within the chronically diseased kidney to urate homeostasis in man, *Am. J. Med.* **43**:876–886.

Stockman, A., Darlington, L. G., and Scott, J. T., 1980, Frequency of chondrocalcinosis in the knees and avascular necrosis of the femoral head in gout: A controlled study, *Ann. Rheum. Dis* **39**:7–11.

Sturge, R. A., Scott, J. T., Kennedy, A. C., Hart, D. P., and W. W. Buchanan, 1977, Serum uric acid in England and Scotland, *Ann. Rheum. Dis* **36**:420–427.

Suki, W. N., Hull, A. R., Rector, F. C., Seldin, D. W., 1967, Mechanism of the effect of thiazide diuretics on calcium and uric acid., *J. Clin. Invest.* **46**:1121 (abstract).

Tak, H. K., Wilcox, W. R., and Cooper, S. M., 1981, The effect of lead upon urate nucleation, *Arthritis Rheum.* **24**:1291–1295.

Talbott, J. H., 1957, *Gout*, Grune & Stratton, New York.

Talbott, J. H., 1959, Gout and blood dyscrasias, *Medicine* **38**:173–205.

Talbott, J. H., 1964, *Gout* 2 ed., Grune & Stratton, New York.

Talbott, J. H., 1981, Solid and liquid nourishment in gout. Selected historical excerpts, largely empiric or fashionable and current scientific concepts in the management of gout and gouty arthritis, *Semin. Arthritis Rheum.* **11**:288–306.

Talbott, J. H., and Lilienfeld, A., 1959, Longevity in gout, *Geriatrics* **14**:409–420.

Talbott, J. H., and Terplan, K. L., 1960, The kidney in gout, *Medicine* **39**:405–468.

Terkeltaub, F., Ginsberg, M. H., 1984, Lipoproteins containing apoprotein B are a major regulator of neutrophil responses to monosodium urate crystals. *J. Clin. Invest.* **73**:1719–1730.

Terkeltaub, F., Ginsberg, M. H., Kozin F., 1983, Plasma protein binding by monosodium urate crystals: Analysis by two-dimensional gel electrophoresis. *Arthritis Rheum* **26**:775–783.

Thompson, G. R., 1968, Calcific tendonitis and soft tissue calcification resembling gout, *JAMA* **203**:464–472.

Tjandramaga, T. B., 1972, Observations on the disposition of probenecid on patients receiving allopurinol, *Pharmacology* **8**:259–272.

Turner, R. E., Frank, M. J., Van Audal, D., and Bollet, A. J., 1960, Some aspects of the epidemiology of gout, sex and race incidence, *Arch. Intern. Med.* **106**:400–406.

Wallace, S. L., 1973, Colchicine: The panacea, *Bull. N.Y. Acad. Med.* **49**:130–135.

Wallace, S. L., Berstein, D., and Diamond, H. 1967, Diagnostic value of colchicine therapeutic trial, *JAMA* **199**:525–528.

Wallace, S. L., Robinson, H., Masi, A. T., and Decker, J. L., 1977, Preliminary criteria for the classification of the acute arthritis of primary gout, *Arthritis Rheum.* **20**:895–900.

Warren, D. J., Leitch, A. G., and Leggett, R. J. E., 1975, Hyperuricemic acute renal failure after epileptic seizures, *Lancet* **2**:385–387.

Weiner, I. M., and Mudge, G. H., 1964, Renal tubular mechanisms for excretion of organic acids and bases, *Am. J. Med.* **36**:743–762.

Weiner, I. M., and Tinker, J. P., 1972, Pharmacology of pyrazinamide: Metabolic and renal function studies related to the mechanism of drug-induced urate retention, *J. Pharmacol. Exp. Ther.* **180**:411–434.

Wilson, J. M., and Kelley, W. N., 1983a, Molecular basis of hypoxanthine-guanine phosphoribosyltransferase deficiency in a patient with the Lesch–Nyhan syndrome, *J. Clin. Invest.* **71**:1331–1335.

Wilson, J. M., and Kelley, W. N., 1983b, Molecular characterization of hypoxanthine–guanine phosphoribosyltransferase deficiency in man, *Clin. Res.* **31**:479A.
Wood, A. W., and Seegmiller, J. E., 1973, Properties of 5-phosphoribosyl-1-pyrophosphate amidotransferase from human lymphoblasts, *J. Biol. Chem.* **248**:138–143.
Wood, M. H., Fox, R. M., Vincent, L., Reye, C., 1972, The Lesch–Nyhan syndrome: Report of three cases, *Aust. N. Z. J. Med.* **1**:57–64.
Woolliscroft, J. O., Colfer, H., and Fox, I. H., 1982, Hyperuricemia in acute illness: A poor prognostic sign, *Am. J. Med.* **72**:58–62.
Wyngaarden, J. B., 1957a, Metabolic and clinical aspects of gout, *Am. J. Med.* **22**:819–814.
Wyngaarden, J. B., 1957b, Overproduction of uric acid as the cause of hyperuricemia in primary gout, *J. Clin. Invest.* **36**:1508–1515.
Wyngaarden, J. B., 1958, The role of the kidney in the pathogenesis and treatment of gout, *Arthritis Rheum.* **1**:191–203.
Wyngaarden, J. B., 1960, Gout, in: *Metabolic Basics of Inherited Disease* (J. B. Stanbury, D. S. Fredrickson, and J. B. Wyngaarden, eds.), McGraw-Hill, New York, pp. 679–760.
Wyngaarden, J. B., 1965, Gout, *Adv. Metab. Dis.* **2**:1–78.
Wyngaarden, J. B., and Stetten, D., Jr., 1953, Uricolysis in normal man, *J. Biol. Chem.* **203**:9–21.
Wyngaarden, J. B., Seegmiller, J. E., Laster, L., and Blair, A. E., 1959, Utilization of hypoxanthine adenine and 4-amino-T-imidazolecarboxamide for uric acid synthesis in man, *Metabolism* **8**:455–464.
Wyngaarden, J. B., Rundles, R. W., and Metz, E. N., 1965, Allopurinol in the treatment of gout, *Ann. Intern. Med.* **62**:842–847.
Young, J. L., Boswell, R. B., and Nies, A. S., 1974, Severe allopurinol hypersensitivity. Association with thiazides and prior renal compromise, *Arch. Intern. Med.* **134**:553–558.
Yu, T.-F., 1965a, Secondary gout associated with myeloproliferative diseases, *Arthritis Rheum.* **8**:765–771.
Yu, T.-F., 1965b, The effect of allopurinol in primary and secondary gout, *Arthritis Rheum.* **8**:905–906.
Yu, T.-F., 1974, Milestones in the treatment of gout, *Am. J. Med.* **56**:676–685.
Yu, T.-F., 1982, The efficacy of colchicine prophylaxis in articular gout—a reappraisal after 20 years, *Semin. Arthritis Rheum.* **12**:256–264.
Yu, T.-F., and Berger, L., 1982, Impaired renal function in gout. Its association with hypertensive vascular disease and intrinsic renal disease, *Am. J. Med.* **72**:95–100.
Yu, T.-F., and Gutman, A. B., 1959, Study of the paradoxical effects of salicylate in low, intermediate and high dosage on the renal mechanisms for excretion of urate in man, *J. Clin. Invest.* **38**:1298–1315.
Yu, T.-F., and Gutman, A. B., 1964, Effect of allopurinol [4-hydroxypyrazolo(3,4-*d*)pyrimidine] on serum and urinary uric acid in primary and secondary gout, *Am. J. Med.* **37**:885–898.
Yu, T.-F., Gutman, A. B., 1967, Uric acid nephrolithiasis in gout: Predisposing factors, *Ann. Intern. Med.* **67**:1133–1148.
Yu, T.-F., Berger, L., Dorph, D. J., and Smith, H., 1979, Renal function in gout. V. Factors influencing the renal hemodynamics, *Am. J. Med.* **67**:766–771.
Zimmer, J. G., and Demis, D. J., 1966, Associations between gout, psoriasis and sarcoidosis: With consideration of their pathologic significance, *Ann. Intern. Med.* **64**:786–796.
Zollner, N., and Griebsch, A., 1974, Diet and gout, in: *Purine Metabolism in Man* (O. Sperling, A. DeVries, and J. B. Wyngaarden, eds.), Plenum Press, New York, pp. 435–442.
Zollner, N., Griebsch, A., and Fink, J. K., 1970, Uber die Wirkung von Benzbromarone auf den Serumharnsaurespiegel und die Harnsaureausscheidung des Gichtkranken, *Deut. Med. Wochenschr.* **95**:2405–2411.

17

Vasculitis

Paul Katz and Anthony S. Fauci

I. INTRODUCTION

Vasculitis refers to the inflammation of and resultant damage to blood vessels, leading to ischemia of distal tissues (Fauci *et al.*, 1978a; Cupps and Fauci, 1981). It is this ischemia with changes in distal tissues that accounts for the manifestions of particular vasculitic syndromes. Vasculitis may be a secondary manifestation of an underlying disease such as rheumatoid arthritis or systemic lupus erythematosus, or it may be the primary or sole clinicopathological expression of a disease such as Wegener's granulomatosis. Additionally, in the former case, therapy of the primary condition may be all that is necessary for control of vascular inflammation, whereas in the latter group, treatment must be directed at the vasculitic process itself.

For years, this heterogeneous group of syndromes has been a problem for clinicians; in part these difficulties have arisen from the confusion in the classification of vasculitic disorders. This point is of more than theoretical importance since the therapy and prognosis of each of these entities are variable and are largely determined by the nature of the process. Thus, it is incumbent on the physician caring for such patients to establish the correct diagnosis as rapidly as possible in order that appropriate treatment may be instituted.

In this chapter, we describe the vasculitic syndromes with regard to pathogenesis, clinical and laboratory manifestations, histology, treatment, and prognosis.

Paul Katz • Department of Medicine, Georgetown University School of Medicine, Washington, D.C. 20007. *Anthony S. Fauci* • Laboratory of Immunoregulation, National Institute of Allergy and Infectious Diseases, National Institutes of Health, Bethesda, Maryland 20205.

II. PATHOGENESIS

The majority of the vasculitic syndromes appear to develop from similar immunopathogenic mechanisms based on an immune complex model (Cochrane and Dixon, 1976). This is similar to the reactions first noted in the Arthus reaction and in experimental serum sickness. With these models, it is possible to develop a scheme applicable to many of these diseases in man. Antigen–antibody complexes formed in a state of relative antigen excess are deposited within blood vessel walls; this process is aided by vasoactive substances liberated from platelets and basophils (Cochrane and Koffler, 1973). Of note, the secondary vasculitis of animal serum sickness can be prevented by pretreatment with antihistamines and antiserotonin agents prior to antigen injection. Immune complex deposition is also increased by blood flow turbulence and hydrostastic forces; additionally, certain characteristics of the complex components may favor or impair localization in vessels.

Blood vessel deposition of immune reactants is followed by activation of the complement cascade via the classical pathway, leading to the generation of chemotactic components, particularly C5a (Fauci *et al.*, 1978a). These factors induce the migration of polymorphonuclear neutrophils from the circulation to the vessel wall. These cells then interact with the antigen–antibody complex by phagocytosis and/or by binding of surface Fc receptors to the antibody component. Lysosomal enzymes, including elastase and collagenase, are liberated and damage the vascular endothelium, eventually inducing hemorrhage, thrombosis, and necrosis, which produce the vasculitic syndrome.

Although immune reactants can often be found in tissue or in the circulation of vasculitis patients as antigen–antibody complexes, a failure to detect these does not preclude an immune complex etiology. One of several mechanisms could account for this, including: (1) Rapid clearance of complexes from the circulation by the reticuloendothelial system; (2) Removal of immune reactants from tissue sites 24 to 48 hr after deposition (Cochrane *et al.*, 1959); and (3) Lack of sensitivity of immunologic techniques to identify components of the complex. It should be noted that the antigen component of the immune complex is only rarely identifiable, an example being the hepatitis B antigen in some cases of polyarteritis nodosa (Sergent *et al.*, 1976). It should also be pointed out, however, that although circulating and even deposited immune complexes have been demonstrated in many of the vasculitic syndromes, the causal relationship of these complexes to the pathophysiological events in most of the vasculitides still remains speculative.

In addition to this model of vasculitis, it is probable that cell-mediated immune reactions also participate in the pathogenesis of certain forms of vasculitis, most notably those in which coexistent granulomatous inflammation is observed (e.g., Wegener's granulomatosis). Under these circumstances, the responsible antigen induces the release of soluble substances (lymphokines) from antigen-sensitized lymphocytes. Mediators such as macrophage migration inhibitory factor attract and activate monocytes, which may in turn release lysosomal enzymes. Alternatively, these cells can evolve into epithelioid cells and eventually into multinucleated giant cells, which comprise part of granulomata (Epstein, 1967). Furthermore, immune complexes themselves can experimentally initiate granuloma formation by direct means (Spector and Heesom, 1969). Therefore, these models demonstrate how similar mechanisms could produce "pure" vasculitis or vasculitis with associated granulomatous inflammation.

III. CLASSIFICATION OF VASCULITIC SYNDROMES

As noted above, much of the difficulty in the approach to the patient with vasculitis has resulted from disagreements in the classification of these syndromes. Many such schemes have been too inclusive, with dissimilar diseases included within the same grouping. Conversely, some classifications have subdivided syndromes into smaller subsets that were probably not legitimately distinct. In this chapter, we utilize a previously reported categorization based on the clinical, histological, and therapeutic features of each syndrome (Fauci *et al.*, 1978a: Cupps and Fauci, 1981). This classification emphasizes differences between syndromes that are largely systemic and those in which cutaneous involvement is dominant. In the former group are those disorders in which irreversible and often life-threatening end-organ dysfunction will develop if the proper therapeutic approach is not instituted; the latter group is comprised of diseases that infrequently result in significant organ dysfunction. In addition, a variety of distinct vasculitic syndromes are recognized by virtue of their characteristic clinicopathological features. The classification scheme that we employ is shown in Table 1.

Table 1. The Clinical Spectrum of Vasculitis[a]

Systemic necrotizing vasculitis (polyarteritis nodosa group)
Classic polyarteritis nodosa
Allergic angiitis and granulomatosis
Polyangiitis "overlap" syndrome
Hypersensitivity vasculitis
Serum sickness and serum-sickness-like reactions
Other drug-related vasculitides
Vasculitis associated with infectious diseases
Henoch–Schönlein purpura
Vasculitis associated with connective tissue diseases
Vasculitis associated with neoplasms (mostly lymphoid)
Vasculitis associated with other underlying diseases
Wegener's granulomatosis
Lymphomatoid granulomatosis
Giant cell arteritides
Cranial or temporal arteritis
Takayasu's arteritis
Other vasculitides
Mucocutaneous lymph node syndrome (Kawasaki's disease)
Vasculitis isolated to the central nervous system
Behcet's disease
Thromboangiitis obliterans (Buerger's disease)
Miscellaneous vasculitides

[a] From Fauci (1982).

A. Systemic Necrotizing Vasculitis Group

The systemic necrotizing vasculitis group is comprised of classic polyarteritis nodosa, allergic angiitis, and granulomatosis (Churg–Strauss syndrome), and the polyangiitis "overlap" syndrome. This broad group has resulted in perhaps the largest amount of confusion surrounding the vasculitides (Fauci *et al.*, 1978a; Cupps and Fauci, 1981). The members of this group are histologically similar in many respects, although, as is detailed below, certain differences exist among them. Left untreated, these diseases are often fatal, which necessitates early and correct diagnosis and prompt therapeutic intervention.

1. Classic Polyarteritis Nodosa

In 1866, Kussmaul and Maier published the case of a young male who had what we would now call classic polyarteritis nodosa (PAN). This disorder is characterized by segmental necrotizing vasculitis of small- and medium-sized muscular arteries, with most lesions developing at vessel bifurcations, with distal arteriolar and adjacent venous involvement (Zeek, 1952, 1953; Rose and Spencer, 1957).

Early in the course of PAN, patients may complain of nonspecific signs and symptoms such as malaise, myalgias, fever, muscle weakness, abdominal pain, and, to a lesser extent, neurological and joint symptoms. The insidious nature and slow progression of the disease, as well as its rarity, may hamper the early diagnosis of PAN.

The major cause of mortality is renal involvement, which is present in approximately 70% of patients. This may be manifested as vessel involvement with secondary glomerular ischemia and/or glomerulonephritis. A major factor contributing to renal dysfunction is hypertension. Although initially felt to be a component of the healing process of renal PAN (Rose and Spencer, 1957), it now appears that this may not always be the case, and hypertension may be present early in the course of the disease prior to renal function impairment. It should be noted that hypertension, apart from the vasculitic process, may be an important contributor to the morbidity and mortality of the disease. Urine analyses may reveal hematuria, cellular casts, and proteinuria.

Primary coronary artery vasculitis may be an important cause of death in PAN (Holsinger *et al.*, 1962). Cardiac disease is clinically apparent in approximately one-third of subjects, whereas autopsy specimens reveal involvement in two-thirds of patients. Clinically, this is manifested as heart failure resulting from coronary arteritis alone or in combination with hypertensive cardiovascular disease. Polyarteritis nodosa may also involve the heart as pericarditis (14% of cases) or as conduction abnormalities secondary to vasculitis of the nutrient arteries supplying this system; additionally, isolated areas of myocardial necrosis without antecedent myocardial infarction may be found (Sheps, 1972).

Up to 75% of patients report gastrointestinal symptoms such as pain, nausea, vomiting, diarrhea, ileus, bleeding, infarction, and perforation of viscera; these are felt to arise from visceral artery vasculitis. Superior mesenteric arteritis may result in abdominal angina and malabsorption with steatorrhea. Other acute presentations may resemble pancreatitis, cholecystitis, or appendicitis. Autopsy series have shown evidence of PAN in the gastrointestinal tract in one-half of cases (Cupps and Fauci, 1981).

As noted above, PAN may be associated with and initiated by the hepatitis B antigen, which can induce liver disease ranging from subclinical involvement with mild increases in transaminase levels to chronic active hepatitis (Sergent *et al.*, 1976). Even in the absence of the hepatitis B antigen, vasculitis of intrahepatic vessels is observed in 50% of cases and may lead to infarction and necrosis (Mowrey and Lundberg, 1967).

Nervous system signs and symptoms are obvious in 80% of patients, with a predilection for the peripheral nervous system (Moore and Fauci, 1981). Peripheral nervous system involvement is seen in 60% of patients as mononeuritis multiplex, extensive mononeuritis, cutaneous neuropathy, or polyneuropathy, which arise secondary to vasa nervorum vasculitis. These manifestations may be relatively recalcitrant to therapy, and affected patients may have residual impairment despite remission in all other systems. Central nervous system abnormalities are present in 40% of subjects as diffuse or focal abnormalities of cortical, brainstem, or cerebellar function. Cranial nerves are usually spared.

Eye involvement occurs secondary to hypertensive changes or retinal vasculitis with cytoid body formation.

By definition, classic PAN spares the pulmonary vasculature; when pulmonary involvement is present, it is usually seen in concert with asthma and eosinophilia and is categorized as allergic angiitis and granulomatosis (Churg–Strauss syndrome, see below) (Churg and Strauss, 1951). Additionally, these two entities may coexist in what we have referred to as the polyangiitis "overlap" syndrome (Fauci *et al.*, 1978a) (see below). However, in the strictest sense, pulmonary vasculitis is not a feature of classic PAN.

Up to 30% of PAN patients develop cutaneous signs of the disease, usually as small muscular arteritis of subcutaneous vessels manifested as tender erythematous nodules or as livedo reticularis (Gilliam and Smiley, 1976). It is unfortunate that the term cutaneous PAN has been used to refer to vasculitis of small subcutaneous arteries in the absence of systemic disease (DeShazo *et al.*, 1977). This entity, unlike its systemic counterpart, usually has a favorable prognosis, although histologically it is similar to classic PAN. We would rather consider this as a form of hypersensitivity vasculitis (see below) or predominantly cutaneous vasculitis than as a component of classic PAN.

Although many patients with PAN will complain of arthralgias, arthritis is unusual. Myalgias may be an initial symptom of the disease secondary to small- and medium-sized muscular arteritis; biopsy of asymptomatic muscles is unlikely to yield abnormal findings. Epididymal and/or testicular pain may also be present early in the course of the illness, and vasculitis of these structures is apparent in 30% of postmortem specimens (Cupps and Fauci, 1981). It should be noted, however, that evidence of vasculitis is only rarely demonstrable with blind biopsy of these organs in the absence of clinical signs or complaints.

The clinical features of classic PAN are outlined in Table 2, and organ system involvement at autopsy is listed in Table 3.

Although there are no laboratory tests that are diagnostic of PAN, there are a number of rather characteristic laboratory abnormalities (Table 4). Not surprisingly, these are indicative of the underlying chronic inflammatory nature of PAN as well as of the end-organ damage resulting from vasculitis. It should be noted that hepatitis B antigenemia is detectable in 30% of classic PAN patients, but this by itself is not diagnostic of this entity (Sergent *et al.*, 1976; Fauci *et al.*, 1979).

The histological diagnosis of PAN rests on the demonstration of necrotizing vasculitis

Table 2. Clinical Profile and Clinical Manifestations in Patients with Classic Polyarteritis Nodosa[a]

Clinical parameter	Value or percent incidence
General considerations	
Age (mean)	45 yr
Sex ratio (male to female)	2.5 to 1
Fever	71
Weight loss	54
Organ system involvement	
Kidney	70
Musculoskeletal system	64
Arthritis/arthralgia	53
Myalgias	31
Hypertension	54
Peripheral neuropathy	51
Gastrointestinal tract	44
Abdominal pain	43
Nausea/vomiting	40
Cholecystitis	17
Bleeding	6
Bowel perforation	5
Bowel infarction	1.4
Skin	43
Rash/purpura	30
Nodules	15
Livedo reticularis	4
Cardiac	36
Congestive heart failure	12
Myocardial infarction	6
Pericarditis	4
Central nervous system	23
Cerebral vascular accident	11
Altered mental status	10
Seizure	4

[a] From Cupps and Fauci (1981), p. 29.

of small- and medium-sized muscular arteries (Fig. 1) in a patient with compatible clinical features of the disease. The decision to biopsy specific sites should be based on clinical and/or laboratory evidence of disease activity and accessibility of involved vessels. As noted above, the diagnosis of PAN is infrequently established by blind biopsy of asymptomatic sites; favored sites have included skin, peripheral nerve, and muscle.

The diagnosis of PAN can also be established angiographically by the demonstration of small "pseudoaneurysms" in renal, hepatic, or visceral vessels (Fig. 2). It should be noted that these findings are not diagnostic of PAN as originally proposed (Bron *et al.*, 1965; Dornfeld *et al.*, 1971); similar abnormalities have been reported in the polyangiitis "overlap" syndrome (Fauci *et al.*, 1978), systemic lupus erythematosus (Longstreth *et al.*, 1974), and fibromuscular dysplasia (Meyers *et al.*, 1974). Nonetheless, these an-

Table 3. Organ System Involvement at Autopsy in Classic Polyarteritis Nodosa[a]

Organ system	Percent
Kidney	85
Heart	76
Liver	62
Gastrointestinal tract	51
Jejunum	37
Ileum	27
Mesentery	24
Colon	20
Duodenum	10
Gallbladder	10
Rectosigmoid	10
Appendix	7
Muscle	39
Pancreas	35
Testes	33
Peripheral nerves	32
Central nervous system	27
Skin	20

[a] From Cupps and Fauci (1981), p. 30.

Table 4. Laboratory Abnormalities in Patients with Classic Polyarteritis Nodosa[a]

Laboratory abnormality	Percent
Erythrocyte sedimentation rate >10 mm/hr	94
Leukocytosis (WBC >10,000 mm^3)	74
Anemia (hematocrit >35%)	66
Thrombocytosis (>400,000/mm^3)	53
Renal function abnormality	70
Proteinuria	64
Hematuria	45
Casts	34
Complement	
Depressed CH50	21
Depressed C3	70
Depressed C4	30
Rheumatoid factor ≧1 : 160	40
Immune complexes present	62.5
Cryoglobulins present	25

[a] From Cupps and Fauci (1981), p. 30.

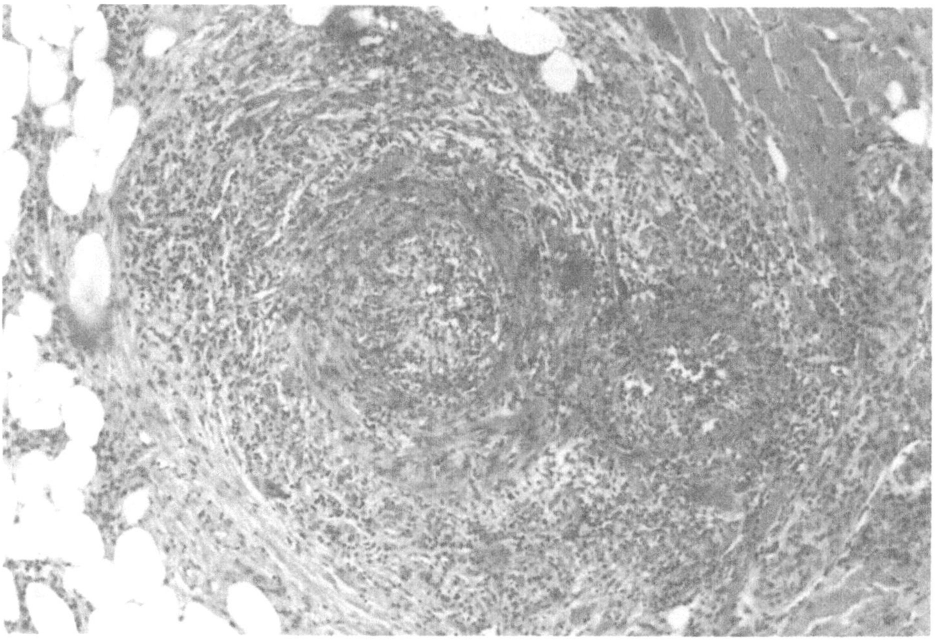

Figure 1. Muscle biopsy of a patient with classic polyarteritis nodosa. Note fibrinoid necrosis of small muscular artery with extensive inflammatory infiltrate and complete obliteration of lumen. Hematoxylin and eosin stain. Magnification $\times 130$.

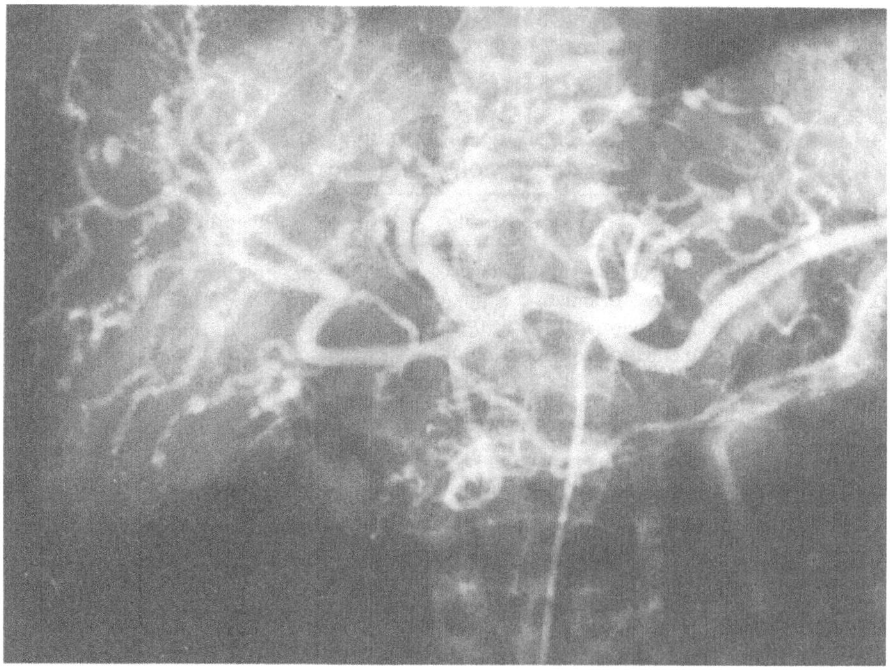

Figure 2. Celiac axis angiogram in a patient with classic polyarteritis nodosa. Multiple small aneurysms are seen throughout the celiac axis vasculature.

giographic findings in a patient with other signs and symptoms of classic PAN would establish this diagnosis.

Without therapy, the prognosis of this syndrome is dismal, with a 13% 5-year survival rate; the advent of corticosteroids improved this, but to a less than acceptable 48% survival at 5 years (Frohnert and Sheps, 1967). It should be noted, however, that these figures were worse for patients with renal disease and/or hypertension. Death in PAN patients usually results from renal failure, cardiovascular events, or gastrointestinal involvement.

The therapy of classic PAN is discussed with that of the other systemic necrotizing vasculitides.

2. *Allergic Angiitis and Granulomatosis (Churg–Strauss Syndrome)*

Allergic angiitis and granulomatosis (AAG) is characterized by granulomatous vasculitis and is similar to classic PAN except that patients with AAG almost invariably have pulmonary vascular involvement (Churg and Strauss, 1951). Furthermore, AAG is characterized by vasculitis of vessels of different sizes and types, granulomatous responses, peripheral blood and tissue eosinophilia, and an association with atopy, usually asthma. This is probably the same disease referred to by Rose and Spencer (1957) as "PAN with pulmonary involvement."

Similar to classic PAN, the early symptoms of AAG are vague; the most specific early signs are those of pulmonary origin such as bronchospasm and fleeting parenchymal infiltrates. Unlike PAN, a higher proportion of patients will have cutaneous disease resulting from small vessel vasculitis. The clinical characteristics of AAG are detailed in Table 5.

Laboratory tests in AAG patients are not diagnostic; most patients will have absolute eosinophilia (>1000 cells/mm^3) and elevated erythrocyte sedimentation rates. Of note, eosinophilia, though not characteristic of PAN, may also be noted in the polyangiitis "overlap" syndrome. Serum immunoglobulin (Ig) E levels may be increased, a not unexpected finding in patients who may have allergic disease.

Eosinophils and granulomata may be observed in and around affected blood vessels of various types in AAG; otherwise, the vascular lesions are similar to those of classic PAN. This histiological picture in combination with appropriate clinical findings is diagnostic of this entity.

Untreated, AAG has a 4% 5-year survival rate, which increases to 60% with corticosteroid treatment (Cupps and Fauci, 1981). The specific protocol for the treatment of AAG is the same as for the other members of this group and is outlined below.

3. *Polyangiitis "Overlap" Syndrome*

It is apparent that a number of patients with systemic necrotizing vasculitis cannot be readily categorized as having classic PAN or AAG; we have referred to this group as the polyangiitis "overlap" syndrome (Fauci *et al.*, 1978a; Cupps and Fauci, 1981). Characteristically, these patients have features of both syndromes; for example, such patients may or may not have atopy, pulmonary involvement, eosinophilia, tissue granulomata, and small vessel vasculitis. Furthermore, patients in this overlap group may have features of PAN and/or AAG together with the small vessel, predominantly cutaneous vasculitis characteristic of "hypersensitivity" vasculitis (see below). This syndrome is truly a sys-

Table 5. Clinical Profile and Manifestations in Allergic Angiitis and Granulomatosis[a]

Category	Value or percent incidence
General considerations	
Age (mean)	44 years
Sex ratio (male to female)	1.3 to 1
Duration (mean) of pulmonary symptoms prior to systemic symptoms	2 years
Fever	Majority of patients
Organ system involvement	
Pulmonary	96
Infiltrate on chest X ray	93
Wheezing	82
Cutaneous	67
Purpura	37
Nodule	35
Peripheral neuropathy	63
Hypertension	54
Gastrointestinal	42
Cardiac	38
Renal	38
Lower urinary tract	10
Arthritis/arthralgia	21

[a] From Cupps and Fauci (1981), p. 45.

temic necrotizing vasculitis with the potential of irreversible end-organ dysfunction and even death. The treatment of the overlap syndrome is identical to that for the other diseases in this group (see below).

4. Treatment of the Systemic Necrotizing Vasculitis Group

As noted, prior to the use of corticosteroids, the prognosis of the systemic necrotizing vasculitides was very poor (Frohnert and Sheps, 1967); even with their use, the 5-year survival is still an unacceptable 50%. It is apparent that some patients will respond to corticosteroids alone, whereas others may have a fulminant downhill course despite the use of these agents; in this latter group are other patients who will respond to combination therapy with corticosteroids plus a cytotoxic drug.

In those individuals without rapidly progressive disease who do not appear at risk of major organ failure, it is prudent to try corticosteroids alone. This is usually instituted as prednisone at a dose of 1 mg/kg per day in divided doses with consolidation over several weeks to a single morning dose (Fauci *et al.*, 1978a). If the patient's course is stable on this schedule for 1 to 2 months, conversion to an alternate-day schedule should be initiated. This regimen should be continued as long as needed with gradual tapering until the drug is no longer necessary or until a dosage level is attained that is required to control signs and symptoms of the disease.

Alternatively, in individuals who do not demonstrate a clinical response to this protocol within 1 month of its inception or in patients with rapidly progressive disease and end-organ functional impairment, cytotoxic drug therapy is warranted. In this regard, we have had excellent results using cyclophosphamide with the protocol originally devised for Wegener's granulomatosis (see below) (Fauci *et al.*, 1978a); this drug is given orally as 2 mg/kg per day in concert with daily prednisone. Prednisone is administered as outlined above until the cyclophosphamide takes effect (generally 2 weeks to 1 month), and the prednisone is then tapered to an alternate-day schedule as quickly as possible; this steroid regimen should be continued for 3 to 6 months until it is discontinued or until a dosage is reached below which symptoms reappear.

Cyclophosphamide dosage is adjusted to maintain the white count at approximately 3000–3500 cells/mm^3 with an absolute neutrophil count of greater than 1000–1500 cells/mm^3 (Fauci *et al.*, 1978a); if these counts are maintained, the risk of infection is minimal. Cyclophosphamide is generally continued for 1 year after complete remission has been achieved by clinical and laboratory criteria; the dose is then tapered in 25-mg decrements every 2 months until the drug has been entirely discontinued.

Other agents such as azathioprine, chlorambucil, and methotrexate have been employed in systemic necrotizing vasculitis, although their efficacy appears to be less than cyclophosphamide. Additionally, results of experimental protocols utilizing single-dose bolus corticosteroids or cyclophosphamide and those employing apheresis have been reported. However, further investigation of these modalities is necessary in order to determine their efficacy.

B. Hypersensitivity Vasculitis

The hypersensitivity vasculitides are a large group of heterogeneous disorders that are characterized by small vessel vasculitis (Winkelmann and Ditto, 1964; Gilliam and Smiley, 1976). The most common histological pattern is that of leukocytoclastic venulitis, and the most common site is the skin, although any organ system may be involved. However, the cutaneous involvement generally dominates the clinical picture. Thus, patients with hypersensitivity vasculitis infrequently have life-threatening disease, although they may have chronic, indolent problems with a cutaneous vasculitis.

The term "hypersensitivity" vasculitis is in many respects an unfortunate one since virtually all of the vasculitides are associated with immunopathogenic mechanisms; however, this term has been employed since this form of vasculitis was initially reported in cases in which a direct antigenic exposure such as a microbe or drug could be implicated (Alarcón-Segovia, 1977). Other terms such as anaphylactoid purpura, microscopic polyarteritis nodosa, leukocytoclastic vasculitis, and allergic vasculitis have been applied to these syndromes, which has undoubtedly contributed to some of the confusion surrounding them.

Although skin manifestations frequently hallmark these entities, systemic signs such as fever, malaise, and myalgia are common. The spectrum of hypersensitivity vasculitis may range from a single, self-limited episode lasting several weeks (e.g., following drug exposure) to a recurrent smoldering course lasting years, particularly when there is no obvious or easily identifiable antigenic stimulus.

Lesions most frequently involve the lower extremities and dependent areas as a result of increased hydrostatic forces in these sites. The most common cutaneous lesion is palpable purpura, although hemorrhage, petechiae, vesicles, urticaria, and nodules may be apparent (Cupps and Fauci, 1981).

Within the hypersensitivity vasculitis group are a number of subgroups that, although clinically distinct, are all characterized by small vessel vasculitis (Table 1). The frequency of extracutaneous vasculitis varies among these subgroups, as is detailed below.

1. Serum Sickness and Serum-Sickness-Like Reactions

These reactions are quite similar to the immune complex vasculitis of animal models (Cochrane and Koffler, 1973; Cochrane and Dixon, 1976). As originally described, serum sickness is uncommon today, since heterologous serum is only rarely employed. The primary agents now responsible are drugs, with the penicillins most frequently implicated (Levine, 1966).

These syndromes represent a prime example of immune-complex-mediated disease; fever, urticaria, lymphadenopathy, and arthralgias are noted 7 to 10 days after antigen exposure. These symptoms are usually antedated by a localized reaction at the injection site 1 to 3 days prior to systemic symptoms. Shorter-duration reactions may be observed 2 to 4 days after antigen challenge when there has been a history of previous antigen exposure. Serum sickness usually resolves spontaneously within 2 weeks of onset; symptoms may be lessened by treatment with antihistamines and/or corticosteroids. Obviously, cessation of exposure to the antigen is integral to resolution.

End-organ involvement other than that noted above is unusual, although proteinuria, carditis, and peripheral neuropathy have been reported (Clark and Kaplan, 1937; De La Pava *et al.*, 1962). These cases have usually occurred in individuals with massive antigen exposure.

2. Henoch–Schönlein Purpura

Henoch–Schönlein purpura (HSP) is an unusual syndrome characterized by nonthrombocytopenic purpura, abdominal symptoms with gastrointestinal bleeding, renal disease, and joint symptoms (Cream *et al.*, 1970), although cutaneous manifestations usually dominate the clinical picture. It is most common in children aged 4 to 7 years, but the disease is well described in adults. Acute episodes of the disease generally last up to 7 days, but several recurrences over months are usual prior to complete remission.

Although the etiology of this syndrome is unknown, most patients have a history of an antecedent upper respiratory tract infection; preceding streptococcal infection is reported in 20% of affected individuals (Cream *et al.*, 1970). Common clinical manifestations include palpable purpura (100% of cases), fever (75%), arthralgias and arthritis (71%), gastrointestinal symptoms (pain, bleeding, intussusception) (68%), and renal involvement (hematuria, proteinuria) (45%) (Cupps and Fauci, 1981).

Of note, elevated serum levels of IgA, IgA-containing immune complexes, and tissue deposits of this Ig are frequently reported in HSP patients (Lowance *et al.*, 1973; Harrington, 1974). Other laboratory tests are generally nonspecific.

Despite its tendency to recur, the prognosis of HSP is excellent, and it usually requires only temporary, supportive care. Very rarely, however, HSP results in end-stage renal failure. Some authors have utilized corticosteroids for recurrences, as these drugs may reduce gastrointestinal and joint symptoms; it is doubtful that such therapy alters the prognosis of patients with abnormal renal function (9% of cases).

3. Vasculitis of Connective Tissue Disease

Although small vessel vasculitis may be seen in a variety of connective tissue diseases, it is most commonly observed in rheumatoid arthritis and systemic lupus erythematosus and is manifested as cutaneous signs and symptoms (Soter, 1976).

Rheumatoid arthritis patients may develop palpable purpura, ulcerations, synovial vasculitis, or rheumatoid nodules as evidence of vasculitis. A less frequent but more dramatic presentation may include a systemic PAN-like vasculitis in patients with more severe disease (Sokoloff and Bunim, 1957). Unfortunately, earlier studies mistakenly concluded that corticosteroid treatment was either responsible for or worsened rheumatoid vasculitis (Kemper *et al.*, 1957; Schmid *et al.*, 1961); it is probable that this association was unwarranted and that these agents may in fact be necessary to treat the vasculitis.

Twenty percent of systemic lupus erythematosus patients develop cutaneous vasculitis during the course of the disease (Estes and Christian, 1971). Although this is usually manifested as palpable purpura, more serious lesions, such as infarction and ulceration, may develop. Small vessel vasculitis may also account for the central nervous system and systemic vasculitides that develop in some lupus patients (Estes and Christian, 1971; Mintz and Fraga, 1965). In addition, a PAN-like illness involving small- and medium-sized muscular arteries of the viscera may be rarely seen in patients with lupus.

In circumstances in which vasculitis develops in the setting of a connective tissue disease, therapy is generally aimed at the primary process; when major organs other than the skin are involved, more aggressive therapy using corticosteroids and/or cytotoxic drugs may be required.

4. Essential Mixed Cryoglobulinemia

Cryoglobulinemia may present in a number of syndromes associated with vasculitis; additionally, it may be present without evidence of an underlying disorder in a syndrome referred to as essential mixed cryoglobulinemia (LoSpalluto *et al.*, 1962; Meltzer and Franklin, 1966). In some instances, the antigen component of the complex may be demonstrable (e.g., hepatitis B antigen), but in most cases this is not possible. Patients with this syndrome usually present with lower extremity purpura in association with constitutional symptoms, arthralgias, and, in some individuals, glomerulonephritis. The serum from these individuals contains a "mixed" cryoglobulin consisting of polyclonal IgG and IgM rheumatoid factor (type II cryoglobulin). Biopsy of skin lesions reveals leukocytoclastic vasculitis with deposits of the cryoglobulin constituents.

The prognosis for affected individuals is good, particularly when cutaneous manifestations predominate. The outcome is less predictable with serious organ involvement such as glomerulonephritis. Therapy in these patients has generally included corticosteroids and cytotoxic drugs, although their efficacy is unproven (Golde and Epstein, 1968). Plasmapheresis may be useful in selected individuals (Capra, 1971).

5. Vasculitis Associated with Malignancy or Other Primary Disorders

Small vessel vasculitis may be associated with certain malignancies, usually of the lymphoreticular system (Sams *et al.*, 1968). This type of vasculitis is most often confined to the skin, although systemic involvement has been reported (Cupps and Fauci, 1982). Of note, the vasculitis may antedate the appearance of the malignancy. Presumably, tumor-related antigens comprise part of the immune complexes responsible for the vasculitis. Therapy should be aimed at treatment of the primary neoplasm.

Hypersensitivity vasculitis may be seen in association with other diseases, including bacterial endocarditis, chronic active hepatitis, ulcerative colitis, retroperitoneal fibrosis, primary biliary cirrhosis, and Goodpasture's syndrome (Gilliam and Smiley, 1976). In general, these are not a major component of the underlying illness; therefore, treatment is directed at the primary disorder.

C. Wegener's Granulomatosis

Wegener's granulomatosis (WG) is hallmarked by the clinical complex of (1) necrotizing granulomatous vasculitis of the upper and lower respiratory tracts; (2) glomerulonephritis; and (3) disseminated small vessel vasculitis (Fauci and Wolff, 1973; Fauci *et al.*, 1983).

The presenting manifestations of this unique syndrome in 85 patients studied at the National Institutes of Health are listed in Table 6 (Fauci *et al.*, 1983). Typically, patients initially develop vague symptoms such as malaise and fatigue with associated upper airway complaints, including rhinorrhea, sinusitis, otitis media, and ulcerations of the nasal mucosa. At this stage, sinus X rays are frequently abnormal, ranging from mucosal thickening to total opacification. The typical saddle-nose deformity may develop following destruction of underlying nasal cartilage. At some time in the course of the disease, most affected individuals develop secondary infection of diseased upper airway structures with *Staphylococcus aureus*. This point is extremely important, since signs and symptoms referable to this area may be misinterpreted as indicative of WG when, in fact, infection may be the etiology.

Without upper respiratory tract signs, pulmonary complaints are rare. When these symptoms do develop, they are usually manifested as cough, hemoptysis, or chest pain. Radiographic studies generally reveal multiple, bilateral nodules, which may cavitate; 20% of patients will have pleural effusions; hilar lymphadenopathy is unusual. Pulmonary function studies may show evidence of airflow obstruction, diminished lung volumes, and decreased diffusing capacity.

Isolated kidney failure is rare in WG; most patients with kidney dysfunction have significant extrarenal disease. Evidence of renal involvement may range from normal renal function with mild urinary sediment abnormalities, as may be seen with mild focal and segmental glomerulonephritis, to progressive renal failure, as might occur with necrotizing glomerulonephritis with proliferative and crescentic changes.

Eye involvement may include changes ranging from mild conjunctivitis to episcleritis and scleritis to scleromalacia performans (Haynes *et al.*, 1977). Secondary proptosis resulting from sinus involvement or retroorbital granulomatous vasculitis may also be noted. Cutaneous lesions are common and generally develop secondary to small vessel

Table 6. Presenting Signs and Symptoms in 85 Patients with Wegener's Granulomatosis[a]

	Patients	
Sign or symptom[b]	*n*	Percent
Pulmonary infiltrates	60	71
Sinusitis	57	67
Joint (arthralgia or arthritis)	37	44
Fever	29	34
Otitis	21	25
Cough	29	34
Rhinitis or nasal symptoms	19	22
Hemoptysis	15	18
Ocular inflammation (conjunctivitis, uveitis, episcleritis, and scleritis)	14	16
Weight loss	14	16
Skin rash	11	13
Epistaxis	9	11
Renal failure	9	11
Chest discomfort	7	8
Anorexia or malaise	7	8
Proptosis	6	7
Shortness of breath or dyspnea	6	7
Oral ulcers	5	6
Hearing loss	5	6
Pleuritis or effusion	5	6
Headache	5	6

[a] From Fauci *et al.* (1983).
[b] Miscellaneous: hoarseness or stridor, saddle-nose deformity, and mastoiditis, three patients each; cranial nerve dysfunction, three; parotid mass or pain, two each; nasolacrimal duct obstruction, thyroiditis, liver function test abnormality, blindness, peripheral neuropathy, ear pinna mass, pedal edema, adenopathy, anosmia, pericarditis, asthma, diabetes insipidus, and Raynaud's phenomenon, one patient each.

vasculitis; these may be manifested as ulcerations, papules, vesicles, or subcutaneous nodules.

The organ system involvement of WG is listed in Table 7; although the airways and kidneys are most frequently involved, multiple other organ systems may also be affected.

Routine laboratory tests are not useful in establishing the diagnosis of WG. Nonetheless, there are certain characteristic laboratory abnormalities that may be helpful. The erythrocyte sedimentation rate is almost always elevated, usually greater than 100 mm/hr. This parameter is perhaps the most useful in determining underlying disease activity even in the absence of clinically apparent disease. Nonspecific findings secondary to the chronic inflammatory nature of the disease include normochromic, normocytic anemia and thrombocytosis. Leukocytosis with a left shift is common. Hyperactivity of the immune system is reflected in the increased levels of IgG and IgA and the presence of rheumatoid factor and circulating immune complexes in some patients. The HLA antigen B8 is found with increased frequency in WG (Katz *et al.*, 1979).

Table 7. Organ System Involvement in Wegener's Granulomatosis[a]

	Patients	
Organ system	*n*	Percent
Lung	80	94
Paranasal sinuses	77	91
Kidney	72	85
Joints	57	67
Nose or nasopharynx	54	64
Ear	52	61
Eye	49	58
Skin	38	45
Nervous system	19	22
Heart	10	12

[a] From Fauci *et al.* (1983).

Histologically, WG is characterized by necrotizing granulomatous vasculitis (Fig. 3). Although the upper airways are easily accessible for biopsy, specimens from these sites may only reveal inflammation and not the characteristic findings of WG. The optimal site for biopsy is the lung, with open procedures preferred to those performed transbronchially, since larger tissue specimens may be obtained by the former means. This procedure also excludes the presence of other diseases included in the differential diagnosis of WG such as pulmonary neoplasms or infectious diseases. The vasculitis usually involves small arteries and veins with granulomata within, adjacent to, or spatially removed from inflamed vessels. Importantly, renal biopsy usually displays a variable pattern from focal and segmental glomerulonephritis to fulminant crescentic glomerulonephritis, with granulomatous vasculitis being relatively uncommon (Horn *et al.*, 1974). Of note, some, but certainly not all, biopsy specimens will have immune complex constituents detectable.

Before cytotoxic drug regimens were initiated, the prognosis for untreated WG was grave, with a particularly malignant course in those patients with renal disease. In these patients, the 1-year mortality was 82%, with a 2-year figure of over 90% (Walton, 1958); corticosteroid therapy alone failed to significantly alter this outcome. It has been clearly demonstrated, however, that chronic low-dose (2 mg/kg per day) cyclosphophamide therapy in concert with alternate-day corticosteroids can induce long-lasting remissions in a high percentage of patients (Fauci and Wolff, 1973; Fauci *et al.*, 1983). In a recently reported series (Fauci *et al.*, 1983), 93% of 85 patients achieved long-term complete remissions, with a substantial number of patients remaining in complete remission following discontinuation of all therapy. The drug is utilized as outlined above for systemic necrotizing vasculitis, and therapy is continued for at least 1 year after induction of remission. The drug is gradually tapered thereafter. In this regard, it is critical to establish the diagnosis of WG early and to initiate therapy as promptly as possible to avoid permanent end-organ dysfunction.

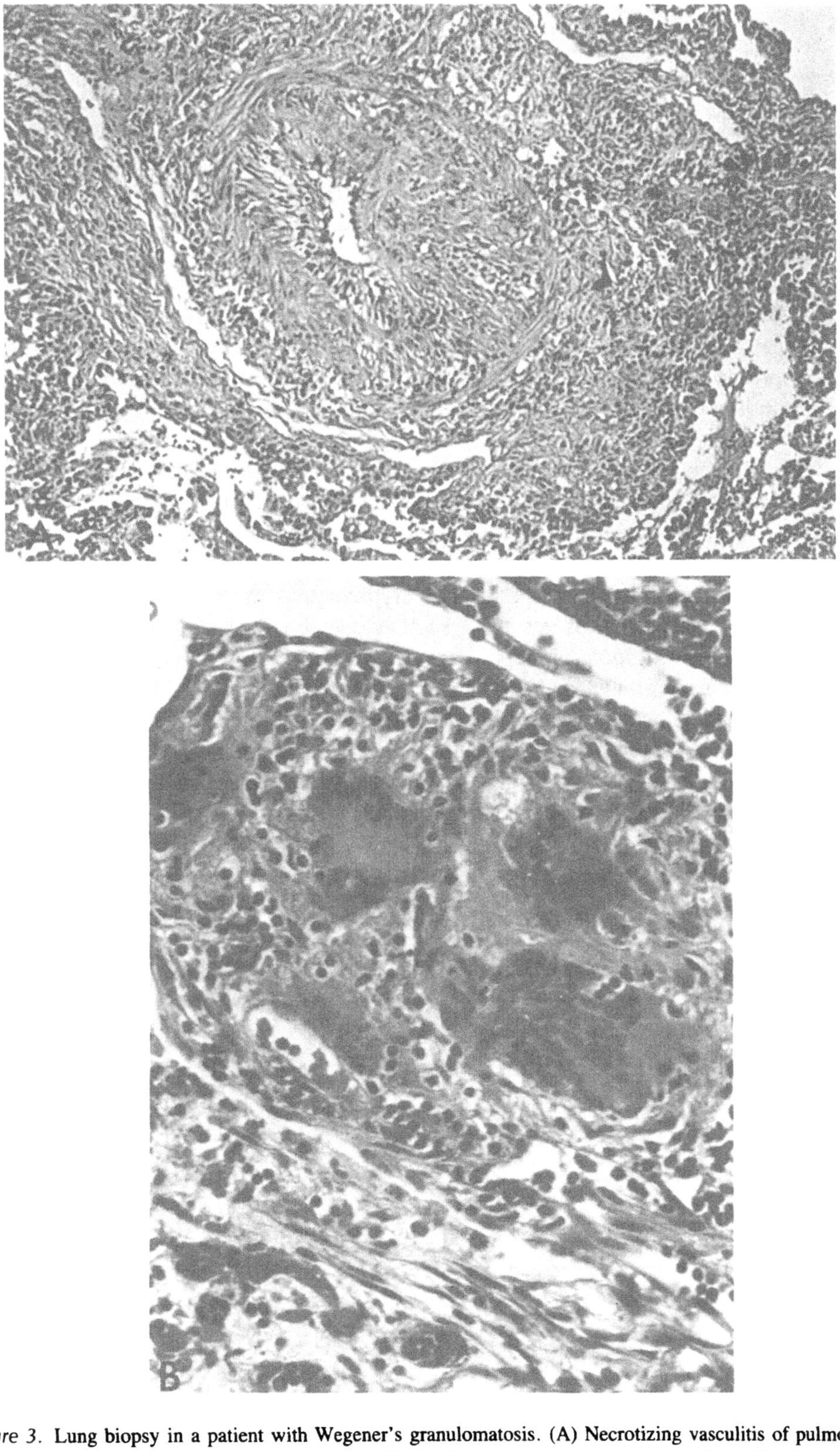

Figure 3. Lung biopsy in a patient with Wegener's granulomatosis. (A) Necrotizing vasculitis of pulmonary artery is seen with extensive mononuclear cell infiltrate. Hematoxylin and eosin stain. Magnification ×150. (B) Several multinucleated giant cells are seen in a section adjacent to the vessel noted in A. Hematoxylin and eosin stain. Magnification ×350.

D. Lymphomatoid Granulomatosis

Lymphomatoid granulomatosis (LG) is an unusual variant of granulomatous vasculitis that is characterized by an angioinvasive infiltration of blood vessels with atypical lymphocytoid and plasmacytoid cells (Liebow *et al.*, 1972). In the truest sense, LG is not really a vasculitis because blood vessels are not inflamed but are invaded by pleomorphic cells; additionally, there has been no evidence to support an immune complex etiology. This disease resembles WG in many respects in that it may involve similar sites, such as lung, skin, and kidneys, which may cause some diagnostic difficulties (Fauci, 1977). Lymphomatoid granulomatosis has characteristics of both a granulomatous vasculitis and a lymphoproliferative disorder with a tendency for lymphomatous transformation. In this regard, one-half of LG patients who fail to respond to a standard treatment protocol (see below) eventually develop non-Hodgkin's lymphoma (Fauci *et al.*, 1982).

Typically, patients develop LG in the fourth or fifth decade and present with ill-defined constitutional symptoms such as malaise, fatigue, fever, and weight loss. Nearly all patients will have signs and symptoms of chest disease such as cough, dyspnea, and chest pain. Roentgenograms usually reveal multiple, bilateral nodular densities. Skin involvement is noted in 40% of patients as erythematous macules or indurated plaques rather than changes typical of vasculitis such as palpable purpura. Renal disease in LG is common, but not as glomerulonephritis; rather, the renal parenchyma is infiltrated with the same atypical mononuclear cells characteristic of this process. Other manifestations may include splenomegaly (18%), hepatomegaly (12%), and lymphadenopathy (8%). The low frequency of these latter findings is somewhat surprising given the tendency for the development of lymphoma. Organ system involvement in LG is outlined in Table 8.

Routine laboratory studies are rarely helpful in LG; 50% of patients will have a leukocytosis, and 20% will be leukopenic. Unlike WG, the erythrocyte sedimentation rate is either normal or minimally elevated. Furthermore, LG patients are frequently

Table 8. Organ or System Involvement in 15 Patients with Lymphomatoid Granulomatosis[a]

Organ or system	No. of patients (%)
Lung	15 (100)
Skin	8 (53)
Kidney	6 (40)
Nodes	6 (40)
Central nervous system	5 (33)
Bone marrow	5 (33)
Liver	4 (27)
Peripheral nervous system	3 (20)
Eyes	3 (20)
Muscle	2 (13)
Paranasal sinuses	1 (7)
Thyroid gland	1 (7)
Epididymis	1 (7)

[a] From Fauci *et al.* (1982).

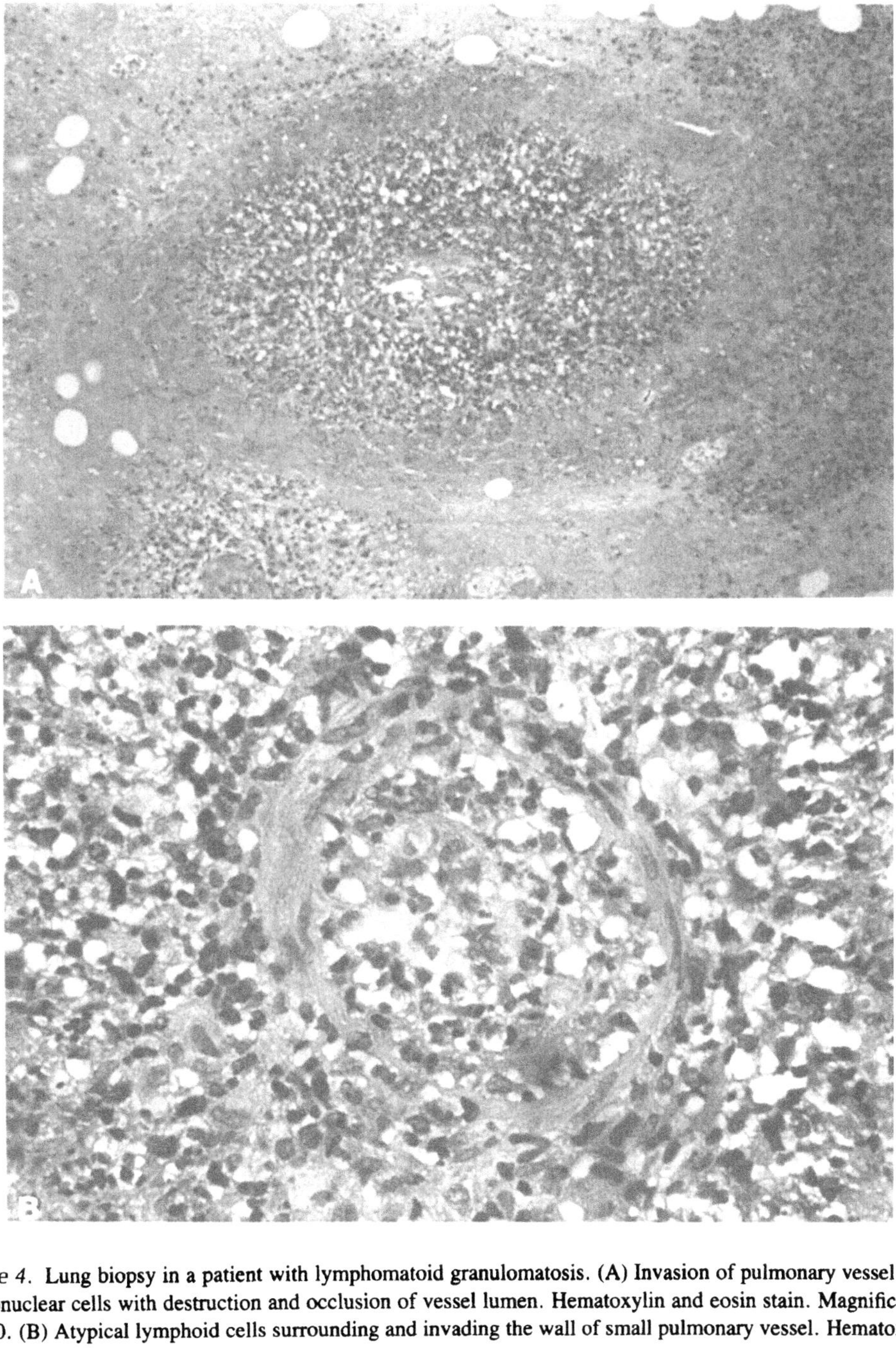

Figure 4. Lung biopsy in a patient with lymphomatoid granulomatosis. (A) Invasion of pulmonary vessel with mononuclear cells with destruction and occlusion of vessel lumen. Hematoxylin and eosin stain. Magnification ×150. (B) Atypical lymphoid cells surrounding and invading the wall of small pulmonary vessel. Hematoxylin and eosin stain. Magnification ×350.

anergic in contradistinction to individuals with WG, who generally maintain cutaneous delayed-type hypersensitivity.

Histologically, LG is characterized by the invasion of arteries and veins with atypical lymphocytes and plasmacytes in which mitotic figures may be apparent (Fig. 4). Unlike WG, the granulomata in LG are less numerous and less distinct. It is extremely important to differentiate pathologically between LG and true lymphoma. This distinction may be aided clinically by the usual lack of bone marrow, splenic, and lymphatic involvement in typical LG.

Left untreated, LG is almost always fatal (Liebow *et al.*, 1972; Katzenstein *et al.*, 1979). Long-lasting remissions were achieved in 50% of LG patients (Fauci *et al.*, 1982) treated with the aforementioned protocol utilized for systemic necrotizing vasculitis; i.e., combined cyclophosphamide and prednisone (Fauci *et al.*, 1978a). The other one-half of LG patients who did not respond to this protocol ultimately developed lymphomas and died. This clearly underscores the necessity for early diagnosis and prompt treatment.

E. Giant-Cell Arteritides

Temporal arteritis (cranial arteritis) and Takayasu's arteritis (pulseless disease) are the two members of the giant-cell arteritis group of vasculitides. These syndromes, although clinically distinct (Table 9), are both characterized by vasculitic involvement of medium- and large-sized arteries with associated granulomatous inflammation and/or giant-cell formation in the vessel walls.

1. Temporal Arteritis

The well-known signs and symptoms of temporal arteritis include fever, elevated erythrocyte sedimentation rate, headache, and anemia, often in concert with polymyalgia rheumatica in individuals over 55 years of age (Hamilton *et al.* 1971; Goodman, 1979). This disease has a predilection for branches of the carotid artery, yet it should be noted that it is in fact a systemic disease that can affect other medium- and large-sized arteries.

This syndrome is common, with 17.4 cases per year 100,000 people over 50 years of age; on occasion, younger individuals, including adolescents, may be affected (Lie *et al.*, 1975). The early signs and symptoms of temporal arteritis include headache (44%), malaise (20%), fatigue (12%), and fever (8%) (Hamilton *et al.*, 1971). Physical examination may reveal tenderness, nodules, and decreased pulses in the temporal arteries in 50% of subjects; however, one-third of patients have no clinical abnormalities of these vessels (Bevan *et al.*, 1968). The dreaded complication of visual impairment is found in 40% of patients, although sudden blindness is distinctly unusual and generally does not occur for 3 to 4 months following disease onset (Goodman, 1979).

One-half of temporal arteritis patients will have the concomitant signs of polymyalgia rheumatica, consisting of morning stiffness, proximal myalgias, and periarticular pain, particularly involving the muscles of the neck, shoulders, lower back, hips, and thighs; likewise, one-half of these individuals will have positive temporal artery biopsies despite a lack of clinical symptoms. The aforementioned nonspecific laboratory findings in the face of a compatible clinical setting should alert the physician to the possibility of temporal

Table 9. Characteristics of the Giant-Cell Arteritides[a]

	Temporal arteritis	Takayasu's arteritis
Patients	Disease of the elderly; women more than men	More prevalent in young women; more common in Orient, but neither racially nor geographically restricted
Blood vessels	Characteristically involves branches of carotid (temporal artery) but is a systemic arteritis and may involve any medium-sized or large artery	Large- and medium-sized arteries with predeliction for aortic arch and its branches; may involve pulmonary artery
Histopathology	Panarteritis; inflammatory mononuclear cell infiltrates; frequent giant-cell formation within vessel wall; fragmentation of internal elastic lamina; proliferation of intima	Panarteritis; inflammatory mononuclear cell infiltrates; intimal proliferation and fibrosis; scarring and vascularization of media; disruption and degeneration of elastic lamina
Manifestations	Classic complex of fever, anemia, high erythrocyte sedimentation rate, muscle aches in an elderly person; headache may be present; strongly associated with polymyalgia rheumatica syndrome	Generalized systemic symptoms; local signs and symptoms related to involved vessels; occlusive phase
Complications	Ocular (sudden blindness)	Related to distribution of involved vessels; death usually occurs from congestive heart failure or cerebrovascular accidents
Diagnosis	Temporal artery biopsy; lesions may be segmental; multiple sections, arteriography, and bilateral biopsy may aid in diagnosis	Arteriography; biopsy of involved vessel
Treatment	Corticosteroids highly effective	Corticosteroids not of proven efficacy; cytotoxic agents currently being tested

[a] From Fauci *et al.* (1978a).

arteritis. Other laboratory abnormalities may include increased acute-phase reactants and serum Ig and elevated liver function tests.

This diagnosis is usually made by the histological demonstration of panarteritis with mononuclear cell infiltration in the temporal artery; associated giant cells and granulomatous inflammation need not necessarily be present. Histochemical studies have found Ig deposition in less than 50% of biopsy specimens, whereas infiltrating T cells appear to be primarily those of the helper/inducer subpopulation (Banks *et al.*, 1983). The focal and segmental nature of the arteritis has led to the suggestion that multiple sections of bilateral temporal artery biopsies should be examined. Angiography of superficial temporal arteries may reveal changes, although these are not specific for temporal arteritis.

Patients are usually quite sensitive to corticosteroid therapy (Hamilton *et al.*, 1971). Treatment is usually initiated with 40 to 60 mg of prednisone daily, which will generally produce clinical improvement in several days. The need for early diagnosis and prompt therapy is underscored by the risk of blindness in untreated patients. Although polymyalgia rheumatica may respond to lower doses (e.g., 15 to 20 mg/day), these levels will not prevent visual abnormalities. Prednisone can be tapered gradually to 7.5 to 10 mg/day with readjustment as dictated by clinical symptoms; therapy for 1 to 2 years has usually been necessary. It is important to note that the erythrocyte sedimentation rate may increase during tapering despite an absence of clinical disease. It is reassuring that tapering can be continued, since recognizable extraocular symptoms usually recur well before visual abnormalities develop. Most patients will eventually be able to discontinue corticosteroids and will remain in remission.

2. Takayasu's Arteritis

Takayasu's arteritis is predominantly a disease afflicting young women and is characterized by vasculitis and stenosis of intermediate- and large-sized arteries. There is a predilection for the aortic arch and its branches (Fraga *et al.*, 1972; Ishikawa, 1978). The disease usually follows a biphasic course with an acute phase manifested by symptoms of systemic inflammatory disease followed by a chronic stage with vascular occlusion and insufficiency. These phases are separated by intervals ranging from several months to several years. Surprisingly, most patients can recall the acute phase, although some may develop ischemic symptoms without antecedent complaints. Physical examination in the late phase may reveal decreased pulses and vascular bruits with symptoms of claudication and Raynaud's phenomenon. Other accompanying findings may include hypertension, syncope, paresthesias, visual changes, cerebral infarction, and cardiac signs such as failure and angina.

The clinical outcome is variable, with remissions and exacerbations common. However, the course of the disease is generally felt to be progressive and ultimately fatal over a period of years. Mortality is commonly a result of congestive heart failure secondary to myocardial infarction in addition to cerebrovascular accidents (Lupi-Herrera *et al.*, 1977).

Arteriography usually establishes the diagnosis with the demonstration of narrowing or occlusion of large arteries; those most frequently involved are the subclavian artery, descending aorta, renal artery, and carotid artery. Biopsy and autopsy specimens reveal panarteritis with mononuclear cell infiltrates.

Although the symptoms of the acute phase can be lessened by corticosteroids, it is uncertain if this alters the eventual outcome. Prospective studies of cytotoxic drug effects on Takayasu's arteritis are in progress.

F. Other Vasculitides

1. Mucocutaneous Lymph Node Syndrome (Kawasaki Disease)

The mucocutaneous lymph node syndrome (MLNS), or Kawasaki disease, is an unusual childhood illness highlighted by prolonged fever, conjunctivitis, oral mucosal and lip involvement, cutaneous changes in distal extremities, truncal exanthem, and cervical lymphadenopathy (Kawasaki *et al.*, 1974). The disease, although initially described in Japan, is now recognized in the United States in children 3 months to 13 years old. The etiology is unknown, and there have been no genetic associations despite the frequency in individuals of Japanese ancestry.

A rare but life-threatening complication is cardiac involvement with cardiomyopathy, mitral or aortic valve insufficiency, and coronary arteritis with aneurysm formation. Late cardiac involvement may result in the 1 to 2% mortality of MLNS. Other signs may include arthralgia, arthritis, abnormal liver function, diarrhea, and aseptic meningitis.

Although usually a self-limited disease, some patients may succumb to the aforementioned cardiac disease. Aspirin at a dose of 30 mg/kg per day in divided doses is the drug of choice and may allay long-term sequelae. Interestingly, preliminary data have suggested that corticosteroids may increase the incidence of cardiac problems; however, this finding has yet to be confirmed.

2. Isolated Central Nervous System Vasculitis

Isolated granulomatous vasculitis of the central nervous system has been reported in the absence of systemic involvement (Cupps *et al.*, 1983). Affected subjects may initially present with headaches, alterations in mental status, and focal neurological abnormalities. Usually, patients lack systemic complaints such as fever.

Cerebrospinal fluid examination may demonstrate increased protein, yet normal fluid does not preclude this diagnosis. Cerebral angiography typically reveals vascular "beading" with narrowing, cut-off, and aneurysms, although this procedure may occasionally be normal. Biopsy may show mononuclear cell infiltration of small arteries and arterioles.

Without therapy, the prognosis is poor. The previously described cyclophosphamide and corticosteroid regimen has improved the long-term outcome in a small number of patients (Cupps *et al.*, 1983).

3. Behcet's Disease

Behcet's disease is an uncommon disorder characterized by oral ulcerations, ocular lesions, genital ulcers, and skin lesions (O'Duffy *et al.*, 1971). Venulitis is most commonly noted histologically, but vessels of any size and type may be involved. The diagnosis is based on the above criteria. Therapy of this entity has been unsatisfactory and has included cytotoxic drugs, colchicine, corticosteroids, and nonsteroidal antiinflammatory agents. However, it has recently been demonstrated that cyclosporin A is effective in the treatment of the ocular involvement of Behcet's disease (Nussenblatt *et al.*, 1983).

4. Thromboangiitis Obliterans (Buerger's Disease)

Thromboangiitis obliterans (Buerger's disease) is an uncommon entity of small- and intermediate-sized arteries and veins of the extremities characterized by inflammation and occlusions. The disease occurs most often in smoking males who frequently present with lower extremity vascular insufficiency or migratory thrombophlebitis. Angiography may display vessel tapering in a segmental fashion. Biopsies of involved vessels reveal acute (neutrophilic invasion and thrombosis), subacute (mononuclear cell infiltration), or chronic (fibrosis and recanalization) changes.

The primary therapy is discontinuation of tobacco with meticulous care of involved tissues. Surgery is not clearly helpful.

Table 10. General Approach to the Patient with Vasculitis

1. Proper categorization of syndrome (specific syndrome; primary versus secondary; localized versus systemic)
2. Determine the extent of disease activity
3. Removal of offending antigen where possible
4. If associated with underlying disease, treat underlying disease where possible
5. Use appropriate therapeutic agents immediately in disease in which efficacy has been clearly demonstrated such as corticosteroids in temporal arteritis and cyclophosphamide plus corticosteroids in Wegener's granulomatosis
6. When feasible, avoid immunosuppressive therapy (corticosteroids or cytotoxic agents) in diseases that do not tend to disseminate, that do not usually result in irreversible organ system dysfunction, and that rarely respond dramatically to such agents
7. Institute a corticosteroid trial immediately in patients with systemic vasculitis; add a cytotoxic agent such as cyclophosphamide if prompt response is not seen or if disease will historically respond only to cytotoxic agents
8. Continually attempt to taper corticosteroids to alternate-day regimen and discontinuation where possible
9. Have a clear-cut understanding of goals and mechanisms of the chronic use of cytotoxic agents in the treatment of nonneoplastic diseases
10. Use other agents where clinical situation dictates (nonsteroidal antiinfflammatory agents, plasmapheresis, etc.) based on results from therapeutic trials

IV. APPROACH TO THE PATIENT WITH SYSTEMIC VASCULITIS

The heterogeneous disorders characterized by vascular inflammation often pose a diagnostic and therapeutic problem for the clinician. In order to effect long-lasting remissions and cures and to avoid significant morbidity, prompt treatment is mandatory. An approach to the patient with systemic vasculitis is presented in Table 10.

REFERENCES

Alarcón-Segovia, D., 1977, The necrotizing vasculitides. A new pathogenetic classification, *Med. Clin. North Am.* **61**:241–260.

Banks, P. M., Cohen, M. D., Ginsburg, W. W., and Hunder, G. G., 1983, Immunohistologic and cytochemical studies of temporal arteritis, *Arthritis Rheum.* **26**:1201–1206.

Bevan, A. T., Dunnill, M. D., and Harrison, M. J. B., 1968, Clinical and biopsy findings in temporal arteritis, *Ann. Rheum. Dis.* **27**:271–278.

Bron, K. M., Stroot, C. A., and Shapiro, A. P., 1965, The diagnostic value of angiographic observations in polyarteritis nodosa, *Arch. Intern. Med.* **116**:450–453.

Capra, J. D., 1971, Clinical and immunologic observations in hypergammaglobulinemic purpura, *Mt. Sinai J. Med.* **38**:375–383.

Churg, J., and Strauss, L., 1951, Allergic granulomatosis, allergic angiitis and periarteritis nodosa, *Am. J. Pathol.* **27**:277–301.

Clark, E., and Kaplan, B. I., 1937, Endocardial, arterial, and other mesenchymal alterations associated with serum sickness in man, *Arch. Pathol.* **24**:458–475.

Cochrane, C. G., and Dixon, F. J., 1976, Antigen–antibody complex induced disease, in: *Textbook of Immunopathology*, 2nd ed., Vol. 1 (P. A. Meischer and H. F. Müller-Eberhard, eds.), Grune & Stratton, New York, pp. 137–154.

Cochrane, C. G., and Koffler, D., 1973, Immune complex disease in experimental animals and man, *Adv. Immunol.* **16:**185–213.

Cochrane, C. G., Weigle, W. O., and Dixon, F. J., 1959, The role of polymorphonuclear leukocytes in the initiation and cessation of the Arthus vasculitis, *J. Exp. Med.* **100:**481.

Cream, J. J., Cumpel, J. M., and Peachy, R. D. G., 1970, Schönlein–Henoch purpura in the adult, *Q. J. Med.* **39:**461–484.

Cupps, T. R., and Fauci, A. S., 1981, *The Vasculitides* 1st ed., W. B. Saunders, Philadelphia.

Cupps, T. R., and Fauci, A. S., 1982, Neoplasm and systemic vasculitis: A case report, *Arthritis Rheum.* **25:**475–477.

Cupps, T. R., Moore, P. M., and Fauci, A. S., 1983, Isolated angiitis of the central nervous system. Prospective diagnostic and therapeutic considerations, *Am. J. Med.* **74:**97–105.

De La Pava, S., Nigogoxyan, G., and Pickren, J. W., 1962, Fatal glomerulonephritis after receiving horse anti-human-cancer serum, *Arch. Intern. Med.* **198:**391–399.

DeShazo, R. D., Levinson, A. I., Lawless, O. F., and Weisbaum, G., 1977, Systemic vasculitis with coexistent large and small vessel involvement. A classification dilemma, *JAMA* **238:**1940–1942.

Dornfeld, L., Lecky, L. W., and Peter, J. B., 1971, Polyarteritis and intrarenal renal artery aneurysms, *JAMA* **215:**1950–1952.

Epstein, W. L., 1967, Granulomatous hypersensitivity, *Prog. Allergy* **11:**36–38.

Estes, D., and Christian, C. L., 1971, The natural history of systemic lupus erythematosus by prospective analysis, *Medicine* **50:**85–95.

Fauci, A. S., 1977, Granulomatous vasculitides: Distinct but related, *Ann. Intern. Med.* **87:**782–783.

Fauci, A. S., 1982, The vasculitic syndromes, in: *Cecil Textbook of Medicine,* 16th ed. (J. B. Wyngaarden and L. H. Smith, Jr., eds.), W. B. Saunders, Philadelphia, pp. 1836–1866.

Fauci, A. S., and Wolff, S. M., 1973, Wegener's granulomatosis: Studies in eighteen patients and a review of the literature, *Medicine* **52:**535–561.

Fauci, A. S., Haynes, B. F., and Katz, P., 1978a, The spectrum of vasculitis: Clinical, pathologic, immunologic, and therapeutic considerations, *Ann. Intern. Med.* **89:**660–676.

Fauci, A. S., Doppman, J. L., and Wolff, S. M., 1978b, Cyclophosphamide-induced remissions in advanced polyarteritis nodosa, *Am. J. Med.* **64:**890–894.

Fauci, A. S., Katz, P., Haynes, B. F., and Wolff, S. M., 1979, Cyclophosphamide therapy of severe systemic necrotizing vasculitis, *N. Engl. J. Med.* **301:**235–238.

Fauci, A. S., Katz, P., Costa, J., Haynes, B. F., and Wolff, S. M., 1982, Lymphomatoid granulomatosis: Prospective clinical and therapeutic experience over 10 years, *N. Engl. J. Med.* **306:**68–74.

Fauci, A. S., Haynes, B. F., Katz, P., and Wolff, S. M., 1983, Wegener's granulomatosis: Prospective clinical and therapeutic experience with 85 patients for 21 years, *Ann. Intern. Med.* **98:**76–85.

Fraga, A., Mintz, G., Valle, L., and Flores-Izquierdo, G., 1972, Takayasu's arteritis: Frequency of systemic manifestations (study of 22 patients) and favorable response to maintenance steroid therapy and adrenocorticosteroids (12 patients), *Arthritis Rheum.* **15:**617–624.

Frohnert, P. P., and Sheps, S. G., 1967, Long-term follow-up study of periarteritis nodosa, *Am. J. Med.* **43:**8–14.

Gilliam, J. N., and Smiley, J. D., 1976, Cutaneous necrotizing vasculitis and related disorders, *Ann. Allergy* **37:**328–339.

Golde, D., and Epstein, W., 1968, Mixed cryoglobulins and glomerulonephritis, *Ann. Intern. Med.* **69:**1221–1227.

Goodman, B. W., 1979, Temporal arteritis, *Am. J. Med.* **67:**839–852.

Hamilton, C. R., Jr., Shelley, W. M., and Tumulty, P. A., 1971, Giant cell arteritis: Including temporal arteritis and polymyalgia rheumatica, *Medicine* **50:**1–27.

Harrington, J. T., 1974, Acute oliguric renal failure with IgA glomerular deposits (Henoch–Schönlein purpura), *N. Engl. J. Med.* **290:**1365–1369.

Haynes, B. F., Fishman, M. L., Fauci, A. S., and Wolff, S. M., 1977, The ocular manifestations of Wegener's granulomatosis. Fifteen years experience and review of the literature, *Am. J. Med.* **63:**131–138.

Holsinger, D. R., Osmundson, P. J., and Edwards, J. E., 1962, The heart in periarteritis nodosa, *Circulation* **25:**610–618.

Horn, R. F., Fauci, A. S., Rosenthal, A. S., and Wolff, S. M., 1974, Renal biopsy pathology in Wegener's granulomatosis, *Am. J. Pathol.* **74:**423–430.

Ishikawa, K., 1978, Natural history and classification of occlusive thromboaortopathy (Takayasu's disease), *Circulation* **57**:617–624.

Katz, P., Alling, D. W., Haynes, B. F., and Fauci, A. S., 1979, Association of Wegener's granulomatosis with HLA-B8, *Clin. Immunol. Immunopathol.* **14**:268–270.

Katzenstein, A.-L. A., Carrington, C. B., and Liebow, A. A., 1979, Lymphomatoid granulomatosis: A clinicopathologic study of 152 cases, *Cancer* **43**:360–373.

Kawasaki, T., Kosaki, F., Okawa, S., Shigematsu, I., and Yanagawa, H., 1974, A new infantile acute febrile mucocutaneous lymph node syndrome (MLNS) prevailing in Japan, *Pediatrics* **54**:271–276.

Kemper, J. W., Baggenstoss, A. H., and Slocumb, C. H., 1957, The relationship of therapy with cortisone to the incidence of vascular lesions in rheumatoid arthritis, *Ann. Intern. Med.* **46**:831–851.

Kussmaul, A., and Maier, K., 1866, Über eine bischer nicht beschreibene eigenthümliche Arterienerkrankung (periarteritis nodosa), die mit Morbus Brightii und rapid fortschreitender allgemeiner Muskellähmung einhergeht, *Deut. Arch. Klin. Med* **1**:484–517.

Levine, B. B., 1966, Immunologic mechanisms of penicillin allergy. A haptenic model for the study of allergic diseases in man, *N. Engl. J. Med.* **275**:1115–1125.

Lie, J. T., Gordon, L. P., and Titus, J. L., 1975, Juvenile temporal arteritis. Biopsy study of four cases, *JAMA* **234**:496–501.

Liebow, A. A., Carrington, C. R. B., and Friedman, P. J., 1972, Lymphomatoid granulomatosis, *Hum. Pathol.* **3**:457–558.

Longstreth, P. L., Lorobkin, M., and Palubinskas, A. J., 1974, Renal microaneurysms in a patient with systemic lupus erythematosus, *Radiology* **113**:65–66.

LoSpalluto, J., Dorward, B., Miller, W., Jr., and Ziff, J., 1962, Cryoglobulinemia based on interaction between a gamma macroglobulin and 7S gamma globulin, *Am. J. Med.* **32**:142–147.

Lowance, D. C., Mullins, J. D., and McPhaul, J. J., 1973, Immunoglobulin A (IgA) associated glomerulonephritis, *Kidney Int.* **3**:167–176.

Lupi-Herrera, E., Sanchez-Torres, G., Marcushamer, J., Mispireta, J., Horwitz, S., and Vela, J. E., 1977, Takayasu's arteritis. Clinical study of 107 cases, *Am. Heart J.* **93**:94–99.

Meltzer, M., and Franklin, E. C., 1966, Cryoglobulinemia—a study of twenty-nine patients. I. IgG and IgM cryoglobulins and factors affecting cryoprecipitability, *Am. J. Med.* **40**:828–838.

Meyers, D. S., Grim, C. E., and Kertzer, W. F., 1974, Fibromuscular dysplasia of the renal artery with medial dissection. A case simulating polyarteritis nodosa, *Am. J. Med.* **56**:412–416.

Mintz, G., and Fraga, A., 1965, Arteritis in systemic lupus erythematosus, *Arch. Intern. Med.* **116**:55–66.

Moore, P. M., and Fauci, A. S., 1981, Neurologic manifestations of systemic vasculitis. A retrospective and prospective study of the clinicopathologic features and responses to therapy in 25 patients, *Am. J. Med.* **71**:517–524.

Mowrey, F. H., and Lundberg, E. A., 1967, The clinical manifestations of essential polyangiitis (periarteritis nodosa) with emphasis on the hepatic manifestations, *Ann. Intern. Med.* **40**:1141–1155.

Nussenblatt, R. B., Palestine, A. G., Rook, A. H., Scher, I., Wacker, W. B., and Gery, I., 1983, Treatment of intraocular inflammatory disease with cyclosporin A, *Lancet* **2**:235–238.

O'Duffy, J. D., Carney, J. A., and Deodhar, S., 1971, Behcet's disease. Report of 10 cases, 3 with new manifestations, *Ann. Intern. Med.* **75**:561–570.

Rose, G. A., and Spencer, H., 1957, Polyarteritis nodosa, *Q. J. Med.* **26**:43–81.

Sams, W. M., Harville, D. D., and Winkelmann, R. K., 1968, Necrotizing vasculitis associated with lethal reticuloendothelial diseases, *Br. J. Dermatol.* **80**:555–567.

Schmid, F. R., Cooper, N. S., Ziff, M., and McEwen, C., 1961, Arteritis in rheumatoid arthritis, *Am. J. Med.* **30**:56–83.

Sergent, J. S., Lockshin, M. D., Christian, D. L., and Gocke, D. J., 1976, Vasculitis with hepatitis B antigenemia: Long-term observations in nine patients, *Medicine* **67**:354–359.

Sheps, S. G., 1972, Vasculitis, in: *Peripheral Vascular Diseases*, 4th ed. (J. F. Fairburn, J. L. Juergens, and J. A. Spittel, eds.), W. B. Saunders, New York, pp. 351–385.

Sokoloff, L., and Bunim, J. J., 1957, Vascular lesions in rheumatoid arthritis, *J. Chron. Dis* **5**:668–687.

Soter, N. A., 1976, Clinical presentations and mechanisms of necrotizing angiitis of the skin, *J. Invest. Dermatol.* **67**:354–359.

Spector, W. G., and Heesom, N., 1969, The production of granulomata by antigen–antibody complexes, *J. Pathol.* **98**:31–39.

Walton, E. W., 1958, Giant-cell granuloma of the respiratory tract (Wegener's granulomatosis), *Br. Med. J.* **2**:265–270.

Winkelmann, R. K., and Ditto, W. B., 1964, Cutaneous and visceral syndromes of necrotizing or "allergic" angiitis: A study of 38 cases, *Medicine* **43**:59–89.

Zeek, P. M., 1952, Periarteritis nodosa. Critical review, *Am. J. Clin. Pathol.* **22**:777–790.

Zeek, P. M., 1953, Periarteritis nodosa and other forms of necrotizing angiitis, *N. Engl. J. Med.* **18**:764–772.

18

Immune Complexes in Human and Experimental Disease

M. Teresa Aguado and Argyrios N. Theofilopoulos

I. INTRODUCTION

Immune Complex (IC) formation occurs as a result of the humoral immune reaction between the response-eliciting antigen and its specific antibody molecules. These ICs possess a wide range of biological activities; they can suppress or augment immune responses, inhibit tumor cell destruction, and accumulate in filtering organs (such as the kidney and other sites) and blood vessel walls, where tissue damage may occur as a result of activation of the complement (C) cascade and attraction of neutrophils and macrophages. Normally, however, IC formation protects the host by facilitating clearance of various antigens and invading microorganisms by the phagocytic system. In this chapter, we discuss the biological functions of ICs and the mechanisms of their deposition onto tissues. Subsequently, the experimental models are analyzed, and, finally, the human diseases associated with ICs and the methods for IC demonstration in tissues and biological fluids are summarized.

II. THE BIOLOGY OF IMMUNE COMPLEXES

On combination with inciting antigens, antibody molecules acquire biological functions not previously inherent, including the ability to interact with serum C proteins and with cellular Fc and C receptors. A variety of factors, including the nature of the antigen and antibody and, more importantly, the ratio of the two reactants (Table 1), have profound influences on the biological activities of ICs.

M. Teresa Aguado and Argyrios N. Theofilopoulos • Department of Immunology, Scripps Clinic and Research Foundation, La Jolla, California 92037.

Table 1. Factors Influencing the Biology of Immune Complexes

Size of antigen
Valence of antigen
Chemical composition of antigen
Amount of antigen and rate of production
Charge of antigen
Class and subclass of antibody
Valence of antibody
Amount of antibody
Affinity of antibody
Charge of antibody
Ratio of antigen to antibody
State of the C system
State of the phagocytic system

Current data suggest that C fixation by soluble ICs containing IgG antibodies requires a structure of more than two or three antibody molecules. Immune complexes activate the C system by both classical and alternative pathways; aggregated or antigen-complexed IgG and IgM activate primarily the classical C pathway, whereas IgA and IgE antibodies activate the alternative pathway (Müller-Eberhard and Schreiber, 1980). Immunoglobulin G_1, IgG_2, and IgG_3 subclasses of human myeloma antibodies can activate C through their Fc portion, but IgG_4 has very limited activating capabilities. Biological activities (Table 2) generated by IC-induced C activation include immune adherence (C3b, C4b), chemotaxis (C5a), anaphylaxis (C3a, C5a), cytotoxicity (direct/indirect) (C5,6,7,8,9), leukocytic response (C3e), macrophage activation (Bb), IC solubilization (C3b), release of cell-bound ICs (C3b) and modification of immune responses (C3a, C5a). Subsequent to these interactions, vasoactive amines are released by platelets, lysosomal enzymes are discharged by neutrophils and macrophages, and phagocytic cell opsonization and ingestion are enhanced.

In addition to complement's well-recognized function as a major effector of antigen–antibody interaction, it has recently been found that physiological concentrations of C can induce profound alterations in the molecular weight, composition, and solubility of ICs (Miller and Nussenzweig, 1975; Takahashi *et al.*, 1980). During the interaction of soluble antigens and their antibodies at or near equivalence, a factor-B-dependent C3 convertase is assembled on the immune precipitate. Subsequent interactions between this complex-bound C3 convertase and serum lead to the continual deposition of activated C3 fragments. These events cause the disruption of some of the primary bonds between antigen and antibody, eventually leading to disaggregation of the complexes. The process results in "solubilized" ICs, which are no longer able to activate C efficiently or bind to cell surface C and Fc receptors.

The precise mode of solubilization is not fully understood. There is increasing evidence, however, that C3 fragments intercalate into the antigen–antibody lattice and disrupt it. In other words, the attachment of C3b to an antibody molecule prevents the reassociation of antibody and antigen through steric hindrance. Indeed, a covalent binding of C3 to the Fd portion of IgG molecules has recently been shown (Takata *et al.*, 1984). It is conceivable that this covalent binding affects the primary antigen–antibody bonds,

Table 2. Possible Effects of Immune Complexes on Biological Functions

- Through complement activation
  - Immune adherence (C3b, C4b)
  - Chemotaxis (C5a)
  - Anaphylaxis (C3a, C5a)
  - Direct and indirect cytotoxicity (C5,6,7,8,9)
  - Leukocyte response (C3e)
  - Macrophage activation (Bb)
  - IC solubilization (C3b)
  - Suppression of humoral immune response (C3a)
  - Enhancement of humoral immune response (C5a)
- On immune response
  - Humoral responses
    - Suppression
      - Through Ag masking or shielding
      - Through interaction with both Ag and Fc receptors on B cells: Ag-specific suppression
      - Through interaction with Fc receptors on B or T cells (release of suppressor factors): non-Ag-specific suppression
      - Effector cell blockade
      - Blockade of T- and B-cell interaction
      - Blockade of T-cell–macrophage interaction
      - Blockade of Ag receptors on T cells or their secreted products
    - Enhancement
      - Enhanced binding of Ag to Ag-receptor-bearing cells
      - Rapid localization of Ag in lymphoid follicles
      - Enhanced processing of Ag by macrophages
      - Enhancement of helper T-cell–B-cell cooperation
      - Processing of Ab and release of Fc fragments with adjuvantlike activities
  - Cellular responses
    - Enhancement or inhibition of Ab-dependent cell-mediated toxicity
    - Blockade of cell-mediated cytotoxicity by lymphocytes and macrophages
    - Blockade of delayed hypersensitivity
    - Altered traffic of lymphocytes

thereby causing solubilization. Immune complexes formed from a wide variety of antigens (proteins, polysaccharides, hapten–protein conjugates) and antibodies of IgG, IgA, and IgM classes from several mammalian species can be solubilized by C from sera of various species.

The C-mediated solubilization of immune precipitates requires activation of C3 via the alternative pathway (Miller and Nussenzweig, 1975; Fujita *et al.*, 1981) but not participation of the late-acting components, C5 through C9 (Takahashi *et al.*, 1976). The classical pathway alone, in the absence of the alternative pathway, is not sufficient to solubilize ICs. However, concomitant participation of both pathways results in much more efficient solubilization than that by the alternative pathway alone. The rate of solubilization depends on many factors, including amount of ICs, properties of antigen and antibody, composition of complexes, and, most importantly, affinity of the complexed antibody for antigen (Czop and Nussenzweig, 1976; Stassen and Beek, 1979). Thus, it appears that the C system is equipped with a control mechanism by which excessive inflammatory reactions can be avoided.

If the solubilization phenomenon is a physiological process, in certain diseases there may be less solubilization of ICs and a resultant increase in tissue injury. Recent studies suggest that this happens in sera and synovial fluids of patients with systemic lupus eryhtematosus (SLE) and rheumatoid arthritis (RA) (Aguado *et al.*, 1981; Dayer *et al.*, 1983). The fact that efficient solubilization proceeds more efficiently in the presence of intact classical and alternative C pathways may explain why IC-mediated diseases are more common in individuals with hereditary deficiencies of early C components (Raum *et al.*, 1980). Such individuals may have an impaired capacity to remove naturally occurring complexes from the circulation. Conversely, IgA-containing complexes and others that preferentially activate the alternative pathway may have a better outcome.

Several cell types express Fc and/or C receptors by which ICs can bind, thereby affecting the cell's functions. Erythrocytes have receptors for C3b and C4b (immune adherence receptors), which play important roles in IC clearance. More recently, these receptors have been found to play an important role (together with factors H and I of the C system) in the degradation of IC-associated C3b to iC3b and subsequently to C3c (released from the complex) and C3dg/C3d (remains covalently bound on the complex) (Medof *et al.*, 1982; Medof and Nussenzweig, 1984). Furthermore, several recent studies have shown decreased C3b (CR1) receptors on red cells of human lupus patients (Miyakawa *et al.*, 1981; Iida *et al.*, 1982), but whether this defect is genetic (Wilson *et al.*, 1982) or an epiphenomenon caused by C3 receptor occupation by ICs (Ross *et al.*, 1984) or other ligands is debatable.

Through their IgG receptors, eosinophils control antibody-dependent cellular cytotoxicity (ADCC) against parasites, and ICs have been found to have strong inhibitory effects in this function (Butterworth *et al.*, 1977). Mast cells and basophils have high-affinity IgE Fc receptors. Degranulation occurs after these cells interact with ICs or with C3a and C5a followed by release of biologically active factors such as heparin, histamine, slow-reacting substances of anaphylaxis, and platelet-activating factor.

B (bone-marrow-derived) and T (thymus-derived) lymphocytes bind ICs through their Fc and C receptors, as do unclassified human lymphocytes (K cells) that mediate ADCC and have high-affinity surface IgG Fc receptors. Virally infected fibroblasts, hepatocytes, placental endothelial cells, epidermal dendritic (Langerhans) cells and human glomerular epithelial cells also interact with IC via Fc and/or C receptors (reviewed by Theofilopoulos and Dixon, 1979).

The ability of ICs to perturb humoral and cellular immune responses is well documented, but the precise mechanisms are not as yet well defined. Depending on the molar ratio of antigen to antibody, the epitope density of the complex, class and affinity of antibody, and C fixing/activation capacity, ICs may suppress or enhance immune functions (Table 2) (Theofilopoulos, 1980).

Suppression of immune responses by ICs or antibody has been observed for several years. A prime example of this phenomenon in man is the therapeutic administration of anti-Rh antibodies, which prevent maternal sensitization by Rh antigens of the fetus (Freda *et al.*, 1966). There are several current explanations for the antibody-induced or IC-induced suppressive effects on humoral immune responses. A simple explanation is that antibody masks antigen and subsequently interferes with cellular recognition of antigenic determinants (Uhr and Moller, 1968). However, since in many systems supression requires the Fc portion of the antibody molecule (Sinclair, 1969), other additional mechanisms have been postulated (reviewed by Theofilopoulos and Dixon, 1979). Thus, ICs could directly block antibody production at the B-cell level through interaction with both antigen and Fc receptors, or they might inhibit immune responses by interacting with IgG Fc receptor-bearing B and T cells, resulting in the release of soluble immune response suppressor factors from these cells.

Other mechanisms proposed for IC-induced suppression of humoral responses include "effector cell blockade" (inhibition at the plasma-cell level), inhibition of T-cell–B-cell or T-cell–macrophage interactions, and blockade of antigen receptors on the surfaces of or secreted by T cells. More recently, suppression of humoral immune responses *in vitro* has been observed in the presence of C3a in the culture medium (Morgan *et al.*, 1982). Thus, IC may suppress immune responses not only directly but also indirectly by their ability to activate the C system.

Immune complexes can have opposite effects (augmentation rather than inhibition) on the humoral immune responses. Several investigators have reported that ICs, especially those in antigen excess, are more immunogenic than free antigens, both for primary and secondary antibody responses *in vivo* and *in vitro* (Morrison and Terres, 1966; Diener and Feldman, 1972). This enhanced responsiveness has been attributed to increased binding of complexed antigens to lymphocytes, to the rapid localization of ICs in lymphoid follicles, and to improved "processing" by macrophages as well as to better cooperation between helper T and B cells. More recently, it has been demonstrated *in vitro* that ICs are initially taken up by macrophages. Thereafter, small Fc fragments derived from the degraded antibody molecules are released and then, either by direct action on B cells or indirectly via helper T cells, stimulate proliferation and differentiation of B cells to plasma cells (Morgan and Weigle, 1980). It has also been shown that binding of C5a anaphylatoxin to macrophages results in augmentation of the primary humoral immune response, presumably via induction of interleukin 1 (IL-1) secretion (Goodman *et al.*, 1982). Interleukin 1 has the capacity to stimulate activated T cells and possibly to directly induce proliferation/differentiation of activated B cells.

Immune complexes may modulate not only humoral immune responses but also several cell-mediated phenomena. For example, depending on their molar ratio, ICs may inhibit or enhance antibody-dependent cell cytotoxicity (ADCC). Thus, in antigen excess, ADCC is inhibited, whereas at antibody excess, "arming" of lymphocytes and enhancement of ADCC occur (Perlmann *et al.*, 1972). "Armed" lymphocytes carrying ICs that have some free antibody valences may attack the cellular target for which the free antibody-combining sites have specificity.

Immune complexes may also interfere with cell-mediated cytolytic reactions mediated by T cells or macrophages. Thus, some sera of humans and animals with malignancies contain substances, termed "blocking factors," that specifically inhibit cell-mediated cytolysis of tumor cells by sensitized lymphocytes (Hellstrom and Hellstrom, 1974). Evidence has been obtained that these blocking factors in cancer sera often represent tumor-antigen–antibody complexes. Additionally, ICs made with tumor antigens and antibodies *in vitro* can specifically block the destruction of tumor cells by sensitized lymphocytes (Gorczynski *et al.*, 1975) and macrophages (Gershon *et al.*, 1974), and putative tumor-antigen–antibody complexes eluted from peripheral mononuclear cells of tumor-bearing patients can inhibit stimulation of the patients' lymphocytes by tumor-related antigens (Hattler and Soehnlen, 1974). Immune complexes have also been postulated to inhibit delayed-type hypersensitivity reactions, possibly because the responsible cells migrate from the circulation to the spleen (Lagrange and Mackaness, 1978). Last, and perhaps related to the above finding, ICs have been observed to affect the traffic patterns of lymphocytes (Stutman, 1973). The results *in toto* strongly suggest that ICs have important direct or indirect effects on various immunocytes and their related functions. The ability of ICs to interfere with immune mechanisms and to enhance or suppress lymphocyte function may represent their most important effects in some diseases.

III. FACTORS DETERMINING IMMUNE COMPLEX PATHOGENICITY AND DEPOSITION

The nature of the antibodies and antigens, as well as their molar ratio, determines the formation, fate, phlogogenicity, and biological activity of circulating ICs, which can instigate pathological sequelae in a variety of tissues regardless of the original antigenic stimuli (Haakenstad and Mannik, 1977).

The immunoglobulin class of the antibody determines its valence for a specific antigen, its binding to cellular Fc receptors, C-system activation capacity, and the association constant for specific antibody–antigen union. Antigen valence, chemical composition, and size are important in IC formation. Lattice construction with corresponding antibodies does not occur for monovalent antigens, which means that the complexes they form circulate for long periods without tissue deposition. Multivalent antigens (polysaccharides, proteins), in contrast, combine with their specific antibodies to form lattices of various compositions depending on the reactants' molar ratio. Some antigens (DNA, lectins) have basement membrane affinity and so provide a mechanism for *in situ* IC disease (Izui *et al.*, 1976; Mannik, 1982).

The antigen : antibody ratio plays a determining role in the fate of circulating ICs; those formed in the presence of antigen excess are small, unable to fix complement, and generally incapable of inciting the inflammatory process. In contrast, those formed in the presence of antibody excess can be large, insoluble, and rapidly phagocytized (which limits their pathogenicity), although they are capable of C activation. Between these two extremes of IC size lies the greatest pathological potential. Immune complexes formed in the presence of a modest antigen excess are medium-sized, soluble, able to fix C, and slowly phagocytized, thereby remaining in the circulation and widely disseminating their phlogogenic effects (Dixon, 1963).

Antigen exposure magnitude and duration also play an important role. Limited duration evokes transient tissue injury and clinical manifestations. Contrastingly, antigen remaining in the circulation for extended periods of time or antigenic material provided continuously (i.e., chronic infections, autoantigens) carries the potential for continuous IC formation and thus IC disease.

Recent studies suggest that the charge of antigens and antibodies that compose an IC may be an important contributing factor in IC deposition to the negatively charged (anionic) glomerular basement membrane (GBM). Thus, it has been shown that ICs prepared with cationized antigen, antibody, or both bound to the anionic sites in the GBM with deposits in the laminae rarae, interna, and externa and the lamina densa (Gallo *et al.*, 1981; Oite *et al.*, 1982; Gauthier *et al.*, 1982). In addition, antibodies to DNA eluted from glomeruli of NZB/W and MRL/1 mice with lupuslike syndromes were found to be more cationic than those in the circulation (Ebling and Hahn, 1980). All of these findings suggest that cationic ICs may preferentially be deposited in anionic subepithelial sites of the GBM.

The state of host phagocytes found in the circulatory and reticuloendothelial systems also determines the fate of circulating ICs. Reduced IC elimination and subsequent tissue deposition and disease result from an overload of this system, Fc and C receptor blockade on macrophages, or presence of an antibody class not interacting with cellular Fc receptors or not fixing C (Frank *et al.*, 1983). Recent studies have shown abnormal Fc receptor function in humans with lupus and other disorders as well as normal individuals, particularly those of the HLA-DR2, -MT1, or -B8/DR3 haplotype (Frank *et al.*, 1979; Kimberly *et al.*, 1983; Lawley *et al.*, 1981). It was initially thought that this was caused by a primary defect in the number or function of receptors for Fc or, secondarily, by occupation of the receptors by circulating ICs (Frank *et al.*, 1979). Other current data, however, indicate that the numbers of IgG Fc receptors on mononuclear cells of lupus and rheumatoid arthritis patients are normal or increased (Fries *et al.*, 1984; Katayama *et al.*, 1981) and that there is no correlation between levels of circulating ICs and degree of clearance defect (Fries *et al.*, 1979; Parris *et al.*, 1982).

Deposition of circulating ICs in tissues is a rare occurrence. Complexes larger than 19 S are required to induce vasculitis. Immune complex deposition requires the release of vasoactive amines (histamine or serotonin from platelets) and increased vascular permeability. Release of vasoactive amines from platelets may arise from any or all of the following three mechanisms: (1) platelet interaction with platelet-activating factor (PAF), a small lipid produced following basophil–IC interaction when the IC contains the antigen and IgE antibodies; (2) indirect or direct platelet lysis by IC-induced C activation; and (3) platelet aggregation following Fc receptor–IC interactions (reviewed by Cochrane and Koffler, 1973). Immune complexes deposited along the basement membranes initiate an inflammatory process depending in large part on the biological activities produced by C activation (particularly C3 and C5 fragments). These biological activities include chemotaxis and immune adherence. Immune adherence caused by binding of ICs bearing C3b to specific receptors on various cell types, including neutrophils and macrophages, results in phagocytosis. Both chemotactic factors (C5a) and anaphylatoxins (C3a, C5a) that directly attract neutrophils and degranulate mast cells promote the influx of inflammatory cells (reviewed by Cochrane and Dixon, 1978). The action of neutrophil-released lysosomal enzymes and possibly macrophages induces the subsequent tissue injury. However, although complement depletion or neutrophil elimination averts necrotizing arteritis, glomerulonephritis (GN) is still possible (Cochrane and Dixon, 1978). Macrophage depletion, in contrast, inhibits IC-induced GN (Holdsworth *et al.*, 1981).

Hemodynamic and anatomic components mediate the deposition of ICs, which tend to localize in vessels with increased blood pressure. This localization may be accounted for by endothelial platelet adherence in areas of vascular turbulence, which may cause increased IC deposition in these areas. Anatomic sites such as the glomerulus, choroid plexus, synovium, skin, and uveal tract are, by virtue of their high blood flow per unit mass of tissue, predisposed to vascular wall IC deposition and subsequent IC disease.

IV. MODELS OF IMMUNE COMPLEX DISEASES

Antigen–antibody interactions occur at three general anatomic sites: (1) ICs arising from the interaction of antibody with soluble circulatory antigens may disseminate and deposit in any large filtering tissues, causing lesions or IC disease; (2) As exemplified in the Arthus reaction, antibody can react with antigen secreted or locally injected into interstitial fluids; (3) Antibodies can react with structural antigens that are part of the cell surface membranes or with fixed intercellular structures such as basement membranes (reviewed by Cochrane and Dixon, 1978).

A. Systemic Immune Complex Disease

1. Acute Serum Sickness

Experimental acute serum sickness is produced by one or several closely spaced relatively large injections of heterologous serum protein. With the initial exposure, there is no preexisting antibody, and the disease develops 1 to 2 weeks after injection; on repeated exposure, the disease develops sooner. In either case, disease appears as antibody formation begins. The essence of serum sickness is the protracted interaction between antigen and antibody in the circulation, with the formation of antigen–antibody complexes in an environment of antigen excess (Wilson and Dixon, 1971).

During the first 2 days, the intravenously injected antigen equilibrates between intra- and extravascular components of the serum protein pool. There follows a relatively slow, nonimmune decline lasting a little more than a week; then the remaining antigen is rapidly eliminated from the circulation within 2 days. The rapid final elimination of circulating antigen is caused by the production of antibody, which combines with circulating antigen, forming antigen–antibody complexes. Initially, very small complexes are formed, but as more antibody becomes available, the complexes enlarge, react with serum C, and finally become so large that they are precipitously removed from the circulation. Simultaneously, the level of serum complement falls abruptly, and acute exudative and proliferative focal inflammatory lesions develop, especially in the kidneys, joints, arteries, and heart.

Apparently, the systemic liberation from platelets of pharmacologically active agents that increase vascular permeability causes circulating complexes to accumulate in vessel walls, particularly in a focal fashion along the internal elastic lamina of arteries and the basement membranes of glomeruli. Polymorphonuclear leukocytes and macrophages accumulate at sites of complex deposition and produce vascular damage and necrosis. By immunohistochemical techniques, antigen, host C, and host γ-globulin, presumably in complex form, localize specifically in tissue lesions and thus appear to be etiologic agents of tissue injury. In time, more antibody is made, the antigen is eliminated, and all ICs disappear from the circulation through phagocytosis by mononuclear cells. The cause of the pathology no longer exists, and the clinical symptoms wane. At this time, free (uncomplexed) antibody is found in the blood.

2. Chronic Serum Sickness

If the antigen is given daily in small amounts, just enough to balance antibody production, nephrotoxic ICs are formed. This experimental model, termed chronic serum sickness, resembles the chronic IC-associated diseases of humans and animals in which there is a continuous supply of antigen in the circulation (Dixon *et al.*, 1961; Wilson and Dixon, 1971). The ratio of antigen to antibody is most important, and, in rabbits, the disease can be turned off or on by changing the dose of antigen. Injecting large amounts of free antigen into the circulation, in fact, can dissolve the glomerular-complex deposits by creating an antigen-excess situation in the glomerulus and can return the kidney to near-normal function and structure. This suggests a possible therapeutic approach to the removal of IC deposits (Mannik and Striker, 1980; Haakenstad *et al.*, 1983).

B. Local Immune Complex Disease

Local IC disease is exemplified in the Arthus reaction, which is induced in actively or passively immunized animals by local injection of antigen (Cochrane and Dixon, 1978). Four to 10 hr after injection, vasculitis appears at the injection site caused by (1) IC formation in small vessel walls; (2) subsequent C activation; and (3) influx of polymorphonuclear cells (2–8 hr) and mononuclear cells (24–28 hr). The reaction can be abrogated by experimental C or polymorphonuclear cell elimination.

Analogously, local IC disease can be induced in certain organs such as joints, lungs, and pleural cavities. One example is the production of antigen-induced arthritis by repeated antigen injection into the joints of rabbits, resulting in prolonged synovitis (Cooke *et al.*, 1975). Injection of heterologous or homologous thyroglobulin into the thyroid, as another example, causes thyroiditis by the formation of ICs in the interstitial spaces as antibodies are synthesized, followed by acute and chronic inflammatory events. Continued thyroglobulin synthesis by follicular cells provides antigens for IC formation (Clagett *et al.*, 1974).

C. Tissue-Fixed Immune Complex Disease

One structural antigen to which autologous and heterologous immune responses are made is glomerular basement membrane (GBM). For example, rabbit antibodies to rat GBM, when injected into rats, circulate only very briefly because they are immediately fixed to the GBM of the rat. They can be identified by immunofluorescence bound in a continuous, linear, homogeneous fashion along the glomerular capillary wall together with host complement. A few hours after the binding of anti-GBM, neutrophils infiltrate the glomerular capillaries, injuring them in a process analogous to the Arthus reaction (Wilson and Dixon, 1973).

Nephrotoxic nephritis takes place in two stages. The first stage (heterologous phase) is the anti-GBM binding to the glomerulus as described above. A few days after injection, however, proteinuria, an indicator of glomerular injury, decreases but later reverts to a high level. This second stage (autologous phase) of glomerular damage is produced as a result of the host antibody response to rabbit IgG bound to the rat GBM. The host antibodies react with the nephrotoxic IgG, which persists bound to the GBM and is now acting as an antigen bound to the glomerulus. The second phase develops slowly and is independent of neutrophils. Animals can also be induced to make antibodies reactive with their own GBM, tubular basement membrane (TBM), or both by immunizing generally with heterologous GBM or TBM (Wilson and Dixon, 1976).

V. CIRCULATING-IMMUNE-COMPLEX-ASSOCIATED DISEASES

Circulating soluble ICs are associated with or causal to a wide variety of human diseases, including autoimmunity, glomerulonephritis (GN), neoplasms, and infectious diseases, which can be triggered by both exogenous and endogenous antigens (Table 3) (reviewed by Theofilopoulos and Dixon, 1979, 1980a,b; Zubler and Lambert, 1977).

A. Autoimmune Diseases

1. Rheumatoid Arthritis

Self-association of IgG anti-γ-globulins or reactions of IgG and IgM rheumatoid factors (RFs) with native IgG invoke IC formation in sera and joint fluids. These ICs seems to play a role in the pathogenesis of RA. Immune complexes of the IgG–IgM RF varieties are often observed in the synovial fluids of RA patients and appear to be responsible for the intraarticular activation of both the classical and alternative C systems. Such ICs are also phagocytized by synovial fluid neutrophils and other synovial fluid phagocytic cells. The IgM RF binding to IgG–IgG RF complexes enhances this process, and such complexes, which have been observed in RA patient sera, may be responsible for the systemic vasculitis associated with this disease.

Table 3. Diseases Associated with Immune Complexes

Autoimmune diseases
Systemic lupus erythematosus, rheumatoid arthritis, Felty's syndrome, Sjogren's syndrome, mixed connective tissue disease, periarteritis nodosa, systemic sclerosis, dermatomyositis
Glomerulonephritis
Exogenous and endogenous antigens
Neoplastic diseases
Solid and lymphoid tumors
Infectious diseases
Bacterial: Infective endocarditis, meningococcal infections, disseminated gonorrheal infection, recurrent infections in children, infected ventriculoatrial shunt, streptococcal infections, leprosy, syphilis
Viral: Dengue hemorrhagic fever, cytomegalovirus infections, viral hepatitis, infectious mononucleosis, subacute sclerosing panencephalitis
Parasitic: Malaria, trypanosomiasis, schistosomiasis, filariasis, toxoplasmosis
Mycosis: Paracoccidioidomycosis
Other conditions
Dermatitis herpetiformis and celiac disease, ulcerative colitis and Crohn's disease, myocardial infarcts, idiopathic interstitial pneumonia, pulmonary eosinophilic granuloma, cystic fibrosis, sarcoidosis, multiple sclerosis, amyotrophic lateral sclerosis, myasthenia gravis, uveitis, otitis media, atopic diseases, arthritis associated with intestinal bypass procedure for morbid obesity, sickle-cell anemia, thrombotic thrombocytopenic purpura, primary biliary cirrhosis, kidney and bone marrow transplantation, pregnancy, preeclamptic and eclamptic syndrome, Lyme arthritis, steroid-responsive nephrotic syndrome, xanthomatosis, vasectomy, oral ulceration and Behcet's syndrome, pemphigus and bullous pemphigoid, IgA deficiency, thyroid disorders, ankylosing spondylitis, diabetes, Henoch–Scholein purpura, hemophilia, cutaneous vasculatis, iatrogenic diseases

2. Systemic Lupus Erythematosus

A variety of antibodies are observed in the sera of SLE patients that react with native or altered autologous antigens, including cytoplasmic or surface antigens of lymphocytes, red cells, platelets, polymorphonuclear cells, neuronal cells, and IgG. Antibodies to nuclear components, the most prominent manifestation of SLE, may be directed toward a variety of antigens, including double- and single-stranded DNA, histones, RNA, and the ribonucleoproteins (RNP, Sm). DNA, Ig, and C deposits in SLE patient kidneys resemble those in animals with experimentally induced nephritis. Similar Ig and C deposits have been observed in the skin and small blood vessels of patients with necrotizing vasculitis, in the choroid plexus of some patients with cerebral involvement, and in the lung. Immunoglobulin eluted from nephritic kidneys of SLE patients is highly enriched for anti-native-DNA and anti-single-stranded-DNA antibodies. Cryoglobulins, which sometimes represent ICs, are also frequent in the sera of SLE patients in quantities correlating with the severity of their diseases. High anti-DNA antibody levels, reduced C, and the presence of C3 breakdown products (C3c and C3d) are also common in these patients. A variety of assays also detect IC-like material. Circulating DNA–anti-DNA complexes have also been found, albeit not in large amounts or uniformly.

3. Other Autoimmune Diseases

Various assays have detected IC-like materials in Sjogren's syndrome, scleroderma, mixed connective tissue disease, and Felty's syndrome. Intermediate IgG–IgG RFs have been identified in the sera of Felty's syndrome patients, and Ig and C inclusions have been observed in the neutrophils of these patients.

B. Neoplastic Disease

Humoral and cell-mediated immune responses are elicited by tumor cells expressing surface membrane antigens that are foreign to the host. Tumor-antigen–antibody ICs can be detected in the sera of patients with malignant disease. Such ICs may occasionally cause GN, which has been observed in association with melanoma, lung, breast, stomach, and colon carcinomas, Burkitt's lymphoma, leukemia, lymphosarcoma, and Hodgkin's disease.

The observed elimination of proteinuria after removal of the primary tumor suggests a definite relationship between neoplastic and renal disease. Immunofluorescence electron microscopy demonstrates IC deposits in the kidneys of 50% of this patient population, and related tumor antigens have been demonstrated in glomerular deposits and eluates.

It has been suggested that circulating tumor-antigen–antibody ICs block cell-mediated tumor cell destruction *in vitro* and could prevent antigen recognition by effector cells by masking, modulating, or shedding tumor antigen. Alternatively, these ICs in antigen excess could react with T-cell receptors and subsequently interfere with effector T-cell function. Positive results in many antigen-nonspecific IC assays have been obtained in the sera of cancer patients, and it is postulated that IC and blocking factor levels correlate with the extent of disease and poor prognosis.

C. Infectious Diseases

1. Infective Endocarditis

Once considered to be a consequence of tissue invasion and injury by the causative microorganism, many of the clinical and histological extravalvular features of infective endocarditis are now considered to be immunologically mediated. Immunoglobulin G and complement granular deposits are regularly observed in the tissue lesions, and circulating ICs, which correlate with the duration of illness, extravascular manifestations, and hypocomplementemia, are observed in more than 90% of these patients. These are generally eliminated by successful antimicrobial or surgical therapy.

2. Other Bacterial Diseases

Allergic complications such as arthritis, vasculitis, and skin lesions occur in meningococcal disease, possibly because of either a Schwartzman reaction or the deposition of ICs containing meningococcal antigens. Immunofluorescence evidence of IC deposition in tissues, low levels of circulating C3, and activation of both the classical and alternative C pathways have been obtained. Similarly, ICs have been found in patients with disseminated gonorrheal infections, in children with recurrent upper respiratory tract infections, and in patients with infected ventriculoatrial shunts surgically implanted for relief of hydrocephalus. The renal injury following infection with nephritogenic streptococci is generally considered to have an IC pathogenesis. Lepromatous leprosy is another example of a chronic infectious process with a large bacillary load and chronic antigenemia. Frequently, such patients develop an acute leprosy reaction, either spontaneously or after treatment with microbicidal drugs. This reaction is characterized by red nodules in the skin and by arthritis and proteinuria resulting from the sudden release of leprosy antigens and their combination with antibodies to form ICs. Glomerulonephritis, presumably caused by ICs, is also sometimes observed in both congenital and secondary syphilis. The GN can be resolved with penicillin therapy because of eradication of the antigenic source.

3. Viral Diseases

Viral infections are frequently associated with the development of ICs and IC disease. The virus is a self-replicating agent that provides a supply of macromolecular antigens in the form of both virions and virus-associated molecules. Both RNA and DNA viruses can cause IC diseases in animals and humans. Examples of human viral diseases associated with ICs are dengue hemorrhagic fever (DHF), viral hepatitis, and cytomegalovirus infections.

Both DHF and shock syndrome are associated with C-system activation by the classical and alternative pathways and with intravascular coagulation and serum ICs. In addition, presumed IC deposits are occasionally demonstrated in tissues and on the surfaces of a small proportion of circulating lymphocytes from these patients. It is of interest to note that *in vitro* ICs formed by IgG nonneutralizing homotypic or heterotypic antibodies to dengue type 2 virus are more efficient in infecting macrophages (the major cell type in which dengue virus replicates) than is the virus alone. This finding may explain the severity of this disease in infants with circulating maternal nonneutralizing heterotypic antidengue antibodies and a primary dengue virus infection.

Hepatitis surface antigen (HBsAg)–antibody complexes have been implicated in the pathogenesis of a vasculitis and arthralgia syndrome seen sometimes as a prodrome in patients with acute viral hepatitis. An association between HBsAg and polyarteritis nodosa has also been recorded. Several histological forms of glomerulonephritis accompany serum hepatitis and are typified by granular deposits of Ig and C as well as electron-dense deposits along the GBM. Moreover, HBsAg is identified occasionally in the glomerular IC deposits examined by immunofluorescence and electron microscopy.

Immune-complex-like materials have also been detected in the sera of 35 to 45% of patients with congenital or natal cytomegalovirus infections. The incidence is highest in children with severe intrauterine infection, and, during the first year of life, it parallels the patterns of viral excretion and humoral immune response. In some patients who die with severe congenital cytomegalovirus infections, granular deposits of Ig and C3 have been detected along the GBM. The circulating ICs appear to contribute to this insidious, progressive disease either by interfering with host defense mechanisms or by direct tissue damage.

Other viral infections associated with glomerular changes are mumps, varicella, infectious mononucleosis, and coxsackievirus B infections.

4. Parasitic Diseases

Because low C levels and circulating ICs have been observed in association with *Plasmodium falciparum* infections, circulating ICs seem to be associated with the immunopathology of malaria. Granular deposits of Ig, C, and malaria antigens accumulate in glomeruli of some humans with transient GN caused by *P. falciparum* or chronic GN and nephrotic syndromes caused by *P. malariae*. Additionally, cryoglobulins, low C3 levels, anti-C activity, and soluble ICs have been detected in the sera of patients with chronic malaria associated with tropical splenomegaly syndrome. Trypanosomiasis, schistosomiasis, onchocerciasis (filariasis), and toxoplasmosis also may be associated with GN and serum- and tissue-deposited ICs.

D. Iatrogenic Diseases

Foreign serum used as a passive antibody and drugs such as penicillamine, sulfa compounds, trimethadione, mercury, gold, and halothane are associated with GN and with electron microscopic and/or immunofluorescent evidence of IC deposition. Immune complexes found in these conditions may contain antibodies against the drug or drug-associated haptenic conjugates or possibly against endogenous antigens released through toxic effects of the drug. Moreover, ICs composed of bovine proteins as antigens and IgG antibodies of maternal origin have been found in the sera of neonates receiving cow's milk.

E. Other Conditions

Circulating IC-like materials and sometimes tissue deposits of Ig and C also have been described in many other conditions (listed in Table 3). Some patients with idiopathic interstitial pneumonias also have circulating and deposited Ig and C along the alveolar walls. Patients given renal or bone marrow allografts sometimes develop ICs together with manifestations of graft-versus-host disease, and in normal pregnancy, maternal antibodies complexed with paternal antigens have been claimed to exist and act as blocking factors against rejection of the fetal allograft.

VI. DISEASES ASSOCIATED WITH LOCALIZED COMPLEX REACTIONS

Classic Arthus reactions may occur in the skin after skin tests with *Aspergillus fumigatus, Candida albicans,* avian serum proteins, and other antigens when precipitating antibodies are present in the blood. Similar reactions were common after repeated antitoxin or antibacterial serum administration and, more recently, have followed insulin injections. In all of these conditions, antigen is deposited in the skin and combines with antibody in the local tissue fluids of previously sensitized individuals. The spontaneous clinical lesion most analogous to the experimental Arthus reaction is that of erythema nodosum leprosum, in which the lesions contain antibody, antigen, C components, and infiltrating polymorphonuclear cells. Similar lesions manifested either as erythema nodosum, nodular vaculitis, or a multiform erythema can be observed after many bacterial, viral, and fungal infections. Recovery without residual lesions is the general rule after removal of the antigen by normal physiological processes or appropriate medical intervention.

Another example of IC formation at a local site is the hypersensitivity pneumonitis that results when inspired air contains a large amount of antigen to which the individual is immune. The IC that forms in the alveoli of the lung produces a severe inflammation with acute respiratory distress. Many clinical cases have been reported in agricultural workers exposed to dusts or particles. Farmer's lung is one such disease that develops on inhalation of dust from hay contaminated with saprophytic fungi. Sugar cane workers develop a similar disease from immunity to antigens contained in the cane.

VII. DISEASES ASSOCIATED WITH IMMUNE RESPONSES TO TISSUE-FIXED ANTIGENS

Many autoimmune responses may develop against tissue antigens and can cause or contribute to diseases. Thus, autoantibodies to red cells, neutrophils, platelets, and lymphocytes bind to these circulating blood cells, readily depleting them from the circulation and thereby causing autoimmune hematologic disorders. It is interesting that some drugs (e.g., phenacetin, quinidine, aspirin, sulfonamides) may combine with red cells or platelets, elicit immune responses, and secondarily cause hemolytic anemias or thrombocytopenias.

The most common structural antigen to which autologous immune responses are made is the basement membrane. Anti-basement-membrane antibody-induced injury in humans is confined largely to the kidneys and lungs. Anti-basement-membrane antibodies cause about 5% of the glomerulonephritides in humans. About two-thirds of these patients may also experience pulmonary hemorrhage, and these combined symptoms are designated anti-GBM antibody-induced Goodpasture's syndrome. By immunofluorescence, linear deposits of IgG and C3 along with GBM can be seen.

VIII. DETECTION OF IMMUNE COMPLEXES

Two main approaches have been used to demonstrate the occurrence of ICs in human or animal diseases. First, the analysis of tissue specimens, and second, the serologic analysis of samples from various biological fluids.

Tissue studies by conventional histological techniques and electron microscopy may lead to the suspicion of an involvement of ICs in the observed lesions on the basis of similarities with experimentally induced IC lesions. On electron microscopy, IC deposits are often observed as electron-dense accumulations in glomerular vessels of the kidney, most frequently in the subepithelial position but also in subendothelial and intramembranous locations. Scattered subepithelial deposits are characteristic of poststreptococcal GN, whereas extensive subepithelial deposits are the hallmark of membranous glomerulopathy. In lupus nephritis, electron-dense deposits are often observed in a subendothelial position, suggesting that the particular antigen–antibody systems involved may form complexes too large to pass through the glomerular basement membrane (GBM). In this disease, however, complexes may exist in subendothelial, mesangial, and subepithelial areas of glomeruli to varying degrees. Immunofluorescence is the most commonly utilized immunohistochemical technique and is dependent on the use of fluorochrome-labeled antibodies (fluorescein isothiocyanate, tetramethylrhodamine isothiocyanate, etc.) for detecting Ig and associated mediator molecules such as C within tissue specimens. This system has recently been improved by use of the avidin–biotin complexes, which further enhance the fluorescence of localized antigens.

The two major antibody-induced forms of glomerular injury (anti-GBM GN, IC GN) have different Ig deposition patterns on immunofluorescence study. Anti-GBM antibodies, which react with antigen distributed throughout the GBM, deposit evenly to produce a smooth, linear pattern. In contrast, ICs depositing in the glomerular filter at random from the circulation are detected as granular, interrupted deposits. In addition, if enough of the diseased tissue is available, deposited ICs can be eluted from it by using low-pH buffers (citrate, HCl–glycine), high-pH buffers, or chaotropic agents (KI, KSCN), after which the antibodies and sometimes the antigens can be recovered, quantified, and identified. One should be aware that eluted antibodies always represent a selected fraction of the complexed molecules and that the elution procedures may alter some antibodies more than others. The amount of immunoglobulins with an identified antibody specificity should be related to the total amount of eluted immunoglobulins to evaluate their relative involvement in the deposited complexes.

A wide array of immunologic techniques have been developed for demonstrating ICs in body fluids. These techniques can be divided into two groups: (1) antigen-specific tests, which detect a specific antigen complexed with antibody; and (2) the larger and more readily applicable antigen-nonspecific tests.

A. Antigen-Specific Methods

The provocative antigen of a pathogenic immune response is rarely known, but when it is, ICs composed of the known antigen and corresponding antibody are easily detected in the circulation. For example, if one suspects a specific viral disease, the serum can be tested for ICs containing the viral antigens by immunoprecipitation with an antiserum to host Ig or antiserum to host C, a reaction that markedly decreases the titers of virus or viral products (determined by radioimmunoassays of LD_{50} titration in experimental animals) in the supernatant.

However, when the viral antigen is present in such large quantities that only a small proportion binds to antibody, circulating titers may not decrease appreciably during immunoprecipitation. In these cases, the precipitation should be preceded by sucrose density gradient fractionation or gel filtration; these preparatory procedures separate molecules according to their size (free antigen has a smaller molecular weight than the combination of antibody plus antigen). The fractions obtained can then be analyzed by methods such as radioimmunoassays for the distribution of the known antigenic substance. Fractions containing antigenic material heavier than free non-Ig-bound antigen should then be separated, and antigen tested for its association with host Ig or C or both. This association becomes evident if the antigen is removed by immunoprecipitation with anti-Ig or anti-C3 or by adsorption to Sepharose-immobilized anti-Ig, anti-C3, or staphylococcal protein A, which has the ability to bind immunoglobulins, especially those of the IgG class.

B. Antigen-Nonspecific Methods

The antigens in the ICs of most spontaneous diseases of animals and humans are unknown, and antigen-specific techniques are of no use in these instances. In such situations, attempts are made to identify ICs by relying on the different physiochemical and biological properties of antigen-complexed Ig versus free Ig. These methods have varying specificity, sensitivity, complexity, clinical applicability, and idiosyncrasies, factors that preclude the detection of all species of ICs. Moreover, materials other than ICs may interfere with the results in the majority of these assays, sometimes leading to false-positive or false-negative results.

Table 4 lists the available procedures for detecting ICs containing unknown antigens in biological fluids. These techniques are based on: (1) physical properties of ICs; (2) interactions of ICs with certain serum factors such as complement, anti-γ-globulins (i.e., rheumatoid factors), and conglutinin; and (3) interactions with cells having Fc and C receptors such as B cells, macrophages, platelets, and red blood cells.

IX. INTERPRETATION OF IMMUNE COMPLEX ASSAYS

Several recent studies suggest that IC measurement may be useful in understanding the pathogenesis of some diseases as well as in prognosis and management. The assays have been used to determine the incidence and amount of circulating ICs in patients with autoimmune disorders, infectious diseases, and various types of malignancies.

In general, there is a good correlation between levels of circulating ICs and disease activity. For example, in patients with SLE, several investigators, using different techniques, have found a close relationship between IC levels and antibodies to DNA, low complement levels, and clinical manifestations. In patients with bacterial endocarditis,

Table 4. Antigen-Nonspecific Methods for Detecting Immune Complexes

Physical techniques:
1. Analytical ultracentrifugation
2. Sucrose density gradient centrifugation
3. Gel filtration
4. Ultrafiltration
5. Electrophoresis and electrofocusing
6. PEG precipitation
7. Cryoprecipitation
8. Nephelometric assays
Methods based on IC biological characteristics
Complement techniques:
1. Microcomplement consumption test
2. Assays based on the interactions of ICs with purified C1q: C1q precipitation in gels, C1q deviation test
3. C1q–PEG assays
4. C1q solid-phase assays
5. Conglutinin assays
6. Anti-C3 solid-phase assays
Antiglobulin techniques:
1. Rheumatoid factor tests
2. Other antiglobulin tests
Cellular techniques:
1. Platelet aggregation test
2. Inhibition of ADCC
3. Intracytoplasmic staining of polymorphonuclear leukocytes
4. Release of enzymes from eosinophils and mast cells
5. Macrophage inhibition assay
6. Rosette inhibition tests
7. Raji cell assay
Binding to staphylococcal protein A

an excellent correlation has been found among circulating IC levels, duration of disease, and extravalvular manifestations. Immune complex levels returned toward normal after appropriate treatment with valvulectomy. High levels of ICs are associated with the cellular form of idiopathic interstitial pneumonia but not with the diffuse fibrosis form. The response to corticosteroid therapy is better in patients with elevated ICs, and the elevated levels return to normal after treatment. Immune complex measurement appears also to be useful in prognosis and management of cancer patients. For example, the median survival time of patients without detectable ICs was more than 18 months in myeloid leukemia, 18 months in acute lymphatic leukemia, and more than $8^1/_2$ months in patients in blastic crisis of chronic myeloid leukemia. The corresponding median survival times of the patients who had elevated IC levels, however, were 64, 135, and 90 days, respectively. A similar correlation between high IC levels and poor prognosis has been described in patients with breast carcinoma, neuroblastoma, lung carcinoma, Hodgkin's disease, and other types of malignancies.

No universal and absolutely specific reagent is yet available for IC detection and quantitation. In general, all IC detection methods described thus far do not differentiate nonspecifically aggregated immunoglobulins from true immune complexes and thus are potential sources of error, particularly in repetitive freezing–thawing and/or heating of samples at more than 56°C prior to testing. Moreover, the C1q-dependent techniques may give false-positive results because of the interference of such substances in the serum sample as DNA or endotoxin. The RF-based tests may be influenced by the presence of endogenous rheumatoid factor in the serum sample and high levels of serum IgG. Cellular techniques may give false-positive results because of the presence of anticellular antibodies frequently found in the sera of patients with autoimmune disorders. Therefore, optimal screening of ICs in human sera may require the use of several tests.

The physician using immune complex assays should appreciate the current state of the art. Available assays will, on occasion, be negative when immune complexes are present, and, conversely, positive tests can result from materials other than immune complexes. An ideal test should be able to analyze the size and constituents of the complex, demonstrate the relevant antigens, and identify the subclasses of the individual participating antibodies. Therefore, we must await the development of assays that are not handicapped by the above problems. This need appears to be fulfilled by a recently developed anti-C3 assay utilizing monoclonal antibodies against determinants expressed on activated C3.

ACKNOWLEDGMENTS. This is Publication No. 3684-IMM from the Immunology Department, Scripps Clinic and Research Foundation, La Jolla, California. Dr. Aguado is the recipient of an Arthritis Foundation Postdoctoral Fellowship.

REFERENCES

Aguado, M. T., Perrin, L. H., Miescher, P. A., and Lambert, P. H., 1981, Decreased capacity to solubilize immune complexes in sera from patients with systemic lupus erythematosus, *Arthritis Rheum.* **24:**1255–1229.

Buttersworth, A. E., Remold, H. G., Houba, V., David, J. R., Franks, D., David, P. H., and Sturrock, R. F., 1977, Antibody-dependent eosinophil-mediated damage to ^{51}Cr-labeled schistosomula of *Schistosoma mansoni*: Mediation by IgG, and inhibition by antigen–antibody complexes, *J. Immunol.* **118:**2230–2236.

Clagett, J. H., Wilson, C. B., and Weigle, W. O., 1974, Interstitial immune complex thyroiditis in mice. The role of autoantibody to thyroglobulin, *J. Exp. Med.* **140:**1439–1456.

Cochrane, C. G., and Dixon, F. J., 1978, Immune complex injury, in: *Immunological Diseases,* Vol. 1, (M. Samter, ed.) Little, Brown, Boston, pp. 210–229.

Cochrane C. G., and Koffler, D., 1973, Immune complex disease in experimental animals and man, *Adv. Immunol.* **16:**185–264.

Cooke, T. D., Hurd, E. R., Jasin, H., Bienenstock, J., and Ziff, M., 1975, Identification of immunoglobulins and complement in rheumatoid articular collagenous tissues, *Arthritis Rheum.* **18:**541–551.

Czop, J., and Nussenzweig, V., 1976, Studies on the mechanism of solubilization of immune aggregates by complement, *J. Exp. Med.* **143:**615–630.

Dayer, E., Gerster, J. C., Aguado, M. T., and Lambert, P. H., 1983, Capacity to solubilize immune complexes in sera and synovial fluids from patients with rheumatoid arthritis, *Arthritis Rheum.* **26:**156–164.

Diener, E., and Feldman, M., 1972, Relationship between antigen and antibody-induced suppression of immunity, *Transplant. Rev.* **8:**76–103.

Dixon, F. J., 1963, The role of antigen–antibody complexes in disease, *Harvey Lect.* **58:**21–52.

Dixon, F. J., Feldman, J. D., and Vazquez, J. J., 1961, Experimental glomerulonephritis: The pathogenesis of a laboratory model resembling the spectrum of human glomerulonephritis, *J. Exp. Med.* **113:**899–920.

Ebling, F., and Hahn, B. H., 1980, Restricted subpopulation of DNA antibodies in kidneys of mice with systemic lupus. Comparison of antibodies in serum and renal eluates, *Arthritis Rheum.* **23**:392–403.
Frank, M. M., Hamburger, M. I., Lawley, T. J., Kimberly, R. P., and Plotz, P. H., 1979, Defective reticuloendothelial system Fc receptor function in systemic lupus erythematosus, *N. Engl. J. Med.* **300**:518–523.
Frank, M. M., Lawley, T. J., Hamburger, M. I., and Brown, E. J., 1983, Immunoglobulin G Fc receptor mediated clearance in autoimmune diseases, *Ann. Intern. Med.* **98**:206–218.
Freda, V. J., Gorman, T. G., and Pollock, W., 1966, Rh factor: Prevention of isoimmunization and clinical trial on mothers, *Science* **151**:828–830.
Fries, L. F., Mullius, W. W., Cho, K. R., Plotz, P. H., and Frank, M. M., 1984, Monocyte receptors for the Fc portion of IgG are increased in systemic lupus erythematosus, *J. Immunol.* **132**:695–700.
Fujita, T., Takata, Y., and Tamura, N., 1981, Solubilization of immune precipitates by six isolated alternative pathway proteins, *J. Exp. Med.* **154**:1743–1751.
Gallo, G. R., Caulin-Glaser, T., and Lamm, M. E., 1981, Charge of circulating immune complexes as a factor in glomerular basement membrane localization, *J. Clin. Invest.* **67**:1305–1313.
Gauthier, V. J., Mannik, M., and Striker, G. E., 1982, Effect of cationized antibodies in preformed immune complexes on deposition and persistence in renal glomeruli, *J. Exp. Med.* **156**:766–777.
Gershon, R. K., Mokyr, M. B., and Mitchell, M. S., 1974, Activation of suppressor T cells by tumor cells and specific antibody, *Nature* **250**:594–596.
Goodman, M. G., Chenoweth, D. E., and Weigle, W. O., 1982, Induction of interleukin 1 secretion and enhancement of humoral immunity by binding of human C5a to macrophage surface C5a receptors, *J. Exp. Med.* **156**:912–917.
Gorczynski, R. M., Kilburn, D. G., Knight, R. A., Norbury, C., Parker, D. C., and Smith, J. B., 1975, Nonspecific and specific immunosuppression in tumor-bearing mice by soluble immune complexes, *Nature* **254**:141–143.
Haakenstad, A. O., and Mannik, M., 1977, The biology of immune complexes, in: *Autoimmunity* (N. Talal, ed.), Academic Press, New York, pp. 278–360.
Haakenstad, A. O., Striker, G. E., and Mannik, M., 1983, Removal of glomerular immune complex deposits by excess antigen in chronic mouse model of immune complex disease, *Lab. Invest.* **48**:323–331.
Hattler, B. G., Jr., and Soehnlen, B., 1974, Inhibition of tumor-induced lymphocyte blastogenesis by a factor or factors associated with peripheral leukocytes, *Science* **184**:1374–1375.
Hellstrom, K. E., and Hellstrom, I., 1974, Lymphocyte-mediated cytotoxicity and blocking serum activity to tumor antigens, *Adv. Immunol.* **18**:209–277.
Holdsworth, S. R., Neale, T. J., and Wilson, C. B., 1981, Abrogation of macrophage-dependent injury in experimental glomerulonephritis in the rabbit. Use of an anti-machrophage serum, *J. Clin. Invest.* **68**:686–698.
Iida, K., Mornaghi, R., and Nussenzweig, V., 1982, Complement receptor (CR1) deficiency in erythrocytes from patients with systemic lupus erythematosus, *J. Exp. Med.* **155**:1427–1438.
Izui, S., Lambert, P.-H., and Miescher, P. A., 1976, *In vitro* demonstration of a particular affinity of glomerular basement membrane and collagen for DNA: A possible basis for a local formation of DNA–anti-DNA complexes in systemic lupus erythematosus, *J. Exp. Med.* **144**:428–443.
Katayama, S., Chia, D., Nasu, H., and Knutson, D. W., 1981, Increased Fc receptor activity in monocytes from patients with rheumatoid arthritis: A study of monocyte binding and catabolism of soluble aggregates of IgG *in vitro*, *J. Immunol.* **127**:643–647.
Kimberly, R. P., Gibofsky, A., Salmon, J. E., and Fotino, M., 1983, Impaired Fc-mediated mononuclear phagocyte system clearance in HLA-DR2 and MT1-positive healthy young adults, *J. Exp. Med.* **157**:1698–1703.
Lagrange, P. H., and Mackaness, G. B., 1978, Site of action of serum factors that block delayed-type hypersensitivity in mice, *J. Exp. Med.* **148**:235–245.
Lawley, T. J., Hall, R. P., Fauci, A. S., Katz, S. I., Hamburger, M. I., and Frank, M. M., 1981, Defective Fc-receptor functions associated with the HLA-B8/DRW3 haplotype: Studies in patients with dermatitis herpetiformis and normal subjects, *N. Engl. J. Med.* **304**:185–192.
Mannik, M., 1982, Pathophysiology of circulating immune complexes, *Arthritis Rheum.* **25**:783–787.
Mannik, M., and Striker, G. E., 1980, Removal of glomerular deposits of immune complexes in mice by administration of excess antigen, *Lab. Invest.* **42**:483–489.
Medof, M. E., and Nussenzweig, V., 1984, Control of the function of substrate-bound C4b–C3b by the complement receptor CR1, *J. Exp. Med.* **159**:1669–1685.

Medof, M. E., Iida, K., Mold, C., and Nussenzweig, V., 1982, Unique role of the complement receptor CR1 in the degradation of C3b associated with immune complexes, *J. Exp. Med.* **156:**1739–1754.

Miller, G. W., and Nussenzweig, V., 1975, A new complement function: Solubilization of antigen–antibody aggregates, *Proc. Natl. Acad. Sci. U.S.A.* **72:**418–422.

Miyakawa, Y., Yamada, A., Kosaka, K., Tsudei, F., Kosugi, E., and Mayumi, M., 1981, Defective immune-adherence (C3b) receptor on erythrocytes form patients with systemic lupus erythematosus, *Lancet* **2:**493–497.

Morgan, E. L., and Weigle, W. O., 1980, Regulation of Fc fragment-induced murine spleen cell proliferation, *J. Exp. Med.* **151:**1–11.

Morgan, E. L., Weigle, W. O., and Hugli, T. E., 1982, Anaphylatoxin-mediated regulation of the immune response. I. C3a-mediated suppression of human and murine humoral immune responses, *J. Exp. Med.* **155:**1412–1426.

Morrison, S. L., and Terres, G., 1965, Enhanced immunologic sensitization of mice by the simultaneous injection of antigen and specific antiserum. II. Effect of varying the antigen–antibody ratio and the amount of immune complex injected, *J. Immunol.* **96:**901–905.

Müller-Eberhard, H. J., and Schreiber, R. D., 1980, Molecular biology and chemistry of the alternative pathway of complement, *Adv. Immunol.* **29:**2–53.

Oite, T., Bhatsford, S. K., Mihatsuh, J. J., Takamiya, H., and Vogt, A., 1982, Quantitative studies of *in situ* immune complex glomerulonephritis in the rat induced by planted, cationized antigen, *J. Exp. Med.* **155:**460–474.

Parris, T. M., Kimberly, R. P., Inman, R. D., McDougal, J. S., Gibofsky, A., and Christian, C. L., 1982, Defective Fc receptor-mediated function of the mononuclear phagocyte system in lupus nephritis, *Ann. Intern. Med.* **97:**526–530.

Perlmann, P., Perlmann, H., and Biberfeld, P., 1972, Specifically cytotoxic lymphocytes produced by preincubation with antibody-complexed target cells, *J. Immunol.* **108:**558–561.

Raum, D., Donaldson, V. H., Alper, C. A., and Rosen, F. S., 1980, Genetics of complement, in: *The Menarini Series of Immunopathology,* Vol. 3 (P. A. Miescher, L. Bolis, and G. Torrigiani, eds.), Schwabe, Basel, pp. 162–183.

Ross, G. D., Walport, M. J., Parker, C. J., Lentine, A. F., Fuller, C. R., Yount, W. J., Myones, B. L., Winfield, J. B., and Lachmann, P. J., 1984, Acquired loss of erythrocyte CR1 (C3b-receptor) in systemic lupus erythematosus and other diseases with autoantibodies and/or complement activation, *Arthritis Rheum.* **27** (Suppl. 4):28.

Sinclair, N. R. St. C., 1969, Regulation of the immune response. I. Reduction in ability of specific antibody to inhibit long-lasting IgG immunological priming after removal of the Fc fragment, *J. Exp. Med.* **129:**1183–1201.

Stassen, F. L., and Beek, C. J., 1979, Complement-mediated solubilization of immune precipitates prepared with antibodies of different avidity, *J. Immunol.* **123:**535–542.

Stutman, O., 1973, Lymphocyte sequestration: Its possible role in tumor immunity, *Transplant. Proc.* **5:**969–973.

Takahashi, M., Czop, J., Ferreira, A., and Nussenzweig, V., 1976, Mechanism of solubilization of immune aggregates by complement. Implications for immunopathology, *Transplant. Rev.* **32:**121–139.

Takahashi, M., Takahashi, S., and Hiroshi, S., 1980, Solubilization of antigen–antibody complexes: A new function of complement as a regulator of immune reactions, *Prog. Allergy* **27:**134–166.

Takata, Y., Tamura, N., and Fujita, T., 1984, Interaction of C3 with antigen–antibody complexes in the process of solubilization of immune precipitates, *J. Immunol.* **132:**2531–2537.

Theofilopoulos, A. N., 1980, Immune complexes in humoral immune responses: Suppressive and enhancing effects, *Immunol. Today* **1:**1–3.

Theofilopoulos, A. N., and Dixon, F. J., 1979, The biology and detection of immune complexes, *Adv. Immunol.* **28:**89–220.

Theofilopoulos, A. N., and Dixon, F. J., 1980a, Immune complexes in human diseases. A review, *Am. J. Pathol.* **100:**531–591.

Theofilopoulos, A. N., and Dixon, F. J., 1980b, Detection of immune complexes: Techniques and implications, *Hosp. Pract.* **15:**107–121.

Uhr, J. W., and Möller, G., 1968, Regulatory effect of antibody on the immune response, *Adv. Immunol.* **8:**81–127.

Wilson, C. B., and Dixon, F. J., 1971, Quantitation of acute and chronic serum sickness in the rabbit, *J. Exp. Med.* **134:**7s–18s.

Wilson, C. B., and Dixon, F. J., 1973, Anti-glomerular basement membrane antibody induced glomerulonephritis, *Kidney Int.* **3**:74–89.

Wilson, C. B., and Dixon, F. J., 1976, The renal response to immunological injury, in: *The Kidney,* Vol. II (B. M. Brenner and F. C. Rector, eds.), W. B. Saunders, Philadelphia, pp. 838–940.

Wilson, J. G., Wong, W. W., Schur, P. H., and Fearon, D. T., 1982, Mode of inheritance of decreased C3b receptors on erythrocytes of patients with systemic lupus erythematosus, *N. Eng. J. Med.* **307**:981–986.

Zubler, R. H., and Lambert, P. H., 1977, Immune complexes in clinical investigation, in: *Recent Advances in Clinical Immunology* (R. A. Thompson, ed.), Churchill Livingston, New York, pp. 125–147.

IV

Pathogenetic Mechanisms

19

Cellular Immune Events in the Joints of Patients with Rheumatoid Arthritis

Nathan J. Zvaifler and Richard M. Silver

I. INTRODUCTION

Our understanding of rheumatology in general, and rheumatoid arthritis in particular, owes much to immunologic studies. In the past three decades, as new technologies and concepts emerged, each in turn has been tested in patients with this disease. In the 1950s and 1960s, emphasis was on the antibodies present in the blood, particularly the antibody to IgG known as rheumatoid factor. Later attention shifted to the inflammatory events mediated by antigen–antibody interactions within the articular cavity. These have been described elsewhere and are not dealt with in this chapter (Silver and Zvaifler, 1985; Zvaifler, 1973). Rather, we review the information on cellular immune findings that has accumulated in the last 10 years and, where appropriate, try to relate it to the immunopathogenesis of rheumatoid synovitis.

The division of the immune system into a cellular arm and a humoral arm has a basis in ontogeny and has been useful in understanding the complex processes of the immune response. However, except for contrived animal experiments and rare clinical situations, such a fine distinction between cellular immunity and humoral immunity cannot be made. Rather, the immune response of the host represents the complex interactions of macrophages, T cells, B cells, and null cells. Macrophages and dendritic cells process and/or present antigens to T lymphocytes; in addition, they release mediators, monokines,

Nathan J. Zvaifler • Department of Medicine, School of Medicine, University of California, San Diego, California 92103. *Richard M. Silver* • Department of Medicine, Medical University of South Carolina, Charleston, South Carolina 29403.

that modulate the immune response. T lymphocytes proliferate in response to antigenic stimulation and produce a variety of soluble products termed lymphokines, which, in turn, regulate in either a positive or negative manner the response. T helper cells, either directly or through soluble mediators, interact with B cells, resulting in their proliferation and differentiation into plasma cells and the synthesis of antibody. Suppressor T cells regulate antibody synthesis by interacting with B cells or with T helper cells. Effector T cells may also be regulated by suppressor T cells. Additionally, the immune response may be modulated by antibodies (particularly antiidiotypes), immune complexes, and cytophilic antibodies.

Thus, the normal host's immune response represents a delicate balance, the result of cellular cooperation, and negative feedback control. In rheumatoid arthritis, this delicate balance appears to be disturbed. Many examples of aberrations in the appropriate responses of lymphocytes from the peripheral blood (PBL) of patients with RA could be cited, but in this review we limit the discussion to the cellular immune events within the rheumatoid joint, the primary focus of the intense immune response in rheumatoid arthritis. Whenever possible, these findings are compared to those in other acute and chronic inflammatory joint diseases. Unfortunately, at this time, these important control observations are limited. Finally, an attempt is made at the end of the chapter to relate the findings in the articular cavity to those in the blood of rheumatoid patients.

II. RHEUMATOID SYNOVIAL LINING CELL POPULATIONS

Synovial lining cells from patients with rheumatoid arthritis can be divided into different populations based on their expression of surface antigens detected by monoclonal antibodies, histochemical staining, conventional morphology, and functional capacities such as adherence to glass or plastic and phagocytosis (Burmester *et al.*, 1983; Poulter *et al.*, 1982; Winchester and Burmester, 1981). One population is comprised of cells with features of the monocyte–phagocyte lineage. These cells have on their membranes detectable molecules of Ia (DR), monocyte differentiation antigens, and appear on microscopy as elongated structures with blunt-ended philopodialike processes at one pole of the cell. A second distinctive cell is most often seen in the lining of patients with RA but usually not in other inflammatory joint diseases. It is nonphagocytic, has abundant surface membrane Ia antigen, but lacks Ig Fc receptors or antigens that distinguish monocytes, B cells, T cells, or fibroblast-associated antigens. These cells may be analogous to the murine dendritic cell or the interdigitating cells of the lymph node. The functional importance of this class of cell is discussed in more detail below. Finally, a third population can be identified that expresses surface antigens found primarily on fibroblasts; these cells are nonphagocytic and lack demonstrable Ia antigens or the differentiation antigens of the monocyte lineage. Because of their remarkable proliferative capacity, they may be the cells so frequently reported as "overgrowing" long-term cultures derived from synovial tissue (Burmester *et al.*, 1983). A subset of synovial lining cells, particularly large, round cells with asteroid projections, have receptors for both the Fc portion of IgG and C3 (Theofilopoulos *et al.*, 1980).

III. HISTOPATHOLOGICAL CHARACTERISTICS OF THE MONONUCLEAR CELLS PRESENT BENEATH THE SYNOVIAL LINING AND IN SYNOVIAL EFFUSIONS OF PATIENTS WITH RHEUMATOID ARTHRITIS

Proliferation of the lining cells and intense inflammation in the stroma beneath the lining cells characterize the synovial lesion of rheumatoid arthritis. The type of inflammatory cell depends, in part, on the chronicity of the lesion. In most established cases of rheumatoid synovitis, large numbers of lymphocytes, plasma cells, and macrophages are present below the lining layer, and, occasionally, lymphoid follicles with germinal centers may be seen (Sokoloff, 1985). In fact, in chronic cases, the rheumatoid synovium has been equated to an ectopic lymphoid organ containing antibody-forming cells as well as lymphocytes (Smiley *et al.*, 1968; Ziff, 1974). The synovial fluid and the synovial membrane of acute rheumatoid arthritis may differ from those of chronic cases (Schumacher and Kitridou, 1972). The synovial fluid leukocyte count in early cases tends to be lower, and lymphocytes rather than polymorphonuclear leukocytes may predominate (Gatter and Richmond, 1975; Schumacher and Kitridou, 1972). Occasionally, the synovial effusion may be noninflammatory, but even in such early cases, inflammation of the synovial membrane is present.

In a histopathological study of the earliest findings in rheumatoid synovitis, lymphocytes were found to be the predominant infiltrating cell, but unlike established cases, they were few in number, lymphoid follicles were not seen, and plasma cells were rare (Schumacher and Kitridou, 1972). Both lymphocytes and granulocytes were located perivascularly, and other evidence of small vessel damage such as endothelial cell injury and erythrocyte extravasation was seen. Electron microscopic examination of chronic rheumatoid synovitis has revealed lymphocytes between the endothelium and perivascular cells and, occasionally, within endothelial cells of veins and venules as they emigrate between the blood and the synovial membrane (Kobayashi and Ziff, 1973). In the majority of cases, three types of lymphoid accumulations have been noted within a single synovial specimen: lymphocyte-rich areas, plasma-cell-rich areas, and transitional areas containing a mixture of cell types (Ishikawa and Ziff, 1976). Perivascular lymphocytes stain almost exclusively for α-naphthylacetate esterase (T lymphocytes), whereas α-naphthylacetate-esterase-negative lymphocytes (possibly B lymphocytes) are found in centers of lymphoid follicles surrounded by plasma cells (Konttinen *et al.*, 1981). This architectural arrangement is typical of germinal centers and indicative of T-lymphocyte-dependent B-cell activation. Occasionally, synovial specimens from unequivocal cases of rheumatoid arthritis show only rare lymphocytes, and macrophage/mononuclear cells or fibroblasts predominate (Young *et al.*, 1984).

Proper interpretation of the histopathological findings in rheumatoid arthritis requires care because there are a number of important variables that are seldom addressed in published reports. Little is known about the reproducibility of synovial morphology. Arthroscopically obtained biopsies have obvious limitations, but even surgical specimens may suffer from sampling errors. Also, the normal synovium is known to have a different morphology in various portions of the joint cavity. Furthermore, it is not clear that the histopathology in one joint, such as a knee, is necessarily similar to the synovium taken simultaneously from a wrist or finger joint. In addition, there is scant information on biopsies from the same joint in the same patient taken over time. Thus, it is not known whether a particular pattern, once established, will persist unchanged. Finally, appropriate controls are often lacking. In many investigations of the rheumatoid synovium, the results are compared to membranes derived from normal individuals or patients with osteoarthritis rather than to other chronic inflammatory joint diseases. This is a most important caveat, since the only study that has conscientiously addressed this issue failed to find significant differences among various forms of synovitis (Lindblad *et al.*, 1983).

IV. IMMUNOPATHOLOGICAL ANALYSIS OF THE MONONUCLEAR CELLS PRESENT BENEATH THE SYNOVIAL LINING AND IN SYNOVIAL EFFUSIONS OF PATIENTS WITH RHEUMATOID ARTHRITIS

Although the predominance of any one cell type may vary from one area of the synovial membrane to another, the majority of lymphocytes in the synovium and the synovial fluid are T lymphocytes. Studies of lymphocytes eluted from rheumatoid synovial membrane by enzymatic digestion with DNAase and collagenase have shown that 70–95% of the lymphocytes are T cells, as defined by the formation of rosettes with sheep erythrocytes (E-rosettes) (Abrahamsen *et al.*, 1975; Bankhurst *et al.*, 1976; Meijer *et al.*, 1980; van Boxel and Paget, 1975). Indirect immunofluorescent staining and histochemical staining have confirmed the predominance of T lymphocytes. Studies of synovial fluid lymphocytes have also demonstrated a preponderance of E-rosette-forming cells, usually higher than that of matched or control peripheral blood (Brenner *et al.*, 1975; Dorwart *et al.*, 1975; Froland *et al.*, 1973; Sheldon *et al.*, 1974; Vernon-Roberts *et al.*, 1974; Winchester *et al.*, 1974). Early observations of these synovial fluid T lymphocytes suggested that they might be activated, based on their tendency to form multiple and dense rosettes with sheep erythrocytes (Galili *et al.*, 1979). Subsequent studies have confirmed these observations (*vide infra*).

Initially there were reports of increased percentages of B lymphocytes in synovial fluid. These probably resulted from a failure to recognize that all cells staining for surface immunoglobulin are not B cells. Antilymphocyte antibodies or rheumatoid factor and IgG-containing immune complexes, which may adhere to mononuclear cells via their Fc receptors, give a similar appearance (Winchester *et al.*, 1974). Since these factors have been taken into account, most investigators have found the percentage of B lymphocytes to be lower in synovial fluid than in peripheral blood (Froland *et al.*, 1973; Meijer *et al.*, 1980; Sheldon *et al.*, 1974; van Boxel and Paget, 1975; Winchester *et al.*, 1974). The presence of reduced numbers of B cells in synovial fluid or synovial eluates may reflect the decreased tendency of B cells to recirculate or the rapid transformation of B lymphocytes to plasma cells within the synovial membrane. When tissue sections are compared with synovial eluates, both plasma cells and B lymphocytes appear to be lost during the elution procedure (Konttinen *et al.*, 1981).

A third population of lymphoid cells that bears no surface immunoglobulin or receptors for sheep erythrocytes has been identified in synovial fluid. Such cells have been designated null cells. One group of investigators found an increase in null cells in synovial fluid from patients with rheumatoid arthritis and other inflammatory joint diseases (Dorwart *et al.*, 1975). Another study found up to 32% of rheumatoid synovial fluid lymphocytes to be null cells (Winchester *et al.*, 1974). Many had receptors for aggregated IgG, and the majority were small lymphocytes. Included within this third population of lymphocytes may be those cells that mediate antibody-dependent cellular cytotoxicity (ADCC) and nonspecific cellular cytotoxicity or natural killing (NK).

Macrophages and cells with a dendritic appearance (long, stellate processes) are the major nonlymphoid cells present beneath the synovial lining of rheumatoid arthritis patients. Mononuclear phagocytes containing lysozyme or α-naphthyl esterase comprise 5–15% of cells in rheumatoid synovial sections or eluates and are diffusely distributed. They are rare in germinal centers (Klareskog *et al.*, 1982a; Konttinen *et al.*, 1981) but are often seen in close contact with T lymphocytes and lymphoblasts of the suppressor/cytotoxic phenotype (Kurosaka and Ziff, 1983). Dendritic-appearing cells are claimed to be prominent in rheumatoid synovial tissue but are infrequently found in synovium from normal individuals or patients with osteoarthritis (Janossy *et al.*, 1981). These stellate-appearing cells are nonlymphoid, nonphagocytic cells. Because of their similarity to the interdigitating cells in lymph nodes or the dendritic cells in blood described by Steinman, they are believed to have a principal role in antigen presentation (Van Voorhis *et al.*, 1983b). There is evidence (*vide infra*) that macrophages play an important role in the biochemical and immunologic processes that characterize the rheumatoid synovium, but the true contribution of dendritic cells will not be known until specific markers for this cell become available.

The development of monoclonal antibodies that can recognize unique cell surface differentiation antigens has allowed further characterization of the lymphocyte subpopulations present in rheumatoid synovium and synovial fluids. Those most commonly employed include antibodies of the OKT and Leu series, which are said to define populations with specific functional capacities; i.e., helper/inducer T lymphocytes have the T4/Leu 3a phenotype, and T8/Leu 2a identifies a cytotoxic/suppressor population. It is important to recognize, however, that function and phenotype are not always equatable. For instance, under certain circumstances, T4/Leu 3a lymphocytes can act as suppressor cells, and cells carrying virus antigens associated with class II MHC antigens can be killed by syngeneic T4 lymphocytes. This caveat may be particularly relevant to the findings in rheumatoid arthritis synovial tissues because studies of isolated synovial fluid lymphocytes suggest a dissociation between function and phenotype (Romain *et al.*, 1982).

Studies with the OKT3 and Leu 4 reagents confirmed that the majority of cells in the rheumatoid synovium are T lymphocytes. Many of the T cells are activated, as shown by expression of Ia or other differentiation antigens. In normal peripheral blood, there are approximately twice as many T4/Leu 3a-bearing T lymphocytes as $T8^+$/Leu 2a cells, but in the rheumatoid synovial membrane a disproportionate percentage of cells show the helper/inducer phenotype, ranging from 4 : 1 to 14 : 1 (Forre *et al.*, 1982c; Janossy *et al.*, 1980; Klareskog *et al.*, 1982b; Malone *et al.*, 1983; Meijer *et al.*, 1982; Young *et al.*, 1984). Very few studies disagree with these findings, but there is considerable divergence of opinion concerning their distribution.

Normally, subpopulations of lymphocytes occupy different microenvironments *in vivo*. For instance, T4 cells are predominant in thymic medulla, blood, tonsillar paracortex, and intestinal lamina propria. T8 cells are mainly located in bone marrow and gut epithelium. In the paracortical area of normal lymph nodes, where antibody-producing B cells are located, T4 lymphocytes are found in juxtaposition to cells that are dendritic in appearance and express strong surface staining with monoclonal antibody to the HLA-DR determinants and stain for membrane ATPase. In rheumatoid arthritis, the synovium often shows a lymphocytic infiltrate with similar phenotypic features, especially in areas with lymphoid follicles or germinal centers (Kurosaka and Ziff, 1983; Meijer *et al.*, 1982; Young *et al.*, 1984). In contrast to the lymph node, where $T8^+$ cells (suppressor/cytotoxic T lymphocytes) are interspersed among the interdigitating cells and the helper/inducer cells, in rheumatoid arthritis the $T8^+$ population is scanty and located peripherally (Forre *et al.*, 1982c; Kurosaka and Ziff, 1983). This had led Janossy and others to propose that in these lymphoid aggregates, dendritic cells are presenting extrinsic or autologous antigen to T helper cells, inducing their proliferation and activation; these, in turn, stimulate B cells to immunoglobulin synthesis. The absence or exclusion of $T8^+$ cells results in the failure of suppressor systems to control this immunostimulatory process (Gatenby and Engleman, 1981; Janossy *et al.*, 1981).

This attractive hypothesis requires that the above-described morphological features be a regular finding in the rheumatoid synovium. Indeed, some workers find this to be the case. Others, however, report that in biopsies from certain patients the lymphocyte populations in areas that lack lymphoid aggregates show T4 and T8 cells interspersed in about equal numbers (Lindblad *et al.*, 1983; Malone *et al.*, 1983; Young *et al.*, 1984). These differences could be explained by sampling errors, but Young *et al.* claim that the patterns in individual patients with rheumatoid arthritis are reproducible and unrelated to other clinical or laboratory parameters (Young *et al.*, 1984). In their study, the supposed typical lymphoid aggregates with well-defined germinal centers—clusters of B cells surrounded by $T4^+$ cells—was only noted in a minority of the patients (Fig. 1). More commonly, T-lymphocyte infiltrates were diffuse and lacked germinal centers (Fig. 2). In some rheumatoid patients, the synovial membranes display a bland appearance with cellular constituents that are almost exclusively synovial fibroblasts, some of which stain with antibody to HLA-DR, and few T cells are present (Fig. 3). Confirmation of the existence of distinctive patterns unique to individual patients would imply that different immunopathogenetic mechanisms may be operating in rheumatoid arthritis.

Natural killer cells are sparse in rheumatoid synovial tissues (Lindblad *et al.*, 1983; Young *et al.*, 1984). Some recent observations suggest that this class of cells may serve to regulate immunoglobulin production (Arai *et al.*, 1983). If these conclusions are correct, their absence could provide an alternative explanation for the exuberant antibody production in the rheumatoid joint.

Compared to the synovial membrane, the analysis of mononuclear cells in rheumatoid synovial fluid is less contentious. In most instances, $T8^+$/Leu 2a lymphocyte populations are increased or comparable to companion blood samples, whereas OKT4/Leu 3a are normal or depressed, with the result that the percentage ratio of helper/inducer to suppressor/cytotoxic cells is lower in synovial fluid than in blood (Duclos *et al.*, 1982; Duke *et al.*, 1983; Fox *et al.*, 1982). This pattern, however, is not unique to patients with rheumatoid arthritis and has been found in most effusions from chronic inflammatory arthritides such as ankylosing spondylitis, nonrheumatoid forms of JRA, and psoriatic arthropathy (Duclos *et al.*, 1982; Nilsson and Biberfeld, 1982). Indeed, Nilsson and Biberfeld found that in acute nonseptic synovitis with duration less than 1 month, the ratio of Leu $3a^+$ to Leu $2a^+$ cells was higher in synovial fluid (4.0) than in blood (1.9), whereas in chronic synovitis (both RA and non-RA), the ratio was significantly lower in

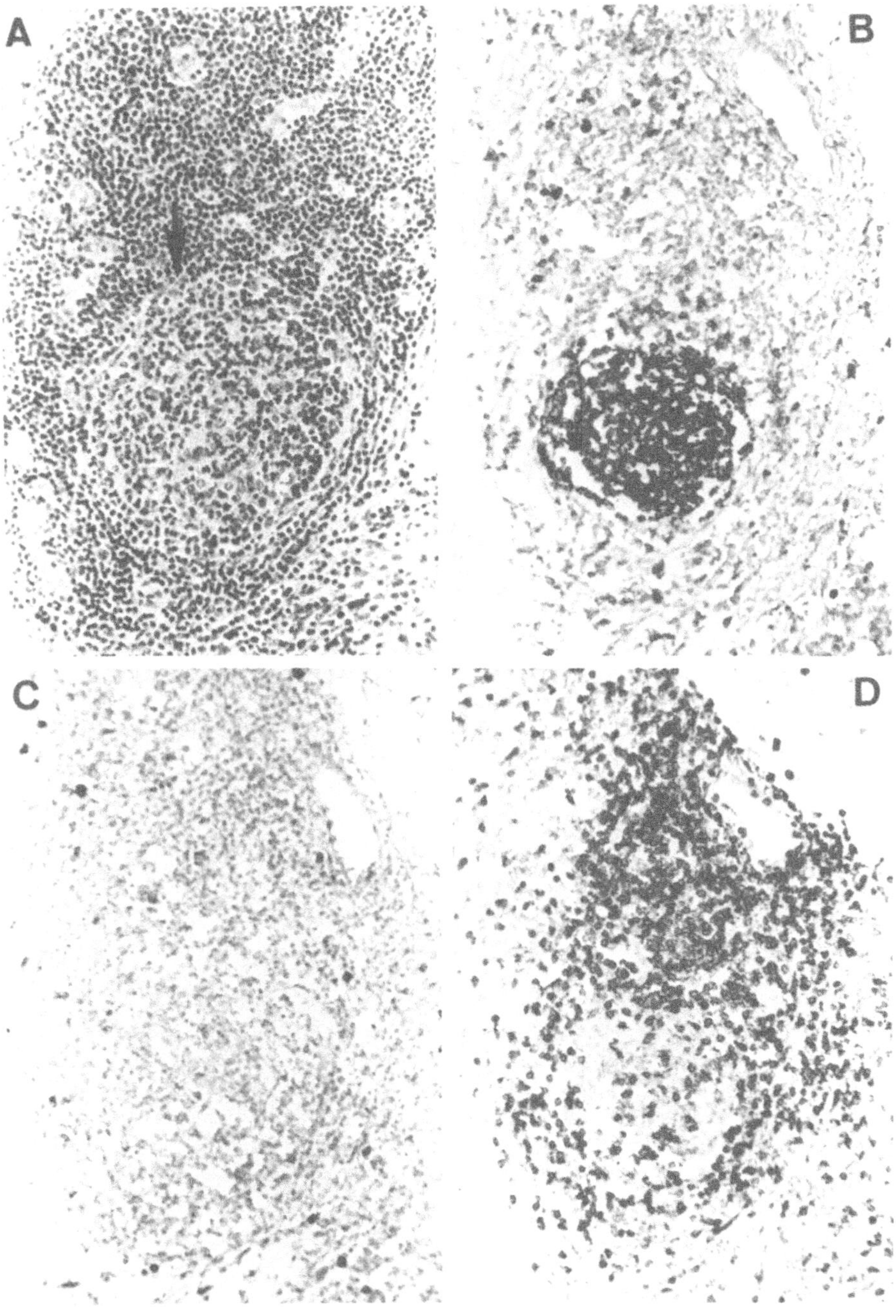

Figure 1. Serial tissue sections of rheumatoid arthritis synovial membrane showing a germinal center pattern (arrow) as detected by hematoxylin–eosin stain (frame A) or immunoperoxidase staining for B cells (frame B) or T cells (frame D). A control using an irrelevant antibody is shown in frame C. (magnification ×50; from Young *et al.*, 1984.)

the effusions (1.1) than in companion blood samples (2.2) (Nilsson and Biberfeld, 1983). These findings suggest that the distribution of T-lymphocyte subsets in synovial fluid may be more related to the duration of synovitis than to its etiology.

In normal peripheral blood, the percentage of Ia^+ T lymphocytes is quite low (<3%). Increased numbers of Ia^+ T lymphocytes are found in the peripheral blood of patients with systemic lupus erythematosus, certain infectious diseases, and following immunization (Yu *et al.*, 1980). Several groups have found increased numbers of Ia^+ T lym-

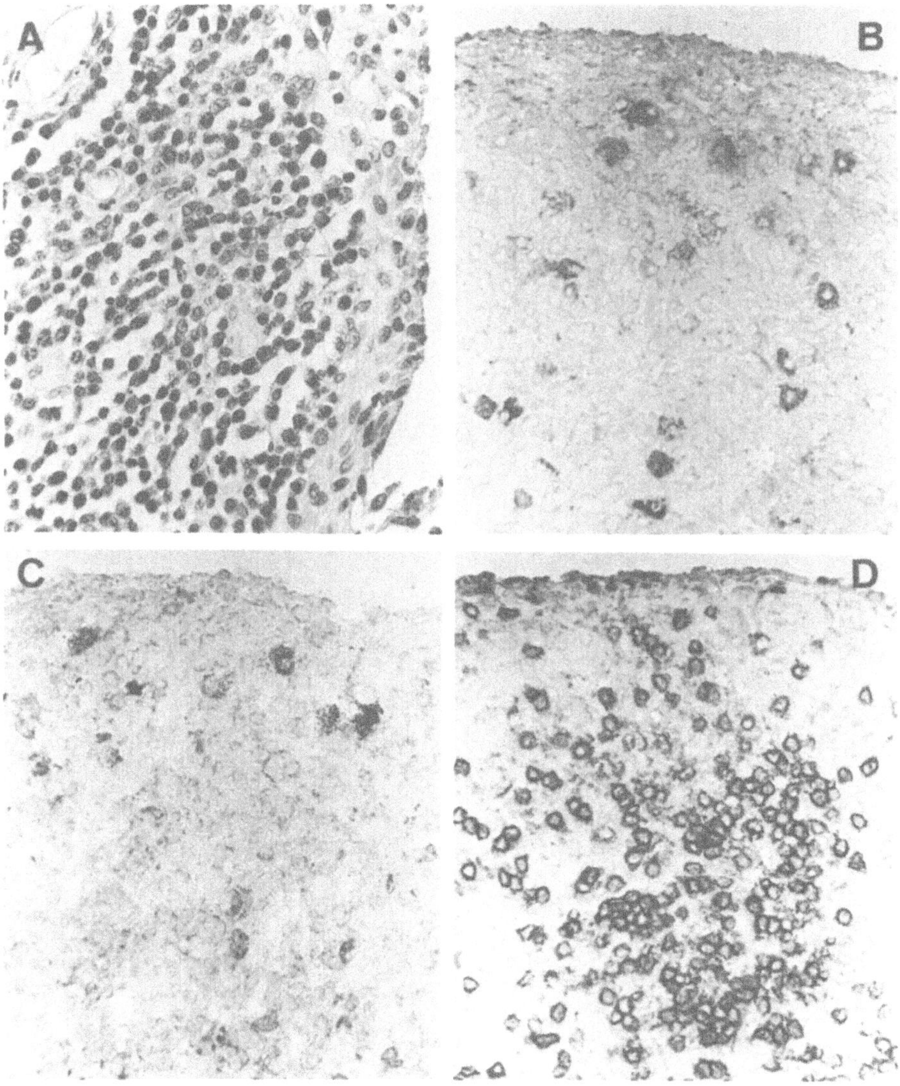

Figure 2. Serial tissue sections of rheumatoid arthritis synovial membrane showing a diffuse T-cell pattern (arrow) as detected by hematoxylin–eosin stain (frame A) or immunoperoxidase staining for B cells (frame B) or T cells (frame D). A control using an irrelevant antibody is shown in frame C. (magnification ×50; from Young *et al.*, 1984).

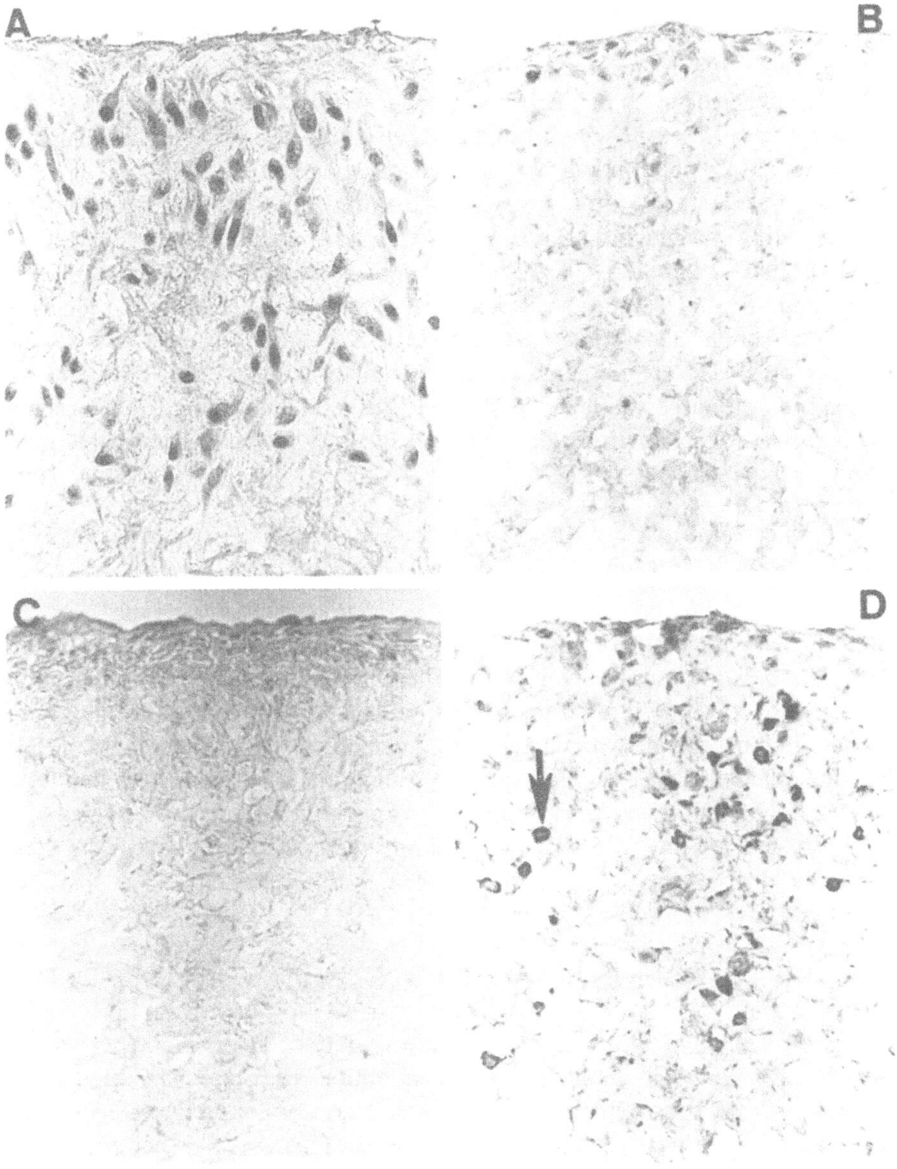

Figure 3. A pattern showing only rare mononuclear cells. Serial tissue sections of rheumatoid arthritis synovial membrane showing only rare mononuclear cells (arrow) as detected by hematoxylin–eosin stain (frame A) or immunoperoxidase staining for B cells (frame B) or T cells (frame D). A control using an irrelevant antibody is shown in frame C. (magnification ×50; from Young *et al.*, 1984.)

phocytes in the peripheral blood of rheumatoid arthritis patients, averaging 15% of the T lymphocytes (Fox *et al.*, 1982, 1983; Yu *et al.*, 1980). The Ia molecules are not merely adsorbed to the T cell surface but are actively synthesized (Pincus *et al.*, 1985). The origin of the circulating Ia^+ T lymphocytes is unknown, but they might come from the synovium, where an average of 40% of the T lymphocytes are Ia^+ (Burmester *et al.*,

1981; Fox *et al.*, 1983; Klareskog *et al.*, 1981; Yu *et al.*, 1980). Similar increases have been noted in the T cells of synovial fluid (Burmester *et al.*, 1981; Forre *et al.*, 1982a; Fox *et al.*, 1982, 1983; Klareskog *et al.*, 1981). Various investigators have found either T4 or T8 lymphocytes to be Ia^+ (Burmester *et al.*, 1981; Meijer *et al.*, 1982). This may reflect sampling differences, or, as suggested by a recent study, activated Ia^+ T lymphocytes may display both phenotypes (Pincus *et al.*, 1985).

As noted above, the normal synovium contains only a few nonlymphoid cells that are Ia^+, including synovial lining cells, endothelial cells, and a few dendritic cells (Janossy *et al.*, 1981; Klareskog *et al.*, 1981; Lindblad *et al.*, 1983). In the rheumatoid synovium, most synovial lining cells are Ia^+, as are the macrophages, and there is a great increase in the number of Ia^+ dendritic appearing cells. The latter are especially abundant in perivascular areas and are frequently in close contact with Ia^+ $T4^+$ lymphocytes. The significance of the large numbers of cells in the joint displaying HLA-D antigens is obvious, given the essential role of these molecules in effective interaction among immunocompetent cells.

V. FUNCTIONAL CHARACTERISTICS OF RHEUMATOID SYNOVIAL MONONUCLEAR CELLS

The state of activity of the cellular constituents of the rheumatoid synovium may be inferred from *in vitro* assays as well as from the phenotypic studies described above. The ability of lymphocytes to proliferate when stimulated by antigens or lectins, to enhance or suppress immunoglobulin production, or to elaborate various factors are all indicative of their functional status. A demonstration of abnormal or exaggerated activity may be relevant to the initiation and perpetuation of rheumatoid inflammation. Once again, the discussion focuses on the cells and the cellular products that occur within the rheumatoid joint.

VI. CYTOKINES (LYMPHOKINES AND MONOKINES)

Cytokines are soluble factors that influence the activity of other cells. Lymphokines and monokines are biologically active nonimmunoglobulin mediators elaborated by lymphocytes and monocyte–macrophages, respectively. They are not produced by resting cells; rather, they are indicative of cell activation or sensitization. Several such soluble products have been isolated from rheumatoid synovial fluids and the supernatants of rheumatoid synovial tissue explants. More than a decade ago macrophage migration inhibition factor (MIF) was shown to be produced by synovial tissue explants from rabbits with antigen-induced arthritis and was found in human joint diseases as well. Migration inhibition factor was present in synovial fluids from 18 of 22 rheumatoid arthritis patients compared with four of 11 other inflammatory synovial fluids and three of 15 osteoarthritis synovial fluids (Stastny *et al.*, 1973, 1975). The same investigators identified two additional substances in most rheumatoid arthritis effusions and in a limited number of osteoarthritis synovial fluids: lymphocyte blastogenic factor, which stimulates proliferation of mouse spleen cells, and a B-cell-stimulating factor, which causes human peripheral blood lymphocytes to synthesize immunoglobulin (Stastny *et al.*, 1975).

Since these early observations, knowledge of the biology and chemistry of cytokines and growth and differentiation factors has expanded dramatically. The sequential interaction of these interleukins ("the lymphokine cascade") is central to the regulation of immunocompetent cells (Oppenheim *et al.*, 1982; Robb, 1984; Smith, 1980). Interleukin 1 (IL-1), a lymphocyte activation factor derived from macrophage/mononuclear cells, provides a necessary signal along with antigen to stimulate the resting T cell. Once activated, T cells elaborate a variety of soluble mediators, including IL-2 (T-cell growth factor), and display cell surface receptors for this growth factor. The engagement of these receptors leads to the proliferation and expansion of both non-antigen- and antigen-specific lymphocytes. Simultaneously, there is the production of factors that control the growth and differentiation of B lymphocytes.

Given the purported immunologic hyperactivity of the rheumatoid joint, it is not surprising that such factors are being found in the synovium or synovial fluid. Small amounts of IL-1 have been identified in RA effusions (Fontana *et al.*, 1982; Nouri *et al.*, 1984; Wood *et al.*, 1983), but similar amounts were also found in fluid from a variety of other joint disease (Fontana *et al.*, 1982; Nouri *et al.*, 1984). Interleukin 1 appears to be the mediator that stimulates the production of collagenase and prostaglandin E_2 by cultured synovial cells and therefore plays a central role in joint destruction (Dayer *et al.*, 1977; Mizel *et al.*, 1981). So far, the exact source of the lymphokine found in synovial fluid has not been determined, since IL-1 can be elaborated by either macrophages or synoviocytes. Both IL-2 and a B-cell growth factor (BCGF) are found in RA effusions (Wilkins *et al.*, 1983). The latter was characterized as a heat-stable 50,000-dalton protein with properties similar to murine BCGF-2 (Cohen *et al.*, 1984). To date, there have been no reports of B-cell differentiation factors in synovial fluids.

Another lymphocyte-derived factor found in synovial fluid that may be important in the pathogenesis of rheumatoid arthritis is a lymphokine capable of suppressing the synthesis of protein and glycosaminoglycans. This factor could explain the suppressed proteoglycan synthesis observed in the antigen-induced experimental model of arthritis and thought to be an early event in cartilage injury (Herman *et al.*, 1981; Lowther *et al.*, 1978).

Explants of rheumatoid synovial tissues spontaneously produce a number of different moieties including blastogenic factors, LIF, and mediators that stimulate the production of collagen and prostaglandin E_2 by cultured synovial cells (Chin *et al.*, 1984; Stastny *et al.*, 1975). γ-Interferon (γ-IFN), an important immunoregulatory lymphokine, was not detectable in supernatants from these synovial explants. This is somewhat surprising, given the fact that activated lymphocytes and natural killer cells are capable of producing γ-IFN and material, with the characteristics of immune interferon has been demonstrated in serum and synovial fluid samples from some patients with RA and other chronic inflammatory joint diseases (Cesario *et al.*, 1983; DeGrere *et al.*, 1983; Husby and Williams, 1984). Husby and Williams were likewise impressed that immunofluorescent staining for IL-2 and γ-IFN in inflamed rheumatoid synovial tissue was weak, especially when compared to other antigens such as OKT4, Ia, and late-acting complement components (Husby and Williams, 1984). These findings are consistent with studies suggesting that RA lymphocytes are defective in their ability to produce these important immunoregulatory molecules (Alcocer-Varela *et al.*, 1984; Combe *et al.*, 1985; Hasler *et al.*, 1983). A paucity of IL-2 in the articular cavity might favor the helper/inducer T cell population, since they can exert their influence without proliferations, whereas suppressor/cytotoxic cells, which need to be expanded to exert an effect, would be less efficient. The net result might be excessive local immunoglobulin production.

VII. LYMPHOCYTE PROLIFERATIVE RESPONSES

Lymphocytes from the blood of patients with rheumatoid arthritis have been subjected to an intense analysis of their cellular function. The results in the simplest models (i.e., the proliferative response of peripheral blood lymphocytes (PBL) to mitogens such as phytohemagglutinin (PHA), which activates all T-cell subsets; or to pokeweed mitogen (PWM), which activates both T and B cells) are generally reported to be normal or slightly depressed. A more striking diminution in the proliferative responses of PBL to concanavalin A (Con A), a mitogen that only stimulates a subpopulation of T cells, is a fairly constant finding (Bluestein, 1984). This apparent defect may not reflect an intrinsic T-cell immune dysfunction, however, since RA serum appears to selectively inhibit the mitogenic response to Con A. Furthermore, there are antilymphocyte antibodies in rheumatoid serum that have enhanced cytotoxic activity against Con-A-activated lymphocytes (Siebert *et al.*, 1978).

Allogeneic lymphoid cells are also potent stimulators of T cells. The antigens provoking the mixed lymphocyte reaction (MLR) are cell membrane molecules coded by genes in the major histocompatibility complex at or near the D locus. T cells from patients with rheumatoid arthritis generally respond near normally in the MLR when the stimulating cells are derived from normal donors, and RA lymphoid cells stimulate normal responses in T cells from healthy subjects (Bluestein, 1984). However, in the autologous mixed lymphocyte reaction in which stimulators and responders from the same individual are recombined *in vitro,* RA T cells show a significantly lower proliferation than do cells from healthy control subjects (Pope *et al.*, 1984; Smith and DeHoratius, 1982). This impairment does not appear to be caused by serum factors but may relate to inability of RA blood T cells to produce or respond to IL-2 (Pope *et al.*, 1984).

Synovial fluid lymphocytes (SFL) usually show an increased spontaneous incorporation of tritiated thymidine but give poor proliferative responses compared with paired PBL (Burmester *et al.*, 1978; Corrigall *et al.*, 1979; Hepburn *et al.*, 1976; Ivanyi *et al.*, 1973; Panayi, 1973; Rawson and Huang, 1974; Reynolds and Abdou, 1973; Sheldon *et al.*, 1974; Silver *et al.*, 1983; Silverman *et al.*, 1976; Stratton and Peter, 1978). The decreased responsiveness of SFL is not caused by factors present in the synovial fluid, as T lymphocytes eluted from synovial tissue also proliferate poorly, and exposure of blood lymphocytes to synovial fluid does not diminish their responsiveness (Abrahamsen *et al.*, 1977; Holborow *et al.*, 1975; Meijer *et al.*, 1980; Petersen *et al.*, 1983; Stratton and Peter, 1978). Neither can the poor response of SFL be explained by an inability to bind lectins, nor does it appear to result from a suppressive mechanism, because the addition of SFL to PBL does not inhibit the proliferative response to PHA, as one might expect if SFL contained a suppressor cell (Holborow *et al.*, 1975; Silver *et al.*, 1983). Finally, a lack of T lymphocytes is not the explanation, since, as noted above, there is an increased percentage of T lymphocytes in synovial fluid compared to blood.

Recent studies indicate that the poor response of rheumatoid SFL may be caused, at least in part by insufficient production of IL-2 (TCGF), since this lymphokine has been shown to be obligatory for the expansion of lectin- or antigen-activated T cells (Robb, 1984; Smith, 1980). In experiments in which IL-2 was added to cultures of rheumatoid SFL, the proliferative response to PHA was partially restored, whereas addition of TCGF to PBL had no significant effect in most cases (Silver *et al.*, 1983). In these studies, the insufficient endogenous production of IL-2 could not be related to drugs, although corticosteroids are known to influence T-cell proliferation by diminishing TCGF production. Nor could the fault be passive adsorption or specific binding of the growth factor by IL-2 receptors on "activated" synovial T cells. Impaired IL-2 production was reported by Combe *et al.*, who also showed that both rheumatoid synovial and blood lymphocytes produced less γ-IFN when treated with IL-2 than did normal blood lymphocytes (Combe *et al.*, 1985). These findings are of interest when coupled with the unexpectedly low levels of these same lymphokines in rheumatoid synovium (*vide supra*). Their true significance, however, awaits the demonstration that they are unique to RA and not merely a consequence of chronic articular inflammation.

VIII. SUPPRESSOR CELL ACTIVITY

The rheumatoid synovium is the site of synthesis of large amounts of immunoglobulin, much of which has rheumatoid factor activity (Sliwinski and Zvaifler, 1970; Smiley *et al.*, 1968). Although the primary stimulus for this polyclonal response is unknown, it has been suggested that perpetuation of the immune response may be the result of a defect in normal immunoregulation. For example, a failure to generate suppressor T lymphocytes might result in unbridled B-cell activity and the formation of autoantibodies. Alternatively, the presence of suppressor T lymphocytes that interfered with the generation of an effective cell-mediated immune response might result in persistent antigenic stimulation and its attendant immunologic consequences.

Studies of nonspecific suppressor cell activity have shown either normal or depressed levels in rheumatoid peripheral blood (Abdou *et al.*, 1981; Bluestein, 1984; Dobloug *et al.*, 1981). In the limited investigations with rheumatoid synovial lymphocytes, suppressor cell function seems to be decreased. Taking advantage of the selective radiosensitivity of suppressor T cells, Biberfeld *et al.* determined the ability of synovial T cells to suppress B-cell differentiation (Biberfeld *et al.*, 1980). They found no enhancement of pokeweed-mitogen-induced immunoglobulin production after irradiation of synovial fluid lymphocytes, suggesting a lack of suppressor activity. Others have confirmed the inability of synovial fluid and synovial-tissue-derived T cells to suppress B-cell differentiation (Chattopadhyay *et al.*, 1979; Romain *et al.*, 1982).

The capacity of synovial T cells to suppress mitogen-induced T-cell proliferation has also been studied. Cells eluted from rheumatoid synovial tissue lacked suppressor activity in a Con-A-activated suppressor system (Chattopadhyay *et al.*, 1979; Romain *et al.*, 1982). In fact, cocultures of Con-A-stimulated synovial T cells with normal allogeneic PBL resulted in an augmented blastogenic response. These data must be interpreted with caution, however, because the generation of Con A suppressor cells requires cell division, and it is well established that synovial T lymphocytes respond poorly to Con A (Burmester *et al.*, 1978; Haynes and Fauci, 1977; Lipsky *et al.*, 1978; Meijer *et al.*, 1980; Stratton and Peter, 1978). Moreover, the augmentation of blastogenesis by synovial T cells, many of which are Ia^+, may reflect an allogeneic MLR rather than deficient suppressor cell activity. And finally, this particular assay measures allogeneic suppressor cell activity and may not be applicable to immune responses occurring within the rheumatoid joint. It is worth pointing out, however, that one type of T suppressor cell that inhibits the MLR in man is controlled by genes in the HLA-D region (Engleman and McDevitt, 1978; McMichael and Sasazuki, 1977). In view of the synovial mononuclear cell MLR data discussed below, and the findings that suggest that MLR-activated suppressor cells inhibit immunoglobulin synthesis (James *et al.*, 1981), the failure to generate such an MLR suppressor cell might be an important determinant of the persistent immune response within the synovium.

Using a purely autologous system, Romain *et al.* found that synovial T lymphocytes, when cocultured with peripheral blood T and B lymphocytes, not only lacked suppressor activity but actually caused an enhancement of mitogen-stimulated immunoglobulin production (Romain *et al.*, 1982). The absence of enhanced suppression in cocultures of synovial and blood T cells suggests that the synovial T-cell suppressor defect is not caused by an absence of the suppressor–inducer $T4^+$ subset. It implies that the abnormality resides in the $T8^+$ population. Thus, synovial fluid T lymphocytes are discordant in terms of phenotype and function. Although they display the $T8^+$ suppressor/cytotoxic cell phenotype, they lack suppressor activity, and they actually augment helper cell activity when cocultured with peripheral blood lymphocytes. A similar augmentation of helper activity was observed in a plaque-forming assay when T cells taken from AMLR cultures at the end of 1 week were added to a mixture of T and B cells (Y. Konttinen and A. Cohen, unpublished data).

IX. MIXED LYMPHOCYTE REACTIVITY

Synovial fluid T cells respond poorly to both allogeneic and autologous non-T cells. The autologous mixed lymphocyte reaction (MLR) is of particular interest because it possesses the features of an immunologic reaction (i.e., memory and specificity), and through the generation of immunoregulatory cells and factors is thought to play an important role in modulating the immune response. Moreover, it has been proposed to be a significant factor in rheumatoid synovial inflammation (Gatenby and Engleman, 1981; Janossy *et al.*, 1981; Silver *et al.*, 1983).

The reason for the impaired response of rheumatoid synovial fluid T lymphocytes to autologous non-T-cell stimulation has not been determined (Beck *et al.*, 1981; Forre *et al.*, 1982b; Romain *et al.*, 1982; Silver *et al.*, 1983). Suppressor cells are not at fault (Romain *et al.*, 1982; Silver *et al.*, 1983), but it may result from a lack of adequate helper cells or factors such as IL-2. This in turn may be a reflection of an altered proportion of IL-2-producing cells, since the major source of this interleukin is T4 cells (Smolen *et al.*, 1981), which are underrepresented in inflammatory synovial fluids. Repetitive stimulation (two or three cycles) of normal peripheral blood T lymphocytes with autologous non-T cells results in an activated state analogous to that of the rheumatoid synovial lymphocyte; i.e., poor responsiveness to further stimulation, which can be only partially restored with exogenous IL-2 (Silver *et al.*, 1983). A similar situation is seen following activation of T cells with lectins such as PHA or antigen. After maximal proliferation, the cells no longer respond to supraoptimal concentrations of IL-2 because of down-regulation of their IL-2 receptors. Exposure of the unresponsive cell to mitogen or antigen leads to reexpression of the IL-2 receptor and ability to proliferate (Robb, 1984). The presence in rheumatoid synovial effusions of activated NK-like cells and a discrepancy between T-cell phenotype and function are other features that can be reproduced by an *in vitro* AMLR culture (Goto and Zvaifler, 1984a). Thus, the suggestion that the cellular defects observed in the joints of patients with rheumatoid arthritis are caused by a continuous exposure to an autologous antigen is attractive.

Although synovial T cells give only minimal autologous responses, the non-T-cell population has remarkable stimulatory potential. In a number of studies, synovial fluid mononuclear cells (SFM) have been shown to stimulate peripheral blood lymphocytes in an AMLR and activate autologous peripheral blood T lymphocytes to a functional state resembling synovial T lymphocytes (Beck *et al.*, 1981; Crout *et al.*, 1976; Galili *et al.*, 1981; Petersen *et al.*, 1983; Silver *et al.*, 1983). Moreover, when rheumatoid SF non-T cells were compared to rheumatoid PB non-T cells for their ability to cause proliferation of autologous T lymphocytes, they proved to be severalfold better stimulators (Silver *et al.*, 1983).

The antigen responsible for the AMLR proliferation remains a matter of dispute. The idea that the reaction is merely a laboratory artifact resulting from exposure to xenoantigens (i.e., sheep erythrocytes in fetal calf serum) used in the isolation of responder and stimulator populations is no longer tenable (Holborow *et al.*, 1975). Pristine T cells can be prepared, and autoreactive T-cell clones exist, that respond to autologous stimuli (Bensussan *et al.*, 1984; Naides *et al.*, 1984). One thing that is clear, however, is the need for Ia-like determinants, because antibody to Ia blocks the autologous MLR (Gottlieb *et al.*, 1979; Huber *et al.*, 1982; Yu *et al.*, 1980). Synovial fluids contain a number of cells that are rich in Ia and thus are candidates to explain this enhanced stimulation. For instance, 20 to 40% of the T cells have Ia^+ on their surface, and Ia-bearing T cells can cause proliferation of autologous T cells (Damle and Gupta, 1982; Forre *et al.*, 1982b).

B cells ordinarily have some surface Ia, but activated B cells display even more, and B lymphocytes infected with Epstein–Barr virus (EBV) show the greatest density of Ia molecules (Bensussan *et al.*, 1984). Evidence that some B cells in rheumatoid effusions may be activated is provided by the observation of increased numbers of spontaneous plaque-forming cells. In addition, there are greater numbers of B cells containing EBV among the lymphocytes from RA effusions than in B cells from other inflammatory joint fluids (McClurg *et al.*, 1983). This need not imply an *in situ* infection; indeed, it seems more likely that EBV-bearing B cells from the circulation regularly traffic through the articular cavity, but for unknown reasons the rheumatoid joint provides a more supportive environment for their growth or retention. In any case, EBV-infected B cells can provoke an unusually intense and prolonged AMLR (Konttinen *et al.*, 1984a; Palacios, 1982).

Some investigators believe that the most potent stimulator of mixed leukocyte reactions is a unique leukocyte with a dendritic appearance (Van Voorhis *et al.*, 1983a). The dendritic cell (DC) differs from a conventional macrophage by being nonphagocytic and lacking surface Fc receptors and cytoplasmic enzymes such as ATPase, nonspecific esterase, and myeloperoxidase (Van Voorhis *et al.*, 1983b). Dendritic cells and macrophages show none of the surface differentiation markers of B, T, and NK cells, but each expresses class I and class II products of the major histocompatibility complex. Although there are a number of macrophage-specific monoclonal antibodies, none have been shown to react with DC. Unfortunately, at least in man, there are no DC-specific monoclonal antibodies, so identification is based primarily on their ability to stimulate mitogenesis and the absence of distinguishing phenotypic markers (Van Voorhis *et al.*, 1983b).

An analysis of the rheumatoid AMLR stimulator population reveals that synovial fluid mononuclear cells can provoke a severalfold greater mitogenic response than companion blood cells (Zvaifler *et al.*, 1985). Treatment of the synovial fluid monocytes with complement and antibodies to macrophage, T-cell, or B-cell surface antigens enhances rather than decreases the proliferative response, which can be eliminated by complement lysis of the synovial stimulators with anti-Ia antibodies. More than 85% of the rheumatoid synovial fluid mononuclear cells are lysed by a mixture of antimacrophage, anti-T-cell, and anti-B-cell monoclonal antibodies and complement. The residual DC-appearing cells (Fig. 4) can be phenotyped or analyzed by electron microscopy. Morphologically, they appear to have a large, irregularly shaped nucleus. Their cytoplasm contains many mitochondria, but lacks the lysosomes and endocytic vacuoles that characterize macrophages (Zvaifler *et al.*, 1985). When studied by indirect immunofluorescence, the synovial fluid DC cells are $OKT3^-$, $OKT6^-$, $BA1^-$, and lack macrophage surface antigens. Their most characteristic feature is very strong immunofluorescence with anti-class-II (Ia) reagents. Based on immunofluorescent analysis and morphology, it is estimated that DCs constitute

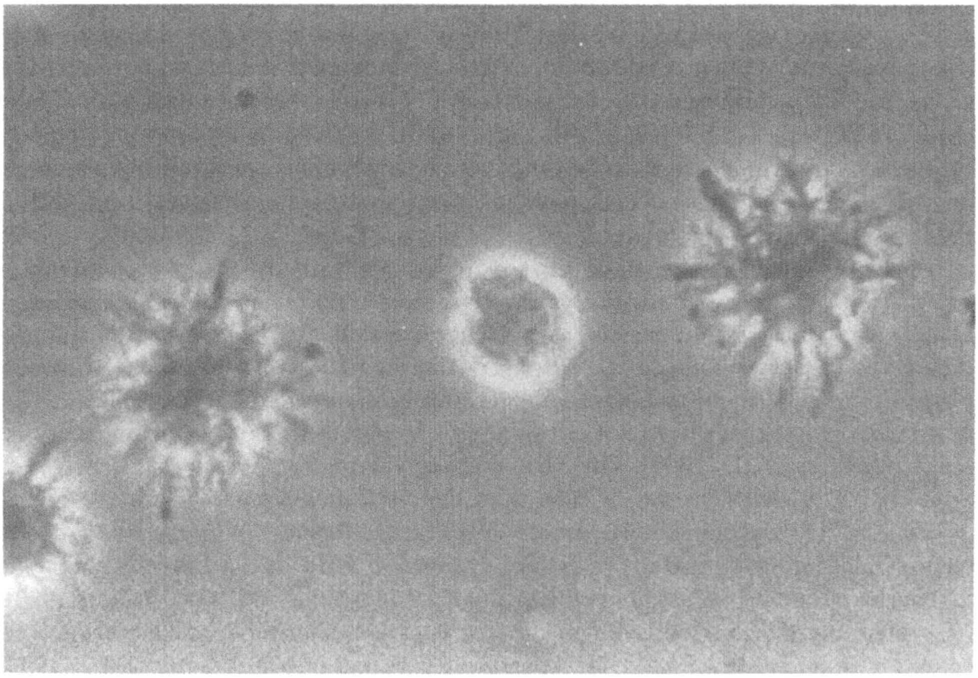

Figure 4. Dendritic-appearing cells that remain after treatment of synovial fluid mononuclear cells by complement lysis using a combination of antimacrophage, anti-T-cell, and anti-B-cell monoclonal antibodies. After treatment, the majority of the viable cells have this appearance. An effete mononuclear cell is included for comparison. (phase-contrast microscopy, ×400 magnification.)

a few percent of the nonpolymorphonuclear leukocyte population in RA effusions. This is five to ten times their concentration in peripheral blood. Currently, there is no explanation for the accumulation of these cells in RA joint fluid. Neither is it known if these DCs are the same as the dendritic-appearing cells in the synovial membrane; nor is there any information concerning their participation in inflammatory joint diseases other than rheumatoid arthritis. Obviously, further experiments will be necessary to define their role in RA synovitis. It is worth reiterating, however, that most of the synoviocytes lining the articular cavity are rich in Ia. An explanation for the enhanced display of these molecules would provide important insights into the origins of rheumatoid synovitis, but even without that understanding, it is obvious that they provide a remarkable reservoir of stimulatory cells to perpetuate autologous T cell proliferation.

X. IMMUNOGLOBULIN PRODUCTION

Plasma cells are abundant in rheumatoid synovium, and immunoglobulin has been demonstrated in rheumatoid synovial fluid and synovial mononuclear cells (Kobayashi and Ziff, 1973; Zvaifler, 1973). Although some of the immunoglobulin in synovial fluid represents transudation from the serum, a significant amount of the IgG is produced locally within the joint (Sliwinski and Zvaifler, 1970). Explants of rheumatoid synovial tissue synthesize immunoglobulins in quantities similar to those of normal spleen and lymph node tissues (Smiley *et al.*, 1968).

The immunoglobulin in the cytoplasm of synovial lining cells consists predominantly of IgG and IgM, both of which may have rheumatoid factor activity (Fish *et al.*, 1966; Mellors *et al.*, 1959; Munthe and Natvig, 1977). Synthesis of IgG and IgM rheumatoid factor has been observed in cultures of isolated rheumatoid synovial cells. The fractions of IgG and IgM with rheumatoid factor activity were greater in synovial cell culture supernatants than in paired serum samples, suggesting a selective synthesis of rheumatoid factor (Wernick *et al.*, 1981). The potential significance of locally produced antiglobulins is discussed in detail elsewhere (Zvaifler, 1973).

Despite the capacity of lymphocytes from the synovium to produce large amounts of immunoglobulins, they show only a minimal specific antibody response when challenged (Abrahamsen *et al.*, 1976; Herman *et al.*, 1971). Such a limited response is consistent with a state of prior commitment of the synovial lymphoid cells or, alternatively, with a defect in the capacity of the synovial T lymphocyte to interact in response to, or in the generation of, signals that govern B-lymphocyte responses.

XI. CELL-MEDIATED CYTOTOXICITY

Antibody-dependent cellular cytotoxicity (ADCC) refers to the lysis of sensitized target cells by mononuclear cells bearing receptors for the Fc portion of IgG. Although an *in vivo* role for ADCC has not been demonstrated, there does appear to be depressed ADCC activity in several rheumatic diseases. Rheumatoid synovial mononuclear cells have depressed ADCC activity compared with paired peripheral blood mononuclear cells (Abrahamsen *et al.*, 1977; Burmester *et al.*, 1978; Corrigall and Panayi, 1978; Diaz-Jouanen *et al.*, 1976). Rheumatoid synovial fluid, as well as sera from rheumatoid arthritis and systemic lupus erythematous patients, is capable of inhibiting ADCC, presumably because of the presence of IgG immune complexes that block the Fc receptors of the effector cells (Diaz-Jouanen *et al.*, 1976; Feldmann *et al.*, 1976). One group has discounted the inhibitory effect of blocking factors such as immune complexes or cytophilic antibodies on the basis of experiments in which preincubation at 37°C or pretreatment with enzymes failed to restore normal ADCC activity (Corrigall and Panayi, 1978). This does not exclude the possibility that synovial fluid mononuclear cells have lost their Fc receptors. In fact, the percentage of T lymphocytes bearing Fc receptors for IgG is low in rheumatoid synovial fluid (Biberfeld *et al.*, 1979; Nakai *et al.*, 1977), and Moretta *et al.* (1978) have shown that binding of IgG immune complexes to the Fc receptor results in an irreversible loss of Fc receptor function accompanied by virtually complete loss of ADCC activity.

Natural killing (NK) refers to spontaneous non-antibody-mediated cellular cytotoxicity and has been implicated in immune surveillance against tumors, viral infections, and foreign tissues (Pross and Baines, 1977). Natural killing is accomplished by a heterogeneous population of cells that morphologically appear as large granular lymphocytes (Herberman, 1982). They differ from classical cytotoxic T lymphocytes both on the basis of function and phenotype. The conventional natural killer present in freshly drawn blood is an Fc-receptor-bearing cell with membrane differentiation antigens detected by monoclonal antibodies OKM1, Leu-7, and Leu-11. A larger constellation of natural cytotoxicity exists, however (Herberman, 1982). The responsible cells are designated by a variety of terms based primarily on the conditions used to produce them. Examples include lymphokine-activated killers, anomalous killers, and NK-like cells generated in the mixed leukocyte reaction (Goto and Zvaifler, 1983; Herberman, 1982). This class of cytotoxic cells consists of T lymphocytes that have a broad range of target specificities, lack Fc receptors, and show a limited number of characteristic cell surface antigens. Typically, they display the 4F2 activation antigen but, unlike conventional NK, lack the Leu-7 marker (Goto and Zvaifler, 1983).

Although there is some disagreement, most studies have shown essentially normal NK activity in rheumatoid peripheral blood (Combe *et al.*, 1984a, 1984b; Dobloug *et al.*, 1982; Goto *et al.*, 1981; Reinitz *et al.*, 1982; Silver *et al.*, 1982), and rheumatoid peripheral blood mononuclear cells (PBM) have not been shown to be cytotoxic toward autologous synovial membrane cells (Burmester *et al.*, 1978; Highton and Panayi, 1980; Neill, 1980). Rheumatoid synovial fluid mononuclear cells (SFM) differ from paired PBM in several respects: (1) SFM have lower NK activity against the NK-sensitive target cell line K562, which may be partially because of an inhibitory factor in synovial fluid; (2) SFM mediate cytotoxicity predominantly by cells that do not bear Fc receptors for IgG; and (3) SFM are capable of killing targets that are resistant to lysis by PBM (Silver *et al.*, 1982). Although Leu-7 cells constitute a portion of the population of synovial fluid lymphocytes, their elimination by treatment with anti-Leu-7 monoclonal antibody and complement had no effect on their cytotoxicity. Neither did killing with the monoclonal antibodies to OKM1 or OKT8. The lysis of both K562 and Raji cell targets, however, was eliminated if the SFM were treated with monoclonal antibodies OKT11 or 4F2 plus complement (Goto and Zvaifler, 1985a). These phenotypic characteristics are identical to those of the NK-like cell produced in the AMLR (Goto and Zvaifler, 1983).

Rheumatoid synovial cytotoxic cells display other unusual features. In contrast to blood NK activity, which is suppressed by activated macrophages, presumably through the release of prostaglandins and superoxide radicals, synovial NK activity is unaffected by incubation with mononuclear cells (Combe *et al.*, 1984b). These differences could reflect either different states of activation of NK cells or the accumulation of unusual cytotoxic cells in synovial fluid of patients with rheumatoid arthritis.

Little is known about the functional significance of the synovial fluid cytotoxic cells. Natural killer and related cytotoxic cells can impair the growth of *in vitro* cultured EBV-infected B lymphocytes, although they cannot eliminate them (Konttinen *et al.*, 1985a). As seen in the left panel of Fig. 5, when EBV-infected B cells are cocultured with autologous E-rosette (E^+) cells from normal individuals previously exposed to the virus (VCA^+), there is an initial proliferation of the E^+ cells. This prolonged and aggressive T-cell stimulation is a response to the increasing amounts of Ia antigen present on the infected autologous B cell (an augmented AMLR) (Konttinen *et al.*, 1985a; Palacios, 1982). During the first week to 10 days in culture, growth factors are elaborated. Interleukin 2, one of these products, expands an $OKM1^+$, $T11^+$ subset of the E^+ population that is the precursor of a cytotoxic cell that is identical to the NK-like cell found in RA synovial effusions (Goto and Zvaifler, 1985a). Although this cell can retard the growth of EBV-infected lymphocytes, their elimination requires a cytotoxic lymphocyte (CTL) (Konttinen *et al.*, 1984a,b). Individuals not previously exposed to the virus (VCA^-, middle panel) show the augmented AMLR and can generate the NK-like cytotoxic cell, but they cannot eliminate the infected B cells because they lack a reservoir of previously sensitized T cells. When synovial fluid E^+ cells from VCA^+ individuals with rheumatoid arthritis are cocultured with EBV-infected B cells, a distinctive picture is seen (right panel). The initial proliferative response is absent because, as noted above, rheumatoid synovial T lymphocytes proliferate poorly to autologous stimulators. Despite this, the infected B

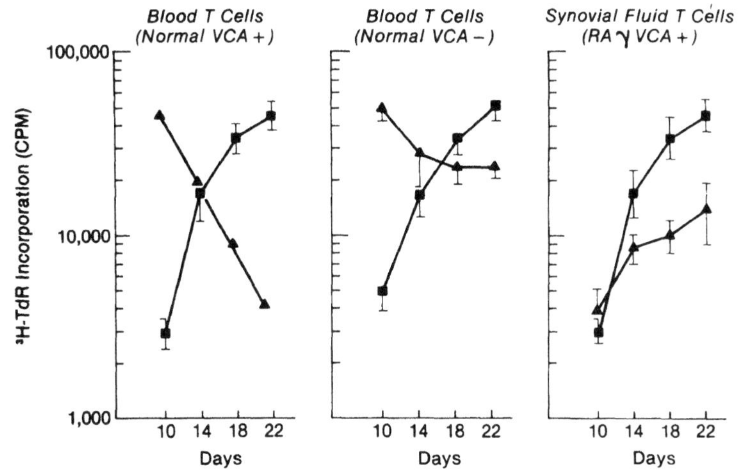

Figure 5. A comparison of the thymidine incorporation observed at various times in cultures of EBV-infected B cells (■) alone or when cocultured with autologous E^+ lymphocyte(s) at a 4 : 1 T : B ratio (▲). The panel at the left shows the pattern observed in normal individuals previously exposed to the Epstein–Barr virus (VCA^+); the middle panel, VCA^- individuals; the right panel, synovial fluid E^+ cells from 3 VCA^+ rheumatoid arthritis patients incubated at a 4 : 1 T : B ratio with autologous EBV-infected B lymphocytes.

cells only grow slowly at first. This initial control is provided by the preexisting activated NK-like cytotoxic cells. By the end of the second week, however, proliferation of the infected B cells is unconstrained.

The failure to eliminate the virus-infected lymphocytes might be explained by either an absence of precursor CTL in rheumatoid synovial effusions or an inability to make sufficient IL-2 to expand them into an effective regulator population. If these *in vitro* experiments can be extrapolated to the joints of patients with rheumatoid arthritis, it might be predicted that, should EBV-infected B cells gain access to the articular cavity, they might be constrained in their growth, but they would not be eliminated. Perhaps more important, the same scenario could apply to any other pathogen that is killed by cytotoxic T cells.

XII. CONCLUSIONS

The information presented in this chapter has focused primarily on the cellular constituents of the rheumatoid joint. Where appropriate, comparisons were made with blood cells of patients with rheumatoid arthritis. In general, the joint fluid immunocytes differ from their circulating counterparts by virtue of their state of activation. Synovial fluid E^+ cells show a higher rate of spontaneous DNA synthesis, formation of stable E-rosettes, and increased natural attachment, all features of activated T cells (Galili *et al.*, 1979, 1981). A large percentage of the E-rosette-positive cells are also Ia^+ and bear other surface membrane activation antigens. The presence in rheumatoid effusions of unusual cytotoxic cells with a broad target specificity that are phenotypical distances from conventional NK cells can be cited as additional evidence.

The reason for the accumulation of these activated cells in the RA articular cavity remains an important unanswered question. Conceivably, as has been suggested, the inflamed joint serves as a sump or trap for the few activated cells in the circulation with exogenous antigen (Fox *et al.*, 1982). Observations on the synovial fluid lymphocytes from other chronic inflammatory diseases are limited, but they seem to show an increase in Ia-bearing T cells and a disproportionate number of $T8^+$ cells (Nilsson and Biberfeld, 1982), lending some credence to this idea. An alternative explanation is that blood mononuclear cells passing through the inflamed joint are activated *in situ*. The demonstration of a variety of mitogenic substances, interleukins, and B-cell growth factors in synovial fluid are consistent with this idea. So too is the finding of a discordance between the phenotype and function of T cells from RA synovial fluids. Obviously, the triggering event is undefined, but the observation that cytotoxic cells from a psoriatic and a colitic effusion have a $T8^+$ phenotype, which would distinguish them from the NK-like cell in RA synovial fluids (Goto and Zvaifler, 1985a), suggests that different activation mechanisms may operate in the various inflammatory rheumatic diseases. As techniques become available for describing the traffic of lymphocytes from the blood into the synovium, it may be possible to demonstrate different patterns of circulation (Butcher, 1985). Such difference might reflect discrete stimuli operating in each of the arthritides.

ACKNOWLEDGMENTS. Supported in parts by grants from the Public Health Service (Training Grant AM14196 and EBV AM25719), the Kroc Foundation, and the Arthritis Foundation. The expert secretarial assistance of Leslye Rucker is greatly appreciated.

REFERENCES

Abdou, N. I., Lindsley, H. B., Racela, L. S., Pascual, E., and Hassanein, K. M., 1981, Suppressor T cell dysfunction and anti-suppressor cell antibody in active early rheumatoid arthritis, *J. Rheumatol.* **8**:9–18.

Abrahamsen, T. G., Froland, S. S., Natvig, J. B., and Pahle, J., 1975, Elution and characterization of lymphocytes from rheumatoid inflammatory tissue, *Scand. J. Immunol.* **4**:823–830.

Abrahamsen, T. G., Froland, S. S., Natvig, J. B., and Pahle, J., 1976, Antigen and unspecific mitogen stimulation of lymphocytes eluted from rheumatoid inflammatory tissue, *Scand. J. Immunol.* **5**:1057–1063.

Abrahamsen, T. G., Froland, S. S., Natvig, J. B., and Pahle, J., 1977, Antibody-dependent cytotoxicity mediated by cells eluted from synovial tissues of patients with rheumatoid arthritis and juvenile rheumatoid arthritis, *Scand. J. Immunol.* **6**:1251–1261.

Abruzzo, L. V., and Rawley, D. A., 1976, Homeostasis of the antibody response: Immunoregulation by NK cells, *Science* **222**:581–585.

Alcocer-Varela, J., Laffon, A., and Alarcón-Segovia, D., 1984, Differences in the production of and/or response to interleukin 2 by T lymphocytes from patients with various connective tissue diseases, *Rheumatol. Int.* **4**:39–44.

Arai, S., Yamamoto, H., Itoh, K., and Kumagi, K., 1983, Suppressive effect of human natural killer cells on pokeweed nitrogen-induced B-cell differentiation, *J. Immunol.* **131**:651–657.

Bankhurst, A. D., Husby, G., and Williams, R. C., Jr., 1976, Predominance of T cells in the lymphocytic infiltrates of synovial tissues in rheumatoid arthritis, *Arthritis Rheum.* **19**:555–562.

Beck, P., Burmester, G. R., Ledwoch, A., Urban, C., and Kalden, J. R., 1981, Autologous and allogeneic MLC-reactivity in patients with rheumatoid arthritis, *J. Clin. Lab. Immunol.* **6**:27–33.

Bensussan, A., Meuer, S. C., Schlossman, S. F., and Reinherz, E. L., 1984, Delineation of an immunoregulatory amplifier population recognizing autologous Ia molecules. Analysis with human T cell clones, *J. Exp. Med.* **159**:559–576.

Biberfeld, G., Nilsson, E., and Biberfeld, P., 1979, T lymphocyte subpopulations in synovial fluid of patients with rheumatic disease, *Arthritis Rheum.* **22**:978–982.

Biberfeld, G., Nilsson, E., and von Stedingk, L. V., 1980, Helper and suppressor activity in synovial fluid lymphocytes of patients with rheumatic disease, in: *Fourth International Congress of Immunology, Paris.*

Bluestein, H. G., 1984, Cellular immunity in rheumatoid arthritis, in: *Rheumatoid Arthritis* (P. D. Utsinger, N. J. Zvaifler, and G. Ehrlich, eds.), J. B. Lippincott, Philadelphia, pp. 251–262.

Brenner, A. I., Scheinberg, M. A., and Cathcart, E. S., 1975, Surface characteristics of synovial fluid and peripheral blood lymphocytes in inflammatory arthritis, *Arthritis Rheum.* **18**:297–303.

Burmester, G. R., Kalden, J. R., Peter, H. H., Schedel, I., Beck, P., and Wittenborg, A., 1978, Immunological and functional characteristics of peripheral blood and synovial fluid lymphocytes from patients with rheumatoid arthritis, *Scand. J. Immunol.* **7**:405–417.

Burmester, G. R., Yu, D. T. Y., Irani, A.-M., Kunkel, H. G., and Winchester, R. J., 1981, Ia^{+} T cells in synovial fluid and tissues of patients with rheumatoid arthritis, *Arthritis Rheum.* **24**:1370–76.

Burmester, G. R., Dimitriu-Bona, A., Waters, S. J., and Winchester, R. J., 1983, Identification of three major synovial lining cell populations by monoclonal antibodies directed to Ia antigens and antigens associated with monocytes–macrophages and fibroblasts, *Scand. J. Immunol.* **17**:69–82.

Butcher, E. C., 1985, Regulation of human and murine lymphocyte traffic, *Curr. Top. Microbiol. Immunol.* (in press).

Cesario, T. C., Andrews, B. S., Martin, D. A., Jason, N., Treadwell, T., Friou, G., and Tilles, J., 1983, Interferon and synovial fluid in the serum of patients with rheumatic diseases, *J. Rheumatol.* **10**:647–650.

Chattopadhyay, C., Chattopadhyay, H., Natvig, J. B., Michaelsen, T. E., and Mellbye, O. J., 1979, Lack of suppressor cell activity in rheumatoid synovial lymphocytes, *Scand. J. Immunol.* **10**:309–318.

Chin, R. C., Chiou, S. S., Multz, C. V., and Allison, A. C., 1984, The absence of gamma interferon and the presence of high levels of inflammatory mediators in the supernatants of rheumatoid arthritis synovial tissue explants, *Fed. Proc.* **43**:947.

Cohen, A. H., Redelman, D., and Zvaifler, N. J., 1984, Characterization of rheumatoid arthritis B cell growth factors, *Arthritis Rheum.* **27**:S35.

Combe, B., Pope, R. M., Darnell, B., Kincaid, W., and Talal, N., 1984a, Regulation of natural killer cell activity by macrophages in the rheumatoid joint and peripheral blood, *J. Immunol.* **133**:709–713.

Combe, B., Pope, R. M., Darnell, B., and Talal, N., 1984b, Modulation of natural killer cell activity in the rheumatoid joint and peripheral blood, *Scand. J. Immunol.* **20**:541–558.

Combe, B., Pope, R. M., Fischbach, M., Darnell, B., Baron, S., and Talal, N., 1985, Interleukin 2 in rheumatoid arthritis. Production of and response to interleukin 2 in rheumatoid synovial fluid, synovial tissue and peripheral blood, *Clin. Exp. Immunol.* **59**:520–528.

Corrigall, V. M., and Panayi, G. S., 1978, Lymphocyte studies in rheumatoid arthritis. II. Antibody-mediated and mitogen-induced lymphocyte cytotoxicity in synovial fluid and peripheral blood, *Ann. Rheum. Dis.* **37**:410–415.

Corrigall, V., Panayi, G. S., and Laurent, R., 1979, Lymphocyte studies in rheumatoid arthritis. III. A comparative study of the responses of peripheral blood and synovial fluid lymphocytes to phytomitogens, *Scand. J. Rheumatol.* **8**:10–16.

Crout, J. E., McDuffie, F. C., and Ritts, R. E., Jr., 1976, Induction of peripheral blood lymphocyte transformation by autologous synovial fluid lymphocytes and synovial fluid, *Arthritis Rheum.* **19**:523–531.

Damle, N. K., and Gupta, S., 1982, Autologous mixed lymphocyte reaction in man. V. Functionally and phenotypically distinct human T cell subpopulations respond to non-T and activated-T cells in AMLR, *Scand. J. Immunol.* **16**:59–68.

Dayer, J.-M., Russell, R. G. G., and Krane, S. M., 1977, Collagenase production by rheumatoid synovial cells: Stimulation by a human lymphocyte factor, *Science* **195**:181–183.

DeGrere, M., Mellbye, O. J., and Klarke-Jenssen, O., 1983, Immune interferon in serum and synovial fluid in rheumatoid arthritis and related disorders, *Ann. Rheum. Dis.* **42**:672–676.

Diaz-Jouanen, E., Bankhurst, A. D., and Williams, R. C., Jr., 1976, Antibody-mediated lymphocytotoxicity in rheumatoid arthritis and systemic lupus erythematosus, *Arthritis Rheum.* **19**:133–141.

Dobloug, J. H., Chattopadhyay, C., Forre, O., Hoyeraal, H. M., and Natvig, J. B., 1981, Con A-induced suppressor cell activity and T-lymphocyte subpopulations in peripheral blood lymphocytes of patients with rheumatoid arthritis and juvenile rheumatoid arthritis, *Scand. J. Immunol.* **13**:367–373.

Dobloug, J. H., Forre, D., Kvien, T. K., and Egeland, T., 1982, Natural killer cell activity of peripheral blood and synovial fluid in synovial tissue lymphocytes in patients with rheumatoid arthritis and juvenile rheumatoid arthritis, *Ann. Rheum. Dis.* **41**:490–494.

Dorwart, B. B., Hebert, J., Schumacher, H. R., and Abdou, N. I., 1975, Cellular and humoral immune parameters of synovial fluid and blood in rheumatoid arthritis, *J. Rheumatol.* **2**:363–372.

Duclos, M., Zeidler, H., Liman, W., Pichler, W. J., Rieber, P., and Peter, H. H., 1982, Characterization of blood and synovial fluid lymphocytes from patients with rheumatoid arthritis and other joint diseases, *Rheumatol. Int.* **2**:75–82.

Duke, E. O., Panayi, G. S., Janossy, G., and Poulter, L. W., 1983, Immunohistologic analysis of the lymphocyte infiltrates of rheumatoid synovial membrane using monoclonal antibodies, *Ann. Rheum. Dis.* **41**:192–195.

Engleman, E. G., and McDevitt, H. O., 1978, A suppressor T cell of the mixed lymphocyte reaction specific for the HLA-D region in man, *J. Clin. Invest.* **61**:828–838.

Feldmann, J.-L., Becker, M. J., Moutsopoulos, H., Fye, K., Blackman, M., Epstein, W. V., and Talal, N., 1976, Antibody-dependent cell-mediated cytotoxicity in selected autoimmune diseases, *J. Clin. Invest.* **58**:173–179.

Fish, A. J., Michael, A. F., Gewurz, H., and Good, R. A., 1966, Immunopathologic changes in rheumatoid arthritis synovium, *Arthritis Rheum.* **9**:267–280.

Fontana, A., Hengartner, H., Weber, E., Fehr, K., Grob, P. J., and Cohen, G., 1982, Interleukin 1 activity in the synovial fluid of patients with rheumatoid arthritis, *Rheumatol. Int.* **2**:49–53.

Forre, D., Dobloug, J. H., and Natvig, J. B., 1982a, Augmented numbers of HLA-DR-positive T lymphocytes in the synovial fluid and synovial tissue of patients with rheumatoid arthritis and juvenile rheumatoid arthritis. *In vivo*-activated T lymphocytes are potent stimulators in the mixed lymphocyte reaction, *Scand. J. Immunol.* **15**:227–231.

Forre, O., Egland, T., Dobloug, J. H., Kvien, T. K., and Natvig, J. B., 1982b, Autologous mixed lymphocyte reactions in patients with rheumatoid arthritis and juvenile rheumatoid arthritis: Both non-T cells and *in vivo* activated T cells can act as stimulator cells, *Scand. J. Immunol.* **16**:173–179.

Forre, O., Thoen, J., Lea, T., Dobloug, J. H., Mellbye, O. J., Natvig, J. B., Pahle, J., and Solheim, B. G., 1982c, The *in situ* characterization of mononuclear cells in rheumatoid tissues using monoclonal antibodies—no reduction of $T8^+$ cells or augmentation of $T4^+$ cells, *Scand. J. Immunol.* **16**:315–319.

Fox, R. I., Fong, S., Sabharwal, U., Carstens, S. A., Kung, P. C., and Vaughan, J. H., 1982, Synovial fluid lymphocytes differ from peripheral blood lymphocytes in patients with rheumatoid arthritis, *J. Immunol.* **128**:351–354.

Fox, R. I., Hueniken, M., Fong, S., Behar, S., Royston, I., Singhal, S. K., and Thompson, L., 1983, A novel cell surface antigen (T305) found in increased frequency on acute leukemic cells and in autoimmune disease states, *J. Immunol.* **131**:762–767.

Froland, S. S., Natvig, J. B., and Husby, G., 1973, Immunological characterization of lymphocytes in synovial fluid from patients with rheumatoid arthritis, *Scand. J. Immunol.* **2**:67–73.

Galili, U., Rosenthal, L., Galili, N., and Klein, E., 1979, Activated T cells in the synovial fluid of arthritic patients: Characterization and comparison with *in vitro* activated human and murine T cells in cooperation with monocytes in cytotoxicity, *J. Immunol.* **122**:878–883.

Galili, U., Rosenthal, L., and Klein, E., 1981, Activated T cells in the synovial fluid of arthritis patients. II. *In vitro* activation of the autologous blood lymphocytes, *J. Immunol.* **127**:430–432.

Gatenby, P. A., and Engleman, E. G., 1981, Immunoregulation in the synovium of rheumatoid arthritis, *Lancet* **2**:1348.

Gatter, R. A., and Richmond, J. D., 1975, Predominance of synovial fluid lymphocytes in early rheumatoid arthritis, *J. Rheumatol.* **2**:340–345.

Goto, M., and Zvaifler, N. J., 1983, Characterization of the killer cell generated in the autologous mixed leukocyte reaction, *J. Exp. Med.* **157**:1309–23.

Goto, M., and Zvaifler, N. J., 1985a, Characterization of the natural killer-like lymphocytes in rheumatoid synovial fluid, *J. Immunol.* **134**:1483–1486.

Goto, M., and Zvaifler, N. J., 1985b, Characterization of the precursors of the NK-like cytotoxic cells generated in the autologous mixed leukocyte reaction and by interleukin 2 activation, (in press).

Goto, M., Tanimoto, K., Chihara, T., and Horiuchi, Y., 1981, Natural cell mediated cytotoxicity in Sjogren's syndrome and rheumatoid arthritis, *Arthritis Rheum.* **24**:1377–82.

Gottlieb, A. B., Fu, S. M., Yu, D. T. Y., and Wang, C. Y., Halper, J., and Kunkel, H. G., 1979, The nature of the stimulatory cell in human allogeneic and autologous MLC reactions; role of isolated IgM-bearing B cells, *J. Immunol.* **123**:1497–1503.

Hasler, F., Bluestein, H. G., Zvaifler, N. J., and Epstein, L. B., 1983, Analysis of the defects responsible for the impaired regulation of EBV-induced B-cell proliferation by rheumatoid arthritis lymphocytes. I. Diminished gamma interferon production in response to autologous stimulation, *J. Exp. Med.* **157**:173–188.

Haynes, B. F., and Fauci, A. S., 1977, Activation of human B lymphocytes. III. Concanavalin A-induced generation of suppressor cells of the plaque-forming cell response of normal human B lymphocytes, *J. Immunol.* **118**:2281–87.

Hepburn, B., McDuffie, F. C., and Ritts, R. E., Jr., 1976, Impaired blastogeneic response of lymphocytes from synovial fluid and peripheral blood of patients with rheumatoid arthritis, *J. Rheumatol.* **3**:118–123.

Herberman, R. B., 1982, *NK and Other Natural Effector Cells,* Academic Press, New York.

Herman, J. H., Bradley, J., Ziff, M., and Smiley, J. D., 1971, Response of the rheumatoid synovial membrane to exogenous immunization, *J. Clin. Invest.* **50**:266–273.

Herman, J. H., Nutman, T. B., Nozoe, M., Mowery, C. S., and Dennis, M. V., 1981, Lymphokine-mediated suppression of chondrocyte glycosaminoglycan and protein synthesis, *Arthritis Rheum.* **24**:824–834.

Highton, J., and Panayi, G. S., 1980, Spontaneous cytotoxicity of rheumatoid and normal peripheral blood mononuclear cells against 4 human lymphoblastoid cell lines, *Ann. Rheum. Dis.* **39**:559–562.

Holborow, E. J., Sheldon, P. J., and Papamichail, M., 1975, Studies on synovial fluid lymphocytes in rheumatoid arthritis, *Rheumatology* **6**:215–218.

Huber, C., Merkenschlager, M., Gattringer, C., Royston, I., Fink, U., and Braunsteiner, H., 1982, Human autologous mixed lymphocyte reactivity is primarily specific for xenoprotein determinants adsorbed to antigen-presenting cells during rosette formation with sheep erythrocytes, *J. Exp. Med.* **155**:1222–1227.

Husby, G., and Williams, R. C., Jr., 1985, Immunohistochemical studies of interleukin 2 and gamma interferon in rheumatoid arthritis, *Arthritis Rheum.* **28**:174–181.

Ishikawa, H., and Ziff, M., 1976, Electron microscopic observations of immunoreactive cells in the rheumatoid synovial membrane, *Arthritis Rheum.* **19**:1–14.

Ivanyi, L., Lehner, T., and Burry, H. C., 1973, The response of synovial fluid lymphocytes to T and B stimulants *in vitro, Immunology* **25**:905–908.

James, S. P., Yenokida, G. G., Graeff, A. S., Elson, C. O., and Strober, W., 1981, Immunoregulatory function of T cells activated in the autologous mixed lymphocyte reaction, *J. Immunol.* **127**:2605–09.

Janossy, G., Tidman, N., Selby, W. S., Thomas, J. A., Granger, S., Kung, P. C., and Golstein, G., 1980, Human T lymphocytes of inducer and suppressor type occupy different microenvironments, *Nature* **288**:81–84.

Janossy, G., Duke, O., Poulter, L. W., Panayi, G., Bofill, M., and Goldstein, G., 1981, Rheumatoid arthritis: A disease of T lymphocyte–macrophage immunoregulation, *Lancet* **2**:839–842.

Klareskog, L., Forsum, U., Tjernlund, U. M., Kabelitz, D., and Wigren, A., 1981, Appearance of anti-HLA-DR-reactive cells in normal and rheumatoid synovial tissue, *Scand. J. Immunol.* **14**:183–192.

Klareskog, L., Forsum, U., Kabelitz, D., Ploen, L., Sundstrom, C., Nilsson, K., Wigren, A., and Wigzell, H., 1982a, Immune functions of human synovial cells. Phenotypic and T cell regulatory properties of macrophage-like cells that express HLA-DR, *Arthritis Rheum.* **25**:488–501.

Klareskog, L., Forsum, U., Wigren, A., and Wigzell, H., 1982b, Relationships between HLA-DR-expressing cells and T lymphocytes of different subsets in rheumatoid synovial tissue, *Scand. J. Immunol.* **15**:501–507.

Kobayashi, I., and Ziff, M., 1973, Electron microscopic studies of lymphoid cells in the rheumatoid synovial membrane, *Arthritis Rheum.* **16**:471–486.

Konttinen, Y. T., Reitamo, S., Ranki, A., Hayry, P., Kankaanapaa, U., and Wegelius, O., 1981, Characterization of the immunocompetent cells of rheumatoid synovium from tissue sections and eluates, *Arthritis Rheum.* **24**:71–79.

Konttinen, Y. T., Bluestein, H. G., and Zvaifler, N. J., 1985a, Regulation of growth of Epstein–Barr virus-infected B cells. I. Growth regression by E-rosetting cells from VCA^+ donors is a combined effect of autologous mixed leukocyte reaction and activation of T8 memory cells, *J. Immunol.* **134**:2287–2293.

Konittinen, Y. K., Bluestein, H. G., and Zvaifler, N. J., 1985b, Regulation of the growth of Epstein–Barr virus infected B cells: II. Temporal profile of the *in vitro* development of cytotoxic cells, *Cell Immunol.* (in press).

Kurosaka, M., and Ziff, M., 1983, Immunoelectron microscopic study of the distribution of T cell subsets in rheumatoid synovium, *Exp. J. Med.* **158**:1191–1210.

Lindblad, S., Klareskog, L., Hedfors, E., Forsum, U., and Sundström, C., 1983, Phenotypic characterization of synovial tissue cells *in situ* in different types of synovitis, *Arthritis Rheum.* **26**:1321–33.

Lipsky, P. E., Ginsburg, W. W., Finkelman, F. D., and Ziff, M., 1978, Control of human B lymphocyte responsiveness: Enhanced suppressor T cell activity after *in vitro* incubation, *J. Immunol.* **120**:902–910.

Lowther, D. A., Sandy, J. D., Santer, V. B., and Brown, H. L. G., 1978, Antigen-induced arthritis: Decreased proteoglycan content and inhibition of proteoglycan synthesis in articular cartilage, *Arthritis Rheum.* **21**:675–680.

Malone, D., Cahill, H., Tsokos, M., Decker, J., and Wilder, R., 1983, Immunohistologic heterogeneity of synovium from patients with clinically active rheumatoid arthritis, *Arthritis Rheum.* **26**:S17.

McClurg, M., Bluestein, H. G., and Zvaifler, N. J., 1983, Epstein–Barr virus infected lymphocytes are in rheumatoid arthritis synovial fluids, *Arthritis Rheum.* **26**:S553.

McMichael, A. J., and Sasazuki, T., 1977, A suppressor T cell in the human mixed lymphocyte reaction, *J. Exp. Med.* **146**:368–380.

Meijer, C. J. L. M., Van de Putte, L. B. A., Lafeber, G. J. M., deHaas, E., and Cats, A., 1980, Membrane and transformation characteristics of lymphocytes isolated from the synovial membrane and paired peripheral blood of patients with rheumatoid arthritis, *Ann. Rheum. Dis.* **39**:75–81.

Meijer, C. J. L. M., de Graaf-Reitsma, C. B., Lafeber, G. J. M., and Cats, A., 1982, *In situ* localization of lymphocyte subsets in synovial membranes of patients with rheumatoid arthritis with monoclonal antibodies, *J. Rheumatol.* **9**:359–365.

Mellors, R. C., Heimer, R., Corcos, J., and Korngold, L., 1959, Cellular origin of rheumatoid factor, *J. Exp. Med.* **110**:875–881.

Mizel, S. B., Dayer, J.-M., Krane, S. M., and Mergenhagen, S. E., 1981, Stimulation of rheumatoid synovial cell collagenase and prostaglandin production by partially purified lymphocyte-activating factor (interleukin-1), *Proc. Natl. Acad. Sci. U.S.A.* **78**:2474–2477.

Moretta, L., Mingari, M. C., and Romanzi, C. A., 1978, Loss of Fc receptors for IgG from human T lymphocytes exposed to IgG immune complexes, *Nature* **272**:618–620.

Munthe, E., and Natvig, J. B., 1971, Characterization of IgG complexes in eluates from rheumatoid tissue, *Clin. Exp. Immunol.* **8**:249–262.

Naides, S. J., Redelman, D., and Zvaifler, N. J., 1984, The role of xenoantigen in the human autologous mixed lymphocyte reaction. Ability to respond in the absence of exposure to xenoantigen depends on the method of T-cell preparation, *Clin. Immunol. Immunopathol.* **34**:216–226.

Nakai, H., Morito, T., Tanimoto, K., and Horiuchi, Y., 1977, Reduced Fc receptor-bearing cells in peripheral bloods of patients with systemic lupus erythematosus and in rheumatoid synovial fluids, *J. Rheumatol.* **4**:405–413.

Neill, W. A., 1980, Cell-mediated cytotoxicity for cultured autologous rheumatoid synovial membrane cells, *Ann. Rheum. Dis.* **39**:570–575.

Nilsson, E., and Biberfeld, G., 1982, Synovial T lymphocyte subpopulations defined by monoclonal antibodies in synovial fluid of patients with rheumatic disease, *J. Clin. Lab. Immunol.* **9**:93–97.

Nilsson, E., and Biberfeld, G., 1983, Synovial T lymphocyte subpopulations in acute and chronic synovitis. Presented at EULAR, Moscow, June 27, Abstract No. 105.

Nouri, A. M. E., Panayi, G. S., and Goodman, S. M., 1984, Cytokines in the chronic inflammation of rheumatoid disease. I. The presence of interleukin 1 in synovial fluid, *Clin. Exp. Immunol.* **55**:295–301.

Oppenheim, J. J., Luger, T., Sztein, M. B., and Steeg, P. S., 1982, Circuit of cytokine cell interactions that regulate immunological and inflammatory reactions, in: *Role of Macrophages in Self Defense Mechanisms* Z. Cohn, and N. Ishida, eds.), Elsevier, Tokyo, pp. 127–136.

Palacios, R., 1982, Epstein–Barr virus increases the proliferative response and the generation of suppressor and cytotoxic T cell functions in autologous mixed lymphocyte reactions, *Scand. J. Immunol.* **15**:17–23.

Panayi, G. S., 1973, Response of rheumatoid synovial fluid lymphocytes to nonspecific mitogens, *Lancet* **2**:512–513.

Petersen, J., Andersen, V., Ingemann-Hansen, T., Halkjaer-Kristensen, J., Wiik, A., and Thyssen, H., 1983, Synovial fluid and blood monocyte influence on lymphocyte proliferation in rheumatoid arthritis and traumatic synovitis, *Scand. J. Rheumatol.* **12**:299–304.

Pincus, S. H., Clegg, D. O., and Ward, J. R., 1985, Characterization of T cells bearing HLA-DR antigens in rheumatoid arthritis, *Arthritis Rheum.* **28**:8–15.

Pope, R. M., McChesney, L., Talal, N., and Fischbach, M., 1984, Characterization of the autologous mixed lymphocyte response in rheumatoid arthritis, *Arthritis Rheum.* **27**:1234–1244.

Poulter, L. W., Duke, O., Hobbs, S., Janossy, G., and Panayi, G., 1982, Histochemical discrimination of HLA-DR positive cell populations in normal and arthritis synovial lining, *Clin. Exp. Immunol.* **48**:381–388.

Pross, H. F., and Baines, M. G., 1977, Spontaneous human lymphocyte-mediated cytotoxicity against tumor target cells, *Cancer Immunol.* **3**:75–85.

Rawson, A. J., and Huang, T. C., 1974, Lymphocytes in rheumatoid arthritis. I. Response to allogeneic cells and to phytomitogens, *Clin. Exp. Immunol.* **16**:41–48.

Reinitz, E., Neighbour, P. A., and Grayzel, A. I., 1982, Natural killer cell activity of mononuclear cells from rheumatoid patients measured by conjugate-binding assay, *Arthritis Rheum.* **25**:1440–44.

Reynolds, M. D., and Abdou, N. I., 1973, Comparative study of the *in vitro* proliferative responses of blood and synovial fluid leukocytes of rheumatoid arthritis patients, *J. Clin. Invest.* **52**:1627–31.

Robb, J., 1984, Interleukin 2: The molecule and its function, *Immunol. Today* **5**:203–209.

Romain, P. L., Burmester, G. R., Enlow, R. W., and Winchester, R. J., 1982, Multiple abnormalities in immunoregulatory function of synovial compartment T cells in patients with rheumatoid arthritis, *Rheumatol. Int.* **2**:121–127.

Schumacher, H. R., and Kitridou, R. C., 1972, Synovitis of recent onset. A clinicopathologic study during the first month of disease. *Arthritis Rheum.* **15**:465–485.

Sheldon, P. J., Papamichail, M., and Holborow, E. J., 1974, Studies on synovial fluid lymphocytes in rheumatoid arthritis, *Ann. Rheum. Dis.* **33**:509–514.

Siebert, F., Kalden, J. R., Fink, P., Fricke, N., and Diecher, H., 1978, The effect of serum and allogeneic antiglobulin preparations on the mitogenic reactivity of peripheral blood lymphocytes from patients with rheumatoid arthritis, *Z. Rheumatol.* **37**:286–295.

Silver, R. M., and Zvaifler, N. J., 1985, Immunologic pathogenesis of rheumatoid arthritis, in: *Rheumatoid Arthritis* (P. D. Utsinger, N. J. Zvaifler and G. Ehrlich eds.), J. B. Lippincott, Philadelphia, pp. 71–89.

Silver, R. M., Redelman, D. D., Zvaifler, N. J., and Naides, S. J., 1982, Studies of rheumatoid synovial fluid lymphocytes. I. Evidence for activated natural killer (NK) cells, *J. Immunol.* **128**:1758–1763.

Silver, R. M., Reddelman, D., and Zvaifler, N. J., 1983, Studies of rheumatoid synovial fluid lymphocytes. II. A comparison of their behavior in the autologous mixed lymphocyte reaction and response to TCGF, *Clin. Immunol. Immunopathol.* **27**:15–27.

Silverman, H. A., Johnson, J. S., Vaughan, J. H., and McGlamory, J. C., 1976, Altered lymphocyte reactivity in rheumatoid arthritis, *Arthritis Rheum.* **19**:509–515.

Sliwinski, A. J., and Zvaifler, N. J., 1970, *In vivo* synthesis of IgG by rheumatoid synovium, *J. Lab. Clin. Med.* **76**:304–310.

Smiley, J. D., Sachs, C., and Ziff, M., 1968, *In vitro* synthesis of immunoglobulin by rheumatoid synovial membrane, *J. Clin. Invest.* **47**:624–632.

Smith, J. B., and DeHoratius, R. J., 1982, Deficient autologous mixed lymphocyte reactions correlated with disease activity and systemic lupus erythematosus in rheumatoid arthritis, *Clin. Exp. Immunol.* **48:**155–162.

Smith, K. A., 1980, T-cell growth factor, *Immunol. Rev.* **51:**337–357.

Smolen, J. S., Luger, T. A., Chused, T. M., and Steinberg, A. D., 1981, Responder cells in the human autologous mixed lymphocyte reaction, *J. Clin. Invest.* **68:**1601–04.

Sokoloff, L., and Hough, A. J., Jr., 1985, Pathology of rheumatoid arthritis and allied disorders, in: *Arthritis and Allied Conditions,* 10th ed. (D. J. McCarty, ed.), Lea & Febiger, Philadelphia. pp. 571–592.

Stastny, P., Cooke, T. D., and Ziff, M., 1973, Production of a macrophage migration inhibitory factor in rabbits with experimental arthritis, *Clin. Exp. Immunol.* **14:**141–147.

Stastny, P., Rosenthal, M., Andreis, M., Cooke, D., and Ziff, D., 1975, Lymphokines in rheumatoid synovitis, *Ann. N.Y. Acad. Sci.* **256:**117–131.

Stratton, J. A., and Peter, J. B., 1978, The responses of peripheral blood and synovial fluid lymphocytes of patients with rheumatoid arthritis to *in vitro* stimulation with mitogens, *Clin. Immunol. Immunopathol.* **10:**233–241.

Theofilopoulos, A. N., Carson, D. A., Tavassoli, M., Slavin, S. F., Speers, W. C., Jensen, F. B., and Vaughan, J. H., 1980, Evidence for the presence of receptors for C3 and IgG Fc on human synovial cells, *Arthritis Rheum.* **23:**1–9.

van Boxel, J. A., and Paget, S. A., 1975, Predominantly T-cell infiltrate in rheumatoid synovial membranes, *N. Engl. J. Med.* **293:**517–520.

Van Voorhis, W. C., Valinsky, J., Hoffman, E., and Steinman, R. M., 1983a, The relative efficacy of human monocytes and dendritic cells as accessory cells for T cell replication, *J. Exp. Med.* **158:**174–191.

Van Voorhis, W. C., Witmer, N. D., and Steinman, R. M., 1983b, The phenotype of dendritic cells and macrophages, *Fed. Proc.* **42:**3114–3118.

Vernon-Roberts, B., Curry, H. L. F., and Perrin, J., 1974, T and B cells in the blood and synovial fluid of rheumatoid patients, *Ann. Rheum. Dis.* **33:**430–434.

Wernick, R., Ziff, M., and Lipsky, P. E., 1981, Rheumatoid factor synthesis by isolated synovial cells, *Clin. Res.* **29:**560A.

Wilkins, J. A., Warrington, R. J., Sigurdson, S. L., and Rutherford, W. J., 1983, The demonstration of interleukin-2-like activity in the synovial fluid of rheumatoid arthritis patients, *J. Rheumatol.* **10:**109–113.

Winchester, R. J., and Burmester, G. R., 1981, Demonstration of Ia antigens on certain dendritic cells and on a novel elongate cell found in human synovial tissue, *Scand. J. Immunol.* **14:**439–444.

Winchester, R. J., Winfield, J. B., Siegal, F., Wernet, P., Bentwich, Z., and Kunkel, H. G., 1974, Analyses of lymphocytes from patients with rheumatoid arthritis and systemic lupus erythematosus. Occurrence of interfering cold-reactive antilymphocyte antibodies, *J. Clin. Invest.* **54:**1082–92.

Wood, D. D., Ihrie, E. J., Dinarello, C. A., and Cohen, P. L., 1983, Isolation of an interleukin 1-like factor from human joint effusions, *Arthritis Rheum.* **26:**975–983.

Young, C. L., Adamson, T. C., Vaughan, J. H., and Fox, R. I., 1984, Immunohistologic characterization of synovial membrane lymphocytes in rheumatoid arthritis, *Arthritis Rheum.* **27:**32–39.

Yu, D. T. Y., Winchester, R. J., Fu, S. M., Gibofsky, A., Ko, H. S., and Kunkel, H. G., 1980, Peripheral blood Ia-positive T cells. Increases in certain diseases and after immunization, *J. Exp. Med.* **151:**91–100.

Ziff, M., 1974, Relation of cellular infiltration of rheumatoid synovial membrane to its immune response, *Arthritis Rheum.* **17:**313–319.

Zvaifler, N. J., 1973, The immunopathology of joint inflammation in rheumatoid arthritis, *Adv. Immunol.* **16:**265–336.

Zvaifler, N. J., Steinman, R., Kaplan, G., and Lau, L., 1985, Immuno stimulatory dendritic cells in synovial effusions of patients with rheumatoid arthritis *J. Clin. Invest.* (in press).

20

Macrophages and Dendritic Cells in Rheumatic Diseases

Øystein Førre, Kristian Waalen, Jørn Thoen, and Torstein Hovig

I. INTRODUCTION

The normal synovial membrane is lined by a double layer of synovial lining cells, which form a multilayer in the rheumatoid synovial membrane. The synovial lining cells have previously been classified according to electron microscopic criteria as A and C cells, which have macrophage characteristics, and B cells, which have fibroblast characteristics. This classification has recently been confirmed using monoclonal antibodies specific for monocyte/macrophage and fibroblast antigens.

Very recently it has been shown that during the rheumatoid inflammation there is extensive infiltration of the synovial membrane by dendritic cells, cells that have characteristic elongated branching processes and strongly express Ia antigens. Dendritic cells lack macrophage, lymphocyte, or fibroblast characteristics. Both the synovial macrophages and dendritic cells are bone marrow derived. In the rheumatoid synovial membrane there is also extensive infiltration with activated T lymphocytes and plasma cells, which sometimes form folliclelike structures. The dendritic cells seem to be the most important accessory cells for the various immune responses, whereas macrophages produce prostaglandins and leukotrienes, which modulate immune responses, collagen deposition, and inflammation. Synovial macrophages also liberate proteolytic enzymes and oxygen radicals, which probably cause the tissue damage seen in rheumatic disorders. Macrophages at different sites also build up the mononuclear phagocyte system, which is responsible

Øystein Førre • Oslo Sanitetsforenings Rheumatism Hospital, Oslo, Norway. *Kristian Waalen and Jørn Thoen* • Institute of Immunology and Rheumatology, Rikshospitalet, The National Hospital, Oslo, Norway. *Torstein Hovig* • Institute for Pathology, Electron Microscopic Laboratory, Rikshospitalet, The National Hospital, Oslo, Norway.

for the clearing of circulating immune complexes. Both synovial macrophagelike cells and dendritic cells are targets for drug therapy in rheumatic diseases.

II. THE ORIGIN AND DEVELOPMENT OF MACROPHAGES AND DENDRITIC CELLS

A. Macrophages

Several studies have shown the bone marrow origin of the macrophages (Coccia *et al.*, 1980; Parwaresch *et al.*, 1981; Radzun *et al.*, 1983; van Furth, 1981). Circulating monocytes migrate into the various tissues and become macrophages (van Furth, 1981). During inflammation, there is an increased turnover of monocytes, which requires augmented proliferation of the progenitors in the bone marrow (van Furth, 1981). This production has recently been shown to be regulated by circulating enhancing and inhibitory factors (Fig. 1) produced at the site of the inflammatory lesion (van Furth, 1981). It has also been shown that very few macrophages proliferate at the inflammatory sites (van Furth, 1981).

The osteoclast can be regarded as a giant macrophage and is probably formed by fusion of several monocytes or macrophages (Teitelbaum and Kahn, 1980; van Furth, 1981). It has also been shown in humans that osteoclasts are bone marrow derived. Thus, a child who was bone marrow transplanted for osteopetrosis had osteoclasts with the phenotypes of the donor after the transplantation (Coccia *et al.*, 1980).

B. Dendritic Cells

Little is known concerning the origin and development of the heterogeneous cell population termed dendritic cells (Steinman and Nussenzweig, 1980). Dendritic cells have a characteristic morphology with many branching cell processes (Steinman and Nussenzweig, 1980). These cells have been identified in many organs and species (Steinman, 1981). The term dendritic cells describes collectively different cell types found in various organs. Lymphoid dendritic cells have been isolated from lymphoid tissue in mice (Spalding *et al.*, 1983; Steinman and Cohn, 1973, 1974; Steinman *et al.*, 1979) and rats (Klinkert *et al.*, 1982). Histologists have identified a population of interdigitating cells in sections of lymphoid tissue, primarily in the thymus-dependent regions (Steinman, 1981). The term "interdigitating" derives from observations that cell processes can indent the outlines of the interdigitating cell (Steinman, 1981). The cytological features of the interdigitating cells are identical to those of lymphoid dendritic cells isolated from the same organ (Steinman, 1981). Langerhans cells are dendritic cells identified in the epidermis (Rowden *et al.*, 1977; Steinman, 1981). Veiled cells are another form of dendritic cells that have been demonstrated in afferent lymph from rodents and man (Balfour *et al.*, 1981; Knight *et al.*, 1982, 1983; Steinman, 1981). In germinal centers, follicular dendritic cells have been identified (Steinman and Nussenzweig, 1980; Steinman, 1981).

Recently, dendritic cells have also been identified in various compartments in humans. Thus, these cells have been identified and isolated from human peripheral blood (Førre *et al.*, 1982a,b; Kuntz-Crow and Kunkel, 1982). Dendritic cells have also been demonstrated in human synovial fluid (Førre *et al.*, 1982a; Førre *et al.*, 1983) and

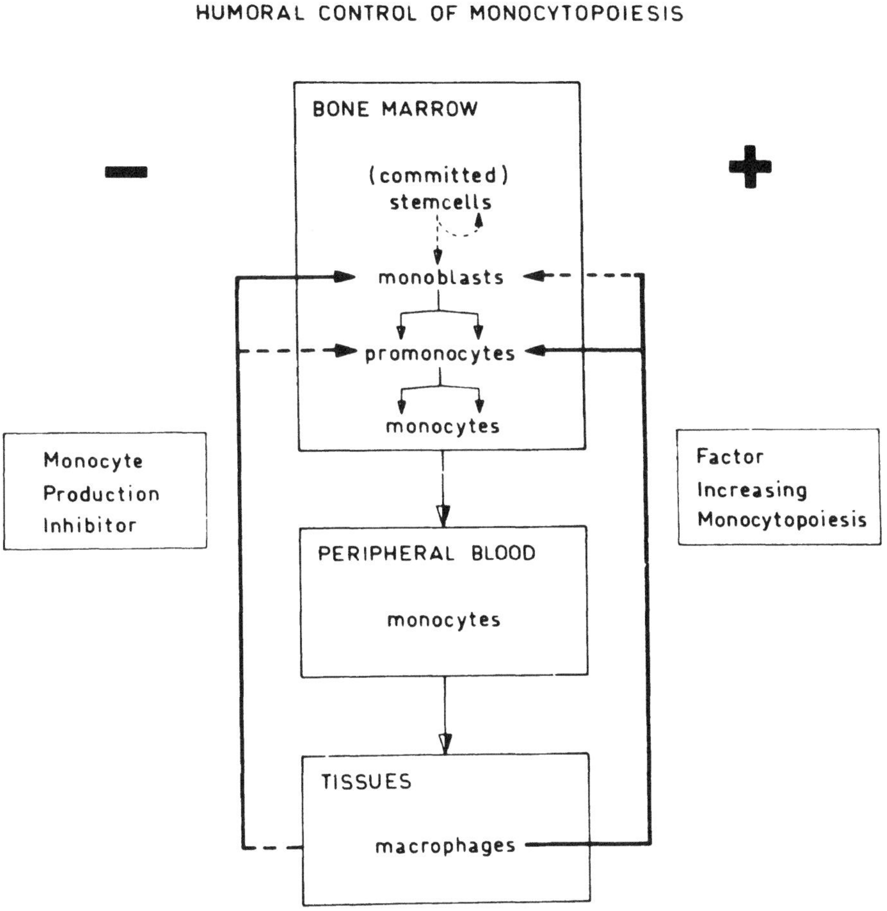

Figure 1. The development of monocytes/macrophages from bone marrow cells. Regulation by enhancing and inhibitory factors produced at sites of inflammation. (From van Furth, 1981, with permission.)

rheumatoid synovial membrane (Burmeister *et al.*, 1983a,b; Føre *et al.*, 1982a; Føre *et al.*, 1983; Janossy *et al.*, 1981; Poulter, 1983; Poulter and Duke, 1983; Poulter *et al.*, 1983; Winchester and Burmeister, 1981).

The various dendritic cell types most probably are bone marrow derived (Steinman and Nussenzweig, 1980). This has clearly been shown to be true for lymphoid dendritic cells (Steinman and Nussenzweig, 1980), for Langerhans cells (Katz *et al.*, 1979), and for dendritic cells in the synovial membrane (Klareskog *et al.*, 1982a).

III. CHARACTERISTICS OF MACROPHAGES, DENDRITIC CELLS, AND SYNOVIAL LINING CELLS

A. Macrophages and Dendritic Cells

Cytochemical and immunologic studies have revealed the characteristics of macrophages and dendritic cells depicted in Table 1. The various types of dendritic cells are strongly

Table 1. Characteristics of Monocyte/Macrophages and Dendritic Cells

Characteristic	Monocyte/macrophage	Dendritic cell
Ia antigen	+	+
Monocyte/macrophage antigen	+	−
B lymphocyte antigen	−	−
T lymphocyte antigen	−	−
Common leukocyte antigen	+	+
IgG Fc Receptor	+	−
C3b Receptor	+	−
Endocytosis	+	−
Nonspecific esterase	+	−
Myeloperoxidase	±	−
ATPase (Ca^{2+},Mg^{2+})	+	−
Adherence to glass and plastic	+	±

Ia-antigen positive (Rowden *et al.*, 1977; Førre *et al.*, 1983; Nussenzweig and Steinman, 1982; Winchester and Burmeister, 1981; van Voorhis *et al.*, 1983). Monocytes and macrophages also express Ia antigens, although to a lesser degree than dendritic cells (Niederhuber, 1978; Rosenthal, 1980; Unanue, 1978; van Voorhis *et al.*, 1983). By means of monoclonal antibodies, it has also recently been possible to define specific monocyte/macrophage (Flotte *et al.*, 1983; Hume *et al.*, 1983; Steinman, 1981; van Voorhis *et al.*, 1983) and dendritic cell markers (Nussenzweig *et al.*, 1982; Parwaresch *et al.*, 1983).

Macrophages and dendritic cells lack specific B-cell and T-cell markers (Steinman, 1981) except for human Langerhans cells, which express a thymocyte antigen (Murphy *et al.*, 1981). It is also possible that a proportion of synovial tissue dendritic cells express a thymocyte marker in humans (unpublished observations). Macrophages also have membrane receptor for IgG Fc and for C3b and exhibit endocytosis, whereas dendritic cells lack these markers (Steinman, 1981). Likewise, macrophages stain for nonspecific esterase, myeloperoxidase, and ATPase, whereas dendritic cells do not (Steinman, 1981). Macrophages and dendritic cells with a few exceptions adhere to glass and plastic surfaces. But whereas dendritic cells loosen after 16 hr the macrophages are still adherent (Steinman, 1981; Steinman and Nussenzweig, 1980). The dendritic cells can be isolated on the basis of their semiadherence to glass and plastic (Steinman, 1981; Steinman and Nussenzweig, 1980).

B. Synovial Lining Cells

The synovial lining cells have, on the basis of electron microscopic studies, been classified into macrophagelike A and C cells and fibroblastlike B cells (Table 2) (Barland *et al.*, 1962; Harris, 1981a,b; van Furth, 1981). The A and C synovial cells are rich in lysosomes, vacuoles, and vesicles, indicating that they are macrophages with phagocytic properties. The B cells have abundant rough endoplasmatic reticulum and golgi complex, indicating that these cells are fibroblasts with the capability of protein synthesis (Harris, 1981a). The synovial lining cells have also been shown to synthesize hyaluronic acid, which is a major component of the synovial fluid. It is probable that both the A and the B cells have the property of producing hyaluronic acid (Harris, 1981a). Synovial lining cells also produces large amounts of fibronectin, which is important in strengthening cell-to-cell contacts and in augmenting phagocytosis (Matsubara *et al.*, 1983; Pommier *et al.*, 1983). The synovial B cells seem to be the major producer of fibronectin (Matsubara *et al.*, 1983). Synovial A and C cells also have membrane receptors for IgG Fc and for C3b, further indicating that these cells are macrophages (Table 2) (Theofilopoulos *et al.*, 1980).

By the staining of synovial tissue sections and eluted adherent synovial tissue cells with anti-Ia reagents, it has recently been shown by many groups that a considerable proportion of the synovial cells are Ia-antigen positive (Burmeister *et al.*, 1983a,b; Førre *et al.*, 1982b; Janossy *et al.*, 1981; Klareskog *et al.*, 1981, 1982 b,c; Meijer *et al.*, 1983; Poulter and Duke, 1983; Poulter *et al.*, 1983; Winchester and Burmeister, 1981). Similarly, monocyte-specific antigens have been demonstrated in synovial tissue sections in the synovial lining layer and around vessels (Förre *et al.*, 1982b; Klareskog *et al.*, 1982b,c). These studies have very recently been extended by staining eluted adherent synovial cells from normals and from patients with rheumatoid arthritis using a panel of monoclonal antibodies specific for monocyte/macrophage antigens, Ia antigen, and fibroblast antigens (Burmeister *et al.*, 1983a,b). In this study, one could discern three major types of synovial lining cells (Table 2). Type I was Ia antigen positive, expressed monocyte/macrophage lineage antigens and receptors for IgG Fc and C3b, and had the property of phagocytosis (Fig. 2). Thus, this cell type is similar to the type A synovial lining cell. Type II cells had abundant Ia antigens only and had a dendritic morphology. This cell type thus represented a noval cell type in the rheumatoid synovial tissue (Fig. 3).

Electronic microscopic studies of eluted synovial tissue dendritic cells have shown that they exhibit small cytoplasmatic veils (Fig. 4). The type III synovial lining cell only expressed fibroblast antigens and was thus similar to the type B cell (Table 2). In the rheumatoid synovial membrane, there are also osteoclasts, which are active in resorbing bone (van Furth, 1981; Teitelbaum and Kahn, 1980). Osteoclasts are Ia antigen positive (Burmeister *et al.*, 1983b), but they lack macrophage markers such as receptors for IgG Fc or C3b (van Furth, 1981). This could, however, be a methodological error. The type I cell constitutes about 30–50%, the type II cell 5–30%, and the type III cell 30–70% of the synovial cells in rheumatoid arthritis (Burmeister *et al.*, 1983b).

Table 2. Characteristics of Synovial Lining Cells[a]

Characteristic	Type I (A and C cells)	Type II (dendritic cell)	Type III (B cell)
Ia antigen	+	+	−
Monocyte antigen	+	−	−
Fibroblast antigen	−	−	+
IgG Fc receptor	+	−	−
C3b	+	−	−
Phagocytosis	+	−	−

[a] Modified after Burmeister *et al.* (1983a).

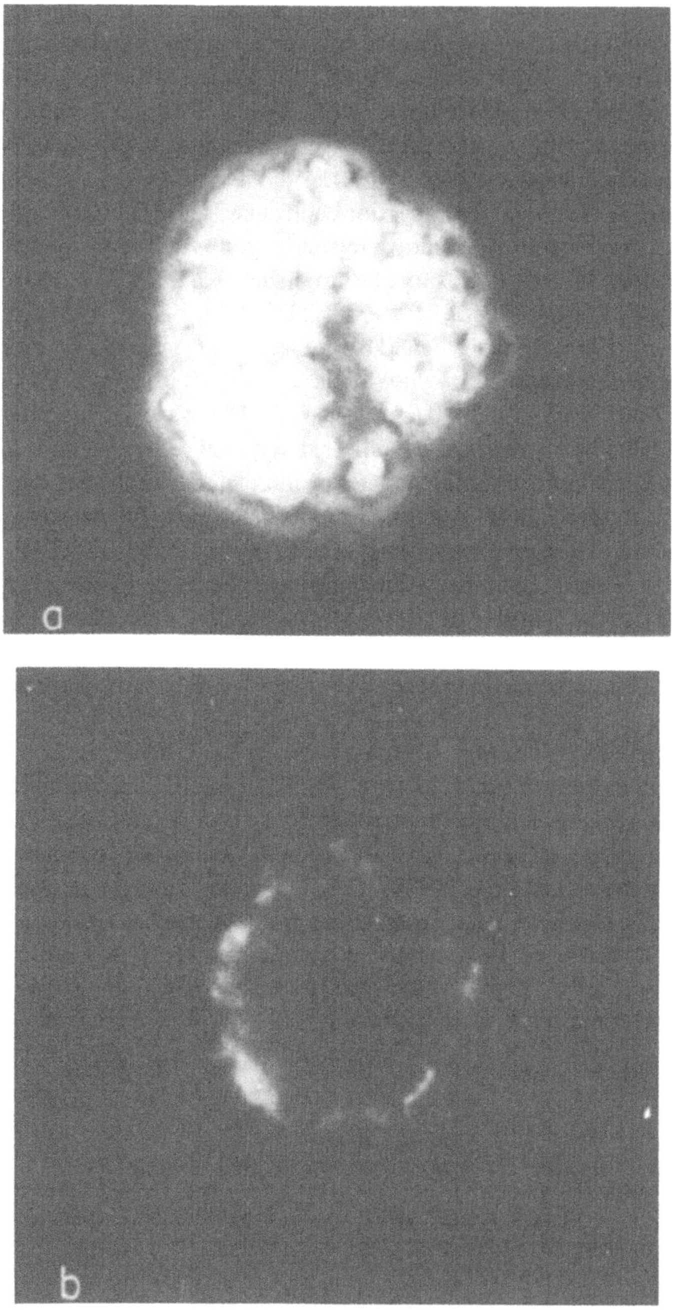

Figure 2. Phagocytic Ia^+ synovial cell. (a) Phase-contrast microscopic picture of a cell that has ingested numerous latex beads. (b) Fluorescent micrograph of the same cell demonstrating Ia antigen expression on a ruffled cell membrane. (From Burmeister *et al.*, 1983a, with permission.)

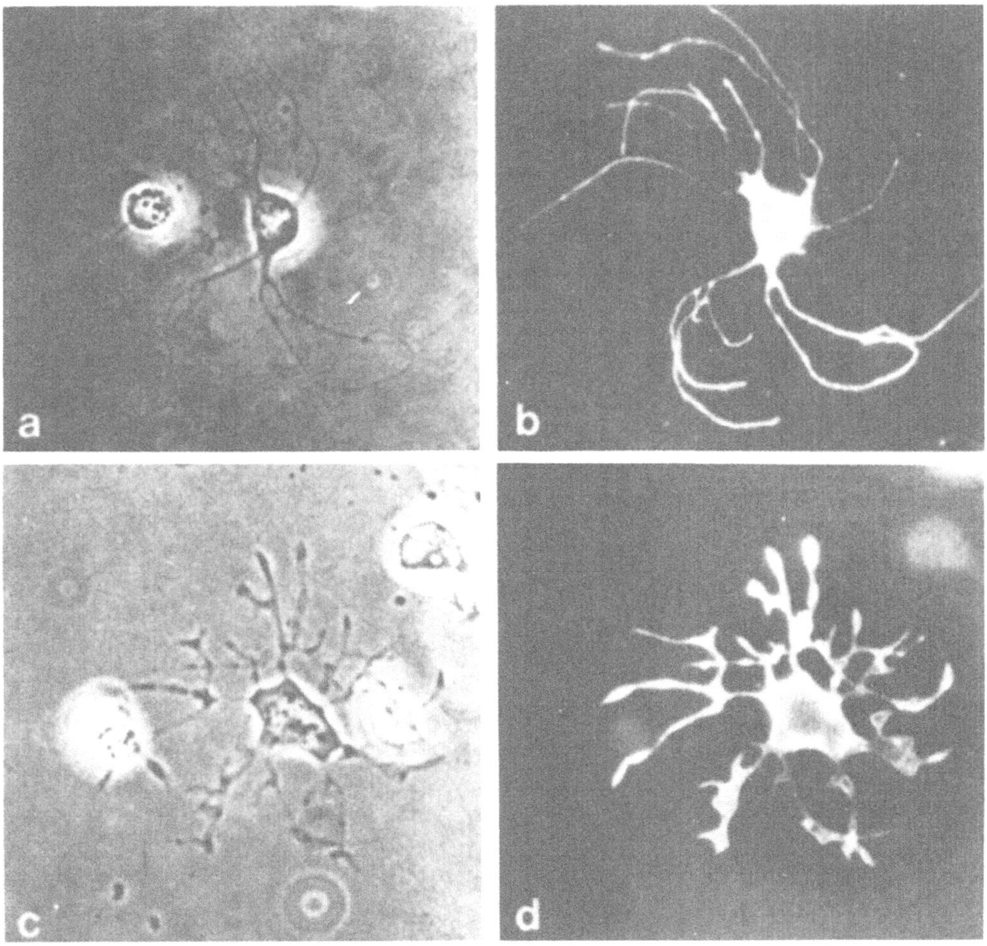

Figure 3. Synovial dendritic cells. (a) Phase microscopy with a monocytoid cell containing lysosomal granules and a binuclear dendritic cell. (b) Fluorescent microscopy demonstrating intense staining of Ia antigens on the dendritic cell. (c) Phase microscopy with two monocytoid cells and a dendritic cell. (d) Fluorescent microscopy demonstrating Ia antigen expression on a scalloped and irregular membrane. (From Winchester and Burmeister, 1981, with permission.)

IV. THE ROLE OF SYNOVIAL CELLS IN THE RHEUMATOID INFLAMMATION

A. Tissue Architecture of Synovial Membranes

In patients with noninflammatory joint diseases, type I cells (A and C cells) represent the major cell proportion of the synovial layer close to the joint cavity (Fig. 5). These cells are also found scattered in the subsynovial tissue and in perivascular areas (Fig. 5). Very few type II cells (dendritic cells) can be identified in synovial membranes from patients with noninflammatory joint diseases (Burmeister *et al.*, 1983a,b). The fibroblastoid type III cells constitute the major cell population in the subsynovial layer in those patients (Fig. 4).

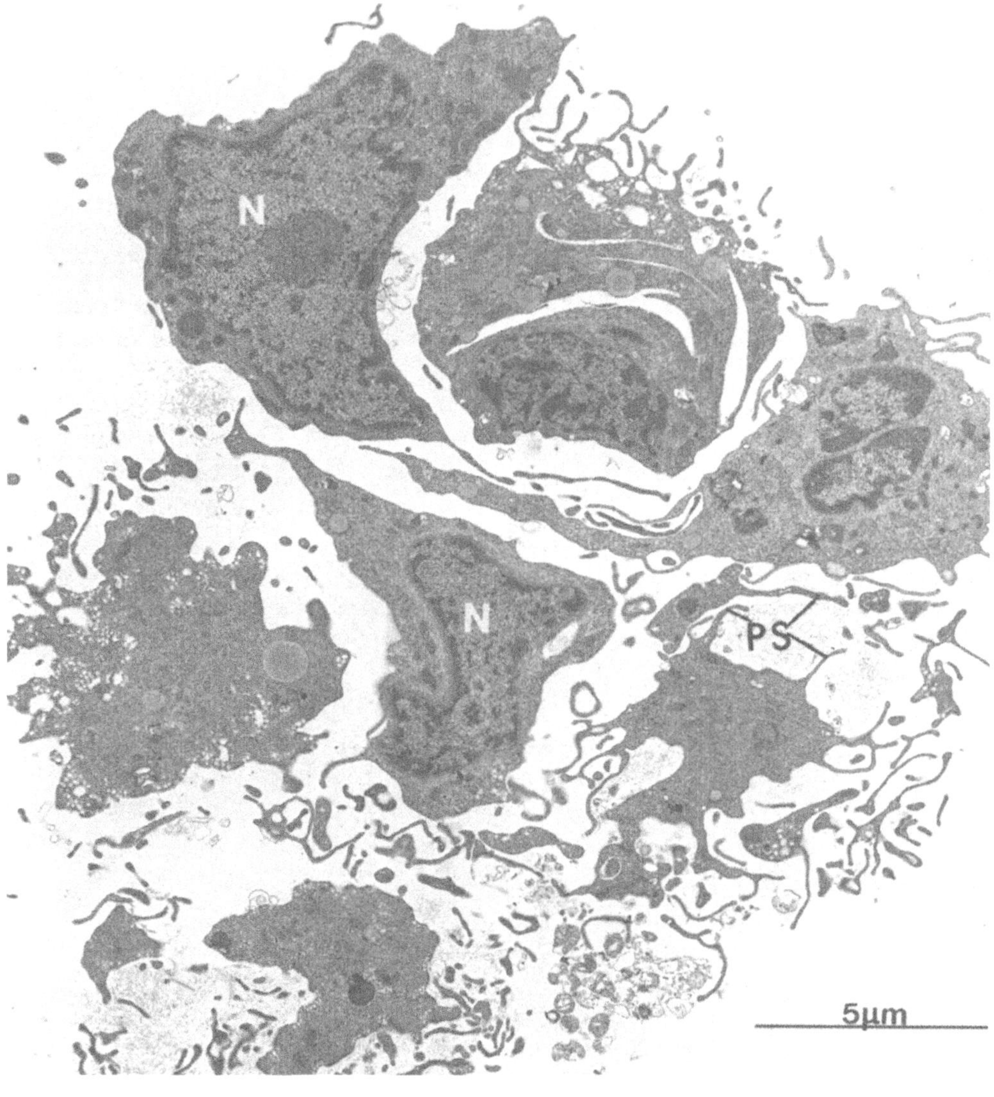

Figure 4. Electron micrograph of dendritic cells isolated from the rheumatoid synovial membrane. The cells show numerous long, slender pseudopods (PS). The cytoplasm contains some mitochondria, lipid droplets, free ribosomes, a few cisternae of granular endoplasmic reticulum, and several filaments 7–10 nm in diameter. The filaments are partly organized as a perinuclear bundle. Langerhans cell granules not observed. Nucleus (N).

In inflammatory joint diseases there is an enormous proliferation of synovial lining cells (Fig. 6). Large numbers of the macrophagelike type I synovial lining cells form a characteristic double configuration with these cells in a layer close to the joint cavity followed by a nonmacrophage layer and a type I cell layer close to the subsynovial tissue (Fig. 5) (Burmeister *et al.*, 1983a,b). In inflammatory disorders, the macrophagelike type I cells can also be demonstrated diffusely in the inflammed subsynovial tissue, in the perivascular regions, and in lymphoid follicles (Fig. 5) (Burmeister *et al.*, 1983a,b).

Type II (dendritic) cells seem to be localized primarily in the broadened layer of the synoviocytes, in perivascular regions, and in the lymphoid follicles (Fig. 5). These findings extend previous observations (Førre *et al.*, 1982b; Janossy *et al.*, 1981; Klareskog *et al.*, 1981, 1982a–c; Poulter and Duke, 1983; Poulter *et al.*, 1983). It has also been shown that macrophagelike (Fig. 7) or dendritic cells in rheumatoid tissues are localized in close contact with T4^{+} helper/inducer T cells, whereas the T8^{+} suppressor (cytotoxic) cells are scattered in between (Førre *et al.*, 1982b; Janossy *et al.*, 1981; Klareskog *et al.*, 1982b,c; Meijer *et al.*, 1983; Poulter and Duke, 1983; Poulter *et al.*, 1983).

In regions with B-cell/plasma-cell infiltration, the functional consequences of this architecture may be immunoglobulin production locally in the diseased joints (Fig. 8) (Janossy *et al.*, 1981): antigens in the tissue are brought to the tissue via the circulation, processed by macrophages, and taken up by dendritic cells (Fig. 8a). The dendritic cells then present the antigens for helper/inducer T cells (Fig. 8b), which again trigger B cells to proliferation and differentiation and immunoglobulin production (Falkoff *et al.*, 1982) (Fig. 8c). The T helper cells also possibly act back on the antigen-presenting dendritic cells (Fig. 8b), thus augmenting their infiltration and Ia antigen positivity (Janossy *et al.*, 1981). It is also probable that the dendritic cells stimulate adjacent T cells in an *in vivo* autologous mixed leukocyte reaction without the need for antigens (Fig. 8b,c) (Førre *et al.*, 1983; Kuntz-Crow and Kunkel, 1982; Klinkert *et al.*, 1982; Steinman *et al.*, 1983). T helper cells might also form clusters around Ia-antigen-positive dendritic cells because the T cells might have antigen-specific receptors for self-Ia (Janossy *et al.*, 1981; Thorsby

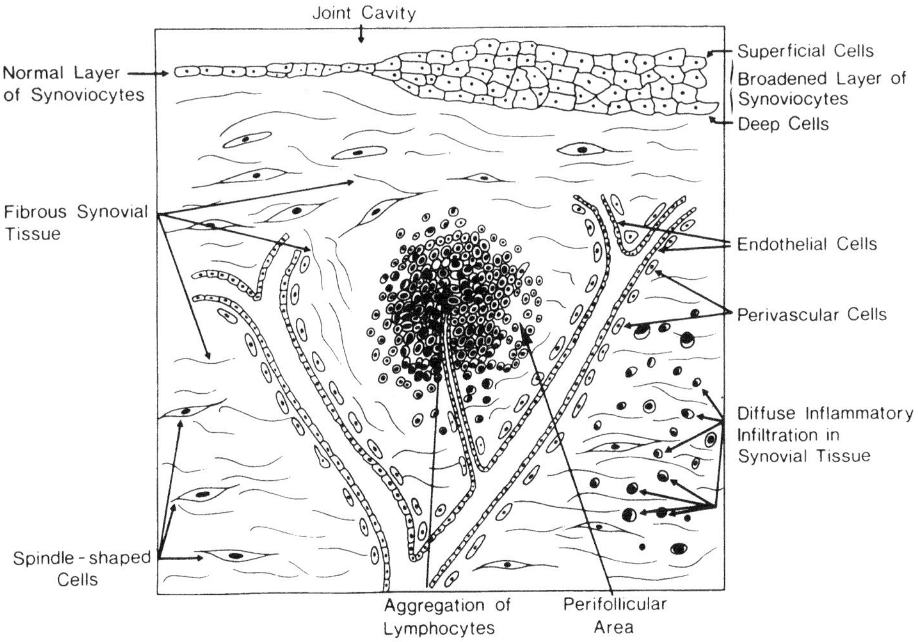

Figure 5. Schematic presentation of a synovial membrane in the noninflamed (left) and inflamed (right) state. (From Burmeister *et al.*, 1983b, with permission.)

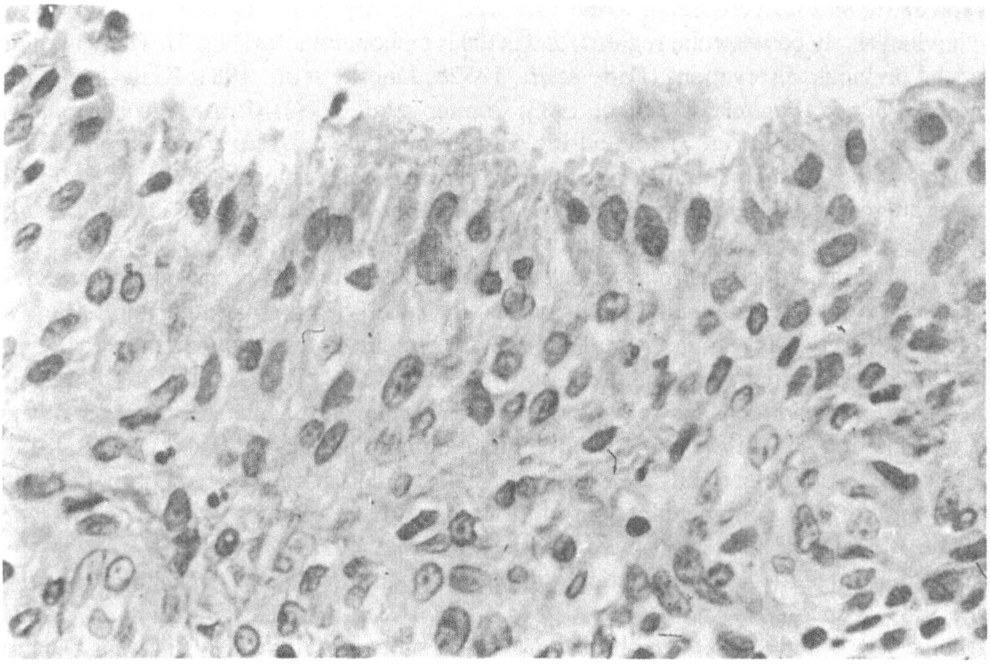

Figure 6. Light microscopic picture of synovial lining cells from a rheumatoid synovial membrane. Synovial cavity upwards.

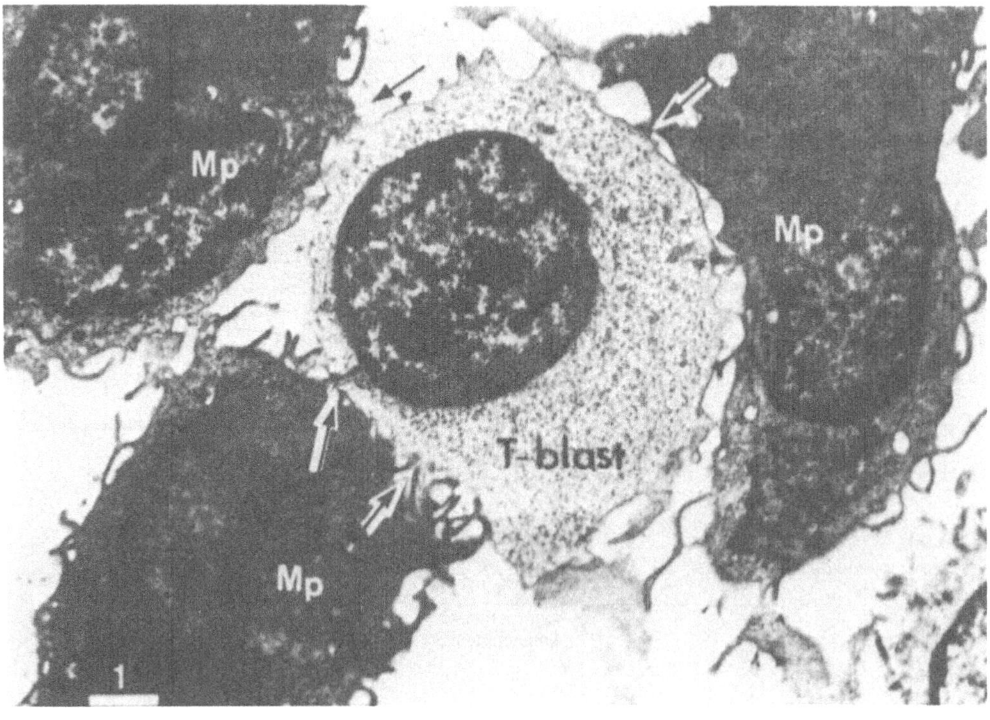

Figure 7. T lymphoblast (T blast) surrounded by three macrophages (Mp). (Provided by H. Ischikawa and M. Ziff, from Harris, 1981, with permission.)

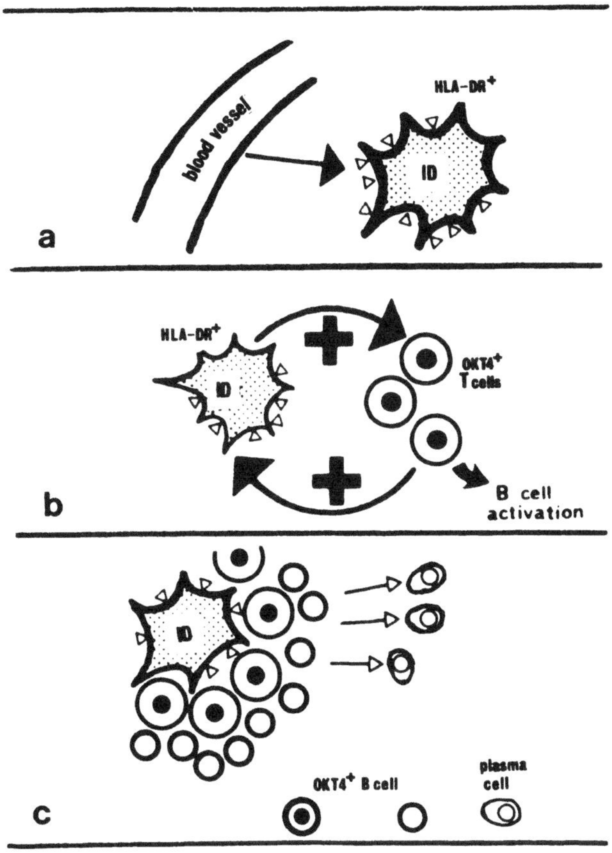

Figure 8. The vicious cycle leading to immunoregulatory disorder in the synovial membrane in rheumatoid arthritis. (a) Antigens (small triangles) are taken up by interdigitating cells (dendritic cells). (b) The antigens are presented for T4$^+$ helper/inducer T cells, which have a positive feedback on the dendritic cells. (c) The T4$^+$ cells trigger the B cells to produce immunoglobulin and rheumatoid factor. (From Janossy *et al.*, 1981, with permission.)

et al., 1982). The close cell-to-cell contact observed for rheumatoid dendritic cells and T helper cells also fits well with the previously observed Ia-antigen restriction for macrophage–dendritic-cell interaction with T cells (Berle *et al.*, 1982; Bergholtz *et al.*, 1980; Hirschberg *et al.*, 1982; Rosenthal, 1980; Thorsby *et al.*, 1982). In preliminary studies we have also observed that rheumatoid dendritic cells presents antigens for T cells in an HLA-D/DR-restricted manner (unpublished observations).

B. Rheumatoid Dendritic Cells as Accessory Cells for Immune Responses

Previously it has been shown that rodent dendritic cells from various compartments and human Langerhans cells and dendritic cells from peripheral blood are very good accessory cells for various immune responses (Berle *et al.*, 1982; Braathen and Thorsby, 1980; Hirscberg *et al.*, 1982; Inoba *et al.*, 1983; Klinkert *et al.*, 1982; Knight *et al.*, 1982, 1983; Kuntz-Crow and Kunkel, 1982; Nussenzweig *et al.*, 1980; Scheynius *et al.*, 1983; Spalding *et al.*, 1983; Steinman and Cohn, 1974; Steinman and Nussenzweig, 1980; Steinman *et al.*, 1983; Sunshine *et al.*, 1983). Macrophages have also been claimed to have good accessory functions (Bergholtz *et al.*, 1980; Librach and Burns, 1983; Niederhuber, 1978; Rosenthal, 1980; Thorsby *et al.*, 1982; Wischer, 1982). Unfractionated adherent synovial cells also stimulate allogeneic T cells and present soluble antigens for autologous T cells in a very efficient way (Klareskog *et al.*, 1982b,c), indicating that these cells must contain cell population(s) with extremely good accessory function(s).

Our group has isolated and purified dendritic cells from peripheral blood, synovial tissue, and synovial fluid from patients with rheumatoid arthritis on the basis of their semiadherence to plastic surfaces (Førre *et al.*, 1982a, 1983). Monocytes/macrophages were further removed from the dendritic cells by incubation on plastic dishes coated with IgG, as these cells are known to express IgG Fc receptors. Our dendritic cells had a purity of more than 85% as assayed by their Ia antigen positivity and lacked Fc receptor positivity and nonspecific esterase positivity. Monocytes with a purity of more than 95% were isolated from peripheral blood using a newly described technique (Bøyum, 1983). The rheumatoid dendritic cells had a much higher stimulating capacity in allogeneic and autologous mixed leukocyte reactions than peripheral non-T cells (mononuclear cells depleted of T cells) and monocytes (Table 3). They also had much more efficient accessory functions for antigen and mitogen responses than non-T cells and monocytes (Table 4). Our findings suggest that rheumatoid dendritic cells, like other types of dendritic cells, are the main accessory cells (Inoba *et al.*, 1983; Klinkert *et al.*, 1982; Kuntz-Crow and Kunkel, 1982; Scheynius *et al.*, 1983; Steinman *et al.*, 1983). Rheumatoid dendritic cells could also present autoantigens such as collagen type II and Fc fragments for autologous T cells in a more efficient way than non-T cells (unpublished observations; Trentham *et al.*, 1978; Weibart *et al.*, 1975). Thus, they are able to act as accessory cells in the synovial membrane for immunoglobulin and other autoantigens, possibly altered by macrophages (Daha *et al.*, 1982).

It has recently been shown that interleukin 1 is a prerequisite for T-cell activation (Lachman *et al.*, 1977; Smith *et al.*, 1980). Interleukin 1 has previously been shown to be produced by macrophages (Lachman *et al.*, 1977; Smith *et al.*, 1980); thus, it is also probably produced by macrophagelike synovial lining cells, as this monokine has been demonstrated in the synovial fluid in large quantities (Fontana *et al.*, 1982; Wood *et al.*, 1983; Ziff, 1981). Recently rheumatoid dendritic cells have also been shown to produce interleukin 1 (Duff *et al.*, 1985). Thus, interleukin 1 production by various types of synovial lining cells can explain the occurrence of fever and the rise in acute-phase reactants often seen in inflammatory joint diseases (Selinger *et al.*, 1980).

Table 3. Comparison of Allogeneic and Autologous Mixed Leukocyte Reaction Responses (Mean cpm and Ranges) Using 10^5 Rheumatoid Non-T Cells, Monocytes, and Dendritic Cells as Stimulator Cells and 10^5 Allogeneic and Autologous T Cells as Responder Cells[a]

Stimulator cells	No.	Allogeneic MLR	No.	Autologous MLR
Non-T cells$_{PB}$	20	16,585 (1,111–83,480)	20	2,112 (354–11,260)
Dendritic cells$_{PB}$	10	58,571 (12,726–135,050)	10	7,755 (1,540–23,292)
Dendritic cells$_{ST}$	5	73,608 (52,676–118,267)	5	25,365 (8,292–49,911)
Dendritic cells$_{SF}$	5	46,202 (12,420–101,156)	5	10,046 (3,320–18,596)
Monocytes$_{PB}$	5	2,828 (688–5,968)	6	810 (156–1,994)

[a] MLR, mixed leukocyte reaction; PB, peripheral blood; ST, synovial tissue; SF, synovial fluid. The responses denote [^{3}H]thymidine incorporation expressed as cpm. The purity of the monocytes was more than 95%, and the purity of dendritic cells was more than 85%.

Table 4. Comparison of PPD and Con A Responses (cpm and Ranges) Using 2.5 × 10^3 Non-T Cells, Monocytes, and Dendritic Cells as Accessory Cells and 10^5 Autologous T Cells as Responder Cells[a]

Accessory cells	No.	PPD responses	No.	Con A responses
Non-T cells$_{PB}$	17	3,841 (119–22,178)	8	5,342 (590–18,199)
Dendritic cells$_{PB}$	10	10,514 (2,165–25,051)	8	13,622 (381–40,226)
Dendritic cells$_{ST}$	5	12,217 (1,873–20,355)	—	—
Dendritic cells$_{SF}$	5	7,453 (2,914–10,783)	—	—
Monocytes$_{PB}$	—	—	4	3,161 (1,577–4,402)

[a] PPD, purified protein derivative of tuberculin; Con A, concanavalin A; PB, peripheral blood; ST, synovial tissue; SF, synovial fluid. The responses denote [^{3}H]thymidine incorporation expressed as cpm. The purity of the monocytes was more than 95%, and the purity of the dendritic cells was more than 85%.

C. Arachidonic Acid Products and Other Regulatory Factors Produced by Macrophagelike Synovial Cells

Membrane phospholipids are converted to arachidonic acid by a lipase in several types of synovial cells. The arachidonate is further enzymatically converted to prostaglandins and thromboxanes by cyclooxygenase and to leukotrienes by a lipoxygenase (Fig. 9) (Bomey *et al.*, 1981; Brune, 1982; Passwell *et al.*, 1979; Pawlowski *et al.*, 1983; Scheinberg *et al.*, 1983; Vaes, 1981; Weissman, 1982, 1983). Phagocytosis of opsonized particles, altered IgG, and immune complexes is probably the main stimulus for the synovial cells to produce prostaglandins and leukotrienes (Panayi, 1981; Roos, 1981; Ziff, 1981). Prostaglandins, throboxanes, and leukotrienes modulate inflammation (Weissman, 1983). It has also been shown that prostaglandins are important regulatory factors for various types of immune responses (Goodwin and Webb, 1980). The lymphocytes also act back on the macrophages and in turn regulate their function (Whitten *et al.*,

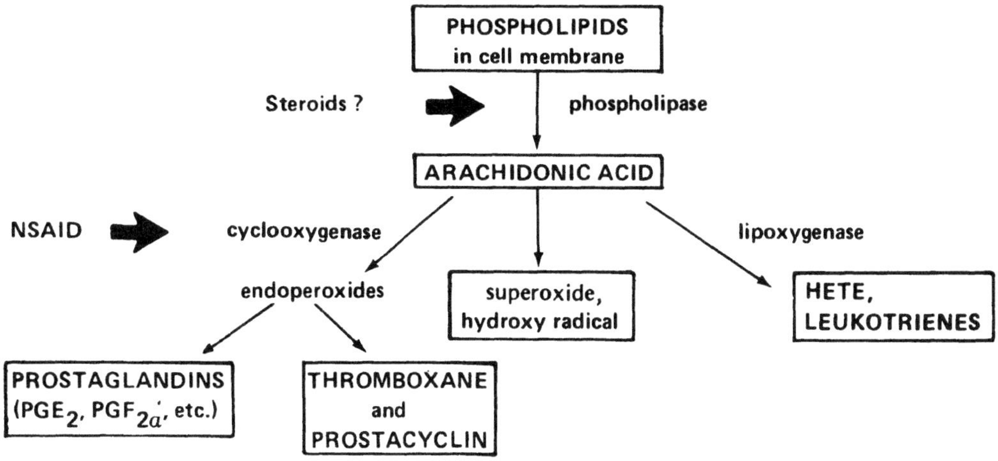

Figure 9. A schematic representation of the arachidonic acid cascade. (From Lombardino, 1983, with permission.)

1983; Wischer, 1982). Prostaglandin E_2 can also stimulate the production of collagenase by macrophages and fibroblastoid dendritic cells in the synovial membrane (Parnham *et al.*, 1981; Wooley, 1978). There are also monokines, including interleukin 1, that regulate the production of collagenase and prostaglandin by rheumatoid synovial cells (Dayer, 1981; Krane *et al.*, 1982). Other monokines probably inhibit collagen synthesis by fibroblasts and fibroblastoid synovial cells (Hart *et al.*, 1983).

D. Production of Enzymes and Oxygen Radicals by Synovial Cells: Role in Tissue Destruction

During phagocytosis or other types of macrophage activation, granular proteolytic enzymes are discharged into phagosomes and serve to kill or digest phagocytized material (Leijh and van Furth, 1981; Roos, 1981). Large amounts of enzymes such as lysozyme, neutral proteinases, and lysosomal hydrolases are also liberated into the surroundings of the phagocytizing cells, where they might cause tissue destruction (Baggiolini, 1981; Roos, 1981; Russel *et al.*, 1981). One of the most important enzymes for the tissue destruction is probably collagenase, which can cleave various types of collagens and which is produced by many types of synovial cells (Krane *et al.*, 1982). Enzymes such as elastases and chymotrypsin may be responsible for the loss of articular cartilage proteoglycan seen in early rheumatoid arthritis in regions remote from the pannus (Krane *et al.*, 1982; Russel *et al.*, 1981; Vaes, 1981).

The resorption of bone seen in rheumatoid arthritis is to a large extent caused by osteoclasts. These cells secrete lytic enzymes that fragment and solubilize organic compounds such as collagen and proteoglycans of the extracellular bone matrix so as to allow endocytosis and further intracellular digestion (Vaes, 1981). Oxygen free radicals are generated during phagocytosis by synovial macrophagelike cells and as a result of tissue destruction (Famey, 1982; Harth *et al.*, 1983; Lunec *et al.*, 1981). It has been suggested that some of the free radicals are able to kill adjacent cells and might therefore play a role in the tissue destruction in rheumatic diseases (Krane *et al.*, 1982).

V. THE MONONUCLEAR PHAGOCYTE SYSTEM IN RHEUMATIC DISEASES

The mononuclear phagocyte system is comprised of mononuclear phagocytes in the spleen, liver, and other lymphoid tissues (Ryan and Hughes, 1982). The most important cells in this system are the macrophages, which have membrane receptors for IgG Fc and for complement factor C3b (Roos, 1981; Johnson *et al.*, 1983). This explains why particles opsonized by IgG and C3b are readily phagocytized. The phagocytosis is enhanced by fibronectin, which is produced in large amounts in the rheumatoid synovial membrane (Harris, 1981a; Pommier *et al.*, 1983). The macrophages in this system are responsible for the clearance of circulating immune complexes (Fields *et al.*, 1983; Ryan *et al.*, 1982; Williams *et al.*, 1979). In patients with systemic lupus erythematosus, it has been shown that there is a defect in monocyte C3b- and Fc-receptor-mediated phagocytosis leading to a reduced clearance of circulating immune complexes (Fields *et al.*, 1983). This is probably an important factor in the pathogenesis of this disorder. Similarly, there is also a defect in monocyte C3b-receptor-mediated phagocytosis in rheumatoid arthritis (Fields *et al.*, 1983; Ryan *et al.*, 1982; Williams *et al.*, 1979). Patients with rheumatoid arthritis and systemic manifestations also have a defect of Fc receptor function. This might lead to the deposition of immune complexes in this disorder (Fields *et al.*, 1983).

VI. MONOCYTES/MACROPHAGES AND DENDRITIC CELLS AS TARGETS FOR DRUG THERAPY

Corticosteroids have many effects on monocytes/macrophages. They inhibit monocyte chemotaxis. Monocytes are also more sensitive to the redistribution effect of corticosteroids than are lymphocytes. The accessory functions of monocytes/macrophages for various immune responses are inhibited by corticosteroids (Cupps and Fauci, 1982). The production of interleukin 1 and other monokines is also inhibited by these drugs (Cupps and Fauci, 1982). It is also probable that corticosteroids have similar effects on the accessory functions of dendritic cells. Thus, corticosteroid-induced effects on accessory cells may indirectly alter the functions of B and T lymphocytes, resulting in altered immune responses (Cupps and Fauci, 1982). Monocyte/macrophage IgG Fc- and C3b-receptor-mediated functions, such as phagocytosis, are modulated by corticosteroids (Cupps and Fauci, 1982). These drugs also inhibit phospholipase A_2, which converts phospholipids into arachidonic acid. This results in reduced production of arachidonate metabolites such as prostaglandins, thromboxanes, and leukotrienes (Fig. 9) (Brune, 1982; Lombardino, 1983; Weissmann, 1982).

Nonsteroidal antiinflammatory drugs inhibit the enzyme cyclooxygenase, which catalyzes the conversion of arachidonic acid to prostaglandins and thromboxanes, thus reducing inflammation and possibly also immune responses in patients with rheumatic diseases (Brune, 1982; Goodwin and Webb, 1980; Weissman, 1982, 1983). It is possible that some of the antiinflammatory drugs also inhibit the liberation of proteolytic enzymes and oxygen radicals from the macrophagelike synovial lining cells and other cell types (Lombardino, 1983; Weissmann, 1982, 1983).

It is probable that the main target cell for the effects of gold salts is the macrophage (Lipsky and Ziff, 1982; Scheinberg *et al.*, 1982). Thus, it has been shown that chemotaxis and IgG Fc- and C3b-receptor-mediated functions are inhibited by gold (Scheinberg *et al.*, 1982). Gold salts are taken up by macrophagelike synovial lining cells during chrysotherapy. This leads to inhibition of lysosomal enzymes (Ziff, 1981) and to inhibition of the accessory capacities of the macrophages (Lipsky and Ziff, 1982).

Antimalarial drugs also primarily act on the macrophages, causing stabilization of lysosomes and inhibition of enzymes (Lombardino, 1983). Cytostatic drugs such as azathioprine, methotrexate, chlorambucil, and cyclophosphamide generally inhibit the DNA synthesis of all dividing cells (Bach, 1975). These drugs thus have many target cells, and they can act on progenitors of both monocyte/macrophages and dendritic cells, which probably proliferate in the bone marrow or at inflammatory sites.

VII. CONCLUDING REMARKS

Until recently the lymphocytes and plasma cells of rheumatoid inflammation have been examined in many studies. However, after the development of monoclonal antibodies and after the discovery of the importance of accessory cells for the various immune responses, attention has also been paid to the rheumatoid macrophages and dendritic cells. Thus, very recent studies have revealed an architecture in the synovial tissue that implies cell-to-cell contact and cooperation between cells leading to local immune reactions.

The synovial cells also produce various types of soluble factors, of which arachidonate products are very important. The prostaglandins were regarded earlier as proinflammatory factors. Recent studies, however, indicate that prostaglandins in fact have antiinflammatory effects. Further studies are therefore needed to clarify the role of macrophages and dendritic cells in rheumatoid inflammation.

ACKNOWLEDGMENTS. The skillful technical assistance of Jorun Grandaunet is gratefully acknowledged. This work was supported by The Norwegian Hydro Company and Pfizer International. We are also grateful to Professor Erik KÅss and Professor Jan Pahle, Oslo Sanitetsforenings Rheumatism Hospital, for providing the material for the study.

REFERENCES

Bach, J. F. (ed.), 1975, *The Mode of Action of Immunosuppressive Agents*, North-Holland/American Elsevier, New York, pp. 93–225.

Baggiolini, M., 1981, Exportable enzymes of phagocytes, *Scand. J. Rheumatol. Suppl.* **40**:42–45.

Balfour, B. M., Drexhage, H. A., Kamperdick, E. W. A., and Hoefsmith, E. M., 1981, Antigen-presenting cells, including Lagerhans cells, veiled cells and interdigitating cells in microenvironments in haemopoietic and lymphoid differentiation, *Ciba Found. Symp.* **84**:281–301.

Barland, P., Novikoff, A. B., and Hamerman, D., 1962, Electron microscopy of the human synovial membrane, *J. Cell. Biol.* **14**:207–212.

Bergholtz, B. D., Thoreson, A. B., and Thorsby, E., 1980, HLA-D/DR restriction of macrophage dependent antigen activation of immune T lymphocytes: Cross-reacting allogeneic HLA-D/DR may partly substitute for self HLA-D/DR, *Scand. J. Immunol.* **11**:541–548.

Berle, E. J., Braathen, L. R., and Thorsby, E., 1982, HLA-D/DR restriction of Langerhans cell-dependent antigen activation of T lymphocytes. The same D/DR determinants are restriction elements on monocytes and Langerhans cells, *Scand. J. Immunol.* **16**:549–552.

Bomey, R. J., Wightman, P. D., Dahlgren, M. E., Humes, J. L., and Davies, P., 1981, The pathways of biosynthesis for prostaglandins by the stimulus triggered macrophage, *Scand. J. Rheumatol. Suppl.* **40**:53–57.

Braathen, L. R., and Thorsby, E., 1980, Studies on human epidermal Langerhans cells, *Scand. J. Immunol.* **11**:401–408.

Brune, K., 1982, Prostaglandins, inflammation and antiinflammatory drugs, *Eur. J. Rheum. Inflam.* **5**:335–349.

Burmeister, G. R., Dimitriu-Bona, A., Waters, S. J., and Winchester, R. J., 1983a, Identification of three major synovial lining cell populations by monoclonal antibodies directed to Ia antigens and antigens associated with monocytes/macrophages and fibroblasts, *Scand. J. Immunol.* **17**:69–82.

Burmeister, G. R., Locher, P., Koch, B., Winchester, R. J., Dimitriu-Bona, A., Kalden, J. R., and Mohr, W., 1983b, The tissue architecture of synovial membranes in inflammatory and non-inflammatory joint diseases. I. The localization of the major synovial cell populations as detected by monoclonal reagents directed towards Ia and monocyte/macrophage antigens, *Rheumatol. Int.* **3**:173–181.

Bøyum, A., 1983, Isolation of human blood monocytes with Nycodenz, a new non-ionic iodinated gradient medium, *Scand. J. Immunol.* **17**:429–431.

Coccia, P. F., Krivit, W., Cervenkea, J., Clomson, C., Kersey, J. H., Kim, T. H., Nesbit, M. E., Ramsay, N. K. C., Warkentin, P. I., and Teitelbaum, S. L., 1980, Successful bone-marrow transplantation for infantile malignant osteopetrosis, *N. Engl. J. Med.* **302:**701–702.

Cupps, T. R., and Fauci, A. S., 1982, Corticosteroid-mediated immunoregulation in man, *Immunol. Rev.* **65:**133–155.

Daha, M. R., vanEs, L. A., Hazevoet, H. M., and Kijlstra, A., 1982, Degradation of soluble immunoglobulin aggregates *in vitro* by monocytes from normal subjects and from patients with systemic lupus erythematosus, *Scand. J. Immunol.* **16:**117–122.

Dayer, J. M., 1981, Some characteristics and functional aspects of the human monokine, MCF, stimulating collagenase and PGE_2 production by rheumatoid synovial cells, *Scand. J. Rheumatol. Suppl.* **40:**88–92.

Duff, G. W., Førre, Ø., Waalen, K., Dickens, E., and Nuki, G., 1985, Rheumatoid arthritis synovial dendritic cells produce interleukin 1. *Brit. J. Rheumatol.* (in press).

Falkoff, R. J. M., Ping Zhu, L., and Fauci, A., 1982, Separate signals for human B cell proliferation and differentiation in response to *Staphylococcus aureus:* Evidence for a two-signal model of B cell activation, *J. Immunol.* **129:**97–102.

Famey, J. P., 1982, Free radicals and activated oxygen, *Eur. J. Rheum. Inflam.* **5:**350–359.

Fields, T. R., Gerardi, E. N., Ghebrehiwet, B., Bennet, R. S., Laley, T. J., Hall, R. P., Plotz, P. H., Karsh, J. R., Frank, M. M., and Hamburger, M. I., 1983, Reticuloendothelial system. Fc-receptor function in rheumatoid arthritis, *J. Rheumatol.* **10:**550–557.

Flotte, T. J., Springer, T. A., and Thorbecke, G. J., 1983, Dendritic cell and macrophage staining by monoclonal antibodies in tissue sections and epidermal sheets, *Am. J. Pathol.* **111:**112–124.

Fontana, A., Hengartner, H., Weber, E., Fehr, K., Grob, P. J., and Cohen, G., 1982, Interleukin 1 activity in the synovial fluid of patients with rheumatoid arthritis, *Rheumatol. Int.* **2:**49–53.

Førre, Ø, Waalen, K., GlennÅs, A., and Thorsby, E., 1982a, Dendritic cells from the rheumatoid synovial membrane as antigen-presenting cells, *Immunobiology* **163:**2/3/4, 115.

Førre, Ø, Thoen, J., Lea, T., Dobloug, J. H., Mellbye, O. J., Natvig, J. B., Pahle, J., and Solheim, B. G., 1982b, *In situ* characterization of mononuclear cells in rheumatoid tissues using monoclonal antibodies. No reduction in T8-positive cells or augmentation of T4-positive cells, *Scand. J. Immunol.* **16:**315–319.

Førre, Ø, Thoen, J., Waalen, K., and Natvig, J. B., 1983, Autologous mixed lymphocyte reactions in rheumatoid arthritis. Characterization of stimulator cells and the recognition unit for autoantigens on the responder cells, in: *The Autologous Mixed Lymphocyte Reaction: A Basic Immune Regulatory Mechanism, Behring Institute Research Communications,* No. 72 (M. E. Weksler, J. R. Kalden, and N. Talal, eds.), Medizinische Verlagsgesellschaft, Marburg, pp. 188–192.

Goodwin, J. S., and Webb, D., 1980, Regulation of the immune response by prostaglandins, *Clin. Immunol. Immunopathol.* **15:**106–122.

Harris, E. D., Jr., 1981a, Biology of the joint, in: *Textbook of Rheumatology* (W. N. Kelley, E. D. Harris, Jr., S. Ruddy, and C. B. Sledge, eds.), W. B. Saunders, Philadelphia, pp. 255–276.

Harris, E. D., Jr., 1981b, Pathogenesis of rheumatoid arthritis in: *Textbook of Rheumatology* (W. N. Kelley, E. D. Harris, Jr., S. Ruddy, and C. B. Sledge, eds.), W. B. Saunders, Philadelphia, pp. 896–927.

Hart, P. H., Powell, L. W., Cooksley, W. G. E., and Holliday, J. W., 1983, Mononuclear cell factors that inhibit fibroblast collagen synthesis. I. *In vitro* conditions determining their production and expression, *Scand. J. Immunol.* **18:**41–49.

Harth, M., Keown, P. A., and Orange, J. F., 1983, Monocyte dependent excited oxygen radical generation in rheumatoid arthritis: Inhibition by gold sodium thiomalate, *J. Rheumatol.* **10:**701–707.

Hirschberg, H., Braathen, L. R., and Thorsby, E., 1982, Antigen presentation by vascular endothelial cells and epidermal Langerhans cells: The role of HLA-DR, *Immunol. Rev.* **66:**57–77.

Hume, D. A., Robinson, A. P., MacPherson, G. G., and Gordon, S., 1983, The mononuclear phagocyte system of the mouse defined by immunohistochemical localization of antigen F4/80. Relationship between macrophages, Langerhans cells, reticular cells and dendritic cells in lymphoid and hematopoietic organs, *J. Exp. Med.* **158:**1522–1536.

Inoba, K., Steinman, R. M., van Voorhis, W. C., and Muramatsu, S., 1983, Dendritic cells are critical accessory cells for thymus-dependent antibody responses in mouse and in man, *Proc. Natl. Acad. Sci. U.S.A.* **80:**6041–6045.

Janossy, G., Duke, O., Poulter, L. W., Panayi, G., Bofill, M., and Goldstein, G., 1981, Rheumatoid arthritis: A disease of T-lymphocyte/macrophage immunoregulation, *Lancet* **2:**839–842.

Johnson, E., Bøgwald, J., Eskeland, T., and Seljelid, R., 1983, Complement (C3) receptor-mediated attachment of agarose beads to mouse peritoneal macrophages and human monocytes, *Scand. J. Immunol.* **17**:403–410.

Katz, S. I., Tamaki, K., and Sachs, D. H., 1979, Epidermal Langerhans cells are derived from cells originating in bone marrow, *Nature* **282**:324–326.

Klareskog, L., Forsum, U., Malmnaes Tjernlund, U., Kabelitz, D., and Wigren, A., 1981, Appearance of anti-HLA-DR-reactive cells in normal and rheumatoid synovial tissue, *Scand. J. Immunol.* **14**:183–192.

Klareskog, L., Forsum, U., and Wigzell, H., 1982a, Murine synovial intima contains I-A-, I-E/C-positive bone-marrow-derived cells, *Scand. J. Immunol.* **15**:509–514.

Klareskog, L., Forsum, U., Scheynius, A., Kabelitz, D., and Wigzell, H., 1982b, Evidence in support of a self-perpetuating HLA-DR-dependent delayed-type cell reaction in rheumatoid arthritis, *Proc. Natl. Acad. Sci. U.S.A.* **79**:3632–3636.

Klareskog, L., Forsum, U., Kabelitz, D., Pløen, L., Sundstrøm, C., Nilsson, K., Wigren, A., and Wiegzell, H., 1982c, Immune functions of human synovial cells. Phenotypic and T cell regulatory properties of macrophage-like cells that express HLA-DR, *Arthritis Rheum.* **25**:488–501.

Klinkert, W. E., LaBadie, J. H., and Bowers, W. E., 1982, Accessory and stimulating properties of dendritic cells and macrophages isolated from various rat tissues, *J. Exp. Med.* **156**:1–19.

Knight, S. C., Balfour, B. M., O'Brien, J., Buttifant, L., Sumerska, T., and Clarke, J., 1982, Role of veiled cells in lymphocyte activation, *Eur. J. Immunol.* **12**:1057–1060.

Knight, S. C., Mertin, J., Stackpoole, A., and Clark, J., 1983, Induction of immune responses *in vivo* with small numbers of veiled (dendritic) cells, *Proc. Natl. Acad. Sci. U.S.A.* **80**:6032–6035.

Krane, S. M., Dayer, J. M., and Goldring, S. R., 1982, Consideration of possible cellular events in the destructive synovial lesion of rheumatoid arthritis, in: *Advances in Inflammation Research,* Vol. 3, *Rheumatoid Arthritis* (S. Gorini, M. Ziff, and G. P. Velo, eds.), Raven Press, New York, pp. 1–16.

Kuntz-Crow, M., and Kunkel, H. G., 1982, Human dendritic cells: Major stimulators of the autologous and allogeneic mixed leukocyte reactions, *Clin. Exp. Immunol.* **49**:338–346.

Lachman, L. B., Hacker, M. P., and Handschumacher, R. E., 1977, Partial purification of human lymphocyte-activating factor (LAF) by ultrafiltration and electrophoretic techniques, *J. Immunol.* **119**:2019–2023.

Leijh, P. C. J., and van Furth, R., 1981, Extracellular stimulation of phagocytes by plasma proteins for optimal intracellular killing of micro-organisms, *Scand. J. Rheumatol. (Suppl.)* **40**:62–64.

Librach, C. L., and Burns, G. F., 1983, Spontaneous reverse haemolytic plaque formation. II. The role of T cells and monocytes in regulating immunoglobulin secretion by human peripheral blood B cells, *Scand. J. Immunol.* **17**:171–181.

Lipsky, P. E., and Ziff, M., 1982, The mechanisms of action of gold and D-penicillamine in rheumatoid arthritis, in: *Advances in Inflammation Research,* Vol. 3, *Rheumatoid Arthritis* (S. Gorini, M. Ziff, and G. P. Velo, eds.), Raven Press, New York, pp. 219–235.

Lombardino, J. G., 1983, Mechanism of action of drugs for treating inflammation and arthritis, *Eur. J. Rheum. Inflam.* **6**:24–35.

Lunec, J., Halloran, S. P., White, A. G., and Dormandy, T. L., 1981, Free-radical oxidation (peroxidation) products in serum and synovial fluid in rheumatoid arthritis, *J. Rheumatol.* **8**:234–245.

Matsubara, T., Spycher, M. A., Ruttner, J. R., and Fehr, K., 1983, The ultrastructural localization of fibronectin in the lining layer of rheumatoid arthritis synovium: The synthesis of fibronectin by type B lining cells, *Rheumatol. Int.* **3**:75–79.

Meijer, C. J. L., de Graaf-Reitsma, C. B., Lafeber, G. J. M., and Cats, A., 1983, *In situ* localization of Lymphocyte subsets in synovial membranes of patients with rheumatoid arthritis with monoclonal antibodies, *J. Rheumatol.* **9**:359–365.

Murphy, G. F., Bhon, A. K., Sato, S., Mihm, M. C., and Harrist, T. J., 1981, A new immunologic marker for human Langerhans cells, *N. Engl. J. Med.* **304**:791–792.

Niederhuber, J. E., 1978, The role of I region gene products in macrophages–T lymphocyte interaction, *Immunol. Rev.* **40**:28–52.

Nussenzweig, M. C., and Steinman, R. M., 1982, The cell surface of mouse lymphoid dendritic cells, *Immunol. Today* **3**:3,65–68.

Nussenzweig, M. C., Steinman, R. M., Gutchinov, B., and Cohn, Z. A., 1980, Dendritic cells are accessory cells for the development of anti-trinitrophenyl cytotoxic T lymphocytes, *J. Exp. Med.* **152**:1070–1084.

Nussenzweig, M. C., Steinman, R. M., Witmer, M. D., and Gutchinov, B., 1982, A monoclonal antibody specific for mouse dendritic cells, *Proc. Natl. Acad. Sci. U.S.A.* **79**:161–165.

Panayi, G., 1981, Substrates for phagocytes in joints, *Scand. J. Rheumatol. (Suppl.)* **40**:32–36.

Parnham, M. J., Shoshan, S., Schoenmarker, H., and Bonta, I. L., 1981, Macrophage regulation of collagen deposition in granuloma tissue *in vivo* and the effect of prostaglandin E_2, *Scand. J. Rheumatol. (Suppl.)* **40**:72–74.

Parwaresch, M. R., Radzun, H. J., and Dommes, M., 1981, The homogeneity and monocytic origin of human peritoneal macrophages evidenced by comparison of esterase polymorphism, *Am. J. Pathol.* **102**:209–218.

Parwaresch, M. R., Radzun, H. J., Hausmann, M. L., and Peters, K. P., 1983, Monoclonal antibody Ki-M4 specifically recognizes human dendritic reticulum cells (follicular dendritic cells) and their possible precursor in blood, *Blood* **62**:585–590.

Passwell, J. H., Dayer, J. M., and Merler, E., 1979, Increased prostaglandin production by human monocytes after membrane receptor activation, *J. Immunol.* **123**:115–120.

Pawlowski, N. A., Kaplan, G., Hamill, A. L., Cohn, Z. A., and Scott, W. A., 1983, Arachidonic acid metabolism by human monocytes. Studies with platelet-depleted cultures, *J. Exp. Med.* **158**:393–412.

Pommier, C. G., Inada, S., Fries, L. F., Takahashi, T., Frank, M. M., and Brown, E. J., 1983, Plasma fibronectin enhances phagocytosis of peripheral blood monocytes, *J. Exp. Med.* **156**:1844–1854.

Poulter, L. W., 1983, Antigen presenting cells *in situ:* Their identification and involvement in immunopathology, *Clin. Exp. Immunol.* **53**:513–520.

Poulter, L. W., and Duke, O., 1983, Dendritic cells of the rhematoid synovial membrane and synovial fluid, in: *Quatrième Cours D'Immunopathologie Articulaire* (J. Clot and J. Sany, eds.), Quick Print, Montpellier, pp. 189–199.

Poulter, L. W., Duke, O., Hobbs, S., Janossy, G., Panayi, G., and Seymour, G., 1983, The involvement of interdigitating (antigen-presenting) cells in the pathogenesis of rheumatoid arthritis, *Clin. Exp. Immunol.* **51**:247–257.

Radzun, H. J., Parwaresch, M. R., and Kreipe, H., 1983, Monocytic origin of human alveolar macrophages, *J. Histochem. Cytochem.* **31**:318–324.

Roos, D., 1981, Molecular events during phagocyte stimulation, *Scand. J. Rheumatol. (Suppl.)* **40**:46–52.

Rosenthal, A., 1980, Current concepts: Regulation of the immune response–role of the macrophage, *N. Engl. J. Med.* **203**:1153–1156.

Rowden, G., Lewis, M. G., and Sullivan, A. K., 1977, Ia antigen expression on human epidermal Langerhans cells, *Nature* **268**:247–248.

Russel, R. G. G., McGuire, M. K. B., Meats, J. E., Ebsworth, N. M., and Beresford, J., 1981, Intercellular messengers in joint tissues in rheumatoid arthritis, *Scand. J. Rheumatol. (Suppl.)* **40**:75–87.

Ryan, P. F. J., and Hughes. G. R. V., 1982, Plasmapheresis and lymphapheresis, in: *Advances in Inflammation Research,* Vol. 3, *Rheumatoid Arthritis* (S. Gorini, M. Ziff, and G. P. Velo, eds.), Raven Press, New York, pp. 271–284.

Scheinberg, M. A., Santos, L. M. B., and Finkelstein, A. E., 1982, The effect of auranofin and sodium aurothiomalate on peripheral blood monocytes, *J. Rheumatol.* **9**:366–369.

Scheinberg, M. A., Rueda, H. O., and Matheus, P. C., 1983, The effect of piroxicam on neutrophil and monocyte–macrophages function, *Eur. J. Rheum. Inflam.* **6**:36–40.

Scheynius, A., Grønvik, K. O., and Andersson, J., 1983, Epidermal Langerhans cells as accessory cells in Con A stimulation of T lymphocytes in the guinea pig, *Scand. J. Immunol.* **17**:283–290.

Selinger, M. J., McAdam, K. P. W. J., Kaplan, M. M., Sipe, J. D., Vogel, S. N., and Rosenstreich, D. L., 1980, Monokine induced synthesis of serum amyloid A protein by hepatocytes, *Nature* **285**:498–500.

Smith, K. A., Lachman, L. B., Oppenheim, J. J., and Fonata, M. F., 1980, The functional relationship of interleukins, *J. Exp. Med.* **151**:1551–1556.

Spalding, D. M., Koopman, W. J., Eldridge, J. H., McGhee, J. R., and Steinman, R. M., 1983, Accessory cells in murine Peyers patch. I. Identification and enrichment of a functional dendritic cell, *J. Exp. Med.* **157**:1646–1659.

Steinman, R. M., 1981, Dendritic cells, *Transplantation* **31**:151–155.

Steinman, R. M., and Cohn, Z. A., 1973, Identification of a novel cell type in peripheral lymphoid organs or mice. I. Morphology, quantitation, tissue distribution, *J. Exp. Med.* **137**:1142–1162.

Steinman, R. M., and Cohn, Z. A., 1974, Identification of a novel cell type in peripheral lymphoid organs of mice. II. Functional properties *in vitro, J. Exp. Med.* **139**:380–397.

Steinman, R. M., and Nussenzweig, M. C., 1980, Dendritic cells: Features and functions, *Immunol. Rev.* **53**:127–147.

Steinman, R. M., Kaplan, G., Witmer, M. D., and Cohn, Z. A., 1979, Identification of a novel cell type in peripheral lymphoid organs of mice. V. Purification of spleen dendritic cells, new surface markers, and maintenance *in vitro, J. Exp. Med.* **149:**1–16.

Steinman, R. M., Gutchinov, B., Witmer, M. D., and Nussenzweig, M. C., 1983, Dendritic cells are the principal stimulators of the primary mixed leukocyte reaction in mice, *J. Exp. Med.* **157:**613–627.

Sunshine, G. H., Gold, D. P., Wortis, H. H., Marrack, P., and Kappler, J. W., 1983, Mouse spleen dendritic cells present soluble antigens to antigen-specific T cell hybridomas, *J. Exp. Med.* **158:**1745–1750.

Teitelbaum, S. L., and Kahn, A. J., 1980, Mononuclear phagocytes, osteoclasts and bone resorption, *Min. Electrolyte Metab.* **3:**2–6.

Theofilopoulos, A. N., Carson, D., Tovassoli, M., Slovin, S. F., Speers, W. C., Jensen, F. B., and Vaughan, J. H., 1980, Evidence for the presence of receptors for C3 and IgG Fc on human synovial cells, *Arthritis Rheum.* **23:**1–9.

Thorsby, E., Berle, E., and Nousiainen, H., 1982, HLA-D region molecules restrict proliferative T cell responses to antigen, *Immunol. Rev.* **66:**39–56.

Trentham, D. E., Dynesius, R. A., Rocklin, R. E., and David, J. R., 1978, Cellular sensitivity to collagen in rheumatoid arthritis, *N. Engl. J. Med.* **299:**327–332.

Unanue, E. R., 1978, The regulation of lymphocyte functions by the macrophage, *Immunol. Rev.* **40:**227–255.

Vaes, G., 1981, Cartilage and bone tissue damage in arthritis: Cellular cooperation and enzymatic mechanisms, *Scand. J. Rheumatol. (Suppl.)* **40:**65–71.

van Furth, R., 1981, The origin of phagocytic cells in the joint and bone, *Scand. J. Rheumatol. (Suppl.)* **40:**13–20.

van Voorhis, W. C., Witmer, M. D., and Steinman, R. M., 1983, The phenotype of dendritic cells and macrophages, *Fed. Proc.* **42:**3114–3118.

Weibart, R. H., Bluestone, R., and Goldberg, L. S., 1975, Cellular immunity to autologous IgG in rheumatoid arthritis and rheumatoid-like disorders, *Clin. Exp. Immunol.* **20:**409–417.

Weissmann, G., 1982, The biochemistry of inflammation: Rheumatoid arthritis and anti-inflammatory drugs, *Eur. J. Rheum. Inflam.* **5:**366–381.

Weissmann, G., 1983, Pathways for arachidonate oxidation to prostaglandins and leucotrienes, *Semin. Arthritis Rheum.* **13**(Suppl. 1)**:**123–129.

Whitten, H. D., Cruse, J. M., and Fudenberg, H. H., 1983, Activation of macrophages by *in vitro* allostimulated T cells, *Scand. J. Immunol.* **17:**335–343.

Williams, B. D., Russel, B. A., Lockwood, C. M., and Cotton, C., 1979, Defective reticuloendothelial system function in rheumatoid arthritis, *Lancet* **1:**1311–1314.

Winchester, R. J., and Burmeister, G. R., 1981, Demonstration of Ia antigens on certain dendritic cells and on a novel elongate cell found in human synovial tissue, *Scand. J. Immunol.* **14:**439–444.

Wischer, T. L., 1982, The possible role of cellular interactions in the pathogenesis of rheumatoid joint lesions, in: *Advances in Inflammation Research,* Vol. 3, *Rheumatoid Arthritis* (S. Gorini, M. Ziff, and G. P. Velo, eds.), Raven Press, New York, pp. 55–64.

Wooley, D. E., 1978, Collagenase localization in cultures of rheumatoid synovial cells, *Science* **200:**773–775.

Wood, D. D., Ihrie, E. J., Dinarello, C. A., and Cohen, P. L., 1983, Isolation of aninterleukin 1-like factor from human joint effusions, *Arthritis Rheum.* **26:**975–983.

Ziff, M., 1981, Phagocytes and substrates in the joint, *Scand. J. Rheumatol. Suppl.* **40:**10–12.

21

Complement Components in Rheumatic Diseases

Peter H. Schur

I. INTRODUCTION

The complement system consists of a group of at least 18 serum proteins that interact sequentially to affect systems of inflammation (Fearon, 1981; Frank and Atkinson, 1975; Muller-Eberhard, 1974; Schur, 1977). Activation of complement is accompanied by a series of specific and limited enzymatic reactions that result in the cleavage of certain components, which subsequently generate new enzymatic activities and lead to the formation of complement complexes that have additional biological activities. Some of these activities are carried out on cells or immune complex surfaces and some in fluid; in some cases, other proteins inhibit these activities, at least in part.

The complement system consists of three pathways: the classic pathway, the alternative (or properdin) pathway, and the terminal attack sequence; into which feed the classic and alternative pathways (Fig. 1). The classic complement pathway consists of components C1, C4, and C2. Component C1 consists of three subunits—C1q, C1r, and C1s—which are held together by calcium but can be dissociated by ethylenediaminetetraacetic acid (EDTA), thus preventing initiation or "activation" of the complement sequence. Immune complexes containing IgM and/or the IgG subclasses IgG1, IgG2, or IgG3 will bind C1q. Such binding leads to the sequential activation of C1r, C1s, C4 and C2 and the eventual cleavage of C3. There are natural controls or modulators of activation of this system. The serum protein C1 esterase inhibitor (C1 INH) regulates the activity of C1s, limiting the cleavage of C4 and C2. C4bp similarily inhibits the action of C4 or C2 by acting with C3b inactivator to cleave C4b.

Peter H. Schur • Division of Rheumatology and Immunology, Brigham and Women's Hospital, Harvard Medical School, Boston, Massachusetts 02115.

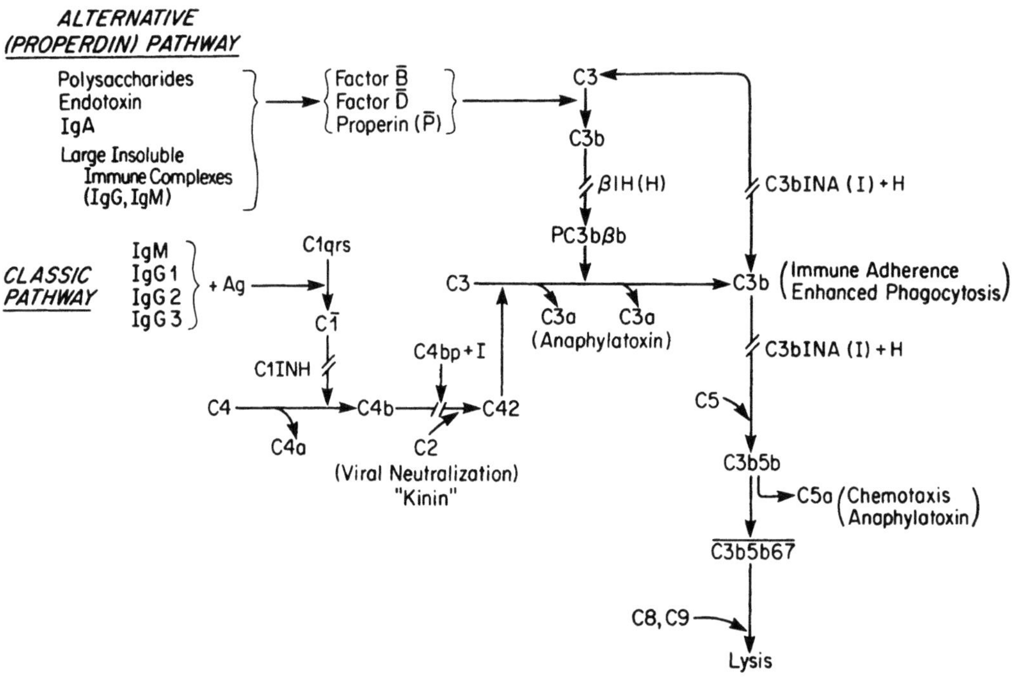

Figure 1. The complement cascade.

Cleavage of C3 can also come about through an alternative pathway, the properdin system. This phylogenetically older system can be activated by immunoglobulins, including aggregated IgA and possibly IgE, and also by polysaccharides, including endotoxin. The pathway consists of a number of proteins (Fig. 1) that interact to cleave C3. The two pathways interact in that activation of the third component splits C3; the larger fragment, C3b, can interact with components of the properdin system, causing further activation and cleavage of C3.

The terminal pathway also begins at C3. Activation of C3 via C3b results in sequential cleavage or activation of C5, C6, C7, C8, and C9. An inactivator of C3b (C3b INA) acting with β-IH can block the hemolytic potential of C3b by cleaving it into two inactive fragments, C3d, which remains bound to the antigen–antibody complex, and C3c, which is released into the fluid. Two proteins that stabilize C3 convertase and thus facilitate the progression of the system are properdin (P) and C3 nephritic factor (C3 NEF). The latter is an IgG directed against part of the C3bBb complex. Deposition on a cell membrane of the multimolecular complex consisting of C5 through C9 leads to the formation of cell membrane defects that cause increased permeability and release of intracellular contents such as hemoglobin. Release of hemoglobin thus provides a means for assaying the sumation of the hemolytic sequence.

Many cells have receptors for complement components or fragments. Their exact properties, interaction with complement, and biological role are just being elucidated (Fearon and Wong, 1983). They appear to have a role in immune complex clearance, enhanced phagocytosis, enhanced ADCC, chemotaxis, respiratory bursts, and secretion. The characteristics of certain receptors are summarized in Table 1.

II. IMMUNOBIOLOGICAL ASPECTS OF THE COMPLEMENT SYSTEM

One important role of complement components is viral neutralization, and C1, C4, and C2 appear to be helpful, if not essential, in this regard (Frank and Atkinson, 1975). A vasoactive peptide results from the interaction of C1 with C4 and C2 and increases local vascular permeability. Two cleavage products of this interaction, C3a and C5a, have anaphylatoxic properties. Subunit C5a is chemotactic for neutrophils, eosinophils, and mononuclear cells.

The presence of C3b on antigen–antibody complexes confers on them the ability to participate in the adherence phenomenon reaction in which the C3b-containing immune complex acts as an opsonin that helps bind to specific receptors on B lymphocytes, monocytes, or polymorphonuclear leukocytes and promotes phagocytosis of these complement complexes with release of lysosomal enzymes. Immune complexes coated with C3b may bind to platelets with subsequent release of vasoactive amines that result in inflammatory reactions. These biological activities of C3b can be blocked by C3b INA.

Receptors for C3b on red blood cells appear to be instrumental in clearing most of the immune complexes from the circulation and presenting them to fixed mononuclear cells in the RE system for phagocytosis (Cornocoff *et al.*, 1983). Deficiencies of red blood cell receptors, as in systemic lupus erythematosus (SLE), may result in an excess of immune complexes in the circulation, and these subsequently deposit in tissues and organs. The biological properties of different complement components are summarized on Table 2.

III. MEASUREMENT OF COMPLEMENT

The complement system can be assessed in a number of ways, including measurement of total hemolytic complement, immunochemical or hemolytic measurement of individual components, measurements of complement breakdown products, determination of complement metabolism, and other indirect methods (Schur, 1977).

Table 1. Types of Complement Membrane Receptors

Receptor type	Specificity	Mol. wt.	Cell type distribution
CR_1	C4b, C3b, iC3b	250,000	Erythrocytes, macrophages, kidney cells, lymphocytes, neutrophils
CR_2	iC3b, C3d-g, C3d	150,000	B lymphocytes
CR_3	iC3b	180,000 and 160,000	Erythrocytes, macrophages, neutrophils, natural killer cells
C1q-R	C1q	?	Lymphocytes, neutrophils, monocytes
H-R	Factor H (β1H)	100,000 and 50,000	Lymphocytes, neutrophils, monocytes
C3a-R	C3a, C4a	?	Mast cells
C3e-R	C3e	?	Neutrophils
C5a-R	C5a, $C5a_{des\text{-}Arg}$	?	Mast cells, monocytes, neutrophils

Table 2. Biological Activities of Complement

Chemotaxis	C5a
Inhibition of macrophage migration	Bb
Opsonization	C3b
Phagocytosis	C3b
Clearance of immune complexes	C4b, C3b
Lysis of immune complexes	C4
Kinin	C4a, C2a
Anaphylatoxin	C3a, C5a
Membrane damage, cell lysis	C5–9
Viral neutralization	C1, C4, C2

The total hemolytic complement level represents the sum of all components of the system. By adding diluted serum to antibody-sensitized sheep erythrocytes, one can measure this level in units that represent the reciprocal of that dilution of serum that causes 50% of cells to lyse (CH_{50}), as determined by the release of hemoglobin.

Complement components are generally measured by immunochemical means—radial immunodiffusion, electroimmunodiffusion, or nephelometry (see Table 3.) Assays depend on the availability of monospecific antisera and standards. However, such determinations yield no information about the functional biological integrity of the components being measured. Besides immunochemical methods, effective molecular titration of individual components is now possible. This functional assay, however, requires that the test serum supply the component being measured in a hemolytic system. The experimental error of these techniques is at least 10%, and since our present technology is limited, not nearly as many sera can be analyzed per day by use of this method as by immunochemical

Table 3. Normal Serum Concentrations

	Range	Mean
CH_{50}	150–250 u/ml	
C1q	35–56 mg/dl	
C1r		3.4 mg/dl
C1s		3.1 mg/dl
C4	26–83 mg/dl	
C2	1.6–3.9 mg/dl	
C3	91–198 mg/dl	
C5	11–23 mg/dl	
C6		6.0 mg/dl
C7		5.5 mg/dl
C8		8.0 mg/dl
C9		16.0 mg/dl
P		2.5 mg/dl
D		0.2 mg/dl
B	19–39 mg/dl	
C1 INH	16–34 mg/dl	
C4bp		25 mg/dl
C3 INA (I)		35 mg/dl
β-IH (H)		36 mg/dl

means. Furthermore, these functional assays, although technically feasible, are much more difficult to perform than are immunochemical methods, and at present they are not done on a routine basis in most clinical laboratories.

In measuring CH_{50} or components, it is important to remember that some components are thermolabile. The CH_{50} will remain relatively stable for a few hours at room temperature or overnight at −20°C; however, samples are best stored at −70°C as soon as possible. Serum stored at room temperature even for a few days is adequate for immunochemical measurement of individual components as proteins (as, for instance, by immunodiffusion), although it is best to store samples as soon as possible at −70°C when one desires to measure the hemolytic levels of individual components. Serum CH_{50} and certain components can be inactivated by heating for 30 min at 56°C.

Activation of the complement system can often be demonstrated by immunoelectrophoresis or counterimmunoelectrophoresis (Arroyaue *et al.*, 1978) of either plasma or serum, with antisera to specific complement components, or by detection of split or conversion products. One should determine whether these fragments arise from specific activation of the complement system of from some other enzymatic split or whether they developed during processing of the blood or on storage.

Complement metabolism is a better way of assessing the dynamic state of individual complement components (Ruddy *et al.*, 1975). However, these studies are rarely performed because of great difficulty in isolating hemolytically and biologically active purified components and in maintaining their activity after radiolabeling.

IV. COMPLEMENT ABNORMALITIES

In view of the apparently different biological functions of components of the complement system, understanding the role of complement in disease requires analysis not only of the whole system, based on total hemolytic complement levels (CH_{50}), but also of the individual components. For instance, a depressed CH_{50} level could be the result of inherited depletion of a single component or acquired depletion of multiple components through immune and nonimmune processes. Furthermore, static measurements of serum CH_{50} levels or of individual complement components should be confirmed whenever possible by serial studies in order to approximate the metabolism of these proteins. Since most disorders of the complement system affect either the classic or the alternative pathway, we recommend that for routine serum analysis serum hemolytic CH_{50} and immunochemical analysis of C1q, C4, C3, and factor B proteins be performed. Late or terminal components are rarely affected unless C3 is affected as well; measurement of C5 protein has been useful in this regard. Generally, when the CH_{50} is decreased, there is also a decrease in C1q, C4, C2, and C3. Similarly, when C1q, C4, C2, or C3 protein is decreased, CH_{50} is decreased. When, on the other hand, CH_{50} levels do not correlate with the levels of these components, one should consider abnormalities of one of the other components or serum handling problems.

V. INHERITED DEFECTS OF COMPLEMENT

Persons who are homozygous deficient in some component generally show virtually no CH_{50} activity; the levels of all other components are normal (Alper and Rosen, 1976;

Glass *et al.*, 1983; Hobart and Lachman, 1976; Schur, 1978). Those who are heterozygous deficient in some component, especially C1, C4, C2, or C3, often have about 50% of normal CH_{50} and normal levels of all components except the deficient component, the level of which is about half normal. One percent of normal persons are heterozygous deficient in C2; CH_{50} is 100 to 150 (i.e., half normal), and C1q, C4, and C3 are normal, but C2 is only half normal. The inherited nature of the defect is confirmed by family studies demonstrating either homozygous or heterozygous defects in other family members. Inheritance of most complement deficiencies is autosomal dominant.

Some persons with isolated complement deficiencies have no clinical problems. In fact, the first person discovered to have such a defect (an immunologist with C2 deficiency) is clinically well (Silverstein, 1960). However, many others with disease have since been discovered to be lacking some component. This not only may reflect a real association but may be because physicians often examine complement levels in patients with rheumatic diseases or recurrent infections. Nevertheless, it appears that there is an association between both C2 and C3b receptor deficiency and systemic lupus erythematosus (SLE) (Schur, 1978; Wilson *et al.*, 1982) as well as between deficiencies of C3, C6, C7, C8, and C3b inactivator and recurrent infection (Table 4) (George and Glass, 1983).

During attacks, patients with hereditary angioedema have low levels of CH_{50}, C4, and C2 and normal levels of C1 and C3 (Rosen and Austen, 1969). During remission, C4 levels often remain decreased. All patients with hereditary angioedema have an inherited deficiency of C1 inhibitor. In 90% of patients, levels of the C1 inhibitor, as assessed immunochemically as protein, are extremely low, whereas in the other 10% protein levels appear to be normal (Rosen and Austen, 1969), but C1 inhibitor is functionally deficient.

Genes that control C2 and C4 levels and the C2, C4, and factor B allotypes are located on the short arm of the sixth chromosome close to the HLA loci (Alper and Rosen, 1976). Genes controlling other complement components appear to be on other, as yet not defined, chromosomes (Hobart and Lachman, 1976). Allotypes of most of the complement components have been described. Some may present as null genes resulting in functional half-normal levels (heterozygous states) or as homozygous states—these are established by family studies. These studies have demonstrated that there are two C4 genes called C4A and C4B (which correspond to the blood groups Chido and Rogers) (O'Neill *et al.*, 1978). There is an increased frequency of C2, C4A, and C4B null genes in patients with SLE (Dawkins *et al.*, 1983). There is also a higher frequency of the F allele of C3 in rheumatoid arthritis (RA) and of C4A4 and C4B2 in the spondylitic form of JRA (George and Glass, 1983).

VI. POSSIBLE MECHANISMS OF INHERITED COMPLEMENT DEFICIENCY DISEASE ASSOCIATION

What is the clinical role of these inherited complement component deficiencies? The association of deficiency of either C3, C5, C6, C7, C8, or C3b inactivator with repeated infections is perhaps easy to understand in view of the importance of these complement components in chemotaxis and phagocytosis, which participate in clearance of bacteria.

The nature of the association between the inherited complement component deficiency, particularly of the early complement components, and SLE is not as clear. These components, including C4 and C2, do play a role in the immune clearance of complexes (Fearon, 1981) and in viral neutralization (Fearon, 1981). However, not all individuals with C4 deficiency and C2 deficiency appear to be afflicted by recurrent infections. Furthermore, the association of immune disease with heterozygous C2 deficiency, where there is adequate complement to participate in the usual complement-dependent reactions, suggests that the C2 deficiency represents primarily a genetic rather than a biological marker and that the association between C2 deficiency and SLE is caused by some other factor(s).

The association between C4 deficiency and C2 deficiency and HLA provides a clue to another possible interrelationship. Since there is increasing evidence that immune response genes may be closely linked to those of HLA, the HLA-linked complement deficiencies may also be linked to immune response genes, which may express themselves as immunologically mediated disease. Deficiency of red cell C3b receptor may result in poor immune complex clearance (Cornocoff *et al.*, 1983), resulting in excessive immune complex tissue deposition in SLE patients. In a sense, then, C2 and C3b receptor deficiency may be only a marker gene for a subset of patients with SLE, although C2 and C3b receptor deficiency may in itself magnify the clinical expression of disease. Observations

Table 4. Clinical Features of Hereditary Complement Deficiencies in Humans

Component	Clinical features	Comment
C1q	SLE	
C1r	Glomerulonephritis	Rare
	SLE	
	Infections and arthritis	
C1s	SLE	Rare
C4	SLE	
C2	SLE	Common
	Normal	1/10,000
	Rheumatoid arthritis	
	Juvenile rheumatoid arthritis	
	Discoid LE	
	Anaphylactoid purpura	
	Dermatomyositis	
C3	Recurrent infections	Rare
C5	SLE	Rare
C6	Normal	
	Recurrent *Neisseria* infection	
C7	Normal	
	Raynaud's disease	
	Recurrent *Neisseria* infection	
C8	Recurrent *Neisseria* infection	
	SLE	
C9	Normal	
C1 INH	Hereditary angiodema	Common
C3b INA (I)	Recurrent infections	

have been made in other rheumatic diseases that microorganisms may induce spondyloarthritis in genetically susceptible HLA-B27 individuals. The interrelationships among inherited complement defects, disease, HLA genes, susceptibility to infection, immune response genes, and immune regulation are not fully understood. Further study should lead to a better understanding of the role of the HLA region in immunity and of the mechanism whereby environmental factors can affect genetically susceptible individuals.

VII. ACQUIRED SERUM COMPLEMENT ABNORMALITIES

Our notions about the role of complement in disease have been derived, for the most part, from examination of serum levels. These static determinations must be viewed as the net result of synthesis and catabolism. Low levels of serum complement have been seen in patients with synthetic defects such as in membranoproliferative glomerulonephritis (MPGN), severe hepatic disease, or nutritional defects. More commonly, elevated levels are seen, as in many acute inflammatory states or infections. High levels have been associated with hepatic disease, surgical manipulation, acute myocardial infarction, cancer, diabetes, pregnancy, sarcoidosis, amyloidosis, thyroiditis, ulcerative colitis, polyarteritis, rheumatoid arthritis, juvenile rheumatoid arthritis, rheumatic fever, typhoid fever, spondylitis, and scleroderma (Schur, 1983).

However, major interest has been focused on low levels of serum complement in association with immune diseases, particularly those with circulating immune complexes. These have included acute poststreptococcal nephritis, serum sickness, SLE, Sjogren's syndrome, vasculitis, rheumatoid arthritis, bacterial endocarditis with nephritis, dengue fever, infected arteriovenous shunts, malaria, acute viral hepatitis with a prodrome of arthritis, fever, and urticaria, cryoglobulinemia, vasculitis preceding the Jarisch–Herxheimer reaction in the treatment of syphilis, and renal graft rejection. These conditions or diseases are thought to depress complement levels primarily through binding to and activation by circulating immune complexes. In addition to low CH_{50}, C4 and C3 levels are usually decreased, and C1 levels (including C1q) may be reduced, especially in association with cryoglobulins (Schur, 1983).

Sometimes patients with nephritis who have low C3 levels also have low levels of properdin factor B, especially in SLE and MPGN. Components of the terminal system are less likely to be decreased, but low C5 levels have been observed in patients with nephritis, MPGN, and SLE.

Finding low complement values is useful in a diagnostic sense, since they help in differentiation of the previously noted conditions from other disorders. For instance, complement levels tend to be low in certain forms of postinfectious nephritis (namely, streptococcal, subacute bacterial endocarditis) but tend to be normal in chronic glomerulonephritis, pyelonephritis, rapidly progressive glomerulonephritis, and Goodpasture's syndrome. However, C1q levels can also occasionally be low in some patients with the nephrotic syndrome; complement levels are also invariably low in MPGN (Lewis, 1971). By analyzing complement components, one can differentiate these disorders to some extent (Table 5). Patients with actue postinfectious nephritis tend to have low levels of C1, C4, and C3; however, after a few weeks, C3 only is low, whereas C5 is rarely low. Patients with MPGN have fairly persistently low levels of C3, factor B, and often C5.

Table 5. Complement Levels in Disease[a]

	CH_{50}	C1q	C1	C2	C4	C3	C5	Factor B
Inherited diseases								
Hereditary angiodema	↓↓	N	N	↓	↓	N	N	N
C2 deficiency	0	N	N	0	N	N	N	N
Renal diseases								
Acute postinfectious glomerulonephritis								
Early	↓	↓	↓	↓	↓	↓	N↓	N↓
Late	↓	N	N	N	N	↓	N	N
Membranoproliferative glomerulonephritis	↓	N	N	N	N	↓	↓	↓
Chronic glomerulonephritis, Goodpasture's syndrome, glomerulonephritis	N	N	N	N	N	N	N	N
Nephrotic syndrome	N↓	N↓	N	N	N	N	N	N
Connective tissue disease								
SLE (active)	↓	↓	↓	N↓	↓	↓	N↓	N↓
Cryoglobulinemia–vasculitis	↓	↓	↓	N↓	↓	N↓	N	N
Rheumatoid arthritis, severe	N↓	N↓	N↓	N	N↓	N↓	N	N
Myositis, scleroderma, rheumatoid arthritis (moderate), periarteritis, sarcoid, gout, rheumatic fever, spondylitis	N/↑	N/↑	N/↑	N/↑	N/↑	N/↑	N/↑	N/↑
Other								
Bacteremia (with shock)	↓	N	N	N	N	↓	↓	↓

[a] N, normal; SLE, systemic lupus erythematosus; ↓, somewhat low levels; ↓↓, very low levels.

Complement levels can also be helpful in the diagnosis of various forms of rheumatic connective tissue disorders (Schur, 1983) (Table 5). The association of high rheumatoid factors with low antinuclear antibody and low complement levels (particularly C1q and C4) usually indicates rheumatoid arthritis, whereas the association of weak rheumatoid factors, high antinuclear antibody (especially anti-DNA), and low complement levels usually means SLE. Low complement, weak rheumatoid factors, and low antinuclear antibody suggest cryoglobulinemia or vasculitis or both. High complement levels usually signal (active) myositis, polyarteritis, or scleroderma and are seen in most patients with rheumatoid arthritis. Low complement levels are seen in vasculitis associated with cryoglobulinemia and necrotizing venulitis (Soter, 1976).

In some cases, complement levels can also be used for follow-up evaluation, since levels will generally be low in the previously mentioned immune-complex-mediated disorders only when a patient has active disease. This is especially true in SLE, nephritis, and vasculitis. As the active inflammation subsides, these levels return to normal, and the disease goes into remission. Serial monitoring of complement levels, immune complexes, and anti-DNA has been of value, particularly in following lupus patients (Table 6) (Lloyd and Schur, 1981).

Low serum complement levels have also been seen occasionally in patients with myasthenia gravis, renal allograft rejection, paroxysmal cold hemoglobinuria, hemolytic anemia, and sickle cell disease (Schur and Austen, 1968). Low levels of CH_{50}, C1, C4, C2, and C1 inhibitor and normal levels of C3 have been found in some patients with varying combinations of lymphoma, 7 S IgM monoclonal gammopathy, and angioedema ("acquired angioedema") (Caldwell, 1972).

VIII. COMPLEMENT IN TRANSUDATES AND EXUDATES

Low-molecular-weight complement components can be detected in transudates. Since high-molecular-weight proteins are less likely to be present in transudates, CH_{50} and complement components are usually very low or absent in these fluids. In exudates, plasma proteins of all sizes are more likely to be present, and CH_{50} levels as well as levels of various components will be closer to serum values. However, CH_{50} or components may then be decreased as a result of enzymatic cleavage or, particularly, immune complex reactions.

Table 6. Ability of Immune Tests to Predict Clinical Exacerbations in SLE

CH_{50}	C3	Anti-DNA	Immune complexes	Clinical evidence
↓ ↓	↓	↑ ↑	Slight ↑	None necessarily
↓ ↓	↓ ↓	↑ ↑ ↑	↑ ↑ ↑	Active nephritis
↓	↓ (not normal)	↑ ↑ ↑	Slight ↑	Active extrarenal
↓ ↓ ↓	↓ ↓ ↓	↑	↑ ↑ ↑	Active nephritis and extrarenal

Table 7. Synovial Fluid Complement[a]

RA	
RF+	↓N
RF-	N↑
JRA	
RF+	↓N
RF-	N↑
SLE	↓N
Gout	↓N↑
Pseudogout	↓N↑
Reiters, spondylitis	↑
Acute bacterial arthritis	↓N↑
Psoriatic arthritis	N
Osteoarthritis	N

[a] ↓, decreased; N, normal; ↑, increased.

In synovial, pleural, and pericardial fluid, CH_{50} and C1q, C4, and C3 proteins are approximately one-third to one-half what they are in the serum of patients with nonimmune fluids (Pekin and Zvaifler, 1970; Schur, 1983; Hunder *et al.*, 1972; Hunder, 1972; Ruddy and Austen, 1970). Therefore, in exudates with inflammation, levels less than one-third of those in serum suggest either enzymatic cleavage or immunologic activation, as in many patients with rheumatoid arthritis and SLE and in some with juvenile rheumatoid arthritis, gout, pseudogout, and bacterial arthritis (see Table 7). Increased fluid levels are seen in patients with juvenile rheumatoid arthritis, gout, pseudogout, Reiter's syndrome, acute polyarthritis, and spondylitis (see Table 7). In addition, conversion products of C3 have been noted, suggesting immune-complex events with fluids.

XI. SYSTEMIC LUPUS ERYTHEMATOSUS

Vaughan *et al.* (1957) were among the first to show that serum complement levels are decreased in patients with SLE. Subsequently, many studies have demonstrated the potential usefulness of CH_{50} and complement components C1q, C4, C2, and C3 as markers for clinical activity (Lloyd and Schur, 1981). Lower levels of CH_{50} have been observed in SLE patients with active nephritis more frequently than in patients with extrarenal manifestations alone. Lupus patients with renal disease tend to have lower mean levels of C1q, C4, and C3 than those without renal disease.

The complement component profile in patients with active lupus nephritis differs somewhat from that seen in other forms of glomerulonephritis. In SLE, there are usually marked depressions of C1q and C4 and less substantial depressions of C3. Although there may be early depressions of C1q and C4 in patients with acute poststreptococcal glomerulonephritis, this disease as well as chronic membranoproliferative glomerulonephritis is characterized by marked depressions of C3 (Lewis *et al.*, 1971).

In a recent study (Lloyd and Schur, 1981), we observed the lowest mean levels of CH_{50}, C1q, C4, and C3 in patients who had both active nephritis and active extrarenal manifestations (Table 8). Of those patients with active renal disease (with or without

Table 8. Clinical Associations of Low Complement Levels in SLE

Low CH_{50}	Rash, proteinuria, anemia, anti-DNA
Low Clq	High BUN, urinary casts, high DNA
Low C4	Anti-NP, urinary casts
Low C3	Anti-ssDNA, urinary casts, leukopenia
Low factor B	High BUN, urinary casts, leukopenia, hematuria, anemia

active extrarenal manifestations), 87% had low CH_{50} levels, 80% had low Clq and C4 levels, and 68% had low C3 levels. By contrast, of those with only active extrarenal manifestations, 50% had low CH_{50} and Clq levels, 62% had low C4 levels, and 37% had low C3 levels. Associations have been noted between low levels of individual components and various facets of SLE (Table 8). Low factor B levels were one of the best complement indicators of active nephritis. Patients with active vasculitis and/or cryoglobulinemia have especially low Clq and C4 levels. A normal C3 level suggested the absence of active renal disease. These studies demonstrate the qualitative and quantitative differences of involvement of the complement system in SLE depending on the presence of active nephritis and active extrarenal disease. However, patients with both renal and extrarenal manifestations tend to have the lowests levels. Patients with only extrarenal manifestations have the fewest and least abnormalities. Some patients (approximately 10%) may have minor depressions of complement components without apparent clinical activity—this is especially true for C4.

Serial measurements of complement parameters (reviewed by Lloyd and Schur, 1981) demonstrated that complement levels increased coincident with clinical improvement. Another important facet of serial studies is to demonstrate which serologic parameters change during the intial phase of clinical exacerbation. From such serial studies, questions relating to monitoring early disease activity by observing the sequence of changing serologic parameters could be better assessed.

In our recent study (Lloyd and Schur, 1981), we noted the importance of C4 depression prior to clinical exacerbation. Low C4 levels were found prior to exacerbation in 25% of patients who developed extrarenal manifestations, in 67% of patients who developed active nephritis alone, and in virtually all patients who developed active nephritis and active extrarenal manifestations. The most significant fall in C4, CH_{50}, and Clq occurred early in exacerbation, whereas C3 continued to decline during the height of clinical illness.

In addition to observing complement abnormalities in association with activity, a number of investigators have focused on the role of antibodies, in pariticular, anti-double-stranded-DNA (dsDNA) antibodies (Lloyd and Schur, 1981; Cameron *et al.*, 1976; Miniter *et al.*, 1979; Hecht *et al.*, 1976; Lightfoot and Hughes, 1976). They have noted that when patients have both low CH_{50} or C4 levels and high levels of anti-dsDNA antibodies, the patients generally had active disease. Exacerbations were often associated, or even preceded by, falls in CH_{50} levels and/or rises in anti-dsDNA antibody levels. Normal C3 and anti-DNA levels were associated with inactive disease and had a good prognosis.

Lupus is considered a prototype of soluble-immune-complex-mediated disease. Certain immune complexes will activate complement. Complement levels, therefore, are an indirect way of measuring the presence of immune complexes. An inverse association between immune complex levels measured by different methods (Levinsky *et al.*, 1977; Nydegger *et al.*, 1974; Pussel *et al.*, 1978) and complement levels has been observed. We have observed (Lloyd and Schur, 1981) an inverse relationship between C1q-binding immune complex levels and CH_{50}, C1q, C4, and C3 levels. Patients with low complement levels, low titers of anti-DNA antibodies, and decreased levels of immune complexes often did not have active disease.

Immunologic tests have been used as a guide to therapy for SLE patients. Lange *et al.* (1965) administered steroid therapy in 15 lupus nephritis patients based on the degree of hypocomplementemia and hypergammaglobulinemia. They observed normalization of γ-globulin, DNA precipitation tests, and CH_{50} by 21 months (Lange *et al.*, 1965). Appel *et al.* (1978), in a prospective study of 25 patients, guided immunosuppressive therapy by changes in CH_{50} and antibody to double-stranded DNA. Follow-up at 2 years revealed that CH_{50} levels correlated better with proteinuria than did anti-DNA. In five patients with persistently low Ch_{50} and anti-DNA, the renal histology became more severe in four and remained severe in one. In contrast, among ten patients who normalized CH_{50}, the histology worsened slightly in two, remained unchanged in five, and improved in three (Appel *et al.*, 1978). The 5-year follow-up suggested that normalization of complement resulted in a trend towards stabilization of renal histology, creatinine clearance, and serum creatinine at a lower final mean dose of prednisone (Jarrett *et al.*, 1981).

In summary, we (Lloyd and Schur, 1981) concluded that an isolated value of any one serologic parameter may assist in diagnosis but is not of any therapeutic consequence. Clinical exacerbations may be predicted by serial monitoring of C4, CH_{50}, C1q binding assay, C3, or anti-DNA antibodies, ranked in that order of usefulness. We feel that different serologic profiles exist for different types of clinical exacerbation. Combinations of serologic tests appear to be more useful in predicting exacerbations and may be useful in guiding therapy: CH_{50}, C4, C3, and C1q binding assays appeared to be most useful.

A. Other SLE Serum Studies

As noted previously, static measurements and even serial measurements of complement may not reflect the metabolism of complement in the individual with SLE. Metabolic studies are the key but are infrequently done because of the difficulty in isolating biologically active complement. In the few studies performed, SLE patients with active disease generally had increased catabolism and increased synthesis of C3 and C4, even though serum levels were normal or decreased (Ruddy *et al.*, 1975; Alper and Rosen, 1967; Sliwinski and Zvaifler, 1972). Several patients were demonstrated to have low synthetic rates of certain complement components (Alper and Rosen, 1967).

Recently, Atkinson *et al.* (1981) described two patients with low CH_{50} levels and low levels of complement components measured by hemolytic assay but normal levels of complement components measured as proteins (antigenically). Plasma had normal complement levels, as did serum incubated at 37°C. These sera could be shown to activate complement *in vitro* at 5°C. These observations reemphasize that not all patients with low complement have active SLE; some may have genetic deficiencies or *in vitro* but not *in vivo* complement activation.

Patients with drug-induced LE-like syndromes generally have normal complement levels (Blomgren *et al.*, 1969). A minority of SLE patients with isolated hemolytic anemia and/or idiopathic thrombocytopenic purpura may have mildly depressed CH_{50} levels.

Complement levels tend to be inversely related to cryoglobulin concentration (Stastny and Ziff, 1969; Gough *et al.*, 1974). These mixed cryoglobulins, which are considered to be cold-precipitable immune complexes, may consist of IgG, IgM, C1q, C4, and/or C3 (Stastny and Ziff, 1969; Schur, 1972).

Although Davis and Bollet (1966) observed an inverse correlation between low complement levels and the presence of rheumatoid factors in patients with lupus nephritis, others, including ourselves, have not been able to confirm this observation.

B. Complement in SLE Cerebrospinal Fluid

Complement levels have been measured in the cerebrospinal fluid (CSF) of SLE patients. Because of the very low protein levels in this fluid, it is impossible to do CH_{50} levels. However, individual components have been measured. Petz *et al.* (1971) noted that CSF hemolytic C4 levels were low in patients with SLE and central nervous system (CNS) involvement, whereas normal levels were found in those SLE patients without CNS involvement. The authors commented on the rapid (7.5%/day) decay of C4 in spinal fluids from normals even when stored at −50°C and thus reported on samples stored for 7 days or less. Hadler *et al.* (1973) found normal levels of CSF hemolytic C4 in both normal individuals and SLE patients with and without CNS involvement. However, when serial C4 levels were determined on patients who went from active CNS involvement into remission, it was apparent that C4 levels went from a low normal value to either normal or high-normal levels, suggesting that serial C4 levels might be of value in evaluating patients with definite or questionable SLE CNS involvement. Hadler's study suggests that these assays must be done within a few hours after spinal tap, as hemolytic activity was nearly all lost within 24 hr of storage of CSF from SLE patients with CNS involvement, although C4 in other CSF decayed less rapidly. Hadler also noted that serum C4 values were not helpful in evaluating his four patients with active SLE CNS involvement.

C. Complement in SLE Tissue

Further evidence for the participation of complement in SLE has been the detection of complement components in inflamed tissue, particularly in the same locations as immunoglobulins and antigens. Complement components detected in renal lesions include C1q, C1s, C4, C2, C3, C5, C6, C9, properdin, and factor B (Lewis *et al.*, 1971; Verroust *et al.*, 1974; Rothfield *et al.*, 1972; Cochrane and Koffler, 1973; Schur, 1975; Koffler and Biesecker, 1983). However, C4 and factor B were seen infrequently despite the fact that serum levels of these components were often low in patients with nephritis. There was no apparent difference in the components deposited in those with predominantly membranous or proliferative nephritis (Schur, 1975). The presence of early, late, and properdin components argues for some involvement of all three pathways, although the classical appears to be most involved.

Similar complement components have been found at the dermal–epidermal junction of patients with skin lesions (Rothfield *et al.*, 1972; Tan and Kunkel, 1966; Provost and Tomasi, 1973; Gilliam *et al.*, 1974).

X. RHEUMATOID ARTHRITIS

Most patients with rheumatoid arthritis (RA) have normal levels of serum complement. However, levels of CH_{50} are somewhat lower in patients with RA having rheumatoid factors (RF). Furthermore, their catabolic rate of C3 appears to be increased (Ruddy *et al.*, 1975), suggesting that complement is being activated in these patients by immune complexes. In addition, in about 4% of RA patients one finds very low levels of CH_{50} (Franco and Schur, 1971). These patients often have rheumatoid vasculitis or very severe highly active RA (Franco and Schur, 1971). However, once they are hospitalized and begun on aggressive therapy, their serum complement levels quickly return to normal with in days, in contrast to the complement abnormalities of the lupus patient, which may take weeks to return to normal. Although C3 levels are usually normal, C1q and C4 levels may be, briefly, markedly depressed (Schur, 1983). These very low levels of complement are usually accompanied by high levels of circulating immune complexes, high titers of rheumatoid factors, and often IgG and/or 7 S IgM rheumatoid factors as well. Complement levels in rheumatoid effusions are decreased, including synovial, pleural, and pericardial fluids. In the RF-positive patient, levels tend to be somewhat lower than in the RF-negative patient; however, in both instances, levels tend to be lower than in patients with osteoarthritis. Hemolytic levels of individual components, especially C1 and C4, are disproportionally even lower than complement protein levels, suggesting that these molecules have participated in an immunologic reaction but are still trapped in the fluid (Ruddy and Austen, 1970). It is for these reasons that it is often valuable to assess complement both hemolytically and as a protein.

XI. VASCULITIS

Complement levels are generally normal in patients with large- or medium-vessel disease (George and Glass, 1983; Schur, 1983) (Table 9). There is little reason to suspect that these may be caused by circulating immune complexes. On the other hand, patients with cutaneous necrotizing venulitis, characterized by either purpura or urticaria (also called leucoclastic angiitis or hypersensitivity vasculitis), often have low complement levels (Soter, 1976). These patients usually have low levels of CH_{50}, C1q, C4, and occasionally

Table 9. Complement Levels in Vasculitis

	CH_{50}	C1q	C4	C3
Necrotising Venulitis	↓↓	↓↓	↓↓	↓↓
with connective tissue disease				
with neutrophil infiltrate	↓↓	↓↓	↓↓	↓
with lymphocyte infiltrate	±↓	±↓	±↓	N
Henoch–Schonlein purpura	N	N	N	N
Polyarteritis				
with hepatitis B	↓↓	↓↓	↓↓	↓↓
without hepatitis B	N	N	N	N
Giant-cell arteritis	N			
Takayasu's	N			

C3. These patients have moderately elevated levels of immune complexes and cryoglobulins, and, pathologically, venules are surrounded by neutrophils. Patients with purpura or urticaria with venulitis with lymphocyte infiltrates tend to have normal complement levels. The low complement levels usually return to normal as clinical evidence for vasculitis—i.e., new skin lesions—abates.

Patients with hepatitis B antigenemia and vasculitis of both venules and small arteries also may have hypocomplementemia. Low CH_{50}, C1q, C4, and C3 levels may persist for a long time, as long as the disease is active (Cohen *et al.*, 1980).

ACKNOWLEDGMENTS. Supported in part by grants AM 11414 and AM 05577 from the National Institutes of Health, the Arthritis Foundation, the Lupus Foundation of America, and the New England Peabody Home.

REFERENCES

Alper, C. A. and Rosen, F. L., 1967, Studies of the *in vivo* behavior of human C3 in normal subjects and patients, *J. Clin. Invest.* **46**:2021–2034.

Alper, C. A., and Rosen, F. S., 1976, Genetics of the complement system, *Adv. Hum. Genet.* **7**:141–188.

Appel, A. E., Sablay, L. B., Golden, R. A., Barlond, P., Grazel, A. I., Bank, N., 1978, The effect of normalization of serum complement and anti-DNA antibody on the course of lupus erythematous, *Am. J. Med.* **64**:274–283.

Arroyaue, C. M., Taylor, D. G., Gallup, P., 1978, Screening test for complement activation by counterimmunoelectrophoresis, *Am. J. Clin. Pathol.* **69**:440.

Atkinson, J. P., Gorman, J. C., Curd, J., Hyla, J. F., Deegan, M. J., Keren, D. F., Abdou, N. I., and Walker, S. E., 1981, Cold dependent activation of complement in discrepancy between clinical and laboratory parameters, *Arthritis Rheum.* **24**:592–601.

Blomgren, S. E., Condemi, J. J., Bignal, M. C., and Vaughan, J. H., 1969, Antinuclear antibody induced by procainamide. A prospective study, *N. Engl. J. Med.* **281**:64–66.

Caldwell, J. R., Ruddy, S., Schur, P. H., 1972, Acquired C1 inhibitor deficiency in lymphosarcoma, *Clin. Immunol. Immunopathol.* **1**:39.

Cameron, J. S., Lessof, M. H., Ogg, C. S., Williams, B. D., and Williams, D. G., 1976, Disease activity in the nephritis of systemic lupus erythematosus in relation to serum complement concentrations, *Clin. Exp. Immunol.* **25**:418–427.

Cochrane, C. G., and Koffler, D., 1973, Immune complex disease in experimental animals and man, *Adv. Immunol.* **16**:186–261.

Cohen, R. D., Conn, D. L., and Ilstrup, D. M., 1980, Clinical features, prognosis, and responses to treatment in polyarteritis, *Mayo Clin. Proc.* **55**:146–155.

Cornocoff, J. B., Herbert, L. H., Smead, W. L., VanAman, M. E., Birmingham, D. J., and Waxman, F. J., 1983, Primate erythrocyte-immune complex-clearing mechanism, *J. Clin. Invest.* **71**:236–247.

Dawkins, R. L., Christiansen, F. T., Kay, P. H., Garlepp, M., McCluskey, J., Hollingsworth, P. N., and Silko, P. J., 1983, Disease associations with complotypes, supratypes and haplotypes, *Immunol. Rev.* **70**:5–22.

Fearon, D. T., 1981, Complement as a mediator of inflammation, *Clin. Immunol. Allergy* **1**:225–242.

Fearon, D. T., and Wong, W. W., 1983, Complement ligand-receptor interactions that mediate biological responses, *Ann. Rev. Imuno..* **1**:243–271.

Franco, A. E., and Schur, P. H., 1971, Hypocomplementemia in rheumatoid arthritis, *Arthritis Rheum.* **14**:231–238.

Frank, M. M., and Atkinson, J. P., 1975, Complement in clinical medicine, *DM* **1975**(Jan.):1–154.

George, D., and Glass, D., 1983, Quantitation of complement proteins in rheumatic disease, *Clin. Rheum. Dis.* **9**:177–198.

Gilliam, J. N., Cheatom, D. E., Hurd, E. R., Stastny, P., and Ziff, M., 1974, Immunoglobulin in clinically uninvolved skin in systemic lupus erythematosus, *J. Clin. Invest.* **53**:1434–1440.

Glass, D., Fearon, D. T., and Austen, K. F., 1983, Inherited abnormalities of the complement system, in: *Metabolic Basis of Inherited Disease*, 5th ed. (J. B. Stanbury and J. B. Wyngaarden, eds.), McGraw-Hill, New York, pp. 1934–1955.

Gough, W., Lightfoot, R. W., and Christian, C. L., 1974, Cryoglobulins and complement in immune complex disease, *Arthritis Rheum.* **17**:497.

Hadler, N. M., Gerwin, R. D., Frank, M. M., Whitaker, J. N., Baker, M., and Decker, J. L., 1973, The fourth component of complement in the cerebrospinal fluid in systemic lupus erythematosus, *Arthritis Rheum.* **16**:507–521.

Hecht, B., Siegel, N., Adler, M., Kashgarian, M., and Hayslett, J. P., 1976, Prognostic indices in lupus erythematosus, *Medicine* **55**:163–164.

Hobart, M. J., and Lachman, P. J., 1976, Allotypes of complement components in man, *Transplant. Rev.* **32**:26–42.

Hunder, G. G., McDuffie, F. C., and Hepper, N. G., 1972, Pleural fluid complement in systemic lupus erythematosus and rheumatoid arthritis, *Ann. Intern. Med.* **76**:357–363.

Hunder, G. G., Mullen, B. J., and McDuffie, F. C., 1974, Complement in pericardial fluid of lupus erythematosus, *Ann. Intern. Med.* **80**:453–548.

Jarrett, M. P., Sablay, L. B., Walter, L., Barland, P., and Grayzel, A. L., 1981, The effect of continuous normalization of serum hemolytic complement on the course of lupus nephritis. A five year prospect study, *Am. J. Med.* **70**:1067–1072.

Koffler, D., and Bieseker, G., 1983, Immunopathogenesis of tissue injury, in: *The Clinical Management of Systemic Lupus Erythematosus* (P. H. Schur, ed.), Grune & Stratton, New York, p. 29–47.

Lange, K., Ores, R., Shauss, W., and Wachstein, M., 1965, Steroid therapy of systemic lupus erythematosus based on immunological considerations, *Arthritis Rheum.* **8**:244–258.

Levinsky, R. I., Cameron, J. S., and Soothill, J. F., 1977, Serum immune complexes and disease activity in lupus nephritis, *Lancet* **1**:564–567.

Lewis, E. J., Carpenter, C. B., and Schur, P. H., 1971, Serum complement components levels in human glomerulonephritis, *Ann. Intern. Med.* **75**:555–560.

Lightfoot, R. W., and Hughes, G. R., 1976, Significance of persisting serologic abnormalities in SLE, *Arthritis Rheum.* **19**:837–843.

Lloyd, W., and Schur, P. H., 1981, Immune complexes, complement and anti-DNA in exacerbations of systemic lupus erythematosus (SLE), *Medicine* **60**:208–217.

Miniter, M. F., Stollar, B. D, and Agnello, V., 1979, Reassessment of the clinical significance of native DNA antibodies in systemic lupus erythematosus, *Arthritis Rheum.* **22**:959–968.

Muller-Eberhard, H. J., 1974, The complement system and nephritis, *Adv. Nephrol.* **4**:3–14.

Nydegger, U. E., Lambert, P. H., Gerber, H., and Miescher, P. A., 1974, Circulating immune complexes in the serum in systemic lupus erythematosus and in carriers of hepatitis B antigen, *J. Clin. Invest.* **54**:297–309.

O'Neill, G. J., Yang, S. Y., Tegoli, J., Berger, R., and Dupont, B., 1978, Chido and Rodgers blood groups are distinct antigenic components of human complement C4, *Nature* **273**:668–670.

Pekin, T. J., Jr., and Zvaifler, N. J., 1970, Synovial fluid findings in systemic lupus erythematosus, *Arthritis Rheum.* **13**:777–785.

Petz, L. D., Sharp, G. C., Cooper, N. R., and Irvin, W. S., 1971, Serum and cerebral spinal fluid complement and serum auto-antibodies in systemic lupus erythematosus, *Medicine* **50**:259–275.

Provost, I. I., and Tomasi, T. B., Jr., 1973, Evidence for complement activation via the alternate pathway in skin diseases, herpes gestationis, systemic lupus erythematosus, and bullous pemphigoid, *J. Clin. Invest.* **52**:1779–1787.

Pussel, B. A., Lockwood, C. M., Scott, D. M., Pinching, A. J., and Peters, D. K., 1978, Value of immune complex assays in diagnosis and management, *Lancet* **2**:359–364.

Rosen, F. S., and Austen, K. F., 1969, The "neurotic edema" (hereditary angioedema), *N. Engl. J. Med.* **280**:1356–1357.

Rothfield, N., Ross, A., Minta, J. O., and Lepow, I. H., 1972, Glomerular and dermal deposition of properdin in systemic lupus erythematosus, *N. Engl. J. Med.* **287**:681–685.

Ruddy, S., and Austen, K. F., 1970, The complement system in rheumatoid synovitis. I. An analysis of complement component activities in rheumatoid synovial fluids, *Arthritis Rheum.* **13**:713–725.

Ruddy, S., Carpenter, C. B., Chin, K. W., Krostmann, J. N., Sorter, N. A., Gotze, O., Muller-Eberhad, H. J., and Austen, K. F., 1975, Human complement metabolism: An analysis of 144 studies, *Medicine* **54**:165–178.

Schur, P. H., 1972, Human gamma G subclasses, *Prog. Clin. Immunol.* **1**:71–104.

Schur, P. H., 1975, Complement in lupus, *Clin. Rheum. Dis.* **1**:519–543.

Schur, P. H., 1977, Complement testing in the diagnosis of immune and autoimmune diseases, *Am. J. Clin. Pathol.* **68**:647–659.

Schur, P. H., 1978, Genetics of complement deficiencies associated with lupus-like syndromes, *Arthritis Rheum.* **21**:5153–5160.

Schur, P. H., 1983, Complement studies of sera and other biologic fluids, *Hum. Pathol.* **14**:338–342.

Schur, P. H., and Austen, K. F., 1968, Complement in human disease, *Annu. Rev. Med.* **10**:1–34.

Silverstein, A. M., 1960, Essential hypocomplementemia: Report of a case, *Blood* **16**:1338–1341.

Sliwinski, A. J., and Zvaifler, N. J., 1972, Decreased synthesis of the third component in hypocomplementemic systemic lupus erythematosus, *Clin. Exp. Immunol.* **11**:21–29.

Soter, N. A., 1976, Clinical presentations and mechanisms of necrotizing angiitis, *J. Invest. Dermatol.* **67**:354–359.

Stastny, P., and Ziff, M., 1969, Cold-insoluble complexes and complement levels in systemic lupus erythematosus, *N. Engl. J. Med.* **280**:1376–1381.

Tan, E. M., and Kunkel, H. G., 1966, An immunofluorescent study of the skin lesions in systemic lupus erythematosus, *Arthritis Rheum.* **9**:37–46.

Vaughan, J. H., Bayles, T. B., and Savour, C. B., 1951, The response of serum gammaglobulin level and complement titer to adrenocorticotrophic hormone therapy in lupus erythematosus disseminatus, *J. Lab. Clin. Med.* **37**:698–702.

Verroust, P. J., Wilson, C. B., Cooper, N. R., Edginton, T. S., and Dixon, F. J., 1974, Glomerular complement components in human glomerulonephritis, *J. Clin. Invest.* **53**:77–84.

Wilson, J. G., Wong, W. W., Schur, P. H., and Fearon, D. T., 1982, Mode of inheritance of decreased C3b receptors on erythrocytes of patients with systemic lupus erythematosus, *N. Engl. J. Med.* **307**:981–986.

22

Immune Complexes, Vasoactive Mediators, and Fibrinoid Necrosis in Connective Tissue Diseases

Allen P. Kaplan

I. INTRODUCTION

Although the inflammatory mechanisms operative in the various connective tissue diseases are all different, there are certain features common to many of them. These include tissue deposition of circulating immune complexes, a vasculopathy, and fibrinoid necrosis of the surrounding tissue. Other chapters in this text deal with immune complexes, activation of complement, and recruitment and activation of neutrophils, all of which are important aspects of immunologically mediated inflammation. This chapter focuses on the tissue deposition of immune complexes, the role of vasoactive factors in the inflammatory response, and the interrelationship of these events with coagulation and fibrinolysis to cause fibrinoid necrosis.

II. CLEARANCE AND DEPOSITION OF IMMUNE COMPLEXES

The localization of immune complexes in tissues is dependent on numerous factors, which are, at present, only partially understood. Two general mechanisms seem to be operative. Immune complexes may be formed within the circulation and then deposited in tissues, or one component of the immune complex may first fix to a tissue site or receptor and then combine with the other component so that the immune complex is formed *in situ*. If one is dealing with a disorder such as Goodpasture's syndrome or certain types of

Allen P. Kaplan • Division of Allergy, Rheumatology, and Clinical Immunology, Department of Medicine, The State University of New York at Stony Brook, Health Sciences Center, Stony Brook, New York 11794.

membranous nephritis, the antibody is directed against a tissue component such as glomerular basement membrane. In this case, the antigenic component of the complex is a tissue element. On the other hand, the immune complex deposition seen in the kidneys in a disorder such as systemic lupus erythematosus may occur as follows. First, circulating free DNA (Steinman, 1984) binds to a DNA receptor (Izui *et al.*, 1976) in the glomerular basement membrane. Then anti-DNA (primarily IgG_1 and IgG_3) binds to the DNA, and an immune complex is formed. This may, in part, account for the preferential localization of DNA–anti-DNA complexes in the kidneys of patients with systemic lupus (Adu and Williams, 1981) even though such complexes seem to be only a small fraction of the total circulating immune complex load. It can also account for the particular site of immune complex localization within the basement membrane; e.g., subendothelial, intramembranous, or subepithelial, depending on the location of receptor sites. Other factors such as size and/or charge of complexes and antibody or complement receptor sites also affect localization of immune complexes; thus, the process is clearly multifactorial.

The tissue deposition of circulating immune complexes is dependent on the circulating blood volume to that tissue, the concentration of the immune complex, and mechanisms by which the immune complex can pass through the vascular barrier. The last parameter is in part a function of the size and charge of the immune complex, and passage into tissues may be facilitated by the generation of factors that are vasodilating or can increase vascular permeability. The concentration of circulating immune complexes is a balance between synthesis and removal by the reticuloendothelial system. Formation of immune complexes as a result of antibody binding to circulating antigenic material is discussed in Chapters 18 and 22; thus, I confine my comments herein to a summary of studies of reticuloendothelial clearance of complexes.

Early work in animal models determined several aspects of immune complex clearance mechanisms using radiolabeled complexes of human serum albumin–antialbumin. Larger complexes of greater than 22 S were cleared rapidly by hepatic Kupffer cells, whereas intermediate-sized complexes (11 S to 22 S) persisted longer, and small complexes (<8 S) were present for a prolonged time (Mannick *et al.*, 1974). Clearance was shown to require interaction of an intact Fc fragment with cell surface Fc receptors (Haakenstad and Mannick, 1974), and the clearance mechanism was saturable. As a result, the administration of aggregated immunoglobulins prolonged the clearance of circulating immune complexes, and increased tissue deposition resulted (Haakenstad and Mannick, 1974). Studies in man have utilized radiolabeled red blood cells coated with IgG or with complement (C3b) in place of antigen. Their respective clearance by splenic macrophages bearing Fc receptors or hepatic Kupffer's cells, which bind C3b (Frank *et al.*, 1977; Schreiber and Frank, 1972), was then determined. It was hoped that the results obtained would reflect clearance of *bona fide* immune complexes. The red blood cells were coated with IgG anti-Rh(D) antibody, which is not complement fixing because the spacing of Rh antigen on the surface is not sufficiently close to form IgG doublets; this is also true of immune complexes of low molecular weight (<8 S), and their inflammatory potential is thereby diminished. For studies of C3b receptors, IgM antibody to blood group A substance was utilized; this fixes complement, and in the absence of IgM receptors, clearance becomes dependent on C3b.

The most convincing data suggesting a relationship between reticuloendothelial clearance mechanisms and tissue immune complex deposition come from studies of systemic lupus erythematosus. In this disorder, a correlation is found among abnormal clearance of IgG-coated red cells, levels of circulating immune complexes, and disease activity (Frank *et al.*, 1979). The most prolonged clearance times were found in the subgroup of patients with glomerulonephritis (Pareis *et al.*, 1982). Clearance of aggregated human serum albumin was normal in such patients, suggesting that splenic macrophages are functional and that the abnormal clearance seen reflects a specific receptor defect. The magnitude of the clearance defect did not correlate with levels of circulatory complement components or anti-DNA levels when pooled data were examined, although these were usually abnormal. With treatment, clearance times shortened in patients who improved clinically (Hamburger *et al.*, 1982). Likewise, short-term intensive plasmapheresis appeared to correct abnormal clearance times and decrease immune complex levels to within normal range concurrent with clinical improvement (Hamburger *et al.*, 1981; Lockwood *et al.*, 1979).

Such studies support the concept of a reversible, saturation-induced, reticuloendothelial cell defect in systemic lupus erythematosus. However, quantitation of IgG Fc receptors on human monocytes in patients with systemic lupus erythematosus revealed an increased number of receptors. This is inconsistent with either a genetically determined defect in receptor number or in receptor saturation as an explanation for the decreased clearance seen (Fries *et al.*, 1984). Thus, further studies regarding the role of complement in immune complex clearance, comparison of fixed macrophages with peripheral monocytes, mononuclear processing of bound immune complexes, etc., are needed before a definitive explanation for this phenomenon is obtained.

Clinical studies of other arthritides or autoimmune disorders have not found a clear relationship among abnormal clearance of coated red cells, immune complex levels, and disease state. In mixed cryoglobulinemia, clearance was normal in the face of high circulating immune complex levels if the patient had no renal disease, but every patient with glomerulonephritis had a defective clearance determination (Hamburger *et al.*, 1979a). Thus, whatever causes the clearance abnormality may predispose to renal disease, although one must consider that the defect could be secondary to the other factors responsible for nephritis. In rheumatoid arthritis, correlation of reticuloendothelial function with disease manifestations could not be made (Fields *et al.*, 1983a), a not surprising result since the critical inflammatory parameters are intraarticular. In Sjogren's syndrome, abnormal clearances were found in patients with widespread disease (extraglandular disease or associated connective tissue disorders) but not in those with disease limited to the exocrine glands (Hamburger *et al.*, 1979b), even though increased complex levels in the two groups were comparable.

Thus, if saturation of Fc receptors were responsible for tissue deposition of complexes, one would have to propose that the physicochemical properties of the complexes in the two circumstances differ or that other factors determine the ability of the reticuloendothelial system to clear complexes in those patients with widespread disease. At least one study suggests genetic control of patients' ability to clear IgG-coated red cells (? immune complexes). Patients with dermatitis herpetiformis were shown to have elevated immune complexes containing IgA antibody but not IgG antibody (Hall *et al.*, 1980), yet half of them had abnormalities of IgG-receptor-dependent clearance of coated red cells. Because of the high association of HLA-B8 and HLA-DRW3 with this disorder and the general association of these genotypes with autoimmune disorders, healthy in-

Table 1. Clearance of Immune Complexes and Disease State or Manifestations

Disorder	Clearance	Correlation
Systemic lupus erythematosus	Prolonged Fc dependent	Disease activity Circulating immune complex levels
	Prolonged C3b dependent	None
Mixed cryoglobulinemia	Prolonged Fc dependent	Nephritis
Rheumatoid arthritis	Prolonged Fc dependent	None
Sjogren's syndrome	Prolonged Fc dependent	Extraglandular manifestations, associated connective tissue disorder
Primary biliary cirrhosis	Prolonged C3b dependent	Normal in other forms of cirrhosis

dividuals bearing these haplotypes were studied, and half had abnormal clearance times (Lawley *et al.*, 1981). Thus, reticuloendothelial function may be under genetic control.

There have been far fewer studies of C3b-dependent clearance. Prolonged clearance times have been described in primary biliary cirrhosis (Jaffe *et al.*, 1978), although other types of cirrhosis lacked the abnormality. About 50% of systemic lupus patients were also abnormal (Miyaka *et al.*, 1981). Such defects could be caused by intrinsic abnormalities of the reticuloendothelial cells of the liver or by receptor saturation by C3b-bearing immune complexes. In separate studies, patients with systemic lupus have been found to have diminished red blood cell levels of the CR_1 receptor (Dobson *et al.*, 1981), which binds C3b and C4b, although the authors differed in interpretation as to whether it is a genetic (Iida *et al.*, 1982) or acquired (Wilson *et al.*, 1982) phenomenon. A similar phenomenon may be observed in patients with rheumatoid arthritis. A summary of the results of these clearance studies is given in Table 1.

III. VASOACTIVE FACTORS AND IMMUNE COMPLEX DEPOSITION

Studies of rabbit models of immune-complex-induced glomerulonephritis first led to the idea that the release of vasoactive factors might be required for the deposition of immune complexes in tissues. Animals were immunized with bovine serum albumin such that elevated levels of circulating albumin–antialbumin complexes resulted, and renal deposition of such complexes resulted in glomerulonephritis. It was found that a combination of antihistamine and antiserotonin agents could prevent renal deposition of complexes and thereby prevent glomerulonephritis although circulating complex levels were unaffected (Knicker and Cochrane, 1968). Thus, it appeared that histamine and serotonin release, at least in rodents, was required for immune complex deposition. It was then shown that the reaction was IgE dependent and associated with mediator release from basophils and platelets (Benveniste *et al.*, 1972). Rabbit platelets contain both histamine and serotonin, and release of both substances was dependent on a factor derived from activated basophils; this was called platelet-activating factor (PAF). The general structure of this factor has been determined to be 1-O-alkyl-2-acetyl-*sn*-glyceryl-3-phophorylcho-

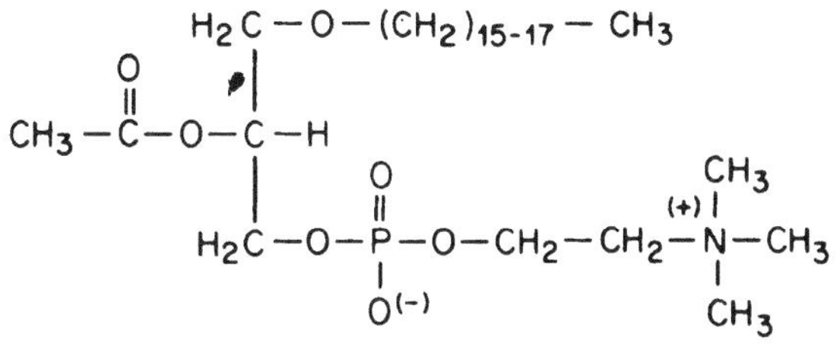

Figure 1. Structure of platelet-activating factor. An alkyl group is in ether linkage to the first carbon, an acetyl group is in ester linkage to the second carbon, and a phosphorylcholine group is linked to the third carbon.

line (Demopoulos) *et al.*, 1979; Hanahan *et al.*, 1980) (AGEPC) (Fig. 1); the alkyl group can be either a 16- or 18-carbon chain.

The relationship between these various mediators in man, however, is different from that seen in rodents. Human basophils contain only histamine, and human platelets contain only serotonin, whereas rodent basophils and platelets each contain both substances. Further, human mast cells have been shown to release AGEPC (MacGlashan *et al.*, 1983), but the data regarding human basophils are unclear (Betz *et al.*, 1980; Camussi *et al.*, 1981; Sanchez *et al.*, 1980).

In summary, these studies suggested a sequence in which IgE antibody to an immunogen caused PAF release from basophils and secondary release of histamine and serotonin from platelets. This was a prerequisite for tissue deposition of immune complexes containing IgG or IgM antibody. With this in mind, it was hoped that by using rodent models of immune-complex-mediated connective tissue diseases, one might prevent nephritis by pretreatment with antihistamine and/or antiserotonin agents. Such studies in the NZB/W mouse model of systemic lupus erythematosus were, however, disappointing in that lupus nephritis was certainly not prevented, and only a small effect on the time of acquisition of renal disease and longevity was seen (Chused and Tarplay, 1973). Nevertheless, the concept is certainly an interesting one, and the results obtained may differ depending on the species tested, the timing of therapy, the particular disease being studied, the relevant mediators released, as well as on the effects of such molecules on the vascular tree and very likely a host of unknown factors.

There are few studies in man that have tested this phenomenon in any fashion. In one report, a diptheria epidemic requiring treatment with horse antitoxin was studied prospectively. A predictable incidence of serum sickness reactions in the recipients was anticipated. Patients receiving antitoxin were divided into two groups, one of which received concomitant therapy with high doses of antihistamines. A significant decrease in incidence of serum sickness was found in the treated group (Knicker, 1972), suggesting an effect of histamine on tissue deposition of immune complexes.

Recent studies have demonstrated the presence of IgE antibody to rheumatoid factor (Zuraw *et al.*, 1981) and DNA (Barone *et al.*, 1981) in patients with rheumatoid arthritis and systemic lupus erythematosus, respectively; however, there has been no demonstration of mediator release from basophils or mast cells as a consequence of this reaction. Since tissue mast cells contain AGEPC, an allergic reaction might cause release of this factor into the circulation. Elevated platelet factor 4 levels in allergic asthmatics (Knauer *et al.*, 1981) (suggesting intravascular platelet degranulation) suggest that such a mechanism is possible. The aforementioned rodent studies also assumed the critical vasoactive factors to be amines and were unaware of the fact the AGEPC has direct vascular effect of its own. When injected intravenously into rabbits, it produces hypotension (Halonen *et al.*

1980), as might be seen during anaphylaxis, and when injected into human skin, it causes vasodilation and increased vascular permeability at molar concentrations 100–1000 times lower than histamine (Humphrey *et al.*, 1982; Pinckard *et al.*, 1980). Thus, AGEPC itself could be an important vasoactive and inflammatory agent that could also contribute to immune complex localization; AGEPC is also released on activation of human neutrophils (Lotner *et al.*, 1980), monocytes (Arnoux *et al.*, 1982; Clark *et al.*, 1980), and endothelial cells (Colman, 1969) so that it can be recruited into inflammatory reactions in many ways.

If we consider that any vasoactive factor released at tissue sites or within the circulation could affect immune complex deposition regardless of whether its formation is IgE dependent, one must then consider the prostaglandins, leukotrienes, and kinins as potential contributors. The arachidonic acid metabolites that possess prominent vasoactive properties include prostaglandin D_2, prostaglandin E_2, prostacyclin (PGI_2), and leukotrienes C and D. Prostaglandin D_2 is of particular interest because it is the main cyclooxygenase product of human mast cells (Lewis *et al.*, 1982; Peters *et al.*, 1984) and is therefore released together with histamine and AGEPC. The hypotensive episodes and flush reaction of systemic mastocytosis have been attributed to release of PGD_2 and/or its metabolites, and partial reversal is obtained with prostaglandin synthesis inhibitors (Roberts *et al.*, 1980). Thus, PGD_2 appears to have significant potential as a vasodilator in man, and it also elicits a wheal and flare response when injected intracutaneously (Flower *et al.*, 1976). Prostaglandin E_2 is a major product of macrophages, synovial cells, and neutrophils, and prostacyclin is a major product of vascular endothelial cells. Both are peripheral vasodilators (Issekutz and Movat, 1982; Williams, 1979; Williams and Peck, 1977).

The leukotrienes C and D (slow-reacting substance of anaphylaxis) (Lewis *et al.*, 1980; Murphy *et al.*, 1979; Orning *et al.*, 1980; Parker *et al.*, 1979) cause venular dilatation and increased vascular permeability (Dahlen *et al.*, 1981; Drazen *et al.*, 1980; Soter *et al.*, 1983; Ueno *et al.*, 1981) and are released from activated basophils (Yecies *et al.*, 1979), mast cells (Peters *et al.*, 1984), and macrophages (Rankin *et al.*, 1984; Rouzer *et al.*, 1980). Although leukotrienes were discovered as a product of activated neutrophils, eosinophils release ten times more per cell (Jorg *et al.*, 1982; Weller *et al.*, 1983). Leukotrienes are likely to be present in the inflammatory reactions seen in connective tissue disorders, as they can be released by most infiltrating cell types. Elevated levels of these lipoxygenase products have been reported in acute gout as well as in the synovial fluid of rheumatoid patients with arthritis and spondyloarthropathies (Klickstein *et al.*, 1980). Prostacyclin and prostaglandin E_1 have also been utilized with some success as therapy for fingertip ulcerations in systemic sclerosis and Raynaud's phenomenon because of their vasodilatory properties (Belch *et al.*, 1983; Martin *et al.*, 1981).

Kinins are polypeptides that cause local peripheral vasodilation, increase vascular permeability, and lead to hypotension when systemic levels are increased. Kinins therefore represent another category of vasoactive substance that could affect immune complex deposition. Most studies have focused on bradykinin, a nine-amino-acid peptide with the sequence Arg-Pro-Pro-Gly-Phe-Ser-Pro-Phe-Arg. Bradykinin is derived from a plasma protein termed kininogen, and its release requires cleavage at two sites (Lys-Arg and Arg-Ser) within the molecule since the bradykinin moiety is internal. The enzymes that cleave kininogen to generate bradykinin are known as kallikreins. There are two general mechanisms by which bradykinin is generated in man, and these involve two different kallikreins and two forms of kininogens. Certain tissues are partially rich in kallikreins; these include salivary glands, pancreas, and kidney (Orstavik *et al.*, 1980), although many other tissues possess cells with kallikreinlike activity. It appears that a prokallikrein may exist, which is converted to an active enzyme within the cell (Nishimura *et al.*, 1980; Spragg, 1983), but the exact mechanism by which this occurs is unclear. When secreted, a large fraction appears already activated.

Plasma, on the other hand, contains a prekallikrein that must be enzymatically cleaved in order to convert it to the enzyme plasma kallikrein. The plasma enzyme is much larger than tissue kallikreins (molecular weight 88,000 vs. ~30,000), and they do not cross react immunologically. Thus, they clearly represent different gene products. The two kininogens in plasma appear to be more closely related. The more plentiful is a kininogen of relatively low molecular weight (~50,000 on SDS gels) (LMW kininogen), which accounts for about 85% of plasma kininogen; the remaining 15% is a high-molecular-weight form (~115,000 on SDS gels) (HMW kininogen). Tissue kallikreins digest both forms of kininogen approximately equally; however, since LMW kininogen is in far excess, most of the kinin formed by tissue kallikrein is derived from this form. However, the product, rather than being bradykinin, is Lys-bradykinin or kallidin, a ten-amino-acid peptide (Webster and Pierce, 1963). An aminopeptidase in plasma can cleave at the N-terminal Lys-Arg group to convert it to bradykinin. The specificity of plasma kallikrein is much greater because it selectively digests the HMW kininogen to form bradykinin. These reactions are summarized in Fig. 2. Studies of the amino acid sequence of high- and low-molecular-weight kininogens have demonstrated that they share a major portion of the molecule, from the N-terminus to just beyond the bradykinin moiety (Kitamura *et al.*, 1983; Thompson *et al.*, 1978), but that the residues subsequent to that point differ.

The level of bradykinin in plasma (and very likely other body fluids) is dependent on the rate of formation of bradykinin and its rate of destruction. The latter process is rapid and of considerable importance but renders the *in vivo* determination of bradykinin as a reflection of kininogen proteolysis difficult. Thus, assessment of the kinin-forming

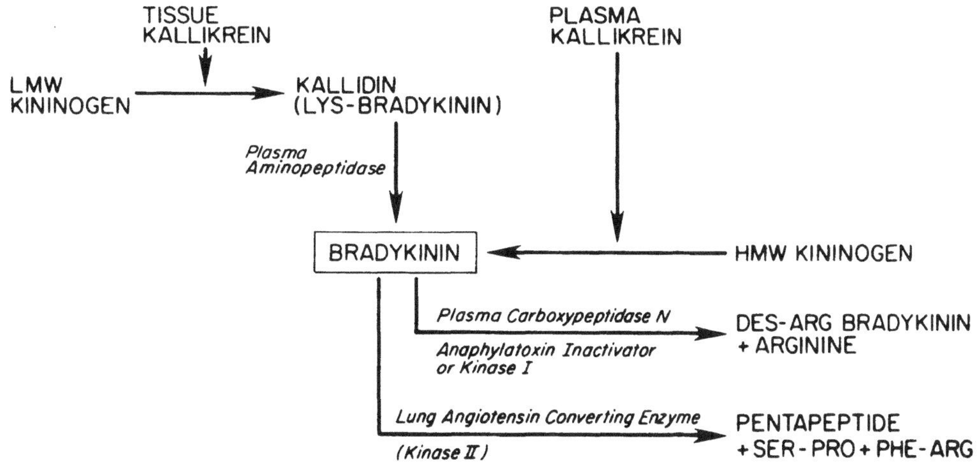

Figure 2. Formation and destruction of bradykinin.

systems in human disease may require determination of kinin degradation products in addition to or perhaps in place of direct kinin assessment. There are two major pathways for *in vivo* bradykinin destruction. In plasma, the major enzyme known as carboxypeptidase N or kininase I (Erdos and Sloane, 1962; Plummer and Horwitz, 1978) removes the C-terminal arginine to leave an inactive octapeptide. This protein is identical to the anaphylatoxin inactivator (Bockish and Muller-Eberhard, 1970), which similarly removes a C-terminal arginine from C3a, C4a, and C5a to cause loss of their contractile and permeability-enhancing properties. The second enzyme is also present in high concentration in the lung, where it rapidly degrades bradykinin in the pulmonary microcirculation. The products are a pentapeptide, Arg-Pro-Pro-Gly-Phe, plus the dipeptides Ser-Pro and Phe-Arg (Sheikh and Kaplan, 1984). This enzyme is better known as the angiotensin-converting enzyme because it also converts angiotensin I to angiotensin II by removal of the dipeptide His-Leu. Radioimmunoassays are available for the determination of plasma bradykinin (Scicli *et al.*, 1982; Talamo *et al.*, 1969). Normal levels appear to be as low as 25 pg/ml (Scicli *et al.*, 1982). Recently, a radioimmunoassay for des-Arg-bradykinin (the kininase I product) has also been reported.

IV. FORMATION OF BRADYKININ IN PLASMA: A PRODUCT OF THE INTRINSIC COAGULATION PATHWAY

Bradykinin formation in plasma requires the interaction of initiating surfaces with three plasma proteins, namely, Hageman factor, prekallikrein, and a high-molecular-weight form of kininogen (HMW-kininogen) (Kaplan, 1983) shown in Fig. 3. These proteins interact in sequence so that once Hageman factor becomes activated, it converts prekallikrein to kallikrein, and kallikrein digests HWM kininogen to liberate bradykinin. In addition, activated Hageman factor converts coagulation factor XI to factor XIa, and factor XIa continues the intrinsic coagulation pathway. Although this scheme is technically correct, it does not indicate the complex manner in which these proteins interact so as to link coagulation with bradykinin formation. First, the substrates of activated Hageman

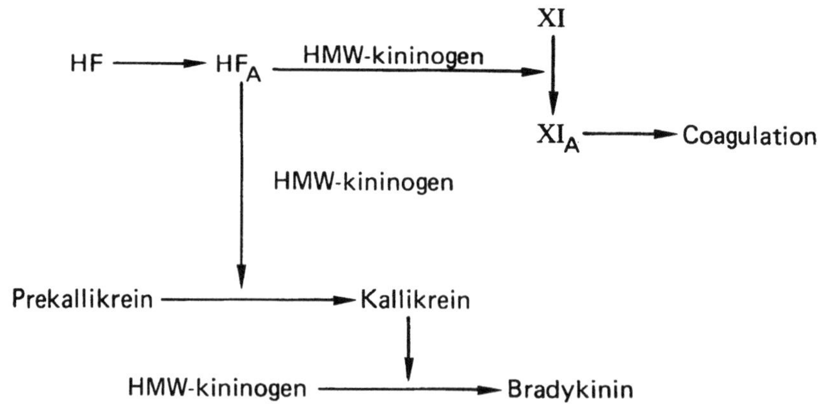

Figure 3. The formation of bradykinin by surface-dependent interaction of Hageman factor, prekallikrein, and high-molecular-weight kininogen.

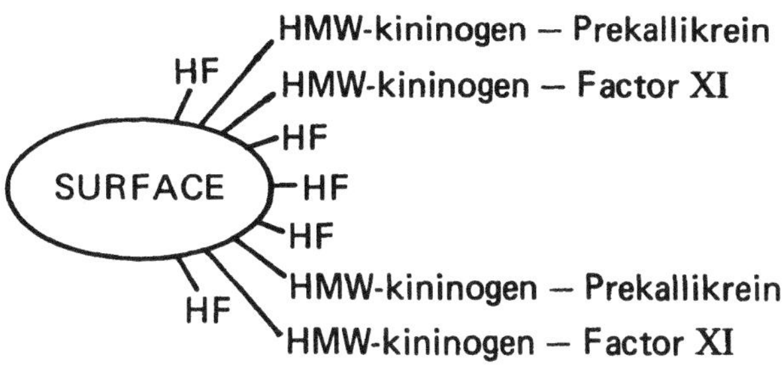

Figure 4. Diagrammatic representation of the interaction of surfaces with those plasma proteins required for "contact activation" of plasma.

factor (i.e., prekallikrein and factor XI), circulate complexed to HMW kininogen (Mandle *et al.*, 1976; Thompson *et al.*, 1977), and it is these complexes that interact with the surface.

This is depicted diagrammatically in Fig. 4. There appears to be approximately twice the concentration of HMW kininogen present in plasma needed to bind all of the prekallikrein and factor XI present. Since the binding constant for each complex is high (Bock and Shore, 1983; Thompson *et al.*, 1979), most of the prekallikrein and factor XI circulate as a complex. Further, it has been shown that HMW kininogen possesses a single binding site that interacts either with prekallikrein or with factor XI but not both. Thus, no trimolecular complex is seen, but instead, two bimolecular complexes are present with a molar ratio of reactants of 1 : 1 (Thompson *et al.*, 1979). When initiating surfaces are added to normal plasma, Hageman factor is bound directly to the surface, where it interacts with the complexes of HWM kininogen–prekallikrein and HMW kininogen–factor XI. The next sections summarize the properties and mechanism of activation of each of these proteins.

A. Hageman Factor

Hageman factor is an 80,000-dalton protein present in normal plasma at a mean concentration of about 35 μg/ml. The protein is a single polypeptide chain that is glycosylated, and some parts of the molecule have now been sequenced (Fujikawa and McMullen, 1983). Although Hageman factor is the initiating protein of the cascade, it is readily cleaved by other proteases, the major one being kallikrein (Cochrane *et al.*, 1973). Thus, a reciprocal interaction exists in which activated Hageman factor converts prekallikrein to kallikrein, and kallikrein activates Hageman factor. When Hageman factor is activated by kallikrein, a single cleavage is initially made at an arginine residue that is located within a disulfide loop (Fig. 5). The resulting molecule of activated Hageman factor (HFa) is thus a two-chain structure comprising a heavy chain of 50,000 daltons derived from the original amino terminus of Hageman factor and a light chain of 28,000 daltons (Revak *et al.*, 1977). This molecule is a serine protease with the active site and catalytic mechanism located in the light chain. Enzymatic activity is readily demonstrated against its natural substrates, prekallikrein or factor XI, and against low-molecular-weight synthetic substrates (Silverberg *et al.*, 1980a). It is also inhibited by the classic serine protease

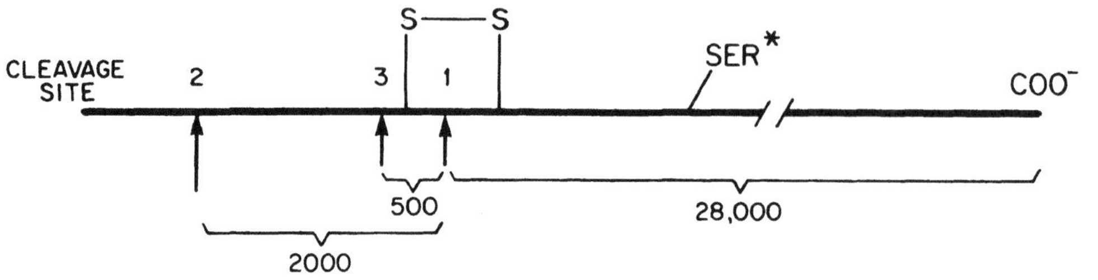

Figure 5. Cleavages required for activation of human Hageman factor. Digestion at site 1 forms HFa, in which a heavy chain of 50,000 molecular weight is disulfide-linked to a light chain of 28,000. Further digestion at sites 2 and then 3 yields the two molecular forms of HFf, an active fragment that is released from the surface and can effectively activate prekallikrein in the fluid phase.

inhibitor diisopropyl fluorophosphate (DFP) as well as by chloromethylketone derivatives of oligopeptides with suitable sequences (Dunn and Kaplan, 1982).

If digestion of Hageman factor by kallikrein continues, two further peptide bonds are cleaved (Fig. 5). The new cleavage sites are located in the heavy chain, outside the disulfide bond that connects the two chains of HFa. The products are two forms of Hageman factor fragment (HFf), which comprise the original light chain of HFa with a small oligopeptide tail connected by a disulfide bond. It appears that the larger form of HFf (mol. wt. 30,000) is formed first and that a subsequent cleavage trims the oligopeptide to produce the smaller form (mol. wt. 28,500) (Dunn and Kaplan, 1982). Both forms remain enzymatically active, as would be expected, since each contains all the catalytic machinery of the original molecule. Thus, HFa and HFf have very similar kinetics of hydrolysis of synthetic substrates (Silverberg *et al.*, 1980a), and both are efficient activators of prekallikrein (Kaplan and Austen, 1970; Revak *et al.*, 1977). A major difference between the two forms of activated Hageman factor is observed when they are assayed by their ability to correct the partial thromboplastin time (PTT) of Hageman-factor-deficient plasma. In this case, it is observed that HFa is an efficient clotting factor but HFf is a very poor one (Kaplan and Austen, 1970, 1971). This difference may be ascribed to their relative abilities to bind to activating surfaces. Thus, HFa binds to the surface, but when the second cleavage occurs, the HFf formed does not remain bound (Revak and Cochrane, 1976). These observations allow us to conclude that the region of Hageman factor that binds to the surface is located on the heavy-chain portion of the molecule (Revak and Cochrane, 1976). On conversion of HFa to HFf, HFf will leave the surface, and it will continue to activate the bradykinin-forming cascade at sites distant from the surface reaction until it is inactivated by a plasma inhibitor.

B. Prekallikrein

Prekallikrein is the precursor of the active serine protease plasma kallikrein. It is a 90,000-dalton protein present in human plasma at a concentration of 25–50 μg/ml. Like Hageman factor, prekallikrein is a single-chain polypeptide that becomes cleaved within a disulfide-bonded loop on activation; the active protein thus has a two-chain structure similar to HFa, and as in HFa, the active site is on the light chain (Mandle and Kaplan, 1977). Purified plasma prekallikrein usually appears on SDS gels as two closely spaced bands

(Mandle and Kaplan, 1976). After reduction of kallikrein, the heterogeneity of the parent protein is reflected in the light chain, which also appears as a doublet of 36,000 and 33,000 daltons (Mandle and Kaplan, 1976). The heavy chain appears to be homogeneous. The source of the heterogeneity has not been determined, but there is no indication that it is caused by proteolysis during purification, since the relative yield of the two bands does not vary from one preparation to another.

The major activator of plasma prekallikrein in normal human plasma is activated Hageman factor (Fig. 2). This apparent paradox, since kallikrein is the major activator of Hageman factor, is discussed in some detail below. Once activated, kallikrein has a number of substrates. These include high-molecular-weight kininogen, as mentioned above, which is cleaved extremely rapidly by kallikrein to liberate bradykinin (Habal *et al.*, 1974; Thompson *et al.*, 1978). This requires two cleavages, since the bradykinin sequence is located internally in the sequence of HMW kininogen.

The sequence at the N-terminal side of bradykinin is unusual in that the cleavage site is a lysine residue; other sites cleaved by kallikrein, and by clotting proteases in general, are arginine residues. Yet kallikrein is inert toward synthetic substrates that are based on peptides of lysine, which suggests that the recognition site in HMW kininogen must involve structural features outside the immediate primary sequence around the cleavage site. Other substrates or potential substrates of plasma kallikrein include plasminogen (Colman, 1969; Mandle and Kaplan, 1977), plasma prorenin (Sealey *et al.*, 1979), and complement components (DiScipio, 1982). Kallikrein may also have other effects in inflammatory reactions since it has chemotactic activity for neutrophils (Kaplan *et al.*, 1972) and can cause neutrophil aggregation (Schapira *et al.*, 1982a,b) and enzyme secretion (Wachtfogel *et al.*, 1983).

C. High-Molecular-Weight Kininogen

The HMW kininogen is a 115,000-dalton protein present in plasma at 80 μg/ml. It contains within it the sequence of bradykinin and thus is a substrate protein for plasma kallikrein. If this were its only function, deficiency of HMW kininogen would not be expected to cause any change in coagulation parameters. In fact, however, plasmas deficient in HMW kininogen show a very marked increase in their PTTs, and studies with purified components show that the rates of activation of prekallikrein, Hageman factor, and factor XI are all very much lower when HMW kininogen is absent (Griffin and Cochrane, 1976; Meier *et al.*, 1977a). After the bradykinin has been liberated, the remainder of the molecule is in the form of a two-chain disulfide-linked protein. This can be reduced and alkylated and the chains separated by chromatography in guanidine hydrochloride. It is remarkable that even after this apparently harsh treatment, coagulation cofactor activity remains and is associated exclusively with the light chain (Thompson *et al.*, 1978). Recent evidence suggests that when HMW kininogen is first cleaved to release bradykinin, the two chains formed are of approximately equal size at about 62,000 daltons (Schiffman *et al.*, 1980). Successive cleavages reduce the size of the light chain to approximately 56,000 and then to 45,000 daltons (Keribiriou and Griffin, 1979; Mori and Nagasawa, 1981; Thompson *et al.*, 1978). The isolated light chains can bind to prekallikrein and factor XI (Thompson *et al.*, 1979) as well as to surfaces and therefore account for the cofactor (coagulant) activity of HMW kininogen.

A longstanding puzzle concerning the structural relationship of the high- and low-molecular-weight forms of plasma kininogen has recently been resolved. The heavy chains of the two species were known to be immunologically indistinguishable from each other (Thompson *et al.*, 1978), but the light chain of the low-molecular-weight form is much smaller and has no coagulant activity (Kato *et al.*, 1976). Low-molecular-weight kininogen is cleaved only slowly by plasma kallikrein but is the primary substrate for tissue kallikrein. It has recently been shown that bovine kininogens are synthesized from a common gene followed by separate coding regions for each light chain separated by noncoding regions (Kitamura *et al.*, 1983). The controlling mechanisms by which the two distinct messenger RNAs are produced remain unknown, but it is now proven that the heavy chains and a short part of the sequence C-terminal to the bradykinin moiety are indeed identical.

D. Surface

The final component of the contact system that has to be considered is the surface. To date there is no unequivocal demonstration of a true physiological surface that can support contact activation, although a number of substances are known, of both organic and nonorganic origin, that are functional. These substances all bear negative charges and are able to form either high-molecular-weight aggregates or are actually particulate. The classic inorganic substances are kaolin and celite, which have been widely used both experimentally and as routine activators for PTT tests; another important inorganic activator is glass (or quartz). There has been continued interest in the development of a soluble activator that would be easier to handle both experimentally and in routine clotting assays. The first such substance proposed was ellagic acid, which is a fused ring structure bearing hydroxyl functional groups (Ratnoff and Crum, 1964). However, recent evidence has shown unequivocally that this material only activates when it is able to form large aggregates in solution by complexing with traces of metal ions (Bock *et al.*, 1981). A more legitimately soluble activator is dextran sulfate; high-molecular-weight forms are very efficient activators but are definitely soluble, where low-molecular-weight species do not activate. Thus, there is a definite requirement for a large particle size, but insolubility *per se* is not apparently necessary.

A recent addition (Fujikawa *et al.*, 1980) to the list of efficient activators is sulfatide, which is a sulfated glycosphingolipid. This is found in brain tissue and presumably does not support contact activation while diluted by other lipids. However, pure preparations of sulfatide are very efficient activators, presumably because they form micelles or vesicles that present a negatively charged surface for Hageman factor to bind to. From consideration of which substances are good activators, one would expect that proteoglycans or their glycosaminoglycan components would also support contact activation. This remains an attractive hypothesis although as yet without confirmation. Earlier reports (Harpel, 1972; Wilner *et al.*, 1968) that collagen activates have not been substantiated by recent work (Fujikawa *et al.* 1980).

Activation of the system can occur on exposure of plasma or purified proteins to monosodium urate and pyrophosphate crystals (Ginsberg *et al.*, 1980; Kellermeyer and Breckenridge, 1965) and the lipid A portion of endotoxin (Morrison and Cochrane, 1974). These results raise the possibility that the contact system may be involved in several pathological states, especially through the generation of bradykinin. This is discussed in more detail in subsequent sections.

E. Initiation by Hageman Factor

The intrinsic coagulation pathway presents a dilemma similar to the activation of C1r subcomponent of the classical complement pathway in that Hageman factor is clearly the initiating protein but it is present in zymogen form and appears to require cleavage to create the activated enzyme (Griffin and Berretta, 1979; Miller *et al.*, 1980; Revak *et al.*, 1977). Yet all of the enzymes that might cleave it require activated Hageman factor for their formation. Hence, the process appears circular, and the starting point is difficult to define. Many proposals have been put forth to explain how initiation occurs, and some of these are described below. At first, it was felt that a conformational change occurs on binding of Hageman factor to certain negatively charged (initiating) surfaces to expose an active site (McMillan *et al.* 1974; Ratnoff and Saito, 1979). However, this concept was questioned because the native uncleaved enzyme does not appear to interact with protease inhibitors, does not incorporate DFP into the bound uncleaved molecule at a rate that is different from the unbound form (Meier *et al.*, 1977a,b), and when rapid DFP incorporation is seen, the molecule is cleaved (Griffin and Berretta, 1979; Miller *et al.*, 1980). On the other hand, it appears clear that surface-bound Hageman factor is more readily cleaved by other enzymes (Griffin, 1978); thus, an initiating surface appears to render Hageman factor a better substrate for proteases but does not form a new site within the uncleaved zymogen.

Alternative proposals have considered the possibility that native uncleaved Hageman factor possesses an active site; i.e., it is not totally unactivated. The very slow uptake of DFP into native Hageman factor has been suggested as evidence of this intrinsic activity (Griffin and Berretta, 1979). Kurachi *et al.* (1980) and Heimark *et al.*, (1980) have presented evidence that uncleaved Hageman factor can activate prekallikrein or factor XI and that the activity present in the zymogen does not differ significantly from that of the cleaved form. In this view, native Hageman factor possesses considerable enzymatic activity, and these authors have considered the possibility that binding of the substrates prekallikrein or factor XI to surfaces causes a conformational change in native Hagemen factor that leads to the expression of such activity. This latter proposal implies a marked difference in the activity of bound and unbound Hageman factor, but the expression of such activity also requires substrate binding.

Our own view differs in that initiation of contact activation appears dependent on the ability of Hageman factor to autoactivate. Such activity was first suggested in studies of rabbit Hageman factor (Wiggins and Cochrane, 1979); DFP-treated Hageman factor appeared to possess residual activity that was a small fraction of that seen with cleaved forms, and this seemed to increase with incubation time. However, the kinetics of activation seen were linear and not consistent with an autoactivation model. A similar conclusion was nevertheless suggested when human Hageman factor was examined (Miller *et al.*, 1980). It appeared that purified Hagemen factor was slowly cleaved on binding to surfaces and such cleavage was not inhibited by agents known to inactivate possible Hageman factor activators (Miller *et al.*, 1980) such as kallikrein (Cochrane *et al.*, 1973), plasmin (Kaplan and Austen, 1971), or factor XIa (Meier *et al.*, 1977b). Further, the rate of HF cleavage appeared to be proportional to the percentage of cleaved (activated) enzyme in the starting material (Miller *et al.*, 1980). In this study, [^{3}H]DFP incorporation was only seen in activated, cleaved Hageman factor, and the percent incorporation was proportional to the percent cleavage.

Studies of autoactivation were greatly facilitated when it was demonstrated that activated Hageman factor will cleave the synthetic substrate D-Pro-Phe-Arg-*p*-nitroanilide (Silverberg *et al.*, 1980a). Using this substrate, we demonstrated that even the most highly purified preparations of Hageman factor possess a small amount of activity. However, this activity appeared to represent traces of activated Hageman factor in the preparation, and even DFP treatment at 40 mM did not completely destroy it. In plastic cuvettes (a noninitiating surface), a linear rate of synthetic substrate cleavage was seen, reflecting the activated HF in the preparation. The slope obtained was proportional to the concentration of activated enzyme present. However, in glass cuvettes, a concave-upward progress curve was seen in which the rate of substrate cleave was continuously increasing; i.e., the reaction accelerated with an increasing rate until the substrate was depleted (Fig. 6). Such a reaction is consistent with an autoactivation mechanism in which activated HF cleaves native HF that is surface bound and the concentration of activated HF continuously increases. To confirm this conclusion, we tested the ability of activated HF to digest native HF. However, activated HF is found in at least two forms, HFa and HFf, so both were tested. When iodinated HF was surface bound and incubated with equimolar quantities of HFa or HFf, cleavage of [^{125}I]HF to form [^{125}I]HFa was obtained with HFa, but HFf had no effect. Thus, HFa appeared to be the molecular species mediating autodigestion and autoactivation (Silverberg *et al.*, 1980a). This is indicated in Fig. 7; however, the source of enzyme for initiation of autoactivation is unclear, and it could be either traces of activated (cleaved) Hageman factor that are always present in the circulation or trace activity in the zymogen.

Because of reports suggesting that native Hageman factor possesses enzymatic activity (Heimark *et al.*, 1980; Kurachi *et al.*, 1980), we attempted to compare the activity

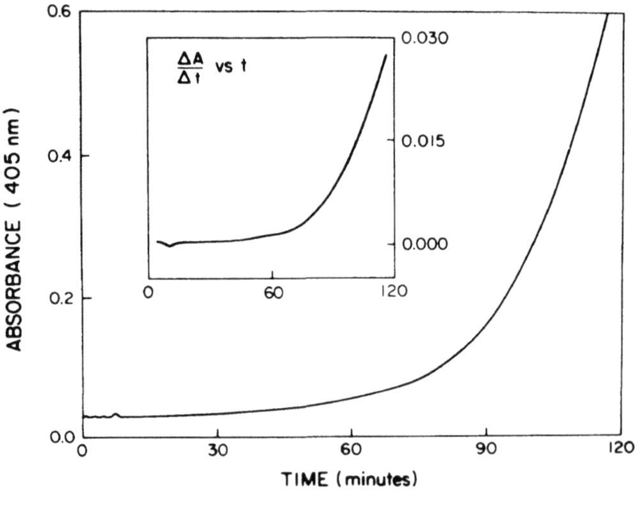

Figure 6. Progress curve demonstrating autoactivation of Hageman factor in a glass cuvette. DFP-treated Hageman factor (0.764 μg/ml) was incubated with D-Pro-Phe-Arg-*p*-nitroanalide, and the release of *p*-nitroanilide was determined at O.D. 405 nm. An accelerating progress curve is seen. The insert shows a plot of the change in absorbance/time vs. time (velocity vs. time), demonstrating that the velocity is increasing; i.e., accelerating.

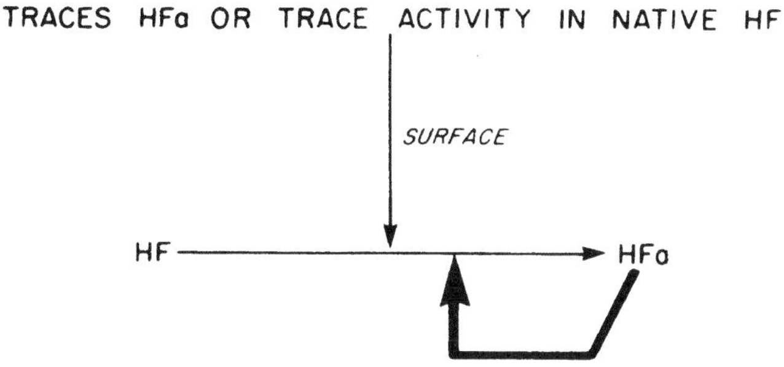

Figure 7. Reaction mechanism indicating that Hageman factor can autoactivate and autodigest. Initiation is either by trace activity present in uncleaved Hageman factor and/or by traces of HFa existing in normal plasma. The surface renders Hageman factor a substrate for itself (as well as other enzymes), and HFa digestion of HF yields more HFa.

of HF and HFa. The time course of inactivation of a preparation containing 4% active enzyme (based on the interaction with D-Pro-Phe-Arg-*p*-nitroanilide in plastic) by Pro-Phe-Arg-chloromethylketone (PPACMK) was performed. We reasoned that if HF possesses activity that is different from HFa, its rate of inactivation would be slower and observable after the 4% HFa had been inactivated.

As shown in Fig. 8, a sharp break in the curve was seen, and because the line is not horizontal (which would imply no residual activity), a second slowly inhibitable site might be present. However, this is at the limits of our ability to reproducibly assay activity, and we estimated that if HF possesses any activity, it is not greater than one four-hundredth the activity of HFa (Silverberg and Kaplan, 1982). This figure is similar

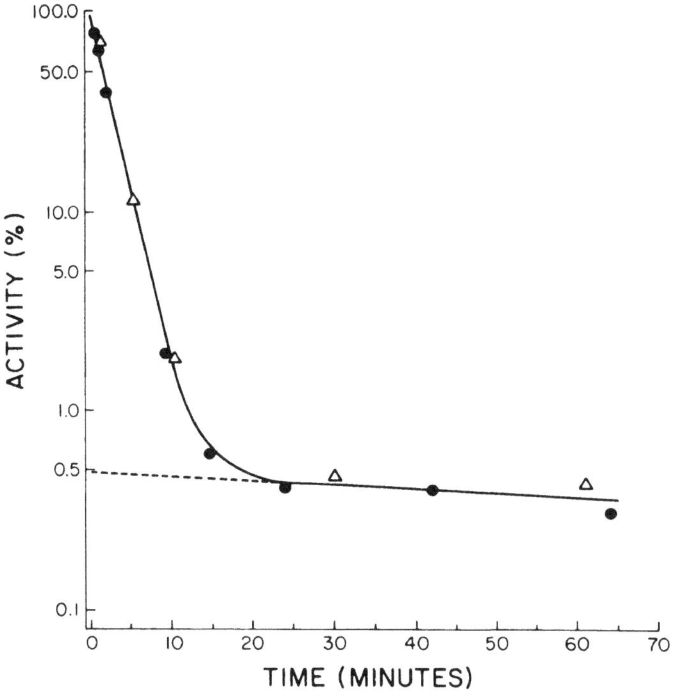

Figure 8. Reaction of Hageman factor at 1.4 ng/ml (■) or 0.3 ng/ml (■) with 5 mM Pro-Phe-Arg-chloromethylketone.

to estimates of the tryptic and chymotryptic activity present in trypsinogen and chymotrypsinogen, respectively (Londsdale-Eccles *et al.*, 1978). Prior estimates of any activity present in HF are far in excess of this, and we suspect that small amounts of HFa present or generated by autoactivation were, in fact, being measured. In the above experiment, after the 4% HFa was inactivated, assay by PTT revealed no depletion of native HF. Thus, no significant amount of PPACMK was bound by the zymogen. We conclude that trace of enzymatic activity in native HF may be sufficient to initiate contact activation or that we really have traces of HFa in the circulation (perhaps about 0.01%). We have not yet distinguished these two possibilities. When the kinetics of prekallikrein activation by surface-bound HF was examined, a brief lag was seen prior to its rapid conversion to kallikrein (Silverberg and Kaplan, 1982). Thus, a rapid substrate-induced conformational change in HF that confers activity similar to that seen in HFa appears unlikely. Two recent studies have confirmed and extended the above observations regarding the kinetics of Hageman factor autoactivation and utilized sulfatides (Tans *et al.*, 1983) or dextran sulfate (Tankersley and Finlayson, 1984) as the initiating surface rather than kaolin.

Since the rate of Hageman factor digestion by kallikrein far exceeds that of the autoactivation reaction (Dunn *et al.*, 1982; Tankersley and Finlayson, 1984), the sequence in normal plasma appears to involve activation of prekallikrein by HFa and then rapid cleavage of residual surface-bound Hageman factor by kallikrein. Quantitatively, this latter reaction accounts for most of the HFa that is generated. This is depicted in Fig. 9, in which Hageman factor activation is depicted as a two-step process, although all the reactions are occurring simultaneously, albeit with differing rates. In the absence of the kallikrein feedback, a slow autoactivation of Hageman factor is seen that may account for the autocorrection of the PTT seen when prekallikrein-deficient plasma (Saito *et al.*, 1974; Weiss *et al.*, 1971; Wuepper, 1973) is incubated with surfaces for a prolonged period. Once HFa is formed (cleavage site 1, Fig. 5), cleavages occur external to the disulfide bond, as indicated at sites 2 and 3 (Fig. 5), to form HFf.

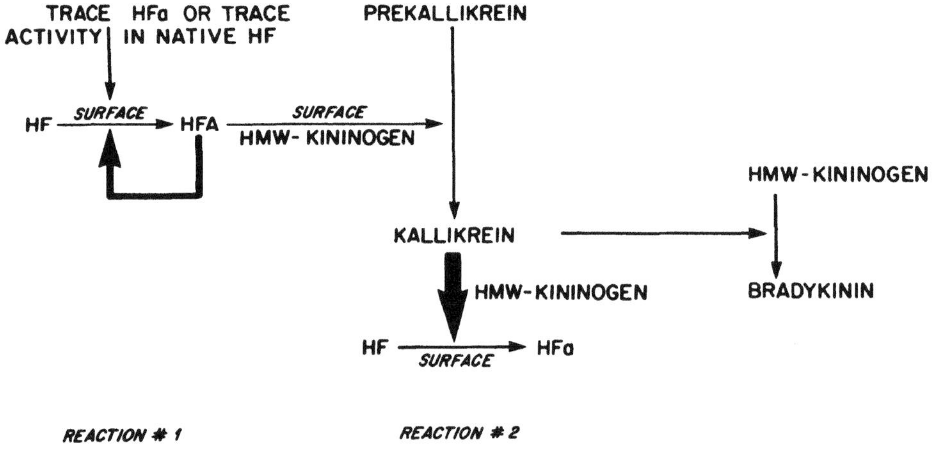

Figure 9. Activation of the intrinsic coagulation–kinin pathway depicting initiation by Hageman factor autoactivation followed by digestion of Hageman factor by kallikrein.

F. The Role of HMW Kininogen

The HMW kininogen not only serves as the substrate from which bradykinin is generated but also is a coagulation cofactor. This was originally determined when a unique coagulation abnormality present in the plasma of patients Flaujeac, Williams, and Fitzgerald was shown to be caused by deficiency of HMW kininogen (Colman *et al.*, 1975; Donaldson *et al.*, 1976; Wuepper *et al.*, 1975). Each of these plasmas generated no bradykinin on contact activation and had a markedly prolonged PTT and abnormal Hageman-factor-dependent fibrinolysis. The mechanism by which HMW kininogen functions as a coagulation cofactor was the subject of numerous investigations, and considerable progress has been made. First, functional studies indicated that surface-dependent activation of prekallikrein and factor XI by HFa was accelerated in the presence of HMW kininogen (Griffin and Cochrane, 1976; Meier *et al.*, 1977a). In addition, the ability of kallikrein to activate HF was likewise shown to be augmented by HMW kininogen (Griffin and Cochrane, 1976; Meier *et al.*, 1977a,b). Later, it was shown that Hageman factor autoactivation differs in that it is not affected by HMW kininogen (Silverberg *et al.*, 1980b). Thus, HMW-kininogen-deficient plasma has not only impaired activation of each of the substrates of HFa (prekallikrein and factor XI) but also impaired activation of Hageman factor. The latter proceeds largely by the initiating autoactivation step with little contribution by the kallikrein "feedback" (see Fig. 9).

Further insight into the role of HMW kininogen was obtained when studies in plasma demonstrated that prekallikrein and factor XI each circulate as 1 : 1 molar complexes with HMW kininogen (Mandle *et al.*, 1976; Thompson *et al.*, 1977). The association constants were found to be 3.4×10^7 M^{-1} and 4.2×10^8 M^{-1}, respectively, for binding of prekallikrein and factor XI to HMW kininogen (Bock and Shore, 1983; Thompson *et al.*, 1979). Since HMW kininogen is present in excess, prekallikrein and factor XI do not compete for binding, and the percentage bound is determined by their concentration in plasma and the association constant. About 10% of plasma prekallikrein remains free (Mandle *et al.*, 1976; Scott and Colman, 1980) and, under test conditions *in vitro*, can partially dissociate from the surface, whereas 99% of factor XI is complexed. Immunologic studies have similarly demonstrated the binding of prekallikrein and factor XI to HMW kininogen (Bouma *et al.*, 1980), although there is some uncertainty as to whether prekallikrein or factor XI binds more firmly to the HMW kininogen binding site (Bouma *et al.*, 1983). The assembly of these molecules on a surface is shown in Fig. 10.

Wiggins *et al.* (1977) studied the binding of prekallikrein and factor XI to a kaolin surface in the presence or absence of HMW kininogen and demonstrated that binding of prekallikrein and factor XI to kaolin is diminished in the absence of HMW kininogen. Activation to kallikrein and to factor XIa was also markedly diminished. However, when binding of prekallikrein and factor XI to kaolin was examined in buffer solutions, binding to kaolin was independent of HMW kininogen (Silverberg *et al.*, 1980a,b; Margalit and Schiffman, 1980). Only in a plasma milieu does HMW kininogen have an effect on the amount bound. Yet activation of prekallikrein and factor XI was abnormal when each was bound directly to the surface in buffers as well as in plasma (Silverberg *et al.*, 1980b). Thus, HMW kininogen appears to be required for binding of prekallikrein and factor XI in a conformation that is susceptible to cleavage by activated HF, and in a plasma milieu, it also augments the quantity bound.

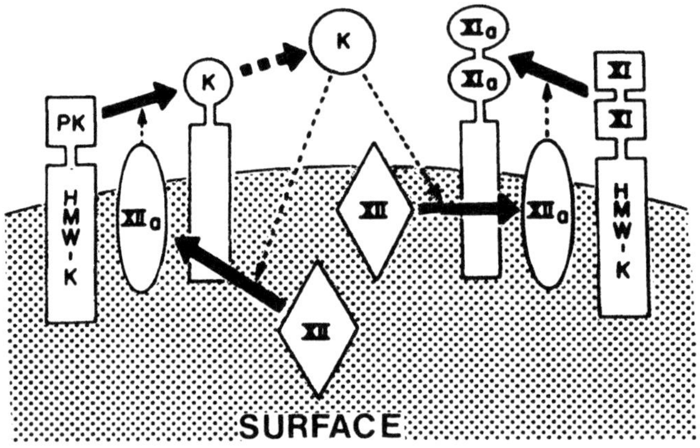

Figure 10. Model of enzymatic events occurring on the surface of a particle, combining the binding interactions and enzymatic reactions described in Figs. 4 and 9.

A recent study by Scott *et al.* (1984b) suggests another explanation for these observations. The binding of HMW kininogen to surfaces was markedly augmented when it was cleaved. Thus, from a coagulation point of view, HMW kininogen is an activatable cofactor similar to factors V and VIII, but in this case the enzyme activator is kallikrein rather than thrombin. It appears likely that some uncleaved HMW kininogen binds first, and as kallikrein is formed, it not only can interact with Hageman factor on adjacent particles but also cleaves adjacent fluid-phase HMW kininogen molecules. Augmented surface binding results, which brings more factor XI and prekallikrein to the particulate surface. This latter reaction may be even more critical for coagulation than kinin formation, since activation of factor XI occurs only on the surface, whereas bradykinin formation can occur via the interaction of HFf, prekallikrein (or kallikrein), and HMW kininogen in the fluid phase.

The effect of HMW kininogen on Hageman factor activation is more difficult to explain, since it does not appear to increase the enzymatic activity of kallikrein, nor does it appear to affect the rate of Hageman factor cleavage by enzymes. Certainly, one of its effects is to convert prekallikrein to kallikrein and thereby create the enzyme that is the major Hageman factor activator. Another relevant observation concerning this reaction is that a fraction of the kallikrein thus formed (~10–20%) dissociates from the HMW kininogen and is available to cleave and activate Hageman factor on adjacent particles (Fig. 10) (Cochrane and Revak, 1980; Silverberg *et al.*, 1980b). In this fashion, contact activation is locally disseminated. Conversely, prekallikrein that is bound directly to surfaces in the absence of HMW kininogen is activated more slowly, and no dissociation occurs. Thus, all of these effects of HMW kininogen appear to increase the effective concentration of kallikrein relative to Hageman factor. Hageman factor activation is therefore indirectly dependent on HMW kininogen, and the effect is mediated via kallikrein formation. Finally, kallikrein complexed to HMW kininogen has been reported to have a longer half-life, i.e., its rate of inactivation by inhibitors is diminished, and this too would augment contact activation (Schapira *et al.*, 1982c). The ability of HMW kininogen to protect kallikrein from inhibition has been questioned by other workers (Van der Graaf *et al.*, 1983a,b), and it appears likely that the magnitude of the effect is small, particularly since kallikrein that is dissociated from HMW kininogen clearly functions to disseminate the reaction (Cochrane and Revak, 1980). These various functions of HMW kininogen on contact activation are summarized in Table 2.

Table 2. Functions of HMW Kininogen (Light Chain) in Contact Activation

1. Forms circulating complexes with prekallikrein and factor XI
2. Attaches prekallikrein and factor XI to initiating surfaces
3. Facilitates conversion of prekallikrein to kallikrein and factor XI to factor XIa
4. Allows dissociation of kallikrein from the surface
5. Inhibits kallikrein inactivation by plasma inhibitors
6. Facilitates activation of Hageman factor by increasing the effective ratio of the [kallikrein]/[Hageman factor] as mediated by items 2–5

V. FIBRINOID NECROSIS: A RECURRENT THEME IN CONNECTIVE TISSUE DISEASES

A. The Coagulation Pathway

From the preceding discussion, it is clear that the three proteins that are obligatory for bradykinin formation (i.e., Hageman factor, prekallikrein, and HMW kininogen) together comprise the initiating factors for this coagulation cascade. The role of this pathway in hemostasis is unclear since it is possible to be deficient in any of the above factors and not have a bleeding diathesis. But as the cascade proceeds, its importance in terms of hemostasis becomes more evident, at least in terms of bleeding as a consequence of aberrant coagulation. Once activated Hageman factor converts factor XI to factor XIa, factor XIa then activates factor IX in the presence of calcium ion and factor VIII (Fig. 11). Patients with deficiency of factor XI have a mild and often variable bleeding disorder, whereas deficiency of either factor IX or factor VIII cause the severe forms of hemophilia. The explanation for these differences in clinical occurrence of bleeding (i.e., increasing severity when a more distal factor is missing) is not understood.

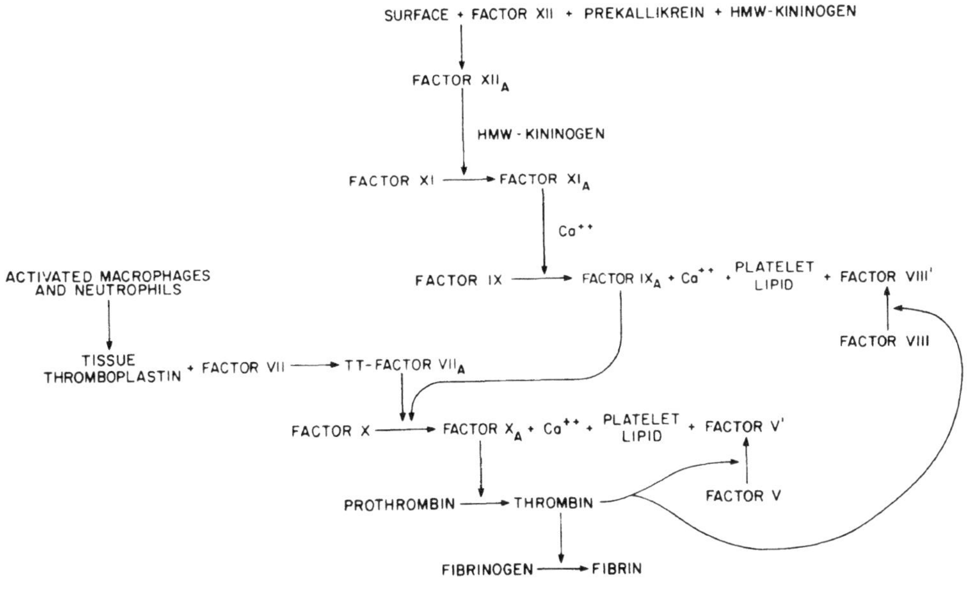

Figure 11. The intrinsic and extrinsic coagulation pathways for formation of fibrin.

The inflammatory reactions caused by immune complex deposition most certainly leads to local blood coagulation. Although a direct demonstration of the steps by which fibrin is formed in this particular circumstance is lacking, one must consider the extrinsic coagulation pathway as the likely mechanism, bearing in mind that contact activation may be more important for bradykinin formation than it is in initiating blood clotting. The extrinsic coagulation pathway is initiated by tissue thromboplastin (tissue factor), a lipoprotein that is released when there is damage to the endothelial surface of blood vessels. It is also released and/or expressed on the surface of activated neutrophils (Niemetz, 1972) or monocytes (macrophages) (Edwards and Rickles, 1980). Tissue factor forms a 1 : 1 molar complex with coagulation factor VII, and this complex converts factor X to factor Xa. As is seen in the intrinsic coagulation pathway, a positive feedback exists in which factor Xa cleaves factor VII, and the factor VIIa formed increases in activity between 50- and 200-fold. Thus, native factor VII (Zur and Nemerson, 1979), or at least the factor-VII–tissue-factor complex, functions as an active zymogen (Broze and Majerus, 1980). However, the two pathways may not function as separately as this figure suggests. As can be seen from Fig. 11, activation of factor X is the branch point of the intrinsic and extrinsic coagulation pathways and is activated by factor IXa. However, factor IX can be activated by factor VIIa (Osterud and Rapaport, 1977) in addition to factor XIa, and at low tissue factor levels activation of factor X by factor IXa rather than direct activation by factor VIIa may be significant (Marler *et al.*, 1982a). In this circumstance, factor IX and the cofactor, factor VIII, would be part of the extrinsic coagulation pathway.

The role of platelets (Holmsen, 1972) in the coagulation cascade is first seen at the factor X activation step. Like the other vitamin-K-dependent factors (factors VII, IX, and prothrombin), factor X contains glutamic acid residues within its amino-terminal domain that possess an extra carboxyl group (γ-carboxyglutamic acid) (Stenflo *et al.*, 1974). Vitamin K acts as a cofactor for the carboxylase enzyme (Larson and Suttie, 1978) that is responsible for catalyzing the addition of these carboxyl groups as a posttranslational modification (Munns *et al.*, 1976). The resultant γ-carboxyglutamic acid chelates calcium ion and binds to calcium-dependent sites on platelet membrane phospholipids (Esmon *et al.*, 1975). Thus, factor X is bound to the platelet membrane, and factor IX or factor IXa may be similarly bound. However, the interactions of factor VIII, factor IX, and factor X at the platelet surface have not been elucidated in great detail.

Coagulation factor VIII is known to be closely associated with plasma Von Willebrand factor, and they circulate as a complex (Mikaelsson *et al.*, 1983; Hoyer, 1981; Weinstein and Chute, 1984). Von Willebrand factor is thought to be required for platelet–endothelial-cell interactions, although the identification of the physiological platelet receptor for Von Willebrand factor is uncertain (Schullek *et al.*, 1984; Fujimoto *et al.*, 1982).

The reactions occurring in the subsequent step in coagulation (i.e., conversion of prothrombin to thrombin) are much better understood. Like factor X, some prothrombin is bound to the platelet surface via γ-carboxyglutamic acid and calcium, and factor V is also weakly bound. Factor V, however, is a true metalloprotein and contains intrinsically bound calcium (Greenquist and Colman, 1975), which is required for cofactor activity. As some factor Xa is formed, prothrombin is converted to thrombin, and thrombin then cleaves and activates factor V. Factor V, like factor VIII and HMW kininogen, is not a proenzyme. Yet, when cleaved, it acts as a cofactor to catalyze the interaction of enzyme and substrate. A high-affinity binding site for factor Va exists at the platelet surface (Miletich *et al.*, 1979) that is independent of γ-carboxyglutamic acid, and the bound factor Va acts as the factor Xa receptor (Kane *et al.*, 1980). A binding site for factor Va also exists on one of the domains of prothrombin (Esmon and Jackson, 1974). Estimates of the ability of this platelet–factor-VaXa complex to convert prothrombin to thrombin in the presence of calcium ion compared to factor Xa alone indicate an augmentation in reaction rate of as much as 300,000-fold (Kane *et al.*, 1980). Thrombin also activates factor VIII (Hultin, 1982), and it seems likely that the platelet, factor IXa, factor VIIIa, and factor X interact in the preceding step in some analogous fashion.

Thrombin, like collagen, epinephrine, and ADP, is also a platelet activator, the consequences of which are: (1) exposure of the phospholipids that catalyze coagulation (Marcus, 1969); (2) platelet aggregation to form a hemostatic plug that may serve to initially limit bleeding of small vessels (Marr *et al.*, 1965); and (3) release of platelet granules that contain factors that help coordinate the coagulation process and have additional effects on the inflammatory process. For example, one of the cationic proteins released appears capable of degranulating mast cells (Weiss, 1975). From the standpoint of blood coagulation, the ADP released serves to further sustain platelet aggregation (Marr *et al.*, 1965); serotonin acts as a small-vessel vasoconstrictor and may facilitate the initial limitation of bleeding by the platelet plug; and the α granule protein thrombospondin (Gartner *et al.*, 1978) may serve to bind platelets together prior to the fusion of their cell membranes to form the more homogeneous final mass.

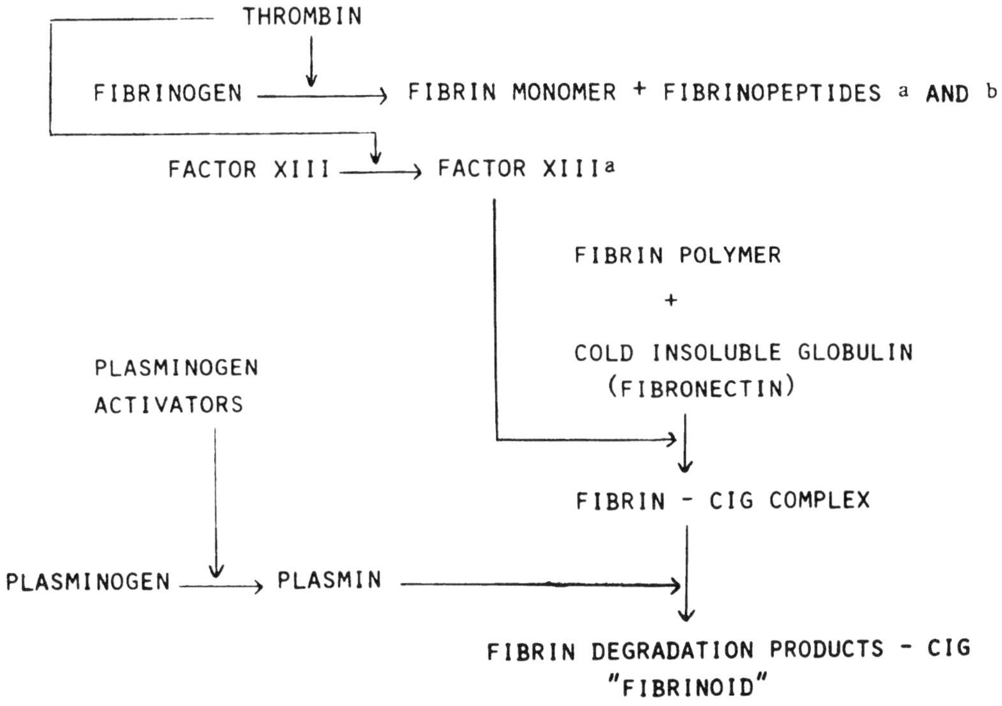

Figure 12. Formation and degradation of fibrinogen to form fibrinoid.

The last step in the blood coagulation pathway involves conversion of fibrinogen to form cross-linked fibrin. Again, the enzyme thrombin is critical to these reactions, which are summarized in Fig. 12. Thrombin cleaves two of the chains of fibrinogen in sequence to release fibrinopeptides A and B, respectively (Blomback *et al.*, 1978). The remaining molecule (fibrin monomer) has exposed sites that result in lateral and end-to-end polymerization to form fibrin. The resultant clot, however, is friable, and stability is conferred on this structure by covalent cross linking of the chains of adjacent fibrin strands. This is accomplished by a unique enzyme (the only nonserine protease in coagulation) known as factor XIIIa or fibrinoligase (Lorand, 1972). Like other coagulation factors, it circulates as a proenzyme that is converted to an active enzyme; the activator is thrombin (Takagi and Doolittle, 1974). Factor XIIIa cross links the γ-carboxy group of glutamine to the ε-amino group of lysine residues to form a peptide bond

$$\text{Glu-COOH}_2 + \text{NH}_2\text{-Lys} \rightarrow \text{Glu-}\overset{\overset{\displaystyle O}{\|}}{C}\text{-}\overset{\overset{\displaystyle H}{|}}{N}\text{-Lys} + H_2O$$

thereby cross-linking the chains (Pisano *et al.*, 1972). Cold-insoluble globulin, a plasma protein that is one of the fibronectinlike molecules in the body (Mosesson and Umfleet, 1980), binds to fibrinogen (fibrin) and is also cross linked to the fibrin matrix by factor XIIIa (Moser, 1976). For a review of fibronectin or cold-insoluble globulin structure and function, see Mosher and Fucht (1981).

Once fibrin is formed, the process for degradation of fibrin (i.e., fibrinolysis) is also set in motion. The final product, plasmin, degrades fibrin to a variety of intermediate products (Budzynski *et al.*, 1974; Marder *et al.*, 1982), and these degradation products, to which cold-insoluble globulin is attached, account for the homogeneous staining material in histological sections of inflamed tissues that is known as "fibrinoid."

B. Fibrinolysis

Since fibrinolytic mechanisms have a role in the formation of "fibrinoid," I now briefly outline some of the critical features of this pathway. Various cells (tissues) contain an enzyme known as tissue plasminogen activator, which rapidly converts plasminogen to plasmin. Like many coagulation factors (e.g., Hageman factor, prekallikrein, or factor X), a single cleavage in plasminogen at an Arg-Val bond within a disulfide bridge (Robbins *et al.*, 1967) converts it from a single chain of molecular weight 92,000 to a two-chain molecule in which a heavy chain of 67,000 is disulfide-linked to a light chain of 25,000. The active site is in the light chain (Summaria *et al.*, 1967). The final product, however, has a molecular weight of only 86,000 (so called Lys-plasmin) because peptides of approximately 8,000 in molecular weight are secondarily cleaved from the amino-terminal end (amino terminus is glutamic acid) of the native molecule (Wiman, 1973). Thus, native Glu-plasminogen or the product Glu-plasmin is cleaved by plasmin to form Lys-plasminogen or Lys-plasmin (Bajaj and Castellino, 1977; Summaria *et al.*, 1975). The net result is that Glu-plasminogen is converted to Lys-plasmin.

The tissue plasminogen activator has been isolated from diverse sources such as uterine tissue or pig heart (Rijken *et al.*, 1979; Cole and Bachman, 1977), but the sources most relevant to this volume are likely from damaged endothelial cells (vascular plasmionogen activator) (Binder *et al.*, 1979; Allen and Pepper, 1981) or secreted by neutrophils (Granelli-Piperno *et al.*, 1977) or macrophages (Vassalli *et al.*, 1976). The latter cells also secrete or express tissue factor activity, and this may be important in coordinating local coagulation and fibrinolysis. Fibrin (but not fibrinogen) appears to possess a strong binding site for tissue plasminogen activator (Thorsen *et al.*, 1972), so that this enzyme can localize at the surface of a clot. Plasminogen also contains a binding site for fibrin at its amino-terminal end; thus, both enzyme and substrate are bound, and the resultant Lys-plasmin will degrade the fibrin.

Plasma also contains an "intrinsic" fibrinolytic cascade that is identical to the sequence of interactions described earlier for the formation of bradykinin. It appears that the main plasminogen activator is kallikrein (Colman, 1969; Mandle and Kaplan, 1977), but contributions are also made by factor XIa and HFa or HFf. Factor XIa is equipotent to kallikrein (Mandle and Kaplan, 1979) on a molar basis, but its plasma concentration is only 10–15% of kallikrein, and its formation is confined to the surface. Thus, its contribution, when compared to kallikrein, is small (Saito, 1980). Likewise, the activity of HFa or HFf (Goldsmith *et al.*, 1978) on plasminogen is only about 5% that of kallikrein. This pathway (kallikrein, in particular) is many thousandfold less effective than well-described plasminogen activators such as urokinase or streptokinase (Goldsmith *et al.*, 1978; Mandle and Kaplan, 1979), and the comparison with tissue plasminogen activator would be similar. Since this is a weak fibrinolytic pathway and the plasma inhibitors or plasmin are potent, it has not been possible to demonstrate fibrinolysis in whole plasma as a consequence of Hageman factor activation. Most systems have utilized diluted, acidified plasma, which serves to inactivate plasma inhibitors of plasmin and of control contact activation. However, by use of synthetic inhibitors of two of these proteins (Miles *et al.*, 1981) (i.e., α_2-antiplasmin and C1 inactivator) one can directly assay plasmin formation in plasma (Miles *et al.*, 1983) as a result of contact activation.

C. Control Mechanisms

One cannot really discuss coagulation and fibrinolytic mechanisms as they may relate to fibrinoid necrosis without at least briefly considering control mechanisms. Clearly, once these cascades are set in motion, there must be a counterbalance so that reactions, once initiated, are not ongoing perpetually. Of course, in some pathological circumstances (e.g., endotoxic shock and/or disseminated intravascular coagulation) this situation is sometimes approached. There are two general types of controls of all plasma proteolytic cascades, intrinsic ones, in which one enzymatic reaction serves to limit another, and extrinsic controls, in which protease inhibitors bind to plasma enzymes and inactivate them.

1. Intrinsic Controls

For the initiating step of contact activation, conversion of HFa to HFf by kallikrein can serve to limit coagulation since factor XI is activated on the surface only by HFa (Bouma and Griffin, 1977; Ratnoff *et al.*, 1961). The HFf, of course, can continue kinin formation in plasma until extrinsic controls take effect. It is also well known that excessive digestion of HMW kininogen by kallikrein leads to progressive destruction of the light chain (Chan *et al.*, 1979) and loss of coagulant activity. A recent abstract suggests that factor XIa can also digest HMW kininogen, and although its bradykinin-forming capability is minimal compared to kallikrein, it may digest the cleaved HMW kininogen light chain and thereby limit its cofactor activity (Scott *et al.*, 1984a). Such mechanisms, i.e.; destruction of coagulation cofactors to slow the reaction rates of their associated enzymes, occur in other steps of coagulation. Factor V and VIII are very susceptible to proteolytic digestion, and, after activation, further cleavage inactivates them. Multiple enzymes may function in this capacity. Thrombin itself can continue to digest factor V and VIII and inactivatethem. A fifth, relatively new vitamin-K-dependent enzyme, however, may be the critical physiological factor and is called protein C (Stenflo, 1976). Protein C is activated by thrombin (Kisiel, 1979), and activated protein C cleaves and inactivates factors V_a and VIII_a (Marler *et al.*, 1982b). An endothelial cell cofactor (thrombomodulin) has been described (Esmon and Owen, 1981) that binds to thrombin at the site of vascular injury and modifies the enzyme so that it no longer activates platelets or clots fibrinogen but augments protein C activation a thousandfold. In some circumstances, factor V_a can also serve as a thrombin cofactor for protein C activation (Salem *et al.*, 1984). In fibrinolytic states, measurable quantities of plasmin circulate, often in addition to activated protein C. Together they can deplete factors V and VIII as has been described in disorders associated with disseminated intravascular coagulation.

Intrinsic controls also exist for the fibrinolytic cascade. At least one plasma protein, histidine-rich glycoprotein, binds to the site on plasminogen that is required for attachment to fibrinogen or fibrin (Lijnen *et al.*, 1980). This serves to limit plasminogen activation by tissue plasminogen activator. Recently, thrombospondin, the secreted platelet factor that has a role in platelet–platelet interactions, has been shown to bind to fibrinogen and to histidine-rich glycoprotein (Leung and Nachman, 1984).

2. *Extrinsic Controls*

A summary of the major plasma inhibitors of each enzyme of the coagulation cascade is given in Table 3. The $C\bar{1}$ inactivator ($C\bar{1}$ INH), the enzyme initially described as the inhibitor of the activated first component of complement, is the main inhibitor of HFa or HFf in plasma (Forbes *et al.*, 1970; Schreiber *et al.*, 1973). The same protein is one of two inhibitors of plasma kallikrein (Gigli *et al.*, 1970). Of particular interest is the disease hereditary angioedema, in which severe, potentially fatal, episodes of swelling occur as a result of the absence of functional $C\bar{1}$ INH. The swelling may be mediated by bradykinin (Fields *et al.*, 1983b), but further activation of the intrinsic coagulation cascade is not seen, presumably because of the effect of other inhibitors acting later in the cascade. The second kallikrein inhibitor in plasma is α_2-macroglobulin (Harpel, 1970). Whereas $C\bar{1}$ INH binds to the active site of enzymes and destroys their activity against any substrate, the effect of α_2-macroglobulin may be steric. Thus, the kallikrein–α_2-macroglobulin complex can still hydrolyze low-molecular-weight synthetic substrates but retains only 1–2% proteolytic activity on protein substrates. The residual activity resists inactivation by $C\bar{1}$ INH; thus, theoretically, traces of kallikrein activity can persist in plasma long after activation has occurred. The significance of this is unknown. Recently, the kinetic constants for kallikrein inhibition by $C\bar{1}$ INH and α_2-macroglobulin have been

Table 3. Inhibitors of Proteases of the Coagulation, Fibrinolytic, and Kinin-Forming Cascades

Enzyme	Main inhibitors
HFa, HFf	$C\bar{1}$ INH
Kallikrein	$C\bar{1}$ INH, α_2-macroglobulin
Factor XIa	α_1-Antitrypsin, $C\bar{1}$ INH
Factor IXa	AT III
Factor Xa	AT III
Tissue factor–factor VII (factor VIIa)	Uncertain
Thrombin	AT III, heparin cofactor II
Plasmin	α_2-Antiplasmin, α_2-macroglobulin

reported (Schapira *et al.*, 1982b,c; Van der Graff, 1983a,b) and confirm earlier reports that, together, they account for over 90% of plasma kallikrein inhibitory activity and are approximately equipotent. The main plasma inhibitor of factor XIa is α_1-antitrypsin (Heck and Kaplan, 1974; Scott *et al.*, 1982); other inhibitors are $C\bar{1}$ INH (Forbes *et al.*, 1970) and antithrombin III (heparin cofactor) (Damas *et al.*, 1973).

Most coagulation proteins, with the possible exception of factor VIIa, are inhibited by antithrombin III (AT III). This is the major plasma inhibitor that is activated by interaction with heparin; the heparin–AT III complex interacts with coagulation factors to form a covalent bond at the active-site serine residue and inactivates them. The enzymes controlled by this protein are factor IXa, Xa, and thrombin. However, when combined with heparin, it also can inactivate HFa, HFf, factor XIa, kallikrein, and plasmin (Damas *et al.*, 1973; Harpel and Rosenberg, 1976; Highsmith and Rosenberg, 1974; Stead *et al.*, 1976). Most studies comparing the activity of AT III with $C\bar{1}$ INH, α_2-macroglobulin, or α_2-antiplasmin have used AT III without added heparin. In the presence of heparin or similar substances, AT III may also contribute to the inactivation of this diverse group of enzymes. For thrombin inactivation by AT III, heparin has been shown to bind to both thrombin and antithrombin, and a ternary complex of thrombin–heparin–antithrombin forms (Nesheim, 1983; Griffith, 1982) in which the role of heparin is to markedly enchance the thrombin/antithrombin affinity (Olson and Shore, 1982). Then, as the stable thrombin–AT III complex forms, heparin is released (Pletcher and Nelsestuen, 1983). Thus, heparin recycles as an enzyme might. The *in vivo* heparin analogue may be heparan sulfate exposed at sites of connective tissue injury (Camussi *et al.*, 1983; Busch and Owen, 1982; Khoory *et al.*, 1980). A second protein, termed heparin cofactor II, is also activatable by heparin or by dermatan sulfate, but it is selective and seems to inhibit only thrombin (Tollefson *et al.*, 1983).

Plasmin is inhibited first by α_2-antiplasmin (Collen, 1976; Moroi and Aoki, 1976; Mullertz and Clemmensen, 1976), which accounts for most of the rapid inhibitory activity of plasma, and then by α_2-macroglobulin. α_2-Antiplasmin binds to fibrin, as do plasminogen and tissue plasminogen activator, so that all of the elements to form plasmin and inactivate it seem to be confined locally. Recently, a separate plasma inhibitor of tissue plasminogen activator has been described (Kruithof *et al.*, 1983; Verheyen *et al.*, 1983).

VI. ADDITIONAL EFFECTS OF THE COAGULATION KININ AND FIBRINOLYTIC PATHWAYS ON INFLAMMATION—RELATION TO RHEUMATIC DISEASES

The Hageman-factor-dependent pathways are among the coagulation factors most closely linked to the inflammatory response. Clearly, the ability of bradykinin to act as a vasodilator, to increase vascular permeability, to cause hypotension, and to increase phospholipase A_2 activity and thereby augment the synthesis of arachidonic acid metabolites accounts for this association. The dramatic swelling characteristic of hereditary angioedema, a consequence of uncontrolled activation of this cascade along with complement, focuses attention on its potential importance.

Over the years, other activities of the proteins involved in contact activation have been described. For example, HFf has been shown to enzymatically activate the C1r subcomponent of complement (Ghebrehiwet *et al.*, 1983). Thus, one can readily demonstrate sequential activation of the complement cascade on addition of HFf to normal plasma (Ghebrehiwet *et al.*, 1981). However, complement-dependent activation of plasma on addition of a surface has not yet been demonstrated. Both HFa and kallikrein can also activate C1 but these are only about 5–10% as potent as HFf on a molar basis. This link between contact activation and complement may be operational whenever complement activation and HFf formation are seen together and is augmented when $C\bar{1}$ INH is absent or dysfunctional. Kallikrein has also been shown to have chemotactic activity for human neutrophils (Kaplan *et al.*, 1972) and monocytes (Gallin and Kaplan, 1974), and, like many other chemotactic factors, it can cause neutrophil aggregation (Schapira *et al.*, 1982a) and secretion (Wachtfogel *et al.*, 1983). Kallikrein also enzymatically activates factor B of the alternative complement pathway (DiScipio, 1982) and can digest C3bi to form a unique degradation product with immunomodulatory capacity (Meuth *et al.*. 1983).

The role of the Hageman-factor-dependent pathways in rheumatic diseases has not been systematically examined, and much work in this area is required. It is not likely to be the primary mediator pathway activated in these disorders, since immune complexes do not appear to directly initiate the cascade (Dahlen *et al.*, 1981), and at least one patient with Hageman factor deficiency has been reported to have rheumatoid arthritis (Donaldson *et al.*, 1972). Although uric acid and pyrophosphate crystals can initiate Hageman factor activation *in vitro* (Kellermeyer and Breckenridge, 1965), this potential contribution to the joint inflammation seen in gout and pseudogout has not been quantitated relative to the other effects of such crystals on complement activation and phagocytosis. The activation of Hageman factor by sodium urate crystals has been examined in plasma and joint fluid of patients with gout. Both HFa and HFf were formed in joint fluid, and Hageman factor cleavage was shown to be dependent on the presence of prekallikrein and HMW kininogen (Ginsberg *et al.*, 1980). The extreme tenderness seen in acute gouty attacks might relate to local kinin formation as well as to the ability of kinins to augment the release of arachidonic acid metabolites.

The observation that exposure to connective tissue elements can initiate the Hageman-factor-dependent pathways requires confirmation, and the specific connective tissue element responsible for such activity needs to be identified. Certainly, if local kinin generation facilitated deposition of immune complexes, and if damaged connective tissue (secondary to inflammation initiated by immune complexes and complement or by cellular immune reactions) could initiate contact activation, perpetuation of the inflammatory response would result.

Of particular interest when one considers the pathogenesis of rheumatoid arthritis are a series of articles in which synovial cells, synovial fibroblasts, or chondrocytes were shown to secrete a procollagenase (Brinckerhoff *et al.*, 1979; Nagase *et al.*, 1981; Ridge *et al.*, 1980) requiring activation in order to yield an active collagenase. (Werb *et al.*, 1977; Vater *et al.*, 1983) Plasmin has been identified as an enzyme that can convert synovial procollagenase to collagenase (Brinckerhoff *et al*, 1979). Subsequently, a 53,000-molecular-weight endogenous activator was isolated from rabbit synovial fibroblast culture medium. Certainly, synovial macrophages secrete plasminogen activator, and plasminogen is present in synovial fluid, so that plasmin is likely to be present. However, when synovial fluid from rheumatoid arthritis patients was fractionated in order to identify the enzyme(s) that could activate procollagenase, the enzyme found had kallikreinlike activity (Sharma *et al.*, 1983). Thus, one function of kallikrein or other enzymes associated with contact activation might be to activate proenzymes secreted from cells, which can then locally degrade connective tissue. This is one of many areas for future investigation regarding a role for this pathway in connective tissue diseases. Prior studies have all been limited in that sensitive assays that could detect only a few percent activation of any of the relevant proteins were not available. Also, the enzyme activity is fleeting because of interaction with plasma inhibitors. Development of double-antibody ELISA assays for enzyme–inhibitor complexes; e.g., kallikrein–$\overline{C1}$ INH (Lewin *et al.*, 1983), may facilitate such studies. Similarly, bradykinin has a very short half-life because of its rapid degradation (Fig. 2), and assays to detect kinin degradation products may be far more revealing.

Platelets are likely to be activated in the vicinity of areas of fibrinoid necrosis, and released products may have other effects on inflammatory reactions that one is only beginning to appreciate. Platelet factor 4, an antiheparin factor contained in α granules and secreted during platelet aggregation, and the platelet-derived growth factor (Deuel *et al.*, 1981, 1982) have been shown to be chemotactic for neutrophils and monocytes. Platelets also appear to secrete cationic proteins (Nachman *et al.*, 1970) that are themselves vasoactive and can increase vascular permeability.

Relevant chemotactic factors can thus be as diverse as arachidonic metabolites such as leukotriene B (Goetzl and Pickett, 1981), platelet-activating factor (Goetzl *et al.*, 1980; Shaw *et al.*, 1981), C5a, kallikrein, PF-4, and platelet-derived growth factor. In addition, collagen degradation fragments (Postlethwaite and Kang, 1976), cleaved elastin (Senior *et al.*, 1980), and cleaved fibronectin (Norris *et al.*, 1982) have been shown to be chemotactic for monocytes, fibrinopeptide b is chemotactic for neutrophils (Kay *et al.*, 1973), and other fibrin degradation products are chemotactic for both neutrophils and monocytes (Richardson *et al.*, 1976; Sueishi *et al.*, 1981). More recently, thrombin has been shown to possess chemotactic activity (Bar-Schavit *et al.*, 1983). Thus, kallikrein and thrombin are the only reported active enzymes to be associated with chemotactic activity. However, it is likely that the other enzymes of the coagulation and fibrinolytic pathways, as well as the many cleavage fragments produced, have additional functions in inflammation that have not yet been examined.

VII. CONCLUDING COMMENTS

Inflammation results from an exceedingly complex interaction of cells and plasma proteins. The number of plasma factors and secreted cell products involved in inflammation is staggering, and for many aspects we are still at a descriptive phase in which all the possible interactions are described. This appears necessary before one can begin to focus and define those that are most important in a particular situation. We may know a great deal about the inflammatory reaction present in the joints in rheumatoid arthritis or gout, the kidney in systemic lupus erythematosus, or the vessel wall in hepatitis-antigen-positive polyarteritis nodsa, but there is still considerable work to be done before one can really describe the sequence of events and the critical reactions for any of these. For other disorders, for example, inflammatory mechanisms in any of the seronegative spondyloarthropathies, we know very little indeed. Further, if one were to try to explain why some patients with lupus nephritis have a proliferative nephritis and others have a membranous or focal nephritis, one can invoke all sorts of notions about differing types of immune complexes, factors governing localization within the kidney, differing effector inflammatory cascades, etc., but an answer based on experimental data is not yet at hand. Our ability to discriminate at this level is actually rather primitive. Thus, it is hoped that this review will serve to outline the present "state of the art" and to stimulate further thought and investigation in areas that appear promising.

REFERENCES

Adu, J., and Williams, D., 1981, DNA–anti DNA circulating complexes in the nephritis of systemic lupus erythematosus, *Clin. Exp. Immunol.* **43:**605–614.

Allen, R. A., and Pepper, D. C., 1981, Isolation and properties of human vascular plasminogen activator, *Thromb. Haemostas.* **45:**43–50.

Arnoux, B., Jouvin-Marche, E., Arnoux, A., and Benveniste, J., 1982, Release of PAF-acether from human blood monocytes, *Agents Actions* **12:**713–716.

Bajaj, S. P., and Castellino, F. J., 1977, Activation of human plasminogen by equimolar levels of streptokinase, *J. Biol. Chem.* **252:**492–498.

Barone, C., Bartolini, C., Jentiloni, N., Greico, A., and Flamini, G., 1981, Systemic lupus erythematosus with only IgE class antinuclear antibodies, *Arthritis Rheum.* **24:**1441–1443.

Bar-Shavit, R., Kahn, A., Fenton, J. W., and Wilner, J. D., 1983, Chemotactic response of monocyte to thrombin, *J. Cell Biol.* **96:**282–285.

Belch, J. J., Drury, J. K., Capell, H., Forbes, C. D., Newman, P., McKenzie, F., Lieberman, P., and Prentice, C. R. M., 1983, Intermittant epoprostenol (prostacyclin) infusion in patients with Raynaud's syndrome, *Lancet* **1:**313–315.

Beneveniste, J., Henson, P. M., and Cochrane, C. G., 1972, Leucocyte-dependent histamine release from rabbit platelets. The role of IgE, basophils, and platelet activating factor, *J. Exp. Med.* **136:**1356–1377.

Betz, S. J., Lotner, G. Z., and Henson, P. M., 1980, Generation and release of platelet-activating factor (PAF) from enriched preparations of rabbit basophils; failure of human basophils to release PAF, *J. Immunol.* **125:**2749–2755.

Binder, B. R., Spragg, J., and Austen, K. F., 1979, Purification and characterization of human vascular plasminogen activator derived from blood vessel pertusates, *J. Biol. Chem.* **254:**1998–2003.

Blomback, B., Hessel, B., Hagg, D., and Therkildsen, L., 1978, A two-step fibrinogen–fibrin transition in blood coagulation, *Nature* **275:**501–505.

Bock, P. E., and Shore, J. P., 1983, Protein–protein interactions in contact activation of blood coagulation. Characterization of a fluorescein-labeled human high molecular weight kininogen light chain as a probe, *J. Biol. Chem.* **258:**15079–15083.

Bock, P. E., Srinivasan, K. R., and Shore, J. D., 1981, Activation of intrinsic blood coagulation by ellagic acid: Insoluble ellagic acid metal ion complexes are the activating species, *Biochemistry* **20:**7258–7266.

Bockisch, V. A., and Muller-Eberhard, H. J., 1970, Anaphylatoxin inactivator of human plasma: Its isolation and characterization as a carboxypeptidase, *J. Clin. Invest.* **49:**2427–2436.

Bouma, B. N., and Griffin, J. N., 1977, Human blood coagulation factor XI. Purification, properties, and mechanism of activation by activated factor XII, *J. Biol. Chem.* **252:**6432–6437.

Bouma, B. N., Keribiriou, D. M., Vlooswijk, R. A. A., and Griffin, J. H., 1980, Immunological studies of prekallikrein, kallikrein, and high molecular weight kininogen in normal and deficient plasmas and in normal plasma after cold-dependent activation, *J. Lab. Clin. Med.* **961:**693–709.

Bouma, B. N., Vlooswijk, R. A. A., and Griffin, J. H., 1983, Immunological studies of human factor XI and its complex with high molecular weight kininogen, *Blood* **62:**1123–1131.

Brinckerhoff, C. E., McMillan, R. M., Fahey, J. V., and Harris, E. D., Jr., 1979, Collagenase production by synovial fibroblasts treated with phorbol myristate acetate, *Arthritis Rheum.* **22:**1109–1116.

Broze, G. J., Jr., and Majerus, P. N., 1980, Purification and properties of human coagulation factor VII, *J. Biol. Chem.* **255:**1242–1247.

Budzynski, A. Z., Marder, V. J., and Schainoff, J. R., 1974, Structure of plasmic degradation products of human fibrinogen. Fibrinopeptide and polypeptide chain analysis, *J. Biol. Chem.* **249:**2294–2302.

Busch, C., and Owen, W. G., 1982, Identification *in vitro* of an endothelial cell surface cofactor for antithrombin III. Parallel studies with isolated perfused rat hearts and microcarrier cultures of bovine endothelium, *J. Clin. Invest.* **69:**726–729.

Camussi, G., Aglietta, M., Coda, R., Bussolino, F., Piacibello, W., and Tetta, C., 1981, Release of platelet activating factor (PAF) and histamine II. The cellular origin of human PAF: Monocytes, polymorphonuclear neutrophils, and basophils, *Immunology* **42:**191–199.

Camussi, G., Aglietta, M., Malavasi, F., Tetta, C., Piacibello, W., Sanavio, F., and Bussolino, F., 1983, The release of platelet-activating factor from human endothelial cells in culture, *J. Immunol.* **131:**2397–2403.

Chan, J. Y. C., Movat, H. Z., and Burrowes, C. E., 1979, High molecular weight kininogen: Its inability to correct the clotting of kininogen deficient plasma after cleavage of bradykinin by plasma kallikrein, plasmin, or trypsin, *Thromb. Res.* **14:**817–824.

Chused, T. M., and Tarplay, T., 1973, Antagonism of vasoactive amines in NZB/W glomerulonephritis. Beneficial effect of methylsergide, *Proc. Soc. Exp. Biol. Med.* **144:**281–283.

Clark, P. O., Hanahan, D. J., and Pinckard, R. N., 1980, Physical and chemical properties of platelet-activating factor obtained from human neutrophils and monocytes and rabbit neutrophils and basophils, *Biochim. Biophys. Acta* **628:**69–75.

Cochrane, C. G., and Revak, S. D., 1980, Dissemination of contact activation in plasma by plasma kallikrein, *J. Exp. Med.* **152:**608–619.

Cochrane, C. G., Wuepper, K. D., Aiken, B. S., Revak, S. D., and Spiegelberg, H. L., 1972, The interaction of Hageman factor and immune complexes, *J. Clin. Invest.* **51:**2736–2745.

Cochrane, C. G., Revak, S. D., and Wuepper, K. D., 1973, Activation of Hagemen factor in solid and fluid phase, *J. Exp. Med.* **138:**1564–1578.

Cole, E. R., and Bachmann, F. W., 1977, Purification of a plasminogen activator from pig heart, *J. Biol. Chem.* **252:**3729–3737.

Collen, D., 1976, Identification and some properties of a new fast-reacting plasmin inhibitor in human plasma, *Eur. J. Biochem.* **69:**209–216.

Colman, R. W., 1969, Activation of plasminogen by human plasma kallikrein, *Biochem. Biophys. Res. Commun.* **35:**273–279.

Colman, R. W., Bagdasarian, A., Talamo, R. C., Scott, C. F., Seavey, M., Guimaraes, J. A., Pierce, J. V., and Kaplan, A. P., 1975, Williams trait: Human kininogen deficiency with diminished levels of plasminogen proactivator and prekallikrein associated with abnormalities of the Hageman factor-dependent pathways, *J. Clin. Invest.* **56:**1650–1662.

Dahlen, S. E., Bjork, J., Hedgvist, P., Arfors, K. E., Hammarstrom, S., Lundgren, J. A., and Samuelsson, B., 1981, Leukotrienes promote plasma leakage and leukocyte adhesion in post capillary venules: *In vivo* effect with relevance to the acute inflammatory response, *Proc. Natl. Acad. Sci. U.S.A.* **78:**3887–3891.

Damas, P. S., Hicks, M., and Rosenberg, R. D., 1973, Anticoagulant activity of heparin, *Nature* **246**:355–357.

Demopoulos, C. A., Pinckard, R. N., and Hanahan, D. J., 1979, Platelet activating factor. Evidence for 1-O-alkyl-2-acetyl-*sn*-glyceryl-3-phosphorylcholine as the active component (a new class of lipid chemical mediators.), *J. Biol. Chem.* **25**:9355–9358.

Deuel, T. F., Senior, R. M., Change, D., Griffin, G. L., Heinrickson, R. L., and Kaiser, E. T., 1981, Platelet factor 4 is chemotactic for neutrophils and monocytes, *Proc. Natl. Acad. Sci. U.S.A.* **78**:4584–4587.

Deuel, T. F., Senior, R. M., Huang, J. S., and Griffin, G. L., 1982, Chemotaxis of monocytes and neutrophils to platelet-derived growth factor, *J. Clin. Invest.* **69**:1046–1049.

DiScipio, R. G., 1982, The activation of the alternative pathway C3 convertase by human plasma kallikrein, *Immunology* **45**:587–595.

Dobson, N. J., Lambris, J. D., and Ross, G. D., 1981, Characteristics of isolated erythrocyte commplement receptor type one (CR_1, C4b–C3b receptor) and CR_1 specific antibodies, *J. Immunol.* **126**:693–698.

Donaldson, V. H., Glueck, H. I., and Fleming, T., 1972, Rheumatoid arthritis in a patient with Hageman trait, *N. Engl. J. Med.* **286**:528–530.

Donaldson, V. H., Glueck, H. I., Miller, M. A., Movat, H. Z., and Habal, F., 1976, Kininogen deficiency in Fitzgerald trait: Role of high molecular weight kininogen in clotting and fibrinolysis, *J. Lab. Clin. Med.* **87**:327–337.

Drazen, J. M., Austen, K. F., Lewis, R. A., Clark, D. A., Goto, G., Marfat, A., and Corey, E. J., 1980, Comparative airway and vascular reactivity of leukotrienes C-1 and D *in vivo* and *in vitro, Proc. Natl. Acad. Sci.* **77**:4354–4358.

Dunn, J. T., and Kaplan, A. P., 1982, Formation and structure of human Hageman factor fragments, *J. Clin. Invest.* **70**:627–631.

Dunn, J. T., Silverberg, M., and Kaplan, A. P., 1982, The cleavage and formation of activated Hageman factor by autodigestion and by kallikrein, *J. Biol. Chem.* **257**:1779–1784.

Edwards, R. L., and Rickles, F. R., 1980, The role of human T cells (and T cell products) for monocyte tissue factor generation, *J. Immunol.* **125**:606–609.

Erdos, E. C., and Sloane, E. M., 1962, An enzyme in human plasma that inactivated bradykinin and kallidins, *Biochem. Pharmacol.* **11**:585–592.

Esmon, C. T., and Jackson, C. M., 1974, The conversion of prothrombin to thrombin. IV. The function of the fragment 2 region during activation in the presence of factor V, *J. Biol. Chem.* **249**:7791–7797.

Esmon, C. T., and Owen, W., 1981, Identification of an endothelial cell cofactor for Thrombin-catalyzed activation of protein C, *Proc. Natl. Acad. Sci. U.S.A.* **78**:2249–2252.

Esmon, C. T., Suttie, J. W., and Jackson, C. M., 1975, The functional significance of vitamin K action. Difference in phospholipid binding between normal and abnormal prothrombin, *J. Biol. Chem.* **250**:4095–4099.

Fields, T. R., Gerardi, E. N., Ghebrehiwet, B., Bennett, R. S., Lawley, T. J., Hall, R. P., Plotz, P., Karsh, J. R., Frank, M. M., and Hamburger, M. I., 1983a, Reticuloendothelial system Fc receptor function in rheumatoid arthritis, *J. Rheumatol.* **10**:550–557.

Fields, T. R., Ghebrehiwet, B., and Kaplan, A. P., 1983b, Kinin formation in hereditary angioedema plasma: Evidence against kinin derivation from C2 and in support of "spontaneous" formation of bradykinin, *J. Allergy Clin. Immunol.* **72**:54–60.

Flower, R. J., Harvey, E. A., and Kingston, W. P., 1976, Inflammatory effects of prostaglandin D_2 in rat and human skin, *Br. J. Pharmacol.* **56**:229–233.

Forbes, C. O., Pensky, J., and Ratnoff, O. D., 1970, Inhibition of activated Hageman factor and activated plasma thromboplastin antecedent by purified C inactivator, *J. Lab. Clin. Med.* **76**:809–815.

Frank, M. M., Schreiber, A. D., Atkinson, J. P., and Jaffe, C. J., 1977, Pathophysiology of immune hemolytic anemia, *Ann. Intern. Med.* **87**:210–222.

Frank, M. M., Hamburger, M. I., Lawley, T. J., Kimberly, R. P., and Plotz, P. H., 1979, Defective reticuloendothelial system Fc-receptor function in systemic lupus erythematosus, *N. Engl. J. Med.* **300**:518–523.

Fries, L. F., Mullins, W. W., Cho, K. R., Plotz, P. H., and Frank, M. M., 1984, Monocyte receptors for the Fc portion of IgG are increased in systemic lupus erythematosus, *J. Immunol.* **132**:685–700.

Fujikawa, K., and McMullen, B. A., 1983, Amino acid sequence of human β factor XIIa, *J. Biol. Chem.* **258**:10924–10933.

Fujikawa, K., Heimark, R. L., Kurachi, K., and Davie, E. W., 1980, Activation of bovine factor XII (Hageman factor) by plasma kallikrein, *Biochemistry* **19**:1322–1330.

Fujimoto, T., O'Hara, S., and Hawiger, J., 1982, Thrombin-induced exposure and prostacyclin inhibition of the receptor for factor VIII/Von Willebrand factor on human platelets, *J. Clin. Invest.* **69:**1212–1222.

Gallin, J. I., and Kaplan, A. P., 1974, Mononuclear cell chemotactic activity of kallikrein and plasminogen activator and its inhibition by $C\bar{1}$ inhibitor and α_2 macroglobulin, *J. Immunol.* **113:**1928–1934.

Gartner, T. K., Williams, D. C., Minion, F. C., and Phillips, D. R., 1978, Thrombin-induced platelet aggregation is mediated by a platelet plasma membrane-bound lectin, *Science* **200:**1281–1283.

Ghebrehiwet, B., Silverberg, M., and Kaplan, A. P., 1981, Activation of the classical pathway of complement by Hageman factor fragment, *J. Exp. Med.* **153:**665–676.

Ghebrehiwet, B., Randazzo, B. P., Dunn, J. T., Silverberg, M., and Kaplan, A. P., 1983, Mechanisms of activation of the classical pathway of complement by Hagemen factor fragment, *J. Clin. Invest.* **71:**1450–1456.

Gigli, I., Mason, J. W., Colman, R. W., and Austen, K. F., 1970, Interaction of plasma kallikrein with the $C\bar{1}$ inhibitor, *J. Immunol.* **104:**574–581.

Ginsberg, M. H., Jaques, B., Cochrane, C. G., and Griffin, J. H., 1980, Urate crystal dependent cleavage of Hageman factor in plasma and synovial fluid, *J. Lab. Clin. Med.* **45:**497–506.

Goetzl, E. J., and Pickett, W. C., 1981, Novel structural determinants of the human neutrophil chemotactic activity of leukotriene B, *J. Exp. Med.* **153:**482–487.

Goetzl, E. J., Derian, C. K., Tauber, A. I., and Valone, F. H., 1980, Novel effects of 1-O-hexadecyl-2-acyl-*sn*-glycero-3-phosphorylcholine mediators in human neutrophil functions: Delineation of the specific roles of the acyl substituents, *Biochem. Biophys. Res. Commun.* **94:**881–888.

Goldsmith, G., Saito, H., and Ratnoff, O., 1978, The activation of plasminogen by Hageman factor (factor XII) and Hageman factor fragments, *J. Clin. Invest.* **62:**54–60.

Granelli-Piperno, P., Vassalli, J. D., and Reich, E., 1977, Secretion of plasminogen activation by human polymorphonuclear leukocytes: Modulation by glucocorticoids and other effectors, *J. Exp. Med.* **146:**1693–1706.

Greenquist, A. C., and Colman, R. W., 1975, Bovine factor V: A calcium-containing metalloprotein, *Blood* **46:**769–782.

Griffin, J. H., 1978, Role of surface in surface-dependent activation of Hageman factor (blood coagulation factor XII), *Proc. Natl. Acad. Sci. U.S.A.* **75:**1998–2002.

Griffin, J. H., and Beretta, G., 1979, Molecular mechanisms of surface-dependent activation of Hageman factor (factor XII), *Adv. Exp. Med. Biol.* **120:**39–51.

Griffin, J. H., and Cochrane, C. G., 1976, Mechanism for the involvement of HMW-kininogen in surface-dependent reactions of Hageman factor, *Proc. Natl. Acad. Sci. U.S.A.* **73:**2559–2563.

Griffith, M. J., 1982, The heparin-enhanced antithrombin III/thrombin reaction is saturable with respect to both thrombin and antithrombin III, *J. Biol. Chem.* **257:**13899–13902.

Haakenstad, A. O., and Mannick, M., 1974, Saturation of the reticuloendothelial system with soluble immune complexes, *J. Immunol.* **112:**1939–1948.

Habal, F. M., Movat, H. Z., and Burrowes, C. E., 1974, Isolation of two functionally different kininnogens from human plasma; separation from proteinase inhibitors and interaction with plasma kallikrein, *Biochem. Pharmacol.* **23:**2291–2302.

Hall, R. P., Lawley, T. J., Heck, J. A., and Katz, S. I., 1980, IgA containing immune complexes in dermatitis herpetiformis, Henoch–Schonlein's purpura systemic lupus erythematosus, and other diseases, *Clin. Exp. Immunol.* **40:**31–37.

Halonen, M., Palmer, J. D., Lohman, I. C., McManus, L. M., and Pinckard, K. N., 1980, Respiratory and circulatory alterations induced by acetyl glyceryl ether phosphorycholine (AGEPC), a mediator of IgE anaphylaxis in the rabbit, *Am. Rev. Respir. Dis.* **122:**915–924.

Hamburger, M. I., Gorevic, P. D., Lawley, T. J., Franklin, E. C., and Frank, M. M., 1979a, Mixed cryoglobulinemia: Association of glomerulonephritis with defective reticuloendothelial system Fc receptor function, *Trans. Assoc. Am. Physicians* **91:**104–112.

Hamburger, M. I., Moutsopoulos, H. M., Lawley, T. J., and Frank, M. M., 1979b, Sjogren's syndrome: A defect in reticuloendothelial system Fc-receptor specific clearance, *Ann. Intern. Med.* **91:**534–538.

Hamburger, M. I., Gerardi, E. N., Fields, T. R., and Bennett, R. S., 1981, Reticuloendothelial system Fc receptor function and plasmapheresis in systemic lupus erythematosus. A preliminary report, *Artif. Organs* **5:**264–268.

Hamburger, M. I., Lawley, T. J., Kimberly, R. P., Plotz, P. H., and Frank, M. M., 1982, A serial study of splenic reticuloendothelial system Fc receptor functional activity in systemic lupus erythematosus, *Arthritis Rheum.* **25**:48–54.

Hanahan, D. J., Demopoulos, C. A., Liehr, J., and Pinckard, R. N., 1980, Identification of platelet-activating factor isolated from rabbit basophils as acetyl glyceryl ether phosphorylcholine, *J. Biol. Chem.* **225**:5514–5516.

Harpel, P. C., 1970, Human plasma alpha 2-macroglobulin. An inhibitor of plasma kallikrein, *J. Exp. Med.* **132**:329–352.

Harpel, P. C., 1972, Studies on the interaction between collagen and a plasma kallikrein-like activity, *J. Clin. Invest.* **51**:1813–1822.

Harpel, P. C., and Rosenberg, R. O., 1976, α_2 Macroglobulin and anti-thrombin–heparin cofactor: Modulators of hemostatic and inflammatory reactions, *Prog. Hemostas. Thromb.* **3**:145–191.

Heck, L. W., and Kaplan, A. P., 1974, Substrates of Hageman factor I. Isolation and characterization of human factor XI (PTA) and inhibition of the activated enzyme by α_1 antitrypsin, *J. Exp. Med.* **140**:1615–1630.

Heimark, R. L., Kurachi, K., Fujikawa, K., and Davie, E. N., 1980, Surface activation of blood coagulation, fibrinolysis, and kinin formation, *Nature* **286**:456–460.

Hibbard, L. S., and Mann, K. G., 1980, The calcium binding properties of bovine factor V, *J. Biol. Chem.* **255**:638–645.

Highsmith, R. F., and Rosenberg, R. D., 1974, The inhibition of human plasma by human anti-thrombin–heparin cofactor, *J. Biol. Chem.* **249**:4335–4338.

Holmsen, H., 1972, The platelet: Its membrane, physiology, and biochemistry, *Clin. Haematol.* **1**:235–266.

Hoyer, L. W., 1981, The factor VIII complex: Structure and function, *Blood* **58**:1–11.

Hultin, M. B., 1982, Role of human factor VIII in factor X activation, *J. Clin. Invest.* **69**:950–958.

Humphrey, D. M., McManus, L. M., Satouchi, K., Hanahan, D. J., and Pinckard, R. N., 1982, Vasoactive properties of acetyl glyceryl ether phosphorylcholine (AGEPC) and AGEPC analogues, *Lab. Invest.* **46**:422–427.

Iida, K., Marnaghi, R., and Nussenzweig, V., 1982, Complement receptor (CR_1) deficiency in erythrocytes from patients with systemic lupus erythematosus, *J. Exp. Med.* **155**:1427–1438.

Issekutz, A. C., and Movat, H. Z., 1982, The effect of vasodilator prostaglandins on polymorphonuclear leucocyte infiltration and vascular injury, *Am. J. Pathol.* **107**:300–309.

Izui, S., Lambert, P. H., and Miescher, P. A., 1976, *In vitro* demonstration of a particular affinity of glomerular basement membrane and collagen for DNA, *J. Exp. Med.* **144**:428–443.

Jaffe, C. J., Vierling, J. M., Jones, E. A., Lawley, T. J., and Frank, M. M., 1978, Receptor specific clearance by the reticuloendothelial system in chronic liver diseases: Demonstration of defective C3b-specific clearance in primary biliary cirrhosis, *J. Clin. Invest.* **62**:1069–1077.

Jorg, A., Henderson, W. R., Murphy, R. C., and Klebanoff, J. J., 1982, Leukotriene generation by eosinophils, *J. Exp. Med.* **155**:390–402.

Kane, W. H., Lindhout, M. J., Jackson, C. M., and Majerus, P. W., 1980, Factor Va dependent binding of factor Xa to platelets, *J. Biol. Chem.* **255**:1170–1174.

Kaplan, A. P., 1983, Hageman factor dependent pathways: Mechanism of initiation and bradykinin formation, *Fed. Proc.* **42**:3123–3127.

Kaplan, A. P., and Austen, K. F. 1970, A prealbumin activator of prehallikrein, *J. Immunol.* **105**:802–811.

Kaplan, A. P., and Austen, K. F., 1971, A prealbumin activator of prekallikrein II. Derivation of activators of prekallikrein from active Hageman factor by digestion with plasmin, *J. Exp. Med.* **133**:696–712.

Kaplan, A. P., Kay, A. B., and Austen, K. F., 1972, A prealbumin activator of prekallikrein III. Appearance of chemotactic activity in human neutrophils by the conversion of human prekallikrein to kallikrein, *J. Exp. Med.* **135**:81–97.

Kato, H., Han, Y. N., Iwanaga, S., Suzuki, T., and Komiya, M., 1976, Bovine plasma HMW and LMW kininogens. Structural differences between heavy and light chains derived from the kinin-free proteins, *J. Biochem.* **80**:1299–1311.

Kay, A. B., Pepper, D. S., and Ewart, M. R., 1973, Generation of chemotactic activity for leukocytes by the action of thrombin on human fibrinogen, *Nature* (*New Biol.*) **243**:56–57.

Kellermeyer, R. W., and Breckenridge, R. T., 1965, The inflammatory process in acute gouty arthritis I. Activation of Hageman factor by sodium urate crystals, *J. Lab. Clin. Med.* **65**:307–315.

Keribiriou, D. M., and Griffin, J. H., 1979, Human high molecular weight kininogen. Studies of structure–function relationships and of proteolysis of the molecule during contact activation of plasma, *J. Biol. Chem.* **254**:12020–12027.

Khoory, M. S., Nesheim, M. E., Bowie, E. J. W., and Mann, K. G., 1980, Circulating heparan sulfate proteoglycan anticoagulant from a patient with a plasma cell disorder, *J. Clin. Invest.* **653:**666–674.

Kisiel, W., 1979, Human plasma protein C. Isolation, characterization, and mechanism of activation by α thrombin, *J. Clin. Invest.* **64:**761–769.

Kitamura, N., Takagaki, Y., Furoto, S., Tanaka, T., Nawa, H., and Nakanishi, S., 1983, A single gene for bovine high molecular weight and low molecular weight kininogens, *Nature* **305:**545–549.

Klickstein, L. B., Shapleigh, C., and Goetzl, E. J., 1980, Lipoxygenation of arachidonic acid as a source of PMN leucocyte chemotactic factors in synovial fluid and tissue in rheumatoid arthritis and spondyloarthritis, *J. Clin. Invest.* **66:**1166–1170.

Knauer, K. A., Lichtenstein, L. M., Adkinson, N. F., and Fish, J. E., 1981, Platelet activation during antigen-induced airway reactions in human asthmatics, *N. Engl. J. Med.* **304:**1404–1406.

Knicker, W. J., 1972, Modulation of the inflammatory response *in vivo:* Prevention or amelioration of immune complex disease, in: *Inflammation—Mechanisms and Control* (P. Ward and I. Lepow, eds.), Academic Press, New York, p. 335–367.

Knicker, W. T., and Cochrane, G. G., 1968, Localization of circulating antigen–antibody complexes in serum sickness: The role of vasoactive amines and hydrodynamic forces, *J. Exp. Med.* **127:**119–130.

Kruithof, E. K. O., Ransijn, A., Tren-Thang, C., and Bachmann, F., 1983, Characteristics of a fast-acting inhibitor of plasminogen activator in human plasma, *Thrombos. Haemostat.* **50:**193.

Kurachi, K., Fujikawa, K., and Davie, E. W., 1980, Mechanism of activation of bovine factor XI by factor XII and factor XIIa, *Biochemistry* **19:**1330–1338.

Larson, A. E., and Suttie, J. W., 1978, Vitamin K-dependent carboxylase: Evidence for a hydroperoxide intermediate in the reaction, *Proc. Natl. Acad. Sci. U.S.A.* **75:**5413–5416.

Lawley, T. J., Hall, R. P., Fauci, A. S., Katz, S. I., Hamburger, M. I., and Frank, M. M., 1981, Defective Fc receptor functions associated with the HLA-B8/DRW3 haplotype, *N. Engl. J. Med.* **304:**185–192.

Leung, L. L. K., and Nachman, R. L., 1984, Complex formation of platelet thrombospondin with fibrinogen, *J. Clin. Invest.* **73:**5–12.

Lewin, M. F., Kaplan, A. P., and Harpel, P. C., 1983, Studies of C$\bar{1}$ Inactivator–plasma kallikrein complexes in purified systems and in plasma. Quantification by an enzyme-linked differential antibody immunosorbent assay, *J. Biol. Chem.* **238:**6415–6421.

Lewis, R. A., Austen, K. F., Drazen, J. M., Clark, D. A., Marfat, A., and Corey, E. J., 1980, Slow reacting substances of anaphylaxis: Identification of leukotrienes C-1 and D from human and rat sources, *Proc. Natl. Acad. Sci. U.S.A.* **77:3710–3714.**

Lewis, R. A., Soter, N. A., Diamond, P. T., Austen, K. F., Oates, J. A., and Roberts, L. J., II, 1982, Prostaglandin D_2 generation after activation of rat and human mast cells with anti IgE, *J. Immunol.* **129:**1627–1631.

Lijnen, H. R., Hoylaerts, M., and Collen, D., 1980, Isolation and characterization of a human plasma protein with affinity for the lysine binding sites in plasminogen, *J. Biol. Chem.* **255:**10214–10222.

Lockwood, C. M., Worlledge, S., Nicholson, A., Cotton, C., and Peters, D. K., 1979, Reversal of impaired splenic function in patients with nephritis or vasculitis (or both) by plasma exchange, *N. Engl. J. Med.* **300:**524–530.

Londsdale-Eccles, J. D., Neurath, H., and Walsh, K. A., 1978, Probes of the mechanism of zymogen catalysis, *Biochemistry* **17:**2805–2809.

Lorand, L., 1972, Fibrinoligase: The fibrin-stabilizing factor system of blood plasma, *Ann. N.Y. Acad. Sci.* **202:**6–30.

Lotner, G. Z., Lynch, J. M., Betz, S. J., and Henson, P. M., 1980, Human neutrophil-derived platelet activating factor, *J. Immunol.* **124:**676–684.

MacGlashan, D. W., Schleimer, R. P., Peters, S. P., Schulman, E. S., Adams, G. K., Sobotka, A. K., Newball, H. H., and Lichtenstein, L. M., 1983, Comparative studies of human basophils and mast cells, *Fed. Proc.* **42:**2504–2509.

Mandle, R. J., and Kaplan, A. P., 1977, Hageman factor substrates: Human prekallikrein. Mechanism of activation by Hageman factor and participation in Hageman factor dependent fibrinolysis, *J. Biol. Chem.* **252:**6097–6104.

Mandle, R. J., Jr., and Kaplan, A. P., 1979, Hageman-factor dependent fibrinolysis: Generation of fibrinolytic activity by the interaction of human activated factor XI and plasminogen, *Blood* **54:**850–862.

Mandle, R. J., Colman, R. W., and Kaplan, A. P., 1976, Identification of prekallikrein and HMW-kininogen as a circulating complex in human plasma, *Proc. Natl. Sci. U.S.A.* **73:**4179–4183.

Manniok, M., Haakenstad, A. D., and Arend, W. P., 1974, The fate and detection of circulating immune complexes, *Prog. Immunol.* **5**:91–101.

Marcus, A. J., 1969, Platelet function, *N. Engl. J. Med.* **280**:1213–1220,1278–1284,1330–1335.

Marder, V. J., Budzynski, A. Z., and James, H. L., 1982, High molecular weight derivative of human fibrinogen produced by plasma III. Their NH_2-terminal amino acids and comparison with NH_2-terminal disulfide knot, *J. Biol. Chem.* **247**:4775–4781.

Margalit, R., and Schiffman, S., 1980, Factor XI adsorption to surfaces: Interaction of high molecular weight kininiogen (HMWK) and a plasma adsorption inhibitor, *Blood* **56**:168–172.

Marler, R. A., Kleiss, A. J., and Griffin, J. H., 1982a, An alternative extrinsic pathway of human blood coagulation, *Blood* **60**:1353–1358.

Marler, R. A., Kleiss, A. J., and Griffin, J. H., 1982b, Mechanism of action of human activated protein C, a thrombin dependent anticoagulant enzyme, *Blood* **59**:1067–1072.

Marr, J., Barboriak, J. J., and Johnson, S. A., 1965, Relationship of appearance of adenosine diphosphate, fibrin formation, and platelet aggregation in the haemostatic plus *in vivo*. *Nature* **205**:259–262.

Martin, M. F., Dowd, P., Ring, E., Cooke, E., Dieppe, P., and Kirby, J., 1981, Prostaglandin E-1 infusions for vascular insufficiency in progressive systemic sclerosis, *Ann. Rheum. Dis.* **40**:350–354.

McMillan, C. R., Saito, H., Ratnoff, O. D., and Walton, A. G., 1974, The secondary structure of human Hageman factor (factor XII) and its alteration by activating agents, *J. Clin. Invest.* **54**:1312–1322.

Meier, H. L., Pierce, J. V., Colman, R. W., and Kaplan, A. P., 1977a, Activation and function of human Hageman factor; the role of HMW-kininogen and prekallikrein, *J. Clin. Invest.* **60**:18–31.

Meier, H. L., Thompson, R. E., and Kaplan, A. P., 1977b, Activation of Hageman factor by factor XIa–HMW-kininogen, *Thromb. Haemostas.* **38**:14.

Meuth, J. L., Morgan, E. L., DiScipio, R. G., and Hugli, T. E., 1983, Suppression of T lymphocyte functions by human C3 fragments I. Inhibition of human T cell proliferative responses by a kallikrein cleavage fragment of human i C3b, *J. Immunol.* **130**:2605–2611.

Mikaelsson, M. E., Forsman, N., and Oswaldsson, D. M., 1983, Human factor VIII: A calcium-linked protein complex, *Blood* **62**:1006–1015.

Miles, L. A., Burnier, J. P., Verlander, M. S., Goodman, M., Kleiss, A. J., and Griffin, J. H., 1981, Inactivation of purified human α_2 antiplasmin and purified human C Inhibitor by synthetic fibrinolytic agents, *Blood* **57**:1015–1024.

Miles, L. P., Rothschild, Z., and Griffin, J. H., 1983, Dextran sulfate-dependent fibrinolysis in whole human plasma, *J. Lab. Clin. Med.* **101**:214–225.

Miletich, J. P., Kane, W. H., Hofmann, S. L., Stanford, N., and Majerus, P. W., 1979, Deficiency of factor X_a–factor V_a binding sites on the platelets of a patient with a bleeding disorder, *Blood* **54**:1015–1022.

Miller, G., Silverberg, M., and Kaplan, A. P., 1980, Autoactivatability of human Hageman factor (factor XII), *Biochem. Biophys. Res. Commun.* **92**:803–810.

Miyaka, Y., Yamada, A., Kosaka, K., Tsuda, F., Kosugi, E., and Mayami, M., 1981, Defective immune adherence (C3b) receptor on erythrocytes from patients with systemic lupus erythematosus, *Lancet* **2**:493–497.

Mori, K., and Nagasawa, S., 1981, Studies on human high molecular weight (HMW) kininogen II. Structural change of HMW-kininogen by the action of human plasma kallikrein, *J. Biochem.* **89**:1465–1473.

Moroi, M., and Aoki, N., 1976, Isolation and characterization of α_2 plasmin inhibitor from human plasma. A novel proteinase inhibitor which inhibits activator-induced clot lysis, *J. Biol. Chem.* **251**:5956–5965.

Morrison, D. C., and Cochrane, C. G., 1974, Direct evidence for Hageman factor (factor XII) activation by bacterial lipopolysaccharides (endotoxins), *J. Exp. Med.* **140**:797–811.

Moser, D. F., 1976, Action of fibrin-stabilizing factor on cold-insoluble globulin and α_2-macroglobulin in clotting plasma, *J. Biol. Chem.* **251**:1639–1645.

Mosesson, M. W., and Umfleet, R., 1980, The cold insoluble globulin of human plasma I. Purification, primary characterization, and relationship to fibrinogen and other cold insoluble fraction components, *J. Biol. Chem.* **245**:5726–5736.

Mosher, D. F., and Fucht, L. J., 1981, Fibronectin: Review of its structure and possible functions, *J. Invest. Dermatol.* **77**:175–180.

Mullertz, S., and Clemmensen, I., 1976, The primary inhibitor of plasmin in human plasma, *Biochem. J.*, **159**:545–553.

Munns, T. W., Johnston, M. F. M., Liszewski, M. K., and Olson, R. E., 1976, Vitamin K-dependent synthesis and modification of precursor prothrombin in cultured H-35 hepatoma cells, *Proc. Natl. Acad. Sci. U.S.A.* **76**:2803–2807.

Murphy, R. C., Hammarstrom, S., and Samuelsson, B., 1979, Leucotriene C: A slow reacting substance from murine mastocytoma cells, *Proc. Natl. Acad. Sci. U.S.A.* **76**:4275–4279.

Nachman, R. L., Weksler, B., and Ferris, B., 1970, Increased vascular permeability produced by human platelet granule cationic extract, *J. Clin. Invest.* **49**:274–281.

Nagase, H., Jackson, R. C., Brickerhoff, C. E., Vater, C. A., and Harris, E. D., Jr., 1981, A precursor form of latent collagenase produced in a cell-free system with RNA from rabbit synovial cells, *J. Biol. Chem.* **256**:11951–11954.

Nesheim, M. E., 1983, A simple rate law that describes the kinetics of the heparin-catalyzed reaction between antithrombin III and heparin, *J. Biol. Chem.* **258**:14708–14717.

Niemetz, J., 1972, Coagulant activity of leukocytes. Tissue factor activity, *J. Clin. Invest.* **51**:307–313.

Nishimura, K., Alhene-Gelas, F., White, A., and Erdos, E. G., 1980, Activation of membrane-bound kallikrein and renin in the kidney, *Proc. Natl. Acad. Sci. U.S.A.* **77**:4975–4978.

Norris, D. A., Clark, R. A. F., Swigart, L. M., Huff, J. C., Weston, W. L., and Howell, S. E., 1982, Fibronectin fragment(s) are chemotactic for human peripheral blood monocytes, *J. Immunol.* **129**:1612–1618.

Olson, S. T., and Shore, J. D., 1982, Demonstration of a two step reaction mechanism for inhibition of α thrombin by antithrombin III and identification of the step affected by heparin, *J. Biol. Chem.* **257**:14891–14895.

Orning, L., Widegran, D., Hammarstrom, S., and Samuelsson, B., 1980, Leucotriene D, a slow reacting substance from rat basophilic leukemia cells, *Proc. Natl. Acad. Sci. U.S.A.* **77**:2014–2017.

Orstavik, J. B., Brandtzaeg, P., Nustad, K., and Pierce, J. V., 1980, Immunohistochemical localization of kallikrein in human pancreas and salivary glands, *J. Histochem. Cytochem.* **28**:557–562.

Osterud, B., and Rapaport, I., 1977, Activation of factor IX by the reaction product of tissue factor and factor VII: Additional pathway for initiating blood coagulation, *Proc. Natl. Acad. Sci. U.S.A.* **74**:5260–5264.

Pareis, T. M., Kimberly, R. P., Inman, R. D., McDougal, S., Gibotsky, A., and Christian, C. L., 1982, Defective Fc receptor-mediated function of the mononuclear phagocyte system in lupus nephritis, *Ann. Intern. Med.* **98**:526–532.

Parker, C. W., Jakschik, B. A., Huber, M. G., and Falkenhein, S. F., 1979, Characterization of slow recting substance as a family of thiolipids derived from arachidonic acid, *Biochem. Biophys. Res. Commun.* **89**:1186–1192.

Peters, S. P., MacGlashan, D. W., Jr., Schulman, E. S., Schleimer, R. P., Hayes, E. C., Rokach, J., Adkinson, N. F., Jr., and Lichtenstein, L. M., 1984, Arachidonic acid metabolism in purified human lung mast cells, *J. Immunol.* **132**:1972–1979.

Pinckard, R. N., Knicker, W. T., Lee, L., Hanahan, D. J., and McManus, L. M., 1980, Vasoactive effects of 1-O-alkyl-2-acetyl-*sn*-glyceryl-3-phosphorylcholine (AGEPC) in human skin, *J. Allergy Clin. Immunol.* **65**:196.

Pisano, J. J., Bronzert, T. J., and Peyton, M. P., 1972, (γ-Glutamyl) lysine cross-links: Determination in fibrin from normals and factor XIII-deficient individuals, *Ann. N.Y. Acad. Sci.* **202**:98–113.

Pletcher, C. H., and Nelsestuen, G. L., 1983, Two substrate reaction model for the heparin-catalyzed bovine antithrombin/protease reaction, *J. Biol. Chem.* **258**:1086–1091.

Plummer, T. H., Jr., and Horwitz, M. Y., 1978, Human plasma carboxypeptidase N. Isolation and characterization, *J. Biol. Chem.* **253**:3907–3912.

Postlethwaite, A. E., and Kang, A. H., 1976, Collagen and collagen peptide induced chemotaxis of human blood monocytes, *J. Exp. Med.* **143**:1299–1307.

Rankin, J. A., Hitchocck, M., Merrill, W. W., Huang, S. S., Brashler, J. R., Bach, M. K., and Askenase, P. W., 1984, IgE immune complexes induce immediate and prolonged release of leukotriene C4 (LTC_4) from rat alveolar macrophages, *J. Immunol.* **132**:1993–1999.

Ratnoff, O. D., and Crum, J. D., 1964, Activation of Hageman factor by solutions of ellagic acid, *J. Lab. Clin. Med.* **63**:359–377.

Ratnoff, O. D., and Saito, H., 1979, Amidolytic properties of single-chain activated Hageman factor, *Proc. Natl. Acad. Sci. U.S.A.* **76**:1461–1463.

Ratnoff, O. D., Davie, E. W., and Mallet, D. L., 1961, Studies on the action of Hageman factor. Evidence that activated Hageman factor in turn activates plasma thromboplastin antecedent, *J. Clin. Invest.* **40**:803–819.

Revak, S. D., and Cochrane, C. G., 1976, The relationship of structure and function in human Hageman factor. The association of enzymatic and binding activities with separate regions of the molecule, *J. Clin. Invest.* **57**:852–860.

Revak, S. D., Cochrane, C. G., and Griffin, J. H., 1977, The binding and cleavage characteristics of human Hageman factor during contact activation, *J. Clin. Invest.* **59**:1167–1175.

Richardson, P. L., Pepper, D. S., and Kay, A. B., 1976, Chemotaxis for human monocytes by fibrinogen-derived peptides, *Br. J. Haematol.* **32**:507–513.

Ridge, S. C., Oronsky, A. L., and Kerwar, S. S., 1980, Induction of the synthesis of latent collagenase and latent neutral protease in chondrocytes by a factor synthesized by activated macrophages, *Arthritis Rheum.* **23**:448–454.

Rijken, D. C., Wijngaards, G., Zaal-de Jong, M., and Wolbergen, J., 1979, Purification and partial characterization of plasminogen activator from human uterus tissue, *Biochim. Biophys. Acta* **580**:140–153.

Robbins, K. C., Summaria, L., Hseih, B., and Shah, R., 1967, The peptide chains of human plasmin. Mechanism of activation of human plasminogen to plasmin, *J. Biol. Chem.* **242**:2333–2342.

Roberts, L. J. II, Sweetman, B. J., Lewis, R. A., Austen, K. F., and Oates, J. A., 1980, Increased production of prostaglandin D_2 in patients with systemic mastocytosis, *N. Engl. J. Med.* **303**:1400–1404.

Rouzer, C. A., Scott, W. A., Hamill, A. L., and Cohn, Z. A., 1980, Dynamics of leukotriene C production by macrophages, *J. Exp. Med.* **152**:1236–1247.

Saito, H., 1980, The participation of plasma thromboplastin antecedent (factor XI) in contact-activated fibrinolysis, *Proc. Soc. Exp. Biol. Med.* **164**:153–157.

Saito, H., Ratnoff, O. D., and Donaldson, V. H., 1974, Defective activation of clotting, fibrinolytic, and permeability enhancing systems in human Fletcher trait plasma, *Circ. Res.* **34**:641–651.

Salem, H. H., Esmon, N. L., Esmon, C. T., and Majerus, P. W., 1984, Effects of thrombomodalin and coagulation factor Va light chain on protein C activation *in vitro, J. Clin. Invest.* **73**:968–972.

Sanchez-Crespo, M., Alonso, F., and Egido, J., 1980, Platelet-activating factor in anaphylaxis and phagocytosis. I. Release from human peripheral polymorphonuclear and monocytes during the stimulation by ionophore A23187 and phagocytosis but not from degranulating basophils, *Immunology* **40**:645–655.

Schapira, M., Despland, E., Scott, C. H., Boxer, L., and Colman, R. W., 1982a, Purified human plasma kallikrein aggregates human blood neutrophils, *J. Clin. Invest.* **69**:1199–1202.

Schapira, M., Scott, C. F., and Colman, R. W., 1982b, Contribution of plasma protease inhibitors to the inactivation of kallikrein in plasma, *J. Clin. Invest.* **69**:462–468.

Schapira, M., Scott, C. F., James, A., Silver, L. D., Kueppers, F., James, H. L., and Colman, R. W., 1982c, High molecular weight kininogen or its light chain protects human plasma kallikrein from inactivation by plasma protease inhibitors, *Biochemistry* **3**:567–572.

Schiffman, S., Mannhalter, C., and Tynerk, D., 1980, Human high molecular weight kininogen. Effects of cleavage by kallikrein on protein structural and procoagulant activity, *J. Biol. Chem.* **255**:6433–6438.

Schreiber, A. D., and Frank, M. M., 1972, The role of antibody and complement in the clearance and destruction of erythrocytes. I. *In vivo* effects of IgG and IgM complement fixing sites, *J. Clin. Invest.* **51**:575–582.

Schreiber, A. D., Kaplan, A. P., and Austen, K. F., 1973, Inhibition by $C\bar{1}$ INH of Hageman factor fragment activation of coagulation, fibrinolysis, and kiningeneration, *J. Clin. Invest.* **52**:1402–1409.

Schullek, J., Jordan, J., and Montgomery, R. R., 1984, Interaction of Von Willebrand factor with human platelets in the plasma milieu, *J. Clin. Invest.* **73**:421–428.

Scicli, A. G., Mindroiu, T., Scicli, G., and Carretero, O. A., 1982, Blood kinins, their concentration in normal subjects and in patients with congenital deficiency in plasma prekallikrein and kininogen, *J. Lab. Clin. Med.* **100**:81–93.

Scott, C. F., and Colman, R. W., 1980, Function and immunochemistry of prekallikreinhigh molecular weight kininogen complex in plasma, *J. Clin. Invest.* **656**:413–421.

Scott, C. F., Schapira, M., James, H. L., Cohen, A. B., and Colman, R. W., 1982, Inactivation of factor XIa by plasma protease inhibitors. Predominant role of α_1 protease inhibitor and protective effect of high molecular weight kininogen, *J. Clin. Invest.* **69**:844–852.

Scott, C. F., Silver, L. D., Purdon, A. D., and Colman, R. W., 1984a, Plasma Factor XIa regulates contact-activated coagulation, *Fed. Proc.* **43**:775.

Scott, C. F., Silver, L. D., Schapira, M., and Colman, R. W., 1984b, Cleavage of human high molecular weight kininogen markedly enhances its coagulant activity. Evidence that this molecule exists as a procofactor, *J. Clin. Invest.* **73**:954–962.

Sealey, J. E., Atlas, S. P., Laragh, J. H., Silverberg, M., and Kaplan, A. P., 1979, Initiation of plasma prorenin activation by Hageman factor dependent conversion of plasma prekallikrein to kallikrein, *Proc. Natl. Acad. Sci. U.S.A.* **76**:5914–5918.

Senior, R. M., Griffin, G. L., and Mecham, R. P., 1980, Chemotactic activity of elastin derived peptides, *J. Clin. Invest.* **66**:859–862.

Sharma, J. N., Zeitlin, I. J., Deodhar, S. D., and Buchanan, W. W., 1983, *Arch. Int. Pharmacodyn.* **262**:279–286.

Shaw, J. O., Pinckard, R. N., Ferrigni, K. S., McManus, L. M., and Hanahan, D. J., 1981, Activation of human neutrophils with 1-O-hexadecyl/octadecyl-2-acetyl-*sn*-glyceryl-3-phosphorylcholine, the active moiety of platelet-activating factor, *J. Immunol.* **127**:1250–1255.

Sheikh, I., and Kaplan, A. P., 1984, Assessment of kallidin, bradykinin, and bradykinin degradation products by high pressure liquid chromatography (HPLC), *Fed. Proc.* **44**:1242 (abstract).

Silverberg, M., and Kaplan, A. P., 1982b, Enzymatic activities of activated and zymogen form of human Hageman factor (factor XII) *Blood* **60**:64–70.

Silverberg, M., Dunn, J. T., Garen, L., and Kaplan, A. P., 1980, Autoactivation of human Hageman factor. Demonstration utilizing a synthetic substrate, *J. Biol. Chem.* **255**:7281–7286.

Silverberg, M., Nicoll, J. E., and Kaplan, A. P., 1980, The mechanism by which the light chain of cleaved HMW-kininogen augments the activation of prekallikrein, factor XI, and Hageman factor, *Thromb. Res.* **70**:173–189.

Soter, N. A., Lewis, R. A., Corey, E. J., and Austen, K. F., 1983, Local effects of synthetic leucotrienes (LT C_4, LT D_4, LT E_4, and LT B_4) in human skin, *J. Invest. Dermatol.* **80**:115–119.

Spragg, J., 1983, Characterization of purified human latent kallikrein, Kinins III, *Adv. Exp. Med. Biol.* **156**:393–398.

Stead, N. W., Kaplan, A. P., and Rosenberg, R. D., 1976, The inhibition of human activated Hageman factor (HF) by human antithrombin-heparin cofactor (AT), *J. Biol. Chem.* **251**:6481–6488.

Steinman, C. R., 1984, Circulating DNA in systemic lupus erythematosus. Isolation and characterization, *J. Clin. Invest.* **73**:832–841.

Stenflo, J., 1976, A new vitamin K-dependent protein. Purification from bovine plasma and preliminary characterization, *J. Biol. Chem.* **251**:355–363.

Stenflo, J., Fernlund, P., Egan, W., and Roepstorff, P., 1974, Vitamin K dependent modifications of glutamic acid residues in prothrombin, *Proc. Natl. Acad. Sci. U.S.A.* **71**:2730–2733.

Sueishi, K., Nanno, S., and Tanaka, K., 1981, Permeability enhancing and chemotactic activities of lower molecular weight degradation products of human fibrinogen, *Thromb. Haemostas.* **45**:90–94.

Summaria, L., Hsieh, B., Groskopf, W. R., and Robbins, K. C., 1967, The isolation and characterization of the S-carboxymethyl β (light) chain derivative of human plasmin. The localization of the active site on the β (light) chain, *J. Biol. Chem.* **242**:5046–5052.

Summaria, L., Arzadon, L., Bernabe, P., and Robbins, K. C., 1975, The activation of plasminogen by urokinase in the presence of the plasmin inhibitor trasylol. The preparation of plasmin with the same NH_2-terminal heavy (A) chain sequence as the parent zymogen, *J. Biol. Chem.* **250**:3486–3995.

Takagi, T., and Doolittle, R. F., 1974, Amino acid sequence studies on factor XIII and the peptide released during its activation by thrombin, *Biochemistry* **13**:750–756.

Talamo, R. C., Haber, E., and Austen, K. F., 1969, A radioimmunoassay for bradykinin in plasma and synovial fluid, *J. Lab. Clin. Med.* **74**:816–827.

Tankersley, D. L., and Finlayson, J., 1984, Kinetics of activation and autoactivation of human factor XII, *Biochemistry* **23**:273–279.

Tans, G., Rosny, J., and Griffin, J. H., 1983, Sulfatide-dependent autoactivation of human blood factor XII, (Hageman factor), *J. Biol. Chem.* **258**:8215–8222.

Thompson, R. E., Mandle, R., Jr., and Kaplan, A. P., 1977, Association of factor XI and high molecular weight kininogen in human plasma, *J. Clin. Invest.* **60**:1376–1380.

Thompson, R. E., Mandle, R., Jr., and Kaplan, A. P., 1978, Characterization of human HMW-kininogen. Procoagulant activity associated with the light chain of kinin-free HMW kininogen, *J. Exp. Med.* **147**:488–499.

Thompson, R. E., Mandle, R., Jr., and Kaplan, A. P., 1979, Studies of the binding of prekallikrein and factor XI to high molecular weight kininogen and its light chain, *Proc. Natl. Acad. Sci. U.S.A.* **76**:4862–4866.

Thorsen, S., Glas-Greenwalt, P., and Astrup, T., 1972, Difference in the binding to fibrin of urokinase and tissue plasminogen activator, *Throm. Pathol. Haemorrh.* **28**:65–74.

Tollefson, D. M., Pestka, C. A., and Monafo, W. J., 1983, Activation of heparin cofactor II by dermatan sulfate, *J. Biol. Chem.* **258**:6713–6716.

Ueno, A., Tanaka, K., Katori, M., Hayashi, M., and Arai, Y., 1981, Species differences in increased vascular permeability by synthetic leukotrienes C_4 and D_4, *Prostaglandins* **21**:637–648.

Van der Graaf, F., Koedam, J. A., and Bouma, B. N., 1983a, Inactivation of kallikrein in human plasma, *J. Clin. Invest.* **71**:149–158.

Van der Graaf, F., Koedam, J. A., Griffin, J. H., and Bouma, B. N., 1983b, Interaction of human plasma kallikrein and its light chain with Cl^- inhibitor, *Biochemistry* **22**:4860–4866.

Vassalli, J. D., Hamilton, J., and Reich, E., 1976, Macrophage plasminogen activator modalation of enzyme production by anti-inflammatory steroids, mitotic inhibitors, and cyclic nucleotides, *Cell* **8**:271–281.

Vater, C. A., Nagase, H., and Harris, E. D., Jr., 1983, Purification of an endogenous activator of procollagenase from rabbit synovial fibroblast culture medium, *J. Biol. Chem.* **258**:9374–9382.

Verheyen, J. H., Chang, G. I. C., and Mullaart, E., 1983, Inhibition of extrinsic (tissue-type) plasminogen activator by human plasma: Evidence for the occurrence a fast-acting plasminogen activator inhibitor, *Thromb. Haemostas.* **50**:294.

Wachtfogel, Y. T., Kuchich, U., James, U. L., Scott, C. H., Schapira, M., Zimmerman, M., Cohen, A. B., and Colman, R. W., 1983, Human plasma kallikrein releases neutrophil elastase during blood coagulation, *J. Clin. Invest.* **72**:1172–1677.

Webster, M. E., and Pierce, J. V., 1963, The nature of kallidins released from human plasma by kallikreins and other enzymes, *Ann. N.Y. Acad. Sci.* **104**:91–105.

Weinstein, M. J., and Chute, L. E., 1984, Two distinct forms of factor VIII coagulant protein in human plasma. Cleavage by thrombin and differences in coagulant activity and association with von Willebrand factor, *J. Clin. Invest.* **73**:307–316.

Weiss, A. S., Gallin, J. I., and Kaplan, A. P., 1971, Fletcher factor deficiency. Abnormalities of coagulation, fibrinolysis, chemotactic activity, and kinin generation attributable to absence of prekallikrein, *J. Clin. Invest.* **53**:622–633.

Weiss, H. J., 1975, Platelet physiology and abnormalities of platelet function, *N. Engl. J. Med.* **293**:531–544.

Weller, P. F., Lee, C. W., Foster, D. W., Corey, E. J., Austen, K. F., and Lewis, R. A., 1983, Generation and metabolism of 5 lipoxygenase pathway leucotrienes by human eosinophils predominant production of leucotriene C4, *Proc. Natl. Acad. Sci. U.S.A.* **80**:7626–7630.

Werb, Z., Mainardi, C. L., Voter, C. A., and Harris, E. D., Jr., 1977, Endogenous activation of latent collagenase by rheumatoid synovial cells, *N. Engl. J. Med.* **296**:1017–1023.

Wiggins, R. C., and Cochrane, C. G., 1979, The autoactivation of rabbit Hageman factor, *J. Exp. Med.* **150**:1122–1133.

Wiggins, R. C., Bouma, B. N., Cochrane, C. G., and Griffin, J. H., 1977, Role of high molecular weight kininogen in surface-binding and activation of coagulation factor XI and prekallikrein, *Proc. Natl. Acad. Sci. U.S.A.* **74**:4636–4640.

Williams, T. J., 1972, Prostaglandins E_2, prostaglandin I_2 and the vascular changes of inflammation, *Br. J. Pharmacol.* **65**:517–524.

Williams, T. J., and Peck, M. J., 1977, Role of prostaglandin-mediated vasodilatation in inflammation, *Nature* **270**:530–532.

Wilner, G. D., Nossel, H. L., and LeRoy, E. C., 1968, Activation of Hageman factor by collagen, *J. Clin. Invest.* **47**:2608–2615.

Wilson, J. G., Wong, W. W., Schur, P. H., and Fearon, D. T., 1982, Mode of inheritance of decreased C3b receptors on erythrocytes of patients with systemic lupus erythematosus, *N. Engl. J. Med.* **307**:981–986.

Wiman, B., 1973, Primary structure of peptides released during activation of human plasminogen by urokinase, *Eur. J. Biochem.* **39**:1–9.

Wuepper, K. D., 1973, Prekallikrein deficiency in man, *J. Exp. Med.* **138**:1345–1355.

Wuepper, K. D., Miller, D. R., and LaCombe, M. J., 1975, Flaujeac trait. Deficiency of human plasma kininogen, *J. Clin. Invest.* **56**:1663–1672.

Yecies, L. D., Wedner, H. J., and Parker, C. W., 1979, Slow reacting substance (SRS) from ionophore A23187-stimulated human leukemia basophils. I. Evidence for a precursor role of arachidonic acid and initial characterization, *J. Immunol.* **123**:2814–2816.

Zur, M., and Nemerson, Y., 1979, The esterase activity of coagulation factor VII. Evidence for intrinsic activity of the zymogen, *J. Biol. Chem.* **253**:2203–2209.

Zuraw, B. L., O'Hair, C. H., Vaughan, J. H., Mathison, D. A., Curd, J. G., and Katz, D. H., 1981, Immunoglobulin E-rheumatoid factor in the serum of patients with rheumatoid arthritis, asthma, and other diseases, *J. Clin. Invest.* **68**:1610–1613.

23

The Role of the Neutrophil in the Inflammatory Response

Marilyn C. Pike and Ralph Snyderman

I. INTRODUCTION

In the latter part of the nineteenth century, Metchnikoff observed the localization of amebocytes around a rose thorn that had penetrated into the coelomic cavity of a transparent starfish larva. He was struck by the "walling off" or engulfment of foreign particles by these motile cells. Based on these and other findings, Metchnikoff (1891) proposed a major role for phagocytic cells in mediating resistance to microbial invasion. The immune system is now known to consist of humoral and cellular components whose complex interactions can protect against microbial invasion and the development and spread of neoplasms. The immunologic recognition of foreign substances results in the production of inflammatory mediators through the activation of enzyme cascade systems such as complement and by the release of soluble products from leukocytes (i.e., lymphokines and arachidonic acid metabolites) (Cohen *et al.*, 1979; Gallin and Quie, 1978; Kuehl and Egan, 1980; Snyderman, 1982). These mediators recruit phagocytes and lymphocytes to sites of immune reactions. Polymorphonuclear leukocytes (PMN) and macrophages are phagocytic cells whose functions are required for the actual degradation of antigens.

The most abundant circulating phagocyte is the neutrophil, whose importance is underscored by the multitude of life-threatening infections that face severely granulocytopenic individuals. Normal neutrophil function is dependent on (1) adequate differentiation of committed stem cells in the bone marrow; (2) release of granulocytes from the bone marrow into the bloodstream; (3) margination and subsequent migration of

Marilyn C. Pike • Departmment of Medicine, Massachusetts General Hospital, Boston, Massachusetts 02115. *Ralph Snyderman* • Laboratory of Immune Effector Function, Howard Hughes Medical Institute, and Division of Rheumatic and Genetic Diseases, Department of Medicine, Duke University Medical Center, Durham, North Carolina 27710.

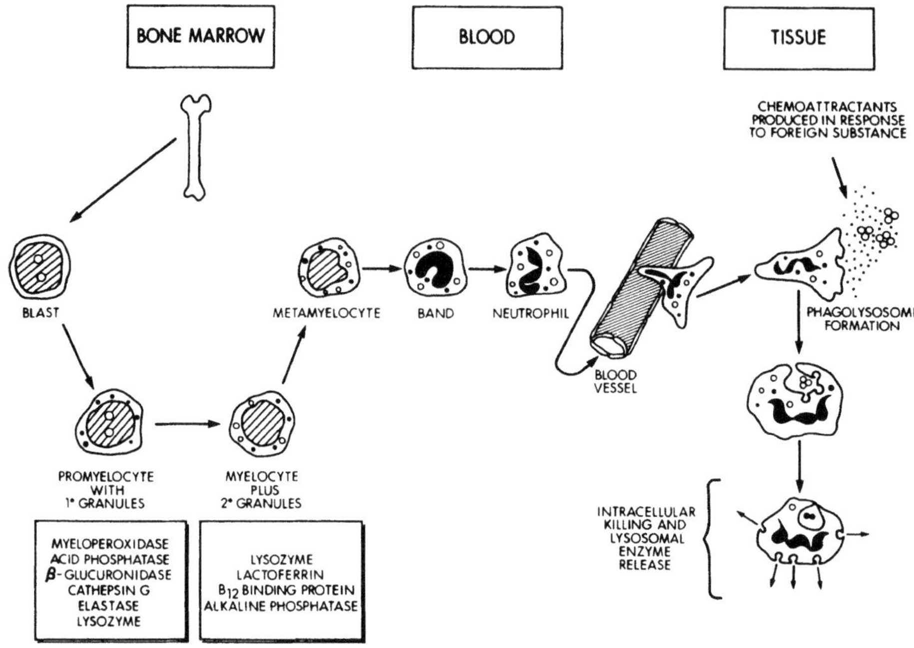

Figure 1. Maturation sequence and functions of leukocytes as mediators of host defense.

neutrophils to sites of inflammation; and (4) destruction of the inciting agents by phagocytosis and/or cidal enzyme systems within the neutrophil (Fig. 1).

The localization of neutrophils at sites of immune reactions occurs by the process of chemotaxis or the directed migration of cells along a concentration gradient of a chemoattractant substance (Snyderman and Goetzl, 1981). The study of neutrophil function has received a great deal of attention over the past several years not only because of its importance in host defense but also because these cells can contribute to the pathogenesis of many rheumatic diseases.

II. DEVELOPMENT AND MORPHOLOGY OF MATURE NEUTROPHILS

A. Myelopoiesis

The formation of granulocytes within the bone marrow proceeds from a myeloid stem cell, which can give rise to precursor cells for erythrocytes, megakaryocytes, monocytes, or granulocytes. Some of these stem cells, termed CFU-C or CFU-G,M (colony forming unit, granulocyte, monocyte), differentiate into a common committed progenitor cell for the neutrophil and monocyte pathway (Cline, 1975; Klebanoff and Clark, 1978; Golde, 1982). The further differentiation of these progenitor cells into granulocytes or monocytes depends on a group of hormones termed colony-stimulating factors (CSF). These are produced primarily by cells of the monocyte–macrophage series and also by activated T cells (Brennan *et al.*, 1980). Complex positive and negative feedback regulation of myelopoiesis by mature monocytes and granulocytes appears to occur (Cline and Golde, 1979).

B. Morphology of Neutrophil Precursors

The myeloblast is the earliest identifiable precursor of the granulocyte series. There are approximately 1 to 3% of these cells in normal bone marrow aspirates. Myeloblasts are characterized morphologically by a large nucleus with prominent nucleoli and dense, evenly distributed chromatin. The cytoplasm is blue and scant. The next cell in the maturation sequence is the promyelocyte, whose nucleus appears similar to that of the myeloblast but whose cytoplasm contains prominent azurophilic or nonspecific (primary) granules (see below). The myelocyte succeeds the promyelocyte and is characterized by a nucleus without prominent nucleoli. In addition to primary granules, the cytoplasm of myelocytes also has secondary or specific granules (see below). The myelocyte is the last cell in the maturation sequence that retains the ability to proliferate. The metamyelocyte, the next cell in the diferentiation process, develops an eccentric, partially indented nucleus with increased chromatin clumping. The cytoplasm contains both primary and secondary granules. These cells further develop into band or stab forms, which have incompletely segmented nuclei and constitute 3 to 5% of the normal circulating leukocyte pool (Golde, 1982).

C. Morphology of Mature Neutrophils

The mature neutrophil contains a nucleus usually composed of three lobes with condensed chromatin; the mature cell ranges in size from 12 to 15 μm in diameter and contains both primary and secondary granules; approximately 10–20% are of the latter type. The azurophilic (primary) granules contain proteases such as cathepsin G, elastase, myeloperoxidase, lysozyme, and acid mucopolysaccharide. The secondary (specific) granules contain lysozyme, lactoferrin, vitamin B_{12}-binding proteins, and alkaline phosphatase (Klebanoff and Clark, 1978). Secondary granules are also thought to contain within their membranes "spare" surface receptors or other components that are involved in the regulation of the chemotactic and respiratory burst responses (Fletcher and Gallin, 1980, 1983) (see below).

III. FUNCTIONS OF NEUTROPHILS

A. Chemotaxis

1. Overview and Historical Aspects

The movement of leukocytes from the bloodstream to local tissue sites appears to depend on their directed migration in response to chemical mediators termed "chemoattractants." The type of chemoattractant produced may vary with the inciting inflammatory agent, as will be discussed. Pfeffer, in 1884, was the first to use the term "chemotaxis" in characterizing the directed migration of plant cells. In 1888, Leber described the migration of leukocytes towards the center of rabbit corneas in response to the injection of extracts of bacteria. Metchnikoff had suggested in 1891 that leukocytes were attracted by bacterial products. The systematic study of chemoattractant substances was hindered by the lack of reproducible, quantitative methodology until 1962, when Boyden developed an *in vitro* technique for measuring leukocyte chemotaxis in plastic chambers. This method utilizes a two-compartment chamber and a porous membrane filter through which the cells can migrate (Snyderman *et al.*, 1968a). The number of cells migrating through to the bottom surface of the filter can be quantified microscopically. Using this technique, Boyden (1962) showed that normal human serum that had been incubated with immune complexes contained a substance that enhanced the directed migration of leukocytes.

2. Chemotactic Factors

Although numerous substances have been described as being chemotactic, few substances have actually been well characterized or have been shown to play a role in leukocyte accumulation *in vivo*.

a. Complement-Derived Chemoattractants. The complement (C) system is an important mediator of the acute inflammatory response. In 1962, Boyden showed that the interaction of immune complexes with fresh but not heat-inactivated serum resulted in the generation of chemotactic activity for PMNs. Subsequently, experiments performed by Ward *et al.* (1966) suggested that this chemotactic activity was associated with the activation of the C system and generation of the macromolecular complex C5b67. Snyderman *et al.* (1968a), however, showed that serum treated with the C activator endotoxin produced a C5-dependent, 15,000-dalton chemoattractant, which was soon identified as the cleavage product of the fifth component of C, C5a (Snyderman *et al.*, 1968b, 1969, 1970; Jensen *et al.*, 1969; Ward and Newman, 1969). Cleavage of highly purified C5 with proteolytic enzymes or with the earlier-acting C components also generated C5a, which had both chemotactic and anaphylatoxic activity (Shin *et al.*, 1968).

Unquestionable evidence now exists that C5a accounts for the vast majority of biologically relevant chemotactic activity produced by C activation (Snyderman *et al.*, 1970; Hugli and Muller-Eberhard, 1978). Although there are reports that a cleavage product of C3, C3a, also has chemotactic activity (Taylor and Ward, 1967; Bokisch *et al.*, 1969), this work has not been substantiated in studies using highly purified C3a (Fernandez *et al.*, 1978). The primary amino acid composition of C3a and C5a has been determined, and the biological effects of these molecules have been studied *in vitro*. Human C5a is a glycoprotein, the polypeptide portion of which contains 74 amino acids, accounting for a mol. wt. of 8200; the carbohydrate portion accounts for 3000 daltons (Fernandez and Hugli, 1976). The most prevalent form of human C5a recovered from serum is $C5a_{desArg}$, a molecule from which the COOH-terminal arginine is removed by carboxypeptidases (Fernandez *et al.*, 1978). $C5a_{desArg}$ is approximately tenfold less potent than the native C5a molecule. C5a has been shown to mediate its chemotactic activity via specific cell surface receptors on neutrophils (Chenoweth and Hugli, 1980).

b. Bacterial Chemotactic Factors and the N-Formylated Peptide Chemoattractants. Culture filtrates of many bacteria are chemotactic for neutrophils (Keller and Sorkin, 1967; Ward *et al.*, 1968; Tempel *et al.*, 1970). Chemotactic factor production is greatest during the log phase of bacterial growth (Ward *et al.*, 1968; Tempel *et al.*, 1970). Until the mid-1970s very little was known about the chemical identity of bacterial chemotactic factors, since the physical properties of the various chemoattractants described by different laboratories were widely divergent. In 1975, however, while studying the nature of bacterial chemotactic factors, Schiffmann *et al.* (1975) made the important discovery that N-terminal-blocked methionyl di- and tripeptides are chemotactic for neutrophils and macrophages. Since formylation of the NH_2 terminus was necessary for the chemotactic activity of these peptides, it was reasoned that the response of mammalian leukocytes to the peptides might provide a simple recognition system for the presence of microbial agents. Prokaryotic cells initiate protein synthesis with a formylmethionyl residue, in contrast to eukaryotic cells, which initiate protein synthesis largely with nonformylated methionine. This hypothesis has apparently been borne out, since Marasco *et al.* (1983) reported that the major chemotactic peptide produced by *E. coli* is formylmethionylleucylphenylalanine (fMet-Leu-Phe), the most potent formylated tripeptide thus far identified (Showell *et al.*, 1976). The N-formylated peptides initiate chemotactic and secretory responses via specific cell surface receptors (Aswanikumar *et al.*, 1977; Williams *et al.*, 1977; Pike and Snyderman, 1982b) that are distinct from those that bind C5a (Williams *et al.*, 1977).

c. Lipid Chemotactic Factors. The observation that oxidized components of polyenoic fatty acids are chemotactic for neutrophils was first made in 1975 by Turner *et al.* Oxidation of arachidonic acid by air exposure or by lipoxygenase treatment resulted in a chemotactic product, 12-L-hydroxy-5,8,10,14-eicosatetraenoic acid (12-HETE). Subsequent studies further defined the biochemistry and activity of the products resulting from lipoxygenation of arachidonic acid. The substance found to be most active as a chemotactic agent for human neutrophils is 5(*S*),12(*R*)-dihydroxy-6,8-*trans*-10,14-*cis*-eicosatetraeonic acid (5,12-diHETE), now known as leukotriene B_4 (LTB_4) (Ford-Hutchinson *et al.*, 1980). This compound is chemotactic for human neutrophils at concentrations as low as 3 ng/ml. Other lipoxygenation products, including 5-HETE, 11-HETE, and 12-HETE, were found to be much less potent for producing chemotactic activity (Goetzl and Pickett, 1980). Slow-reacting substance of anaphylaxis (leukotriene C) and several platelet-derived trihydroxytetraenoic acids produced only marginal chemotactic activity (Ford-Hutchinson *et al.*, 1981). In human PMNs, LTB_4 is a poor stimulant of lysosomal enzyme secretion, producing less than a third of the maximal secretion of β-glucoronidase and lysozyme as seen with C5a and the formylated peptides (Ford-Hutchinson, 1980). Like these former chemoattractants, however, LTB_4 binds to specific cellular receptors on neutrophils (Goldman and Goetzl, 1982, 1984; Kreisle and Parker, 1983).

d. Cell-Derived Chemotactic Factors. In 1972, it was shown that human lymphocytes from tuberculin-sensitive donors, when incubated with purified protein derivative, produced a 12,500-dalton molecule with chemotactic activity for human monocytes (Snyderman *et al.*, 1972). The same substance, also produced when lymphocytes are incubated with mitogens, has been termed lymphocyte-derived chemotactic factor (LDCF) (Snyderman *et al.*, 1972, 1977a). This factor is isoelectrically and antigenically distinct from C5a (Altman *et al.*, 1975) and does not require cell division for its production but does depend on new protein synthesis (Snyderman *et al.*, 1977a). Supernatants of mixed leukocyte cultures from HLA-nonidentical individuals also contain LDCF. The importance of this chemoattractant *in vivo* is suggested by studies that have demonstrated that LDCF appears at sites of delayed hypersensitivity reactions just prior to the local influx of macrophages (Postlethwaite and Snyderman, 1975).

A cell-derived chemotactic factor termed crystal-induced chemotactic factor (CCF) has been characterized by Spilberg *et al.* (1976). Phagocytosis by human polymorphonuclear leukocytes of sodium urate or calcium pyrophosphate crystals results in the formation of an 8400-mol wt glycoprotein with chemotactic activity for PMNs and monocytes. Since intraarticular injection of monosodium urate or calcium pyrophosphate crystals precipitates acute attacks of gout and pseudogout, respectively, it was hypothesized that the CCF is a primary mediator of inflammation in these diseases. Subsequent studies showed that injection of purified CCF intraarticularly in rabbits resulted in arthritis as measured by synovial inflammation and accumulation of PMNs in the joint fluid (Spilberg *et al.*, 1977).

e. Platelet-Derived Products as Chemotactic Agents. Platelets are prominent components of the inflammatory response, and their various functions, including adhesion, aggregation, and mediator release, have been intensively studied. Platelet factor 4 (PF4), a heparin-binding protein released from α-granules following adherence of platelets to vascular endothelial cells, stimulates directed migration of neutrophils and monocytes *in vitro* at concentrations found in normal human serum (Deuel *et al.*, 1981). Another factor produced by platelets, platelet-derived growth factor (PDGF), also reportedly is chemotactic for human neutrophils and monocytes (Deuel *et al.*, 1982; Williams *et al.*, 1983). This 32,000-dalton polypeptide is a potent mitogen for fibroblasts, vascular smooth muscle cells, and giant cells. It is released from the α-granules of stimulated platelets and is thought to stimulate fibroblast growth and thus wound healing.

f. Chemotactic Factors Associated with the Kinin- and Clot-Forming Systems Chemotactic activity has been attributed to products derived from the kinin-forming system as well as from the fibrinolytic and clotting systems. For example, conversion of prekallekrein to kallekrein by prekallekrein activator is associated with the production of chemotactic activity for neutrophils, which appears to reside in kallekrein itself (Kaplan *et al.*, 1972). The interaction of thrombin with human fibrinogen also produces chemotactic activity, which has been attributed to release of fibrinopeptide B (McKenzie *et al.*, 1975). Fibrin split products produced by the addition of plasmin to fibrin clots are reportedly chemotactic for neutrophils (Stetcher and Sorkin, 1972). Recent studies have shown that human α-thrombin is a potent chemoattractant, with maximal activity *in vitro* occurring at 10 nM (Bar-Shavit *et al.*, 1983). Analysis of the chemotactic activity of certain chemically modified thrombins indicated that the regions responsible for chemotaxis are distinct from the catalytic site and from exosites required for clotting. Chemotactic products derived from the kinin-forming and fibrin-forming systems and fibrinolytic pathways may function to attract leukocytes to areas of clot formation and may be important for subsequent wound healing.

3. Molecular Mechanisms of the Chemotactic Response

The chemotaxis of leukocytes is the culmination of a complex series of biochemical events including binding of chemoattractants to cell surface receptors (Williams *et al.*, 1977; Aswanikumar *et al.*, 1977; Niedel *et al.*, 1979), alterations in ion fluxes (Gallin and Rosenthal, 1974; Boucek and Snyderman, 1976; Naccache *et al.*, 1977), stimulation of energy-producing pathways, changes in membrane lipid composition (Pike and Snyderman, 1980, 1981a; Pike *et al.*, 1979), rearrangement of cytoskeletal structures (Gallin *et al.*, 1978a; Anderson *et al.*, 1982; Schliwa *et al.*, 1982), and transmethylation reactions (Pike *et al.*, 1978; Pike and Snyderman, 1981a,b; O'Dea *et al.*, 1978). The availability of purified chemoattractants labeled to high specific radioactivity has allowed the characterization of specific cell surface receptors for the formylated oligopeptides (Williams *et al.*, 1977; Aswanikumar *et al.*, 1977), C5a (Chenoweth and Hugli, 1980), LTB_4 (Kreisle and Parker, 1982; Goldman and Goetzl, 1982), and CCF (Spilberg *et al.*, 1977; Spilberg and Mehta, 1979). The N-formyl peptide receptor exists in two affinity states, the expression of which is regulated by guanine nucleotides and presumably a guanine nucleotide regulatory protein (Koo *et al.*, 1982, 1983; Snyderman *et al.*, 1984). The biological relevance of this observation is discussed below.

It is important to appreciate that chemoattractant receptors for C5a and N-formylated peptides induce not only directed migration but also stimulation of the respiratory burst and secretion of lysosomal enzymes (Goldstein *et al.*, 1973; Klebanoff and Clark, 1978). Interestingly, doses of chemoattractants required for initiating chemotaxis are generally only a tenth to 1/15 of those required for the stimulation of secretory functions (Showell *et al.*, 1976; Lehmeyer *et al.*, 1979; Yuli *et al.*, 1982). These observations suggest different regulatory mechanisms for the migratory and secretory activities of chemoattractant receptors. This contention is borne out by pharmacological manipulation of the N-formyl oligopeptide receptor on neutrophils. These studies have shown that conditions that enhance the affinity of chemoattractant receptors (i.e., mild membrane fluidization) inhibit their stimulation of the oxidative burst and secretion of lysosomal enzymes (Yuli *et al.*, 1982). Chemotactic responsiveness, on the other hand, is enhanced by such conditions. Conversely, pharmacological manipulation of neutrophils that lowers the affinity of chemoattractant receptors increases stimulated degranulation of specific granules but inhibits the chemotactic response (Lohr and Snyderman, 1982).

Thus, it appears that a higher-affinity state of the oligopeptide chemoattractant receptor favors the mediation of chemotaxis whereas a lower-affinity state mediates secretion and superoxide anion production (Snyderman *et al.*, 1984). Studies have shown that the degranulation response itself may regulate N-formylated peptide receptor expression on the cell surface (Gallin *et al.*, 1978c; Fletcher and Gallin, 1980; Fletcher *et al.*, 1982). Limited release of secondary neutrophil granules causes an increase in chemoattractant receptor numbers on the cell surface with a concomitant decrease in receptor affinity (Fletcher *et al.*, 1982). The fusion of granule membranes with the plasma membrane of PMN during chemotaxis could provide additional surface receptors at the leading fronts of migrating leukocytes.

The biochemical events that mediate transduction of the signal from the occupied chemoattractant receptor through the PMN membrane leading to polarized cellular movement are a subject of intense investigation. Leukocytes treated with chemotactic factors rapidly remodel their plasma membrane (Hoffstein *et al.*, 1982). This results from the presumed activation of phospholipase C (Pike and Snyderman, 1981b, 1982b), which converts phosphatidylinositol and phosphatidylinositol polyphosphates (PIP_1, PIP_2) to myoinositol phosphate, inositol polyphosphates, and diacylglycerol (Volpi *et al.*, 1983; Yano *et al.*, 1983; Lapetina, 1984). This latter compound can then be rapidly metabolized to phosphatidic acid by diacylglycerol kinase or to glycerol and long-chain fatty acids (i.e., arachidonate) via the action of diacylglycerol lipase. Arachidonate is itself an activator of protein kinase C (McPhail *et al.*, 1984) and also serves as the precursor of prostaglandins and hydroxyendoperoxides formed by the lipoxygenase enzyme pathway. These agents are mediators of inflammatory reactions (Kuehl and Egan, 1980; Weissmann, 1983). In addition, inositol-4,5-bisphosphate is a potent mobilizer of calcium (Ohsako and DeGuchi, 1981; Serhan *et al.*, 1981) and could thereby act as a "second messenger" for the chemoattractant receptor (Fig. 2).

Transmethylation reaction mediated by S-adenosylmethionine are required for the chemotactic response of both neutrophils and mononuclear phagocytes (Pike *et al.*, 1978; Pike and Snyderman, 1982b; O'Dea *et al.*, 1978; Snyderman *et al.*, 1980). Inhibition of transmethylation reactions causes a marked decrease in chemotaxis. Although it is unclear

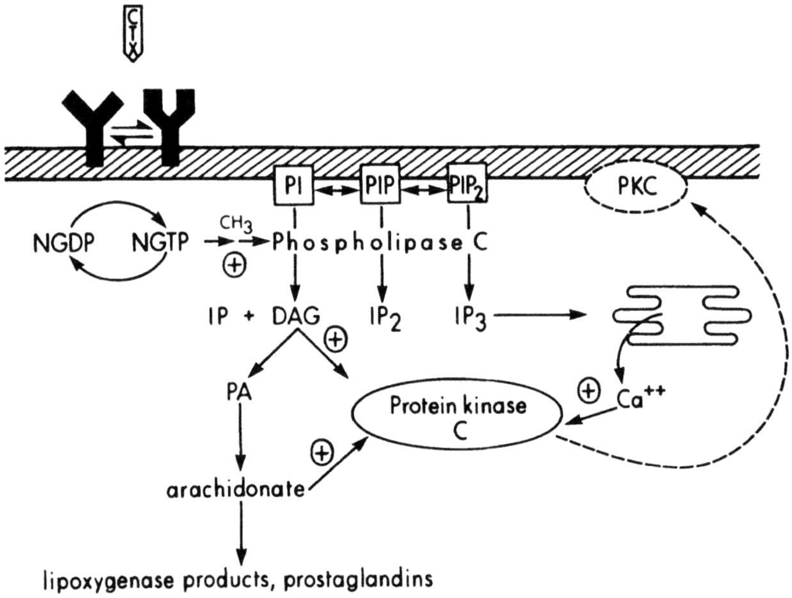

Figure 2. A current hypothesis regarding transduction of chemoattractant receptor-mediated signals in leukocytes. A chemoattractant (CTX) binds to a specific cell surface receptor, which exists in high- and low-affinity states modulated by a guanine-nucleotide-activated regulatory protein (N). Binding of the chemoattractant to the receptor results in activation of phospholipase C, whose optimal activity is dependent on a transmethylation reaction (CH_3). The enzyme converts phosphatidylinositol (PI), phosphatidylinositol 4-phosphate (PIP), and phosphatidylinositol-4,5-biphosphate (PIP_2) into diacylglycerol (DAG) and the corresponding phosphoinositide (IP, IP_2, IP_3). These latter compounds produce release of intracellular Ca^{2+} stores. Protein kinase C (PKC) in the cytosol or loosely bound to the membrane is activated by Ca^{2+}, DAG, and arachidonate. The ultimate action of the chemoattractant on PKC is to increase the kinase activity of the enzyme associated with the membrane. (Adapted from Pike and Snyderman, 1984.)

which methylation reactions are required for chemotaxis, it has been demonstrated that chemotactic factors inhibit the methylation of phosphatidylethanolamine at the leading front membrane of migrating leukocytes (Pike *et al.*, 1979; Pike and Synderman, 1981a). In addition, inhibition of methylation reactions in guinea pig macrophages decreases the affinity of the oligopeptide chemoattractant receptor (Pike and Snyderman, 1982a). The consequence of this inhibition is a decrease in the phosphatidylcholine: phosphatidylethanolamine ratio, which may produce microviscosity changes or alterations in lipid–protein interactions. These changes may be necessary for sustained directed cellular migration. Chemoattractants also produce a transient, rapid increase in intracellular cAMP (Simchowitz *et al.*, 1980) but do not activate adenylate cyclase in leukocyte membrane preparations (Verghese and Snyderman, 1983). It has recently been postulated that chemoattractants may cause transient phosphodiesterase inhibition and thereby cause the cAMP increase in neutrophils (Verghese and Snyderman, 1984).

Protein kinase C is a calcium- and lipid-dependent enzyme that is present in many tissues of the body (Nishizuka, 1984). Tumor-promoting phorbol esters bind to protein kinase C and, in so doing, translocate the enzyme from cytosolic to membrane cellular fractions of yolk sac parietal cells (Kraft and Anderson, 1983). A similar phenomenon is seen in human monocytes, where the appearance of protein kinase C activity in the monocyte membrane is correlated with activation of superoxide anion production by phorbols (Myers *et al.*, 1984). Chemoattractants, in the presence of cytochalasin B, also cause the appearance of protein kinase C activity in human leukocyte membrane preparations (McPhail *et al.*, 1984). This effect correlates with leukocyte responses that are initiated by high doses of chemoattractants such as superoxide production and lysosomal enzyme release. Protein kinase C may thus be involved in the transduction of those chemoattractant receptor signals that mediate stimulation of secretion and the oxidative burst (Fig. 2).

B. Phagocytosis

Phagocytosis, or the ingestion of particulate matter by neutrophils, results from the movement of the cellular membrane and cytoplasm around an ingestible particle. This is followed by fusion of the plasma membrane, resulting in internalization of the particle along with a portion of the cell membrane, which now lines the phagocytic vesicle. Lysosomal granules migrate to the newly formed vesicle and fuse with it, thereby forming a phagolysosome (Fig. 1; Klebanoff and Clark, 1978). Under normal conditions, this series of events leads to digestion of the foreign substance. The phagocytic signal at the neutrophil membrane can be initiated by (1) F_c receptor binding to the appropriate immunoglobin coating the foreign substance (Ward and Enders, 1933; LoBuglio *et al.*, 1967; Huber *et al.*, 1968); (2) C3b or $C3b_i$ receptor binding to its ligand on the surface of the foreign material (Nelson, 1965; Johnston *et al.*, 1969; Henson, 1976); or (3) nonspecific membrane interactions (Lerner, 1956; Smith and Wood, 1958). During early studies of phagocytosis, it was found that when serum was added to bacteria, their ingestion by phagocytes was enhanced (Wright and Douglas, 1903). This "opsonic" activity of serum was composed of a heat-stable and a heat-labile component, now known to be immunoglobin and complement, respectively. Thus, interaction of foreign substances with immunoglobulin results in complement activation, C5a release, chemotaxis of neutrophils to the area of penetration by foreign substances, and engulfment of materials, which frequently have immunoglobulin and C3b bound to their surface.

Opsonins are particularly important for the phagocytosis of encapsulated organisms such as *Streptococcus pneumoniae* and *Hemophilus influenzae*. Fully encapsulated (smooth) pneumococci are more virulent than noncapsulated forms, and components of the pneumococcal capsule can directly inhibit the phagocytic response of neutrophils (Ward and Enders, 1933; Rothbard, 1948; Hirsch and Church, 1960). Enzymatic removal or neutralization with specific antibody directed against the capsular carbohydrate promotes phagocytosis of smooth strains and thus reduces their virulence. The pathological importance of the antiphagocytic nature of the capsule of these organisms and its neutralization by specific antibody are underscored by the clinical observation that agammaglobulinemic and hypogammaglobulinemic individuals have recurrent infections only with encapsulated organisms (Klebanoff and Clark, 1978). Other types of organisms produce antiphagocytic activity. The protein A exoprotein produced by coagulase-positive *Staphylococcus aureus* inhibits phagocytes by binding to the F_c portion of immunoglobin, thus blocking attachment of neutrophil F_c receptors to the organism (Forsgren and Quie, 1974). The antiphagocytic activity of group A streptococci resides in two surface components, the M protein and the hyaluronic acid capsule (Rothbard, 1948; Hirsch and Church, 1960). The capsule of *Cryptococcus neoformans* also contains antiphagocytic activity (Kozel, 1977). Virulent colonies of *Neisseria gonorrheae* are more resistant to phagocytosis by neutrophils than avirulent colony types (Rosenthal *et al.*, 1977).

The phagocytic process of neutrophils is an energy-requiring process, the ATP for which is generally thought to be generated by anaerobic glycolysis but not by oxidative phosphorylation (Allison *et al.*, 1963; Stossel *et al.*, 1972; Sbarra and Karnovsky, 1959). These conclusions were made by studies showing that glycolytic inhibitors such as deoxyglucose, fluoride, and arsenate inhibit phagocytosis whereas hypoxia and inhibitors of oxidative phosphorylation such as dinitrophenol have no effect on the ingestion process.

Changes in neutrophil microfilament activity and in contractile proteins are an absolute requirement for the phagocytic response of neutrophils (Malawista *et al.*, 1971; Zurier *et al.*, 1973). Substances that prevent the polymerization of actin microfilaments (i.e., cytochalasins) inhibit the phagocytic response of leukocytes. Drugs that inhibit microtubule assembly (i.e., colchicine, vinca alkaloids) have no effect on phagocytosis (DeChatelet *et al.*, 1971; Malawista, 1971). It has been postulated that contact of ingestible objects with the phagocyte membrane alters the association of an "actin-binding protein" with cellular F actin, which promotes cross linking of F-actin polymers (Stossel and Hartwig, 1975; Stossel, 1977). The altered interaction of actin-binding protein with actin mediates the gel–sol transformation of the cytoplasm of neutrophils undergoing the phagocytic response. The cellular movement accompanying the phagocytic response is most likely dependent on a myosin Mg^{2+}-ATPase-based energy transduction system. Myosins similar to those found in smooth muscle have been isolated from neutrophils (Hartwig and Stossel, 1976). The importance of contractile proteins in the phagocytic response is evidenced by studies describing a patient with recurrent bacterial infections and failure to produce purulent exudates. *In vitro* studies of the patient's neutrophils showed decreased phagocytosis and normal actin levels but a defect in actin polymerization (Boxer *et al.*, 1974; Southwick and Stossel, 1981).

C. Microbicidal and Cytotoxic Activities

Neutrophils have potent antimicrobial activity that is dependent on oxidative and nonoxidative processes. Biochemical changes occur in the leukocyte as a result of binding to chemoattractants or opsonized particles that enhance microbicidal potential. These include increased glycolysis, a burst of oxygen consumption (respiratory burst), and generation of superoxide anion, which is then metabolized to other toxic oxygen radicals as well as to H_2O_2 (Baldridge and Gerard, 1933; Iyer *et al.*, 1961; Klebanoff, 1971, 1972; Fridovich, 1972). The enzyme responsible for the respiratory burst and production of superoxide is a NADPH oxidase that, when activated, is associated with the plasma membrane (Babior *et al.*, 1976; Henson *et al.*, 1977; McPhail and Snyderman, 1984). The enzyme activity is not detectable in unstimulated neutrophils but increases dramatically following contact of the cells with opsonized particles or chemoattractants.

The NADPH oxidase appears to be a multicomponent enzyme consisting of a flavoprotein, cytochrome b, and perhaps a ubiquinone (McPhail *et al.*, 1976; Babior and Kipnis, 1977; Cunningham *et al.*, 1982; Segal *et al.*, 1983). This NADPH oxidase activity is missing in patients with chronic granulomatous disease (see below). The general reaction for the production of superoxide (O_2^-) catalyzed by NADPH oxidase is as follows:

$$\text{NADPH} + O_2 \rightarrow \text{NADP} + O_2^-$$

Superoxide is then further metabolized to hydroxyl radical ($\cdot OH$), OH^-, and H_2O_2, all of which have bactericidal activity (Johnston *et al.*, 1975a; Rosen and Klebanoff, 1979). Myeloperoxidase and a halide such as Cl^- also provide important antimicrobial activity by leading to the formation of hypochlorous ion (OCl^-) (Klebanoff, 1967a, 1975; Weiss *et al.*, 1982). Neutrophils also contain nonoxidative antimicrobial mechanisms dependent in large part on the cationic proteins and enzymes (i.e., lysozyme) that are present in lysosomal granules (Okamura *et al.*, 1979, 1982; Weiss *et al.*, 1982; Spitznagel, 1984). Following particle ingestion, fusion of both primary and secondary granules with the phagosome occurs, converting this structure to a phagolysosome (Lockwood and Allison, 1963). The enzyme contents of the granules as well as their products are now in contact with the foreign substance. The pH of the phagocytic vesicle falls, with resultant activation of acid hydrolases and of the myeloperoxidase enzyme system (Rous, 1925; Klebanoff, 1967b, 1968).

In addition to release of granule contents into the phagolysozyme, extracellular degranulation can occur following the phagocytic response. β-Glucurondiase, lysozyme, cathepsin, myeloperoxidase, acid phosphatase, and alkaline phosphatase are found in the extracellular fluid following treatment of neutrophils with phagocytic stimuli as well as with high doses of chemotactic agents (Weissmann *et al.*, 1964; Woodin and Wieneke, 1966; Goldstein *et al.*, 1973). This extracellular release of toxic products is thought to play an important role in the tissue destruction seen in the rheumatoid joint (Weissmann *et al.*, 1969; Zvaifler, 1983). Ingestion of rheumatoid factor complexes by neutrophils in joint fluid results in the release of degradative enzymes that can destroy synovial tissues and cartilage. Studies have shown that the injection of neutrophil granules into the joints of rabbits produces acute inflammation, with repeated intraarticular injections producing hypertrophy and hyperplasia of synovial lining cells and subsequent pannus formation (Weissmann *et al.*, 1969).

IV. EFFECTS OF PHARMACOLOGICAL AGENTS ON NEUTROPHIL FUNCTION

A. Glucocorticosteroids

Glucocorticosteroids have numerous affects on neutrophil function. Administration of corticosteroids produces a neutrophilia that peaks after approximately 4 to 6 hr and is attributable to both accelerated release of the pool of mature cells from the bone marrow and reduced neutrophil margination to and migration through vascular endothelium (Fauci *et al.*, 1976).

Perhaps the most important effect of corticosteroids on neutrophil function *in vivo* is inhibition of leukocyte accumulation at inflammatory sites. Studies performed in multiple species using the Rebuck skin window technique have demonstrated decreased accumulation of neutrophils and monocytes following a single dose of hydrocortisone (Boggs *et al.*, 1964; Bishop *et al.*, 1968). Corticosteroids inhibit granulocyte adherence to vascular endothelium (Ebert and Barclay, 1952) and at very high doses (i.e., *ca.* 10^{-4} M) inhibit *in vitro* chemotaxis (Shea and Morse, 1978). Alternate-day therapy reduces the inhibitory effect of steroids on leukocyte accumulation *in vivo* (Dale *et al.*, 1974). Corticosteroids also suppress both phagocytic and bactericidal activities of human neutrophils; however, the concentrations of drug used in these studies were much higher than those thought to be achievable with steroid therapy (Hirsch and Church, 1961; Mandell *et al.*, 1970). Granulocytes from patients receiving corticosteroids have decreased nitroblue tetrazolium reduction but otherwise normal phagocytic and microbicidal activity (Chretien and Garagusi, 1971).

It has been proposed, largely on the basis of *in vitro* studies, that neutrophil lysosomal membranes are "stabilized" by corticosteroids (Persellin and Ku, 1974). This effect may reduce the amount of inflammatory enzymes released by neutrophils *in vivo*. *In vitro* steroid treatment reduces leukocytic pyrogen production (Dillard and Bodel, 1970) and their capacity to produce procoagulant (tissue factor) activity in response to such inflammatory stimuli as endotoxins, complement-activated plasma, or antigen–antibody complexes (Muhlfelder *et al.*, 1982). Steroids reduce prostaglandin levels in intact cells and in isolated organs (Tashjian *et al.*, 1975; Floman and Zor, 1976). This action of steroids is caused by inhibition of the release of polyunsaturated fatty acid precursors for both the cyclooxygenase and lipoxygenase pathways (Hong and Levine, 1976). This steroid effect requires glucocorticoid receptor occupancy as well as RNA and protein synthesis (Danon and Assouline, 1978; Russo-Marie *et al.*, 1979). The synthesized proteins that are stimulated by corticosteroids apparently inhibit the phospholipase-induced deacylation of arachidonate. The synthesis of proteins that inhibit phospholipase has been described in rat macorphages (macrocortin) (Blackwell *et al.*, 1980), rabbit neutrophils (lipomodulin) (Hirata *et al.*, 1980), and rat renomedullary interstitial cells (renocortins) (Rothhut *et al.*, 1983).

B. Nonsteroidal Antiinflammatory Agents

Several nonsteroidal antiinflammatory agents (NSAIAs) affect the function of neutrophils *in vitro* (Table 1), but little is known about the biologically relevant effects that these agents produce *in vivo*. Indomethacin, which interferes with prostaglandin production through inhibition of cyclooxygenase and also inhibits phospholipase A_2 activity, blocks leukocyte aggregation, lysosomal enzyme release, and superoxide generation in response to chemotactic peptides (O'Flaherty *et al.*, 1979; Smolen and Weissmann, 1980). These effects have been noted at high *in vitro* drug concentrations, far in excess of those necessary to inhibit cyclooxygenase and phospholipase A_2 activity. Indomethacin at high doses does interfere with chemotactic peptide binding to neutrophil surface receptors (Cost *et al.*,

Table 1. Drug Effects on Neutrophil Function

Drug	Effect
1. Glucocorticosteroids	Neutrophilia
	↓ Migration *in vivo*
	↓ Adherence
	↓ Nitroblue tetrazolium reduction
	Stabilization of lysosomes
	↓ Procoagulant activity
	Lipomodulin production
	Inhibition of phospholipase A_2
2. Nonsteroidal antiinflammatory agents	↓ Aggregation[a]
Indomethacin	↓ Lysosomal enzyme release[a]
	↓ Superoxide production[a]
	↓ Chemoattractant binding[a]
	↑ cAMP[a]
3. Antifungal agents	↓ Chemotaxis
Amphotericin B	↓ Phagocytosis
Nystatin	↓ Chemoattractant binding
4. Antitubulins	↓ Chemotaxis
Colchicine	
Vinblastine	
Vincristine	
5. Antibacterial agents	↓ Bactericidal activity
Aminoglycosides	↓ Phagocytosis
Doxycycline	
Tetracycline	
6. Sulfonamides	↓ Fungicidal activity
Sodium sulfadiazine	↓ Myeloperoxidase mediated
Sodium sulfacetamide	bacterial killing
Sulfathiazole	
Sulfisoxazole	
7. Gold compounds	↓ Phagocytic activity
Gold salts	↓ Superoxide production
Triethylphosphine gold	↓ Chemiluminescence

[a] Effect is at higher doses than those achievable therapeutically.

1981), which is probably a result of nonspecific hydrophobic interactions among the drug, the chemotactic peptide, and the receptor. High *in vitro* concentrations of indomethacin also cause increased cAMP levels in neutrophils (Mikulikova and Trnovsky, 1982). Since elevations in this nucleotide are known to inhibit various neutrophil functions, this has been postulated as a mechanism for indomethacin effects on neutrophil function *in vivo*. Piroxicam has been shown to inhibit chemotactic-peptide-induced superoxide anion generation and lysosomal enzyme secretion, whereas ibuprofen inhibits only enzyme secretion, leaving O_2^- production intact (Edelson *et al.*, 1982). It remains to be determined whether all of the antiinflammatory effects of the NSAIAs can be explained by inhibition of cyclooxygenase.

C. Antifungal Agents

Amphotericin B and nystatin are polyene antibiotics that bind to ergosterol in the plasma membrane of fungi, thus resulting in damage to the osmotic barrier and lysis of the organisms (Lampen, 1969; Andreoli, 1973). The extreme toxicity of these agents for humans lies in their ability to also bind cholesterol, an integral component of cell membranes. Amphotericin B and nystatin markedly decrease the chemotactic responsiveness of neutrophils *in vitro* at concentrations that are attainable by therapeutic regimens currently used to treat fungal disease in humans (Table 1) (Bjorksten *et al.*, 1976; Boxer *et al.*, 1981). This defect in chemotaxis is attributable to altered chemoattractant receptor activity on the surface of the neutrophil in the presence of the drugs (Lohr and Snyderman, 1982). Polyene antibiotics do not depress the ability of neutrophils to produce superoxide anion or to secrete lysozyme (Lohr and Snyderman, 1982; Snyderman, 1983), but several studies report decreased phagocytic activity in the presence of the drugs (Chan and Balish, 1978). Other antifungal agents including griseofulvin, 5-flucytosine, and miconazole have not been shown to inhibit human neutrophil function (Mandell, 1982).

D. Vinca Alkaloids and Colchicine

The vinca alkaloids vincristine and vinblastine as well as colchicine depress *in vitro* neutrophil chemotaxis but not migration *per se* (Table 1) (reviewed by Gallin *et al.*, 1978a). These agents disrupt or otherwise interfere with the microtubule function of neutrophils, which is required for sustained chemotactic migration. Therapeutic doses of colchicine for gout do not, however, depress neutrophil migration *in vivo* (Fordham *et al.*, 1981). *In vitro* colchicine treatment inhibits lysosomal enzyme release by stimulated neutrophils.

E. Antibacterial Agents

Aminoglycosides such as gentamicin, tetramycin, skomicin, amikacin, and ribostamycin inhibit the bactericidal activity of human neutrophils, with gentamicin being the most toxic (Table 1) (Ferrari *et al.*, 1980). Doxycycline, chlorotetracycline, and tetracycline hydrochloride all inhibit neutrophil phagocytic activity *in vitro,* and cells isolated from donors after oral deoxycycline and tetracycline likewise showed decreased phagocytic capacity (Forsgren *et al.*, 1974). Sulfonamides including sulfadiazine, sulfacetamide, sulfathiazole, and sulfisoxazole substantially reduce the ability of normal PMNs to kill strains of *Candida albicans* and *Candida tropicalis* (Lehrer, 1971). The sulfonamides also decrease bactericidal activity in cell-free systems containing purified myeloperoxidase, suggesting that those compounds directly affect this enzyme-mediated bactericidal response (Mandell, 1982). Interestingly, in contrast to normal PMNs, sulfisoxazole increases the bactericidal capacity of neutrophils from patients with chronic graunlomatous disease (CGD) (Johnston *et al.*, 1975b). The mechanism of this augmentation of abnormal bactericidal activity by sulfisoxazole in CGD remains unknown.

F. Gold Compounds

In vivo and *in vitro* studies have shown that gold salts inhibit the phagocytic activity of human neutrophils as well as monocytes and macrophages (Davis *et al.*, 1983). Triethylphosphine gold inhibits superoxide radical formation and chemiluminescence by human neutrophils (Davis *et al.*, 1983). At therapeutic concentrations, auranofin, a new oral gold compound, inhibits neutrophil chemotaxis, phagocytosis, secretion, and superoxide production (Hafstrom *et al.*, 1984).

V. ABNORMALITIES OF NEUTROPHIL FUNCTION

A. Clinical Aspects

Functional defects in neutrophil chemotaxis, lysosomal enzyme secretion and bactericidal activity occur in humans (Table 2). The predominant presenting symptoms associated with these defects are recurrent bacterial and/or fungal infections, most commonly with *Staphylococcus aureus* or *Hemophilus influenzae*. Recurrent cutaneous abscesses occur frequently, as do pneumonia, otitis media, bronchitis, and sinusitis. In patients with severe abnormalities of chemotaxis, the symptoms of infection resemble those of neutropenic individuals.

B. Disorders of Neutrophil Chemotaxis

Abnormalities in chemotactic factor production or chemotactic responsiveness of leukocytes can all be associated with abnormalities of the inflammatory response in certain human diseases.

1. Abnormalities of Humoral Factors That Result in Chemotactic Defects

The production of C5a is dependent on the activation of the classical and alternative complement pathways (Shin *et al.*, 1968; Snyderman *et al.*, 1968a,b). It has been demonstrated that an agammaglobulinemic individual had defective production of chemotactic activity by inflammatory stimuli (Steerman *et al.*, 1971; Gallin, 1975). Defective chemotactic factor production has also been noted in individuals with deficiencies of the complement system, including the components C2, C1r, C3, and C5 (Gewurz *et al.*, 1967; Miller and Nilsson, 1970; Rosenfield and Leddy, 1974; Alper *et al.*, 1970). Individuals with deficiencies of the early components (C1r or C2) have an increased incidence of inflammatory diseases manifested by dermatomyositis or systemic lupus ery-

Table 2. Abnormalities of Neutrophil Function

Function	Associated disease or condition
A. Chemotaxis	
1. Abnormal humoral factors	
Defects in recognition and chemoattractant production	Agammaglobulinemia
	C1r, C2, C3, C5 deficiencies
	C3b inactivator deficiency
Circulating inhibitors of chemoattractants	Hemodialysis
	Glomerulonephritis
	Hodgkin's disease
	Sarcoid
	Leprosy
	Cirrhosis
	Systemic lupus erythematosus
2. Cellular abnormalities	Rheumatoid arthritis
Cell-directed inhibitors	Bone marrow transplant
Intrinsic cellular defects	Chediak–Higashi syndrome
	Lazy-leukocyte syndrome
	Specific granule deficiency
	Kartagener's syndrome
	Glutathione synthetase deficiency
	Juvenile periodontitis
	Hyper-IgE syndrome
	Diabetes mellitus
	Actin dysfunction
B. Lysosomal degranulation	Chediak–Higashi syndrome
	Specific granule deficiency
	Thermal injury
C. Microbicidal activity	Chronic granulomatous disease
	Myeloperoxidase deficiency

thematosus (Gewurz *et al.*, 1967; Day *et al.*, 1972; Ruddy *et al.*, 1972). Not all individuals with C5 deficiencies have difficulties with severe recurrent infections, however. Snyderman *et al.*, (1979) identified a woman with recurrent *Neisserial* infections and C5 deficiency whose identical twin, likewise C5 deficient, was perfectly healthy. A functional deficiency of C3 produced by hypercatabolism of this component as a result of lack of C3b inactivator was found in a patient with severe recurrent infections (Alper *et al.*, 1970). Serum from this individual did not generate chemotactic activity *in vitro* because the activation of C3 is necessary for clevage of C5.

Several diseases have been associated with increased levels of circulating inhibitors of the chemoattractants, thereby producing functional chemotactic defects. The first humoral inhibitor of chemotactic factors was described by Gewurz *et al.* (1967), who demonstrated that the plasma from patients with glumerulonephritis contained a heat-labile inhibitor of chemotactic activity. This factor disappeared following renal transplantation or nephrectomy. Inhibitors of chemotactic factors have also been described in patients undergoing chronic hemodialysis (Goldblum *et al.*, 1979). Circulating inhibitors of chemotactic factors have also been described in other groups of patients who suffer from an increased incidence of infection, including those with Hodgkin's disease (Ward and Berenberg, 1974), sarcoidosis (Maderazo *et al.*, 1976), lepromatous leprosy (Ward *et al.*, 1976), or cirrhosis of the liver (Maderazo *et al.*, 1975). Several studies have shown that patients with systemic lupus erythematosus have an abnormality in the ability of their serum to generate C5a chemotactic activity (Clark *et al.*, 1974). Subsequent reports indicated that sera from patients with SLE contain an inhibitor of C5a chemotactic activity (Perez *et al.*, 1978).

2. Cell-Derived Inhibitors of Chemotaxis

Humoral substances that directly inhibit the chemotaxis of neutrophils have been described as being present in certain human disease states. The depressed chemotaxis that has been noted in some patients with rheumatoid arthritis has been attributed to rheumatoid factor–immunoglobulin complexes (Mowat and Baum, 1971; Kemp *et al.*, 1979; Hanlon *et al.*, 1980). A patient with recurrent infections and abnormal neutrophil chemotaxis has been described in whom an IgG inhibitor was found that bound directly to neutrophils and inactivated their motility response (Kramer *et al.*, 1980). Patients with bone marrow transplants have difficulties with bacterial and fungal infections. In a study involving 34 bone marrow recipients, it was found that a portion of these patients had decreased neutrophil chemotactic activity (Clark *et al.*, 1976). The presence of graft-versus-host syndrome and treatment with antithymocyte globulin correlated with the depressed chemotactic response. A circulating inhibitor of chemotaxis was found in the serum of these patients and was characterized as antithymocyte globulin, suggesting that the material contains antineutrophil antibody. Thus, treatment of graft-versus-host disease with antithymocyte globulin must be weighed against the potentially deleterious effects of this substance on neutrophil function.

3. Intrinsic Cellular Defects of the Chemotactic Response

An inherited abnormality of neutrophil adhesion has been described in a male child with recurrent bacterial infections (Crowley *et al.*, 1980). This defect was associated with the absence of 110,000-dalton protein that was normally present in the particulate fraction of neutrophils. Decreased levels of this protein were noted in the neutrophils of the patient's mother and sister but not father, suggesting an X-linked mode of genetic transmission. Abnormalities of cellular deformability have been shown to contribute to chemotactic defects in the "lazy-leukocyte" syndrome (Miller, 1979). This is a rare disease of children characterized by pronounced neutropenia, severe recurrent infections, periodontitis, and dermatitis. The cells of these individuals exhibit normal phagocytosis, and their sera generate normal amounts of chemotactic activity. Although the exact metabolic defect is currently unknown, the cells appear to lack the mechanisms for diapedesis, since the bone marrow of these patients contains normal amounts of mature neutrophils. Another familial syndrome characterized by a neutrophil chemotactic defect, icthyosis and recurrent infections, has been described by Miller *et al.* (1973). This condition differs from the lazy-leukocyte syndrome in that the patients are not neutropenic and the neutrophils exhibit normal random motility.

Neutrophil chemotactic defects stemming from abnormal microtubule assembly have been described in several diseases. The first is the Chediak–Higashi syndrome, which is a rare autosomal recessive disorder characterized by oculocutaneous albinism, severe recurrent infections, neutropenia, and giant lysosomal granules in all granule-containing cells (Clark and Kimball, 1971; Wolf *et al.*, 1972). Patients with Chediak–Higashi syndrome frequently develop a lymphomalike illness, which has been termed the accelerated phase of the disease. In addition to the chemotactic defect, neutrophils from these patients show decreased lysosomal enzyme release in response to phagocytic stimuli and delayed bactericidal activity (Padgett, 1967). The neutrophils display a concanavalin-A-induced membrane receptor-capping response that resembles that of normal cells following treatment with colchicine (Oliver *et al.*, 1975). From these studies, it was suggested that the primary defect in these cells was in the microtubule system. Ultrastructural studies reveal a decreased number of centriole-associated microtubules (Oliver, 1976), and more recently, Nath *et al.* (1982) demonstrated decreased tyrosylation of tubulin in the leukocytes of two brothers with Chediak–Higashi syndrome. In addition to the microtubular defect, abnormal membrane microviscosity (Haak *et al.*, 1979) and increased intracellular levels of cAMP (Boxer *et al.*, 1976) have been noted in the neutrophils from patients with this disease.

Another condition characterized by abnormal microtubule function is Kartagener's syndrome, an autosomal recessive disorder characterized by chronic sinusitis, nasal polyps, recurrent respiratory infections, situs inversus, and male infertility (Caleb *et al.*, 1977; Afzelius *et al.*, 1980). The latter problem stems from the immobility of spermatozoa, which has been attributed to the lack of dynein arms, a protein that binds microtubules to cilia and flagellae. Several groups have demonstrated a neutrophil chemotactic defect (Gallin *et al.*, 1980; Afzelius *et al.*, 1980) in patients with this disease, and Gallin *et al.* (1980) have noted a mild defect in hydrogen peroxide formation in the cells after stimulation with opsonized staphylococci. These investigators speculated that the chemotactic defect of the neutrophils in this disorder contributes to the recurrent infections.

Abnormal chemotaxis has been described in two other patients with microtubule defects. One of these individuals had a deficiency of glutathione synthetase, and it was postulated that reduced levels of glutathione lead to increased oxidative damage to microtubules (Boxer, 1980). A child with excessive numbers of microtubules in her neutrophils had very high levels of cGMP and was found to have a neutrophil chemotactic defect (Gallin *et al.*, 1978b). In addition, neutrophil adherence, bactericidal activity, and lymphocyte function were abnormal in this patient.

Neutrophil and monocyte chemotactic defects have also been described in patients who suffer from a syndrome characterized by dermatitis, coarse facial features, elevated serum IgE, and recurrent cold staphylococcal abscesses of the skin and lungs (Davis *et al.*, 1966; Buckley *et al.*, 1972; Hill and Quie, 1974; Snyderman *et al.*, 1977b; Gallin *et al.*, 1980, 1983; Donabedian and Gallin, 1983). The neutrophil chemotactic defect is not present in all patients with this syndrome and is variably present in other patients. For this reason, this defect may not be the cause of the recurrent infections. The mechanism of the chemotactic abnormality in this syndrome remains unclear. It does not appear that the IgE itself causes the defect since incubation of normal leukocytes with IgE does not depress chemotaxis. It has been suggested that histamine released by IgE-dependent mechanisms leads to the chemotactic defect, since this mediator does inhibit cell migration *in vitro* (Hill *et al.*, 1976). The role of increased IgE with subsequent histamine release must be questioned as being the cause of the chemotactic defect, since many other conditions characterized by increased levels of this immunoglobulin are not associated with chemotactic defects.

Defects in chemotaxis have been associated with both congenital and acquired defects of neutrophil-specific granules (Davis *et al.*, 1980; Breton-Gorius *et al.*, 1980; Gallin *et al.*, 1982). As discussed above, it has been postulated that release of specific granules in the presence of chemotactic agents provides new cell surface membrane chemoattractant receptors (Fletcher and Gallin, 1983; Fletcher *et al.*, 1982). This replenishment of receptors at the leading front of the migrating cell is thought to be necessary for preservation of chemoattractant gradient sensing along the surface of the neutrophil. A child with recurrent infections and a specific neutrophil granule deficiency characterized by absent intracellular lactoferrin and vitamin-B_{12}-binding proteins was found to have decreased PMN and monocyte accumulation into Rebuck skin windows (Gallin *et al.*, 1982). Chemotaxis to several chemoattractants *in vitro* was abnormal, and the patient's cells exhibited decreased binding of the peptide fMet-Leu-[^{3}H]Phe. In addition, the cells did not show the characteristic increase in cell surface receptors following treatment with secretagogues. Defects in neutrophil bactericidal activity, superoxide generation, and NBT reduction were also noted in this patient. Acquired neutrophil-specific granule deficiency has been noted in burn patients approximately 2 weeks following severe thermal injury (Davis *et al.*, 1980; Till, 1983). This is associated with a neutrophil chemotactic defect, impaired bacterial killing, elevated serum lysozyme levels, and correspondingly decreased neutrophil lysozyme levels. The onset of these neutrophil dysfunctions following thermal injury occurs at the same time that these patients have problems with severe infections.

Several groups have described abnormally increased chemotactic responsiveness in the neutrophils from patients with Behcet's syndrome (Fordham *et al.*, 1982). Phagocytic and adherent activities of the cells are not changed. The increased chemotactic response is most prominent in those patients with ocular involvement. Defective neutrophil chemotaxis has also been described in individuals with juvenile periodontal disease (Cianciola, 1977; Van Dyke *et al.*, 1980; Genco *et al.*, 1980). This defect, which is not encountered in patients with the adult form of the disease, is usually intrinsic to the cell, although circulating cell-directed inhibitors have been described in several patients (Lavine *et al.*, 1979). It appears that a genetic predisposition to the disease may exist in that unaffected family members of these individuals also have depressed chemotaxis (Genco *et al.*, 1980).

C. Defects in Lysosomal Degranulation

Stimulated lysosomal enzyme release is decreased in neutrophils from patients with Chediak–Higashi syndrome (Padgett, 1967) and the selective specific granule deficiencies (Davis *et al.*, 1980; Gallin *et al.*, 1982) described above. In addition, some patients with leukemia have been found to have a selective decrease in certain neutrophil granule populations (Klebanoff and Clark, 1978).

D. Defects in Microbicidal Activity

Defective microbicidal activity can result from decreased oxidative metabolism as seen in chronic granulomatous disease, granule dysfunction, or myeloperoxidase deficiency.

1. Chronic Granulomatous Disease

Chronic granulomatous disease is a rare disease of infants and children, the most common form of which exhibits X-linked genetic transmission (Janeway *et al.*, 1954; Quie *et al.*, 1968; Klebanoff and Clark, 1978; Gallin *et al.*, 1983). Variants of the disease occur as autosomal recessive disorders. Chronic granulomatous disease is characterized by severe, repeated infections with *Staphylococcus aureus,* certain gram-negative bacteria, and fungal pathogens, most commonly *Candida albicans* and *Aspergillus* strains. Chronic suppurative lymphadenitis is the most common feature of the disease, with stomatitis, conjunctivitis, persistent rhinitis, pneumonitis, and lung abscesses occurring frequently. Pathologicaly, the lesions are characterized by multiple abscesses, granulomas, and lipid-filled macrophages.

The pathogenesis of CGD is related to the inability of these patients' neutrophils to kill certain bacteria intracellularly (Quie *et al.*, 1968; Good *et al.*, 1968). Patients generally do not have problems with catalase-negative organisms such as streptococci and pneumococci, since the myeloperoxidase bacterial killing system is intact. In contrast to the killing defect, the chemotaxis and phagocytic activity of CGD neutrophils are normal (Bridges *et al.*, 1959; Snyderman *et al.*, 1975). Various molecular lesions of CGD neutrophils have been described to account for the microbial defect. These include leukocyte NADPH oxidase deficiency (Holmes and Good, 1972), glutathionine peroxidase deficiency (in the autosomal recessive form) (Holmes *et al.*, 1970), and an absence of cytochrome b_{245} (Segal *et al.*, 1983). In a recent multicenter evaluation of CGD in which 27 patients and their families were studied, it was found that cytochrome b_{245} was undetectable in all males with the X-linked form of the disease (Segal *et al.*, 1983). Heterozygous female relative carriers had reduced levels of the cytochrome. In contrast, all patients with a probable autosomal recessive inheritance of CGD had normal levels of cytochrome b in their neutrophils; however, it was nonfunctional. In these patients, no defect in the cytochrome itself could be detected by several criteria except that it did not undergo reduction on cellular stimulation. It was therefore speculated that the defect in the autosomal recessive form of the disease could be an as yet undetected abnormality of the activation system, the absence or malfunction of a proximal electron donor, or an abnormality in the cytochrome itself.

2. Myeloperoxidase Deficiency

Neutrophil myeloperoxidase deficiency has been described in both congenital and acquired forms. The congenital defect is thought to follow an autosomal recessive mode of inheritance, and patients with the disease commonly have increased infections with *Candida* or bacterial pathogens, although most are in good health (Grignaschi *et al.*, 1963). Neutrophils from these patients have decreased fungicidal and bactericidal activity, but in contrast to CGD neutrophils, there is no decrease in superoxide production or phagocytosis-induced NBT reduction (Klebanoff and Clark, 1978). Acquired myeloperoxidase deficiency has been noted in some patients with severe bacterial infections (Graham, 1920), acute myelogenous leukemia (Schmalzl *et al.*, 1970), and the blast crisis phase of granulocytic leukemia (Catovsky *et al.*, 1972).

REFERENCES

Afzelius, B. A., Ewetz, L., Palmblad, C., Jr., Uden, A. M., and Venizeros, N., 1980, Structure and function of neutrophil leukocytes from patients with the immotile-cilia syndrome, *Acta Med. Scand.* **208**:145–154.

Allison, F., Lancaster, M. G., and Crosthwaite, J. L., 1963, Studies on the pathogenesis of acute inflammation. V. An assessment of factors that influence *in vitro* the phagocytic and adhesive properties of leukocytes obtained from rabbit peritoneal exudates, *Am. J. Pathol.* **43**:775–795.

Alper, C. A., Abramson, N., Johnston, R. B., Jr., Jondl, J. H., and Rosen, F. S., 1970, Increased susceptibility to infection associated with abnormalities of complement-mediated functions and of the third component of complement (C3), *N. Engl. J. Med.* **282**:349–354.

Altman, L. C., Chassey, B., and Mackler, B. F., 1975, Physicochemical characterization of chemotactic lymphokines produced by human T and B lymphocytes, *J. Immunol.* **110**:18–21.

Anderson, D. C., Wible, L. J., Hughes, B. J., Smith, C. W., and Brinkley, B. R., 1982, Cytoplasmic microtubules in polymorphonuclear leukocytes: Effects of chemotactic stimulation and colchicine, *Cell* **31**:719–729.

Andreoli, T. E., 1973, On the anatomy of amphotericin B-cholesterol pores in lipid bilayer membranes, *Kidney Int.* **4**:337–345.

Aswanikumar, S., Corcoran, B., Schiffman, E., Day, A. R., Freer, R. J., Showell, H. J., and Pert, C. G., 1977, Demonstration of a receptor on rabbit neutrophils for chemotactic peptides, *Biochem. Biophys. Res. Commun.* **74**:810–817.

Babior, B. M., and Kipnis, R. S., 1977, Superoxide forming enzyme from human neutrophils: Evidence for a flavin requirement, *Blood* **50**:517–524.

Babior, B. M., Curnette, J. T., and McMurrich, B. J., 1976, The particulate superoxide-forming system from human neutrophils. Properties of the system and further evidence supporting its participation in the respiratory burst, *J. Clin. Invest.* **58**:989–996.

Baldridge, C. W., and Gerard, R. W., 1933, The extra respiration of phagocytosis, *Am. J. Physiol.* **103**:235–236.

Bar-Shavit, R., Kahn, G., and Wilner, G. D., 1983, Monocyte chemotaxis: Stimulation by specific exosite region in thrombin, *Science* **220**:728–731.

Bishop, C. R., Athens, J. W., and Boggs, D. R., 1968, Leukokinetic studies. XIII. A new-steady state kinetic evaluation of the mechanism of cortisone-induced granulocytosis, *J. Clin. Invest.* **47**:249–260.

Bjorksten, B., Ray, B., and Quie, P. G., 1976, Inhibition of human neutrophil chemotaxis and chemiluminescence by amphotericin B, *Infect. Immun.* **14**:315–320.

Blackwell, G. J., Carnuccio, R., DiRosa, M., Flower, R. J., Parente, L., and Persico, P., 1980, Macrocortin: A polypeptide causing the anti-phospholipase effect of glucocorticoids, *Nature* **287**:147–149.

Boggs, D. R., Athens, J. W., and Cartwright, G. E., 1964, The effect of adrenal glucocorticoids upon the cellular composition of inflammatory exudates, *Am. J. Pathol.* **44**:763–773.

Bokisch, V. A., Muller-Eberhard, H. J., and Cochrane, C. G., 1969, Isolation of a fragment (C3a) of the third component of human complement containing anaphylatoxin and chemotactic activity and description of an anaphylatoxin inactivator of human serum, *J. Exp. Med.* **129**:1109–1130.

Boucek, M. M., and Snyderman, R., 1976, Calcium influx requirement for human neutrophil chemotaxis: Inhibition by lanthanum chloride, *Science* **193**:905–907.

Boxer, L. A., 1980, Vitamin E and oxidant damage, *Ann. Intern. Med.* **93**:330–346.

Boxer, L., Hedley-Whyte, E. T., and Stossel, T. P., 1974, Neutrophil actin dysfunction and abnormal neutrophil behavior, *N. Engl. J. Med.* **291**:1093–1099.

Boxer, L. A., Wantanabe, A. M., Rister, M., Besch, H. R., Jr., Allen, J., and Baehner, R. L., 1976, Correction of leukocyte function in Chediak Higashi syndrome by ascorbate, *N. Engl. J. Med.* **295**:1041–1045.

Boxer, L. A., Ingraham, L. M., Allen, J., Oseas, R. S., and Baehner, R. C., 1981, Amphotericin B promotes leukocytes aggregation of nylon-wood-fiber-treated polymorphonuclear leukocytes, *Blood* **58**:518–525.

Boyden, S., 1962, The chemotactic effects of mixtures of antibody and antigen on polymorphonuclear leukocytes, *J. Exp. Med.* **115**:453–466.

Brennan, J. K., Lichtman, M. A., DiPersio, J. F., and Abboud, C. N., 1980, Chemical mediators of granulopoiesis: A review, *Exp. Hematol.* **8**:441–464.

Breton-Gorius, J., Mason, D. Y., Buriot, D., Vilde, J. L., and Griscelli, C., 1980, Lactoferrin deficiency as a consequence of a lack of specific granules in neutrophils from a patient with recurrent infections, *Am. J. Pathol.* **99**:413–428.

Bridges, R. A., Berendes, H., and Good, R. A., 1959, A fatal granulomatous disease of childhood: The clinical, pathological and laboratory features of a new syndrome, *J. Dis. Child.* **97**:387–408.

Buckley, R. H., Wrag, B. B., and Belmaker, E. Z., 1972, Extreme hyperimmunoglobulinemia E and undue susceptibility to infection, *Pediatrics* **49**:59–70.

Caleb, M., Lecks, H., South, M. A., and Norman, M. E., 1977, Kartagener's syndrome and abnormal cilia, *N. Engl. J. Med.* **297**:1012–1013.

Catovsky, D., Galton, D. A. G., and Robinson, J., 1972, Myeloperoxidase-deficient neutrophils in acute myeloid leukemia, *Scand. J. Hematol.* **9**:142–148.

Chan, C. K., and Balish, E., 1978, Inhibition of granulocyte phagocytosis of *Candida albicans* by amphotericin B, *Can. J. Microbiol.* **24**:363–364.

Chenoweth, D. E., and Hugli, T. E., 1980, Human C5a and C5a analogs as probes of the neutrophil C5a receptor, *Mol. Immunol.* **17**:151–161.

Chretien, J. H., and Garagusi, V. F., 1971, Suppressed reduction of nitroblue tetrazolium by polymorphonuclear neutrophils from patients receiving steroids, *Experientia* **27**:1343.

Cianciola, L. J., Genco, R. J., Patters, M. J., McKenna, J., and Van Oss, C. J., 1977, Defective polymorphonuclear leukocyte function in human periodontal disease, *Nature* **265**:445–449.

Clark, R. A., and Kimball, H. R., 1971, Defective granulocyte chemotaxis in the Chediak–Higashi syndrome, *J. Clin. Invest.* **50**:2645–2652.

Clark, R. A., Kimball, H. R., and Decker, J. L., 1974, Neutrohil chemotaxis in systemic lupus erythematosus, *J. Clin. Invest.* **33**:167–172.

Clark, R. A., Johnson, F. L., and Klebanoff, S. J., 1976, Defective neutrophil chemotaxis in bone marrow transplant patients, *J. Clin. Invest.* **58**:22–31.

Cline, M. J., 1975, *The White Cell*, Harvard University Press, Cambridge.

Cline, M. J., and Golde, D. W., 1979, Cellular interactions in hematopoiesis, *Nature* **277**:177–179.

Cohen, S., Pick, E., and Oppenheim, J. J., 1979, *Biology of the Lymphokines*, Academic Press, New York.

Cost, H., Gospach, C., and Abita, J. P., 1981, Effect of indomethacin on the binding of the chemotactic peptide formyl-Met-Leu-Phe on human polymorphonuclear leukocytes, *FEBS Lett.* **132**:85–88.

Crowley, C. A., Curnutte, J. T., Rosin, R. E., Andre-Schwartz, J., Gallin, J. I., Klempner, M., Snyderman, R., Southwick, F. S., Stossel, T. P., and Babior, B. M., 1980, An inherited abnormality of neutrophil adhesion, its genetic transmission and its association with a missing protein, *N. Engl. J. Med.* **302**: 1163–1168.

Cunningham, C. C., DeChatelet, L. R., Spach, P. I., Parce, W., Thomas, M. J., Lees, C. J., and Shirley, P. S., 1982, Identification and quantification of electron transport components in human polymorphonuclear neutrophils, *Biochim. Biophys. Acta* **682**:430–435.

Dale, D. C., Fauci, A. S., and Wolff, S. M., 1974, Alternate day prednisone: Leukocyte kinetics and susceptibility to infections, *N. Engl. J. Med.* **291**:1154–1158.

Danon, A., and Assouline, G., 1978, Inhibition of prostaglandin biosynthesis by corticosteroids requires RNA and protein synthesis, *Nature* **273**:552–554.

Davis, J. M., Dineen, P., and Gallin, J. I., 1980, Neutrophil degranulation and abnormal chemotaxis after thermal injury, *J. Immunol.* **124**:1467–1471.

Davis, P., Johnson, C., Miller, C. L., and Wong, K., 1983, Effects of gold compounds on the function of phagocytic cells: II. Inhibition of superoxide radical generation by tripeptide-activated polymorphonuclear leukocytes, *Arthritis Rheum.* **26**:82–86.

Davis, S. D., Schaller, J., and Wedgewood, R. J., 1966, Job's syndrome: Recurrent "cold," staphylococcal abscesses, *Lancet* **1**:1013–1015.

Day, N. K., Geiger, H., Stroud, R., DeBrocco, M., Mancadq, B., Windhorst, D., and Good, R. A., 1972, C1r deficiency: An unborn error associated with cutaneous anergy and renal disease, *J. Clin. Invest.* **51**:1102–1108.

DeChatelet, L. R., Cooper, M. R., and McCall, C. E., 1971, Dissociation by colchicine of the hexose monophosphate shunt activation from the bactericidal activity of the leukocyte, *Infect. Immun.* **3**:66–72.

Deuel, T. F., Senior, R. M., Chang, D., Griffin, G. L., Heinrikson, R. L., and Kaiser, E. T., 1981, Platelet factor 4 is chemotactic for neutrophils and monocytes, *Proc. Natl. Acad. Sci. U.S.A.* **78**:4584–4587.

Deuel, T. F., Senior, R. M., Huang, J. S., and Griffin, G. L., 1982, Chemotaxis of monocytes and neutrophils to platelet derived growth factor, *J. Clin. Invest.* **69**:1046–1049.

Dillard, G. M., and Bodel, P., 1970, Studies on steroid fever II. Pyrogenic and anti-pyrogenic activity *in vitro* of some endogenous steroids of man, *J. Clin. Invest.* **49**:2418–2426.

Donabedian, H., and Gallin, J. I., 1983, The hyperimmunoglobulin E recurrent infection (Job's) syndrome. A review of the NIH experience and the literature, *Medicine* **62**:195–208.

Ebert, R. H., and Barclay, W. R., 1952, Changes in connective tissue reactions induced by cortisone, *Ann. Intern. Med.* **37**:506–518.

Edelson, H. S., Kaplan, H. B., Korchak, H. M., and Weissmann, G., 1982, Differing effects of nonsteroidal anti-inflammatory agents (NSAIA) on neutrophil functions, *Clin. Res.* **30**:469A.

Fauci, A. S., Dale, D. C., and Balow, J. E., 1976, Glucocorticoid therapy: Mechanisms of action and clinical considerations, *Ann. Intern. Med.* **84**:304–315.

Fernandez, H. N., and Hugli, T. E., 1976, Partial characterization of human C5a anaphylatoxin. I. Chemical description of the carbohydrate and polypeptide portions of human C5a, *J. Immunol.* **177**:1688–1694.

Fernandez, H. N., Henson, P. M., Otani, A., and Hugli, T. E., 1978, Chemotactic response to human C3a and C5a anaphylatoxins: I. Evaluation of C3a and C5a leukotaxis *in vitro* and under stimulated *in vivo* conditions, *J. Immunol.* **120**:109–115.

Ferrari, F. A., Pagani, A., Marconi, M., Stefanoni, R., and Siccardi, A. G., 1980, Inhibition of candidacidal activity of human neutrophil leukocytes by aminoglycoside antibiotics, *Agents Chemother.* **17**:87–88.

Fletcher, M. P., and Gallin, J. I., 1980, Degranulating stimuli increase the availability of receptors on human neutrophils for the chemoattractant fMet-Leu-Phe, *J. Immunol.* **124**:1585–1588.

Fletcher, M. P., and Gallin, J. I., 1983, Human neutrophils contain an intracellular pool of putative receptors for the chemoattractant N-formylmethionylleucylphenylalanine, *Blood* **62**:792–799.

Fletcher, M. P., Seligmann, B. E., and Gallin, J. I., 1982, Correlation of human neutrophil secretion, chemoattractant receptor mobilization and enhanced functional capacity, *J. Immunol.* **128**:941–948.

Floman, Y., and Zor, U., 1976, Mechanism of steroid action in inflammation: Inhibition of prostaglandin synthesis and release, *Prostaglandins* **12**:403–413.

Fordham, J. N., Kirwan, J., Cason, J., and Currey, H. L. F., 1981, Prolonged reduction in polymorphonuclear adhesion following oral colchicine, *Ann. Rheum. Dis.* **40**:605–608.

Fordham, R. N., Davies, P. G., Kirk, A., and Cuney, H. L. F., 1982, Polymorphonuclear leukocyte function in Bechet's syndrome, *Ann. Rheum. Dis.* **41**:421–425.

Ford-Hutchinson, A. W., Bray, M. A., Doig, M. V., Shipley, M. E., and Smith, M. J. H., 1980, Leukotriene B_4, a potent chemokinetic and aggregating substance released from polymorphonuclear leukocytes, *Nature* **286**:264–265.

Ford-Hutchinson, A. W., Bray, F. M., Cunningham, F. M., Davidson, E. M., and Smith, M. J. H., 1981, Isomers of leukotriene B_4 possess different biological potencies, *Prostaglandins* **21**:143–161.

Forsgren, A., and Quie, P. G., 1974, Effects of staphyloccocal protein A on heat-labile opsonins, *J. Immunol.* **112**:1177–1180.

Forsgren, A., Schmeling, D., and Quie, P. G., 1974, Effect of tetracycline on the phagocytic function of human leukocytes, *J. Infect. Dis.* **130**:412–415.

Fridovich, I., 1972, Superoxide radical and superoxide dismutase, *Accts. Chem. Res.* **5**:321–326.

Gallin, J. I., 1975, Abnormal chemotaxis: Cellular and humoral components, in: *The Phagocytic Cell in Host Resistance* (J. A. Bellanti and D. H. Dayton, eds.), Raven Press, New York, pp. 227–248.

Gallin, J. I., and Quie, P. G., 1978, *Leukocyte Chemotaxis: Methods, Physiology and Clinical Implications*, Raven Press, New York.

Gallin, J. I., and Rosenthal, A. S., 1974, The regulatory role of divalent cations in human granulocyte chemotaxis: Evidence for an association between calcium exchanges and microtubule assembly, *J. Cell. Biol.* **62**:594–609.

Gallin, J. I., Gallin, E. K., Malech, H. L., and Cramer, E. B., 1978a, Structural and ionic events during leukocyte chemotaxis, in: *Leukocyte Chemotaxis* (J. I. Gallin and P. G. Quie, eds.), Raven Press, New York, pp. 123–141.

Gallin, J. I., Malech, H. L., Wright, D. G., Whisnant, J. K., and Kirkpatrick, C. H., 1978b, Recurrent severe infections in a child with abnormal leukocyte function: Possible relationship to increased microtubule assembly, *Blood* **51**:919–933.

Gallin, J. I., Wright, D. G., and Schiffmann, E., 1978c, Role of secretory events in modulating human neutrophil chemotaxis, *J. Clin. Invest.* **62**:1364–1374.

Gallin, J. I., Wright, D. G., Malech, H. L., Davis, J. M., Klempner, M. S., and Kirkpatrick, C. H., 1980, Disorders of phagocyte chemotaxis, *Ann. Intern. Med.* **92**:520–538.

Gallin, J. I., Fletcher, M. P., Seligmann, B. E., Hoffstein, S., Cehrs, K., and Mounessa, N., 1982, Human neutrophil-specific granule deficiency: A model to assess the role of neutrophil-specific granules in the evolution of the inflammatory response, *Blood* **59**:1317–1329.

Gallin, J. I., Buescher, E. S., Seligmann, B. E., Nath, J., Gaither, T., and Katz, P., 1983, Recent advances in chronic granulomatous disease, *Ann. Intern. Med.* **99**:657–674.

Genco, R. J., Van Dyke, T. E., Park, B., Ciminelli, M., and Horoszewicz, H., 1980, Neutrophil chemotaxis impairment in juvenile periodontitis: Evaluation of specificity adherence, deformability and serum factors, *J. Reticuloendothel. Soc.* **28**:81s–91s.

Gewurz, H. A., Page, A. R., Pickering, R. J., and Good, R. A., 1967, Complement activity and neutrophil exudation in man. Studies in patients with glomerulonephritis, essential hypocomplementemia and agammaglobulinemia, *Int. Arch. Allergy Appl. Immunol.* **32**:64–90.

Goetzl, E. J., and Pickett, W. C., 1980, The human PMN leukocyte chemotactic activity of complex hydroxyeicosatetraenoic acids (HETES), *J. Immunol.* **125**:1789–1791.

Goldblum, S. E., Van Epps, D. E., and Reed, W. P., 1979, Serum inhibitor of C5 fragment-mediated polymorphonuclear leukocyte chemotaxis associated with chronic hemodialysis, *J. Clin. Invest.* **64**:255–264.

Golde, D. W., 1982, Development and morphology of granulocytes and macrophages, in: *Cecil Textbook of Medicine* (J. B. Wyngaarden and L. H. Smith, eds.), W. B. Saunders, Philadelphia, pp. 902–905.

Goldman, D. W., and Goetzl, E. J., 1982, Specific binding of leukotriene B_4 to receptors on human polymorphonuclear leukocytes, *J. Immunol.* **129**:1600–1604.

Goldman, D. W., and Goetzl, G. J., 1984, Heterogeneity of human polymorphonuclear leukocyte receptors for leukotriene B_4. Identification of a subset of high affinity receptors that transduce the chemotactic response, *J. Exp. Med.* **159**:1027–1041.

Goldstein, I., Hoffstein, S., Gallin, J., and Weissmann, G., 1973, Mechanisms of lysosomal enzyme release from human leukocytes: Microtubule assembly and membrane fusion induced by a component of complement, *Proc. Natl. Acad. Sci. U.S.A.* **70**:2916–2920.

Good, R. A., Quie, P. G., Windhorst, D. B., Page, A. R., Rodey, G. E., White, J., Wolfson, J. J., and Holmes, B. H., 1968, Fatal chronic granulomatous disease of childhood: A hereditary defect of leukocyte function, *Semin. Hematol.* **5**:215–254.

Graham, G. S., 1920, The neutrophilic granules of the circulating blood in health and in disease. A preliminary report, *N.Y. State J. Med.* **20**:46–55.

Grignaschi, V. I., Sporperato, A. M., Etcheverry, M. J., and Macario, A. J. L., 1963, Un neuvo cuadro cito quimico: Negatividad. Ispontanea de las reacciones de peroxidasas, oxidasas y lipido en la progenie neutrofike y en los monacitos de dos hermanos, *Rev. Assoc. Med. Argent.* **77**:218–221.

Haak, R. A., Ingraham, L. M., Baehner, R. L., and Boxer, L. A., 1979, Membrane fluidity in human and mouse Chediak–Higashi leukocytes, *J. Clin. Invest.* **64**:138–144.

Hafstrom, I., Seligmann, B. E., Friedman, M. M., and Gallin, J. I., 1984, Auranofin affects early events in human polymorphonuclear neutrophil activation by receptor mediated stimuli, *J. Immunol.* **132**:2007–2014.

Hanlon, S. M., Panagi, G. S., and Laurent, R., 1980, Defective polymorphonuclear leukocyte chemotaxis in rheumatoid arthritis associated with serum inhibitor, *Ann. Rheum. Dis.* **39**:68–74.

Hartwig, J. H., and Stossel, T. P., 1976, Interactions of actin, myosin and an actin binding protein of rabbit pulmonary macrophages. III. Effects of cytochalasin B, *J. Cell. Biol.* **71**:295–303.

Henson, D., DeChatelet, L. R., Spitznagel, J. K., and Wang, P., 1977, Comparison of NADH and NADPH oxidase activities in granules isolated from human polymorphonuclear leukocytes with a fluorimetric assay, *J. Clin. Invest.* **59**:282–288.

Henson, P. M., 1976, Membrane receptors on neutrophils, *Immunol. Commun.* **5**:757–774.

Hill, H. R., and Quie, P. G., 1974, Raised serum IgE levels and defective neutrophil chemotaxis in three children with eczema and recurrent bacterial infections, *Lancet* **1**:183–187.

Hill, H. R., Estensen, R. D., Hogan, N. A., and Quie, P. G., 1976, Severe staphylococcal disease associated with allergic manifestations, hyperimmunoglobulinemia E and defective neutrophil chemotaxis, *J. Lab. Clin. Med.* **88**:796–806.

Hirata, F., Schiffmann, E., Venkatasubramanian, K., Solomon, B., and Axelrod, J., Jr., 1980, A phospholipase A_2 inhibitory protein in rabbit neutrophils induced by glucocorticoids, *Proc. Natl. Acad. Sci. U.S.A.* **77**:2533–2536.

Hirsch, J. G., and Church, A. B., 1960, Studies of phagocytosis of group A streptocci by polymorphonuclear leukocytes *in vitro, J. Exp. Med.* **111**:309–322.

Hirsh, J. G., and Church, A. B., 1961, Adrenal steroids and infection: The effect of cortisone administration on polymorphonuclear leukocyte functions and on serum opsonins and bactericidins, *J. Clin. Invest.* **40**:794–798.

Hoffstein, S. T., Friedman, R. S., and Weissmann, G., 1982, Degranulation, membrane addition, and shape change during chemotactic factor-induced aggregation of human neutrophils, *J. Cell. Biol.* **95**:234–241.

Holmes, B., and Good, R. A., 1972, Metabolic and functional abnormalities of human neutrophils, in: *Phagocytic Mechanisms in Health and Disease* (B. Williams and H. Fudenberg, eds.), Intercontinental Medical Book Corporation, New York, pp. 51–66.

Holmes, B., Park, B. H., Malawista, S. E., Quie, P. G., Nelson, D. L., and Good, R. A., 1970, Chronic granulomatous disease in females. A deficiency of leukocyte glutathione peroxidase, *N. Engl. J. Med.* **283**:217–221.

Hong, S. C. L., and Levine, L., 1976, Inhibition of arachidonic acid release from cells as the biochemical action of anti-inflammatory corticosteroids, *Proc. Natl. Acad. Sci. U.S.A.* **73**:1730–1734.

Huber, H., Pulley, M. J., Linscott, W. D., Fudenberg, H. H., and Muller-Eberhard, H. J., 1968, Human monocytes: Distinct receptor sites for the third component of complement and for immunoglobulin G, *Science* **162**:1281–1283.

Hugli, T. E., and Muller-Eberhard, H. J., 1978, Anaphylatoxins, *Adv. Immunol.* **26**:1–53.

Iyer, G. Y. N., Islam, D. M. F., and Quaster, J. H., 1961, Biochemical aspects of phagocytosis, *Nature* **192**:535–541.

Janeway, C. A., Craig, J., Davidson, M., Downey, W., Gitlin, D., and Sullivan, J. C., 1954, Hypergammaglobulinemia associated with severe recurrent and chronic nonspecific infection, *Am. J. Dis. Child.* **88**:388–389.

Jensen, J., Snyderman, R., and Mergenhagen, S. E., 1969, Chemotactic activity: a property of guinea pig C5 anaphylatoxin, in: *Cellular and Humoral Mechanisms in Anaphylaxis and Allergy,* S. Karger, Basel, pp. 265–278.

Johnston, R. B., Jr., Klemperer, M. R., Alper, C. A., and Rosen, F. S., 1969, The enhancement of bacterial phagocytosis by serum. The role of complement components and two cofactors, *J. Exp. Med.* **129**:1275–1290.

Johnston, R. B., Jr., Keele, B. B., Jr., Misra, H. P., Lehmeyer, J. E., Webb, L. S., Baehner, R. L., and Rajagopalan, K. V., 1975a, The role of superoxide anion generation in phagocytic bactericidal activity. Studies with normal and chronic granulomatous disease leukocytes, *J. Clin. Invest.* **55**:1357–1372.

Johnston, R. B., Jr., Wilfert, C. M., Buckley, R. H., Webb, L. S., DeChatelet, L. R., and McCall, C. E., 1975b, Enhanced bactericidal activity of phagocytes from patients with chronic granulomatous disease in the presence of sulphisoxazole, *Lancet* **1**:824–827.

Kaplan, A. P., Kay, A. B., and Austen, K. F., 1972, A prealbumin activator of prekallekrein III. Appearance of chemotactic activity for human neutrophils by the conversion of prekallekrein, *J. Exp. Med.* **135**:81–97.

Keller, H. U., and Sorkin, E., 1967, Studies on chemotaxis V. On the chemotactic effect of bacteria, *Int. Arch. Allergy Appl. Immunol.* **31**:505–517.

Kemp, A. S., Roberts-Thompson, P., Nooh, S. H., and Brown, S., 1979, Inhibition of neutrophil migration by sera from patients with rheumatoid arthritis, *Clin. Exp. Immunol.* **36**:423–429.

Klebanoff, S. J., 1967a, A peroxidase mediated antimicrobial system in leukocytes, *J. Clin. Invest.* **46**:1078–1083.

Klebanoff, S. J., 1967b, Iodination of bacteria: A bactericidal mechanism, *J. Exp. Med.* **126**:1063–1078.

Klebanoff, S. J., 1968, Myeloperoxidase–halide–hydrogen peroxide anti-bacterial system, *J. Bacteriol.* **95**:2131–2138.

Klebanoff, S. J., 1971, Intraleukocytic microbicidal defects, *Annu. Rev. Med.* **22**:39–62.

Klebanoff, S. J., 1972, Relationship of metabolism to function in the polymorphonuclear leukocyte, in: *The Molecular Basis of Electron Transport* (D. Schultz and K. Cameron, eds.), Academic Press, New York, pp. 275–295.

Klebanoff, S. J., 1975, Antimicrobial mechanisms in neutrophilic polymorphonuclear leukocytes, *Semin. Hematol.* **12:**117–142.

Klebanoff, S. J., and Clark, R. A., 1978, *The Neutrophil; Function and Clinical Disorders,* North-Holland, Amsterdam.

Koo, C., Lefkowitz, R. J., and Snyderman, R., 1982, The oligopeptide chemotactic factor receptor on human polymorphonuclear leukocyte membranes exists in two affinity states, *Biochem. Biophys. Res. Commun.* **106:**442–449.

Koo, C., Lefkowitz, R. J., and Snyderman, R., 1983, Guanine nucleotides modulate the binding affinity of the oligopeptide chemoattractant receptor on human polymorphonuclear leukocytes, *J. Clin. Invest.* **72:**748–753.

Kozel, T. R., 1977, Non-encapsulated variant of *Cryptococcus neoformans.* II. Surface receptors for cryptococcal polysaccharide and their role in inhibition of phagocytosis by polysaccharide, *Infect. Immun.* **16:**99–106.

Kraft, A. S., and Anderson, W. B., 1983, Phorbol esters increase the amount of Ca^{+2}· phospholipid-dependent protein kinase associated with plasma membrane, *Nature* **301:**621–623.

Kramer, N., Perez, H. D., and Goldstein, I. M., 1980, An immunoglobulin (Ig6) inhibitor of polymorphonuclear leukocyte mobility in a patient with recurrent infection. *N. Engl. J. Med.* **27:**1253–1258.

Kreisle, R. A., and Parker, C. W., 1982, Specific binding of leukotriene B_4 to a receptor on human polymorphonuclear leukocytes, *J. Exp. Med.* **157:**628–641.

Kuehl, F. A., Jr., and Egan, R. W., 1980, Prostaglandins, arachidonic acid and inflammation, *Science* **210:**978–984.

Lampen, J. O., 1969, Amphotericin B and other polyenic antifungal antibiotics, *Am. J. Clin. Pathol.* **52:**138–146.

Lapetina, E., 1984, Prostacyclin inhibition of phosphatidic acid synthesis in human platelets is not mediated by protein kinase C, *Biochem. Biophys. Res. Commun.* **120:**37–44.

Lavine, W. S., Maderazo, E. G., Stolman, J., Ward, P. A., Cogen, R. B., Greenblatt, I., and Robertson, P. B., 1979, Impaired neutrophil chemotaxis in patients with juvenile and rapidly progressing periodontitis, *J. Periodont. Res.* **14:**10–19.

Leber, T., 1888, Uber die Entstehung der Entzundung und die Wirkung dur entzundungerregenden Schadlichkeiten, *Forsch. Med.* **4:**460.

Lehmeyer, J. E., Snyderman, R., and Johnston, R. B., Jr., 1979, Stimulation of neutrophil oxidative metabolism by chemotactic peptides: Influence of calcium ion concentration and cytochalasin B and comparison with stimulation by phorbol myristate acetate, *Blood* **54:**35–39.

Lehrer, R. I., 1971, Inhibition by sulfonamides of the candidacidal activity of human neutrophils, *J. Clin. Invest.* **50:**2498–2505.

Lerner, E. M. II, 1956, Phagocytosis of bacteria in the absence of antibody and the effect of physical surface. A reinvestigation of surface "phagocytosis," *J. Exp. Med.* **104:**233–243.

LoBuglio, A. F., Cotran, R. S., and Jande, J. H., 1967, Red cells coated with immunoglobulin G: Binding and sphering of mononuclear cells in man, *Science* **158:**1582–1585.

Lockwood, W. R., and Allison, F., 1963, Electronmicrographic studies of phagocytic cells I. Morphological changes of the cytoplasm and granules of rabbit granulocytes associated with ingestion of rough pneumococcus, *Br. J. Exp. Pathol.* **44:**593–600.

Lohr, K. M., and Snyderman, R., 1982, Amphotericin B alters the affinity and functional activity of the oligopeptide chemotactic factor receptor on human polymorphonuclear leukocytes, *J. Immunol.* **129:**1594–1599.

Maderazo, E., Ward, P. A., and Quintiliani, R., 1975, Defective regulation of chemotaxis in cirrhosis, *J. Lab. Clin. Med.* **85:**621–630.

Maderazo, E., Ward, P. A., Woronick, C. L., Kubik, J., and DeGraff, A. C., Jr., 1976, Leukotactic dysfunction in sarcoidosis, *Ann. Intern. Med.* **84:**414–419.

Malawista, S. E., 1971, Vinblastine: Colchicine like effects on human blood leukocytes during phagocytosis, *Blood* **37:**519–529.

Malawista, S. E., Gee, J. B. L., and Bensch, K. G., 1971, Cytochalasin B reversibly inhibits phagocytosis: Functional, metabolic and ultrastructural effects in human blood leukocytes and rabbit alveolar macrophages, *Yale J. Biol. Med.* **44:**286–300.

Mandell, G. L., Rubin, W., and Hock, E. W., 1970, The effect of a NADH oxidase inhibitor (hydrocortisone) on polmorphonuclear leukocyte bactericidal activity. *J. Clin. Invest.* **49:**1381–1388.

Mandell, L. A., 1982, Effects of antimicrobial and antineoplastic drugs on the phagocytic and microbicidal function of the polymorphonuclear leukocyte, *Rev. Infect. Dis.* **4:**683–697.

Marasco, W. A., Krutzsch, H., Showell, H. J., Feltner, D. E., Nairn, R., Becker, E. L., and Ward, P. A., 1983, Purification and identification of formyl-methionyl-leucyl-phenylalanine as the major peptide neutrophil chemotactic factor produced by *E. coli.*, in: *Satellite Symposium of the 5th International Congress of Immunological Sciences.*
McKenzie, R., Pepper, D. S., and Kay, A. B., 1975, The generation of chemotactic activity for human leukocytes by the action of plasmin on human fibronogen, *Throm. Res.* **6**:1–8.
McPhail, L., and Snyderman, R., 1984, Direct activation of protein kinase C in human polymorphonuclear leukocytes by arachidonic acid, *Science* **224**:622–625.
McPhail, L. C., DeChatelet, L. R., and Shirley, P. S., 1976, Further characterization of NADPH oxidase activity of human polymorphonuclear leukocytes, *J. Clin. Invest.* **58**:774–780.
McPhail, L., Wolfson, M., Clayton, C., and Snyderman, R., 1984, Protein kinase C and neutrophil activation: Differential effects of chemoattractants and phorbol myristate acetate, *Fed. Proc.* **43**:1661.
Metchnikoff, E., 1891, Lecture on phagocytosis and immunity, *Br. Med. J.* **1**:213–217.
Mikulikova, D., and Trnovsky, K., 1982, The effect of indomethacin and its ester on lysosomal enzyme release from polymorphonuclear leukocytes and intracellular levels of cAMP and cGMP after phagocytosis of urate crystals, *Biochem. Pharmacol.* **31**:460–463.
Miller, M. E., 1979, Cell elastimetry in the study of normal and abnormal movement of human neutrophils, *Clin. Immunol. Immunopathol.* **14**:502–510.
Miller, M. E., and Nilsson, U. F., 1970, A familial deficiency of the phagocytosis-enhancing activity of serum related to a dysfunction of the fifth component of complement (C5), *N. Engl. J. Med.* **282**:354–358.
Miller, M. E., Norman, M. G., Klobenzer, P. J., and Schonauer, T., 1973, A new familial defect of neutrophil movement, *J. Lab. Clin. Med.* **82**:1–8.
Mowat, A. G., and Baum, J., 1971, Chemotaxis of polymorphonuclear leukocytes from patients with rheumatoid arthritis, *J. Clin. Invest.* **50**:2541–2549.
Muhlfelder, T. W., Niemetz, J., and Kang, S., 1982, Glucocorticoids inhibit the generation of leukocyte procoagulant (tissue factor) activity, *Blood* **60**:1169–1172.
Myers, M. A., McPhail, L. C., and Snyderman, R., 1984, Protein kinase C activity in human lymphocytes and monocytes: Phorbol myristate acetate stimulation shifts activity from cytosol to membrane components, *Clin. Res.* **32**:353A.
Naccache, P. H., Showell, H. J., Becker, E. L., and Sha'afi, R. I., 1977, Transport of sodium, potassium, and calcium across rabbit polymorphonuclear leukocyte membranes: Effect of chemotactic factor, *J. Cell. Biol.* **73**:428–444.
Nath, J., Flavin, M., and Gallin, J. I., 1982, Tubulin tyrosinolation in human polymorphonuclear leukocytes: Studies in normal subjects and in patients with the Chediak–Higashi syndrome, *J. Cell Biol.* **95**:519–526.
Nelson, D. S., 1965, Immune adherence, *Ciba Found. Symp.* pp. 222–241.
Niedel, J. E., Kahane, I., and Cuatrecasas, P., 1979, Receptor-mediated uptake and degradation of ^{125}I chemotactic peptide by human neutrophils, *J. Biol. Chem.* **254**:10700–10706.
Nishizuka, Y., 1984, The role of protein kinase C in cell surface signal transduction and tumor promotion, *Nature* **308**:693–698.
O'Dea, B. F., Viveros, O. H., Aswanikumar, S., Schiffmann, E., Chang, P. K., Cantoni, G. L., and Axelrod, J., 1978, A protein carboxymethylation stimulated by chemotactic peptides in leukocytes, *Fed. Proc.* **37**:1656.
O'Flaherty, J. T., Showell, H. J., Becker, E. L., and Ward, P. A., 1979, Role of arachidonic acid derivatives in neutrophil aggregation: A hypothesis, *Prostaglandins* **17**:915–927.
Ohsaka, S., and Deguchi, T., 1981, Stimulation of phosphatidic acid of calcium influx and cyclic GMP synthesis in neuroblastoma cells, *J. Biol. Chem.* **256**:10945–10948.
Okamura, N., Ishibashi, S., and Takano, T., 1979, Evidence for bactericidal activity of polymorphonuclear leukocytes without phagocytosis, *J. Biochem.* **86**:469–475.
Oliver, J. M., 1976, Impaired microtubule function correctable by cyclic GMP and cholinergic agonists in the Chediak Higashi syndrome, *Am. J. Pathol.* **85**:395–418.
Oliver, J. M., Zurier, R. B., and Berlin, R. D., 1975, Concanavalin A cap formation on polymorphonuclear leukocytes of normal and beige (Chediak–Higashi) mice, *Nature* **253**:471–473.
Padgett, G. A., 1967, Neutrophilic function in animals with the Chediak–Higashi syndrome, *Blood* **29**:906–915.
Perez, H. D., Lipton, M., and Goldstein, I. M., 1978, A specific inhibitor of complement (C5)-derived chemotactic activity in serum from patients with systemic lupus erythematosus, *J. Clin. Invest.* **62**:29–38.

Persellin, R. H., and Ku, L. C., 1974, Effects of steroid hormones on human polymorphonuclear leukocyte lysosomes, *J. Clin. Invest.* **54**:919–925.

Pfeffer, W., 1884, Locomotorische Richtungsbewegungen durch Chemische Reize, *Untersuch. Bot. Inst. Tubingen* **1**:363.

Pike, M. C., and Snyderman, R., 1980, Lipid requirements for leukocyte chemotaxis and phagocytosis: Effects of inhibitors of phospholipid and cholesterol synthesis, *J. Immunol.* **124**:1963–1969.

Pike, M. C., and Snyderman, R., 1981a, Alterations of new methylated phospholipid synthesis in the plasma membranes of macrophages exposed to chemoattractants, *J. Cell. Biol.* **91**:221–226.

Pike, M. C., and Snyderman, R., 1981b, Transmethylation reactions are required for initial morphologic and biochemical responses of human monocytes to chemoattractants, *J. Immunol.* **127**:1444–1449.

Pike, M. C., and Snyderman R., 1982a, Transmethylation reactions regulate affinity and functional activity of chemotactic factor receptors on macrophages, *Cell* **28**:107–114.

Pike, M. C., and Snyderman, R., 1982b, Chemoattractant–receptor interactions in leukocytes, in: *Advances in Inflammation Research,* Vol. 4 (G. Weissmann, ed.), Raven Press, New York, pp. 109–130.

Pike, M. C., and Snyderman, R., 1984, Chemoattractant receptors, in: *The Receptors,* Vol. 1 (M. Conn, ed), Academic Press, New York pp. 223–259.

Pike, M. C., Kredich, N. M., and Snyderman, R., 1978, Requirement of S-adenosyl-L-methionine-medicated methylation for human monocyte chemotaxis, *Proc. Natl. Acad. Sci. U.S.A.*, **75**:3928–3932.

Pike, M. C., Kredich, N. M., and Snyderman, R., 1979, Phospholipid methylation in macrophages is inhibited by chemotactic factors, *Proc. Natl. Acad. Sci. U.S.A.* **76**:2922–2926.

Postlethwaite, A., and Snyderman, R., 1975, Characterization of chemotactic activity produced *in vivo* by a cell mediated immune reaction in the guinea pig, *J. Immunol.* **114**:274–278.

Quie, P. G., Kaplan, E. L., Page, A. R., Grusky, F. L., and Malawista, S. E., 1968, Defective polymorphonuclear leukocyte function and chronic granulomatous disease on two female children, *N. Engl. J. Med.* **278**:976–980.

Rosen, H., and Klebanoff, S. J., 1979, Hydroxyl radical generation by polymorphonuclear leukocytes measured by electron spin resonance spectroscopy, *J. Clin. Invest.* **64**:1725–1729.

Rosenfield, S. I., and Leddy, J. P., 1974, Hereditary deficiency of the fifth component of complement of man, *Clin. Res.* **22**:162A.

Rosenthal, R. S., Fulbright, R. S., Eads, M. E., and Sawyer, W. D., 1977, Ethylenediaminetetraacetic acid sensitive anti-phagocytic activity of *Neisseria gonorrhoeae, Infect. Immun.* **15**:817–827.

Rothbard, S., 1948, Protective effect of hyaluronidase and type-specific anti-M serum on experimental group A *Streptococcus* infections in mice, *J. Exp. Med.* **88**:325–3411.

Rothhut, B., Cloix, J. F., and Russo-Marie, F., 1983, Dexamethasone induces the synthesis of "renocortins," two antiphospholipase proteins in rat renomedullary interstitial cells in culture, *"Adv. Prostaglandin Thromboxane Leukotriene Res."* **12**:51–56.

Rous, P., 1925, The relative reaction within living mammalian tissues. II. On the mobilization of acid materials within cells and the reaction as influenced by the cell state, *J. Exp. Med.* **41**:399–411.

Ruddy, S., Gigli, I., and Austen, K. F., 1972, The complement system of man, *N. Engl. J. Med.* **287**:592–596.

Russo-Marie, F., Paing, M., and Duval, D., 1979, Involvement of glucocorticoid receptors in steroid induced inhibition of prostaglandin secretion, *J. Biol. Chem.* **254**:8498–8504.

Sbarra, A. J., and Karnovsky, M. L., 1959, The biochemical basis of phagocytosis. I. Metabolic changes during the ingestion of particles by polymorphonuclear leukocytes, *J. Biol. Chem.* **234**:1355–1362.

Schiffmann, E., Corcoran, B. A., and Wahl, S. M., 1975, N-Formylmethionyl peptides as chemoattractants for leukocytes, *Proc. Natl. Acad. Sci. U.S.A.* **72**:1059–1062.

Schliwa, M., Pryzwansky, K. B., and Eutenwer, U., 1982, Centrosome splitting in neutrophils: An unusual phenomenon related to cell activation and motility, *Cell* **31**:705–717.

Schmalzl, F., Lederer, B., and Braunsteiner, H., 1970, Atypical myeloblastic leukemia with differentiation into "paraneutrophils," *Blut* **20**:337–349.

Segal, A. W., Cross, A. R., Garcia, R. C., Borregaard, N., Valerius, N. H., Scothill, J. F., and Jones, O. T. G., 1983, Absence of cytochrome b_{245} in chronic granulomatous disease, *N. Engl. J. Med.* **308**:245–251.

Serhan, C. N., Fridovich, J., Goetzl, E. J., Dunham, P. B., and Weissmann, G., 1981, Leukotriene B_4 and phosphatidic acid are calcium ionophores. Studies employing arsenazo III in liposomes, *J. Biol. Chem.* **256**:4746–4752.

Shea, C., and Morse, E. D., 1978, Inhibition of human neutrophil chemotaxis by corticosteroids, *Ann. Clin. Lab. Sci.* **8**:30–33.
Shin, H. S., Snyderman, R., Friedman, E., Mellors, A., and Mayer, M. D., 1968, Chemotactic and anaphylatoxic fragment, cleaved from the fifth component of guinea pig complement, *Science* **162**:361–363.
Showell, H. J., Freer, R. J., Zigmond, S. H., Schiffmann, E., Aswanikumar, S., Corcoran, B. A., and Becker, E. L., 1976, The structure–activity relations of synthetic peptides as chemotactic factors and inducers of lysosomal enzyme secretion for neutrophils, *J. Exp. Med.* **143**:1154–1169.
Simchowitz, L., Fishbein, L. C., Spilberg, I., and Atkinson, J. P., 1980, Induction of a transient elevation in intracellular levels of adenosine-3',5'-cyclic monophosphate by chemotactic factors: An early event in human neutrophil activation, *J. Immunol.* **124**:1482–1491.
Smith, M. R., and Wood, W. B., Jr., 1958, Surface phagocytosis. Further evidence of destructive action upon fully encapsulated pneumococci in the absence of type-specific antibody, *J. Exp. Med.* **109**:1–12.
Smolen, J. E., and Weissmann, G., 1980, Effects of indomethacin, 5,8,11,14-eicosatetraenoic acid and *p*-bromophenacyl bromide on lysosomal enzyme release and superoxide anion generation by human polymorphonuclear leukocytes, *Biochem. Pharmacol.* **29**:533–538.
Snyderman, R., 1982, Mechanisms of inflammation and tissues: Destruction in the rheumatic diseases, in: *Cecil Textbook of Medicine*, (L. H. Smith and J. B. Wyngaarden, eds.), W. B. Saunders, Philadelphia, pp. 1832–1839.
Snyderman, R., 1983, Pharmacologic manipulation of leukocyte chemotaxis, present knowledge and future trends, *Am. J. Med.* **75**:10–18.
Snyderman, R., and Goetzl, E. J., 1981, Molecular and cellular mechanisms of leukocyte chemotaxis, *Science* **213**:830–837.
Snyderman, R., Gewurz, H., and Mergenhagen, S. E., 1968a, Interactions of the complement system with endotoxic lipopolysaccharide. Generation of a factor chemotactic for polymorphonuclear leukocytes, *J. Exp. Med.* **128**:259–275.
Snyderman, R., Shin, H. S., Phillips, J. K., Gewurz, H., and Mergenhagen, S. E., 1968b, A neutrophil chemotactic factor derived from C5 upon interaction of guinea pig serum with endotoxin, *J. Immunol.* **103**:413–422.
Snyderman, R., Shin, H. S., Phillips, J. K., Gewurz, H., and Mergenhagen, S. E., 1969, A neutrophil chemotactic factor derived from C5 upon interaction of guinea pig serum with endotoxin, *J. Immunol.* **103**:413–418.
Snyderman, R., Phillips, J. K., and Mergenhagen, S. E., 1970, Polymorphonuclear leukocyte chemotactic activity in rabbit and guinea pig serum treated with immune complexes: Evidence for C5a as the major chemotactic factor, *Infect. Immun.* **1**:521–525.
Snyderman, R., Altman, L. C., Hausman, M. S., and Mergenhagen, S. E., 1972, Human mononuclear leukocyte chemotaxis: A quantitative assay for mediators of humoral and cellular chemotactic factors, *J. Immunol.* **108**:857–860.
Snyderman, R., Pike, M. C., and Altman, L. C., 1975, Abnormalities of leukocyte chemotaxis in human disease, *Ann. N.Y. Acad. Sci.* **256**:386–401.
Snyderman, R., Meadows, L., and Amos, D. B., 1977a, Characterization of human chemotactic lymphokine production induced by mitogens and mixed leukocyte reactions using a new microassay, *Cell. Immunol.* **30**:225–235.
Snyderman, R., Rogers, E., and Buckley, R. H., 1977b, Abnormalities of leukotaxis in atopic dermatitis. *J. Allergy Clin. Immunol.* **60**:121–126.
Snyderman, R., Durack, D. T., McCarty, G. A., Ward, F. E., and Meadows, L., 1979, Deficiency of the fifth component of complement in humans: Clinical, genetic and immunological studies in a large kindred, *Am. J. Med.* **67**:638–645.
Snyderman, R., Pike, M. C., and Kredich, N. M., 1980, Role of transmethylation reactions in cellular motility and phagocytosis, *Mol. Immunol.* **17**:209–218.
Snyderman, R., Pike, M. C., Edge, S., and Lane, B., 1984, A chemoattractant receptor on macrophages exists in two affinity states regulated by guanine nucleotides, *J. Cell. Biol.* **98**:444–448.
Southwick, F. S., and Stossel, T. P., 1981, Neutrophil actin dysfunction: An autosomal recessive genetic disorder of actin molecules, *Clin. Res.* **29**:397A.
Spilberg, I., and Mehta, J., 1979, Demonstration of a specific neutrophil receptor for a cell derived chemotactic factor, *J. Clin. Invest.* **63**:85–88.

Spilberg, I., Gallacher, A., Mehta, J., and Mandell, B., 1976, Urate crystal induced chemotactic factor, isolation and partial characterization, *J. Clin. Invest.* **58**:815–819.

Spilberg, I., Rosenberg, D., and Mandell, B., 1977, Induction of arthritis by purified cell-derived chemotactic factor: Role of chemotaxis and vascular permeability, *J. Clin. Invest.* **59**:582–585.

Spitznagel, J. K., 1984, Nonoxidative antimicrobial reactions of leukocytes, in: *Contemporary Topics in Immunobiology*, Vol. 14 (R. Snyderman, ed.), Plenum Press, New York, pp. 283–343.

Steerman, R. L., Snyderman, R., Leiken, S. L., and Colten, H. R., 1971, Intrinsic defect of the polymorphonuclear leukocyte resulting in impaired chemotaxis and phagocytosis, *Clin. Exp. Immunol.* **9**:939–946.

Stetcher, V. J., and Sorkin, E., 1972, The chemotactic activity of fibrin lysis products, *Int. Arch. Allergy Appl. Immunol.* **43**:879–886.

Stossel, T. P., 1977, Contractile proteins in phagocytosis: An example of cell surface-to-cytoplasm communication, *Fed. Proc.* **36**:2181–2184.

Stossel, T. P., and Hartwig, J. H., 1975, Interactions between actin, myosin, and an actin-binding protein from rabbit alveolar macrophages. Alveolar macrophage myosin Mg^{+2}-adenosine triphosphatase requires a cofactor for activation by actin, *J. Biol. Chem.* **250**:5706–5712.

Stossel, T. P., Mason, R. J., Hartwig, J., and Vaughn, M., 1972, Quantitative studies of phagocytosis by polymorphonuclear leukocytes: Use of emulsions to measure the initial rate of phagocytosis, *J. Clin. Invest.* **5**:615–624.

Tashjian, A. H., Jr., Voelkel, E. F., McDonough, J., and Levine, L., 1975, Hydrocortisone inhibits prostaglandin production by mouse fibrosarcoma cells, *Nature* **258**:739–741.

Taylor, F. B., and Ward, P. A., 1967, Generation of chemotactic activity in rabbit serum by plasminogen–streptokinase mixtures, *J. Exp. Med.* **126**:149–158.

Tempel, T. R., Snyderman, R., Jordan, H. V., and Mergenhagen, S. E., 1970, Factors from saliva and oral bacteria, chemotactic for polymorphonuclear leukocytes: Their possible role in gingival inflammation, *J. Periodon.* **41**:3/71–12/80.

Till, G. O., 1983, The cellular and humoral defense systems and inflammatory mechanisms in thermal injury, *Clin. Lab. Med.* **3**:801–815.

Turner, S. R., Cambell, J. A., and Lynn, W. S., 1975, Polymorphonuclear leukocyte chemotaxis towards oxidized lipid components of cell membranes, *J. Exp. Med.* **141**:1437–1441.

Van Dyke, T. E., Horoszewiez, L. J., Cianciola, L. J., and Genco, R. J., 1980, Neutrophil chemotaxis dysfunction in human periodontitis, *Infect. Immun.* **27**:124–132.

Verghese, M. W., and Snyderman, R., 1983, Hormonal regulation of adenylate cyclase in macrophage membranes is regulated by guanine nucleotides, *J. Immunol.* **180**:869–873.

Verghese, M., and Snyderman, R., 1984, Inhibition of phosphodiesterase by chemoattractants in human neutrophils (PMNs): A potential new mechanism for receptor-mediated enhancement of cAMP, *Clin. Res.* **32**:471A.

Volpi, M., Yassin, R., Naccache, P. H., and Sha'afi, R. I., 1983, Chemotactic factor causes rapid decreases in phosphatidylinositol-4,5-biphosphate and phosphatidylinositol 4-monophosphate in rabbit neutrophils, *Biochem. Biophys. Res. Commun.* **112**:957–964.

Ward, H. K., and Enders, J. F., 1933, An analysis of the opsonic and tropic action of normal and immune sera based on experiments with pneumococcus, *J. Exp. Med.* **57**:527–547.

Ward, P. A., and Berenberg, J. L., 1974, Defective regulation of inflammatory mediators in Hodgkins disease, *N. Engl. J. Med.* **290**:76–80.

Ward, P. A., and Newman, L. J., 1969, A neutrophil chemotactic factor from human CS. *J. Immunol.* **102**:93–99.

Ward, P. A., Cochrane, C. G., and Muller-Eberhard, H. J., 1966, Further studies on the chemotactic factor of complement and its formation *in vivo*, *Immunology* **11**:141–145.

Ward, P. A., Lepow, I. H., and Newman, L. J., 1968, Bacterial factors chemotactic for polymorphonuclear leukocytes, *Am. J. Pathol.* **52**:725–736.

Ward, P. A., Goralnick, S., and Bullock, W. E., 1976, Defective leukotaxis in patients with lepromatous leprosy, *J. Lab. Clin. Med.* **87**:1025–1032.

Weiss, S. J., Klein, R., Slivka, A., and Wei, M., 1982, Chlorination of taurine by human neutrophils. Evidence for hypochlorous acid generation, *J. Clin. Invest.* **70**:598–607.

Weissmann, G., 1983, Pathways of arachidonate oxidation to prostaglandins and lekotrienes, *Semin. Arthritis Rheum.* **13**(Suppl. 1):123–129.

Weissmann, G., Becher, B., and Thomas, L., 1964, Studies on lysosomes V. The effects of streptolysins and other hemolytic agents on isolated leukocyte granules, *J. Cell. Biol.* **22**:115–126.

Weissmann, G., Spilberg, I., and Krakauer, K., 1969, Arthritis induced in rabbits by lysates of granulocyte lysosomes, *Arthritis Rheum.* **12**:103–116.

Williams, L. T., Snyderman, R., Pike, M. C., and Lefkowitz, R. J., 1977, Specific receptor sites for chemotactic peptides on human polymorphonuclear leukocytes, *Proc. Natl. Acad. Sci. U.S.A.* **74**:1204–1208.

Williams, L. T., Antoniades, H. N., and Goetzl, E. J., 1984, Platelet-derived growth factor stimulates mouse 3T3 cell mitogenesis and leukocyte chemotaxis through different structural determinants, *J. Clin. Invest.* **72**:1759–1763.

Wolf, S. M., Dale, D. C., Clark, R. A., Root, R. K., and Kimball, H. R., 1972, The Chediak–Higashi syndrome: Studies of host defense, *Ann. Intern. Med.* **76**:293–306.

Woodin, A. M., and Wieneke, A. A., 1966, The secretion of protein by the polymorphonuclear leukocyte treated with streptolysin O, *Exp. Cell. Res.* **43**:319–331.

Wright, A. E., and Douglas, S. R., 1903, An experimental investigation of the role of the blood fluids in connection with phagocytosis, *Proc. R. Soc. (London)* **72**:357–370.

Yano, K., Nakashima, S., and Yoshinori, N., 1983, Coupling of polyphoinositide breakdown with calcium efflux in formyl-methionyl-leucyl-phenylalanine stimulated rabbit neutrophils, *FEBS Lett.* **161**:296–300.

Yuli, I., Tomonaga, A., and Snyderman, R., 1982, Chemoattractant receptor functions in human polymorphonuclear leukocytes are divergently altered by membrane fluidizers, *Proc. Natl. Acad. Sci. U.S.A.* **79**:5906–5910.

Zurier, R. B., Hoffstein, S., and Weissmann, G., 1973, Cytochalasin B: Effect on lysosomal enzyme release from human leukocytes, *Proc. Natl. Acad. Sci, U.S.A.* **70**:844–848.

Zvaifler, N. J., 1983, Pathogenesis of the joint disease of rheumatoid arthritis, *Am. J. Med.* **75**:3–8.

24

Drug-Related Rheumatic Diseases

Basic Mechanisms

Evelyn V. Hess and Allen Litwin

I. DRUG-RELATED LUPUS

A. Introduction

The most important and most common drug-related rheumatic disease is drug-related lupus. The first case of a probable drug-related lupus (DRL) was described by Hoffman (1945) and incriminated the antibiotic sulfadiazine. Other reports during the 1950s related to other sulfonamides and penicillin. It is possible that these were accidental occurrences or that the patients had idiopathic systemic lupus erythematosus (SLE).

The first definite occurrence was reported in association with the use of hydralazine, an antihypertensive agent (Morrow *et al.*, 1953). Since this was one of the few drugs available at that time for the treatment of hypertension, this new syndrome represented a significant handicap for many patients. Indeed, the more severe the hypertension, especially the accelerated form, and the higher the hydralazine dose employed for blood pressure control, the greater was the occurrence of this undesirable side effect (Perry, 1973). Since then, many other drugs have been implicated in this syndrome, thus limiting their usefulness in treatment. The most important lupus-related drug now in use is procainamide (Spiegel *et al.*, 1967).

B. Incriminated Drugs

Including the drugs mentioned above, a total of over 40 drugs have been implicated in published reports to the present time (Hess, 1981). Many of these reports are single

Evelyn V. Hess and Allen Litwin • Department of Medicine, University of Cincinnati Medical Center, Cincinnati, Ohio 45267.

associations, others of serologic changes only. Most lack controlled prospective data. It is appropriate to classify these drug associations as follows:

1. Those for which there is definite proof of association and appropriate controlled prospective studies have been completed. Drugs in this group include hydralazine, procainamide, isoniazid, methyldopa, and chlorpromazine. With the latter two drugs, the studies confirm serologic conversion of negative to positive ANF; there have been few patients with clinical symptoms, although there have been reports of various types of arthralgias and arthritis occurring with isoniazid.
2. Those with a possible association. Included are (1) the β blockers (reported to date are practolol, atenolol, metoprolol, oxprenolol, acebutolol); (2) anticonvulsants (included are diphenylhydantoin, mephenyltoin, trimethadione, and ethosuximide); (3) antithyroid drugs (reported to date are propylthiouracil and methimazole); (4) quinidine; (5) penicillamine; (6) captopril; (7) lithium carbonate; and (8) phenelzine.
3. The third group includes drugs that have unlikely or as yet unproven associations. Included are phenylbutazone, gold salts, the oral contraceptives, griseofulvin, penicillin, and the sulfonamides.

There have been a number of agents, many constituents of drugs, and therapeutic modalities that are also suspect. Aromatic amines or hydrazine compounds are common substrates and are present in the food supply and environment. Hydrazines can be detected in a natural state in tobacco, tobacco smoke, mushrooms, and in *Penicillium*. They are used in industry, agriculture, and medicine. The aromatic amines are used in the cosmetic industry and can be found in various hair-curling solutions. Burry (1969) noted the possible relationship between eosin in lipstick and lupus. Reidenburg (1983) has reported on a lupuslike illness related to hydrazine. There have been recent observations on the possible exacerbation of SLE (Roberts and Hayashi, 1983) and also on a lupuslike disease in monkeys related to a nonprotein amino acid, L-canavanine (Malinow *et al.*, 1982). This material is found in alfalfa seeds and sprouts and many other leguminous plants.

Drug-related lupus continues to be an annoying and persistent clinical problem even though other drugs have been developed that can substitute for those related to the lupus syndrome. However, for the immunologist/rheumatologist, the most intriguing aspect of this problem is the fact that simple, low-molecular-weight compounds can induce autoimmunity with or without clinical disease in a large number of seemingly immunologically normal individuals either in the form of autoantibodies or clinical disease. A reasonable expectation is that knowledge of the mechanisms by which these compounds induce lupus or autoimmunity should have a major impact on our understanding of the pathogenesis of "idiopathic" systemic lupus.

It appears that lupus syndromes caused by drugs are becoming more common, thus uncovering new populations for the expression of lupus. The evidence to the present time that SLE itself is exacerbated or worsened by the giving of various DRL drugs is unconvincing. Much important information has been obtained from the study of patients receiving these drugs, but studies directed toward uncovering the pathogenetic processes by which these drugs cause autoimmunity have not yet provided the answers despite the efforts of many investigators.

C. Criteria for DRL

Diagnostic criteria for DRL have not yet been defined. The American Rheumatism Association criteria for the classification of SLE are useful, and the revised second edition is recommended (Tan *et al.*, 1982). Of these 11 criteria, four are needed for consideration of SLE. In the diagnosis of DRL by these criteria, some cases may be only probable. For example, a patient may have only two criteria; e.g., arthritis and a positive ANA. There must be prior administration of a drug that is followed by remission of symptoms on withdrawal and recurrence on its readministration. The latter circumstance is rarely indicated clinically and therefore seldom fulfilled. The remission of symptoms after drug withdrawal may not occur in all patients, and in some, symptoms and signs can persist for a long period of time after drug withdrawal before remission occurs (Hildreth *et al.*, 1960). Recurrence of symptoms after readministration of the drug does not invariably reinduce lupus (Perry, 1973).

D. Role of the Acetylator Phenotype in DRL

Figure 1 illustrates the structure of two of the most common lupus-related drugs, hydralazine and procainamide. Their only chemical commonality is the possession of either an aromatic amine or a hydrazine group. This suggests that the metabolism of these drugs could play an important role in the causation of the lupus syndrome. At least with procainamide and hydralazine, patients who are slow acetylators of these drugs (i.e., have low levels of acetyltransferase activity in their livers, intestines, and kidneys) develop antinuclear antibodies sooner, with higher titers, and are much more prone to develop clinical lupus (Perry, 1973; Woosley *et al.*, 1978). In a prospective study of patients on procainamide, the time required for 50% of slow and rapid acetylator patients to develop a positive ANA test was 2.9 and 7.3 months, respectively (Woosley *et al.*, 1978). Approximately 30% of these patients developed a lupus syndrome that appeared at 12 ± 5 months for slow acetylators and 48 ± 22 months for rapid acetylators.

Prospective studies (Litwin *et al.*, 1981a) of patients receiving hydralazine further emphasized this point. Autoantibodies to poly(A), poly(A–U), and single-stranded DNA were detected soon after hydralazine therapy was initiated but occurred almost exclusively in patients who were slow acetylators (Table 1). These autoantibodies increased in quantity with continued drug exposure but, again, only in the slow acetylator patients. Only one

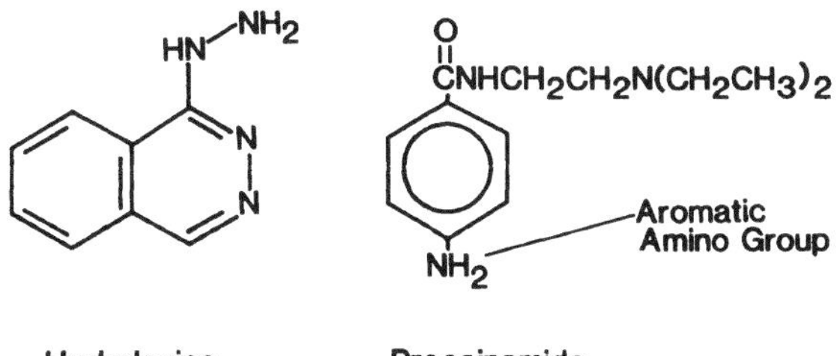

Figure 1. The hydralazine and procainamide molecules.

Table 1. Humoral Results in Hydralazine Treated and Control Groups

	Hydralazine group (number positive/ total number)	Control group (number positive/ total number)
Latex test	4/27	3/19
Coombs test	Negative	Negative
Ig levels	WNL[a]	WNL
C'3, C'4 levels	WNL	WNL
ANA	4/27	0/19
Poly(A) antibodies	10/13 Slow acetylators[b] 3/9 Rapid acetylators	0/19
Poly(A–U) antibodies	10/13 Slow acetylators 3/9 Rapid acetylators	0/19
ss-DNA antibodies	8/13 Slow acetylators 3/9 Rapid acetylators	0/19
Lymphocytotoxic antibodies	3/4 Slow acetylators 0/3 Rapid acetylators	2/7
Hydralazine antibodies	0/27	0/19

[a] WNL, within normal limits.
[b] Acetylation rate not determined in five hydralazine patients. In these five, 1/5 had antibodies to ss-DNA, 2/5 to poly(A), and 1/5 to poly(A–U).

patient in this series developed DRL, and he was a slow acetylator. Earlier, Perry *et al.* (1970) had pointed out that DRL in hydralazine-treated patients occurred primarily in slow acetylator patients. It might be expected that if enough drug is given to maintain a constant blood level of parent drug, almost as many rapid as slow acetylator patients should develop DRL if these previous metabolic studies are correct. One such study has been done with procainamide (Sonnhag *et al.*, 1979). When the dose of procainamide was increased to maintain a similar blood level in slow and rapid acetylator patients, the incidence of DRL was similar.

Further proof for the role of acetylation in DRL would be that the acetylated form of the drug would not induce symptoms, and, as a corollary, its administration to patients with DRL would result in relief of their symptoms. The acetylated forms of hydralazine and isoniazid are pharmacologically inactive. However, N-acetylprocainamide (Fig. 2) has the antiarrhythmic properties of the parent compound, but its administration to patients does not result in either a positive ANA or antibodies to ss-DNA nearly as rapidly as procainamide itself (Lahita *et al.*, 1979; Stec *et al.*, 1979; Roden *et al.*, 1980). Figure 3 shows that N-

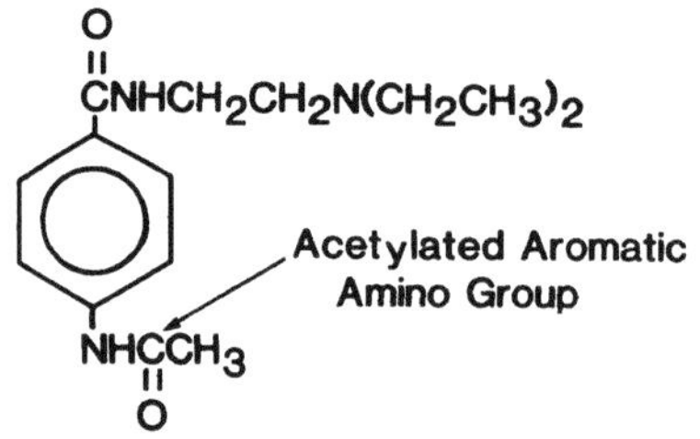

Figure 2. The acetylprocainamide molecule.

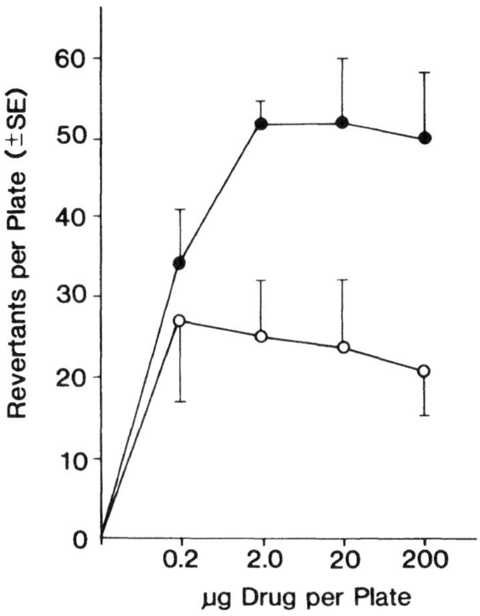

Figure 3. Comparison of the reactivity of procainamide (●) and N-acetylprocainamide (○) in the Ames test. Data represent the mean ± S.E. number of revertants above the spontaneous reversion rate. (From Uetrecht *et al.*, 1981.)

acetylprocainamide produced a smaller number of revertants in the Ames test than procainamide (Uetrecht *et al.*, 1981). Its use in patients with procainamide DRL resulted in alleviation of symptoms (Stec *et al.*, 1979). That N-acetylprocainamide has any autoimmunity-inducing potential at all is probably related to its *in vivo* deacetylation by potent deacetylating enzymes in the serum. Part of the more profound effect of hydralazine in slow acetylators as compared to procainamide may be because of the higher first-pass hepatic metabolism of hydralazine than of procainamide (Uetrecht and Woosley, 1981).

An important question is whether the parent drug itself or an oxidative nonacetylated metabolite of the parent drug is responsible for the DRL syndrome. The concept of a reactive metabolite capable of binding to macromolecules and/or membranes would be intellectually most attractive. The only supportive evidence for this concept is based on the observation that a reactive nonacetylated metabolite of procainamide produced by incubating procainamide with liver microsomes was capable of both covalently binding to liver macromolecules and causing a positive Ames test (i.e., was mutagenic) which implies binding and/or altering of nucleic acids (Freeman *et al.*, 1979).

E. Role of the Acetylator Phenotype in SLE

Another important and intriguing question is the possible role of acetylator phenotype in patients with SLE. Does acetylator phenotype have a similar importance in disease causation in these patients as it does for those with DRL? Before considering this problem, it is necessary to consider whether these two entities are the same disease. There are a number of differences:

1. Drug-related lupus does not have the female dominance of SLE. In SLE, 80–90% of patients are female compared to 60% or less in DRL. Basically, the disease for which the patient is being treated provides the determinant factor for the sex

and also the age of the patient with DRL. Examples include DRL occurring in older men treated with various drugs used in the treatment of heart disease and hypertension; DRL in children may be caused by the anticonvulsants commonly used.

2. Central nervous system disease does not occur in DRL, and there is a relative paucity of cases with renal disease, with only 13 biopsy-proven cases (Sheikh *et al.*, 1981). This has been explained in part as reflecting the lack of development of antibodies to ds-DNA in DRL. Such antibodies can play a major role in the renal disease found in SLE (Koffler *et al.*, 1967).
3. Pleural and pericardial disease is a major feature of DRL. Goldberg *et al.* (1984) have described a procainamide lupus patient with pulmonary disease in whom bronchoalveolar lavage showed a flux of neutrophils into the lung. Serial studies showed that the alveolitis continued although all other features of the disease cleared. The particular mechanism for this neutrophil inflammatory action has not yet been defined, although it is of interest that *in vivo* fixation of ANA in the pleura has been reported (Chandrasekhar *et al.*, 1978).
4. There is less occurrence of skin and mucosal involvement and adenopathy in DRL. This may in part reflect the use of these lupus-related drugs in older patients in whom SLE itself may have a different clinical expression.
5. There are serologic differences such as the aforementioned paucity of antibodies to ds-DNA and SM antigen in DRL and the infrequent depression of complement or any of its individual components. However, DRL patients do share in common with SLE patients antibody responses to ss-DNA, histones, ribonucleoprotein, poly(A), poly(A–U), lymphotoxic antibodies, and on occasions a false-positive serology. The immune response to histones is of special interest. Initially, Fritzler and Tan (1978) demonstrated by an elution procedure in the immunofluorescent ANA slide test that 90% of DRL patients had ANA antibodies directed toward the histone moiety of the desoxyribonucleoprotein (DNA–histone complex) whereas only 30% of SLE patients had histones as the principal antigen. In a more recent study employing a solid-phase radioimmunoassay, Rubin *et al.* (1982) found a less distinct difference between the two groups, as half the SLE and three-fourths of the DRL patients had antihistone antibodies. This high incidence of antihistone antibodies probably accounts for the striking incidence of LE cells in DRL patients. Portanova *et al.* (1982) noted differences in the histones involved in DRL caused by hydralazine and procainamide. It should be noted that more of these histone responses have been observed in procainamide than in hydralazine DRL. The histone subclass in DRL is most frequently the H2A–H2B subclass. Portanova *et al.* (1982) suggested that the antibody to these particular histone subclasses could be reacting with either a junctional or conformationally dependent determinant that is expressed on this particular subclass but not on the uncomplexed H2A–H2B. This same group have shown that hydralazine sera have antihistone activity to H1, H2A–H2B, and H3–H4. Another important difference is that with hydralazine most of the antibodies are of the IgM class, whereas with procainamide they are of both IgM and IgG classes. A study by Grossman and Barland (1981) showed that symptomatic DRL patients had antihistone antibodies, whereas the asymptomatic subjects did not.

6. There appear to be genetic differences. There is an increased prevalence of HLA-DR2 and HLA-DR3 in SLE, whereas HLA-DR4 is increased in hydralazine-related lupus, at least in Great Britain (Batchelor *et al.*, 1980). This has recently been challenged (Brand *et al.*, 1984).
7. Blacks in the United States rarely develop DRL, in contrast to their rather high incidence of SLE.

If DRL represents a different target population with certain intriguing differences to SLE, then it is valid to consider the role of acetylator phenotype in SLE. The first report of an increased prevalence of slow acetylator phenotype in SLE was by Reidenberg and Martin (1974). They reported that ten of 14 patients were slow acetylators. In a similar study, Foad *et al.* (1977) found that 17 of 25 patients (68%) were slow acetylators, a difference that was greater than the expected 52% but not statistically significant. When clinical and serologic features were compared in this series, no differences were noted between the two patient groups except for possibly lower complement levels in the slow acetylator SLE group. This slight difference in complement levels was noted by another group (Vansant *et al.*, 1978). In subsequent studies, other investigators have noted no obvious clinical or serologic differences between slow and rapid acetylator SLE patients.

By 1980, several more studies of acetylator phenotype in SLE had been reported from the United States, Israel, Europe, and Mexico. These studies were reviewed (Reidenberg *et al.*, 1980) in detail. Five studies reported an increased prevalence of slow acetylators, and two did not. Because of the difficulty in obtaining a sufficient number of patients to achieve statistical significance when 52% of normal individuals are slow acetylators, Reidenberg performed a χ^2 analysis of all the studies reported up to that time. He obtained a significance level of $P < 0.001$. It must be noted that these studies included patient populations from many countries and that historical controls were used in several. It is possible that acetylation rates could vary in different ethnic groups within each country. Studies by Spencer-Green and Hess (1984) have shown that among first-degree relatives of patients with SLE, 17 of 20 family members from nine propositi were slow acetylators. Of the nine lupus patients, seven were slow acetylators. Since 1980, there has been at least one additional study reported from Japan in which no increase in slow acetylators was found in SLE. This Japanese experience is of special interest as only 11.5% of normal Japanese are slow acetylators (Tanaka *et al.*, 1982) although the prevalence of SLE in Japan is similar to that found in Europe and the United States (Fukase, 1976).

If it is assumed that the correlation between slow acetylation and idiopathic lupus is significant, could acetylator status play a pathophysiological role in SLE? Reidenberg (1981) has proposed that environmental amines act as the lupus-related drugs do; i.e., as inciting agents to induce disease. This would not be a causal factor for all lupus patients but only for a subset. Among the environmental candidates he has suggestd are azo dyes, hair dyes, tobacco and tobacco smoke, mushrooms, and *Penicillium*. Tartrazine (FDC yellow #5) in the rat undergoes cleavage by gut microflora of the azo linkage, and the aminopyrazalone ring results in a hydrazine, 4-sulfophenylhydrazine. Absorption of this hydrazine in a slow acetylator could produce an active metabolite that could then induce lupus in a genetically predisposed individual. Hein and Weber (1982) have provided evidence that a wide variety of hydrazines as well as primary amines are polymorphically

N-acetylated. Drayer *et al.* (1982) have added another line of evidence to indirectly support Reidenberg's hypothesis. They found that patients with SLE have higher rates of oxidative metabolism measured by pentobarbital oxidation, implying than an oxidative metabolite of an environmental amine could be produced in a slow acetylator, genetically lupus-predisposed individual, which could then act as the inciting agent for that patient to develop lupus.

F. Animal Models

It is critical to be able to investigate these problems in an animal model. Such models would lend themselves to the considerable experimental manipulation required to study how various drugs initiate disease. Unfortunately, the animal studies to date have been minimally informative with many conflicting results.

1. Dogs

Dogs as a species are extremely poor acetylators with low levels of acetyltransferase. This fact was unknown to early investigators. In the first attempt to use a lupus-related drug in this animal, or indeed in any animal, Comens (1956) reported the production of positive LE cells, renal glomerular lesions (wire-loop), and some hematological changes as well as cachexia, convulsions, and death in dogs receiving oral hydralazine. Symptoms occurred within a few weeks to a few months of starting hydralazine. Seven of the eight dogs had LE cells. In two of the dogs, the LE cells were confirmed by Hargraves himself. However, neither Gardner (1957) nor Dubois *et al.* (1961) were able to reproduce this experiment except for toxic reactions and some hematological abnormalities observed by the former; LE-like cells were observed by Gardner but were very atypical, still retaining some nuclear structure. Recently Balázs *et al.* (1981) induced antinuclear antibodies in two of 12 dogs treated with oral hydralazine. They also found antibodies to native and denatured DNA and desoxyribonucleoprotein. Lymphocytes from one of the two responding dogs showed a proliferative response to DNA and to hydralazine. However, no alterations were detected in serum proteins or in the hemogram, and all the dogs remained clinically healthy.

Similar equivocal or negative results have been obtained by a host of other investigators in attempts to create an animal model of DRL using pigs, guinea pigs, and mice. In some experiments, undoubtedly, antinuclear antibodies were induced, but in no study did clear-cut clinical lupus occur. One factor contributing to these negative results is probably the unknown acetylator phenotype of the experimental animal, which is of such critical significance in human DRL. It is known that guinea pigs, hamsters, dogs, mice, and syngeneic strains of mice have monomorphic rather than dimorphic acetylator phenotypes for procainamide.

2. Mice

Initial studies to develop a rodent model are reported by Roberts *et al.* (1984). The rate of *in vivo* procainamide (PA) acetylation was determined in seven strains of laboratory mice, five strains of laboratory rats, and in a population of wild rats. There was no evidence of PA acetylator polymorphism among wild rats, and differences among strains of laboratory mouse and laboratory rat were too small to provide the basis for polymorphism. A sex difference in *in vivo* PA acetylation was observed for Sprague-Dawley rats but not for SHR/N or Wistar rats. Measurement of *in vitro* hepatic PA acetylation confirmed the sex difference in *in vivo* acetylation as well as the absence of PA acetylator polymorphism among wild rats. Weber and Tannen (1981) did consider the possible requirement for dimorphic acetylator status in the species to be studied. They used procainamide in A/J and C57BL/65 strains of mice. A/J mice are slow and C57BL/65 rapid acetylators of sulfamethazine. However, both strains monomorphically acetylate procainamide. Although they found that A/J mice developed a higher incidence of ANA than did C57BL/6Js, no mouse developed clinical lupus. They found a statistical difference in computing the "whole life score" ANA, but considerable numbers of the rapid acetylator strain mouse, C57BL/6J, had positive ANA.

The only strain of laboratory animal that has dimorphic acetylation for procainamide is the rabbit, and no feeding experiments have been attempted with them. Experiments employing injection of immunogenic forms of hydralazine such as hydralazine–human-serum-albumin conjugates into rabbits (Yamauchi *et al.*, 1975) and hydralazine–bovine-serum-albumin conjugates (Carpenter *et al.*, 1980) into guinea pigs did succeed in inducing anti-DNA antibodies but not clinical disease. Such experiments, of course, bypass the acetylating enzymes but are based on several assumptions, among which are that the etiologic agent is the parent drug rather than an oxidative metabolite and that it acts as a hapten rather than in a pharmacological manner in effecting the immune response.

Antibodies to histone have also been reported in NZB/NZW mice. These studies, utilizing monoclonal antibodies, suggested that perhaps a relatively large fraction of antibodies that react with nucleoproteins in these mice are also directed against histones. There are certainly differences among the various murine strains, suggesting that these responses may be caused by differences of IR genes and/or Ig variable genes of the individual murine strains. The possibility suggested by Laskov *et al.* (1984) is that there may be a quite different etiology and pathogenesis in the different strains of mice. These continued studies in murine models and the application of the monoclonal antibodies to studies of humans with these disorders will provide important information in the near future.

G. Pathophysiological Mechanisms

The most intriguing aspects of DRL relate to the pathophysiological mechanisms, which so far remain unknown despite many experimental attempts. It has been noted that the oxidative, nonacetylated metabolites of drugs rather than parent compounds are more likely candidates as initiators. However, there exist data supporting a number of hypotheses by which either a parent drug or a nonacetylated oxidative metabolite of that drug could induce DRL.

The first hypothesis is that the metabolite or parent drug may be cross reactive with a nucleic acid, resulting in tolerance to the nucleic acids being broken either at the T- or B-cell level. Hydralazine is a phthalazine with a reactive hydrazine group that specifically reacts with pyrimidine moieties of DNA. These bases are modified by hydralazine and are later removed from nucleosides. The purine nucleosides are not effective. Dubroff *et al.* (1981) have proposed a model of hydralazine-related lupus based on the fact that hydralazine may interfere with its own metabolic conversion by modifying the specific acetylases, thus increasing hydralazine concentration.

There is a strong chemical resemblance between hydralazine and adenine (Fig. 4), and antibodies induced to adenine can be inhibited by hydralazine (Cameron and Erlanger, 1976). In the studies of Yamauchi *et al.* (1975), rabbits that had been hyperimmunized with a hydralazine–human-serum-albumin complex produced high titers of antibodies highly cross reactive with ss-DNA and to some extent with ds-DNA. However, the animals did not acquire lupus. In the prospective study of hydralazine-treated hypertensive patients, antibodies were not detected to hydralazine, nor were titers of antibodies to ss-DNA, poly(A), or poly(A–U) inhibited by hydralazine or hydralazine–human-serum-albumin compounds (Litwin *et al.*, 1981a). In another prospective study of hydralazine-treated patients (Carpenter *et al.*, 1980) similar results were obtained except that antihydralazine antibodies were detected in a few patients. These antibodies were not cross reactive with DNP. However, it is possible that cross reactivity could occur at the T-cell level alone and produce a T-cell bypass that could then activate B-cell clones directed toward nucleic acids. According to Weigle (1980), such active B-cell clones are continually arising in normal individuals and are directed toward various self-antigens but are not activated because of the persistently tolerant state of T cells directed toward the same antigens. However, if T cells lose their tolerance, then autoimmunity can ensue. In the prospective study of hydralazine-treated patients (Litwin *et al.*, 1981a), significant lymphocyte transformation to hydralazine–human-serum-albumin compounds was noted in some of the patients who were producing autoantibodies. This implies the induction of T cells, possibly helper cells, directed toward hydralazine as the antigen. As noted already, antibodies induced to adenine cross react with hydralazine, and, therefore, by implication, T cells reactive to hydralazine could also respond to nucleic acid or at least to their bases. The fact that patients with DRL have antibodies to ss-DNA (i.e., involving the DNA bases) further supports this hypothesis. Definitive proof awaits further work on the nature of the T-cell receptor. Only with this knowledge can cross reactivity at the T-cell level be adequately tested.

The intriguing histone antibody story and their animal and human relationships have already been mentioned and are of particular importance to the cross-reactive hypothesis.

A second hypothesis states that the cells involved in immunoregulation are directly affected by either the parent drug or an oxidative nonacetylated metabolite of the drug. These compounds, particularly a reactive metabolite, could bind to a cell membrane, causing function alteration. Gilmore Harris (1983) has recently reviewed the data and

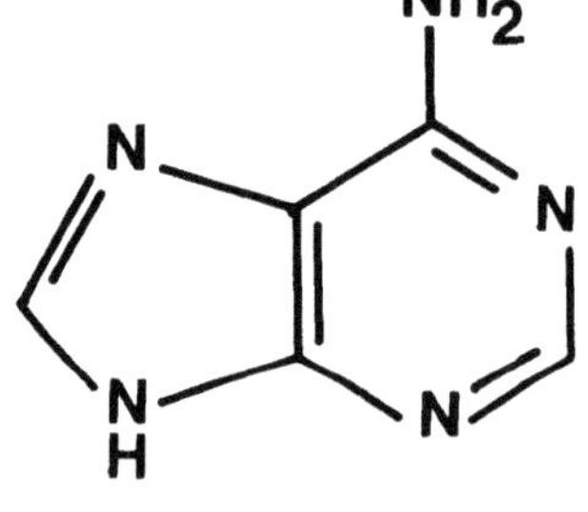

Figure 4. The adenine molecule.

concepts relating to DNA damage and repair in immunologically active cells. This is highly recommended reading for those with a further interest in this particular aspect of DRL.

The known effect of UV radiation on DNA is well accepted. Some recent intriguing observations relevant to environmental factors in SLE and DRL are provided in a study (Hersey *et al.*, 1983) of a controlled exposure to UV irradiation on the human immune system. These studies showed that in the exposed subjects there was a reduced skin test response to DNCB, a relative increase in OKT-3, mostly because of an increase in OKT-8 suppressor/cytotoxic phenotype subset of T cells. The OKT-4 helper/inducer phenotype T cells were reduced, and there was a significant decrease in the $T4^+/T8^+$ cell ratio. Other observations showed an increase in suppressor T-cell activity against *in vitro* production of IgG and also a depression of natural killer cell activity. The cells involved in these various reactions could include macrophages or other antigen-presenting cells, T helper cells, T supressor cells, B cells, or multiple populations of these cells. In addition, a group of lymphokines and/or monokines could also be involved. In SLE, abnormalities have been found in all of these different cell populations.

Evidence supporting this hypothesis is fragmentary and somewhat contradictory. Miller and Salem (1982) found T-helper-cell function to be increased nonspecifically in procainamide-treated patients who were normal clinically; i.e., did not have DRL. Ochi *et al.* (1983) found *in vitro* that normal B cells incubated with procainamide were not increased in number but were induced to become immunoglobulin-secreting cells, a form of polyclonal B-cell activation. They supplied some evidence that at least part of this effect was caused by the inhibition of suppressor T cells. The same group also reported the opposite event occurring *in vivo* in procainamide-treated patients, namely, that fewer antibody-secreting B cells were found compared to the control population.

A number of other drugs have been reported to have effects on immunologic function. Phenytoin inhibits lymphocyte transformation (MacKinney and Booker, 1972), as do local anesthetics (Ferguson *et al.*, 1976). These same authors showed that chlorpromazine could inhibit cytoxic murine T cells. It should be noted that this anesthetic class of agents are lipid-soluble drugs that are incorporated into and usually exert their effect on cell membranes. Procainamide, local anesthetics, many tranquilizers, the anticonvulsants, and the antiarrhythmics are all included in this class of compounds. This may provide a unifying theme, at least for this group of drugs, in their ability to relate to drug lupus.

The work of Scorza-Smeraldi *et al.* (1983) has shown that the adrenergic mediators dopamine and norepinephrine bind to adrenergic receptors and can interfere with the specific absorption of anti-HLA antibodies to HLA-A1 and to a lesser extent to other cross-reacting specificities. They have also shown that chlorpromazine and propranolol were also interfered with by such antigens and bound poorly to cell membrane receptors. Bluestein *et al.* (1981) have noted that procainamide could alter the *in vitro* proliferative response of normal human lymphocytes to both mitogenic and antigenic stimulation.

Lymphocytotoxic antibodies have been noted in some patients with procainamide DRL (Bluestein *et al.*, 1981) and in another study (Litwin *et al.*, 1981b) were found with similar frequency in slow and rapid acetylators of hydralazine. These antibodies are also a reflection of lymphocyte immune alteration.

A third hypothesis suggests the alteration by the drug or an oxidative metabolite of a nucleic acid(s), which could then enhance the nucleic acids' low order of immunogenicity. Chemically modified DNA has been shown to be a potent immunogen (Stollar, 1973). Incubation of DNP with hydralazine alters its physicochemical properties but not its antigenicity (Tan, 1974). However, immunologic studies have not been done with this compound. Blomgren *et al.* (1972) could not demonstrate enhanced immunogenicity of UV light adducts of procainamide and ss-DNA, nor did these procainamide–ss-DNA compounds bind more antibody from sera of procainamide-induced lupus patients than did ss-DNA alone. It has been shown that slow acetylators have a greater rate of DNA repair than rapid acetylators. Cavalgia (1980) has shown that hydralazine can induce sister-chromatid exchanges both in cultured lymphocytes and in base substitutions in bacteria. There is, then, the possibility that damage to DNA by the various agents could initiate various cellular events. Other possibilities include drugs or oxidative metabolites acting as adjuvants, particularly as polyclonal B-cell activators. This might better explain the variety of autoantibodies found in patients with DRL.

H. Conclusions

It is quite possible that these various hypotheses for pathophysiological mechanisms may well require a genetic factor for the expression of the autoimmune response and the clinical disease. Unfortunately, there have been relatively few studies on the role of the IR genes. Batchelor *et al.* (1980) showed a 73% frequency of HLA-DR4 in hydralazine-related lupus, particularly in women. Kincaid-Smith and Whitworth (1983) have reported four hydralazine-related glomerulonephritis patients from Australia who were all female, slow acetylators, and two were HLA-DR4. Another study has shown an increased frequency of HLA-DW44 in psychiatric patients on chlorpromazine. Forty-six percent of this group, contrasted to a normal Caucasian frequency of 19%, was noted to have DW44 (Canoso *et al.*, 1982). Gold and *d*-penicillamine nephropathy have been noted to be associated with HLA-B8 and HLA-DRW3 (Wooley *et al.*, 1980).

A number of the clinical features both of DRL and SLE are very similar to those induced by virus infection. The possibility of the activation of a latent virus, perhaps as a result of the abnormalities of immunoregulation induced by the drugs or their metabolites or even the possibility of a more metabolic action, must also be considered.

These proposed mechanisms need not be mutually exclusive, and it is highly likely that more than one could coexist simultaneously. It is now realized that various agents may themselves be multifunctional; for example, poly(I–C) can act both as an adjuvant and as an immunogen (Jacobs *et al.*, 1972). Those readers interested in more detailed information on this fascinating topic are referred to the Kroc Foundation publication on drug-related lupus, which appears as a special supplement of *Arthritis and Rheumatism*, August, 1981, Vol. 24, No. 8.

II. DRUG-RELATED RHEUMATIC DISEASES OTHER THAN LUPUS

A. Corticosteroids

Since 1957, corticosteroids have been associated with a number of rheumatic diseases, including avascular necrosis, myopathy, and a "pseudoarthritis" when patients receiving long-term corticosteroid therapy are withdrawn from the drug. Spontaneous rupture of tendons in patients receiving local or systemic steroids is well recognized. The precise pathogenesis of these syndromes remains unknown except for the possible involvement of fat emboli in avascular necrosis. In one study of corticosteroid-associated avascular necrosis, 12 of 20 patients had evidence for intravascular fat emboli in bone specimens (Jones, 1979). There are some animal studies that support this human observation (Fisher, 1978).

B. Penicillamine

Penicillamine is a drug of many contradictions. Even the observation that stimulated its original use, the depolymerization of macroglobulins, seems unrelated to its immunomodulating properties in the treatment of rheumatoid arthritis. Although it seems an effective modality in the management of rheumatoid arthritis, its use is associated with the evolution of an extraordinary variety of drug-related diseases, many of which are themselves likely to be present on an autoimmune basis (Stein *et al.*, 1980). These include a lupuslike syndrome, proteinuria associated with a membranous type of glomerulonephritis, thrombocytopenia and aplastic anemia, Goodpasture's syndrome, dermatomyositis, myasthenia gravis, worsening of the patient's arthritis with perhaps a superimposed arthritis, obliterative bronchiolitis, and a wide variety of skin rashes. A rare reaction is elastosis perforens serpiginosa. These syndromes can also occur in Wilson's disease and cystinuria, although less frequently. Reports of recrudescence of penicillamine-induced polymyositis by penicillin, though few in number, require explanation (Jaffe, 1975). Penicillamine used to be contaminated by trace amounts of penicillin but is now produced synthetically, thereby eliminating this possibility.

The exact mode of action of penicillamine in the treatment of rheumatoid arthritis is unknown. Evidence has been presented to indicate that, at least in some patients, it causes a reduction in rheumatoid factors (Wernick *et al.*, 1983) and in the level of circulating immune complexes, interferes with cellular immunologic reaction that lead to immunoglobulin synthesis, and, in *in vivo* experiments with rats, increases the response of spleen and lymph node cells to concanavalin A (Binderup *et al.*, 1980a–c). Many of these effects, including those on immune complexes, have been related to an effect of penicillamine on macrophages. According to Binderup and Arrigoni-Martelli (1979), it preferentially binds the membrane of macrophages but not the lymphocytes. It also enhances the uptake of glucosamine by macrophages as well as increasing phagocytosis of aggregated γ-globulin (Binderup *et al.*, 1978). Since macrophages are a primary antigen-presenting cell, it is conceivable that the processing of a number of cell antigens by macrophages under the influence of penicillamine could result in these cell antigens becoming antigenic rather than tolerogenic. This is theoretical and unproven but nevertheless attractive.

Another effect of *d*-penicillamine on macrophages has been observed in adjuvant arthritis. The response to the T-cell mitogen Con A and to the B-cell mitogen LPS is blunted in rats with active disease and may be related to suppressor macrophages. Suppressor activity can be revived by treatment of the rats with *d*-penicillamine (Binderup *et al.*, 1980c). Normal rats treated with penicillamine showed a self-limited increase in Con A responsiveness in lymph nodes and spleen cells. The effect was dependent on the presence of functionally intact macrophages.

Lipsky (1984), using short-term incubation with penicillamine has found somewhat different results. The target cell of penicillamine seems to be the T lymphocyte, and he has shown that PHA stimulation of lymphocytes is inhibited by penicillamine in the presence of cupric sulfate or ceruloplasmin. This inhibition is seemingly mediated in part by hydrogen peroxide. Monocyte lysates exerted a protective effect through a heat-labile azide-sensitive soluble factor.

C. Other Drug Associations

Rhabdomyolosis and intravascular coagulopathy have been recognized as consequences of intravenous amphetamine administration, and similar conditions occur with heroin and phencyclidine usage. Skin changes suggestive of scleroderma and also pulmonary fibrosis have been associated with bleomycin therapy. Those exposed to polyvinyl chloride can have similar changes and also manifest acroosteolysis. Levamisole is associated with a severe arthritis when given to Crohn's disease patients. Prazosin is associated with an acute febrile polyarthritis. Methysergide given for headache has been associated with retroperitoneal fibrosis, as has atenolol, a β blocker. A number of drugs used in the treatment of thyroid disease, including carbimazole, can induce arthropathy and a lupus syndrome. A recent report from Japan (Hirata *et al.*, 1980) describes a significant percentage of patients with an autoimmune insulin syndrome who had received methimazole treatment for thyrotoxicosis. Another recent report (Blackshear *et al.*, 1983) describes a patient who developed symptomatic hypoglycemia with antiinsulin antibodies of the IgG type in the same year that she developed a lupus syndrome when on procainamide and hydralazine. Chloroquine has been associated with myopathies and neuromyopathies.

Hemolytic anemia occurs in about 1% of patients taking methyldopa, but the drug does not act as a hapten in this situation. Another intriguing association is with the drug venocuran, which is used in Europe for the treatment of venous disease. These patients develop a DRL-like syndrome but have antimitochondrial and not antinuclear antibodies. A Sjögrenlike syndrome has been reported following the use of practolol, which can also cause DRL syndrome. It has been noted already that chlorpromazine, which is related to a lupus syndrome, also produces an inhibitor to coagulation factor VIII, and a similar abnormality occurs in association with penicillin. Parker (1981) has suggested that an antipenicillin antibody may cross react with factor VIII molecules.

The very common associations of drug-induced crystal arthropathies and the many drugs associated with the serum sickness syndromes and other hypersensitivity reactions really need no detailing in this chapter.

D. Other Agents

An intriguing new syndrome called the "toxic syndrome" has recently been reported from Spain (Mateo *et al.*, 1985). This is a disorder of multisystemic character related to the ingestion of adulterated rapeseed oil. Patients manifest a nonnecrotizing vasculitis, various types of hepatic injury, and/or a combination of musculoskeletal manifestations. Forty-six percent of this latter group have had positive antinuclear antibodies. Female sex and haplotype HLA-DR3 and/or DR4 may provide a possible explanation why 15% of the 20,000 affected patients in Spain actually developed these chronic syndromes. Work is currently under way to determine possible pathogenetic mechanisms for these intriguing observations.

REFERENCES

Balázs, T., Robinson, C. J. G., and Balter, N., 1981, Hydralazine-induced antinuclear antibodies in beagle dogs, *Toxicol. Appl. Pharmacol.* **57**:452–456.

Batchelor, J. R., Welsh, K. I., Tinoco, R. M., Collery, C. T., Hughes, G. R. V., Bernstein, R., Ryan, P., Naish, P. F., Aber, G. M., Binz, R. F., and Russell, G. I., 1980, Hydralazine-induced systemic lupus erythematosus: Influence of HLA-DR and sex on susceptibility, *Lancet* **1**:1102–1109.

Binderup, L., and Arrigoni-Martelli, E., 1979, [^{14}C]D-Penicillamine: Uptake and distribution in rat lymphocytes and macrophages, *Biochem. Pharmacol.* **28**:189.

Binderup, L., Bramm, E., and Arrigoni-Martelli, E., 1978, D-Penicillamine and macrophages: Modulation of lymphocyte transformation by concanavalin A, *Scand. J. Immunol.* **7**:259–264.

Binderup, L., Bramm, E., and Arrigoni-Martelli, E., 1980a, D-Penicillamine *in vivo* enhances lymphocyte DNA synthesis: Role of macrophages, *Scand. J. Immunol.* **11**:23–28.

Binderup, L., Bramm, E., and Arrigoni-Martelli, E., 1980b, Effect of *d*-penicillamine *in vitro* and *in vivo* on macrophage phagocytosis, *Biochem. Pharmacol.* **29**:2273–2278.

Binderup, L., Bramm, E., and Arrigoni-Martelli, E., 1980c, Immunological effects of *d*-penicillamine during experimentally induced inflammation in rats, *Scand. J. Immunol.* **12**:239–247.

Blackshear, P. J., Rotner, H. E., Kriauciunas, K. A. M., and Kahn, C. R., 1983, Reactive hypoglycemia and insulin autoantibodies in drug-induced lupus erythematosus, *Ann. Intern. Med.* **99**:182–183.

Blomgren, S. E., Condemi, J. J., and Vaughan, J. H., 1972, Procainamide-induced lupus erythematosus. Clinical and laboratory observations, *Am. J. Med.* **52**:338–348.

Bluestein, H. G., Redelmen, D., and Zvaifler, N., 1981, Procainamide–lymphocyte reactions, *Arthritis Rheum* **24**(8):1019–1023.

Brand, C., Davidson, A., Littlejohn, G., and Ryan, P., 1984, Hydralazine induced lupus: No association with HLA-DR4, *Lancet* **1**:462.

Burry, J. N., 1969, Lipstick and lupus erythematosus, *N. Engl. J. Med.* **281**:620–621.

Cameron, D. J., and Erlanger, B. F., 1976, Nucleic acid-reactive antibodies of restricted heterogeneity, *Immuno. Chem.* **13**:263–269.

Canoso, R. P., Lewis, M. E., and Yunis, E. J., 1982, Association of HLA BW44 with chlorpromazine induced autoantibodies, *Clin. Immunol. Immunopathol.* **25**:278–282.

Carpenter, J. R., McDuffie, F. C., Sheps, S. G., Spiekerman, R. E., Brumfield, H., and King, R., 1980, Prospective study of immune response to hydralazine and development of anti-desoxyribonucleoprotein in patients receiving hydralazine, *Am. J. Med.* **69**:395–400.

Cavaglia, A. M., 1980, *In vitro* induction of sister-chromatid and human peripheral lymphocytes by hydralazine, *Mutat. Res.* **77**:383–385.

Chandrasekhar, A. J., Robinson, J., and Barr, L., 1978, Antibody deposition in the pleura: A finding in drug-induced lupus, *J. Allergy Clin. Immunol.* **61**:399–402.

Comens, P., 1956, Experimental hydralazine disease and its similarity to disseminated lupus erythematosus, *J. Lab. Clin. Med.* **471**:444–454.

Drayer, D. E., Lorenzi, B., Lahita, R. G., Robbins, W. C., and Reidenberg, M. D., 1982, Microsomal hydroxylation as measured by pentobarbital elimination in patients with systemic lupus erythematosus, *Clin. Pharmacol. Ther.* **32**:195–200.

Dubois, E. L., Katz, Y. J., Freeman, V., and Garbak, F., 1961, Chronic toxicity studies of hydralazine (Apresoline) in dogs with particular reference to the production of the "hydralazine syndrome," *J. Lab. Clin. Med.* **50**:119–126.

Dubroff, L. M., Reid, R., Jr., and Papalian, M., 1981, Molecular models for hydralazine-related systemic lupus erythematosus, *Arthritis Rheum.* **24**(8):1092–1085.

Ferguson, R. M., Schmidtke, J. R., and Simnons, R. L., 1976, Inhibition of mitogen produced lymphocyte transformation by local anesthetics, *J. Immunol.* **116**:627–634.

Fisher, D. E., 1978, The role of fat embolism in the etiology of corticosteroid-induced avascular necrosis, *Clin. Orthoped.* **130**:68–80.

Foad, B., Litwin, A., Zimmer, H., Hess, E. V., 1977, Acetylator phenotype in systemic lupus erythematosus, *Arthritis Rheum.* **20**:815–818.

Freeman, R. W., Woosley, R. L., Oates, J. H., and Harbison, R. D., 1979, Evidence for the biotransformation of procainamide to a reactive metabolite, *Toxicol. Appl. Pharmacol.* **50**:9–16.

Fritzler, M. J., and Tan, E. M., 1978, Antibodies to histones in drug-induced and idiopathic lupus erythematosus, *J. Clin. Invest.* **62**:560–567.

Fukase, M., 1976, Epidemiology of SLE, *Saishin Igaku* **32:**2–11.
Gardner, D. L., 1957, The response of the dog to oral 1-hydrazinophthalazine (hydralazine), *Br. J. Exp. Pathol.* **38:**227–235.
Goldberg, S., Lipschutz, J., Ricketts, R., and Fine, A., 1984, Procainamide induced lupus lung disease characterized by neutrophil alveolitis, *Am. J. Med.* **76:**146–150.
Grossman, L., and Barland, P., 1981, Histone reactivity of drug induced anti-nuclear antibodies, *Arthritis Rheum.* **24:**927–931.
Harris, G., 1983, DNA damage and repair in immunologically active cells, *Immunol. Today,* **4**(4)**:**109–112.
Hersey, P., Hasic, E., Edwards, A., Bradley, M., Haran, G., and McCarthy, W. H., 1983, Immunological effects of solarium exposure, *Lancet* **1:**545–548.
Hess, E. V., 1981, Introduction to drug-related lupus, *Arthritis Rheum.* **24**(8)**:**6–10.
Hein, D. W., and Weber, W. W., 1982, Polymorphic N-acetylation of phenelzine and monoacetylhydrazine by highly purified rabbit liver isoniazid N-acetyltransferase, *Drug Metab. Dispos.* **10:**225–229.
Hildreth, E. A., Biro, C. E., and McCreary, I. A., 1960, Persistence of the "hydralazine syndrome." A follow-up study of eleven cases, *JAMA* **173:**657–660.
Hirata, Y., Omori, Y., Takei, M., and Nakazawa, M., 1980, Autoimmunity in diabetes mellitus, *Gunma Symp. Endocrinol.* **17:**81–91.
Hoffman, B. J., 1945, Sensitivity to sulfadiazine resembling acute disseminated lupus erythematosus, *Arch. Dermatol. Syph.* **51:**190–192.
Jacobs, M. E., Steinberg, A. D., Gordon, J. K., and Talal, N., 1972, Adjuvant effects of poly I · poly C in New Zealand mice, *Arthritis Rheum.* **15:**201–207.
Jaffe, J. A., 1975, Penicillamine treatment of rheumatoid arthritis: Effect on immune complexes, *Ann. N.Y. Acad. Sci.* **256:**330.
Jones, J. P., Jr., 1979, Osteonecrosis, in: *Arthritis and Allied Conditions,* 9th ed. (D. J. McCarthy, ed.), Lea & Febiger, Philadelphia, p. 1121.
Kincaid-Smith, P., and Whitworth, P. A., 1983, Hydralazine-associated glomerulonephritis, *Lancet* **2:**348.
Koffler, D., Schur, P. H., and Kunkel, H. G., 1967, Immunological studies concerning the nephritis of systemic lupus erythematosus, *J. Exp. Med.* **126:**607–623.
Lahita, R., Kluger, J., Drayer, D. E., Koffler, D., and Reidenberg, M. D., 1979, Antibodies to nuclear antigens in patients treated with procainamide or acetylprocainamide, *N. Engl. J. Med.* **301:**1382–1385.
Laskov, R., Muller, S., Hochberg, M., Giloh, H., Van Regenmortel, M., and Eilat, D., 1984, Monoclonal autoantibodies to histones from autoimmune NZB/NZW F_1 mice, *Eur. J. Immunol.* **14:**74–81.
Lipsky, P., 1984, Immunosuppression by *d*-penicillamine *in vitro.* Inhibition of human T lymphocyte proliferation by copper- or ceruloplasmin-dependent generation of hydrogen peroxide and protection by monocytes, *J. Clin. Invest.* **73:**53–65.
Litwin, A., Adams, L. E., Zimmer, H., Foad, B., Loggie, J. H. M., and Hess, E. V., 1981a, Prospective study of immunologic effects of hydralazine in hypertensive patients, *Clin. Pharmacol. Ther.* **29:** 447–456.
Litwin, A., Adams, L. E., Zimmer, H., and Hess, E. V., 1981b, Immunologic effects of hydralazine in hypertensive patients, *Arthritis Rheum.* **24**(8)**:**1074–1077.
MacKinney, A. A., and Booker, H. E., 1972, Diphenylhydantoin effect on human leukocytes *in vitro* and *in vivo, Arch. Intern. Med.* **129:**988.
Malinow, M. R., Bardana, E. J., Jr., Pirofsky, B., Craig, S., and McLaughlin, P., 1982, Systemic lupus erythematosus-like syndrome in monkeys fed alfalfa sprouts: Role of a non-protein amino acid, *Science* **216:**415–427.
Mateo, I. M., Izquierdo, M., Fernandez-Dapica, M. P., Navas, J., Cabello, A., and Gomez-Reino, J. J., 1985, Toxic epidemic syndrome: Musculoskeletal manifestations, *J. Rheumatol.* (in press).
Miller, E. B., and Salem, D., 1982, Immune regulatory abnormalities produced by procainamide, *Am. J. Med.* **73:**487–492.
Morrow, J. D., Schroeder, H. A., and Perry, H. M., Jr., 1953, Studies on the control of hypertension by hyphex. II. Toxic reactions and side effects, *Circulation* **8:**829–839.
Ochi, T., Goldings, E. A., Lipsky, P. E., and Ziff, M., 1983, Immunomodulatory effect of procainamide in man. Inhibition of human suppressor T-cell activity *in vitro, J. Clin. Invest.* **71:**36–45.
Perry, H. M., Jr., 1973, Late toxicity to hydralazine resembling systemic lupus erythematosus or rheumatoid arthritis, *Am. J. Med.* **54:**58–72.

Perry, H. M., Jr., Tan, E. M., Carmody, S., and Sakamoto, H., 1970, Relationship of acetyl transferase activity to antinuclear antibodies and toxic symptoms in hypertensive patients treated with hydralazine, *J. Lab. Clin. Med.* **76:**114–124.

Portanova, J. P., Rubin, R. L., Joslin, F. G., Agnello, V. D., and Tan, E. M., 1982, Reactivity of anti-histone antibodies induced by procainamide and hydralazine, *Clin. Immunol. Immunopathol.* **25:** 67–79.

Reidenberg, M. M., 1981, The chemical induction of systemic lupus erythematosus and lupus-like illnesses, *Arthritis Rheum.* **24:**1004–1008.

Reidenberg, M. M., 1983, Aromatic amines and the pathogenesis of lupus erythematosus, *Am. J. Med.* **75:**1037–1042.

Reidenberg, M. M., and Martin, J. H., 1974, Acetylator phenotype of patients with systemic lupus erythematosus, *Drug Metab. Dispos.* **2:**71–73.

Reidenberg, M. M., Levy, M., Drayer, D. E., Zylber-Katz, E., and Robbins, W. C., 1980, Acetylator phenotype in idiopathic systemic lupus erythematosus, *Arthritis Rheum.* **23:**569–573.

Roberts, J. L., and Hayashi, J. A., 1983, Exacerbation of SLE associated with alfalfa ingestion, *N. Engl. J. Med.* **308:**1361.

Roberts, S. M., Budinsky, R. A., Adams, L. E., Litwin, A., and Hess, E. V., 1985, Procainamide acetylation in strains of rat and mouse. *Drug Metab. Dispos.* (in press).

Roden, D. M., Reele, S. B., Higgins, S. B., Wilkinson, G. R., Smith, R. F., Oates, J. H., and Woosley, R. L., 1980, Anti-arrhythmic efficiency, pharmacokinetics and safety of N-acetylprocainamide in human subjects: Comparison with procainamide, *Am. J. Cardiol.* **46:**463–468.

Rubin, R. L., Joslin, F. G., and Tan, E. M., 1982, Specificity of antihistone antibodies in systemic lupus erythematosus, *Arthritis Rheum.* **25:**779–782.

Scorza-Smeraldi, R., Sabbadini Villa, M. G., Fabio, G., Bonara, P., Vanoli, M., Resele, L., and Zanussi, C., 1983, HLA antigens and the reactivity of lymphocytes to some drugs and PHA, *Int. J. Immunopharmacol.* **5:**145–149.

Sheikh, T. K., Charron, R. C., and Katz, A., 1981, Renal manifestations of drug-induced systemic lupus erythematosus, *Am. J. Clin. Pathol.* **75:**755–762.

Sonnhag, C., Karlsson, E., and Hed, J., 1979, Procainamide-induced lupus erythematosus-like syndrome in relation to acetylator phenotype and plasma levels of procainamide, *Acta Med. Scand.* **206:**245–251.

Spencer-Green, G., Adams, L. E., Hurtubise, P., Kravatz, G., and Hess, E. V., 1985, Familial alterations of immunoregulation in systemic lupus erythematosus, *J. Rheumatol.* (in press).

Spiegel, M., Lee, S. L., and Peress, N. S., 1967, The epidemiology of drug-induced systemic lupus erythematosus, *Arthritis Rheum.* **10:**407–415.

Stec, G. P., Lertoro, J. J. L., Atkinson, A. J., Jr., Nevin, M. J., Kushner, W., Jones, C., Schmid, F. R., and Askennzi, J., 1979, Remission of procainamide-induced lupus erythematosus with N-acetylprocainamide therapy, *Ann. Intern. Med.* **90:**799–801.

Stein, H. B., Patterson, A. C., Offer, R. C., Atkins, C. J., Teufel, A., and Robinson, H. S., 1980, Adverse effects of *d*-penicillamine in rheumatoid arthritis, *Ann. Intern. Med.* **92:**24–29.

Stollar, B. D., 1973, Nucleic acid antigen, in: *The Antigens,* Vol. I (M. Sela, ed.), Academic Press, New York, pp. 1–85.

Tan, E. M., 1974, Drug-induced autoimmune disease, *Fed. Proc.* **33:**1894–1897.

Tan, E. M., Cohen, A. S., Fries, J. F., Masi, A. T., McShane, D. J., Rothfield, N. F., Schaller, J. G., Talal, N., and Winchester, R. J., 1982, The 1982 revised criteria for the classification of systemic lupus erythematosus, *Arthritis Rheum.* **25:**1271–1277.

Tanaka, K., Shozaburo, J., Kajiyama, K., Nighigouri, S., Kameda, S., Toshiyuki, Y., Yamaguchi, M., Matsuyama, K., and Iguchi, S., 1982, Increased hydrazine excretion associated with systemic lupus erythematosus, *Clin. Immunol. Immunopathol.* **22:**55–59.

Uetrecht, J. P., and Woosley, R. L., 1981, Acetylator phenotype and lupus erythematosus, *Clin. Pharmacokinet.* **6:**118–134.

Uetrecht, J. P., Freeman, R. W., Woosley, R. L., 1981, The implications of procainamide metabolism to its induction of lupus, *Arthritis Rheum.* **24:**994–999.

Vansant, J., Woosley, R. L., John, J. T., and Sergent, J. S., 1978, Normal distribution of acetylator phenotypes in systemic lupus erythematosus, *Arthritis Rheum.* **21:**192–195.

Weber, W. W., and Tannen, R. H., 1981, Pharmacogenetic studies on the drug-related lupus syndrome.

Differences in antinuclear antibody development and drug-induced DNA damage in rapid and slow acetylator animal models, *Arthritis Rheum.* **24:**979–985.

Weigle, W. O., 1980, Analysis of autoimmunity through experimental models of thyroiditis and allergic encephalomyelitis, *Adv. Immunol.* **30:**159–273.

Wernick, R., Merryman, P., Jaffe, I., and Ziff, M., 1983, IgG and IgM rheumatoid factors in rheumatoid arthritis. Quantitative response to penicillamine therapy and relationship to disease activity, *Arthritis Rheum.* **26:**593–598.

Wooley, P. H., Griffin, J., Panayi, G. S., Batchelor, J. R., Welsh, K. I., and Gibson, T. J., 1980, HLA-DR antigens and toxicity to sodium aurothiomalate and penicillamine in rheumatoid arthritis, *N. Engl. J. Med.* **303:**300–302.

Woosley, R. L., Drayer, D. E., Reidenberg, M. D., Nies, A. S., Carr, K., and Oates, J. A., 1978, Effect of acetylator phenotype on the rate at which procainamide induces antinuclear antibodies and the lupus syndrome, *N. Engl. J. Med.* **298:**1157–1159.

Yamauchi, Y., Litwin, A., Adams, L. E., Zimmer, H., and Hess, E. V., 1975, Induction of antibodies to nuclear antigens in rabbits by immunization with hydralazine-human serum albumin conjugates, *J. Clin. Invest.* **56:**958–969.

25

Psychoneuroimmunologic Contributions to the Study of Rheumatic Diseases

Robert Ader

I. INTRODUCTION

Psychosocial factors are related to the predisposition to and the precipitation and/or perpetuation of a variety of pathophysiological processes, including those involving immunologic defense mechanisms. That is not to say that psychosocial factors cause disease. I know of no organic disease that is directly "caused" by psychological or social conditions. There is abundant evidence, however, that psychosocial variables contribute to the development and progression of disease—not just some diseases, those referred to as "psychosomatic," but, to a greater or lesser extent, virtually all diseases. One can adopt this position without denying the existence of "germs." In the real world, however, individuals are rarely exposed to pathogens in a dose or via a route that unconditionally elicits clinical disease. Health, rather than illness, is the norm, and it is not uncommon to observe large individual differences among individuals exposed to common pathogenic stimuli.

As Dubos (1959) has so eloquently argued, biomedical research is modeled after the successful approach taken by Koch, Pasteur, and a following generation of scientists who designed and conducted their experiments in order to minimize any "extraneous" factors that might influence the phenomena that they were studying. Such a strategy, however, minimizes the myriad factors that do, in reality, influence the behaving individual in his adaptation to the real world. Therefore, to "model" a disease process in a laboratory animal and selectively impose conditions that do not provide the latitude for the expression of variables that may contribute to the development and progression of

Robert Ader • Division of Behavioral and Psychosocial Medicine, Department of Psychiatry, University of Rochester School of Medicine and Dentistry, Rochester, New York 14642.

disease as these occur in the real world serve only to identify conditions that may be necessary but that may not be sufficient for the expression of disease. The incompleteness of the classic biomedical model and alternative strategies that emphasize the host and consider the multifactorial causality of disease have been discussed by several authors (Ader, 1981a; Engle, 1977; Weiner, 1978).

A similar point of view has been expressed by Smith and Steinberg (1983) with respect to autoimmune disease. These authors argue that Koch's postulates are not applicable to all diseases and that one can no longer restrict the study of autoimmune disorders to the search for single causative agents. It is the characteristics of the host that are of paramount importance in the multifactorial etiology of many autoimune diseases. It is argued that autoimmune diseases result from some disruption of the normal functioning of immunoregulatory circuits. They also emphasize that many (and, perhaps, all) diseases are mediated by alterations in immune function and are sensitive to genetic and environmental influences. Smith and Steinberg do not elaborate on the kinds of environmental factors that could influence the expression of autoimmune disease through their effects on immunoregulatory functions. I may be going well beyond what Smith and Steinberg meant to imply, but the point that is being raised in the present chapter is that immune function is, indeed, subject to environmental influences and that many (and, perhaps, the most important) of these effects act through the central nervous system.

Given a biological vulnerability, environmental circumstances that are perceived as "stressful" or as constituting a threat to the psychological or biological integrity of the individual and the multidetermined capacity of that individual to adapt or cope with the demands and events in the environment are some of the psychobiological factors that determine the response to superimposed pathogenic stimuli as well as the biological (and immunologic?) state of the organism. Theoretically, conditions would be optimal for the expression of disease (in response to superimposed pathogenic stimulation or as a consequence of a disruption of immunoregulatory functions, for example) if there exists a high biological predisposition, if the person's personality structure or existing psychophysiological state is such that environmental circumstances are perceived as threatening or "stressful," and if the individual is unable or no longer able to cope effectively with such circumstances. For any given pathophysiological process or in any given individual, however, we are not yet able to determine the relative contribution of each of these factors.

A great deal of research has been directed to the physiological mechanisms that may mediate the effects of psychosocial factors on alterations in the susceptibility to and recovery from disease. For some diseases (and, perhaps, for a growing number of diseases), the underlying mechanisms may involve immune processes. Such a hypothesis, however, is predicated on documentation of a functional relationship between the immune system and the brain. Indirect data in support of such an hypothesis have existed for years, and data bearing directly on the hypothesis are accumulating rapidly (Adler, 1981b). Several studies, for example, have documented the effects of "stress" on susceptibility to what are, or what are presumed to be, immunologically mediated diseases, and in recent years, research has been initiated to delineate the effects of "stress" on various measures of immunologic reactivity *per se*. Recent studies have also shown that immunologic reactivity may be modified by conditioning (learning). With respect to "hard" data, it will have to suffice here to simply refer to selected studies that provide evidence for central-nervous-system–immune-system interactions. Lesions and electrical stimulation of the hypothalamus, for example, result in alterations in humoral and cell-mediated immunity (Stein *et al.*, 1981), and, conversely, elicitation of an immune response influences electrical and neuroendocrine output from the hypothalamus (e.g., Besedovsky *et al.*, 1977). The prominence of the hypothalamus in regulating neuroendocrine functions implies a role for hormones and neurotransmitters in the modulation of immune responses. Indeed, there is a vast literature on such effects, reinforced by the identification of receptors for hormones and neurotransmitter substances on lymphocytes (e.g., Ahlqvist, 1981; Comsa *et al.*, 1982; Hall and Goldstein, 1981). The existence of neurochemical channels of communication between the central nervous system and the immune system is supported by other studies that have documented the innervation of lymphoid tissue (e.g., Bulloch and Moore, 1981; Felten *et al.*, 1981).

Such data provide the foundation and the rationale for expecting functional relationships between the brain and the immune system. For all its complexity and capacity for self-regulation, the immune system is a homeostatic defense mechanism that is integrated with other physiological systems of defense and, therefore, ultimately subject to regulation or modulation by the brain. As such, central-nervous-system-mediated alterations in immunoregulatory functions could be responsible for many of the effects of behavioral factors on the maintenance of health and the development of disease. The present chapter confines itself to an illustration of the role of behavioral factors in altering disease susceptibility and immunologic reactivity, emphasizing the data on autoimmune disease and the role of conditioning in modifying development of autoimmune disease in experimental animals.

II. PSYCHOSOCIAL FACTORS AND DISEASE

A. Studies in Humans

From a behavioral perspective, most of the literature implicating the central nervous system in the modulation of immune processes comes from clinical studies in humans and experimental studies in animals of the effects of psychosocial factors on susceptibility to disease processes that involve immunologic defense mechanisms and studies of immune responses to "stress." Infectious disease processes, for example, illustrate the ubiquitous observation that despite a common exposure to potentially pathogenic agents, only a relatively small proportion of infected individuals actually manifest clinical disease.

The likelihood of developing disease as well as the progression of disease appear to be sensitive to the perception of and response to major life events (e.g., Dohrenwend and Dohrenwend, 1974; Gunderson and Rahe, 1974; Rabkin and Struening, 1976). Meyer and Haggerty (1962) followed several families for a year and found that rating scale reports for "chronic stress" were associated with increased susceptibility to streptococcal disease. Jacobs *et al.* (1970) observed greater problems of adjustment among college students who sought medical attention for symptoms of respiratory illness than among a symptom-free sample of students. In terms of recovery, Boyce *et al.* (1977) found that the duration of respiratory illness was prolonged among children who scored high on a scale of life event changes, and Greenfield *et al.* (1959) reported a relatonship between "ego strength" as measured by a standard personality inventory and recovery from infectious mononucleosis in college students. Similar data exist for allergic conditions (e.g., Engels and Wittkower, 1975) and for autoimmune disorders (discussed below).

As part of a more extensive study of viral respiratory infections, Jackson *et al.* (1960) made some observations on the induction of "cold" symptoms that are relevant to the data on conditioned immunopharmacological responses described below. A sample of control subjects who were treated with placebo nasal drops showed a linear relationship between their previous susceptibility to colds and the development of cold symptoms following the inhalation of an isotonic salt solution. For example, 26% of those who reported having had five or more colds per year developed "cold" symptoms following the placebo treatment, whereas fewer than 10% of those who reported having had only one or two colds per year developed such "cold" symptoms. Also, "susceptible" individuals were more likely to believe that emotional states could influence physical health and to report their concern about personal problems that existed at the time of the experiment. Although personality factors influenced the report of "cold" symptoms in response to placebo treatment, "susceptible" and "nonsusceptible" subjects did not differ in response to an inoculation of virus.

One of the more extensive studies of psychosocial factors in infectious disease was conducted with over 1000 cadets from the West Point Military Academy (Kasl *et al.*, 1979). This prospective study concentrated on identifying risk factors predictive of the clinical expression and course of infectious mononucleosis among susceptible students who were known to be infected with Epstein–Barr virus (EBV). Initially, approximately two-thirds of the students were found to be immune to infection (i.e., had EBV antibody). Among the nonimmune population, approximately 20% became infected ("seroconverted"), and 25% of these seroconverters developed infectious mononucleosis. The risk that EBV infection would be expressed was increased among highly motivated students, those with poor academic performance, and those with "overachieving" fathers. These same risk factors also predicted elevated antibody titers among seroconverters without apparent disease and the length of hospitalization among those with clinical disease. Other recent studies (Kiecolt-Glaser *et al.*, 1984) have demonstrated decreased stimulation of B lymphocytes by EBV and lower antibody levels to EBV and other herpes viruses among seropositive medical students in response to the "stress" of examinations. A more extensive review of the potential influence of psychosocial factors on susceptibility to or recovery from infectious disease in humans has been prepared by Jemmott and Locke (1984).

Clinical studies and case reports also implicate psychosocial factors and the capacity to cope with "stress" as predisposing factors in the development of autoimmune disease (Weiner, 1977). Rheumatoid arthritis has been one of the most frequently examined disease processes in this regard (Moos, 1963). Descriptions of patients with rheumatoid arthritis based on extensive interview material have purported to uncover distinctive personality patterns and (ineffective) coping styles. In addition to the disparate personality profiles that have been described, there are the ubiquitous observations of real or threatened losses that precede the onset of disease (e.g., Ellman and Mitchell, 1936; Ludwig, 1955; Robinson, 1957). More recent and extensive observations of rhematoid arthritis patients (Shocket *et al.*, 1969) confirm the suggestion of a relationship between major life events, particularly those involving separation experiences, and the onset or exacerbation of symptoms. Hendrie *et al.* (1971) were unable to discern differences in "life change" scores between arthritis patients and controls but did find higher scores among those arthritis patients who had higher immunoglobulin levels.

Some of the most comprehensive studies of the personality characteristics of rheumatoid arthritis patients were conducted by Moos and Solomon (1964a, 1965a,b). The control group was comprised of that sister closest in age to the female patient with arthritis. These authors failed to confirm many of the personality profiles previously described but uncovered other outstanding characteristics in their patient populations. Compared to their healthy sisters, the rheumatoid arthritis patients were more conscientious, more masochistic and self-sacrificing, and tended to deny hostility. Although there was reasonable agreement between siblings in their descriptions of their parents (indicating that these retrospective reports were not simply a function of their physical condition), the arthritis patients perceived a greater degree of rejection by their parents than their sisters did. Meyerowitz *et al.* (1968) evaluated the role of psychosocial factors in the development of disease in monozygotic twins discordant for rheumatoid arthritis. No consistent developmental or health status differences were observed before the onset of arthritis. In four of the five adult twin sets that were studied in detail, however, there was evidence of a common "stressful" experience that preceded the development of disease in each of the affected twins.

The studies by Moos and Solomon also revealed an association between rheumatoid arthritis and longstanding "stressful" circumstances. Almost every patient linked the development of her disease with some acute or chronic "stress" varying from an unwanted move to a new home to the death of a relative. In attempting to relate psychological variables to the course of rheumatoid arthritis, Moos and Solomon (1964b) suggest that those patients with the most rapidly progressing disease were experiencing feelings of ego disintegration and an accompanying anxiety and depression that reflected their inability to maintain previously effective modes of coping. Rimon (1969), too, observed that "stressful" life events were more prevalent among rheumatoid arthritis patients with rapid onset and progression of the disease than among those whose disease progressed more slowly. Recognizing the need for a finer analysis of the relationship between personality and disease variables, several investigators (e.g., Crown *et al.*, 1975; Rimon, 1973) obtained psychometric data from arthritis patients with and without rheumatoid factor in their sera. These studies indicated that the seropositive (RF^+) patients were less aggressive and had lower anxiety scores than other arthritis patients. In studying the healthy relatives of patients with rheumatoid arthritis, Solomon and Moos (1965) found that those with rheumatoid factor were better adjusted psychologically than those who lacked this factor. These authors suggested that, given the biological predisposition to rheumatoid disease, it is those individuals who are unable to deal effectively with certain "stressful" life events that are likely to manifest clinical disease.

Dramatic illustrations of the potential impact of psychosocial factors in the onset of autoimmune disease are also provided by studies on juvenile onset arthritis. An increase in the frequency of important life events (e.g., hospitalization, significant psychological losses), for example, has been reported to precede the development of arthritis in children (Heisel, 1972). Henoch *et al.* (1978) compared 88 children with juvenile rheumatoid arthritis with a random pediatric population from the same geographic area. In the arthritis group there was a high (28%) incidence of parents who were divorced, separated, or widowed compared to the controls (11%), and in half of these cases, the loss of one parent occurred near the time of disease onset. Adoption, too, was three times more prevalent among the children with arthritis than among the control population. Rimon *et al.* (1977) were unable to abstract any common element with respect to family interactions among juvenile arthritis patients but did note personality characteristics that were similar to those described in adult patients with rheumatoid arthritis.

In reviewing the literature on the psychosocial influences and personality characteristics associated with rheumatoid arthritis, several authors (e.g., Solomon, 1981; Spergel *et al.*, 1977; Weiner, 1977) have commented on the complexity of the issues and the difficulties in conducting controlled studies, the limitations of correlative data, the inherent problems in retrospective analyses, and, perhaps as a consequence, the essential similarity of the data on the personality profile in patients with rheumatoid arthritis and patients with other disorders having autoimmune features such as ulcerative colitis (e.g., Engel, 1953), multiple sclerosis (e.g., Grinker and Robbins, 1954), Graves' disease (e.g., Mandelbrote and Wittkower, 1955; Morillo and Gardner, 1979), and systemic lupus erythematosus (McClary *et al.*, 1955; Otto and McKay, 1967).

With respect to an analysis of the predisposing personality characteristics that may interact with biological factors to influence the onset and course of rheumatoid arthritis, a recent study by Vollhardt *et al.* (1982) controlled some of the confounding variables indentified in previous research. These investigators compared RF^+ rheumatoid arthritis patients, RF^- arthritis patients, and a mixed group of chronic nonrheumatoid arthritis patients. The groups were carefully defined in terms of their disease classification and matched for chronicity of disease, functional impairment, and psychosocial and demographic variables. In addition to the biological (the American Rheumatologic Association diagnostic criteria for rheumatoid arthritis) and demographic data collected, standard instruments for the assessment of a variety of mood states and feelings and for subjectively perceived distress were administered.

None of the psychometric tests scores differentiated between the RF^- and mixed group of patients; both of these groups, however, differed significantly from the RF^+ group of arthritis patients. Based on the several scales that yielded statistically reliable differences, the RF^+ group could be described as showing less psychopathology. A factor analysis that included the biological, demographic, and psychological data yielded four independent factors, one of which was comprised exclusively of psychometric socres. Although rheumatoid arthritis is a heterogeneous entity, a considerable homogeneity exists among those with adult onset, RF^+ arthritis. Likewise, this seropositive group shows homogeneity with respect to a variety of psychometric indices. As a result, Vollhardt *et al.* could, on the basis of the psychometric measures alone, correctly categorize patients with rheumatoid arthritis into their diagnostic subgroups. That is, 63% of the mixed group, 65% of the RF^- group, and 100% of the RF^+ group could be correctly classified. The association between biological and psychological characteristics observed by Vollhardt *et al.* is consistent with the previously reported association between the presence of rheumatoid factor and low psychopathology scores among rheumatoid arthritis patients (Crown *et al.*, 1975; Gardner, 1980; Rimon, 1973) or their relatives (Solomon and Moos, 1965). It would not be unreasonable to anticipate the extension of these data to the design of prospective studies of individuals who may be at risk for rheumatoid arthritis.

The central nervous system involvement in SLE results in neurological dysfunctions and behavioral abnormalities (e.g., Carr *et al.*, 1978; Ganz *et al.*, 1972) that have yet to be systematically described or organized (Kassan and Lockshin, 1979). Under these circumstances, it is particularly difficult to evaluate the psychosocial and personality factors that may predispose to or precipitate the onset of disease symptoms. Even so, clinical observations have indicated that emotional situations, notably the real or threatened loss of important interpersonal relationships, preceded the onset of the disease in 13 of 14 SLE patients in one study (McClary *et al.*, 1955) and in all 28 patients of another (Otto and McKay, 1967).

The influence of psychobiological factors in SLE is most dramatically illustrated, perhaps, by a clinical vignette. Kirkpatrick (1981) described a documented case of lupus in a young Phillippine–American woman that was cured by witchcraft. Sustained, high-dose prednisone and cyclophosphamide treatment was recommended when a biopsy revealed membraneous and focal glomerulonephritis and immune complex disease. The woman chose, instead, to return to the Phillippine village where she was born. While she was there, a witch doctor removed a curse that had been placed on her by a former suitor. She returned to the United States 3 weeks later free of symptoms and "normal." Two years later she gave birth to a healthy child. Even though placebo therapy can be effective and voodoo deaths have been amply documented, "how," asked Kirkpatrick, "did the machinations of an Asian medicine man cure active lupus nephritis, change myxedema into euthyroidism, and allow precipitous withdrawal from corticosteroid treatment without symptoms of adrenal insufficiency?"

B. Studies in Animals

Most of the experimental data on the relationship between "stress" and disease comes from animal research, some of which is of potential relevance within the context of the present volume. For example, stimulation generally considered to be "stressful" has been reported to increase susceptibility to herpes simplex (Rasmussen *et al.*, 1957), Coxsackie B (Johnson *et al.*, 1959), polyoma (Chang and Rasmussen, 1964), and vesicular stomatitis (Jensen and Rasmussen, 1963; Yamada *et al.*, 1964) viruses in mice. Paralleling a not uncommon clinical situation (e.g., Holmes *et al.*, 1951), Friedman *et al.* (1965) found that neither "stress" nor an inoculum of Coxsackie B virus, alone, was sufficient to induce manifest disease in adult mice. The combination of "stress" and virus inoculation, however, did elicit symptoms of disease.

In contrast to the above results, Jensen (1968) found that "stress" decreased susceptibility to Rauscher leukemia virus in mice, and Levine *et al.* (1962) found that physical restraint but not a cold bath exposure suppressed development of allergic encephalomyelitis in rats. Johnson and Rasmussen (1965) found that "stress" increased susceptibility to poliomyelitis virus in mice, whereas Marsh *et al.* (1963) found that the same kind of environmental demands (avoidance conditioning) decreased susceptibility to polio in monkeys. The incidence of tumors induced by Moloney sarcoma virus was increased by physical restraint (Seifter *et al.*, 1973), whereas Amkraut and Solomon (1972) found that fighting and electric shock stimulation experienced before the introduction of virus decreased tumor size; electric shock experience after inoculaton of virus increased tumor size.

With respect to parasitic infection, both fighting (Weinmann and Rothman, 1967) and exposure to a predator (Hamilton, 1974) have been found to decrease resistance to

Hymenolepsis nana in mice. Resistance to *Plasmodium berghei,* a rodent malaria, however, is increased in rats maintained under "stressful" environmental circumstances (Friedman *et al.*, 1973).

A further illustration of the complex relationship between "stress" and disease comes from studies in which the social interactions among animals is manipulated. The simplest of these have dealt with differential housing (but referred to as studies of the effects of "crowding" or "isolation"). In summary, group housing or other experimental interventions that increase the social intercourse among animals have been found to increase susceptibility to some infectious processes such as trichinosis (Davis and Read, 1958), rabies virus (Soave, 1964), and malaria (Plaut *et al.*, 1969) but to decrease susceptibility to others, e.g., encephalomyocarditis virus (Friedman *et al.*, 1969) and *Escherichia coli* (Gross and Siegel, 1965). Still other studies (e.g., Tobach and Bloch, 1956; Edwards *et al.*, 1980) demonstrate that the effects of differential housing are determined by interactions involving gender and/or the conditions of housing before and/or after initiation of the infectious process.

Only a few studies have examined the effects of "stress" on autoimmune disease. The clinical literature (Solomon, 1981) suggests that rheumatoid arthritis patients tend to be hyperactive and that the development of arthritis often occurs when activity is thwarted. Based on such observations, Solomon *et al.* (1964) attempted to induce arthritis in rats by first eliciting and then blocking their high activity levels. Rats were trained to use activity wheels in order to obtain food, and the number of revolutions per unit of time required to procure the same food ration was gradually increased. Subsequently, wheel running was completely blocked, and then animals were subjected to an alternating schedule of permissible and impermissible activity for a period of 1 month. No evidence of joint inflammation could be observed. It was noticed, however, that the paws and digits of the animals subjected to this experimental regimen seemed to be cooler and paler than those of control animals, although temperature measurements failed to confirm these impressions. These investigators then measured peripheral vasoconstriction in response to "cold stress." They found lower temperatures and a slower adaptation to repeated cold exposures among animals subjected to the above regimen in which wheel running was blocked than in animals that were not trained to be active.

Although the frustration of an acquired pattern of behavior (in this case, wheel running), was not sufficient, in itself, to induce vasoconstriction, it was capable of pontentiating the effects of cold. In keeping with these data—and the argument outlined at the outset of this chapter regarding psychobiological interaction—it is hardly surprising that a nondebilitating behavioral intervention alone would not be sufficient to induce a pathophysiological state without a constitutional or experientially determined biological vulnerability on which it might be capable of exerting some effect. The superimposition of "stress," or the frustration of activity if that constitutes a particularly salient experience, on subthreshold treatment with known inducers of arthritis (e.g., complete Fruend's adjuvant or collagen) or in genetically prone mice might be an appropriate experimental model for studying the psychobiological processes involved in the pathogenesis of arthritis.

Rogers *et al.* (1980b) examined the effects of "stress" on collagen-induced arthritis. Groups of outbred rats were either moved from their colony housing and exposed to a cat, merely transported from the colony room and handled for an equivalent amount of time, or left totally unmanipulated. These interventions were imposed four times daily beginning 3 days before and continuing for 10 days after immunization with type II collagen. As expected, the incidence of arthritis in untreated animals was 40%. Only one of 39 rats exposed to a cat developed arthritis, and only four of 39 "handled" animals showed evidence of disease. Although both "stress" experiences reduced susceptibility to arthritis, defecation scores, taken as an index of emotionality, were higher among animals exposed to a cat than among those that experienced only a comparable duration of stimulation from the experimenters.

To the extent that group housing can be considered "stressful," these results appear inconsistent with the observation of more rapid onset and severity of adjuvant-induced arthritis in group- than in pair-housed male rats (Amkraut *et al.*, 1971). However, in another study (Rogers *et al.*, 1980a), rats exposed to a 100-db noise every 5 min for an hour each day beginning before and continuing after immunization with type II collagen showed an accelerated development of arthritis.

It is clear, even from this limited overview, that psychosocial factors are capable of altering pathophysiological processes that are (or may be) mediated by immunologic defense mechanisms. It is equally clear, however, that the effects of "stress" are not unitary; that is, they are neither uniformly detrimental nor beneficial to the organism. These and other studies using other disease models indicate that the impact of environmental events, whether or not they are labeled as being "stressful," depends on the psychophysiological state of the individual on whom such events are superimposed. The effects of "stress," in turn, contribute to the (experientally determined) state of the organism on which potentially pathogenic stimuli are constantly impinging. The variety of environmental interventions and the variety of pathophysiological processes that have been studied yield a seemingly contradictory pattern of results that preclude any generalizations regarding the effects of "stress." The observed effects depend, to a large extent, on the nature of the environmental circumstances and the nature of the disease process under study. More elaborate discussion of the relationship between "stress" and disease and the heuristic value of the concept of "stress" are available elsewhere (Ader, 1980, 1981a).

III. BEHAVIORAL INFLUENCES ON THE IMMUNE SYSTEM

A. Effects of "Stress"

Experiential as well as genetic factors are capable of influencing specific and nonspecific immune mechanisms. Host factors such as age (e.g., Makinodan and Yunis, 1977) and nutrition (e.g., Gross and Newberne, 1980) are among the more obvious ones. Environmental circumstances that are perceived as threatening to the psychological or biological well-being of the individual (i.e., "stressful" environmental circumstances) elicit a variety of psychobiological changes within the organism, and it is becoming evident that changes in immunocompetence are among the psychophysiological alterations that are induced by such events. At the very least, alterations in immunocompetence are a consequence of other neural or endocrine changes that occur in response to "stress" or represent one aspect of the process of adapting to the demands of the environment. The impact of "stress" and behavioral processes of adaptation on immune function, then, is receiving growing attention.

Several attempts have been made to relate personality factors and the efficacy of coping behaviors to immune function in humans (Jemmott and Locke, 1984). For the most part, these studies are quite preliminary in nature. Provocative results, however, have been reported. For example, one major life event that is regarded as psychobiologically disruptive is the death of one's spouse. Bartrop *et al.* (1977) found that bereavement was accompanied by a depression in mitogen-induced lymphocyte proliferation that was independent of the hormonal responses that were measured at the same time. Similar observations have been made and are being extended by Schleifer *et al.* (1983). A depression of immunologic reactivity in response to separation experiences has also been observed in monkeys (Coe *et al.*, 1984; Laudenslager *et al.*, 1982; Reite *et al.*, 1981), rats (Michaut *et al.*, 1981), and mice (Keller, *et al.*, 1983a).

Studies in animals have described "stress-induced" increases as well as decreases in humoral and cell-mediated immunity (Monjan, 1981). "Stressful" stimulation has been reported to increase contact sensitivity reactions to topically applied agents (Guy, 1952; Mettrop and Visser, 1969). A variety of "stressful" stimuli reduce inflammatory as well as cell-mediated immune responses (Amkraut *et al.*, 1973; Christian and Williamson, 1958; Gauci *et al.*, 1981; Funk and Jensen, 1967; Rasmussen *et al.*, 1959; Smith *et al.*, 1960; Pitkin, 1965; Treadwell and Rasmussen, 1961; Wistar and Hildemann, 1960). Mice subjected to the "stress" of acceleration in a centrifuge or etherization show a suppression of lymphocyte function depending on the strain of animal used (Gisler *et al.*, 1971).

Electric shock stimulation also suppresses lymphocyte function (Granata *et al.*, 1978; Keller *et al.*, 1981) and reduces leukocyte migration into the peritoneal cavity in response to an inflammatory agent (Bassett and Tait, 1981). In addition, electric shock and other "stresssful" stimuli (e.g., immobilization) decrease macrophage activity (Pavlidas and Chirigos, 1980; Teshima *et al.*, 1981). More sophisticated approaches to the study of "stress" effects suggest that the organism's capacity to cope with environmental circumstances determines the ultimate response. Rats that are able to escape from electric shock stimulation do not show a shock-induced depression of mitogen-induced lymphocyte proliferation (Laudenslager *et al.*, 1983).

Other noxious stimuli, including the manipulation of social interactions among animals, can increase or decrease primary and secondary antibody responses to different antigens in several species (Edwards *et al.*, 1980; Glenn and Becker, 1969; Hill *et al.*, 1967; Solomon, 1969; Vessey, 1964). Also, certain kinds of early life experiences that can chronically alter subsequent behavioral and physiological reactivity are capable of influencing animals' subsequent immunologic reactivity (Keller *et al.*, 1983a; Laudenslager *et al.*, 1982; Michaut *et al.*, 1981; Monjan and Mandell, 1980; Solomon *et al.*, 1968).

Most often, these "stress-induced" alterations in immune function are attributed to an elevation in adrenocortical steroids (whether or not measurements of steroids were included in the study). The complex relationship between steroids and immune function (e.g., Comsa *et al.*, 1982) is beyond the scope of this review. Suffice it to say that the extent to which there is a correlation between immunologic and adrenocortical activity depends on the chronicity of the "stressful" circumstances (e.g., Monjan and Collector, 1977), and too few parametric studies of the effects of "stress" are yet available to characterize this relationship. Nevertheless, some of the observed effects of "stress" probably are related to corticosteroid elevations; others are not. The results obtained by Blecha *et al.* (1982), for example, indicate that adrenal corticosteroids are involved in the immobilization-induced suppression of delayed-type hypersensitivity but can not account for the immobilization-induced enhancement of a contact sensitivity reaction. Gisler and Schenkel-Hulliger (1971) were able to mimic the *in vitro* immunologic effects of acceleration and etherization by treating animals with ACTH. However, the *in vivo* immunologic effects of these stimuli could not be reproduced by ACTH (Solomon and Amkraut, 1981). Similarly, Zweifach (1960) was unable to reproduce with ACTH the pattern of immunologic changes induced by a series of "stressful" stimuli. Keller *et al.* (1981) observed a reduction in lymphocyte reactivity *in vitro* related to the degree or intensity of environmental stimulation. These findings were repeated in a second study and were not abolished by adrenalectomy (Keller *et al.*, 1983b).

Psychosocial manipulations and "stressful" stimulation are capable of altering humoral and cell-mediated immune responses *in vitro* and *in vivo*. As with the data on disease susceptibility, however, there is considerable variability in the results, which, again, raises the question about the heuristic value of classifying all environmental perturbations under the general and nonspecific rubric of "stress." The effects of "stress" on immune function are determined by (1) the quality and quantity of environmental stimulation; (2) the quality and quantity of immunogenic stimulation; (3) the temporal relationship between "stress" and immunogenic stimulation; (4) the species, strain, age, gender, nutritional status, and other host factors on which "stress" and immunogenic stimuli are superimposed; (5) the immune process and sampling procedures that are chosen for measurement; and (6) the interactions among any or all of these variables.

B. Condition Alterations in Immunologic Reactivity

Learning is the primary means by which higher organisms adapt to their environment. It is also a primary function of brain activity—the most complex, perhaps, of all central nervous system functions. One of the most dramatic and compelling illustrations of the role of the central nervous system in the modulation of immune function, then, comes from the demonstration that one is able to modify immune responses by conditioning (Ader, 1981c; Ader and Cohen, 1981).

Historically, the conditioning of physiological responses dates from the work of Pavlov (1928). The classical or Pavlovian conditioning paradigm involves the selection of a stimulus, such as food, that unconditionally elicits a specific response, such as salivation. Food, then, is the unconditioned stimulus (UCS), and salivation is the unconditioned response (UR). If one repeatedly pairs a neutral stimulus such as the sound of a bell (i.e., a stimulus that does not unconditionally induce the unconditioned response in which the experimenter happens to be interested) with an unconditioned stimulus (food), the neutral stimulus will subsequently be able to evoke salivation when it is presented without food. The neutral stimulus has become a conditioned stimulus (CS) for salivation, and salivation in response to the CS is designated as a conditioned response. Similarly, if a light or a tone (the CS) is repeatedly associated with an electric shock that unconditionally elicits a flexion of the stimulated leg, leg flexion will eventually occur in response to the CS alone.

In the classical conditioning paradigm, a predictable temporal contingency is established among the CS, the UCS, and the UR. In contrast, instrumental or operant conditioning involves the reward or reinforcement of some desired response when it occurs in the context of some specific signal or set of environmental circumstances. A hungry rat may be rewarded with food for turning left in a maze, or a thirsty animal may be reinforced with a drop of water when it depresses a lever in its cage. Each such reinforcement strengthens or increases the probability of occurrence of the immediately preceding response.

Both classical and instrumental conditioning paradigms have been used to alter physiological as well as behavioral states. Interest in visceral and autonomic conditioning and the physiological concomitants of the acquisition and extinction of conditioned responses has received a great deal of attention over the past several years as a result of studies (e.g., Miller, 1969; DiCara, 1970) indicating that autonomic responses, previously thought to be involuntary, could be brought under experimental control using instumental as well as classical conditioning procedures. For technical reasons, primarily, most of this work has concentrated on cardiovascular responses, and research on the conditioning of endocrine responses is now receiving some attention. A great deal of research is being directed to the conditioning of a variety of pharmacological responses (Eikelboom and Stewart, 1982). Evidence is accumulating, for example, that the response (tolerance) to opiates involves conditioned responses (e.g., Siegel, 1977).

One especially effective conditioning paradigm is referred to as taste aversion learning (e.g., Garcia *et al.*, 1974). This is a passive avoidance conditioning situation in which consumption of a novel, distinctively flavored drinking solution (the CS) is paired with a stimulus (most frequently a pharmacological agent) that produces some noxious internal effects (the UCS). If, for example, water-deprived rats are provided with a saccharin-flavored drinking solution and then injected with lithium chloride, which causes temporary gastrointestinal upset, the rats learn in a single trial to avoid consuming saccharin-flavored water. Any number of conditioned stimuli (e.g., coffee, tea, or spice-flavored water solutions) and unconditioned stimuli (e.g., apomorphine, *d*-amphetamine, ethanol, cyclophosphamide, or radiation) are effective for studying illness-induced taste aversons. As is true of other situations, taste aversion learning is probably not a pure instance of either classical or instrumental learning but contains components of both. Also, depending on the procedures adopted, the taste aversion paradigm contains an element of conflict. If, for example, water-deprived conditioned animals are reexposed to the CS by providing them with a single drinking bottle containing the flavored solution previously associated with noxious drug affects, avoidance of the drinking solution is modified by the need to ingest fluid. In addition to the ease and rapidity with which they are established, taste aversions are retained over long periods of time (e.g., 3 months), and, in contrast to other learning paradigms, associations between gustatory cues and gastrointestinal consequences can be established with intervals of several hours between presentation of the CS and presentation of the UCS.

Using the illness-induced taste aversion paradigm, Ader and Cohen (1975) showed that reexposing conditioned animals to a CS previously paired with an immunosuppressive drug resulted in an aversion to saccharin and an attentuation of immunologic reactivity. The basic experimental protocol involved conditioning animals by providing them with a novel sodium saccharin drinking solution during a regularly scheduled drinking period to which they have been adapted. After consuming the novel solution, conditioned animals were injected with cyclophosphamide (CY), an unconditioned stimulus for suppression of the antibody response. Nonconditioned animals also receive CY, but CY was not paired with the consumption of saccharin. When subsequently immunized with sheep red blood cells (SRBC), some conditioned animals were injected with CY to define the unconditioned immunosuppressive effects of the drug, others were provided only with plain water to control for the effects of prior conditioning *per se,* and the critical experimental group was reexposed to the CS. Nonconditioned animals that never experienced saccharin paired with CY were similarly reexposed to the CS. Evidence for conditioning was provided by the observation that conditioned rats reexposed to the CS showed a depressed antibody response to SRBC relative to nonconditioned animals or conditioned animals that were not reexposed to the CS.

The phenomenon of conditioned immunosuppression has been observed repeatedly and under a variety of experimental conditions. The data shown in Fig. 1, for example, come from a study in which conditioned animals were reexposed to the CS before immunization with SRBC (Ader *et al.,* 1982). Also, these animals were reexposed to the CS (saccharin) in a preference-testing procedure in which two drinking bottles were

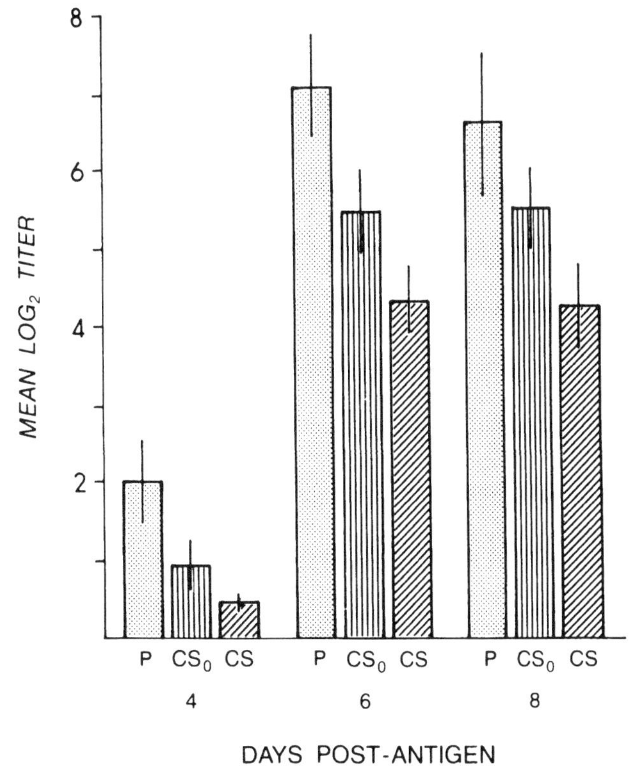

Figure 1. Hemagglutinating antibody titers (means ± S.E.) obtained 4, 6, and 8 days after injection of SRBC from independent groups of nonconditioned (placebo-treated) rats (P), conditioned animals that were not reexposed to conditioned stimuli (CS_0), and those that were reexposed to conditioned stimuli (CS) during the interval between conditioning and immunization. (Reprinted from Ader *et al.,* 1982, with permission from the American Psychological Association, Inc.)

provided to the animals: one contained saccharin and the other contained plain water. Under these conditions, one observes an aversion to saccharin, but total fluid consumption is constant for experimental and control groups. Several investigators have now documented behaviorally conditioned immunosuppression of antibody responses in rats and in mice (Ader and Cohen, 1981; Ader *et al.*, 1979; Cohen *et al.*, 1979; Gorczynski *et al.*, 1984; Rogers *et al.*, 1976; Wayner *et al.*, 1978). A conditioned enhancement of antibody production has also been reported (Jenkins *et al.*, 1983).

Conditioning is also capable of modulating cell-mediated immune responses. After the repeated grafting of allogeneic skin, conditioned mice responded to the stimulus conditions associated with grafting in the absence of the immunogenic stimulus (Gorczynski *et al.*, 1982). It is especially interesting that only half the animals that were tested in each of several replications of this study showed the conditioned response. When "responders" were divided into subgroups, those that received additional conditioning trials showed conditioned enhancement of immunologic reactivity on retesting, whereas none of those original "responders" that received extinction trials (unreinforced presentations of the CS) showed a change in responsivity.

Acquisition and extinction of a conditioned suppression of a graft-versus-host (GvH) response have been demonstrated by Bovbjerg *et al.* (1982, 1984). Three low-dose injections of CY introduced during initiation of a GvH response are capable of suppressing the popliteal lymph node response of female Lewis × Brown Norwegian rats in response to the injection of Lewis splenic leukocytes. A single-low-dose injection of CY, however, is only minimally immunosuppressive. In rats conditioned 7 weeks before immunogenic stimulation, reexposure of conditioned animals to the CS plus a single low-dose injection of CY suppressed the GvH response to a greater extent than a single low-dose injection of CY in conditioned animals that were not reexposed to the CS or in nonconditioned animals. Suppression of the GvH response in the experimental group did not differ from that in animals subjected to three low-dose injections of the drug. Further, repeated unreinforced exposures to the CS during the 7-week interval between conditioning and injection of cells resulted in extinction of the conditioned immunosuppressive response (Fig. 2).

Further confirmation of behaviorally conditioned suppression of cell-mediated reactivity comes from a study by Kusnecov *et al.* (1983), who used antilymphocyte serum rather than CY as the unconditioned stimulus. Also, preliminary data reported by Smith and McDaniels (1983) suggest that *in vivo* delayed-type hypersensitivity reactions to tuberculin can be attenuated in human subjects by using a conditioning paradigm.

Of particular relevence to the subject matter of this volume is the recent study by Klosterhalfen and Klosterhalfen (1983), who applied the conditioning of immunosuppression to the reduction of peripheral joint inflammation in an animal model of rheumatoid arthritis. Using the taste aversion conditioning paradigm, induction of an inflammatory response by injection of Freund's complete adjuvant in a hind paw was accompanied by reexposure to a saccharin-vanilla taste stimulus previously paired with CY. Swelling normally occurs in the injected paw within 24 hrs, and the contralateral paw becomes inflamed about 12 days later. Although there were no group differences in the swelling that occurred in the injected paw, reexposure to the CS in conditioned animals obviated external signs of inflammation in the contralateral paw. As these investigators suggest, these findings may be a function of the dose of CY. The use of subthreshold immunogenic

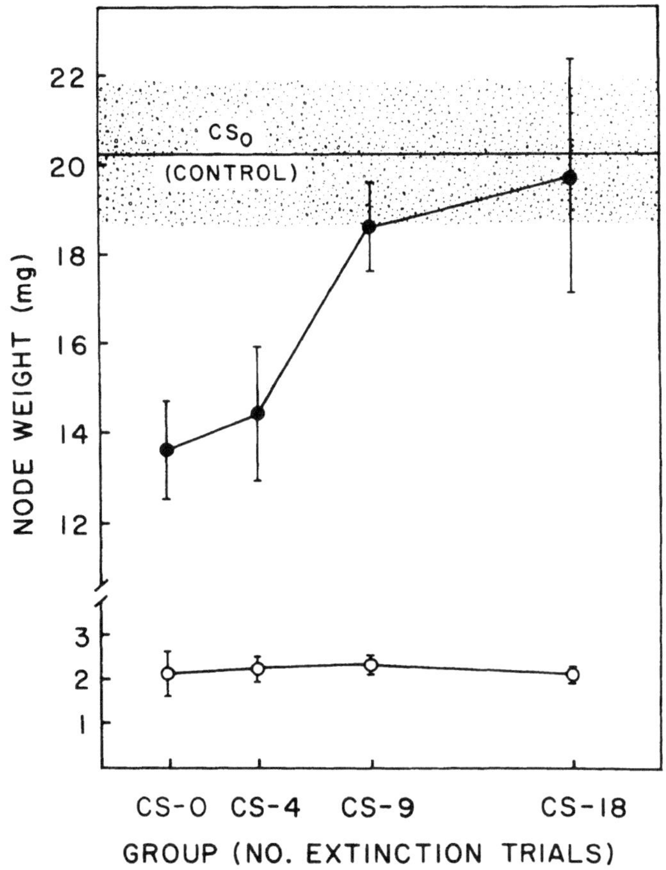

Figure 2. Effects of extinction trials on conditioned suppression of a GvH response. Results represents mean (±S.E.) weights of draining (filled circles) and unstimulated (open circles) popliteal lymph nodes. (Reprinted from Bovbjerg *et al.*, 1984, with permission from *The Journal of Immunology*.)

stimulation in a manner analogous to the use of subthreshold pharmacological stimulation by Bovbjerg *et al.* (1982) as suggested above with respect to the precipitation of arthritis represents an additional strategy that might yield dramatic effects.

These several studies on the acquisition and extinction of conditioned changes in humoral and cell-mediated immune responses support the notion that associative processes are involved in the behavioral modulation of immunity. The mechanisms underlying these effects remain to be determined. It seems likely that (conditioned) neuroendocrine changes may be involved. Considering the complexity of endocrine–immune system interactions (e.g., Ahlqvist, 1981; Comsa *et al.*, 1982) and the conditioning data that are currently available (Ader and Cohen, 1975; Ader *et al.*, 1979), it should be noted that it does not appear that nonspecific (i.e., "stress-induced") or conditioned elevations in adrenocortical steroids can account for the observed alterations in humoral or cell-mediated responses (Ader and Cohen, 1985).

C. Behavioral Conditioning in the Chemotherapy of Autoimmune Disease in Mice

For the most part, the studies of conditioning described above have yielded relatively small effects. It has been the consistency rather than the magnitude of the effects that has made the data on conditioning so persuasive. But is there any significance to relatively small conditioned effects?

In order to evaluate the biological impact of conditioned immunosuppressive responses, we chose a model wherein a suppression of immunologic reactivity would operate in the interests of the organism. The development of a disease related to systemic lupus erythematosus (SLE) in female (NZB × NZW)F_1 mice seemed to meet our requirements (Steinberg *et al.*, 1981; Theofilopoulos and Dixon, 1981; Talal, 1976), since treatment with cyclophosphamide prolongs survival in these mice, which would otherwise develop a lethal glomerulonephritis between 8 and 14 months of age (Casey, 1968; Hahn *et al.*, 1975; Lehman *et al.*, 1976; Morris *et al.*, 1976; Russell and Hicks, 1968; Steinberg *et al.*, 1975). Since we had demonstrated that immunologic reactivity could be suppressed by conditioning techniques, we hypothesized that the substitution of conditioned stimulus for immunosuppressive drug in conditioned animals would delay the development of proteinuria and mortality relative to nonconditioned animals treated with the same amount of drug (Ader and Cohen, 1982).

Individually caged (NZB × NZW)F_1 female mice were maintained under a 12-hr light–dark cycle and provided with food and water *ad libitum*. Chemotherapy was begun when the animals were 4 months of age. Each week, all animals were administered a solution of sodium saccharin (SAC) by pipette. Cyclophosphamide (30 mg/kg) was injected i.p. according to the following schedule outlined in Table 1.

The group that was treated under a standard or traditional protocol (group C100) received an injection of CY once each week immediately after tasting the SAC solution. Saccharin and CY were presented at the same time and the same day each week. This group was intended to define the effects of a standard 8-week course of immunosuppressive therapy. This regimen of chemotherapy was sufficient to prolong survival but was not sufficient to prevent the ultimate development of SLE in these mice.

The critical experimental group of conditioned mice (Group C50) received SAC weekly, but SAC was followed by an injection of CY on only half of these occasions; on half the trials they were injected with saline. The SAC and CY pairing occurred randomly in each of the two 4-week periods.

Table 1. Experimental Protocol

Group	Week 1	2	3	4	8
C100	SAC + CY[a]	SAC + CY	SAC + CY	SAC + CY	SAC + CY
C50	SAC + CY	SAC + sal[a]	SAC + sal	SAC + CY	SAC + CY
NC50	H_2O + CY SAC	H_2O + sal SAC	H_2O + CY SAC	H_2O + sal SAC	H_2O + CY SAC
P	H_2O + sal SAC	H_2O + sal SAC	H_2O + sal SAC	H_2O + sal SAC	H_2O + sal SAC

[a] SAC, saccharin; CY, cyclophosphamide; sal, saline.

Nonconditioned animals (group NC50) also received SAC weekly and received the same schedule of injections of CY and saline as group C50. In this group, however, SAC and CY (or saline) were never paired; that is, these stimuli were presented on different days of the same week.

Control animals (group P) received no immunosuppressive therapy. They were subjected to weekly presentations of SAC and injections of saline administered in a noncontingent manner.

Mice treated with CY weekly were expected to show symptoms of SLE and die more slowly than any of the other groups. Group NC50, nonconditioned mice that received half the cumulative amount of immunosuppressive drug given to group C100, were expected to develop SLE and die sooner than mice that were treated weekly. Group C50 also received only half the amount of drug administered to Group C100. However, to the extent that reexposure to the conditioned stimulus (SAC) in conditioned animals is capable of eliciting an immunosuppressive response, it was hypothesized that mice in group C50 would develop SLE more slowly than nonconditioned mice treated with the same amount of drug.

The results conformed precisely to these predictions. Weekly treatment with CY delayed the onset of proteinuria and prolonged survival. As noted above, this dose and duration of chemotherapy did not prevent the ultimate development of disease. Therefore, the longer one monitors the progression of disease, the less likely one would be to discern group differences. There were, in fact, overall differences based on the total population of each group. The treatment effects are particularly striking, however, when one uses as a reference point the rate of development of proteinuria for the initial half of each group that developed SLE (Fig. 3) or the rate at which the first half of each group died (Fig. 4).

Mice treated with CY weekly developed proteinuria more slowly than any of the other animals. Nonconditioned mice treated with half the CY administered under the standard chemotherapeutic regimen did not differ from mice that were not treated with CY. Conditioned mice that were also treated with half the amount of drug as animals in group C100 developed proteinuria more slowly than untreated controls. The critical comparison between groups C50 and NC50 indicated that conditioned animals developed proteinuria significantly more slowly than nonconditioned animals treated with the same amount of drug.

With respect to mortality, nonconditioned mice did not differ from placebo-treated control animals. Group C50, however, survived significantly longer than untreated controls and did not differ statistically from group C100, animals that received twice as much drug. Again, the critical comparison is between groups C50 and NC50, mice that received the same amount of drug. Mortality was significantly delayed in conditioned relative to nonconditioned animals.

Significant within-group correlations between development of proteinuria and mortality and a relatively constant interval between the development of proteinuria and mortality indicate that the progression of disease followed a similar course in all groups. There was, nonetheless, a dramatic difference in the onset of SLE that could be attributed to the treatment regimens imposed.

In conditioning terms, the therapeutic protocol in this initial study was comprised of a series of conditioning trials in which CS presentations were pharmacologically

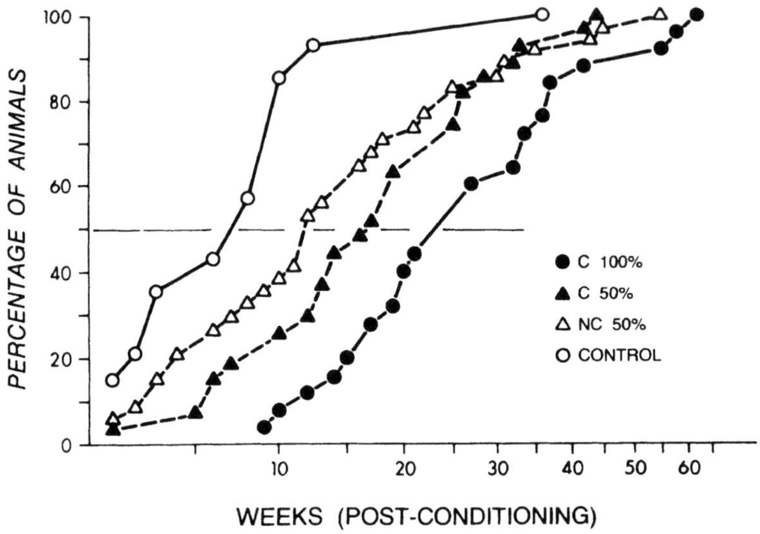

Figure 3. Rate of development of an unremitting proteinuria in (NZB × NZW)F_1 mice under different chemotherapeutic regimens. Group C100 received saccharin and CY weekly; group C50 received saccharin weekly and CY paired with saccharin on 50% of the trials; group NC50 received the same amount of saccharin and CY as group C50 but in an unpaired manner; control mice received no CY. (Reprinted from Ader and Cohen, 1982, with permission from the American Association for the Advancement of Science.)

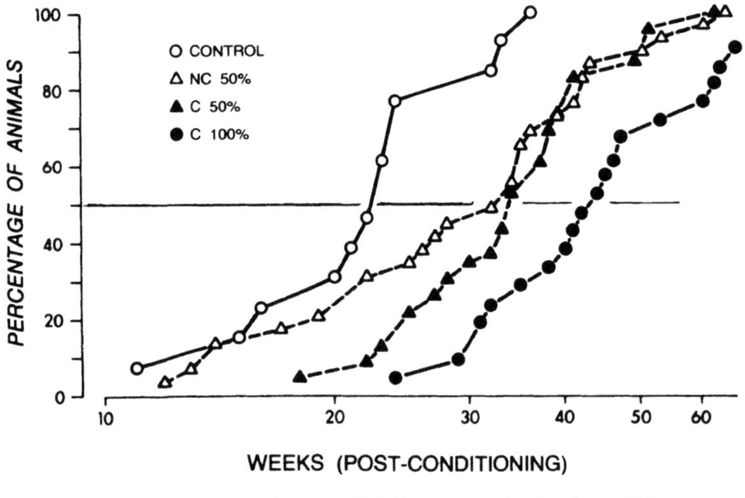

Figure 4. Cumulative mortality rate in (NZB × NZW)F_1 mice maintained on different chemotherapeutic regimens. Group treatments are as described in Fig. 3. (Reprinted from Ader and Cohen, 1982, with permission from the American Association for the Advancement of Science.)

reinforced by injections of CY (the UCS) on either 100% or 50% of the weekly trials. Experimental extinction, on the other hand, is operationally defined as unreinforced presentations of the CS; i.e., CS presentations that are not followed by the UCS. Repeated unreinforced presentations of the CS result in a gradual diminution and, ultimately, elimination (extinction) of the conditioned response. Preliminary data on the effects of extinction procedures were obtained in a second experiment.

During an initial period of chemotherapy, this experiment was identical to the first except that the critical experimental group (group C33) received CY following only one-third of the weekly SAC presentations. Nonconditioned mice (group NC33) received the same SAC and CY presentations in a noncontingent manner. At the end of the therapy period, each group was subdivided into those that (1) continued to receive SAC and CY on the same schedule as existed during the therapy period; (2) received SAC but no CY; and (3) received neither SAC nor CY. If learning processes are involved in the pharmacotherapeutic process, unreinforced presentations of the CS should influence the development of autoimmune disease in conditioned but not in nonconditioned animals. Again, the results confirmed the predictions.

Among the animals trained under a continuous schedule of chemotherapy (group C100), mortality was delayed in mice that continued to receive chemotherapy compared to mice that were deprived of CY (Fig. 5). Those mice that continued to receive CS presentations (saccharin plus i.p. injections of saline) after the termination of CY treatment, however, died more slowly than mice that were deprived of all "medication." Moreover, there was no difference between the mortality rate of mice that continued to receive CS presentations without CY and those that continued to receive both SAC and CY.

Among the mice conditioned under a 33% reinforcement schedule (group C33), those that were subsequently deprived of CY died more rapidly than mice that continued to receive the immunosuppressive drug. Conditioned animals that were deprived of CY but continued to receive weekly presentations of the CS died more slowly than mice deprived of both SAC and CY, and, at least for the initial half of these populations, the mortality rate of the animals that received only the CS did not differ from that in animals that continued to receive drug treatment (Fig. 6). Continued SAC presentations in nonconditioned animals, however, were without effect. The mortality rate in these animals

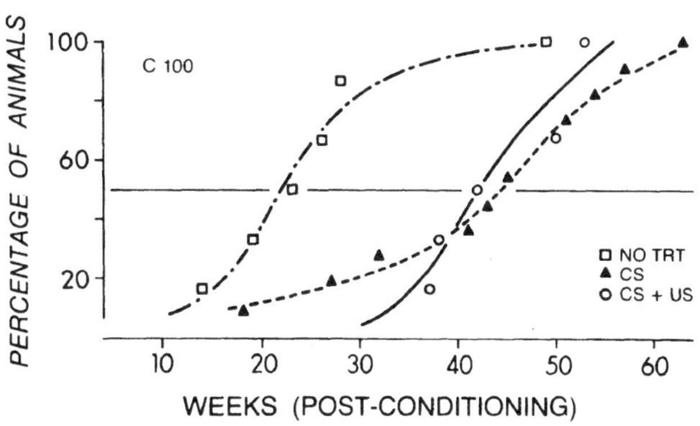

Figure 5. Mortality rate in (NZB × NZW)F_1 mice treated with saccharin and CY weekly and then continued on a regimen of saccharin and CY (group CS + US; $N = 6$), continued on saccharin alone (group CS; $N = 11$), or deprived of both saccharin and CY (no treatment; $N = 6$). (Reprinted from Ader, 1985, with permission from The Guilford Press.)

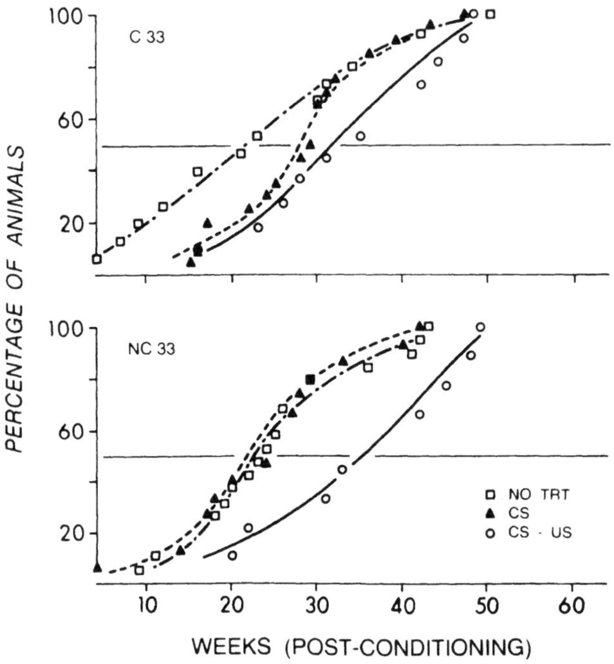

Figure 6. Mortality rate in conditioned (C33) and nonconditioned (NC33) (NZB × NZW)F_1 mice that continued to receive saccharin and CY (group CS + US), continued to receive only saccharin (group CS), or received neither saccharin nor CY (no treatment); $N = 11$ to 20 per subgroup. (Reprinted from Ader, 1985, with permission from The Guilford Press.)

was no different from that in animals that received neither SAC nor CY. (The obvious comparison of resistance to extinction between animals trained under continuous and partial schedules of reinforcement was not possible in this initial experiment since mice provided with continuous chemotherapy received three times as much CY as mice in group C33.)

It might be argued that an elevation in adrenocortical steroid levels might account for the observed differences. Novel stimuli, including gustatory stimuli such as saccharin, can elicit an adrenocortical response; so can an i.p. injection of CY or saline. Conditioned and nonconditioned mice, however, received the same number of such stimuli. As a matter of fact, the effects of combining environmental stimuli are not additive (Friedman and Ader, 1967). Indeed, one could argue that, compared to conditioned animals, nonconditoned mice subjected to SAC and i.p. injections on different days experienced twice as many stimuli capable of eliciting an adrenocortical response. In conditioning a taste aversion, it is posible to condition an elevation in plasma corticosterone level in water-deprived rats (Ader, 1976). It is not likely that the present results are caused by conditioned elevations in corticosteroids, however, since 30 mg/kg CY is insufficient to induce a taste aversion in (NZB × NZW)F_1 or C57BL/6 mice.

Although these experiments do not constitute direct evidence of conditioned immunosuppression (autoantibodies, for example, were not measured), the results are consistent with previous data indicating that the pairing of saccharin and cyclophosphamide would enable saccharin, acting as a CS, to attenuate an immune response. These findings are also consistent with the predicted effects that would result from the superimposition of such a conditioning protocol on a chemotherapeutic regimen designed to delay the development of autoimmune disease in (NZB × NZW)F_1 mice, namely, that reexposure to a conditioned stimulus paired with CY could be substituted for some proportion of actual drug and thereby delay the onset of autoimmune disease under a regimen of chemotherapy that was not, in itself, sufficient to influence the development of disease.

Finally, these observations suggest that there may be some heuristic value in viewing some pharmacotherapeutic regimens in terms of conditioning principles (Ader, 1985). It might be hypothesized, for example, that the imposition of extinction procedures (unreinforced exposures to the CS) would extend the pharmacotherapeutic effects of a partial schedule of reinforcement to a greater extent than a continuous schedule of reinforcement (i.e., the standard pharmacotherapeutic protocol) among animals treated with the same amount of drug. As noted above, the extinction data described here do not meet this criterion; mice trained under continuous pharmacological reinforcement received three times as much drug as those under the partial reinforcement schedule. This hypothesis, then, remains to be tested. Nonetheless, these preliminary observations of the effects of extinction procedures provide additional evidence for the operation of associative processes in the (conditioned) immunopharmacological modification of the development of autoimmune disease in (NZB $\times$ NZW)F_1 mice.

Human SLE may actually represent one appropriate clinical model in which to evaluate this alternative pharmacotherapeutic strategy. Current treatment practices evidently vary widely depending upon the indiosynchratic characteristics of each case (Wasner and Fries, 1980). There is striking agreement among clinicians in some instances and striking disagreement in others. There is agreement, for example, that high doses of prednisone should be used in cases of CNS lupus despite the fact that there are few studies that demonstrate the efficacy of such treatment. In other instances, it is argued that corticosteroid therapy should be used very selectively, if at all. Under these circumstances, the possibility of applying conditioning principles to titrate drug dose in a manner that might optimize therapeutic effects and reduce deleterious side effects might be considered.

IV. GENERAL DISCUSSION

The data reviewed in this chapter provide clinical and experimental evidence of an association between psychosocial factors and the susceptibility and/or the response to disease, including pathophysiological processes that are presumed to involve immunologic defense mechanisms. Data are also cited to indicate that psychosocial factors and "stress" are capable of influencing immunologic reactivity *in vitro* and *in vivo*. Finally, research on conditioned alterations of immunologic reactivity is described. The biological significance of conditioned immunosuppressive responses is seen in the results of studies in which a conditioning paradigm was applied to the chemotherapy of autoimmune disease in (NZB $\times$ NZW)F_1 mice. As a result of the conditioning processes that may accompany all pharmacotherapeutic protocols, the onset of SLE was delayed in conditioned animals receiving a dose of immunosuppressive drug that was not, by itself, sufficient to alter the development of disease. These behavioral studies represent only one of the converging lines of research that document a central nervous system involvement in the regulation or modulation of the immune system.

There is probably no major organ system or homeostatic defense mechanism that is not subject to the influences exerted by the interaction between psychosocial and physiological events. The complexity of the mechanisms underlying these interactions, however, is imperfectly understood, and the most imperfectly understood, perhaps, are those involving the brain and the immune system. Nevertheless, an understanding of the relationship between central nervous system function and immune function could contribute substantially to an understanding of the pathogenesis of autoimmune diseases. Viewed as a physiological phenomenon (e.g., Dixon, 1982), a genetic predisposition may be necessary but is not a sufficient condition for the development of SLE except, perhaps, with advancing age. Of the several endogenous and exogenous factors that appear to be capable of modifying the onset of clinical disease, the available data, limited though they may be, suggest that psychological factors play a role that has not been sufficiently appreciated or examined. The fact that brain processes have been implicated in the regulation or modulation of immune processes reinforces the hypothesis that behaviorally induced changes in immunoregulatory functions are of relevance to an understanding of the development and progression of autoimmune disease.

A consideration of central-nervous-system–immune-system interactions takes on added significance when one considers that the disruptions of immunoregulatory processes that occur in autoimmune disease have also been implicated in the pathogenesis of other disease states. Accini and Dixon (1979), for example, have suggested that there are immunologic components in the development of coronary artery disease leading to myocardial infarction in lupus-prone mice, and Lattime and Strausser (1977) have demonstrated that the arteriosclerosis that occurs in multiply-bred ("stressed") rats is associated with suppression of T-cell function. In short, an understanding of the interactions between the central nervous system and the immune system mediating the behavioral effects on the onset and course of autoimmune disease may have important implications for a variety of pathophysiological processes.

ACKNOWLEDGMENTS. Preparation of this chapter was supported by a Research Scientist Award (K5MH-06318) from the National Institute of Mental Health, United States Public Health Service. The author wishes to thank Dr. Nicholas Cohen and Dr. Shmuel Livnat for their constructive comments on an earlier draft of this chapter.

REFERENCES

Accini, L., and Dixon, F. J., 1979, Degenerative vascular disease and myocardial infarction in mice with lupus-like syndrome, *Am. J. Pathol.* **96**:477–492.

Ader, R., 1976, Conditioned adrenocortical steroid elevations in the rat, *J. Comp. Physiol. Psychol.* **90**:1156–1163.

Ader, R., 1980, Presidential address: Psychosomatic and psychoimmunologic research, *Psychosom. Med.* **42**:307–322.

Ader, R., 1981a, Animal models in the study of brain, behavior, and bodily disease, in: *Brain, Behavior, and Bodily Disease* (H. Weiner, M. A. Hofer, and A. J. Stunkard, eds.), Raven Press, New York, pp. 11–26.

Ader, R. (ed.), 1981b, *Psychoneuroimmunology*, Academic Press, New York.

Ader, R., 1981c, A historical account of conditioned immunobiologic responses, in: *Psychoneuroimmunology* (R. Ader, ed.), Academic Press, New York, pp. 321–354.

Ader, R., 1985, Conditioned immunopharmacologic effects in animals: Implications for a conditioning model of pharmacotherapy, in: *Placebo: Clinical Phenomena and New Insights* (L. White, B. Tursky, and G. E. Schwartz, eds.), Guilford, New York (in press).

Ader, R., and Cohen, N., 1975, Behaviorally conditioned immunosuppression, *Psychosom. Med.* **37**:333–340.

Ader, R., and Cohen, N., 1985, CNS-immune system interactions: Conditioning phenomena. *Behav. Brain Sci.* **8**:379–426.

Ader, R., and Cohen, N., 1981, Conditioned immunopharmacologic responses, in: *Psychoneuroimmunology* (R. Ader, ed.), Academic Press, New York, pp. 281–320.

Ader, R., and Cohen, N., 1982, Behaviorally conditioned immunosuppression and murine systemic lupus erythematosus, *Science* **215**:1534–1536.

Ader, R., Cohen, N., and Grota, L. J., 1979, Adrenal involvement in conditioned immunosuppression, *Int. J. Immunopharmacol.* **1**:141–145.

Ader, R., Cohen, N., and Bovbjerg, D., 1982, Conditioned suppression of humoral immunity in the rat, *Comp. Physiol. Psychol.* **96**:517–521.

Ahlqvist, J., 1981, Hormonal influences on immunologic and related phenomena, in: *Psychoneuroimmunology* (R. Ader, ed.), Academic Press, New York, pp. 355–403.

Amkraut, A., and Solomon, G. F., 1972, Stress and murine sarcoma virus (Moloney)-induced tumors, *Cancer Res.* **32**:1428–1433.

Amkraut, A. A., Solomon, G. F., and Kraemer, H. C., 1971, Stress, early experience and adjuvant-induced arthritis in the rat, *Psychosom. Med.* **33**:203–214.

Amkraut, A. A., Solomon, G. F., Kasper, P., and Purdue, P., 1973, Stress and hormonal intervention in the graft-versus-host response, in: *Microenvironmental Aspects of Immunity* (B. D. Jankovic and K. Isakovic, eds.), Plenum Press, New York, pp. 667–674.

Bartrop, R. W., Lazarus, L., Luckhurst, E., Kiloh, L. G., and Penny, R., 1977, Depressed lymphocyte function after bereavement, *Lancet* **1**:834–836.

Bassett, J. R., and Tait, N. N., 1981, The effect of stress on the migration of leukocytes into the peritoneal cavity of rats following injection of an inflammatory agent, *Aust. J. Exp. Biol. Med. Sci.* **59**:651–666.

Besedovsky, H. O., Sorkin, R., Felix, D., and Haas, H., 1977, Hypothalamic changes during the immune response, *Eur. J. Immunol.* **7**:325–328.

Blecha, F., Kelley, K. W., and Satterlee, D. G., 1982, Adrenal involvement in the expression of delayed-type hypersensitivity to SRBC and contact sensitivity to DNFB in stressed mice, *Proc. Soc. Exp. Biol. Med.* **169**:247–252.

Bovbjerg, D., Ader, R., and Cohen, N., 1982, Behaviorally conditioned immunosuppression of a graft-vs-host response, *Proc. Natl. Acad. Sci. U.S.A.* **79**:583–585.

Bovbjerg, D., Ader, R., and Cohen, N., 1984, Acquisition and extinction of conditioned suppression of a graft-vs-host response in the rat, *Immunology* **132**:111–113.

Boyce, W. T., Cassel, J. C., Collier, A. M., Jensen, E. W., Ramey, C. T., and Smith, A. H., 1977, Influence of life events and family routines on childhood respiratory tract illness, *Pediatrics* **60**:609–615.

Bulloch, K., and Moore, R. Y., 1981, Innervation of the thymus gland by brainstem and spinal cord in mouse and rat, *Am. Anat.* **163**:157–166.

Carr, R. I., Shucard, D. W., Hoffman, A., Bardana, E. J., and Harbeck, R., 1978, Neuropsychiatric involvement in systemic lupus erythematosus, *Birth Defects* **14**:209–235.

Casey, T. P., 1968, Immunosuppression by cyclophosphamide in NZB/NZW mice with lupus nephritis, *Blood* **32**:436–444.

Chang, S., and Rasmussen, A. J., Jr., 1964, Stress-induced suppression in interferon production in virus-infected mice, *Nature* **205**:623–624.

Christian, J. J., and Williamson, H. O., 1958, Effect of crowding on experimental granuloma formation in mice, *Proc. Soc. Exp. Biol. Med.* **99**:385–387.

Coe, C. L., Wiener, S. G., Rosenberg, L. T., and Levine, S., 1985, Endocrine and immune responses to separation and maternal loss in nonhuman primates, in: *Psychobiology of Attachments* (M. Reite and T. Field, eds.), Academic Press, New York (in press).

Cohen, N., Ader, R., Green, N., and Bovbjerg, D., 1979, Conditioned suppression of a thymus-independent response, *Psychosom. Med.* **41**:487–491.

Comsa, J., Leonhardt, H., and Wekerle, H., 1982, Hormonal coordination of the immune response, *Rev. Physiol. Biochem. Pharmacol.* **92**:115–189.

Crown, S., Crown, J. M., and Fleming, A., 1975, Aspects of the psychology of and epidemiology of rheumatoid disease, *Psychol. Med.* **5**:291–299.

Davis, D. E., and Read, C. P., 1985, Effect of behavior on development of resistance in trichinosis, *Proc. Soc. Exp. Biol. Med.* **98**:269–272.

DiCara, L. V., 1970, Learning in the autonomic nervous system, *Sci. Am.* **222**(1):31–39.
Dixon, F. J., 1982, Murine SLE models and autoimmune disease, *Hosp. Pract.* **17**:63–73.
Dohrenwend, B. P., and Dohrenwend, B. S. (eds.), 1974, *Stressful Life Events: Their Nature and Effects,* Wiley, New York.
Dubos, R., 1959, *Mirage of Health,* Harper & Row, New York.
Edwards, E. A., Rahe, R. H., Stephens, P. M., and Henry, J. P., 1980, Antibody response to bovine serum albumin in mice: The effects of psychosocial environmental change, *Proc. Soc. Exp. Biol. Med.* **164**:478–481.
Eikelboom, R., and Stewart, J., 1982, Conditioning of drug-induced physiological responses, *Psychol. Rev.* **89**:507–528.
Ellman, P., and Mitchell, S. D., 1936, The psychological aspects of chronic rheumatoid joint disease, in: *Reports of Chronic Rheumatoid Disease* (C. W. Buckley, ed.), Macmillan, New York, pp. 109–119.
Engel, G., 1953, Studies of ulcerative colitis: III. The nature of the psychologic process, *Am. Med.* **19**:231–256.
Engel, G. L., 1977, The need for a new medical model: A challenge for biomedicine, *Science* **196**:129–136.
Engels, W. D., and Wittkower, E. D., 1975, Psychophysiological allergic and skin disorders, in: *Comprehensive Textbook of Psychiatry, II* (A. M. Freedman, H. J. Kaplan, and B. J. Sadock, eds.), Williams & Wilkins, Baltimore, pp. 1685–1694.
Friedman, S. B., and Ader, R., 1967, Adrenocortical response to novelty and noxious stimulation. *Neuroendocrinology* **2**:209–212.
Felten, D. L., Overhage, J. M., Felten, S. Y., and Schmedtje, J. F., 1981, Noradrenergic sympathetic innervation of lymphoid tissue in the rabbit appendix: Further evidence for a link between the nervous and immune systems, *Brain Res. Bull.* **7**:595–612.
Friedman, S. B., Ader, R., and Glasgow, L. A., 1965, Effects of psychological stress in adult mice inoculated with Coxsackie B viruses, *Psychosom. Med.* **27**:361–368.
Friedman, S. B., Glasgow, L. A., and Ader, R., 1969, Psychosocial factors modifying host resistance to experimental infections, *Ann. N.Y. Acad. Sci.* **164**:381–392.
Friedman, S. B., Ader, R., and Grota, L. J., 1973, Protective effect of noxious stimulation in mice infected with rodent maleria, *Psychosom. Med.* **35**:535–537.
Funk, G. A., and Jensen, M. M., 1967, Influence of stress on granuloma formation, *Proc. Soc. Exp. Biol. Med.* **124**:653–655.
Ganz, V. H., Gurland, B. J., Deming, W. E., and Fisher, B., 1972, The study of the psychiatric symptoms of systemic lupus erythematosus. A biometric study, *Psychosom. Med.* **34**:207–220.
Garcia, J., Hankins, W. G., and Rusiniak, K. W., 1974, Behavioral regulation of the milieu interne in man and rat, *Science* **185**:824–831.
Gardner, B. M., 1980, Psychological aspects of rheumatoid arthritis, *Psychol. Med.* **10**:159–163.
Gauci, L., Gerber, M., Dubois, J. B., and Serrou, B., 1981, Stress, immunity and local irradiation, in: *Immunopharmacologic Effects of Radiation Therapy* (J. B. Dubois, B. Serrou, and C. Rosenfeld, eds.), Raven Press, New York, pp. 7–21.
Gisler, R. H., and Schenkel-Hulliger, L., 1971, Hormonal regulation of the immune response. II. Influence of pituitary and adrenal activity on immune responsiveness *in vitro, Cell Immunol.* **2**:646–657.
Gisler, R. H., Bussard, A. E., Mazie, J. C., and Hess, R., 1971, Hormonal regulation of the immune response: I. Induction of an immune response *in vitro* with lymphoid cells from mice exposed to acute systemic stress, *Cell. Immunol.* **2**:634–645.
Glenn, W. G., and Becker, R. E., 1969, Individual versus group housing in mice: Immunological response to time-phased injections, *Physiol. Zool.* **42**:411–416.
Gorczynksi, R. M., Macrae, S., and Kennedy, M., 1982, Conditioned immune response associated with allogeneic skin grafts in mice, *J. Immunol.* **129**:704–709.
Gorczynski, R. M., Macrae, S., and Kennedy, M., 1984, Factors involved in the classical conditioning of antibody responses in mice, in: *Breakdown in Human Adaptation to Stress: Towards a Multidisciplinary Approach* (R. Ballieux, J. Fielding, and A. L'Abbatte, eds.), Martinus Nijhoff, The Hague, pp. 704–712.
Granata, A. L., Vecchi, C., and Corsi, A., 1978, Activity of the reticuloendothelial system following exposure to electric stress and thymectomy, *Experientia* **34**:591–592.
Greenfield, N. S., Roessler, R., and Crosley, A. P., 1959, Ego strength and length of recovery from infectious mononucleosis, *J. Nerv. Ment. Dis.* **128**:125–128.
Grinker, R. R., Jr., and Robbins, F. P., 1954, *Psychosomatic Case Book,* Blakeston, New York.
Gross, R. L., and Newberne, P. M., 1980, Role of nutrition in immunologic function, *Physiol. Rev.* **60**:188–302.

Gross, W. B., and Siegel, H. S., 1965, The effect of social stress on resistance to infection with *Escherechia coli* or *Mycoplasma gallisepticum, Poult. Sci.* **44:**98–1001.

Gunderson, E. K., and Rahe, R. H. (eds.), 1974, *Life Stress and Illness,* Charles C Thomas, Springfield, IL.

Guy, W. B., 1952, Neurogenic factors in contact dermatitis, *Arch. Dermatol. Syphil.* **66:**1–8.

Hahn, B. D., Knotts, L. N. M., and Hamilton, T. R., 1975, Influence of cyclophosphamide and other immunosuppressive drugs on immune disorders and neoplasia in NZB/NZW mice. *Arthritis Rheum.* **18:**145–152.

Hall, N. R., and Goldstein, A. L., 1981, Neurotransmitters and the immune system, in: *Psychoneuroimmunology* (R. Ader, ed.), Academic Press, New York, pp. 521–543.

Hamilton, D. R., 1974, Immunosuppressive effects of predator induced stress in mice with acquired immunity to *Hymenolepsis nana, J. Psychosom. Res.* **18:**143–153.

Heisel, J. S., 1972, Life changes as etiologic factors in juvenile rheumatoid arthritis, *Arthritis Rheum.* **16:**411–420.

Hendrie, H. C., Paraskevas, F., Barabar, F. D., and Adamson, J. D., 1971, Stress, immunoglobulin levels and immunological processes, *J. Psychosom. Res.* **15:**337–342.

Henoch, M. J., Batson, J. W., and Baum, J., 1978, Psychosocial factors in juvenile rheumatoid arthritis, *Arthritis Rheum.* **21:**229–233.

Hill, C. W., Greer, W. E., and Felsenfeld, O., 1967, Psychological stress, early response to foreign protein, and blood cortisol in vervets, *Psychosom. Med.* **29:**279–283.

Holmes, T. H., Trueting, T., and Wolff, H. G., 1951, Life situations, emotions and nasal disease: Evidence on summative effects exhibited in patients with "hay fever," *Psychosom. Med.* **13:**72–82.

Jackson, G. G., Dowling, H. F., Anderson, T. O., Riff, L., Saporta, M. S., and Turck, M., 1960, Susceptibility and immunity to common upper respiratory viral infections—the common cold, *Ann. Intern. Med.* **53:**719–738.

Jacobs, M. A., Spilken, A. Z., Norman, M. M., and Anderson, L. S., 1970, Life stress and respiratory illness, *Psychosom. Med.* **32:**233–242.

Jemmott, J. B., and Locke, S. E., 1984, Psychosocial factors, immunologic mediation, and human susceptibility to infectious diseases: How much do we know? Psychol. Bull. **95:**78–108.

Jensen, M. M., 1968, The influence of stress on murine leukemia virus infection, *Proc. Soc. Exp. Biol. Med.* **127:**610–614.

Jensen, M. M., and Rasmussen, A. F., Jr., 1963, Stress and susceptibility to viral infections: II. Sound stress and susceptibility to vesicular stomatitis virus, *J. Immunol.* **90:**21–23.

Jenkins, P. E., Chadwick, R. A., and Nevin, J. A., 1983, Classically conditioned enhancement of antibody production. *Bull. Psychon. Soc.* **21:**485–487.

Johnson, T., and Rasmussen, A. F., Jr., 1965, Emotional stress and susceptibility to poliomyelitis virus infection in mice, *Arch. Ges. Virusforsch.* **18:**392–397.

Johnson, T., Lavender, J. F., and Marsh, J. R., 1959, The influence of avoidance learning stress on resistance to Coxsackie virus in mice. *Fed. Proc.* **18:**575.

Kasl, S. V., Evans, A. S., and Neiderman, J. C., 1979, Psychosocial risk factors in the development of infectious mononucleosis, *Psychosom. Med.* **41:**445–466.

Kassan, S. S., and Lockshin, M. D., 1979, Central nervous system lupus erythematosus, Arthritis Rheum. **22:**1382–1385.

Keller, S. E., Weiss, J., Schleiffer, S. J., Miller, N. E., and Stein, M., 1981, Supression of immunity by stress: Effects of a graded series of stressors on lymphocyte stimulation in the rat, *Science* **213:**1397–1400.

Keller, S. E., Ackerman, S. H., Schleifer, S. J., Shindledecker, R., Camerino, M., Hofer, M., Weiner, H., and Stein, M., 1983a, Effect of premature weaning on lymphocyte stimulation in the rat, *Psychosom. Med.* **45:**75.

Keller, S. E., Weiss, J. M., Schleifer, S. J., Miller, N. E., and Stein, M., 1983b, Stress-induced suppression of immunity in adrenalectomized rats, *Science* **221:**1301–1304.

Kiecolt-Glaser, J. K., Speicher, C. E., Holliday, J. E., and Glaser, R., 1984, Stress and the transformation of lymphocytes by Epstein–Barr virus, *J. Behav. Med.* **7:**1–12.

Kirkpatrick, R. A., 1981, Witchcraft and lupus erythematosus, *JAMA* **245:**1937.

Klosterhalfen, W., and Klosterhalfen, S., 1983, Pavlovian conditioning of immunosuppression modifies adjuvant arthritis in rats, *Behav. Neurosci.* **97:**663–666.

Kusnecov, A. W., Sivyer, M., King, M. G., Husband, A. J., Cripps, A. W., and Clancy, R. L., 1983, Behaviorally conditioned suppression of the immune response by antilymphocyte serum, *J. Immunol.* **130:**2117–2120.

Lattime, E. C., and Strausser, H. R., 1977, Arteriosclerosis: Is stress-induced immune suppression a risk factor? *Science* **198**:302–303.

Laudenslager, M. L., Reite, M., and Harbeck, R. L., 1982, Suppressed immune response in infant monkeys associated with maternal separation, *Behav. Neural. Biol.* **36**:40–48.

Laudenslager, M. L., Ryan, S. M., Drugan, R. C., Hyson, R. L., and Maier, S. F., 1983, Coping and immunosuppression: Inescapable but not escapable shock suppresses lymphocyte proliferation, *Science* **221**:568–570.

Lehman, D. H., Wilson, C. B., and Dixon, F. J., 1976, Increased survival times of New Zealand hybrid mice immunosuppressed by graft-versus-host reactions, *Clin. Exp. Immunol.* **25**:297–302.

Levine, S., Strebel, R., Wenk, E. J., and Harman, P. J., 1962, Suppression of experimental allergic encephalomyelitis by stress, *Proc. Soc. Exp. Biol. Med.* **109**:294–298.

Ludwig, A. O., 1955, Psychiatric considerations in rheumatoid arthritis, *Arthritis Rheum.* **6**:166–171.

Makinodan, T., and Yunis, E. (eds.), 1977, *Immunology and Aging*, Plenum Press, New York.

Mandelbrote, B. M., and Wittkower, E. D., 1955, Emotional factors in Graves' disease, *Psychosom. Med.* **17**:109–117.

Marsh, J. T., Lavender, J. F., Chang, S., and Rasmussen, A. F., Jr., 1963, Poliomyelitis in monkeys: Decreased susceptibility after avoidance stress, *Science* **140**:1415–1416.

McClary, A. R., Meyer, E., and Weitman, D. J., 1955, Observation on role of mechanism of depression in some patients with disseminated lupus erythematosus, *Psychosom. Med.* **17**:311–321.

Mettrop, P. J. G., and Visser, P., 1969, Exteroceptive stimulation as a contingent factor in the induction and elicitation of delayed-type hypersensitivity reactions to 1-chloro-2,4-dinitrobenzene in guinea pigs, *Psychophysiology* **5**:385–388.

Meyer, R. J., and Haggerty, R. J., 1962, Streptococcal infections in families: Factors altering individual susceptibility, *J. Pediatr.* **29**:339–349.

Meyerowitz, S., Jacox, R. F., and Hess, D. W., 1968, Monozygotic twins discordant for rheumatoid arthritis: A genetic, clinical and psychological study of 8 sets, *Arthritis Rheum.* **11**:1–21.

Michaut, R. J., DeChambre, R. P., Doumerc, S., Lesourd, B., Devillechabrolle, A., and Moulias, R., 1981, Influence of early maternal deprivation on adult humoral immune response in mice, *Physiol. Behav.* **26**:189–191.

Miller, N. E., 1969, Learning of visceral and glandular responses, *Science* **163**:434–445.

Monjan, A. A., 1981, Stress and immunologic competence: Studies in animals, in: *Psychoneuroimmunology* (R. Ader, ed.), Academic Press, New York, pp. 185–229.

Monjan, A. A., and Collector, M. I., 1977, Stress-induced modulation of the immune response, *Science* **196**:307–308.

Monjan, A. A., and Mandell, W., 1980, Fetal alcohol and immunity: Depression of mitogen-induced lymphocyte blastogenesis, *Neurobehav. Toxicol.* **2**:213–215.

Moos, R. H., 1963, Personality factors associated with rheumatoid arthritis: A review, *J. Chron. Dis.* **17**:41–55.

Moos, R. H., and Solomon, G. F., 1964a, Minnesota Multiphasic Personality Inventory response patterns in patients wiht rheumatoid arthritis, *J. Psychosom. Res.* **8**:17–23.

Moos, R. H., and Solomon, G. F., 1964b, Personality correlates of the rapidity of progression of rheumatoid arthritis, *Ann. Rheum. Dis.* **23**:145–151.

Moos, R. H., and Solomon, G. F., 1965a, Psychologic comparisons between women with rheumatoid arthritis and their nonarthritic sisters: I. Personality test and interview rating data, *Psychosom. Med.* **27**:135–149.

Moos, R. H., and Solomon, G. F., 1965b, Psychologic comparisons between women with rheumatoid arthritis and their nonarthritic sisters: II. Content analysis of interviews, *Psychosom. Med.* **27**:150–164.

Morillo, E., and Gardner, L. I., 1979, Bereavement as an antecedent factor in thyrotoxicosis of childhood: Four case studies with survey of possible metabolic pathways, *Psychosom. Med.* **41**:454–555.

Morris, A. D., Esterly, J., Chase, G., and Sharp, G. C., 1976, Cyclophosphamide protection in NZB/NZB disease, *Arthritis Rheum.* **19**:49–55.

Otto, R., and McKay, R., 1967, Psychosocial and emotional disturbance in systemic lupus erythematosus, *Med. J. Aust.* **2**:488–493.

Pavlidas, N., and Chirigos, M., 1980, Stress-induced impairment of macrophage tumoricidal function, *Psychosom. Med.* **42**:47–54.

Pavlov, I. P., 1928, *Lectures on Conditioned Reflexes*, Liverwright, New York.

Pitkin, D. H., 1965, Effect of physiological stress on the delayed hypersensitivity reaction, *Proc. Soc. Exp. Biol. Med.* **120**:350–351.

Plaut, S. M., Ader, R., Friedman, S. B., and Ritterson, A. L., 1969, Social factors and resistance to malaria in the mouse: Effects of group vs. individual housing on resistance to *Plasmodium berghei* infection, *Psychosom. Med.* **31**:536–552.

Rabkin, J. G., and Struening, E. L., 1976, Life events, stress, and illness, *Science* **194**:1013–1020.

Rasmussen, A. F., Jr., Marsh, J. R., and Brill, N. C., 1957, Increased susceptibility to herpes simplex in mice subjected to avoidance-learning stress or restraint, *Proc. Soc. Exp. Biol. Med.* **96**:183–189.

Rasmussen, A. F., Jr., Spencer, E. S., and Marsh, J. T., 1959, Decrease in susceptibility of mice to passive anaphylaxis following avoidance-learning stress, *Proc. Soc. Exp. Biol. Med.* **100**:878–879.

Reite, M., Harbeck, R., and Hoffman, A., 1981, Altered cellular immune response following peer separation, *Life Sci.* **29**:1133–1136.

Rimon, R. A., 1969, Psychosomatic approach to rheumatoid arthritis. A clinical study of 100 female patients, *Acta Rheum. Scand. (Suppl.)* **13**:1–154.

Rimon, R. A., 1973, Rheumatoid factor and aggression dynamics in female patients with rheumatoid arthritis, *Scand. J. Rheumatol.* **2**:119–122.

Rimon, R., Belmaker, R. H., and Ebstein, R., 1977, Psychosomatic aspects of juvenile rheumatoid arthritis, *Scand. J. Rheumatol.* **6**:1–10.

Robinson, C. E., 1957, Emotional factors in rheumatoid arthritis, *Can. Med. Assoc. J.* **34**:533–547.

Rogers, M. P., Reich, P., Strom, T. B., and Carpenter, C. B., 1976, Behaviorally conditioned immunosuppression: Replication of a recent study, *Psychosom. Med.* **38**:447–451.

Rogers, M. P., Trentham, D. E., Dynesius, R. A., Reich, P., and David, J. R., 1980a, Exacerbation of type II collagen-induced arthritis by auditory stress, *Clin. Res.* **28**:508.

Rogers, M. P., Trentham, D. E., McCune, W. J., Ginsberg, B. I., Rennke, H. G., Reich, P., and David, J. R., 1980b, Effect of psychological stress on the induction of arthritis in rats, *Arthritis Rheum.* **23**:1337–1342.

Russell, P. J., and Hicks, J. D., 1968, Cyclophosphamide treatment of renal disease in (NZB × NZW)F_1 hybrid mice. *Lancet* **i**:440–446.

Schleifer, S. J., Keller, S. E., Camerino, M., Thornton, J. C., and Stein, M., 1983, Supression of lymphocyte stimulation following bereavement, *JAMA* **250**:374–377.

Seifter, E., Rettura, G., Zisblatt, M., Levenson, S. M., Levine, N., Davidson, A., and Seifter, J., 1973, Enhancement of tumor development in physically-stressed mice incubated with an oncogenic virus, *Experientia* **29**:1379–1382.

Shocket, B. R., Lisansky, E. T., Schubart, A. F., Fiocco, V., Kurland, S., and Pope, M., 1969, A medical psychiatric study of patients with rheumatoid arthritis, *Psychosomatics* **10**:271–279.

Siegel, S., 1977, Morphine tolerance acquisition as an associative process, *Exp. Psychol. Anim. Behav. Proc.* **3**:1–13.

Smith, G. R., and McDaniels, S. M., 1983, Psychologically mediated effect on the delayed hypersensitivity reaction to tuberculin in humans, *Psychosom. Med.* **45**:65–70.

Smith, H. R., and Steinberg, A. D., 1983, Autoimmunity—a perspective, *Annu. Rev. Immunol.* **1**:175–210.

Smith, L. W., Molomut, N., and Gottfried, B., 1960, Effect of subconvulsive audiogenic stress in mice on turpentine induced inflammation, *Proc. Soc. Exp. Biol.* **103**:370–372.

Soave, O. A., 1964, Reactivation of rabies virus infection in the guinea pig due to the stress of crowding, *Am. Vet. Res.* **25**:268–269.

Solomon, G. F., 1969, Stress and antibody in rats, *Int. Arch. Allergy* **35**:97–104.

Solomon, G. F., 1981, Emotional and personality factors in the onset and course of autoimmune disease, particularly rheumatoid arthritis, in: *Psychoneuroimmunology* (R. Ader, ed.), Academic Press, New York, pp. 159–182.

Solomon, G. F., and Amkraut, A. A., 1981, Psychoneuroendrocinological effects on the immune response, *Annu. Rev. Microbiol.* **35**:155–184.

Solomon, G. F., and Moos, R. H., 1965, The relationship of personality to the presence of rheumatoid factor in asymptomatic relatives of patients with rheumatoid arthritis, *Psychosom. Med.* **27**:350–360.

Solomon, G. F., Moos, R. H., Stone, G. C., and Fessel, W. J., 1964, Peripheral vasoconstriction induced by emotional stress in rats, *Angiology* **15**:362–365.

Solomon, G. F., Levine, S., and Kraft, J. K., 1968, Early experience and immunity, *Nature* **220**:821–822.

Spergel, P., Ehrlich, G. E., and Glass, D., 1977, The rheumatoid arthritis personality: A psychodiagnostic myth, *Psychosomatics* **19**:79–85.

Stein, M., Schleifer, S. J., and Keller, S. E., 1981, Hypothalamic influences on immune responses, in: *Psychoneuroimmunology* (R. Ader, ed.), Academic Press, New York, pp. 429–447.

Steinberg, A. D., Gelfand, M. C., Hardin, J. A., and Lowenthal, D. T., 1975, Therapeutic studies in NZB/W mice. III. Relationship between renal status and efficacy of immunosuppressive drug therapy, *Arthritis Rheum.* **18**:9–14.

Steinberg, A. D., Huston, D. P., Taurog, J. D., Cowdery, J. S., and Raveche, E. S., 1981, The cellular and genetic basis of murine lupus, *Immunol. Rev.* **55**:121–154.

Talal, N., 1976, Disordered immunologic regulation and autoimmunity, *Transplant. Rev.* **31**:240–263.

Teshima, H., Kubo, C., Nagata, S., Imada, Y., and Ago, Y., 1981, *Jpn. J. Psychol.* **21**:99–103.

Theofilopoulos, A. N., and Dixon, F. J., 1981, Etiopathogenesis of murine SLE, *Immunol. Rev.* **55**:179–216.

Tobach, E., and Bloch, H., 1955, A study of the relationship between behavior and susceptibility to tuberculosis in rats and mice, *Adv. Tuberc. Res.* **6**:62–89.

Treadwell, P. E., and Rasmussen, A. F., Jr., 1961, Role of the adrenals in stress-induced resistance to anaphylactic shock, *J. Immunol.* **87**:492–497.

Vessey, S. H., 1964, Effects of grouping on levels of circulating antibodies in mice, *Proc. Soc. Exp. Biol. Med.* **115**:252–255.

Vollhardt, B. R., Ackerman, S. H., Grayzel, A. I., and Barland, P., 1982, Psychologically distinguishable groups of rheumatoid arthritis patients: A controlled, single blind study, *Psychosom. Med.* **44**:353–358.

Wasner, C. K., and Fries, J. H., 1980, Treatment decisions in systemic lupus erythematosus, *Arthritis Rheum.* **23**:283–286.

Wayner, E. A., Flannery, G. R., and Singer, G., 1978, Effects of taste aversion conditioning on the primary antibody response to sheep red blood cells and *Brucella abortus* in the albino rat, *Physiol. Behav.* **21**:995–1000.

Weiner, H., 1977, *Psychobiology and Human Disease*, Elsevier/North-Holland, Amsterdam, New York.

Weiner, H., 1978, The illusion of simplicity: The medical model revisited, *Am. J. Psychiatry* **135**(Suppl.):27–33.

Weinmann, C. J., and Rothman, A. H., 1967, Effects of stress upon acquired immunity to the dwarf tapeworm *Hymenolepsis nana*, *Exp. Parasitol.* **21**:61–67.

Wistar, R., Jr., and Hildemann, W. H., 1960, Effect of stress on skin transplantation immunity in mice, *Science* **131**:159–160.

Yamada, A., Jensen, M. M., and Rasmussen, A. F., Jr., 1964, Stress and susceptibility to viral infections: III. Antibody response and viral retention during avoidance learning stress, *Proc. Soc. Exp. Biol. Med.* **116**:677–680.

Zweifach, B. W., 1960, The contribution of the reticuloendothelial system to the development of tolerance to experimental shock, *Ann. N.Y. Acad. Sci.* **88**:203–212.

V

Therapy

26

Immunopotentiators and Rheumatic Diseases

Gerard Renoux and Micheline Renoux

I. INTRODUCTION

A number of disparate therapeutic modalities have been utilized in the medical management of rheumatic diseases. Traditionally, treatments have developed empirically utilizing distinct classes of therapeutic modalities. Nonspecific antiinflammatory drugs and corticosteroids exert antipyretic, antiinflammatory, and analgesic effects and thus offer symptomatic relief, yet they have not been shown to prevent the development of damage to bone or cartilage or to alter the course of the disease. The second group includes diverse unrelated drugs such as gold compounds, *d*-penicillamine, and antimalarials. They have been shown to have the potential to affect the progress of the disease, inducing remissions in some patients and limiting disease-induced tissue damages at the expense of numerous side or toxic effects. Cytotoxic and immunosuppressive drugs are also utilized with variable efficacy and significant toxicity. Although all of these drugs have a variety of pharmacological activities, a common property for their partial effectiveness has not yet been clearly elucidated.

The prominent role of host defense mechanisms has been somewhat neglected during the flourishing years of chemotherapy. Not enough attention was paid to drug-induced immunosuppression, which might have aggravated the fundamental immune defect underlying the disease, which deleterious influence could be blamed for the only limited effectiveness.

Recent developments in clinical and experimental immunology have provided evidence that rheumatic diseases are always associated with immunodeficiency or immune dysfunction. These many abnormalities have fostered the impression that immunologic

---

Gerard Renoux and Micheline Renoux • Laboratoire d'Immunologie, Faculté de Médecine, F-37032 Tours Cedex, France.

disturbances might play a key role in the pathogenesis and natural history of these conditions. Currently found abnormalities thought to be of clinical relevance are covered fully elsewhere in the present volume and therefore are not summarized here.

The concept of pharmacological regulation of the immune system presents a new and exciting therapeutic approach to treat diseases associated with immunologic imbalance. This opportunity became apparent with our initial observation that an antihelminthic agent, levamisole, exerts various effects on the immune system. Subsequently, the drug has been extensively investigated, providing detailed understanding of the potential, mode of action, and problems associated with immunotherapeutic agents (reviewed by Renoux, 1978, 1980, 1984).

Agents other than levamisole have also been clinically employed, almost entirely in rheumatoid arthritis.

II. LEVAMISOLE

A. General Activities and Properties

The antihelminthic drug levamisole (2,3,5,6-tetrahydro-6-phenylimidazo[2,1-b]thiazole hydrochloride) is used in many parts of the world to eliminate roundworms in human subjects and animals. Studying the immune response to bacterial vaccines, we observed erratic responses in different groups of experimental animals and came to the conclusion that in the groups dewormed with levamisole, antibody responses were greatly enhanced (Renoux and Renoux, 1971). Carrying this a step further, we demonstrated a profound augmentation of delayed-type hypersensitivity and stimulation of T-cell function, including graft rejection in normal animals (Renoux and Renoux, 1973, 1974; Renoux *et al.*, 1976b). This initiated enthusiastic clinical testing, as levamisole was the first chemically defined agent endowed with immunoenhancing activities; it opened a new field in immunotherapy. The oral administration of levamisole was also a practical advantage over many other immunotherapies, as many patients prefer to receive pills instead of injections that might be painful. From recent reviews the main features of interest follow (Renoux, 1978, 1980, 1984).

1. Pharmacology and Toxicology

The primary pharmacological effects of levamisole were reported as central nervous system and neuromuscular stimulatory properties in vertebrates, in contrast to its paralyzing effect on roundworms. Levamisole is a potent inhibitor of some alkaline phosphatases and a modifier of inducible arylhydroxylases. The median lethal doses (LD_{50}) are shown in Table 1. In rats, daily oral administration of 100 mg/kg levamisole for 3 months did not produce any adverse effect, but prolonged treatment with doses above 20 mg/kg produced convulsions in dogs and sheep. Levamisole has no direct effect on fungi, bacteria, or viruses, is not cytotoxic to normal or tumor cells in concentrations up to 100 μg/ml, and does not appear to be an interferon inducer.

No carcinogenic effect or adverse hematological modifications were observed in a 12 to 18-month survey in rats and dogs. For doses between 5 and 150 mg/kg, levamisole

Table 1. Acute Toxicity of Levamisole (LD_{50}, mg/kg)

	Route of administration		
	Intravenous	Subcutaneous	Oral
Mice	28	121	285
Rats	28	89	345

was devoid of teratogenic or toxic effects on rabbit or rat fetuses, nor does it modify male or female fertility.

2. Influences on the Immune System: Experimental

Levamisole exerts numerous effects on immune functions of healthy animals, including responses to heteroantigens (Renoux and Renoux, 1971, 1974), to bacterial vaccines (Renoux and Renoux, 1973), delayed-type hypersensitivity and graft rejection (Renoux *et al.*, 1976b), lymphocyte responses to T-cell mitogens (Renoux, 1978), macrophage phagocytosis, and listericidal activity (Renoux *et al.*, 1976a). The agent modifies mouse immune responses to various viral, rickettsial, or bacterial infections (Renoux and Renoux, 1972; Renoux *et al.*, 1974; Fischer *et al.*, 1975; Irwin and Knight, 1975; Kenyon *et al.*, 1976).

In vitro enhancement of murine spleen cell blastogenesis, increased responsiveness to PHA or Con A, and augmented activities of macrophages have been reported (Woods *et al.*, 1974; Hadden *et al.*, 1975; Merluzzi *et al.*, 1975; Douglas *et al.*, 1976).

All in all, the data give evidence for stimulant effects of levamisole on immune functions of healthy animals. These effects explain the reported efficacy of the agent in "anergic" subjects.

3. Mode of Action

Review of the effects of levamisole on clinical testing reveals conflicting results. However, they could have been predicted from experimental data. The effectiveness of the agent is critically dose dependent. This variation ranges from marked potentiation to inhibition of the immune response (Renoux and Renoux, 1974; Renoux, 1978, 1980; Dieppe *et al.*, 1976; Trabert *et al.*, 1976). In addition, levamisole was found able to interfere with the spread and development of neoplasia. Timing of administration and dose were critical (Fidler and Spitler, 1975; Johnson *et al.*, 1975; Sampson *et al.*, 1977; Gordon and Prager, 1978), and a dose of levamisole increasing the response to sheep red blood cells enhanced the "take" incidence of transplanted leukemia (Mantovani and Spreafico, 1975). The response to levamisole has been seen to vary among different strains of mice (Renoux *et al.*, 1980), and such variation may occur in other species, including man. This suggestion is supported by the observation that levamisole is extensively metabolized in the liver by various pathways, some of which include enzymes prone to genetic variation (Renoux, 1978, 1980).

Further attempts to reconcile the rather conflicting findings of some studies have focused on the immunologic activities of the various parts of the levamisole molecule

(Renoux *et al.*, 1977b). At least two groups have been identified, each possessing distinctive actions on the immune system. The first is the sulfur-containing moiety, the activities of which were studied using sodium diethyldithiocarbamate (Imuthiol®, DTC). This has been shown to induce the development of a serum factor that promotes the acqusition of T-cell surface markers, even in athymic *nu/nu* mice, and a factor generated in these mice by levamisole therapy is able, *in vitro,* to induce the development of T-cell markers on precursor cells (Renoux and Renoux, 1977a). The factor is without effect on B cells or their precursors and apparently affects the T-cells by acting at a surface receptor.

The second active group of levamisole resides in the imidazole ring. Imidazole has cholinergic activity and can alter intracellular cyclic nucleotide levels, seemingly in a direct fashion without the mediation of a surface receptor. Cyclic-GMP levels are increased, whereas cAMP levels are decreased. This change in the cyclic nucleotide balance promotes cellular proliferative activity (Hadden *et al.*, 1975) while inhibiting maturation (Scheid *et al.*, 1978). Imidazole does not induce the development of T-cell markers or enhance delayed hypersensitivity reactions *in vivo* and triggers cells to either increased or inhibited responses (Renoux *et al.*, 1977b; Renoux, 1981). Imidazole and levamisole have common activities *in vitro,* whereas levamisole has in common with imuthiol some of the *in vivo* influence of the latter agent. The overall activity of levamisole *in vivo* represents a balance between these effects. Levamisole, as well as azathioprine or other thioimidazoles, is readily metabolized to an imidazole, and imidazoles are known immunosuppressants, particularly under repeated administration (reviewed in Renoux, 1985). One can therefore envision the ambivalent activity of levamisole as the result of a conflict between differentiation promoted by its sulfur moiety and indiscriminate proliferation caused by its imidazole moiety.

B. Levamisole and Rheumatoid Arthritis

1. Clinical Findings

Schuerman (1975) and Basch *et al.* (1975) reported subjective and objective improvement in pilot studies of levamisole efficacy in the treatment of rheumatoid arthritis.

In the first reported controlled trial, 34 patients were studied, 12 receiving at least 6 months' treatment with levamisole in a dose of 50 mg three times daily, 12 receiving penicillamine, 250 mg daily for 2 weeks and increasing thereafter at 2-week intervals by 250 mg daily up to a total daily dose of 1 g, and ten receiving placebo (Huskisson *et al.*, 1976). Levamisole was superior to placebo and comparable in efficacy to penicillamine, with a plateau effect achieved after 4–6 months of treatment. The findings were confirmed in a multicenter study carried out under the auspices of the European League against Rheumatism (Multicentre Study Group, 1978) and comparing two dosage regimens, 150 mg given on three or seven consecutive days each week. In these studies levamisole relieved pain, reduced the duration of morning stiffness, and improved the articular index and other clinical criteria as well as reducing ESR and the titer of rheumatoid factor. There was also a demonstrable reduction in the need for symptomatic remedies including corticosteroids.

In a well-conducted although open study, Veys and Mielants (1977) showed that disease activity was completely suppressed or markedly improved in 18 patients, whereas three patients showed no improvement. Overall, statistically significant improvement was obvious after 6 months of treatment with 150 mg/day levamisole, 4 days per week. Continuation of the treatment gave another gain in improvement as compared to the initial evaluation. The beneficial effect of levamisole therapy occurred slowly, reaching a maximum after 6 months, as in the above studies. However, it soon became apparent that there were major differences in efficacy and toxicity of different dosage regimes. Indeed, in double-blind studies involving 21 and 30 patients, respectively, Runge *et al.* (1977, 1979) utilized levamisole, 100 mg/day, on four consecutive days per week. In the first series, the levamisole group was compared to a placebo group; in the second series, the code was broken after 16 weeks, and the placebo group then received levamisole. Almost one-third of the patients who responded initially developed recurrent disease while on continued treatment, in contrast with patients treated with a 150-mg dosage (Huskisson *et al.*, 1976; Veys and Mielants, 1977; Multicentre Study Group, 1978).

A double-blind crossover evaluation of levamisole was performed on 20 patients: ten were randomly selected for levamisole, 150 mg daily, for the initial 16 weeks and placebo for the second 16 weeks, while the other ten patients received therapy on the reverse schedule (Miller *et al.*, 1980). For each variable tested except joint count, ring size, and 50-foot walking time, the degree of improvement from week 0 to 16 was significantly greater in the levamisole group than in the placebo group. The arthritis of the ten patients who started with levamisole became worse after blinded crossover to placebo but remained better than at week 0. Two patients did not complete the study because of adverse effects, and no patients achieved a full remission. Combining these results and those carried out by the Multicentre Study Group (1978, 1982), it seems that the optimal dosage of levamisole is 150 mg weekly; 50 mg weekly is clearly less effective. The use of 150 mg on 3 or 7 days of each week produces little if any increase in efficacy (Veys and Mielants, 1978).

2. *Influence on Immunologic Parameters*

Assessments of the possible relationships between the clinical effectiveness and the influence of levamisole on immunologic parameters are scarce. In one study, there was a tendency for patients on levamisole to show increased responsiveness to tuberculin, and a statistically significant correlation was found between changes in skin test and pain relief (Huskisson *et al.*, 1976), although the skin test to keyhole limpet hemocyanin yielded no significant difference between the group on levamisole and the group on placebo (Miller *et al.*, 1980). A negative correlation between enhanced skin test reactions to four antigens and clinical improvement was noted by Runge *et al.* (1979).

Humoral antibody responses to tetanus, typhoid, and keyhole limpet antigens increased by similar magnitudes in levamisole- and placebo-treated patients (Miller *et al.*, 1980).

No significant changes in absolute numbers or in percentages of T cells or B cells were observed in any groups of controlled studies. A tendency to evoke a normal OKT4 : OKT8 ratio was found by Dr. Corke after one administration of 150 mg levamisole in patients with active disease and elevated OKT4 : OKT8 ratio (Fig. 1).

After 16 weeks of levamisole therapy, there was a greater enhancement over base line for the response to PHA in patients with good clinical response than in those with poor or no clinical response (Miller *et al.*, 1980). A relationship between increase in response to PHA

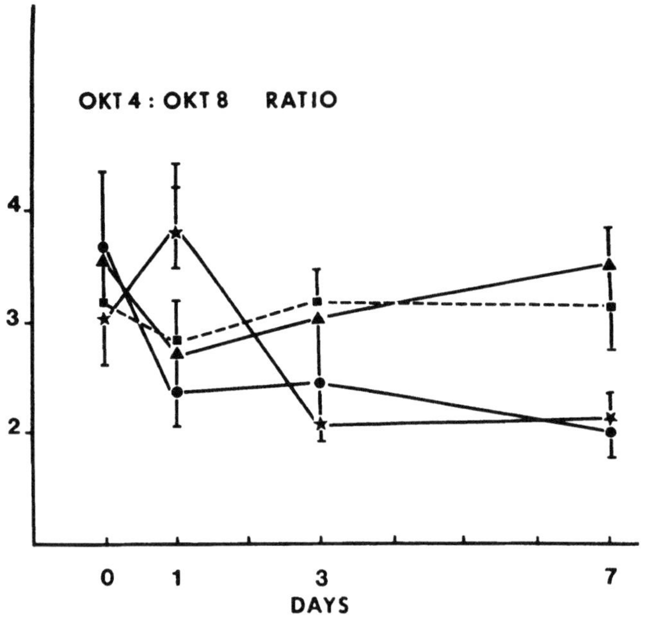

Figure 1. The ratio of OKT4- to OKT8-positive peripheral blood mononuclear cells. Sequential sampling following treatment on day 0 with imuthiol (●), TP5 (▲), levamisole (★), or placebo (■). Vertical bars represent standard errors.

and clinical improvement was also noted by Runge *et al.* (1979). Depressed initial responses to mitogens and subsequent improvement might be secondary features in RA patients because of "normalization" of cellular function rather than primary changes in cellular immune function caused by drug therapy, as the increase in PHA responsiveness was a slowly appearing phenomenon. The hypothesis that the clinical efficacy of levamisole in rheumatoid arthritis might be unrelated to its actions on the immune system has been put forth. The levamisole molecule may be cleaved to form OPMI [*dl*-2-oxo-3-(2-mercaptoethyl)-5-phenylimidazolidine]. This compound has been shown to act as a scavenger of free radicals and to react with tubulin sulfhydrils (De Brabander *et al.*, 1978). It has been suggested that this effect might be responsible for the effect of levamisole in rheumatoid arthritis. However OMPI was found to be endowed with antimitotic activities as effective as vinblastine or colcemide (Otterness and Bliven, 1980).

3. *Adverse Reactions*

Although the different dosage regimens, above 100 mg/day, of levamisole may make little difference to its efficacy in rheumatoid arthritis, they profoundly influence the frequency and nature of adverse reactions. They have recently been reviewed in comparison with other drugs (Franchimont *et al.*, 1978; Veys *et al.*, 1981a). The toxicity of levamisole is dominated by neutropenia, allergic reactions, and neurological side effects. Neutropenia has been reported in 5–10% of patients treated with levamisole in a dose of 150 mg daily on either 3 or 7 days of each week and has frequently been associated with the HLA-B27 haplotype. A few fatalities have been associated with levamisole-induced neutropenia, and its prevention is a major aim of weekly treatment. It is important to recognize that the patients thus afflicted had also been treated with various combinations of prednisolone, ACTH, phenylbutazone, hydroxychloroquine, disalicyclic acid, indomethacin, penicillamine, and ketoprofene before or concomitant with levamisole. There may thus be a peculiar sensitivity of the granulocytes of some of the individuals with rheumatoid arthritis who were treated with immunosuppressive or antiinflammatory drugs and levamisole. In addition, the concomitant use of levamisole and immunosuppressive agents, especially antimitotic drugs, could be deleterious since levamisole induces lymphocyte proliferation and chemotherapeutic agents kill young and replicating cells (Renoux, 1978). Weekly blood counts in levamisole-treated patients are nevertheless required, especially if other drugs, including aspirin, are simultaneously administered. Neutropenia resolves spontaneously on cessation of treatment. Early detection is possible by leukocyte count performed 10 to 14 hr after drug administration.

Vasculitis and other allergic reactions, including urticaria, erythematous and lichenoid reactions, or mouth ulcers, have been described in patients receiving levamisole on 3 or 7 days each week for some months. Typical lesions of vasculitis appear on the lower limb and may be multiple. Very extensive lesions and ulceration may occur, requiring skin grafting. The reactions were often associated with fever and flulike symptoms and sometimes with shivering, myalgia, arthralgia, malaise, chest pain, flushing, and nausea. These reactions usually occur repeatedly with each exposure to the drug and demand withdrawal of treatment.

Diverse neurological side effects including insomnia, sensory stimulation, and a hyperalert state have been reported in about 8% of levamisole-treated patients. Other minor side effects such as headache or dizziness have also been reported with placebo.

An overall assessment indicates that 50% of patients experienced side effects on levamisole, whereas the incidence on placebo was 29%. The increased incidence of side effects on levamisole over controls thus amounted to 20% and was related entirely to reactions of immunologic origin likely linked with its phenol and thiazole sensitizing moieties. However, the adverse effects of levamisole on about 40% of patients, which necessitated 18% withdrawal, must be compared with those of other drugs used in the treatment of RA. For example, *d*-penicillamine triggers 66% adverse effects and 32% withdrawals, and gold salts 32% adverse effects and 22% withdrawals. The seriousness of retinopathy, infections, cholestasis, membranous glomerulonephritis, and neurological complication occurring with gold salts, chloroquine, antimitotics, or penicillamine therapies is far greater than the potential dangers of levamisole.

Rheumatoid arthritis thus seems to be the disease in which the most encouraging results are obtained with levamisole, supporting favorable comparison with penicillamine in regard to both patient improvement and side effects. The longer the treatment, the better were the results in patients uninterruptedly treated with one single weekly dose of 150 mg, accurately supervised, and responding within 3 months, inasmuch as a high frequency of relapses has been noted after too early an interruption of treatment.

C. Miscellaneous Rheumatic Diseases and Levamisole

1. Spondylarthropathies

Open studies concluded that levamisole was possibly effective in ankylosing spondylitis (SSA) and Reiter's syndrome but was associated with minor side effects in 13 of 23 patients in one study and 27 of 44 patients in the other (Trabert *et al.*, 1975; Rosenthal *et al.*, 1976a,b).

In a randomized controlled crossover study (Goebel *et al.*, 1977), 37 male patients affected with SSA were treated with levamisole, 150 mg/day 3 days per week, or placebo. Each period ran for 4 months. Clinical response was measured in terms of morning stiffness, pain index, joint index, and radiologic and joint scanning with [^{99} Tc]pyrophosphate. Laboratory studies included blood tests, hepatic and renal function tests, fluorescent antinuclear antibodies, sensitized sheep-cell agglutination, and HLA profiles. Immunologic tests included active E-rosettes, immunoglobulin determination, serum antitoxic activity, and leukocyte migration inhibition to a soluble synovial protein as antigen.

The results apparently did not depend upon the clinical diagnosis (18 patients had classical ankylosing spondititis, 14 had Reiter's disease, and five psoriasic arthritis). Nine patients on levamisole were withdrawn from the study because of either maculopapular rash or transient agranulocytosis, with pneumonia in one case.

Twenty-eight patients completed the trial. After 12 weeks, the cumulative degree of joint inflammation showed a mean decrease of 50% compared with a mean increase up to 55% during the placebo period ($P < 0.003$). Morning stiffness showed a significant improvement relative to values during placebo treatment ($P < 0.005$). Decrease in pain was observed, although it was not statistically significant. Lower back flexibility was significantly increased during levamisole treatment and was unchanged with placebo ($P < 0.006$). Joint radiology and scanning revealed no progress in the disease during levamisole therapy. Except for IgM levels, which fell significantly under levamisole ($P < 0.01$), the laboratory values remained unchanged.

2. Systemic Lupus Erythematosus

The effect of levamisole alone on NZB/w mice, the experimental model for SLE, is unclear (Russel, 1976). Depending on the dose, levamisole alone may have a detrimental effect on animals with higher levels of anti-DNA antibodies at the beginning of treatment. However, levamisole treatment, 125 μg/mouse on 2 consecutive days each week for a total of 16 weeks, administered after a treatment of 4 weeks with 50 mg/kg body weight of cyclophosphamide twice weekly, delayed the reappearance of antibodies to DNA and decreased glomerular immunoglobulin deposition (Zulman *et al.*, 1978).

Sixteen consecutive patients meeting American Rheumatism Association criteria for the diagnosis of SLE have been treated with levamisole (Gordon and Yanagihara, 1977). All were suffering an active disease as shown by an obligate requirement for corticosteroids and/or cytostatic–immunosuppressive drugs such as azathioprine, cyclophosphamide, or chlorambucil. Patients were started on 450 mg levamisole administered over 3 days every second week irrespective of their weight. If needed, the dosage was raised to 300 mg 2 days each week, then to 450 mg administered over 3 days each week. Patients were continued on intermittent levamisole for periods from 200 to 597 days, then discontinued. During the observation time up to 4 to 8 months after arrest of levamisole, arthritis regressed or disappeared, as did other SLE stigmata such as antinuclear antibodies. Levamisole exerted a significant steroid-sparing effect on all patients. No sequelae of levamisole treatment were noted in this series of patients. No deaths were recorded. Parameters of overall T-cell activity did not appear to be affected significantly in SLE patients on levamisole therapy. The favorable influence of levamisole on the clinical course of SLE, on reduction in dosage of steroid and cytostatic drugs, and on the immunologic responses was also observed in two other cases (Renoux, 1978).

Many other open studies report long-term clinical improvement and normalization of laboratory parameters such as responsiveness of lymphocytes to mitogens or serum complement levels (Smolen *et al.*, 1977; Rosling *et al.*, 1978; Scherak *et al.*, 1978, 1980; Shaposhinov and Gorbunov, 1979; Ogawa *et al.*, 1979; Rovensky *et al.*, 1982). However, 150 mg levamisole once weekly was of no benefit in a double-blind study on patients affected with active SLE (Hadidi *et al.*, 1981).

3. Behcet's Disease

From 1978 to 1982, three studies repeatedly reported a favorable influence of levamisole on the clinical course of Behcet's syndrome accompanied by a decrease in immune complexes, although the regimen of levamisole administration was different (Sampson, 1978; de Merieux *et al.*, 1981; Hamza *et al.*, 1982).

4. Chronic Brucellosis

Five patients affected by rheumatism for 2 to 10 years had been treated unsuccessfully with every known treatment for arthritis or arthrosis. A diagnosis of chronic brucellosis was established from a battery of tests. Levamisole, 150 mg/day, was prescribed daily for a week then 3 consecutive days per week for a month in association with tetracycline, an antibiotic to which patients have not responded when it was given alone. Symptoms worsened for about a week, 10–15 days after initiation of levamisole. Continuation of therapy resulted in remission of all symptoms, immunorestoration, and negativity of serologic tests during follow-up of more than 1 year (Renoux and Renoux, 1977c). Remission of all symptoms, preceded by transient exacerbation, was also reported in 43 of 55 patients with chronic brucellosis (Willoughby and Wood, 1979).

All in all, levamisole exerted a beneficial influence in rheumatic diseases other than rheumatoid arthritis and in which abnormal immunologic function existed.

III. IMUTHIOL

A. General Activities and Properties

The development of imuthiol (sodium diethyldithiocarbamate, DTC) resulted from the search for a chemically defined compound devoid of the ambivalent effect of levamisole on T cells, which adverse effects derived from the cholinergiclike influence of the imidazole nucleus and sensitization induced by thiazole or benzole rings (Renoux and Renoux, 1977b; Renoux, 1985).

1. Pharmacology and Toxicology

Imuthiol was employed as a chelating agent to treat nickel poisoning (Dithiocarb) and as a tool to study metalloenzymes (Albert, 1973; Panel on Nickel, 1975; Sunderman, 1979). Taken from recent reports (Renoux, 1982; Renoux and Renoux, 1984) the main features of interest follow. Imuthiol is a nonsensitizing, nonpyrogenic, nonmutagenic, and noncarcinogenic agent that protects liver cells against drug-induced damage and prevents or cures chemically induced malignant tumors. It also protects against the lethal effects of ionizing radiation. Administration of imuthiol inhibits the toxicity of *cis*-platinum without altering its antitumor efficacy. Imuthiol has *in vivo* and *in vitro* antibiotic effects against a variety of bacteria, fungi, and parasites. It has a fast elimination rate, so that it will not interfere with other drugs such as barbiturates if administered after a 3-hr interval. Purified and lyophilized imuthiol (Institut Mérieux) is essentially devoid of toxicity and side effects for use as an immunopotentiator. The acute toxicity by the intravenous route is above 1500 mg/kg. Chronic i.v. administration of up to 250 mg/kg daily for months did not trigger toxic effects.

2. Experimental Influences on the Immune System

As a biological response modifier, imuthiol demonstrates a unique efficacy on the T-cell lineage. It is not a polyclonal activator and does not modify the number of splenic B cells. Administration of imuthiol elicited a marked increase in T-cell-associated events: specific primary IgG antibody production, increased lymphoproliferative responses to PHA and Con A and to alloantigens, and enhanced and long-term sustained delayed-type hypersensitivity reactions (Renoux and Renoux, 1977b, 1979, 1981, 1984; Renoux *et al.*, 1984a; Neveu, 1978; Neveu *et al.*, 1982), which effects were associated with augmented numbers of Thy-1^+ cells in the spleen of normal mice (Renoux and Renoux, 1980c; Renoux *et al.*, 1979b) as well as in Lyt-1^+ and Qa-1^a cells (Renoux and Renoux, 1984). Administration of imuthiol was also found to increase NK reactivity against YAC-1 cells without production of endogenous interferon and at a time period when interferon and interferon inducers were inactive (Renoux *et al.*, 1982). Chronic administration induced stimulated responses at a magnitude identical to that observed after a single administration without inducing spleno or hepatomegaly. Imuthiol was found able to restore to normality the T-cell responses inhibited or abrogated by chronic concomitant treatments with azathioprine or cortisone and partially restored those responses suppressed by cyclophosphamide (Renoux and Renoux, 1980a). Oral and systemic administrations were equally active.

Current studies also indicate that imuthiol increased cytotoxic T-cell activities against P815 or EL4 tumor cells and restored to normality the T-cell function altered by aging (M. Bruley-Rosset, unpublished data).

3. Pharmacotoxicology in Man

Informed volunteer patients were entered in phase I–II studies. They were treated once or chronically, either orally or intravenously, with 1 to 40 mg/kg imuthiol. No untoward side effects, irrespective of dose, occurred in individuals treated via the intravenous route, provided a slow injection, over at least 40 min, was given. Oral treatment was equally well accepted when pills where swallowed with a large glass of water and before a meal, preferentially breakfast. An antialcohol, antabuselike effect was frequently observed. No effects other than a tendency to a return to normal values were observed in hematological or biochemical parameters (Renoux, 1981; Renoux *et al.*, 1983a). Current studies indicate that oral or intravenous administration for more than 4 years was devoid of toxicity or side effects requiring interruption of the treatment. The data confirm those gained in therapeutic assays of sodium diethyldithiocarbamate against nickel poisoning (Sunderman, 1979).

4. Immunologic and Clinical Testing in Man

A treatment prior to surgery prevented the immunodepression associated with surgical trauma and anesthesia in patients already immunosuppressed by cancer and restored to normal levels the responses of peripheral blood lymphocytes to T-cell mitogens. In patients afflicted with chronic pulmonary infection, the responses to PHA and Con A that were impaired prior to treatment returned to normal values within 2 days. The percentage of T cells returned to normal values when the figure was either abnormally high or low before treatment. Imuthiol did not affect the percent of B(sig^+) cells, autologous rosette-forming cells, or the levels of IgA, IgM, and IgG (Renoux *et al.*, 1983a; Renoux and Renoux, 1981). A regulatory influence of imuthiol on the T4 : T8 ratio and on delayed-hypersensitivity responses in cancer patients was repeatedly observed (Renoux *et al.*, 1983a). Imuthiol was also found to cure postsurgery infections (G. Champeault, personal communication) or tuberculosis in those patients in whom usual antibiotherapy was ineffective (B. Martin-Lalande, personal communication).

Recently, it was found that cultures of peripheral blood lymphocytes from healthy humans in imuthiol (10^{-5} μg/ml)-conditioned medium resulted in a significant increase above control values of $OKT3^+$, $OKT4^+$, and $HLA\text{-}DR^+$ T cells (Pompidou *et al.*, 1985), which findings demonstrate that the agent could activate T cells. Flow cytometric analyses revealed that cultures for 5 days of patient's lymphocytes in the presence of imuthiol restored impaired T4 : T8 ratios to normal or near-normal values, an influence similar to that observed after treatment (Renoux *et al.*, 1984b). In all the studies summarized above, no changes in B-cell numbers were observed.

5. Mode of Action

In short-term induction assays using the Komuro–Boyse technique (1973), imuthiol was unable to promote T- or B-cell differentiation from precursors (Renoux and Renoux, 1977a, 1980c). In apparent contrast, the agent induced significant changes in the T-cell cell-surface markers in long-term induction assays, which changes were likely modulated by monocytes (Pompidou *et al.*, 1985). A series of experiments demonstrated that the early efficacy of imuthiol on the T-cell lineage was mediated through an increased production in euthymic mice or a *de novo* synthesis in congenitally athymic animals of hormonelike factors specific for T cells. The factor(s), in turn, induced *in vivo* and *in vitro* recruitment and activation of T cells from undifferentiated precursor cells and even across the species barrier. All in all, the findings strongly suggest that imuthiol was able to trigger a T-cell-specific extrathymic factor (Renoux, 1982, 1984; Renoux and Renoux, 1977a, 1980c, 1983; Renoux *et al.*, 1979b, 1980b, 1984a). Imuthiol was also found able to induce a late (3 to 5 days after treatment) increase in IL-2 production followed by a second-step increase of IL-1 levels (Chung *et al.*, 1983).

The anabolic influence of imuthiol on endotoxin-induced wasting disease concomitant with its hormone-mediated efficacy on the T-cell lineage led to the hypothesis that the central nervous system could be involved (Renoux and Renoux, 1979). A series of experiments demonstrated a role for the brain neocortex in the control of T-cell responses. Imuthiol acts as a modifier of a cascade of events that start in the neocortex and, likely through the hypothalamo–pituitary axis, modulate the release of thymic and extrathymic hormones that trigger T cell recruitment and differentiation (Bizière *et al.*, 1982; Renoux *et al.*, 1980d, 1983b, 1984a).

Available data thus indicate that imuthiol induces the recruitment and regulation of cells of the T-cell lineage, likely through increased synthesis of hormones and lympholines. As the immunologic system is an intricate network of interacting cells, imuthiol would also act indirectly on B cells and monocyte–macrophages. These actions occur in the absence of events initiated by other triggering influences and contrast with those of other immunomodulators known to act as promoters to increase an already evoked immune event or as adjuvants to augment the responses to an antigen, which are known also to be immunosuppressive agents at prolonged or high dosages. As imuthiol is a nontoxic agent at immunopotentiating doses, it could be a drug effective to treat syndromes and diseases in which the underlying defect is a T-cell deficiency or dysfunction. It might be able, as in the case of athymic mice, to correct a genetically determined immunodeficiency disease. As imuthiol is effective equally well via the oral route or by intravenous administration, the clinician is able to choose the most suitable preparation.

B. Imuthiol and Rheumatoid Arthritis

The excellent toxicology record of imuthiol in both animal and human studies and the immunologic activities of the agent justified a pilot study, which was undertaken by Dr. Charles F. Corke (Department of Rheumatology, Dr. E. C. Huskisson, St. Bartholomew's Hospital, London, U.K.). We are greatly indebted to Dr. Corke for permission to utilize parts of his data prior to his own publication.

1. Clinical Study

As imuthiol has not previously been used in rheumatoid arthritis, a pilot study was designed to detect toxicity and to obtain a gross impression of any clinical response over a period of 6 months. An oral dose of 250 mg once weekly was arbitrarily chosen. Twelve patients with advanced destructive diseases, all of whom had previously received *d*-penicillamine and other "second-line" agents (gold, chlorambucil, azathioprine, thymopoietin, or levamisole), were evaluated. The placebo group comprised 20 patients who had entered in a previous double-blind study against *d*-penicillamine. Although the placebo group was far from ideal, as most initial values for clinical parameters were much below those in the treated group, the data have provided help in clarifying the changes found in the imuthiol-treated group.

Clinical assessment was performed by a single blind observer. Blood tests were performed by personnel who were unaware of the treatment administered. Pharmacotoxicity was evaluated by full urinalysis and blood tests (SGOT, alkaline phosphatase, bilirubin, albumin, creatinine, urea, calcium, phosphate, platelet counts, red and white cell counts, hemoglobin). In addition, erythrocyte sedimentation rate (ESR), serum immunoglobulins (IgA, IgM and IgG), and rheumatoid factors (latex and rheumatoid arthritis haemagglutination) were employed to detect clinical efficacy. Changes over the period of evaluation within each group were statistically analyzed by the Mann–Whitney *U* test.

The nature of the study was fully explained to all patients who were offered the opportunity to choose their treatment group.

The observed changes can be briefly summarized as follows. The articular index improved significantly over the 6 months of treatment ($P < 0.01$), whereas no change was observed in the placebo group. The pain score was decreased significantly at 3 months ($P < 0.05$) and remained low at 6 months. There was no significant change in the placebo group. A trend towards reduced morning stiffness was observed in the imuthiol-treated patients, which did not occur in the placebo-treated patients. The ERS dropped over the 6 months in the treated patients; no corresponding reduction was observed in the placebo group. The hemoglobulin level did not change significantly in either group of patients, although there was a small rise in the imuthiol-treated group and a small fall in the placebo group.

In one patient (no. 10) who did not respond to a 4-month treatment with *d*-penicillamine followed by 3 months of chlorambucil, a dramatic improvement occurred following the treatment with imuthiol. Other tests were not significantly modified by imuthiol treatment, implying that the drug is well tolerated and not associated with serious side effects.

All patients volunteered to remain on the treatment.

From this pilot controlled study, there is evidence that a dose of 250 mg of imuthiol once weekly exerts a beneficial effect on both clinical and laboratory parameters of rheumatoid disease activity. Inasmuch as a majority of patients had longstanding severely destructive disease and all patients had previously been treated unsuccessfully with *d*-penicillamine and other "second line" anti-rheumatic agents, it is reasonable to suppose that these patients might be less responsive to imuthiol therapy than patients previously untreated.

2. *Immunologic Study*

The influence of a single dose of thymopoietin (TP5, 50 mg i.v., Ortho, Raritan, NJ, USA), levamisole (150 mg, oral), or imuthiol (250 mg, oral, Institut Mérieux, Lyon, France) on the T-cell subsets was evaluated the day before and 24 hr, 3 and 7 days after treatment on eight patients in each treated group and compared to 11 patients on placebo. All patients were suffering from active disease as evaluated by the ARA criteria and had an initially high OKT4 : OKT8 ratio. No treatment apart from nonsteroidal antiinflammatory drugs was administered to these patients.

Figure 1 depicts the results. No significant changes occurred in the percentage or absolute numbers of cell subsets and in the OKT4 : OKT8 ratio between samples obtained from control patients. There was no significant change in the number of $OKT8^+$ or $OKT4^+$ cells following thymopoietin treatment. A fall in the number of $OKT3^+$ (from 1.54×10^9 to 1.18), $OKT4^+$ (from 1.2×10^9 to 0.8), and $OKT8^+$ (0.4 to 0.23×10^9) cells was observed 1 day after levamisole therapy, raising the OKT4 : OKT8 ratio significantly above controls ($P < 0.001$). Similar changes over a short time course have been observed and related to the flulike syndrome assessed with intermittent levamisole (Suykens *et al.*, 1983). However, the T4 : T8 ratio was significantly reduced in comparison to controls ($P < 0.05$) 7 days later. An increase in the number of T ($OKT3^+$) cells and significant enhancement of both percentages ($P < 0.01$) and absolute numbers ($P < 0.05$) of $OKT8^+$ cells without quantitative changes in the $OKT4^+$ population were observed in imuthiol-treated patients. This resulted in OKT4 : OKT8 ratios significantly lower than initial or control values ($P < 0.05$).

As summarized above, a return to normality has been observed in patients with depressed OKT4 : OKT8 ratios who were treated with imuthiol. The effect was obtained either by increasing the OKT4$^+$ subset or decreasing excessive numbers of OKT8$^+$ cells. A comparison of the data with those found in rheumatoid patients gives evidence for the regulatory influence of imuthiol on T-cell function.

The absence of toxicity and the effect on the clinical course and on T cells in this pilot study support further studies to elucidate the efficacy of imuthiol following other timing of administration or dose levels. Patients in an early stage of disease could be entered in such studies, as there are no grounds to restrict treatment to advanced cases.

IV. THYMOPOIETIN

A. General Properties and Activities

A number of factors have been isolated from thymus or blood as a consequence of the concept that the thymus epithelium secretes hormones to control T-cell differentiation (Miller, 1961). Four groups of factors have been extensively studied: (1) thymosins (Low *et al.*, 1979); (2) thymus humoral factor (Trainin *et al.*, 1975); (3) facteur thymique sérique (FTS), and zinc-containing thymulin (Bach and Dardenne, 1972; Dardenne *et al.*, 1981); and (4) thymopoietin and its synthetic pentapeptide TP5 (Goldstein and Manganaro, 1971; Basch and Goldstein, 1974; Goldstein *et al.*, 1979).

Thymopoietin was first described under the name of thymin as a thymic polypeptide acting on the neuromuscular junction (Goldstein and Manganaro, 1971) and then as a thymic hormone inducing T-cell differentiation *in vitro* (Basch and Goldstein, 1974). Purification of the crude peptide led to thymopoietin, a 49-amino-acid polypeptide (Schlesingerd *et al.*, 1975), and to the synthesis of the pentapeptide TP5 (Goldstein *et al.*, 1979).

The biological attributes of thymopoietin and TP5 can be summarized as follows. Both have the capacity to induce *in vitro* differentiation of T and B cells from precursors and to enhance allogeneic or cytotoxic responses and spontaneous DNA synthesis, which effects have been linked to cyclic guanosine monophosphate mediation and are blocked by imidazole or indomethacin (Basch and Goldstein, 1974; Lay and Goldstein, 1980; Scheid *et al.*, 1978; Sunshine *et al.*, 1978; Twomey and Kouttab, 1982). *In vivo* effectiveness on murine cells was attained on T and B cells after daily administration for 10 to 14 days (Scheid *et al.*, 1975; Goldstein *et al.*, 1979).

Similarly, thymopoetin restored T-cell-mediated activities of human cells in tests *in vitro,* whereas its efficacy to treat diverse immune disorders remained questionable (reviews in Friedman, 1975, 1979; Beers and Basset, 1980; Klein *et al.*, 1983).

B. Thymopoietin and Rheumatic Diseases

In a 6-month trial (Thrower *et al.*, 1982), 36 patients were randomly allocated to one of the following treatment groups: thymopoietin (TP5), 50 mg intravenously weekly; levamisole, 150 mg orally weekly; or *d*-penicillamine, 250–750 mg orally daily. Diverse side effects (rash, itching, gastrointestinal, or herpes) were observed in five out of 12 TP5-treated patients versus three in the levamisole group and ten in the penicillamine group. Efficacy was comparable to that of levamisole and penicillamine, although re-

Table 2. Global Responses at 6 Months in a Double-Blind Comparison of the Effectiveness of 1 mg TP5 Intramuscularly or 50 mg TP5 Intravenously

Global response	Controls (n = 20)	TP5 (1 mg i.m.; n = 18)	TP5 (50 mg i.v.; n = 44)
Marked improvement	0	1	8
Moderate improvement	11	10	28
Deterioration	5	4	8
Withdrawn for inefficacy	4	3	0

duction in ESR was small and there were no significant changes in rheumatoid factor. The time course of the response to thymopoietin was similar to that to penicillamine and levamisole.

In a second study, 92 patients were divided into three groups, namely, placebo (1 ml saline intramuscularly), TP5 (1 mg i.m. once weekly), and TP5 (50 mg intravenously) and were evaluated for disease activity at the beginning of the study and at 3 and 6 months (Veys *et al.*, 1982a). One patient in the 1-mg-TP5 group experienced fever; two patients reported skin rash; one reported herpes zoster; and one reported diarrhea in the 50-mg-TP5 group. No adverse reactions were reported in the control groups.

Global responses at 6 months are indicated on Table 2. Intramuscular thymopoietin in a single weekly dose of 1 mg was not superior to placebo, whereas intravenous thymopoietin 50 mg weekly produced clinical effects comparable to those of gold or penicillamine.

Although thymopoietin was introduced with the thought that it would reproduce the effects of levamisole, the effects in individual patients fail to support the view of a common mode of action. On the one hand, no tests for overall immunologic activity were reported in these two studies; apparently, an i.v. injection of 50 mg TP5 did not modify the absolute numbers and percentages of the OKT subsets (see Section III.B, Imuthiol and Rheumatoid Arthritis). Thrower *et al.* (1982) found that such parameters as morning stiffness, joint size, articular index, and ESR were significantly more reduced in the levamisole group, whereas TP5 was more active than levamisole in reducing pain. Hemoglobin levels fell in patients receiving TP5 and rose in those receiving levamisole; the difference was highly significant ($P < 0.005$).

The major drawback at the present time is the need to give thymopoietin by intravenous or intramuscular injection, and further development should await the availability of a more convenient mode of administration inasmuch as there were no obvious advantages over levamisole or penicillamine.

V. INOSIPLEX

A. General Activities and Properties

Inosiplex (Methisoprinol, Delimmun, Immunoviral, Isoprinosine, Isoprinosina, Pranosina, Prinosine, Viruxan) is a complex between inosine and N,N-dimethylamino-2-propanol-*p*-acetamidobenzoic acid on a 1 : 3 molar basis. It is a virtually nontoxic drug apart a degree of hyperuricemia, which results from metabolism of the inosine moiety. It has no deleterious effects on reproductive function, and no abnormalities were detected in offspring. Inosiplex is likely to be a nonmutagenic agent, as it is unable to induce chromatid and chromosome abnormalities of human lymphocytes (Weh *et al.*, 1980). Mild to moderate or significant efficacy has been reported in subacute sclerosing panencephalitis, herpes simplex, influenza, and rhinovirus infection (Glasky *et al.*, 1975; Hadden *et al.*, 1976; Simon and Glasky, 1978). It is rapidly becoming obvious that the antivirus efficacy is not associated only with a direct effect on the compound on virus replication, because the dosage active *in vivo* was far less than the amount needed in tests *in vitro*. In light of this background, inosiplex was found by us and others to be an inducer of lymphocyte differentiation and a modulator of lymphocyte and macrophage function.

Administration of inosiplex (0.05–50 mg/kg) at the time of SRBC immunization or as pretreatment for 7 days, as well as oral doses (10–100 mg/kg), augmented spleen IgM and IgG plaque-forming cells two- to threefold (Renoux *et al.*, 1977b, 1979a). Inosiplex, 0.5, 5, and 50 mg/kg i.p., augmented the response to Con A of mouse splenocytes at day 1 and 3 after the last injection, which effect was lost by day 5, and these treatments did not modify NK and ADCC responses or the response to a thymus-independent antigen (Vecchi *et al.*, 1978). Oral inosiplex treatment (0.6 mg/kg daily) of influenza-virus-infected mice reverted the viral-induced suppression of the response to Con A (Simon and Glasky, 1978). Inosiplex is not an interferon inducer, but it enhanced the *in vivo* antiviral effects of exogenous interferon against encephalomyocarditis virus and against 180/TG sarcoma (Chany and Cerutti, 1977a,b; Cerruti *et al.*, 1979).

Inosiplex was found to be active against rodent neoplasias (Hadden and Giner-Sorolla, 1981). However, inosiplex-treated C3H (H-2^k) mice showed progressive takes of transplanted incompatible (H-2^d) L 1210 leukemia, a tumor cell line to which C3H mice are usually resistant (Vecchi *et al.*, 1978). A similar tumor-promoting influence has been observed with other immunomodulators, such as levamisole, BCG, *C. parvum*, and pyran copolymer.

The effectiveness of inosiplex to increase the recruitment and function of lymphocytes was confirmed by clinical testing. The agent increased mitogen-induced lymphoproliferation (Bradshaw and Summer, 1977; Waldman and Ganguly, 1977), and impaired E-rosettes (Wybran, *et al.*, 1978). Long-term administration is likely to increase the percentage of $OKT8^+$ cells without affecting the $OKT4^+$ subset (A. Pompidou, personal communication).

The *in vivo* effects have been amply conformed by assays *in vitro*. Inosiplex enhanced the human lymphocyte proliferation induced by PHA (Hadden *et al.*, 1976a) and the response to allogeneic antigens (Wybran *et al.*, 1978) or to tetanus toxoid (Morin *et al.*, 1980), although the agent was not mitogenic in itself. Addition of inosiplex to mouse spleen cells augmented the response to PHA and to Con A (Renoux *et al.*, 1979a).

In the mouse system, inosiplex was as active as Con A to increase suppressor T-cell activity (Renoux *et al.*, 1979d), whereas Touraine *et al.* (1980) showed that inosiplex enhanced the Con-A-induced suppressor activity but was inactive alone on human peripheral blood cells. In addition to T-cell induction, inosiplex has effects on B cells. Added to cell suspensions, the agent increased the number of plaque-forming cells in the Mishell–Dutton assay (Glasky *et al.*, 1975), activated the pokeweed influence on B cells (Morin *et al.*, 1980), and induced an augmented number of B cells, revealed by the complement receptor marker (Hadden and Giner-Sorolla, 1981). Inosiplex was also found effective on macrophage activities such as phagocytosis of yeast (Wybran *et al.*, 1978) and phagocytosis and killing of *L. monocytogenes* (Hadden *et al.*, 1979).

The mechanisms of inosiplex's action are not yet fully understood, as is true for most immunomodulators. A single injection of inosiplex to athymic nude mice induced 4 days later 10 to 18% Thy-1$^+$-bearing spleen cells (Renoux *et al.*, 1979d), and a direct effect of inosiplex to induce T-cell differentiation *in vitro* has been evidenced (Hadden and Giner-Sorolla, 1981).

Inosiplex was found to modify nuclear refringence of lymphocytes (Pompidou *et al.*, 1980), which effect reflects the state of chromatin activation (Pompidou *et al.*, 1979), suggesting that one pathway of inosiplex activity might be related to RNA metabolism. Inosiplex may also act by giving to lymphocytes the inosine these cells need for life and development. Indeed, in congenital defects of the enzymes adenosine deaminase and nucleoside phosphorylase, which are involved in the purine salvage pathway, normal development of cell systems other than the lymphoid is observed. In addition, immune stimulation afforded by polyinosinic:polycytidilic acid strengthens the hypothesis that products of the purine pathway, such as inosine, may play a role in the natural history of lymphocytes.

In brief, the profiles of inosiplex activity are essentially those of a promoter of events initiated by other triggering influences.

B. Trials on Rheumatic Diseases

In an open study, inosiplex was given to 15 rheumatoid arthritis patients, 3 g daily until improvement occurred, and the dosage was then reduced to 1 or 2 g daily. The drug was discontinued in those cases in which no response was observed. Subjective and objective evaluations of symptoms were done at the onset of treatment and repeated every 2 weeks according to the criteria of the American Rheumatism Association (Wybran *et al.*, 1981).

After 2 months, the results were judged as excellent in four patients, good in one patient, and moderate in four patients. Aggravation of symptoms or lack of effects were observed in six cases even after 3 months of treatment. No side effects, toxic symptoms, or pathological levels of uricemia were recorded. Long-term assessment for improvement was not determined. A mild to excellent response to inosiplex therapy was therefore found in nine out of 15 patients in this preliminary series (Wybran *et al.*, 1981).

The results of two other open studies contrast with the above findings. They involve nine and 14 patients, respectively. In one study (Alcalay *et al.*, 1981), patients were treated with 50 mg/kg inosiplex for 5 consecutive days each 2 weeks, and in the other (Segond *et al.*, 1981), six patients were treated with 50 mg/kg for 5 consecutive days each 2 weeks, eight received 50 mg/kg daily, and three received 500 mg/day irrespective of weight; some patients were treated successively by two schedules. All treatments were given for 3 months.

Inosiplex was well tolerated, but no clinical improvement was observed other than a mild effect in four out of 23 patients. In addition, there were no significant changes in immunologic parameters (enumeration of T or B cells, proliferative responses to PHA and Con A, skin tests to PPD, *Candida,* and *Streptococcus*) evaluated on nine patients before and after treatment (Alcalay *et al.*, 1981). The preliminary assays of inosiplex on rheumatoid arthritis do not appear encouraging for further study.

VI. HUMAN PLACENTA-ELUTED γ-GLOBULINS

A. General Activities and Properties

Placenta-eluted γ-globulins (PEGG) were prepared from large pools of human placenta extensively washed to discard retroplacental blood. Tissues were teased, and PEGG was obtained by multiple fractionation and elutions at various pH, purified by preparative chromatography, and finally concentrated to a final protein content of 37 g/liter (Bonneau *et al.*, 1973).

Placenta-eluted γ-globulins contain blood group antigens at trace levels, very low amounts of antibodies to various bacteria, viruses, and parasites, and also to HLA A, B, and C antigens; PEGG are free of HBs antigen. They contain less than 3 pg/ml of steroid hormones. There was no rheumatoid factor activity, and PEGG were found to inhibit *in vitro* stimulating cells in mixed lymphocyte cultures (MLR) at a concentration of 100 μg/ml, suggesting that they might contain polyspecific anti-HLA-DR antibodies.

B. Trials on Rheumatoid Diseases

It has been advocated that the immunologic disturbances in rheumatoid arthritis could possibly be related to HLA-DR phenotypes (Stastny, 1974). Since PEGG have shown inhibitory activities in MLR, clinical trials were undertaken on the assumption that such an activity might modify the course of the disease.

Four groups of hospitalized patients were studied (Sany *et al.*, 1982). Groups A, B, and C were treated with PEGG. Each patient received a slow intravenous perfusion (5 hr) of 1500 mg of PEGG diluted in 250 ml of sterile saline. In group A (case 1), the treatment was given discontinuously: 1500 mg once a week for 4 weeks (the follow-up period after treatment in this case was 16 months). Group B included four patients (cases 2, 3, 4, and 5) who received 1500 mg daily for 7 days, and in one patient (no. 4), a second therapeutic period (4 bis) with the same dosage took place 3 months after the first trial. The follow-up periods after the end of perfusions in this group were 22 months (case 2), 12 months (case 3), 15 months (case 4), and 10 months (case 5). Group C comprised five patients (cases 6, 7, 8, 9, and 10) who received 1500 mg of PEGG daily for 7 days each month. Treatment is still continuing in three patients (7, 8, and 10) with follow-up periods of 5 months (case 7), 4 months (case 8), and 2 months (case 10). Treatment was interrupted because of a clinical failure (after five therapeutic sequences) in case 6 and because of renal side effects in case 9. Group D (control group) included three patients who received 1500 mg of veinoglobulin (Institut Mérieux) daily for a week. The same patients were treated by PEGG after a period of 51, 56, and 46 days, respectively, after the arrest of veinoglobulin treatment, and are referred to as patients 7, 8, and 9 in group C, above. Veinoglobulin did not contain appreciable amounts of anti-HLA-DR activity.

Clinical evaluation of patients was made prior to treatment and after eacn 7-day period of treatment by the same blind investigator, who was not aware of the treatment. Clinical assessment included pain evaluation, morning stiffness (in minutes), time needed for a 15-m walk (in seconds), and Lee's and Ritchie's indices. The data were analyzed by arbitrarily scoring the above evaluations and applying Student's *t* test to recorded paired values before and after each 7-day period of perfusion. Biological parameters were assessed before and until 4 months after treatments. These included erythrocyte sedimentation rate (ESR), red blood cell, white blood cell, and platelet counts, blood urea and creatinine, urinary protein, Waaler–Rose test, total complement, C3 and C4 components, total plasma proteins, protein electrophoresis, serum IgG, IgA, and IgM levels, and antinuclear and anti-DNA antibodies. Immunologic tests employed were immune complexes, E-rosettes, B cells (sIg^+), and Fc-receptor-bearing cells, responses to phytohemagglutinin (PHA), concanavalin A (Con A), pokeweed mitogen (PWM), and alloantigens (MLR).

Table 3 summarizes the clinical assessments (Sany *et al.*, 1982). From 1 to 8 months of improvement were attained in five of the eight patients whose treatment was terminated at the time of report (Sany *et al.*, 1982). The good result observed in patient 3 at 3 months after arrest of treatment is likely a spontaneous remission, as rheumatoid arthritis is a disease with a variable natural history and long-term spontaneous remissions (Duthie *et al.*, 1957; Hart, 1976). Most immunologic parameters remained unchanged with the exceptions of active E-rosette counts, which were significantly increased above initial and control values in patients 2 to 5 ($P < 0.01$), and Fc-receptor-bearing cell counts, which decreased within 1 month of treatment. Responses to PHA, Con A, and PWM were found enhanced ($P < 0.05$) for 1 month after treatment and significantly decreased ($P < 0.01$) afterwards. Inhibition of MLR by patients' sera occurred in a few tests, but only with serum collected less than 8 days post-treatment.

Table 3. Clinical Assessment of the Influence of PEGG in Ten Cases of Rheumatoid Arthritis[a]

	Improvement				
Patient	Initial day[b]	Duration (months)	Mean percentage change[c]	D/O[d]	*P* values[e]
1	None	—	—	—	—
2	None	—	—	—	—
3	90	8	−66.5	−14.5	0.05
4	5	2	−75.3	−15.5	0.02
4 bis	8	1	−55.1	−18.2	0.05
5	8	1	−50.8	−16.3	0.05
6	None	—	—	—	—
7	16	Still under treatment	−52.9	−9.0	0.01
8	None	—	—	—	—
9	10	3	−70.1	−71.2	0.02
10	8	Still under treatment	−72.3	−46.2	0.01

[a] Patients 7, 8, and 9 previously served as controls. Control patients (veinoglobulin treatment) did not show clinical improvement during 46 to 56 days of survey.
[b] Earliest time of a statistically significant change, calculated from clinical scoring.
[c] Mean percentage of decrease in clinical scores.
[d] Mean difference of clinical scores between the day (*D*) of improvement and day 0 (0).
[e] *P* value (Student's *t* test) for paired values and related to the mean in differences.

Side effects were observed in five out of ten patients: nausea (three patients), headache (one patient), and edema of the upper lip (one patient). Treatment had been interrupted in two cases (2 and 9) because of intercurring nephropathy. No toxic or side effects were reported from the three control patients. Although all patients have shown transient immunologic changes, it is difficult to assess a relationship between such changes and clinical effectiveness of PEGG infusion or to determine from the data whether the agent influenced either HLA-DR amounts or immune complexes. This preliminary assay of PEGG, involving few patients and even fewer controls, does not appear encouraging for further studies.

VII. DISCUSSION

Conventional therapies for rheumatic diseases have only partial effectiveness and induce remissions but not cures, at the price that more than 50% of patients withdraw because of serious adverse effects. They cannot therefore be considered the ultimate therapeutic response. An alternative was possible, since immunologic abnormalities have been demonstrated in patients affected with rheumatic diseases: the attempt to utilize therapeutic agents able to restore immunologic balance. Such an opportunity was presented by the discovery of the immunomodulating influence of levamisole.

Levamisole has not proved a particularly satisfactory agent in rheumatologic practice because of its side effects. However levamisole is clinically effective, and the clinical toxicity associated with levamisole therapy has to some extent been overestimated by the high incidence of side effects associated with the continuous therapy initially employed and other concomitant treatments. The dosage interval and optimal dose of levamisole have proved difficult to determine, particularly because it is unclear which immunologic parameter should be monitored. But levamisole has provided evidence that immunomodulation might offer a useful therapeutic approach to rheumatoid arthritis.

Levamisole also made it possible to express the concept that chemically defined compounds can modulate lymphocyte function in a way that could be better controlled than by the use of ill-defined biologicals. As a prototype of a new class of agents, levamisole has revealed the complexities of the biological pathways underlying the clinical effectiveness of agents proposed as immunomodulators and the role of host factors in modulating their influence.

The bimodal influence of levamisole, which can either stimulate or inhibit immune responses, has been linked to the role of the imidazole ring as an immunosuppressant. Thioimidazoles such as levamisole, azathioprine, niridazole, and thiabendazole readily metabolize to an imidazole and show a dose- and time-dependent effectiveness when this effect was tested for. The underlying mechanism is likely mediated by the increase in cGMP levels produced by the cholinergic activity of imidazole and inhibition of cell differentiation. A drug such as imidazole that liberates *in vivo* a metabolite known to be an activator of cGMP cannot be recommended as a safe drug for prolonged administration, particularly in the immunocompromized host.

The development of imuthiol stemmed from the studies of levamisole's activities and represents the second generation of drugs. It is reasonable to anticipate from a pilot controlled study that the agent will be more effective in clinical use and associated with

Table 4. Main Differences between Levamisole and Imuthiol

Test	Response: Levamisole	Response: Imuthiol
In vitro short-term induction assay	Yes[a]	No
Mitogenic effect	Yes[a]	No
Inhibitory influence	Yes[a]	No
Increase in cGMP levels	Yes[a]	NT
Long-term (5 days) *in vitro* induction assay	NT	Yes
Direct influence on B-cell or macrophage function	Yes	No
Evidence for nonresponders *in vivo*	Yes	No
Production of a general lymphocyte activator	Yes	No
Sensitization	Yes	No
Low-dose toxicity	Yes	No
Antibiotic activity	No	Yes
Possible direct anticancer effect	No	Yes

[a] Shared with imidazole; NT, not tested.

less untoward effects and toxicity (Table 4). Preliminary data suggest that it could be a useful agent in inflammatory rheumatisms.

Further clinical trials with other proposed agents are not supported by available data.

VIII. FUTURE TRENDS

Until recently, immunomodulating agents have been clinically tested before being sufficiently well known. Attention to adverse effects, either general or on the immune system, has been drawn more from clinical studies than from systematic experimental assays. A benefit from immunotherapy has, however, been noted, and not only in rheumatic diseases, despite the empirical approach.

Insofar as the immune system is directly involved in the natural history of rheumatic diseases and immunologic disturbance contributes to their pathogenesis, the use of cytotoxic drugs should be avoided, as they will aggravate the fundamental immune defect underlying the disease. A drug restoring a normal or near-normal balance to the faltering immune system seems a more appropriate treatment. After all, the idea of treating a dysfunctional or failing immune system parallels that of many other organ systems for which we have therapies for dysfunction.

Progress in clinical immunology such as the recent use of monoclonal antibodies to identify human lymphocyte subsets will facilitate useful comparisons between experimental approaches and clinical findings. We hope that analyses of changes among subsets of immune cells may facilitate rational application of immunotherapy. Progress in cooperative immunopharmacology, immunotoxicology, pharmacology, and pharmacokinetics will provide the immunotherapeutist with pertinent data to make his decision for application of a biological response modifier (BRM).

From a reflection on the pioneers' work, a rational, scientifically based approach could be now envisioned for the efficacious utilization of well-defined BRMs. These agents are administered to patients and not to healthy individuals. The general guideline is, therefore, a careful evaluation of the disease state, the benefit for the patient, and the risk of the drug. As a consequence, the clinician should be provided with as much of the available experimental data as possible prior to the design of clinical testing.

An overall appreciation of the reports on BRMs led us to conceptualize the following specifications for candidates to be suitable agents for clinical trials. The agent should have defined influences on sets or subsets of immunocompetent cells as its essential activity. These influences should have been assessed *in vivo* so as not to be distorted by nonspecific effects, and because a man, and even a mouse, is not a test tube. The agent should have demonstrated that it has no immunosuppressive effects under prolonged administration, as it is a drug proposed for chronic therapy. Known toxic levels and pharmacological effects will delineate the range of doses and help to predict most adverse effects. The absence of carcinogenicity, of tumor-promoting influence, and of antigenicity or sensitizing effect is an essential prerequisite, as the agent will be administered for long periods of time to patients already at risk. Such requirements would likely eliminate most of the inconsistencies that have dampened confidence in most BRMs. They will also prevent nosocomial diseases that may be induced by insufficiently studied compounds.

An agent should not be introduced in clinical trials unless it has fulfilled the above requirements.

Immunologic tests should be performed in conjunction with clinical evaluation, as the final aim is to provide reasonable evidence that BRM-induced clinical changes correlate with immunologic modifications. Otherwise, the data would suggest the agent has direct, nonimmunologic influences on the disease, thus allowing for new developments in other directions.

Both to select a BRM and to monitor its efficacy, the clinician will have to consider all those parameters displaying an important role in modifying the immune system. Among these are genetic factors, sex, age, nutrition, intercurrent diseases, and associated therapies. The immune system is exquisitely sensitive to nutritional requirements, hormones, and neurotransmitters. It embodies a complex network of regulatory circuits so that modification at one point of the system might indirectly result in changes of other immune functions, and a minor modification on the activity of a cell subset may be revealed by a major change in an overall response through the many amplification circuits in the immune system. This is thus a plea for carefully controlled clinical testing.

The pharmacological regulation of the immune system through nontoxic and specific agents is a new and exciting approach to treating diseases presently considered permanently chronic ailments open only to symptomatic relief. One might expect, for example that a treatment of systemic lupus erythematosus with corticoids will be considered faulty and erroneous because corticoids destroy suppressor cells already insufficient in such patients. Immunorestoration is one of the most promising types of therapy biomedical research has yet offered to treat and even to prevent rheumatic diseases. Still in its infancy, the future of immunotherapy is great, particularly, if a closer discourse between clinicians and basic researchers, already established, is fostered.

ACKNOWLEDGMENTS. Personal work has been supported by grants from INSERM, PIRMED (CNRS) and grants-in-aid from Janssen Pharmaceutica (levamisole), Newport Pharmaceuticals International and Laboratoires Delalande (Isoprinosine), and Institut Mérieux (imuthiol). We are indebted to Mrs. Patricia Galmard for excellent typing.

REFERENCES

Albert, A., 1973, Metal-binding substances, in: *Selective Toxicity,* ed. 5, Chapman and Hall, London, pp. 334–391.

Alcalay, M., Vincent, F., Alcalay, D., Ziegler, J. E., Brigeon, B., and Bontoux, D., 1981, Traitement de la polyarthrite rhumatoide par l'isoprinosine. Echec d'une posologie discontinue de 50 mg/kg, *Rhumatologie* **33**:343–344.

Bach, J. F., and Dardenne, M., 1972, Thymus dependency of rosette forming cells. Evidence for a circulating thymic hormone, *Transplant. Proc.* **4**:345–350.

Basch, M. E. S., Spitler, E. P., and Engleman, E. P., 1975, The effects of levamisole on rheumatoid arthritis, *Arthritis Rheum.* **18**:385–388.

Basch, R. S., and Goldstein, G., 1974, Induction of T-cell differentiation *in vitro* by thymin, a purified polypeptide hormone of the thymus, *Proc. Natl. Acad. Sci. U.S.A.* **71**:1474–1478.

Beers, R. F., Jr., and Basset, E. G., 1980, *Polypeptide Hormones,* Raven Press, New York.

Bizière, K., Renoux, M., and Renoux, G., 1982, Modulation of cellular immunity by the cerebral neocortex, *Neuroscience* **7**:528.

Bonneau, M., Latour, M., Revillard, J. P., Robert, M., and Traeger, J., 1973, Blocking antibodies eluted from human placenta, *Transplant. Proc.* **5**:589–592.

Bradshaw, L. J., and Summer, H. L., 1977, *In vitro* studies of cell-mediated immunity in patients treated with inosiplex for herpes virus infection, *Ann. N.Y. Acad. Sci.* **284**:190–196.

Cerutti, I., Chany, C., and Schlumberger, J. P., 1979, Isoprinosine increases the antitumor action of interferon, *Int. J. Immunopharmacol.* **1**:59–63.

Chany, C., and Cerutti, I., 1977a, Effet stimulant de l'isoprinosine sur l'action antivirale de l'interferon, *C.R. Acad. Sci. (Paris) (D)* **284**:499–501.

Chany, C., and Cerutti, I., 1977b, Enhancement of antiviral protection against encephalomyocarditis virus by a combination of isoprinosine and interferon, *Arch. Virol.* **55**:225–231.

Chung, V., Florentin, I., and Renoux, G., 1983, Action du diethyldithiocarbamate (DTC) chez des souris normales et immunodeficientes sur la production d'interleukines 1 et 2, *Bull. Soc. Fr. Immunol.* **25**:7a.

Dardenne, M., Pleau, J. M., Lefrancier, P., and Bach, J. F., 1981, Role du zinc et d'autres métaux dans l'activité biologique du FTS (thymuline), *C.R. Acad. Sci. (Paris) (D)* **292**:793–795.

De Brabander, M., Aerts, F., Geuens, G., Wan de Weire, R., and Van Belle, K., 1978, O.M.P.I. A sulfhydril metabolite of levamisole than interact with microtubules, *Chem. Biol. Interact.* **28**:45–49.

de Merieux, P., Spitler, L. E., and Paulus, H. E., 1981, Treatment of Behcet's syndrome with levamisole, *Arthritis Rheum.* **24**:64–70.

Dieppe, P. A., Willoughby, D. A., Stevens, C., Kirby, J. D., and Huskisson, E. C., 1976, Specific therapy in new and conventional animal models, *Rheum. Rehabil.* **15**:201–206.

Douglas, S. D., Schmidt, M. E., and Daughaday, C. C., 1976, Effects of levamisole on monocyte–macrophage immunoprotein receptors and *in vitro* function, *Fed. Proc.* **35**:335.

Duthie, J. J. R., Brown, P. E., Knox, J. D. E., and Thompson, M., 1957, Course and prognosis in rheumatoid arthritis, *Ann. Rheum. Dis.* **16**:411–425.

Fidler, I. J., and Spitler, L. E., 1975, Effect of levamisole on *in vivo* and *in vitro* murine host response to syngeneic transplantable tumors, *J. Natl. Cancer Inst.* **55**:1107–1112.

Fischer, G. W., Podgore, J. K., Bass, J. W., Kelley, J. L., and Kobayashi, G. Y., 1975, Enhanced host defense mechanisms with levamisole in suckling rats, *J. Infect. Dis.* **132**:578–581.

Franchimont, P., Heynen, G., and Hauwaert, C. H., 1978, Adverse reactions to the principal drugs used in rheumatoid arthritis, *J. Rheumatol.* **5**(Suppl. 4):85–92.

Friedman, H., 1975, Thymus factors in immunity, *Ann. N.Y. Acad. Sci.* **249**:547.

Friedman, H., 1979, Subcellular factors in immunity, *N.Y. Acad. Sci.* **332**:625.

Glasky, A. J., Pfadenhauer, E. H., Settineri, R., and Ginsberg, T., 1975, Isoprinosine, a purine derivative: Metabolic, immunological and antiviral effects, in: *Combined Immunodeficiency Disease and Adenosine Deaminase Deficiency, a Molecular Defect,* (H. J. Meuwissen, ed.), Academic Press, New York, pp. 157–172.

Goebel, K. M., Goebel, F. D., Schubotz, R., Hahn, E., and Neurath, F., 1977, Levamisole-induced immunostimulation in spondylarthropathies, *Lancet* **1**:214–217.

Goldstein, G., and Manganaro, A., 1971, A thymic polypeptide causing the neuromuscular block of myasthemia gravis, *Ann. N.Y. Acad. Sci.* **183**:230–240.

Goldstein, G., Scheid, M. P., Boyse, E. A., Schlesinger, D. H., and Van Wauve, J., 1979, A synthetic pentapeptide with biological activity characteristic of the thymic hormone, thymopoietine, *Science* **204:**1309–1310.

Gordon, B. L., and Yanagihara, R., 1977, Treatment of systemic lupus erythematosus with the T-cell immunopotentiator levamisole: A follow-up report of 16 patients under treatment for a minimum period of four months, *Ann. Allergy* **39:**227–236.

Gordon, W. C., and Prager, M. D., 1978, Effects of levamisole on normal and malignant murine lymphocytes, *J. Natl. Cancer Inst.* **61:**415–421.

Hadden, J. W., and Giner-Sorolla, A., 1981, Isoprinosine and NPT 15392: Modulators of lymphocyte and macrophage development and function, in: *Augmenting Agents in Cancer Therapy: Current Status and Future Prospects,* (E. M. Hersh and M. A. Chirigos, eds.), Raven Press, New York, pp. 497–522.

Hadden, J. W., Coffey, R. G., Hadden, E. M., Lopez-Corrales, E., and Sunshine, G. H., 1975, Effects of levamisole and imidazole on lymphocyte proliferation and cyclic nucleotide levels, *Cell. Immunol.* **20:**98–103.

Hadden, J. W., Hadden, E. M., and Coffey, R. G., 1976, Isoprinosine augmentation of phytohemagglutinin-induced lymphocyte proliferation, *Infect. Immun.* **13:**382–387.

Hadden, J. W., Englard, A., Sadlik, J. R., and Hadden, E. M., 1979, The comparative effects of isoprinosine, levamisole, muramyl-dipeptide and SM 1213 on lymphocyte and macrophage proliferation and activation *in vitro, Int. J. Immunopharmacol.* **1:**17–27.

Hadidi, T., Decker, J. L., El-Nagdy, L., and Sany, M., 1981, Ineffectiveness of levamisole in systemic lupus erythematosus: A controlled trial, *Arthritis Rheum.* **24:**60–63.

Hamza, M., Ayed, K., and Ben Ayed, H., 1982, Treatment of Behcet's disease with levamisole, *Arthritis Rheum.* **25:**714–715.

Hart, F. D., 1976, History of the treatment of rheumatoid arthritis, *Br. Med. J.* **1:**763–765.

Huskisson, E. C., Dieppe, P. A., Scott, J., Trapnell, J. Balme, H. W., and Willoughby, D. A., 1976, Immunostimulant therapy with levamisole in rheumatoid arthritis, *Lancet* **1:**393–395.

Irwin, M. R., and Knight, H. D., 1975, Enhanced resistance to *Corynebacterium pseudotuberculosis* infections associated with reduced serum immunoglobulin levels in levamisole-treated mice, *Infect. Immun.* **12:**1098–1103.

Johnson, R. K., Houchens, D. R., Gaston, M. R., and Goldin, A., 1975, Effects of levamisole (NCS-17702) and tetramisole (NSC-102063) in experimental tumor systems, *Cancer Chemother. Rep.* **59:**697–705.

Kenyon, A. J., Kassel, R., Notani, G., and Hahn, E. C., 1976, Separation of aleutian disease antibody response from induction of gammapathy with levamisole, *Fed. Proc.* **35:**569.

Klein, T., Specter, S., Friedman, H., and Szentivanyi, A., 1983, *Biological Response Modifiers in Human Oncology and Immunology,* Plenum Press, New York.

Komuro, K., and Boyse, E. A., 1973, *In vitro* demonstration of thymic hormone in the mouse by conversion of precursor cells into lymphocytes, *Lancet* **1:**740–743.

Lay, C. Y., and Goldstein, G., 1980, Functional effects of thymopoietin on cytotoxic lymphocyte precursor units, *J. Immunol.* **124:**1861–1863.

Low, T. L. K., Thurman, G. B., Chincharini, C., McClure, J. E., Marshall, G. D., Hu, S. K., and Goldstein, A. L., 1979, Current status of thymosin research: Evidence for the existence of a family of thymic factors that control T-cell maturation, *Ann. N.Y. Acad. Sci.* **332:**33–48.

Mantovani, A., and Spreafico, F., 1975, Allogeneic tumor enhancement by levamisole, a new immunostimulatory compound: Studies on cell-mediated immunity and humoral antibody response, *Eur. J. Cancer* **11:**537–544.

Merluzzi, V. J., Badger, A. M., Kaiser, C. W., and Copperband, S. R., 1975, *In vitro* stimulation of murine lymphoid cell cultures by levamisole, *Clin. Exp. Immunol.* **22:**486–492.

Miller, B., De Merieux, P., Srinivasan, R., Clements, P., Levy, J., and Paulus, H. E., 1980, Double-blind placebo controlled cross over evaluation of levamisole, in rheumatoid arthritis, *Arthritic Rheum.* **23:**172–182.

Miller, J. F. A. P., 1961, Immunological function of the thymus, *Lancet* **2:**748–750.

Morin, A., Touraine, J. L., Renoux, G., and Hadden, J. W., 1980, Isoprinosine as an immunomodulating agent, in: *New Trends in Human Immunology and Cancer Immunotherapy,* (B. Serrou and C. Rosenfeld, eds.), Doin, Paris, pp. 1021–1031.

Morin, A., Touraine, J. L., Renoux, G., and Hadden, J. W., 1980, Isoprinosine as an immunomodulating agent, in: *New Trends in Human Immunology and Cancer Immunotherapy,* (B. Serrou and C. Rosenfeld, eds.), Doin, Paris, pp. 1021–1031.

Multicentre Study Group, 1978, Levamisole in rheumatoid arthritis. A randomised double-blind study comparing two dosage regimens of levamisole with placebo, *Lancet* **2:**1007–1012.
Multicentre Study Group, 1982, Levamisole in rheumatoid arthritis. Final report on a randomised double-blind study comparing a single weekly dose of levamisole with placebo, *Ann. Rheum. Dis.* **41:**159–163.
Neveu, P. J., 1978, The effect of the thiol moiety of levamisole on both cellular and humoral immunity during the early response to the hapten–carrier complex, *Clin. Exp. Immunol.* **32:**419–422.
Neveu, P. J., Perdoux, D., and Lafleur, L., 1982, *In vivo* enhancement of mitogen induced lymphocyte DNA synthesis by sodium diethyldithiocarbamate (DTC), *Int. J. Immunopharmacol.* **4:**9–13.
Ogawa, K., Sano, T., Hisano, G., and Tsubura, E., 1979, Levamisole in systemic lupus erythematosus, *Ann. Allergy* **43:**187–189.
Otterness, I. G., and Bliven, M. L., 1980, Comparative stimulating and anti-mitotic effects of levamisole and its metabolite BMPI on thymocytes, *Int. J. Immunopharmacol.* **2:**23–29.
Panel on Nickel, 1975, Nickel, a report to the committee on medical and biological effects of environmental pollutants, *Proc. Natl. Acad. Sci. U.S.A.* 113–123.
Pompidou, A., Touraine, J. L., Macé, B., Ananthakrishan, R., and Hadden, J. M., 1979, Role of nucleic acid and cytosqueleton in nuclear refringence phenomena of human blood lymphocytes, *Int. J. Immunopharmacol.* **2:**29–32.
Pompidou, A., Macé, B., Esnous, D., and Michel, P., 1980, The nuclear refringence test: A new method for the evaluation of blood lymphocyte nucled response *in vitro* to lectins and immunomodulators in man, in: *New Trends in Human Immunology and Cancer Immunotherapy*, B. Serrou and C. Rosenfeld, eds.), Doin, Paris, pp. 696–703.
Pompidou, A., Macé, B., Ducher, N., Coutance, F., Cooper, M. D., Hadden, J. W., and Renoux, G., 1985, A selective effect of sodium diethyldithiocarbamate (imuthiol) on human T cells, *Int. J. Immunopharmacol.* (in press).
Renoux, G., 1978, Modulation of immunity by levamisole, *Pharmacol. Ther.* **2:**397–423.
Renoux, G., 1980, The general immunopharmacology of levamisole, *Drugs* **19:**89–99.
Renoux, G., 1982, Immunopharmacologie et pharmacologie du diethyldithiocarbamate de sódium, DTC, *J. Pharmacol. (Paris)* **13:**95–134.
Renoux, G., 1984, The mode of action of imuthiol (sodium diethyldithiocarbamate). A new role for the brain neocortex and the endocrine liver in the regulation of the T-cell lineage in: *Immune Modulation Agents and their Mechanisms* (R. L. Ferichel and M. A. Chirigos eds.), Marcel Dekker, New York pp. 607–624.
Renoux, G., 1985, Studies with prototype immunotoxic agents, in: *Toxicology of the Immune System* (J. Dean, ed.), Raven Press, New York (in press).
Renoux, G., and Renoux, M., 1971, Effet immunostimulant d'un imidothiazole sur l'immunisation des souris par *Brucella abortus, C.R. Acad. Sci. (Paris) (D)* **269:**1467–1469.
Renoux, G., and Renoux, M., 1972, Antigenic competition and nonspecific immunity after a rickettsial infection in mice: Restoration of antibacterial immunity by phenyl-imidothiazole treatment, *J. Immunol.* **109:**761–765.
Renoux, G., and Renoux, M., 1973, Stimulation of anti-*Brucella* vaccination in mice by tetramisole, a phenylimidothiazole salt, *Infect. Immun.* **8:**544–548.
Renoux, G., and Renoux, M., 1974, Modulation of immune reactivity by phenylimidazole salts in mice immunized by sheep red blood cells, *J. Immunol.* **113:**779–790.
Renoux, G., and Renoux, M., 1977a, Thymus-like activities of sulphur derivatives on T-cell differentiation, *J. Exp. Med.* **145:**466–471.
Renoux, G., and Renoux, M., 1977b, Roles of the imidazole or thiol moiety on the immunostimulant action of levamisole, in: *Control of Neoplasia by Modulation of the Immune System,* (M. A. Chirigos, ed.), Raven Press, New York, pp. 67–80.
Renoux, M., and Renoux, G., 1977c, Brucellosis, immunodepression and levamisole, *Lancet* **1:**372.
Renoux, G., and Renoux, M., 1979, Immunopotentiation and anabolism induced by sodium diethyldithiocarbamate, *J. Immunopharmacol.* **1:**247–267.
Renoux, G., and Renoux, M., 1980a, The effects of sodium diethyldithiocarbamate, azathioprine, cyclophosphamide or hydrocortisone acetate administered alone or in association for 4 weeks on the immune responses of BALB/c mice, *Clin. Immunol. Immunopathol.* **15:**21–32.
Renoux, G., and Renoux, M., 1980c, Administration of DTC evidences a role of the thymus in the control and regulation of factors inducing thymocyte differentiation in the mouse, *Thymus* **2:**139–146.
Renoux, G., and Renoux, M., 1981, Immunologic activity of DTC: Potential for cancer therapy, in: *Augmenting*

Agents in Cancer Therapy: Current Status and Future Prospects (E. M. Hersh and M. A. Chirigos, eds.), Raven Press, New York, pp. 427–440.

Renoux, G., and Renoux, M., 1983, DTC, a T-cell specific agent in *nu/nu* mice, in: *Current Drugs and Methods of Cancer Treatment* (G. Mathé, E. Mihich, and P. Reizenstein, eds.), Masson, Paris, New York, pp. 171–173.

Renoux, G., and Renoux, M., 1984, Diethyldithiocarbamate (DTC). A biological augmenting agent specific for T cells, in: *Immune Modulation Agents and their Mechanisms* (R. L. Fenichel and M. A. Chinigos, eds.), Marcel Dekker, New York, Basel, pp. 6–20.

Renoux, G., Renoux, M., and Guillaumin, J. M., 1974, Suppression par le tetramisole de la tolerance des souris à une fraction de *Brucella melitensis, Ann. Immunol.* **125C**:550–551.

Renoux, G., Renoux, M., and Aycardi, D., 1976a, Levamisole promotes the killing of *Listeria monocytogenes* by macrophages, *Fed. Proc.* **3**:336.

Renoux, G., Renoux, M., Teller, M. N., McMahon, S., and Guillaumin, J. M., 1976b, Potentiation of T-cell mediated immunity by levamisole, *Clin. Exp. Immunol.* **25**:288–296.

Renoux, G., Kassel, R. A., Renoux, M., Fiore, N. C., Guillaumin, J. M., and Palat, A., 1977a, Immunomodulation by levamisole in normal and leukemic mice. Evidence for a serum transfer, in: *Modulation of Host Immune Resistance in the Prevention or Treatment of Induced Neoplasias, 1974,* (M. A. Chirigos, ed.), Fogarty International Center Proceedings No. 28, U.S. Government Printing Office, Washington, pp. 45–51.

Renoux, G., Renoux, M., and Guillaumin, J. M., 1977b, Un agent antiviral, l'isoprinosine, stimule les responses immunes, *Ann. Immunol. Inst. Pasteur.* **128c**:40.

Renoux, G., Renoux, M., and Guillaumin, J. M., 1979a, Isoprinosine as an immunopotentiator, *J. Immunopharmacol.* **1**:337–356.

Renoux, G., Renoux, M., Guillaumin, J. M., and Gouzien, C., 1979b, Differentiation and regulation of lymphocyte populations: Evidence for immunopotentiator-induced T cell recruitment, *J. Immunopharmacol.* **1**:415–422.

Renoux, G., Renoux, M., and Guillaumin, J. M., 1979c, Genetic and epigenetic control of levamisole-induced immunostimulation, *Int. J. Immunopharmacol.* **1**:43–48.

Renoux, G., Renoux, M., and Degenne, D., 1979d, Suppressor cell activity after isoprinosine treatment of lymphocytes from normal mice, *Int. J. Immunopharmacol.* **1**:239–241.

Renoux, G., Renoux, M., Gyenes, L., and Guillaumin, J. M., 1980a, A comparison of the *in vivo* T-cell recruiting capacity of DTC, serum of DTC-treated mice, and two synthetic "thymic hormones," *J. Immunopharmacol.* **2**:167.

Renoux, G., Touraine, J. L., and Renoux, M., 1980b, Induction of differentiation of human null cells into T lymphocytes by the serum of mice treated with sodium diethyldithiocarbamate, *J. Immunopharmacol.* **2**:49–59.

Renoux, G., Renoux, M., Greco, J., Baudoin, J., Lavandier, M., and Lemarié, E., 1980c, Phase I–II studies of sodium diethyldithiocarbamate, DTC, in: *New Trends in Human Immunology and Cancer Immunotherapy* (B. Serrou and C. Rosenfeld, eds.), Doin, Paris, pp. 974–985.

Renoux, G., Bizière, K., Renoux, M., and Guillaumin, J. M., 1980d, Le cortex cérébral règle les réponses immunes des souris, *C.R. Acad. Sci. (Paris) [D]* **290**:719–722.

Renoux, G., Bardos, P., Degenne, D., and Musset, M., 1982, Sodium diethyldithiocarbamate (DTC)-induced modifications of NK activity in the mouse, in: *NK Cells and other Natural Effector Cells* (R. B. Herberman, ed.), Academic Press, New York, pp. 443–448.

Renoux, G., Renoux, M., Lemarié, E., Lavandier, M., Greco, J., Bardos, P., Lang, J. M., Boilletot, A., Oberling, F., Armand, J., Musset, M., and Biron, G., 1983a, Sodium diethyldithiocarbamate (imuthiol) and cancer, in: *Biological Response Modifiers (BRM) in Human Oncology and Immunology* (T. Klein, S. Specter, and H. Friedman, eds.), Plenum Press, New York, pp. 223–239.

Renoux, G., Bizière, K., Renoux, M., Guillaumin, J. M., and Degenne, D., 1983b, A balanced brain asymmetry modulates T cell-mediated events, *J. Neuroimmunol.* **5**:227–238.

Renoux, G., Renoux, M., Bizière, K., Guillaumin, J. M., Bardos, P., and Degenne, D., 1984a, Involvement of brain neocortex and liver in the regulation of T cells: The mode of action of sodium diethyldithiocarbamate (imuthiol), *Immunopharmacology* **7**:89–100.

Rosenthal, M., Trabert, U., and Mueller, W., 1976a, Immunotherapy with levamisole in rheumatic diseases, *Scand. J. Rheumatol.* **5**:216–220.

Rosenthal, M., Trabert, U., and Müler, W., 1976b, The effect of levamisole on peripheral blood lymphocyte subpopulations in patients with rheumatoid arthritis and ankylosing spondylitis, *Clin. Exp. Immunol.* **25**:493–496.

Rosling, A. E., Rhodes, E. L., and Watson, B., 1978, Removal of a blocking factor from the sera of patients with systemic lupus erythematosus with levamisole, *Clin. Exp. Dermatol.* **3**:39–42.

Rovensky, J., Cebecauer, L., Zitman, D., Lukac, J., and Ferencik, M., 1982, Levamisole treatment of systemic lupus erythematosus, *Arthritis Rheum.* **25**:470–471.

Runge, L. A., Pinals, R. S., Lourie, S. H., and Tomar, R. H., 1977, Treatment of rheumatoid arthritis with levamisole: A controlled trial, *Arthritis Rheum.* **20**:1445–1448.

Runge, L. A., Pinals, R. S., and Tomar, R. H., 1979, Treatment of rheumatoid arthritis with levamisole: Long-term results and immune changes, *Ann. Rheum. Dis.* **38**:122–127.

Russel, A. S., 1976, Therapeutic trials with levamisole and other agents in NZB/W mice, *J. Rheumatol.* **3**:380–383.

Sampson, D., 1978, Studies on levamisole, a potentially useful drug in the treatment of Behcet's syndrome, *J. Oral Pathol.* **7**:383–386.

Sampson, D., Peters, T. G., Lewis, J. S., Metzig, J., and Kurtz, B. E., 1977, Dose dependence of immunopotentiation and tumor regression induced by levamisole, *Cancer Res.* **37**:3526–3529.

Sany, J., Clot, J., Bonneau, M., and Andary, M., 1982, Immunomodulating effect of human placenta-eluted gamma globulins in rheumatoid arthritis, *Arthritis Rheum.* **25**:17–24.

Scheid, M. P., Goldstein, G., and Boyse, E. A., 1975, Differentiation of T cells in nude mice, *Science* **190**:1211–1213.

Scheid, M. P., Goldstein, G., and Boyse, E. A., 1978, The generation and regulation of lymphocyte populations. Evidence for differentiative induction systems *in vitro, J. Exp. Med.* **147**:1727–1743.

Scherak, O., Smolen, J., Kolarz, G., Kojer, M., and Menzel, J., 1978, Clinical experience with levamisole treatment of patients with systemic lupus erythematosus, *Wien, Klin. Wochenschr.* **91**:758–762.

Scherak, O., Smolen, J. S., Menzel, E. J., Kojer, M., and Kolarz, G., 1980, Effect of levamisole on immunological parameters in patients with systemic lupus erythematosus, *Scand. J. Rheumatol.* **9**:106–112.

Schuerman, Y., 1975, Levamisole in rheumatoid arthritis, *Lancet* **1**:111.

Segond, P., Sallière, D., Clerc, D., Bisson, M., and Massias, P., 1981, Isoprinosine et polyarthrite rheumatoide; resultat d'une étude ouverte, *Rev. Rhum. Mal. Osteoartic.* **49**:45–49.

Shaposhinov, O. K., and Gorbanov, V. F., 1979, Diagnosis of T-immunodeficiencies in lupus erythematosus and patient treatment with levamisole, *West. Dermatol. Vener.* **3**:3–6.

Simon, L., and Glasky, A., 1978, Isoprinosine: An overview, *Cancer Treat. Rep.* **62**:1963–1970.

Smolen, J., Scherak, O., Menzel, J., Kojer, M., and Kolarz, G., 1977, Levamisole in systemic lupus erythematosus, *Arthritis Rheum.* **20**:1558–1559.

Stastny, P., 1974, Mixed lymphocyte culture typing cells from patients with rheumatoid arthritis, *Tissue Antigens* **4**:571–579.

Sunderman, P. W., 1979, Efficacy of sodium diethyldithiocarbamate (Dithiocarb) in acute nickel carbonyl poisoning, *Ann. Clin. Lab. Sci.* **9**:1–10.

Sunshine, G. H., Basch, R. S., Coffey, R. G., Cohen, K. W., Goldstein, G., and Hadden, J. W., 1978, Thymopoietin enhances the allogeneic response and cyclic GMP levels of mouse peripheral, thymus-derived lymphocytes, *J. Immunol.* **120**:1594–1597.

Suykens, S., Veys, E. M., Hermanns, P., Mielants, H., and Verbruggen, G., 1983, The mechanisms of flu-like syndrome induced by levamisole can be the base of its mode of action in rheumatoid arthritis, *Clin. Rheumatol.* **2**:106.

Thrower, P. A., Dayle, D. V., Scott, J., and Huskisson, E. C., 1982, Thymopoietin in rheumatoid arthritis, *Rheumatol. Rehabil.* **21**:72–77.

Touraine, J. L., Serrou, B., Hadden, J. W., Morin, A., and Touraine, P., 1980, Isoprinosine-induced suppressor activity, in: *New Trends in Human Immunology and Cancer Immunotherapy* (B. Serrou and C. Rosenfeld, eds.), Doin, Paris, pp. 1032–1037.

Trabert, U., Rosenthal, M., Müller, W., Müller, S., and Wurm, K., 1975, Levamisol bei der Behundlung entzündlish-rheumatischer Enkrankungen und der Sarcoidose, *Deutsch. Med. Wochenschr.* **44**:2297–2298.

Trabert, U., Rosenthal, M., and Muller, W., 1976, The effects of levamisole on adjuvant arthritis in the rat, *J. Rheumatol.* **3**:165–174.

Trainin, N., Small, M., Zipori, D., Umiel, T., Kook, A. I., and Rotter, V., 1975, Characteristics of THF, a thymic hormone, in: *Biological Activity of Thymic Hormones* (D. W. Van Bekkum, ed.), Kooyler Scientific, Rotterdam, pp. 117–144.

Twomey, J. J., and Kouttab, N. M., 1982, Selected phenotypic induction of null lymphocytes from mice with thymic and nonthymic agents, *Cell. Immunol.* **72**:186–194.

Vecchi, A., Sironi, M., and Spreafico, F., 1978, Preliminary characterization in mice of the effect of isoprinosine on the immune system, *Cancer Treat. Rep.* **62**:1975–1979.

Veys, E. M., and Mielants, H., 1977, Longterm evaluation of intermittent levamisole treatment in rheumatoid arthritis, *J. Rheumatol.* **4**:27–34.

Veys, E. M., and Mielants, H., 1978, Experience and recommendations for treatment schedule of levamisole in rheumatoid arthritis, *J. Rheumatol.* **5**(Suppl. 4):31–45.

Veys, E. M., Mielants, H., Verbruggen, G., Dhondt, E., Goethals, L., Cherontre, L., and Buelens, H., 1981a, Levamisole as basic treatment of rheumatoid arthritis: Longterm evaluation, *J. Rheumatol.* **8**:45–56.

Veys, E. M., Hermanns, P., Goldstein, G., Kung, P., Schindler, J., and Van Wauve, J. V., 1981b, Determination of T-lymphocyte subpopulations by monoclonal antibodies in rheumatoid arthritis. Influence of immunomodulating agents, *Int. J. Immunopharmacol.* **3**:313–319.

Veys, E. M., Huskisson, E. C., Rosenthal, M., Vischer, T. L., Mielants, H., Thrower, P. A., Scott, J., Ott, H., Scheijgrond, M., and Symoens, J., 1982a, Clinical response to therapy with thymopoietin pentapeptide (TPS) in rheumatoid arthritis, *Ann. Rheum. Dis* **41**:441–443.

Veys, E. M., Hermanns, P., Schindler, J., Kung, P. C., Goldstein, G., Symoens, J., and Van Wauve, J. V., 1982b, Evaluation of T-cell subsets with monoclonal antibodies in patients with rheumatoid arthritis, *J. Rheumatol.* **9**:25–29.

Waldman, R. M., and Ganguly, R., 1977, Therapeutic efficacy of inosiplex (isoprinosine) in rhinovirus infection, *Ann. N.Y. Acad. Sci.* **284**:153–160.

Weh, M. J., Bernheim, A., and Berger, R., 1980, Isoprinosine et chromosomes humains, *Pathol. Biol.* **28**:319–322.

Willoughby, D. A., and Wood, C., 1979, Forum in immunotherapy. Levamisole in infectious diseases, *R. Soc. Med. (London)* **2**:11.

Woods, W. A., Fliegelman, M. J., and Chirigos, M. A., 1974, *In vitro* stimulation of spleen cell cultures by poly I : poly C and levamisole, *Cell. Immunol.* **14**:327–331.

Wybran, J., Govaerts, A., and Appelboom, J., 1978, Inosiplex, a stimulation agent for human T cells and normal leukocytes, *J. Immunol.* **121**:1184–1187.

Wybran, J., Famaey, J. P., and Appelboom, T., 1981, Inosiplex: A novel treatment in rheumatoid arthritis, *J. Rheumatol.* **8**:643–646.

Zulman, J., Michalski, J., McCombs, C., Greenspan, J., and Talal, N., 1978, Levamisole maintains cyclophosphamide-induced remission in murine lupus erythematosus, *Clin. Exp. Immunol.* **31**:321–327.

27

Thymic Hormones and Rheumatoid Arthritis

J. F. Bach and M. Dardenne

I. INTRODUCTION

T-cell differentiation proceeds under the command of several signals, among which thymic hormones (TH) play a central role. A number of T-cell abnormalities have been described in rheumatoid arthritis (RA), both by marker and functional studies. One may raise the question of thymic hormone production in RA and in related immunologic diseases such as systemic lupus erythematosus (SLE). Additionally, since thymic hormones can modulate T-cell functions, one may attempt to improve the clinical status of RA patients by using pharmacological doses of the hormones independently of a preexisting abnormality of thymic hormone production.

II. THYMIC HORMONES

A. Chemistry and Biology

Several immunopharmacologically active peptides have been isolated from the thymus. We shall not discuss here nonpurified or partially purified preparations, which in fact, from a theoretical viewpoint, have no more interest than indicating the existence in the thymus of unidentified substance(s) with a given activity, with the important reservation that no evidence is generally provided that the substance(s) in question is (are) really specifically produced by the thymus (they may be also synthesized in other organs). As far as chemically well-defined peptides are concerned, one is confronted with a series of molecular entities with no apparent relationship. One may presently place in this series four distinct peptides: thymopoietin, thymosin α 1, thymic humoral factor (THF), and

J. F. Bach and M. Dardenne • INSERM U 25, Hopital Necker, 75015 Paris, France.

thymulin (formerly called FTS) with molecular weights ranging from 800 to 5500. To date, only three of them have been synthesized: thymopoietin, thymosin α 1, and thymulin (Table 1).

1. Thymopoietin

Thymopoietin, a polypeptide hormone of the thymus, was isolated by its neuromuscular effects rather than by its action on the immune system. The development of experimental models of myasthenia gravis led to the detection of a thymic hormone influence on neuromuscular transmission, and electromyographic assays were used to monitor the fractionation of thymic extracts (Goldstein, 1974). By this means, thymopoietin was isolated, and the biochemically homogeneous polypeptide was shown to be active in the neuromuscular assay. Thymopoietin was also shown to be capable of inducing various T-cell-specific alloantigens *in vitro* (Basch and Goldstein, 1974).

Thymopoietin is a 49-amino-acid polypeptide. The complete amino acid sequence of thymopoietin has been determined (Goldstein, 1975). The two forms (termed thymopoietin I and II) differ only by two amino acid substitutions (Schlesinger and Goldstein, 1975). A synthetic pentapeptide has the complete activity of thymopoietin and is selective

Table 1. Summary of the Main Characteristics of Current Thymic Preparations

Preparation	Biochemistry Molecular weight	Functional assay	Main properties
Thymosin (fraction 5)[a]	Heterogeneous mixture of more than 25 polypeptides (two peptides sequenced) 1000–12,000 α1 = 3,107 β4 = 4,982	Thy-l induction (rosettes) E-rosette induction	Suppressor T cells, GVH, MLC, skin graft rejection (fraction 5)
Thymopoietin (formerly thymin)[b]	Two pure entities, Tp and TpII, Sequence known, 5562 (TpII)	Neuromuscular transmission	Antibody affinity in aged mice, Thy-l induction, suppressor T cells
THF (Thymic humoral factor)[c]	Peptide not yet completely characterized 2–4000	GVH *in vitro* cAMP synthesis	Helper T cells, GVH, MLC
Thymulin (formerly FTS for facteur thymique sérique)[d]	Nonapeptide, sequence known, synthesis made 847	Thy-l induction Mouse rosette forming cells	Allogeneic cytotoxicity, MSV sarcoma rejection, suppressor T cells (NZB + normal mice), skin graft rejection, helper T cells IgA deficiency

[a] Goldstein *et al.* (1972, 1977).
[b] Goldstein (1975).
[c] Trainin and Small (1970).
[d] Bach (1983).

for T-cell differentiation *in vitro* (Goldstein *et al.*, 1979). Thymopoietin or its pentapeptide fragment (TP-5) has been shown to enhance several T-cell functions *in vivo* (rejection of carcinoma, prevention of autoimmunity in mice, and generation of cytotoxic T cells; Goldstein and Lau, 1980). Recently, a polypeptide related to thymopoietin has been isolated from the spleen. This polypeptide, which only differs at one residue from thymopoietin, promotes differentiation of both B and T cells.

2. *Thymosin α 1*

Thymosin α 1 was the first peptide isolated from thymosin fraction 5 and sequenced. It consists of 28 amino acid residues and has a molecular weight of 3108 (A. L. Goldstein *et al.*, 1977). It increases mitogenic responses of murine lymphocytes, enhances production of the macrophage migration inhibition factor, and augments the number of Thy-1^+Lyt 123^+ cells in thymocytes (Ahmed *et al.*, 1979). It also modulates the appearance of deoxynucleotidyltransferase in prothymocytes and thymocytes and its disappearance in mature T cells (Wetzel *et al.*, 1980). The *in vitro* treatment of thymocytes with thymosin α 1 results in increased percentage of glucocorticoid-resistant cells (Osheroff, 1981). Moreover, the *in vitro* incubation of lymphocytes with thymosin α 1 enhances the production of lymphokines (Thurman *et al.*, 1977), stimulates the specific release of prostaglandin E_2 (PGE_2) from splenic lymphocytes and thymocytes (Rinaldi-Garaci *et al.*, 1983), and increases the ability to form E-rosettes (Low *et al.*, 1979).

Although in some of these assay systems, thymosin α 1 seems to have a higher specific activity than thymosin fraction 5, it is difficult to determine the role of thymosin α 1 among biologically active thymosin fraction 5 peptides.

3. *Thymulin (FTS)*

Thymulin, formerly called FTS (for *facteur thymique serique*), is a nonapeptide initially prepared from porcine serum (Pleau *et al.*, 1977) but also isolated to purity from human serum and calf thymus. Thymulin binds zinc with a dissociation constant of 10^{-7} M (as evaluated by equilibrium chromatography) (Gastinel *et al.*, 1984), and the presence of zinc is necessary for its biological activity (Dardenne *et al.*, 1982b). More than 40 analogues of thymulin have been synthesized and immunologically evaluated (in bioassays and receptor assays), permitting the localization of the molecule's activity on the seven terminal amino acids (Bach, 1983). Some analogues have been shown to bind to the receptor and to inhibit thymulin activity, behaving like antihormones (Pleau *et al.*, 1979).

Thymulin is exclusively produced by the thymic epithelium as demonstrated by different approaches including its isolation from thymic extracts (Dardenne *et al.*, 1980) and the demonstration of its exclusive presence in thymic epithelial cells by immunochemistry using xenoantisera (Monier *et al.*, 1980; Jambon *et al.*, 1981) and specific monoclonal antibodies (Savino *et al.*, 1982). Recent studies using these antithymulin monoclonal antibodies have shown that the number of thymulin-containing cells increases after peripheral depletion of the hormone either by active immunization against the peptide or by injection of an antithymulin monoclonal antibody. Conversely, the increase in thymulin-containing cells normally noted in cultured thymic epithelial cells is slowed down by the addition of synthetic thymulin (Savino *et al.*, 1983b; Cohen *et al.*, 1983). These data suggest the existence of a feedback regulation of thymulin secretion, thymulin itself being the inhibitory signal.

Thymulin circulates in the blood partly bound to a 40- to 60,000-molecular-weight carrier molecule. It is subjected to the action of several inhibitors (Bach, 1983).

Thymulin apparently acts exclusively on T cells. It binds to T-cell membrane receptors with a high affinity (there are two sites with respective K_ds of 10^{-9} M and 10^{-7} M without negative cooperativity; Pleau *et al.*, 1980). Thymulin does not clearly stimulate cAMP synthesis but has been shown to enhance prostaglandin E_2 production by human lymphocytes (Gualde *et al.*, 1982). As far as its biological activity is concerned, thymulin has been shown to enhance the function of the various T-cell subsets (Table 2). The hormone is mostly active in recipients with the putative postthymic target cells (but may also be active in mature T cells) when the simultaneous effects of supressor and helper (or effector) cells do not counterbalance each other. Interestingly, thymulin shows a preferential action on suppressor T cells at high doses, particularly in normal recipients. At low doses or in immunodeficient patients, it is more difficult to predict which T-cell subset will be preferentially stimulated.

B. Evaluation of the Thymic Endocrine Function

The thymic epithelium endocrine function is generally evaluated by measuring TH serum levels. More recently, and essentially in experimental animals, it has become possble to study directly the TH-producing cells.

1. Measurement of TH Serum Levels

Several bioassays and radioimmunoassays have been developed for the quantitation of TH levels in murine and human blood.

a. Bioassays. The first of these bioassays was described in our laboratory (Dardenne and Bach, 1975). It is based on the changes induced by TH on a minority of spleen cells from adult thymectomized (ATx) mice that form spontaneous rosettes with sheep erythrocytes. The assay consists of detecting the smallest serum concentration that renders spleen rosette-forming cells (RFC) sensitive to anti-Thy-1 serum or to azathioprine, the widely used immunosuppressive agent that inhibits rosette formation at a low concentration in normal mice but loses this property in ATx mice. In selected cases, the relationship between the activity detected and thymulin may be verified by passing the serum on an immunoadsorbent prepared with an antibody raised against synthetic thymulin or by preincubating the serum with an antithymulin monoclonal antibody. The strict thymic dependence of the activity detected by the rosette assay is demonstrated by its total absence in the sera from nude or Tx mice and in patients with DiGeorge's syndrome and its reappearance in all these individuals after thymus grafting.

A similar method was described in 1977 by Twomey *et al.* (1977) using a cytotoxic assay. This bioassay measures the induction of the Thy-1 thymus-specific antigen on the membranes of null lymphocytes from the spleens of germ-free athymic mice. The assay is performed in the presence of ubiquitin, which inhibits nonspecific T-cell induction and increases the sensitivity of the assay. The activity is determined from the percentage of indicator cells induced to express Thy-1 antigen. Results are expressed as equivalent inductive capacity in comparison with known amounts of thymopoietin per milliliter.

Table 2. Effects of Thymulin on T-Cell Functions

Proliferation	
PHA-induced	Mouse, mice Tx[a] at 3 weeks Rat, ATx rats Human, immunodeficiencies
Autologous mixed lymphocyte reaction (lupus)[b]	
Cytotoxicity and delayed hypersensitivity	
Allogeneic cytotoxicity	ATx mice
Anti-TNP cytotoxicity	Normal thymocytes[b]
Graft-versus-host reaction	Normal mice
Rejection of MSV-induced sarcoma (low dose)	B mice
Stimulation of delayed-type hypersensitivity	ATx mice
Helper T cells	
Antibody production (SRBC)	Aging mice
Induction of IgA (and IgE) synthesis	Ataxia telangiectasia and variable immunodeficiency
Production of interleukin-2	Normal thymocytes and nude mouse spleen cells
Increase in anti-DNA IgG autoantibodies	Young B/W mice (females)
Suppressor T cells	
Retardation of skin allograft rejection	Normal mice
Depression of antibody production	
SRBC	Normal mice
PVP	NZB mice
DNA	B/W mice (males)
Depression of T-cell-mediated cytotoxicity	Normal mice
Depression of delayed-type hypersensitivity	Normal mice
Stimulation of Con-A-induced suppression	Lupus patients Normal subjects
Other effects	
Increase of NK cell activity (*in vitro* and *in vivo*) in humans and in mice	
Stimulation of colony-forming unit (CFU-S) entry into DNA synthesis in Tx mice after thymus-dependent antigen treatment	
Alteration of the migration capacity of fetal hemopoietic precursor cells[b]	
Increased resistance to *Salmonella typhimurium*	
Enhancement of LPS-induced polyclonal B-cell responses *in vitro* of CBA/N mice	
Increase in "early" null radiation-induced leukemias in Tx AKR mice	
Decrease in TdT expression in the mouse[b] and in the human[b]	

[a] Tx, thymectomized.
[b] *In vitro* experiment.

Interestingly, thymulin, whose effects are inhibited by ubiquitin, is not active in the test. Expression of results in nanogram equivalents of thymopoietin does not fully take into account molecules other than thymopoietin that could be active in the test or interfering molecules (carrier proteins, inhibitors). As for the rosette assay, the specificity of the Twomey assay is assessed by its negativity with the sera from nude and Tx mice and sera from patients with DiGeorge's syndrome.

b. Radioimmunoassays. Radioimmunoassays (RIA) have been described for three well-defined thymic peptides: thymosin α 1 (McClure *et al.*, 1981), thymulin (Pleau *et al.*, 1981), thymulin (Pleau *et al.*, 1978), and thymopoietin (Goldstein, 1976); RIA have not yet been successfully applied to the evaluation of thymulin or thymopoietin in serum samples, essentially because of unsolved interference by serum proteins. More conclusive results have been reported for thymosin α 1. McClure *et al.* (1981) have recently succeeded in developing a RIA for serum thymosin α 1. Antiserum to synthetic thymosin α 1 was produced in rabbits by immunization with the synthetic peptide coupled to hemocyanin by means of glutaraldehyde. By using a highly purified synthetic thymosin α 1 standard, a calibration curve was generated that provided a minimal detectable dose of 30 to 50 pg. However, one still awaits the unequivocal demonstration of the total absence of RIA-positive material in the serum of thymectomized animals or humans compared with normal individuals, as has been obtained for two bioassays mentioned above.

c. Study of TH-Containing Cells. Several antibodies have been raised against some of the TH listed in Table 1. Thus, polyclonal antisera have been produced against thymosin α 1 and thymopoietin, and several monoclonal antibodies have been obtained against synthetic and natural thymulin (Dardenne *et al.*, 1982a; Berrih *et al.*, 1984). These antibodies have successfully been used to visualize TH-containing cells in the thymus by indirect immunofluorescence. The strict specificity of immunofluorescence has been demonstrated in various ways including negative fluorescence of nonthymic tissues and inhibition of antibody binding to the thymus by incubation with synthetic hormone.

C. Physiological Age-Dependent Decline in Thymic Hormone Production

Before we discuss abnormal TH production, it is worthwhile to outline the physiological age-dependent decline of serum TH levels, which is accompanied by a decrease in the intrathymic content of the hormones. As we first showed in 1972, the thymulin serum level is maximal at birth, remains constant until the age of 15 to 20 years, and then declines progressively (Bach *et al.*, 1972), a finding that has now been confirmed by other investigators (Fabris, 1980; Garaci *et al.*, 1978; Iwata *et al.*, 1983). This progressive age-dependent decline of thymulin blood levels is paralleled in mice by a decrease in the number of thymulin-containing cells in the thymus (Savino *et al.*, 1983a).

An identical age-dependent decline of serum thymopoietinlike activity was reported by Twomey *et al.* (1977). At variance with these data, the serum level of thymosin α 1, assessed by RIA, was reported to be highest *in utero,* to sharply decline after birth, and to remain stable thereafter (McClure *et al.*, 1981). The number of thymosin α 1-containing cells has also been shown to decrease with age in humans (Hirokawa *et al.*, 1982).

D. Thymulin Production in Autoimmunity

1. Systemic Lupus Erythematosus

An accelerated decline of TH production occurs in human and murine lupus. Thus, 2-month-old NZB and B/W mice as well as young SLE patients exhibit low thymulin levels compared to age-matched controls (Bach *et al.*, 1973). Autoimmune mice also exhibit a precocious thymic atrophy. More recently, we observed that the rapid decline in thymulin levels noted in young NZB mice was paralleled by a decrease in the number of thymulin-containing cells (Savine *et al.*, 1983b).

A similar pattern has been observed in other autoimmune strains such as MRL/1 (M. A. Bach and Charreire, 1979), Swan (Dardenne *et al.*, 1983), and *db/db* diabetic mice (Dardenne *et al.*, 1983b). The presence of thymulin in thymic crystalline structures has suggested that autoimmune states could be associated with abnormal thymulin storage (Schmitt *et al.*, 1982). Several weeks after thymulin disappearance, autoimmune mice show a deficit in their production of T-cell factors both of the suppressor type (SIRS) and of the helper type (IL-2) (reviewed by Bach, 1982). The relationship between these anomalies and thymic failure is plausible, especially since TH have been shown to influence suppressor T-cell function and IL-2 production. Although it is true that the pathogenetic role of the abnormal production of these lymphokines has not been established, it may be hypothesized that IL-2-associated differentiation of regulatory T cells is faulty in autoimmune mice.

The defect of T-cell regulation in autoimmunity has, in the past, been the source of a number of therapeutic attempts, particularly in NZB and B/W mice. The use of TH in autoimmune mice was suggested by the favorable effect of thymic grafting on the autoimmune hemolytic anemia of NZB mice (see Bach, 1982) and the pharmacological stimulatory effect of thymic hormones on suppressor T cells. Crude thymic extracts have been used in NZB mice without favorable results. Conversely, positive data have been obtained with thymulin in NZB and B/W mice (M. A. Bach *et al.*, 1980; Israel-Biet *et al.*, 1983). However, the effects of thymulin were not consistently favorable. Table 3 summarizes the results obtained to date. It is interesting and somewhat paradoxical that the disease can either be improved or aggravated according to the recipient mouse and the autoimmune manifestations considered. These data may be explained by the variable thymic dependence of autoimmune parameters as well as by the different T-cell subset alterations present in various autoimmune mice. Young female B/W or NZB mice have marked deficiencies in suppressor T cells that prevent the induction by TH of efficient suppressor-cell function, whereas helper T cells, which are longer lived (they are more resistant to adult thymectomy), persist in these mice and are more readily stimulated than suppressor cells by thymic hormones. In contrast, old male B/W mice probably still possess thymic-hormone-responsive suppressor T cells.

In addition, IgG anti-DNA antibodies are highly thymus dependent (their production is prevented by neonatal thymectomy), and it may be assumed that, as far as their sensitivity to thymic hormones is concerned, the stimulation of helper T cells overwhelms the potential beneficial effect of suppressor cell stimulation. Conversely, in other systems

Table 3. Effects of Thymulin in NZB and B/W Mice

	NZB		B/W	
	Young ♀	Old ♀	Young ♀	Old ♂
PVP antibody production	Decrease	Enhancement		
Sjögren	Improvement	Improvement	Improvement	NT[a]
Hemolytic anemia	Improvement	NT	NT	NT
Anti-DNA antibodies (glomerulonephritis)	No effect	NT		Suppression

[a] NT, not tested.

that are less thymus dependent, such as PVP antibody production, suppression is more easily detected, at least when suppressor cells or suppressor-cell precursors are available.

2. Rheumatoid Arthritis

Thymic hormone level was determined in two series of patients with RA using the biological rosette-inhibition assay previously described. The levels in RA were high in most cases (between 1/8 and 1/64) irrespective of age. However, a few patients with juvenile RA had low thymulin levels, and a minority of them even had a very low thymulin level as noted for SLE. WHen patients were compared with age-matched controls, a significant difference ($P < 0.01$) was found for subjects over 50 years with higher levels than controls (Bach *et al.*, 1975).

However, high thymulin values found in RA could be caused not by hyperthymic secretion but by the presence in the serum of factors unrelated to thymulin activity. It is known that factors secreted by activated T cells may in some cases look like thymulin in the rosette assay (Dardenne and Bach, 1977). These allogeneic factors do not have the same electric charge and do not bind to carboxymethylcellulose as thymulin does. Moreover, their activity is not inhibited by specific antithymulin monoclonal antibodies.

In a recent study involving 30 RA patients, the nature of the factor under study was investigated by incubating the RA sera with a specific antithymulin immunoadsorbent prepared by coupling rabbit antithymulin IgG to sepharose beads or by incubating the RA sera with an antithymulin monoclonal antibody. In all cases, the specific immunoadsorbent or monoclonal antibody was not able to remove all the thymulinlike activity present in RA sera, as they do in normal sera, suggesting that the factor measured is not thymulin itself, whose exlusive thymic origin has been demonstrated by thymectomy experiments. The nature of the factor in question is still unknown. It could be related to inflammation mediators produced in RA. Its presence prevents a satisfactory evaluation of actual thymulin serum levels in RA.

E. The Effect of Thymic Hormones on RA Lymphocytes

The study of T-cell subsets by use of monoclonal antibodies has revealed in a large percentage of RA patients with active disease an increase of the $OKT4^+/OKT8^+$ ratio, resulting essentially from a decrease in the percentage of suppressor/cytotoxic T cells ($OKT8^+$) or, more rarely, from an increase of the percentage of helper/inducer T cells ($OKT4^+$) (Pfrendschuh *et al.*, 1981; Veys *et al.*, 1981, 1982a,b; Duclos *et al.*, 1982; Faure *et al.*, 1982). This observation is in keeping with previous ones based on other T-cell markers established on a much less firm basis (lower reproducibility and consistency, dubious significance).

Several authors, using different thymic preparations, have attempted to correct the T-cell subset imbalance (as evaluated by E-rosette formation or monoclonal antibodies) by incubating RA lymphocytes with thymic hormone for short-term period. Using thymosin fraction V, Moutsopoulos *et al.* (1976) reported an increase in E-rosette number in a minority of RA patients with decreased E-rosette level. Using the thymopoietin synthetic fragment TP-5, Auteri *et al.* (1980a,b) obtained a similar result *in vitro* and *in vivo*. More strikingly, Faure *et al.* (1985), using synthetic thymulin, have reported that thymulin normalized the $OKT4^+/OKT8^+$ ratio in four patients with initially increased ratios as a result of an increase of $OKT8^+$ cells, a decrease of $OKT4^+$ cells, or both. The ratio remained normal or slightly decreased in two patients who initially had normal ones. No alteration of $OKT3^+$ cell number was observed except in one patient, where it was reduced and increased under thymulin treatment. Interestingly, one of the four patients, sensitive to thymulin, was under steroid treatment, which indicates that steroids do not prevent the thymulin effect on T cells. These results resemble those obtained by the same authors (Bene *et al.*, 1982) with lymphocytes from immunodeficient children. One should add that similar results were obtained after *in vivo* treatment with thymosin TP-5 (1/4) or thymulin (G. Faure, unpublished data), although the effect proved to be less consistent than that in *in vitro* studies.

These results indicate that thymic peptides can alter T-cell membranes and tend to normalize the subtle abnormalities present in RA patients. They also show that RA patients' lymphocytes express receptors for thymic hormones. Whether these effects indicate that T-cell functions are also normalized is still open to further investigation. This will not be easy, inasmuch as there is no clear-cut, consistent anomaly of T-cell function in RA. In any case, taken together with the effect of thymic hormones in experimental autoimmune diseases, these data have prompted the undertaking of thymic hormone clinical trials in RA.

F. Preliminary Clinical Trials of Thymic Hormones in RA

Two synthetic peptides have been used in therapeutic clinical trials in RA. Thymopoietin was used in the form of the synthetic fragment TP-5. Initial clinical studies using a small intramuscular dose showed little effect. Subsequently, a dose–response study on E-rosette-forming cells in normal elderly subjects and patients with minor pathology showed a single intravenous dose of 50 mg to give the most highly significant effect. This was also found to be the optimum dose in RA patients: it restored the number of E-rosette-forming cells to normal after 12 hr, and the effect lasted 6 to 7 days (Auteri *et al.*, 1980b; Laghi-Pasini *et al.*, 1980). In an open study involving 36 RA patients with active disease, TP-5 (50 mg i.v. weekly) for 6 months was compared to levamisole and penicillamine; TP-5 produced a statistically significant reduction in pain, duration of morning stiffness, articular index, and joint size with little or no effect on biological parameters (ESR, rheumatoid factor, Ig levels). Penicillamine and levamisole provided comparable improvements, but reduction in pain was greatest with TP-5. Minor side effects were noted (two cases of skin rashes with TP-5; Thrower *et al.*, 1982). In another trial, TP-5 (1 mg weekly) was compard in a double-blind protocol to a placebo. No effect was noted at 3 months, but a significant decrease in the number of swollen joints, morning stiffness, and pain was noted at 6 months with TP-5. However, patients in the placebo group also improved, making differences between TP-5 and placebo not significant. Finally, in a third trial (Veys *et al.*, 1982a), TP-5 (50 mg weekly) was compared to the placebo group of the previous study. Clinical improvement was detected at 3 months—significantly better than in the placebo group or in the 1-mg TP-5 group, again without effect on ESR.

Thymulin (FTS-Zn) was submitted to three clinical trials. The first was an open trial on six patients with recent onset RA (G. Faure, unpublished data). Four of these patients had proven to be sensitive to thymulin *in vitro*, as described above. Although it is difficult

Table 4. Clinical Parameters at the Beginning of the Trial and Mean Changes after 4 Months of Therapy with Thymulin

	Thymulin, 150 μg (n = 8)		Thymulin, 1 mg (n = 8)	
Parameters[a]	Before trial	Mean change after 4 months	Before trial	Mean change after 4 months
Morning stiffness (min)	136 (107)[d]	−42 (128)	151 (117)	−52.2 (90.6)
Articular index (Ritchie)	12.9 (5.7)	+0.63 (5.9)	13.4 (4.6)	−5.4 (3.2)
Swollen joints (number)	17.3 (6.8)	−1.38 (3.4)	17.6 (8.5)	−5.0 (4.9)[b]
Grip strength (mm Hg)	257 (130)	+44.4 (63.4)[c]	258 (195)	−6.8 (205)
PIP circumference (mm)	593 (26.0)	−8.9 (11.4)[c]	617 (56)	−9.6 (9.5)[b]
Pain (mm)	71.8 (17.8)	−1.63 (19.9)	54.9 (36.6)	−6.5 (23)
Functional index (Lee)	12.1 (3.2)	+0.25 (1.8)	13.4 (3.8)	−0.9 (1.8)
ESR (mm/hr)	53.1 (14.5)	+3.1 (6.8)	58.0 (27.2)	−7.5 (22.7)

[a] PIP, Proximal interphalangeal joint; ESR, erythrocyte sedimentation rate.
[b] $P < 0.05$.
[c] $P < 0.10$.
[d] Standard deviations.

to give a final interpretation of the results obtained because of the lack of an adequate placebo control group, striking effects were observed, with rapid decrease of pain, swollen joints, and physical inability. Amor *et al.* (1984) conducted two trials with thymulin in patients with active disease of late onset. The first was open, using daily doses of 150 μg or 1 mg s.c. In the 150-μg group, the only changes observed were enhancement of grip strength and reduction of IPP circumference. With 1 mg, a significant improvement was observed for the Ritchie index, the number of swollen joints, and IPP circumference (Table 4). In a more recent randomized double-blind trial, Amor *et al.* showed that thymulin, 1 and 5 mg 3 times weekly, provided an improvement of most clinical parameters that, however, was only significantly better than in the placebo group for the 5-mg dose.

III. CONCLUSION

In conclusion, it appears that TP-5 and thymulin may improve the clinical status of RA patients, particularly when they are used at relatively high doses (50 mg once weekly for TP-5, 5 mg three times weekly for thymulin). The recent thymulin randomized double-blind trial has now confirmed in a statistically satisfactory fashion the favorable impression gained in open trials (no such double-blind trial is presently available for TP-5). If these results are confirmed, they will provide a new harmless treatment for active RA. Thymic peptides are physiological and natural mediators without known side effects. The only foreseeable problem relates to the necessary use of intravenous or subcutaneous injections. One may hope in that regard that clinical pharmacology studies will provide us an easier means of drug administration. The use of long-lasting analogues that have been synthesized for thymulin could represent a possible approach permitting us to space the doses.

REFERENCES

Ahmed, A., Wong, D. M., Thurman, G. B., Low, T. L. K., and Goldstein, A. I., 1979, T-lymphocyte maturation cell surface markers and immune function, induced by T-lymphocyte cell free products and thymosin polypeptides, *Ann. N.Y. Acad. Sci.* **332:**81–94.

Amor, B., Dougados, M., Mery, C., de Gery, A., Choay, J., Dardenne, M., and Bach, J. F., 1984, Thymulin (FTS) in rheumatoid arthritis, *Arthritis Rheum.* **27:**117–118.

Auteri, A., Laghi Pasini, F., Pasque, A. L., Bilenchi, R., and Di Perri, T., 1980a, Azione della timopoietina pentapeptide sulla formazione di rosette lifocitarie E di pazienti affetti da artrite reumatoide I. Studio *in vitro, Boll. Soc. Ital. Biol. Sper.* **4:**308–311.

Auteri, A., Laghi Pasini, F., Pasqui, A. L., Bilenchi, R., and Di Perri, T., 1980b, Azione della timopoietina pentapeptide sulla formazione di rosette linfociatarie E di pazienti affetti da artrite reumatoide II. Studio *in vivo, Boll. Soc. Ital. Biol. Sper.* **4:**312–315.

Bach, J. F., 1982, Thymic factors and immunoregulation role in autoimmune diseases, in: *Regulation of the Immune Response* (D. N. Jacobs and P. L. Ogra, eds.), Karger, Basel, pp. 20–29.

Bach, J. F., 1983, Thymulin (FTS-Zn), *Clin. Immunol. Allergy* **3:**133–157.

Bach, J. F., Dardenne, M., Papiernik, M., Barois, A., Levasseur, P., and Le Brigand, H., 1972, Evidence for a serum factor produced by the human thymus, *Lancet* **1:**1056–1058.

Bach, J. F., Dardenne, M., and Salomon, J. C., 1973, Studies on thymus products. IV. Absence of serum "thymic activity" in adult NZB and (NZB × NZW) F_1 mice, *Clin. Exp. Immunol.* **14:**247–256.

Bach, J. F., Dardenne, M., and Clot, J., 1975, Evaluation of serum thymic hormone and of circulating T cells in rheumatoid arthritis and in systemic lupus erythematosus, *Rheumatology* **6:**242–250.

Bach, M. A., and Charreire, J., 1979, Role of a circulating thymic factor in self recognition and self tolerance, *Ann. N.Y. Acad. Sci.* **332:**55–63.

Bach, M. A., Droz, D., Noël, L. H., Blanchard, D., Dardenne, M., and Peking, A., 1980, Effect of long-term treatment with circulating thymic factor on murine lupus, *Arthritis Rheum.* **23:**1351–1358.

Basch, R. S., and Goldstein, G. 1974, Induction of T-cell differentiation *in vitro* by thymin, a purified polypeptide hormone of the thymus, *Proc. Natl. Acad. Sci. U.S.A.* **71:**1474–1478.

Bene, M. C., Faure, G., Bordigoni, P., Olive, S., and Duheille, J., 1982, *In vitro* induction of monoclonal antibody-defined T-cell markers in lymphocytes from immunodeficient children by synthetic serum thymic factor (FTS), *Clin. Exp. Immunol.* **48:**423–428.

Berrih, S., Savino, W., Azoulay, M., Dardenne, M., and Bach, J. F., 1984, Production of anti-thymulin (FTS) monoclonal antibodies by immunization against hyman thymic epithelial cells, *J. Histochem. Cytochem.* **32:**432–438.

Cohen, S., Berrih, S., Dardenne, M., and Bach, J. F., 1983, Régulation in vitro de la secrétion de thymuline par les cellules épithéliales thymiques humaines. *C. R. Acad. Sci. (Paris) (D)* **297:**63–65.

Dardenne, M., and Bach, J. F., 1975, The sheep cell rosette assay for the evaluation of thymic hormones, in: *Biological Activity of Thymic Hormones,* (D. van Bekkum ed.), Kooyker Science, Rotterdam, pp. 235–243.

Dardenne, M., and Bach, J. F., 1977, Demonstration and characterization of a serum factor produced by activated T cells, *Immunology* **33:**643.

Dardenne, M., Monier, J. C., Biozzi, G., and Bach, J. F., 1974, Studies on thymus products. V. Influence of genetic selection based on antibody production of thymic hormone production, *Clin. Exp. Immunol.* **17:**339–344.

Dardenne, M., Pleau, J. M., Blouquit, J. Y., and Bach, J. F., 1980, Characterization of facteur thymique sérique (FTS) in the thymus II. Direct demonstration of the presence of FTS in thymosin fraction V. *Clin. Exp. Immunol.* **42:**477–482.

Dardenne, M., Pleau, J. M., Savino, W., and Bach, J. F., 1982a, Monoclonal antibody against the serum thymic factor (FTS), *Immunol. Lett.* **48:**61–69.

Dardenne, M., Pleau, J. M., Nabarra, B., Lefrancier, P., Derrien, M., Choay, J., and Bach, J. F., 1982b, Contribution of zinc and other metals to the biological activity of the serum thymic factor, *Proc. Natl. Acad. Sci. U.S.A.* **79:**5370–5373.

Dardenne, M. Savino, W., Gastinel, L. N., Nabarra, B., and Bach, J. F., 1983, Thymic dysfunction in the mutant diabetic (*db/db*) mouse, *J. Immunol.* **130**(3)**:**1195–1199.

Duclos, M., Zeidler, H., Liman, W., Pichler, W. J., Rieber, P., and Peter, H. H., 1982, Characterization of blood and synovial fluid lymphocytes from patients with rheumatoid arthritis and other joint diseases by monoclonal antibodies (OKT series) and acid alpha-naphtyl esterase staining, *Rheumatol. Int.* **2:**75–82.

Fabris, N., 1980, Serum thymic factor determination in different human pathologies, *Int. J. Immunopharmacol* **2**:157–160.

Faure, G., Bach, M. A., Bene, M. C., Kahn, M. F., Bach, J. F., and Gaucher, A., 1982, Etude des sous-populations lymphocytaires T au cours des rheumatismes inflammatoires chroniques, *Rev. Rhum.* **49**:439–445.

Faure, G., Bene, M. C., Tamisier, J. N., Gaucher, A., and Duheille, J., 1984, Thymulin (FTS-Zn) induced *in vitro* modulation of T cell subsets markers on lymphocytes from rheumatoid arthritis and systemic lupus erythematosus patients, *Int. J. Immunopharmacol.* **6**:381–388.

Garaci, E., Ronchetti, R., Del Gobbio, V., Tramutoti, G., Rinaldi-Garaci, C., and Imperato, C., 1978, Decreased serum thymic activity in asthmatic children, *J. Allergy Clin. Immunol.* **62**:357–362.

Gastinel, L. N., Dardenne, M., Pleau, J. M., and Bach, J. F., 1984, Studies on the zinc binding to the serum thymic factor, *Biochim. Biophys. Acta.* **797**:147–155.

Goldstein, A. L., Guha, A., Zatz, M. M., Hardy, A., and White, A., 1972, Purification and biological activity of thymosin, a hormone of the thymus gland, *Proc. Natl. Acad. Sci. U.S.A.* **69**:1800–1804.

Goldstein, A. L., Low, T. L. K., McAdoo, M., McLure, J., Thurman, G. B., Rossio, J. J., Lai, C. Y., Chang, D., Wang, S. S., Harvey, C., Ramel, A. H., and Meienhoffer, J., 1977, Thymosin α1: Isolation and sequence analysis of an immunologically active thymic polypeptide, *Proc. Natl. Acad. Sci. U.S.A.* **74**:725–729.

Goldstein, G., 1974, Isolation of bovine thymin: A polypeptide hormone of the thymus, *Nature,* **247**:11–14.

Goldstein, G., 1975, The isolation of thymopoietin (thymin), *Ann. N.Y. Acad. Sci.* **249**:177–183.

Goldstein, G., 1976, Radioimmunoassay for thymopoietin, *J. Immunol.* **117**:690–692.

Goldstein, G., and Lau, C., 1980, Thymopoietin and immunoregulation, in: *Polypeptide Hormones* (R. F. Beers, Jr., and E. G. Bassett, eds.), Raven Press, New York, pp. 459–465.

Goldstein, G., Scheid, M. P., Boyse, E. A., Schlesinger, D. H., and Van Vauwe, J., 1979, A synthetic pentapeptide with biological activity characteristic of the thymic hormone thymopoietin, *Science* **204**:1309–1310.

Gualde, N., Rigaud, M., and Bach, J. F., 1982, Stimulation of prostaglandin synthesis by the serum factor (FTS), *Cell Immunol.* **70**:363–366.

Hirokawa, K., McClure, J. E., and Goldstein, A. L., (1982) Age related changes in localization of thymosin in the human thymus, *Thymus* **4**:19–29.

Israel-Biet, D., Noël, L. H., Bach, M. A., Dardenne, M., and Bach, J. F., 1983, Reversal of the autoimmune disease of (NZB × NZW) F_1 mice by cyclosporin A and thymulin (FTS-Zn), Clin. Exp. Immunol. **54**:359–365.

Iwata, T., Incefy, G. S., Good, R. A., Cunningham-Rundles, S., Dardenne, M., Kapoor, N., Kirkpatrick, D., and O'Reilly, R. J., 1983, Circulating thymic hormone levels in severe combined immunodeficiency, *Clin. Exp. Immunol.* **53**:1–9.

Jambon, B., Montagne, P., Bene, M. C., Brayes, M. P., Faure, G., and Duheille, J., 1981, Immunohistologic localization of "facteur thymique sérique (FTS)" in human thymic epithelium, *J. Immunol.* **127**:2055–2059.

Laghi-Pasini, F., Auteri, A., Pasqui, A. L., and Di Petro, T., 1980, Immunokinetics of a single dose of thymopoietin pentapeptide, *Int. J. Immunopharmacol.* **2/3**:154–155.

Low, T. L. K., Thurman, G. B., Chincarini, C., McClure, J. E., Marshall, G. D., Hu, S. K., and Goldstein, A. L., 1979, Current status of thymosin research: Evidence for the existence of a family of thymic factors that control T-cell maturation, *Ann. N.Y. Acad. Sci.* **332**:33.

McLure, J. E., Lameris, N., Wara, D. W., and Goldstein, A. L., 1981, Immunochemical studies on thymosin: Radioimmunoassay of thymosin α1, *J. Immunol.* **128**:368–375.

Monier, J. C., Dardenne, M., Pleau, J. M., Schmitt, D., Deschaux, P., and Bach, J. F., 1980, Characterization of the facteur thymique sérique (FTS) in the thymus. I. Fixation of anti-FTS antibodies on thymic reticulo-epithelial cells, *Clin. Exp. Immunol.* **42**:470–476.

Moutsopoulos, H., Fye, K. H., Sawada, S., Becker, M. J., Goldstein, A., and Talal, N., 1976, *In vitro* effect of thymosin on T-lymphocyte rosette formation in rheumatic diseases, *Clin. Exp. Immunol.* **26**:563–573.

Osheroff, P. L., 1981, The effect of thymosin on glucocorticoid receptors in lymphoid cells, *Cell. Immunol.* **60**:376.

Pfreudschuh, M., Michel, H., Parino, G., Stock, C., Gause, A., and Hunstein, W., 1981, T-lymphocyte subpopulations in rheumatoid arthritis. II. Definition by monoclonal antibodies, *Z. Rheumatol.* **40**:245–249.

Pleau, J. M., Dardenne, M., Blouquit, Y., and Bach, J. F., 1977, Structural study of circulating thymic factor: A peptide isolated from pig serum. II. Amino acid sequence, J. Biol. Chem. **252**:8045–8047.

Pleau, J. M., Pasques, D., Bach, J. F., Gros, E., and Dray, F., 1978, Dosage radioimmunologique du facteur thymique sérique (FTS), in: *Radioimmunoassay and Related Procedures in Medicine,* Vol. II. International Atomic Energy Agency, Vienna. pp. 505–510.

Pleau, J. M., Dardenne, M., Blanot, D., Bricas, I., and Bach, J. F., 1979, Antagonistic analogue of serum thymic factor (FTS) interacting with the FTS cellular receptor, *Immunol. Lett.* **1**:179–182.

Pleau, J. M., Fuentes, V., Morgat, J. L., and Bach, J. F., 1980, Specific receptors for the serum thymic factor (FTS) in lymphoblastoid cultured cell lines. *Proc. Natl. Acad. Sci. U.S.A.* **77**:2861–2865.

Rinaldi-Garaci, C., Garaci, E., DelGobbo, V., Favalli, C., Jezzi, T., and Goldstein, A. L., 1983, Modulation of endogenous prostaglandins by thymosin α1 in lymphocytes, *Cell. Immunol.* **80**:57–65.

Savino, W., Dardenne, M., Papiernik, M., and Bach, J. F., 1982, Thymic hormone containing cells, characterization and localization of serum thymic factor in young mouse thymus studied by monoclonal antibodies, *J. Exp. Med.* **156**:628–634.

Savino, W., Dardenne, M., and Bach, J. F., 1983a, Thymic hormone containing cells II. Evolution of cells containing the serum thymic factor (FTS or thymulin) in normal and autoimmune mice, as revealed by anti-FTS monoclonal antibodies. Relationship with Ia bearing cells, *Clin. Exp. Immunol.* **52**:1–6.

Savino, W., Dardenne, M., and Bach, J. F., 1983b, Thymic hormone containing cells. III. Evidence for a feed-back regulation of the secretion of the serum thymic factor (FTS) by thymic epithelial cells, *Clin. Exp. Immunol.* **52**:7–12.

Schlesinger, D. H., and Goldstein, G., 1975, The amino acid sequence of thymopoietin II, *Cell* **5**:361–366.

Schmitt, D., Monier, J. C., Dardenne, M., Pleau, J. M., and Bach, J. F., 1982, Location of FTS (facteur thymique sérique) in the thymus of normal and autoimmune mice, *Thymus* **4**:221–231.

Thrower, P. A., Doyle, D. V., Scott, J., and Huskisson, E. C., 1982, Thymopoietin in rheumatoid arthritis, *Rheum. Rehabil.* **21**:72–77.

Thurman, G. B., Rossio, J. L., and Goldstein, A. L., 1977, Thymosin-induced enhancement of MIF production by peripheral blood lymphocytes of thymectomized guinea pigs, in: *Regulatory Mechanisms in Lymphocyte Activation* (D. O. Lucas, ed.), Academic Press, New York, pp. 629–631.

Trainin, N., and Small, M., 1970, Studies on some physicochemical properties of a thymus humoral factor conferring immunocompetence on lymphoid cells, *J. Exp. Med.* **132**:885–889.

Twomey, J. J., Goldstein, G., Lewis, V. M., Bealmear, P. M., and Good, R. A., 1977, Biossay determinations of thymopoietin and thymic hormone levels in human plasma, *Proc. Natl. Acad. Sci. U.S.A.* **74**:2541.

Veys, E. M., Hermans, P., Goldstein, G., Kung, P. C., Schlinder, J., and Van Wauwe, J., 1981, Determination of T lymphocyte subpopulations by monoclonal antibodies in rheumatoid arthritis. Influence of immunomodulating agents, *Int. J. Immunopharmacol.* **3**:312–319.

Veys, E. M., Hermans, P., Schindler, J., Kung, P. C., Goldstein, G., Symoens, J., and Van Wauwe, J., 1982a, Evaluation of T cell subsets with monoclonal antibodies in patients with rheumatoid arthritis, *J. Rheumatol.* **9**:25–29.

Veys, E. M., Huskisson, E. C., Rosenthal, M., Vischer, T. L., Mielants, H., Thrower, P. A., Scott, J., Ott, H., Scheijgrond, H., and Symoens, J., 1982b, Clinical response to therapy with thymopoietin pentapeptide (TP-5) in rheumatoid arthritis, *Ann. Rheum. Dis.* **41**:441–443.

Wetzel, R., Heyweker, H. L., Goeddel, D. V., Jhurani, P., Shapiro, J., Crea, R., Low, T. L. K., McClure, J. E., Thurman, G. B., and Goldstein, A. L., 1980, Production of biologically active N alpha desacetyl thymosin α1 in *Escherichia coli* through expression of a chemically synthesized gene, *J. Biol. Chem.* **19**:6096–6104.

28

Plasmapheresis

J. R. Kalden

I. INTRODUCTION

The idea of plasmapheresis was introduced in 1914 by Abel *et al.* in an account of their attempt to develop an artificial kidney. In 1944, Co Tui *et al.* used this technique for the preparation of blood plasma. Skoog and Adams (1959) and Solomon and Fahey (1963) successfully applied plasma exchange in patients with Waldenström's macroglobulinemia, demonstrating a striking improvement of symptoms of hyperviscosity and a reduction in macroglobulin serum level.

With the replacement of the conventional multibag procedure by highly efficient separation and filtration techniques capable of separating plasma from cellular elements and different cellular elements from one another, the therapeutic application of plasmapheresis increased dramatically from year to year starting in the mid-1970s. Besides plasma exchange (plasmapheresis and plasmaperfusion), therapeutic apheresis (the Greek term *apharesis* refers to "removal") now also includes the separation of different cellular components from the circulation.

Plasma exchange will be most effective in situations in which a circulating agent (i.e., a toxin) is no longer being produced by or introduced into the body. However, in autoimmune and chronic inflammatory diseases with a continuous formation of autoaggressive antibodies and/or autoaggressive cellular components, the beneficial effect of plasmapheresis depends on the duration of the disease tending to produce possible irreversible damage of the target organ by the autoimmune process and on the rate of antibody synthesis possibly followed by immune complex formation. Plasmapheresis is not capable of reversing already established damage of target organs. Factors such as antibody synthesis and immune complex formation are especially of importance with regard to the number of therapeutic plasmaphereses performed and to the concomitant drug regimens.

J. R. Kalden • Institut und Poliklinik Für Klinische Immunologie, und Rheumatologie der Universität Erlangen-Nürnberg, D-8520 Erlangen, Federal Republic of Germany.

Although the number of therapeutic plasmaphereses increased significantly within recent years, some rather important questions are still open. These include the nonselectiveness and lack of specificity existing with regard to tissue-offending agents, the exact mode of action of plasmapheresis, the question of exchange media, ethical considerations with the introduction of control groups of sham-treated patients, and, finally, the problem of the cost-to-benefit ratio.

In the present chapter, some of the theoretical aspects of plasmapheresis are summarized, followed by a discussion of the current status of therapeutic plasmapheresis in systemic lupus erythematosus, rheumatoid arthritis, polymyositis, and progressive systemic sclerosis.

II. THEORETICAL ASPECTS OF PLASMAPHERESIS

A. Plasma Exchange Techniques

The principal types of plasma-cell separators, the continuous-flow system (e.g., IBM Aminco) and the semicontinuous system (e.g., Haemonetics), are both adapted for plasma separation. The disadvantages of the continuous flow system (high costs and complicated reassembly of the reusable centrifuge bowl) and of the semicontinuous system (fluctuating hematocrit, especially in patients with a low hemoglobin) have now been eliminated. Centrifugal plasma separation is usually performed by connecting the patient to a separator by two venipunctures. Anticoagulants are introduced into the blood extracted from the body before it flows into the centrifuge, where it is separated into plasma and the cellular fractions (for technical details see Calabrese *et al.*, 1980; Borberg, 1981; Hester *et al.*, 1979; Kellog and Hester, 1981).

The development of a technique for plasma separation by membrane filtration has given a further boost to its clinical application (Castino *et al.*, 1976, 1981; Gurland *et al.*, 1981, 1983; Solomon *et al.*, 1978; Sieberth and Glöckner, 1981). With regard to efficacy in removing serum constituents, centrifugal plasma separation and plasmapheresis by membrane filtration have been reported to be comparable (Gurland *et al.*, 1981). However, filtration efficiency remains to be optimized, and the possible activating effect on the complement system has to be carefully studied (Sieberth and Glöckner, 1981). Plasma membrane filtration usually needs a high bood flow (80 ml/min), which in general requires access to the central vein (Gurland *et al.*, 1981). In our own experience, the use of a jugularis catheter (Shaldon catheter) has proven to be most suitable. By applying a special steering system, both centrifugal plasma separation and plasma membrane filtration can now be performed by a single-needle technique using only one venous puncture. In certain acute fulminating disease situations, an arterial–venous shunt seems to be necessary. Although this method provides excellent blood flow and is well tolerated by the patients, shunts are a potent site for infection in immune-suppressed patients. As with the centrifugal devices, anticoagulants in the membrane filtration system (usually heparin with an initial dose of 3000 units followed by 1000 units/hr) are introduced into the tube after the blood has left the patient. A scheme of the plasma separation technique is illustrated in Fig. 1.

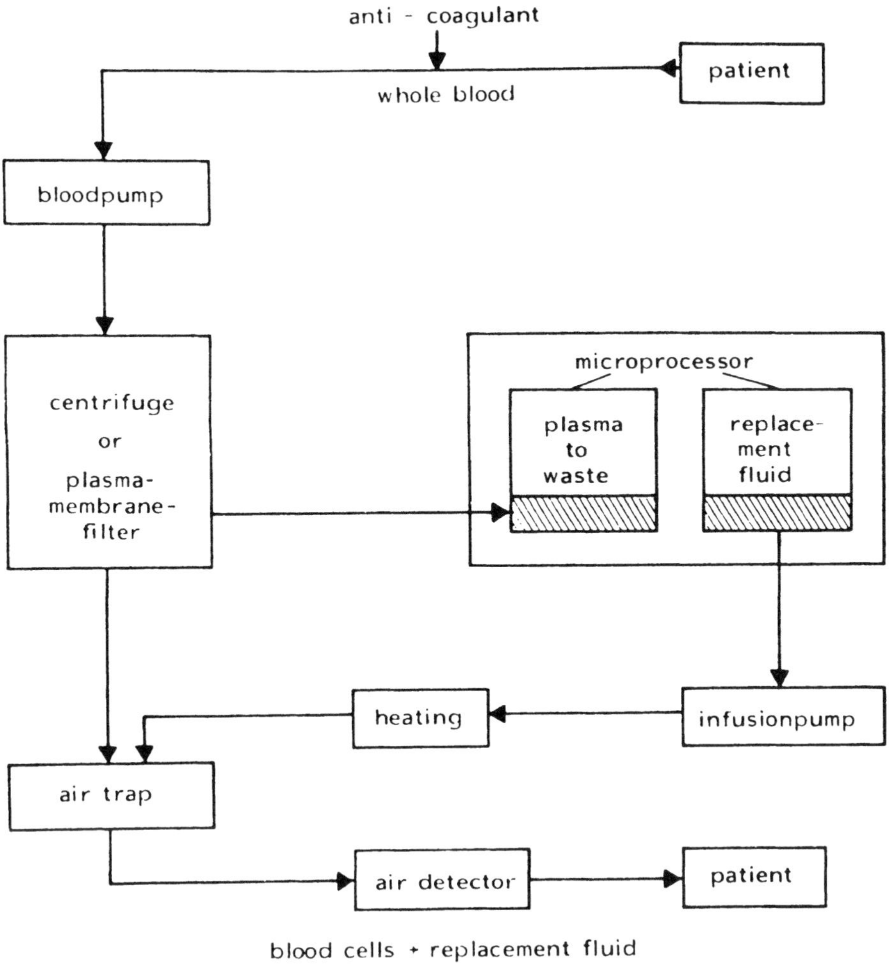

Figure 1. A scheme of plasma separation techniques using either cell centrifugation or plasma membrane filtration. By applying an additional special steering system, both plasma separation procedures can now be performed by single-needle technique using only one venous puncture.

B. Plasma Substitution

Therapeutic plasmapheresis with a separated plasma volume of more than 500 ml requires an isovolumetric substitution. In addition to the restoration of plasma volume and oncotic pressure, secondary factors such as clotting factors, immunoglobulins, complement components, and other serum proteins have to be considered.

Three types of replacement fluid are presently available. Human serum albumin, a 5% or 2.5% isotonic solution, rapidly restores volume and pressure while avoiding the additional risk of hepatitis (Borberg, 1981; Gurland and Samtleben, 1983; Seiler *et al.*, 1981). However, using albumin, one has to be aware of the lack of coagulating factors and globulins. Studies on the effect of albumin on normal serum constituents in plasmapheresed patients (Flaum *et al.*, 1979; Orlin and Berkman, 1980; Miller and Nussenzweig, 1975) demonstrate a prolongation of prothrombin time associated with a reduction in fibrinogen, clotting factors, and platelet counts as well as a significant decrease in plasma levels of various hormones. With the exception of fibrinogen, the serum complement component C3, and the immunoglobulins IgG and IgM, all other plasma constituents recover within 48 hr. Plasma protein fraction (PPF) containing a prekallikrein activator with vasodilatator properties might lead to hypotension.

Fresh frozen plasma (FFP) represents the most physiological replacement fluid containing clotting factors, immunoglobulins, complement components, and other serum proteins. The substitution with complement components may additionally increase the solubilization of tissue-fixed immune complexes (Miller and Nussenzweig, 1975). However, FFP carries the risk of transferring infectious diseases such as hepatitis B, non-A, non-B hepatitis, cytomegalovirus infections, etc. Furthermore, sensitization to serum proteins and to HLA antigens derived from damaged blood cells cannot be completely excluded.

Finally, a standardized, stabilized plasma preserve can be applied, containing albumin and immunoglobulins in physiological concentrations but only minute amounts of complement components and clotting factors. The rapid replacement of immunoglobulins, especially when purified immunoglobulin preparations are used, may additionally exert a nonspecific suppressive effect on a possible plasmapheresis-induced antibody feedback mechanism (Kalden *et al.*, 1982; Taylor, 1982).

In our hands, a combination of 2.5% albumin solution and a standardized stabilized plasma preserve have proven to be most effective as a replacement fluid during plasmapheresis. In certain situations (e.g., in systemic lupus erythematosus and certain forms of nephritis associated with hypocomplementemia) FFP may be valuable if given at the end of a plasma exchange in order to restore clotting factors and complement components.

C. Volume and Frequency

The intensity and frequency of plasma exchange are in part dependent on the severity of the disease, the pathogenic mechanisms involved, and the desired therapeutic effect. An exchange of the total plasma volume removes approximately 60 to 70% of a substance confined to the circulation (Calabrese *et al.*, 1980; Borberg, 1981; Gurland *et al.*, 1981). By extending the exchanges, no further significant effect on the removal of an intravascular component can be achieved. This is exemplified by a study by Calabrese *et al.* (1980) demonstrating that the removal of 2 liters of plasma from an individual with a plasma volume of 3 liters will remove approximately 50% of the intravascular component, and extension of the exchanged volume to 4 liters will eliminate only a further 5%. Based on these findings, many centers now apply therapeutic plasmapheresis two to three times a week over a total period of 14 days, exchanging 2 to 3 liters each time (Calabrese *et al.*, 1980; Borberg, 1981; Gurland *et al.*, 1981; Kalden *et al.*, 1982; Pinching, 1980; Vogler, 1983).

The determination of the frequency of plasmapheresis is also dependent on the distribution of plasma proteins in the extra- and intravascular compartments and on the resynthetic rate of plasma proteins following plasma exchange. Both reactions will also be influenced by the applied replacement fluid. Short-term effects of plasmapheresis result mainly from the ratio of the redistribution and diffusion of plasmaproteins between the extra- and intravascular compartments, which might be altered in certain disease states such as vasculitis syndromes, including SLE.

With regard to immunoglobulins, in the absence of a systemic inflammation, IgG molecules reequilibrate with a half-life of 24 to 48 hr between the extra- and intravascular space, which is dependent on the fact that only 45 to 52% of the IgG immunoglobulins are present in the intravascular compartment. A similar half-life can be expected for the redistribution of the IgA molecules. However, since 70 to 74% of the IgM immunoglobulin is contained in the intravascular compartment, plasmapheresis is most effective in eliminating this antibody class. The third complement component (C3) is distributed between extra- and intravascular compartments in a ratio of 1 : 3 (Charlesworth *et al.*, 1974). However, whether the extravascular C3 component is readily available for redistribution or the reequilibration of the C3 component occurs by rapid resynthesis following plasma exchange is still an open question (Lockwood *et al.*, 1979a,b). This problem of differentiating whether the reequilibration of plasma proteins occurs by redistribution or rapidly occurring resynthesis also applies to many other serum proteins.

Long-term effects of plasma exchange are additionally dependent on the rate of resynthesis of plasma proteins, especially autoantibodies. With regard to plasma proteins, a consistent hypoalbuminemia, which increases the synthesis of lipoproteins (Roseman *et al.*, 1956), could also stimulate the synthesis of acute-phase reactants (Pinching, 1980).

From earlier animal studies (Bystryn *et al.*, 1971), it was concluded that the synthesis of specific antibodies depends, at least in part, on the level of serum antibody. Depletion of circulating antibody led to an increased antibody synthesis. On the other hand, more recent animal experiments by Hall *et al.* (1977), Klaus (1978), and Taylor (1982) suggest that specific antibody synthesis needs the presence of antibody in circulation. If feedback mechanisms act on antibody resynthesis following therapeutic plasma exchange, in the first case concomitant immunosuppressive therapy would be of utmost importance, especially in diseases with autoaggressive autoantibody formations, whereas in the second situation, plasma exchange alone might be sufficient to suppress antibody resynthesis. In spite of the increasing number of therapeutic plasma exchanges, the real effect of plasmapheresis on the rate of antibody synthesis is still unknown, which is also true for the effect on the antiidiotype network of immunoregulation. The fact, however, is that approximately 50% of plasmapheresed SLE patients without concomitant immunosuppressive therapy exhibited evidence of an antibody rebound phenomenon with severe clinical deterioration in some (Jones, 1982a,b). A similar observation that was also made in patients with Goodpasture's syndrome undergoing plasmapheresis therapy (Swanson *et al.*, 1978) is suggestive of a stimulating effect of plasma exchange on the resynthesis of antibodies.

With regard to the effect of plasmapheresis on the assembly of immune complexes, plasma exchange might, apart from the removal of preformed antigen–antibody complexes, influence the relationship between free antigen and free antibody, and, therefore, the physicochemical nature of immune complexes might be changed.

D. Side Effects of Plasmapheresis

Hazards of plasma exchange are related to (1) vascular problems; (2) adverse reactions during; and (3) complications following plasmapheresis therapy.

Plasmapheresis via a central venous catheter may rarely be complicated by the perforation of the blood vessel, a pneumothorax, or a venous thrombosis (Sutton *et al.*, 1981). Arteriovenous shunts can be a source of infections, especially in immunosuppressed individuals. Adverse reactions during plasmapheresis are almost entirely caused by the materials and methods employed rather than by the process of plasma exchange itself. Most of the complications observed can be attributed to the replacement fluid used. Side reactions that range from 4 to 24% in different centers are demonstated in Table 1. Hypocalcemia will occur especially in patients receiving citrate as anticoagulant, and FFP as replacement fluid can be substituted with calcium. Allergic reactions, which may manifest when FFP is used as a replacement fluid, can also rarely be encountered in patients substituted with albumin because of the presence of microaggregates and prekallikrein activators. Cardiologic problems such as tachycardia and extrasystole have been reported in 2.6% of patients, probably caused by changes in the concentrations of plasma electrolytes (Sutton *et al.*, 1981). Thus far, three fatal complications during plasmapheresis have been reported: in two of the patients, death was attributed to the development of pulmonary edema (Aufeuvre *et al.*, 1980); one patient died of cardiac arrest of unknown origin (Sutton *et al.*, 1981). Other complications following plasmapheresis are partly to be explained by low serum level of antithrombin III following plasmapheresis, which carries a higher risk of thrombosis.

The known side effects that may occur during plasmapheresis therapy clearly indicate that this procedure cannot be regarded as a routine therapeutic approach, and, furthermore, patients undergoing this type of treatment have to be monitored carefully with regard to the heart situation as well as major changes in plasma factors such as clotting factors and electrolytes.

III. PLASMAPHERESIS IN RHEUMATIC DISEASES

A. General Considerations

Rheumatic disorders in which plasma exchange has been applied are listed in Table 2. Mechanisms that are postulated to be responsible for a successful therapeutic plasma-

Table 1. Incidence (%) of Side Effects during Therapeutic Plasma Exchange

Investigators	Number of plasmaphereses	Hypotension	Allergic reactions	Fever	Hypocalcemia	Heart problems
Aufeuvre *et al.* (1980)	3431	—	—	5.3	—	—
Fabre *et al.* (1980)	616	0.5	12	0.7	9	—
Samtleben *et al.* (1980)	120	4.2	8.3	—	5	—
Borberg (1981)	205	1.5	—	9.8	1.5	—
Sutton *et al.* (1981)	887	6.5	—	3.2	—	2.6
Tindall *et al.* (1982)	130	8.5	1.5	—	—	—
Own observations	161	2.4	1.8	3.1	—	—

Table 2. Rheumatic Diseases in Which Plasma Exchange Has Been Used

I. Disorders successfully treated by plasma exchange
   A. Systemic lupus erythematosus
   B. Non-SLE immune-complex vasculitis
   C. Rheumatoid arthritis with vasculitis (lymphoplasmapheresis)
   D. Wegener's granulomatosis
   E. Mixed cryoglobulinemia
II. Disorders in which benefit following plasma exchange is uncertain
   A. Rheumatoid arthritis without vasculitis
   B. Polymyositis
   C. Systemic progressive sclerosis
   D. Panarteritis
   E. Mixed connective tissue disease

pheresis, especially in SLE but also in other rheumatic diseases that benefit from plasma separation, are summarized in Table 3.

1. Removal of Noxious Autoantibodies

The role that autoantibodies play in the pathogenesis of some of the clinical manifestations of SLE has been firmly established. Thus, anti-DNA antibodies have been identified as the major antibody–antigen complex found in the glomeruli of patients with diffuse renal involvement (Koffler *et al.*, 1974). With regard to complex deposition in the glomeruli, evidence has been obtained that in the membranous form of nephritis immune complexes are formed *in situ* (Couser and Salant, 1980; Tung *et al.*, 1981) because of the affinity of DNA for the glomerular basement membrane (Izui *et al.*, 1976). In contrast, in diffuse proliferative glomerulonephritis, immune complexes formed in the circulation are deposited in the kidney (Jarrett *et al.*, 1981; Lloyd and Schur, 1981). The repeated removal of the DNA antibody in an acute disease situation will, therefore, most likely affect the reassembly of DNA–anti-DNA immune complexes systemically or locally provided that stimulated DNA antibody synthesis following plasmapheresis is prevented.

Bluestein *et al.* (1981) recently published evidence for the pathogenic role of brain reactive antibodies in CNS disease in SLE patients. Although the authors also speculated on local antibody synthesis and immune complex formation, the removal of the brain reactive antibodies by plasmapheresis may at least partly explain the beneficial effect of this treatment regimen in patients with the organic brain syndrome.

Table 3. Postulated Effects of Therapeutic Plasmapheresis in Rheumatic Diseases

1. Removal of noxious autoantibodies (e.g., SLE: autoantibodies against ds-DNA, brain, T-suppressor lymphocytes)
2. Removal of circulating immune complexes (e.g., SLE, RA, non-SLE immune-complex vasculitis)
3. Increase in RES clearance (e.g., SLE, non-SLE immune-complex vasculitis, RA)
4. Modification of immunoregulation

2. Removal of Circulating Immune Complexes

The detection of circulating immune complexes in the vast majority of SLE patients, as demonstrated mainly by C1q binding or the Raji-cell assay (Lambert *et al.*, 1978; Krapf *et al.*, 1982), has added further evidence for their role in the generation of tissue injury in SLE. However, with regard to the detection of serum immune complexes, it has to be considered that circulating immune complexes might differ from the injurious complexes deposited in the tissue. Thus, Winfield *et al.* (1977) reported that DNA antibodies eluted from the kidneys of SLE patients were of high avidity in contrast to low-avidity serum anti-DNA antibodies found in NZB/W mice, as shown by Steward *et al.* (1978). Furthermore, as demonstrated in our thus far unpublished experiments, besides C1q-binding circulating immune complexes, sera of SLE patients also contain IgE-containing immune complexes or other complexes that are not detected by the C1q binding assay or other test systems that are based on the interaction with the C1q complement component. Immune complexes containing IgE have been clearly shown to be involved in the pathogenesis of various vasculitis syndromes such as the Churg–Strauss vasculitis (Krapf *et al.*, 1983). Although circulating immune complexes may well be directly responsible for tissue injury in some clinical situations, they can merely reflect an active state of disease rather than taking part in tissue destructive mechanism. In the latter situation, plasma exchange will obviously be less or not effective.

3. Increase in RES Clearance

Tissue fixation of immune complexes is determined not only by the rate of formation but also by the rate of clearance from the circulation by the reticuloendothelial system (Barcelli *et al.*, 1981; Haakenstad and Mannik, 1974). With regard to the RES clearance function, patients with active systemic lupus erythematosus were shown to have a decreased Fc-receptor-mediated clearance of autologous IgG-coated erythrocytes (Frank *et al.*, 1979a; Hamburger *et al.*, 1982) that was correlated to serum levels of immune complexes as measured by the C1q binding assay and to disease activity. As the disease improved and levels of immune complexes fell, RES function tended to return to normal (Parris *et al.*, 1981). Likewise, as in patients with nephritis and/or vasculitis (Lockwood *et al.*, 1979a,b), the impaired Fc-mediated clearance function also rapidly improved in SLE patients following therapeutic plasmapheresis (Hamburger *et al.*, 1981a). In contrast, however, Kabbash *et al.* (1982) did not find an overall defect of Fc receptor clearance function in SLE with the exception of a slightly decreased clearance in patients with active lupus nephritis. The beneficial effect of plasmapheresis in some patients suffering from rheumatoid arthritis (Skoog and Adams, 1959; Goldman *et al.*, 1979) has also been claimed to be at least partly attributable to the restoration of a defective RES clearance function (Hamburger *et al.*, 1981b). Obviously, more studies are needed to establish whether the abnormal clearance function in some SLE patients is caused by an overload of the RES by immune complexes, as suggested by a close follow-up study of DNA antibody and immune complex serum levels and C3d activity following plasmapheresis (Fig. 2), or whether other factors, such as drugs, are additionally active. Corticosteroids, for example, are known to effect RES functions in a nonspecific manner both in men and animals (Lahnborg *et al.*, 1979; Gotjamos, 1970), depressing RES receptor clearance function in guinea pigs (Atkinson *et al.*, 1973).

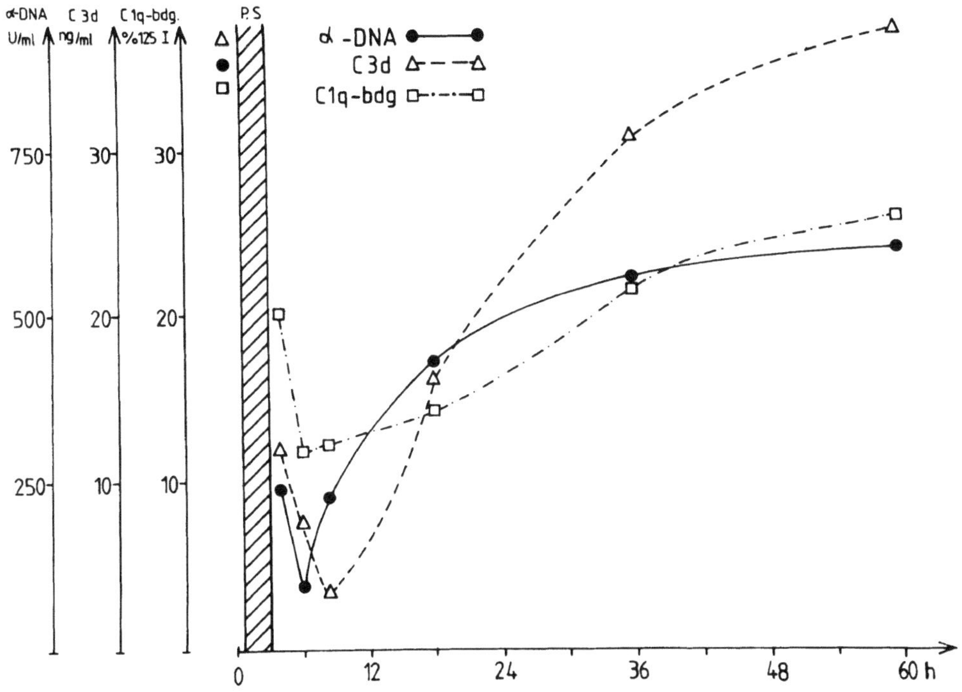

Figure 2. Serum DNA-antibody, immune complex, and C3d serum levels after therapeutic plasmapheresis (exchange volume 2.5 liters) in a patient with SLE. Within the first 6 hr following plasma exchange, the determined serum parameters continued to decrease, indicative of a reassembly of circulating immune complexes and their reuptake by the RES. Sixty hours after plasma exchange, the C3d serum level was equal to that observed before plasmapheresis, whereas DNA antibodies and circulating immune complexes reached only 60% of preplasmapheresis concentrations. (From Krapf *et al.*, 1985.)

It was reported in earlier studies that nonspecific clearance of aggregated human albumin or colloidal lipid, which are thought to be immunologically inert particles (Frank *et al.*, 1979b; Jaffe *et al.*, 1978; Salky *et al.*, 1965), was not different from that in controls. However, our own recent experiments using microaggregated human serum albumin with a size smaller than 80 nm and labeled with 1 mCi ^{99m}Tc also revealed a defective RES clearance function in SLE patients (Löw *et al.*, 1985), which could be correlated to the presence of circulating immune complexes and to clinical activity. This decreased clearance significantly improved after plasmapheresis (Fig. 3).

4. Modification of Immunoregulation

In active SLE, antibodies reactive with suppressor T-lymphocyte populations but also with T-helper cells, B-lymphocytes, and monocytes have been demonstrated (Sakane *et al.*, 1979; Morimoto *et al.*, 1980; Okudaira *et al.*, 1979, 1982). Whether the removal of these antibodies by plasma-exchange therapy interferes with immunoregulatory mechanisms, for example, inducing an improvement of T-suppressor lymphocytes as reported by Abdou *et al.* (1981) in SLE patients, appears doubtful. Studies by Tsokos *et al.* (1982) in SLE patients did not reveal a significant alteration in T-lymphocyte numbers, prolif-

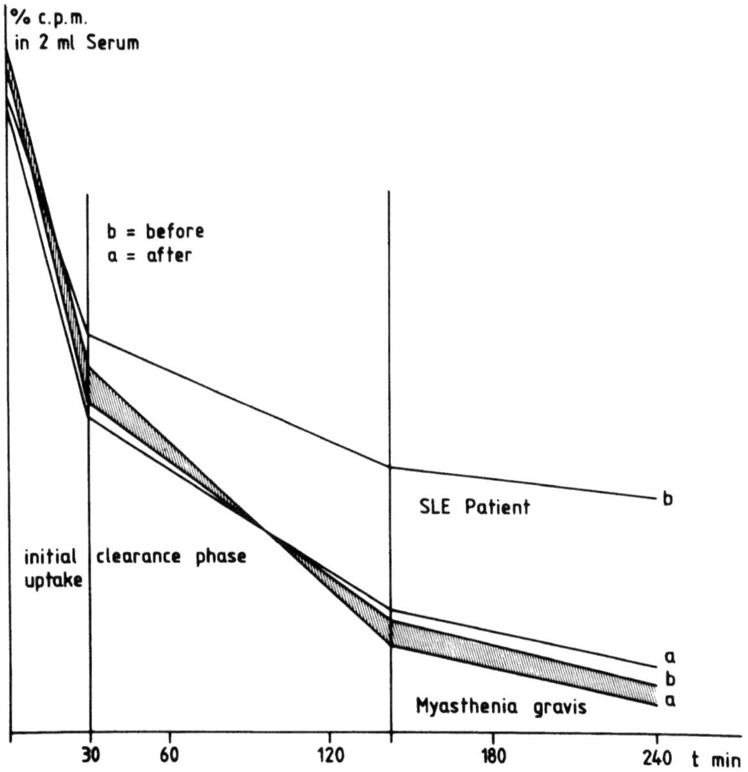

Figure 3. Reticuloendothelial system clearance function in a patient with SLE as compared to a patient with myasthenia gravis using 0.5 mg of a human albumin microcolloid labeled with 1 mCi ^{99m}Tc. Serum activity was measured before and 30, 60, 120, 180, and 240 min following the therapeutic plasma exchange. The clearance rate is given in percent of the serum activity obtained 5 min after the intravenous injection of the labeled microcolloid. In contrast to the patient with myasthenia gravis, the patient suffering from SLE demonstrated a marked increase in clearance rate after plasma exchange. When a series of SLE patients was investigated, the clearance rate of the labeled microcolloid after plasmapheresis correlated with the decrease in serum DNA antibody and immune complex levels (Löw *et al.*, 1985).

erative responses to mitogens or alloantigens, cell-mediated lympholysis, or in spontaneous as well as pokeweed-mitogen-induced *in vitro* immunoglobulin synthesis after plasmapheresis as compared to controls. Similar data were obtained by our group that failed to show a significant effect of plasma exchange on the presence of spontaneous and Con-A-activated suppressor cells in the peripheral blood of SLE patients or in the distribution of different lymphocyte subsets (Tables 4, 5). In similar studies in some patients with severe rheumatoid arthritis, plasmapheresis was followed by an improved phagocytic activity as tested by chemiluminescence (Kayashima *et al.*, 1982).

As in the case of the removal of circulating antibodies, the removal of serum immune complexes may also result in a modification of immune function. Circulating immune complexes might interefere with antibody synthesis (Klaus, 1978). Furthermore, immune complexes are often thought capable of modulating the function of polymorphonuclear leukocytes, different T-lymphocyte subsets, B cells, and macrophages, presumably by

Table 4. Cell Marker Analysis (%) in PBL from SLE Patients Before and After Therapeutic Plasmapheresis

	Pat. P.H.		Pat. H.E.		Pat U.V.		Pat H.C.	
Marker	Before	After	Before	After	Before	After	Before	After
T_3	63	67	59	63	57	60	59	57
T_4	41	40	39	43	34	40	37	39
T_8	22	21	31	31	18	21	31	29
22C6[a]	17	21	17	19	59	19	18	16
S39[b]	19	15	11	12	35	21	9	11
B_1[c]	12	12	7	6	—	—	11	14

[a] Anti-Ia.
[b] Antimonocyte.
[c] Anti-B-cell.

their interaction with Fc membrane receptors. With regard to SLE sera, a considerable amount of work (reviewed by Raveche and Steinberg, 1979) has shown that SLE sera interfere with normal T-lymphocyte proliferative responses to antigens, alloantigens, and mitogens as well as with mitogen-induced T-cell suppressor functions. Since, however, immune complexes in general exhibit an inhibitory effect on Fc-receptor-bearing cells (Williams, 1980), the removal of immune complexes may lead to an improvement of cell function, which, in the case of autoimmune diseases, might not necessarily result in a beneficial effect as has been reported in tumor situations (Bansal *et al.*, 1980).

B. Plasmapheresis in SLE

The first reports of plasmapheresis in SLE patients were those of Jones *et al.* (1976, 1979). In these studies, eight of 14 patients with SLE showed evidence of either clinical improvement or improvement of immunologic parameters during plasma-exchange therapy. Following the original application by Jones *et al.*, a steadily increasing number of reports describing the effect of plasma-exchange therapy in SLE patients have been recorded (Jones, 1982b); these can be divided into three groups according to the therapy regimens that were performed concomitant to the plasma exchange.

Table 5. Concanavalin-A-Activated and Spontaneous Suppressor T-Lymphocyte Activity Before and After Therapeutic Plasmapheresis

		Con-A-activated suppression		Spontaneous suppression	
Patient		Before	After	Before	After
P.H.	PHA	−33%	+25%	−46%	−69%
H.E.	PHA	+19%	−39%	−27%	−67%
U.V.	PHA	+17%	+13%	−87%	+14%
H.C.	PHA	−20%	−57%	+94%	+58%

1. Plasma Exchange Alone

There have been five communications on plasma exchange in a total of 12 SLE patients without concomitant immunosuppressive therapy (Jones *et al.*, 1979, 1981b; Schlansky *et al.*, 1981; Kater *et al.*, 1981; Hamilton *et al.*, 1980). Plasmapheresis was performed over a period of 2 to 8 weeks with a plasma removal volume of 2 to 6 liters per week. Improvement of the clinical situation was recorded in half of the patients with only a brief response that lasted 10 days to 1 month in most of the patients. Studies in some of the plasmapheresed patients established a fall in the serum levels of circulating immune complexes and DNA autoantibodies that was not seen in sham-apheresed patients (Huston *et al.*, 1981). A rebound phenomenon, a severe clinical and immunologic deterioration, was seen in six of the 12 patients within 1 month following therapeutic plasma exchange.

2. Plasmapheresis with Glucocorticosteroids

With regard to a combined therapy of plasmapheresis and different concomitant drug regimens, no control trials have been reported so far, although these appear to be necessary to separate the effect of plasmapheresis from that of various immunosuppressive agents concomitantly used.

Including seven of our own observations, 41 patients with SLE have been treated concomitantly by plasmapheresis and corticosteroids (Lockwood *et al.*, 1979a; Abdou *et al.*, 1981; Jones *et al.*, 1979, 1981b; Kater *et al.*, 1981; Dequeker *et al.*, 1980; Wallace *et al.*, 1980; Wei *et al.*, 1981; Young *et al.*, 1980; Hubbard and Portnoy 1979; Moran *et al.*, 1977; Rossen *et al.*, 1977). Plasma exchange was performed over a period of 2 to 8 weeks with a plasma removal rate of 2 to 10 liters per week. Eighty percent of the patients were reported to have improved clinically or clinically and immunochemically, with a remission period following plasma exchange between 2 months and 2 years. The daily dose of prednisone given ranged between 10 and 200 mg, not exceeding 60 mg per day in most of the studies. All patients responded to plasmapheresis with a fall in serum immune complexes and DNA autoantibody levels. In none of the studies was a rebound phenomenon observed. Figure 4 and Table 6 describe six patients with SLE who underwent plasmapheresis six times over a period of 14 days. In these cases, 2 to 3 liters of plasma were removed three times a week. Concomitant therapy was a high-pulse glucocorticosteroid treatment (1 g/day) administered on the days between the plasma exchanges. All patients included in this group underwent plasmapheresis because of involvement of CNS, heart, lungs, or kidneys refractory to other treatment schedules. With only one exception, a long-lasting (2- to 24-month) remission period was achieved.

3. Plasmapheresis with Glucocorticosteroids Combined with Purine Antagonists or Cytotoxic Drugs

Of a total of 14 patients, eight improved under plasmapheresis combined with glucocorticosteroids and purine antagonists or cytotoxic drugs (Calabrese *et al.*, 1980; Lockwood *et al.*, 1979a; Jones *et al.*, 1979, 1981b; Wallace *et al.*, 1980; Moran *et al.*, 1977; Rossen *et al.*, 1977; Schilderman *et al.*, 1979). The longest remission periods of 18 months (Lockwood *et al.*, 1979a; Schilderman *et al.*, 1979) and 4 years, respectively (Jones *et al.*, 1981b), were seen in patients treated additionally with cyclophosphamide.

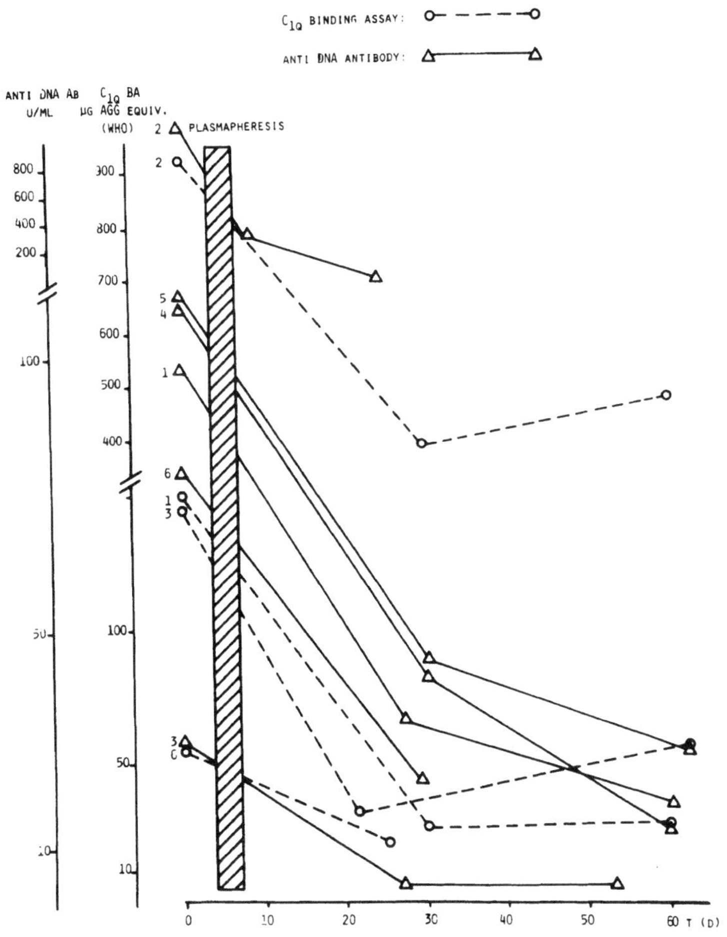

Figure 4. Comparison of the effects of six plasmaphereses (exchange volume 2 to 3 liters each time) on different clinical manifestations, DNA antibody, and immune complex serum levels in six patients with SLE. Over an observation period of 2 months, only one patient with kidney and heart involvement (patient 2), who could not be treated concomitantly with glucocorticosteroids, developed a rebound phenomenon.

The daily dose of cyclophosphamide ranged between 50 and 100 mg. Prednisone was administered in a dose between 10 and 100 mg/day.

To summarize the available data on the effect of plasma exchange on patients with SLE, plasmapheresis alone appears to produce only a transient improvement in disease activity. Moreover, in 50% of patients treated by plasmapheresis alone, a severe clinical and immunochemical deterioration may occur within 4 weeks after plasma exchange. Plasmapheresis with a concomitant prednisone treatment may improve the clinical as well as immunochemical situation in up to 80%, but again the effect is of rather short duration. Best results appear to be possible when plasmapheresis is combined with glucocorticosteroids and cytotoxic drugs such as cyclophosphamide. If purine antagonists are used instead of alkylating agents, the extent and duration of the clinical improvement seem to be rather short and most likely related to the concomitant therapy with glucocorticosteroids.

Table 6. The Effect of Plasmapheresis and Corticosteroid Treatment on the Clinical Course of SLE Patients with Different Clinical Manifestations

Patient	Clinical manifestation	Effect of plasmapheresis
1	Diffuse proliferative nephritis (biopsy proven)	Normalization of serum creatinine, proteinuria, and hematuria
2	Diffuse proliferative nephritis (biopsy proven)	Normalization of serum creatinine, proteinuria, and hematuria
	Perimyocarditis	Significant EKG improvement
3	Factor VIII anticoagulant	Abrogation of bleeding problems, normalization of prothrombin time
4	Pancreatitis	Long-term normalization of serum amylase
5	Organic brain syndrome	Complete recovery
	Pneumonitis	Normalization of lung X ray
6	Pneumonitis	Normalization of lung X-ray

The decision for plasma-exchange therapy should be dependent on the involvement of CNS, heart, lung, kidneys, or severe generalized vasculitis resistant to other therapy regimens. If necessary, a course of six to eight plasmaphereses may be repeated. Therapy should be controlled by clinical and immunochemical parameters such as serum levels of DNA antibodies, serum immune complexes, and complement components. The monitoring of therapeutic plasma exchange by the measurement of serum complexes alone may not be sufficient, since levels of serum complexes do not necessarily correlate with the activity of the disease state (Pary *et al.*, 1981).

With regard to the effect of therapeutic plasma exchange on diseases complicating the clinical course of SLE, a beneficial effect has been reported on thrombocytopenic purpura in a 17-year-old girl (Oen *et al.*, 1980). Similarly, plasma exchange combined with cyclophosphamide induced a long remission period in a girl suffering from SLE with pneumonitis, acute renal failure, and red blood cell hypoplasia (Isbister *et al.*, 1981). Finally, in a young woman who had developed severe SLE during her second pregnancy, a third pregnancy was well managed by plasmapheresis so that she could give birth to a healthy child (Hubbard and Portnoy, 1979).

In patients with a severe systemic vasculitis including the involvement of visceral organs but without any evidence for systemic lupus erythematosus (e.g., no DNA serum antibodies and no DNA-containing serum immune complexes) plasmapheresis may also be used in a combination with glucocorticosteroids and cytotoxic drugs. Our observations on four patients with a high level of C1q-binding material and the clinical syndrome of a therapy-resistant severe vasculitis indicate that this form of therapy may induce a sustained clinical improvement (Fig. 5).

C. Plasmapheresis in Rheumatoid Arthritis

Rheumatoid arthritis (RA) is characterized by an immunologically mediated inflammation, mainly localized within the synovial tissue. Recent studies on the mononuclear cell infiltration of the inflamed synovium suggest that these mononuclear cells play a critical part in the joint-destructive mechanism (Burmester *et al.*, 1980; Galili *et al.*, 1981; Janossy *et al.*, 1981; Burmester *et al.*, 1983) including the local synthesis of rheumatoid factor (Smiley *et al.*, 1968; Munthe and Natvig, 1972). In addition, 20–30% of RA patients develop symptoms of a systemic vasculitis with the presence of serum rheumatoid factor, immune complexes, nodules, and erosive joint disease (Scott *et al.*, 1981a; Erhardt *et al.*, 1979; Quismorio *et al.*, 1983). Although RA can often take a mild clinical course, it may also develop a progressive and unremitting disease that only poorly responds to conventional therapy. Therefore, attempts were made to look for an alternative therapy regimen. As early as 1963, the first report of plasmapheresis in RA was published (Jaffe, 1963), which was followed in 1976 by the first communication on the effect of extracorporal irradiation of thoracic duct lymphocytes as an immune-suppressive treatment (Edgren *et al.*, 1976). Since then, a number of reports have been published describing the effect of plasmapheresis, lymphapheresis, and lymphoplasmapheresis in rheumatoid arthritis.

Based on the findings by Jaffe (1963) and Edgren *et al.* (1976) indicating the therapeutic efficacy of plasma exchange as well as ductus thoracicus drainage, and based on the hypothesis that rheumatoid arthritis is at least in part an immune complex disease, several groups of investigators began investigations of the role of therapeutic apheresis in rheumatoid arthritis.

1. Plasmapheresis Alone

Plasmapheresis alone has been thought to be of benefit as adjunct therapy in rheumatoid vasculitis (Calabrese *et al.*, 1980; Goldman *et al.*, 1979; Scott *et al.*, 1981b) and in some refractory cases of rheumatoid arthritis (Wallace *et al.*, 1979). In the study by Calabrese *et al.* (1980), a sustained remission was seen in three and a transient beneficial effect in one patient with additional symptoms of vasculitis. Plasmapheresis was followed by a rapid decrease of circulating imune complexes, although a rebound phenomenon was observed in the majority of patients at follow-up examinations. Similar findings were obtained in the study by Goldman *et al.* (1979), who treated with plasmapheresis four patients in whom conventional therapy had been ineffective. Again, in all the patients, a transient clinical improvement was seen in parallel to a rapidly decreasing level of circulating immune complexes. Finally, Scott *et al.* (1981b), applying plasmapheresis to the management of nine patients with rheumatoid vasculitis, reported an arrest of clinical progression in seven of them. Four patients received a relatively short course of 3 to 5 days because of poor venous access. From that, the authors noted that treatment response did not seem to correlate with the extent of plasma exchange.

Kosaka and Salomon (1980) and Baron *et al.* (1982) showed that plasmapheresis was effective in a life-threatening hyperviscosity syndrome complicating RA. Finally, Wallace *et al.* (1982a), summarizing their experience, concluded that ideal patient candidates for plasma exchange are those with life-threatening complications such as cryoglobulinemia, hyperviscosity syndrome, vasculitis, and Felty's syndrome, patients with functional class 3 disease who were seropositive and had failed to respond to conventional drug therapy. In contrast to these findings, Rothwell *et al.* (1980), comparing the effect of plasma-exchange therapy in ten RA patients on conventional therapy with a clinically matched group of ten patients, did not find an additional clinical benefit from plasma exchange. Similarly, in a controlled double-blind crossover trial, Dwosh *et al.* (1983) also failed to show that plasmapheresis was effective in chronic rheumatoid arthritis in spite of impressive laboratory changes. Twenty-six patients with rheumatoid arthritis who were unresponsive to antiinflammatory and slow-acting antirheumatic drugs received ten true and ten sham plasmaphereses. No information is given, however, about whether the patients were additionally suffering from systemic vasculitis. Recently, one report has been published demonstrating a beneficial effect of plasmapheresis on a D-penacillamine-induced thrombotic thrombocytopenic purpura in a RA patient (Trice *et al.*, 1983).

Since rheumatoid arthritis is a disease that is characterized by "spontaneous" phases and remissions, and since there is a good chance to have favorable placebo effects in the treatment (Jones *et al.*, 1981a; Russel *et al.*, 1981), further double-blind control studies with clinically comparable groups of patients seem to be necessary to adequately evaluate the effectiveness of plasmapheresis (Bennett and Hamburger, 1982). The experience obtained up to now shows that phasmapheresis in RA should be limitied to patients with severe extraarticular involvement.

2. *Leukapheresis*

Following reports on the effect of thoracic duct drainage on the clinical course of RA (Edgren *et al.*, 1976; Paulus *et al.*, 1977; Uedo *et al.*, 1979) indicating a significant although transient amelioration of disease activity, leukapheresis was introduced as an alternative in the treatment of RA.

With a continuous cell separator, a 3-hr run yields about 0.9×10^{10} lymphocytes (range 0.5 to 2.0×10^{10}). In three runs per week, 2.7×10^{10} cells will be removed. Since the intravascular lymphocyte count is about 10^{10} cells, it appears obvious that depletion is readily obtained in a short term period (Wright *et al.*, 1981). The number of monocytes removed is in general about 10 to 45% of the number of lymphocytes.

With regard to immunologic parameters, the absolute percentage of T lymphocytes as defined by a rosetting technique appeared to decrease more rapidly than other lymphocyte subpopulations; T-lymphocyte proliferation to mitogens was also found to be decreased after lymphapheresis. Although serum IgM levels dropped, the rheumatoid factor did not change. None of the observed changes that occurred within the first week of treatment correlated with the beneficial effect of lymphapheresis (Karsh *et al.*, 1979). Wilder *et al.* (1982), on the basis of a double-blind study, published evidence that in six out of seven patients with an abnormal response to recall antigens, leukapheresis was followed by a significant increase in lymphocyte proliferation to the applied antigen preparations. This procedure was accompanied by a significant improvement of the clinical situations. In four patients who did not exhibit disturbed lymphocyte activity towards recall antigens before leukapheresis, no significant effect on the clinical course was observed.

In their initial pilot studies, Karsh *et al.* (1979) provided evidence that 40 patients with severe seropositive RA, when treated with leukapheresis for a period of 5 weeks, experienced a rapid decrease in the articular index within the first week of apheresis, with further improvement continuing more slowly over the following 4 to 5 weeks. Although the improvement continued after leukapheresis, the disease suddenly relapsed after a mean of 19 weeks. In a following double-blind randomized (leukapheresis verus sham-apheresis) (Karsh *et al.*, 1979; Wilder *et al.*, 1982) study, leukapheresed patients showed a substantial clincial improvement within the first 7 to 14 days. The control patients improved after 21 to 34 days. The clinical improvement in both groups persisted for a variable period with an average of about 3 months. From a comparison of the two studies (Wilder *et al.*, 1982), it was obvious that the clinical improvement in the open study was greater than the one observed in the double-blind investigation.

To summarize the therapeutic efficiency of leukapheresis in severe rheumatoid arthritis based on the available data, the results suggest that about 50% of randomly selected patients will show a mild to modest improvement and that 10 to 25% of the patients exhibit a substantial improvement with a 40% decrease in articular index. Twenty-five to 40% of the patients will not improve or will show only a minimal improvement with less than 10% change in the articular index. The duration of improvement varies widely with an average of 3 months. Significant side effects are usually uncommon. Because of an unresponsiveness to this treatment in some patients, because of the usually brief period of substantial amelioration following leukapheresis, and because of the considerable costs associated with this procedure, leukapheresis cannot yet be regarded as a therapeutic modality for general application. Further studies seem to be necessary with regard to the modulating effect on the immune system.

3. Lymphoplasmapheresis

Lymphoplasmapheresis applied to RA patients (Wallace *et al.*, 1979, 1982a) also produced a transient but significant beneficial effect on the clinical situation in open studies. Anemia, thrombocytopenia, hypocalcemia, and hypokalemia were the side effects observed. Plasma constituents such as IgG, IgM, IgA, the complement component C3, rheumatoid factor, and circulating immune complexes were reported to decrease by 40 to 80% during the first 3 weeks of therapy. In a recently published double-blind control study in 14 RA patients, Wallace *et al.* (1982b) demonstrated a significantly improved morning stiffness in the plasmapheresed group versus the sham-treated group.

Although synovitis as assessed by the Ritchie index improved in both groups of patients, the improvement was significantly greater in the lymphoplasmapheresed group than in the sham-treated group. A significant fall in serum levels of immune complexes as well as the serum complement component C3 and the immunoglobulins were only noted in the treated group of patients.

From the studies so far available, lymphoplasmapheresis appears to be the most effective apheresis procedure in patients with severe RA.

D. Plasmapheresis in Other Rheumatic Diseases

In an uncontrolled clinical trial, plasmapheresis combined with prednisone and cyclophosphamide was reported to produce a clinical improvement in 14 of 15 scleroderma patients with skin and internal organ involvement (Dau, 1981). All improved patients exhibited relaxation of skin contractures and healing of cutaneous ulcers when present. Gastrointestinal syndromes were ameliorated, and a severe polymyositis was largely reversed in two patients. Antinuclear antibodies declined relatively more than the IgG levels in six of nine patients; in 11 out of 15 patients, a significant reduction in endothelial cell cytotoxic activity was found. Two patients died during the period of study; in the other patients, stabilization in the disease activity was recorded for a period of 2 to 23 months. The mechanism by which this combined treatment was influencing the clinical course of scleroderma is still unknown, and more studies seem to be necessary to prove the possible place of a combination of plasmapheresis with immunosuppressive drug therapy in the management of patients with moderate to severe scleroderma.

In contrast to reports by Dau (1981, 1982) and Dau *et al.* (1981) describing a beneficial effect of plasma exchange on the clinical course of idiopathic polymyositis with a substantial decrease in the serum creatinine phosphate kinase activity, Wallace *et al.* (1982a) found that lymphoplasmapheresis or plasmapheresis alone was not beneficial in dermatomyositis. As in the report by Wallace *et al.*, in our hands, extensive plasmapheresis did not induce an amelioration in the clinical situation of patients with severe polymyositis despite a significant fall in the serum creatinine kinase phosphate. Plasmapheresis was combined with immunosuppressive therapy with glucocorticosteroids and cyclophosphamide. From the data available, plasmapheresis and lymphoplasmapheresis do not seem to provide a valuable adjunctive form of therapy in the management of myositis or dermatositis.

To date, only a few case reports attest to the benefits of therapeutic apheresis in patients with renal involvement of Wegner's granulomatosis and panarteritis nodosa (Lockwood *et al.*, 1979; Kincaid-Smith and d'Apice, 1978). Wallace *et al.* (1982a) reported evidence that a patient suffering from Wegner's disease did benefit from plasmapheresis but not from lymphoplasmapheresis.

In mixed cryoglobulinemia, plasmapheresis was reported to be successful in combination with immunosuppressive therapy that included glucocorticosteroids and cytotoxic drugs (Getner *et al.* 1981; Cloarec *et al.*, 1983).

IV. CONCLUSIONS

Therapeutic plasmapheresis, lymphapheresis, and lymphoplasmapheresis are expensive, time-consuming procedures not without risk. Therefore, the application should be used critically and should mainly be restricted to those circumstances in which effectiveness has been shown before, preferably in controlled trials. Therapeutic plasma exchange, however, can be important in life-threatening complications of acute SLE or severe vasculitis syndromes that do not respond to conventional therapy, including vasculitis associated with rheumatoid arthritis.

With the obvious increasing demand for plasma exchange, it has become necessary to look for less expensive and more specific alternatives (reviewed by Pineda, 1982; Saal and Gordon, 1982). In that respect, for rheumatic disease the application of plasma filtration, filters, or affinity columns coated with immobilized sorbents has already shown promising results. These techniques have the additional advantage of permitting the use of the patient's own plasma as replacement solution, which is more physiological and less costly. Thus, McLeod and Sasseti (1980) reported in patients with cryoglobulinemia therapeutic plasma exchange with the return of cryoglobulin-depleted autologous plasma. Similar results were published by Krakauer *et al.* (1982), who demonstrated that five patients with cryoglobulinemia who were successfully treated with lymphoplasmapheresis similarly responded to selective plasma-exchange therapy. Terman *et al.* (1979) showed that plasmapheresis in a patient with SLE-using a DNA collodium charcoal column—resulted, after the removal of 4000 ml of plasma, in a reduction of immune complexes and in the normalization of serum C3 levels. Matus *et al.* (1983), applying plasmapheresis combined with immunoadsorption using purified *Staph.* portein A and low-prednisone therapy, induced a sustained remission in a dog with SLE. The application of protein A as immunoadsorbent might also be used for the elimination of specific serum antibodies. Thus, Besinger *et al.* (1981) reported a depletion of antibodies to blood groups A and B in a patient undergoing bone marrow transplantation from ABO-incompatible donors. Besa *et al.* (1981) treated patients with chronic lymphocytic leukemia and severe autoimmune hemolytic anemia using a cell separator and protein A. Finally, using a similar device, Nilson *et al.* (1981) removed high titers of factor IX antibodies by an extracorporal protein-A–sepharose adsorption.

In spite of the first successful attempts to specifically remove plasma components, the technical devices have to be improved further, including the development of techniques for the removal of specific cell populations from the circulation. As soon as those techniques become available for clinical application, specific aphereses will have to be studied in controlled double-blind, crossover trials.

ACKNOWLEDGMENTS. The expert editorial help of Mrs. U. Rath and Dr. G. R. Burmester is thankfully acknowledged. Some of the experimental work presented in this chapter was supported by the grant of the Deutsche Forschungsgemeinschaft KA 325-9.

REFERENCES

Abdou, N. J., Lindsley, H. B., Pollock, A., Stechschulte, D. J., and Wood, G., 1981, Plasmapheresis in active systemic lupus erythematosus: Effects on clinical, serum and cellular abnormalities. Case report, *Clin. Immunol. Immunopathol.* **19:**44–54.

Abel, J. J., Rowntree, L. G., and Turner, B. B., 1914, Plasma removal with return of corpuscles (plasmapheresis), *J. Pharmacol. Exp. Ther.* **5:**625–641.

Atkinson, J. P., Schreiber, A. S., and Frank, M. M., 1973, Effects of corticosteroids and splenectomy on the immune clearance and destruction of erythrocytes, *J. Clin. Invest.* **52:**1509–1517.

Aufeuvre, J. P., Morin-Hertel, F., Cohen-Solal, M., Lefloch, A., and Baudelot, J., 1980, Hazards of plasma exchange. A nationwide study of 3431 exchanges in 592 patients, in: *Plasma Exchange* (H. G. Sieberth, ed.), Schattauer, Stuttgart, pp. 149–155.

Bansal, S. C. Bansal, B. R., Thomas, H. L., Siegel, P. D., Rhoads, J. E., Jr., Cooper, D. R., Terman, D. S., and Mark, R., 1980, *Ex vivo* removal of serum IgG in a patient with colon carcinoma: Some biochemical, immunological and histological observations, *Cancer* **42:**1–11.

Barcelli, U., Rademacher, R., Ooi, Y. M., and Oi, B. S., 1981, Modification of glomerular immune complex deposition in mice by activation of the reticuloendothelial system, *J. Clin. Invest.* **67:**20–27.

Baron, M., Fam, A. G., Elkan, I., and Underdown, B., 1982, Hyperviscosity syndrome in rheumatoid arthritis, *J. Rheumatol.* **9:**843–849.

Bennett, R. S., and Hamburger, M. I., 1982, A critical review of therapeutic apheresis in the treatment of severe rheumatoid arthritis, in: *Therapeutic Apheresis and Plasmaperfusion* (R. S. A. Tindall, ed.), Alan R. Liss, New York, pp. 33–48.

Besa, E. C., Ray, P. K., Swami, V. K., Idiculla, A., Rhoads, J. E., Bassett, J. G., Joseph, R. R., and Cooper, D. R., 1981, Specific immunoadsorption of IgG antibody in a patient with chronic lymphocytic leukemia and autoimmune hemolytic anemia: A new form of therapy for the acute critical stage, *Am. J. Med.* **71:**1035–1040.

Besinger, W. I., Baker, D. A., Buckner, C. D., Clift, R. A., and Thomas, E. D., 1981, Immunoadsorption for removal A and B blood group antibodies, *N. Engl. J. Med.* **404**:160–162.

Bluestein, H. G., Williams, G. W., and Steinberg, A. D., 1981, Cerebrospinal fluid antibodies to neuronal cells: Association with neuropsychiatric manifestations of systemic lupus erythematosus, *Am. J. Med.* **70**:240–246.

Borberg, H., 1981, Problems of plasma exchange therapy in: *Therapeutic Plasma Exchange* (H. J. Garland, V. Heinze, and H. A. Lee, eds.), Springer, Berlin, Heidelberg, New York, pp. 191–195.

Burmester, G. R., Yu, D. T. Y., Iranai, A., Kunkel, H. G., and Winchester, R. J., 1981, Ia^+ T cells in synovial fluid and tissues of patients with rheumatoid arthritis, *Arthritis Rheum.* **24**:1370–1376.

Burmester, G. R., Locher, P., Koch, B., Winchester, R. J., Dimitriu-Bona, A., Kalden, J. R., and Mohr, W., 1983, The tissue architecture of synovial membranes in inflammatory and non inflammatory joint diseases. I. The localization of the major cell populations as detected by monoclonal reagents directed towards Ia and monocytes antigens, *Rheum. Int.* **3**:173–181.

Bystryn, J. C., Schenken, J., and Uhr, J. H. W., 1971, A model for regulation of antibody synthesis by serum antibody, in: *Progress in Immunology* (B. Amos, ed.), Academic Press, New York, pp. 630–645.

Calabrese, L. H., Clough, J. D., Krakauer, R. S., and Hoeltge, G. A., 1980, Plasmapheresis therapy of immunologic disease, *Cleve. Clin. Q.* **47**:53–72.

Castino, F., Scheucher, K., Malchesky, P. S., Koshino, I., and Nose, Y., 1976, Microemboli-free blood detoxification utilizing plasma filtration, *Trans. Am. Soc. Artif. Intern. Organs* **22**:637–645.

Castino, F., Friedman, J., Wiltbank, T. B., Daniels, J. R., Grapka, B., and Solomon, B. A., 1981, Plasma separation by membrane filtration, in: *Plasma Exchange Therapy* (H. Borberg, and P. Reuther, eds.), Thieme-Stratton, Stuttgart, New York, pp. 11–19.

Charlesworth, J. A., Gwyn Williams, D., Sherington, E., Lachman, P. J., and Peters, D. K., 1974, Metabolic studies of the third complement component and blue glycine-rich beta glycoprotein in patients with hypocomplementaemia, *J. Clin. Invest.* **53**:1578–1587.

Cloarec, M., Graisely, G., Dumas, R., Caillard, P., Wurm, M., Le Morine, C., Solvay, H., and Kahn, M., 1983, Gangrenes parcellaires distales, *J. Mal. Vasc.* **8**:83–86.

Co Tui, T. C., Bartter, F. C., Wright, A. M., and Holt, R. B., 1944, Red cell reinfusion and the frequency of plasma donations: Preliminary report of multiple donations in eight weeks by each of six donors, *JAMA* **124**:331–339.

Couser, W. G., and Salant, D. J., 1980, *In situ* immune complex formation and glomerular injury, *Kidney Int.* **17**:1–13.

Dau, P. C., 1981, Plasmapheresis in idiopathic inflammatory myopathy: Experience with 35 patients, *Arch. Neurol.* **38**:544–552.

Dau, P. C., 1982, The role of plasma exchange in treatment of idiopathic polymyositis, in: *Therapeutic Apheresis and Plasmaperfusion* (R. S. A. Tindall, ed.), Alan R. Liss, New York, pp. 223–232.

Dau, P. C., Kahalel, M. B., and Sabebiel, W., 1981, Plasmapheresis and immunosuppressive therapy in scleroderma, *Arthritis Rheum.* **24**:1128–1136.

Dequeker, J., Geusens, P., and Wielands, L., 1980, Short- and longterm experience with plasmapheresis in connective tissue diseases, *Biomedicine* **32**:189–194.

Dwosh, I. L., Giles, A. R., Ford, P. M., Pater, J. L., Anastassiades, T. P., and the Queen's University Plasmapheresis Study Group, 1983, Plasmapheresis therapy in rheumatoid arthritis. A controlled double-blind cross over study, *N. Engl. J. Med.* **308**:1124–1129.

Edgren, J., Klockars, M., Weber, T., Anders, W., Lindstrom, B., Streusand, K., Petersson, T., Diska, H., Kajander, A., and Wigelius, O., 1976, Extracorporal irradiation of thoracic duct lymph as immunosuppressive treatment in rheumatoid arthritis, *Scand. J. Rheumatol.* **5**:108–114.

Erhardt, C. C., Mumford, P., and Maini, R. N., 1979, The association of cryoglobulinemia with nodules, vasculitis and fibrosing alveolitis in rheumatoid arthritis and their relationship to serum C1q binding activity and rheumatoid factor, *Clin. Exp. Immunol.* **38**:405–413.

Fabre, M., Andreu, G., and Mannoni, P., 1980, Some biological modifications and clinical hazards observed during plasma exchange, in: *Plasma Exchange* (H. G. Sieberth, ed.), Schattauer, Stuttgart, New York, pp. 143–149.

Flaum, M. A., Cuneo, R. A., Appelbaum, F. R., Deisseroth, A. B., Engel, W. K., and Gralnick, H. R., 1979, The hemostatic imbalance of plasma-exchange transfusion, *Blood* **54**:694–702.

Frank, M. M., Hamburger, M. I., Lawley, T. J., Kimberly, R. P., and Plotz, P. H., 1979a, Defective reticuloendothelial system Fc-receptor function in systemic lupus erythematosus, *N. Engl. J. Med.* **300**:518–523.

Frank, M. M., Hamburger, M. I., Lawley, T. J., Kimberly, R. P., and Plotz, P. H., 1979b, Defective reticuloendothelial system Fc receptor function in systemic lupus erythematosus, *N. Engl. J. Med.* **300**:518.

Galili, A., Rosenthal, L., and Klein, E., 1981, Activated T cells in the synovial fluid of arthritic patients. II. *In vitro* activation of autologous blood lymphocytes, *J. Immunol.* **127**:430–432.

Geltner, D., Kohn, R. W., Gorevic, P., and Franklin, E. C., 1981, The effect of combination therapy (steroids, immunosuppressives and plasmapheresis) on 5 mixed cryoglobulinemia patients with renal, neurologic and vascular involvement, *Arthritis Rheum.* **24**:1121–1127.

Goldman, J. A., Casey, H. L., Mellwain, H., Kirby, J., Wilson, C., Jr., and Miller, S. B., 1979, Limited plasmapheresis in RA with vasculitis, *Arthritis Rheum.* **22**:1146–1150.

Gotjamos, T., 1970, Alterations in reticuloendothelial organ structure and function following cortisone administration in mice, *J. Reticuloendothel. Soc.* **8**:433–439.

Gurland, H. J., and Samtleben, W., 1983, Klinische Einsatzmöglichkeiten und technische Durchführung der Plasmapherese, *Internist* **24**:14–26.

Gurland, H. J., Samtleben, W., Blumenstein, M., Randerson, D. H., and Schmidt, B., 1981, Clinical applications of macromolecular separations, *Trans. Am. Soc. Artif. Intern. Organs* **27**:356–363.

Haakenstad, A. O., and Mannik, M., 1974, Saturation of the reticuloendithelial system with soluble immune complexes, *J. Immunol.* **112**:1939–1948.

Hall, C. L., Colvin, R. B., Carey, K., and McCluskey, R. T., 1977, Passive transfer of autoimmune disease with isologous IgG_1 and IgG_2 antibodies to tubular basement membrane in strain XIII guinea pigs, *J. Exp. Med.* **146**:1246–1260.

Hamburger, M. I., Gerardi, E. H., Fields, J. R., and Bennett, R. S., 1981a, Reticuloendothelial system Fc-receptor function and plasmapheresis in systemic lupus erythematosus: A preliminary report, *Artif. Organs* **5**:264–68.

Hamburger, M. I., Gerardi, E. H., Fields, T. R., Bernstein, M. L., and Bennett, R. S., 1981b, Lymphoplasmapheresis and reticuloendothelial system (RES) Fc-receptor function in rheumatoid arthritis (RA), *Arthritis Rheum.* **24**:98.

Hamburger, M. I., Lawley, T. J., Kimberly, R. P., Plotz, P. H., and Frank, M. M., 1982, A serial study of systemic reticuloendothelial system Fc-receptor functional activity in systemic lupus erythematosus, *Arthritis Rheum.* **25**:48–54.

Hamilton, W. A. P., Vergani, D., Bevis, L. O., Tee, D. E. H., Zilkva, U. J., and Colton, L. T., 1980, Plasma exchange in SLE, *Lancet* **1**:1249.

Hester, J. P., Kellog, R. M., Mulzet, A. P., Krager, V. R., McGredie, K. B., and Freireich, E. J., 1979, Principles of blood separation and component extraction in a disposable continuous flow single-stage channel, *Blood* **54**:254–268.

Hubbard, H. C., and Portnoy, B., 1979, Systemic lupus erythematosus in pregnancy treated with plasmapheresis, *Br. J. Dermatol.* **101**:87–89.

Huston, D. P., Wei, N., Klima, E., Hall, R. P., Lawley, T. J., Kippel, J. H., Balow, J. E., Plotz, P. H., Steinberg, A. D., and Decker, J. L., 1981, Immunochemical effects of plasmapheresis in systemic lupus erythematosus, *Arthritis Rheum.* **24**:892.

Isbister, J. R., Ralston, M., Hayes, J. M., and Wright, R., 1981, Fulminant lupus pneumonitis with acute renal failure and RBC aplasia. Successful management with plasmapheresis and immunosuppression, *Arch. Intern. Med.* **141**:1081–1083.

Izui, S., Lambert, P. H., and Miescher, P. A., 1976, *In vitro* demonstration of a particular affinity of glomerular basement membrane and collagen for DNA. A possible basis for local formation of DNA–anti-DNA complexes in systemic lupus erythematosus, *J. Exp. Med.* **144**:428–443.

Jaffe, C. J., Vierling, J. M., Jones, E. A., Lawley, T. J., and Frank, M. M., 1978, Receptor specific clearance by the reticuloendothelial system in chronic liver diseases: Demonstration of defective C3b-specific clearance in primary biliary cirrhosis, *J. Clin. Invest.* **62**:1069.

Jaffe, I. A., 1963, Comparison of the effect of plasmapheresis and penicillamine on the level of circulating rheumatoid factor, *Ann. Rheum. Dis.* **22**:71–76.

Janossy, G., Duke, D., Poulter, L. W., Panayi, G., Bofill, M., and Goldstein, G., 1981, Rheumatoid arthritis: A disease of T lymphocyte/macrophage immunoregulation, *Lancet* **1**:839–921.

Jarrett, M. P., Sablay, L. B., Walter, L., Barland, P., and Grayzel, A. I., 1981, The effect of continuous normalization of serum hemolytic complement on the course of lupus nephritis. A five year prospective study, *Am. J. Med.* **70**:1067–1072.

Jones, J. V., 1982a, The application of plasmapheresis in systemic lupus erythematosus, in: *Therapeutic Apheresis and Plasmaperfusion* (R. S. A.. Tindall, ed.), Alan R. Liss, New York, pp. 81–89.

Jones, J. V., 1982b, Plasmapheresis in SLE, *Clin. Rheum. Dis.* **8**:243–260.

Jones, J. V., Cumming, R. H., Bucknal, R. C., Asplin, C. M., Fraser, I. D., Bothamley, J., Davis, P., and Hamblin, T. J., 1976, Plasmapheresis in the management of acute systemic lupus erythematosus? *Lancet* **1**:709–711.

Jones, J. V., Cumming, R. H., Bacon, P. A., Evers, J., Fraser, I. D., Bothamley, J., Tribe, C. R., Davis, P. G., and Hughes, G. R. V., 1979, Evidence for a therapeutic effect of plasmapheresis in patients with systemic lupus erythematosus, *Q. J. Med.* **48**:555–576.

Jones, J. V., Clough, J. D., Klinenberg, J. R., and Davis, P., 1981a, The role of therapeutic plasmapheresis in the rheumatic diseases, *J. Lab. Clin. Med.* **97**:589–598.

Jones, J. V., Robinson, M. F., Parciany, R. K., Layfer, L. F., and McLeod, B., 1981b, Therapeutic plasmapheresis in systemic lupus erythematosus: Effect on immune complexes and antibodies to DNA, *Arthritis Rheum.* **24**:1113–1120.

Kabbash, L., Brandwein, S., Eschaule, J., Danoff, D., Fuks, A., and Shuster, J., 1982, Reticuloendothelial system Fc-receptor function in systemic lupus erythematosus, *J. Rheumatol.* **9**(3):374–379.

Kalden, J. R., Schranz, W., Lösch, G., Krapf, F., and Bartels, O., 1982, Neue Indikationsgebiete zur hochdosierten Immunglobulintherapie: Therapeutischer Plasmaaustausch, *Autoimmunopathien. Beitr. Infusionsther. Klin. Ernaehr.* **9**:48–59.

Karsh, J., Wright, D. J., Klippel, J. H., Decker, J. L., Deisseroth, A. B., and Flye, M. W., 1979, Lymphocyte depletion by continuous flow cell centrifugation in rheumatoid arthritis. Clinical effects, *Arthritis Rheum.* **22**:1055–1059.

Karsh, J., Klippel, J. H., Plotz, P. H., Decker, J. L., Wright, D. C., and Flye, M. W., 1981, Lymphapheresis in rheumatoid arthritis. A randomized trial, *Arthritis Rheum.* **24**:867–873.

Kater, L., Derksen, R. H. W. M., Houwert, F. A., Hene, R. J., Struyvenberg, A., Gmelig Meyling, F. H. J., and Verroust, P., 1981, Effect of plasmapheresis in active systemic lupus erythematosus, *Neth. J. Med.* **24**:209–216.

Kayashima, K., Smith, J. W., Barna, R., Matsubara, S., Abe, Y., Ueno, M., Katsume, C., Valenzuela, R., Clough, J. D., Melchesky, P. S., and Nose, Y., 1982, Improved white blood cell functions: Additional effects of membrane plasmapheresis, *Trans. Am. Soc. Artif. Intern. Organs* **28**:312–317.

Kellog, R. M., and Hester, J. P., 1981, Plasma exchange by continuous flow centrifugation, in: *Plasma Exchange Therapy* (H. Borberg, and P. Reuther, eds.), Thieme-Stratton, Stuttgart, New York, pp. 5–10.

Kincaid-Smith, P., and d'Apice, A. F., 1978, Plasmapheresis in rapidly proliferative glomerulonephritis, *Am. J. Med.* **65**:564.

Klaus, G. G. B., 1978, Antigen-antibody complexes elicit anti-idiotypic antibodies to self idiotypes, *Nature* **272**:265–266.

Koffler, D., Agnello, V., and Kunkel, H. G., 1974, Polynucleotide immune complexes in serum and glomeruli of patients with systemic lupus erythematosus, *Am. J. Pathol.* **74**:109–124.

Kosaka, M., and Salomon, A., 1980, Hyperviscosity syndrome associated with an idiopathic monoclonal IgA rheumatoid factor, *Am. J. Med.* **60**:145–151.

Krakauer, R. S., Asanuma, Y., and Zawicki, C., 1982, Circulating immune complexes in rheumatoid arthritis: Selective removal by cryogelation with membrane filtration, *Arch. Intern. Med.* **142**:395–397.

Krapf, F. E., Renger, D., Schedel, J., Leiendecker, K., Leyssens, H., and Deicher, H., 1982, A PEG-precipitation laser nephelometer technique for detection and characterization of circulating immune complexes in human sera, *J. Immunol. Methods* **54**:107–117.

Krapf, F. E., Manger, B., Krauledat, P., and Kalden, J. R., 1983, IgE containing immune complexes in human sera: Quantification and analysis, *Immunobiology* **165**:305.

Krapf, P., Manger, B., Koch, B., Krauledat, P., Kalden, J. R., 1985, The estimation of circulating immune complexes, C3D, and levels anti-ds-DNA-antibody serum levels in a monitoring of therapeutic plasmapheresis in a patient with systemic lupus erythematous. A case report, *Clin. Exp. Rheum.* **3**:159–162.

Lahnborg, G., Berghem, L., Ahlgreen, T., Groth, C. G., Lundgren, G., and Tillegard, A., 1979, Reticuloendothelial function in human renal allograft recipients, *Transplantation* **28**:111–115.

Lambert, P. H., Dixon, F. J., Zubler, R. H., Agnello, V., Cambiaso, C., Casali, P., Clarke, J., Concery, J. S., McDuffie, F. C., Hay, F. C., MacLennan, I. C. M., Masson, P., Muller-Eberhard, H. J., Pettinen, K., Smith, M., Tappeiner, G., Theofilopoulos, A. N., and Verroust, P., 1978, A WHO collaborative study for the evaluation of eighteen methods for detecting immune complexes in serum, *J. Clin. Lab. Immunol.* **1**:1–15.

Lloyd, W., and Schur, P. H., 1981, Immune complexes, complement, and anti-DNA in exacerbations of systemic lupus erythematosus (SLE), *Medicine (Baltimore)* **60**:208–212.

Lockwood, C. M., Pussel, B., Wilson, C. B., and Peters, D. K., 1979a, Plasma exchange in nephritis, *Adv. Nephrol.* **8**:383–418.

Lockwood, C. M., Worlledge, S., Nicolas, A., Cotton, C., and Peters, D. K., 1979b, Reversal of impaired splenic function in patients with nephritis or vasculitis (or both) by plasma exchange, *N. Engl. J. Med.* **300**:524–530.

Löw, A., Hotze, A., Krapf, F. E., Schranz, W., Mahlstedt, J., Wolf, F., and Kalden, J. R., 1985, Assessment of RES clearance function in autoimmune diseases before and after therapeutic plasma exchange, *Rheum. Int.* **5**:69–72.

Matus, R. E., Scott, R. C., Saal, S., Gordon, B. R., and Hurvits, A. I., 1983, Plasmapheresis—immunoadsorption for treatment of systemic lupus erythematosus in a dog, *J. Am. Vet. Med. Assoc.* **182**:499–502.

McLeod, B. C., and Sasseti, R. J., 1980, Plasmapheresis with return of cryoglobulin-depleted autologous plasma in cryoglobulinemia, *Blood* **55**:866–870.

Miller, C. W., and Nussenzweig, V. A., 1975, New complement function: Solubilisation of antigen–antibody aggregates, *Proc. Natl. Acad. Sci. U.S.A.* **72**:428.

Moran, C. J., Parry, H. F., Mowbray, J., Richards, J. D. M., and Goldstone, A. H., 1977, Plasmapheresis in systemic lupus erythematosus, *Br. Med. J.* **1**:1573–1574.

Morimoto, C., Reinherz, E. L., Abe, T., Homma, M., and Schlossman, S. F., 1980, Characteristics of anti-T cell antibodies in systemic lupus erythematosus: Evidence for selective reactivity with normal suppressor cells defined by monoclonal antibodies, *Clin. Immunol. Immunopathol.* **16**:474–484.

Munthe, E., and Natvig, J. B., 1972, Immunoglobulin classes, subclasses and complexes of IgG rheumatoid factor in rheumatoid plasma cells, *Clin. Exp. Immunol.* **12**:55–70.

Nilson, I. M., Jonsson, S., Sundquist, S.-B., Ahlberg, A., and Bergentz, S.-E., 1981, A procedure for removing high titer antibodies by extracorporal protein-A–sepharose adsorption in hemophilia: Substitution therapy and surgery in a patient with hemophilia B and antibodies, *Blood* **58**:38–44.

Oen, K. Pelty, R. E., Schroeter, M. Z., Briggs, E. J., and Bishop, A. J., 1980, Thrombotic, trombocytopenic purpura in a girl with systemic lupus erythematosus, *J. Rheumatol.* **7**:727–729.

Okudaira, K., Nakai, H., Hayakawa, T., Kashiwado, T., Tanimoto, K., Horiuchi, Y., and Juji, T., 1979, Detection of antilymphocyte antibody with two-color method in systemic lupus erythematosus and its heterogeneous specificities against human T-cell subsets, *J. Clin. Invest.* **64**:1213–1220.

Okudaira, K., Searles, R. P., Ceuppens, J. L., Goodwin, J. S., and Williams, R. C., 1982, Anti-Ia reactivity in sera from patients with systemic lupus erythematosus, *J. Clin. Invest.* **69**:17–24.

Orlin, J. B., and Berkman, E. M., 1980, Partial plasma exchange using albumin replacement. Removal and recovery of normal constituents, *Blood* **56**:1055–1059.

Parris, T. M., Kimberley, R. P., and Inman, R. D., 1981, Dynamics of reticuloendothelial function in systemic lupus erythematosus: Changes associated with disease activity, *Arthritis Rheum.* **24**(Suppl.):1208–1214.

Pary, H. F., Moran, C. J., Svaible, M. C., Richards, J. D., Goldstone, A. H., Nineham, L. J., Hay, F. C., Morrow, W. J., and Roitt, I. M., 1981, Plasma exchange in systemic lupus erythematosus, *Ann. Rheum. Dis.* **40**:224–228.

Paulus, H. E., Machleder, H. I., Levine, S., Yu, D. T., and McDonald, N. S., 1977, Lymphocyte involvement in rheumatoid arthritis. Studies during thoracic duct drainage, *Arthritis Rheum.* **20**:1249–1262.

Pinching, A. J., 1980, Plasma exchange in immunologically mediated disease, in: *Recent Advances in Clinical Immunology*, Vol. 2 (R. A. Thomson, ed.), Churchill-Livingstone, London, pp. 313–341.

Pineda, A. A., 1982, Methods for selective removal of plasma constituents, in: *Therapeutic Apheresis and Plasma Perfusion* (R. S. A. Tindall, ed.), Alan R. Liss, New York, pp. 361–373.

Quismorio, F. P., Beardmore, T., Kaufman, R. L., and Mongan, E. S., 1983, IgG rheumatoid factors and anti-nuclear antibodies in rheumatoid vasculitis, *Clin. Exp. Immunol.* **52**:333–340.

Raveche, E. S., and Steinberg, A. D., Lymphocytes and lymphocyte function in systemic lupus erythematosus, *Semin. Hematol.* **16**:344–370.

Roseman, R. H., Friedman, M., and Byers, S. O., 1956, The causal role of plasma albumin deficiency in experimental nephrotic hypolipidaemia and hypocholesterinaemia, *J. Clin. Invest.* **35**:522–527.

Rossen, R. D., Hersh, E. M., Sharp, J. T., McCredie, K. B., Gyorkey, F., Suki, W. N., Eknoyan, G., and Reisberg, M. A., 1977, Effect of plasma exchange on circulating immune complexes ana antibody formation in patients treated with cyclophosphamide and prednisone, *Am. J. Med.* **63**:674–682.

Rothwell, R. S., Davis, P., Gordon, P. A., Dasgupta, M. K., Johny, K. V., Russel, A. S., and Percey, J. S., 1980, A controlled study of plasma exchange in the treatment of severe rheumatoid arthritis, *Arthritis Rheum.* **23**:785–790.

Russel, A. S., Davis, P., and Percey, J. S., 1981, Editorial, *J. Rheumatol.* **8**:3.

Saal, S. D., and Gordon, B. R., 1982, Extracorporal modification of plasma and whole blood, in: *Therapeutic Apheresis and Plasma Perfusion,* (R. S. A. Tindall, ed.), Alan R. Liss, New York, pp. 375–384.

Sakane, T., Steinberg, A. D., Reeves, J. P., and Green, I., 1979, Studies of immune functions of patients with systemic lupus erythematosus: Complement dependent IgM anti-T cell antibodies preferentially inactivate suppressor cells, *J. Clin. Invest.* **63**:945–965.

Salky, N. K., Mills, D., and DiLuzio, N. R., 1965, Activity of the reticuloendothelial system in diseases of altered immunity, *J. Lab. Clin. Med.* **66**:952–960.

Samtleben, W., Hillebrand, G., Krumme, D., and Gurland, H. J., 1980, Membrane plasma separation: Clinical experience with more than 120 plasma exchanges, in: *Plasma Exchange* (H. G. Sieberth, ed.), Schattauer, Stuttgart, New York, pp. 173–181.

Schilderman, B., Dequeker, J., and van de Putte, I., 1979, Plasmapheresis combined with corticosteroids in uncontrolled active systemic lupus erythematosus, *J. Rheumatol.* **6**:687–690.

Schlansky, R., Dehoratius, R. J., Pincus, T., and Tung, K. S. K., 1981, Plasmapheresis in systemic lupus erythematosus. A cautionary note, *Arthritis Rheum.* **24**:49–53.

Scott, D. G. L., Bacon, P. A., and Tribe, C. R., 1981a, Systemic vasculitis: A clinical and laboratory study of 50 cases, *Medicine* **60**:288–297.

Scott, D. G. L., Bacon, P. A., Bothamley, J. E., Allen, C., Elson, C. J., and Wallington, T. B., 1981b, Plasma exchange in rheumatoid vasculitis, *J. Rheumatol.* **8**:433–439.

Seiler, F. R., Karges, H., Geursen, R., and Sedlacek, H. H., 1981, Possibilities, problems and hazards with blood plasma substitution therapy, in: *Plasma Exchange Therapy* (H. Borberg and R. Reuther, eds.), Thieme-Stratton, Stuttgart, New York, pp. 37–42.

Sieberth, H. G., and Glöckner, W. M., 1981, Separation of cells from plasma in man using hollow-fiber-membranes of large pore size, in: *Plasma Exchange Therapy* (H. Borberg and P. Reuther, eds.), Thieme-Stratton, Stuttgart, New York, pp. 20–25.

Skoog, W. A., and Adams, W. S., 1959, Plasmapheresis in case of Waldenström's macroglobulinaemia, *Clin. Res.* **7**:96–101.

Smiley, J. D., Sachs, C., and Ziff, M., 1968, *In vitro* synthesis of immunoglobulin by rheumatoid synovial membrane, *J. Clin. Invest.* **47**:624–632.

Solomon, A., and Fahey, J. L., 1963, Plasmapheresis therapy in macroglobulinaemia, *Ann. Intern. Med.* **58**:780–800.

Solomon, B. A., Castino, F., Lysaght, M. J., Colton, C. K., and Friedman, L. I., 1978, Continuous flow membrane filtration of plasma from whole blood, *Trans. Am. Soc. Artif. Intern. Organs* **24**:21–26.

Steward, M. W., Katz, F. E., and West, N. J., 1978, The role of low affinity antibody in immune complex disease. The quantity of anti-DNA antibodies in NZB/W hybrid mice, *Clin. Exp. Immunol* **21**:121.

Sutton, D. M. C., Cardella, C. J., Uldall, P. R., and Deveber, G. A., 1981, Complications of intensive plasma exchange, *Plasma Ther.* **2**:19–25.

Swanson, C. F., Robson, J. S., Urbaniak, S. F., Keller, A. J., and Kay, A. B., 1978, Treatment of Goodpasture's disease by plasma exchange and immunosuppression, *Clin. Exp. Immunol.* **32**:233–248.

Taylor, R. B., 1982, Regulation of antibody responses by antibody towards the immunogen, *Immunol. Today* **3**:47–48.

Terman, D. S., Buffaloe, G., Maltioli, C., Cook, G., Tillquist, R., Sullivan, M., and Ayus, J. C., 1979, Extracorporal immunoadsorption: Initial experience in human systemic lupus erythematosus, *Lancet* **2**:824–827.

Tindall, R. S. A., Walker, J. E., Ehle, A. L., Near, L., Rollins, J., and Bekker, D., 1982, Plasmapheresis in multiple sclerosis: Prospective trial of pheresis and immunosuppression versus immunosuppression alone, *Neurology (New York)* **32**:739–743.

Trice, J. M., Pinals, R. S. and Plitman, G. I., 1983, Thrombotic thrombocytopenic purpura during penicillamine therapy in rheumatoid arthritis, *Arch. Intern. Med.* **143**:1487–1488.

Tsokos, G. G., Balow, J. E., Huston, D. P., Wei, N., and Decker, J. L., 1982, Effect of plasmapheresis on T and B lymphocyte functions in patients with systemic lupus erythematosus: A double blind study, *Clin. Exp. Immunol.* **48**:449–457.

Tung, K. S. K., Dehoratius, R. S., and Williams, R. C., 1981, Study of circulating complex size in systemic lupus erythematosus, *Clin. Exp. Immunol.* **43**:615–625.

Uedo, T., Tanaka, S., Tominaja, Y., Ogawa, H., Sakumari, T., 1979, The effect of thoracic duct drainage on lymphocytic dynamics and clinical symptoms in patients with rheumatoid arthritis, *Arthritis Rheum.* **22**:1405.

Vogler, W. R., 1983, Therapeutic apheresis: Where we've been and where we are going, in: *Therapeutic Apheresis and Plasma Perfusion* (R. S. A. Tindall, ed.), Alan R. Liss, New York, pp. 1–13.

Wallace, D. J., Goldfinger, D., Gatti, R., Lowe, C. Fan, P., Bluestone, R., and Klinenberg, J. R., 1979, Plasmapheresis and lymphoplasmapheresis in the management of rheumatoid arthritis, *Arthritis Rheum.* **22**:703–710.

Wallace, D. J., Goldfinger, D., Thompson-Breton, R., Martin, V., Lowe, C. M., Bluestone, R., and Klinenberg, J. R., 1980, Advances in the use of therapeutic apheresis for the management of rheumatic disease, *Semin. Arthritis Rheum.* **10**:81–91.

Wallace, D. J., Goldfinger, D., and Klinenberg, J. R., 1982a, The current status of therapeutic apheresis in the management of rheumatoid arthritis, in: *Therapeutic Apheresis and Plasmaperfusion* (R. S. A. Tindall, ed.), Alan R. Liss, New York, pp. 27–32.

Wallace, D. J., Goldfinger, D., Lowe, C., Nichols, S., Weiner, J., Brachman, M., and Klinenberg, J. R., 1982b, A double-blind controlled study of lymphoplasmapheresis versus sham apheresis in rheumatoid arthritis, *N. Engl. J. Med.* **306**:1406–1410.

Wei, N. Huston, D. P., Lippel, H. J., Balow, J. E., Dawley, T. J., Hall, R. P., Plotz, R. M., Steinberg, A. D., and Decker, J. L., 1981, A randomized trial of plasmapheresis in systemic lupus erythematosus, *Arthritis Rheum.* **24**(Suppl.):299.

Wilder, R., Wahl, S., Katona, J., Wahl, L., Allen N., Wei, N., Scher, J., and Decker, J. L., 1982a, Depletion of a functionally abnormal population of mononuclear cells by leukapheresis in rheumatoid arthritis. Correlation with clinical improvement, *Arthritis Rheum.* **25**(Suppl):60.

Wilder, R. L., Yarboro, C. H., and Decker, J. L., 1982b, The effects of repeated leukapheresis in patients with severe refractory rheumatoid arthritis, in: *Therapeutic Apheresis and Plasmaperfusion* (R. S. A. Tindall, ed.), Alan R. Liss, New York, pp. 49–59.

Williams, R. C., 1980, Immune Complexes, in: *Clinical and Experimental Medicine*, Harvard University Press, Cambridge, pp. 486–491.

Winfield, J. B., Faiferman, I., and Koffer, D., 1977, Avidity of anti-DNA antibodies in serum and IgG glomerular eluates from patients with systemic lupus erythematosus. Association of high avidity anti-native DNA antibody with glomerulonephritis, *J. Clin. Invest.* **59**:90–96.

Wright, D. G., Karsh, J., Fauci, A. S., Klippel, J. U., Decker, J. L., O'Donnel, J. F., and Deisseroth, A. B., 1981, Lymphocyte depletion and immunosuppression with repeated leukapheresis by continuous flow centrifugation, *Blood* **58**:451–458.

Young, D. W., Thompson, R. A., and Mackie, P. H., 1980, Plasmapheresis in hereditary angioneurotic edema and systemic lupus erythematosus, *Arch. Intern. Med.* **140**:127–128.

29

Immunoregulatory Drugs

Michael L. Miller and Alfred D. Steinberg

I. INTRODUCTION

Immunoregulatory drugs are now commonly used to treat patients with diverse clinical disorders including malignancies and a variety of nonmalignant immune-mediated diseases. The rationale for their use is that modulation of the abnormal immune reactivity found in these conditions will alleviate if not eliminate associated clinical manifestations. This chapter reviews the current concepts of normal immunoregulation, specific and nonspecific immune suppression and enhancement, and the pharmacology of specific immunoregulatory medications.

II. IMMUNOREGULATION

Basic research over the last 20 years has allowed a sophisticated understanding of immunoregulation to emerge, which has provided a rationale for the use of immunoregulatory agents already in use, such as prednisolone, as well as the introduction of new immunoregulatory drugs. It has been shown that the immune response to antigens can be initiated by the presentation of antigen by accessory cells to T cells, which trigger antigen-specific B cells to differentiate and secrete specific antibody. In addition to the antigen-specific signals, antigen-nonspecific growth and differentiation factors are critical to the ultimate immune response. The magnitude and duration of antibody production are determined by numerous factors, including prior exposure to the antigen (causing memory B-cell production), magnitude of T-cell help and suppression, and modulation of B-cell

Michael L. Miller and Alfred D. Steinberg • National Institutes of Health, National Institute of Arthritis, Diabetes, and Digestive and Kidney Diseases, Arthritis and Rheumatism Branch, Cellular Immunology Section, Bethesda, Maryland 20205.

responsiveness by feedback mechanisms, both specific (including antibody, antiidiotype, and antigen) and nonspecific (such as by soluble mediators produced by numerous cell populations including macrophages and lymphocytes).

The immune response results from an interacting network of lymphoid cell populations and their products (Jerne, 1974). If immune-mediated diseases could be characterized by specific abnormalities localized to portions of the network, immunoregulatory agents could theoretically be used to correct or alleviate these abnormalities. However, even if agents with such specific actions could be defined, they might have effects contrary to those desired. This might occur because alterations at one part of the network might result in the opposite effect at a more distant location. For example, "immunosuppressive" agents might actually lead to increased immune responsiveness if they inhibit suppressor cells more than helper cells (Taliaferro and Taliaferro, 1954; Dixon and McConahey, 1963). The converse might hold for "immune enhancers," resulting in suppression (Tripodi, *et al.*, 1973; Pross and Eldinger, 1974; Brodeur and Merigana, 1975). Immunoregulatory agents need to be considered in the context of their overall action on the immune system as well as of their specific effects.

Actions of immunoregulatory agents are dependent on other factors as well. The schedule of administration of some agents may determine their effect on the cell cycle of some cell populations. An agent may be an immune enhancer and suppress tumor growth in one schedule but enhance tumor growth in another. In addition, the ability of drugs to enhance or suppress different immune responses will depend on the cell populations with which they directly interact as well as other populations that are indirectly affected because of disruption of normal feedback control mechanisms.

III. IMMUNOREGULATORY DRUGS

There are now a large number of drugs capable of immunoregulation. These include those given specifically for immunoregulation as well as those with secondary immunologic effects. The latter group includes antihistamines, polypeptide hormones, cardioactive glycosides, foods and food additives, anticonvulsants, antiarrhythmics, and other medications. "Immunoregulatory" drugs are usually meant to be those given because of their specific immunoregulatory properties. Many of these were initially developed for chemotherapy of malignancies and subsequently used in nonmalignant diseases (Sack and Peppercorn, 1983; Kovarsky, 1983).

A. Cell Cycle

A brief description of the relationship of the cell cycle to lymphocyte function will facilitate an understanding of how many immunoregulatory agents work. The modulation of lymphocyte commitment towards either proliferation or differentiation is an important determinant of the nature of the immune response. This commitment is determined as part of the cell cycle (Table 1). G_0-to-G_1 transition corresponds to activation of the cell. During this phase, RNA and new protein synthesis occur, and membrane receptors allowing proliferation or differentiation at a future stage are formed. Interactions of these receptors with their ligands determine whether the cell will proceed towards proliferation ($S + G_2 + M$) or differentiation (resulting, for example, in B-cell secretion of immu-

Table 1. The Cell Cycle and Immunoregulatory Agents

Phase	Cellular Activity	Agents active during this phase
G_1	Interphase	Vinblastine
S	DNA synthesis	Methotrexate
		Hydroxyurea
		Thioguanine
		Cyclophosphamide (also acts throughout the cell cycle)
G_2	Postsynthetic rest	Daunorubicin
M	Mitosis	Vincristine, vinblastine (cells must first be exposed in S phase)

noglobulin). With regard to B cells, interaction with antigen induces receptors for B-cell growth factors, which interact with ligands, exposing B-cell differentiation factor receptors. In addition, powerful soluble factors can take a resting B cell to S phase of the cell cycle without the need for antigen. The latter is, however, necessary for specific antibody production. Various "nutrients" necessary for growth, such as insulin and transferrin, appear to work by triggering specific receptors. In fact, the transferrin receptor appears to be critical to the proliferation of all cells under discussion.

Different cytotoxic and cytostatic drugs interfere with cellular events involved in proliferation. However, most of these have been developed as antineoplastic agents and are not specific for receptors responsible for triggering cells to differentiate or proliferate. The antineoplastic drugs tend to either kill cells or prevent their subsequent division (Table 2). Future attempts at immunoregulation should be directed towards receptors specific for stages in G_1. This would allow more direct control over commitment of lymphocytes towards differentiation or proliferation, resulting in greater control over the

Table 2. Mechanism of Action of Immunoregulatory Agents

Type of Agent	Mechanism	Examples
Purine analogues	Inhibition of purine synthesis	Azathioprine
		6-Mercaptopurine
		6-Thioguanine
		Deoxycoformycin
Alkylating	Binding to DNA, RNA, and proteins	Nitrogen mustard
		Cyclosphamide
		Chlorambucil
Folic acid antagonists	Interference with one-carbon transport for purine and protein synthesis	Methotrexate
	Interfere with methylation of deoxyuridylic acid	
Pyrimidine analogues	Inhibition of ribo-/deoxyribonucleotide synthesis	5-Fluorouracil
Hydroxyureas	Killing of cells in S phase by inhibition of ribonucleotide reductase	Hydroxyurea
	Prevents cells from entering S phase	
Alkaloids	Inhibition of mitotic spindle formation, resulting in metaphase arrest	Vinblastine
		Vincristine
Antibiotics	Inhibition of DNA-dependent RNA polymerase and of DNA synthesis	Daunorubicin
		Actinomycin D

immune response. A few such antireceptor agents are currently under preliminary investigation.

Drugs such as methotrexate that are primarily active during the S phase kill rapidly dividing cells and have minimal effects on resting cells. Other drugs act throughout the cell cycle and kill resting as well as proliferating cells. A drug that induces nonlethal chromosomal damage in a resting cell prevents the cell from dividing and therefore appears to have a greater effect on proliferating cells.

Most purine and pyrimidine analogues, because they are given in small doses, have access to cells in all phases of the cell cycle. However, methotrexate and certain alkylating agents may be more effective when given in large doses intermittently. Unfortunately, this is not always possible because of toxicity for nonlymphoid cell populations. Therefore, the usefulness of a particular therapeutic regimen depends on the relative sensitivities of the different tissues as well as on the regenerative capacities of the cell populations affected.

B. Effects on Lymphocyte Subpopulations

Another means of understanding the mode of action of immunoregulatory agents is the study of lymphocyte subpopulations in tissues or the circulation of treated patients. These populations are altered by the diseases themselves, and, when a patient is under treatment, it is often difficult to know whether observed changes are caused by a direct effect of the therapeutic agent on lymphoid cells or by the underlying disease process. Furthermore, peripheral blood changes may reflect recirculation patterns rather than total body alterations and give little insight into the composition and function of lymph nodes, spleen, bone marrow, Peyer's patches, and thymus.

Nonetheless, it appears that different drugs affect different types of cells. For example, cyclophosphamide appears to cause greater reduction in small lymphocytes than in larger mononuclear cells. Azathioprine tends preferentially to reduce large mononuclear cells. Furthermore, B-cell-mediated functions are lost before T-cell-mediated immunity on initiation of cyclophosphamide therapy, although both B and T cells are affected by the drug. In contrast, both azathioprine and corticosteroids reduce T-cell functions before B-cell functions.

In the final analysis, the rationale for the use of immunoregulatory drugs in many diseases remains empirical. These medications were generally introduced to treat diseases mediated by abnormal interactions within the immune system, a reason that remains valid but simplistic. The abnormalities emphasized were often excessive antibody production or lymphoid cell proliferation, and immunoregulatory agents were used to modulate these excesses. The mechanisms by which such modulation occurs may be only in part related to immunosuppression. There are most likely several mechanisms through which each medication results in modulation of disease processes. More complete understanding of these mechanisms awaits future research.

IV. IMMUNOSUPPRESSION

Immunosuppression can be antigen specific or nonspecific. Specific suppression may be achieved through the use of specific antigen or antibody. Nonspecific suppression is the more common result of immunoregulatory therapy, although it may be difficult to distinguish these effects from those resulting in specific suppression. Examples include removal of lymphoid tissues or their products through such procedures as splenectomy, thoracic duct drainage, or leukapheresis. Physical (e.g., irradiation), chemical (medications), biological (e.g., antibodies), and living agents (e.g., BCG) may result in either antigen-specific or nonspecific immunosuppression depending on whether they are given with specific antigens or have unique specificities. For example, large doses of cyclophosphamide given with an antigen tend to suppress antibody response to that antigen to a greater extent than responses to unrelated antigens. This kind of specific suppression is dependent on timing of administration of these agents. Some immunoregulatory agents act in synergy when given together. Synergistic effects have been noted in primary immune responses (Friedman *et al.*, 1971), tolerance (Hyman *et al.*, 1975), and treatment of autoimmune disease (Gelfand *et al.*, 1972; Steinberg *et al.*, 1975).

A variety of mechanisms result in nonspecific suppression of immune responses. These include such procedures as total-body irradiation or use of large doses of cyclophosphamide prior to bone marrow transplantation. Such methods are used to reduce certain immune functions without eliminating the ability of the immune system to fight infections, especially through maintenance of adequate granulocyte and phagocytic function.

Another method that causes nonspecific suppression while allowing specific immune responses is physical removal of part of the immune system. Thus, splenectomy results in reduced autoantibody production in various autoimmune states including systemic lupus, idiopathic thrombocytopenic purpura, and autoimmune hemolytic anemia. Splenectomy reduces removal of antibody-coated cells by the mononuclear phagocytic system but does little to impair granulocyte function; there is, however, a decreased ability to eliminate antibody-coated bacteria. Certain infections, such as pneumococcal septicemia, are more difficult to combat. Appropriate immunization (e.g., with pneumococcal vaccines) may reduce many of the risks that follow splenectomy.

Thoracic duct drainage results in removal of lymphocytes, particularly T cells. T-cell-mediated disorders such as rheumatoid arthritis (Paulus *et al.*, 1977; Machleder and Paulus, 1978) can, in certain circumstances, be effectively treated in this manner; the risk of infection and difficulty of long-term drainage have led to leukapheresis as an alternative (Oon and Hobbs, 1975). The use of a machine able to separate cells allows lymphocytes and monocytes to be preferentially removed from peripheral veins and other circulating cells and plasma to be returned to the body. Although not particularly time and cost effective, this procedure could be used in many patients if it were effective and long-lasting. Nevertheless, controlled studies will be needed to demonstrate the efficacy of leukapheresis in the diseases for which it has been tried.

Total lymphoid irradiation (Sutherland *et al.*, 1983) combines some of the benefits of splenectomy and thoracic duct drainage. It involves irradiation of the spleen and most peripheral lymph nodes with shielding of the mediastinum and spine. Initially designed for treatment of lymphoid malignancies, it shows promise in being effective in treating patients with rheumatoid arthritis (Kotzin *et al.*, 1981; Trentham *et al.*, 1981) and systemic lupus (Tanay *et al.*, 1984). Since the benefit may come from induction of suppressor cells as well as lymphoid depletion, a smaller dose of irradiation may induce the former and be sufficient therapeutically. As with leukapheresis, future controlled trials will determine the most appropriate patients for whom this treatment will be of benefit.

There are theoretical means of producing nonspecific immunosuppression that have yet to be developed. For instance, drugs could be developed that preferentially augment suppressor T-cell function. Nonspecific suppressor factors could someday be produced either from T-cell hybridomas or by genetic engineering. *In vivo* administration to patients with immune-mediated diseases could result in modulation of excessive immune responses.

V. NONSPECIFIC IMMUNE ENHANCEMENT

Immune responses to a variety of antigens can be augmented by administration of immune adjuvants with antigens. This is commonly done in the course of immunizations. In addition to specific enhancement of antibody production, nonspecific enhancement can be obtained through administration of polyclonal B-cell activators. Polyclonal activators include naturally occurring materials such as oligonucleotides, bacterial endotoxin, and certain viruses. Synthetic polynucleotides and certain drugs can also result in nonspecific stimulation of B cells. T cells can be similarly stimulated by a variety of agents. However, these agents may cause changes in the immune network that can counteract the stimulation.

The most widely used adjuvant in experimental immunology is Freund's adjuvant, which consists of a combination of killed mycobacteria, paraffin oil, and an emulsifying agent. Administration of antigen emulsified in Freund's adjuvant results in marked augmentation of specific antibody production as well as delayed hypersensitivity (Freund, 1947). This material is prohibitively toxic and is not used in humans. A synthetic drug that gives similar results is N-acetylmuramyl-L-alanyl-D-isoglutamine (muramyl dipeptide) (Chedid *et al.*, 1976), which is effective when administered orally (Audibert *et al.*, 1976). Water-soluble preparations of peptidoglycan isolated from Freund's adjuvant are able to stimulate delayed hypersensitivity (Adam *et al.*, 1972; Hiu, 1972). However, consideration of their use is limited by potential severe toxic side effects. There are a variety of agents capable of enhancement of immune responses. Theoretically, they might be of benefit in treating diseases characterized by deficient numbers or function of lymphoid populations. The exact role of such enhancers remains to be determined.

VI. SPECIFIC IMMUNOREGULATORY AGENTS

A. 6-Mercaptopurine and Azathioprine

6-Mercaptopurine (6MP) is the analogue of hypoxanthine in which the hydroxyl group on the sixth carbon atom is replaced by a thiol group. Azathioprine is 6MP with an imidazole group attached to the sulfur atom. Although azathioprine is broken down to produce 6MP *in vivo*, there are differences between the two drugs that appear to be important. For example, the imidazole group of azathioprine gives it different rates of passage through cell membranes and conversion to active products as compared with 6MP. Azathioprine and 6MP also differ in predilection for various tissues.

Both drugs are absorbed after oral administration. Typical doses give peak blood levels of 0.1 to 2.0 μg/ml; however, large intravenous doses may yield levels as high as

25 μg/ml (Loo *et al.*, 1968; Coffey *et al.*, 1972, Elion, 1972). Although drug levels may vary after oral doses (Zimm *et al.*, 1983), absolute neutrophil counts have correlated well with thioguanine metabolite levels (Herber, *et al.*, 1982). The plasma half-life of 6MP is less than 90 min in adults and is even shorter in children. Both drugs are metabolized and excreted by degradation, tissue uptake, and urinary excretion. Most of the 6MP given orally is oxidized to nontoxic thiouric acid by xanthine oxidases. Allopurinol, a xanthine oxidase inhibitor, cannot be given with 6MP, particularly in the oral form (Zimm *et al.*, 1983), or azathioprine without reducing the dose of the antimetabolite by about 75%.

After administration, small amounts of 6MP are converted to the ribonucleotides of 6MP, 6-methylmercaptopurine, and 6-thioguanine (6TG) by the enzymes of the purine metabolic pathways (Hamilton and Elion, 1954; Skipper, 1954; Yeh and Phang, 1983). These ribonucleotides inhibit DNA synthesis by several processes. For example, 6MP ribonucleotide (thioinosinic acid) competitively inhibits the enzymes that convert (1) inosinic acid to xanthylic and adenylosuccinic acids; and (2) adenylosuccinic acid to adenylic acid (Elion, 1967; Zimmerman, 1974). In addition, 6-methylmercaptopurine ribonucleotide causes feedback inhibition of the formation of 5-phosphoribosylamine, which inhibits DNA synthesis. 6-Thioguanine is incorporated into DNA as an abnormal base, leading to errors in transcription and replication (Scannell and Hitchings, 1966).

In humans, azathioprine and 6MP suppress both antibody production and cell-mediated immunity only when drug is given after antigen (Hersh *et al.*, 1966; Abdou, *et al.*, 1973). Azathioprine is not as suppressive of anti-sheep-red-blood-cell responses in mice as is 6MP (Medzihradsky *et al.*, 1982). Induction of specific tolerance (with regard to antibody production) to subsequent immunization was achieved by treatment with antigen and 6MP followed by antigen challenge 1 day after stopping 6MP (Levin *et al.*, 1964).

Standard oral doses of azathioprine result in only small reductions of *in vitro* responses to mitogens and antigens. There is no effect on delayed skin hypersensitivity if prior sensitization has occurred. In contrast, induction of primary sensitization is inhibited in some. Survival of organ grafts, such as kidney, is prolonged by either medication.

The usual method of administration of azathioprine is in a dose of 2 to 5 mg/kg per day orally. The major toxicity of both medications is on bone marrow. Neutropenia has been correlated with both 6MP and 6TG levels 2 weeks after initiation of therapy in children with leukemia (Lennard *et al.*, 1983). Leukopenia has been noted more frequently than thrombocytopenia or significant anemia. Sudden onset of peripheral leukopenia accompanied by a central maturation arrest of white cells in marrow, resembling an idiosyncratic reaction, has been seen in some patients within a week of beginning the drug. Occasional cases of red cell aplasia have occurred during long-term use of azathioprine; this may respond to cyclophosphamide (Old *et al.*, 1978). 6-Mercaptopurine and azathioprine administration has also been associated with hepatitis. As mentioned, toxicity can result when full doses of either drug are given in conjunction with allopurinol. The risk of toxicity can be alleviated by reducing the 6MP or azathioprine drug dose by 75% or by giving 6-thioguanine, which is metabolized through a different pathway. Case reports of overdosage of 6MP (Hendrick and Mirkin, 1984) and azathioprine (Carney *et al.*, 1974) suggest that acute toxicity is limited to mild, transient hepatic dysfunction.

There is an increased incidence of lymphoreticular malignancies (particularly intracerebral) in kidney transplant patients who are placed on purine analogue immunosuppression (Hoover and Fraumeni, 1973). Epithelial tumors, especially of the skin and uterine cervix, are also noted more frequently in patients receiving azathioprine even if they have not received transplants. Whether the incidences of other malignancies are increased has not been accurately determined. However, leukemia and intracerebral reticulum cell sarcoma have been seen in rheumatoid arthritis and systemic lupus erythematosus patients who have received azathioprine.

As with other immunosuppressive drugs, purine analogues predispose patients to common infections as well as to infections by organisms not usually pathogenic (such as *Pneumocystis carinii* and *Candida*). These infections can occur in the absence of severe leukopenia, raising the possibility of abnormal T-cell–macrophage defenses. This is supported by a report of normal neutrophil function in patients receiving azathioprine (Losito *et al.*, 1978).

B. Adenosine Deaminase Inhibitors

Adenosine deaminase inhibitors have been used as immunosuppressive agents because of the association of adenosine deaminase deficiency with severe combined immune deficiency in children. One such inhibitor, deoxycoformycin, a deoxyadenosine analogue, is being studied for its ability to serve as an immunosuppressive medication (Smyth, 1979).

C. Alkylating Agents

These drugs contain an alkyl radical substituted with at least one reactive end group, usually chlorine. These reactive end groups can covalently bind with other molecules. The presence of two or more reactive groups allows binding to two or more different molecules, which can result in cross linking to a large molecule such as DNA. Because cross-linked DNA cannot replicate, alkylating agents impair cellular division (Roberts *et al.*, 1971). These agents also affect major cellular proteins and ribonucleic acids. Potential toxicities include predisposition to lymphoreticular malignancies including leukemia (Steinberg *et al.*, 1978; Grunwald and Rosner, 1979).

D. Nitrogen Mustard

Nitrogen mustard, a bifunctional alkylating agent, interferes with cell replication and other cellular processes by mechanisms noted above. It acts through all stages of the cell cycle. Clearance from the blood after intravenous administration is rapid: 90% is cleared within the first minute. The drug is detoxified and then cleared through the urine.

Typical doses are 0.4 to 0.6 mg/kg given intravenously every 3 to 4 weeks. Thrombosis and phlebitis may result from direct contact of the medication with the intima of the injected vein. Nausea and emesis may be alleviated by appropriate premedication. Leukopenia and thrombocytopenia are common, often within days of initiation of therapy; they may last as long as 3 weeks after a single dose. The therapeutic index of nitrogen mustard in experimental animals is much lower than that of cyclophosphamide with regard to immunosuppressive effects.

E. Cyclophosphamide

Cyclophosphamide, a cyclic phosphoramide mustard, contains a ring structure that renders the drug essentially inert by reducing the reactivity of the terminal chlorine atoms. It is metabolized, primarily by the liver, to several alkylating, and, unlike other alkylating agents, phosphorylating metabolites (Brock *et al.*, 1971). Low doses of oral cyclophosphamide may be more completely metabolized than large intravenous boluses.

After a single large intravenous dose, the serum half-life is about 5 hr. Approximately 15% of the unmetabolized drug is excreted by the kidney; an additional 60% is excreted by the kidney in metabolized form. Since renal clearance is impaired in patients with renal insufficiency, drug doses need to be reduced to reduce risks of toxicity (Bagley *et al.*, 1973; Cohen *et al.*, 1970; Mouridsen and Jacobsen, 1975). Drugs that affect hepatic enzymes (mixed-function oxidases) that metabolize cyclophosphamide may alter its metabolism. These include steroids, phenobarbital, and many other drugs that act on the mixed-function oxidases (Gershwin *et al.*, 1974). Allopurinol may also enhance toxicity by mechanisms that are unclear.

Cyclophosphamide acts primarily during the S phase of the cell cycle, resulting in inactivation of rapidly proliferating cells. Nonproliferating populations are also affected, often to an extent that prevents self-repair. Therefore, cyclophosphamide tends to reduce antibody production when given at the same time as antigen or when given after antigen (Turk and Parker, 1982). This is one of the reasons for its use in preparing patients for bone marrow grafting (Camitta *et al.*, 1976) and, in smaller doses, for kidney transplantation (Starzl *et al.*, 1971). In addition to these actions, cyclophosphamide has antiinflammatory properties (Stevens and Willoughby, 1969).

The toxicity of cyclophosphamide includes bone marrow suppression and, in high doses, predisposition to infection. Leukopenia appears to be dose related; however, a previously tolerated dose may lead to marked leukopenia as much as 1 or 2 years after initiation of treatment, as the marrow loses its capacity to regenerate rapidly. Alopecia, usually resulting from high doses, is generally reversible on reduction of or discontinuing the medication.

One of the most serious toxicities of cyclophosphamide is damage to the urinary tract, resulting from damage to transitional epithelium by metabolites of the drug. This process is enhanced in the bladder, where there are high concentrations of metabolites for long periods. Cystitis, bladder fibrosis, intractable hemorrhage, and bladder carcinoma may result (Johnson and Meadows, 1971; Ansell and Castro, 1975). The risk of some of these toxicities may be lessened by the concurrent intravenous administration of large volumes of fluid and by frequent emptying of the bladder. Acetylcysteine may someday prove effective in preventing bladder complications. Cyclophosphamide may also cause other malignancies, especially lymphomas and leukemias (Puri and Campbell, 1977; Krause, 1982). This may be in part a result of chronic changes in bone marrow stem cells; for instance, cyclophosphamide caused decreased long-term suppression of granulocyte colony formation in rheumatoid arthritis patients (Thomas *et al.*, 1983). In one series, 19 of 2006 patients with rheumatologic diseases who received cyclophosphamide developed leukemia; the rate was greater than 20 times that expected (Kahn *et al.*, 1979). Because of similar reports, some investigators believe that the use of cyclophosphamide in patients with nonmalignant diseases should be reserved for life-threatening complications (Grunwald and Rosner, 1979; Kovarsky, 1983).

As with other alkylating agents, cyclophosphamide can damage the germinal epithelium, resulting in azoospermia within a year in males, although libido and potency are unaffected, as are Leydig and Sertoli cells (Lazowski *et al.*, 1982). Damage to prepubertal testes may be reversible following withdrawal of the drug if duration of treatment and dosage have been modest. In women, cyclophosphamide can inhibit thecal cell proliferation, preventing follicular formation as well as formation of ova. Amenorrhea often occurs in premenopausal women within a few years of initiation of therapy; estrogen levels are reduced. The possible secondary immunoregulatory effects of cyclophosphamide mediated by sex hormone changes have not been explored.

Very large doses may result in myocardial or pulmonary toxicity. Moderate doses can induce an antidiuretic-hormone-like effect (DeFronzo *et al.*, 1973), requiring the administration of saline in addition to glucose solutions to avoid hyponatremia. Prophylatic treatment with antiemetics can reduce the nausea and vomiting that accompany intravenous administration of large doses. Intermittent intravenous doses of cyclophosphamide (0.5 g/m^2 to 1.0 g/m^2) every 3 to 4 weeks with large volumes (>4 liters for adults) of intravenous fluids appear to increase the efficacy and reduce the toxicity of cyclophosphamide (Carette *et al.*, 1983).

F. Chlorambucil

Chlorambucil, a bifunctional alkylating agent, is structurally related to nitrogen mustard; the methyl group is replaced by phenylbutyric acid. It is metabolized by the β-oxidation of the butyric acid to 2(4-N, N-bis-2-chloroethylaminophenyl)acetic acid, which is probably responsible for most of the cytotoxic activity of the drug (McLean *et al.*, 1976).

At low doses, chlorambucil appears to exert a stronger effect on lymphopoiesis than on granulopoiesis (Stukov, 1976). Higher doses suppress all stem cells of the hematopoietic system. In combination chemotherapy, it synergizes with other drugs in its action on lymphopoiesis but not on granulocytopoiesis (Stukov, 1976). The effectiveness of chlorambucil is said to be enhanced without increasing toxicity by giving it conjugated to anti-T-lymphocyte globulin. Chlorambucil can be bound to antibody to target organs without reducing the alkylating activity of the drug (Ghose *et al.*, 1977).

The usual dosage is 0.05 to 0.20 mg/kg per day orally. The most worrisome toxicity is bone marrow depression. Either leukopenia or thrombocytopenia may occur during the course of therapy. Although these usually are rapidly reversible on early withdrawal of drug, occasional patients fail to recover marrow function. This has been reported in several patients with rheumatologic diseases (Rudd *et al.*, 1975). Overdosage has been reported to cause renal failure and seizures (Blank *et al.*, 1983).

Additional problems include nausea, vomiting, hepatitis (perhaps a hypersensitivity reaction), infertility in both sexes (as in cyclophosphamide therapy; Lazowski, 1982), and mutagenicity. The exact risk of develoment of lymphoreticular malignancy is unknown; however, chlorambucil treatment seems to be particularly associated with various types of leukemia and lymphoma (Cameron, 1977; Chaplin, 1982; Greene, *et al.*, 1982;

Albanin *et al.*, 1983), especially if treatment extends beyond 3 years (Kahn and deSeze 1975). Chromosomal damage, as measured by sister chromatid exchange (Clare *et al.*, 1982), was found in one study to be related to dosage and duration of therapy, particularly in a patient who died because of leukemia (Palmer *et al.*, 1984). It is possible that monitoring of sister chromatid exchange may allow more accurate determination of the risk of developing malignancy.

G. Methotrexate

Methotrexate is an analogue of folic acid whose binding to folic reductase has an affinity 10^5 times that of the natural substrate, dihydrofolic acid. This binding blocks conversion of dihydrofolic acid to tetrahydrofolic acid and then to N^5,N^{10}-methylenetetrahydrofolic acid. This in turn prevents one-carbon transfer required for thymidine synthesis, preventing synthesis of DNA. In this manner, methotrexate is able to kill proliferating, but not resting, cells. Proliferating cells not yet irreversibly damaged by methotrexate can be rescued by administration of folinic acid (N^5-formyltetrahydrofolic acid), which overcomes the metabolic block.

Methotrexate may be given orally or parentally. Oral administration results in only 60% absorption. Serum proteins bind half of the circulating drug, which can be displaced by other drugs such as salicylates and sulfonamides. The plasma half-life is about 2 hr (Henderson *et al.*, 1965). Most of the medication is excreted in the urine unchanged within 24 hr. Despite substantial biliary excretion, nearly complete intestinal reabsorption results in little fecal excretion of methotrexate.

Immunosuppression depends on dosage and schedule (Pinedo *et al.*, 1977; Eichholtz and Trott, 1980; Groff *et al.*, 1983; Jolivet *et al.*, 1983). Daily methotrexate is more effective than weekly administration in suppressing antibody formation (Berenbaum, 1962; Santos *et al.*, 1964; Swanson and Schwartz, 1967). Immunosuppression results whether antigen is given at the initiation of treatment or during the course of therapy. No suppression is observed when methotrexate is given prior to the antigen (Hersh *et al.*, 1966).

Toxic effects include leukopenia, thrombocytopenia, stomatitis, nausea, vomiting, and diarrhea. These are reduced by folinic acid (Gorgun and Watne, 1966; Mitchell *et al.*, 1969). Leukemia has been reported (Advani *et al.*, 1983). Long-term daily treatment or treatment of patients with underlying liver diseases may lead to cirrhosis. Toxic effects are seen more commonly when methotrexate is administered daily.

Methotrexate may be given orally in three divided doses separated by 12 hr each weekend, or it may be given parenterally once a week. Adult dosages range from 5 to 40 mg per week. Use of the drug during the first 3 months of pregnancy is associated with a high risk of teratogenesis. The increased toxicity of methotrexate in renal failure may be reduced by decreasing the dosage. Increased risk of malignancy has not been documented in patients who have taken the drug.

H. 5-Fluorouracil

5-Fluorouracil, a pyrimidine analogue that competes with uracil in intermediary metabolic pathways, is converted into fluorodeoxyuridine rather than thymidine. This results in inhibition of thymidylate synthetase, a rate-limiting enzyme required for DNA synthesis. The drug is effective at all phases of the cell cycle. Most metabolism and excretion is hepatic rather than renal. Major toxicity is generally seen with daily administration rather than intermittent bolus therapy. The earliest side effect may be mucocutaneous erythema; ulcerative stomatitis and gastrointestinal ulcerations may ensue. Other side effects include nausea and vomiting, thrombocytopenia, granulocytopenia, alopecia, erythematous dermatitis, and cerebellar ataxia.

I. Hydroxyurea

Hydroxyurea kills cells in S phase and prevents other cells form entering that phase. Oral administration, resulting in peak blood levels 1 to $2^1/_2$ hr later, is followed by rapid renal excretion of more than half the dose within 8 hr. Side effects include thrombocytopenia and leukopenia, both of which can be seen during the first 2 days after administration, with recovery occurring over the following week. Other toxic effects include oral and gastrointestinal ulcerations, nausea and vomiting, and a maculopapular rash.

J. Vincristine

Vincristine, an alkaloid extracted from the periwinkle plant *Vinca rosea,* irreversibly interferes with the assembly of the protein subunits of the mitotic spindle. The drug is therefore specific for the M phase of the cell cycle. However, arrest at M phase can result from exposure to vincristine during earlier phases.

Most of the drug is cleared from the blood within 30 min of parenteral administration. Most excretion is hepatic. The drug can suppress bone marrow function within 12 to 18 hr after injection; recovery occurs by about 36 hr. Marrow suppression can result in leukopenia or thrombocytopenia, particularly at high doses or after prolonged therapy. Thrombocytosis has been observed after short-term therapy. Neurotoxicity is the major side effect. Peripheral neuropathy, which may be manifested by severe paresthesias and muscle weakness, can result in wasting. Vocal cord paralysis can cause hoarseness, and cranial nerve palsies (bilateral ptosis, diplopia), cerebellar signs, convulsions, coma, and depression may also occur. Urinary incontinence may be secondary to bladder atony. Furthermore, patients may develop severe constipation and even paralytic ileus. For this reason, adequate hydration is important, and prophylactic stool softeners should be given.

Toxicity can also result in alopecia, patchy liver necrosis, oral and gastrointestinal ulcerations, rash, nausea and vomiting, mutagenicity, orthostatic hypotension, and inappropriate secretion of ADH. Extravasation from injection sites causes severe, painful inflammatory reactions; if extensive, this can lead to phlebitis and cellulitis. Because of hepatobiliary excretion, hepatic damage or biliary obstruction can contribute to more severe neurotoxicity.

K. Vinblastine

Vinblastine, an alkaloid related to vincristine, binds more reversibly to the mitotic spindle. Neurotoxicity is usually not as severe; more significant side effects, such as paralytic ileus, are less likely to occur. Vinblastine bound to platelets has been used to treat idiopathic thrombocytopenia (Ahn *et al.*, 1978).

L. Levamisole

This three-ringed antihelminthic drug has a molecular weight of about 241. Although stable in aqueous solutions in acid, it is hydrolyzed in alkaline solutions. Readily absorbed from the gastrointestinal tract, it has a plasma half-life of about 4 hr. Peak blood levels occur 2 hr after an oral dose (Symoens and Rosenthal, 1977). Following hepatic metabolism, it is excreted primarily through the urine. Small amounts of the unmetabolized drug may be found in urine, breast milk, tears, and respiratory secretions.

Levamisole amplifies nonspecific inflammatory functions by increasing neutrophil and monocyte chemotaxis and phagocytosis (Snyderman *et al.*, 1978; Rabson *et al.*, 1977), particularly when these functions are impaired. However, several studies have failed to show improved host defenses against infections (Wright *et al.*, 1977; Hogan and Hill, 1978; Donabedian *et al.*, 1982). In general, the drug increases resistance to secondary infections to a much greater extent than to primary infections.

In addition to its inflammatory effects, levamisole has a more direct action on early stages of T-cell function, resulting in increased helper, amplifier, cytotoxic, and suppressor T-cell functions (Sampson and Luir, 1976). It can reverse skin anergy and increase numbers of circulating T cells in patients with decreased numbers, usually with a decrease in non-T, non-B cells (suggesting maturation of pre-T cells) (Rosenthal *et al.*, 1976). As a result of these actions, an indirect stimulatory effect on antibody production has been described (Miller *et al.*, 1980). It may be more effective when combined with appropriate lymphocyte-depleting agents (Zulman *et al.*, 1978). The multiple effects of levamisole may explain its ability to improve some experimental autoimmune diseases and worsen others.

Levamisole has been used to treat malignancies, aphthous stomatitis, herpes labialis, Crohn's disease, rheumatoid arthritis, and systemic lupus (Lehner *et al.*, 1976; Symoens and Brugmans, 1974; Kint and Verlinden, 1974; Segal *et al.*, 1977; Runge *et al.*, 1977; Scott *et al.*, 1978; Miller *et al.*, 1980). Unfortunately, there are many side effects. The most dangerous is granulocytopenia, frequent in patients with rheumatic diseases (Symoens and Brugmans, 1974; Miller *et al.*, 1980). Agranulocytosis may be particularly common in patients with HLA B27 (Schmidt and Mueller-Eckhardt, 1977; Veys *et al.*, 1978). Although corticosteroids have been recommended for protection against this complication, three deaths have been reported in patients receiving both drugs (Clara and Germanes, 1977).

Other side effects include nausea and vomiting, fatigue and drowsiness, urticarial skin rash, and drug fever. Levamisole stimulates both sympathetic and parasympathetic systems, has positive chronotropic and inotropic effects on the heart, and inhibits alkaline phosphatases. In summary, despite some favorable results in patients with rheumatoid arthritis, the side effects may outweigh the benefits.

M. Steroid Hormones

Sex hormones have been shown to be immunoregulatory. For instance, androgens can suppress numerous immune responses in animals (Eidinger and Garrett, 1972; Castro *et al.*, 1973; Terres *et al.*, 1968, Batchelor, 1971; Wasi and Block, 1961; Steinberg *et al.*, 1978) as well as improve the manifestations of spontaneous autoimmune disease (Steinberg *et al.*, 1978; Raveche *et al.*, 1976; Roubinian *et al.*, 1977; Duvic *et al.*, 1978; Melez,

1978 a,b). Androgens probably cause these effects by multiple mechanisms, although they have not been well studied. It appears that androgens affect a variety of gene expressions in such processes as hypothalamic imprinting, thymocyte maturation, stem-cell maturation, and clearance of immune complexes. However, the toxicities of androgens make their use in autoimmune disease problematic despite the use of danazol in hereditary angioneurotic edema (Spaulding, 1960; Davis *et al.*, 1974; Sheffer *et al.*, 1977; Gelfand *et al.*, 1976).

Corticosteroids at high doses suppress the induction of both cellular and humoral immune responses. However, there may be great differences between the high daily doses given in the past and the generally lower doses currently used. Furthermore, bolus therapy may have effects not observed with lower daily doses. Additional effects on human lymphocytes include suppression of stem-cell differentiation, stimulation of B-cell differentiation without proliferation, and direct and indirect effects on macrophages. Therefore, it is often difficult to know the mechanisms of action by which a given drug dose may work.

N. Cyclosporin A

Although originally used as an antifungal agent, cyclosporin has proven to be more useful as an immunoregulator. Because it is a cyclic peptide with N-methylated amino acids (Borel *et al.*, 1976), it is resistant to the acid pH found in the stomach as well as to proteolytic enzymes secreted into the small intestine. The drug is active without further metabolism but is poorly soluble in water (a consideration for parenteral use).

Probably because cyclosporin is effective in reducing T-cell function (Navarro and Touraine, 1983) without major marrow suppression, it has been found especially effective in preventing rejection of transplanted kidneys (Starzl *et al.*, 1981; White and Calne, 1982) and other transplanted organs (Canafax and Ascher, 1983). In fact, cyclosporin appears to be ushering in an era of increased boldness in nonrenal organ transplantation because of its effectiveness in suppressing T-cell functions (White and Calne, 1982).

The exact mechanism of action of the drug is under active investigation. It seems to interfere with early stages in T cell activation that are dependent on interleukin 2 (Larsson, 1980; White and Calne, 1982; Bendtzen *et al.*, 1983). Since this results in reduction of helper T-cell function, it might be anticipated that cyclosporin would also reduce T-cell-dependent B-cell functions; evidence for this has been reported (Cammisuli, 1981). In addition, cyclosporin inhibits early B-cell activation (Muraguchi *et al.*, 1983). It has been suggested that the drug might have a direct effect on a B-cell subset (Kunkel and Klaus, 1980). Despite this, the net effect of therapy is increased serum IgG concentrations (White and Calne, 1982).

Cyclosporin has proven useful in alleviating graft-versus-host (GVH) disease in patients receiving bone marrow transplantation. This is because of the ability of the drug to impair T-cell-mediated GVH without injuring rapidly dividing stem cells of transplanted marrow. The utility of cyclosporin in rheumatic diseases is not yet proven, although such diseases as polymyositis and rheumatoid arthritis might be favorably treated. Clinical trials have yet to support this enthusiasm.

Despite its lack of marrow suppression, cyclosporin has other major side effects. Nephrotoxicity can be severe, an especial problem in patients receiving renal allografts, but also in other patients. Activation of Epstein–Barr virus and lymphoma development have been noted. Other side effects include gum hypertrophy, transient hirsutism, and liver function test abnormalities. However, bacterial infections have not been reported as a side effect.

O. Dapsone

This sulfone (4,4′-diaminodiphenylsulfone) has been used for a long time for the treatment of leprosy. It has recently been reported as effective in treating bullous skin diseases, especially those characterized by granulocyte infiltration such as in dermatitis herpetiformis (Katz *et al.*, 1980), erythema elevatum diutinum (Katz *et al.*, 1977), and the uncommon bullous eruptions of patients with lupus (Hall *et al.*, 1982). It is absorbed well after oral administration, and the plasma half-life is approximately 1 day (Mandell and Sande, 1980). It is acetylated in the liver and excreted primarily through the kidney.

Dapsone therapy is begun at doses of 50 to 100 mg daily, with increases up to 200 to 400 mg per day. Side effects, dose related, include hemolysis and methemoglobinemia, which may be tolerable if mild. Other side effects include gastrointestinal intolerance and occasionally peripheral neuropathy, nervousness, insomnia, and headache.

P. Other Drugs

Certain drugs used in rheumatic diseases, such as colchicine and indomethacin, vitamins, and even heavy metals (Koller *et al.*, 1976), may modulate immune responses by a variety of mechanisms. Because of the variety of cells involved in immune responses and the various feedback control mechanisms, many of these agents may decrease immune responses under some circumstances and increase them in others. In addition, a large number of cytotoxic or cytostatic drugs used in cancer chemotherapy to the exclusion of autoimmune diseases have immunoregulatory effects.

Recently, interleukin-2 (IL-2) and γ-interferon (IFN) have been used in preliminary studies to treat patients with the acquired immune deficiency syndrome (AIDS) (Lane *et al.*, 1984). AIDS is a recently described syndrome caused by a retrovirus with a tropism for human T cells; there is no known cure. The clinical manifestations include opportunistic infections (particularly by cytomegalovirus, *Candida*, and *Pneumocystis carinii*) and Kaposi's sarcoma (Fauci, 1984). It affects predominantly homosexual or bisexual males but has also been reported in intravenous drug users, Haitians, and hemophiliacs. Patients with AIDS lack functional cellular immune responses because of a loss of helper/inducer T cells (Gottleib *et al.*, 1981; Stahl *et al.*, 1982). Interleukin 2 has been shown to enhance the depressed *in vitro* natural killer and cytomegalovirus-specific cytotoxicities of AIDS lymphocytes (Rook *et al.*, 1983). Clinical trials of IL-2 or γ-IFN have not yet shown beneficial effects *in vivo*.

VII. IMMUNOSUPPRESSION BY PHYSICAL AGENTS

A. Ionizing Radiation

The interaction of X rays and γ rays with atoms in living tissues will result in ejection of electrons from irradiated atoms. If the irradiation is of sufficient energy, ejected electrons will ionize surrounding atoms, resulting in the formation of reactive free radicals. These radicals, in turn, can damage a variety of organic molecules important to cellular function, especially nuclear DNA. It is for this reason that radiation has the greatest effect on rapidly dividing cells such as those found in the immune system, bone marrow, and intestinal epithelium. Irradiated lymphocytes have high mortality rates without having to undergo division (interphase death); most other cells die only after one or two postirradiation mitoses (mitotic death). Furthermore, T- and B-cell subsets vary in their sensitivity to low doses of irradiation: precursor cells, particularly suppressor precursors, have greater sensitivity to low doses of radiation. B cells prior to terminal clonal proliferation are more sensitive than are helper T cells, probably because they require more divisions to become functional.

Among B-cell subsets that vary in radiation sensitivity, those that bear surface immunoglobulin are more sensitive than those with surface receptors for complement (Rand *et al.*, 1978). However, B cells are more radioresistant to ultraviolet radiation than are T cells (Horowitz *et al.*, 1974). The effect of irradiation on the immune response is dose dependent: responses may be increased at low doses and decreased at high doses because of varying radiosensitivities of lymphocyte subpopulations (Macario and Conway de Macario, 1978). In addition, effects on the immune system will depend on the frequency of administration of radiation because of differences in the abilities of lymphocyte subsets to repair radiation damage.

Total-body irradiation leads to marked side effects, and it has generally been reserved in clinical practice for preparation for bone marrow transplantation. A modification of this procedure, called total lymphoid irradiation (TLI), is used in the treatment of lymphoid malignancies. Total lymphoid irradiation involves the irradiation of lymph nodes and spleen with shielding of nonlymphoid tissues as completely as possible. Although the heart and spine are well shielded, the lungs cannot be completely shielded; thus, at high doses of TLI, pneumonitis can be a complication.

Recent studies suggest that TLI may be of benefit for patients with severe rheumatoid arthritis that is refractory to more conventional treatment including immunosuppressive medications (Trentham *et al.*, 1981; Kotzin *et al.*, 1981). Preliminary studies in mice with lupus and with a few patients with lupus (Tanay *et al.*, 1984) have also suggested benefit. Side effects have been noted; in one center, several serious infections in rheumatoid arthritis patients were reported, and two of ten patients died after TLI. Therefore, this procedure remains experimental; future controlled trials will determine the best role for TLI in the treatment of nonmalignant autoimmune disease. It is possible that lower doses than have been studied will be as effective in these diseases, since lower doses may still result in induction of suppressor cells, which may be the reason for the effectiveness of TLI.

Although not well studied, ultraviolet light may also prove to be useful in the treatment of nonmalignant immune diseases. It is possible that the benefits of warm climates for rheumatoid arthritis patients result in part from increased exposure to ultraviolet radiation. In animal studies, UV radiation has been shown to reduce numbers of Ia^+ macrophages. In studying the usefulness of UV light in patients, its potential adverse effects will have to be considered.

B. Physical Removal of Cells or Soluble Plasma Substances

Physical removal of antibody has been used in the treatment of the hyperviscosity syndrome of Waldenstrom's macroglobulinemia, either by itself or as an adjunct to medical treatment (Bloch and Maki, 1973). This has been accomplished by means of plasma exchange through continuous-flow centrifugation (Russell *et al.*, 1977). This has been reported to be useful in the treatment of autoimmune thrombocytopenia, autoimmune hemolytic anemia, myasthenia gravis, multiple sclerosis, Goodpasture's syndrome, other forms of glomerulonephritis, and severe rhesus disease (Branda *et al.*, 1975; Lockwood *et al.*, 1977; Dau *et al.*, 1977; Graham-Pole *et al.*, 1977; Pusey and Lockwood, 1982; Hauser *et al.*, 1982; Valbonesi *et al.*, 1982, Valbonesi and Garelli, 1983; Dau, 1982; Shumak and Rock, 1984). Plasmapheresis may also be useful in removing serum factors that inhibit tumor rejection and in reducing circulating immune complexes in autoimmune diseases such as rheumatoid arthritis (Karsh *et al.*, 1981; Bennett and Hamburger, 1982) and systemic lupus erythematosus (Jones *et al.*, 1976; Terman *et al.*, 1977b), although its efficacy was not shown in a well-controlled trial in which sham pheresis was also studied (Wei *et al.*, 1983). This treatment suffers from the theoretical disadvantage of rebound in antibody production to levels higher than pretreatment, possibly as a result of removal of suppressive factors and antibodies. This type of rebound seems to be more of a problem with primary than secondary responses (Branda *et al.*, 1975). However, adjunctive treatment with immunosuppressive drugs may prevent such rebound (L'Abbate *et al.*, 1983). It is possible that plasmapheresis could result in preferential removal of specific antibodies such as those against DNA (Terman *et al.*, 1977a).

VIII. IMMUNOREGULATION IN SPECIFIC DISEASES

The use of immunoregulation in individual human disorders depends on the ability of an agent to arrest or ameliorate the disease process without causing significant immediate or long-term toxicities as well as on the availability of alternative therapies. Furthermore, patients with particular diseases vary greatly; their therapy should be individualized to a certain extent. Therefore, it is not possible to outline here the uses of immunoregulatory agents in particular disorders without qualifying each with regard to individual involvement, severity, reversibility, and other factors. The rapid progress being made in the study of immunoregulation in animals and humans permits the hope that newer approaches will soon be available. Nonetheless, it is useful to illustrate some of the applications of particular immunoregulatory therapies to a variety of diseases. Although some of these applications are widespread despite the lack of evidence of established efficacy by randomized trials, there are many therapies that are effective and whose use has been proven to be better than preexisting treatments. Finally, there are treatments not yet widespread whose efficacy may soon be established by appropriate trials. This category includes the use of intermittent boluses of cyclophosphamide in patients with life-threatening active systemic lupus.

Some diseases in which immunoregulatory therapy may be of benefit are listed in Table 3. This list is neither exhaustive nor a recommendation for therapy. Additional diseases could have been included. The list does indicate that drugs initially used for treatment of neoplasms are now used for numerous nonmalignant diseases. Future studies should be directed at additional modalities such as antiidiotype or other antireceptor antibodies, immunoregulatory molecules, drug-bound monoclonal antibodies (Feinerman *et al.*, 1983), drug-containing liposomes (Yatvin and Lelkes, 1982), and combinations of therapies. The possibility that cells can be cloned and give rise to immunosuppressive

Table 3. Immunoregulatory Therapy of Some Rheumatologic Diseases[a]

Disease	Therapy	References
Rheumatoid arthritis	Azathioprine	Currey *et al.*, 1974; Abel *et al.*, 1978; Whisnant and Pelkey, 1982; Groff *et al.*, 1983; Iannuzzi *et al.*, 1983; Willkens, 1983
Systemic lupus erythematosus	Nitrogen mustard Azathioprine Cyclophosphamide Pulse methylprednisolone	Donadio *et al.*, 1972; Hahn, 1973; Donadio *et al.*, 1978; Dosa, 1978 ; Klippel, 1979; Kimberly *et al.*, 1981; Liebling *et al.*, 1982; Wallace *et al.*, 1982; Carette *et al.*, 1983
Dermatomyositis	Methotrexate	Metzger *et al.*, 1974; Henriksson and Sandstedt, 1982; Winkelmann, 1982
Psoriatic arthritis	Methotrexate Azathioprine	Willkens, 1983
Wegener's granulomatosis	Cyclophosphamide	Fauci *et al.*, 1983

[a] This list is neither exhaustive nor conclusive. The references listed are selective; they include reviews and clinical trials. Many additional studies have been published. Additional information concerning long-term response to and toxicity from the immunoregulatory therapies listed will result in changes in this list.

factors holds out the promise of nontoxic or less toxic immunosuppression. Additional studies of immune enhancement should be directed at subsets of cells and involve agents less toxic than those currently used (such as levamisole).

For the present, we must rely on the drugs mentioned in this review. The guidelines listed in Table 4 may provide a basis for determining whether a patient is a candidate for immunosuppression. If a patient has a disorder without a demonstrated effective agent, potential new drugs for the disorder are best studied as part of randomized trials in which they are compared to standard therapy.

Table 4. Guidelines for the Use of Immunoregulatory Agents in Rheumatologic Diseases

1. The disease should be life-threatening (e.g., severe lupus nephritis) or severely debilitating (e.g., severe rheumatoid arthritis).
2. Conventional therapy has proven unable to stabilize the disease in the absence of intolerable toxicity.
3. Disease manifestations are considered reversible.
4. The patient has no infections (if agent used suppresses host defenses).
5. Clearly defined clinical parameters are carefully monitored before, during, and after therapy to determine efficacy of treatment. Parameters include those that are subject to toxic effects of therapy.
6. If part of study, a protocol is used that is approved by peer review and includes informed consent. If very few patients with a particular disease are available, multicenter studies should be considered.
7. Before use of treatment, patients should be screened for contraindications (e.g., liver disease or alcohol intake excludes methotrexate). The ability of patients to comply with the treatment regimen in terms of their psychosocial situations should be considered.
8. The effects of withdrawal (i.e., flare-up of disease) should be anticipated if the agent needs to be discontinued because of toxicity. Alternative treatment should be planned.
9. Drug interactions need to be considered (e.g., allopurinol and azathioprine).
10. Periodic reevaluation of treatment will allow medications to be tapered or discontinued when treatment goals have been attained or when toxicities are more severe than benefits of treatment.

REFERENCES

Abdou, N. I., Zweiman, B., and Casella, S. R., 1973, Effects of azathioprine therapy on bone marrow-dependent and thymus-dependent cells in man, *Clin. Exp. Immunol.* **13**:55–64.

Abel, T., Urowitz, M. B., Smythe, H. A., Keystone, E. C., and Norman, C. B., 1978, Long-term effects of azathioprine in rheumatoid arthritis, *Arthritis Rheum.* **21**:539–543.

Adam, A., Ciobraru, R., Petit, J. F., and Lederer, E., 1972, Isolation and properties of a macromolecular water soluble, immuno-adjuvant fraction from the cell wall of *Mycobacterium smegmatis, Proc. Natl. Acad. Sci. U.S.A.* **69**:851–854.

Advani, S. H., Doval, D. C., Gopal, R., Nair, C. N., and Kutty, P. M., 1983, Therapy-related leukemia. A report of five patients and a review of the literature, *Oncology* **40**:268–272.

Ahn, Y. S., Byrnes, J. J., Harrington, W. J., Cayer, M. L., Smith, D. S., Brunskill, D. E., and Pall, L. M., 1978, The treatment of idiopathic thrombocytopenia with vinblastine-loaded platelets, *N. Engl. J. Med.* **298**:1101–1107.

Albanin, K. S., LeBeau, M. M., Vardiman, J. W., Golomb, H. M., and Rowley, J. D., 1983, Development of dysmyelopoietic syndrome in a hairy cell leukemia patient treated with chlorambucil: Cytogenetic and morphologic evaluation, *Cytogenetics* **8**:107–115.

Ansell, I. D., and Castro, J. E., 1975, Carcinoma of the bladder complicating cyclophosphamide therapy, *Br. J. Urol.* **47**:413–418.

Audibert, F., Chedid, L., Lefrancier, P., and Chory, J., 1976, Distinctive adjuvanticity of synthetic analogs of mycobacterial water-soluble components, *Cell. Immunol.* **21**:243–249.

Bagley, C. M., Jr., Bostick, F. W., and Devita, V. T., 1973, Clinical pharmacology of cyclophosphamide, *Cancer Res.* **33**:226–233.

Batchelor, J. R., 1971, Hormonal control of antibody formation, in: *Regulation of the Antibody Response* (B. Cinander, ed.), Charles C. Thomas, Springfield, IL, pp. 276–293.

Bendtzen, K., Petersen, J., and Soeberg, B., 1983, Effects of cyclosporin A (CyA) and methylprednisolone (MP) on the immune response. I. Further studies of the monocyte-T cell interactions leading to lymphokine production, *Acta Pathol. Microbiol. Immunol. Scand.* **91**:159–167.

Bennett, R. S., and Hamburger, M. I., 1982, A critical review of therapeutic apheresis in the treatment of severe rheumatoid arthritis, *Prog. Clin. Biol. Res.* **106**:33–48.

Berenbaum, M. C., 1962, The effect of cytotoxic agents on the production of antibody to TAB vaccine in the mouse, *Biochem. Pharmacol.* **11**:29–44.

Blank, D. W., Nanji, A. A., Schreiber, D. H., Hudman, C., and Sanders, H. D., 1983, Acute renal failure and seizures associated with chlorambucil overdose, *J. Toxicol. Clin. Toxicol.* **20**:361–365.

Bloch, K. J., and Maki, D. G., 1973, Hyperviscosity syndromes associated with immunoglobulin abnormalities, *Semin. Haematol.* **10**:113–124.

Borel, J. F., Feurer, C., Gubler, H. U., and Stahelin, H., 1976, Biological effects of cyclosporin A: A new antilymphocytic agent, *Agents Actions* **6**:468–475.

Branda, R. F., Moldow, C. F., McCullough, J. J., and Jacobs, H. S., 1975, Plasma exchange in the treatment of immune disease, *Transfusion* **15**:570–576.

Brock, N., Gross, R., Hohorst, H. J., Klein, H. O., and Schneider, B., 1971, Activation of cyclophosphamide in man and animals, *Cancer* **27**:1512–1529.

Brodeur, B. R., and Merigan, T. C., 1975, Mechanism of the suppressive effect of interferon on antibody synthesis *in vivo, J. Immunol.* **114**:1323–1328.

Cameron, S., 1977, Chlorambucil and leukemia, *N. Engl. J. Med.* **296**:1065.

Camitta, B. M., Thomas, E. D., and Nathan, D. G., 1976, Severe aplastic anemia: A prospective study of the effect of early marrow transplantation on acute mortality, *Blood* **48**:63–70.

Cammisuli, S., 1981, Inhibition of a secondary homoral immune response by cyclosporin A, *Transplant. Clin. Immunol.* **13**:15–19.

Canafax, D. M., and Ascher, N. L., 1983, Cyclosporine immunosuppression, *Clin. Pharmacol.* **2**:515–524.

Carette, S., Klippel, J. H., Decker, J. L., Austin, H. A., Plotz, P. H., Steinberg, A. D., and Balow, J. E., 1983, Controlled studies of oral immunosuppressive drugs in lupus nephritis, *Ann. Intern. Med.* **99**:1–8.

Carney, D. M., Zukosi, C. F., and Ogden, D. A., 1974, Massive azathioprine overdose: Case report and review of the literature, *Am. J. Med.* **56**:133–136.

Chedid, L., Audibert, F., Lefrancier, P., Chory, J., and Lederer, E., 1976, Modulation of the immune response by a synthetic adjuvant and analogs, *Prov. Natl. Acad. Sci. U.S.A.* **73**:2472–2475.

Clara, R., and Germanes, J., 1977, Levamisole and agranulocytosis, *Lancet* **1**:47–48.

Clare, M. G., Jones, W. G., and Taylor, J. H., 1982, Sister chromatid exchanges in human lymphocytes exposed to single cytotoxic drugs *in vivo* or *in vitro*, *Eur. J. Cancer Clin. Oncol.* **18**:979–989.

Coffey, J. J., White, C. A., Lesk, A. B., Rogers, W. I., and Serpick, A. A., 1972, Effect of allopurinol on the pharmacokinetics of 6-mercaptopurine (NCS-755) in cancer patients, *Cancer Res* **32**:1283–1289.

Cohen, J. L., Jao, J. Y., and Jusko, W. J., 1970, Pharmacokinetics of cyclophosphamide in man, *Br. J. Pharmocol.* **43**:677–680.

Currey, H. L. F., Harris, J. R. M., Mason, R. M., Woodland, J., Beveridge, T., Roberts, C. J., Vere, D. W., Dixon, A. S. J., Davies, J., and Owen-Smith, B., 1974, Comparison of azathioprine, cyclophosphamide and gold in treatment of rheumatoid arthritis, *Br. Med. J.* **3**:763–768.

Dau, P. C., 1982, Plasmapheresis in myasthenia gravis, *Prog. Clin. Biol. Res.* **88**:265–285.

Dau, P. C., Lindstrom, J. M., Cassel, C. K., Denys, E. H., Shev, E. E., and Spitler, L. E., 1977, Plasmapheresis and immunosuppressive drug therapy in myasthenia gravis, *N. Engl. J. Med.* **297**:1134–1140.

Davis, P. J., Davis, F. B., and Charache, P., 1974, Long-term therapy of hereditary angioedema (HAE), *Johns Hopkins Med. J.* **135**:391–398.

DeFronzo, R. A., Braine, H., and Colvin, O. M., 1973, Water intoxication in man after cyclophosphamide therapy. Time course and relation to drug activation, *Ann. Intern. Med.* **78**:861–869.

Dixon, F. J., and McConahey, P. J., 1963, Enhancement of antibody formation whole body X-irradiation, *J. Exp. Med.* **117**:833–848.

Donabedian, H., Alling, D. W., and Gallin, J. I., 1982, Levamisole is inferior to placebo in the hyperimmunoglobulin E recurrent-infection (Job's) syndrome, *N. Engl. J. Med.* **307**:290–292.

Donadio, J. V., Jr., Holley, K. E., and Wagoner, R. D., 1972, Treatment of lupus nephritis with prednisone and combined prednisone and azathioprine, *Ann. Intern. Med.* **77**:829–835.

Donadio, J. V., Jr., Holley, K. E., Ferguson, R. H., and Illstrup, D. M., 1978, Treatment of diffuse proliferative lupus nephritis with prednisone and combined prednisone and cyclphosphamide, *N. Engl. J. Med.* **299**:1151–1155.

Dosa, S., Cairns, S. S., and Lawler, W., 1978, Treatment of lupus nephritis by methyl prednisolone pulse therapy, *Postgrad. Med. J.* **54**:628–632.

Duvic, M., Steinberg, A. D., and Klassen, L. W., 1978, Effect of the anti-estrogen, Nafoxidine, on NZB/W autoimmune disease, *Arthritis Rheum.* **21**:414–417.

Eichholtz, H., and Trott, K.-R., 1980, Effect of methotrexate concentration and exposure time on mammalian cell survival *in vitro*, *Br. J. Cancer* **41**:277–284.

Eidinger, D., and Garrett, T. J., 1972, Studies of the regulatory effects of sex hormones on antibody formation and stem cell differentiation, *J. Exp. Med.* **136**:1098–1116.

Elion, G. B., 1967, Biochemistry and pharmacology of purine analogues, *Fed. Proc.* **26**:898–903.

Elion, G. B., 1972, Significance of azathioprine metabolites, *Proc. R. Soc. Med.* **65**:257–260.

Fauci, A. S., Moderator, 1984, Acquired immunodeficiency syndrome: Epidemiologic, clinical, immunologic, and therapeutic considerations, *Ann. Intern. Med.* **100**:92–106.

Fauci, A. S., Haynes, B. F., Katz, P., and Wolff, S. M., 1983, Wegener's granulomatosis: Prospective clinical and therapeutic experience with 85 patients for 21 years, *Ann. Intern. Med.* **98**:76–85.

Feinerman, B., Paul, R. D., and Feinerman, G., 1983, Treatment of a murine leukemia with chlorambucil bound monoclonal antibodies, *Adv. Exp. Med. Biol.* **166**:59–66.

Freund, J., 1947, Some aspects of active immunization, *Annu. Rev. Microbiol.* **1**:291–308.

Friedman, E. A., Gelfand, M. C., and Bernheimer, H. P., 1971, Synergism in immunosuppression. I. Effect of combination immunosuppressive drugs on tetanus antitoxin production in the mouse, *Transplantation* **11**:479–486.

Gelfand, J. A., Sherrins, R. J., Alling, D. W., and Frank, M. M., 1976, Treatment of hereditary angioedema with Danazole. Reversal of clinical and biochemical abnormalities, *N. Engl. J. Med.* **295**:1444–1448.

Gelfand, M. C., Steinberg, A. D., Nagle, R., and Knepshield, J. H., 1972, Therapeutic studies in NZB/W mice. I. Synergy of azathioprine, cyclophosphamide and methylprednisolone in combination, *Arthritis Rheum.* **15**:239–246.

Gershwin, M. E., Goetzl, E. J., and Steinberg, A. D., 1974, Cyclophosphamide: Use in practice, *Ann. Intern. Med.* **80**:531–540.

Ghose, T., Norvell, S. T., Gluclu, A., Bodurtha, A., Tai, J., and MacDonald, A. S., 1977, Immunochemotherapy of malignant melanoma with chlorambucil-bound antimelanoma globulins: Preliminary results in patients with disseminated disease, *J. Natl. Cancer Inst.* **58**:845–852.

Gorgun, B., and Watne, A. L., 1966, Skin homograft survival in cancer chemotherapy patients, *Cancer* **19:**1316–1320.

Gottlieb, M. S., Schroff, R., Schanker, H. M., Weisman, J. D., Fan, P. T., Wolf, R. A., and Saxon A., 1981, *Pneumocystis carinii* pneumonia and mucosal candidiasis in previously healthy homosexual men: Evidence of a new acquired cellular immunodeficiency, *N. Engl. J. Med.* **305:**1425–1431.

Graham-Pole, J., Barr, W., and Willoughby, M. L., 1977, Continuous-flow plasmapheresis in management of severe rhesus disease, *Br. Med. J.* **1:**1185–1188.

Greene, M. H., Boice, J. D., Jr., Greer, B. E., Blessing, J. A., and Dembo, A. J., 1982, Acute nonlymphocytic leukemia after therapy with alkylating agents for ovarian cancer: A study of five randomized clinical trials, *N. Engl. J. Med.* **307:**1416–1421.

Groff, G. D., Shenberger, K. N., Wilke, W. S., and Taylor, T. H., 1983, Low dose oral methotrexate in rheumatoid arthritis: An uncontrolled trial and review of the literature, *Semin. Arthritis Rheum.* **12:**333–347.

Grunwald, H. W., and Rosner, F., 1979, Acute leukemia and immunosuppressive drug use. A review of patients undergoing immunosuppressive therapy for nonneoplastic diseases, *Arch. Int. Med.* **139:**461–466.

Hahn, B., Bagby, M. K., Hamilton, T. R., and Osteroland, C. K., 1973, Comparison of therapeutic and immunosuppressive effects of azathioprine, prednisolone, and combined therapy in NZB/NZW mice, *Arthritis Rheum.* **16:**162–170.

Hall, R. P., Lawley, T. J., Smith, H. R., and Katz, S. I., 1982, Bullous eruption of systemic lupus erythematosus, *Ann. Intern. Med.* **97:**165–170.

Hamilton, L., and Elion, G. B., 1954, The fate of 6-mercaptopurine in man, *Ann. N.Y. Acad. Sci.* **60:**304–314.

Hauser, S. L., Fosburg, M., Kervy, S., and Weiner, H. L., 1982, Plasmapheresis, lymphocytapheresis, and immunosuppressive drug therapy in multiple sclerosis, *Prog. Clin. Biol. Res.* **106:**239–254.

Henderson, F. S., Adamson, R. H., and Oliverio, V. T., 1965, The metabolic rate of tritiated methotrexate. II. Absorption and excretion in man, *Cancer Res.* **25:**1018–1024.

Hendrick, D., and Mirkin, B. L., 1984, Metabolic disposition and toxicity of 6-mercaptopurine after massive overdose, *Lancet* **1:**277.

Henriksson, K. G., and Sandstedt, P., 1982, Polymyositis—treatment and prognosis. A study of 107 patients, *Acta Neurol. Scand.* **65:**280–300.

Herber, S., Lennard, L., Lilleyman, J. S., and Maddocks, J., 1982, 6-mercaptopurine: Apparent lack of relation between prescribed dose and biological effect in children with leukaemia, *Brit. J. Cancer* **46:**138–141.

Hersh, E. M., Carbone, P. O., and Freireich, E. J., 1966, Recovery of immune responsiveness after drug suppression in man, *J. Lab. Clin. Med.* **67:**566–572.

Hiu, I. J., 1972, Water-soluble and lipid-free fraction from BCG with adjuvant and antitumor activity, *Nature (New Biol.)* **238:**241–242.

Hogan, N. A., and Hill, H. R., 1978, Enhancement of neutrophil chemotaxis and alternation of levels of cellular cyclic nucleotides by levamisole, *J. Infect. Dis.* **138:**437–444.

Hoover, R., and Fraumeni, J. F., Jr., 1973, Risk of cancer of renal-transplant recipients, *Lancet* **2:**55–57.

Horowitz, S., Cripps, D., and Hong, R., 1974, Selective T cell killing of human lymphocytes by ultraviolet radiation, *Cell. Immunol.* **14:**80–86.

Hyman, L. R., Kovacs, K., and Steinberg, A. D., 1975, Drug-induced tolerance: Selective induction with immunosuppressive drugs and their synergistic interaction, *Int. Arch. Allergy Appl. Immunol.* **48:**248–260.

Iannuzzi, L., Dawson, N., Zein, N., and Kushner, I., 1983, Does drug therapy slow radiographic deterioration in rheumatoid arthritis? *N. Engl. J. Med.* **309:**1023–1028.

Jerne, N. K., 1974, Towards a network theory of the immune system, *Ann. Immunol.* **125C:**373–389.

Johnson, W. W., and Meadows, D. C., 1971, Urinary bladder fibrosis and telangiectasia associated with long term cyclophosphamide therapy, *N. Engl. J. Med.* **284:**290–294.

Jolivet, J., Cowan, K. H., Curt, G. A., Clendeninn, N. J., and Chabner, B. A., 1983, The pharmacology and clinical use of methotrexate, *N. Engl. J. Med.* **309:**1094–1104.

Jones, J. V., Cumming, R. H., and Bucknall, R. C., 1976, Plasmapheresis in the management of acute systemic lupus erythematosus, *Lancet***1:**709–711.

Kahn, M. F., and deSeze, S., 1975, Surveillance cancerologique on long cours des patients traités par les immunodepresseurs (chlorambucil) en rheumatologie, *Scan. J. Rheumatol.* **4:**(Suppl. 8):9–23.

Kahn, M. F., Arlet, J., and Bloch-Michel, H., 1979, Leucémies aigues apres traitement par agents cytotoxiques en rheumatologie—19 observations chez 2006 patients, *Nouv. Presse Med.* **8:**1393–1397.

Karsh, J., Klippel, J. H., Decker, J. L., Wright, D. G., and Flye, M. W., 1981, Lymphapheresis in rheumatoid arthritis. A randomized trial, *Arthritis Rheum.* **24:**867–873.

Katz, S. I., Gallin, J. I., Hertz, K. C., Fauci, A. S., and Lawley, T. J., 1977, Erythema elevatum diutinum: Skin and systemic manifestations, immunologic studies and successful treatment with dapsone, *Medicine* **56**:443–455.

Katz, S. I., Hall, R. P., Lawley, T. J., and Strober, W., 1980, Dermatitis herpetiformis: The skin and the gut, *Ann. Intern. Med.* **93**:857–874.

Kimberly, R. P., Lockshin, M. D., and Sherman, R. L., 1981, High dose intravenous methylprednisolone pulse therapy in systemic lupus erythematosus, *Am. J. Med.* **70**:817–824.

Kint, A., and Verlinden, L., 1974, Levamisole for recurrent herpes labialis, *N. Engl. J. Med.* **291**:308.

Klippel, J. H., 1979, Studies in the treatment of lupus nephritis, *Ann. Intern. Med.* **91**:599–602.

Koller, L. D., Exon, J. H., and Roan, J. G., 1976, Humoral antibody response in mice after single dose exposure to lead or cadmium, *Proc. Soc. Exp. Biol. Med.* **151**:339–342.

Kotzin, B. L., Strober, S., Engleman, E. G., Calin, A., Hoppe, R. T., Kansas, G. S., Terrell, C. P., and Kaplan, H. S., 1981, Arthritis with total lymphoid irradiation, *N. Engl. J. Med.* **305**:969–976.

Kovarsky, J., 1983, Clinical pharmacology and toxicology of cyclophosphamide: Emphasis on use in rheumatic diseases, *Semin. Arthritis Rheum.* **12**:359–372.

Krause, J. R., 1982, Chronic idiopathic thrombocytopenic purpura (ITP): Development of acute non-lymphocytic leukemia subsequent to treatment with cyclophosphamide, *Med. Pediatr. Oncol.* **10**:61–65.

Kunkel, A., and Klaus, G. G. B., 1980, Selective effects of cyclosporin A on functional B cell subsets in the mouse, *J. Immunol.* **125**:2526–2531.

L'Abbate, A., Magiore, Q., Caccamo, A., Bartolomeo, F., and Misefari, V., 1983, Suppression of post-apheresis autoantibody rebound in cryoglobulinemia and cold agglutinin hemolytic anemia, *Int. J. Artif. Organs* **6**(Suppl. 1):51–56.

Lane, H. C., Masur, H., Rook, A. H., Quinnan, G. V., Gelmann, E., Steis, R., Longo, D., Palestine, A., Macher, A., and Fauci, A. S., 1984, Treatment of patients with the acquired immunodeficiency syndrome with interleukin-2 or interferon, *Fed. Proc.*

Larsson, E. L., 1980, Cyclosporin A and dexamethasone suppress T cell responses by selectively acting at distant sites of the triggering process, *J. Immunol.* **124**:2828–2833.

Lazowski, Z., Janczewski, Z., and Polowiec, Z., 1982, The effect of alkylating agents on the reproductive and hormonal testicular function in patients with rheumatoid arthritis, *Scand. J. Rheumatol.* **11**:49–54.

Lehner, T., Wilton, J. M. A., and Ivanyi, L., 1976, Double blind crossover trial of levamisole in recurrent aphthous ulteration, *Lancet* **2**:926–929.

Lennard, L., Rees, C. A., Lilleyman, J. S., and Maddocks, J. L., 1983, Childhood leukaemia: A relationship between intracellular 6-mercaptopurine metabolites and neutropenia, *Br. J. Clin. Pharmacol.* **16**:359–363.

Levin, R. H., Landy, M., and Frei, E., 1964, The effect of 6-mercaptopurine on immune response in man, *N. Engl. J. Med.* **271**:16–21.

Liebling, M. R., McLaughlin, K., and Boonsue, S., 1982, Monthly pulses of methylprednisolone in SLE nephritis, *J. Rheumatol.* **9**:543–548.

Lockwood, C. M., Rees, A. J. Russell, B., and Peters, D. K., 1977, Experience of the use of plasma exchange in the management of glomerulonephritis and SLE, *Exp. Hematol.* **5**(Suppl.):117–136.

Loo, T. L., Luce, J. K., Sullivan, M. P., and Frei, E. III, 1968, Clinical pharmacologic observations on 6-mercaptopurine, *Clin. Pharmacol. Ther.* **9**:180–194.

Losito, A., Williams, D. G., and Harris, L., 1978, The effects on polymorphonuclear leukocyte function of prednisolone and azathioprine *in vivo* and prednisolone, azathioprine and 6-mercaptopurine *in vitro, Clin. Exp. Immunol.* **32**:423–428.

Macario, A. J. L., and Conway de Marcario, E., 1978, Enhancement and inhibition of immunological mechanisms by immunosuppressive agents. I. Dose effect on priming and generation of memory to a bacterial antigen, *Clin. Exp. Immunol.* **31**:281–290.

Machleder, H. I., and Paulus, H., 1978, Clinical and immunological alterations observed in patients undergoing long-term thoracic duct draining, *Surgery* **84**:157–165.

Mandell, G. L., and Sande, M. A., 1980, Antimicrobial agents. Drugs used in the chemotherapy of tuberculosis and leprosy, in: *The Pharmacologic Basic of Therapeutics,* ed. 6 (L. S. Goodman and A. Gilman, eds.), Macmillan, New York, pp. 965–978.

McLean, A., Newell, D., and Baker, G., 1976, The metabolism of chlorambucil, *Biochem. Pharmacol.* **29**:2039–2047.

Medzihradsky, J. L., Klein, C., and Elion, G. B., 1982, Differential interference by azathioprine and 6-

cercaptopurine with antibody-mediated immunoregulation: Synergism of azathioprine and antibody in the control of an immune response, *J. Immunol.* **129:**145–149.

Melez, K., Reeves, J. P., and Steinberg, A. D., 1978a, Modification of NZB/NZW disease by sex hormones, *J. Immunopharmacol.* **1:**27–42.

Melez, K., Reeves, J. P., and Steinberg, A. D., 1978b, Modification of murine lupus by sex hormones, *Ann. Immunol.* **129C:**707–712.

Metzger, A. L., Bohan, A., and Goldberg, L. A., 1974, Polymyositis and dermatomyositis: Combined methotrexate and corticosteroid therapy, *Ann. Intern. Med.* **81:**182–189.

Miller, B., DeMerieux, P., and Srinivasan, R., 1980, Double-blind placebo controlled crossover evaluation of levamisole in rheumatoid arthritis, *Arthritis Rheum.* **23:**172–182.

Mitchell, M. S., Wade, W. E., DeConti, R. C., Bertino, J. R., and Calabresi, P., 1969, Immunosuppressive effects of cytosine arabinoside and methotrexate in man, *Ann. Intern. Med.* **70:**535–547.

Mouridsen, H. T., and Jacobsen, E., 1975, Pharmacokinetics of cyclophosphamide in renal failure, *Acta Pharmacol. Toxicol.* **36:**409–414.

Muraguchi, A., Butler, J. L., Kehrl, J. H., Falkoff, R. J., and Fauci, A. S., 1983, Selective suppression of an early step in human B cell activation by cyclosporin A, *J. Exp. Med.* **158:**690–702.

Navarro, J., and Touraine, J. L., 1983, Comparative study of cyclomunine cyclosporin A on human lymphocyte proliferation *in vitro.* The lack of an immunosuppressive effect by specific clonal deletion, *Int. J. Immunopharmacol.* **5:**157–162.

Old, C. W., Flannery, E. P., Grogen, I. M., Stone, W. H., and San Antonio, R. P., 1978, Azathioprine-induced pure red blood cell aplasia, *JAMA* **240:**552–554.

Oon, C. J., and Hobbs, J. R., 1975, Review: Clinical application of the continuous-flow separator machine, *Clin. Exp. Immunol.* **20:**1–16.

Palmer, R. G., Dore, C. J., and Denman, A. M., 1984, Sister chromatid exchanges in lymphocytes, *Lancet* **2:**174.

Paulus, H. E., Machleder, H. I., Levine, S., Yu, D. T. Y., and Macdonald, N. S., 1977, Lymphocyte involvement in rheumatoid arthritis. Studies during thoracic duct drainage, *Arthritis Rheum.* **20:**1249–1262.

Pinedo, H. M., Zaharko, D. S., Bull, J., and Chabner, B. A., 1977, The relative contribution of drug concentration and duration of exposure to mouse bone marrow toxicity during continuous methotrexate infusion, *Cancer Res.* **37:**445–450.

Pross, H. F., and Eidinger, D., 1974, Antigenic competition: A review of nonspecific antigen induced suppression, *Adv. Immunol.* **18:**133–168.

Puri, H. C., and Campbell, R. A., 1977, Cyclophosphamide and malignancy, *Lancet* **1:**1306.

Pusey, C. D., and Lockwood, C. M., 1982, Plasma exchange and immunosuppressive drugs in the management of severe glomerulonephritis, *Prog. Clin. Biol. Res.* **106:**91–104.

Rabson, A. R., Whiting, D. A., Anderson, R., Glover A., and Koornhof, H. J., 1977, Depressed neutrophil motility in patients with recurrent herpes simplex virus infection: *In vitro* restoration with levamisole, *J. Infect. Dis.* **135:**113–116.

Rand, R. J., Kenkins, D. M., and Blumer, R., 1978, T- and B-lymphocyte subpopulations following radiotherapy for invasive squamous cell carcinoma of the uterine cervix, *Clin. Exp. Immunol.* **33:**159–165.

Raveche, E. S., Klassen, L. W., and Steinberg, A. D., 1976, Sex differences in formation of anti-T cell antibodies, *Nature* **263:**415–416.

Roberts, J. J., Brent, T. P., and Crathorn, A. R., 1971, Evidence for the inactivation and repair of the mammalian DNA template after alkylation by mustard gas and half mustard gas, *Eur. J. Cancer* **7:**515–524.

Rook, A. H., Masur, H., Lane, C., Frederick, W., Kasahara, T., Macher, A. M., Djeu, J. Y., Manischewitz, J. F., Jackson, L., Fauci, A. S., and Quinnan G. V., Jr., 1983, Interleukin-2 enhances the depressed natural killer and cytomegalovirus-specific cytotoxic activities of lymphocytes from patients with the acquired immune deficiency syndrome, *J. Clin. Invest.* **72:**398–403.

Rosenthal, M., Trabert, U., and Mueller, W., 1976, The effect of levamisole on peripheral blood lymphocyte subpopulations in patients with rheumatoid arthritis and ankylosing spondylitis, *Clin. Exp. Immunol.* **25:**493–496.

Roubinian, J. R., Papoian, R., and Talal, N., 1977, Androgenic hormones modulate autoantibody responses and improve survival in murine lupus, *J. Clin. Invest.* **59:**1066–1070.

Rudd, P., Fried, J. F., and Epstein, W. V., 1975, Irreversible bone marrow failure with chlorambucil, *J. Rheumatol.* **2:**421–429.

Runge, L. A., Pinals, R. S., Lourie, S. H., and Tomar, R. H., 1977, Treatment of rheumatoid arthritis with levamisole. A controlled trial, *Arthritis Rheum.* **20**:1445–1448.

Russell, J. A., Toy, J. L., and Powles, R. L., 1977, Plasma exchange in malignant paraproteinanemias, *Exp. Haematol.* **5**(Suppl. 1):105–109.

Sack, D. M., and Peppercorn, M. A., 1983, Drug therapy of inflammatory bowel disease, *Pharmacotherapy* **3**:158–176.

Sampson, D., and Lui, A., 1976, The effect of levamisole on cell-mediated immunity and suppressor-cell function, *Cancer Res.* **36**:952–955.

Santos, G. W., Owens, A. H., and Sensenbrenner, L. L., 1964, Effects of selected cytotoxic agents on antibody production in man, *Ann. N.Y. Acad. Sci.* **114**:404–423.

Scannell, J. P., and Hitchings, G. H., 1966, Thioguanine in Deoxyribonucleic acid from tumors of 6-Mercaptopurine-treated mice, *Proc. Soc. Exp. Biol. Med.* **122**:627–629.

Schmidt, K. L., and Mueller-Eckhardt, C., 1977, Agranulocytosis, levamisole, and HLA-B27, *Lancet* **2**:85.

Scott, J., Dieppe, P. A., and Huskisson, E. C., 1978, Continuous and intermittent levamisole, *Ann. Rheum. Dis.* **37**:259–261.

Segal, A. W., Levi, A. J., and Loewi, G., 1977, Levamisole in the treatment of Crohn's disease, *Lancet* **2**:382–385.

Sheffer, A. L., Fearon, D. T., and Austen, K. F., 1977, Methyltestosterone therapy in hereditary angioedema, *Ann. Intern. Med.* **86**:306–308.

Shumak, K. H., and Rock, G. A., 1984, Therapeutic plasma exchange, *N. Engl. J. Med.* **310**:762–771.

Skipper, H. E., 1954, On the mechanism of action of 6-mercaptopurine, *Ann. N.Y. Acad. Sci.* **60**:315–321.

Smyth, J., 1979, Treatment of lymphoid malignancy with adenosine deaminase inhibitors, *Ciba Found. Symp.* **68**:263–279.

Spaulding, W. B., 1960, Methyltestosterone therapy for hereditary episodic edema (hereditary angioneurotic edema), *Ann. Intern. Med.* **53**:739–744.

Stahl, R. E., Friedman-Kien, A., Dubin, R., Marmor, M., and Zolla-Pazner, S., 1982, Immunologic abnormalities in homosexual men: Relationship to Kaposi's sarcoma, *Am. J. Med.* **73**:171–178.

Starzl, T. E., Putnam, C. W., Halgrimson, C. G., Schroter, G. T., Martinequ, G., Lavnois, B., Corman, J. L., Penn, I., Booth, A. S., Groth, C. G., and Porter, K. A., 1971, Cyclophosphamide and whole organ transplantation in human beings, *Surg. Gynecol. Obstet.* **133**:981–991.

Starzl, T. E., Klintmalm, G. B. G., Weil, R. III, Porter, K. A., Watsurki, S., Schroter, G. P., Fernandez-Bueno, C., and MacHugh, N., 1981, Cyclosporin A and steroid therapy in sixty-six cadaver kidney recipients, *Surg. Gyn. Obstet.* **153**:486–494.

Steinberg, A. D., Gelfand, M. C., Hardin, J. A., and Lowenthal, D. T., 1975, Therapeutic studies in NZB/W mice. III. Relationship between renal status and efficacy of immunosuppressive drug therapy, *Arthritis Rheum.* **18**:9–14.

Steinberg, A. D., Klassen, L. W., Raveche, E. S., Gerber, N. L., Reinertsen, J. L., Krakauer, R. S., Ranney, D. F., Gershwin, M. E., Kovacs, K., Williams, G. W., and Reeves, J. P., 1978, Study of the multiple factors in the pathogenesis of autoimmunity in New Zealand mice, *Arthritis Rheum.* **21**:S190–201.

Stevens, J. E., and Willoughby, D. A., 1969, The anti-inflammatory effect of some immunosuppressive agents, *J. Patholol.* **97**:367–373.

Stukov, A. N., 1976, Experimental study of the combined effect of leukeran, degranol, and prednisolone, *Neoplasma* **22**:181–184.

Sutherland, D. E. R., Ferguson, R. M., Simmons, R. L., Kim, T. H., Slavin, S., and Najarian, J. S., 1983, Total lymphoid irradiation, *Urol. Clin. North Am.* **10**:277–288.

Swanson, M. A., and Schwartz, R. S., 1967, Immunosuppressive therapy. The relations between clinical response and immunologic competence, *N. Engl. J. Med.* **277**:163–170.

Symoens, J., and Brugmans, J., 1974, Treatment of recurrent aphthous stomatitis and herpes with levamisole, *Br. Med. J.* **4**:592.

Symoens, J., and Rosenthal, M., 1977, Levamisole in the modulation of the immune response: The current experimental and clinical state, *J. Reticuloendothel. Soc.* **21**:175–221.

Synderman, R., and Pike, M. C., 1978, Pathophsiologic aspects of leukocyte chemotaxis: Identification of a specific chemotactic factor binding site on human granulocytes and defects of macrophage function associated with neoplasia, in: *Leukocyte Chemotaxis: Methods, Physiology, and Clinical Implications* (J. I. Gallin and P. G. Quie, eds.), Raven Press, New York, pp. 174–195.

Taliaferro, W. H., and Taliaferro, L. G., 1954, Effect of X-rays on hemolysin formation following various immunization and irradiation procedures, *J. Infect.* **95:**117–133.

Tanay, A. S., Field, E. H., and Strober, S., 1984, Opposite effects of total lymphoid irradiation (TLI) on serum levels of autoantibodies in patients with rheumatoid arthritis (RA) and systemic lupus erythematosus (SLE) nephritis, *Arthritis Rheum.* **275:**61.

Terman, D. S., Petty, D., and Harbeck, R., 1977a, Specific removal of DNA antibody *in vivo* by extracorporeal circulation over DNA immobilized in collodion charcoal, *Clin. Immunol. Immunopathol.* **8:**90–96.

Terman, D. S., Petty, D., Ogden, D., Pefley, C., and Buffaloe, G., 1977b, Specific extraction of antigens *in vivo* by extracorporeal circulation over antibody immobilized in collodioncharcoal, *J. Immunol.* **117:**1971–1975.

Terres, G., Morrison, S. L., and Habicht, G. S., 1968, A quantitative difference in the immune response between male and female mice, *Proc. Soc. Exp. Biol. Med.* **127:**664–667.

Thomas, M. R., Robinson, W. A., Boyle, D. J., Entringer, M. A., and Steigerwald, J. F., 1983, Longterm effects of cyclophosphamide on granulocyte colony formation in patients with rheumatoid arthritis, *J. Rheumatol.* **10:**778–783.

Trentham. D. E., Belli, J. A., Anderson, R. J., Buckley, J. A., Goetzl, E. J., David, J. R., and Austen, K. F., 1981, Clinical and immunologic effects of fractionated total lymphoid irradiation in refractory rheumatoid arthritis, *N. Engl. J. Med.* **305:**976–982.

Tripodi, D., Parks, L. C., and Brugmans, J., 1973, Drug-induced restoration of cutaneous delayed hypersensitivity in anergic patients with cancer, *N. Engl. J. Med.* **289:**354–357.

Turk, J. L., and Parker, D., 1982, Effect of cyclophosphamide on immunological control mechanisms, *Immunol. Rev.* **65:**99–113.

Valbonesi, M., and Garelli, S., 1983, Plasma exchange in neurological diseases. A critical approach, *Vox Sang.* **44:**65–80.

Valbonesi, M., Garelli, S., Zerbi, D., Forlani, G., Cornelio, F., and Pelucchetti, D., 1982, Plasma exchange combined with cytotoxic drugs and lymphocytapharesis for myasthenia gravis, *Vox Sang.* **43:**142–146.

Veys, E. M., Mielants, H., and Verbruggen, G., 1978, Levamisole-induced adverse reactions in HLA-B27-positive rheumatoid arthritis, *Lancet* **1:**148.

Wallace, D. J., Podell, T. E., Weiner, J. M., Cox, M. B., Klinenberg, J. R., Forouzesh, S., and Dubois, E. L., 1982, Lupus nephritis. Experience with 230 patients in a private practice from 1950 to 1980, *Am. J. Med.* **72:**209–220.

Wasi, P., and Block, M., 1961, The histopathologic study of the development of the irradiation-induced leukemia in C57BL mice and of its inhibition by testosterone, *Cancer Res* **21:**463–473.

Wei, N., Klippel, J. H., Huston, D. P., Hall, R. P., Lawley, T. J., Balow, J. E., Steinberg, A. D., and Decker, J. L., 1983, Ramdomised trial of plasma exchange in mild systemic lupus erythematosus, *Lancet* **1:**17–22.

Whisnant, J. K., and Pelkey, J., 1982, Rheumatoid arthritis: Treatment with azathioprine (Imuran®). Clinical side-effects and laboratory abnormalities, *Ann. Rheum. Dis.* **41S:**44–47.

White, D. J. G., and Calne, R. Y., 1982, The use of cyclosporin A immunosuppression in organ grafting, *Immunol. Rev.* **65:**115–131.

Wilkens, R. F., 1983, Reappraisal of the use of methotrexate in rheumatic disease, *Am. J. Med.* **75:**19–25.

Winkelmann, R. K., 1982, Dermatomyositis in childhood, *Clin. Rheum. Dis.* **8:**353–368.

Wright, D. G., Kirkpatrick, C. H., and Gallin, J. I., 1977, Effects of levamisole on normal and abnormal leukocyte locomotion, *J. Clin. Invest.* **59:**941–950.

Yatvin, M. B., and Lelkes, P. I., 1982, Clinical prospects for liposomes, *Med. Phys.* **9:**149–175.

Yeh, G. C., and Phang, J. M., 1983, Pyrroline-5-carboxylate stimulates the conversion of purine antimetabolites to their nucleotide forms by a redox-dependent mechanism, *J. Biol. Chem.* **258:**9774–9779.

Zimm, S., Collins, J. M., O'Neill, D., Chabner, B. A., and Poplack, D. G., 1983, Inhibition of first-pass metabolism in cancer chemotheraphy: Interaction of 6-mercaptopurine and allopurinol, *Clin. Pharmacol. Ther.* **341:**810–817.

Zimmerman, T. P., Chu, L-C., Bugge, C. J. L., Nelson, D. J., Lyon G. M., and Elion, G. B., 1974, Identification of 6-methylmercaptopurine ribonucleoside 5'-diphosphate and 5'-triphosphate as metabolites of 6-mercaptopurine in man, *Cancer Res.* **34:**221–224.

Zulman, J., Michalski, J., McCombs, C., Greenspan, J., and Talal, N., 1978, Levamisole maintains cyclophosphamide-induced remission in murine lupus erythematosus, *Clin. Exp. Immunol.* **31:**321–327.

30

Total Lymphoid Irradiation

Brian L. Kotzin and Samuel Strober

I. INTRODUCTION

There remains a great need in medicine for new immunosuppressive therapies that are capable of suppressing disease activity but are not associated with the complications of general cytotoxicity and nonselective immunosuppression. Currently available immunosuppressive drugs are too frequently associated with serious and sometimes lethal complications. We review here the relatively unique immunologic changes associated with total lymphoid irradiation (TLI) and the development of this form of radiotherapy as an immunosuppressive treatment for rheumatic diseases.

II. INITIAL OBSERVATIONS OF THE USE OF TLI IN HODGKIN'S DISEASE

The rationale for using total lymphoid irradiation (TLI) as an immunosuppressive treatment originated from studies of patients with Hodgkin's disease, where TLI has been an accepted form of therapy for over 15 years. Figure 1 shows the radiation ports used to administer TLI to patients with Hodgkin's disease (Kaplan, 1980). The supradiaphragmatic tissues irradiated ("mantle" field) include the cervical, axillary, supraclavicular, and mediastinal lymph nodes as well as the thymus. Subdiaphragmatic tissues irradiated ("inverted Y" field) include the paraaortic, iliac, and inguinal–femoral lymph nodes. Most Hodgkin's disease patients are splenectomized before radiotherapy, and only the splenic pedicle is irradiated. All tissues not in the ports (i.e., lungs, kidneys, bone marrow, central nervous system, etc.) are shielded with lead or are outside of the perimeter of the

Brian L. Kotzin • Department of Medicine, University of Colorado Health Sciences Center, and Rheumatology Section, Veterans Administration Medical Center, Denver, Colorado 80220. *Samuel Strober* • Department of Medicine, Division of Immunology, Stanford University Medical Center, Stanford, California 94305.

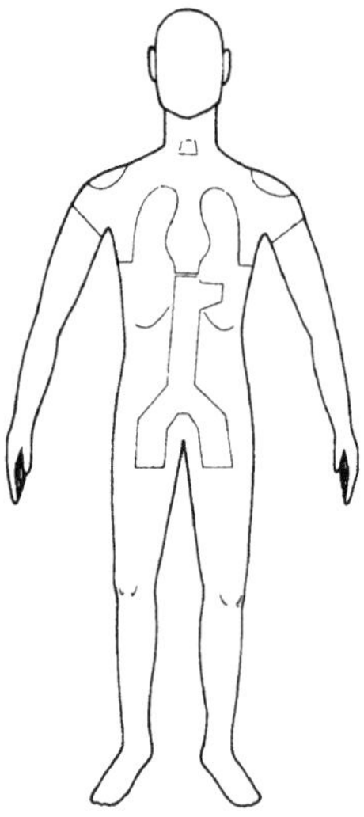

Figure 1. Total lymphoid irradiation (TLI) in man. Shaded areas show ports for irradiation.

X-ray beam. Irradiation is given to the mantle field in doses of 150–250 rads per fraction until a total dose of 4400 rads is achieved over a period of 4 to 6 weeks (Kaplan, 1980). A similar course of fractionated radiotherapy is then administered to the subdiaphragmatic fields to complete the regimen. The radiation source used at most centers is a linear accelerator.

This radiotherapy regimen was noted to induce profound long-lasting immunologic defects in patients with Hodgkin's disease (Fuks *et al.*, 1976). After treatment with TLI, patients were noted to have a marked decrease in the number of circulating total lymphocytes and T cells. Although the total count had fully recovered by 2 years after TLI, the T lymphocytopenia persisted for at least 10 years after treatment. After radiotherapy, peripheral blood lymphocytes from patients with Hodgkin's disease showed a markedly reduced proliferative response to the T-cell mitogen phytohemagglutinin (PHA) and to allogeneic cells (mixed leukocyte reaction, MLR) compared to pretreatment levels. Although the reduced PHA response also persisted for at least 10 years after radiotherapy, proliferation in MLR slowly recovered such that normal responses were uniformly observed 5 or more years after radiotherapy. Of those untreated patients who demonstrated a delayed hypersensitivity response to dinitrochlorobenzene (DNCB), almost all lost their skin reactivity immediately after the completion of TLI. Approximately one-third of these patients remained anergic for at least 8 years after radiotherapy.

Despite the potent and long-lasting immunosuppression induced by TLI, it is an outpatient procedure that has been associated with few serious complications. Fewer than 1% of Hodgkin's disease patients given TLI to a total dose of 4400 rads required hospitalization for irradiation complications (Kaplan, 1980). Severe thrombocytopenia or leukopenia (less than 50% of base line) that persisted beyond 2 months after treatment was observed in fewer than 1% of patients. The incidence of severe bacterial infection requiring hospitalization was less than 1% and was not significantly increased above that associated with splenectomy performed at the time of staging of disease. Approximately 20–30% of patients treated with TLI developed herpes zoster within 2 years after completion of therapy, but fewer than 1% of this group progressed to dissemination requiring hospitalization (Kaplan, 1980). There have been no cases of acute leukemia or non-Hodgkin's lymphoma in several hundred patients treated for Hodgkin's disease with TLI alone at Stanford and followed for up to 10 years (Coleman *et al.*, 1977; Kirkorian *et al.*, 1979). This low incidence of second malignancies in patients given radiotherapy alone has been confirmed at other large oncology centers (Baccarini *et al.*, 1980; Valagussa *et al.*, 1980).

III. IMMUNOLOGIC CHANGES IN EXPERIMENTAL ANIMALS TREATED WITH TLI: THE DEVELOPMENT OF SUPPRESSOR CELLS AND TOLERANCE

The above studies of patients with Hodgkin's disease suggested that TLI might be an effective and safe immunosuppressive regimen. Therefore, immunologic changes in experimental animals treated with TLI were studied. Irradiation ports were designed to treat adult mice and rats such that all the major lymph nodes, the spleen, and the thymus were included within the radiation fields (Slavin *et al.*, 1976, 1977). The major bone marrow areas (skull, tail, and hindlimbs) and lungs were shielded with lead. The radiotherapy regimen usually consisted of 17 fractions of 200 rads each, given to the supra- and subdiaphragmatic fields simultaneously.

Immediately after TLI, few lymphocytes remained in the peripheral blood, and T lymphocytes could not be detected until the second month after TLI (Slavin *et al.*, 1977). Although the total lymphocyte count returned to normal by about 3 months after irradiation, the decrease in peripheral blood T cells persisted for as long as the animals were followed. The proliferative responses of murine peripheral blood lymphocytes to the mitogens phytohemagglutinin (PHA) and concanavalin A (Con A) were eliminated immediately after the completion of TLI (Slavin *et al.*, 1977), and the response to PHA remained depressed even after long-term follow-up. The *in vitro* response of murine peripheral blood lymphocytes to allogeneic cells (MLR) was also markedly reduced shortly after TLI (Slavin *et al.*, 1977). Recovery of this response was observed by 2 to 3 months after treatment.

The effect of TLI on antibody responses was studied by immunizing mice with various antigens at different time intervals after completion of radiotherapy. Markedly different effects were observed depending on whether the injected antigen induced a T(helper)-cell-dependent or T(helper)-cell-independent antibody response (Tanay and Strober, 1984). When mice were immunized 30 days after completion of TLI, the T-cell-dependent antibody response to the dinitrophenylated heterologous protein keyhole limpet hemocyanin (DNP-KLH) in complete Freund's adjuvant was diminished 100-fold. In contrast, the T-cell-independent antibody response to the trinitrophenylated polysaccharide antigen *Brucella abortus* (TNP-BA) was enhanced five- to tenfold compared to that of control animals. Spleen cells from animals treated with TLI were then compared to cells from normal mice in the ability to restore the antibody response in whole-body-irradiated recipients (syngeneic primary adoptive transfer system) (Table 1). The IgG anti-DNP-KLH response of hosts given cells from TLI-treated donors was 1000-fold below that of

Table 1. Effect of TLI on the Ability of Spleen Cells to Restore the Primary Adoptive Response to DNP-KLH or TNP-BA[a]

	Increase in antibody respone (relative units)			
	DNP-KLH		TNP-BA	
Donor spleen cells[b]	IgM	IgG	IgM	IgG
Normal	15	>1000	2–3	2
TLI	~1	<1	12	>500

[a] Adapted from Tanay and Strober (1984). Recipient BALB/c mice were given 500 rad of whole body irradiation and then 5×10^6 spleen cells from syngeneic donors 1 day later. On the following day, the adoptive hosts were immunized with either DNP-KLH in complete Freund's adjuvant (which results in a T-cell-dependent antihapten antibody response) or TNP-BA (which results in a T-cell-independent antihapten response). The antibody response was determined 14 days after immunization.

[b] Spleen cells were obtained from syngeneic donors 30 days after TLI or from unirradiated controls.

[c] Relative units = [antibody response with donor cells (units, ELISA assay)]/ [antibody response of nonreconstituted mice (units, ELISA assay)].

hosts given cells from untreated donors. In marked contrast, the IgG anti-TNP-BA response was at least 200-fold higher using cells from TLI-treated donors.

The early recovery phase after TLI is characterized by a rapid repopulation of the peripheral lymphoid tissues with large immature cells, probably originating from the shielded bone marrow. These cells, which bear the "null" (non-T, non-B) surface phenotype, appear to be capable of suppressing a variety of immune functions. (King *et al.*, 1981; May *et al.*, 1983). For example, in coculture studies, spleen cells from TLI-treated BALB/c mice suppressed the response of BALB/c (H-2^d) responder cells to C57BL/Ka (H-2^b) stimulator cells by nearly 90% as compared to control cultures (King *et al.*, 1981). The suppressor cells were shown to be specific for neither the responder nor the stimulator cells. Spleen cells from BALB/c mice given 550 rad of whole-body irradiation (WBI) did not suppress the MLR at any time. This "nonspecific" suppressor activity was only detectable in the first few weeks after completion of TLI. Functional and phenotypic characteristics of these TLI-induced suppressor cells appeared to be similar to those "natural" suppressor cells found in neonatal spleen and adult bone marrow (Okada and Strober, 1982; May *et al.*, 1983; Oseroff *et al.*, 1984).

Another unique characteristic of TLI as an immunosuppressive regimen relates to its ability to allow for the induction of antigen-specific tolerance. TLI-treated mice responded normally to immunization with bovine serum albumin (BSA) in complete Freund's adjuvant (CFA); however, if, after TLI, mice were first given an injection of nondeaggregated BSA in saline, they made a minimal antibody response to an immunizing dose of the same antigen (i.e., BSA in CFA) (Zan-Bar *et al.*, 1978). These mice appeared to be permanently tolerized to the antigen BSA. Unirradiated mice or WBI-treated mice could not be similarly tolerized. Tolerance was shown to be specific for BSA, since mice given TLI and then BSA in saline responded normally to bovine γ-globulin (BGG) in CFA. Similarly, mice given TLI and then BGG in saline responded poorly to BGG in CFA but made a normal response to BSA in CFA. In adoptive transfer studies, tolerance appeared to be mediated by antigen-specific suppressor T cells (Zan-Bar *et al.*, 1978).

In transplantation experiments, specific tolerance to allogeneic antigens could be induced after TLI. BALB/c (H-2^d) mice were given TLI and an intravenous injection of bone marrow cells from C57BL/Ka (H-2^b) donors 1 day later (Slavin *et al.*, 1977; Gottlieb *et al.*, 1981). Skin grafts from the donors were also placed on the recipients at the same time. Approximately 90% of the TLI-treated recipients became stable chimeras as judged by the presence of donor-type lymphocytes in the peripheral blood more than 100 days after bone marrow transplantation. Although allogeneic bone marrow engraftment was achieved, no clinical evidence of graft-versus-host disease (GVHD) was observed in the recipients. In contrast, nearly all mice prepared with single-dose lethal WBI developed GVHD and were dead by 60 days after bone marrow transplantation. Stable chimeras prepared with TLI permanently accepted skin grafts from the marrow donor strain but rejected skin grafts from third-party (C3H, H-2^k) donors (Slavin *et al.*, 1977). Thus, the chimeras were specifically tolerant to the alloantigens of the bone marrow donor. Similar results were obtained in rats and dogs given TLI and allogeneic bone marrow (Slavin *et al.*, 1978; Gottlieb *et al.*, 1980).

In cotransfer studies designed to investigate the mechanism of allograft tolerance after TLI, nonspecific suppressor cells from BALB/c mice given TLI (see above) were able to suppress GVHD *in vivo* (King *et al.*, 1981). Thus, when C57BL/Ka bone marrow cells in combination with spleen cells from TLI-treated BALB/c donors were cotransferred to lethally whole-body-irradiated BALB/c recipients, approximately 90% of the recipients survived, and half became stable chimeras. If allogeneic bone marrow cells alone were transferred, all the recipients died of typical features of GVHD. The cotransfer of normal BALB/c spleen cells with allogeneic bone marrow cells allowed about half of the recipients to survive 100 days, but none of the survivors was chimeric. Only the spleen cells from TLI-treated mice allowed the allogeneic cells to repopulate the host lymphoid tissues and also prevented the development of GVHD.

As noted above, allograft tolerance in stable long-term TLI chimeras was antigen specific in that these animals were capable of rejecting third-party grafts. Furthermore, donor-type cells isolated from long-term chimeras (i.e., C57BL/Ka → BALB/c chimeras) were shown to be capable of mediating lethal GVHD in third-party (i.e., C3H, H-2^k) recipients but not in host-strain (BALB/c) recipients (Gottlieb *et al.*, 1981). These results indicate that the chimeric donor cells are immunocompetent and specifically tolerant of the alloantigens of the chimeric hosts. Recent laboratory experiments have suggested a link between the early development of the nonspecific suppressor cells and the long-term development of specific mutual host and donor tolerance in chimeric mice. In the MLR, both antigen-specific killer cells and antigen-specific suppressor T cells are generated simultaneously by responder cells (Hess and Tutschka, 1980). In coculture experiments, nonspecific suppressor cells blocked the generation of cytotoxic effector cells in the MLR but did not block the generation of alloantigen-specific suppressor cells (Okada and Strober, 1982). Thus, the nonspecific suppressor cells may first help to prevent rejection of bone marrow in the period immediately after transplantation by suppressing the generation of host cytotoxic T cells directed against donor alloantigens. In addition, the same suppressor cells may block GVHD by inhibiting the generation of donor-derived cytotoxic T cells directed against the host. On the other hand, the development of mutual tolerance can be explained by the accumulation of antigen-specific suppressor cells derived from both the host and donor.

IV. THE USE OF TLI IN THE AUTOIMMUNE DISEASE OF EXPERIMENTAL ANIMALS

A. Suppression of the Lupuslike Disease of NZB/NZW Mice

NZB/NZW F_1 mice spontaneously develop an autoimmune disease characterized by antinuclear antibodies and a fatal immune-complex glomerulonephritis and are considered to be experimental models of human systemic lupus erythematosus (SLE) (Howie and Helyer, 1968). A large group of NZB/NZW female mice (mean age 6.0 months) with established nephritis and proteinuria were randomly allocated to treatment (TLI) or control groups (Kotzin and Strober, 1979). Total lymphoid irradiation resulted in a marked improvement in survival such that at 12 months of age over 90% of the treated animals were alive, whereas 75% of the control animals were dead ($P < 0.0001$). This improvement in survival was secondary to suppression of the lupuslike nephritis. Thus, whereas there were no renal deaths in the TLI group, 90% of the control group deaths were associated with histological evidence of severe or end-stage glomerulonephritis. Anti-native-DNA antibody levels were also noted to be suppressed in the TLI-treated group, suggesting that anti-native-DNA production in NZB/NZW mice is a T-helper-cell-dependent process (see above). The mice tolerated the irradiation well, and no complications of therapy were noted.

Surprisingly, in further studies, single-dose WBI (500 rads) also induced a prolonged remission in the disease activity of adult female NZB/NZW mice (Kotzin *et al.*, 1983b). Mice treated with WBI were noted to have significant improvement in survival, retarded progression of proteinuria, and suppression of anti-native-DNA antibodies compared to control animals. Suppression of disease was, however, greater and longer lasting after TLI than after WBI.

The mechanism by which irradiation suppresses NZB/NZW disease remains unclear. In recent studies, disease remissions after TLI lasted far longer than the recovery of both cell-mediated and humoral immunity (B. L. Kotzin, S. Okada, and S. Strober, unpublished observations). Furthermore, the disease could not be reestablished in irradiated hosts by transferring large numbers of cells from donors with active disease (Kotzin *et al.*, 1983b). Although defects in suppressor cell generation have been described in NZB/NZW mice, nonspecific suppressor cells of the MLR (see above) were easily demonstrated in the spleens of TLI-treated mice (B. L. Kotzin, S. Okada, and S. Strober, unpublished observations). As in studies of nonautoimmune mice given TLI, these suppressor cells were not detectable longer than 6 weeks after TLI and were not detected at any time after WBI. Attempts to transfer suppression of disease with spleen cells from TLI-treated mice to unirradiated littermate recipient animals were unsuccessful. The above experiments suggest that irradiation does not merely deplete the immunocompetent cells that mediate this autoimmune disease. However, at this time, there is no definite evidence that suppressor cells induced after TLI play a role in disease suppression.

B. Suppression of the Autoimmune Disease of MRL/l Mice

MRL-lpr/lpr (MRL/1) mice also spontaneously develop an autoimmune disease with antinuclear antibodies and glomerulonephritis (Andrews *et al.*, 1978). In addition, these animals develop a marked nonmalignant T-cell proliferation with massive lymph node and spleen enlargement. Approximately 50% of untreated animals will be dead by 5 to 6 months of age. Of such mice, 100% given TLI at the clinical onset of disease and 82% given WBI (300 rads) remained alive at 9 months of age, when the experiment was terminated (Theofilopoulos *et al.*, 1980). At that age, 92% of unirradiated controls were dead with massive lymph node hyperplasia, splenomegaly, and severe glomerulonephritis. In contrast, none of the TLI or WBI animals had enlarged lymph nodes or splenomegaly, and only 10 to 15% developed glomerulonephritis. Levels of anti-native-DNA antibodies were minimally reduced in irradiated animals as compared to controls, and anti-single-stranded-DNA antibodies were the same in all groups.

There is recent evidence to suggest that accelerated autoimmune disease in MRL/l mice (compared to MRL/n, which do not demonstrate lymphoproliferation) is secondary to the proliferation of helper T cells and an enhanced helper effect on autoantibody production. (Prud'homme *et al.*, 1983). In this regard, TLI- and WBI-treated mice had tenfold fewer lymphocytes in their lymph nodes than did unmanipulated diseased mice, which was secondary to the lack of T-cell proliferation. Interestingly, at 6 months post-irradiation, helper T-cell activity in the lymphoid tissues of irradiated mice on a cell-per-cell basis was much below that of the controls, whereas suppressor T-cell function was normal (Theofilipoulos *et al.*, 1980).

C. Suppression of Adjuvant Arthritis in Rats

Rats can be induced to develop arthritis by the subcutaneous injection of complete Freund's adjuvant (mineral oil with *Mycobacteria butyricum*). Injected animals were randomized to receive no treatment, TLI alone, paw irradiation alone, or both TLI and paw irradiation, and treatments were initiated after the appearance of arthritis (Schurman *et al.*, 1981). Animals were evaluated by clinical arthritis scores and by radiographic joint destruction. The most dramatic improvement in joint inflammation and deformity was recorded in rats treated with both TLI and paw irradiation. The arthritis scores decreased markedly during this combined treatment and remained at the posttreatment level for the remainder of the study (significantly different compared to pretreatment scores or scores of untreated animals, $P < 0.001$). The group receiving TLI alone demonstrated significantly less arthritis at the conclusion of irradiation. However, improvement was not long lasting, and the arthritis scores of the TLI group subsequently worsened to pretreatment levels. These mice then stabilized at a modestly improved level compared to untreated controls. The severity of inflammation and deformity in the rats treated with only local paw irradiation was only slightly decreased.

D. Suppression of Experimentally Induced Nephritis in Rats

Current evidence suggests that the majority of glomerulonephritides are mediated by immunologic processes. However, treatment of these diseases with conventional immunosuppressive drugs (e.g., azathioprine or cyclophosphamide) has been mostly unsuccessful. The potential therapeutic efficacy of TLI as an immunosuppressive therapy in immune glomerular disease was explored in two experimentally induced animal models (Lowry *et al.*, 1984a,b). In the accelerated autologous form of nephrotoxic serum nephritis

(AA-NTSN), rats previously sensitized to heterologous (i.e., sheep) immunoglobulin are given a subnephritogenic dose of sheep anti-rat-glomerular-basement-membrane antibodies. Within a few days post-injection, animals manifest significant proteinuria associated with histological glomerulonephritis. Glomerular damage appears to be strongly related to the host antibody response directed at the "planted" heterologous immunoglobulin (Lowry *et al.*, 1984a). Rats with established AA-NTSN were randomized to either control or TLI groups (Lowry *et al.*, 1984b); TLI resulted in a significant reduction in proteinuria, which was still apparent 4 months after completion of TLI. Histological abnormalities in the TLI group were confined to two of the nine rats, which had the highest 24-hr protein excretion rates when TLI was initiated. In contrast, kidney sections from eight of nine control animals were abnormal. Total lymphoid irradiation also resulted in decreased levels of circulating antibody to heterologous (sheep) immunoglobulin early post-TLI.

Rats were immunized with a subcellular preparation of crude renal tubular extract in adjuvant in order to induce autologous immune complex (Heymann's) nephritis (AICN) (Lowry *et al.*, 1984b). Although this was initially thought to be secondary to deposition of circulating immune complexes, more recent evidence suggests an immunopathogenic role for direct binding of host antibody to glomerular capillary wall nephritogenic antigens (Neale and Wilson, 1982). The glomerulonephritis that develops has morphological and immunopathological similarities to human membranous nephropathy. Administration of TLI to rats with established AICN resulted in significant reduction of proteinuria, serum creatinine, and incidence of lipemia compared to controls.

V. THE TREATMENT OF INTRACTABLE RHEUMATOID ARTHRITIS WITH TLI

A. Clinical Results of Initial Feasibility Studies

Approximately 20 to 30% of patients with progressive rheumatoid arthritis will not respond to treatment with gold compounds or penicillamine either because of lack of efficacy or unacceptable side effects. Although cytotoxic drugs such as azathioprine or cyclophosphamide have been demonstrated to be efficacious in many of these patients, these drugs are frequently associated with serious complications. In a literature comparison, TLI appeared to result in more potent, longer lasting, and uniquely more selective immunosuppressive changes compared to these cytotoxic drugs. Furthermore, the toxicity associated with the use of TLI in the treatment of Hodgkin's disease appeared to be less than that associated with the chronic use of these drugs in rheumatoid arthritis. We therefore initiated an uncontrolled feasibility study investigating the potential efficacy and toxicity of TLI in rheumatoid arthritis patients who were considered candidates for cytotoxic drugs (Kotzin *et al.*, 1981). Eleven patients with severe, destructive rheumatoid arthritis were entered into the study. The mean duration of disease prior to entry was 16 years, and all patients had previously been treated with multiple nonsteroidal antiinflammatory drugs, gold compounds, and penicillamine. In addition, eight patients had already received treatment with azathioprine without benefit. Ten patients had been receiving low-dose prednisone for a mean duration of 11 years.

Patients were treated with TLI as described above for the treatment of Hodgkin's disease. However, evidence from large animal studies (Gottlieb *et al.*, 1980) indicated that potent immunosuppression could be achieved with a lower total dose (2000 rad) than that used for Hodgkin's disease (4400 rad). Furthermore, more complete shielding of certain radiosensitive structures (i.e., lung and thyroid) was attempted to further limit toxicity. The spleen was not removed prior to irradiation and was included in the subdiaphragmatic field.

Clinical parameters used to follow patients included duration of morning stiffness, total joint scores for tenderness and swelling, and global composite score, which is a composite index of joint and patient function. Most patients began to show clinical improvement by 3 months after therapy. The magnitude of improvement continued to increase over the next several months and then stabilized at about 6 months after completion of irradiation (Kotzin *et al.*, 1981; Field *et al.*, 1983). When clinical evaluation scores at the last observation point (13 to 28 months after TLI) were compared to scores before irradiation, marked improvement was apparent. For each clinical parameter, the mean absolute scores for the entire group of 11 patients at last observation were significantly different ($P < 0.001$) from their scores before TLI. If a favorable response to therapy is defined as a decrement greater than 35% in each of these parameters, then nine of the 11 patients were classified as responders (Kotzin *et al.*, 1981; Field *et al.*, 1983). Although occasional transient flares of disease were noted in a few patients, no trend to relapse was observed during the follow-up period. Reduction of the daily dosage of prednisone was begun 6 months after therapy if a patient showed persistent clinical improvement. Ten of the patients were receiving prednisone at entry into the study (mean daily dose of 9.25 mg). The mean daily dose has been reduced to 4.3 mg, and two patients have had steroids discontinued.

Nearly all patients experienced one or more constitutional side effects (e.g., fatigue, anorexia, nausea) during the administration of TLI. These symptoms subsided within 2 months of treatment. Three patients had irradiation treatments interrupted because of neutropenia (<2000 neutrophils/mm^3). In two cases, the neutrophil count returned to normal within 4 weeks without complications. A diagnosis of Felty's syndrome was made in the third patient, who had persistent neutropenia and fevers, and the white blood cell count returned to normal within 3 days after splenectomy. Other complications observed more than 2 months after therapy included herpes zoster (confined to a single dermatome) in two patients, transient clinical pericarditis in two patients, and severe restrictive rheumatoid lung disease in one patient. The latter patient had documented rheumatoid lung disease before TLI and had a marked flare 3 months after radiotherapy when her joint disease was clinically quiescent. No new side effects have been identified during the last 12 months of follow-up.

In another uncontrolled feasibility study, ten patients with refractory rheumatoid arthritis were given TLI (total dose 3000 rads) (Trentham *et al.*, 1981). Although considerable initial improvement was noted in eight of ten patients, a partial recrudescence of disease activity was noted 1 year after irradiation. However, with follow-ups ranging from 15 to 40 months after TLI (Helfgott *et al.*, 1983), six of the ten patients continued to be improved compared to pre-TLI evaluations. Furthermore, significant improvement was still apparent for the group overall in morning stiffness, number of swollen joints, 50-foot walking time, and ARA functional class. There appeared to be a greater number of side effects from the TLI compared to the above Stanford studies. Seven patients experienced severe xerostomia, with four patients losing teeth; four patients had weight loss greater than 10 kg; three patients developed herpes zoster; and three patients developed hypothyroidism. In addition, three patients developed *Staph.* septicemia more than 1 year after TLI.

The difference in clinical results in the two feasibility studies remains to be explained. However, the difference in radiotherapy techniques is notable. The radiotherapy techniques used by the Harvard group (Trentham *et al.*, 1981; Helfgott *et al.*, 1983) differed from those used at Stanford (Kotzin *et al.*, 1981; Field *et al.*, 1983) in that radiation fields were divided into three regions instead of two, the total dose was 3000 rads instead of 2000, and the duration of therapy was 14 weeks instead of 5.

B. Clinical Results from a Controlled Study

In order to determine the efficacy of TLI in a controlled trial, 26 patients with intractable rheumatoid arthritis were randomized to receive either high-dose (total dose, 2000 rads; 200 rads per fraction) or low-dose (200 rads total; 20 rads per fraction) irradiation (Strober *et al.*, 1985a). Patients and observers were blinded with regard to the treatment group. Of the patients entered, 13 completed high-dose and 11 completed low-dose therapy. The patients in the two groups were well matched prior to treatment in regard to age, duration of disease, disease activity (i.e., morning stiffness, joint scores, and global composite score), prednisone dose, functional class (American Rheumatism Association), and rheumatoid factor titer.

Significant improvement in morning stiffness, joint tenderness, joint swelling, and global composite scores were observed in the high-dose group at 3 and 6 months after TLI as compared to pretreatment values. No significant change was observed in any parameter in the low-dose group. When the percentage improvement in the high- and low-dose groups was compared, the former showed significantly greater improvement in three of the four clinical parameters. Both patients given high-dose and low-dose irradiation experienced constitutional symptoms during TLI, which resolved within 2 months after TLI. Furthermore, three patients in each group developed herpes zoster. Other complications observed in the high-dose group included transient severe leukopenia with white cell counts less than 2000/mm^3 (three patients), transient thrombocytopenia (one patient), pleuritis (one patient), and gastric ulcer (one patient). Two deaths in the high-dose group 9 and 18 months after TLI (secondary to myocardial infarction and pulmonary embolism) appeared to be unrelated to radiotherapy.

C. Laboratory Studies

1. Lack of Changes in the Serum Level of Autoantibodies

Despite the improvement in joint disease activity after TLI, there was no appreciable change in serum rheumatoid factor titer or in antinuclear antibodies (Kotzin *et al.*, 1981; Trentham *et al.*, 1981; Field *et al.*, 1983; Tanay and Strober, 1984). The effect of TLI on T-cell-dependent and -independent humoral immune responses in patients with rheumatoid arthritis was further studied by Tanay *et al.*, (1984). As previously demonstrated in rodents, TLI appeared to selectively decrease T-helper-cell-dependent antibody responses [i.e, antibodies to diptheria (DT) and tetanus (TT) toxoids] in patients with rheumatoid arthritis while leaving intact or augmenting T-helper-cell-independent antibody responses [i.e., antibodies to pneumococcal polysaccharide (PPS)].

Thus, experiments showing no decrease in the serum levels of rheumatoid factors and antinuclear antibodies after TLI were most consistent with these autoantibodies being relatively independent of T-helper-cell function. Furthermore, in light of the clinical improvement observed after TLI, it seems unlikely that T-cell-independent autoantibody responses alone maintain the joint disease activity in rheumatoid arthritis.

2. *Changes in the Absolute Number and Proportions of T-Cell Subsets after TLI*

As expected, irradiation resulted in a profound decrease in the peripheral blood absolute lymphocyte count in all 11 patients (Kotzin *et al.*, 1981, 1983a). The mean count dropped precipitously during therapy and was less than 250/mm^3 at its completion. Six months after TLI, the count had risen to nearly 600/mm^3, but little further increment occurred up to 18 months after TLI.

Lymphocyte subsets were studied using monoclonal antibodies and the fluorescence-activated cell sorter (FACS) (Table 2) (Kotzin *et al.*, 1981, 1983a; Field *et al.*, 1983). In active RA patients prior to TLI, the percentage of lymphocytes that bear the pan-T-cell antigen Leu-1 was slightly lower than in controls. Interestingly, the percentage of Leu-2 cells (which mediate predominantly suppressor/cytotoxic functions) was slightly lower than in controls, and the percentage of Leu-3 cells (which mediate predominantly helper/inducer functions) slightly higher. This resulted in a lower than normal Leu-2/Leu-3 ratio (0.39 vs. 0.60, $P < 0.02$) (Table 2). However, because the absolute lymphocyte count in these patients was below the normal range, the absolute numbers of total T, Leu-2, and Leu-3 cells were lower than normal.

After TLI, there was a marked decrease in the percentage of Leu-1 cells and Leu-3 cells but an increase in the percentage of Leu-2 cells in the peripheral blood (Table 2).

Table 2. Changes in Lymphocyte Subsets after TLI[a]

	Absolute number of lymphocytes/mm^3	Percentage of cells bearing different surface antigens[b]			
		Leu-1	Leu-2	Leu-3	Leu-2/Leu-3[d]
Controls ($N = 21$)	2038 ± 73	71 ± 1.6	24 ± 1.7	42 ± 2.1	0.60 ± 0.09
RA Before TLI ($N = 14$)	1278 ± 120	64 ± 2.8	17 ± 1.9	48 ± 2.9	0.39 ± 0.06
RA After TLI ($N = 15$)[c]	667 ± 66	47 ± 4.7	33 ± 3.9	21 ± 1.9	1.73 ± 0.23
RA After drug response ($N = 9$)	1878 ± 241	78 ± 2.5	25 ± 4.0	54 ± 3.8	0.52 ± 0.12

[a] Adapted from Kotzin *et al.* (1983a).
[b] Value shown is the mean ± S.E. of the individual values for the number of patients indicated.
[c] Patients were studied from 1 to 18 months (mean ± S.E. = 7.0 ± 1.5 months) after completion of TLI.
[d] The mean of the Leu-2/Leu-3 ratios may not equal the ratio of the mean percentages.

These changes were reflected in a dramatic fourfold increase in the Leu-2/Leu-3 ratio. The mean absolute number of Leu-1 cells fell to less than one-half of the pretreatment value, which could be accounted for by the absolute decrease in number of Leu-3 cells. There was little change in the absolute number of Leu-2 cells after treatment with TLI. The preferential decrease in Leu-3 cells has persisted for up to 2 years following radiotherapy. These changes were not observed in rheumatoid arthritis patients who had experienced clinical improvement from various remittive drugs including azathioprine (Table 2) (Kotzin *et al.*, 1983a).

We performed kinetic studies to understand the mechanism by which TLI induces these T-cell-subset alterations. Interestingly, we found that TLI did not selectively deplete the Leu-3 population (Kotzin *et al.*, 1983a). During TLI, there was a dramatic acute decrease in the numbers of total T, Leu-3, and Leu-2 cells and little change in the Leu-2/Leu-3 ratio (Table 3). Shortly thereafter, the number of circulating cells bearing the Leu-2 antigen increased rapidly while there was little recovery of the Leu-3 population. This resulted in a marked increase in the ratio of Leu-2/Leu-3 cells (Table 3). These studies suggested that the two major T-cell subsets have different rates of repopulation after TLI.

3. *Changes in T-Cell Proliferative Responses*

Total lymphoid irradiation also resulted in marked alterations of *in vitro* lymphocyte function (Kotzin *et al.*, 1981; Field *et al.*, 1983). The proliferative responses of peripheral blood lymphocytes to the mitogens phytohemagglutinin (PHA), concanavalin A (Con A), and pokeweed mitogen (PWM) were profoundly decreased after TLI as compared to pretreatment and control responses. There was also a marked decrease in the response to allogeneic cells (MLR) after TLI. These alterations in immune responses have so far shown kinetics similar to those reported in patients treated for Hodgkin's disease (Field *et al.*, 1983). Thus, the proliferative responses to mitogens remained depressed throughout the observation period, whereas the proliferative response in the MLR showed some recovery during the third year after TLI.

To determine whether an intrinsic deficit in helper/inducer (Leu-3) cell proliferation contributed to the decreased proliferative responses of whole PBL, Leu-3 cells were

Table 3. Kinetic Studies of T-Cell-Subset Changes after TLI[a]

	Percentage Leu-1	Percentage Leu-2	Percentage Leu-3	Leu-2/Leu-3
Patient 1				
Pre-TLI	65	24	39	0.62
At completion of TLI	13	10	19	0.53
3 months post-TLI	60	55	16	3.4
Patient 2				
Pre-TLI	80	16	66	0.24
At completion of TLI	8.3	4.5	8.2	0.55
3 months post-TLI	68	59	23	2.6

[a] Adapted from Kotzin *et al.* (1983a). Data are shown for two representative patients of four studied.

purified from the peripheral blood of patients before and afer TLI (Field *et al.*, 1984a). The purified Leu-3 cells obtained after TLI showed a marked reduction in [^{3}H]thymidine incorporation in response to PHA, Con A, allogeneic cells, and several protein antigens (tetanus toxoid, diptheria toxoid, herpes zoster, and herpes simplex antigens) as compared to that by cells obtained from the same patients before TLI. Thus, TLI induces both a prolonged reduction in the absolute number of circulating Leu-3 cells and a reduction in the proliferative capacity of Leu-3 cells. It is possible that the proliferative defect itself contributes to the inability of the Leu-3 cells to repopulate the lymphoid tissues after TLI.

4. Suppression of in Vitro Immunoglobulin Secretion

Peripheral blood lymphocytes (PBL) were also tested for their ability to secrete immunoglobulin *in vitro* after stimulation with pokeweed mitogen (PWM) (Kotzin *et al.*, 1981, 1984; Field *et al.*, 1983). This *in vitro* system requires the interaction of T cells, B cells, and monocytes and, furthermore, is regulated by helper and suppressor T cells (Keightley *et al.*, 1976; Fauci *et al.*, 1980; Rosenberg and Lipsky, 1979; Reinherz *et al.*, 1980). The PWM system has been used by many investigators to study defects in the human immune system in both autoimmune and immunodeficiency diseases. Peripheral blood lymphocytes were obtained from normal controls and patients before and after treatment with TLI and were then stimulated in culture with PWM (Table 4). Lymphocytes from patients with RA before TLI generated approximately 60% of the normal level of immunoglobulin-secreting cells. An additional tenfold reduction of both IgM and IgG secretion was observed after treatment with TLI (Table 4) (Kotzin *et al.*, 1984). Ten of 12 patients post-TLI showed a response below the normal range (for both IgM and IgG), whereas only one of 14 patients before TLI had such a low response. No tendency for the secretory response to recover was observed during extended follow-up periods (Field *et al.*, 1983).

This impaired ability of post-TLI PBL to produce immunoglobulin was associated with the presence of suppressor cells in coculture studies (Kotzin *et al.*, 1984). In an allogeneic coculture system, PBL from patients were tested for their ability to suppress immunoglobulin synthesis of responder cells obtained from normal individuals. Figure 2

Table 4. Pokeweed-Mitogen-Stimulated Immunoglobulin Production in Patients Before and After TLI[a]

	Plaque-forming cells/10^6 Cells[b]		Percentage of control response[d]
	IgM	IgG	
Control (N = 12)	19,000 ± 3,600	18,200 ± 6,100	—
Pre-TLI (N = 14)	11,387 ± 3,033	11,547 ± 1,904	61
Post-TLI (N = 12)[c]	1,185 ± 561	1,265 ± 550	7

[a] Adapted from Kotzin *et al.* (1984).
[b] Values shown are the number of plaque-forming cells (PFC) per 10^6 responder cells originally placed into culture and are the mean ± S.E. of the independent means of the number of patients indicated.
[c] Patients were studied 5.7 ± 3.8 months (mean ± S.D.) after completion of TLI.
[d] The mean of the percentage control response for IgM and IgG production is indicated.

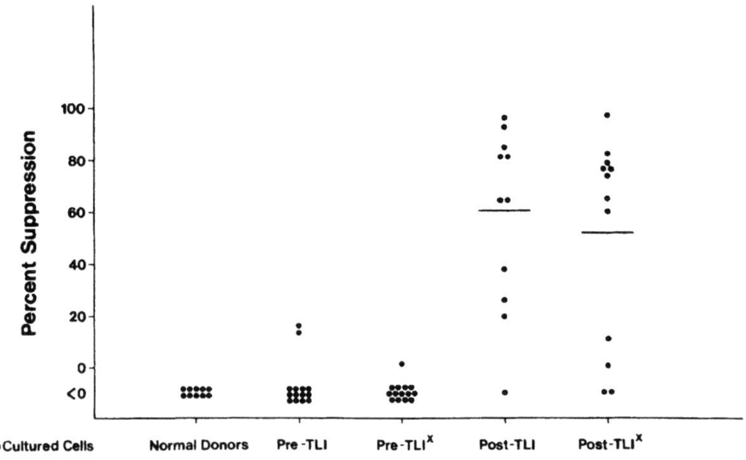

Figure 2. Suppression of PWM-stimulated immunoglobulin synthesis by PBL obtained from patients before and after TLI: allogeneic system. The data are presented as percentage suppression of the control response (compared with responder cells without allogeneic cocultured cells). Each point represents the mean of the percentage suppression for IgM and IgG production for an individual patient. The lines indicate the mean percentage suppression for the respective groups. Patients were studied 5.5 ± 4.3 months (mean ± S.D.) after completion of TLI. ^xCells irradiated to 1000 R *in vitro* prior to culture. (Adapted from Kotzin *et al.*, 1984.)

shows that the addition of cells from normal individuals or from rheumatoid arthritis patients before TLI actually enhanced immunoglobulin production by normal allogeneic cells. Irradiation of the cocultured cells (1000 R) to eliminate contributions by this population to the PFC response did not change the pattern of results. In contrast, the addition of PBL from eight of 12 patients after TLI resulted in greater than 50% suppression of both the IgM and IgG secretory response as compared with the responder cells without cocultured cells.

Peripheral blood lymphocytes from four of seven patients studied after TLI also demonstrated suppression in an autologous system using responder cells cryopreserved before TLI. In no case did cells obtained from the same patients before TLI demonstrate suppression in the autologous system. The presence or absence of suppression in the autologous and allogeneic systems correlated in every case.

When cell subsets were isolated from patients after TLI, suppressor cells were demonstrated in the Leu-2^+ T-cell fraction (Kotzin *et al.*, 1984). Despite the fact that only PBL obtained after TLI exerted suppression, Leu-2^+ cells from TLI-treated patients were no more potent on a cell-per-cell basis than purified Leu-2^+ cells obtained before TLI. Additional experiments suggested that the suppression by T cells after TLI is related to the increased ratio of Leu-2 to Leu-3 cells observed after radiotherapy. In one half of the patients studied, suppressor cells were also found in the non-T fraction and were probably monocytes.

VI. CONCLUSIONS

The results of initial feasibility studies and a recent controlled study indicate that TLI results in long-lasting suppression of disease activity in patients with refractory rheumatoid arthritis. Initial feasibility studies of TLI in the treatment of refractory lupus nephritis have been equally encouraging (Strober *et al.*, 1985b). We are also currently involved in studies of TLI in the treatment of polymyositis, progressive systemic sclerosis, and autoimmune demyelinating polyneuropathy. Although the future clinical role of TLI in these autoimmune diseases remains unclear, results thus far indicate that TLI is a unique immunosuppressive regimen when compared to currently used immunosuppressive drugs. Whereas these drugs show little selectivity with relatively short-lived effects, TLI results in a selective and long-lasting reduction in the number and function of helper T cells; TLI also is uniquely associated with the appearance of antigen-nonspecific suppressor cells and appears to allow for the induction of antigen-specific tolerance.

REFERENCES

Andrews, B. S., Eisenberg, R. A., Theofilipoulous, A. N., Izui, S., Wilson, C. B., McConahey, P. J., Murphy, E. D., Roths, J. B., and Dixon, F. J., 1978, Spontaneous murine lupus-like syndromes: Clinical and immunopathological manifestations in several strains, *J. Exp. Med.* **148:**1198–1215.

Baccarini, M., Bosi, A., and Papa, G., 1980, Second malignancy in patients treated for Hodgkin's disease, *Cancer* **46:**1735–1740.

Coleman, C. N., Williams, C. J., Flint, A., Glatstein, E., Rosenberg, S. A., and Kaplan, H. S., 1977, Hematologic neoplasia in patients treated for Hodgkin's disease, *N. Engl. J. Med.* **297:**1249–1252.

Fauci, A. S., Whalen, G., and Burch, C., 1980, Activation of human B lymphocytes. XVI. Cellular requirements, interactions, and immunoregulation of pokeweed mitogen-induced total-immunoglobulin producing plaque-forming cells in peripheral blood, *Cell. Immunol.* **54:**230–240.

Field, E. H., Strober, S., Hoppe, R. T., Calin, A., Engleman, E. G., Kotzin, B. L., Tanay, A. S., Calin, H. J., Terrell, C. P., and Kaplan, H. S., 1983, Sustained improvement of intractable rheumatoid arthritis after total lymphoid irradiation, *Arthritis Rheum.* **26:**937–946.

Field, E. H., Engleman, E. G., Terrell, C. P., and Strober, S., 1984a, Reduced *in vitro* immune responses of purified human Leu-3 (helper/inducer phenotype) cells after total lymphoid irradiation. *J. Immunol.* **132:**1031–1035.

Fuks, Z., Strober, S., Bobrove, A. M., Sasazuki, T., McMichael, A., and Kaplan, H. S., 1976, Long-term effects of radiation on T and B lymphocytes in peripheral blood of patients with Hodgkin's disease, *J. Clin. Invest.* **58:**803–814.

Gottlieb, M., Strober, S., Hoppe, R. T., Grumet, F. C., and Kaplan, H. S., 1980, Engraftment of allogeneic bone marrow without graft-versus-host disease in mongrel dogs using total lymphoid irradiation, *Transplantation* **29:**487–491.

Gottlieb, M., Strober, S., and Kaplan, H. S., 1981, Cellular basis of graft versus host tolerance in chimeras prepared with total lymphoid irradiation (TLI), *J. Exp. Med.* **152:**736–741.

Helfgott, S., Brahn, E., Trentham, D., Belli, J., Anderson, R., Reinherz, E., Schlossman, S., and Austin, K. F., 1983, Long-term effects of total lymphoid irradiation in refractory rheumatoid arthritis, *Arthritis Rheum.* **26:**S7.

Hess, A. D., and Tutschka, P. J., 1980, Effect of cyclosporin A on human lymphocyte responses *in vitro*. 1. Cs A allows for the expression of alloantigen-activated suppressor cells while preferentially inhibiting the induction of cytolytic effector lymphocytes in MLR, *J. Immunol.* **124:**2601–2608.

Howie, J. B., and Helyer, B. J., 1968, The immunology and pathology of NZB mice, *Adv. Immunol.* **9:**215–284.

Kaplan, H. S., 1980, *Hodgkin's Disease*, ed. 2, Harvard University Press, Cambridge, Massachusetts.

Keightley, R. G., Cooper, M. D., and Lawton, A. R., 1976, The T cell dependence of B cell differentiation induced by pokeweed mitogen, *J. Immunol.* **117:**1538–1544.

King, D. P., Strober, S., and Kaplan, H. S., 1981, Suppression of the mixed leukocyte response and of graft-versus-host disease by spleen cells following total lymphoid irradiation (TLI), *J. Immunol.* **126:**1140–1145.

Kotzin, B. L., and Strober, S., 1979, Reveral of NZB/NZW disease with total lymphoid irradiation, *J. Exp. Med.* **150:**371–378.

Kotzin, B. L., Strober, S., Engleman, E. G., Calin, A., Hoppe, R. T., Kansas, G. S., Terrell, C. P., and

Kaplan, H. S., 1981, Treatment of intractable rheumatoid arthritis with total lymphoid irradiation, *N. Engl. J. Med.* **305**:969–976.

Kotzin, B. L., Kansas, G. S., Engleman, E. G., Hoppe, R. T., Kaplan, H. S., and Strober, S., 1983a, Changes in T-cell subsets in patients with rheumatoid arthritis treated with total lymphoid irradiation, *Clin. Immunol. Immunopathol.* **27**:250–260.

Kotzin, B. L., Ward, R., and Strober, S., 1983b, Failure of NZB/NZW spleen cells to re-establish disease in irradiated syngeneic recipients, *Arthritis Rheum.* **26**:S75.

Kotzin, B. L., Strober, S., Kansas, G. S., Terrell, C. P., and Engleman, E. G., 1984, Suppression of pokeweed mitogen stimulated immunoglobulin production in patients with rheumatoid arthritis after treatment with total lymphoid irradiation, *J. Immunol.* **132**:1049–1055.

Krikorian, J. G., Burke, J. S., Rosenberg, S. A., and Kaplan, H. S., 1979, Occurrence of non-Hodgkin's lymphoma after therapy for Hodgkin's disease, *N. Engl. J. Med.* **300**:452–458.

Lowry, R. P., Forbes, R. D., and Blackburn, J. H., 1984a, Immune reactivity and immunosuppressive intervention (TLI) in experimental nephritis. 1. Immunopathologic correlates in the accelerated autologous form of nephrotoxic serum nephritis, *J. Immunol.* **132**:1001–1006.

Lowry, R. P., Forbes, R. D., Carpenter, C. B., Gurley, K. E., and Merrill, J. P., 1984b, Immune reactivity and immunosuppressive intervention in experimental nephritis. 11. Effect of TLI on the course of two models of nephritis in the inbred rat, *J. Immunol.* **132**:1007–1012.

May, R. D., Slavin, S., and Vitetta, E. S., 1983, The partial characterization of suppressor cells in the spleens of mice conditioned with fractionated total lymphoid irradiation (TLI), *J. Immunol.* **131**:1108–1114.

Neale, T. J., and Wilson, C. B., 1982, Glomerular antigens in Heymann's nephritis: Reactivity of eluted and circulating antibody, *J. Immunol.* **128**:323–330.

Okada, S., and Strober, S., 1982, Spleen cells from adult mice given total lymphoid irradiation (TLI) or from newborn mice have similar regulatory effects in the mixed leukocyte reaction (MLR). 1. Generation of antigen-specific suppressor cells in the mixed leukocyte reaction after the addition of spleen cells from adult mice given total lymphoid irradiation, *J. Exp. Med.* **156**:522–538.

Oseroff, A., Okada, S., and Strober, S., 1984, Natural suppressor (NS) cells found in the spleen of neonatal mice and of adult mice given total lymphoid irradiation (TLI) express the null surface phenotype, *J. Immunol.* **132**:101–110.

Prud'homme, G. J., Park, C. L., Feiser, T. M., Kofler, R., Dixon, F. J., and Theofilopoulos, A. N., 1983, Identification of a B cell differentiation factor(s) spontaneously produced by proliferating T cells in murine lupus strains of the lpr/lpr genotype, *J. Exp. Med.* **157**:730–742.

Reinherz, E. L., Morimoto, C., Penta, A. C., and Schlossman, S. F., 1980, Regulation of B cell immunoglobulin secretion by functional subsets of T lymphocytes in man, *Eur. J. Immunol.* **10**:570–572.

Rosenberg, S. A., and Lipsky, P. E., 1979, Monocyte dependence of pokeweed mitogen-induced differentiation of immunoglobulin-secreting cells from human peripheral blood mononuclear cells, *J. Immunol.* **122**:926–931.

Schurman, D. J., Hirshman, P., and Strober, S., 1981, Total lymphoid irradiation and local joint irradiation in the treatment of adjuvant arthritis, *Arthritis Rheum.* **24**:38–44.

Slavin, S., Strober, S., Fuks, Z., and Kaplan, H. S., 1976, Long-term survival of skin allografts in mice treated with fractionated total lymphoid irradiation, *Science* **193**:1252–1255.

Slavin, S., Strober, S., Fuks, Z., and Kaplan, H. S., 1977, Induction of specific tissue transplantation tolerance using fractionated total lymphoid irradiation in adult mice: Long-term survival of allogeneic bone marrow and skin grafts, *J. Exp. Med.* **146**:34–48.

Slavin, S., Reitz, B., Bieber, C. P., Kaplan, H. S., and Strober, S., 1978, Transplantation tolerance in adult rats using total lymphoid irradiation: Permanent survival of skin, heart and marrow allografts, *J. Exp. Med.* **147**:700–707.

Strober, S., Tanay, A., Field, E., Hoppe, R. T., Calin, A., Engleman, E. G., Kotzin, B. L., Brown, B. W., and Kaplan, H. S., 1985a, Efficacy of total lymphoid irradiation in intractable rheumatoid arthritis: A double-blind randomized trial, *Ann. Intern. Med.* **102**:441–449.

Strober, S., Field, E., Hoppe, R. T., Kotzin, B. L., Shemesh, O., Engleman, E., Ross, J. C., and Meyers, B. D., 1985b, Treatment of intractable lupus nephritis with total lymphoid irradiation, *Ann. Intern. Med.* **102**:450–458.

Tanay, A., and Strober, S., 1984, Opposite effects of total lymphoid irradiation on T cell dependent and T cell independent antibody responses, *J. Immunol.* **132**:979–984.

Tanay, A., Strober, S., Logue, G. L., and Schiffman, G., 1984, Use of total lymphoid irradiation (TLI) in studies of the T cell dependence of autoantibody production in rheumatoid arthritis, *J. Immunol.* **132:**1036–1040.

Theofilopoulos, A. N., Balderas, R., Schawler, D. L., Izui, S., Kotzin, B. L., Strober, S., and Dixon, F. J., 1980, Inhibition of T cell proliferation and SLE-like syndrome of MRL/l mice by whole body or total lymphoid irradiation, *J. Immunol.* **125:**2137–2142.

Trentham, D. E., Belli, J. A., Anderson, R. J., Buckley, J. A., Goetzl, E. J., David, J. R., and Austen, K. F., 1981, Clinical and immunologic effects of fractionated total lymphoid irradiation in refractory rheumatoid arthritis, *N. Engl. J. Med.* **305:**976–982.

Valagussa, P., Santoro, A., Kenda, R., Fossati Bellani, F., Franchi, F., Banfi, A., Rilke, F., and Bonadonna, G., 1980, Second malignancies in Hodgkin's disease: A complication of certain forms of treatment, *Br. Med. J.* **280:**216–219.

Zan-Bar, I., Slavin, S., and Strober, S., 1978, Induction and mechanism of tolerance to bovine serum albumin in mice given total lymphoid irradiation (TLI), *J. Immunol.* **121:**1400–1404.

Index

GPSR Compliance

The European Union's (EU) General Product Safety Regulation (GPSR) is a set of rules that requires consumer products to be safe and our obligations to ensure this.

If you have any concerns about our products, you can contact us on ProductSafety@springernature.com

In case Publisher is established outside the EU, the EU authorized representative is:

Springer Nature Customer Service Center GmbH
Europaplatz 3
69115 Heidelberg, Germany

Batch number: 10684222

Printed by Printforce, the Netherlands

Michael Englbrecht, Oliver Pehnke

SAP®-Schnittstellenprogrammierung

Rheinwerk
Publishing

Liebe Leserin, lieber Leser,

SAP-Landschaften sind komplex, und wir alle wissen, wie schnell sich Technologien und Anforderungen in der IT-Welt ändern. Genau da setzt SAP PRESS an: mit Büchern, die nicht nur Theorie vermitteln, sondern konkret im Alltag helfen.

In diesem Buch finden Sie direkt umsetzbare Ratschläge, praktische Beispiele und Lösungen für drängende Herausforderungen. Unsere Autorinnen und Autoren sind Profis, die wissen, wo der Schuh drückt – und wie man Probleme effizient löst. Mit ihrer Erfahrung an Ihrer Seite können Sie Ihre SAP-Projekte gezielter angehen, fundiertere Entscheidungen treffen und die vielen Facetten von SAP besser meistern.

Ob Sie gerade erst beginnen oder schon lange im SAP-Umfeld tätig sind: Wir sind davon überzeugt, dass dieses Buch Ihnen hilfreiche Anleitungen und Tipps an die Hand gibt, um Ihre täglichen Aufgaben und Projekte erfolgreich zu meistern.

Wir freuen uns stets über Lob, aber auch über kritische Anmerkungen, die uns helfen, unsere Bücher zu verbessern. Zögern Sie also nicht, sich bei mir zu melden; Ihr Feedback ist jederzeit willkommen.

Wir wünschen Ihnen viele Aha-Momente und eine erfolgreiche Umsetzung mit diesem Buch!

Ihre Janina Schweitzer
Senior-Lektorin SAP PRESS

janina.schweitzer@rheinwerk-verlag.de
www.rheinwerk-verlag.de
Rheinwerk Verlag · Rheinwerkallee 4 · 53227 Bonn

Auf einen Blick

Wir hoffen, dass Sie Freude an diesem Buch haben und sich Ihre Erwartungen erfüllen. Ihre Anregungen und Kommentare sind uns jederzeit willkommen. Bitte bewerten Sie doch das Buch auf unserer Website unter **www.rheinwerk-verlag.de/feedback**.

An diesem Buch haben viele mitgewirkt, insbesondere:

Lektorat Janina Schweitzer
Korrektorat Claudia Lötschert, Neuss
Herstellung Stefanie Häb
Typografie und Layout Vera Brauner
Einbandgestaltung Bastian Illerhaus
Coverbild Unsplash: Meriç Dagli
Satz SatzPro, Krefeld
Druck Beltz Grafische Betriebe, Bad Langensalza

FSC www.fsc.org MIX Papier | Fördert gute Waldnutzung FSC® C089473

Dieses Buch wurde gesetzt aus der TheAntiquaB (9,35/13,7 pt) in FrameMaker.

Gedruckt wurde es mit mineralölfreien Farben auf chlorfrei gebleichtem, FSC®-zertifiziertem Offsetpapier (90 g/m²).

Hergestellt in Deutschland.

Bibliografische Information der Deutschen Nationalbibliothek:
Die Deutsche Nationalbibliothek verzeichnet diese Publikation in der Deutschen Nationalbibliografie; detaillierte bibliografische Daten sind im Internet über *http://dnb.dnb.de* abrufbar.

ISBN 978-3-367-10329-4

5., aktualisierte und erweiterte Auflage 2025

Rheinwerk Verlag GmbH • Rheinwerkallee 4 • 53227 Bonn
service@rheinwerk-verlag.de

Informationen zu unserem Verlag und Kontaktmöglichkeiten finden Sie auf unserer Verlagswebsite **www.rheinwerk-verlag.de**. Dort können Sie sich auch umfassend über unser aktuelles Programm informieren und unsere Bücher und E-Books bestellen.

Inhalt

TEIL III SAP-Schnittstellenprogrammierung in der Cloud

Einleitung

In dieser fünften, aktualisierten und erweiterten Auflage unseres Handbuchs zur SAP-Schnittstellenprogrammierung finden Sie detaillierte technische Informationen darüber, wie SAP-Systeme untereinander und mit externen Systemen kommunizieren können. Diese Informationen werden mit lauffähigen und ausprogrammierten Programmierbeispielen illustriert, die Ihnen die Umsetzung in der Praxis erleichtern. Hier lassen wir unsere Erfahrungen als Trainer und Schnittstellenentwickler einfließen. Dabei berücksichtigen wir die fünf wichtigen Programmiersprachen ABAP, C/C++, Java, C# und JavaScript.

Zielgruppe

Dieses Buch wendet sich an Entwickler, die ihre Programme mit SAP-Systemen integrieren möchten, an technische Berater, die ihren Kunden Integrationsmöglichkeiten empfehlen möchten, und an SAP-Kunden, die einen fundierten Einblick in die Integrationsprogrammierung wünschen.

Aufbau

Der Aufbau des Buchs ist wie folgt:

- **Kapitel 1**, »Grundlagen der SAP-Schnittstellenprogrammierung«, beginnt mit einem Überblick über die gesamte Thematik und führt die Beispielanwendung ein, die uns während des ganzen Buchs begleiten wird. Mit dieser Beispielanwendung werden Bestellungen von Buchhändlern an Großhändler und von Großhändlern an Verlage verwaltet.
- In **Kapitel 2**, »Grundlagen der Schnittstellenprogrammierung auf der SAP Business Technology Platform«, führen wir in die SAP Business Technology Platform (SAP BTP) ein. Wir gehen auf deren Positionierung und Konzepte sowie auf die Themen Sicherheit und Integration ein.
- In **Kapitel 3** bis **Kapitel 6** geht es dann um Remote Function Calls (RFCs). Dies ist eine SAP-Schnittstellentechnologie, mit der Funktionsbausteine in anderen Systemen aufgerufen werden können. **Kapitel 3**, »Remote Function Call mit ABAP«, beleuchtet das Thema aus der Perspektive von ABAP, **Kapitel 4**, »Remote Function Call mit C/C++«, erläutert die Programmierung mit C, **Kapitel 5**, »Remote Function Call mit Java«, die Programmierung mit Java und **Kapitel 6**, »Remote Function Call mit C#«, die Programmierung mit C# und dem SAP Connector for Microsoft .NET. Auch die Entwicklung und Verwendung von Business Application Programming Interfaces (BAPIs) werden in diesen Kapiteln erklärt.
- **Kapitel 7**, »IDocs und Application Link Enabling«, erläutert das Application Link Enabling (ALE). Diese SAP-Technologie erlaubt es Anwendun-

gen, Informationen in Form von Intermediate Documents (IDocs) auszutauschen. Sie baut selbst wieder auf RFC auf.

- Nach den SAP-Technologien RFC und ALE wendet sich **Kapitel 8**, »SOAP-Webservices«, dem Protokoll SOAP zu. Dieser offene Webstandard ermöglicht es Anwendungen, Informationen in Form von XML-Dokumenten über HTTP oder andere Protokolle auszutauschen, und wird heutzutage von nahezu allen Entwicklungsplattformen unterstützt, wie wir am Beispiel von Java und C# zeigen werden. Neben dem Inside-Out-Ansatz, der von vorhandenen Funktionsbausteinen ausgeht, erläutern wir auch den Outside-In-Ansatz. Bei diesem Ansatz beschreiben Sie zuerst die Schnittstellen, generieren dann aus der Schnittstellenbeschreibung heraus die Klassen, die die technische Kommunikation realisieren, und nutzen dann diese Klassen bei der Implementierung der Anwendung.
- In **Kapitel 9**, »SAP Gateway und OData«, erläutern wir die Entwicklung von OData-Services mit ABAP und deren Verwendung mit SAPUI5 und C#. Das OData-Protokoll ermöglicht den Austausch von Informationen über HTTP in Form von JSON- oder XML-Dokumenten.
- In **Kapitel 10**, »SAP HANA und ABAP Core Data Services«, beschreiben wir das als ABAP-Programmiermodell für SAP Fiori bekannte Programmiermodell und dessen Bezug zu SAP HANA. Wir erläutern die Bereitstellung von OData-Services über Core-Data-Service-(CDS-)Views.
- Neu in dieser Auflage ist **Kapitel 11**, »ABAP RESTful Application Programming Model und OData«. In diesem Kapitel führen wir in das derzeit von SAP für SAP S/4HANA empfohlene Programmiermodell ein. Dieses Modell ist zukunftsweisend für die Implementierung von OData-Services auf SAP S/4HANA. Wir implementieren in diesem Kapitel einen OData-Service mit lesenden und ändernden Operationen.
- In **Kapitel 12**, »ABAP Channels«, geht es um Kommunikationskanäle, mit denen die ABAP-Plattform Push-Nachrichten an Clients schicken kann. Hier zeigen wir Ihnen, wie Sie in ABAP das WebSocket Protocol nutzen können, um Nachrichten an einen Webclient zu schicken.
- Mit dem ebenfalls neuen **Kapitel 13**, »SAP Cloud Application Programming Model und OData«, beschreiben wir erstmalig die Entwicklung von OData-Diensten für die SAP BTP. Wir zeigen, wie man mit diesem Programmiermodell OData-Dienste implementiert und diese auf der SAP BTP zur Verfügung stellt.
- Ein weiteres neues Kapitel ist **Kapitel 14**, »SAP Business Accelerator Hub«. Hier geben wir Ihnen einen Überblick über diese für Integrationsszenarien wichtige Webanwendung. Wir zeigen Ihnen, wie man mit dem

SAP Business Accelerator Hub arbeitet und welche Möglichkeiten er bietet, um investitionssichere Integrationsszenarien zu implementieren.

- Den Abschluss des Buchs bildet das neue **Kapitel 15**, »Echtzeitkommunikation mit Event-driven Architecture«, in dem wir SAP Event Mesh und die SAP Integration Suite als wegweisende neue Werkzeuge für die Integration vorstellen. Wir zeigen, wie Sie mit diesen Werkzeugen eine Event-driven Architecture (EDA) aufbauen können, und erläutern dies anhand von Programmbeispielen in JavaScript.

Für diese fünfte Auflage haben wir den gesamten Text und alle Programmierbeispiele überarbeitet und auf den neuesten Stand gebracht.

Zusatzinformationen

Wichtige Hinweise und Zusatzinformationen werden in Form von Infokästen gesondert hervorgehoben. Diese Kästen haben unterschiedliche Schwerpunkte und sind mit verschiedenen Symbolen markiert:

- [!] Seien Sie bei der Durchführung einer Aufgabe oder eines Schritts, der mit einem *Ausrufezeichen* markiert ist, besonders vorsichtig.
- [«] Wird das besprochene *Thema erläutert und vertieft*, macht ein Doppelpfeil Sie darauf aufmerksam.
- [+] Nützliche *Tipps*, die Ihnen die Arbeit erleichtern, sind mit einem Pluszeichen gekennzeichnet.

Systemvoraussetzungen

Das Buch eignet sich sowohl als Nachschlagewerk als auch als Lehrbuch bei der Programmierung von Schnittstellen zwischen SAP- und Nicht-SAP-Systemen. Es stellt grundlegende Techniken der Schnittstellenprogrammierung vor und erläutert sie praxisnah. Die jeweiligen Systemvoraussetzungen für die Installation der benötigten Software entnehmen Sie den entsprechenden Download-Seiten der einzelnen Produkte in der SAP Community (*https://community.sap.com/*).

- Die ABAP-Beispiele wurden in einem SAP-S/4HANA-System 2022 implementiert.
- Um die Stand-alone-Java-Beispiele nachzuvollziehen, können Sie jede Java-Entwicklungsumgebung verwenden. Die Programmierbeispiele liegen im Download-Material jedoch als Eclipse- und IntelliJ-Projekte vor, sodass sich die Verwendung dieser IDEs anbietet.
- Für die C#- und C/C++-Beispiele haben wir Microsoft Visual Studio 2022 in der frei verfügbaren Community Edition verwendet.
- Für die JavaScript-Beispiele kam das SAP Business Application Studio zum Einsatz.

Beispiele zu diesem Buch

Alle Codebeispiele können Sie sich auf der Verlagshomepage unter *http://www.sap-press.de/5955* herunterladen.

Danksagung

Dieses Buch beruht auf vielen öffentlich zugänglichen Quellen von SAP: der Online-Hilfe auf *http://help.sap.com* sowie den Blogs, Diskussionsforen und White Papers der SAP Community. Ein herzliches Dankeschön geht an dieser Stelle an die SAP SE für die großartige Software und an alle Menschen, die sie entwickelt oder dabei geholfen haben. Ebenfalls möchten wir unseren herzlichen Dank Michael Wegelin aussprechen, der in den zurückliegenden Auflagen ein großartiger Mitautor war.

Großer Dank gilt auch unserer Lektorin Janina Schweitzer und dem gesamten Team beim Rheinwerk Verlag. Ein riesengroßes Dankeschön geht an das Team der eXXcellent solutions: ein fantastisches Team mit fantastischen Kolleginnen und Kollegen.

Michael Englbrecht möchte Michaela, Domenik und Sophie für ihr Verständnis und ihre Geduld danken. Eingespannt in viele im Arbeitskontext stattfindende Themen geben die drei mir die wichtigen Impulse, auch mal die Seele baumeln zu lassen und achtsam zu sein.

Oliver Pehnke möchte allen danken, die dieses Buch ermöglicht haben. Es war eine spannende Reise, Neues und Altes neu zu entdecken, auch wenn es viel Zeit und Energie kostete.

Michael Englbrecht
Principal Managing Consultant, Portfolio Manager SAP und
Business Manager bei eXXcellent solutions GmbH, Ulm

Oliver Pehnke
Senior Architekt bei der eXXcellent solutions GmbH, Ulm

TEIL I

Grundlagen

Kapitel 1
Grundlagen der SAP-Schnittstellenprogrammierung

In diesem Kapitel finden Sie in komprimierter Form das Grundlagenwissen, das Sie für die SAP-Schnittstellenprogrammierung benötigen: Informationen zur Architektur der ABAP-Plattform, zum Aufbau von ABAP-Programmen und zu den unterstützten Anwendungsprotokollen.

Dieses erste Kapitel gibt Ihnen eine Übersicht über die Architektur der ABAP-Plattform (SAP NetWeaver Application Server ABAP) und stellt dabei insbesondere die Komponenten heraus, die für die Kommunikation mit externen Systemen verantwortlich sind. Sie erhalten eine kurze Einführung in die Programmierung mit ABAP und lernen die Werkzeuge der ABAP Workbench kennen. Daran schließt sich eine erste Auflistung der Schnittstellen an, die von der ABAP-Plattform unterstützt werden. Zusätzlich werden Bibliotheken und Konnektoren für die Programmiersprachen C, Java und C# beschrieben, die für die Schnittstellenprogrammierung benötigt werden.

1.1 Die ABAP-Plattform

In diesem Abschnitt stellen wir Ihnen die Architektur der ABAP-Plattform vor. Dabei konzentrieren wir uns auf die Komponenten, die für die Schnittstellenprogrammierung besonders wichtig sind. Dazu gehören vor allem die Komponenten der Applikationsschicht, die für die Ausführung der ABAP-Programme verantwortlich sind.

1.1.1 Anwendungsserver für SAP S/4HANA

Die ABAP-Plattform dient als Anwendungsserver für SAP S/4HANA. Es handelt sich um eine Technologieplattform für alle Geschäftsanwendungen in SAP S/4HANA, z. B. das Finanzwesen, die Logistikanwendungen und SAP HCM for SAP S/4HANA.

SAP NetWeaver Application Server

In der klassischen SAP-Architektur ist der *SAP NetWeaver Application Server* ein portabler Anwendungsserver, der auf vielen verschiedenen Hardware-,

Betriebssystem- und Datenbankplattformen läuft. Er unterstützt Anwendungen, die in ABAP oder Java geschrieben sind. Er besteht demnach im Prinzip aus zwei Anwendungsservern, die entweder separat (Single Stack) oder im Verband (Double Stack) installiert werden können.

Client-Server-Architektur

Der SAP NetWeaver Application Server bildet ebenso wie die heutige APAP-Plattform die mittlere Schicht einer klassischen dreischichtigen *Client-Server-Architektur*. Diese Architektur besteht aus der Datenschicht, der Applikationsschicht und der Präsentationsschicht. Abbildung 1.1 zeigt diese Architektur.

- **Datenschicht**
  Die Datenschicht besteht aus einer relationalen Datenbank. Bei SAP S/4HANA ist das SAP HANA. Klassischerweise konnten beliebige Datenbanksysteme wie z. B. Oracle oder Microsoft SQL Server mit SAP eingesetzt werden. In den Datenbanktabellen sind die betriebswirtschaftlichen Stamm- und Bewegungsdaten sowie Systemdaten gespeichert. Innerhalb der Datenbank sind die Schemata für den ABAP- und den Java-Teil strikt voneinander getrennt. Das heißt, dass ABAP-Anwendungen nicht direkt auf Daten im Java-Teil der Datenbank zugreifen können und umgekehrt.
- **Applikationsschicht**
  Die Applikationsschicht besteht aus Prozessen, die die Anwendungsprogramme ausführen, die entweder in ABAP oder in Java geschrieben sind. In der Applikationsschicht werden auch die grafischen Benutzerdialoge erzeugt, die von der Präsentationsschicht angezeigt werden. Der SAP NetWeaver Application Server besteht aus zwei Technologie-Stacks: dem ABAP-Stack (dunkel in Abbildung 1.1) und dem Java-Stack. Bei der Installation eines SAP NetWeaver Application Servers können entweder nur der ABAP-Stack (SAP NetWeaver AS ABAP) oder nur der Java-Stack (SAP NetWeaver AS Java) oder beide Stacks zusammen installiert werden (Double-Stack-System). Technologie-Stack für SAP S/4HANA ist lediglich die ABAP-Plattform. Den Java-Stack erwähnen wir an dieser Stelle lediglich der Vollständigkeit halber. Im weiteren Verlauf dieses Kapitels werden wir ihn jedoch nicht weiter betrachten.
- **Präsentationsschicht**
  In der Präsentationsschicht werden die Ergebnisse der Applikationsschicht für den Benutzer visualisiert. Sie nimmt die Eingaben eines Benutzers entgegen und leitet seine Befehle an die Applikationsschicht weiter. Die Präsentationsschicht wird durch das SAP Graphical User Interface (SAP GUI) oder einen HTML-Browser realisiert. Diese Programme werden

auf den Desktop-PCs der Benutzer installiert, die mit den Anwendungen auf einem SAP NetWeaver Application Server arbeiten möchten.

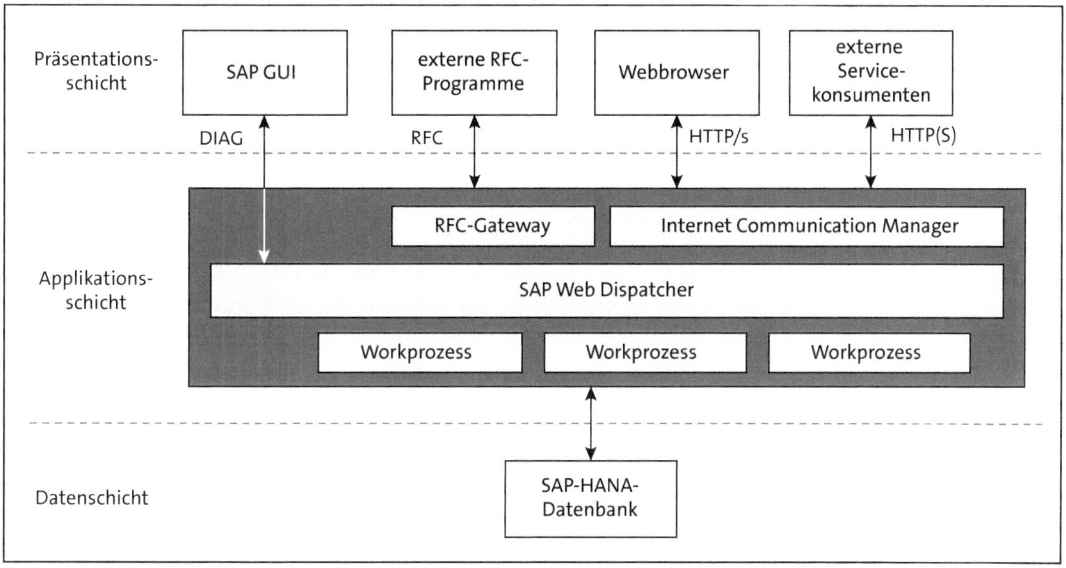

Abbildung 1.1 Dreischichtige Architektur eines SAP-Systems

1.1.2 SAP NetWeaver Application Server ABAP

Die meisten und wichtigsten SAP-Lösungen sind in ABAP realisiert, dies gilt auch für SAP S/4HANA. Es ist daher besonders wichtig, die Architektur und das Laufzeitverhalten des SAP NetWeaver Application Server ABAP zu kennen, der in SAP S/4HANA von der ABAP-Plattform fortgeführt wird. Falls Sie bisher noch nie mit einem SAP-System gearbeitet haben, erfahren Sie im nächsten Abschnitt, wie Sie sich am System anmelden und zwischen den Anwendungen navigieren können, bevor Sie dann den ABAP-Applikationsserver im Detail kennenlernen.

Wir gehen davon aus, dass Sie Zugriff auf einen vollständig installierten ABAP-Applikationsserver haben. Im SAP Developer Center (*https://developers.sap.com/trials-downloads.html*) finden Sie z. B. eine Testversion (Trial-Version), die Sie kostenlos herunterladen können.

Anmeldung und Navigation mit dem SAP GUI

Um mit einem ABAP-System zu arbeiten, starten Sie auf Ihrer lokalen Workstation das SAP Graphical User Interface (SAP GUI). Dies ist eine Windows-Anwendung, die über das DIAG-Kommunikationsprotokoll (Dynamic Information and Action Gateway) mit dem SAP NetWeaver AS ABAP kommunizieren kann. Neben dem SAP GUI für Windows gibt es auch ein SAP GUI für Java und eines für HTML.

Benutzersitzung Wenn Sie das SAP GUI starten, verbindet es sich mit einem SAP NetWeaver AS ABAP der Applikationsschicht. Während einer solchen Benutzersitzung, die mit der Anmeldung beginnt und mit der Abmeldung endet, arbeiten Sie immer mit genau einem SAP NetWeaver AS ABAP eines ganzen Systems. Dieser Server wird dem SAP GUI beim Start angegeben, oder er wird vom Message-Server des SAP-Systems über einen Lastverteilungsmechanismus zugeteilt.

Anmeldung Nach dem Start des SAP GUI sehen Sie einen Anmeldebildschirm wie in Abbildung 1.2. Zur Anmeldung müssen Sie vier Angaben machen:

- **Mandant (Client)**
  SAP-Systeme sind mandantenfähig. Damit ist es möglich, innerhalb eines SAP-Systems betriebswirtschaftlich voneinander unabhängige Daten zu speichern. Dies wird dadurch ermöglicht, dass die erste Spalte jeder betriebswirtschaftlichen Tabelle die dreistellige Mandantennummer enthält. Die Datenbankschnittstelle des SAP NetWeaver AS ABAP ergänzt die `WHERE`-Klausel jeder Datenbankabfrage mit dem aktuellen Anmeldemandanten des Benutzers. Damit sehen und bearbeiten Sie als Benutzer immer nur die Daten des Mandanten, mit dem Sie sich angemeldet haben. In der Praxis wird dies hauptsächlich auf Qualitätssicherungs- und Testsystemen genutzt, um unterschiedliche Testdatenbestände voneinander zu trennen.
- **Benutzer (User)**
  Damit Sie sich als Anwender am System anmelden können, muss für Sie ein mandantenbezogener Benutzerstammsatz angelegt sein. Sie identifizieren sich durch einen Benutzernamen, der innerhalb des Mandanten eindeutig ist. Bei der Anmeldung wird dieser Benutzername angegeben.
- **Passwort (Password)**
  Die Anmeldung ist nur dann erfolgreich, wenn Sie das für Sie gültige Passwort eingeben.
- **Sprache (Language)**
  SAP-Systeme sind mehrsprachig. Alle Texte, die auf der grafischen Benutzeroberfläche angezeigt werden, können von den Entwicklern in verschiedene Sprachen übersetzt werden. Die bei der Anmeldung angegebene Sprache legt fest, in welcher Sprache diese Texte ausgegeben werden.

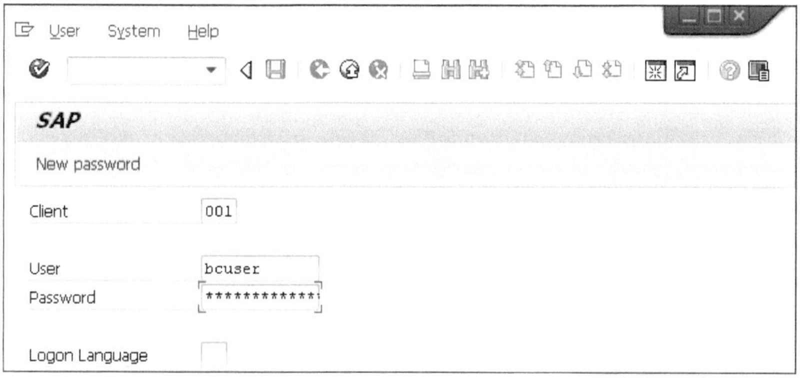

Abbildung 1.2 Anmeldebildschirm des SAP GUI

Bildschirmaufbau

Nach der Anmeldung öffnet sich der SAP-Easy-Access-Bildschirm. Wie es in Abbildung 1.3 zu sehen ist, ist der Bildschirm in verschiedene Bereiche aufgeteilt:

- **Menüleiste**
  In der obersten Zeile des Bildschirms sind Drop-down-Menüs zu finden, mit denen Anwendungsfunktionen ausgelöst werden. Diese Menüleiste enthält für jede Anwendung unterschiedliche Funktionen. Lediglich die beiden letzten Menüpunkte, **System** und **Hilfe**, sind für alle Anwendungen gleich.
- **Systemfunktionsleiste**
  Die Systemfunktionsleiste unterhalb der Menüleiste ist für alle Anwendungen gleich und bietet Zugriff auf wichtige Systemfunktionen wie **Eingabeprüfung**, **Befehlseingabe**, **Speichern**, **Zurückgehen**, **Beenden**, **Abbrechen**, **Drucken**, **Suchen** und **Blättern in Listen**.

  Das erste Icon in der Systemfunktionsleiste, ein weißes Häkchen über einem grünen Ball, löst eine Überprüfung der Benutzereingaben aus. Fehleingaben führen dazu, dass die fehlerhaften Eingabefelder rot angezeigt werden und in der Statuszeile am unteren Bildschirmrand eine Fehlermeldung erscheint.
- **Kommandofeld**
  Das Kommandofeld für die direkte Eingabe von Kommandos ist nach der ersten Anmeldung in der Regel nicht zu sehen, wird aber eingeblendet, wenn Sie auf das kleine graue Dreieck in der Systemfunktionsleiste klicken. Über Eingaben im Kommandofeld können Sie Transaktionen (ABAP-Programme) starten und beenden. Tabelle 1.1 listet die wichtigsten Befehle auf.

Kommando	Funktion
/n	Beendet die laufende Transaktion.
/nxxxx	Beendet die laufende Transaktion und startet Transaktion xxxx.
/i	Löscht den aktuellen externen Modus.
/o	Listet alle externen Modi auf. Aus dem Dialog kann ein neuer externer Modus gestartet werden.
/oxxxx	Startet einen neuen externen Modus mit Transaktion xxxx.

Tabelle 1.1 Wichtige Kommandos für das Kommandofeld in der Systemfunktionsleiste

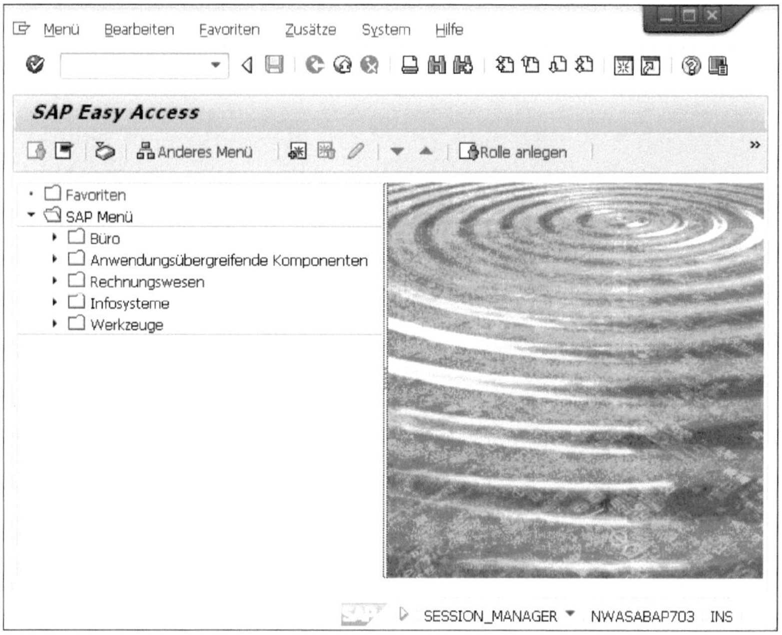

Abbildung 1.3 SAP Easy Access – Standardeinstiegsbildschirm

- **Titelleiste**
  Unter der Systemfunktionsleiste wird der Titel des gerade ausgeführten Programms angezeigt.
- **Anwendungsfunktionsleiste**
  Unterhalb der Titelleiste befindet sich die Anwendungsfunktionsleiste. Hier können Sie die wichtigsten anwendungsspezifischen Funktionen per Mausklick auslösen.

- **Bildschirmbild**
  Den größten Teil des Bildschirms nimmt eine Fläche ein, in die Sie als Anwender Daten eintragen und auf der Sie Funktionen auswählen oder Listen anschauen können. Bei der Anwendung SAP Easy Access befindet sich im rechten Fensterbereich ein Logo. Der linke Fensterbereich enthält einen Baum, das **SAP-Menü**, aus dem heraus die betriebswirtschaftlichen Programme gestartet werden können.
- **Statusleiste**
  Ganz unten befindet sich die Statusleiste. Hier werden Systemmeldungen (Fehler, Warnungen und Informationen) angezeigt. Dort sind auch weitere Informationen wie etwa die System-ID, der Anmeldemandant, der Benutzername, der Transaktionscode der gerade ausgeführten Anwendung oder der Hostname des Applikationsservers zu finden. Auch diese Zusatzinformationen können sich zunächst hinter einem kleinen grauen Dreieck verbergen.

Externer Modus

Während einer Benutzersitzung kommunizieren Sie (als Benutzer) über das SAP GUI immer mit demselben SAP NetWeaver AS ABAP und können bis zu sechs Fenster öffnen, die sogenannten *externen Modi*. In diesen Fenstern können unterschiedliche Programme laufen, zwischen denen Sie wechseln können. Der gesamte Benutzerkontext innerhalb einer Sitzung wird vom SAP NetWeaver Application Server gespeichert.

ABAP-Instanz

Innerhalb eines SAP-Systems gibt es auf der Datenschicht nur einen einzigen Datenbankprozess, aber auf der Applikationsschicht kann es mehrere ABAP-Instanzen geben, die ABAP-Programme ausführen. Jede Instanz besteht ihrerseits aus verschiedenen Prozessen, die genau abgegrenzte Aufgaben übernehmen. Eine Instanz wird durch die Angabe von drei Parametern eindeutig identifiziert:

- **System-ID**
  Die System-ID identifiziert ein SAP-System eindeutig innerhalb eines Systemverbunds. Die System-ID ist ein Identifizierer, der aus drei Stellen (Buchstaben und Ziffern) besteht, z. B. SD1. In der Regel wird als Name für die Datenbank eines SAP-Systems die System-ID verwendet.
- **Hostname**
  Alle Prozesse einer SAP-Instanz laufen auf demselben Host. Es kann aber mehrere SAP-Instanzen innerhalb eines Systems geben, die in der Regel auf verschiedenen Hosts laufen. Daher muss zur Identifizierung einer SAP-Instanz der Hostname angegeben werden.

- **Systemnummer**
  Auf einem Host können aber auch mehrere SAP-Instanzen laufen. Zur eindeutigen Unterscheidung verschiedener Instanzen auf demselben Host ist daher eine dritte Angabe notwendig: die zweistellige Systemnummer. Diese Systemnummer kann jeden beliebigen Wert zwischen »00« und »99« annehmen. Die Systemnummern zweier SAP-Instanzen auf demselben Host müssen unterschiedlich sein, selbst dann, wenn diese SAP-Instanzen zu verschiedenen SAP-Systemen gehören.

Der Name einer SAP-Instanz setzt sich demnach aus drei Bestandteilen zusammen: `<SID>_<HOST>_<SYSNR>`. Dabei ist `<SID>` die dreistellige System-ID, `<HOST>` der Hostname des Applikationsservers und `<SYSNR>` die zweistellige Systemnummer der SAP-Instanz. So lautet etwa der vollständige Instanzname der Instanz mit der Systemnummer `50` des Systems mit der System-ID `UL0`, die auf dem Host `saphost` läuft, `ul0_saphost_50`.

Kommunikationsprotokolle

Eine SAP-Instanz kann über verschiedene Anwendungsprotokolle mit externen Programmen kommunizieren. Diese Anwendungsprotokolle werden über das Transaction Control Protocol (TCP) transportiert. Für jedes Anwendungsprotokoll öffnet eine Komponente der SAP-Instanz einen TCP-Port auf ihrem Host. Diese drei Protokolle werden von der SAP-Basis unterstützt:

- **Dynamic Information and Action Gateway (DIAG)**
  DIAG ist ein Anwendungsprotokoll, mit dessen Hilfe SAP GUI und SAP-Instanz miteinander kommunizieren. Über dieses Protokoll sendet die SAP-Instanz Bildschirmbilder und Listen an das SAP GUI und nimmt Benutzerbefehle entgegen.

  Dieses Protokoll wird vom Dispatcher innerhalb der SAP-Instanz implementiert. Für die Kommunikation mit DIAG öffnet der Dispatcher den TCP-Port mit der Nummer **32<SYSNR>** auf dem Host. Da die Portnummern eindeutig sein müssen, muss jede Instanz auf einem Host eine andere Portnummer haben. In der Services-Datei von Rechnern, die über diesen Port mit einer SAP-Instanz kommunizieren, wird ihm der Servicename `sapdp<SYSNR>` zugewiesen.

  Bei der Installation des SAP GUI auf einem Rechner erfolgen die Einträge der Servicenamen und der zugehörigen Portnummern in die Services-Datei automatisch. Auf Windows-Systemen ist die Services-Datei unter **<WINDIR>/system32/drivers/etc** zu finden. Listing 1.1 zeigt einen Ausschnitt aus dieser Services-Datei.

```
# Copyright (c) 1993-2004 Microsoft Corp.
#
# Diese Datei enthält die Portnummern für
# bekannte Dienste gemäß IANA.
#
# Format:
#
# <Dienstname>  <Portnummer>/<Protokoll>  [Alias...]
echo                   7/tcp
echo                   7/udp
discard                9/tcp    sink null
#...
sapdp00             3200/tcp
sapdp01             3201/tcp
sapdp02             3202/tcp
#...
sapgw00             3300/tcp
sapgw01             3301/tcp
sapgw02             3302/tcp
#...
```

Listing 1.1 Zuordnungen von Servicenamen zu Portnummern in der Services-Datei

- **Remote Function Call (RFC)**
  RFC ist ein Anwendungsprotokoll von SAP, mit dem externe Programme Funktionsbausteine in der SAP-Instanz aufrufen können. Dabei können Parameter an den Funktionsbaustein übergeben und von diesem empfangen werden.

  RFC wird vom Gateway implementiert. Dazu öffnet das Gateway den TCP-Port mit der Nummer **33<SYSNR>** auf dem Host; der dazugehörige Servicename lautet `sapgw<SYSNR>`.
- **Hypertext Transfer Protocol (HTTP)**
  Seit Release 6.10 bietet die SAP-Basis mit HTTP ein weiteres Anwendungsprotokoll an. Dieses Protokoll wird vom Internet Connection Manager (ICM) implementiert. Der ICM nimmt HTTP-Anfragen entgegen und leitet sie an entsprechende Anwendungen weiter. Der Standardport für den HTTP-Dienst ist 80, aber der Administrator eines SAP-Systems kann einen beliebigen anderen TCP-Port für diesen Dienst wählen.
- **WebSockets**
  Ab SAP NetWeaver 7.4 SP05 können Webclients auch über das WebSocket Protocol mit einem ABAP-Server kommunizieren. Über eine WebSocket-

Verbindung ist eine bidirektionale Kommunikation möglich. Damit kann ein ABAP-Server auch Push-Nachrichten an einen Webclient schicken. Implementiert wird dieses Protokoll ebenfalls durch den ICM, der Anfragen an eine Handler-Klasse weiterleitet.

Workprozesse

Innerhalb einer SAP-Instanz nimmt der Dispatcher eine zentrale Rolle ein. Er nimmt Anfragen entgegen und leitet sie zur Ausführung an den nächsten freien Workprozess weiter.

[»]

Optimale Ressourcennutzung durch Dispatching an Workprozesse

Es gibt in der Regel sehr viel weniger Workprozesse innerhalb einer SAP-Instanz, als es aktive Benutzeranmeldungen an dieser Instanz gibt. Der Grund dafür ist, dass zwischen zwei Anfragen eines Benutzers üblicherweise viel Zeit vergeht – aus Sicht des Computers jedenfalls. Während der Zeit, in der ein Benutzer die Ausgaben eines Bildschirms liest und Eingaben vornimmt, kann der Workprozess die Anfrage eines anderen Benutzers bearbeiten.

Dadurch, dass nur einige Workprozesse die Anfragen von vielen Benutzern bearbeiten, können Ressourcen auf dem Application Server optimal genutzt werden. Es laufen deutlich weniger Prozesse, und es gibt auch deutlich weniger Verbindungen zur Datenbank, als dies der Fall wäre, wenn jedem Benutzer ein eigener Workprozess zugeteilt würde.

Allerdings hat dies auch deutliche Auswirkungen auf das Transaktionskonzept, wie wir es in diesem Abschnitt unter der Überschrift »ABAP-Transaktionskonzept« zeigen.

Typen von Workprozessen

Die Workprozesse, die vom Dispatcher einer SAP-Instanz verwaltet werden, sind von unterschiedlichem Typ und jeweils durch einen der Buchstaben D, B, S, V oder E gekennzeichnet.

- **Dialog-Workprozesse (D)**
  Dialog-Workprozesse führen sowohl ABAP-Programme im Benutzerdialog als auch über RFC aufgerufene Funktionsbausteine aus.
- **Background-Workprozesse (B)**
  Background-Workprozesse führen ABAP-Programme aus, die für die Hintergrundverarbeitung eingeplant wurden. Diese ABAP-Programme nehmen keinen Benutzerdialog vor, und die notwendigen Eingaben werden bereits zum Zeitpunkt ihrer Einplanung spezifiziert.
- **Spool-Workprozesse (S)**
  Spool-Workprozesse sind für das Ausdrucken von Listen verantwortlich.
- **Verbuchungs-Workprozesse (V)**
  Diese Workprozesse führen Programme aus, die Änderungen in die be-

triebswirtschaftlichen Datenbanktabellen schreiben. Diese Programme werden aus Dialogprogrammen heraus angestoßen, wie wir es in Abschnitt 1.3.5, »Verbuchungsbausteine«, noch genauer besprechen.

- **Sperrverwaltungs-Workprozesse (E)**
  Das Buchstabenkürzel E leitet sich von dem Begriff *Enqueue* ab (etwa: an eine Warteschlange anstellen). Innerhalb eines SAP-Systems gibt es genau eine Instanz, die genau einen Sperrverwaltungsprozess hat. Über diesen Prozess setzen und lösen ABAP-Programme Datensatzsperren. Es ist wichtig, dass zu einer Zeit immer nur einer der vielen Dialogprozesse der unterschiedlichen Server eine bestimmte Sperre setzen kann. Daher darf es nur einen E-Prozess im gesamten SAP-System geben, und die Sperranfragen müssen in eine einzige Warteschlange eingereiht werden. Dieses Konzept schauen wir uns unter der Überschrift »Sperrobjekte« in diesem Abschnitt genauer an.

Speicherbereiche

Neben diesen Workprozessen verfügt eine Instanz vor allem über Speicherbereiche, die von allen Workprozessen gemeinsam genutzt werden. Dazu gehören unter anderem:

- **Pufferbereich für Datenbankinhalte**
  Daten, die von einem Workprozess von der Datenbank gelesen wurden, können in diesem Pufferbereich gespeichert werden und stehen danach allen Workprozessen zur Verfügung. Damit wird der lesende Zugriff auf solche Daten beschleunigt.
- **Rollbereich für Benutzerkontexte**
  In diesem Speicherbereich werden die Kontexte der angemeldeten Benutzer gespeichert. Dazu gehören insbesondere die Zustände der Programme, die gerade für einen Benutzer ausgeführt werden.

Lastverteilung durch den Message-Server

In einem SAP-System gibt es genau eine Instanz, die mit dem Message-Server einen weiteren zentralen Dienst zur Verfügung stellt. Der Message-Server dient der Kommunikation zwischen den Dispatchern aller SAP-Instanzen eines SAP-Systems. Über den Message-Server finden die Workprozesse einer Instanz z. B. den Enqueue-Prozess statt, der für die Sperrverwaltung zuständig ist.

Eine weitere wichtige Aufgabe des Message-Servers ist die Lastverteilung zwischen den SAP-Instanzen. Die SAP-Instanzen eines SAP-Systems können vom Administrator in mehrere Logon-Gruppen aufgeteilt werden. Um die Last zwischen den SAP-Instanzen einer Logon-Gruppe zu verteilen, kann das SAP GUI so konfiguriert werden, dass es sich beim Start zunächst einmal an den Message-Server wendet, um einer SAP-Instanz einer bestimmten Logon-Gruppe zugeteilt zu werden. Aufgrund der periodischen

Meldungen der SAP-Instanzen an den Message-Server über ihre momentane Belastung ist dieser in der Lage, eine geeignete SAP-Instanz aus der angeforderten Logon-Gruppe auszuwählen und dem SAP GUI für die Anmeldung zuzuweisen.

Das SAP GUI und die Dispatcher kommunizieren mit dem Message-Server ebenfalls über TCP. Der Administrator eines SAP-Systems ordnet dem Message-Server eine Portnummer zu. Als Servicename wird `sapms<SID>` gewählt und in die Services-Dateien eingetragen.

Damit haben das SAP GUI und andere Client-Programme zwei Möglichkeiten, um sich mit einer SAP-Instanz zu verbinden: direkt über die Angabe des Hostnamens des Applikationsservers und der Systemnummer oder indirekt über die Angabe des Hostnamens und des Servicenamens des Message-Servers. Diese beiden Möglichkeiten sind in Tabelle 1.2 zusammengefasst.

Verbindungsart	Notwendige Angaben
ohne Lastverteilung	▪ Hostname oder IP-Adresse des Anwendungsservers ▪ Systemnummer der ABAP-Instanz Bei RFC-Verbindungen können zusätzlich noch der Hostname und der Servicename eines alternativen Gateways angegeben werden, falls nicht mit dem Gateway des angegebenen Applikationsservers gearbeitet werden soll.
mit Lastverteilung	▪ Hostname oder IP-Adresse des Message-Servers des SAP-Systems ▪ Servicename des Message-Servers ▪ Logon-Gruppe

Tabelle 1.2 Angaben, die ein Client für die Verbindung zum SAP NetWeaver AS ABAP machen muss

Firewalls und SAP-Router

Zwei Verbindungsmöglichkeiten

Externe Clients haben in der Regel keinen direkten Zugriff über TCP/IP auf eine SAP-Instanz, sondern sind durch Firewalls und mindestens einen, in der Regel aber zwei SAP-Router von dieser getrennt, wie es in Abbildung 1.4 dargestellt ist.

Ein SAP-Router bündelt Client-Anfragen an mehrere SAP-Instanzen. Damit muss in der Firewall vor dem SAP-Router nur die Route auf die IP-Adresse und den Port des SAP-Routers freigegeben werden. Als TCP-Port wählt der Administrator bei der Installation des SAP-Routers in der Regel **3299/tcp**.

Dies ist die höchste mögliche Portnummer für einen Dispatcher, und es ist daher unwahrscheinlich, dass dieser Port schon von einem Dispatcher einer SAP-Instanz verwendet wird.

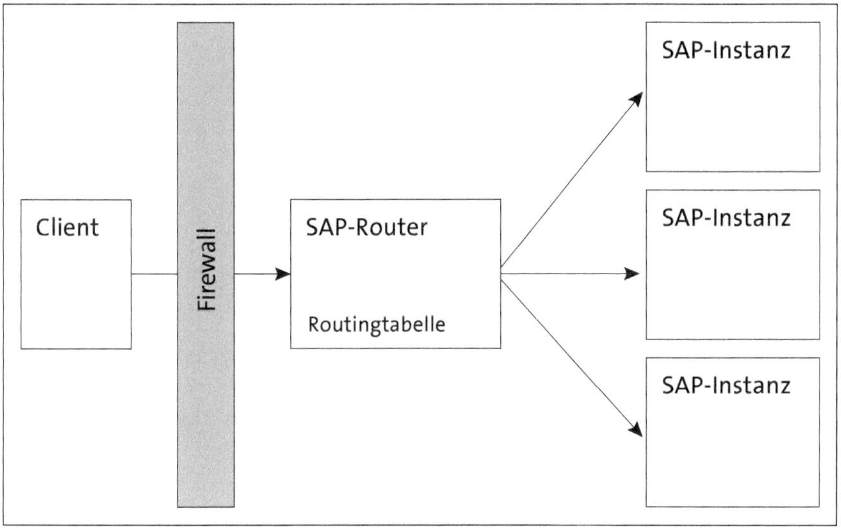

Abbildung 1.4 Firewall und SAP-Router – sicherer Zugriff auf SAP-Instanzen

Der SAP-Router enthält eine Tabelle, in der Routen von Clients (identifiziert über deren IP-Adresse) zu SAP-Instanzen (identifiziert über deren IP-Adresse und Systemnummer) vom Administrator freigegeben oder gesperrt werden.

SAP-Router-String

Möchte ein Client sich mit einer SAP-Instanz verbinden, muss er daher außer dem Hostnamen des Applikationsservers und der Systemnummer der Instanz zusätzlich den Hostnamen oder die IP-Adresse des SAP-Routers und dessen Portnummer angeben. Diese Angabe wird im sogenannten *SAP-Router-String* vorgenommen, der dem Hostnamen des Applikationsservers vorangestellt wird:

```
/H/<routerhost>/S/<routerport>/H/
```

Dabei ist `<routerhost>` der Hostname oder die IP-Adresse des SAP-Routers und `<routerport>` seine Portnummer.

Dialogverarbeitung

Abbildung 1.5 zeigt schematisch, wie eine Dialogtransaktion abläuft. Dabei startet der Benutzer am SAP GUI eine SAP-Transaktion, z. B. durch die Eingabe des Transaktionscodes in das Kommandofeld der Systemfunktionsleiste.

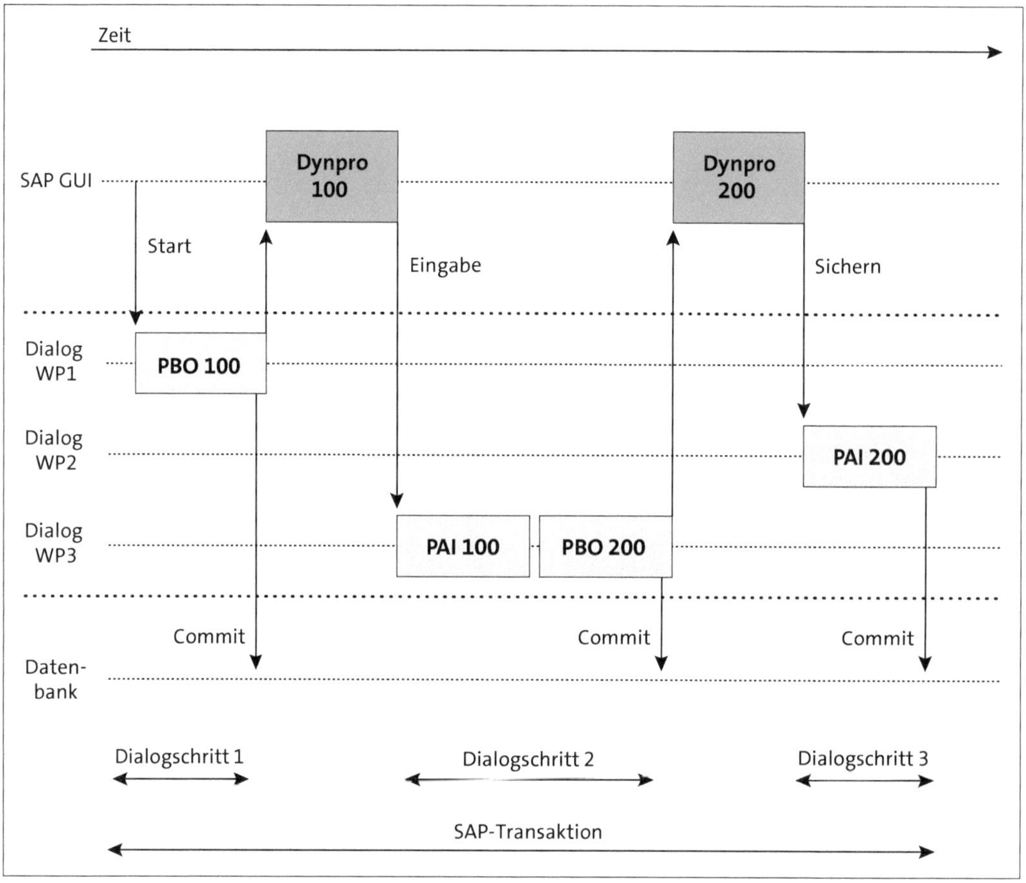

Abbildung 1.5 Ablauf einer SAP-Dialogtransaktion

In Abbildung 1.5 werden Ihnen als Benutzer im Lauf der Transaktion zwei Bildschirmbilder gezeigt, die Dynpros 100 und 200. Im Dynpro 100 werden Benutzereingaben vorgenommen, z. B. der Schlüssel des zu bearbeitenden Datensatzes eingegeben. Im Dynpro 200 wird der Datensatz geändert und seine Sicherung ausgelöst.

Dialogschritte

Aus Sicht des Anwendungsservers ist diese SAP-Transaktion in drei Dialogschritte aufgeteilt, die von drei verschiedenen Dialog-Workprozessen ausgeführt werden können. Bei der Dialogverarbeitung in SAP-Systemen wird die Ablauflogik mit dem Bildschirm definiert. Nachdem der Benutzer seine Eingaben im SAP GUI eingetragen hat, werden die PAI-Module (Process After Input) abgearbeitet. Bevor der Bildschirm im SAP GUI angezeigt wird, werden die PBO-Module (Process Before Output) abgearbeitet. Ein Dialogschritt besteht somit aus den PAI-Modulen eines Bildschirms und den PBO-Modulen des Folgebildschirms.

[«]

Ein Dialog-Workprozess für viele Benutzer

Nachdem ein Dialog-Workprozess einen Dialogschritt abgearbeitet hat, steht er sofort wieder für den nächsten Benutzer zur Verfügung. Dies ist möglich, weil die Dialog-Workprozesse im Vergleich zur Arbeitsgeschwindigkeit der Benutzer sehr schnell arbeiten. Damit können mit wenigen Dialog-Workprozessen und einem relativ geringen Ressourcenverbrauch auf dem Applikations- und dem Datenbankserver viele Benutzer bedient werden.

Impliziter Datenbank-Commit

Da ein Workprozess nacheinander völlig unzusammenhängende Dialogschritte ausführt, muss er nach jedem Dialogschritt einen Commit auf der Datenbank absetzen. Dies wird von der SAP-Basis ohne weiteres Zutun des ABAP-Entwicklers ausgelöst. Das bedeutet, dass auch ohne ein explizites Statement `COMMIT WORK` des ABAP-Entwicklers nach jedem Dialogschritt die Datenbankänderungen, die in diesem Dialogschritt vorgenommen wurden, auf der Datenbank festgeschrieben werden.

Programmieren Sie als ABAP-Entwickler einen expliziten `ROLLBACK WORK`, wird dieser Rollback natürlich auch an die Datenbank weitergereicht. Somit funktioniert ein Rollback auf der Datenbank immer nur bis zum Anfang des aktuellen Dialogschritts. Ein Rollback auf der Datenbank über mehrere Dialogschritte hinweg ist mit datenbanktechnischen Mitteln nicht möglich.

Erstreckt sich eine Benutzertransaktion daher über mehrere Dialogschritte, müssen besondere Vorkehrungen getroffen werden, damit im Fehlerfall oder beim Abbruch durch den Benutzer ein Rollback möglich wird.

ABAP-Transaktionskonzept

Eine Benutzertransaktion, die sich auch über mehrere Dialogschritte erstrecken kann, wird auch *SAP-Transaktion* oder *SAP Logical Unit of Work* (SAP-LUW) genannt und so von der *Datenbanktransaktion* oder *Database Logical Unit of Work* (DB-LUW) unterschieden. Wie Sie im vorangegangenen Abschnitt erfahren haben, müssen bei einer SAP-Transaktion besondere Vorkehrungen getroffen werden, um einen Abbruch durch den Benutzer oder im Fehlerfall einen Rollback zu erlauben. Dies trifft insbesondere auf ändernde Transaktionen zu, die Stamm- oder Bewegungsdaten in der Datenbank anlegen, ändern oder löschen.

Sperren

Eine ändernde SAP-Transaktion beginnt in der Regel damit, dass Sie (als Benutzer) im Eingangsbildschirm den Datensatz auswählen, den Sie ändern möchten. Im ersten Dialogschritt setzt der Dialog-Workprozess eine Sperre auf diesen Datensatz. Dazu kommuniziert er mit dem Enqueue-Workprozess, von dem in jedem SAP-System genau einer läuft. Ist noch keine Sperre auf den angeforderten Datensatz gesetzt, trägt der Enqueue-Workprozess die Sperre in seine Sperrtabelle ein. Ist bereits eine Sperre gesetzt, muss der Dialog-Workprozess eine entsprechende Fehlermeldung an den Benutzer ausgeben und darf mit der vorgesehenen Änderung nicht fortfahren.

In den folgenden Dialogschritten sammelt der Dialog-Workprozess im Dialog mit dem Benutzer die Änderungen, die am Datensatz vorgenommen werden sollen. Diese Änderungen werden nicht sofort durchgeführt, sondern zur Vormerkung gesammelt.

Asynchrone Verbuchung

Dazu stellt die SAP-Basis die Technik der sogenannten *Verbuchungsfunktionsbausteine* zur Verfügung. Dies sind Funktionsbausteine, in denen der Entwickler die ändernden Datenbank-Statements `UPDATE`, `INSERT` und `DELETE` kapselt und die vom Entwickler als Verbuchungsfunktionsbausteine markiert worden sind. Während die Änderungen gesammelt werden, ruft das Dialogprogramm diese Funktionsbausteine auf und übergibt ihnen die zu ändernden Daten über deren Schnittstelle. Das SAP-System führt diese Funktionsbausteine nicht sofort aus, sondern speichert den Namen des Funktionsbausteins und die übergebenen Daten in der sogenannten *Verbuchungstabelle* für die spätere Ausführung.

Commit und Rollback

Somit können Sie als Benutzer die SAP-Transaktion jederzeit einfach abbrechen. In diesem Fall, oder falls während der SAP-Transaktion ein Fehler auftritt, muss das Dialogprogramm einfach das Statement `ROLLBACK WORK` ausführen. Das SAP-System verwirft dann alle Einträge in der Verbuchungstabelle und löscht die gesetzten Sperren.

Beenden Sie die SAP-Transaktion mit der Aufforderung zum Speichern, führt das Dialogprogramm das Statement `COMMIT WORK` aus. In diesem Fall startet das SAP-System asynchron einen neuen Task in einem Verbuchungs-Workprozess. Der Verbuchungs-Workprozess führt die vorgemerkten Funktionsbausteine in der Reihenfolge aus, in der sie in die Verbuchungstabelle eingetragen wurden, und übergibt ihnen dabei die Daten, die ebenfalls in der Verbuchungstabelle gespeichert wurden. Erst jetzt führen die Funktionsbausteine die Datenbankänderungen tatsächlich aus.

Läuft alles fehlerfrei ab, setzt der Verbuchungs-Workprozess auf der Datenbank einen Commit ab und löscht die gesetzten Sperren. Tritt irgendwo in einem der Funktionsbausteine ein Fehler auf, setzt der Verbuchungs-Workprozess auf der Datenbank einen Rollback ab und informiert den Benutzer. Der Rollback über mehrere Funktionsbausteine ist möglich, weil der Verbuchungs-Workprozess innerhalb einer einzigen Datenbank-LUW arbeitet.

1.2 Sicherheit

Heterogene, integrative Landschaften müssen ein hohes Maß an Sicherheit bieten. Gerade bei der Schnittstellenprogrammierung ist dies ein wichtiger Aspekt. Wenn Sie externen Anwendungen Zugriff auf Ihre SAP-Systeme geben, müssen Sie dafür sorgen, dass diese externen Systeme nur die Daten sehen und vor allem auch nur die Daten ändern, die sie sehen und ändern dürfen; und Sie müssen dafür sorgen, dass nur einwandfrei identifizierte Anwendungen Zugriff auf Ihr Netzwerk erhalten.

Facetten der Sicherheit

Das höchste Maß an Sicherheit kann nur dann gegeben sein, wenn es aus unterschiedlichen Facetten besteht. Dies sind unter anderem die Authentifizierung und Autorisierung von Benutzern und die Verschlüsselung von Nachrichten. Der folgende Abschnitt beschreibt, wie diese Facetten theoretisch aussehen, um im Anschluss die Umsetzung von Sicherheitskonzepten zu diskutieren.

1.2.1 Sicherheit in heterogenen Landschaften

Sicherheit spielt in heterogenen Landschaften, die ein hohes Maß an Integration besitzen, eine wichtige Rolle. Durch den Integrationscharakter kann Sicherheit aber nicht mit einem Wundermittel erreicht werden. Zudem müssen Sie sich darüber im Klaren sein, dass es eine hundertprozentige Sicherheit niemals gibt; Sie können es Angreifern letztlich nur schwerer machen, ihr Ziel zu erreichen.

Es gibt zwei grundlegende Arten von Sicherheit im Unternehmen:

- **Infrastrukturelle Sicherheit**
  Zum einen ist da die infrastrukturelle Sicherheit. Damit bezeichnet man die Sicherheit, die z. B. durch Firewalls oder Backup-Konzepte erreicht werden kann. Es handelt sich dabei weniger um Software als vielmehr um Hardware, die eingesetzt wird, um die Daten und die Infrastruktur selbst zu schützen.
- **Anwendungssicherheit**
  Zum anderen gibt es die Anwendungssicherheit. Diese Art der Sicherheit erreichen Sie dadurch, dass Sie Programmiermittel verwenden, um ein möglichst hohes Maß an Sicherheit zu gewährleisten. Darauf konzentrieren wir uns in diesem Abschnitt.

Natürlich können infrastrukturelle und Anwendungssicherheit auch kombiniert werden. Ein Beispiel dafür ist die Zutrittskontrolle in Unternehmen.

Anforderungen an sicherheitskritische Systeme

Generell können Sie, wie bei allen Systemen, auch bei integrativen Landschaften gewisse sicherheitsrelevante Anforderungen an die Landschaft beschreiben:

- **Systemsicherheit**
  Konzepte des Monitorings
- **Datensicherheit**
  Vertraulichkeit, Integrität und Verbindlichkeit der Daten
- **Zugriffssicherheit**
  Authentifizierung und Autorisierung von Benutzern

Diese mehrstufige Sicherheit zeigt, dass ein Zusammenspiel aus unterschiedlichen Komponenten und Konzepten das Sicherheitsmaß im System erhöht.

Vertraulichkeit der Daten

Verschlüsselungsverfahren

Die Datensicherheit enthält Konzepte für die Vertraulichkeit der Daten, d. h. den Schutz vor unerlaubtem Zugriff auf Informationen, die zwischen Systemen ausgetauscht werden. Diese wird mithilfe von Verschlüsselungskonzepten gewährleistet. Dabei gibt es unterschiedliche Konzepte. Die beiden bekanntesten Konzepte sind die *Public-Key-Kryptografie* und die *Private-Key-Kryptografie*. Man spricht auch von asymmetrischen und symmetrischen Verfahren.

- **Symmetrische Verschlüsselung**
  Symmetrische Verfahren arbeiten mit lediglich einem kryptografischen Schlüssel. Der Schlüssel wird sowohl für das Verschlüsseln als auch für das Entschlüsseln der Daten verwendet. Symmetrische Verfahren sind besonders bei der Verschlüsselung von Kommunikationsdaten nur sehr schwer direkt einzusetzen, da der Schlüssel vor der Kommunikation ausgetauscht werden muss.
- **Asymmetrische Verschlüsselung**
  Asymmetrische Verfahren verwenden bei kryptografischen Operationen zwei korrespondierende Schlüssel: den öffentlichen und den privaten Schlüssel. Alle Operationen, die mit dem einen Schlüssel durchgeführt werden, können durch den anderen Schlüssel rückgängig gemacht bzw. verifiziert werden. Sicherheit wird dadurch erreicht, dass ein Rückschluss von einem der Schlüssel auf den anderen nur mit einem hohen Zeitaufwand möglich ist.

SSL

Neben der rein symmetrischen bzw. asymmetrischen Kryptografie gibt es Mischformen beider Varianten (*hybride Verfahren*). Eine der wohl bekanntesten Mischformen ist *Secure Sockets Layer* (SSL). SSL funktioniert wie folgt:

- Zwei Kommunikationspartner (System A und B) möchten sicher miteinander kommunizieren. System B ist die Datenquelle und System A der Anfragensteller.
- System B ist im Besitz eines asymmetrischen Schlüsselpaars und in der Lage, symmetrische Schlüssel zu erzeugen. System A ist im Besitz des öffentlichen Schlüssels von System B.
- Stellt nun A eine Anfrage an B, erzeugt B einen symmetrischen Schlüssel und verschlüsselt diesen mit seinem privaten Schlüssel. B übersendet die chiffrierte Information an System A.
- System A erhält das Datenpaket und entschlüsselt dieses mit dem öffentlichen Schlüssel von B.
- Beide sind nun im Besitz des symmetrischen Schlüssels und können mit diesem die Kommunikation verschlüsseln.

Der Vorteil dieses Verfahrens zur Sicherung der Kommunikation liegt darin, dass der Schlüssel zur Sicherung der Kommunikation erst zum Austausch der Nachricht generiert und nach der Verwendung sofort wieder gelöscht wird. Durch dieses Vorgehen wird die Möglichkeit des Kompromittierens des Schlüssels reduziert, wenn nicht sogar völlig ausgeschlossen. Aber wie immer im Kontext der Sicherheit – nichts ist unmöglich.

Integrität der Daten

In Integrationsszenarien spielt neben der Vertraulichkeit auch die Integrität der Daten eine wichtige Rolle. Bei der Integrität geht es prinzipiell darum, dass Daten, die zwischen zwei Kommunikationsteilnehmern ausgetauscht werden, während des Transports nicht verändert werden oder Änderungen zumindest festgestellt werden können.

Hash-Funktionen

Für die Integrität der Daten wird der sogenannte *Hash-Wert* verwendet. Der Hash-Wert ist das Resultat der Verarbeitung einer Hash-Funktion. Hash-Funktionen werden überall dort eingesetzt, wo eine verkürzte, möglichst eindeutige Darstellung einer Information benötigt wird. Hash-Funktionen sind sogenannte *Einwegfunktionen*. Rückschlüsse von einem Hash-Wert auf die verkürzt dargestellte Information dürfen nicht möglich sein.

Nun stellt sich zudem die Frage, woran der Empfänger erkennen kann, ob die Daten beim Übertragen verändert wurden. Um die Veränderung aufzudecken, muss der Ist-Zustand mit dem Soll-Zustand verglichen werden. Die Information muss deshalb eigentlich zweimal übertragen werden. Der Sender einer Information erzeugt vor dem Versenden einen Hash-Wert aus der Information, die übertragen werden soll. Danach sendet er zum einen die Information selbst und zum anderen deren Hash-Wert. Der Empfänger kann dann aus den empfangenen Daten den Hash-Wert berechnen und im Anschluss daran einen Vergleich mit der Information durchführen, die er empfangen hat.

Verbindlichkeit von Informationen

Zu guter Letzt müssen Daten, die zwischen zwei Kommunikationsteilnehmern ausgetauscht werden, verbindlich sein. Die Verbindlichkeit von Informationen kann, wie im »richtigen Leben«, durch eine Unterschrift gewährleistet werden.

Digitale Signaturen

Digitale Signaturen werden in heterogenen Systemen auf unterschiedliche Weise verwendet. Die Erstellung der digitalen Signatur ist denkbar einfach. Für eine Information, die digital signiert werden soll, wird der Hash-Wert berechnet. Der Hash-Wert, zusammen mit dem privaten Schlüssel des Unterzeichners, wird als Eingabe für einen Algorithmus zur digitalen Signatur verwendet. Zum Abschluss kann dann die Information zusammen mit der digitalen Signatur sowie dem Hash-Wert an den Empfänger übertragen werden.

Gemäß dem Grundsatz der asymmetrischen Kryptografie muss der Empfänger einer digitalen Signatur diese mit dem öffentlichen Schlüssel des Senders prüfen. Dies stellt auch kein Sicherheitsproblem dar, denn der öffentliche Schlüssel kann ohne Bedenken zwischen Kommunikationsteilnehmern ausgetauscht werden. Die Voraussetzung für den problemlosen Austausch öffentlicher Schlüssel ist jedoch, dass die privaten Schlüssel absolut sicher aufbewahrt werden. Denn wenn der private Schlüssel des Senders kompromittiert ist, könnte sich ein Angreifer den privaten Schlüssel verschafft haben und nun Daten im Namen eines anderen unterschreiben. Daher muss ein möglichst zentrales Schlüsselmanagement etabliert werden.

Schlüsselmanagement

Der Begriff des *Schlüsselmanagements* schließt die Erzeugung von Schlüsselpaaren, die Verwaltung sogenannter Sperrlisten, die Zertifizierung von Schlüsseln sowie das Anbieten eines Verzeichnisdiensts ein. Die Schlüsselmanagementstelle ist die zentrale Anlaufstelle für alle Dienste im Zusammenhang mit dem Schlüsselmaterial. Sie ist zudem dafür zuständig, dass alle Kommunikationspartner dem Schlüsselmaterial vertrauen können. Innerhalb der Sperrliste werden jene Schlüssel von Kommunikationsteilnehmern gelistet, die kompromittiert wurden. Gerade bei integrativen Szenarien ist es wichtig, dass z. B. ein eingehendes Angebot tatsächlich von dem Absender stammt, der auf dem Angebotsschreiben angegeben ist. Diese Sicherheit kann nur erreicht werden, wenn eine gemeinsame Stelle eingerichtet wird, die sich dafür verantwortlich zeichnet, dass das Schlüsselmaterial und die entsprechende Infrastruktur über ein hohes Maß an Sicherheit verfügen. Diese zentrale Stelle muss die öffentlichen Schlüssel der Kommunikationspartner als vertrauenswürdig kennzeichnen. Dies geschieht mithilfe von Zertifikaten.

Zertifikate

Digitale Zertifikate sind nichts anderes als ein Nachweis darüber, dass der öffentliche Schlüssel zu einer bestimmten Identität – und zwar nur zu dieser – gehört. Zertifikate können nicht nur für natürliche Personen ausgestellt werden, sondern auch für Rechner oder Anwendungen, und stellen somit auch eine Möglichkeit für die Authentifizierung dar. Mittels eines Zertifikats bestätigt die zentrale Verwaltungsstelle durch eine digitale Signatur, dass ein Schlüssel zu einer Identität gehört. Problematisch ist hier die Signatur selbst bzw. deren Prüfung. Der Empfänger benötigt für die Prüfung der Korrektheit einer Signatur den öffentlichen Schlüssel des Signierenden. Diesen besorgt er sich, wie bereits angesprochen, mithilfe des Zertifikats des Unterzeichners, wobei er wiederum die Signatur des Unterzeichners jenes Zertifikats prüfen muss.

Dieses Durchprüfen der öffentlichen Schlüssel kann sehr komplex und langwierig sein. Aus diesem Grund entscheidet der Kommunikationsteilnehmer bzw. die Anwendung, ab welchem Grad einer sogenannten *Vertrauensstellung* der Schlüssel als sicher eingestuft werden kann. Infrastrukturen, die solche Vertrauensstellungen darstellen und die für die Verwaltung zuständig sind, nennt man *Public-Key-Infrastrukturen* (PKI). Wir gehen hier nicht vertiefend auf PKIs ein, stellen aber fest, dass durch ihre Verwendung ein hoher Aufwand im Unternehmen entstehen kann.

1.2.2 Authentifizierung und Autorisierung

Nachdem wir nun die Grundlagen des Schlüsselmanagements diskutiert haben, wendet sich dieser Abschnitt den Aspekten der Authentifizierung und Autorisierung zu, die wir in Abschnitt 1.2.1, »Sicherheit in heterogenen Landschaften«, bereits kurz angesprochen haben. Wir werden sowohl die Konfiguration von Single Sign-on (SSO) zwischen einem Konsumenten und einem ABAP-System als auch die Konfiguration von Secure Network Communication (SNC) besprechen.

Authentifizierung

Besonders, aber nicht nur in heterogenen und verteilten Integrationsszenarien, muss sichergestellt werden, dass nur jene Identitäten Zugriff auf Informationen besitzen, denen ausdrücklich das Recht für den Zugriff eingeräumt wurde. Die zugreifende Identität muss für den Zugriff autorisiert sein. Damit die Autorisierung des Zugreifenden geprüft werden kann, muss er im ersten Schritt authentifiziert werden. Sowohl die Authentifizierung als auch die nachgeschaltete Autorisierung sind zwei Mechanismen, die in keinem System fehlen dürfen und bei jedem Zugriff erfolgen müssen.

Multiple Sign-on

Authentifizierungskonzepte reichen von der Abfrage einer Kombination des Benutzernamens und eines Passworts bis hin zur Prüfung von biometrischen Merkmalen. Welches Konzept zur Authentifizierung verwendet wird, hängt von der vorhandenen Infrastruktur bzw. den vorhandenen Produkten ab. Die meisten Systeme bieten nicht nur eine Art der Authentifizierung an, sondern lassen dem Benutzer die Wahl, sich für die Variante zu entscheiden, die sich am besten in die Infrastruktur integrieren lässt. Ein Problem bleibt jedoch bei dieser Vielfalt an Möglichkeiten bestehen: Es besteht die Gefahr, dass der Benutzer bei einer heterogenen, vielschichtigen Landschaft mehrmals täglich (immer wenn er auf ein anderes System zugreifen möchte) aufgefordert wird, sich zu authentifizieren. Besitzt er dann auch noch unterschiedliche Benutzerkennungen und Passwörter für die verschiedenen Systeme, ist es nur noch sehr schwer oder nur durch Aufschreiben der Zugangsdaten möglich, den Überblick zu behalten.

Vereinfachung der Login-Prozedur

Das wiederholte Anmelden bei einem Systemwechsel kann durch die Nutzung von Single Sign-on verhindert werden. SSO-Lösungen helfen dabei, dass Benutzer sich nur an einem System anmelden müssen, am besten am Betriebssystem beim Systemstart. Wechselt ein Benutzer dann zwischendurch das System, delegiert das zentrale System seine Identität. Durch den Aufbau einer »Vertrauensbeziehung« zwischen den unterschiedlichen Systemen spart der Benutzer Zeit.

Nachteile von SSO-Lösungen

Leider haben SSO-Lösungen auch Nachteile. Der erste, rein auf die Infrastruktur bezogene Nachteil ist, dass die Benutzeridentitäten homogenisiert werden müssen. Der Benutzer `mmayer` muss auf allen Systemen dieselbe User-ID besitzen, in diesem Beispiel `mmayer`. Ein zweiter Nachteil ist, dass diese einzelne Zugangsberechtigung ein Sicherheitsrisiko darstellt. Sollte ein potenzieller Angreifer im Besitz der einzigen Zugangs-ID sein, stehen ihm alle Türen zum System offen. Abschließend lässt sich deshalb sagen, dass ein hohes Maß an Sicherheit nur durch eine sinnvolle Kopplung verschiedener Sicherheitsfunktionen erreicht werden kann. Dazu gehören auch Entscheidungen darüber, wo und wie SSO eingesetzt wird.

1.2.3 Sichere Integration externer Systeme

Nachdem wir die reine SAP-Integration besprochen haben, betrachten wir nun die Möglichkeiten, Systeme aus einer externen SAP-Landschaft sicher zu verwenden. Bei der Integration solcher Systeme stellt sich oftmals die Frage, wie die Authentifizierung durchgeführt werden kann. Es gibt verschiedene Techniken, die von der reinen Konfiguration bis hin zur Programmierung von Authentifizierungsmechanismen reichen.

Sicherheit auf der Transportschicht

Der geschützte Datenzugriff nützt nicht viel, wenn der Datenaustausch selbst im »Klartext« erfolgt. Der Angreifer kann dann nämlich ganz einfach auf dem Netzwerk »lauschen«, um auf die vertraulichen Informationen zuzugreifen. Daher beschäftigen wir uns nun mit der Nutzung der Sicherheit auf der Transportschicht. Dies umfasst die Authentizität der Kommunikationspartner, die Datenintegrität und die Vertraulichkeit der Daten.

SNC oder SSL

Für die Sicherung der Kommunikation zwischen den SAP-NetWeaver-Komponenten werden zwei verschiedene Sicherheitsprotokolle unterstützt:

- Secure Sockets Layer (SSL) für die Sicherung von HTTP
- Secure Network Communication (SNC) für die Sicherung von RFC und DIAG

SSL und SNC arbeiten beide auf der Basis von Zertifikaten. Wir betrachten im Folgenden die Verwendung von SNC genauer und erläutern, wie dessen Infrastruktur aufgesetzt wird.

Einführung in Secure Network Communication

Secure Network Communication wird zur Sicherung der Kommunikation zwischen zwei SAP-NetWeaver-Kommunikationspartnern verwendet. SNC beschreibt dabei eigentlich nur eine Schicht in der SAP-NetWeaver-Systemarchitektur, die eine Schnittstelle für die Integration externer Sicherheitsprodukte definiert. Genauer gesagt, wird über SNC die Schnittstelle zwischen der SAP-System-Kernel-Schicht und einer Bibliothek (Implementierung) eines externen Herstellers beschrieben. Hersteller der Bibliothek müssen dabei die sogenannte GSSAPI V2 (Generic Security Services Application Programming Interface Version 2) implementieren. Sie wird während der Initialisierungsphase von SNC dynamisch geladen.

Stufen der Sicherheit mit SNC

SAP selbst bietet für die Nutzung von SNC eine eigene Implementierung einer solchen externen Bibliothek an: *SAP Cryptolib*. Die Herangehensweise bei SNC ist vergleichbar mit dem beschriebenen PAM-Konzept von JAAS. Wie bereits erwähnt, adressiert SNC drei Bereiche der Sicherheit:

- nur Authentifizierung
- Schutz der Integrität
- Schutz der Daten durch Verschlüsselung

Als Benutzer von SNC können Sie somit Sicherheit in mehreren Stufen erreichen. Bei der Nutzung der Authentifizierung stellt das System lediglich die Identität des Kommunikationspartners sicher. Zur Sicherung der Kommunikation während des Transits zwischen den Kommunikationspartnern sollten Sie aber zwingend sowohl die Integrität der Daten als auch den Schutz der Daten durch Verschlüsselung verwenden. Dies wird über Profilparameter im Instanzprofil des Applikationsservers konfiguriert.

SNC arbeitet, wie bereits angesprochen, mit Zertifikaten. Der eine Kommu nikationspartner muss im Besitz des digitalen Zertifikats des anderen Kommunikationspartners sein und ihm ein gewisses Maß an Vertrauen entgegenbringen. Die Schlüsselinformationen müssen dabei in einer Form vorliegen, die einen Missbrauch erschweren. Im Rahmen der Speicherung von Schlüsselinformationen wird das Personal Security Environment eingesetzt. PSE-Dateien enthalten neben einer Zertifikatsliste jener Zertifikate, denen vertraut wird, auch die eigenen Schlüsselinformationen.

Szenarien der Vertrauensstärke

Die Stärke des Vertrauens wird innerhalb von SNC mithilfe zweier Szenarien beschrieben:

- **Szenario 1: Alle Kommunikationspartner, die mit dem ABAP-System über SNC kommunizieren, verwenden dasselbe PSE.**

  Der Vorteil bei diesem Szenario ist die sehr viel einfachere Verwaltung im ABAP-Stack. Zusätzlich ist der Aufwand, bevor sicher kommuniziert werden kann, wesentlich geringer. Dies liegt daran, dass nicht für jeden Kommunikationspartner ein neues PSE erzeugt und somit in den ABAP-Stack das Zertifikat des Partners importiert werden muss.

  Der Nachteil dieser Vorgehensweise ist jedoch auch nicht außer Acht zu lassen: Es kann vorkommen, dass ein Angreifer in den Besitz der PSE-Datei gelangt und der Aufwand für das Schließen der Sicherheitslücke – je nach Anzahl der Kommunikationspartner – enorm hoch ausfallen kann. Außerdem sollten Sie bedenken, dass es nur schwer möglich ist, Kommunikationsprobleme eines Partners zu lokalisieren, denn man kann kaum herausfinden, welche SNC-Verbindung fehlerhaft ist.

- **Szenario 2: Jeder Kommunikationspartner erhält ein individuelles PSE.**

  Was bei Szenario 1 ein großer Vorteil war, wird in diesem Szenario zu einem großen Problem: Der initiale Administrationsaufwand ist größer und eine spontane Kommunikation damit nicht möglich. Bevor Kommunikation stattfinden kann, müssen beide Partner ihr digitales Zertifikat aus dem PSE exportieren und das Zertifikat des anderen importieren.

Mischformen

Mischformen der beiden Szenarien sind auch denkbar, indem z. B. mehrere Gruppen von Systemen gebildet werden und jede Systemgruppe dasselbe PSE verwendet.

Installation von SAP Cryptolib

Bevor Sie mit der Konfiguration der SNC-Kommunikation anfangen können, benötigen Sie die SAP Cryptolib für den SAP NetWeaver AS ABAP. Für den Download rufen Sie die Seite *http://s-prs.de/v1032900* im Portal *SAP for Me* auf. Sie finden unter dieser Adresse die Bibliotheken für alle von SAP unterstützten Plattformen als SAR-Dateien. Da die Beispiele in diesem Buch auf Microsoft Windows entwickelt wurden, entscheiden Sie sich für die Nutzung der Windows-Plattform. In der Datei finden Sie drei Ordner für die jeweilige Ausprägung einer Windows-Plattform. Jeder dieser Ordner enthält die Datei **sapcrypto.dll** und eine Version des Werkzeugs **sapgenpse.exe**. Zusätzlich finden Sie, neben einer Reihe von Textdateien, eine Datei mit dem Namen **ticket**. Diese Datei stellt das Lizenzzertifikat für die Erzeugung eigener Zertifikate bereit.

Installationspfad

Um die SAP Cryptolib zu installieren, kopieren Sie die Dateien einfach in die entsprechenden Verzeichnisse, **exe** und **sec**, des Applikationsservers. Maßgeblich für den Ablageort der Dateien ist der Konfigurationsparameter `DIR_INSTANCE`. Er zeigt unter Windows auf **<Laufwerk>\usr\sap\<SID>\<instance>**. Der Parameter wird allen Profilparametern vorangestellt, um das Installationsverzeichnis der Serverinstanz anzugeben.

Kopieren Sie die Dateien **sapcrypto.dll** und **sapgenpse.exe** in das im Profilparameter `DIR_EXECUTABLE` angegebene Verzeichnis. Unter Windows zeigt der Parameter normalerweise auf **DIR_INSTANCE\exe**. Danach legen Sie die Datei mit dem Ticket im Unterverzeichnis **DIR_INSTANCE\sec** ab. Sollte in diesem Verzeichnis bereits eine Datei mit dem Namen **ticket** vorhanden sein, erzeugen Sie ein Unterverzeichnis und legen die Datei dort ab.

Umgebungsvariable »SECUDIR«

Zum Abschluss der Installation setzen Sie die Betriebssystem-Umgebungsvariable `SECUDIR` in das Unterverzeichnis **sec**, in dem das Ticket abgelegt ist, also auf **DIR_INSTANCE\sec** bzw. in das von Ihnen erzeugte Unterverzeichnis. Dabei müssen Sie beachten, dass die Umgebungsvariable unter dem Benutzer gesetzt wird, unter dem der Applikationsserver später ausgeführt werden soll. Durch das Setzen der Variablen teilen Sie der Laufzeitumgebung mit, wo die vertrauenswürdigen Tickets zu finden sind.

Konfiguration des Applikationsservers für die Verwendung von Secure Network Communication

Nachdem die SAP Cryptolib installiert wurde, wenden wir uns der SNC-Konfiguration zu. Im ersten Teil der Konfiguration müssen Sie dem Applikationsserver die nötigen Informationen über die Ablaufparameter für SNC mitteilen. Dies geschieht über das Instanzprofil. Dazu starten Sie Transaktion RZ10. Im Anschluss öffnen Sie das Instanzprofil im Modus **Erweiterte Pflege**.

Über [⇧] + [F8] wechseln Sie in den Editiermodus und beginnen mit dem Hinzufügen der Parameter. Dies kann entweder über den Button **Parameter** oder über die Taste [F5] erfolgen. Tabelle 1.3 zeigt die zu setzenden Parameter und ihre Bedeutung.

Parametername	Wert	Beschreibung
`snc/enable`	1	aktiviert die Nutzung von SNC
`snc/gssapi_lib`	$(DIR_EXECUTABLE)\sapcrypto.dll	verweist auf die Implementierung der GSSAPI
`snc/identity/as`	p:CN=AOU, OU=IT, O=ADO, C=DE	eindeutige Identifizierer des Applikationsservers
`snc/data_protection/max`	3	maximale Sicherheitsunterstützung
`snc/data_protection/min`	1	minimale Sicherheitsunterstützung
`snc/data_protection/use`	3	zu verwendende Sicherheitsunterstützung
`snc/accept_insecure_cpic`	1	Zugriff ohne SNC per CPIC-Verbindung erlaubt

Tabelle 1.3 Übersicht über die SNC-Profilparameter und ihre Bedeutung

Parametername	Wert	Beschreibung
snc/accept_insecure_gui	1	1 = Zugriff ohne SNC erlaubt per SAP GUI
snc/accept_insecure_r3int_rfc	1	1 = SAP-systeminterner Zugriff ohne SNC erlaubt
snc/accept_insecure_rfc	1	1 = Zugriff über RFC auch ohne SNC erlaubt
sec/libsapsecu	$(DIR_EXECUTABLE)\sapcrypto.dll	Dateiname der SAP Cryptographic API, die beim Start des Servers geladen werden soll
ssf/ssfapi_lib	$(DIR_EXECUTABLE)\sapcrypto.dll	Dateiname der SAP Cryptographic Library
ssf/name	SAPSECULIB	Angabe der Betriebssystem-Umgebungsvariablen

Tabelle 1.3 Übersicht über die SNC-Profilparameter und ihre Bedeutung (Forts.)

Wie Sie in der Tabelle im Beschreibungsfeld sehen, sind die Parameter so eingestellt, dass eine unsichere Kommunikation mit dem ABAP-System immer noch möglich ist. Zum Abschluss der Konfiguration setzen Sie den Parameter `snc/enable` auf den Wert »1«. Im Anschluss sollten Sie den Server neu starten.

[!]

Installation und Einstellungen genau prüfen

Achten Sie darauf, dass der Parameter `snc/enable` erst dann auf den Wert »1« gesetzt wird, wenn Sie sich sicher sind, dass die Installation der SAP Cryptolib vollständig ist und alle Parameter der Tabelle 1.3 richtig gesetzt sind. Bei einer fehlerhaften Installation und Konfiguration der Bibliothek startet der Applikationsserver nicht mehr.

Erzeugung des SNC-PSE-Containers

Nachdem der Server erfolgreich hochgefahren wurde, können Sie mit dem Abschluss der serverseitigen Konfiguration beginnen. Da SNC auf der Public-Key-Kryptografie unter der Verwendung von digitalen Zertifikaten basiert, muss jeder Kommunikationspartner ein vertrauenswürdiges Zertifikat vorweisen.

Um die Vertrauensbeziehungen im ABAP-System zu konfigurieren, starten Sie Transaktion STRUSTSSO2. Nach dem Start der Transaktion sehen Sie in Ihrem System auf der linken Seite des Bildschirmbilds einen rot markierten Eintrag: **SNC (SAP Cryptolib)**. Durch einen Klick auf den Eintrag wählen Sie über das Kontextmenü den Menüpunkt **Anlegen** aus. In dem erscheinenden Fenster geben Sie denselben Wert an wie im Profilparameter `scn/identity/as` (siehe Tabelle 1.3). Sie erzeugen damit eine serverseitige PSE-Datei für Ihren Applikationsserver.

Nachdem Sie dies bestätigt haben, werden Sie aufgefordert, ein Passwort für den soeben angelegten SNC-PSE-Eintrag zu erstellen. Über den Button **Kennwort** (siehe Abbildung 1.6) erzeugen Sie ein Passwort, mit dem der Zugriff auf die PSE-Datei geschützt wird. Nun wird der Eintrag **SNC (SAP Cryptolib)** nicht mehr rot, sondern mit einer grünen Ampel gekennzeichnet.

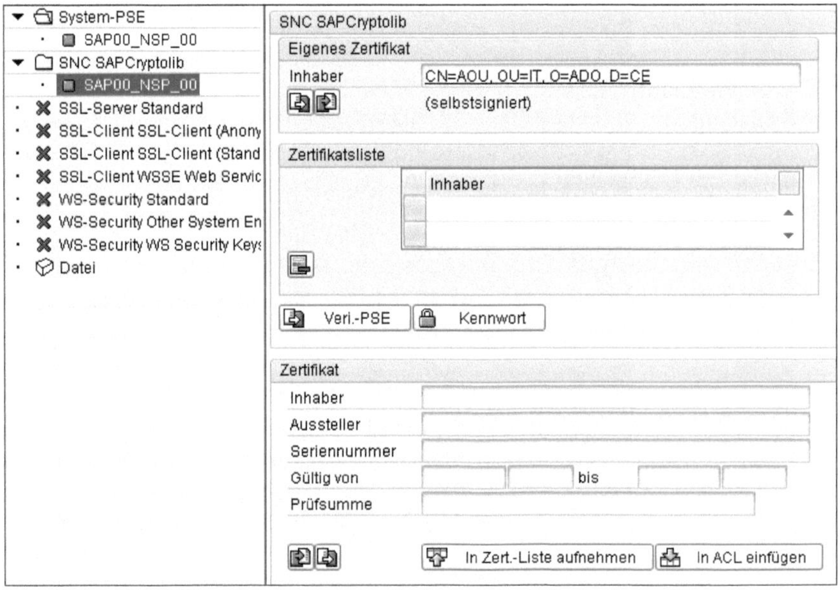

Abbildung 1.6 Transaktion STRUSTSSO2 mit SNC-PSE-Datei

Testen der Konfiguration

Leider gibt es keine integrierte Möglichkeit, um zu testen, ob Installation und Konfiguration der SNC-Umgebung erfolgreich waren. Sie müssten warten, bis die SNC-Umgebung z. B. aus einem RFC-Client verwendet wurde. Bei einem Fehler wissen Sie dann im schlimmsten Fall allerdings nicht, was die Fehlerursache ist: die Konfiguration, der Client selbst oder das Client-Zertifikat.

Testprogramm

Mit den SAP-Hinweisen 800240 und 912405 wird Ihnen jedoch ein Programm an die Hand gegeben, das Sie sich über Transaktion SE80 in Ihr ABAP-System kopieren können. Das Programm trägt den Namen ZSSF_TEST_PSE und prüft, ob die SNC-Konfiguration erfolgreich durchgeführt wurde.

1.3 Programmierung auf der ABAP-Plattform

Im Folgenden entwickeln wir eine kleine Anwendung in ABAP, die wir in Kapitel 3, »Remote Function Call mit ABAP«, bis Kapitel 9, »SAP Gateway und OData«, immer wieder als Beispiel heranziehen werden. Die Beispielanwendung verwaltet Kundenaufträge und Lieferantenbestellungen eines Buchgroßhändlers. Wir werden diese Anwendung mit eingehenden Schnittstellen (für Kundenaufträge von Buchhandlungen) und ausgehenden Schnittstellen (für Lieferantenaufträge an Verlage) in verschiedenen Schnittstellentechnologien versehen:

- Remote Function Call (RFC) in Abschnitt 3.1, »RFC-Funktionsbausteine in ABAP«
- Business Application Programming Interface (BAPI) in Abschnitt 3.4, »Background-RFC«
- Application Link Enabling (ALE) in Kapitel 7, »IDocs und Application Link Enabling«
- Service-Oriented Architecture Protocol (SOAP) in Kapitel 8, »SOAP-Webservices«
- SAP Gateway und OData Protocol (OData) in Kapitel 9, »SAP Gateway und OData«

Die hier aufgezählten Schnittstellentechnologien werden in Abschnitt 1.4, »Überblick über die Schnittstellentechnologien von SAP«, genauer vorgestellt und in den angegebenen Abschnitten bzw. Kapiteln mit ausprogrammierten Beispielen erläutert. Dabei werden auch die entsprechenden ausgehenden Schnittstellen bei der Buchhandlung und die eingehenden Schnittstellen beim Verlag in den Programmiersprachen C/C++, Java und C# realisiert. Abbildung 1.7 zeigt die grundsätzlich beteiligten Systeme im Überblick.

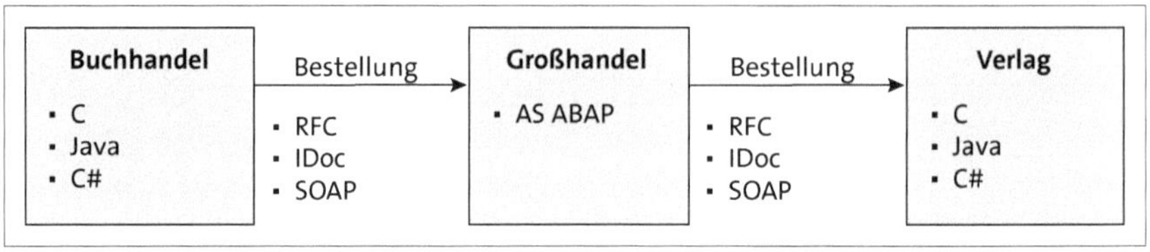

Abbildung 1.7 Beispielanwendung

1.3.1 ABAP Dictionary

Die Anwendung besteht aus zwei Datenbanktabellen mit Kopfdaten und Positionsdaten von Bestellungen:

- `ZIFPORDER`
  Diese Tabelle enthält Angaben über die Bestellungen.
- `ZIFPORDERPOS`
  Diese Tabelle enthält Informationen über die Positionen einer Bestellung.

Dabei werden Kundenaufträge und Lieferantenbestellungen in denselben Tabellen gespeichert und durch den Inhalt des Felds `TYPE` voneinander unterschieden. Bei Kundenaufträgen enthält dieses Feld den Wert »SO« (für Sales Order), bei Lieferanteneinträgen den Wert »PO« (für Purchase Order).

Pakete

Sie ordnen alle Repository-Objekte dem Paket `ZIFP` zu, das mit der ABAP Workbench SE80 angelegt wird. Dazu starten Sie Transaktion SE80 und wählen aus der Drop-down-Liste den Eintrag **Paket** aus. Geben Sie `ZIFP` als Namen des Pakets an, und klicken Sie auf den Button mit der Brille, um sich die Objekte anzeigen zu lassen, die diesem Paket zugeordnet sind. Da das Paket noch nicht existiert, wird Ihnen angeboten, das Paket zu erzeugen. Generieren Sie dabei auch gleich einen neuen Transportauftrag für die neu zu erstellenden Repository-Objekte.

Datenbanktabellen

Felder der Beispieltabellen

Nachdem Sie das Paket erstellt haben, können Sie entweder direkt aus dem Object Navigator oder mit Transaktion SE11 die beiden transparenten Tabellen definieren. Die Felder der Tabelle `ZIFPORDER`, deren Datenelemente (betriebswirtschaftliche Datentypen), Längen und Beschreibungen sind in Tabelle 1.4 aufgelistet, die Angaben zu Tabelle `ZIFPORDERPOS` in Tabelle 1.5.

Feld	Datenelement	Datentyp	Länge	Beschreibung
MANDT	MANDT	CLNT	3	Mandant
ORDERID	ZIFPORDERID	NUMC	10	Bestellnummer
TYPE	ZIFPORDERTPYE	CHAR	2	Bestelltyp
REFID	ZIFPREFID	NUMC	10	Referenznummer
BUYER	ZIFPBUYER	CHAR	50	Käufer
SELLER	ZIFPSELLER	CHAR	50	Lieferant
DATE	ZIFPORDERDATE	DATS	8	Bestelldatum

Tabelle 1.4 Spalten der Tabelle »ZIFPORDER«

Feld	Datenelement	Datentyp	Länge	Beschreibung
MANDT	MANDT	CLNT	3	Mandant
ORDERID	ZIFPORDERID	NUMC	10	Bestellnummer
ORDERPOS	ZIFPPOS	NUMC	5	Bestellposition
MATID	ZIFPMATID	CHAR	20	Materialnummer
MATTEXT	ZIFPMATTEXT	CHAR	40	Materialtext
ORDERCOUNT	ZIFPCOUNT	INT4	–	Anzahl
PRICE	ZIFPPRICE	CURR	8,4	Preis
CURRENCY	ZIFPCURRENCY	CUKY5	5	Währung

Tabelle 1.5 Spalten der Tabelle »ZIFPORDERPOS«

Abbildung 1.8 zeigt die Definition der Tabelle ZIFPORDERPOS im ABAP Dictionary (DDIC).

Fremdschlüssel

Die Schlüsselfelder der Tabelle ZIFPORDER sind MANDT und ORDERID. Die Schlüsselfelder der Tabelle ZIFPORDERPOS sind hingegen MANDT, ORDERID und ORDERPOS. Das Feld MANDT in beiden Tabellen ist ein Prüffeld mit der Prüftabelle T000, die die Mandanten enthält. Das Feld ORDERID der Tabelle ZIFPORDERPOS ist ein Prüffeld mit der Prüftabelle ZIFPORDER. Der Fremdschlüssel in der Tabelle ZIFPORDERPOS, der eindeutig einen Eintrag aus der Tabelle ZIFPORDER festlegt, besteht aus den Feldern ZIFPORDER-MANDT und ZIFORDER-ORDERID. Mithilfe dieser Fremdschlüsselbeziehungen kann das System später automatische Eingabeprüfungen auf Dynpros vornehmen, die die Prüffelder verwenden.

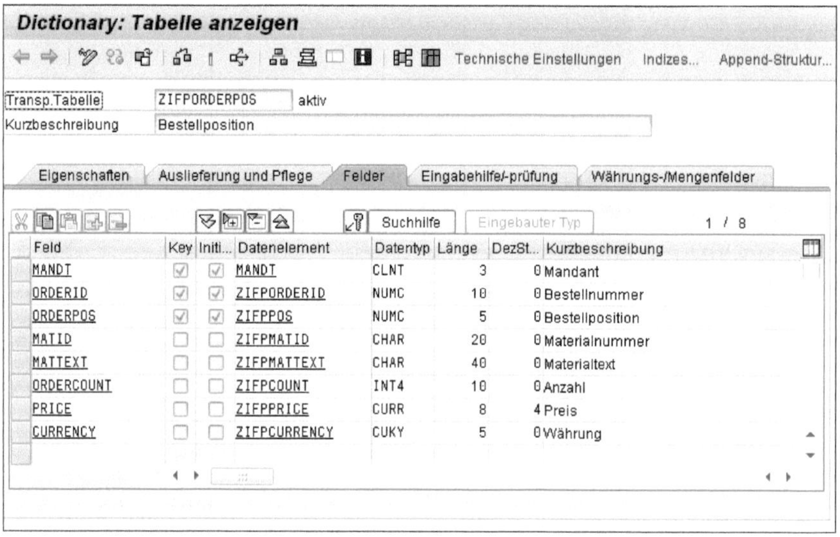

Abbildung 1.8 Tabelle »ZIFPORDERPOS« im ABAP Dictionary

Tabellenpflege

Bei der Definition der Tabellen können Sie über eine Drop-down-Liste auf der Registerkarte **Auslieferung und Pflege** festlegen, ob eine Tabellenpflege erlaubt sein soll. Lassen Sie diese zu, damit Sie mit den Transaktionen SE16 und SA16 die Inhalte der Tabellen pflegen können.

Bei den technischen Eigenschaften, die Sie über den Menüpfad **Springen • Technische Einstellungen** erreichen, legen Sie für beide Tabellen fest, dass sie Stamm- und Bewegungsdaten enthalten. In diesem Dialog stellen Sie auch die Größenkategorie 0 ein. Da die beiden Tabellen Bewegungsdaten enthalten, sollten sie nicht gepuffert werden. Sobald Sie die Tabellendefinitionen aktivieren, werden die entsprechenden Datenbanktabellen angelegt. Mit Transaktion SE16 oder SA16 können Sie nun die ersten Testdaten in die Tabellen eintragen.

Suchhilfen

Sammelsuchhilfen

Da wir die Tabelle `ZIFPORDER` bei der Besprechung des Business-Objekts `Helpvalues` in Abschnitt 3.5.3, »Business-Objekt ›Helpvalues‹«, benötigen, legen wir zwei elementare Suchhilfen und eine Sammelsuchhilfe für diese an:

- `ZIFPORDERA`
  Diese elementare Suchhilfe dient zur Suche nach Bestellungen über den Namen des Käufers.

- ZIFPORDERB
  Diese elementare Suchhilfe dient zur Suche nach Bestellungen über den Namen des Verkäufers.
- ZIFPORDER
  Diese Sammelsuchhilfe umfasst die elementaren Suchhilfen ZIFPORDERA und ZIFPORDERB.

Suchhilfen werden mit dem ABAP Dictionary (Transaktion SE11) angelegt. Sie dienen dazu, die Wertehilfe (F4-Hilfe) für die Anzeige gültiger Eingabewerte komfortabler zu gestalten.

Suchhilfen für Bestellungen

Die Suchhilfe ZIFPORDERA, die in Abbildung 1.9 zu sehen ist, bezieht ihre Daten von der Datenbanktabelle ZIFPORDER. Dies ist die sogenannte *Selektionsmethode* der Suchhilfe, die die vier Suchhilfeparameter ORDERID, TYPE, BUYER und SELLER umfasst. Diese vier Parameter werden in der Trefferliste der Suchhilfe dargestellt (in der Spalte **LPos** in Abbildung 1.9). Die ersten drei dieser Parameter, ORDERID, TYPE und SELLER, werden im Selektionsbild der Suchhilfe abgebildet (in der Spalte **SPos** in Abbildung 1.9). Das Selektionsbild einer Suchhilfe ist ein Benutzerdialog, in dem der Anwender Selektionskriterien angeben kann, die die Trefferzahl einschränken. Soll die Suchhilfe z. B. nur Kundenbestellungen auflisten, geben Sie im Selektionsbild im Selektionsfeld TYPE den Wert »SO« ein.

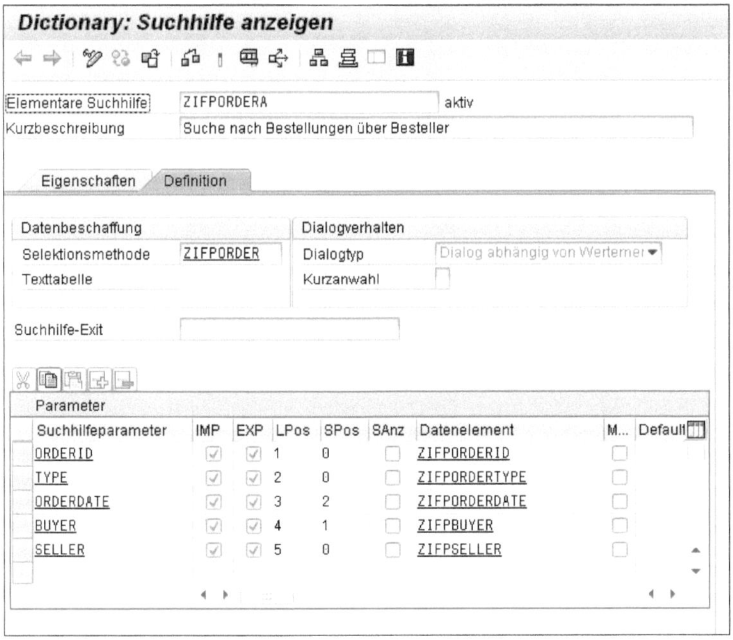

Abbildung 1.9 Elementare Suchhilfe »ZIFPORDERA«

Anbindung von Suchhilfen

Suchhilfen können Sie an Prüftabellen, Tabellenfelder oder Datenelemente anbinden. Der häufigste Fall ist die Anbindung an Prüftabellen. Wenn Sie in einem Prüffeld mit einer Prüftabelle die Wertehilfe (F4-Hilfe) anfordern, wird die daran angebundene Suchhilfe gezogen. In diesem Beispiel binden Sie die Suchhilfe ZIFPORDER an die Prüftabelle ZIFPORDER an. Wenn Sie dann in einem Prüffeld der Prüftabelle ZIFPORDER nach einer gültigen Bestellnummer suchen, verwendet das System diese Suchhilfe.

Die beiden elementaren Suchhilfen ZIFPORDERA und ZIFPORDERB werden in der Sammelsuchhilfe ZIFPORDER inkludiert. Diese Sammelsuchhilfe wird an die Prüftabelle ZIFPORDER und außerdem an das Feld ORDERID dieser Tabelle angebunden.

Sperrobjekte

Bei der Entwicklung einer ABAP-Anwendung müssen Sie beachten, dass viele Benutzer gleichzeitig mit einem SAP-System arbeiten können. Daher muss vor dem Löschen oder Ändern von Datensätzen ermittelt werden, ob gerade ein anderer Benutzer mit dem Datensatz arbeitet. Dazu wird zunächst eine Schreibsperre auf den betreffenden Datensatz gesetzt. Kann die Sperre nicht erfolgreich gesetzt werden, weil der Datensatz bereits von einem anderen Benutzer bearbeitet wird, muss die Verarbeitung abgebrochen werden. Kann die Sperre gesetzt werden, darf der Datensatz gelöscht oder verändert werden.

Entwicklung von Sperrobjekten

Um Sperren setzen zu können, entwickeln Sie in Transaktion SE11 ein Sperrobjekt. Damit Sie mit einer Bestellung auch all ihre Positionen sperren können, entwickeln Sie ein Sperrobjekt EZIFPORDER mit den Feldern ORDERID und ORDERPOS. Das Sperrobjekt bezieht sich auf die primäre Tabelle ZIFPORDER und die sekundäre Tabelle ZIFPORDERPOS. Beim Anlegen des Sperrobjekts mit Transaktion SE11 geben Sie diese beiden Tabellen an.

Sperrbausteine

Bei der Aktivierung des Sperrobjekts werden die beiden Funktionsbausteine ENQUEUE_EZIFPORDER und DEQUEUE_EZIFPORDER generiert, mit denen Sperren gesetzt und entfernt werden können. Diese beiden Funktionsbausteine haben die Importparameter ORDERID und ORDERPOS, mit denen der zu sperrende Datensatz aus der Tabelle ZIFPORDERPOS eindeutig bestimmt werden kann. Es können auch generisch alle Positionen einer Bestellung gesperrt werden, indem für das Sperrargument ORDERID nichts übergeben wird. Die restlichen Importparameter von ENQUEUE_EZBOOK regeln Details des Sperrmechanismus, sind aber mit Standardwerten vorbelegt, die für unsere Zwecke ausreichen.

1.3.2 Authentifizierung und Autorisierung

Bei der Anmeldung über das SAP GUI authentifiziert sich ein Benutzer durch die Angabe von Benutzername, Passwort und Mandant. Diese drei Angaben müssen mit den Daten übereinstimmen, die beim Anlegen eines Benutzerstammdatensatzes mit Transaktion SU01 vergeben werden. Ob ein authentifizierter Benutzer jedoch auch autorisiert ist, bestimmte Aktionen auszuführen, muss die Anwendung selbst feststellen. Dazu vergleicht sie mit der Anweisung `AUTHORITY-CHECK`, ob in den Profilen des Benutzers Berechtigungen mit bestimmten, von der Anwendung festgelegten Werten hinterlegt sind.

Berechtigungsobjekte

Dazu erzeugen Sie aus dem Object Navigator (Transaktion SE80) oder Transaktion SU21 das Berechtigungsobjekt `ZIFPORDER` mit dem Feld `ACTVT` (für Activity = Aktivität). Das Feld `ACTVT` kann die Werte »01« (Hinzufügen oder Erzeugen), »02« (Ändern), »03« (Anzeigen) und »06« (Löschen) annehmen.

Um nun einem Benutzer z. B. das Recht zu geben, Bestellungen anzuzeigen, müssen Sie (als Administrator) mit Transaktion SU03 eine Berechtigung zu diesem Berechtigungsobjekt anlegen, bei der dem Feld `ACTVT` der Wert »03« zugewiesen wird. Diese Berechtigung wird dann mit Transaktion SU02 einem Profil zugeordnet, das wiederum schließlich mit Transaktion SU01 den entsprechenden Benutzern zugewiesen wird.

Berechtigungsprüfung

Bevor eine Anwendung dem Benutzer nun Bestellungen anzeigt, muss sie überprüfen, ob er in seinen Profilen tatsächlich eine Berechtigung für das Berechtigungsobjekt `ZIFPORDER` hat, in der das Feld `ACTVT` den Wert »03« annimmt. Ist dies nicht der Fall, darf die Anwendung dem Benutzer die Daten nicht anzeigen. Listing 1.2 zeigt den ABAP-Code für diese Prüfung.

```
* Berechtigung zum Anzeigen prüfen
AUTHORITY-CHECK OBJECT 'ZIFPORDER' ID 'ACTVT' FIELD '03'.
CHECK SY-SUBRC EQ 0.
* Hier geht es nur weiter, wenn SY-SUBRC = 0 ist.
* Daten anzeigen.
```

Listing 1.2 Prüfen der Berechtigung zum Anzeigen von Bestellungen

1.3.3 Nummernkreise

Damit für neu angelegte Bestellungen Order-IDs automatisch erzeugt werden können, muss mit Transaktion SNRO (Nummernkreispflege) ein Nummernkreisobjekt angelegt werden. Dieser Nummernkreis erhält den Namen ZIFPORDER. Für die Nummernlänge dieses Nummernkreisobjekts wird die Domäne ZIFPORDERDOM verwendet.

Nummernkreisintervalle

Nach dem Erzeugen und Speichern des Nummernkreisobjekts kann dazu passend ein Nummernkreisintervall angelegt werden. Dies geschieht im Einstiegsbildschirm von Transaktion SNRO über den Button **Nummernkreise** in der Anwendungsfunktionsleiste. Von dort können Sie über den Button **Intervalle ändern** neue Intervalle anlegen oder bestehende ändern. Abbildung 1.10 zeigt ein Intervall dieses Nummernkreises. Um aus diesem Intervall eine Nummer zu ziehen, wird der Funktionsbaustein NUMBER_GET_NEXT verwendet.

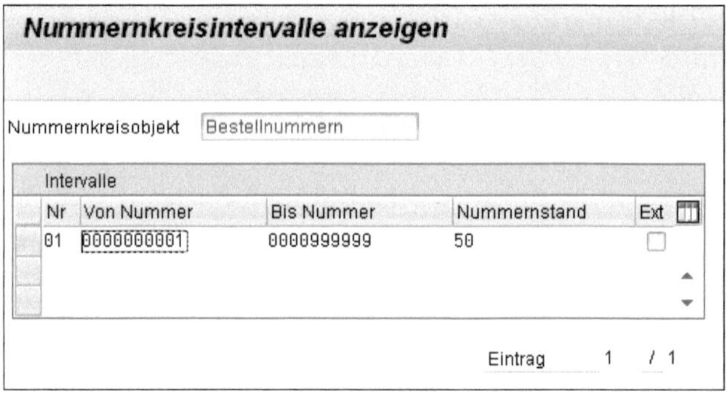

Abbildung 1.10 Nummernkreisintervall des Nummernkreisobjekts »ZIFPORDER« für Bestellnummern

1.3.4 Funktionsbausteine

Funktionsbausteine sind Modularisierungseinheiten der Programmiersprache ABAP. Sie enthalten ausführbaren Code und können aus ABAP-Programmen über die ABAP-Anweisung CALL FUNCTION aufgerufen werden. Sie haben eine wohldefinierte Schnittstelle für die Übergabe und Entgegennahme von Daten. Die Schnittstelle definiert dabei sowohl den Typ der Parameter als auch die Übergaberichtung. Daten können nur über diese Schnittstelle an den Funktionsbaustein übergeben und von ihm entgegengenommen werden.

Dieser Abschnitt befasst sich mit dem, was allen Funktionsbausteinen gemein ist. Im Folgenden begegnen Sie konkreten Funktionsbausteinen, insbesondere in Abschnitt 1.3.5, »Verbuchungsbausteine«, und Abschnitt 1.4.2, »Remote Function Call (RFC)«, sowie in Kapitel 3, »Remote Function Call mit ABAP«.

Function Builder

Funktionsbausteine erstellen Sie mit dem Function Builder (Transaktion SE37). Neben dem Quelltext werden mit dem Function Builder auch die Schnittstelle und die Eigenschaften des Funktionsbausteins festgelegt.

Funktionsgruppen

Jeder Funktionsbaustein ist Teil einer Funktionsgruppe. Eine Funktionsgruppe ist ein Programm (vom Typ F), das wie jedes andere Programm globale Daten, Dynpros, Module und andere Bestandteile enthalten kann. Der Funktionsbaustein DDIF_FIELDINFO_GET etwa gehört zur Funktionsgruppe SDIFRUNTIME. Diese Funktionsgruppe enthält für den Zugriff auf das ABAP Dictionary noch weitere Funktionsbausteine, wie z. B. DDIF_NAMETAB_GET, DD_INT_UPDATE_DDFTX und DDIF_FIELDLABEL_GET.

Jeder Funktionsbaustein einer Funktionsgruppe kann auf die globalen Daten dieser Funktionsgruppe zugreifen. Dabei wird für jedes aufrufende Programm eine neue Instanz der globalen Daten der Funktionsgruppe angelegt; die Inhalte der globalen Daten einer Funktionsgruppe sind demnach für jedes aufrufende Programm unterschiedlich. Ruft ein Programm zwei Funktionsbausteine einer Funktionsgruppe auf, kann der erste Funktionsbaustein Daten in die globalen Daten der Funktionsgruppe schreiben, die der zweite Funktionsbaustein dann lesen und verwenden kann. Auf diese Art können die Aufrufe von Funktionsbausteinen zustandsbehaftet (stateful) werden.

Schnittstelle eines Funktionsbausteins

Mit dem aufrufenden Programm kann der Funktionsbaustein Daten lediglich über seine Schnittstelle austauschen. Die Schnittstelle besteht aus fünf Teilen:

- **Import**
  Über Importparameter werden Daten an den Funktionsbaustein übergeben. Die Aktualparameter können dabei nicht vom Funktionsbaustein geändert werden. Importparameter können einfach oder strukturiert und zudem als optional gekennzeichnet sein. In diesem Fall wird bei der Parameterdefinition auch ein Vorschlagswert festgelegt.
- **Export**
  Über Exportparameter werden Daten vom Funktionsbaustein entgegengenommen, nachdem er seine Ausführung beendet hat. Exportparameter können einfach oder strukturiert sein.
- **Changing**
  Changing-Parameter sind eine Kombination aus Import- und Exportparametern: Über die Changing-Parameter können dem Funktionsbaustein Daten übergeben werden, die er dann ändert und wieder zurückgibt.
- **Tabellen**
  Import-, Export- und Changing-Parameter dürfen bis Release 6.40 nur

einfach oder strukturiert sein. Um interne Tabellen (Arrays) zu übergeben, werden Tabellenparameter verwendet. Tabellenparameter werden immer per Referenz übergeben. Sie dienen sowohl zur Übergabe an den Funktionsbaustein als auch zur Rückgabe von Werten aus dem Funktionsbaustein. Welche dieser beiden Funktionen ein Tabellenparameter erfüllt, müssen Sie der Funktionsbaustein-Dokumentation entnehmen, die Sie im Einstiegsbild des Function Builders mit [F9] aufrufen können. In ABAP wurden Tabellenparameter in Funktionsbausteinen mit ABAP-Release 7.40 SP02 als obsolet markiert. Stattdessen sollen Tabellentypen als `IMPORTING`/`EXPORTING`-Parameter oder als `CHANGING`-Parameter verwendet werden. Wir behandeln das Thema trotzdem noch in diesem Buch, da es sein kann, dass Tabellenparameter im individuellen Kontext noch verwendet werden.

- **Ausnahmen**
  Auch mögliche Ausnahmezustände werden in der Schnittstelle des Funktionsbausteins definiert. Falls ein Fehler auftritt, löst der Funktionsbaustein eine der definierten Ausnahmen durch das Schlüsselwort `RAISE` aus. Der Aufrufer ist dafür verantwortlich, den Returncode des Funktionsbausteins auszuwerten. Ist eine Ausnahme aufgetreten, ist der Returncode ungleich null.

Jeder Funktionsbaustein hat eine solche Schnittstelle. Neben der Schnittstelle besitzt ein Funktionsbaustein weitere Eigenschaften. Der nächste Abschnitt befasst sich mit Verbuchungsbausteinen, während es in Kapitel 3, »Remote Function Call mit ABAP«, um RFC-Funktionsbausteine geht.

1.3.5 Verbuchungsbausteine

Aufgrund des in Abschnitt 1.1.2, »SAP NetWeaver Application Server ABAP«, erläuterten Transaktionskonzepts sollten Anwendungsprogramme Datenbankänderungen nicht direkt über `INSERT`-, `UPDATE`- und `DELETE`-Statements programmieren, da diese Datenbankänderungen sofort nach jedem Dialogschritt über einen impliziten Datenbank-Commit auf der Datenbank festgeschrieben werden. Stattdessen sollten die Anwendungsprogramme spezielle Funktionsbausteine mit dem Zusatz `IN UPDATE TASK` aufrufen. Diese Funktionsbausteine sind bei den Eigenschaften als Verbuchungsbausteine gekennzeichnet. Sie werden nicht direkt beim Aufruf ausgeführt, sondern erst, wenn das Anwendungsprogramm den Befehl `COMMIT WORK` absetzt. Erst dann werden diese Verbuchungsbausteine in einem separaten Workprozess vom Typ `V` asynchron ausgeführt und schreiben die Daten, die ihnen zum Zeitpunkt des Aufrufs übergeben wurden, in die Datenbank. Durch dieses Konzept ist es möglich, auch eine SAP-LUW, die aus mehreren Dialogschritten besteht, durch ein ROLLBACK WORK abzubrechen, ohne dass die geänderten Daten auf der Datenbank festgeschrieben werden.

Massenverbuchung

Verbuchungsbausteine zur Erzeugung von Datensätzen sollten die ihnen übergebenen Daten zunächst einmal in einer internen Tabelle innerhalb der Funktionsgruppe speichern und dann ein Unterprogramm mit dem Zusatz ON COMMIT aufrufen, das die eigentliche Verbuchung mit Array-Insert-Techniken vornimmt. Mit auf diese Weise programmierten Verbuchungsbausteinen ist es möglich, innerhalb einer Transaktion mehrere Objekte performant zu erzeugen. Das Unterprogramm, das die eigentliche Verbuchung vornimmt, wird nur einmal ausgeführt und schreibt alle Datensätze in einem einzigen Datenbankzugriff. Dies ist besonders dann wichtig, wenn Massendaten eingelesen werden sollen.

Listing 1.3 zeigt den Verbuchungsbaustein z_ifp_v_create_order. Er schreibt den übergebenen Parameter für Kopf- und Positionsdaten zunächst in die internen Tabellen it_orderheader_buffer und it_orderpos_buffer, die im globalen Datenbereich der Funktionsgruppe ZIFP definiert wurden. Danach ruft er das Unterprogramm buffersave mit dem Zusatz ON COMMIT auf. Aufgrund dieses Zusatzes wird das Unterprogramm im Verbuchungsprozess tatsächlich nur einmal ausgeführt.

```
FUNCTION z_ifp_v_create_order.
*"----------------------------------------------------------------
*"*"Verbuchungsfunktionsbaustein:
*"*"Lokale Schnittstelle:
*"  IMPORTING
*"     VALUE(IM_ORDERHEADER) TYPE  ZIFPORDER
*"  TABLES
*"      IM_ORDERPOS STRUCTURE  ZIFPORDERPOS
*"----------------------------------------------------------------
" Die übergebenen Daten zunächst in Buffer-Tabelle speichern.
  APPEND im_orderheader TO it_orderheader_buffer.
  IF sy-subrc NE 0.
    MESSAGE a601(zifp) WITH im_orderheader-orderid.
  ENDIF.
  APPEND LINES OF im_orderpos TO it_orderpos_buffer.
  IF sy-subrc NE 0.
    MESSAGE a602(zifp) WITH im_orderheader-orderid.
  ENDIF.
  " Die ganze Tabelle beim Commit abspeichern.
  PERFORM buffersave ON COMMIT.
ENDFUNCTION.
```

```
FORM buffersave.
  INSERT zifporder FROM TABLE it_orderheader_buffer.
  IF sy-subrc NE 0.
    MESSAGE a603(zifp).
  ENDIF.
  INSERT zifporderpos from table it_orderpos_buffer.
  IF sy-subrc NE 0.
    MESSAGE a604(zifp).
  ENDIF.
ENDFORM.                    "buffersave
```

Listing 1.3 Verbuchungsbaustein »z_ifp_v_create_order«

1.3.6 Anwendungsfunktionalität und Benutzeroberflächen

Bis hierher haben Sie die Datenzugriffsschicht der Beispielanwendung mit transparenten Tabellen, Suchhilfen, Sperrobjekten, Berechtigungsobjekten und Verbuchungsbausteinen programmiert. Als Nächstes müssten nun die Anwendungsfunktionalität und die Benutzeroberfläche der Anwendung entwickelt werden. Für unsere Zwecke ist dies jedoch nicht notwendig, und die Vorgehensweise ist in anderen Büchern hinreichend beschrieben. Hier skizzieren wir daher nur die grobe Vorgehensweise.

Kapselung der Funktionalität

Damit eine Anwendung mit alternativen Benutzeroberflächen versehen oder auch von externen Programmen über Schnittstellen genutzt werden kann, ist es sinnvoll, die Anwendungsfunktionalität in Funktionsbausteinen zu kapseln. Dies werden Sie in Kapitel 3, »Remote Function Call mit ABAP«, sehen. Die dort entwickelten Funktionsbausteine dienen als Grundlage für ALE- und SOAP-Schnittstellen in Kapitel 7, »IDocs und Application Link Enabling«, und Kapitel 8, »SOAP-Webservices«. Soll eine Anwendung schnittstellenfähig sein, ist daher weniger die verwendete Interprozess-Kommunikationstechnologie ausschlaggebend als vielmehr die sinnvolle Zerlegung der Anwendungsfunktionalität in elementare Bausteine, die von verschiedenen Verwendern genutzt werden können.

Grafische Benutzeroberflächen

Ist die Anwendungsfunktionalität erst einmal so gekapselt, ist es auch leicht, grafische Benutzeroberflächen mit unterschiedlichen Techniken zu erstellen. Dazu gibt es in SAP-Umgebungen mehrere Möglichkeiten, z. B:

- **SAPUI5**

  SAPUI5 ist ein User-Interface-Framework (UI-Framework) für die Entwicklung von Webanwendungen. Es bildet die Grundlage für die Entwicklung von *SAP-Fiori-Anwendungen*. SAP Fiori ist die Designsprache von SAP und sorgt für eine einheitliche User Experience. SAP Fiori dient ebenfalls als Basis für das Framework *SAP Fiori Elements*. Bei SAP Fiori Elements handelt es sich um eine Technologie zur Implementierung von SAP-Fiori-Anwendungen auf Basis von UI-Template-Klassen. Diese Template-Klassen definieren UI-Vorlagen zur Einhaltung der SAP-Fiori-Designregeln. SAPUI5 und SAP Fiori werden in anderen Werken in der Tiefe behandelt (siehe z. B. Englbrecht/Pflugrad: Das neue SAPUI5-Handbuch, SAP PRESS 2020, und Englbrecht: SAP Fiori, SAP PRESS 2020).

- **Reports**
  Reports sind ABAP-Programme vom Typ `1`, die im Wesentlichen Daten auf der Datenbank selektieren und in Form von Listen im SAP GUI ausgeben.
- **Modulpools**
  Modulpools sind ABAP-Programme vom Typ `M`, die aus einzelnen Dynpros bestehen. Sie werden über Transaktionscodes aufgerufen.
- **Business Server Pages**
  Business Server Pages (BSP) sind HTML-Seiten mit eingebettetem ABAP-Code. Diese Anwendungen werden nicht über das SAP GUI, sondern über einen Webbrowser verwendet (siehe z. B. Plantiko: BSP-Praxisbuch, dpunkt 2007). Die Nutzung von BSP wird von SAP unterstützt, allerdings ist es nicht mehr die für die Entwicklung von Webanwendungen empfohlene Technologie. Anstelle von BSP sollte SAPUI5 für Neuimplementierungen verwendet werden.
- **Web Dynpro ABAP**
  Dies ist ein Framework zur Entwicklung von Webanwendungen. Hier wird die Oberfläche nicht direkt in HTML entwickelt, sondern mit grafischen Werkzeugen für die Web-Dynpro-Laufzeitumgebung beschrieben (siehe z. B. Schwaiger und Ofenloch, *Web Dynpro ABAP*, 2014). Web Dynpro ABAP kann weiterhin auch unter SAP S/4HANA für die Entwicklung von browserfähigen Anwendungen verwendet werden, allerdings wird für Neuentwicklungen empfohlen, SAPUI5 und SAP Fiori Elements zu verwenden.

Benutzeroberflächen ohne ABAP entwickeln

Darüber hinaus ist es natürlich auch denkbar, Benutzeroberflächen ganz ohne ABAP zu entwickeln, z. B. mit Web Dynpro ABAP, ASP.NET (Active Server Pages), SAPUI5, Angular und vielen weiteren Technologien.

1.4 Überblick über die Schnittstellentechnologien von SAP

In diesem Abschnitt stellen wir Ihnen die wichtigsten Schnittstellentechnologien vor, die von ABAP-Programmen verwendet werden:

- die Dateischnittstelle zum Lesen und Schreiben von Dateien (siehe Abschnitt 1.4.1, »Dateischnittstelle«)
- Remote Function Call (RFC) zum Remote-Aufruf von Funktionsbausteinen, siehe Abschnitt 1.4.2, »Remote Function Call (RFC)«
- Business Application Programming Interfaces (BAPIs), die eine objektorientierte Sicht auf Anwendungsfunktionen bieten (siehe Abschnitt 3.5, »Business-Objekte und BAPIs«)
- die ALE-Schnittstelle (Application Link Enabling) zum asynchronen Austausch von Nachrichten (siehe Kapitel 7, »IDocs und Application Link Enabling«)
- SOAP, ein Protokoll, das auf den Internetstandards HTTP und XML aufsetzt (siehe Kapitel 8, »SOAP-Webservices«)
- OData, ein von Microsoft entwickeltes Protokoll, das die Internetstandards Atom Syndication und Atom Publishing erweitert (siehe Kapitel 9, »SAP Gateway und OData«)

In diesem Abschnitt erklären wir Ihnen die grundlegenden Zusammenhänge und zeigen Ihnen die wichtigsten Transaktionen zur Administration der Schnittstellen.

1.4.1 Dateischnittstelle

Eine auch in der Praxis wichtige Methode, Daten zwischen zwei Systemen auszutauschen, ist deren Senden über das Dateisystem. Das sendende System schreibt Daten in eine Datei, die dann in ein Verzeichnis des Zielsystems transportiert wird. Diese Datei wird vom Zielsystem gelesen und in die Datenbank importiert.

Importprogramme

Bei SAP-Systemen gibt es bereits fertige Programme für den Import wichtiger Arten von Daten. Diese Programme erwarten allerdings die Datei in einem festgelegten Format. Die Datei wird gelesen, und die Daten werden auf eine von drei Arten in die Datenbanktabellen geschrieben:

- **Call-Transaction-Programm**
  Die Programmiersprache ABAP kennt das Schlüsselwort `CALL TRANSACTION`, mit dem eine SAP-Transaktion aufgerufen werden kann. Dieser Transaktion werden die einzugebenden Daten in Form einer sogenannten *Batch-Input-Tabelle* übergeben. Für jedes Eingabefeld der Dynpros der aufgerufenen Transaktion stehen in der Batch-Input-Tabelle die einzugebenden Daten. Außerdem enthält die Tabelle für jedes Dynpro den Funktionscode, mit dem die Eingabe beendet und zum nächsten Dynpro navigiert werden soll.

Ein Call-Transaction-Programm liest die Datei mit den einzugebenden Daten, baut für jeden Datensatz eine Batch-Input-Tabelle auf und übergibt diese Tabelle per `CALL TRANSACTION` an die SAP-Transaktion (die normalerweise im Dialog ausgeführt wird), um einen neuen Datensatz anzulegen. Die aufgerufene Transaktion wird im Hintergrund abgespielt; die Dynpros werden daher nicht angezeigt. Es finden natürlich alle Eingabeprüfungen statt, die in der SAP-Transaktion programmiert sind. Damit ist gewährleistet, dass über die Call-Transaction-Technik nur gültige und konsistente Daten in die Datenbank gelangen.

- **Batch-Input**
  Der erste Schritt verläuft beim Batch-Input-Programm wie beim Call-Transaction-Programm: Die Datei mit den einzugebenden Daten wird gelesen, und für jeden Datensatz wird eine Batch-Input-Tabelle erzeugt. Diese Batch-Input-Tabelle wird jedoch nicht direkt an die SAP-Transaktion weitergegeben, sondern in einer sogenannten *Batch-Input-Mappe* in der Datenbank gespeichert. Diese Batch-Input-Mappe wird später durch den Batch-Input-Monitor (Transaktion SM35) gelesen, und die darin enthaltenen Batch-Input-Tabellen werden an die SAP-Transaktion übergeben. Man sagt, die Batch-Input-Mappe wird »abgespielt«.

  Beim Abspielen wird ein Protokoll erstellt, das später mit dem Batch-Input-Monitor analysiert werden kann. Im Fehlerfall haben Sie die Möglichkeit, die Daten zu korrigieren und die Mappe erneut abzuspielen. Diese Möglichkeit der Fehlerkontrolle und Fehlerkorrektur ist der wesentliche Vorteil des Batch-Input-Verfahrens gegenüber der Call-Transaction-Technik.

- **Direct Input**
  Insbesondere für Massendatenübernahmen können die beiden genannten Techniken zu langsam sein. Für manche Datenarten, insbesondere für Finanzbuchhaltungsbelege, gibt es daher Direct-Input-Programme. Diese Programme lesen die Datei mit den einzugebenden Daten, prüfen die Daten und speichern sie direkt per `UPDATE` in der Datenbank. Hier werden aus Gründen der Performance die vorhandenen Dialogtransaktionen nicht verwendet.

»CALLTRANSACTION«

Manchmal werden diese drei Techniken der programmgesteuerten Dateneingabe innerhalb von Funktionsbausteinen gekapselt. Die einzugebenden Daten werden dabei über `TABLES`-Parameter des Funktionsbausteins übergeben. Der Funktionsbaustein kann dann per `CALL TRANSACTION` oder über Direct Input die Daten in die Datenbanktabellen schreiben oder eine Batch-Input-Mappe zum späteren Abspielen aufbauen. Insbesondere die Verwendung von `CALL TRANSACTION` in einem selbst geschriebenen Funktionsbaustein ist nützlich, wenn kein geeignetes BAPI zur Verfügung steht.

1.4.2 Remote Function Call (RFC)

Über das Anwendungsprotokoll *Remote Function Call* können ABAP-Funktionsbausteine auch von externen Programmen aufgerufen werden. RFC-fähige Funktionsbausteine sind in ihren Eigenschaften speziell als remotefähig gekennzeichnet.

Abbildung 1.11 zeigt z. B. die Eigenschaften des Funktionsbausteins `DDIF_FIELDINFO_GET`, mit dem Sie Eigenschaften von Datenbankfeldern aus dem ABAP Dictionary lesen können. Im Abschnitt **Ablaufart** ist er als remotefähiger Funktionsbaustein gekennzeichnet, kann demnach von externen Programmen aufgerufen werden.

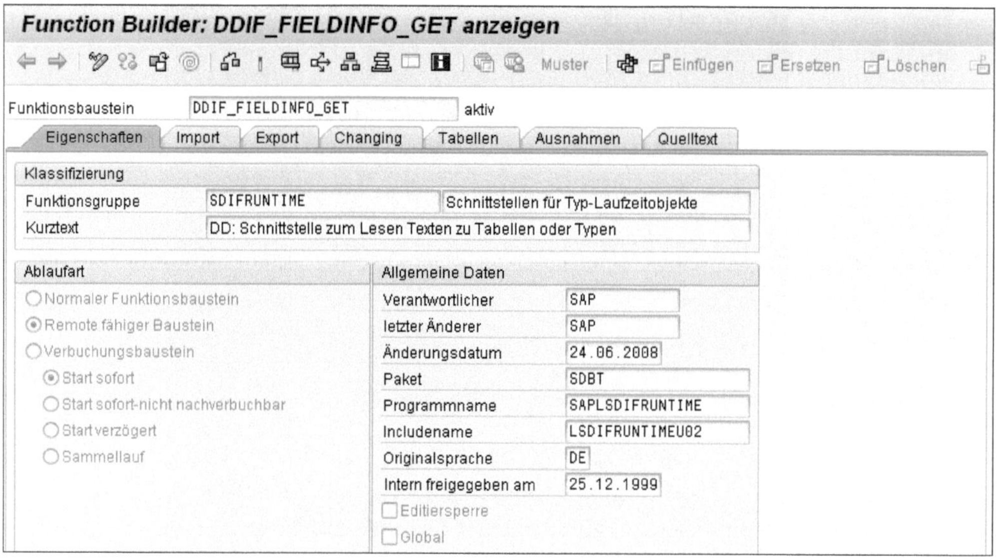

Abbildung 1.11 RFC-Funktionsbaustein »DDIF_FIELDINFO_GET«

Typisierung der Parameter

Bei remotefähigen Bausteinen müssen sämtliche Parameter mit Bezug zum ABAP Dictionary typisiert sein, und die Übergabeart für Import- und Exportparameter muss immer **Wertübergabe** sein. Das heißt, Sie müssen bei allen Parametern das Auswahlfeld **Wertübergabe** ankreuzen. Remotefähige Funktionsbausteine dürfen außerdem erst seit Release 6.40 Changing-Parameter besitzen.

RFC-Destinationen

RFC-Verbindungstypen

Aus einem ABAP-Programm wird ein Funktionsbaustein mit dem Befehl `CALL FUNCTION` aufgerufen. Soll der Funktionsbaustein in einem anderen System ausgeführt werden, wird der Zusatz `DESTINATION <dest>` verwendet, wobei `<dest>` ein Bezeichner ist, der mit Transaktion SM59 (RFC-Destinationen) gepflegt wird. Über diese Transaktion werden mit dem Bezeichner die technischen Informationen gepflegt, die vom rufenden System benötigt werden, um das Zielsystem zu erreichen.

Zwei RFC-Verbindungstypen sind für uns besonders interessant:

- Verbindungstyp `3`: Das Zielsystem ist ein SAP-System.
- Verbindungstyp `T`: Das Zielsystem ist ein externes System.

ABAP-Zielsystem

Ist das Zielsystem ein SAP-System, gehören zu den technischen Informationen, die Sie beim Anlegen einer RFC-Destination pflegen, die Angaben über den Application Host oder den Message-Server, das zu verwendende Gateway und die Angaben für den Logon im Zielsystem.

Um eine RFC-Destination mittels Transaktion SM59 anzulegen, klicken Sie auf den Button **Anlegen** auf der Anwendungsfunktionsleiste. Sie sehen dann einen Dialog, in dem Sie die allgemeinen Attribute der Destination eingeben können. Dazu gehören der Bezeichner, eine Kurzbeschreibung und vor allem der Typ der Destination.

Für eine Verbindung zu einem SAP-System wählen Sie **Verbindungstyp 3**. Sobald Sie die [↵]-Taste drücken, ändert sich das Aussehen des Bildschirms (siehe Abbildung 1.12). Über die Optionsfelder **Lastverteilung ja/nein** können Sie auswählen, ob der Message-Server des Zielsystems beim Verbindungsaufbau einen Anwendungsserver festlegen soll oder ob Sie mit einem bestimmten Anwendungsserver kommunizieren möchten. Im ersten Fall müssen Sie den Hostnamen oder die IP-Adresse des Message-Servers, die System-ID und die Logon-Gruppe angeben, im zweiten Fall den Hostnamen oder die IP-Adresse des Anwendungsservers sowie die Systemnummer der SAP-Instanz.

Schließlich müssen Sie noch angeben, unter welchem Mandanten, mit welchem Benutzer und Passwort und in welcher Sprache Sie sich am Zielsystem anmelden möchten. Über den Button **Verbindungstest** auf der Anwendungsfunktionsleiste können Sie prüfen, ob eine Verbindung zum anderen System aufgenommen werden kann. Wenn Sie auf den Button **Remote Login** klicken, wird eine neue SAP-GUI-Sitzung mit dem anderen System gestartet.

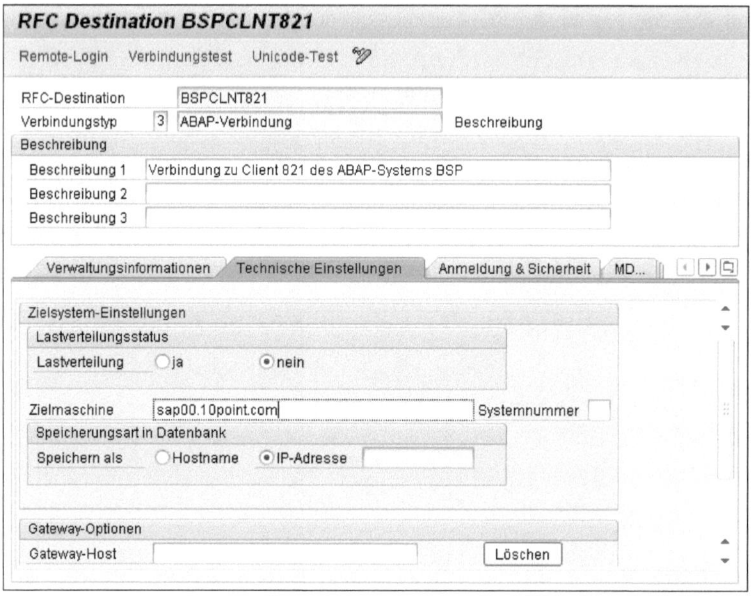

Abbildung 1.12 RFC-Destination vom Typ »3«

Externes Zielsystem

Ist das Zielsystem dagegen ein externes System, müssen Sie in Transaktion SM59 angeben, wie dieses externe System erreicht werden kann. Eine RFC-Destination zu einem externen System ist vom Verbindungstyp T. Sobald Sie den Namen, den Verbindungstyp und die Beschreibung der Destination eingegeben haben, drücken Sie auf die [↵]-Taste. Der Bildschirm sieht dann aus, wie in Abbildung 1.13 dargestellt.

Zugriff auf externes System

Es gibt vier Möglichkeiten, wie Sie ein externes System erreichen können:

- **Start auf dem Applikationsserver**
  Wählen Sie die Option **Anstarten auf Applikationsserver**. Im Eingabefeld **Programm** geben Sie den Pfad zu einem RFC-Serverprogramm auf dem Applikationsserver an. Das Programm muss auf dem Applikationsserver liegen, auf dem das ABAP-Programm ausgeführt wird, das den Befehl `CALL FUNCTION` absetzt. Beim Aufruf wird das angegebene Programm auf dem Applikationsserver gestartet und führt die gewünschte Funktion aus.
- **Start auf explizitem Host**
  Wählen Sie die Option **Anstarten auf explizitem Host**. In den Eingabefeldern **Zielmaschine** und **Programm** geben Sie den Hostnamen und den Pfad zu einem RFC-Serverprogramm auf diesem Host an. Beim Aufruf wird das angegebene Programm auf dem angegebenen Host gestartet und führt die gewünschte Funktion aus.

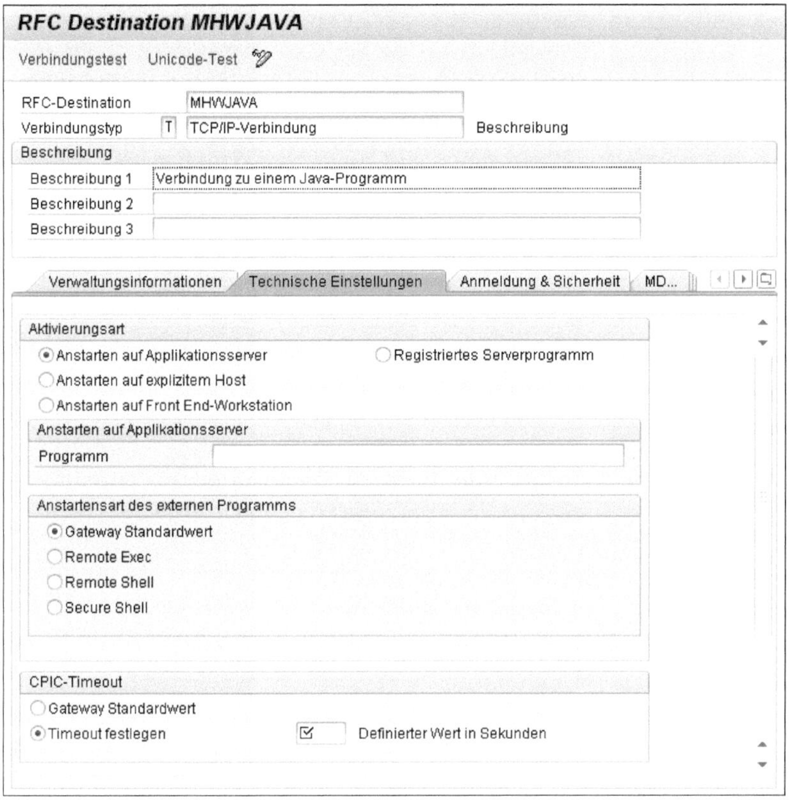

Abbildung 1.13 RFC-Destination vom Typ »T« mit Registrierung

- **Start auf dem Präsentationsserver**
  Hier geben Sie den Pfad zu einem RFC-Serverprogramm auf dem Präsentationsserver an. Dazu wählen Sie die Option **Anstarten auf Frontend-Workstation**. Im Eingabefeld **Programm** geben Sie den Pfad zu einem RFC-Serverprogramm auf der Frontend-Workstation an. Das Programm muss auf der Workstation des Benutzers liegen, die das ABAP-Programm mit dem Befehl `CALL FUNCTION` ausführt. Beim Aufruf wird das angegebene Programm auf der Workstation des Benutzers gestartet und führt die gewünschte Funktion aus.

- **Registrierung**
  Hier geben Sie eine sogenannte *Programm-ID* an, unter der sich das externe Programm an einem SAP Gateway registriert. Das externe Programm muss daher unabhängig von der Ausführung von `CALL FUNCTION` bereits vorher gestartet worden sein. Die Programm-ID ist wie der Bezeichner für die Destination case sensitive, Groß- und Kleinschreibung sind daher wichtig. Wichtig ist zudem, dass Sie auch das Gateway ange-

ben, an dem sich das externe Programm registriert hat. Dafür geben Sie die Namen des Gateway-Hosts und des Gateway-Service in den beiden Feldern **Gateway-Host** und **Gateway-Service** ein. Der Gateway-Service hat immer den Namen **sapgw<SYSNR>**, wobei **<SYSNR>** die zweistellige Systemnummer der SAP-Instanz ist, zu der das Gateway gehört.

Die Registrierung ist in der Praxis wahrscheinlich der wichtigste Schritt und wird daher auch in Abbildung 1.13 dargestellt. Das externe Programm wird unabhängig gestartet, z. B. durch einen Windows-Service oder einen Unix-Daemon, und registriert sich unter einer Programm-ID an einem Gateway. Ab diesem Zeitpunkt können die Funktionen des externen Programms aus einem ABAP-Programm heraus genutzt werden.

Destinationsangabe beim Aufruf

Sobald Sie eine Destination gepflegt haben und der Verbindungstest erfolgreich war, können Sie aus einem ABAP-Programm heraus Funktionsbausteine mit `CALL FUNCTION ... DESTINATION ...` aufrufen. Hinter dem Schlüsselwort `DESTINATION` geben Sie den Namen der RFC-Destination so an, wie Sie ihn mit Transaktion SM59 gepflegt haben.

Test im Function Builder

Auch ohne ein ABAP-Programm zu schreiben, kann der Aufruf im fremden System mit Transaktion SE37, dem Function Builder, getestet werden. Geben Sie im Einstiegsbild des Function Builders den Namen des Funktionsbausteins ein, und klicken Sie auf den Button **Einzeltest** ([F8]) in der Anwendungsfunktionsleiste. Im dann erscheinenden Dialog zur Eingabe der Übergabeparameter können Sie auch den Bezeichner für die Destination eingeben. Vorsicht, dieser Bezeichner ist case sensitive; Groß- und Kleinschreibung sind also auch hier wichtig.

RFC-Arten

Im Lauf der Zeit hat SAP die folgenden fünf Spielarten des Remote Function Calls entwickelt:

- **Synchroner RFC (sRFC) zum Lesen**
  Diese normale Ausführung des RFC dient zum Lesen von Daten im gerufenen System. Abbildung 1.14 zeigt das Ablaufschema beim synchronen RFC. Der Client ruft den Funktionsbaustein auf und wartet so lange, bis der Funktionsbaustein abgearbeitet ist. Danach wird das Client-Programm direkt nach dem Aufruf weitergeführt und kann die Ausnahmen und Rückgabeparameter des Funktionsbausteins auswerten.

  Im Client erfolgt beim Aufruf des Funktionsbausteins ein impliziter Datenbank-Commit, da der Aufruf einen neuen Dialogschritt beginnt und den alten beendet. Auch im Zielsystem erfolgt nach der Abarbeitung des

Funktionsbausteins ein impliziter Datenbank-Commit. Der Funktionsbaustein wird demnach innerhalb einer einzigen Datenbank-LUW ausgeführt; der synchrone RFC wird in der Regel eingesetzt, um Daten zu lesen.

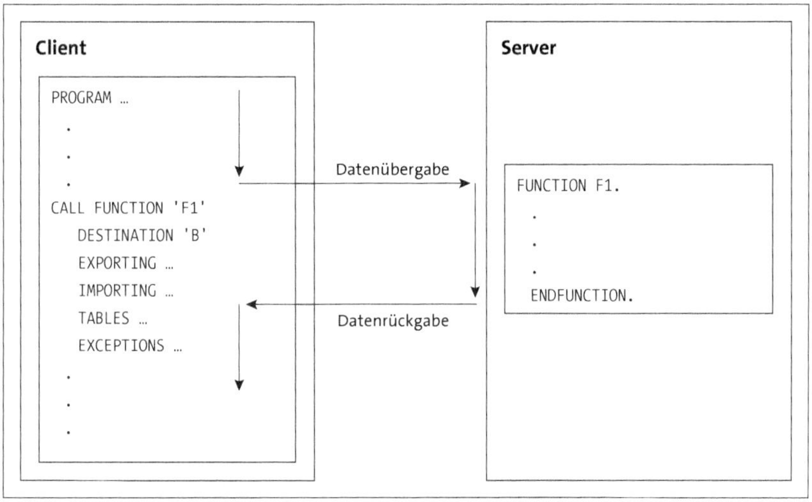

Abbildung 1.14 Ablaufschema des synchronen RFC

- **Asynchroner RFC (aRFC) zur Lastverteilung**
  Beim asynchronen RFC wird das Client-Programm direkt nach dem Aufruf des Funktionsbausteins fortgesetzt, ohne das Ablaufen des gerufenen Funktionsbausteins abzuwarten. Damit können Aufgaben parallelisiert werden.

  Abbildung 1.15 zeigt das Ablaufschema beim asynchronen RFC. Das Client-Programm wird direkt nach dem Aufruf des Funktionsbausteins fortgesetzt, ohne das Ablaufen des gerufenen Funktionsbausteins abzuwarten. Es kann daher weder die Rückgabeparameter noch die spezifischen Ausnahmen des Funktionsbausteins entgegennehmen und auswerten. Allerdings besteht die Möglichkeit, beim Aufruf ein FORM-Unterprogramm zu registrieren, das nach Abarbeitung des Funktionsbausteins vom System aufgerufen wird und in dem die Rückgabeparameter des Funktionsbausteins empfangen werden können.

  Auch hier erfolgt im Client nach dem Aufruf ein impliziter Datenbank-Commit, und auch hier läuft der Funktionsbaustein im Zielsystem in einer eigenen Datenbank-LUW ab. Der asynchrone RFC dient dazu, Aufgaben zu parallelisieren. Er steht nur ABAP-Programmen, nicht aber externen Programmen zur Verfügung.

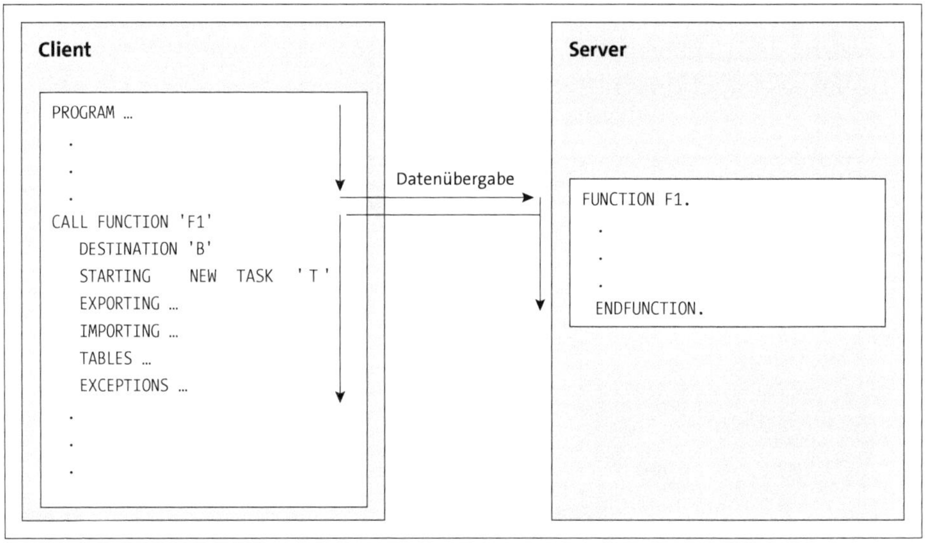

Abbildung 1.15 Ablaufschema des asynchronen RFC

- **Transaktionaler RFC (tRFC) zum Schreiben**
  Bei dieser Art des RFC wird beim Aufruf des Funktionsbausteins mit den Importparametern auch eine Transaktions-ID (TID) mitgegeben. Die Ausführung erfolgt auf dem Server garantiert nur einmal.

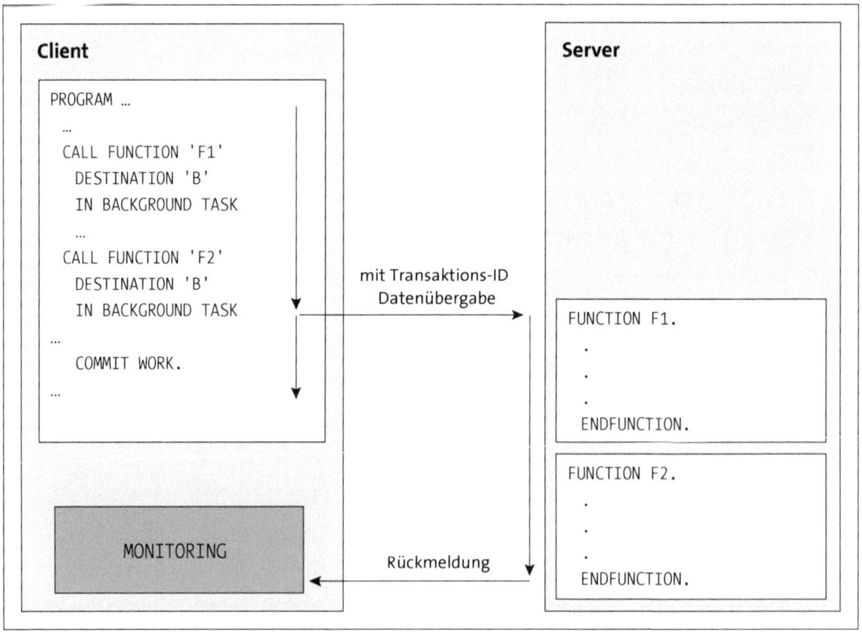

Abbildung 1.16 Ablaufschema des transaktionalen RFC

Abbildung 1.16 zeigt das Ablaufschema beim transaktionalen RFC. Beim Empfang der TID überprüft das gerufene System, ob Daten mit dieser TID schon einmal verarbeitet wurden. Es führt den aufgerufenen Funktionsbaustein nur aus, wenn dies nicht der Fall ist. Damit ist garantiert, dass Daten mit derselben TID nur einmal verarbeitet werden.

Der Client kann bei einem System- oder Verbindungsfehler die Daten zusammen mit der TID speichern und zu einem späteren Zeitpunkt noch einmal senden. Selbst wenn die Daten auf dem gerufenen System schon verarbeitet worden wären, z. B. weil der Verbindungsfehler erst bei der Rückmeldung aufgetreten ist, kann der Client die Daten mit dieser TID beliebig oft senden. Es ist sichergestellt, dass sie nur ein einziges Mal verarbeitet werden.

Wie beim asynchronen RFC erhält auch hier der Client die Rückgabeparameter des Funktionsbausteins nicht zurück. Beim Aufruf eines Funktionsbausteins auf dem Client wird kein impliziter Datenbank-Commit abgesetzt. Erst wenn das explizite `COMMIT WORK` erfolgt, ist der Dialogschritt auf dem Client beendet. Auf dem Server werden die gerufenen Funktionsbausteine in einer einzigen Datenbank-LUW abgearbeitet. Der tRFC wird eingesetzt, um Daten zu schreiben oder zu ändern.

- **Queued RFC (qRFC)**
  Abbildung 1.17 zeigt das Ablaufschema des qRFC. Dabei wird sichergestellt, dass zwei tRFC-Pakete, die vom Client hintereinander abgesetzt worden sind, auch vom Server nacheinander abgearbeitet werden.

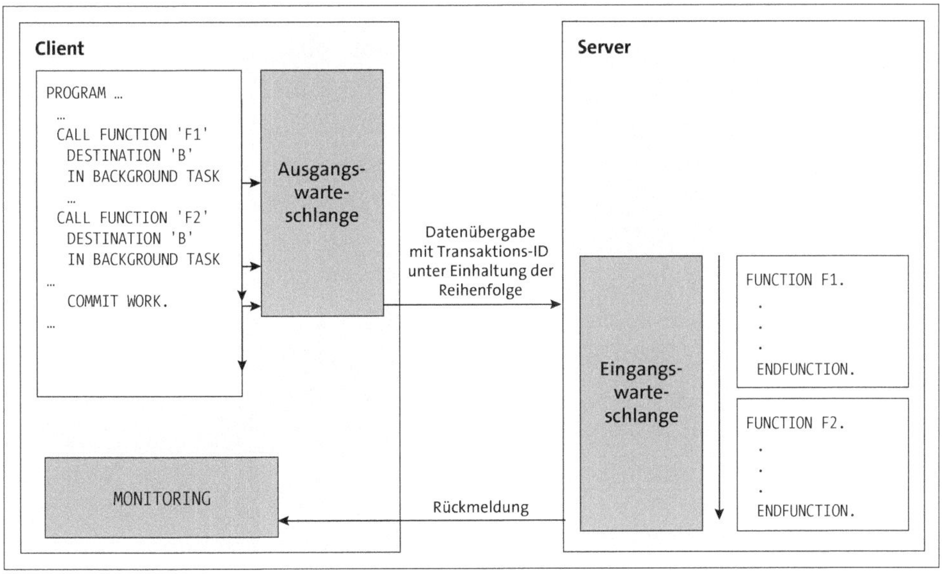

Abbildung 1.17 Ablaufschema des qRFC

Dazu werden die tRFC-Pakete vom Sender in eine Queue (Ausgangswarteschlange) geschrieben. Die Pakete in dieser Queue werden dann per tRFC in der Reihenfolge an den Empfänger geschickt, in der sie in die Queue geschrieben wurden. Die Verwendung von tRFC stellt sicher, dass ein tRFC-Paket auch im Fehlerfall genau einmal verarbeitet wird. Ein Paket aus der Queue wird erst dann an den Empfänger geschickt, wenn das vorangegangene Paket sicher beim Empfänger angekommen ist. Nur dadurch kann gewährleistet werden, dass die Verarbeitungsreihenfolge erhalten bleibt.

- **Background RFC (bgRFC)**
  Der bgRFC ist eine neue Implementierung des tRFC und des qRFC, der mit dem SAP NetWeaver Application Server ABAP 7.0 EHP 1 (Support Package Stack 4) parallel zu den beiden älteren Spielarten eingeführt wurde und diese allmählich ablösen soll.

Berechtigungen beim RFC

Innerhalb von Funktionsbausteinen finden, ebenso wie innerhalb jedes anderen ABAP-Programms, Berechtigungsprüfungen statt. Es wird überprüft, ob der ausführende Benutzer in einem der Profile, die seinem Benutzerstammdatensatz zugeordnet sind, eine Berechtigung mit den notwendigen Feldinhalten besitzt.

Berechtigungsobjekt

Eine Berechtigung ist eine Instanz eines Berechtigungsobjekts. Das Berechtigungsobjekt definiert Felder und die möglichen Werte dieser Felder. Ein Feld eines Berechtigungsobjekts könnte z. B. `ACTVT` (für »Activity«) heißen, und die möglichen Feldinhalte könnten »01« zum Anzeigen, »02« zum Erzeugen und »03« zum Ändern sein. Ein weiteres Feld könnte z. B. `BUKRS` heißen, und die möglichen Feldinhalte könnten die Buchungskreisnummern sein. Wenn Sie als Benutzer z. B. eine Berechtigung mit den Feldwerten `ACTVT` = »01« und `BUKRS` = »1000« haben, dürfen Sie sich die Daten zum Buchungskreis 1000 anzeigen lassen.

Als ABAP-Programmierer überprüfen Sie innerhalb Ihres Programms mit dem ABAP-Statement `AUTHORITY CHECK`, ob der Benutzer über die erforderliche Berechtigung verfügt, um die gewünschte Aktion auszuführen. Wenn ja, wird das Programm fortgesetzt, anderenfalls wird es mit einer Fehlermeldung abgebrochen.

Berechtigungsobjekt für Funktionsgruppen

Zusätzlich zu den Berechtigungsprüfungen, die im Funktionsbaustein stattfinden, überprüft das ABAP-Laufzeitsystem auch das Berechtigungsobjekt `S_RFC`. Dieses Berechtigungsobjekt enthält drei Felder:

- **RFC_NAME**
  Dieses Feld enthält den Namen einer Funktionsgruppe.
- **ACTVT**
  Dieses Feld kann nur den Wert »16« (Ausführen) haben.
- **RFC_TYPE**
  Dieses Feld enthält immer den Wert »FUGR« (Funktionsgruppe).

Über das Berechtigungsobjekt `S_RFC` kann gesteuert werden, ob ein RFC-Benutzer Funktionsbausteine einer bestimmten Funktionsgruppe ausführen darf. Eine Beschränkung auf bestimmte Funktionsbausteine einer Funktionsgruppe ist derzeit leider nicht möglich.

Einem RFC-Benutzer sollten nur diejenigen Berechtigungen gegeben werden, die er unbedingt benötigt, um den oder die Funktionsbausteine ausführen zu können, die für die Aufgabe notwendig sind. Ihm sollte daher keinesfalls das Berechtigungsprofil `SAP_ALL` zugeordnet werden. Um herauszufinden, welche Berechtigungen für ein bestimmtes Schnittstellenszenario benötigt werden, kann der Profilparameter `auth/authorization_trace` in der Profildatei der SAP-Instanz auf den Wert »y« gesetzt werden. Bei dieser Einstellung schreibt das System die durchgeführten Berechtigungsprüfungen und deren Ergebnis in die Tabelle `USOBX`. Dies ist in SAP-Hinweis 0543164 genauer beschrieben.

Monitoring und Troubleshooting

RFC-Aufrufe überwachen

Innerhalb eines SAP-Systems gibt es einige Werkzeuge, um die Ausführung von RFC-Aufrufen zu beobachten und damit Hinweise auf Fehler zu erhalten.

- **Transaktion ST22**
  Mit Transaktion ST22 können ABAP-Kurz-Dumps aufgelistet und analysiert werden, die von RFC-Funktionsbausteinen ausgelöst wurden. Ein ABAP-Kurz-Dump enthält Informationen über einen aufgetretenen Fehler, über die Programmstelle, an der der Fehler aufgetreten ist, die Inhalte von Systemvariablen, die Kette der Aufrufer (*Call Stack*) und weitere nützliche Informationen.
- **Gateway-Monitor**
  Über den Gateway-Monitor (Transaktion SMGW) kann ein Gateway-Trace angezeigt werden. Dazu wählen Sie die Menüfolge **Springen • Trace • Gateway • Datei anzeigen**.
- **RFC-Tracing**
  Mit Transaktion ST05 kann das RFC-Tracing für einen Benutzer eingeschaltet werden. Bis zum Ausschalten wird für diesen Benutzer ein RFC-

Trace mitgeschrieben, der anschließend mit Transaktion ST05 analysiert werden kann. RFC-Traces können auch, bezogen auf eine Destination, mitgeschrieben werden. Dazu wird beim Pflegen der Destination mit Transaktion SM59 das Kennzeichen **Trace** gesetzt. Über die Menüfolge **RFC • Trace anzeigen** können Sie sich diesen Trace dann anzeigen lassen.

1.4.3 Business Application Programming Interface (BAPI)

Komponenten von Business-Objekten

Die sogenannten *Business-Objekte* bieten eine objektorientierte Sicht auf einen großen Teil der betriebswirtschaftlichen Daten und Transaktionen eines SAP-Systems. Die Objekttypen der Business-Objekte werden im Business Object Repository (BOR) mit den Transaktionen SWO1 und SWO gepflegt. Die Komponenten eines solchen Objekttyps sind:

- **Grunddaten**
  Dabei handelt es sich um die technischen Daten des Objekttyps, wie etwa die interne Bezeichnung, das Release oder Transportdaten.
- **Interfaces**
  Dies sind die Schnittstellen, die vom Objekttyp implementiert werden.
- **Schlüsselfelder**
  Schlüsselfelder sind Felder, deren Inhalte eine Instanz des Objekttyps eindeutig identifizieren. Dies sind oft Felder der Datenbanktabellen, in denen die Objekte persistent gespeichert werden.
- **Attribute**
  Das sind die Eigenschaften des Objekttyps, entweder Referenzen auf Datenbankfelder oder auf andere Business-Objekte.
- **Methoden**
  Über Methoden werden Transaktionen oder Funktionsbausteine aufgerufen.
- **Ereignisse**
  In Workflow-Definitionen können Ereignisse verwendet werden. Ereignisse werden über Nachrichten oder Zustandsänderungen ausgelöst.

Methoden von Business-Objekten

Einige Methoden eines Objekttyps können als Business Application Programming Interfaces (BAPIs) gekennzeichnet sein. BAPIs sind immer als RFC-Funktionsbausteine implementiert und können daher wie andere RFC-Funktionsbausteine verwendet werden. Darüber hinaus haben BAPIs weitere Eigenschaften:

- **BAPIs haben eine stabile Schnittstelle.**
  SAP garantiert, dass die Schnittstelle eines veröffentlichten BAPIs in einem höheren Release nicht inkompatibel geändert wird. Das bedeutet,

dass in einem höheren Release höchstens optionale Parameter hinzukommen. In der Regel aber bleibt in höheren Releases das BAPI unangetastet. Bei Funktionsänderungen oder Erweiterungen stellt SAP ein neues BAPI mit einem neuen Namen bereit. So gibt es etwa zum Anlegen von Kundenaufträgen die BAPIs BAPI_SALESORDER_CREATEFROMDATA und BAPI_SALESORDER_CREATE_FROMDAT1. Die obsolet gewordenen BAPIs werden noch für mindestens zwei Releases beibehalten, damit auch alte Clients mit dem neuen Release arbeiten können.

- **BAPIs haben keine Präsentationsschicht.**
  BAPIs rufen keine Dynpros mit CALL SCREEN auf. Sie kommunizieren ausschließlich über die Schnittstelle ihres implementierenden Funktionsbausteins. Sollen die Ergebnisse des BAPIs visualisiert werden, ist der Aufrufer dafür selbst verantwortlich. BAPIs können daher auch in Programmen verwendet werden, in denen ohne Benutzereingriff zwischen zwei Maschinen kommuniziert werden soll.
- **BAPIs lösen keine Ausnahmen aus.**
  Für Rückmeldungen über Erfolg, Warnungen und Fehler verwenden BAPIs den Exportparameter RETURN. Je nach BAPI ist dieser Parameter eine Struktur des Typs BAPIRETURN, BAPIRETURN1, BAPIRET1 oder BAPIRET2 bzw. eine interne Tabelle mit diesen Zeilentypen. All diesen Strukturen sind die beiden folgenden wichtigen Felder gemeinsam:
  - TYPE
    Dieses Feld kann die Werte »S« (Success), »E« (Error), »W« (Warning) oder »I« (Information) annehmen. Im Erfolgsfall kann dieses Feld auch initial sein; es enthält dann einen Space.
  - MESSAGE
    Dabei handelt es sich um einen Nachrichtentext mit einem Fehlerhinweis.
- **Datenbankaktualisierungen erfolgen im Verbucher.**
  BAPIs führen Datenbankaktualisierungen stets über den Aufruf eines Verbuchungsbausteins mit CALL FUNCTION IN BACKGROUND TASK aus. Innerhalb des BAPIs wird kein COMMIT WORK oder ROLLBACK WORK programmiert. Um die Datenbankaktualisierung tatsächlich durchzuführen bzw. zu verwerfen, stehen die beiden folgenden BAPIs zur Verfügung:
  - BAPI_TRANSACTION_COMMIT
    Führt alle vorgemerkten Verbucher aus. In einem Importparameter dieses BAPIs kann festgelegt werden, ob die Verbuchung synchron oder asynchron erfolgen soll.
  - BAPI_TRANSACTION_ROLLBACK
    Verwirft die vorgemerkten Datenbank-Updates.

Standard-BAPIs Die meisten Business-Objekte stellen die folgenden Standard-BAPIs bereit:

- `GetList`
  Diesem BAPI können in der Regel Suchkriterien übergeben werden. Als Ergebnis wird eine Tabelle mit den Schlüsseln aller Objekte zurückgegeben, die diesen Suchkriterien entsprechen.
- `GetDetail`
  Dieses BAPI verlangt den Schlüssel eines Objekts als Importparameter und gibt die anderen Attribute des Objekts zurück.
- `Change`
  Mit diesem BAPI können unter Angabe eines Objektschlüssels und der neuen Attribute die bisherigen Attribute des Objekts geändert werden.
- `CreateFromData`
  Diesem BAPI können die Attribute eines neu zu erzeugenden Objekts mitgegeben werden. Zurückgeliefert wird der Schlüssel des neu angelegten Objekts.

Transaktion BAPI Mittels Transaktion BAPI können Sie sich eine Liste aller Business-Objekte und ihrer BAPIs anzeigen lassen. Die Anzeige erfolgt entweder gegliedert nach Anwendungsbereichen oder alphabetisch geordnet nach Business-Objekten. Zu jedem Business-Objekt, seinen BAPIs und deren Parametern liefert Transaktion BAPI eine ausführliche Dokumentation. Aus der Transaktion können auch die Werkzeuge aufgerufen werden, mit denen die BAPIs getestet und verwaltet werden können.

Transaktion BAPI unterscheidet zwischen instanzabhängigen und instanzunabhängigen BAPIs:

- Um instanzabhängige BAPIs aufzurufen, muss der Schlüssel eines Business-Objekts angegeben werden. Die Standard-BAPIs `Get-Detail` und `Change` sind Beispiele für instanzabhängige BAPIs.
- Instanzunabhängige BAPIs benötigen im Gegensatz dazu keine Schlüsselangabe. Sie arbeiten unabhängig von einer Objektinstanz. Beispiele sind die Standard-BAPIs `GetList` und `CreateFromData`.

1.4.4 Application Link Enabling (ALE)

Application Link Enabling stellt innerhalb von SAP-Systemen Dienste und Werkzeuge bereit, um Nachrichten zwischen Anwendungen in verschiedenen Systemen auszutauschen. Der Austausch erfolgt in der Regel durch das Versenden und den Empfang elektronischer Dokumente, den *Intermediate Documents* (IDocs). Zweck dieses Nachrichtenversands ist es, verteilte Geschäftsprozesse zu realisieren. Mit ALE können Customizing-Daten, Stammdaten und Applikationsdaten auf verschiedene Systeme verteilt werden.

Ein Beispiel wäre die Auslieferung von Kundenbestellungen in SAP ERP. Sobald feststeht, wann welche Waren an welche Kunden geliefert werden, schickt das SAP-System einen Lieferauftrag an ein externes Warenlager. Dort werden die Waren auf Paletten und in Lkw geladen. Sobald der Lkw mit der Lieferung losfährt, wird eine Auftragsbestätigung an das SAP-System zurückgeschickt. Außer Lieferaufträgen und Auftragsbestätigungen müssen in diesem Szenario auch noch Kunden- und Materialstammdaten ausgetauscht werden.

ALE-Architektur

Abbildung 1.18 zeigt schematisch die Architektur von ALE. Die sendende Anwendung ist dafür verantwortlich, das IDoc aufzubauen, gegebenenfalls die Empfänger zu ermitteln und das IDoc an die ALE-Schicht zu übergeben.

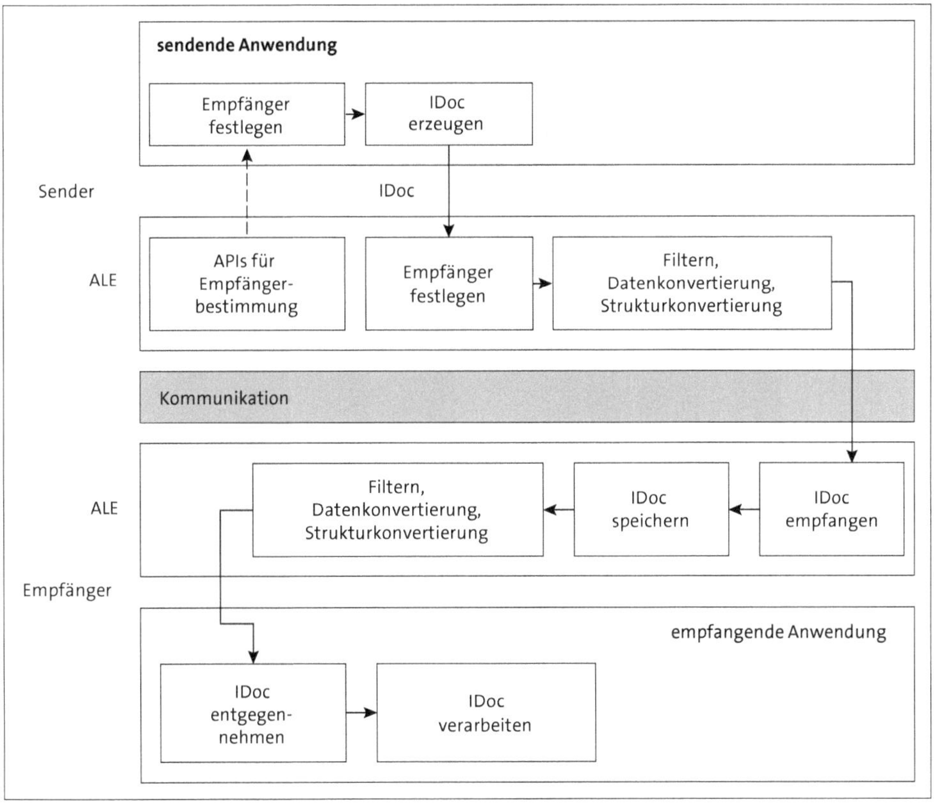

Abbildung 1.18 Architektur von ALE

Nach der Entgegennahme des IDocs ermittelt die ALE-Schicht die Empfänger, falls diese nicht schon von der sendenden Applikation festgelegt wurden. Das IDoc wird dann nach einstellbaren Regeln weiterbearbeitet: Einzelne Felder oder Segmente können gefiltert werden, Daten können konvertiert oder die Struktur des IDocs an die Struktur älterer Releases angepasst werden. Für jeden Empfänger wird dabei ein IDoc erzeugt, das zum Weitertransport an die Kommunikationsschicht übergeben wird.

Die Kommunikationsschicht leitet das IDoc an das Zielsystem weiter. In der Regel wird dazu über tRFC der Funktionsbaustein IDOC_INBOUND_ASYNCHRONOUS im Zielsystem aufgerufen. Es können aber auch andere Transportmechanismen konfiguriert werden, wie z. B. die Übergabe über das Dateisystem.

Im Zielsystem wird das IDoc nach dem Empfang gespeichert und an die ALE-Schicht weitergegeben. In der ALE-Schicht kann das empfangene IDoc, ähnlich wie im Sender, weitere Verarbeitungsschritte durchlaufen, bevor es an einen Funktionsbaustein der empfangenden Anwendung weitergegeben wird.

Logische Systeme

Bei ALE werden Sender und Empfänger als *logische Systeme* bezeichnet. Die logischen Systeme werden über Namen identifiziert, die zehn Zeichen lang sind. Die Namen der logischen Systeme werden mit Transaktion SALE im Rahmen des ALE-Customizings gepflegt. Neben einem Namen wird dort auch eine kurze Beschreibung für das logische System hinterlegt. Jeder Mandant in einem SAP-System erhält einen logischen Namen. Dieser setzt sich in der Regel aus der System-ID und dem Mandanten zusammen, etwa ULOCLNT800 für das logische System, das dem Mandanten 800 im System ULO entspricht.

Nachrichten

Bei ALE werden Nachrichten zwischen den logischen Systemen ausgetauscht. Die Namen der möglichen Nachrichten werden zusammen mit einer Kurzbeschreibung in Transaktion WE81 gepflegt. Zum Beispiel steht die Nachricht MATMAS (Material Master) für einen Austausch von Materialstammdaten, und die Nachricht DELVRY (Delivery) beschreibt einen Austausch von Lieferaufträgen.

IDocs

Die Nachrichten zwischen zwei logischen Systemen werden in Form von Intermediate Documents (IDocs) verschickt. Diese Dokumente beinhalten die Daten, die ausgetauscht werden sollen.

IDoc-Segmente

Ein IDoc besteht aus Datensätzen, die auch *Segmente* genannt werden. Jedes Segment beginnt mit einem Header von 63 Byte Länge, danach kommen die eigentlichen Daten mit bis zu 1.000 Byte Länge. Der Header hat in jedem Segment den gleichen Aufbau, und das gesamte IDoc folgt einer hierarchischen Struktur: Jedes Segment kann auf ein Elternsegment verweisen, das in der Hierarchie über dem betreffenden Segment steht (siehe Tabelle 1.6).

Feld	Länge	Bedeutung
SEGNAM	30	Typname des Segments, der die Struktur des Datenfelds SDATA festlegt
MANDT	3	Nummer des SAP-Mandanten
DOCNUM	16	eindeutige Nummer des IDocs, zu dem dieses Segment gehört
SEGNUM	6	laufende Nummer des Segments innerhalb des IDocs
PSGNUM	6	laufende Nummer des Elternsegments
HLEVEL	2	Hierarchiestufe dieses Segments
SDATA	1.000	die eigentlichen Anwendungsdaten

Tabelle 1.6 Aufbau eines IDoc-Segments

IDoc-Segmente werden mit Transaktion WE31 definiert. Dort werden ein Name und eine Kurzbeschreibung für die Segmente vergeben. Vor allem aber wird die Struktur des Felds SDATA genauer beschrieben.

Ein IDoc-Segment kann in mehreren IDoc-Typen vorkommen. IDoc-Typen werden mit Transaktion WE30 definiert. Dabei wird festgelegt, welche Segmente in dem IDoc-Typ vorkommen, ob das betreffende Segment optional ist, wie viele Segmente dieses Typs maximal vorkommen können und welches die Kindsegmente des Segments in diesem IDoc-Typ sind.

Nachrichtentypen

Ein IDoc-Typ ist einem oder mehreren Nachrichtentypen zugeordnet. Zum Beispiel kann das IDoc ORDERS04 dazu verwendet werden, Nachrichten vom Typ ORDER (Bestellung) oder ORDRSP (Bestellbestätigung) zu transportieren. Die Zuordnung einer Nachricht zu einem IDoc-Typ wird mit Transaktion WE82 vorgenommen. Dabei bestimmen das Release des SAP NetWeaver Application Server ABAP und der Nachrichtenname den IDoc-Typ eindeutig. Ab dem Release 3.0 wird der IDoc-Typ ORDERS01, ab Release 3.0D der IDoc-Typ ORDERS02, ab Release 4.0A der IDoc-Typ ORDERS03, ab Release 4.5A der Typ ORDERS04 und seit Release 4.6A der Typ ORDERS05 verwendet.

ALE-Verteilungsmodell

Welche Nachrichten von einem Sender an welche Empfänger geschickt werden, wird im Rahmen des ALE-Customizings in einem sogenannten *Verteilungsmodell* festgelegt. Das Verteilungsmodell hat eine hierarchische Struktur mit dem Sendersystem als Wurzel. Unter dem Sendersystem werden die Empfängersysteme aufgelistet, darunter die Nachrichten und darunter die Filter, die auf die Nachrichten angewandt werden sollen.

ALE-Konfiguration

Die Einstellungen im ALE-System werden mit Transaktion SALE gepflegt. Diese Transaktion stellt eine Untermenge des SAP Implementation Guides dar, den Sie in der Projektverwaltung (Transaktion SPRO) über den Button **SAP Reference Implementation Guide** erreichen können. In dieser Transaktion werden die notwendigen Schritte aufgelistet, um das ALE-System einzustellen. Im einfachsten Fall sind dies folgende Schritte:

- **Benennung der logischen Systeme**
  In diesem Schritt werden die logischen Systeme benannt.
- **Zuordnung der logischen Systeme zu Mandanten**
  Jeder SAP-Mandant erhält einen logischen Systemnamen.
- **Pflege von Destinationen**
  Mit Transaktion SM59 werden tRFC-Destinationen für die logischen Systeme angelegt. Damit in einem späteren Schritt weitere Definitionen automatisch generiert werden können, sollte die Destination für ein logisches System genauso benannt werden wie das logische System selbst.
- **Pflege des Verteilungsmodells**
  Hier wird festgelegt, an welche Empfänger welche Nachrichten mit welchen Filtern geschickt werden. Aus der Pflege des Verteilungsmodells heraus können sogenannte *Partnerprofile* generiert werden. Partnerprofile kontrollieren die Verarbeitung von eingehenden und ausgehenden IDocs.
- **Überprüfung des Partnerprofils**
  Zum Schluss prüfen Sie die automatisch generierten Partnerprofile. Wichtige Parameter eines Verteilungsprofils sind:
  - **Ausgangsport**
    Der Ausgangsport legt fest, wie ein Partner erreicht werden kann. Die Ports werden bei der Generierung der Partnerprofile automatisch angelegt, wenn die logischen Systeme und die dafür angelegten tRFC-Destinationen den gleichen Namen haben.
  - **Versende- und Verarbeitungsmodus**
    IDocs können entweder sofort verschickt bzw. verarbeitet oder so

lange gesammelt werden, bis ein Paket mit einer festgelegten Anzahl von IDocs entstanden ist. Die IDocs in diesem Paket werden dann zusammen versendet und verarbeitet.

- **Paketgröße**
  Die Größe der zu versendenden und zu verarbeitenden Pakete kann festgelegt werden.

Daneben bietet Transaktion SALE Zugriff auf viele weitere Funktionen zur Konfiguration der IDoc-Verarbeitung und des IDoc-Monitorings.

BAPIs und ALE

BAPIs asynchron aufrufen

Es gibt auch die Möglichkeit, BAPI-Aufrufe asynchron über ALE vorzunehmen. Es ist sogar so, dass alle neuen asynchronen Schnittstellen (IDocs) auf BAPIs beruhen sollten. Für ein gegebenes BAPI können Sie die notwendigen Definitionen mit Transaktion BDBG generieren:

- **Nachrichtentyp**
  Für ein BAPI wird ein Nachrichtentyp generiert.
- **IDoc-Typ**
  Für die Exportparameter des BAPIs werden Segmente und ein IDoc-Typ generiert, mit dem diese Parameter transportiert werden können. Der IDoc-Typ wird dem generierten Nachrichtentyp zugeordnet.
- **Ausgehender Funktionsbaustein**
  Dieser Funktionsbaustein hat dieselben Importparameter wie das BAPI und wird von der sendenden Anwendung anstelle des BAPIs aufgerufen. Er baut aus den Übergabeparametern ein IDoc auf und übergibt es an die ALE-Dienste zur Weiterverarbeitung.
- **Eingehender Funktionsbaustein**
  Die ALE-Dienste verwenden diesen Funktionsbaustein, um das eingehende IDoc zu verarbeiten. Er extrahiert die Daten aus dem IDoc und ruft das entsprechende BAPI im Empfängersystem auf.

ALE-BAPI-Schnittstelle

Der generierte Nachrichtentyp kann dann wie jeder andere Nachrichtentyp bei der Erstellung eines ALE-Verteilungsmodells verwendet werden. Möchte eine Applikation BAPIs in externen Systemen aufrufen, geht sie folgendermaßen vor:

- **Abfrage der Filter**
  Der Funktionsbaustein `ALE_BAPI_GET_FILTEROBJECTS` wird aufgerufen, um für ein bestimmtes BAPI die Filterobjekte zu ermitteln, die bei der Pflege des Verteilungsmodells angelegt wurden.

- **Abfrage der Empfänger**
  Der Funktionsbaustein `ALE_ASYNC_BAPI_GET_RECEIVER` wird aufgerufen, um aus den Verteilungsmodellen eine Liste der logischen Empfängersysteme zu erhalten. Dazu muss die rufende Applikation die Tabelle der Filterobjekte übergeben.
- **Asynchroner Aufruf des BAPIs**
  Nun wird der generierte ausgehende Funktionsbaustein aufgerufen, dem außer den BAPI-Importparametern die Liste der Empfängersysteme mitgegeben wird.
- **COMMIT WORK**
  Schließlich muss über den ABAP-Befehl `COMMIT WORK` dafür gesorgt werden, dass das generierte IDoc an die ALE-Schicht weitergegeben wird.

Durch diese Vorgehensweise können BAPI-Aufrufe als IDocs von einer Anwendung zur anderen geschickt werden.

1.4.5 SOAP

Seit Release 6.20 können mit dem SAP NetWeaver Application Server ABAP auch SOAP-Services und -Clients realisiert werden. Bei SOAP über HTTP schickt der SOAP-Client eine Anfrage in Form eines XML-SOAP-Dokuments an einen SOAP-Server, der mit einem XML-SOAP-Dokument antwortet.

Internet Connection Manager

Der SAP NetWeaver AS ABAP ruft einen SOAP-Webservice über HTTP-POST auf. Der Aufruf wird zunächst vom Internet Connection Manager (ICM) entgegengenommen. Mit Transaktion SMICM kann die Konfiguration des ICMs betrachtet und verändert werden. Über den Menüpfad **Springen • Services** können Sie sehen, auf welchem TCP-Port der ICM HTTP-Anfragen entgegennimmt. Über den Menüpfad **Springen • HTTP-Server • Daten anzeigen** sehen Sie die konfigurierten Ports des J2EE-Servers (bei einem Double-Stack-System) und eine Tabelle der URL-Präfixe (Uniform Resource Locator). Fordert ein HTTP-Client eine URL an, die mit einem dieser Präfixe beginnt, leitet der ICM die Anfrage an das Internet Communication Framework (ICF) auf dem ABAP-Stack weiter, sonst an den konfigurierten J2EE-Server.

Internet Communication Framework

Die konfigurierten Services im ICF sehen Sie in Transaktion SICF. Auf dem Selektionsbild, das beim Start der Transaktion erscheint, wählen Sie **Service** als **Hierarchietyp** aus. Ihnen wird dann eine Liste aller HTTP-Services angezeigt, die im ICF konfiguriert sind. SOAP-Webservices werden über die Services unterhalb des Knotens **/sap/bc/srt** implementiert. Direkt unter diesem Knoten sehen Sie z. B. die Knoten **IDoc** (SOAP-Eingang für IDoc), **rfc** (SOAP-Runtime für RFC) und **xip** (SOAP-Runtime für XI-Message-Interface).

Wenn Sie z. B. doppelt auf den Eintrag **srt** klicken, sehen Sie auf der Registerkarte **Handler-Liste** die ABAP-Klasse `CL_SOAP_HTTP_EXTENSION` als Handler für Anfragen, deren URL-Pfad mit **/sap/bc/srt/rfc** beginnt. Das ICF analysiert den URL-Pfad der Anfrage und leitet sie an die entsprechende Handler-Klasse weiter.

Webservice

In Kapitel 8, »SOAP-Webservices«, zeigen wir Ihnen, wie Sie einen Webservice im Object Navigator erzeugen können. Dabei haben Sie prinzipiell zwei Möglichkeiten:

- **Entwicklung nach dem Inside-Out-Ansatz**
  Hier gehen Sie von vorhandener ABAP-Funktionalität in Form von Funktionsbausteinen aus, für die Sie nachträglich einen Webservice und die WSDL dafür generieren.
- **Entwicklung nach dem Outside-In-Ansatz**
  Hier beschreiben Sie zuerst den Webservice im Enterprise Services Repository von SAP NetWeaver PI, generieren daraus einen Webservice im AS ABAP und programmieren die Funktionalität ganz zum Schluss.

Nach der Erzeugung muss ein Webservice für die SOAP-Laufzeitumgebung mit Transaktion SOAMANAGER freigegeben werden. Mit dieser Transaktion können Sie auch die WSDL-Datei (Web Service Description Language) eines Webservice abrufen und einen Webservice testen. Für diesen Test stellt SAP auf jedem AS Java die Anwendung `wsnavigator` bereit. Dieser Anwendung kann eine URL an die WSDL des Webservice übergeben werden. Sie erzeugt dann aus der WSDL eine grafische Benutzeroberfläche, über die der Webservice getestet werden kann.

1.4.6 OData

Leichtgewichtiges Protokoll für mobile Clients

Ähnlich wie SOAP ermöglicht das *Open Data Protocol*, kurz OData, den Aufruf von serverseitigen Funktionen über HTTP. OData ist jedoch leichtgewichtiger als SOAP, implementiert das Programmierparadigma *Representational State Transfer* (REST) besser und kann neben XML-Dokumenten auch Dokumente im Format der *JavaScript Object Notation* (JSON) austauschen. Das Protokoll eignet sich daher besonders gut für die Implementierung mobiler Clients.

OData wurde von Microsoft veröffentlicht und basiert auf den älteren Atom-Syndication- und Atom-Publishing-Protokollen. SAP stellt mit SAP Gateway eine Implementierung dieses Protokolls bereit. Ab Release 7.3 des SAP NetWeaver AS ABAP ist diese Implementierung in den ABAP-Kernel integriert. Vorher musste SAP Gateway entweder als Add-on oder auf einem separaten ABAP-Server installiert werden.

In Kapitel 9, »SAP Gateway und OData«, zeigen wir Ihnen, wie Sie mit SAP Gateway OData-Services entwickeln können und wie Sie diese mit SAPUI5- und C#-Clients konsumieren. In Kapitel 11, »ABAP RESTful Application Programming Model und OData«, zeigen wir dann, wie in SAP S/4HANA OData-Services mit dem Programmiermodell *ABAP RESTful Application Programming Model* implementiert werden. In Kapitel 13, »SAP Cloud Application Programming Model und OData«, zeigen wir die Implementierung von OData-Services unter Verwendung des *SAP Cloud Application Programming Models*.

1.4.7 ABAP Channels

Seit ABAP NetWeaver 7.4 SP05 kann ein ABAP-Server auch Push-Nachrichten an Clients schicken. Im ABAP Channels Framework stellt der Server dazu zwei Arten von Kommunikationskanälen zur Verfügung:

- **ABAP Message Channels (AMC)**
  Über ABAP Message Channels können Push-Nachrichten an andere Dialogprozesse innerhalb desselben Systems verschickt werden.
- **ABAP Push Channels (APC)**
  ABAP Push Channels sind eine Implementierung des WebSocket Protocols, mit dem Push-Nachrichten an Webclients geschickt werden können.

ABAP Channels stellen wir in Kapitel 12, »ABAP Channels«, vor.

Kapitel 2
Grundlagen der Schnittstellenprogrammierung auf der SAP Business Technology Platform

Cloud-Infrastrukturen spielen eine zentrale Rolle bei der Integration von Systemen und Anwendungen. Mit der SAP Business Technology Platform steht eine zentrale SAP-Plattform in der Cloud zur Verfügung.

Die Zukunft der IT liegt in der Cloud. Mit der SAP Business Technology Platform (SAP BTP) stellt SAP eine eigene Cloud-Plattform für die Bereitstellung von Diensten und Anwendungen über die Cloud zur Verfügung. Dieses Kapitel gibt eine Einführung in die Grundlagen der SAP BTP und legt die Basis für die Entwicklung von Schnittstellen in der SAP BTP. Nach einer Einführung in die SAP BTP in Abschnitt 2.1 befassen wir uns in Abschnitt 2.2 mit deren Infrastruktur. Hier erläutern wir u. a., wie der Cloud Connector eine nahtlose Verbindung zwischen der SAP BTP und bestehenden On-Premise-Systemen ermöglicht. In Abschnitt 2.3 gehen wir auf die Sicherheitsaspekte der SAP BTP ein. Wir zeigen Ihnen das Objektmodell und zeigen, wie Benutzerberechtigungen für den Zugriff auf SAP-BTP-Dienste konfiguriert werden. In Abschnitt 2.4 wird schließlich das SAP Business Application Studio vorgestellt – das Entwicklungswerkzeug für die Entwicklung moderner SAP-Cloud- und SAP-Fiori-Anwendungen.

2.1 Einführung in die SAP Business Technology Platform

Grundlegende Services

Die SAP Business Technology Platform ist eine vielseitige Plattform, die es Unternehmen ermöglicht, ihre Abläufe im digitalen Zeitalter zu innovieren, zu integrieren und zu transformieren. Mit einer Reihe von Werkzeugen und Services versetzt die Plattform Unternehmen in die Lage, sich von ihren Mitbewerbern abzuheben, den Geschäftswert zu steigern und eine hervorragende Kundenerfahrung zu schaffen. SAP BTP bietet eine Reihe grundlegender Services in den folgenden Bereichen:

- Anwendungsentwicklung
- Automatisierung
- Integration
- Daten und Analysen
- künstliche Intelligenz

Diese Services sind so konzipiert, dass sie nahtlos zusammenarbeiten und Unternehmen in die Lage versetzen, innovative Anwendungen zu entwickeln, unterschiedliche Systeme zu verbinden und aus ihren Daten verwertbare Erkenntnisse zu gewinnen.

Erstellung personalisierter Lösungen

Was die SAP BTP so leistungsfähig macht, ist die Tatsache, dass sie die Werkzeuge für die Erstellung personalisierter Lösungen bietet. Sie können damit Ihre eigenen Anwendungen erstellen oder bestehende Anwendungen und Dienste erweitern und integrieren, um diese an Ihre individuellen Geschäftsanforderungen anzupassen. Dank Low-Code-/No-Code-Lösungen, die ebenfalls über die SAP BTP angeboten werden, können Geschäftsanwender Aufgaben automatisieren, Workflows einrichten und ihre eigenen maßgeschneiderten Schnittstellen erstellen. Ein weiteres bemerkenswertes Merkmal ist die Fähigkeit, sowohl Cloud-native als auch hybride Lösungen aus der Cloud zu unterstützen und gleichzeitig die Integration mit On-Premise-Systemen zu gewährleisten. Durch diese Flexibilität können Unternehmen sich an veränderte Geschäfts- und Infrastrukturanforderungen anpassen, ohne die Sicherheit oder Leistung der Lösung zu beeinträchtigen. Dabei sind Anwendungsentwicklung, Automatisierung, Integration, Daten und Analysen sowie künstliche Intelligenz die Eckpfeiler der SAP BTP. Sie bieten Unternehmen die Werkzeuge und Fähigkeiten, die sie benötigen, um ihre Geschäftsprozesse zu digitalisieren, schnell zu innovieren und außergewöhnliche Kundenerlebnisse im digitalen Zeitalter zu schaffen.

Anwendungsentwicklung

Der erste Aspekt – die Anwendungsentwicklung – konzentriert sich darauf, Entwickler in die Lage zu versetzen, Anwendungen effizient zu erstellen, einzusetzen und zu verwalten. Die SAP BTP bietet verschiedene Entwicklungswerkzeuge und -dienste, die unterschiedliche Programmiersprachen und Entwicklungsansätze unterstützen. Ein zentrales Werkzeug ist *SAP Build Code*, das speziell für die Erstellung und Erweiterung von Geschäftsanwendungen auf der SAP BTP entwickelt wurde. SAP Build Code stellt Entwicklern eine kollaborative, cloudbasierte Umgebung mit vorkonfigurierten Werkzeugen und Services für die Anwendungsentwicklung zur Verfügung und ermöglicht so schnellere und effizientere Entwicklungszyklen. Durch die Integration von KI-Funktionen werden Entwickler zusätzlich unterstützt und in ihrer Arbeit optimiert. SAP BTP unterstützt auch die Low-Code-Entwicklung, sodass Fachanwender Anwendungen ohne umfangreiche Programmierkenntnisse erstellen können. Ein konkretes Beispiel aus der Praxis wäre ein

Fahrradgeschäft, in dem Mitarbeiter eine auf ihre spezifischen Geschäftsanforderungen zugeschnittene Anwendung mit einfachem Zugriffslink entwickeln können.

Automatisierung

Die Automatisierung innerhalb der SAP BTP ermöglicht es Unternehmen, sich wiederholende Aufgaben zu rationalisieren, die Effizienz zu steigern und manuelle Eingriffe in Geschäftsprozesse zu reduzieren. Ein wichtiges Werkzeug hierfür ist *SAP Build Process Automation* für die Automatisierung von Routineaufgaben wie Dateneingabe oder Rechnungsbearbeitung. Die SAP BTP bietet außerdem Funktionen zur Workflow-Automatisierung, die es Unternehmen ermöglichen, komplexe Geschäftsabläufe einfach zu gestalten, auszuführen und zu überwachen. Durch die Automatisierung alltäglicher Aufgaben und Arbeitsabläufe können Unternehmen Ressourcen freisetzen, Fehler minimieren und sich auf strategisch bedeutsame Aktivitäten konzentrieren, die das Unternehmenswachstum fördern. Nehmen wir noch einmal unser Beispiel zur Hand: Wenn das Fahrradgeschäft neue Teile bestellen möchte, bevor sie zur Neige gehen, könnte es diesen Prozess automatisieren. Sobald das System beispielsweise feststellt, dass bestimmte Teile nicht mehr auf Lager sind, könnte eine Bestellung beim Hersteller ausgelöst werden.

Integration

Integration ist ein wichtiger Aspekt der SAP BTP, der eine nahtlose Kommunikation und den Datenaustausch zwischen verschiedenen Systemen, Anwendungen und Datenquellen ermöglicht. Die SAP BTP bietet die *SAP Integration Suite*, um die Konnektivität zwischen On-Premise- und Cloud-Umgebungen sowie mit externen Partnern und Kunden zu erleichtern. Außerdem gibt es Ressourcen für die API-Verwaltung und vorgefertigte Geschäftsinhalte für sofort einsatzbereite Lösungen. Mit der Integration in der SAP BTP können Unternehmen Datensilos aufbrechen, Geschäftsprozesse rationalisieren und das volle Potenzial ihres digitalen Ökosystems ausschöpfen. Wenn unser Fahrradladen eine Verbindung zum System des Herstellers herstellen muss, kann er entweder im SAP Business Accelerator Hub nach vorhandenen APIs suchen oder mit SAP Integration Suite APIs erstellen.

Daten und Analytik

Die Daten- und Analysefunktionen der SAP BTP versetzen Unternehmen in die Lage, Erkenntnisse aus ihren Daten zu gewinnen, fundierte Entscheidungen zu treffen und Geschäftsergebnisse zu erzielen. Dazu gehören Services für Data Warehousing, Datenmodellierung und erweiterte Analysen. Die SAP BTP bietet außerdem Datenvisualisierungsfunktionen und Services für maschinelles Lernen, mit denen Unternehmen verborgene Muster, Trends und Chancen in ihren Daten aufdecken können. Durch die Nutzung der Leistungsfähigkeit von Daten und Analysen in SAP BTP können Unternehmen Wettbewerbsvorteile erzielen, ihre Abläufe optimieren und mit Zuversicht Innovationen einführen. Im Hinblick auf unser Beispiel: Das Fahrradgeschäft sammelt die Daten von Lieferanten, Kunden und Verkäufen. Diese Daten können mit SAP-BTP-Datenmanagementprodukten wie SAP Analytics Cloud, SAP Datasphere, SAP HANA Cloud und anderen gespeichert, verwaltet und visualisiert werden.

Künstliche Intelligenz

SAP BTP bietet ein umfassendes Angebot an KI-Technologien und -Services, z. B. *SAP AI Business Services* und *Generative AI Hub*. Damit können Unternehmen die Leistungsfähigkeit künstlicher Intelligenz nutzen, um Innovationen voranzutreiben, die Effizienz zu steigern und ihren Kunden einen Mehrwert zu bieten. Durch die Nutzung dieser KI-Funktionen können Unternehmen der Konkurrenz einen Schritt voraus sein und sich in der heutigen digitalen Wirtschaft erfolgreich behaupten. Nehmen wir ein letztes Mal das Beispiel zur Hand: Die Kunden unseres fiktiven Fahrradladens können KI-gestützte personalisierte Empfehlungen erhalten, um das für sie am besten geeignete Produkt zu finden und von einem verbesserten Kundenerlebnis zu profitieren.

2.1.1 Planung für den Einsatz der SAP BTP

SAP Discovery Center

Die SAP BTP ist die Zielplattform von SAP. Um den Zugang zu Informationen und Vorgehensweisen strukturiert und relativ niederschwellig zu gewährleisten, bietet SAP das *SAP Discovery Center* an. Das SAP Discovery Center finden Sie unter *https://discovery-center.cloud.sap/*. Nach dem Aufruf der Webseite öffnet sich die Startseite, die in Abbildung 2.1 zu sehen ist. Auf der Startseite werden folgende Kategorien angezeigt:

- **Missions**: Unter Missions versteht SAP die Schritt-für-Schritt-Anleitungen für die Implementierung eines konkreten Anwendungsfalls bzw. Szenarios. Ein Beispiel wäre hierfür das Aufsetzen der SAP Business Technology Platform).
- **Reference Architectures**: In diesem Bereich zeigt SAP, wie die von SAP empfohlene Architektur für einen konkreten Anwendungsfall (d. h. eine Mission) aussehen sollte.
- **SAP BTP Services**: Dieser Bereich bietet den Zugriff zu Informationen über die von SAP angebotenen Services auf der SAP BTP.
- **SAP Business AI Features**: Dies ist (Stand: Dezember 2024) ein noch relativ neuer Bereich im SAP Discovery Center. Hier können sich Kunden über Dienste und Anwendungen informieren, die mit künstlicher Intelligenz ausgestattet sind oder diese nutzen.

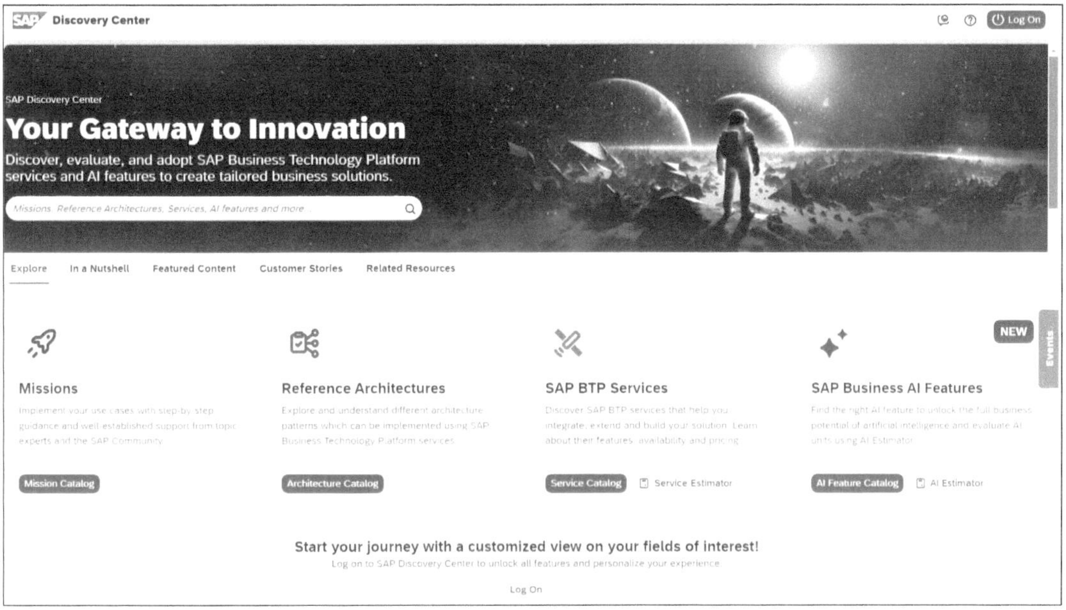

Abbildung 2.1 Startseite des SAP Discovery Centers

Die Anmeldung am SAP Discovery Center erfolgt über Ihren S-User. Nach der Anmeldung erhalten Sie personalisierten Zugriff auf das Center, wie in Abbildung 2.2 gezeigt. Über die Karte **My Started Missions** haben Sie zudem Zugriff auf die von Ihnen begonnen Missionen.

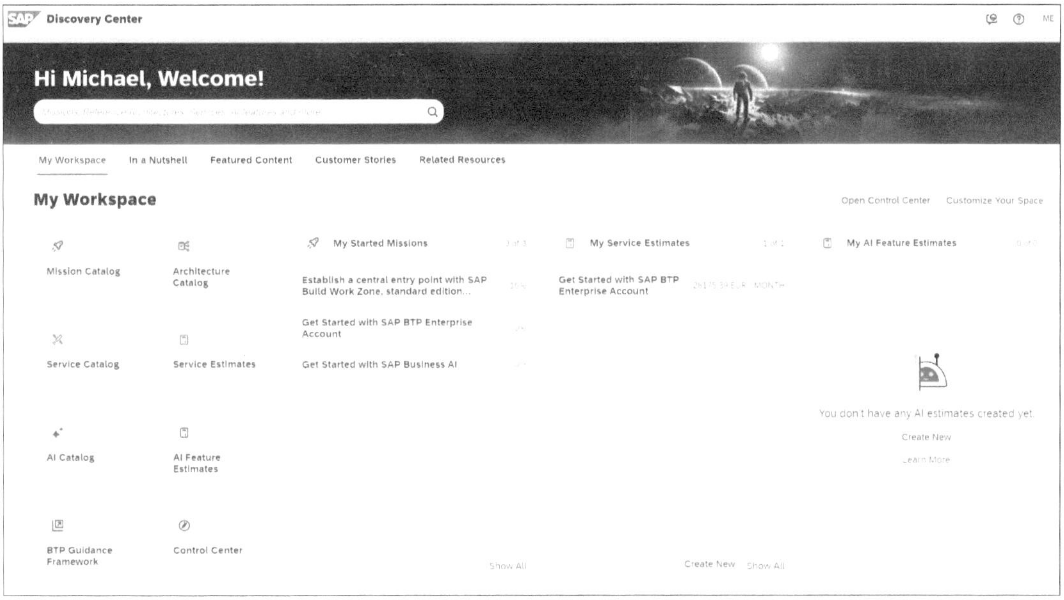

Abbildung 2.2 Persönlicher Arbeitsbereich im SAP Discovery Center

Mission »Get Started with SAP BTP Enterprise Account«

Im Rahmen der Mission gibt SAP in der Overview zunächst eine Übersicht über die Mission und deren Bestandteile. Auf der Registerkarte **Project Board** sehen Sie, welche Aspekte für den Einstieg in die SAP BTP bearbeitet werden müssen, welche empfohlen oder optional sind (siehe Abbildung 2.3). Hinter den einzelnen Kacheln stellt SAP weiterführende Informationen bereit, darunter Videos und Anleitungen, die beim Einrichten der SAP BTP helfen. Wie in der Abbildung zu sehen, sind auch optionale Themen im Projektplan enthalten. Abhängig von den Zielen kann es notwendig sein, sich beispielsweise mit der ABAP-Umgebung in der SAP BTP auseinanderzusetzen, insbesondere wenn ein Clean-Core-Ansatz Teil Ihrer SAP-Strategie ist.

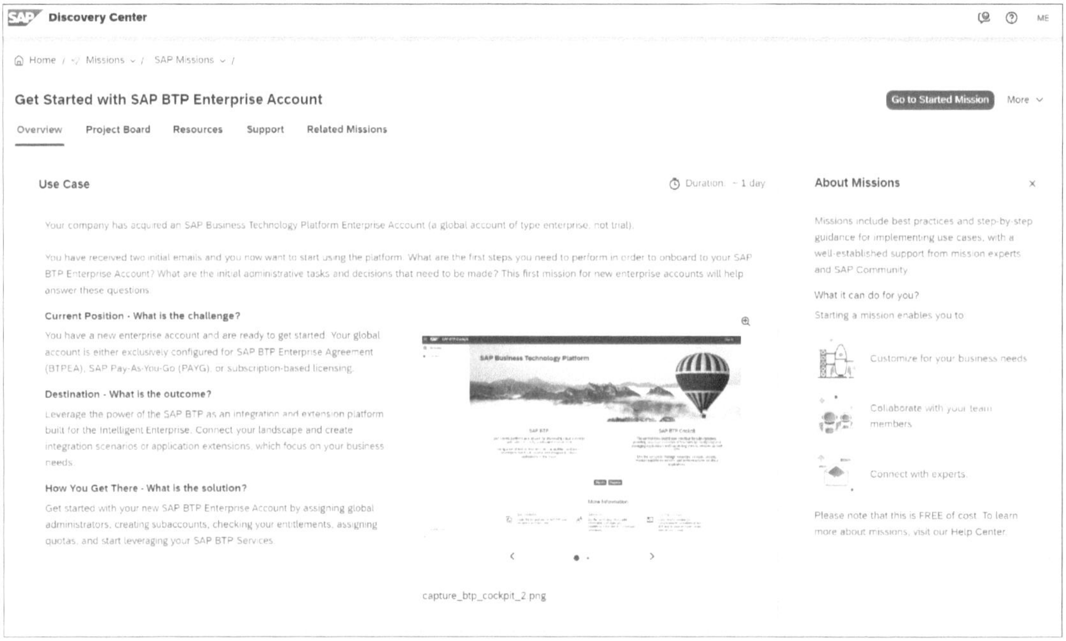

Abbildung 2.3 Übersicht über die Mission »Get Started with SAP BTP Enterprise Account«

Project Board

SAP bietet im SAP Discovery Center für die Mission **Get Started with SAP BTP Enterprise Account** weiterführende Informationen an. Abbildung 2.4 zeigt das Project Board für diese Mission.

Im Bereich **Resources** stehen je nach Mission weiterführende Dokumente zur Verfügung. Besonders wichtig ist der Bereich **Support**, in dem Sie nach dem Start der Mission einen direkten Kommunikationskanal zu den Experten von SAP erhalten. Über eine Chat-Funktion können Sie hier direkt Fragen stellen. Zusätzlich bietet die Support-Seite häufig gestellte Fragen (FAQs) zu den am meisten auftretenden Problemen.

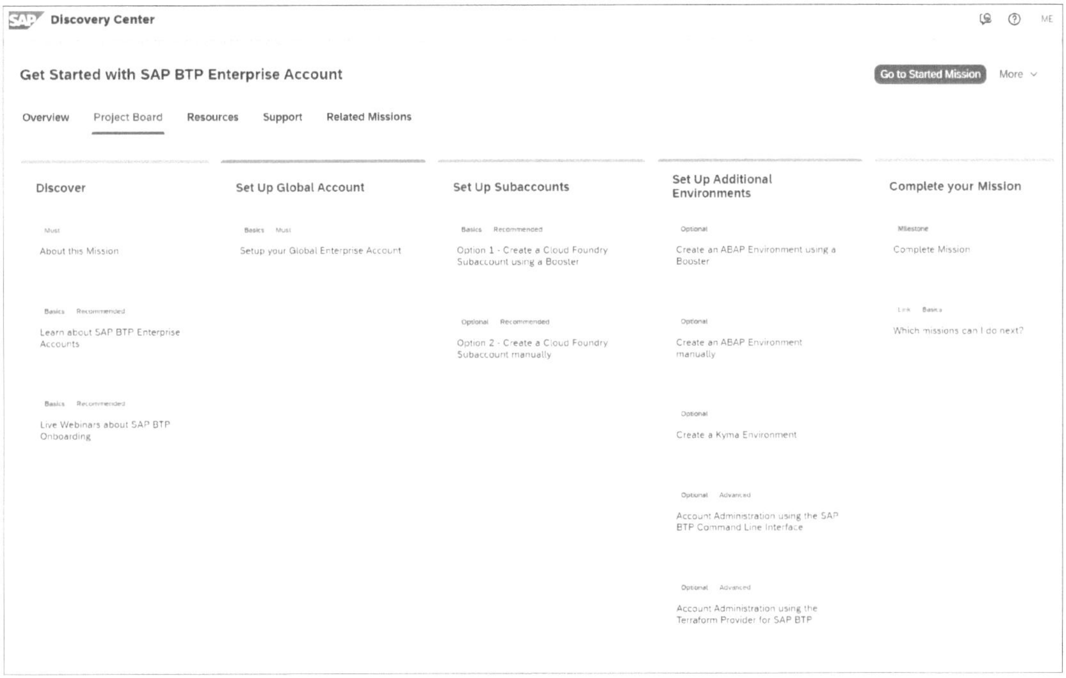

Abbildung 2.4 Project Board der Mission »Get Started with SAP BTP Enterprise Account«

Weiterführende Missionen

Nach dem Motto »Nach der Mission ist vor der Mission« finden Sie im Bereich **Related Missions** weitere Missionen, die nach Abschluss der aktuellen Mission für Sie von Interesse sein könnten. Im Falle der hier betrachteten Mission könnten dies z. B. folgende Missionen sein:

- Get Started on SAP BTP with SAPUI5/Fiori - Create a Hello World App
- Get Started with Integration Suite
- Get Started with SAP BTP, ABAP environment

Beachten Sie, dass die verschiedenen Missionen im SAP Discovery Center sowie das Einrichten und Aktivieren von Diensten in der SAP BTP in der Regel mit Kosten verbunden sind.

2.1.2 SAP-BTP-Bezahlmodell

Drei Bezahlmodelle

Wenn Sie als Unternehmen planen, die SAP BTP zu nutzen, müssen Sie die richtige Lizenzierung für Ihre Bedürfnisse wählen. Um einen Vertrag abzuschließen, nutzen Sie den SAP Store oder wenden sich an Ihren SAP-Vertriebsmitarbeiter. SAP bietet drei kommerzielle Modelle an:

- Pay-As-You-Go (PAYG)
- SAP BTP Enterprise Agreement (SAP BTPEA)
- Verbrauchsbasiertes Modell und Cloud Credits

Diese Modelle repräsentieren ein zunehmendes Engagement für die SAP-BTP-Services, von einem begrenzten Engagement bei PAYG bis zu einem hohen Engagement bei Subscription.

Pay-As-You-Go

Das PAYG-Modell ermöglicht es Ihnen, Cloud-Services in Ihrer Produktionsumgebung zu nutzen – ohne Vorabkosten, ohne Mindestnutzungsanforderungen und ohne finanzielle Verpflichtungen. Mit Pay-As-You-Go für die SAP BTP können Sie klein anfangen und ohne Einschränkungen wachsen. Sie können dieses kommerzielle Modell ganz einfach über den SAP Store nutzen. Pay-As-You-Go for SAP BTP ermöglicht es Ihnen, Anwendungen in Ihrer Produktionsumgebung zu erstellen und nur für das zu bezahlen, was Sie nutzen.

SAP BTP Enterprise Agreement

Wenn Ihnen das PAYG-Modell nicht mehr ausreicht, können Sie zum *SAP BTP Enterprise Agreement* wechseln, sobald Sie eine vorhersehbare Nutzung erreicht haben. Damit können Sie schnell und zuverlässig auf sich ändernde Geschäftsanforderungen reagieren, indem Sie produktive Anwendungen bereitstellen und diese schnell skalieren. Da es keine Mindestnutzungsanforderungen gibt, können Sie eine übermäßige Bereitstellung vermeiden.

Verbrauchsbasiertes Modell und Cloud Credits

Beim *verbrauchsbasierten Bezahlmodell* inklusive der Cloud Credits zahlen Kunden nur für die tatsächlich Nutzung der SAP-BTP-Dienste. Bei den *Cloud Credits* handelt es sich um eine Art Währung. Kunden erwerben eine bestimmte Menge an Cloud Credits und können diese flexibel für die Nutzung der SAP-BTP-Dienste nutzen.

Zugang zu kostenlosen Tier-Serviceplänen, um Services ohne Kosten in Ihrer produktiven Umgebung zu testen, bietet die *Free-Tier-Option* an.

Kosten im Blick

Im SAP Discovery Center erhalten Sie direkt beim jeweiligen SAP-BTP-Service auch Informationen über die Kosten bei der Nutzung des Service. Nachdem Sie einen Service ausgewählt haben, können Sie sich im Bereich **Pricing** einen Überblick über die anfallenden Kosten verschaffen. Über die Auswahlliste **Commercial Model** können Sie zwischen den Bezahlmodellen wechseln und erhalten dann Preisinformationen für das Modell. In Abbildung 2.5 sehen Sie beispielhaft die Preisindikation für den SAP-BTP-Service *SAP Integration Suite, advanced event mesh*. Wie in der Abbildung zu sehen ist, werden die Preise für das Bezahlmodell SAP BTPEA gelistet.

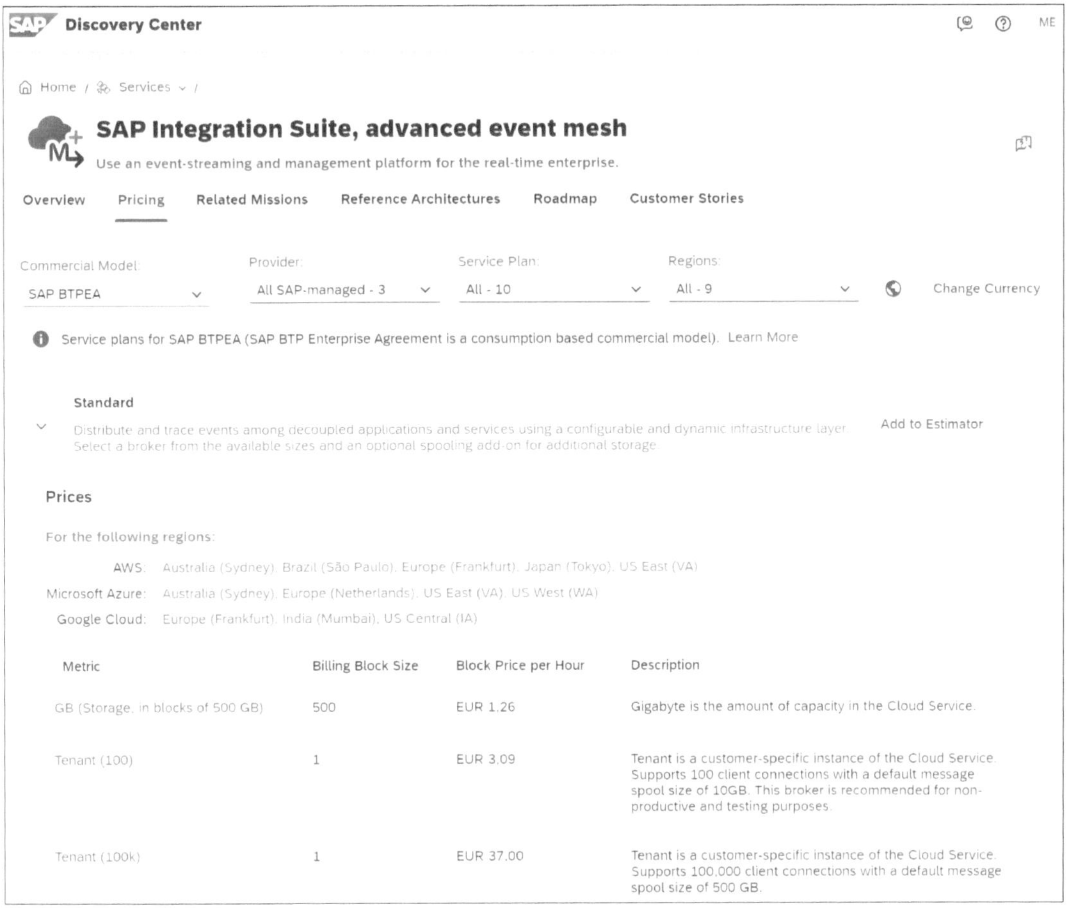

Abbildung 2.5 Beispiel für ein Preismodell der SAP Integration Suite

Schätzen der Kosten

In den Regel werden nicht nur einzelne Services aus der SAP BTP für ein Cloud-Szenario benötigt. Oft benötigen Unternehmen mehr als einen Service aus der SAP BTP, um Unternehmensprozesse abzubilden. Um einen Überblick über die möglichen Gesamtkosten zu erhalten, enthält das SAP Discovery Center ein Werkzeug zur Berechnung bzw. Schätzung der zu erwartenden Kosten: die Karte **My Service Estimates** im persönlichen Arbeitsbereich. Über den Button **Create New** können Nutzer eine neue Kostenschätzung erstellen. Nach dem Klick auf die Schaltfläche gelangt man in die initiale Maske zur Erstellung einer neuen Kalkulation. Über den Button **Add Service** können SAP-BTP-Dienste aus einer Liste ausgewählt und der Berechnung hinzugefügt werden. Abbildung 2.6 zeigt eine beispielhafte Berechnung für die Nutzung von SAP Build Work Zone inklusive SAP Business Application Studio zur Entwicklung von SAP-Fiori-Anwendungen und dem SAP Cloud Identity Service zur Benutzer- und Gruppenverwaltung. Wie Sie der Abbildung entnehmen können, ist es möglich, dass der Kunde noch Konfigurationseinstellungen bei einem konkreten Service durchführen kann. Beispielsweise in welcher Region, also in welchem Rechenzentrum, der Service gehostet werden soll und wie viele Mandaten benötigt werden.

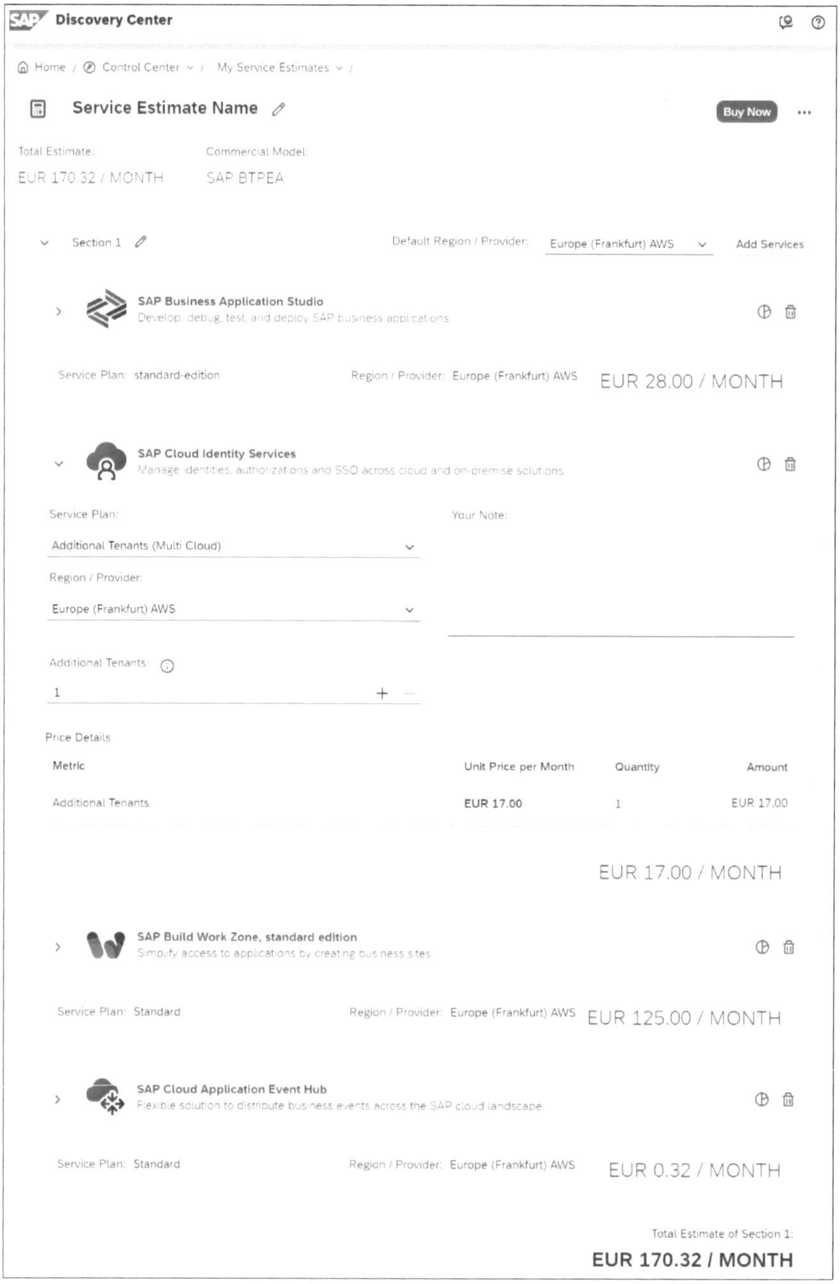

Abbildung 2.6 Kostenschätzung

2.2 Aufbau der Infrastruktur

Nachdem wir im vorangegangenen Abschnitt eine kurze Einführung in die Positionierung der SAP Business Technology Platform und dem SAP Discovery Center gegeben haben, wendet sich dieser Abschnitt nun der Arbeit mit der SAP BTP zu.

2.2.1 Account-Konzept der SAP BTP

Für die Nutzung der SAP BTP benötigen Sie einen Zugang von SAP. Dieser erfolgt durch die Einrichtung eines sogenannten *Global Accounts* in der SAP BTP. Der globale Account stellt sicher, dass der Zugang zur SAP BTP auf einer vertraglichen Basis zwischen SAP und dem Kunden erfolgt. Global Accounts sind unabhängig von Regionen und Umgebungen. Es kann jedoch auch Fälle geben, in denen sichergestellt werden muss, dass die Datenverarbeitung in einer bestimmten Region stattfindet. Wenn Kunden beispielsweise aufgrund von DSGVO-Vorgaben die Anforderung haben, ihre Daten ausschließlich in Europa zu verarbeiten, ist dies ebenfalls möglich.

Subaccounts

Innerhalb eines Global Accounts können Kunden sogenannte *Subaccounts* erstellen, die zur Strukturierung und Organisation der Cloud-Landschaft dienen. Dabei gibt es keine Begrenzung hinsichtlich der Anzahl der Subaccounts, die in einem Global Account angelegt werden können. Anzahl und Struktur der Subaccounts können je nach Unternehmensorganisation und individuellen Anforderungen variieren. Subaccounts werden immer in einer bestimmten Region angelegt. Eine Region bezeichnet ein geografisches Gebiet, in dem sich das Rechenzentrum mit der entsprechenden Cloud-Infrastruktur befindet. Diese Infrastruktur wird entweder direkt von SAP oder von einem Infrastructure-as-a-Service-Partner (IaaS) wie Amazon Web Services (AWS), Microsoft Azure, Google Cloud oder Alibaba Cloud bereitgestellt. Während die Infrastruktur von den jeweiligen Partnern betrieben wird, ist SAP für die Plattformebene und die Verwaltung von Cloud Foundry zuständig. Abbildung 2.7 veranschaulicht ein Beispiel eines Global Accounts mit drei Subaccounts. Kunden sind dabei nicht an eine bestimmte Region gebunden, sondern können je nach Anforderungen eine passende Region auswählen. In der Abbildung sind alle drei Subaccounts im Rechenzentrum in Frankfurt gehostet. Die drei Subaccounts sind Multi-Cloud-Umgebungen, die von AWS gehostet werden.

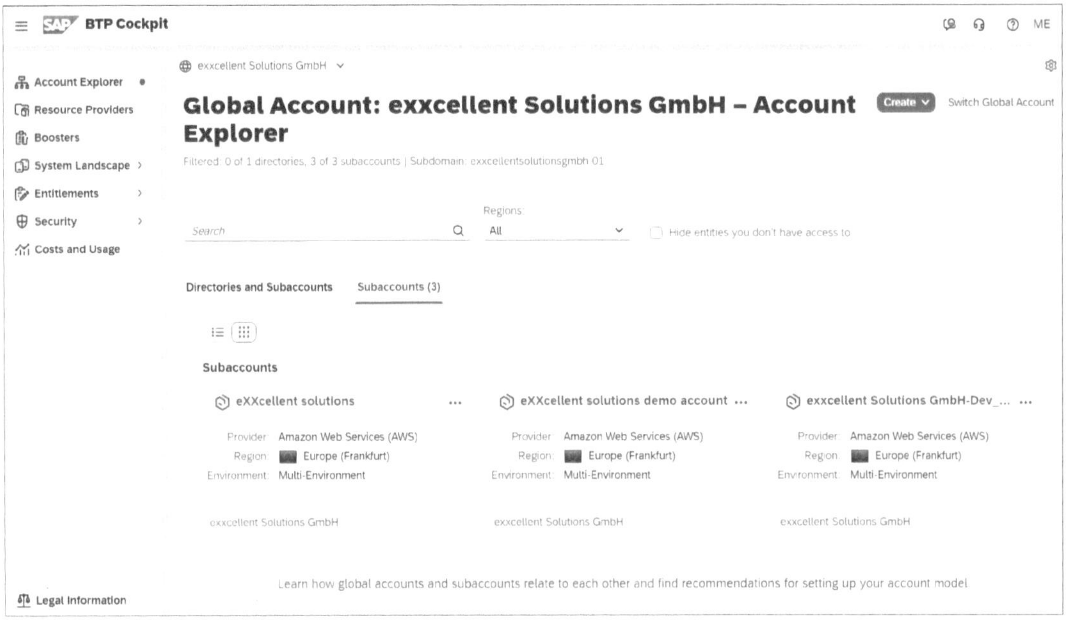

Abbildung 2.7 Account-Übersicht in der SAP BTP

Subaccounts agieren unabhängig von dem Global Account, in dem sie erstellt wurden. Sie ermöglichen die Nutzung aktivierter Cloud-Dienste sowie die Bereitstellung von Anwendungen. Um einen neuen Subaccount innerhalb eines Global Accounts zu erstellen, klicken Sie oben rechts auf das Drop-down-Menü **Create**. In der Auswahlliste können Sie auswählen, ob Sie einen initialen Subaccount, einen Subaccount auf Basis eines bestehenden oder aber ein Verzeichnis anlegen möchte. Wenn Sie den Eintrag **Subaccount** auswählen, öffnet sich ein Dialogfeld zur Eingabe der Subaccount-Details. Abbildung 2.8 zeigt ein Beispiel mit ausgefüllten Feldern.

Geben Sie im Feld **Display Name** den Namen des Subaccounts ein und wählen Sie anschließend aus der Drop-down-Liste die gewünschte Region samt Plattformanbieter aus. Sollten Sie einen Subaccount für produktive Zwecke anlegen, können Sie im Bereich **Advanced** die Option **Used for production** aktivieren. Diese Einstellung verändert zwar nicht die Funktionalität des Subaccounts, erleichtert jedoch die Verwaltung, indem produktive Subaccounts entsprechend markiert werden können. Die SAP BTP wird kontinuierlich weiterentwickelt. Als Teil dieses Prozesses stellt SAP Testversionen von noch nicht freigegebenen Funktionen zur Verfügung. Wenn Sie diese sogenannten Beta-Features im Subaccount testen möchten, können Sie im Bereich **Advanced** die Option **Enable beta features** aktivieren. In Fällen, in denen eine große Anzahl von Subaccounts in einem Global Account vorhanden ist, kann es schwierig sein, den benötigten Subaccount zu finden. Um die Übersicht zu verbessern oder Subaccounts zu gruppieren, lassen sich sogenannte *Labels* hinzufügen. Ein Label besteht aus einem Schlüssel und einem oder mehreren Werten. Diese Merkmale können im Label-Bereich des Dialogs festgelegt werden.

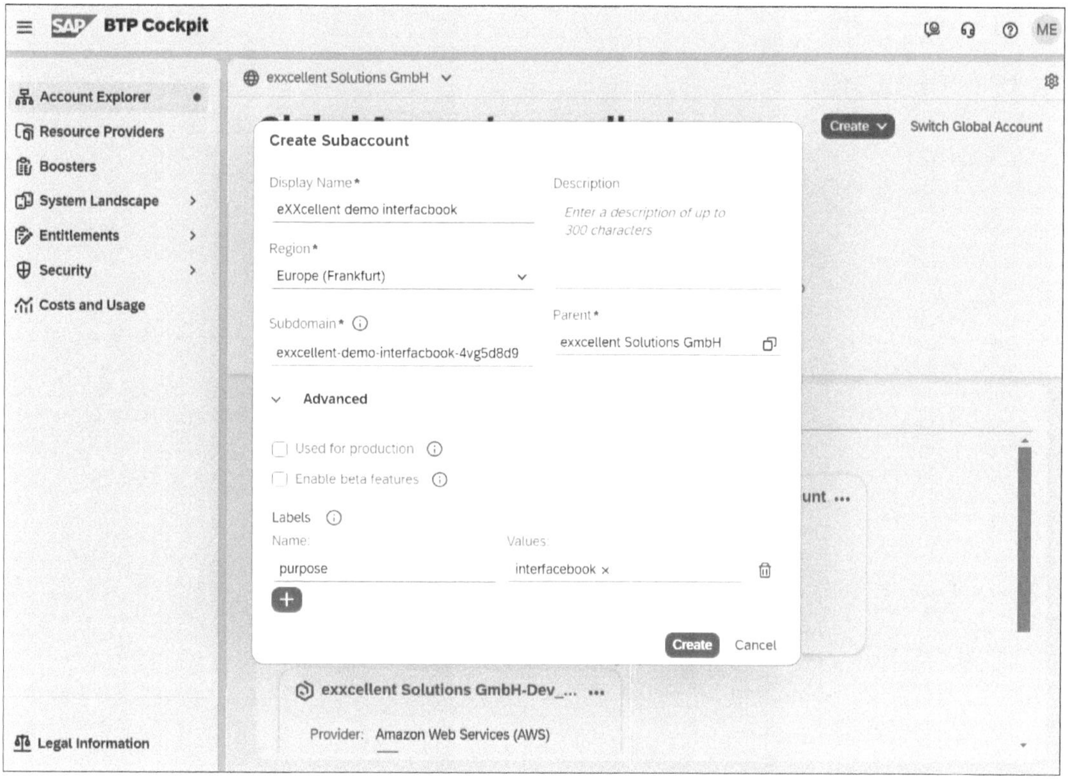

Abbildung 2.8 Anlegen eines neuen Subaccounts

Nach der Erstellung eines Subaccounts werden diese automatisch bestimmten Dienste zugewiesen. Die Berechtigung zur Nutzung dieser Dienste wird als *Entitlement* bezeichnet. In Abbildung 2.9 ist ein neu erstellter Subaccount dargestellt. Wie der Abbildung zu entnehmen ist, werden in der Subaccount-Übersicht im Abschnitt **Entitlements** verschiedene Dienste aufgelistet.

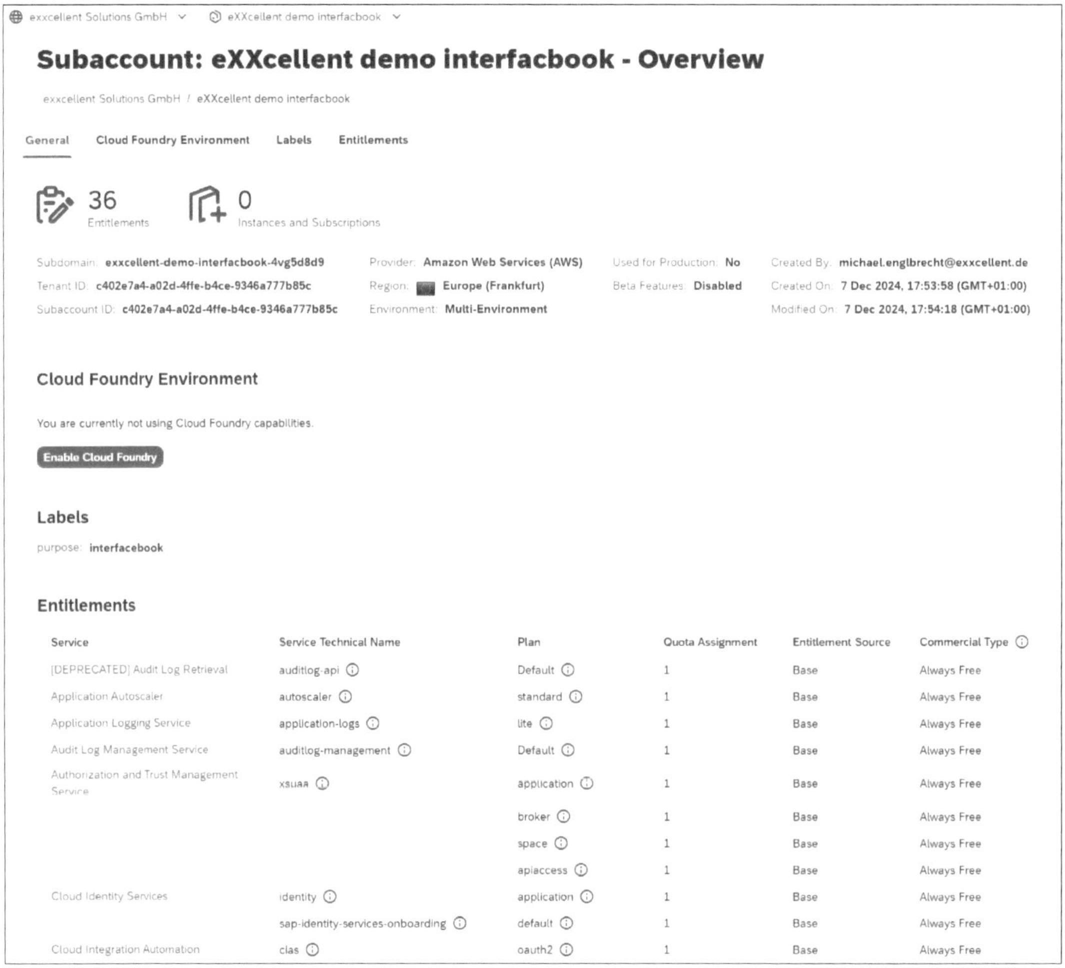

Abbildung 2.9 Neu angelegter Subaccount

2.2.2 Verzeichnisse

SAP entwickelt die SAP BTP und die zugehörigen Cloud-Management-Tools kontinuierlich weiter. Im Zuge dieser Verbesserungen werden die Accounts schrittweise auf die neuen Tools umgestellt. Dabei unterscheidet SAP zwischen zwei Versionen der Cloud-Management-Werkzeuge: *Feature Set A*, das die erste Version repräsentiert, und *Feature Set B*, das die neuen Management-Werkzeuge umfasst. Um herauszufinden, welches Feature Set in Ihrem Global Account aktiv ist, navigieren Sie im Menü zu **About**. Daraufhin öffnet sich ein Dialog, wie in Abbildung 2.10 dargestellt. In diesem Beispiel zeigt der Dialog, dass der Global Account auf Feature Set B basiert. Weitere Details zur Thematik der Feature Sets finden Sie in SAP-Hinweis 3027721.

Mit Verzeichnissen arbeiten

Große Unternehmen können eine Vielzahl von Subaccounts haben, was die Übersicht und Verwaltung erschweren kann. Um eine klarere Struktur zu schaffen, gibt es die Möglichkeit, *Verzeichnisse* (Directories) zu verwenden. Diese Funktion steht jedoch nur in Global Accounts mit aktiviertem Feature Set B zur Verfügung. Um zu überprüfen, welches Features Set man in seinem Global Account verwendet, rufen Sie über das Benutzermenü in der rechten oberen Ecke mit Ihren Initialen den Menüpunkt **About** auf. Abbildung 2.10 zeigt, dass in diesem Global Account das Feature Set B verwendet wird. Weitere Informationen zu den Feature Sets erhalten Sie über den Link, der im About-Dialog angezeigt wird.

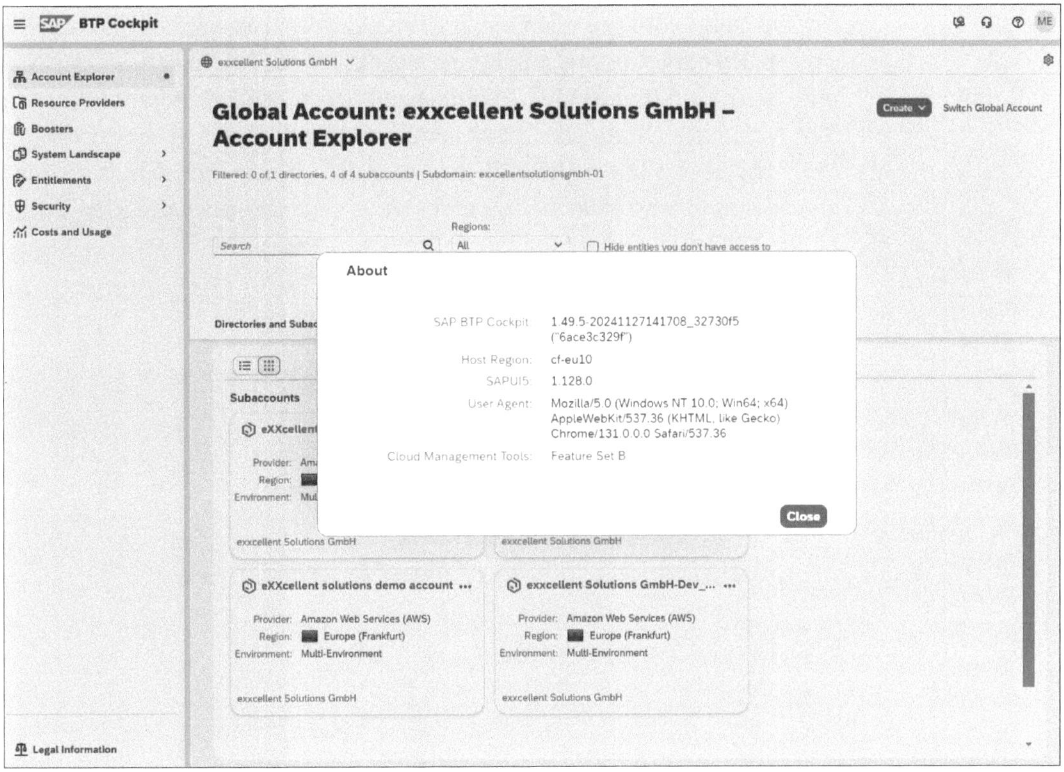

Abbildung 2.10 Informationen zum Feature Set

Um die Verzeichnisansicht aufzurufen, wechseln Sie einfach zur Registerkarte **Directories and Subaccounts** (siehe Abbildung 2.11).

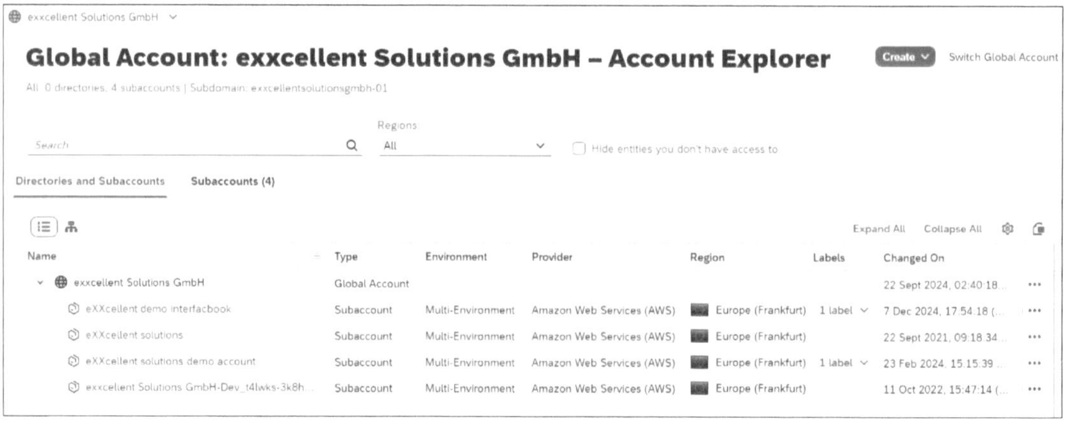

Abbildung 2.11 Directory-Übersicht im Global Account

Um ein Verzeichnis zu erstellen, wählen Sie in der Auswahlliste **Create** die Option **Directory** aus. Anschließend erscheint ein Dialog, in dem Sie den Namen des neuen Verzeichnisses eingeben können. Im Feld **Parent** legen Sie fest, auf welcher Ebene das Verzeichnis erstellt werden soll. Sie haben die Möglichkeit, das Verzeichnis direkt unter dem Wurzelverzeichnis anzulegen oder es in ein bereits bestehendes Unterverzeichnis zu integrieren. Abbildung 2.12 zeigt den Dialog mit ausgefüllten Feldern.

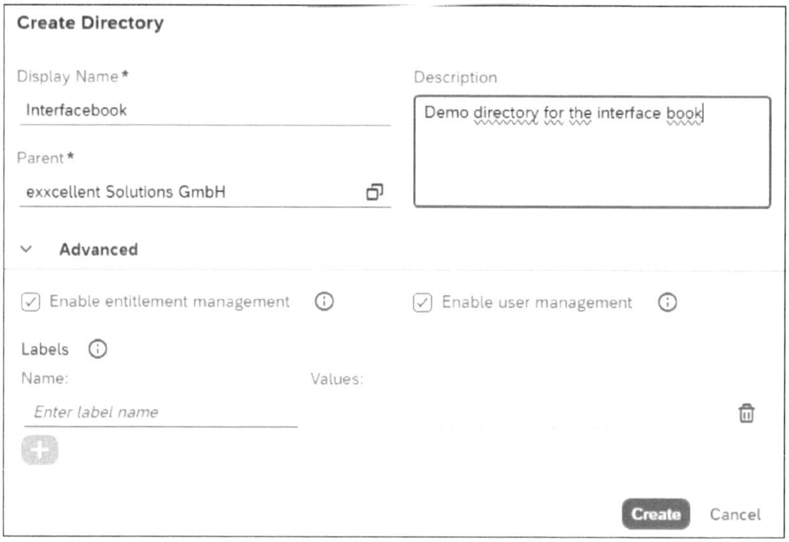

Abbildung 2.12 Erstellung eines neuen Verzeichnisses

Wie in der Abbildung zu sehen ist, gibt es im Bereich **Advanced** zusätzlich die Möglichkeit, zu wählen, ob die Nutzerverwaltung auf Verzeichnisebene erfolgen soll. Über die Option **Enable entitlement management** können Sie festlegen, ob bereits auf der Verzeichnisebene voreingestellt werden soll, welche Berechtigungen in den darunterliegenden Subaccounts vergeben werden. Ebenso wie bei Subaccounts können auch für Verzeichnisse **Labels** eingerichtet werden, um eine bessere Organisation zu ermöglichen. Nachdem Sie den Dialog mit dem Button **Create** bestätigt haben, wird das neue Verzeichnis erstellt. Wie in Abbildung 2.13 zu sehen ist, erscheint in der Spalte **Type** für das neu angelegte Verzeichnis der Eintrag **Directory** mit dem Zusatz (**Managed**) in Klammern.

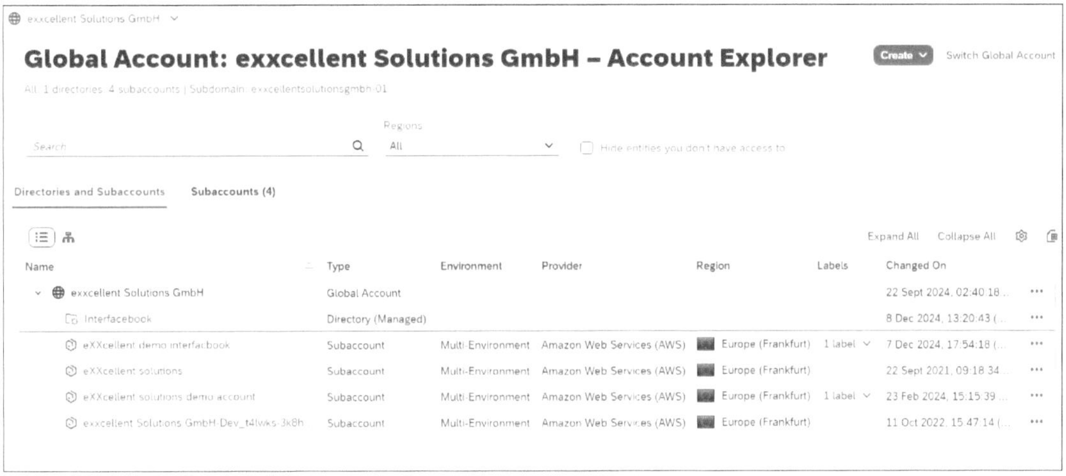

Abbildung 2.13 Verwaltetes Verzeichnis in einem Global Account

Verwalten von Verzeichnissen

Verzeichnisse können optional mit Funktionen zur Berechtigungs- und Benutzerverwaltung ausgestattet werden. Wie in Abbildung 2.14 dargestellt, enthält ein verwaltetes Verzeichnis die Menüpunkte **Users** und **Entitlements**. Im Bereich **Users** lässt sich festlegen, welche Benutzer, wie z. B. die Role Collection *Directory Administrator*, die Berechtigung zur Verwaltung des Verzeichnisses erhalten. Wenn man den Menüeintrag **Entitlements** erweitert, öffnet sich der Zugang zu den beiden weiteren Menüpunkten **Entity Assignment** und **Service Assignment**.

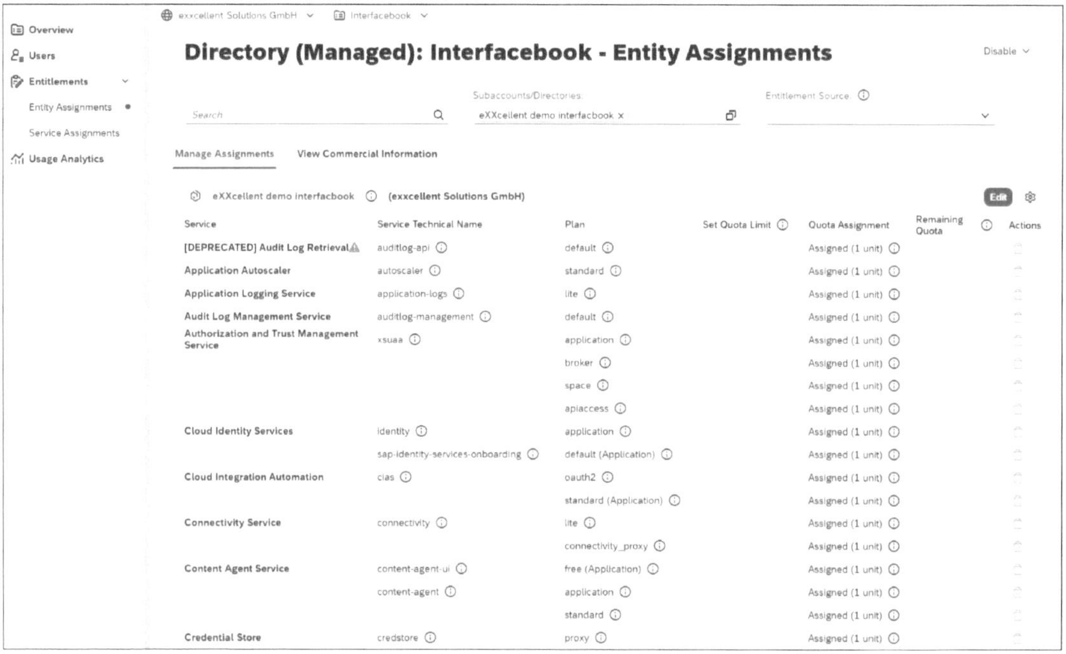

Abbildung 2.14 Entitlement-Verwaltung in einem Verzeichnis

2.2.3 Einführung in den Cloud Connector

Cloud Connector

Damit die Dienste aus der SAP BTP auf Systeme der On-Premise-Landschaft zugreifen können, müssen diese für die SAP BTP erreichbar sein. Dies kann entweder durch direkte Erreichbarkeit des Systems über das Internet erfolgen, was jedoch in den meisten Fällen nicht bevorzugt wird, oder durch einen Mittler zwischen der SAP BTP und den On-Premise-Systemen. Dieser Mittler ist der *Cloud Connector*. Der Cloud Connector fungiert als Bindeglied zwischen der SAP-BTP-Landschaft und den On-Premise-Systemen. Die Verbindung ist bidirektional, sodass sowohl die SAP BTP mit den On-Premise-Systemen als auch umgekehrt eine Kommunikation zwischen den On-Premise-Systemen und der SAP BTP ermöglicht wird. Auch wenn dieses Kapitel hauptsächlich die Kommunikation von der SAP BTP zu den On-Premise-Systemen behandelt, sollte beachtet werden, dass die Kommunikation auch in umgekehrter Richtung – von On-Premise zu Cloud-Diensten – initiiert werden kann. Der Cloud Connector wird in der On-Premise-Landschaft installiert. Für jeden Subaccount in der SAP BTP, der mit der On-Premise-Landschaft verbunden werden soll, werden im Connector die entsprechenden Subaccount-Konfigurationen erstellt. In dieser Konfiguration werden die für den Subaccount benötigten Backend-Systeme definiert.

Der zentrale Punkt für die Kommunikation aus Sicht der SAP BTP ist der *SAP Destination Service*. Über die Administrationsoberfläche dieses Diensts werden Verbindungen zu externen Systemen oder Diensten eingerichtet und konfiguriert. Jede Verbindung erhält einen eindeutigen Namen, über den sie dann aus der SAP BTP heraus angesprochen werden kann. Anwendungen und SAP-BTP-Dienste können mithilfe einer API, der sogenannten Destination API, auf die konfigurierten Destinationen zugreifen.

Zugriff auf Destinationen

Aufgrund der zentralen Bedeutung des Cloud Connectors für die Systemlandschaft ist seine hohe Verfügbarkeit unerlässlich. Ein Ausfall oder eine Fehlfunktion des Cloud Connectors könnte im schlimmsten Fall das gesamte Unternehmen stark beeinträchtigen. Aus diesem Grund hat SAP die Möglichkeit geschaffen, den Cloud Connector im Master- und Shadow-Betrieb zu betreiben. Dabei wird eine Hauptinstanz des Cloud Connectors (Master) installiert, während weitere Instanzen als sogenannte Shadow-Instanzen fungieren. Diese Shadow-Instanzen überwachen die Hauptinstanz und übernehmen deren Funktion im Falle eines Ausfalls.

Hochverfügbarkeit

Installation

Bevor der Cloud Connector installiert werden kann, ist es wichtig, sicherzustellen, dass alle erforderlichen Voraussetzungen erfüllt sind. Dazu gehören die Hardwareanforderungen, das Betriebssystem sowie infrastrukturelle Bedingungen. Weitere Informationen dazu finden Sie im SAP Help Portal unter *http://s-prs.de/v1032901*.

Der Cloud Connector kann über die Webseite *https://tools.hana.ondemand.com/#cloud* heruntergeladen werden. Um zum Downloadbereich zu gelangen, klicken Sie nach dem Aufrufen der Seite auf den Menüpunkt **CLOUD**. Wie in Abbildung 2.15 zu sehen ist, wird der Cloud Connector für die Betriebssysteme Linux, Windows und Mac OS in zwei Varianten angeboten: als portable Version und als Installationspaket. Die portable Version kann nach dem Download einfach entpackt und, sofern alle Voraussetzungen erfüllt sind, direkt manuell gestartet werden. Das Installationspaket erfordert eine Installation, bei der der Cloud Connector als Service im Betriebssystem registriert wird. Nach einem Neustart des Systems wird der Service automatisch gestartet. Die portable Version hat jedoch Einschränkungen: Sie verfügt nicht über einen automatisierten Upgrade-Prozess und kann nicht als Service im Betriebssystem ausgeführt werden. Daher empfiehlt SAP diese Version nicht für den Einsatz in produktiven Szenarien.

Download

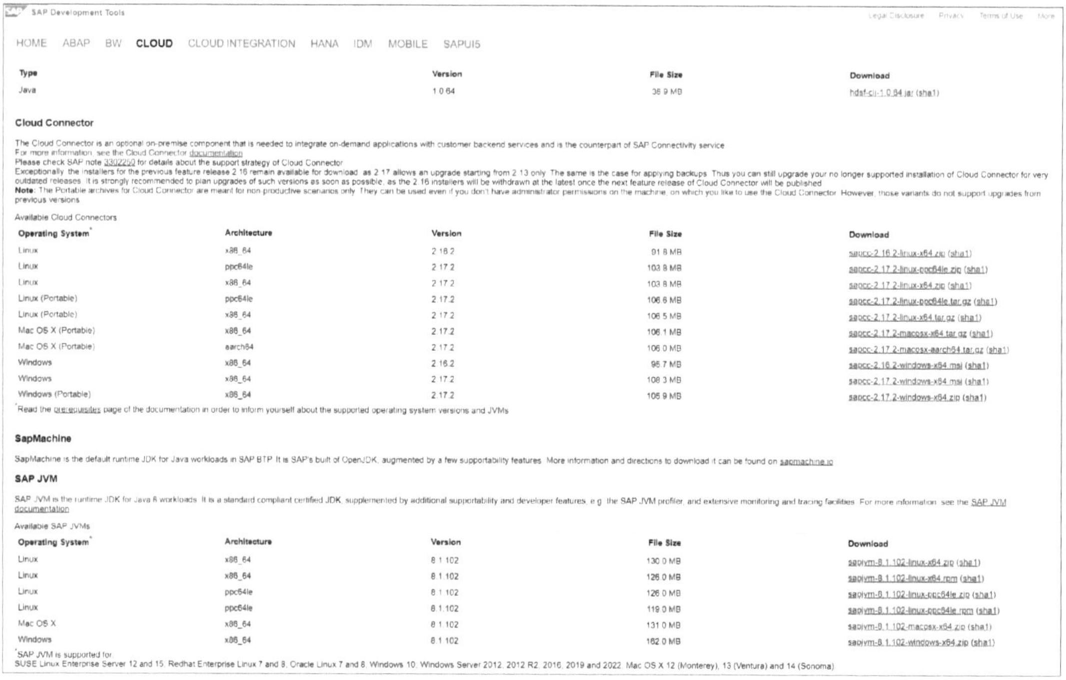

Abbildung 2.15 Downloadseite des Cloud Connectors

Für die Demonstration des Cloud Connectors in diesem Buch ist es für uns ausreichend, die portable Version des Produkts zu verwenden. Nach dem Download und dem Entpacken haben wir die in Abbildung 2.16 gezeigte Verzeichnisstruktur auf der Festplatte.

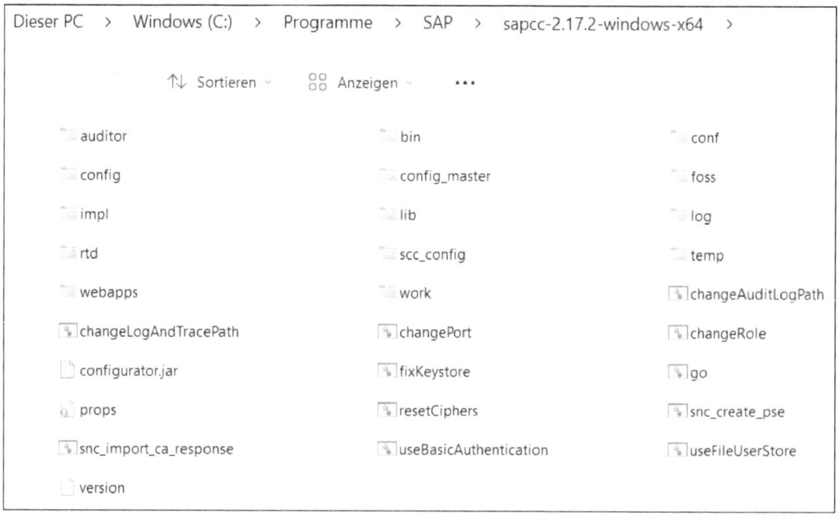

Abbildung 2.16 Verzeichnisstruktur des Cloud Connectors nach dem Entpacken

JVM

2

Der Cloud Connector basiert auf dem Tomcat-Webserver, einem etablierten Produkt, das bereits seit vielen Jahren auf dem Markt ist. Da Tomcat auf Java-Technologie basiert, ist es erforderlich, dass auf dem Zielrechner eine Java Virtual Machine (JVM) installiert ist, um den Cloud Connector zu betreiben. Aktuell werden die 64-Bit-Versionen der folgenden JVMs unterstützt: SAP JVM 1.8, Oracle JDK 8 und SapMachine in Version 17.

Bevor Sie den Cloud Connector verwenden können, stellen Sie sicher, dass eine der genannten Java-Versionen installiert ist. Wie in Abbildung 2.15 gezeigt, stellt SAP die eigene Java VM in Version 1.8 direkt auf der Tools-Seite zum Download bereit. Alternativ können Sie die unterstützte Version der SapMachine unter *https://sap.github.io/SapMachine/* herunterladen und installieren.

Umgebungsvariable »JAVA_HOME«

Nach der Installation der Java VM ist es wichtig, die Umgebungsvariable `JAVA_HOME` korrekt zu setzen. Diese Variable muss den Pfad zum Installationsverzeichnis der Java VM enthalten. Falls die Umgebungsvariable bereits auf dem Zielrechner existiert, aber auf eine nicht unterstützte Version verweist, müssen Sie sicherstellen, dass der Cloud Connector mit dem richtigen Pfad arbeitet. Sie erreichen das am einfachsten, indem Sie im Startprogramm `go.bat` die Variable `JAVA_HOME` entsprechend für die unterstützte Version setzen. Für den Start öffnen Sie ein Eingabeaufforderung und wechseln in das Installationsverzeichnis des Cloud Connectors. Rufen Sie nun das Startprogramm `go.bat` auf.

Cloud Connector starten

Nach dem Aufruf startet der Cloud Connector. Wie Sie Abbildung 2.17 entnehmen können, ist es bei der portablen Version des Cloud Connectors wichtig, dass bei der Verwendung der Anwendung das ausführende Fenster nicht geschlossen wird.

[«]

Port ändern

Der Cloud Connector nutzt standardmäßig den Port 8443. Falls dieser Port bereits auf Ihrem Rechner verwendet wird, können Sie den Port einfach über das Programm **changeport.bat** ändern. Es befindet sich im Installationsverzeichnis des Cloud Connectors. Für die Änderung des Ports rufen Sie das Programm auf und übergeben den von Ihnen gewünschten Port. Beispielsweise für den Port 9000 rufen Sie das Programm wie folgt auf: `changeport 9000`.

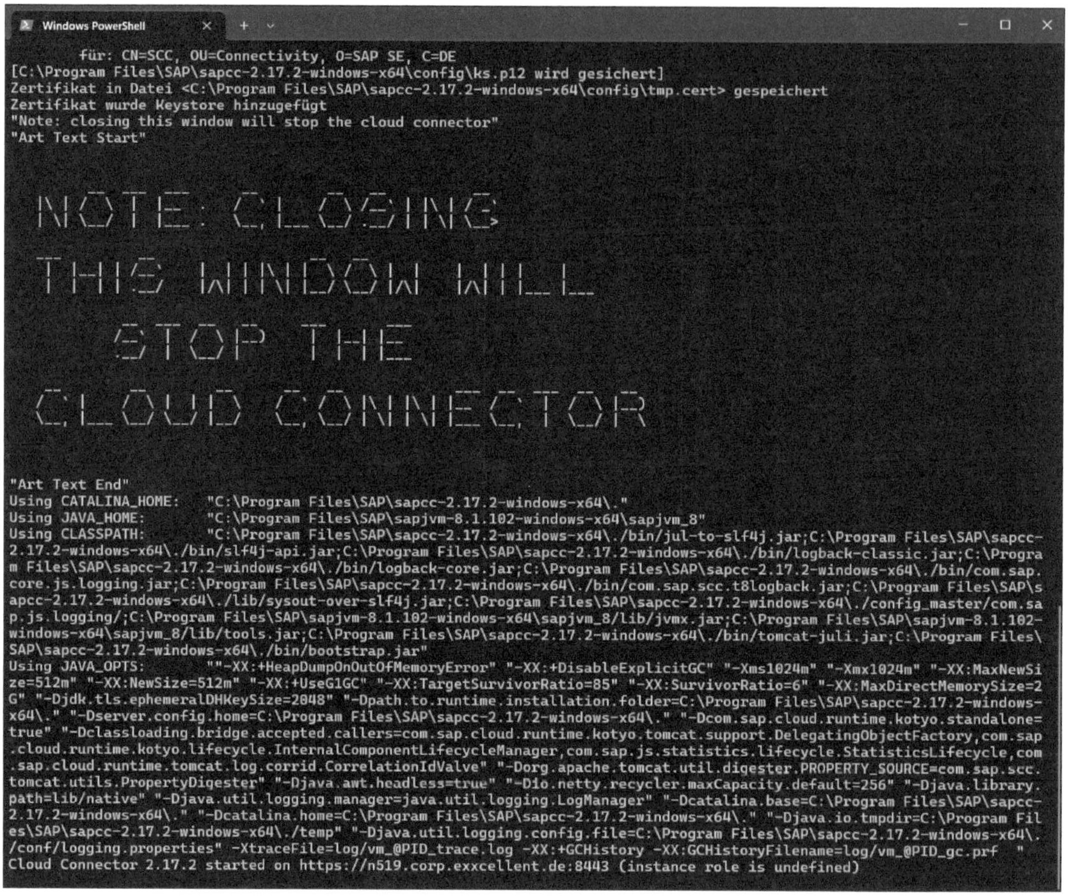

Abbildung 2.17 Startbildschirm des Cloud Connectors

Grundkonfiguration

Nach der Installation können Sie mit der grundlegenden Konfiguration beginnen. Der Cloud Connector wird, wie zuvor erläutert, mit mindestens einem Subaccount des SAP-BTP-Global-Accounts verbunden. Für die Einrichtung dieser Verbindung sind zwei Informationen erforderlich: die Region, in der sich Ihr Subaccount befindet, sowie die sogenannte *Subaccount-ID*. Beide Informationen finden Sie im SAP BTP Cockpit. Im Startbildschirm des SAP BTP Cockpits werden alle verfügbaren Subaccounts angezeigt. Um die benötigten Informationen abzurufen, wählen Sie den gewünschten Subaccount aus und klicken auf das Drei-Punkte-Symbol. Im daraufhin angezeigten Menü wählen Sie den Eintrag **More Info** aus. Wie in Abbildung 2.18 dargestellt, werden Ihnen nun zusätzliche Details angezeigt. Notieren Sie sich den Wert im Feld **Region** und kopieren Sie die Subaccount-ID in die Zwischenablage.

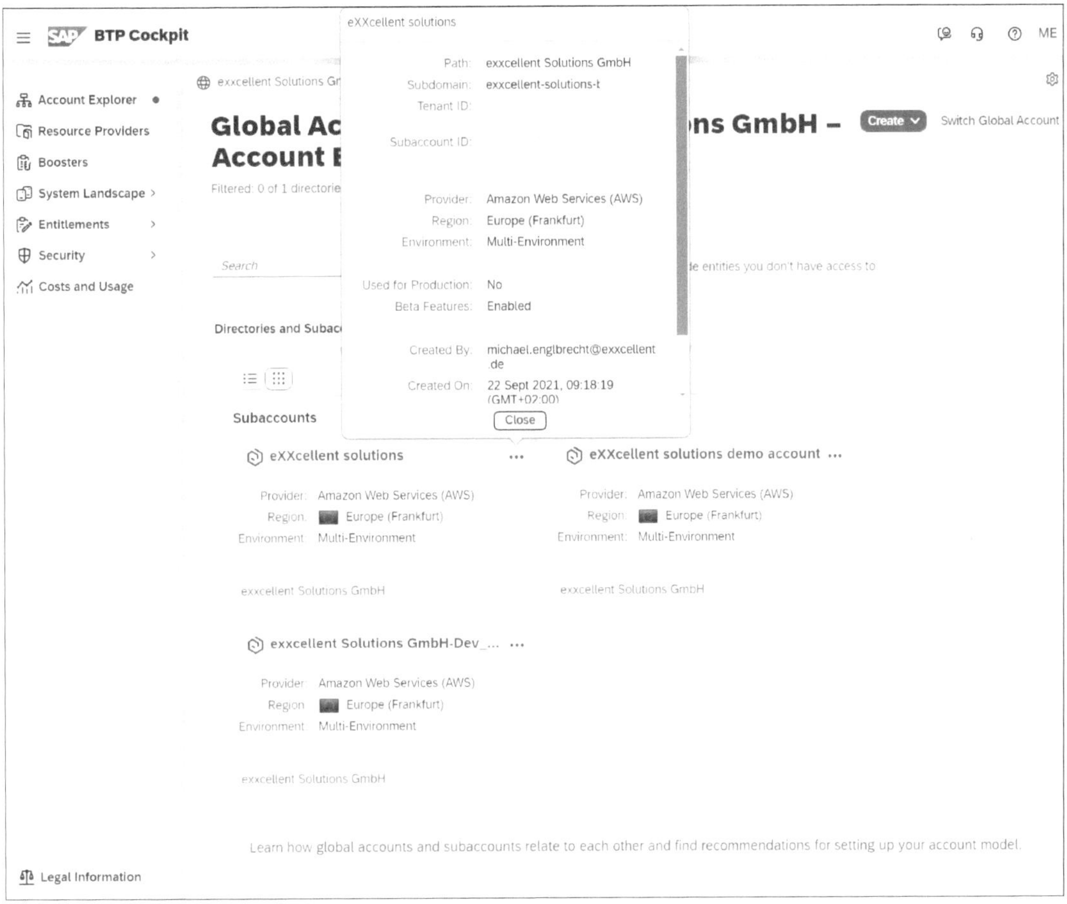

Abbildung 2.18 Anzeige der Subaccount-Details

Administrationsberechtigungen

Damit die Konfiguration erfolgreich durchgeführt werden kann, muss sichergestellt sein, dass der Benutzer, der die Verbindung zwischen dem Cloud Connector und dem Subaccount in der SAP BTP herstellt, über die erforderlichen Berechtigungen verfügt. Benutzer, die eine solche Verbindung einrichten möchten, benötigen die Role Collection **Cloud Connector Administrator**. Um die Berechtigungen zu überprüfen, melden Sie sich zunächst im entsprechenden Subaccount der SAP BTP an. Navigieren Sie anschließend zu **Security • Role Collections**, um die in der SAP BTP verfügbaren Role Collections einzusehen. Es wird Ihnen eine Übersicht angezeigt, die ähnlich wie in Abbildung 2.19 aussieht.

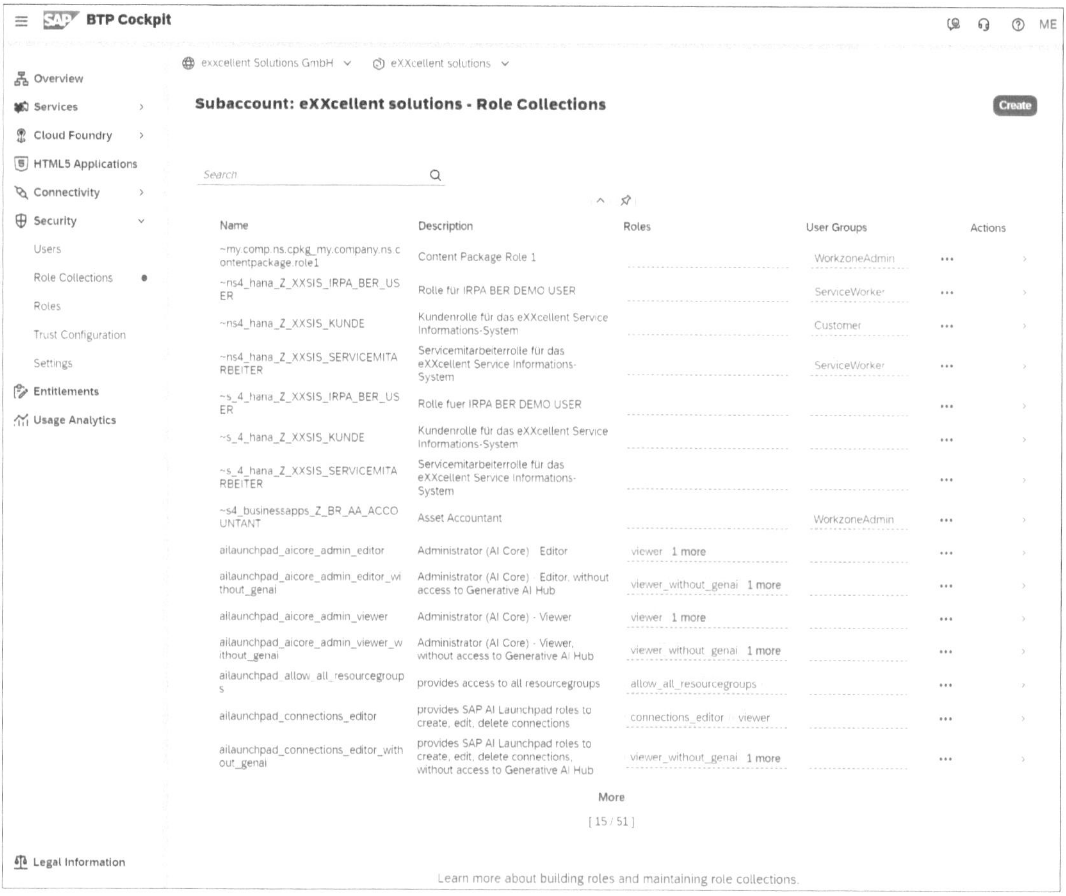

Abbildung 2.19 Vorhandene Role Collections eines Subaccounts

Wählen Sie anschließend die Role Collection **Cloud Connector Administrator** aus. Auf der rechten Seite werden die Details zu dieser Role Collection angezeigt. Überprüfen Sie dort, ob der entsprechende Benutzer in der Liste **Users** aufgeführt ist. Sollte der Benutzer fehlen, klicken Sie auf **Edit**, um die erforderlichen Änderungen vorzunehmen. Tragen Sie die E-Mail-Adresse des Benutzers in die Felder **ID** und **E-Mail** ein. Wählen Sie anschließend den passenden **Identity Provider** für Ihre Umgebung aus. In der in diesem Buch beschriebenen Landschaft verwenden wir den **Default identity provider** von SAP (siehe Abbildung 2.20). Klicken Sie abschließend auf **Save**.

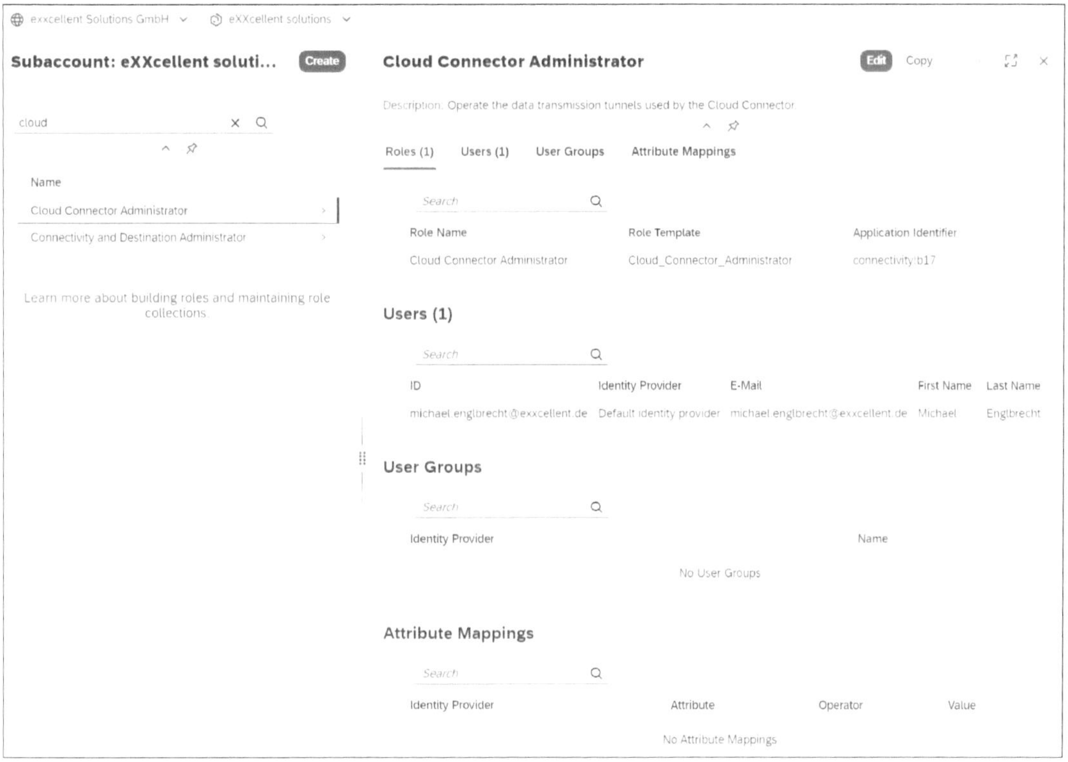

Abbildung 2.20 Konfiguration der Role Collection »Cloud Connector Administrator«

Initiale Passwortänderung

Nachdem alle erforderlichen Informationen für die initiale Konfiguration des Cloud Connectors vorliegen, können wir mit der eigentlichen Konfiguration beginnen. Öffnen Sie dazu ein neues Browserfenster und geben Sie die URL *https://localhost:8443* ein. Es erscheint die in Abbildung 2.21 gezeigte Anmeldemaske.

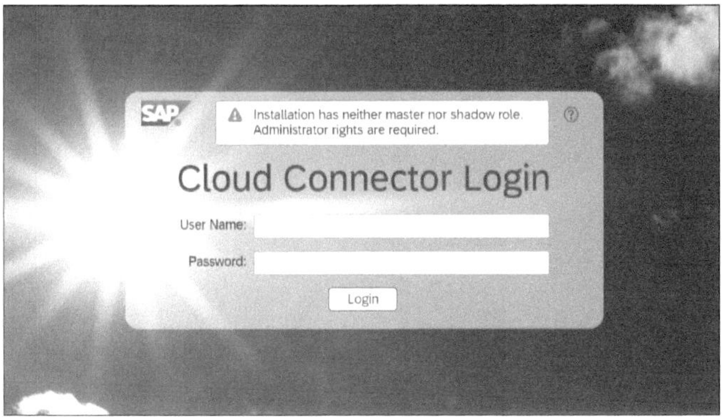

Abbildung 2.21 Anmeldemaske einer neu installierten Cloud-Connector-Instanz

Tragen Sie im Feld **User Name** den Wert »Administrator« und im Feld **Password** das anfängliche Administrator-Passwort »manage« ein. Klicken Sie anschließend auf **Login**. Nach der erfolgreichen Anmeldung müssen Sie im nächsten Schritt das initiale Passwort des Benutzers Administrator ändern. Geben Sie im Feld **Current Password** das ursprüngliche Passwort »manage« ein. Tragen Sie im Feld **New Password** das neue Passwort für den Administrator-Benutzer ein und wiederholen Sie es im Feld **Repeat New Password** (siehe Abbildung 2.22). Bestätigen Sie die Passwortänderung, indem Sie auf **Save** klicken.

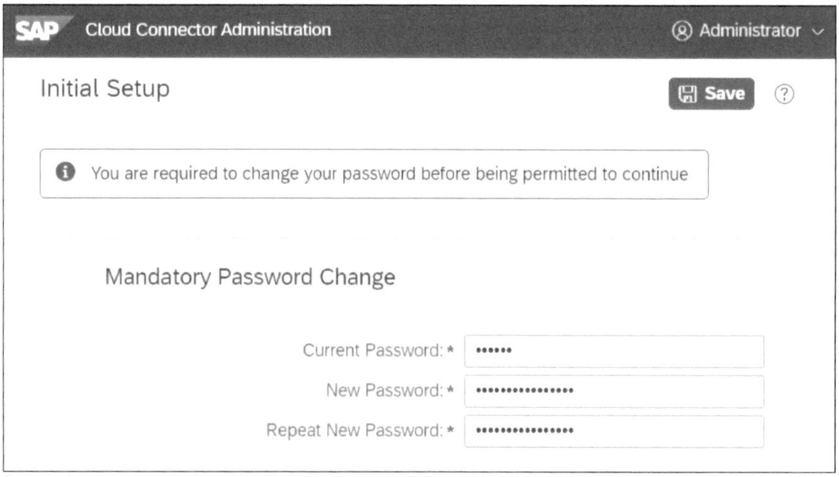

Abbildung 2.22 Initiale Passwortänderung im Cloud Connector

Instanz konfigurieren

Nach der Passwortänderung müssen wir im zweiten Schritt festlegen, ob wir eine Hauptinstanz oder eine Backup-Instanz konfigurieren. In unserem Beispiel konfigurieren wir eine Hauptinstanz und belassen daher die Auswahl auf **Master (Primary Installation)**. Wir bestätigen die Maske mit **Save**. Im Anschluss werden wir zur Konfigurationsmaske **Define Subaccount** weitergeleitet (siehe Abbildung 2.23). Hierüber müssen wir nun den Cloud Connector mit einem Subaccount auf der SAP BTP verbinden.

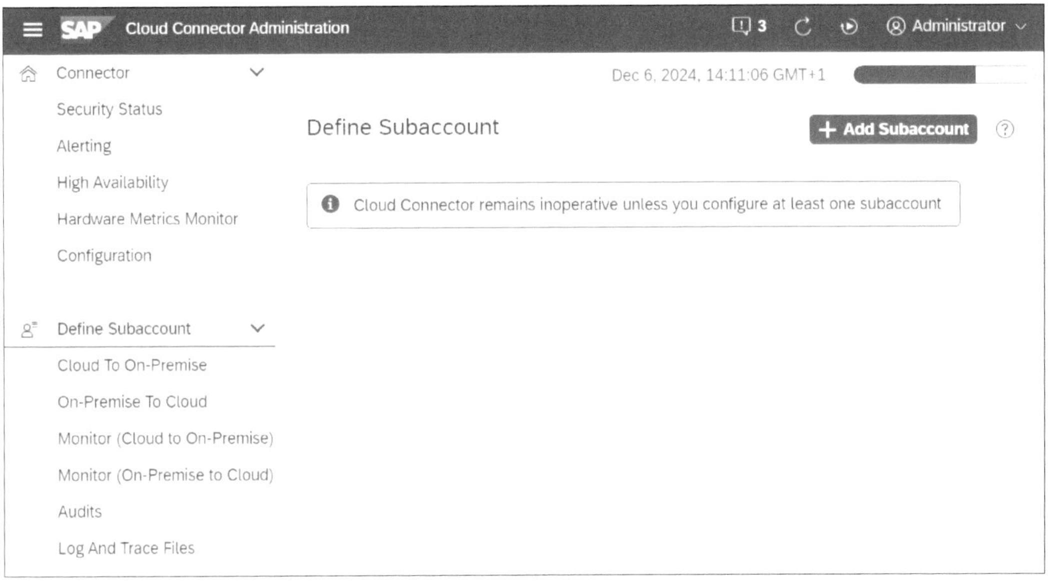

Abbildung 2.23 Einstiegsbild zur Konfiguration eines ersten Subaccount

Subaccount anlegen

Um einen Subaccount anzulegen, klicken Sie auf die Schaltfläche **Add Subaccount**. Sie werden zunächst gebeten, eine etwaige Proxy-Konfiguration anzugeben. Abhängig von Ihrer Infrastruktur geben Sie die relevanten Proxyinformationen ein und bestätigen den Konfigurationsschritt mit **Next**. Im nächsten Schritt werden Sie gebeten, auszuwählen, ob Sie die Subaccount-Konfiguration manuell oder aber eine zuvor exportierte Datei nutzen möchten. In unserem Fall belassen wir die Auswahl auf **Configure manually** und bestätigen wieder mit **Next**. Im letzten Schritt können wir nun die Subaccount-Verbindungsinformationen eintragen.

Wählen Sie zunächst im Feld **Region** die Region aus, in der Ihr Subaccount gehostet wird. Geben Sie anschließend die Subaccount-ID in das entsprechende Feld ein. Tragen Sie im Feld **Login E-Mail** die E-Mail-Adresse ein, die der Role Collection **Connector Administrator** zugewiesen wurde, und geben Sie im Feld **Password** das zugehörige Passwort ein. Speichern Sie Ihre Eingaben, indem Sie auf **Save** klicken. Eine beispielhafte Konfiguration ist in Abbildung 2.24 dargestellt.

Sobald die Verbindung zum Subaccount in der SAP BTP erfolgreich hergestellt wurde, wird Ihnen, wie in Abbildung 2.25 dargestellt, eine entsprechende Erfolgsmeldung angezeigt.

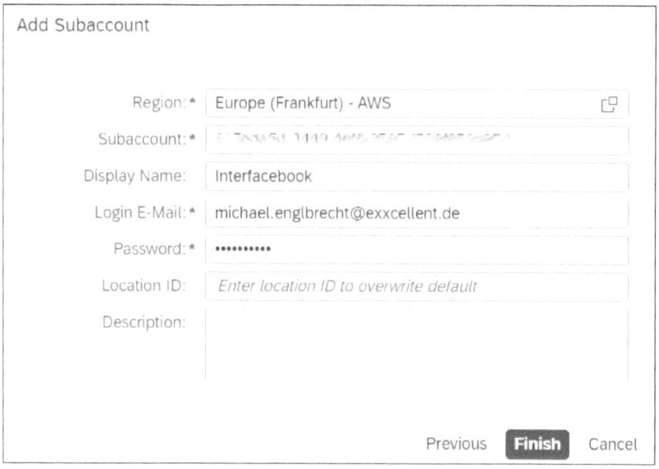

Abbildung 2.24 Beispielkonfiguration für einen Subaccount im Cloud Connector

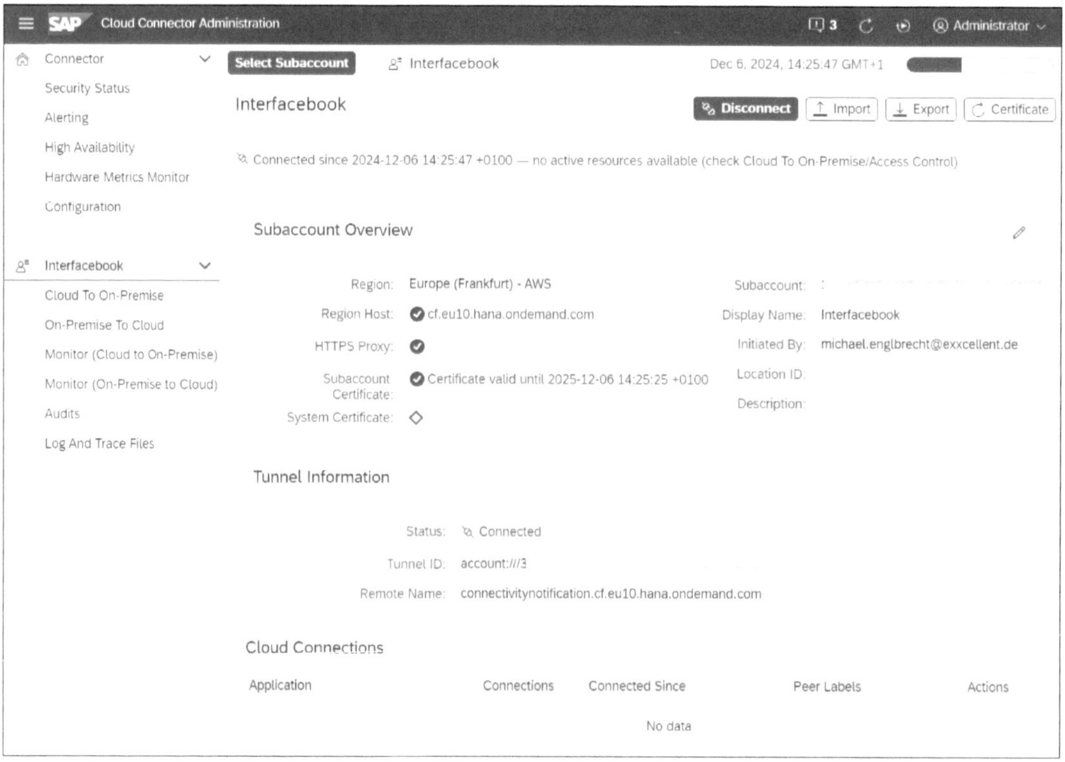

Abbildung 2.25 Übersicht des neu hinzugefügten Subaccounts im Cloud Connector

Verbindung prüfen

Auch im Subaccount der SAP BTP lässt sich überprüfen, ob die Verbindung erfolgreich hergestellt wurde. Melden Sie sich dazu in der SAP BTP an und navigieren Sie zu dem verwendeten Subaccount. Wählen Sie anschließend **Connectivity • Cloud Connectors** aus. Sie erhalten nun eine Übersicht der aktuell bestehenden Cloud-Connector-Verbindungen (siehe Abbildung 2.26).

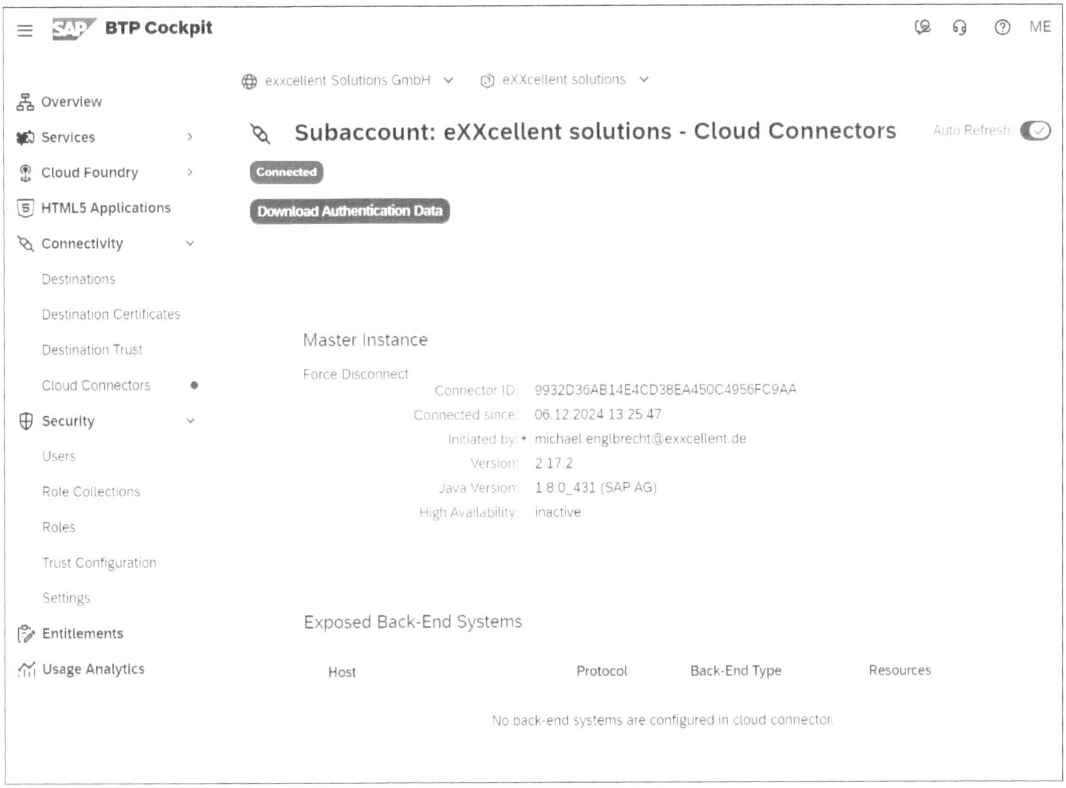

Abbildung 2.26 Verbundener Cloud Connector in der SAP BTP

Vertrauensstellung zwischen SAP-System und Cloud Connector herstellen

Sicherheitskonfiguration

Der Cloud Connector hat als zentraler Kommunikationspunkt zwischen der SAP BTP und den angebundenen SAP-Systemen eine besondere Stellung. Dadurch ist Sicherheit ein sehr wichtiger Aspekt. Standardmäßig vertraut der Cloud Connector keinem angebunden SAP-System, dies ist für eine sichere Kommunikation über HTTPS über den Cloud Connector allerdings notwendig.

Um uns diese im Detail anzusehen, rufen Sie den Cloud Connector wie bereits beschrieben auf und melden sich mit dem Benutzer **Administrator** am

System an. Als Nächstes rufen Sie im Menü den Eintrag **Configuration** auf und im angezeigten Fenster die Registerkarte **ON PREMISE**. Scrollen Sie nun zum Bereich **Backend Trust Store** (siehe Abbildung 2.27). Wie Sie erkennen können, wird die Meldung **No trusted backend are configured – HTTPS communication is not possible** angezeigt. Die Konfigurationsoption **Determining Trust Trough Allowlist** steht auf **On**. Dies bedeutet, dass ein System, mit dem der Cloud Connector kommunizieren soll, zunächst in die Erlaubnisliste aufgenommen werden muss. Wenn Sie es sich leicht machen möchten, könnten Sie den Schieberegler einfach auf **OFF** schieben. Dies ist allerdings nicht zu empfehlen, da dadurch keine sichere Kommunikation stattfindet.

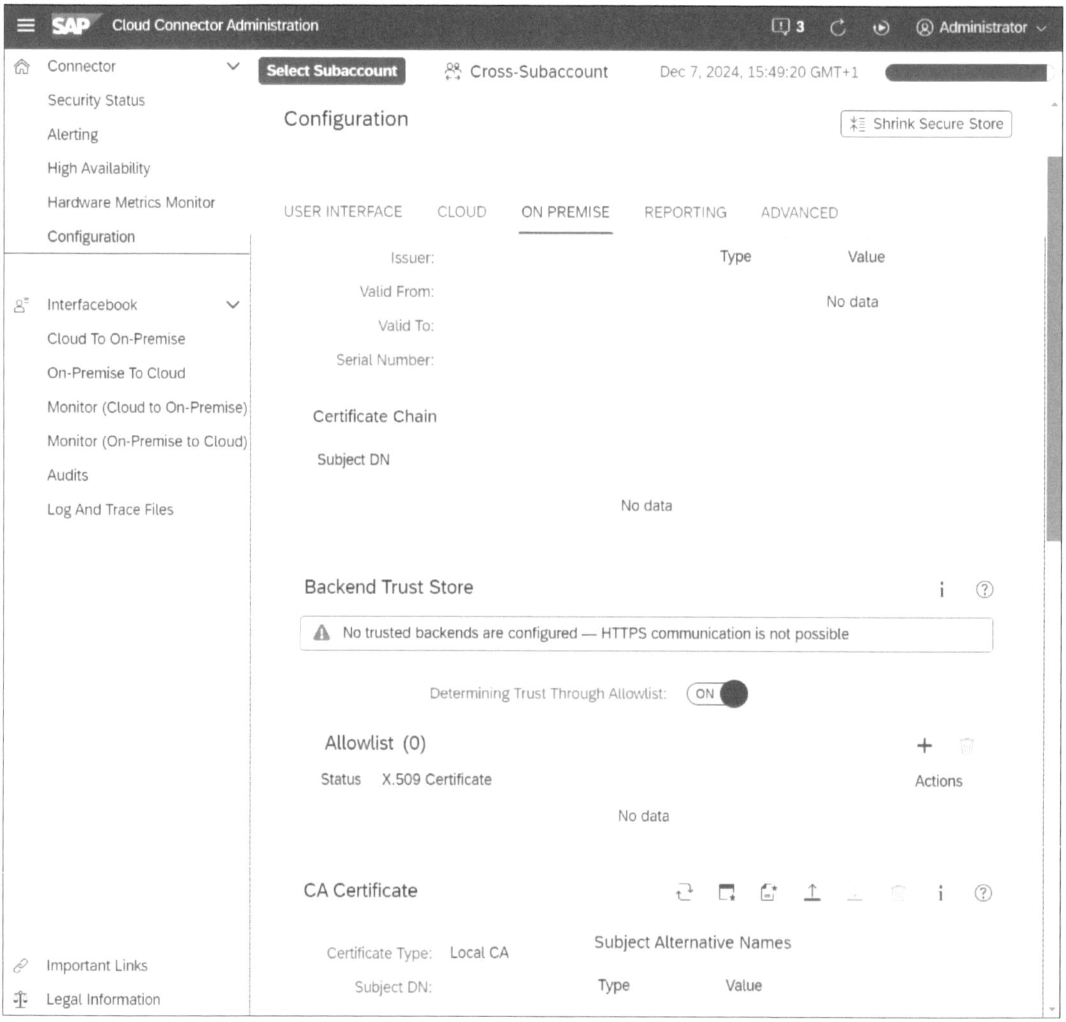

Abbildung 2.27 Backend Trust Store im Cloud Connector

Für die sichere Kommunikation ist es notwendig, das Zertifikat des SAP-Systems entsprechend in die Erlaubnisliste des Cloud Connectors aufzunehmen. Das Zertifikat aus dem SAP-System erhalten Sie über den *Trust Manager*. Melden Sie sich daher an Ihrem SAP-System an und rufen Sie nach der erfolgreichen Anmeldung Transaktion STRUST auf. Wählen Sie im Baum, falls nicht standardmäßig ausgewählt, den Eintrag **System PSE** aus. Als Nächstes wählen Sie, wie in Abbildung 2.28 gezeigt, das Zertifikat Ihres SAP-Systems aus. Nach der Auswahl klicken Sie auf das Icon (**Zertifikat exportieren**) und exportieren das Zertifikat im DER-Format auf Ihre Festplatte.

SAP-System in Erlaubtliste hinzufügen

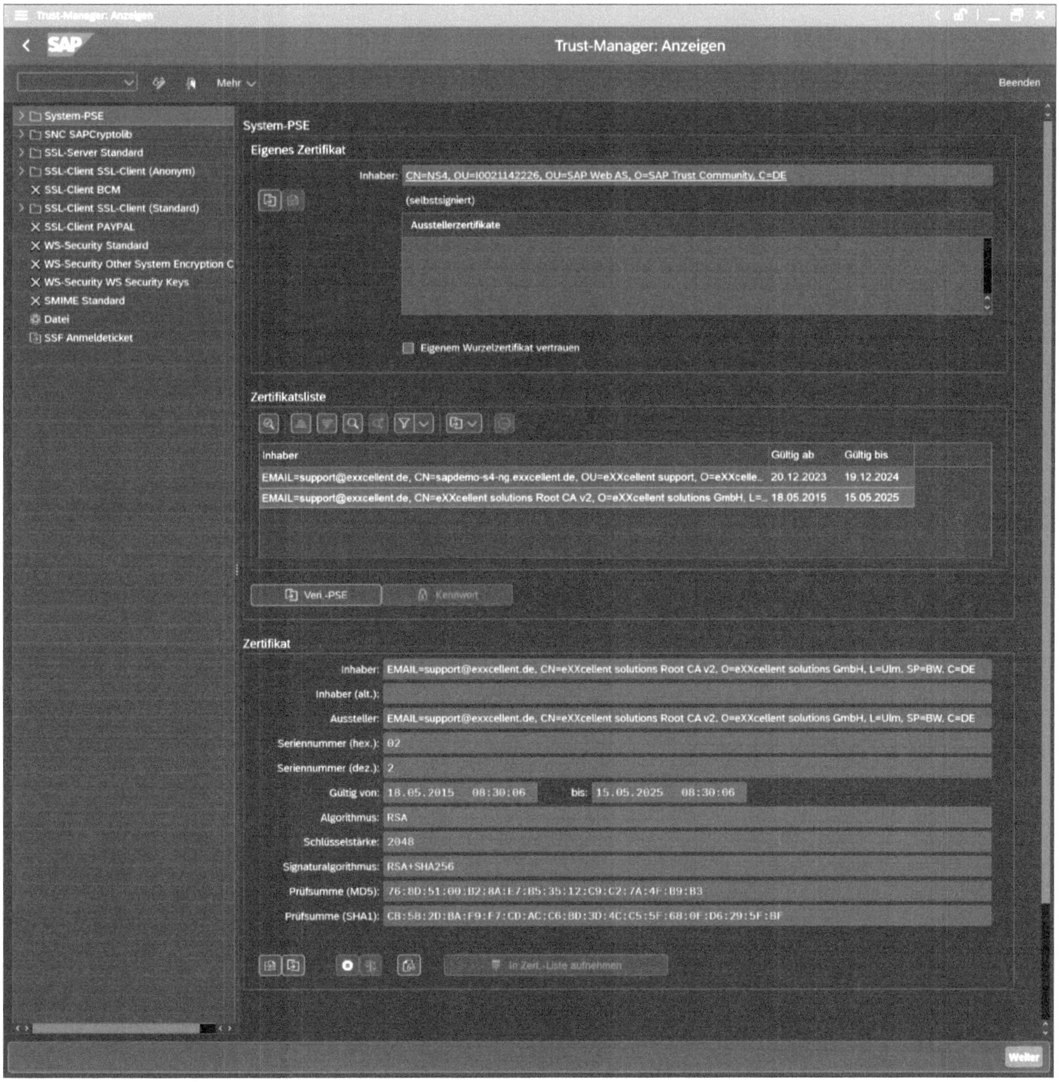

Abbildung 2.28 Trust Manager

Nach dem Export wechseln Sie wieder zurück in den Cloud Connector und klicken auf das Plus-Icon (+) im Bereich der Erlaubtliste. Im sich öffnenden Dialog klicken Sie auf die Schaltfläche **Browse** und wählen das zuvor exportierte Zertifikat aus. Abbildung 2.29 zeigt den Dialog mit ausgewähltem Zertifikat. Im Anschluss bestätigen Sie den Dialog mit **Save**.

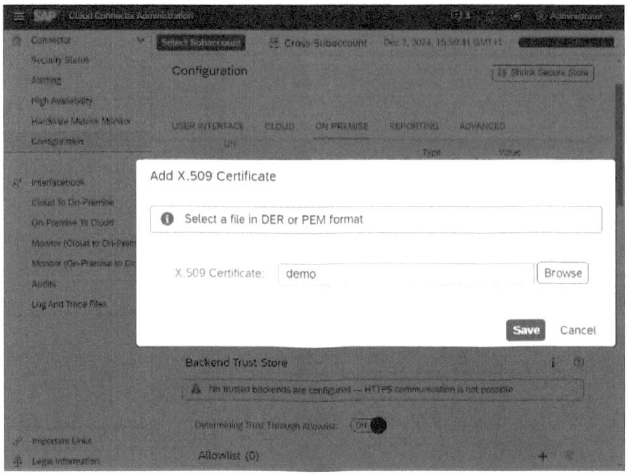

Abbildung 2.29 Hinzufügen eines SAP-Zertifikats zur Erlaubnisliste

Nachdem Hinzufügen des Zertifikats wird das Zertifikat, wie in Abbildung 2.30 gezeigt, in die Erlaubnisliste aufgenommen.

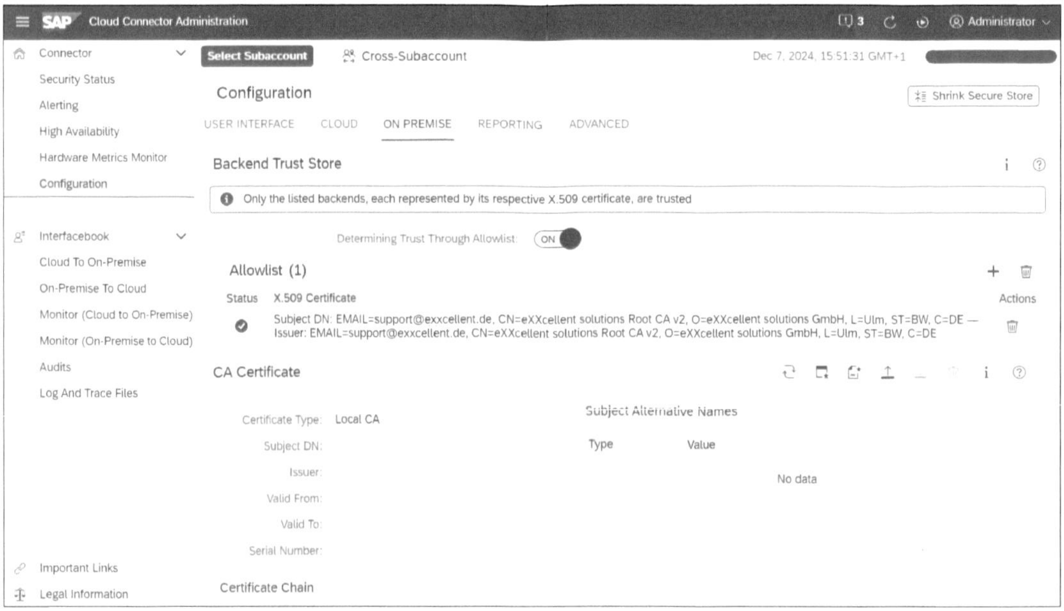

Abbildung 2.30 Die Erlaubnisliste mit hinzugefügtem Zertifikat

Konfiguration von Verbindungen

Nachdem die erste Verbindung zwischen dem Cloud Connector und dem SAP-BTP-Subaccount hergestellt wurde, kann die eigentliche Konfiguration eines Kommunikationskanals entweder zwischen dem SAP-BTP-Subaccount und einem spezifischen On-Premise-System oder umgekehrt erfolgen. In diesem Abschnitt werden wir nach einer kurzen Einführung in die Konfigurationsoptionen eine Verbindung zwischen einem SAP-BTP-Subaccount und einem SAP-S/4HANA-System einrichten.

Anwendungsfälle für die Systemintegration

Wie bereits eingeführt, unterstützt der Cloud Connector zwei Anwendungsfälle für die Systemintegration. Im ersten Fall wird aus der SAP BTP auf ein On-Premise-System zugegriffen. Dies könnte beispielsweise der Fall sein, wenn eine auf der SAP BTP bereitgestellte Anwendung Daten über einen On-Premise-OData-Service konsumieren muss. Der zweite Anwendungsfall betrifft die entgegengesetzte Richtung, bei der ein On-Premise-System einen Service aus der SAP BTP nutzen möchte. In diesem Szenario kann der Cloud Connector als Proxy für das On-Premise-System dienen. Ein Beispiel hierfür wäre, wenn eine Cloud-Anwendung eine SAP-HANA-Datenbank auf der SAP BTP mit Daten versorgt, die anschließend auch On-Premise genutzt werden sollen.

Konfiguration eines System-Mappings

Wir starten die Konfiguration der Verbindung, indem wir ein System-Mapping im Cloud Connector bereitstellen. Dazu navigieren wir in der zuvor konfigurierten Subaccount-Verbindung zum Menüpunkt **Cloud To On-Premise** (siehe Abbildung 2.31).

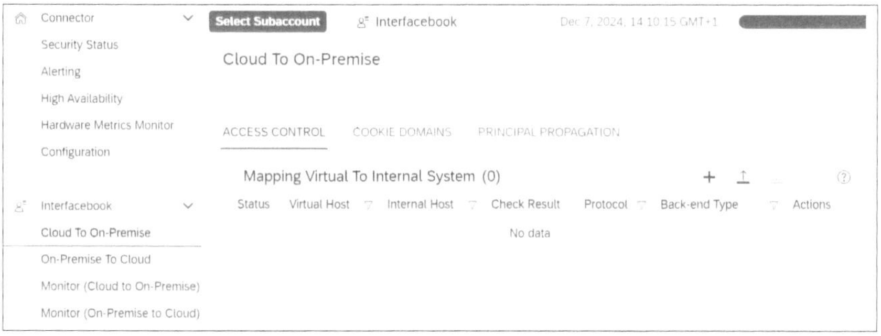

Abbildung 2.31 Konfigurationsseite für Cloud-To-On-Premise-Verbindungen

Systemzuordnung erstellen

Um eine neue Systemzuordnung zu erstellen, klicken Sie auf das Plus-Symbol in der Werkzeugleiste. Daraufhin öffnet sich der Dialog, der in Abbildung 2.32 dargestellt ist. Zunächst müssen Sie den Backend-Typ auswählen. Der Cloud Connector bietet eine Vielzahl von Systemarten an. Je nach gewählter Systemart werden in den folgenden Schritten unterschiedliche Konfigurationsoptionen angeboten. Da Sie ein S/4HANA-System integrieren möchten, wählen Sie, wie in der Abbildung gezeigt, den Eintrag **ABAP System** aus.

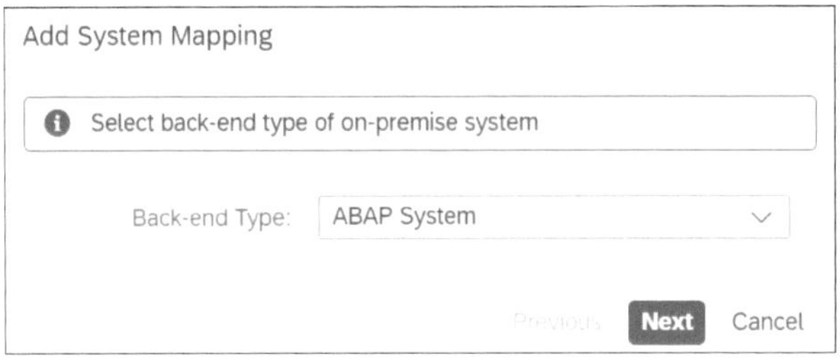

Abbildung 2.32 Auswahl des Backend-Typs

Protokoll wählen

Bestätigen Sie die Auswahl, indem Sie auf **Next** klicken. Im nächsten Schritt, wie in Abbildung 2.33 gezeigt, werden Sie aufgefordert, das Kommunikationsprotokoll auszuwählen. In unserem Fall verwenden Sie HTTPS als Protokoll. Daher wählen Sie den entsprechenden Eintrag aus und bestätigen mit **Next**.

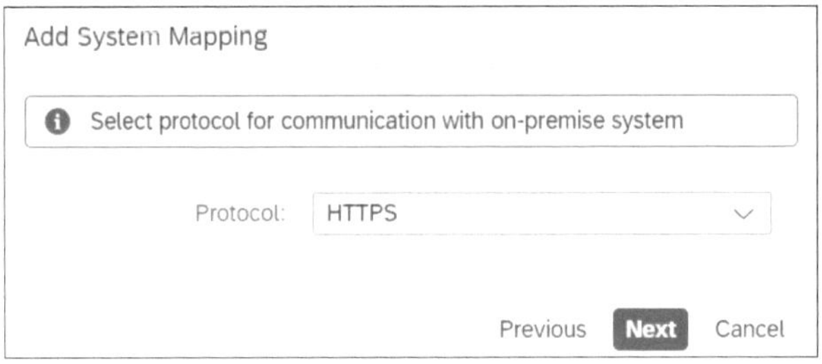

Abbildung 2.33 Protokoll auswählen

Interner Host

Im nächsten Schritt geben Sie den internen Hostnamen des SAP-Systems sowie den entsprechenden HTTPS-Port an. Falls in der vorherigen Auswahl ein anderes Protokoll, wie z. B. HTTP, gewählt wurde, geben Sie den entsprechenden Port für dieses Protokoll an. Nachdem Sie die richtigen Parameter für Ihre Umgebung eingegeben haben, bestätigen Sie den Dialog, der in Abbildung 2.34 gezeigt wird, mit **Next**.

Virtueller Host

Im nächsten Dialogschritt werden Sie aufgefordert, den virtuellen Hostnamen sowie den virtuellen Port anzugeben. Die eingegebenen Werte sind fiktiv und müssen nicht mit tatsächlichen Host- oder Port-Informationen übereinstimmen. Diese Werte dienen lediglich der Registrierung des konfigurierten Systems in der SAP BTP und werden entsprechend verwendet. Füllen Sie die beiden Eingabefelder, wie in Abbildung 2.35 dargestellt, aus und bestätigen Sie mit **Next**.

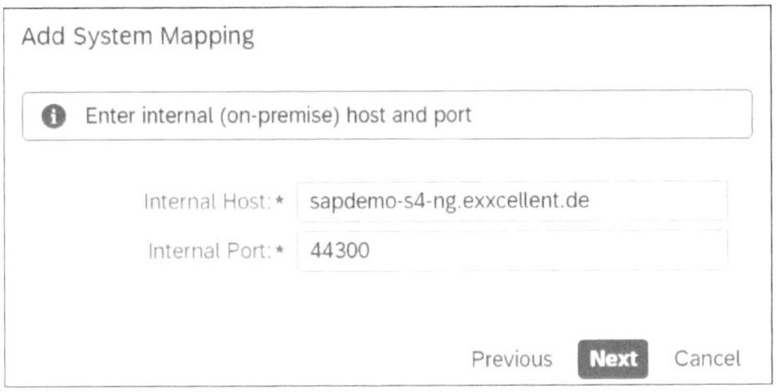

Abbildung 2.34 Konfiguration des internen SAP-Systems

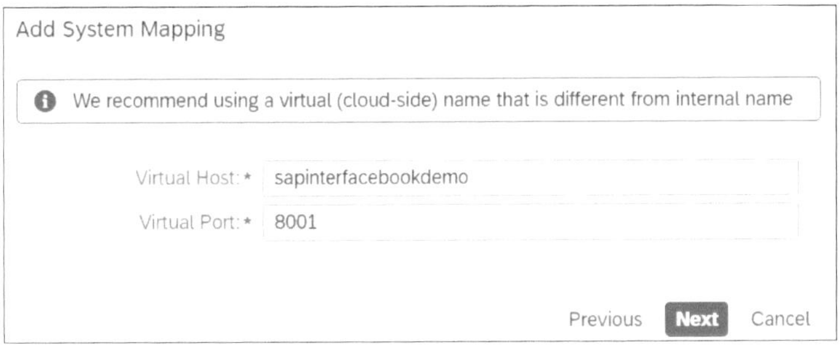

Abbildung 2.35 Virtuellen Host konfigurieren

Bestätigen Sie die nächsten Dialogschritte jeweils mit **Next**, bis Sie zu dem in Abbildung 2.36 gezeigten Abschlussdialog kommen. Im letzten Dialogschritt können Sie die von Ihnen gemachten Eingaben prüfen. Schließen Sie den Dialog ab, indem Sie auf **Finish** klicken.

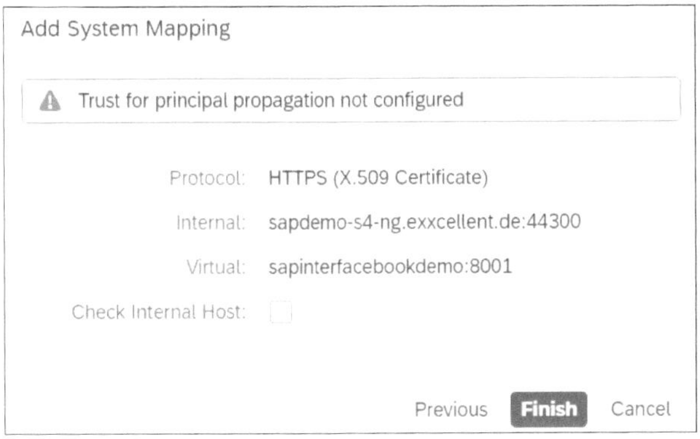

Abbildung 2.36 Überblick über die Konfigurationsangaben

Verbindung testen

Nach Abschluss der Eingaben wird das Mapping wie in Abbildung 2.37 angezeigt. Um zu überprüfen, ob das System mit den unter **Internal Host** und **Protocol** angegebenen Informationen erreichbar ist, können Sie einen Verbindungstest durchführen, indem Sie auf den Button mit dem -Icon (**Check availability of internal host**) klicken. Das Testergebnis wird in der Spalte **Check Result** angezeigt.

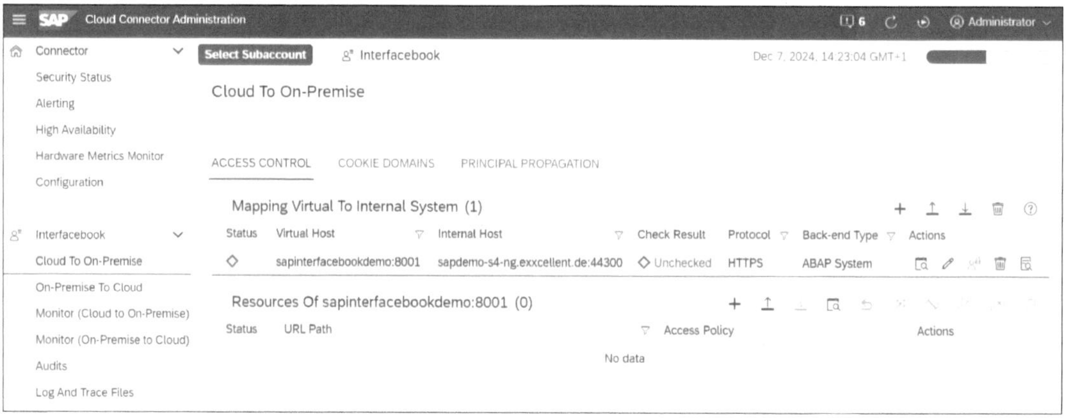

Abbildung 2.37 Vorläufig konfiguriertes System-Mapping

Endpunkte konfigurieren

Wie in Abbildung 2.37 gezeigt, wird in der Spalte **Status** ein graues Symbol angezeigt. Wenn Sie mit dem Mauszeiger über das Icon fahren, erscheint der Tooltip **There are no accessible resources.** Dieser Hinweis signalisiert, dass Konsumenten das System in der SAP BTP zwar grundsätzlich sehen können, jedoch noch keine Endpunkte erreichen, die auf dem System verfügbar sind. Wir müssen uns daher auf der Ebene der Verbindungen genauer damit befassen, auf welche Endpunkte Konsumenten zugreifen können. In diesem Zusammenhang sprechen wir von *ICF-Endpunkten* (siehe folgender Hinweiskasten zum Internet Communication Framework).

Je nach den Anforderungen des jeweiligen Anwendungsfalls sind unterschiedliche Endpunkte erforderlich. In Tabelle 2.1 wird aufgeführt, welche ICF-Endpunkte für eine Embedded- oder Hub-Installation freigegeben werden müssen. Da die zugrunde liegende Infrastruktur in diesem Buch ein Embedded-SAP-S/4HANA-System ist, werden wir die entsprechenden Ressourcen für dieses Szenario konfigurieren.

ICF-Endpunkt	Backend	Embedded Client
/sap/bc/bsp/sap/	*/sap/bc/bsp/sap/*	*/sap/bc/bsp/sap/*
/sap/bc/lrep/	*/sap/bc/gui/*	*/sap/bc/gui/*
/sap/bc/ui2/app_index/	*/sap/bc/ui5_ui5/sap/*	*/sap/bc/lrep/*
/sap/bc/ui2/cdm3/	*/sap/bc/webdynpro/*	*/sap/bc/ui2/app_index/*
/sap/bc/ui2/flp/	*/sap/opu/odata/*	*/sap/bc/ui2/cdm3/*
/sap/bc/ui5_ui5/sap/	*/sap/public/bc/uics/*	*/sap/bc/ui2/flp/*
/sap/bc/ui5_ui5/ui2/	*/sap/public/bc/ur/*	*/sap/bc/ui5_ui5/sap/*
/sap/opu/odata/	*/sap/public/bc/webdynpro/*	*/sap/bc/ui5_ui5/ui2/*
/sap/public/bc/ui5_ui5	*/sap/public/icmandir/its/*	*/sap/bc/webdynpro/*
/sap/public/bc/uics/	*/sap/bc/nwbc/*	*/sap/opu/odata/*
/sap/public/bc/ui2	*/sap/bc/bsp/srmnxp/*	*/sap/public/bc/ui5_ui5*
–	–	*/sap/public/bc/uics/*
–	–	*/sap/public/bc/ur/*
–	–	*/sap/public/bc/webdynpro/*
–	–	*/sap/public/icmandir/its/*
–	–	*/sap/bc/nwbc/*
–	–	*/sap/bc/bsp/srmnxp/*
–	–	*/sap/public/bc/ui2*

Tabelle 2.1 Übersicht über die zur Basiskonfiguration gehörenden freizugebenden Ressourcen

[«]

Internet Communication Framework

Das *Internet Communication Framework* (ICF) ist eine API, die auf Interfaces und Klassen basiert und es ABAP-Programmen ermöglicht, mit dem Internet zu kommunizieren. Es unterstützt die Protokolle HTTP, HTTPS und SMTP. Jeglicher Datenaustausch zwischen ABAP und dem Internet, der auf diesen Protokollen basiert, wird über das ICF abgewickelt.

ICF-Endpunkt erstellen

Um einen ICF-Endpunkt im Cloud Connector freizugeben, klicken Sie auf den Plus-Button ([+]). Im daraufhin geöffneten Dialog (siehe Abbildung 2.38) fügen Sie in das Feld **URL Path** den ersten Eintrag aus der Tabelle ein und wählen die Option **Path And All Sub-Paths** aus. Damit geben Sie an, dass auch alle Unterknoten freigegeben werden. Bestätigen Sie die Eingabe mit **Save** und wiederholen Sie den Vorgang für alle Pfade in der Spalte **Embedded Client** aus Tabelle 2.1.

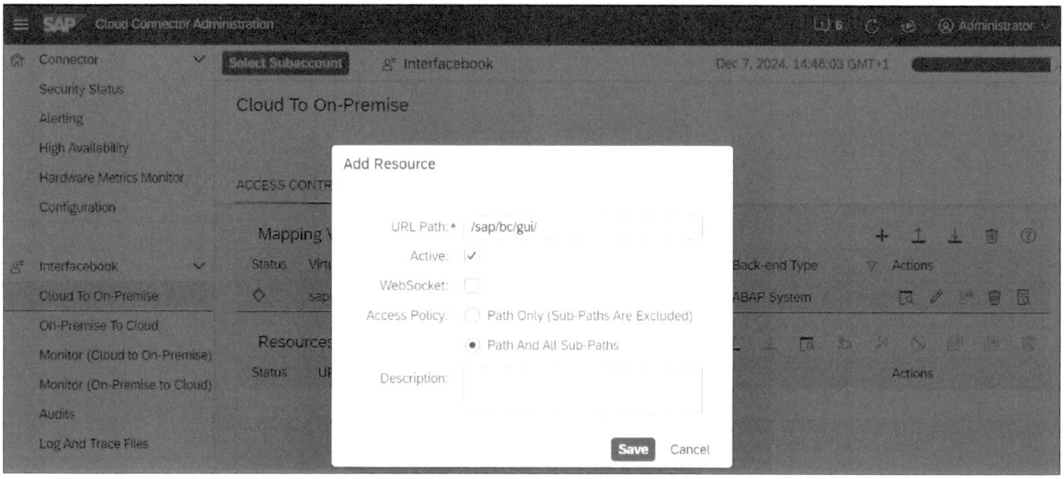

Abbildung 2.38 Konfiguration einer Ressource

Nachdem Sie alle Pfade erfasst haben, wird das System-Mapping vollständig konfiguriert (siehe Abbildung 2.39).

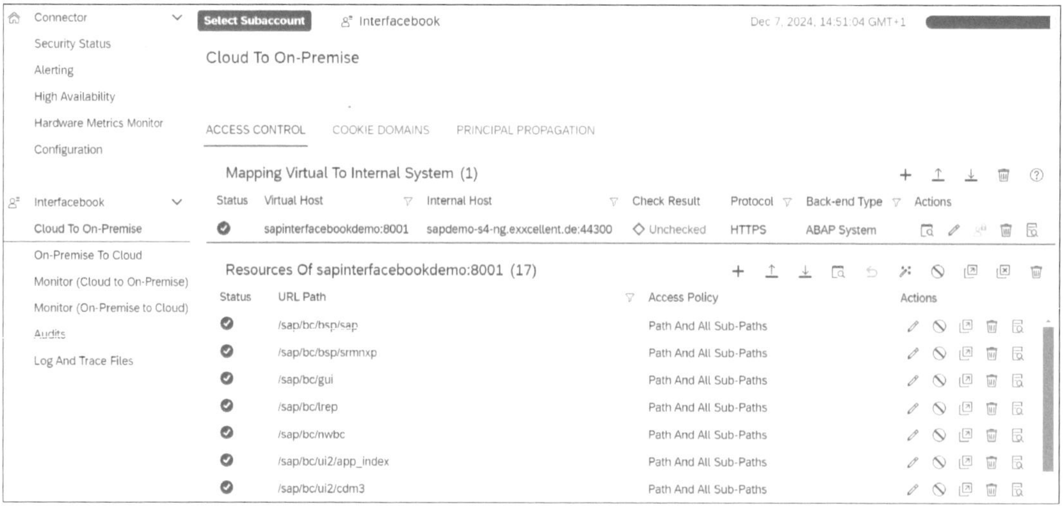

Abbildung 2.39 Vollständig konfigurierte Verbindung

Melden Sie sich nun im Subaccount der SAP BTP an, mit dem Sie sich dem Cloud Connector verbunden haben. Navigieren Sie im Menü über **Connectivity • Cloud Connectors** und Ihnen werden, wie in Abbildung 2.40 dargestellt, der virtuelle Systemname und der virtuelle Port angezeigt. In der Spalte **Resources** wird angezeigt, dass der Cloud Connector über konfigurierte Ressourcen verfügt. Ob diese jedoch korrekt und vollständig für den jeweiligen Anwendungsfall eingerichtet sind, kann an dieser Stelle noch nicht garantiert werden. Dies lässt sich erst bei der tatsächlichen Nutzung aus der SAP BTP heraus feststellen.

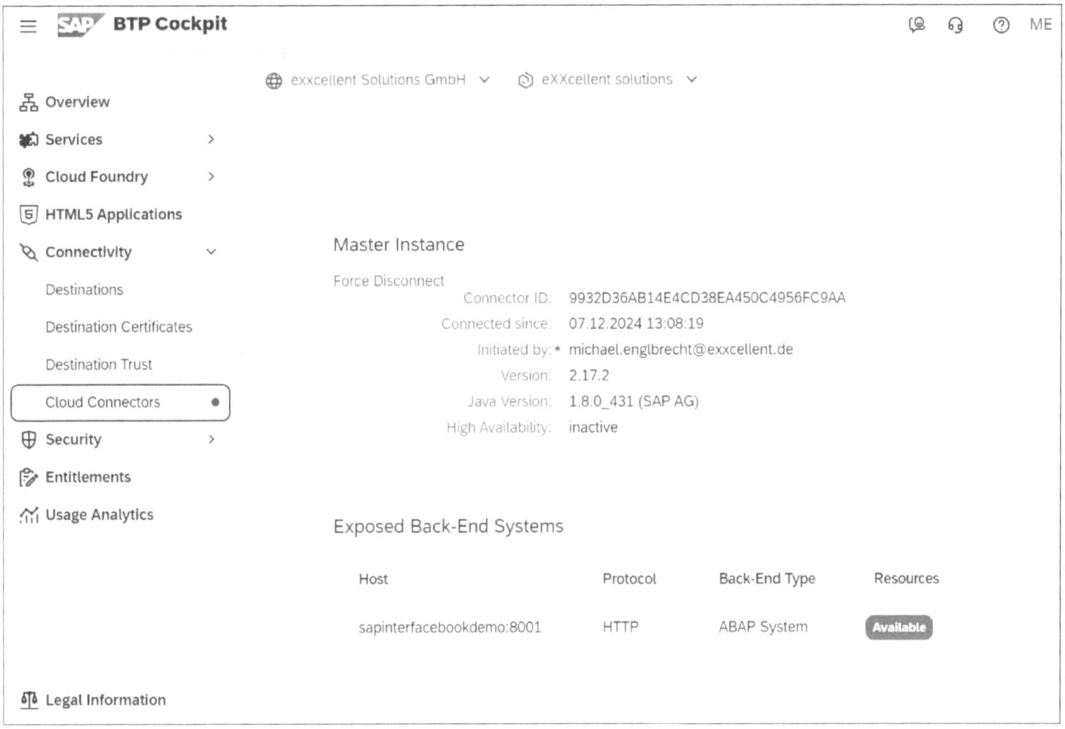

Abbildung 2.40 Verbundener Cloud Connector

Konfiguration einer Destination

Destinations bereitstellen

Nachdem die Einrichtung des Cloud Connectors abgeschlossen ist und Sie im letzten Schritt überprüft haben, ob das im Connector veröffentlichte System in der SAP BTP angezeigt wird, widmen wir uns in diesem Abschnitt der Konfiguration einer Destination in der SAP BTP. SAP stellt in der SAP BTP den SAP Destination Service bereit, der sowohl von SAP-eigenen BTP-

Diensten als auch von kundenspezifischen Anwendungen genutzt werden kann, die in der SAP BTP installiert und den Nutzern zur Verfügung gestellt werden. Der Ausgangspunkt für die Nutzung des SAP Destination Service ist die Bereitstellung von konfigurierten Destinations in der SAP BTP. Um dies einzurichten, navigieren Sie im SAP BTP Cockpit im Seitenmenü über **Connectivity • Destinations** in die Übersichtsseite der Destinations (siehe Abbildung 2.41).

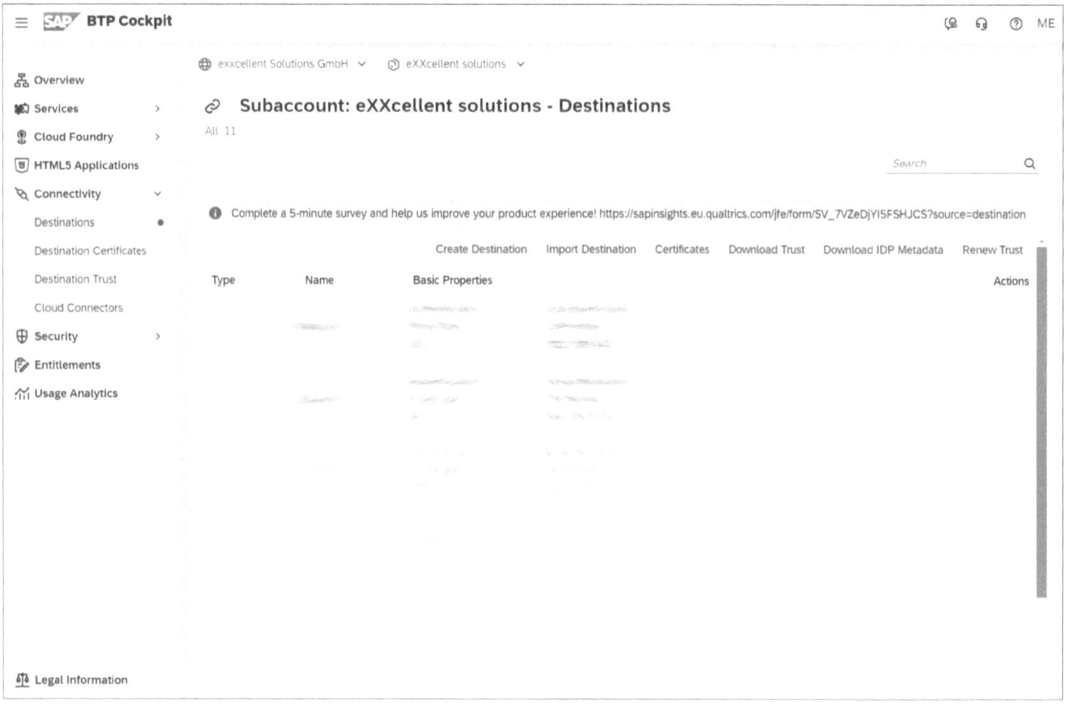

Abbildung 2.41 Destination-Konfigurationsbereich

Verbindung anlegen

Um eine neue Verbindung anzulegen, klicken Sie auf den Button **Create Destination**. Daraufhin wird die leere Erfassungsmaske angezeigt, die in Abbildung 2.42 zu sehen ist. Die Maske lässt sich in zwei Hauptbereiche unterteilen: Der obere Teil dient der Eingabe der Verbindungsdaten, während der untere Bereich, der mit **Additional Properties** überschrieben ist, zur Eingabe von Eigenschaften verwendet wird, die von den SAP-BTP-Diensten benötigt werden, um korrekt zu funktionieren.

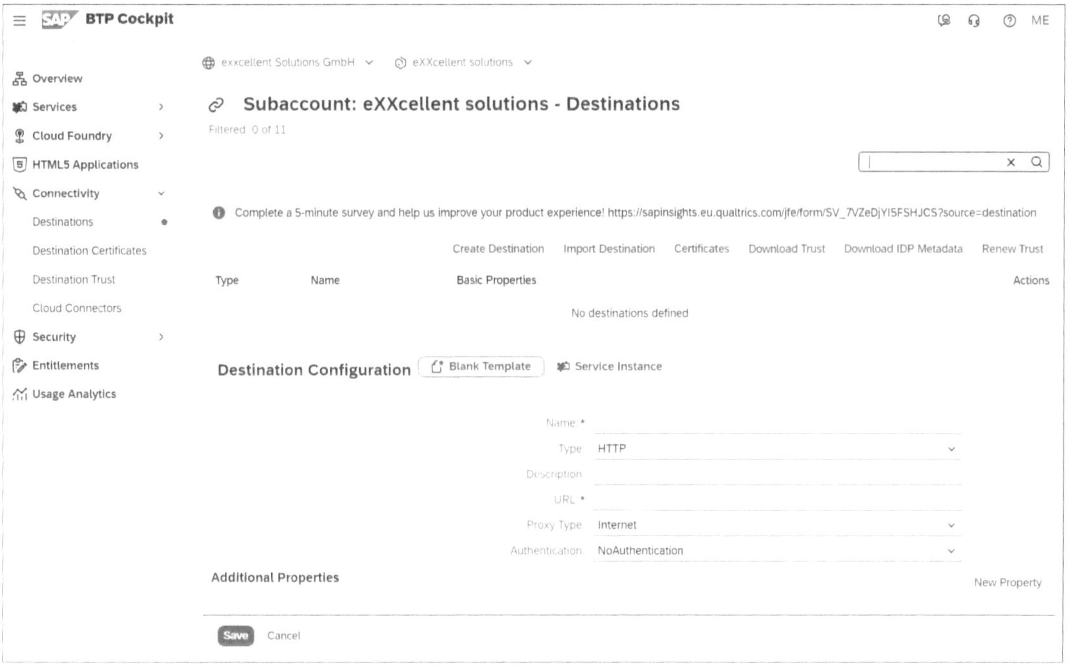

Abbildung 2.42 Vorlage für die Konfiguration einer Destination

Verbindung konfigurieren

Im nächsten Schritt geben wir die erforderlichen Parameter für unsere Verbindung ein. In das Feld **Name** tragen Sie den Namen der Verbindung ein, der später von den SAP-BTP-Diensten verwendet wird, die auf diese Verbindung zugreifen möchten. Wählen Sie aus der Auswahlliste **Type** das Kommunikationsprotokoll aus, wobei derzeit die Optionen **HTTP**, **LDAP**, **MAIL** und **RFC** verfügbar sind. Im Feld **URL** geben Sie die URL des durch den Cloud Connector freigegebenen Systems ein. Diese Information können wir aus dem Menü **Connectivity • Cloud Connectors** (siehe Abbildung 2.43) entnehmen bzw. kopieren. Die URL setzt sich aus dem gewählten Protokoll, dem virtuellen Hostnamen und der Portangabe zusammen. Aus der Auswahlliste **Proxy Type** wählen Sie **OnPremise** aus. Im Feld **Authentication** legen Sie fest, welche Authentifizierungsmethode verwendet werden soll. Zu Beginn wählen Sie **NoAuthentication**. Dies führt dazu, dass Benutzer und Passwort bei der Nutzung der Destination abgefragt werden. Da wir die Master-Instanz des Cloud Connectors verwenden, können wir das Feld **Location ID** leer lassen.

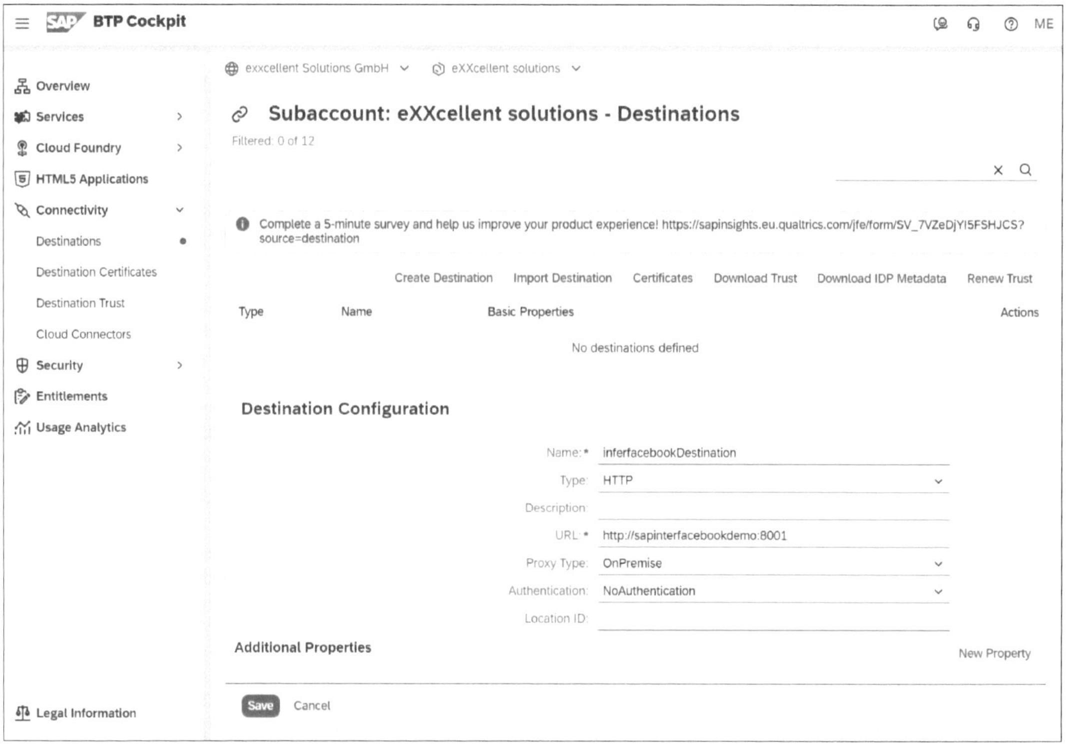

Abbildung 2.43 Konfiguration einer Destination

Als Nächstes müssen Sie noch weitere Eigenschaften hinzufügen (siehe Tabelle 2.2). Hierbei gehen wir davon aus, dass die Destination vom SAP Business Application Studio genutzt werden soll. Um eine neue Eigenschaft hinzuzufügen, klicken wir zunächst auf den Button **New Property**.

Eigenschaft	Wert	Erläuterung
HTML5.DynamicDestination	true	–
HTML5.Timeout	60000	Zeitangabe, wie lange auf eine Antwort gewartet werden soll
sap-client	100	SAP-Mandant
WebIDEEnabled	true	–

Tabelle 2.2 Eigenschaften für die Konfiguration einer SAP-BTP-Destination

Eigenschaft	Wert	Erläuterung
WebIDEUsage	odata_abap,ui5_execute_abap,dev_abap,bsp_execute_abap	–

Tabelle 2.2 Eigenschaften für die Konfiguration einer SAP-BTP-Destination (Forts.)

Nachdem die Eigenschaften gepflegt sind, erhalten wir die in Abbildung 2.44 gezeigt Konfiguration.

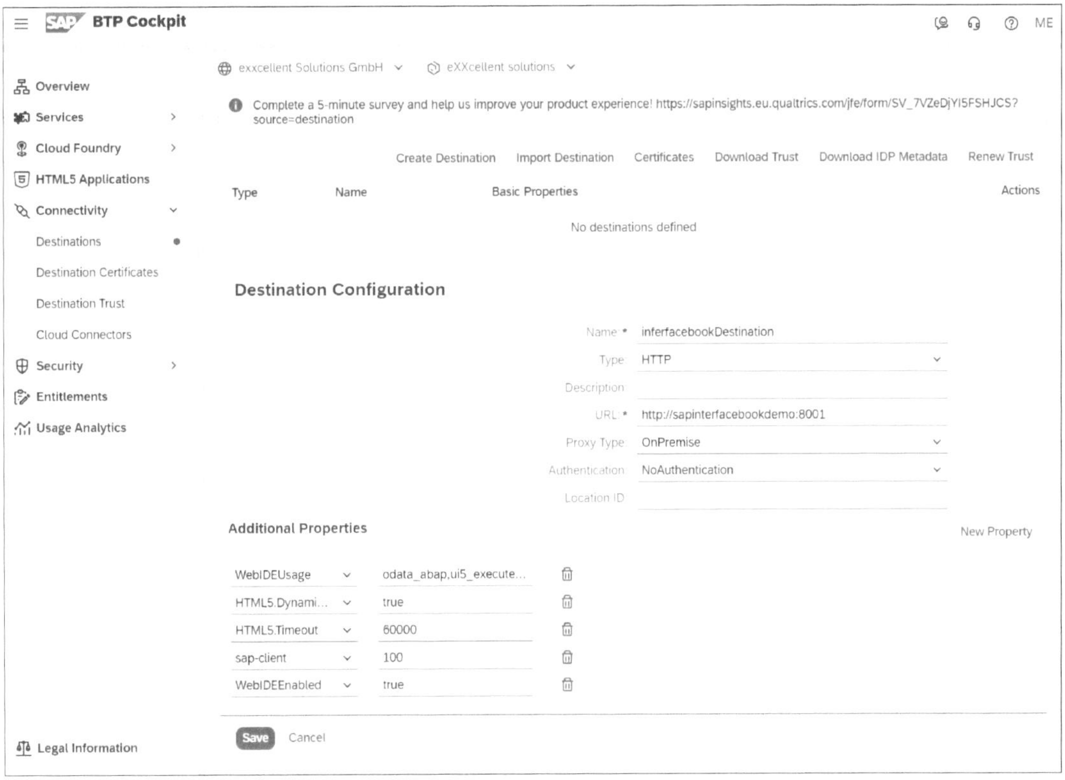

Abbildung 2.44 Vollständig konfigurierte Destination

Verbindung prüfen

Nachdem Sie die zusätzlichen Eigenschaften eingegeben haben, speichern Sie Ihre Angaben mit **Save**. Zum Abschluss der Konfiguration klicken wir auf die Schaltfläche **Check Connection**. Diese Funktion überprüft, ob das angebundene System erreichbar ist. Sie testet jedoch nicht, ob das System tatsächlich für die Nutzung eines bestimmten SAP-BTP-Service bereitgestellt werden kann. In unserem Beispiel wird also nicht überprüft, ob das System tatsächlich vom SAP Business Application Studio verwendet werden kann oder ob die bei **WebIDEUsage** angegebenen Parameter korrekt sind. Abbildung 2.45 zeigt das Ergebnis des erfolgreichen Verbindungstests.

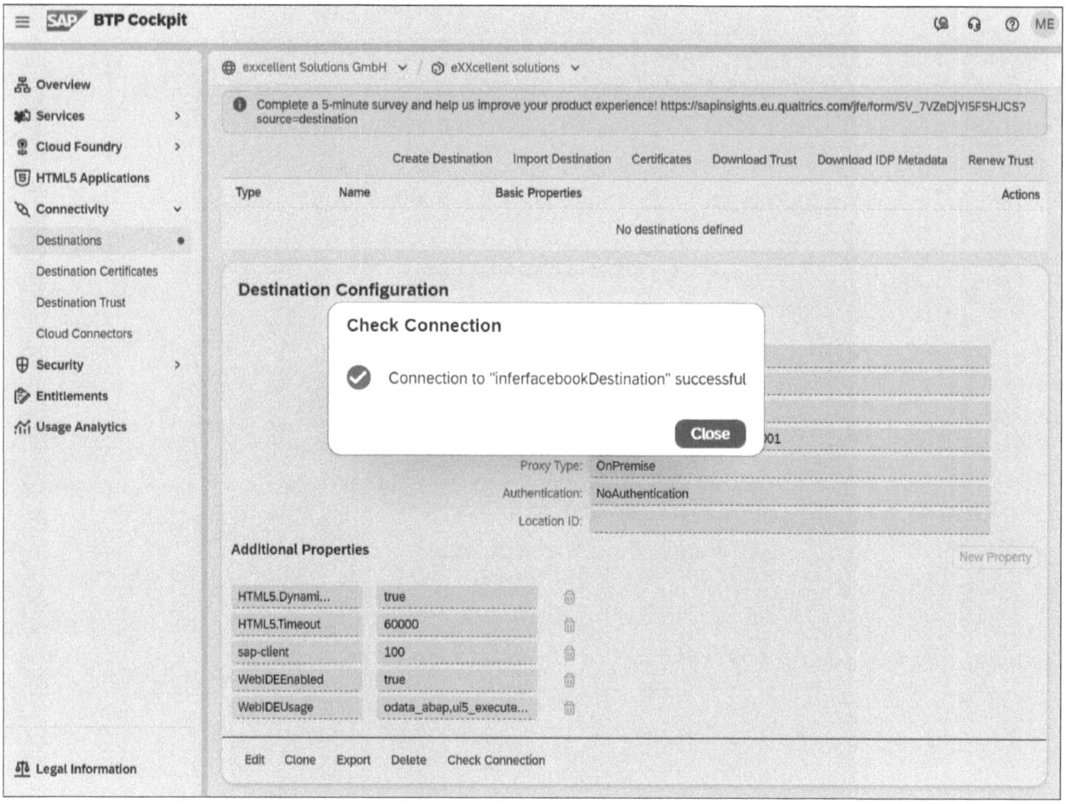

Abbildung 2.45 Erfolgreiche Verbindungsprüfung

2.3 Sicherheit

Nachdem wir im vergangenen Abschnitt die Verbindung zwischen der SAP BTP und On-Premise-Systemen mit dem Cloud Connector erläutert haben, behandeln wir in diesem Abschnitt das Thema Sicherheit in der SAP BTP. Dabei geben wir jedoch nur einen Überblick über die wichtigsten Aspekte. Weitere Informationen finden Sie unter *https://pages.community.sap.com/topics/btp-security*.

2.3.1 Benutzer

Der zentrale Aspekt beim Zugriff auf den Global Account bzw. den Subaccounts ist, dass für den Zugriff ein Benutzer benötigt wird. Benutzer können entweder direkt in der SAP BTP administriert oder über einen externen Identity Provider bereitgestellt werden. Für den Global Account werden die Benutzer über **Security • Users** gepflegt.

Benutzerverwaltung

Abbildung 2.46 zeigt die Maske zur Verwaltung von Benutzern im Global Account. Wie Sie aus der Abbildung entnehmen können, können neue Benutzer über den Button **Create** angelegt werden. Um einen existierenden Benutzer zu pflegen, wählt man diesen aus und kann in der Detailansicht entsprechend in den Bearbeitungsmodus wechseln.

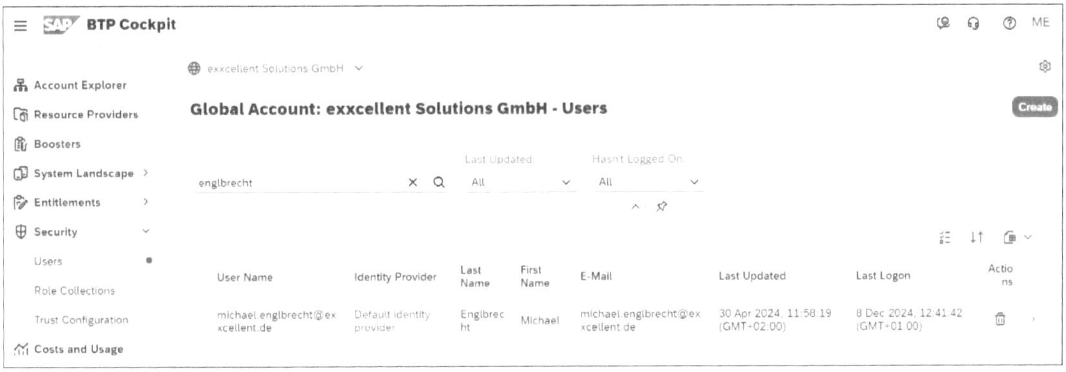

Abbildung 2.46 Benutzerverwaltung des Global Accounts

Analog zur Benutzerverwaltung auf Global-Account-Ebene ist auf Subaccount-Ebene die Verwaltung ebenfalls über den Menüeintrag **Security • Users** möglich.

2.3.2 Application Roles und Role Collections

Entitlement

Für die Nutzung eines SAP-BTP-Service ist zunächst ein sogenanntes *Entitlement* erforderlich. Dies bedeutet, dass der gewünschte SAP-BTP-Service dem Subaccount zugewiesen werden muss.

Role Collection

Nachdem der Service zugewiesen ist, ist es notwendig, SAP-BTP-Benutzer für die Nutzung des Diensts zu berechtigen. Der Zugriff auf SAP-BTP-Dienste wird zunächst grundsätzlich über Anwendungsrollen (*Application Roles*) gesteuert. Dabei werden Benutzer nicht direkt einer Rolle, sondern einer *Role Collection* zugewiesen. Eine Role Collection kann eine oder mehrere Anwendungsrollen enthalten. Rollen sind Instanzen sogenannter *Role Templates*. Diese Role Templates werden im Rahmen der Entwicklung eines SAP-BTP-Service durch den Entwickler definiert. Abbildung 2.47 zeigt den Zusammenhang zwischen *Role Templates*, *Role* und *Role Collection*.

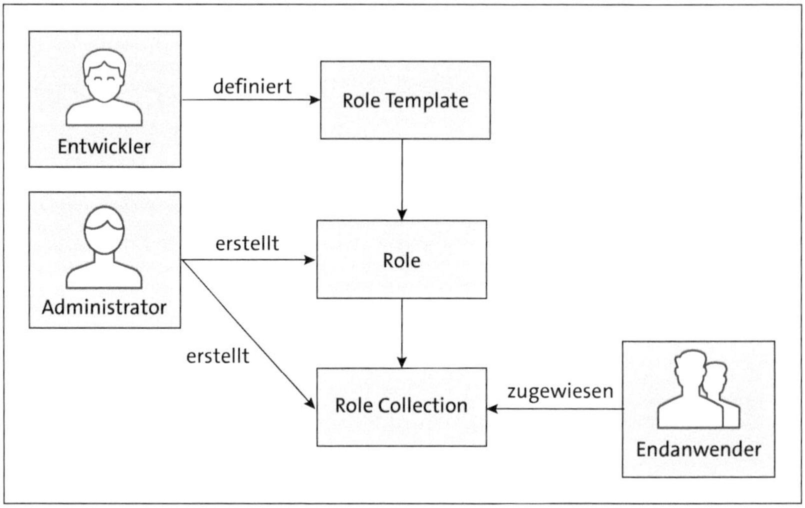

Abbildung 2.47 Veranschaulichung des Berechtigungskonzepts

Rollen verwalten Die Rollen-Administration können Sie sowohl im Global Account als auch im Subaccount über die Menüeinträge **Security • Roles** aufrufen. Abbildung 2.48 zeigt die Ansicht der Rollenverwaltung in einem Subaccount.

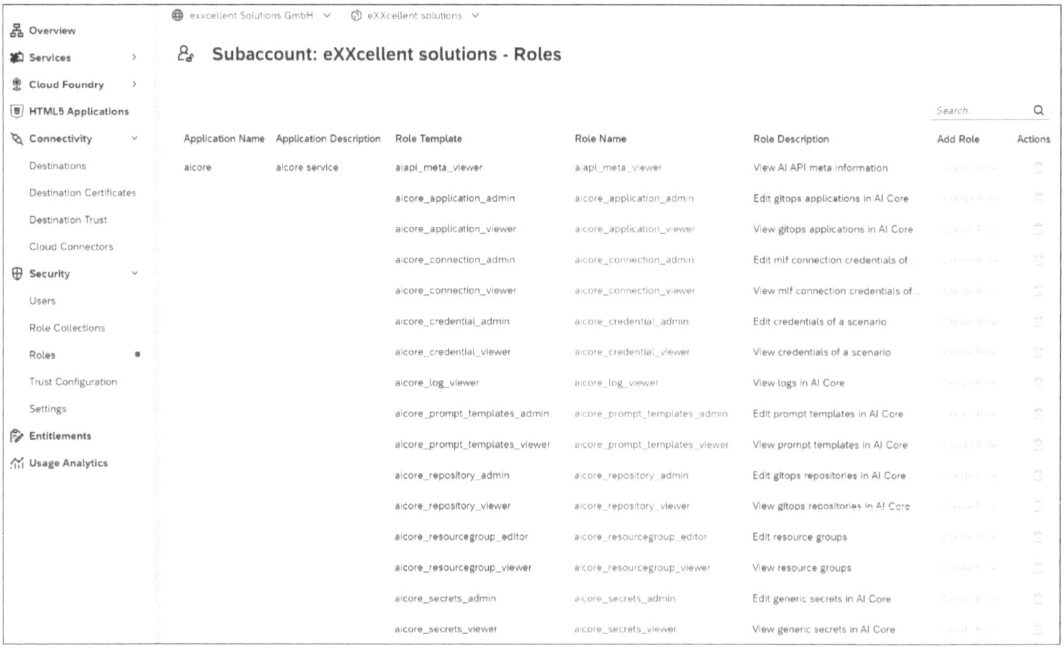

Abbildung 2.48 Rollenverwaltung in einem Subaccount

Wie Sie aus der Abbildung entnehmen können, enthält die Liste in der ersten Spalte die Anwendung, in der die Rolle definiert ist, genauer gesagt das Template der Rolle. Die dritte Spalte enthält den Namen des Templates. Die vierte Spalte enthält den Rollennamen. Dieser ist als Link dargestellt. Über den Link gelangen Sie zu den Details der Rolle.

Abbildung 2.49 zeigt die Details der Rolle **Cloud Connector Administrator**. Wie Sie sehen, ist die Rolle Cloud Connector aktuell drei Role Collections zugeordnet.

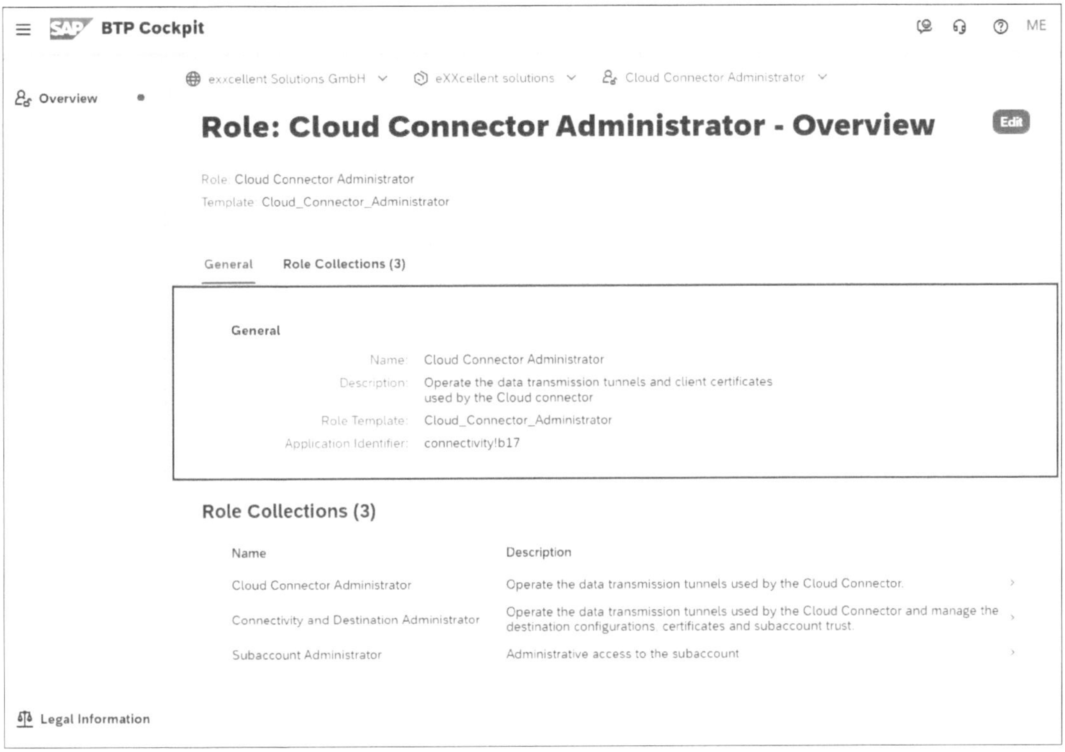

Abbildung 2.49 Rollendetails zur Rolle Cloud Connector Administrator

Role Collections werden im Administrationsbereich **Security • Role Collections** verwaltet. Abbildung 2.50 zeigt diesen Bereich. Über die Schaltfläche **Create** können eigene Role Collections erstellt werden. Durch die Auswahl einer bestehenden Collection gelangen Sie in das Detailbild der Collection. Hierüber können Sie beispielsweise einen neuen Benutzer einer Rolle zuordnen.

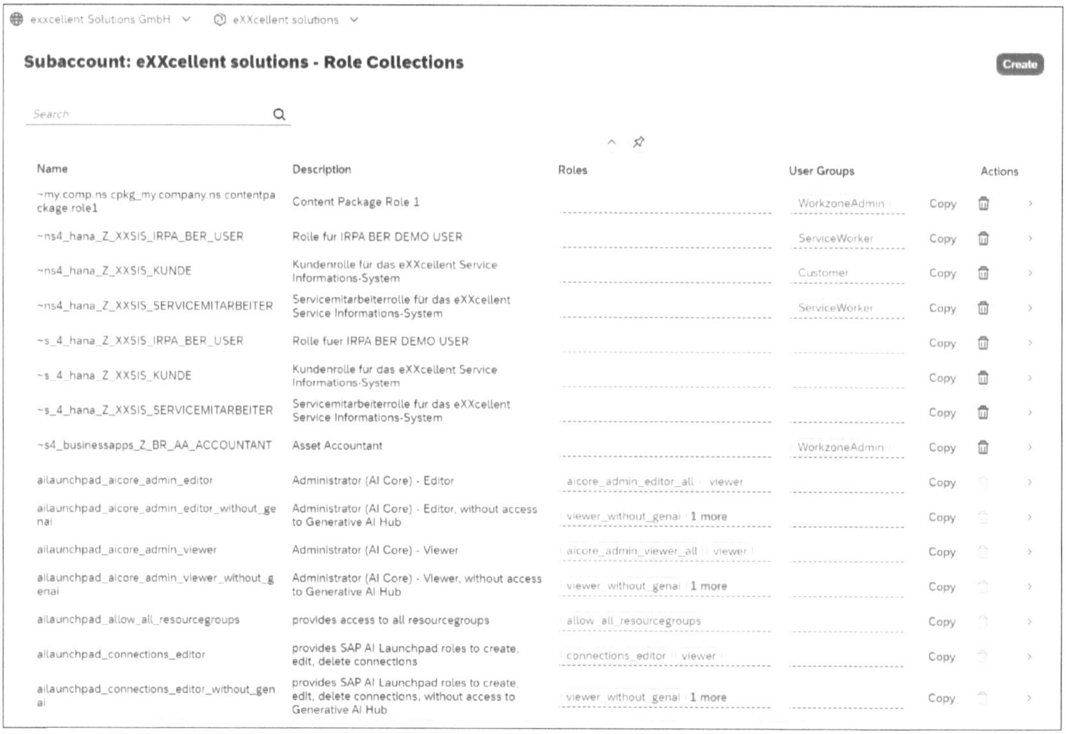

Abbildung 2.50 Verwaltung von Role Collections

2.3.3 Identity Provider

Die Anforderungen an die Sicherheitsinfrastruktur sind auch für Cloud-Plattformen von zentraler Bedeutung. Dabei ist entscheidend, dass die Plattform eine einheitliche Grundlage für Cloud-Dienste und die darauf bereitgestellten Anwendungen bietet. SAP ermöglicht die Bereitstellung von Authentifizierungsfunktionen durch den Einsatz sogenannter *Identity Provider*. Die SAP BTP stellt standardmäßig den *SAP ID Service* als integrierten Identity Provider bereit. Dieser vorkonfigurierte, öffentliche Provider besitzt eine Vertrauensbeziehung zu allen SAP-BTP-Subaccounts innerhalb eines globalen Accounts und wird zentral von SAP verwaltet. In diesem Service werden alle Benutzerkonten – darunter S-, P-, D- und I-Benutzer – administriert, die auch für die SAP-Entwickler- und Partnergemeinschaft sowie die offizielle SAP-Website genutzt werden.

Identity Provider verwalten

Im SAP BTP Cockpit können die für einen globalen Account konfigurierten Identity Provider über den Menüpunkt **Security • Trust Configuration** eingesehen werden. Abbildung 2.51 zeigt den entsprechenden Bereich im SAP

BTP Cockpit. Auf dieser Ebene wird standardmäßig der voreingestellte Identity Provider von SAP angezeigt. Die Verwaltung solcher Vertrauensbeziehungen kann entweder auf Ebene des globalen Accounts oder auf Subaccount-Ebene erfolgen.

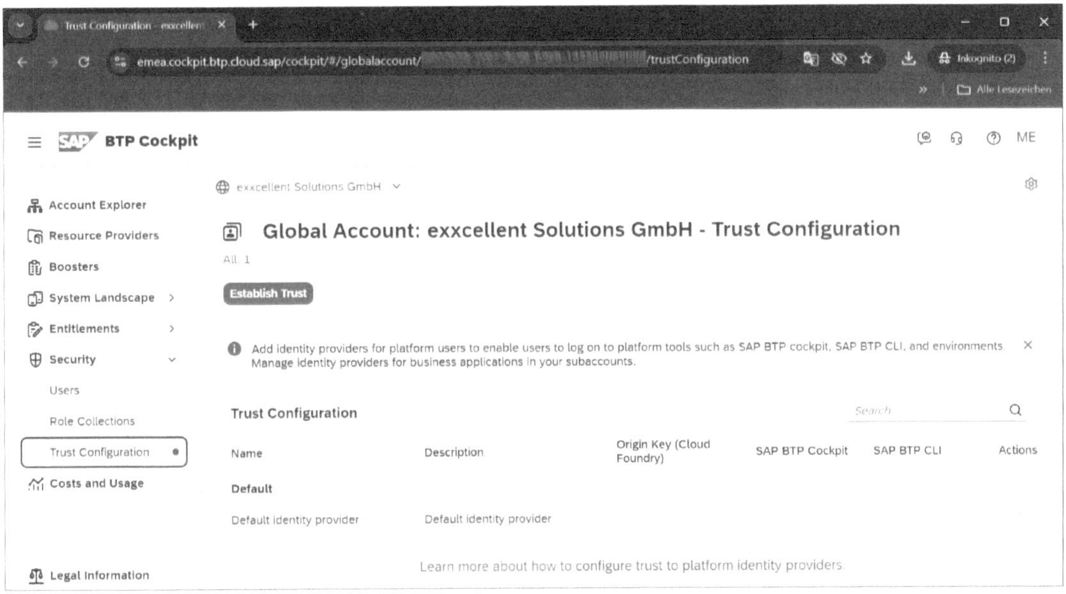

Abbildung 2.51 Trust-Konfiguration eines Global Accounts

2.3.4 Vertrauensbeziehung aufbauen

Um einen Identity Provider in der SAP BTP nutzen zu können, muss zunächst eine Vertrauensbeziehung eingerichtet werden. Dazu öffnen wir die Administrationsoberfläche für Vertrauensbeziehungen über den Menüpunkt **Security • Trust Configuration**. Nach dem Laden der Seite erscheint die in Abbildung 2.52 dargestellte Ansicht. Wie dort zu erkennen ist, ist derzeit nur der standardmäßige Default Identity Provider konfiguriert.

Vertrauensbeziehung einrichten

Um eine neue Vertrauensbeziehung einzurichten, klicken Sie auf den Button **Establish Trust**. Daraufhin öffnet sich ein Dialog, der Sie, wie in Abbildung 2.53 gezeigt, Schritt für Schritt durch die Konfiguration führt. Im ersten Schritt der Konfiguration wählen Sie den Tenant aus, auf dem unser Identity Provider bereitgestellt wird (siehe Abbildung 2.53). In unserem Beispiel ist die Auswahl unkompliziert, da in unserer Cloud-Infrastruktur nur ein Tenant vorhanden ist. Markieren Sie diesen Tenant. Nach der Auswahl wird der **Next**-Button aktiviert. Durch Klicken auf **Next** gelangen Sie zum zweiten Schritt der Konfiguration.

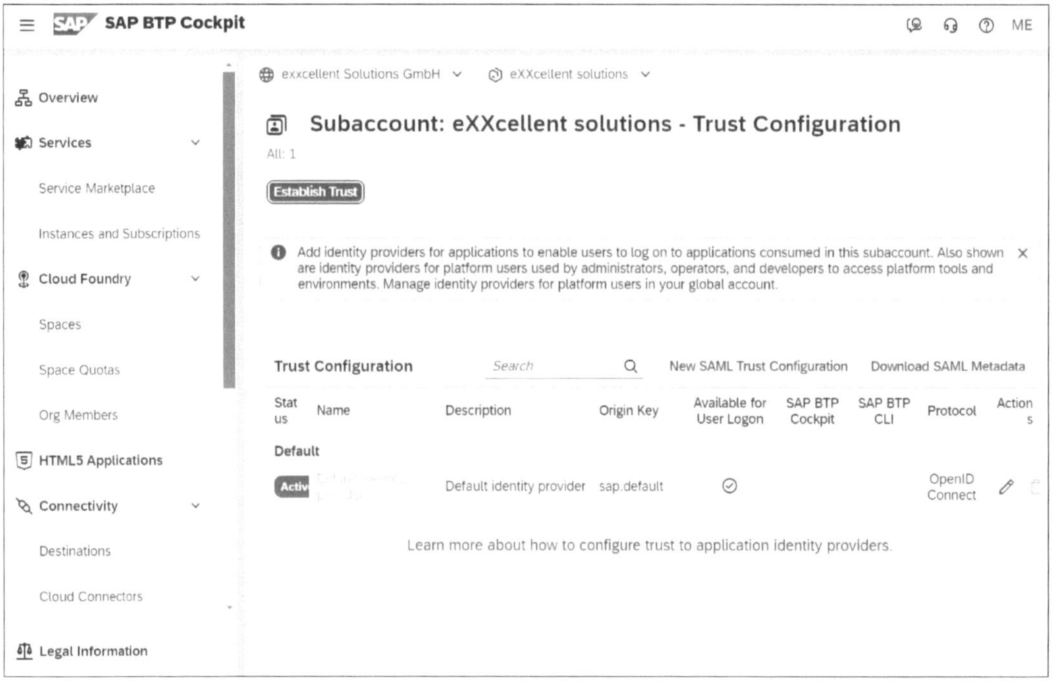

Abbildung 2.52 Konfigurationsoberfläche für Vertrauensbeziehungen

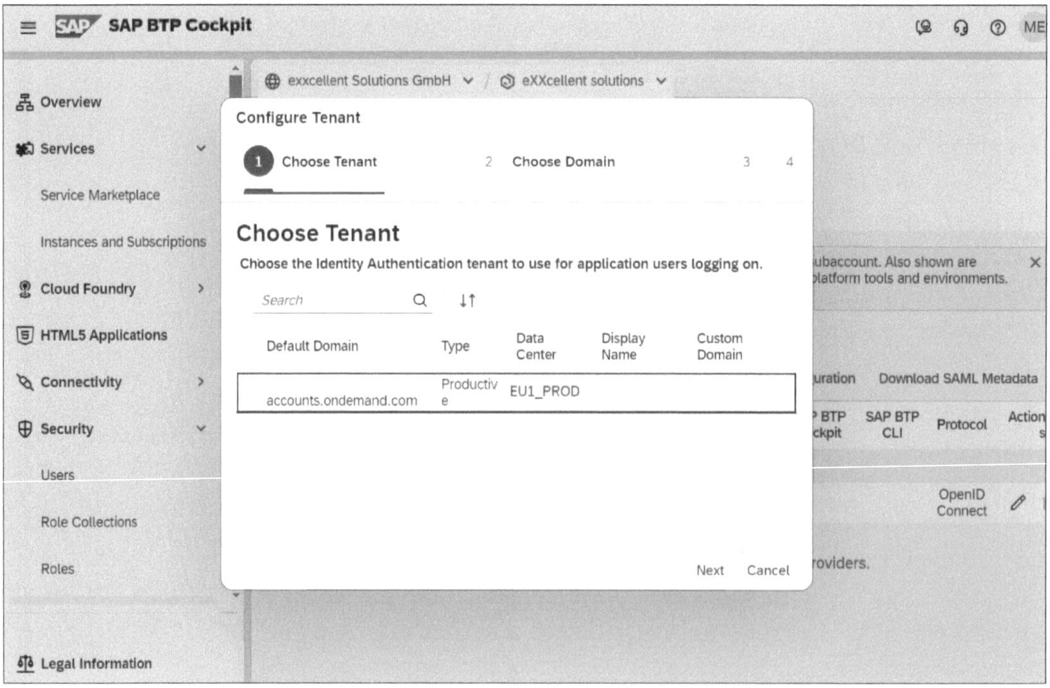

Abbildung 2.53 Auswahl des Identity-Provider-Tenants

Tenant einrichten

Im zweiten Schritt wählt man die Domäne Ihres *Tenants* aus (siehe Abbildung 2.54). Wir wählen diese aus und bestätigen mit **Next**.

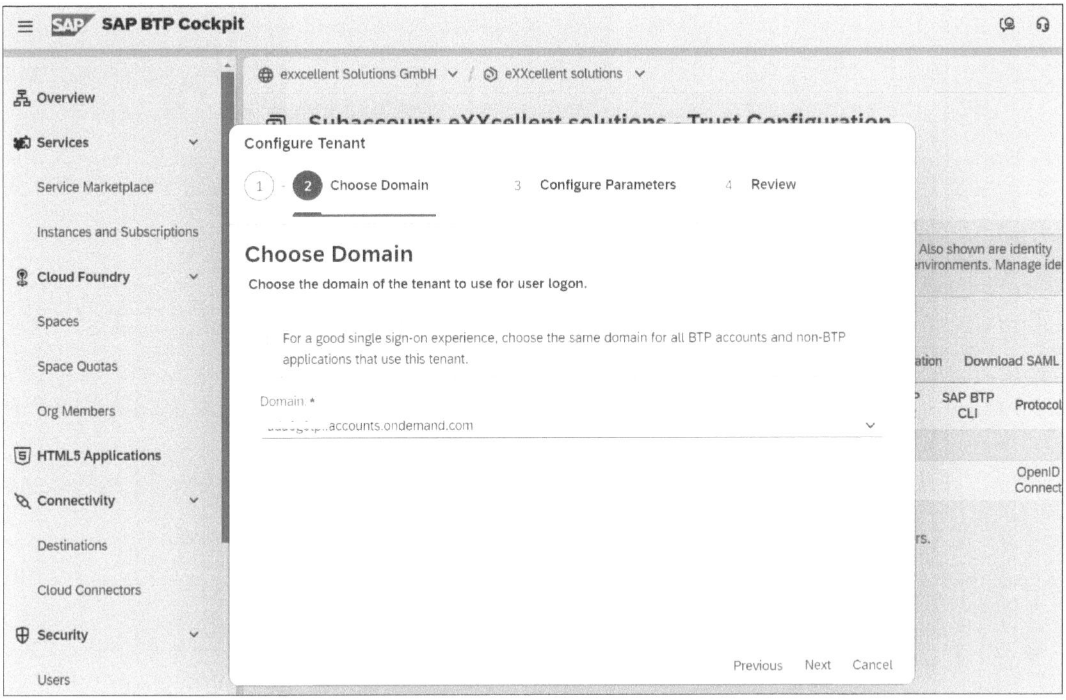

Abbildung 2.54 Auswahl der Tenant-Domäne

Parameter festlegen

Im dritten und vorletzten Schritt der Konfiguration müssen Sie einige Parameter festlegen, die sowohl in der Übersicht der Vertrauenskonfiguration angezeigt werden als auch bei der Anmeldung an den jeweiligen SAP-BTP-Dienst relevant sind. Die Felder sind standardmäßig mit vordefinierten Werten ausgefüllt, können jedoch nach Bedarf angepasst oder übernommen werden. Im ersten Feld, **Name**, legen Sie den Namen der Konfiguration fest. Dieser Wert wird in der Spalte **Name** der Liste der konfigurierten Vertrauensbeziehungen angezeigt. Im zweiten Feld, **Description**, können Sie eine Beschreibung für die Konfiguration hinzufügen. Der dritte Parameter, **Origin Key**, gibt an, wer die Konfiguration erstellt hat. Standardmäßig ist das Feld mit dem Wert **sap.custom** belegt. Der letzte Parameter, **Link text for user logon**, enthält den Text, der später bei der Benutzeranmeldung in der Auswahlliste der Identity Provider angezeigt wird. Wie in Abbildung 2.55 dargestellt, übernehmen wir die meisten Standardwerte. Passen Sie lediglich den **Link text for user logon** wie gezeigt an.

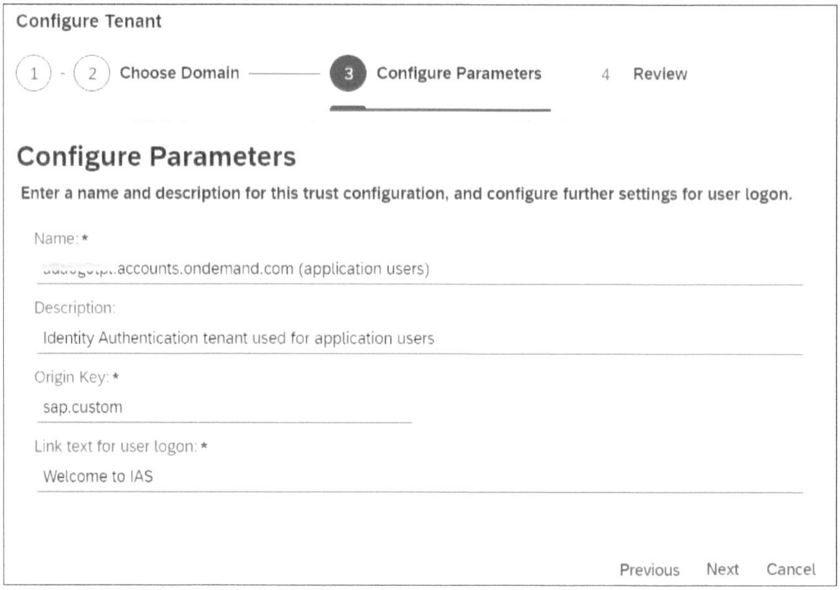

Abbildung 2.55 Festlegen von Parametern für die Identity-Provider-Konfiguration

Bestätigen Sie die Eingaben mit **Next** und Sie erhalten im letzten Schritt eine Übersicht unserer festgelegten Konfigurationsparameter zur Prüfung. Bestätigen Sie zum Abschluss der Konfiguration den Dialog mit einem Klick auf **Finish**.

Trust Configuration

Nachdem die konfigurierte Vertrauensbeziehung angelegt wurde, wird diese wie in Abbildung 2.56 gezeigt aufgelistet.

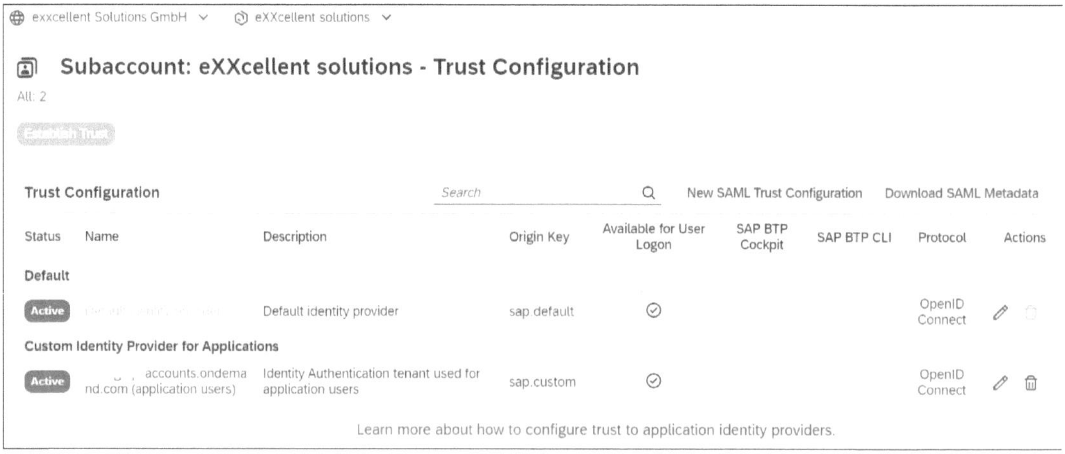

Abbildung 2.56 Liste der konfigurierten Vertrauensbeziehungen

Durch einen Klick auf den als Link dargestellten Namen gelangen wir zur Konfiguration des soeben angelegten kundenspezifischen Identity Providers. Wie in Abbildung 2.57 dargestellt, erhalten wir dabei eine Übersicht über die zuvor angegebenen Konfigurationsparameter sowie über Parameter, die erst nach der Erstellung der Vertrauensbeziehung angepasst werden können. Ein Beispiel für einen solchen Parameter ist **Create Shadow Users on User Logon**, der standardmäßig auf **Yes** gesetzt ist. Dieser Parameter bestimmt, ob bei der Erstanmeldung eines Benutzers, der im angebundenen Identity Provider verwaltet wird, automatisch ein Schattenbenutzer in der Benutzerliste der SAP BTP erstellt werden soll.

Schattenbenutzer

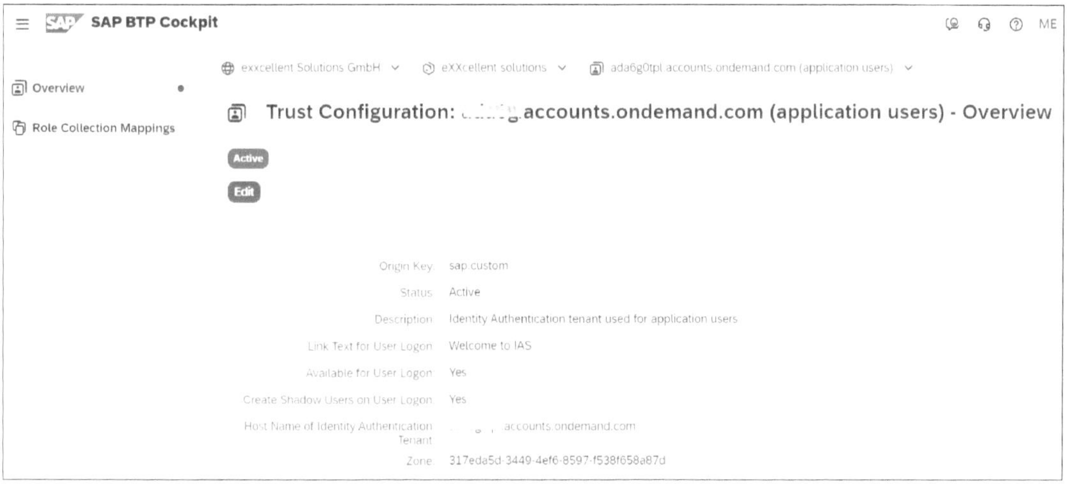

Abbildung 2.57 Übersicht der konfigurierten Vertrauensbeziehung

Die durchgeführte Konfiguration hat nicht nur Auswirkungen auf die SAP BTP. Die durchgeführte Konfiguration führt ebenfalls dazu, dass in den *SAP Cloud Identity Services* nun in der Liste der vertrauenswürdigen Anwendungen die SAP BTP aufgelistet wird. Über den Menüpunkt **Applications & Resources • Applications** gelangen Sie in die Übersicht der registrierten Anwendungen. Abbildung 2.58 zeigt den registrierten SAP-BTP-Subaccount.

Liste der vertrauenswürdigen Anwendungen

Nachdem die Konfiguration abgeschlossen ist, sehen Sie beim Aufrufen von SAP-BTP-Diensten den in Abbildung 2.59 dargestellten Auswahlbildschirm. Der erste Eintrag **Welcome to IAS** bezieht sich auf den von Ihnen konfigurierten Identity Provider. Der zweite Eintrag stellt, wie der Name bereits vermuten lässt, den Standard-Identity-Provider von SAP dar. Je nach Auswahl muss man sich mit dem Benutzer aus dem jeweiligen Identity Provider anmelden. Es ist dabei wichtig zu beachten, dass die Berechtigungen im Fall des eigenen Identity Providers nicht über das SAP BTP Cockpit verwaltet werden, sondern über die SAP Cloud Identity Services.

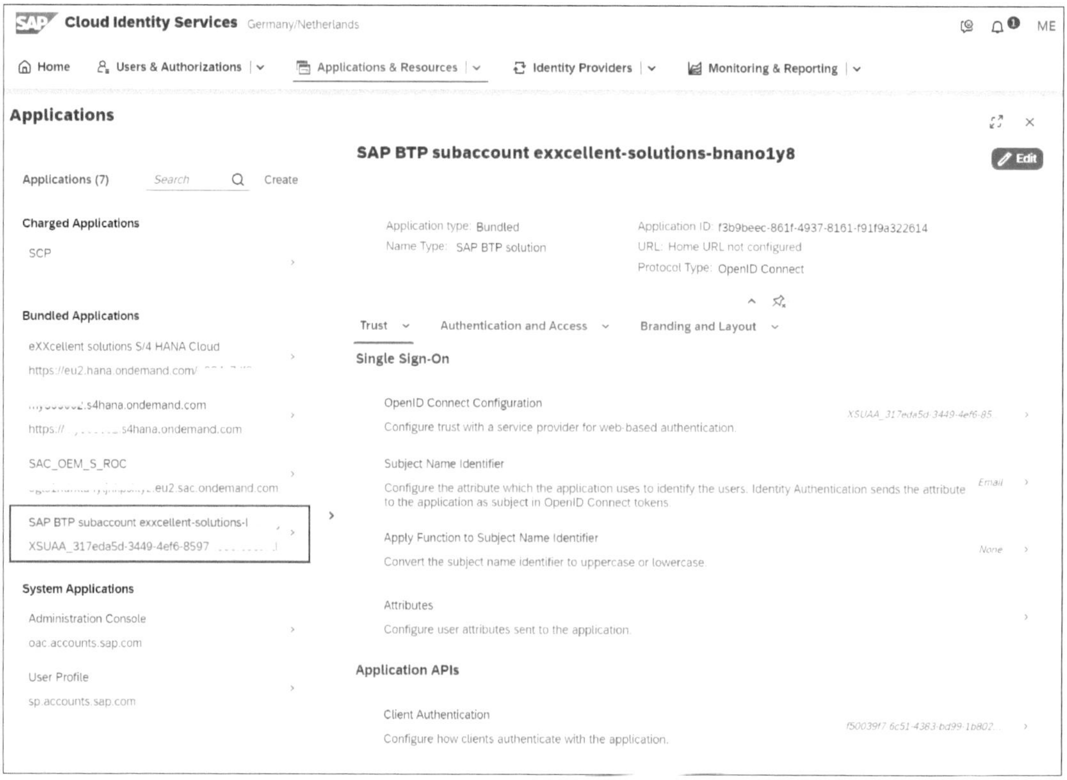

Abbildung 2.58 Registrierter SAP-BTP-Subaccount in den SAP Cloud Identity Services

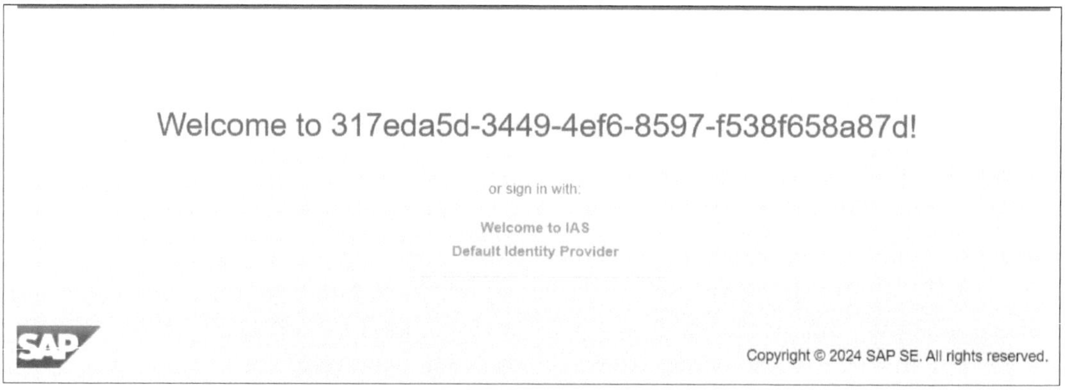

Abbildung 2.59 Auswahl des Identity Providers

2.4 Entwicklungsinfrastruktur aufsetzen

SAP bietet seit Jahren die unterschiedlichsten Entwicklungswerkzeuge für die Implementierung und Erweiterung von kundenindividuellen und SAP-eigenen Lösungen an. So auch für die SAP-Cloud- und On-Premise-Entwicklung. In diesem Abschnitt führen wir in das Entwicklungswerkzeug SAP Business Application Studio ein.

2.4.1 SAP Business Application Studio als Entwicklungsumgebung bereitstellen

Für die Entwicklung von Nicht-ABAP-basierten Lösungen für die Cloud und on-premise stehen grundsätzlich zwei Entwicklungswerkzeuge zur Verfügung:

- SAP Business Application Studio
- Visual Studio Code von Microsoft mit entsprechenden Erweiterungen für die Entwicklung von SAP Cloud Application Programming Model und SAP Fiori bzw. SAPUI5-Anwendungen

SAP Business Application Studio

Das *SAP Business Application Studio* ist ein Entwicklungswerkzeug von SAP, das in der SAP BTP als SAP-BTP-Service angeboten wird. Voraussetzung für die Verwendung der Entwicklungsumgebung ist daher ein Zugang zur SAP BTP. Hier kann sowohl ein kostenpflichtiger Zugang als auch ein sogenannter Free-Tier-Zugang verwendet werden. Der Free-Tier-Zugang ist kostenlos und wird von SAP zu Testzwecken und zum Kennenlernen des SAP-Angebots zur Verfügung gestellt. Es ist jedoch nicht gestattet, produktiv genutzte Anwendungen mit dem Free-Tier-Angebot zu implementieren. Zusätzlich gibt es kleinere Einschränkungen im Funktionsumfang. Weiterführende Informationen zum Angebot und dem Preismodell des SAP-BTP-Service finden Sie im SAP Discovery Center unter *http://s-prs.de/v1032902*.

Nachdem Aufruf der URL gelangen Sie auf die in Abbildung 2.60 gezeigte Informationsseite zum SAP Business Application Studio. Über die Registerkarte **Pricing** liefert SAP einen Preisindikationen für die Verwendung des Entwicklungswerkzeugs.

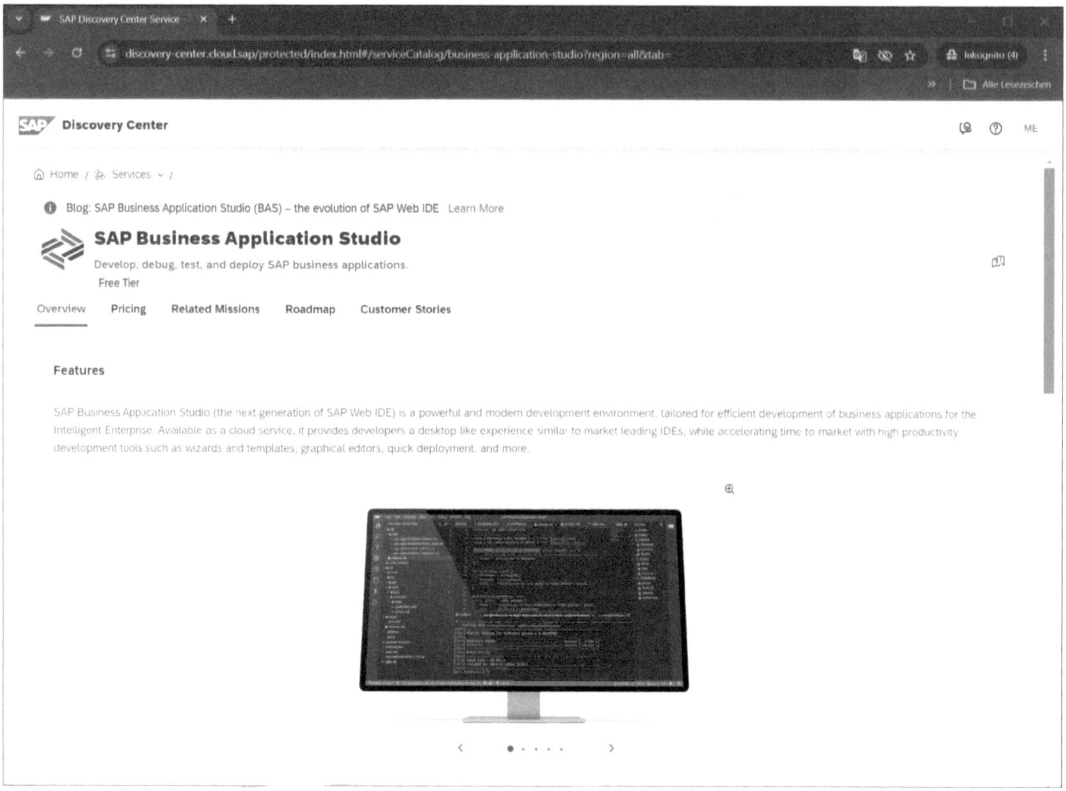

Abbildung 2.60 Informationen zum SAP Business Application Studio im SAP Discovery Center

2.4.2 Voraussetzung für die Verwendung des SAP Business Application Studios

Die Verwendung des SAP Business Application Studios in der SAP BTP setzt voraus, dass der SAP-BTP-Service zunächst in unserem Subaccount aktiviert wird. Voraussetzung für die Aktivierung ist, dass der Service für den Subaccount zur Verfügung steht. Für das SAP Business Application Studio ist dies normalerweise standardmäßig der Fall. Zur Sicherheit überprüfen wir jedoch, ob das sogenannte Entitlement auch vorliegt. Hierzu rufen Sie in Ihrem Subaccount, wie in Abbildung 2.61 gezeigt, den Menüeintrag **Entitlements** auf. Im Anschluss prüfen Sie, ob das SAP Business Application Studio in den vorhandenen Entitlements vorhanden ist. Wie in Abbildung 2.61 erkennbar, ist dies bei uns der Fall.

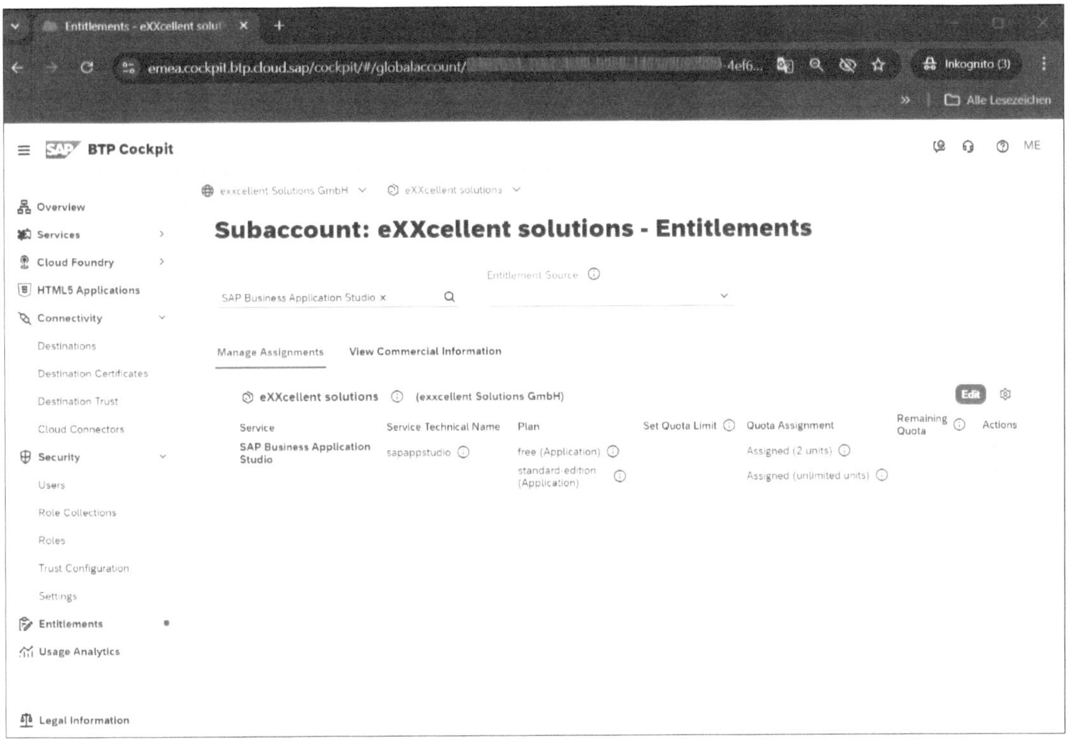

Abbildung 2.61 Entitlement für das SAP Business Application Studio

SAP Business Application Studio abonnieren

Bevor Sie in SAP Business Application Studio arbeiten können, muss der Account Administrator in Ihrem Subaccount das SAP Business Application Studio abonnieren. Das Abonnieren eines SAP-BTP-Service erfolgt über den Menüeintrag **Services • Instances and Subscriptions**. Nachdem die Seite geladen ist, klicken Sie auf den Button **Create**. Es öffnet sich der in Abbildung 2.62 gezeigte Dialog. Hier wählen wir wie in der Abbildung zu sehen zunächst im Feld **Service** den Service **SAP Business Application Studio** aus. Als Nächstes wählen wir aus der Auswahlliste **Plan** den für uns relevanten Serviceplan aus. Falls Sie das Free-Tier-Angebot von SAP nutzen wollen, wählen Sie **free**, falls Sie den nicht kostenlosen Zugriff nutzen wollen, wählen Sie **standard-edition**. Bestätigen Sie die nächsten Dialogschritte jeweils mit **Next** bzw. zum Abschluss mit **Create**.

Nachdem der Plan hinzugefügt und der Service aktiviert wurde, wird dieser, wie in Abbildung 2.63 gezeigt, in der Liste der Subscriptions dargestellt.

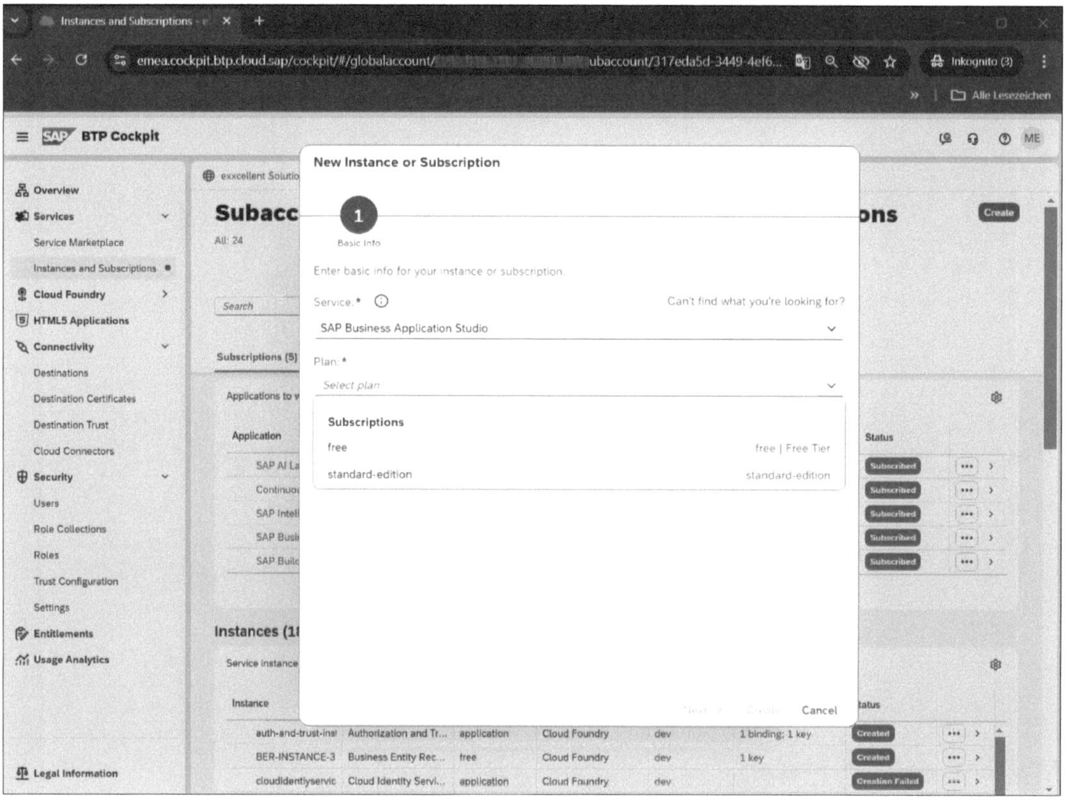

Abbildung 2.62 SAP-Business-Application-Studio-Servicepläne hinzufügen

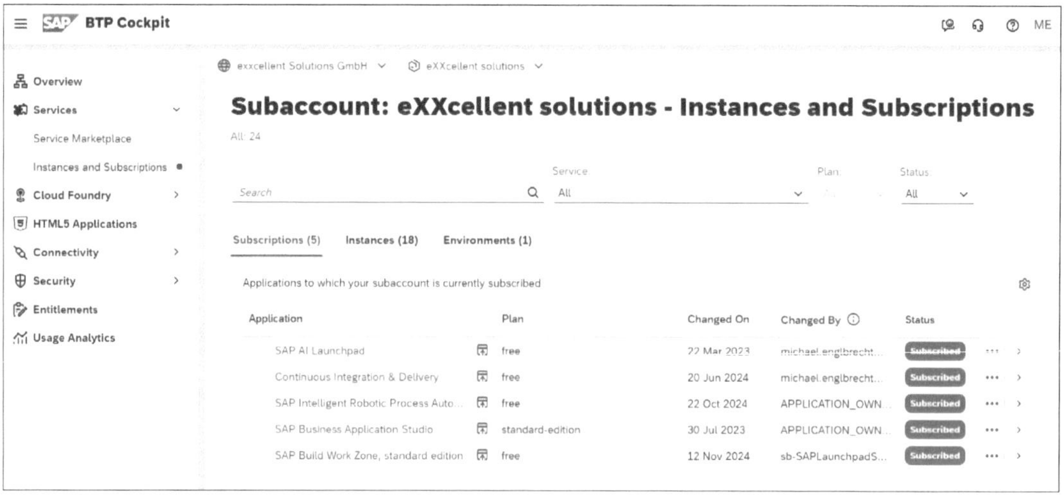

Abbildung 2.63 Aktivierter SAP-Business-Application-Studio-Service

Berechtigungen einrichten

Die Aktivierung des SAP-Business-Application-Studio-Service reicht noch nicht zur Verwendung des Diensts aus. Nachdem der Service aktiv ist, müssen wir die Nutzer noch für die Verwendung des Diensts berechtigen. Um uns zunächst einen Überblick über die vorhandenen Role Collections zu verschaffen, wechseln wir über den Menüpunkt **Security • Role Collection** in die Administration der Role Collections. Im Anschluss filtern Sie, wie in Abbildung 2.64 gezeigt, die Liste aller zur Verfügung stehenden Role Collections, nach dem Begriff »business_Ap«. Wie Sie in Abbildung 2.64 sehen können, gibt es im Moment drei Role Collections die im Zusammenhang mit dem SAP Business Application Studio stehen. Für die Entwicklung sind die beiden Rollen `Business_Application_Studio_Developer` und `Business_Application_Studio_Extension_Deployer` zu verwenden, für administrative Tätigkeiten die Rolle `Business_Application_Studio_Administrator`.

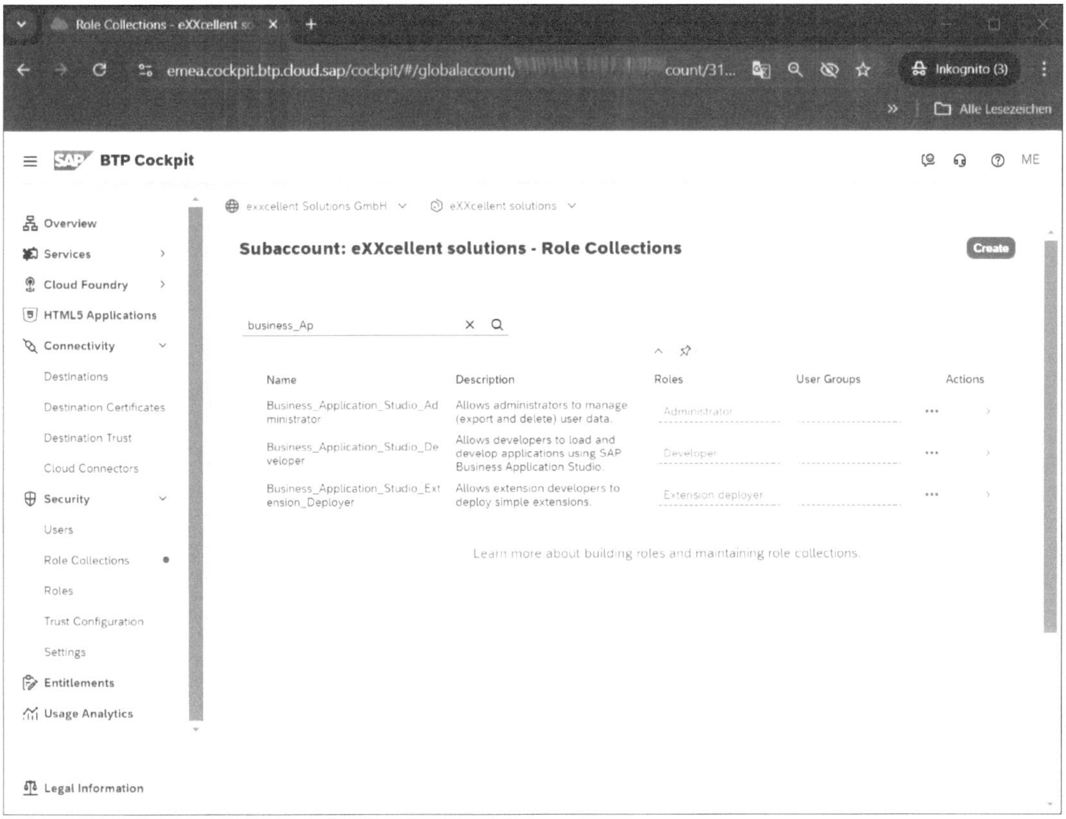

Abbildung 2.64 Role Collections für die Verwendung des SAP Business Application Studios

Die Zuweisung der Role Collection zum Benutzer kann entweder direkt in der Role Collection oder über den Benutzer erfolgen. Wechseln Sie über **Security • Users** zur Administration der SAP-BTP-Benutzer und suchen Sie nach dem entsprechenden Benutzer. Nach der Auswahl werden die Details des Benutzers wie in Abbildung 2.65 gezeigt dargestellt. Wie Sie sehen können, wurde in diesem Beispiel ein Filter bei den zugewiesenen Role Collections angewandt. Der Hintergrund ist, dass der gezeigte Benutzer bereits über eine Vielzahl von Berechtigungen verfügt und es sonst etwas unübersichtlich wäre.

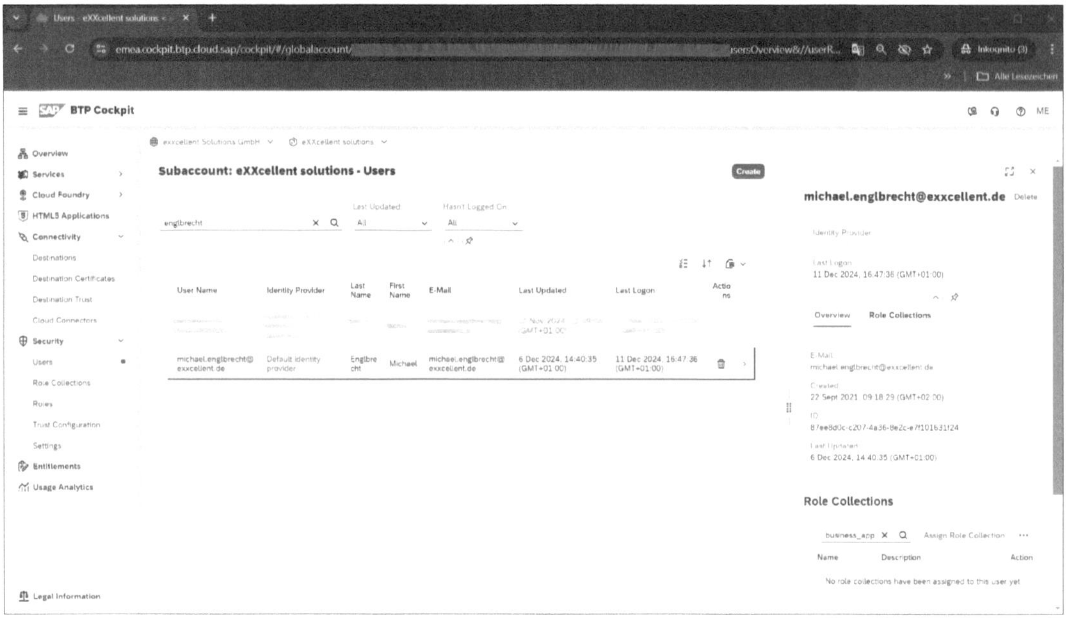

Abbildung 2.65 Benutzer-Details in der SAP BTP

Role Collection zuweisen

Für das Zuweisen von Role Collections klicken Sie auf die Schaltfläche **Assign Role Collection**. Es öffnet sich, wie in Abbildung 2.66 gezeigt, ein Auswahldialog für die verfügbaren Role Collections. Filtern Sie die Liste und wählen Sie im Anschluss, wie in der Abbildung zu sehen, die drei für das SAP Business Application Studio relevanten Role Collections aus. Zum Abschluss klicken Sie auf den Button **Assign Role Collection**.

Nachdem die Role Collections hinzugefügt sind, werden diese wie in Abbildung 2.67 gezeigt in der Role-Collection-Liste des Benutzers angezeigt.

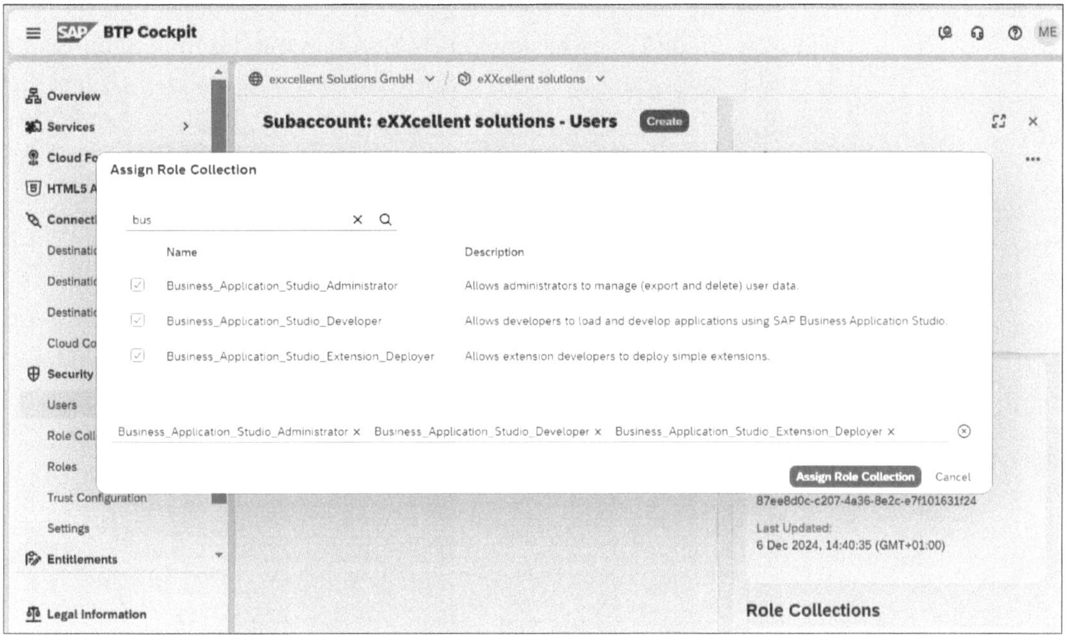

Abbildung 2.66 Auswahldialog für Role Collections

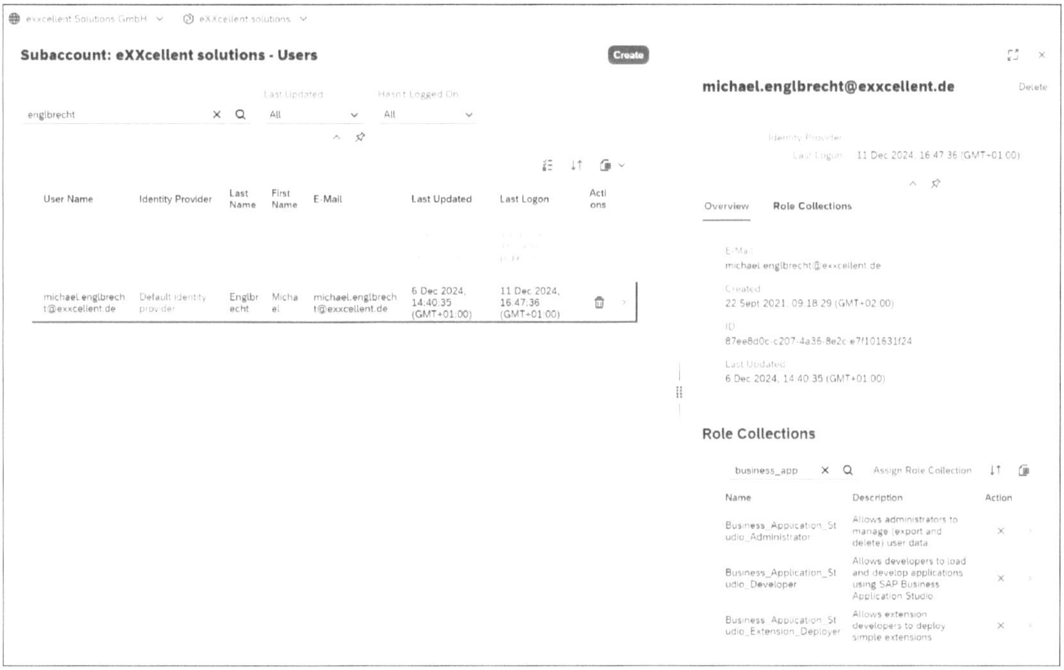

Abbildung 2.67 Zugewiesene Role Collections für die Verwendung des SAP Business Application Studios

Service aufrufen

Nachdem die Berechtigungen vergeben sind, können die so berechtigten Benutzer auf den Service zugreifen. Zusammen mit der in Abschnitt 2.2.3, »Einführung in den Cloud Connector«, durchgeführten Cloud-Connector-Konfiguration kann der Nutzer nun aus dem SAP Business Application Studio auf die über den Cloud Connector angebundenen SAP-Systeme zugreifen.

TEIL II
Schnittstellenprogrammierung auf der ABAP-Plattform

Kapitel 3
Remote Function Call mit ABAP

Dieses Kapitel beschreibt detailliert die Schnittstellenprogrammierung in ABAP mit RFCs und BAPIs. Sie lernen, wie Sie RFC-Funktionsbausteine zum Lesen, Schreiben und Ändern von Datensätzen entwickeln können, und nutzen diese Funktionsbausteine bei der Entwicklung eines Business-Objekts und seiner BAPIs.

Der *Remote Function Call* (RFC) ist die SAP-Schnittstellentechnologie, mit der Funktionsbausteine in einem anderen System aufgerufen werden können. In diesem Kapitel erläutern wir die in Abschnitt 1.4.2, »Remote Function Call (RFC)«, vorgestellten Spielarten des RFC und gehen auf Business-Objekte und ihre Business Application Programming Interfaces (BAPIs) als spezielle RFC-Funktionsbausteine ein. Wir zeigen anhand des Beispiels, das wir in Abschnitt 1.3, »Programmierung auf der ABAP-Plattform«, eingeführt haben, die Programmierung von RFC-Clients und RFC-Servern mit der Programmiersprache ABAP. Funktionsbausteine und die hier beschriebenen BAPIs stellen eine etablierte und gut dokumentierte Technologie da, die oft nötig ist, um mit älteren SAP-Systemen oder Legacy-Code zu arbeiten.

3.1 RFC-Funktionsbausteine in ABAP

Kundenbestellungen bearbeiten

Im Folgenden entwickeln Sie einige Funktionsbausteine in ABAP, mit denen Sie Kundenbestellungen anlegen, ändern und löschen können. Diese Funktionsbausteine sollen von externen Systemen verwendbar, also RFC-fähige Funktionsbausteine sein. Sie legen für diese Funktionsbausteine die Funktionsgruppe `ZIFP` im Kundennamensraum an. Zur Erinnerung: Funktionsgruppen sind ein spezieller Typ von ABAP-Programmen, die Funktionsbausteine enthalten.

3.1.1 Funktionsbausteine zum Lesen

Zuerst legen Sie Funktionsbausteine zum Lesen von Kundenaufträgen und Lieferantenbestellungen an. Jede Bestellung ist eindeutig durch ihre `ORDERID` definiert. Dem Besteller ist diese `ORDERID` jedoch in der Regel nicht bekannt, da sie beim Anlegen eines Kundenauftrags auf Lieferantenseite erstellt wird. Daher benötigen Sie zunächst einmal einen Funktionsbaustein, der Ihnen eine Tabelle sämtlicher Bestellnummern (ORDERID) bei gegebenem Bestelltyp und optionaler REFID (die Kundenbestellnummer) liefert. Wird nur der Bestelltyp angegeben, gibt der Funktionsbaustein alle Bestellnummern dieses Typs zurück. Wird die REFID angegeben, gibt der Funktionsbaustein die Lieferantenbestellnummer zu einer Kundenbestellnummer zurück. Listing 3.1 zeigt den Quellcode des Funktionsbausteins Z_IFP_ORER_GETLIST, der diese Aufgabe erledigt.

```
FUNCTION z_ifp_order_getlist.
*"----------------------------------------------------------
*"*"Lokale Schnittstelle:
*"  IMPORTING
*"     VALUE(IM_ORDERTYPE) TYPE  ZIFPORDERTYPE DEFAULT 'SO'
*"     VALUE(IM_REFID)     TYPE  ZIFPREFID OPTIONAL
*"  TABLES
*"      TA_ORDERS STRUCTURE  ZIFPORDER
*"  EXCEPTIONS
*"      NOT_AUTHORIZED
*"      NO_DATA
*"----------------------------------------------------------
  AUTHORITY-CHECK OBJECT 'ZIFPORDER' ID 'ACTVT' FIELD '03'.
  IF sy-subrc NE 0.
    RAISE not_authorized.
  ENDIF.
  IF NOT im_refid IS INITIAL.
* Bestellungen mit gegebener REFID selektieren
    SELECT * FROM zifporder INTO TABLE ta_orders WHERE
      type  = im_ordertype AND
      refid = im_refid.
  ELSE.
* Bestellungen ohne REFID selektieren
    SELECT * FROM zifporder INTO TABLE ta_orders WHERE
      type  = im_ordertype.
  ENDIF.
  IF sy-subrc NE 0.
    RAISE no_data.
  ENDIF.
ENDFUNCTION.
```

Listing 3.1 Funktionsbaustein »Z_IFP_ORDER_GETLIST«

Dieser Funktionsbaustein definiert in seiner Schnittstelle die beiden optionalen Importparameter IM_ORDERTYPE und IM_REFID. IM_ORDERTYPE ist mit dem Vorschlagswert »SO« (für Sales Order, Kundenauftrag) versehen, sodass der Funktionsbaustein nach Kundenaufträgen sucht, falls IM_ORDERTYPE beim Aufruf nicht explizit mit 'PO' (für Purchase Order, Lieferantenbestellung) belegt wird. Die gefundenen Bestellungen schreibt der Funktionsbaustein in den Tabellenparameter TA_ORDERS.

Berechtigungsprüfung

Der Funktionsbaustein prüft zunächst, ob der Aufrufer die Berechtigung hat, Bestellungen zu lesen. Darf der Aufrufer keine Bestellungen lesen, löst der Funktionsbaustein die Ausnahme NOT_AUTHORIZED aus. Danach liest der Funktionsbaustein über einen SELECT-Befehl Bestellungen aus der Datenbank und berücksichtigt dabei in der WHERE-Klausel die Importparameter. Findet er keine Daten, löst er die Ausnahme NO_DATA aus.

Bestellungsdetails

Der nächste Funktionsbaustein, Z_IFP_ORDER_GETDETAIL, liefert Details zu einer Bestellung bei bekannter ORDERID. Listing 3.2 zeigt den Quellcode dieses Funktionsbausteins. Die Schnittstelle definiert einen Importparameter für die ORDERID, einen Exportparameter für den Bestellkopf, einen Tabellenparameter für die Bestellpositionen sowie die Ausnahmen NOT_AUTHORIZED und NO_DATA.

```
FUNCTION z_ifp_order_getdetail.
*"------------------------------------------------------------
*"*"Lokale Schnittstelle:
*"  IMPORTING
*"     VALUE(IM_ORDERID)    TYPE  ZIFPORDERID
*"  EXPORTING
*"     VALUE(EX_ORDERHEAD) TYPE  ZIFPORDER
*"  TABLES
*"     TA_ORDERPOS STRUCTURE  ZIFPORDERPOS
*"  EXCEPTIONS
*"     NOT_AUTHORIZED
*"     NO_DATA
*"------------------------------------------------------------
  AUTHORITY-CHECK OBJECT 'ZIFPORDER' ID 'ACTVT' FIELD '03'.
  IF sy-subrc NE 0.
    RAISE not_authorized.
  ENDIF.
* Bestellkopf lesen
  SELECT SINGLE * FROM zifporder INTO ex_orderhead
    WHERE orderid = im_orderid.
  IF sy-subrc NE 0.
    RAISE no_data.
```

```
  ELSE.
* Bestellpositionen lesen
    SELECT * FROM zifporderpos INTO TABLE ta_orderpos
      WHERE orderid = im_orderid.
  ENDIF.
ENDFUNCTION.
```

Listing 3.2 Funktionsbaustein »Z_IFP_ORDER_GETDETAIL«

Skalare und strukturierte Parameter

Der Importparameter IM_ORDERID muss beim Aufruf die ORDERID der gewünschten Bestellung enthalten. Der Importparameter ist vom Typ ZIFPORDERID, bezieht sich demnach direkt auf ein Datenelement. Daher ist er ein sogenannter *skalarer Parameter*. Der Exportparameter EX_ORDERHEAD enthält nach dem Aufruf die Kopfdaten der Bestellung und der Tabellenparameter TA_ORDERPOS die Bestellpositionen.

Wird im Importparameter IM_ORDERID eine nicht vorhandene ORDERID eingegeben, wird die Ausnahme NO_DATA ausgelöst, und Export- und Tabellenparameter bleiben initial. Der Exportparameter ist vom Typ ZIFPORDER; er bezieht sich demnach auf eine transparente Tabelle im ABAP Dictionary. Er ist ein *strukturierter Parameter.*

Übergabe per Wert

Sowohl Import- als auch Exportparameter eines RFC-fähigen Funktionsbausteins müssen per Wert übergeben werden. Eine Referenzübergabe ist nicht möglich. Achten Sie auch bei den Funktionsbausteinen darauf, dass bei den Eigenschaften das Optionsfeld **Remote** ausgewählt ist.

3.1.2 Aufruf per sRFC

»CALL FUNCTION ... DESTINATION«

Listing 3.3 zeigt den Quelltext eines Reports, der die beiden Funktionsbausteine über sRFC aufruft. Dies läuft über die ABAP-Anweisung CALL FUNCTION ... DESTINATION p_dest ... ab. Die Variable p_dest wurde mit der PARAMETERS-Anweisung deklariert und ist vom Typ RFCDEST. Die PARAMETERS-Anweisung sorgt dafür, dass für den Report ein Selektionsbild generiert wird, das beim Start angezeigt wird. Das Selektionsbild enthält ein Eingabefeld, in das der Benutzer einen Wert für die Variable p_dest eingeben kann. Der Wert muss der Name einer gültigen RFC-Destination sein, die mittels Transaktion SM59 gepflegt wurde.

```
REPORT  zifp_orders_read.
DATA:
  it_orderhead TYPE STANDARD TABLE OF zifporder,
  wa_orderhead TYPE zifporder,
  it_orderpos  TYPE STANDARD TABLE OF zifporderpos,
```

```
  wa_orderpos  TYPE zifporderpos,
  msg_text(80) TYPE c.
PARAMETERS:
  p_dest TYPE rfcdest.
START-OF-SELECTION.
* ORDERID-Liste besorgen
  CALL FUNCTION 'Z_IFP_ORDER_GETLIST'
    DESTINATION p_dest
    TABLES
      ta_orders             = it_orderhead
    EXCEPTIONS
      not_authorized        = 1
      no_data               = 2
      system_failure        = 3  MESSAGE msg_text
      communication_failure = 4  MESSAGE msg_text
      OTHERS                = 5.
  IF sy-subrc <> 0.
    WRITE:/ msg_text.
  ENDIF.
* alle Bestellungen ausgeben
  LOOP AT it_orderhead INTO wa_orderhead.
    WRITE:/
      wa_orderhead-orderid COLOR COL_KEY,
      wa_orderhead-type,
      wa_orderhead-refid,
      wa_orderhead-buyer,
      wa_orderhead-seller,
      wa_orderhead-orderdate.
* Bestelldetails besorgen
    CALL FUNCTION 'Z_IFP_ORDER_GETDETAIL'
      DESTINATION p_dest
      EXPORTING
        im_orderid            = wa_orderhead-orderid
*   IMPORTING
*     EX_ORDERHEAD            =
      TABLES
        ta_orderpos           = it_orderpos
    EXCEPTIONS
      not_authorized          = 1
      no_data                 = 2
      system_failure          = 3  MESSAGE msg_text
      communication_failure   = 4  MESSAGE msg_text
      OTHERS                  = 5.
```

```
    IF sy-subrc <> 0.
      WRITE:/ msg_text.
    ENDIF.
* Bestelldetails ausgeben
    LOOP AT it_orderpos INTO wa_orderpos.
      WRITE:/
        wa_orderpos-orderid COLOR COL_KEY,
        wa_orderpos-orderpos COLOR COL_KEY,
        wa_orderpos-matid,
        wa_orderpos-mattext,
        wa_orderpos-ordercount,
        wa_orderpos-price,
        wa_orderpos-currency.
    ENDLOOP.
    ULINE.
  ENDLOOP.
```

Listing 3.3 Report »ZIFP_ORDERS_READ«

Systemausnahmen

Wie der Quellcode in Listing 3.3 veranschaulicht, sollte der Aufrufer nicht nur auf Ausnahmen reagieren, die in der Schnittstelle der Funktionsbausteine definiert werden, sondern zusätzlich auch auf die beiden Systemausnahmen `system_failure` und `communication_failure`. Die Ausnahme `system_failure` wird bei Systemfehlern z. B. dann ausgelöst, wenn der aufgerufene Funktionsbaustein im Zielsystem nicht existiert. Die Ausnahme `communication_failure` wird bei Kommunikationsfehlern ausgelöst, z. B. wenn das Zielsystem nicht erreichbar ist oder die angegebene Destination nicht gepflegt wurde. Bei beiden Fehlern kann über den `MESSAGE`-Zusatz die Systemnachricht in einer Variablen vom Typ `C` gespeichert werden, um damit Systeminformationen über den Fehler anzeigen zu können.

Standarddestinationen

Neben den Destinationen, die mit Transaktion SM59 gepflegt werden, gibt es noch die drei Standarddestinationen `SPACE`, `'NONE'` und `'BACK'`. Ist `p_dest` initial bzw. wird stattdessen die Konstante `SPACE` verwendet, wird der Funktionsbaustein lokal aufgerufen. Enthält `p_dest` den Wert »NONE«, wird der Funktionsbaustein ebenfalls lokal aufgerufen. Allerdings wird der Aufruf zum Gateway der aktuellen SAP-Instanz geleitet und so behandelt, als ob er von außen käme. Steht Ihnen nur ein System zur Verfügung, können Sie diese Destination für einen RFC-Test verwenden. Möchten Sie aus einem RFC-Baustein einen Funktionsbaustein im rufenden System aufrufen, können Sie dazu die Destination `'BACK'` verwenden. Sie dient zum Rückruf in den Aufrufer.

Impliziter Datenbank-Commit

Nach jedem CALL FUNCTION erfolgt auf dem rufenden System implizit ein Commit auf der Datenbank. Änderungen an der Datenbank, die vor dem Funktionsaufruf mit INSERT, UPDATE, MODIFY oder DELETE vorgenommen wurden, können danach nicht mehr rückgängig gemacht werden. Auch im aufgerufenen System findet ein impliziter Commit in der Datenbank statt, d. h., jeder RFC-Funktionsaufruf entspricht einem Dialogschritt. Daher eignet sich der synchrone RFC in dieser Form nur zum Lesen, nicht aber dazu, systemübergreifende Transaktionen zu realisieren.

3.1.3 Funktionsbausteine zum Löschen und Ändern

Bestelldaten ändern

Listing 3.4 zeigt den Quellcode des Funktionsbausteins Z_IFP_ORDER_CHANGE, mit dessen Hilfe die Daten einer Bestellung geändert werden können.

```
FUNCTION z_ifp_order_change.
*"----------------------------------------------------------
*"*"Lokale Schnittstelle:
*"  IMPORTING
*"     VALUE(IM_ORDERHEADER)  TYPE  ZIFPORDER
*"     VALUE(IM_ORDERHEADERX) TYPE  ZIFPORDERX
*"     VALUE(IM_TESTRUN)      TYPE  CHAR1 DEFAULT SPACE
*"     VALUE(IM_COMMIT)       TYPE  CHAR1 DEFAULT SPACE
*"  TABLES
*"      TA_ORDERPOS  STRUCTURE  ZIFPORDERPOS
*"      TA_ORDERPOSX STRUCTURE  ZIFPORDERPOSX
*"  EXCEPTIONS
*"      NOT_AUTHORIZED
*"      NO_DATA
*"      NO_LOCK
*"----------------------------------------------------------
  DATA:
    orderheader_old TYPE zifporder,
    orderpos_old    TYPE zifporderpos,
    orderpos_new    TYPE zifporderpos,
    orderposx       TYPE zifporderposx.
  AUTHORITY-CHECK OBJECT 'ZIFPORDER' ID 'ACTVT' FIELD '02'.
  IF sy-subrc NE 0.
    RAISE not_authorized.
  ENDIF.
* Sperre setzen
  CALL FUNCTION 'ENQUEUE_EZIFPORDER'
    EXPORTING
```

```
        orderid = im_orderheader-orderid
      EXCEPTIONS
        OTHERS   = 1.
    IF sy-subrc <> 0.
      RAISE no_lock.
    ENDIF.
*   Kopfdaten lesen
    SELECT SINGLE * FROM zifporder
      INTO orderheader_old
      WHERE orderid = im_orderheader-orderid.
    IF sy-subrc <> 0.
*   nichts gefunden: Sperre entfernen
      CALL FUNCTION 'DEQUEUE_EZIFPORDER'
        EXPORTING
          orderid = im_orderheader-orderid.
      RAISE no_data.
    ELSE.
      IF im_testrun IS INITIAL.
*   Änderungen in Kopfdaten vornehmen
        IF NOT im_orderheaderx-type IS INITIAL.
          orderheader_old-type      = im_orderheader-type.
        ENDIF.
        IF NOT im_orderheaderx-refid IS INITIAL.
          orderheader_old-refid     = im_orderheader-refid.
        ENDIF.
        IF NOT im_orderheaderx-buyer IS INITIAL.
          orderheader_old-buyer     = im_orderheader-buyer.
        ENDIF.
        IF NOT im_orderheaderx-seller IS INITIAL.
          orderheader_old-seller    = im_orderheader-seller.

        ENDIF.
        IF NOT im_orderheaderx-orderdate IS INITIAL.
          orderheader_old-orderdate =
            im_orderheader-orderdate.
        ENDIF.
*   Verbuchungsbaustein für Kopfdaten aufrufen
        CALL FUNCTION 'Z_IFP_V_UPDATE_ORDER'
          IN UPDATE TASK
          EXPORTING
            im_orderheader = orderheader_old.
      ENDIF.
    ENDIF.
```

```
* Schleife über die zu ändernden Bestellpositionen
  LOOP AT ta_orderpos INTO orderpos_new.
    READ TABLE ta_orderposx INTO orderposx INDEX sy-index.
* Bestellposition von Datenbank lesen
    SELECT SINGLE * FROM zifporderpos
      INTO orderpos_old
      WHERE
      orderid  = orderpos_new-orderid AND
      orderpos = orderpos_new-orderpos.
    IF sy-subrc <> 0.
* nichts gefunden: Sperre lösen
      CALL FUNCTION 'DEQUEUE_EZIFPORDER'
        EXPORTING
          orderid = im_orderheader-orderid.
      ROLLBACK WORK.
      RAISE no_data.
    ELSE.
      IF im_testrun IS INITIAL.
* Bestellposition wie gewünscht ändern
        IF NOT orderposx-matid IS INITIAL.
          orderpos_old-matid      = orderpos_new-matid.
        ENDIF.
        IF NOT orderposx-mattext IS INITIAL.
          orderpos_old-mattext    = orderpos_new-mattext.
        ENDIF.
        IF NOT orderposx-ordercount IS INITIAL.
          orderpos_old-ordercount = orderpos_new-ordercount.
        ENDIF.
        IF NOT orderposx-price IS INITIAL.
          orderpos_old-price      = orderpos_new-price.
        ENDIF.
        IF NOT orderposx-currency IS INITIAL.
          orderpos_old-currency   = orderpos_new-currency.
        ENDIF.
* Verbuchungsbaustein für Bestellposition aufrufen
        CALL FUNCTION 'Z_IFP_V_UPDATE_ORDERPOS'
          IN UPDATE TASK
          EXPORTING
            im_orderpos = orderpos_old.
      ENDIF.
    ENDIF.
  ENDLOOP.
```

```
* falls gewünscht, COMMIT WORK absetzen
  IF im_commit = 'X'.
    COMMIT WORK.
    CALL FUNCTION 'DEQUEUE_ALL'.
  ENDIF.
ENDFUNCTION.
```

Listing 3.4 Funktionsbaustein »Z_IFP_ORDER_CHANGE«

Der Funktionsbaustein hat den strukturierten Importparameter IM_ORDER_HEADER für die Kopfdaten und den Tabellenparameter TA_ORDERPOS für die Positionsdaten der Bestellung. Über das Feld IM_ORDER_HEADER-ORDERID wird die Bestellung eindeutig identifiziert. Der Funktionsbaustein nimmt die Datenbankänderungen nicht direkt vor, sondern ruft die Verbuchungsbausteine aus Abschnitt 1.3.5, »Verbuchungsbausteine«, mit dem Zusatz IN UPDATE TASK auf. Der optionale Importparameter IM_COMMIT steuert, ob der Funktionsbaustein selbst ein COMMIT WORK absetzt.

X-Parameter mit Änderungskennzeichen

Für jeden Importparameter mit den zu ändernden Daten hat der Funktionsbaustein einen zweiten Importparameter. In diesem zweiten Parameter kann der Aufrufer angeben, welche der übergebenen Daten im ersten Parameter tatsächlich geändert werden sollen. Dies ist notwendig, da ABAP keine »NULL«-Werte kennt und deshalb einem RFC-Funktionsbaustein keine »NULL«-Werte in den Parametern übergeben werden können. Ist ein Importparameter initial, kann daher der Funktionsbaustein nicht entscheiden, ob der Aufrufer den entsprechenden Wert in der Datenbank auf den Initialwert ändern möchte oder ob die Daten nicht geändert werden sollen.

Der Funktionsbaustein hat daher die beiden zusätzlichen Parameter IM_ORDERHEADERX und TA_ORDERPOSX. Der Importparameter IM_ORDERHEADERX ist vom Typ ZIFPORDERX. Dieser Typ hat bis auf MANDT und ORDERID die gleichen Komponenten wie die transparente Tabelle ZIFPORDER; allerdings sind alle Komponenten vom Typ CHAR1. Eine Komponente des Parameters IM_ORDERHEADERX ist mit 'X' belegt, wenn der Wert der jeweiligen Komponente des Bestellkopfs durch den Wert im Importparameter IM_ORDERHEADER ersetzt werden soll. Entsprechendes gilt für den Importparameter TA_ORDERPOSX, der vom Zeilentyp ZIFPORDERPOSX ist.

Exklusive Schreibsperre

Zunächst prüft der Funktionsbaustein, ob der Aufrufer die Berechtigung zum Ändern von Bestellungen hat. Falls nicht, löst er die Ausnahme NOT_AUTHORIZED aus. Ist der Aufrufer berechtigt, eine Bestellung zu ändern, setzt der Funktionsbaustein eine exklusive Schreibsperre auf die Bestellung und all ihre Positionen. Schlägt das Setzen der Sperre fehl, wird die Ausnahme NO_LOCK ausgelöst, und es werden keine Änderungen vorgenommen. Konnte die Sperre erfolgreich gesetzt werden, werden die Änderungen vorgenommen.

Vor dem Aufruf der Verbuchungsbausteine prüft der Funktionsbaustein, ob die Bestellung und die Bestellpositionen existieren. Falls nicht, wird die Sperre wieder gelöscht, ein ROLLBACK WORK initiiert und die Ausnahme NO_DATA ausgelöst.

Am Schluss überprüft der Funktionsbaustein den Importparameter IM_COMMIT. Falls dieser Parameter mit 'X' belegt wird, führt der Funktionsbaustein ein COMMIT WORK aus und löst die gesetzten Sperren. Auf diese Art und Weise können mehrere Änderungen in einer Logical Unit of Work (LUW) vorgenommen werden. Erst der letzte Funktionsbaustein in der Änderungsserie muss dann mit IM_COMMIT = 'X' versorgt werden. Die Verwendung von Verbuchungsbausteinen innerhalb einer SAP-LUW haben wir in Abschnitt 1.3.5, »Verbuchungsbausteine«, erläutert.

Daten löschen

Die Funktionsbausteine Z_IFP_ORDER_DELETE und Z_IFP_ORDER_DELETEPOS zum Löschen einer Bestellung und zum Löschen einer Bestellposition sind analog aufgebaut, nur werden diesmal nicht die kompletten Daten übergeben, sondern lediglich die ORDERID und die ORDERPOS. Diese identifizieren die zu löschenden Datensätze eindeutig. Listing 3.5 zeigt den Funktionsbaustein Z_IFP_ORDER_DELETE.

```
FUNCTION Z_IFP_ORDER_DELETE.
*"----------------------------------------------------------
*"*"Lokale Schnittstelle:
*"  IMPORTING
*"     VALUE(IM_ORDERID) TYPE  ZIFPORDERID
*"     VALUE(IM_COMMIT)  TYPE  CHAR1 DEFAULT SPACE
*"  EXCEPTIONS
*"      NOT_AUTHORIZED
*"      NO_DATA
*"      NO_LOCK
*"----------------------------------------------------------
  AUTHORITY-CHECK OBJECT 'ZIFPORDER' ID 'ACTVT' FIELD '06'.
  IF sy-subrc NE 0.
    RAISE not_authorized.
  ENDIF.
* Sperre setzen
  CALL FUNCTION 'ENQUEUE_EZIFPORDER'
    EXPORTING
      orderid = im_orderid
    exceptions
```

```
      others   = 1.
    IF sy-subrc <> 0.
      RAISE no_lock.
    ENDIF.
* Datensatz lesen
    SELECT SINGLE COUNT( * ) FROM zifporder
      WHERE orderid = im_orderid.
    IF sy-subrc <> 0.
* nicht gefunden: Sperre lösen
      CALL FUNCTION 'DEQUEUE_EZIFPORDER'
        EXPORTING
          orderid = im_orderid.
      RAISE no_data.
    ELSE.
* Verbuchungsbaustein zum Löschen aufrufen
      CALL FUNCTION 'Z_IFP_V_DELETE_ORDER'
        IN UPDATE TASK
        EXPORTING
          im_orderid = im_orderid.
    ENDIF.
    IF im_commit = 'X'.
* falls gewünscht, COMMIT WORK absetzen und Sperre lösen
      COMMIT WORK.
      CALL FUNCTION 'DEQUEUE_ALL'.
    ENDIF.
ENDFUNCTION.
```

Listing 3.5 Funktionsbaustein »Z_IFP_ORDER_DELETE«

Aufruf über sRFC

Der Aufruf dieser drei Funktionsbausteine kann mit dem synchronen RFC vorgenommen werden. Im Fall der Exception `communication_failure` kann der Aufruf später problemlos wiederholt werden. Denn selbst wenn die Funktionsbausteine trotz des Kommunikationsfehlers auf dem Zielsystem ausgeführt wurden, ändert ein nochmaliger Aufruf nichts am Zustand der Datenbank im Zielsystem. Im schlechtesten Fall wird der Datensatz unnötigerweise nochmals geändert, d. h., es wird versucht, einen schon gelöschten Datensatz nochmals zu löschen.

3.2 Transaktionaler RFC

Aufruf über tRFC

Wie Abschnitt 3.1, »RFC-Funktionsbausteine in ABAP«, erläutert, ist es problematisch, Datensätze in einem entfernten System mittels sRFC zu ändern oder zu löschen. Das Anlegen von Datensätzen per sRFC ist noch heikler, da nun im Fehlerfall der Aufruf nicht einfach wiederholt werden kann, weil sonst möglicherweise Datensätze doppelt angelegt würden.

Besser ist es daher, die Funktionsbausteine, die Daten ändern oder neu anlegen, mit einem transaktionalen RFC aufzurufen. Transaktional bedeutet in diesem Fall, dass im aufrufenden System die übergebenen Parameter gespeichert werden und der Aufruf mit Transaktion SM58 nochmals wiederholt werden kann.

»IN BACKGROUND TASK«

Einen tRFC-Aufruf realisieren Sie dadurch, dass Sie beim Aufruf den Zusatz `IN BACKGROUND TASK` verwenden. Dieser Zusatz muss vor dem `DESTINATION`-Zusatz stehen. Zum Zeitpunkt des Aufrufs wird der Funktionsbaustein auf dem Zielsystem noch nicht ausgeführt, sondern der Aufruf wird mitsamt seinen Parametern und einer Transaktions-ID in den Tabellen `ARFCSSTATE` und `ARFCSDATA` im lokalen System gespeichert. Erst beim `COMMIT WORK` erfolgt der Aufruf im Zielsystem. Ist der Aufruf erfolgreich, werden die Einträge in den Vormerktabellen `ARFCSSTATE` und `ARFCSDATA` gelöscht.

Verhalten im Fehlerfall

Ist das Zielsystem nicht erreichbar, kann automatisch ein Job erzeugt werden, der den Aufruf mit derselben Transaktions-ID wiederholt. Die Anzahl der Wiederholungsversuche und die Länge des Intervalls zwischen den Wiederholungen werden bei der Pflege der Destination mit Transaktion SM59 bei den tRFC-Optionen hinterlegt. Es empfiehlt sich jedoch eher, die tRFC-Statustabellen mit Transaktion SM58 regelmäßig zu überwachen und abgebrochene Aufrufe von dort aus manuell zu wiederholen, nachdem das Kommunikationsproblem beseitigt worden ist.

Bricht der Remote-Funktionsbaustein mit einem Fehler ab, führt das Zielsystem automatisch den Befehl `ROLLBACK WORK` aus. Auf dem aufrufenden System wird kein Job zur Wiederholung des Aufrufs eingeplant. Der Fehler, der im Zielsystem aufgetreten ist, wird in den tRFC-Statustabellen protokolliert. Auch in diesem Fall kann der abgebrochene Aufruf aus Transaktion SM58 wiederholt werden.

Falls mit dem Befehl `COMMIT WORK` auch die lokale Verbuchung angestoßen wird, wird die LUW im Zielsystem nur dann ausgeführt, wenn die lokale Verbuchung fehlerfrei abgeschlossen wurde. Beim Aufruf mit dem Zusatz `IN BACKGROUND TASK` können Sie weder den Zusatz `EXPORTING` verwenden noch auf Ausnahmen hin testen, die in der Schnittstelle des Funktionsbausteins definiert wurden. Beides steht erst fest, wenn der Funktionsbaustein im Zielsystem tatsächlich ausgeführt wurde, und dies ist frühestens nach dem `COMMIT WORK` der Fall.

Spezielle Funktionsbausteine

Alle Funktionsbausteine, die im Quellsystem mit dem Zusatz IN BACKGROUND TASK aufgerufen werden, bilden im Zielsystem eine LUW. Sie werden im Zielsystem innerhalb einer einzigen Datenbanktransaktion abgearbeitet. Bricht ein Funktionsbaustein ab, erfolgt automatisch ein ROLLBACK im Zielsystem. Die LUW wird durch eine Transaktions-ID identifiziert. Diese Transaktions-ID kann im aufrufenden System über den Funktionsbaustein ID_OF_BACKGROUNDTASK ermittelt werden, der vor dem COMMIT WORK aufgerufen werden muss. Mit dem Funktionsbaustein STATUS_OF_BACKGROUNDTASK kann unter Angabe der Transaktions-ID der Ausführungsstatus der LUW ermittelt werden. Dieser Funktionsbaustein muss im lokalen System nach dem COMMIT WORK aufgerufen werden. Soll die LUW im Zielsystem nicht sofort ausgeführt werden, können Sie vor dem COMMIT WORK Datum und Uhrzeit der Ausführung über den Funktionsbaustein START_OF_BACKGROUNDTASK festlegen.

Bei den beiden vorliegenden Funktionsbausteinen kann der Fall eintreten, dass der betreffende Datensatz gesperrt ist. Dann brechen die beiden Funktionsbausteine mit einem RAISE ab. Wie beschrieben, können Sie in Transaktion SM58 die LUW nochmals ausführen lassen. Alternativ könnten Sie aber auch den Funktionsbaustein RESTART_OF_BACKGROUNDTASK aufrufen, damit im rufenden System der Job wieder eingeplant wird.

Funktionsbausteine zum Anlegen

Listing 3.6 zeigt einen Funktionsbaustein, mit dem eine Bestellung angelegt werden kann. Als Importparameter werden die Details der neu anzulegenden Bestellung übergeben. Der Funktionsbaustein prüft wie üblich, ob der Aufrufer eine Bestellung anlegen kann. Danach erzeugt er eine Bestellnummer, die er im Exportparameter EX_ORDERID zurückgibt.

```
FUNCTION z_ifp_order_create.
*"----------------------------------------------------------
*"*"Lokale Schnittstelle:
*"  IMPORTING
*"     VALUE(IM_ORDERHEADER) TYPE  ZIFPORDER
*"     VALUE(IM_TESTRUN)     TYPE  CHAR1 DEFAULT SPACE
*"     VALUE(IM_COMMIT)      TYPE  CHAR1 DEFAULT SPACE
*"  EXPORTING
*"     VALUE(EX_ORDERID)     TYPE  ZIFPORDERID
*"  TABLES
*"     TA_ORDERPOS STRUCTURE  ZIFPORDERPOS
*"  EXCEPTIONS
*"     NOT_AUTHORIZED
*"     NO_NUMBER
*"     NO_LOCK
```

```
*"----------------------------------------------------------
  AUTHORITY-CHECK OBJECT 'ZIFPORDER' ID 'ACTVT' FIELD '01'.
  IF sy-subrc NE 0.
    RAISE not_authorized.
  ENDIF.
  CALL FUNCTION 'NUMBER_GET_NEXT'
    EXPORTING
      nr_range_nr = '01'
      object      = 'ZIFPORDER'
    IMPORTING
      number      = im_orderheader-orderid
    EXCEPTIONS
      OTHERS      = 1.
  IF sy-subrc <> 0.
    RAISE no_number.
  ENDIF.
  CALL FUNCTION 'ENQUEUE_EZIFPORDER'
    EXPORTING
      orderid     = im_orderheader-orderid
    EXCEPTIONS
      OTHERS  = 1.
  IF sy-subrc <> 0.
    RAISE no_lock.
  ENDIF.
  IF im_testrun IS INITIAL.
    CALL FUNCTION 'Z_IFP_V_CREATE_ORDER'
      IN UPDATE TASK
      EXPORTING
        im_orderheader = im_orderheader
      TABLES
        im_orderpos    = ta_orderpos.
    IF im_commit = 'X'.
      COMMIT WORK.
      CALL FUNCTION 'DEQUEUE_ALL'.
    ENDIF.
ENDIF.
  ex_orderid = im_orderheader-orderid.
ENDFUNCTION.
```

Listing 3.6 Funktionsbaustein »Z_IFP_ORDER_CREATE«

Aufruf über tRFC

Funktionsbausteine zum Anlegen von Datensätzen werden in der Regel per transaktionalem RFC aufgerufen, wie Listing 3.7 zeigt. Der Report ZIFP_

ORDER_CREATE liest einen Lieferantenauftrag aus der lokalen Datenbank, um mit diesen Daten eine Kundenbestellung im Lieferantensystem anzulegen. Der Aufruf erfolgt transaktional, da der Aufrufer im Fall eines communication_failure nicht weiß, ob der Datensatz im Zielsystem bereits angelegt wurde. Bei einem erneuten Aufruf würde dann nämlich ein zweiter Datensatz erzeugt. Wird der Funktionsbaustein jedoch transaktional aufgerufen, werden im aufrufenden System die übergebenen Parameter gespeichert, und der Aufruf kann bei einem communication_failure mit Transaktion SM58 problemlos nochmals wiederholt werden. Es ist auf jeden Fall sichergestellt, dass der Funktionsbaustein im Zielsystem nur einmal ausgeführt wird.

```
REPORT  zifp_order_create.
PARAMETERS:
  pa_id  TYPE zifporder-orderid,
  p_dest TYPE rfcdes-rfcdest value check.
DATA:
  orderheader  TYPE zifporder,
  it_orderpos  TYPE STANDARD TABLE OF zifporderpos,
  msg_text(80) TYPE c.
AT SELECTION-SCREEN.
* Prüfen, ob es die ausgewählte Lieferantenbestellung gibt
  SELECT SINGLE * FROM zifporder
  INTO orderheader
  WHERE
    orderid   = pa_id AND
    type      = 'PO'.
  IF sy-subrc <> 0.
    Message e001(zifp).
  endif.
START-OF-SELECTION.
* Lieferantenbestellung aus Quelle als Kundenauftrag an Ziel
*   Bestelltyp auf Kundenauftrag setzen
    orderheader-type  = 'SO'.
*   ORDERID auf REFID setzen
    orderheader-refid = orderheader-orderid.
*   Positionsdaten lesen
    SELECT * FROM zifporderpos INTO TABLE it_orderpos
    WHERE
      orderid = pa_id.
*   Kundenauftrag im Zielsystem erzeugen
    CALL FUNCTION 'Z_IFP_ORDER_CREATE'
      IN BACKGROUND TASK
```

```
    DESTINATION p_dest
    EXPORTING
      im_orderheader        = orderheader
      im_commit             = 'X'
    TABLES
      ta_orderpos           = it_orderpos
    EXCEPTIONS
      system_failure        = 1  MESSAGE msg_text
      communication_failure = 2  MESSAGE msg_text
      OTHERS                = 3.
  IF sy-subrc <> 0.
    WRITE:/ msg_text.
    ROLLBACK WORK.
  ENDIF.
  COMMIT WORK.
```

Listing 3.7 Report »ZIFP_ORDER_CREATE«

Exportparameter nicht zugänglich

Beim Aufruf des Funktionsbausteins über den transaktionalen RFC erhalten Sie jedoch weder die Exportparameter noch eine eventuell im Funktionsbaustein ausgelöste Ausnahme zurück. Sie wissen hier daher nicht, welche ORDERID der erzeugte Kundenauftrag im Zielsystem erhalten hat bzw. ob der Auftrag überhaupt erzeugt werden konnte. Daher wird dem Kundenauftrag im Feld REFID die Nummer der ursprünglichen Lieferantenbestellung mitgegeben. Mit dem Funktionsbaustein Z_IFP_ORDER_GETLIST können Sie über die REFID nach den Kundenaufträgen suchen und damit die ORDERID ermitteln.

Transaktionsmodell bei BAPIs

Ein etwas anderer Weg wird z. B. bei BAPIs beschritten. Hier werden auch ändernde oder erzeugende Funktionsbausteine per sRFC aufgerufen. Damit kann das rufende System Exportparameter und Ausnahmen sofort erfahren. Der RFC-Funktionsbaustein nimmt die Verbuchung jedoch nicht unmittelbar vor, sondern ruft einen Verbuchungsbaustein mit dem Zusatz IN UPDATE TASK auf. Damit im Zielsystem die Verbuchung angestoßen wird, ruft das lokale System das BAPI BAPI_COMMIT_WORK im Zielsystem auf. Dieses BAPI enthält im Wesentlichen die Codezeile COMMIT WORK und löst damit die Verbuchung im Zielsystem aus. Unsere Funktionsbausteine Z_IFP_ORDER_CHANGE, Z_IFP_ORDER_DELETE und Z_IFP_ORDER_CREATE sind so gestaltet, dass sie für eine BAPI-Implementierung wiederverwendet werden können.

Bestellposition erzeugen

Der Funktionsbaustein Z_IFP_ORDER_CREATEPOS in Listing 3.8 beinhaltet als Abschluss der Implementierungsarbeiten den ABAP-Code zur Erzeugung einer einzelnen Bestellposition.

```
FUNCTION Z_IFP_ORDER_CREATEPOS.
*"----------------------------------------------------------
*"*"Lokale Schnittstelle:
*"  IMPORTING
*"     VALUE(IM_ORDERPOS) TYPE  ZIFPORDERPOS
*"     VALUE(IM_TESTRUN)  TYPE  CHAR1 DEFAULT SPACE
*"     VALUE(IM_COMMIT)   TYPE  CHAR1 DEFAULT SPACE
*"  EXCEPTIONS
*"      NOT_AUTHORIZED
*"      NO_ORDER
*"      NO_LOCK
*"      DUPLICATE_POS
*"----------------------------------------------------------
  DATA:
    wa_orderpos TYPE zifporderpos.
  AUTHORITY-CHECK OBJECT 'ZIFPORDER' ID 'ACTVT' FIELD '01'.
  IF sy-subrc NE 0.
    RAISE not_authorized.
  ENDIF.
  SELECT SINGLE orderid FROM zifporder
    INTO wa_orderpos-orderid
    WHERE orderid = im_orderpos-orderid.
  IF sy-subrc NE 0.
    RAISE no_order.
  ENDIF.
  SELECT SINGLE orderid orderpos FROM zifporderpos
    INTO (wa_orderpos-orderid, wa_orderpos-orderpos)
    WHERE
      orderid  = im_orderpos-orderid AND
      orderpos = im_orderpos-orderpos.
  IF sy-subrc EQ 0.
    RAISE duplicate_pos.
  ENDIF.
  CALL FUNCTION 'ENQUEUE_EZIFPORDER'
    EXPORTING
      orderid = im_orderpos-orderid
    EXCEPTIONS
      OTHERS  = 1.
  IF sy-subrc <> 0.
    RAISE no_lock.
  ENDIF.
  IF im_testrun IS INITIAL.
    CALL FUNCTION 'Z_IFP_V_CREATE_ORDERPOS'
```

```
        IN UPDATE TASK
        EXPORTING
          im_orderpos = im_orderpos.
      IF im_commit = 'X'.
        COMMIT WORK.
        CALL FUNCTION 'DEQUEUE_ALL'.
      ENDIF.
    ENDIF.
ENDFUNCTION.
```

Listing 3.8 Der Funktionsbaustein »ZIFP_ORDER_CREATEPOS«

3.3 Queued RFC

Logical Units of Work, die über tRFC erstellt wurden, werden im Zielsystem unabhängig voneinander ausgeführt. Insbesondere bei Netzwerkproblemen ist damit nicht garantiert, dass die Reihenfolge des Aufrufs der Funktionsbausteine im lokalen und die ihrer Abarbeitung im Zielsystem dieselbe ist. Um diese Reihenfolge zu gewährleisten, kann der *queued RFC* (qRFC) eingesetzt werden.

qRFC-Architektur

Der qRFC ist eine Erweiterung des tRFC. Diese Erweiterung besteht aus einer zusätzlichen Schicht zwischen der sendenden bzw. der empfangenden Anwendung und der tRFC-Schicht. Das qRFC-Kommunikationsmodell unterscheidet drei Szenarien, die in Abbildung 3.1 dargestellt sind:

- **tRFC**
  Dieses Szenario können Sie verwenden, wenn die Daten von hintereinander ausgeführten Funktionsbausteinen nicht miteinander verbunden sind. Die rufende Anwendung im Client-System verwendet tRFC, um sicherzustellen, dass die Daten im Serversystem nur einmal verarbeitet werden. Die Reihenfolge, in der die gerufenen Funktionsbausteine abgearbeitet werden, ist nicht garantiert. Falls Übertragungsfehler auftreten, kann es durchaus sein, dass später abgesetzte tRFC-Funktionsaufrufe im Empfangssystem früher abgearbeitet werden.
- **qRFC mit Ausgangswarteschlange**
  In diesem Szenario verwendet das sendende System eine Ausgangswarteschlange (Outbound Queue), um die Serialisierung der Daten sicherzustellen. Die aufgerufenen Funktionsmodule werden in der Ausgangswarteschlange des sendenden Systems gespeichert. Damit ist garantiert, dass sie genau einmal und genau in der Aufrufreihenfolge im empfangenden System abgearbeitet werden. Die Ausgangswarteschlange wird

von einem Standardprozess, dem QOUT-Scheduler, regelmäßig geleert. Das Empfangssystem hat keine Kenntnis von der Existenz der Ausgangswarteschlange im sendenden System. Dieses Szenario kann daher auch mit externen tRFC-Servern eingesetzt werden. Der Code im externen tRFC-Server muss dazu nicht geändert werden.

- **qRFC mit Ausgangs- und Eingangswarteschlange**
  Hier gibt es zusätzlich zur Ausgangswarteschlange im sendenden System auch eine Eingangswarteschlange (Inbound Queue) im empfangenden System. Selbst wenn das empfangende System eine Eingangswarteschlange bereitstellt, gibt es im sendenden System immer eine Ausgangswarteschlange, weil diese dazu dient, die Aufrufe zu serialisieren. Die Eingangswarteschlange im empfangenden System trennt hingegen die Übertragung der Aufrufe von deren Verarbeitung. Die übertragenen Aufrufe werden so lange in der Eingangswarteschlange gespeichert, bis die Anwendung oder ein Standardprozess, der QIN-Scheduler, die Verarbeitung anstößt. Die RFC-Bibliothek stellt Funktionen zur Verfügung, mit denen externe Clients per tRFC Funktionsaufrufe in eine Eingangswarteschlange eines empfangenden SAP-Systems einstellen können.

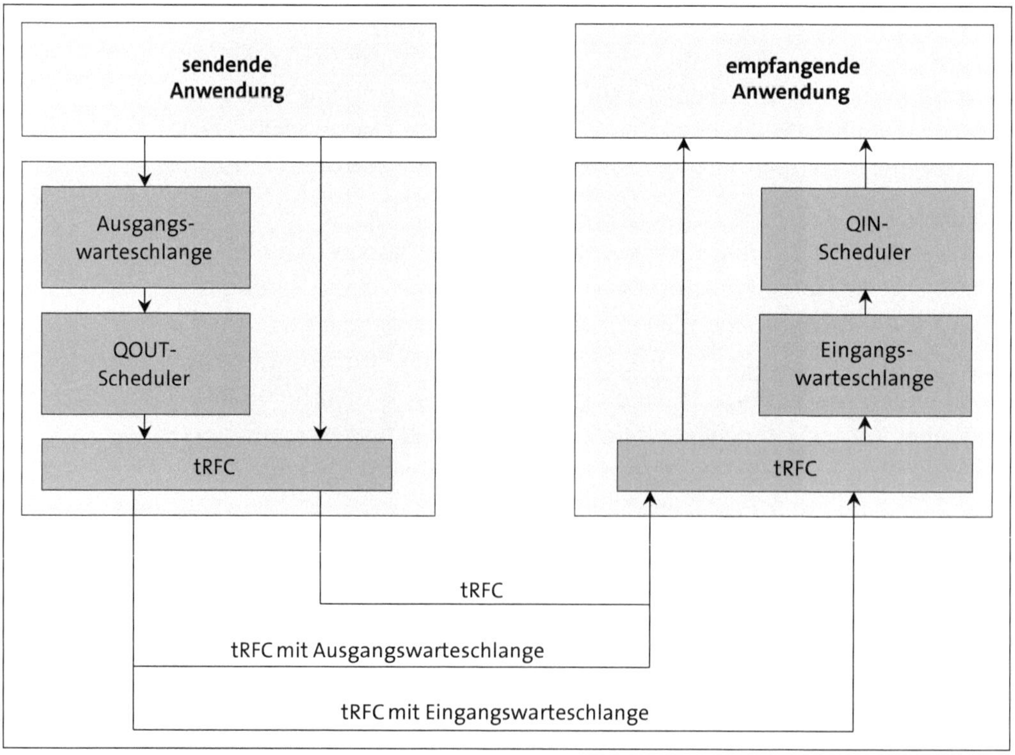

Abbildung 3.1 qRFC-Kommunikationsszenarien

3.3.1 qRFC mit Ausgangswarteschlange

Funktionsbaustein »TRFC_SET_QUEUE_NAME«

Um eine qRFC-LUW in eine Ausgangswarteschlange zu stellen, müssen Sie vor dem qRFC-Aufruf den Namen der Ausgangswarteschlange angeben, indem Sie den Funktionsbaustein TRFC_SET_QUEUE_NAME lokal aufrufen. Mit COMMIT WORK schließen Sie dann die LUW ab. Listing 3.9 zeigt ein Beispiel, das eine qRFC-LUW in eine Queue mit dem Namen ZIFPQUEUE stellt. Die LUW besteht aus mehreren Aufrufen des Funktionsbausteins Z_IFP_ORDER_CREATE.

```
REPORT  zifp_qrfc.
DATA:
  orderheader    TYPE zifporder,
  it_orderheader TYPE STANDARD TABLE OF zifporder,
  it_orderpos    TYPE STANDARD TABLE OF zifporderpos.
SELECT-OPTIONS:
  so_id FOR orderheader-orderid.
PARAMETERS:
  p_dest TYPE rfcdes-rfcdest VALUE CHECK.
AT SELECTION-SCREEN.
* prüfen, ob die Lieferantenbestellungen existieren
  SELECT * FROM zifporder
  INTO TABLE it_orderheader
  WHERE
    orderid IN so_id AND
    type    = 'PO'.
  IF sy-subrc <> 0.
    MESSAGE e001(zifp).
  ENDIF.
START-OF-SELECTION.
* qRFC initialisieren
  CALL FUNCTION 'TRFC_QUEUE_INITIALIZE'.
  CALL FUNCTION 'TRFC_SET_QUEUE_NAME'
    EXPORTING

      qname              = 'ZIFPQUEUE'
    EXCEPTIONS
      invalid_queue_name = 1
      OTHERS             = 2.
  CHECK sy-subrc EQ 0.
* für jede Lieferantenbestellung einen
* Kundenauftrag erzeugen
  LOOP AT it_orderheader INTO orderheader.
    orderheader-type  = 'SO'.
    orderheader-refid = orderheader-orderid.
```

```
* Positionen zum Auftrag lesen
    SELECT * FROM zifporderpos INTO TABLE it_orderpos
    WHERE
      orderid = orderheader-orderid.
* Kundenauftrag im Zielsystem anlegen
    CALL FUNCTION 'Z_IFP_ORDER_CREATE'
      IN BACKGROUND TASK
      DESTINATION p_dest
      EXPORTING
        im_orderheader        = orderheader
        im_commit             = ' '
      TABLES
        ta_orderpos           = it_orderpos.
  ENDLOOP.
  COMMIT WORK.
```

Listing 3.9 qRFC mit Ausgangswarteschlange

QOUT-Scheduler

Die Abarbeitung der Ausgangswarteschlangen wird durch den QOUT-Scheduler veranlasst, den Sie mit Transaktion SMQS überwachen können. Sobald eine LUW im sendenden System abgeschlossen wurde, geschieht zweierlei:

- Die Zieldestination wird beim QOUT-Scheduler registriert.
- Der QOUT-Scheduler wird aktiviert und arbeitet die Warteschlangen zu dieser Zieldestination ab.

[+]

Überwachung der Ausgangswarteschlange

Damit Sie mit der Monitoring-Transaktion SMQ1 für die Überwachung der ausgehenden Warteschlangen im Normalfall überhaupt etwas sehen, müssen Sie zu einem kleinen Trick greifen: In Transaktion SMQS für den QOUT-Scheduler klicken Sie auf den Button **Deregistrierung**, um Ihre Zieldestination beim QOUT-Scheduler zu deregistrieren. Wenn Sie dann den Report ZIFP_QRFC in Listing 3.9 ausführen, sehen Sie die Ausgangswarteschlange ZIFPQUEUE in Transaktion SMQ1, dem qRFC-Monitor für die Ausgangswarteschlangen. Wählen Sie diese Ausgangswarteschlange in Transaktion SMQ1, und lassen Sie sich die Details anzeigen.

LUW einer Ausgangswarteschlange

Wenn Sie den im Kasten beschriebenen Trick anwenden, sehen Sie sämtliche LUWs einer Ausgangswarteschlange. Wenn Sie eine LUW auswählen und sich wiederum die Details anzeigen lassen, sehen Sie die Funktionsbausteine in dieser LUW (siehe Abbildung 3.2). Aus diesem Bildschirm können Sie dann die Ausgangswarteschlange manuell an das Zielsystem senden.

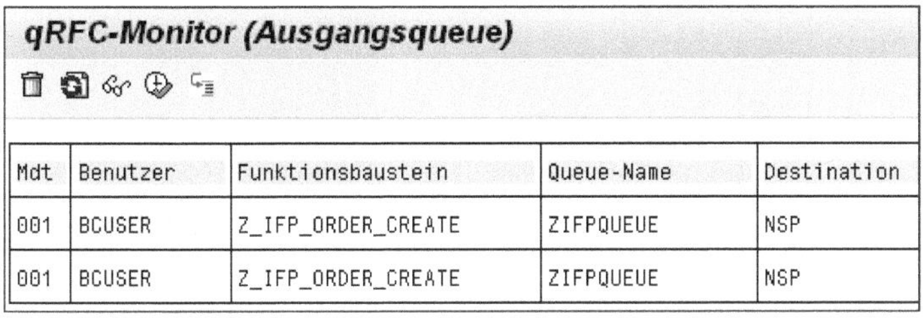

Mdt	Benutzer	Funktionsbaustein	Queue-Name	Destination
001	BCUSER	Z_IFP_ORDER_CREATE	ZIFPQUEUE	NSP
001	BCUSER	Z_IFP_ORDER_CREATE	ZIFPQUEUE	NSP

Abbildung 3.2 Funktionsbausteine in Ausgangswarteschlange

Zieldestination registrieren

Normalerweise registrieren Sie jedoch die Zieldestination manuell oder automatisch beim QOUT-Scheduler. Dieser arbeitet dann die Ausgangswarteschlange sofort ab, sobald die LUW mit einem `COMMIT WORK` abgeschlossen wird.

3.3.2 qRFC mit Ausgangs- und Eingangswarteschlange

Funktionsbaustein »TRFC_SET_QIN_PROPERTIES«

Um eine tRFC-LUW im empfangenden System zunächst in eine Eingangswarteschlange zu stellen, muss vor jedem einzelnen tRFC-Aufruf im sendenden System der Name der Eingangswarteschlange durch einen lokalen Aufruf des Funktionsbausteins `TRFC_SET_QIN_PROPERTIES` angegeben werden. Optional kann mit diesem Parameter auch der Name der Ausgangswarteschlange angegeben werden, der sonst gleich dem Namen der Eingangswarteschlange gewählt wird. Listing 3.10 zeigt ein Beispiel.

```
REPORT zifp_qrfc_in.
DATA:
  orderheader    TYPE zifporder,
  it_orderheader TYPE STANDARD TABLE OF zifporder,
  it_orderpos    TYPE STANDARD TABLE OF zifporderpos.
SELECT-OPTIONS:
  so_id FOR orderheader-orderid.
PARAMETERS:
  p_dest TYPE rfcdes-rfcdest VALUE CHECK.
AT SELECTION-SCREEN.

* prüfen, ob Lieferantenbestellungen existieren
  SELECT * FROM zifporder
  INTO TABLE it_orderheader
```

```
  WHERE
    orderid IN so_id AND
    type    = 'PO'.
  IF sy-subrc <> 0.
    MESSAGE e001(zifp).
  ENDIF.
START-OF-SELECTION.
* qRFC initialisieren
  CALL FUNCTION 'TRFC_QUEUE_INITIALIZE'.
* zu jeder Lieferantenbestellung einen Kundenauftrag
* im Zielsystem anlegen

  LOOP AT it_orderheader INTO orderheader.
    orderheader-type  = 'SO'.
    orderheader-refid = orderheader-orderid.
* Bestellpositionen zum Auftrag lesen
    SELECT * FROM zifporderpos INTO TABLE it_orderpos
    WHERE
      orderid = orderheader-orderid.
* Eigenschaften der Eingangswarteschlange setzen
    CALL FUNCTION 'TRFC_SET_QIN_PROPERTIES'
      EXPORTING
       qout_name                = 'ZIFPQUEUE'
       qin_name                 = 'ZIFPQUEUE'
      EXCEPTIONS
       invalid_queue_name       = 1
       OTHERS                   = 2.
    CHECK sy-subrc EQ 0.
* Kundenauftrag im Zielsystem anlegen
    CALL FUNCTION 'Z_IFP_ORDER_CREATE'
      IN BACKGROUND TASK
      DESTINATION p_dest
      EXPORTING
        im_orderheader        = orderheader
        im_commit             = ' '
      TABLES
        ta_orderpos           = it_orderpos.
  ENDLOOP.
  COMMIT WORK.
```

Listing 3.10 qRFC mit Eingangswarteschlange

Eine tRFC-LUW wird in eine Ausgangswarteschlange mit dem Namen ZIFPQUEUE gestellt. Im empfangenden System wird diese LUW nicht sofort abgearbeitet, sondern in eine Eingangswarteschlange mit dem Namen ZIFPQUEUE gestellt. Die LUW besteht wiederum aus mehreren Aufrufen des Funktionsbausteins Z_ORDER_CREATE. Vor jedem Aufruf wird der Name der Eingangswarteschlange mit TRFC_SET_QIN_PROPERTIES angegeben.

Monitoring

Die Abarbeitung der Eingangswarteschlange erfolgt nicht automatisch. Daher sehen Sie in Transaktion SMQ2, dem qRFC-Monitor für Eingangswarteschlangen, auch sofort einen Eintrag für ZIFPQUEUE im Zielsystem, nachdem Sie den Report ZIFP_QRFC_IN aus Listing 3.10 im Sendesystem ausgeführt haben. Wählen Sie diese Eingangswarteschlange in Transaktion SMQ2, und lassen Sie sich die Details anzeigen. Sie sehen dann sämtliche LUWs in dieser Eingangswarteschlange. Wenn Sie eine LUW auswählen und sich wiederum die Details anzeigen lassen, sehen Sie die Funktionsbausteine in dieser LUW wie in Abbildung 3.3. Aus diesem oder dem vorangegangenen Bild können Sie dann die Abarbeitung der Eingangswarteschlange im Zielsystem veranlassen.

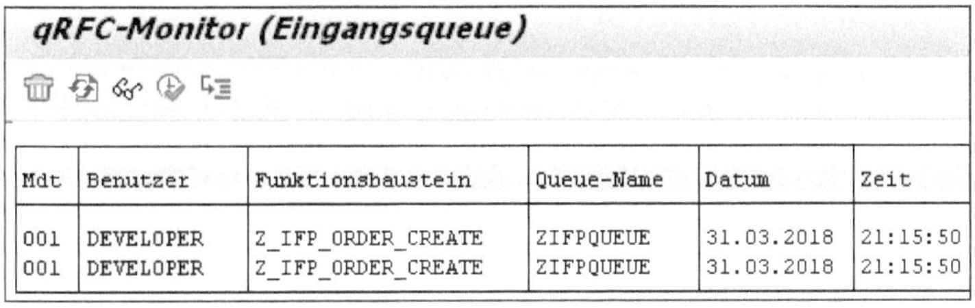

Mdt	Benutzer	Funktionsbaustein	Queue-Name	Datum	Zeit
001	DEVELOPER	Z_IFP_ORDER_CREATE	ZIFPQUEUE	31.03.2018	21:15:50
001	DEVELOPER	Z_IFP_ORDER_CREATE	ZIFPQUEUE	31.03.2018	21:15:50

Abbildung 3.3 Funktionsbausteine in Eingangswarteschlange

Abarbeitung mit »TRFC_QIN_RESTART«

Die Verarbeitung der Funktionsbausteine in der Eingangswarteschlange erfolgt nicht automatisch, sondern kann durch den Aufruf des Funktionsbausteins TRFC_QIN_RESTART von der Anwendung selbst angestoßen werden. Dieser Funktionsbaustein kann entweder aus einem Batch-Programm im Empfängersystem oder per RFC aus dem Sendersystem aufgerufen werden. Diesem Funktionsbaustein muss der Queue-Name übergeben werden.

QIN-Scheduler

Damit nicht jede qRFC-Anwendung ihren eigenen Scheduler zum Anstoß der Queue-Verarbeitung schreiben muss, gibt es einen QIN-Scheduler, der registrierte Queues automatisch abarbeitet. Die Registrierung einer Eingangs-Queue erfolgt dabei entweder programmatisch über den Funktionsbaustein QIWK_REGISTER oder von Hand über den qRFC-Monitor für den QIN-Scheduler (Transaktion SMQR). Abbildung 3.4 zeigt diese Transaktion nach der Registrierung der Eingangswarteschlange ZIFPQUEUE.

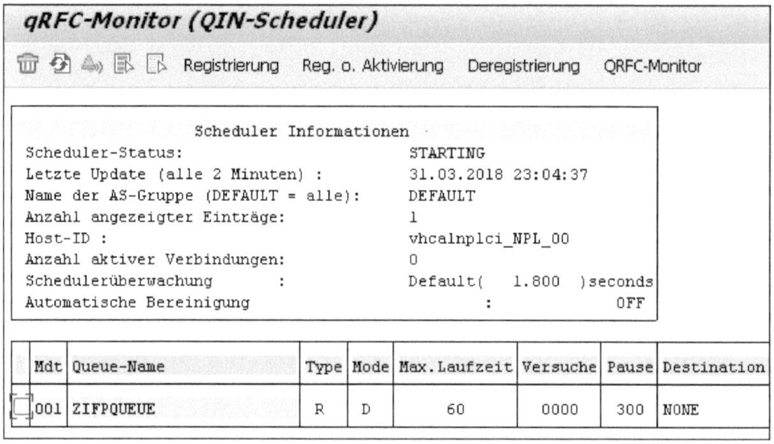

Abbildung 3.4 Registrierung einer Eingangswarteschlange

Parallelisierung mit dem aRFC

Der asynchrone RFC (aRFC) dient der Verteilung von Aufgaben auf mehrere SAP-Systeme. Mit dem Zusatz `STARTING NEW TASK t` kann ein Funktionsbaustein asynchron auf einem anderen System gestartet werden. Dabei ist `t` ein zeichenartiges Datenobjekt, mit dem der Programmierer dem Task einen Namen gibt. Unter Angabe dieses Namens kann er später Informationen zum Task abfragen. Auch beim aRFC können zum Zeitpunkt des Aufrufs keine Exportparameter und Ausnahmen entgegengenommen werden. Da aRFC aber für externe Systeme nicht zur Verfügung steht, spielt er bei der Schnittstellenprogrammierung keine Rolle.

3.4 Background-RFC

Parallel zum besprochenen tRFC, qRFC und aRFC gibt es zusätzlich den Background-RFC (bgRFC). Alles, was Sie bislang mit tRFC, qRFC oder aRFC realisiert haben, können Sie auch mit dem neueren bgRFC erreichen. Der bgRFC bietet jedoch darüber hinaus verbesserte Leistungsfähigkeit, ein vereinheitlichtes objektorientiertes Programmiermodell sowie erweiterte Funktionen für Programmierer und Administratoren. SAP empfiehlt, für neue Anwendungen den bgRFC einzusetzen und alte Anwendungen, die noch tRFC und qRFC verwenden, nach und nach zu migrieren.

bgRFC-Szenarien

Der bgRFC kennt zwei Szenarien, die auch miteinander kombiniert werden können:

- **Outbound-Szenario**
  Die Aufrufe der Funktionsbausteine werden im rufenden System aufgezeichnet und nach dem Abschluss der LUW durch `COMMIT WORK` zu einem

anderen System transportiert, in dem sie in der Reihenfolge des Aufrufs ausgeführt werden.

- **Inbound-Szenario**
  Die Aufrufe der Funktionsbausteine werden ebenfalls im rufenden System aufgezeichnet. Sie werden nach Abschluss der LUW durch `COMMIT WORK` zu einem Anwendungsserver *in demselben* System transportiert, auf dem sie in der Reihenfolge des Aufrufs ausgeführt werden.

Das Inbound-Szenario dient demnach lediglich der Lastverteilung innerhalb eines Systems und ersetzt den aRFC. Damit ist das Inbound-Szenario für die Kommunikation mit entfernten Systemen nicht relevant; daher schauen wir uns hier nur das Outbound-Szenario an, das den tRFC und den qRFC für die Kommunikation mit fremden Systemen ersetzt.

3.4.1 Programmierung mit bgRFC

bgRFC-Client

Ein ABAP-Client, der bgRFC verwenden möchte, geht in fünf Schritten vor:

1. **Ein Destinationsobjekt erzeugen**
   Dazu ruft der Client die Klassenmethode `CREATE` der Klasse `CL_BGRFC_DESTINATION_OUTBOUND` auf.
2. **Ein Unit-Objekt erzeugen**
   Dazu ruft der Client die Methode `CREATE_TRFC_UNIT` oder `CREATE_QRFC_UNIT` des soeben erzeugten Destinationsobjekts auf.
3. **Das Unit-Objekt gegebenenfalls einer Queue zuweisen**
   Dazu ruft der Client die Methode `ADD_QUEUE_NAME_OUTBOUND` des soeben erzeugten Unit-Objekts auf.
4. **Die Funktionsbausteine aufrufen**
   Dazu verwendet der Client den Zusatz `IN BACKGROUND UNIT` und gibt dabei das zuvor erzeugte Unit-Objekt an.
5. **Die LUW abschließen**
   Dazu ruft der Client `COMMIT WORK` auf.

Bestellung mit bgRFC erzeugen

Listing 3.11 zeigt ein ABAP-Client-Programm für einen bgRFC mit derselben Funktionalität wie das Client-Programm aus Listing 3.9, das qRFC verwendet. Beide Programme erzeugen in einem fremden System Bestellungen, indem sie den Funktionsbaustein `Z_IFP_ORDER_CREATE` aufrufen. Beide Programme gehen nach demselben Schema vor und unterscheiden sich nur durch die verwendete API.

```
REPORT  zifp_bgrfc.
DATA:
  orderheader     TYPE zifporder,
```

```
  it_orderheader TYPE STANDARD TABLE OF zifporder,
  it_orderpos    TYPE STANDARD TABLE OF zifporderpos,
  r_destination  TYPE REF TO if_bgrfc_destination_outbound,
  r_unit         TYPE REF TO if_qrfc_unit_outbound,
  dest_name      TYPE bgrfc_dest_name_outbound,
  queue_name     TYPE qrfc_queue_name.
SELECT-OPTIONS:
  so_id FOR orderheader-orderid.
PARAMETERS:
  p_dest TYPE rfcdes-rfcdest VALUE CHECK.
AT SELECTION-SCREEN.
* prüfen, ob die Lieferantenbestellungen existieren
  SELECT * FROM zifporder
  INTO TABLE it_orderheader
  WHERE
    orderid IN so_id AND
    type    = 'PO'.
  IF sy-subrc <> 0.
    MESSAGE e001(zifp).
  ENDIF.
START-OF-SELECTION.
  TRY.
* bgRFC-Destination anlegen
    dest_name = p_dest.
    r_destination =
      cl_bgrfc_destination_outbound=>create( dest_name ).
  CATCH cx_bgrfc_invalid_destination.
    MESSAGE e101(bc).
  ENDTRY.
* bgRFC-Unit anlegen
  r_unit = r_destination->create_qrfc_unit( ).
  TRY.
* bgRFC-Queue-Namen hinzufügen
    r_unit->add_queue_name_outbound( 'ZIFPQUEUE' ).
  CATCH cx_qrfc_duplicate_queue_name.
    MESSAGE e101(bc).
  ENDTRY.
* alle Lieferantenbestellungen als Kundenaufträge
* im Zielsystem anlegen
  LOOP AT it_orderheader INTO orderheader.
    orderheader-type = 'SO'.
    orderheader-refid = orderheader-orderid.
* Bestellpositionen zum Auftrag lesen
```

```
    SELECT * FROM zifporderpos INTO TABLE it_orderpos
    WHERE
      orderid = orderheader-orderid.
* Kundenauftrag per bgRFC im Zielsystem anlegen
    CALL FUNCTION 'Z_IFP_ORDER_CREATE'
      IN BACKGROUND UNIT r_unit
      EXPORTING
        im_orderheader        = orderheader
        im_commit             = ' '
      TABLES
        ta_orderpos           = it_orderpos.
  ENDLOOP.
  COMMIT WORK.
```

Listing 3.11 Report, der bgRFC anstelle von qRFC verwendet

Auswahl der qRFC-Version in Transaktion SM59

Im Selektionsbild des Reports in Listing 3.11 müssen Sie eine RFC-Destination angeben, die beim bgRFC registriert ist. Dazu ändern Sie in Transaktion SM59 Ihre Destination. Wählen Sie die Registerkarte **Spezielle Optionen**, und stellen Sie in der Drop-down-Liste **Übertragungsprotokoll** die Option **1 klassisch mit bgRFC** ein, wie Abbildung 3.5 zeigt.

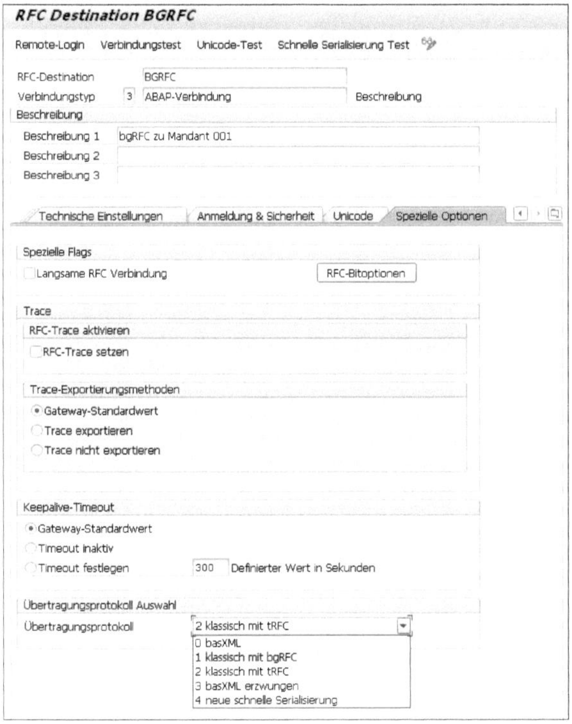

Abbildung 3.5 Auswahl der qRFC-Version in Transaktion SM59

bgRFC-Monitor

Mit Transaktion SBGRFCMON können Sie verfolgen, wie Ihre bgRFC-Aufrufe abgearbeitet werden. Abbildung 3.6 zeigt den bgRFC-Monitor, nachdem das Programm `ZIFP_BGRFC` aus Listing 3.11 dreimal ausgeführt wurde. Der Monitor listet auf der linken Seite die Destinationen und darunter die Queues auf. Rechts sind dann zu einer Queue die Units zu sehen. Die erste Unit, die um 22:14:26 hinzugefügt wurde, ist zur Ausführung bereit. Die beiden anderen Units, die später hinzugefügt wurden, sind noch gesperrt.

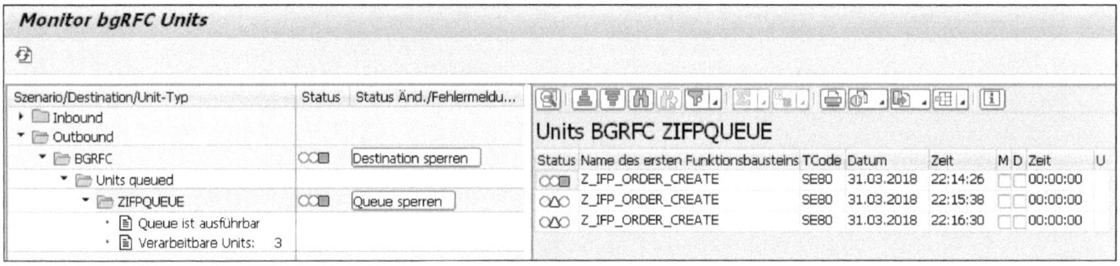

Abbildung 3.6 bgRFC-Monitor

3.4.2 Konfiguration des bgRFC

Damit die Daten nun auch an das Fremdsystem geschickt werden, müssen Sie mit Transaktion SBGRFCCONF einen oder mehrere Scheduler einrichten. Im Gegensatz zum qRFC gibt es beim bgRFC keinen zentralen Scheduler, sondern Sie können nun je Anwendungsserver und sogar je Destination beliebig viele Scheduler einrichten, die parallel arbeiten. Konflikte zwischen parallel arbeitenden Schedulern löst die Implementierung des bgRFC-Systems von selbst, indem sie Sperren verwendet.

Zur Konfiguration der bgRFC-Scheduler führen Sie folgende Schritte im Mandanten 000 durch. Davon ist nur der erste Schritt zwingend notwendig; alle anderen Schritte sind optional:

1. Legen Sie die Supervisor-Destination an.
2. Passen Sie die Systemeinstellungen an.
3. Passen Sie die Standardkonfiguration für alle Scheduler an.
4. Legen Sie die applikationsserverspezifischen Scheduler-Konfigurationen an.
5. Definieren Sie die Inbound-Destinationen.
6. Legen Sie die destinationsspezifischen Scheduler-Konfigurationen an.

Die einzelnen Schritte beschreiben wir im Folgenden:

Supervisor-Destination

Die Supervisor-Destination ist eine RFC-Destination, die vom bgRFC verwendet wird, um die Konfiguration der Inbound- und Outbound-Destinationen zu lesen und die notwendigen Scheduler auf den beteiligten Applikationsservern nach Bedarf zu starten oder zu stoppen. Sie legen die Supervisor-Destination mit Transaktion SBGRFCCONF auf der Registerkarte **Supervisor Dest. pflegen** an. Klicken Sie dazu auf den Button **Anlegen**, und geben Sie im Dialog **RFC Destination für Supervisor anlegen** den gewünschten Namen für die Destination sowie den Namen und das gewünschte Passwort für den Supervisor-Benutzer an (siehe Abbildung 3.7).

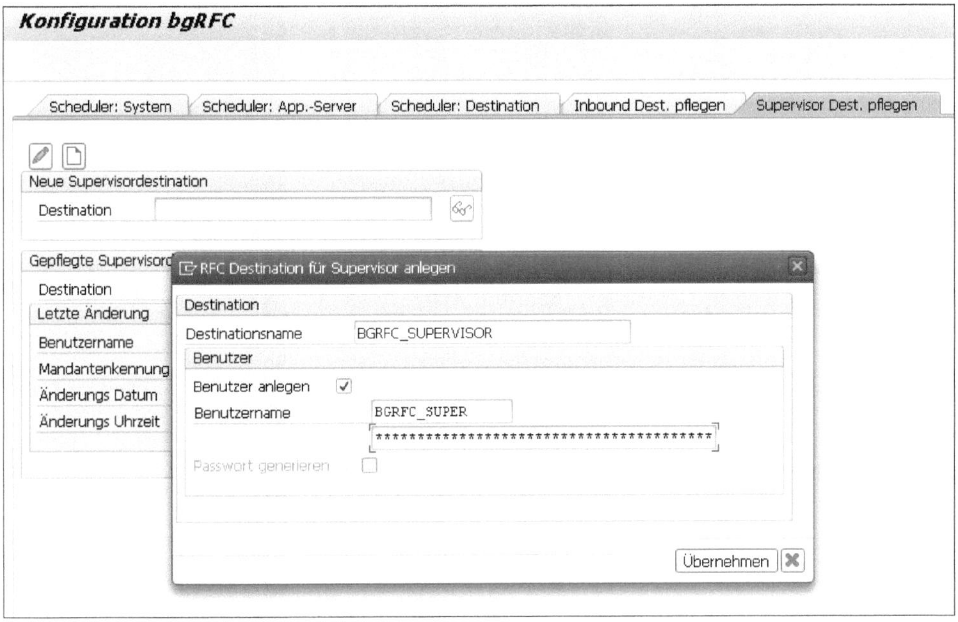

Abbildung 3.7 Anlegen der Supervisor-Destination

Wenn Sie auf **Übernehmen** klicken, wird ein Benutzer mit dem angegebenen Namen und Passwort angelegt. Dieser Benutzer ist der PFCG-Rolle SAP_BC_BGRFC_SUPERVISOR zugeordnet. Außerdem wird eine RFC-Destination mit dem gewünschten Namen angelegt. Bei den technischen Einstellungen dieser Destination sind keine Angaben hinterlegt, d. h., es ist weder der Lastausgleich noch ein spezifischer Anwendungsserver angegeben. Auf der Registerkarte **Anmeldung & Sicherheit** werden der Supervisor-Benutzer, dessen Passwort, der Mandant und die aktuelle Anmeldesprache hinterlegt. Auf der Registerkarte **Spezielle Optionen** ist in der Drop-down-Liste **Übertragungsprotokoll** der Eintrag **tRFC** ausgewählt.

Systemeinstellungen

Auf der Registerkarte **Scheduler: System** können Sie nun die folgenden systemweiten Einstellungen pflegen, die Sie in Abbildung 3.8 sehen.

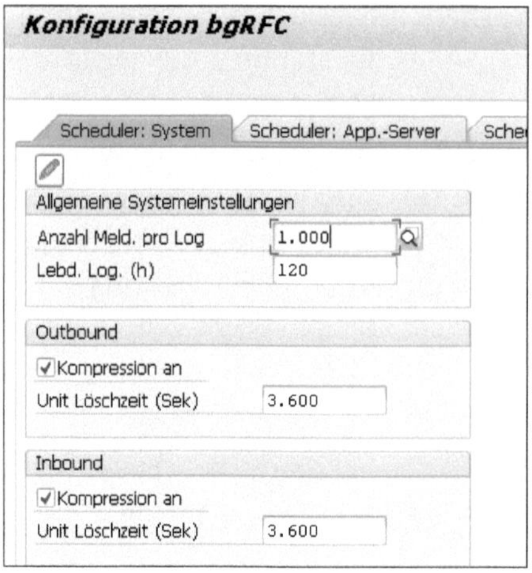

Abbildung 3.8 Systemweite Einstellungen für den bgRFC

Standardkonfiguration für alle Scheduler

Auf der Registerkarte **Scheduler App.-Server** können Sie die Standardeinstellungen für alle Scheduler definieren. Dort sehen Sie in der Liste **Applikationsserver** schon einen Eintrag mit dem Namen **Defaulteintrag**. Wenn Sie diesen auswählen, sehen Sie rechts die Einstellungen für die Outbound- und Inbound-Scheduler. Wenn Sie auf das **Editieren**-Icon (Stift) klicken, können Sie diese Einstellungen auch ändern (siehe Abbildung 3.9).

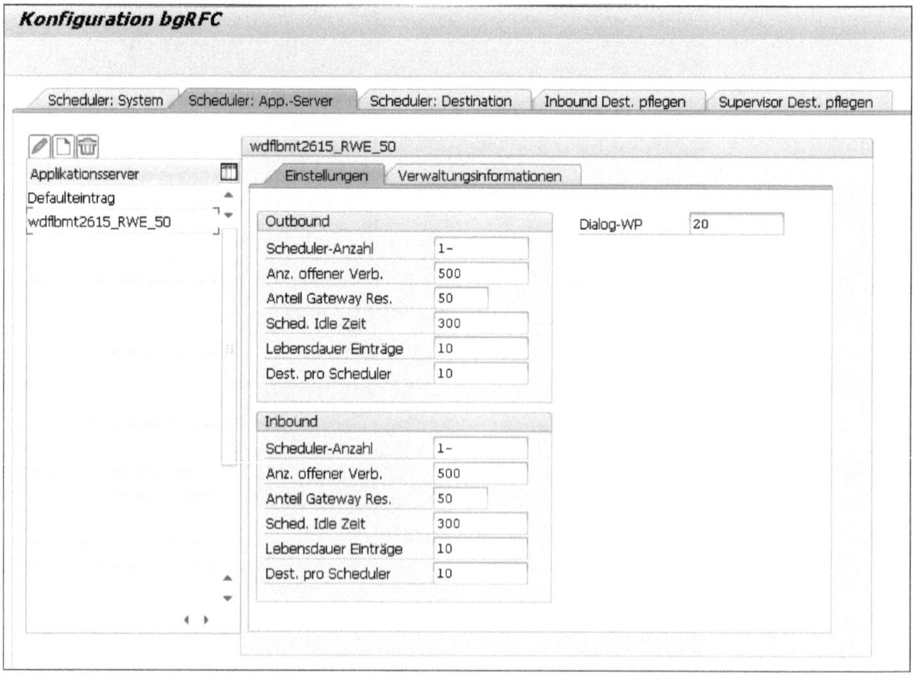

Abbildung 3.9 Standardkonfiguration und serverspezifische Konfiguration

Serverspezifische Konfiguration

Wenn Sie für einzelne Applikationsserver in Ihrem System andere Scheduler-Konfigurationen benötigen, klicken Sie auf das **Anlegen**-Icon und geben den betreffenden Applikationsserver an. Er wird dann in der Liste Anwendungsserver eingetragen, und Sie können die Einstellungen für alle Scheduler auf diesem Server ändern. Auch dies sehen Sie in Abbildung 3.9.

Inbound-Destinationen

Wenn Sie Inbound-Szenarien implementieren wollen, müssen Sie Inbound-Destinationen anlegen und konfigurieren. Gehen Sie dazu in Transaktion SBGRFCCONF zur Registerkarte **Define Inbound Dest.**, und legen Sie dort für jede Anwendung eine Destination an. Für jede Inbound-Destination können Sie dort einen Server oder eine Servergruppe festlegen, die für die Abarbeitung der aufgezeichneten LUWs verantwortlich sind. Mithilfe eines *Queue-Präfix* können Sie steuern, welche Inbound-Destination zur Verarbeitung der bgRFC-Inbound-Unit herangezogen wird. Hierzu wird das am besten passende Queue-Präfix zum verwendeten Queue-Namen der Unit gesucht. Falls kein passendes Queue-Präfix vorliegt, wird die Transaktion im klassischen qRFC verarbeitet. Abbildung 3.10 zeigt ein Beispiel.

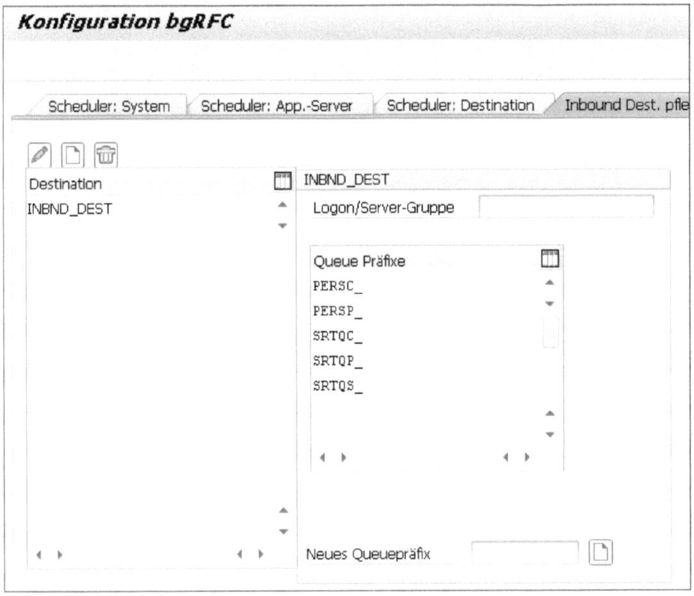

Abbildung 3.10 Inbound-bgRFC-Destinationen

Outbound-Destinationen

Im Gegensatz zu den Inbound-Destinationen müssen Sie die Outbound-Destinationen nicht in Transaktion SBGRFCCONF definieren. Hier genügt die Definition einer entsprechenden RFC-Destination in Transaktion SM59. Damit die aufgezeichneten bgRFC-Units aber auch abgearbeitet werden, müssen Sie in Transaktion SBGRFCCONF zumindest die Supervisor-Destination definieren.

Destinationsspezifische Konfiguration

Für einzelne Destinations – egal ob Inbound oder Outbound – können Sie mit Transaktion SBGRFCCONF auch abweichende Scheduler-Konfigurationen definieren. Wechseln Sie dazu zur Registerkarte **Scheduler: Destination**. Klicken Sie auf das **Anlegen**-Icon, um eine Inbound- oder Outbound-Destination hinzuzufügen und dann die Scheduler-Konfiguration für diese Destination festzulegen. Dies wird in Abbildung 3.11 gezeigt.

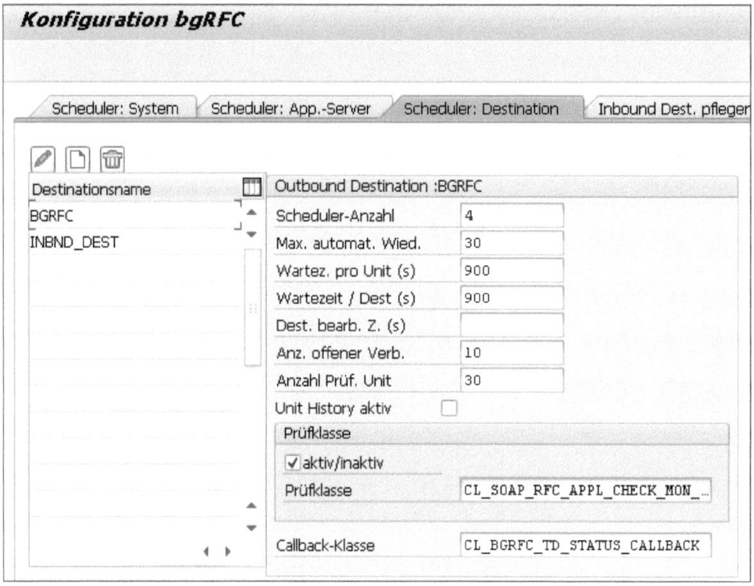

Abbildung 3.11 Destinationsspezifische Konfiguration

3.5 Business-Objekte und BAPIs

Business Application Programming Interfaces (BAPIs) sind Methoden von Business-Objekten. Beispiele für Business-Objekte in SAP ERP sind Customer, Employee oder Material. In der Regel entwickeln SAP-Kunden keine eigenen Business-Objekte, sondern verwenden oder erweitern die BAPIs von SAP-Business-Objekten. Lediglich für Eigenanwendungen kann es interessant sein, eigene Business-Objekte zu definieren.

3.5.1 Entwicklung von Business-Objekten

Business-Objekttyp anlegen

Business-Objekttypen definieren Sie mit Transaktion SWO1 (Business Object Builder). Starten Sie dazu diese Transaktion, und geben Sie den Namen Z_BUS4500 in das Feld **Objekttyp/Interfacetyp** ein. Wählen Sie **Anlegen** ([F5]). Geben Sie die Informationen aus Tabelle 3.1 in die Dialogbox **Objekttyp anlegen** ein.

Bildschirmfeld	Eingabe	Bemerkung
Objektname	Order	Dies ist ein beschreibender englischer Name zur Anzeige der Business-Objekte im Business Object Repository (BOR).
Bezeichnung	Order (IFP example)	Diese Bezeichnung sollte aussagekräftig genug sein, um darüber eine Auswahl des Objekttyps vornehmen zu können.
Kurzbeschreibung	Bestellbeispiel für IFP	–
Programm	Z_BUS4500	Wird vom System vorgeschlagen.
Anwendung	Z	Kundenprogramme

Tabelle 3.1 Anlegen eines Business-Objekts

Attribute von Business-Objekten

Das neu erzeugte Business-Objekt besteht aus fünf Komponenten (Interfaces, Schlüsselfelder, Attribute, Methoden und Ereignisse), die Sie bereits in Abschnitt 1.4.3, »Business Application Programming Interface (BAPI)«, kennengelernt haben.

Werte der Schlüsselfelder

Markieren Sie als Nächstes den Eintrag **Schlüsselfelder**, und wählen Sie **Anlegen** (F5). Beantworten Sie die Frage **Anlegen mit ABAP/4 Dictionary Feldvorgaben?** mit **Ja**, und wählen Sie aus der Tabelle ZIFPORDER das Feld ORDERID aus. Legen Sie mithilfe dieser Auswahl das Schlüsselfeld orderid des Objekttyps an. Ihr Objekttyp sollte jetzt wie in Abbildung 3.12 aussehen.

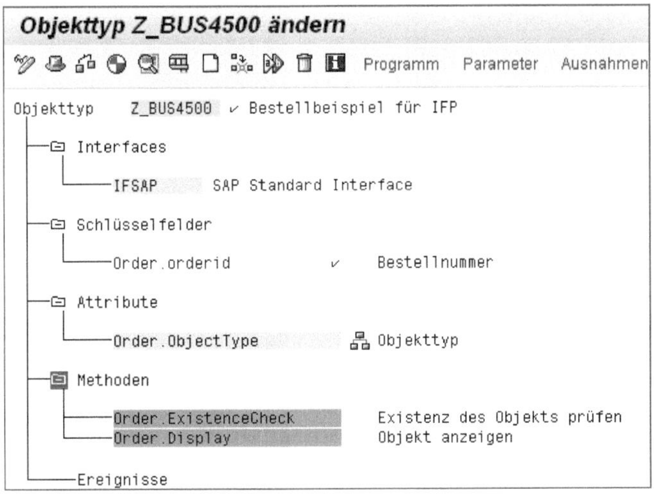

Abbildung 3.12 Business-Objekt »Order«

Wählen Sie den Menüeintrag **Bearbeiten • Freigabestatus ändern • Objekttyp • implementiert**, und generieren Sie dann den Objekttyp über **Generieren** ([Strg] + [F3]).

3.5.2 Entwicklung von BAPIs

Im nächsten Schritt entwickeln Sie die BAPIs und ordnen diese dem Objekttyp zu. Dabei definieren Sie zunächst im ABAP Dictionary die benötigten Domänen, Datenelemente und Strukturen für die BAPI-Parameter. Danach implementieren Sie den RFC-Funktionsbaustein für das BAPI mit dem Function Builder. Diesen Funktionsbaustein ordnen Sie anschließend als API-Methode dem Business-Objekt im Object Builder zu.

Konventionen für BAPIs

BAPIs müssen einige Konventionen einhalten:

- Für Standard-BAPIs sollten die generischen Namen verwendet werden:
  - `Create` und `CreateFromData`
    Diese BAPIs erzeugen neue Business-Objekt-Instanzen. Sie sind instanzunabhängig.
  - `Change`
    Dieses instanzabhängige BAPI ändert den Zustand einer existierenden Instanz eines Business-Objekts. Die Instanz wird dabei über die Werte der Schlüsselfelder identifiziert.
  - `Delete`
    Dieses instanzabhängige BAPI löscht eine Instanz eines Business-Objekts aus der Datenbank. Die Instanz wird dabei über die Werte der Schlüsselfelder identifiziert.
  - `GetList`
    Dieses instanzunabhängige BAPI liefert eine Tabelle von Schlüsselwerten zurück, die Instanzen des Business-Objekts identifizieren.
  - `GetDetail`
    Dieses instanzunabhängige BAPI liefert Details einer Instanz eines Business-Objekts zurück. Die Instanz wird dabei über die Werte der Schlüsselfelder identifiziert.
- Die Methodennamen sollten gemäß der von SAP festgelegten Konvention für BAPIs in englischer Sprache vergeben werden und dürfen maximal 30 Zeichen lang sein.
- Unterstriche sind in BAPI-Namen nicht erlaubt. Falls sich ein BAPI-Name aus mehreren Wörtern zusammensetzt, sollte das sogenannte *Camel Case* verwendet werden, d. h., jedes Wort beginnt mit einem Großbuch-

staben, wie z. B. in `GetDetail`. Bei den Namen zugeordneter Funktionsbausteine wird dann die Camel-Case-Schreibweise durch Unterstriche zwischen den Wörtern ersetzt, z. B. `GET_DETAIL`.

Konventionen für Parameter

Auch für die Parameter müssen einige Konventionen eingehalten werden:

- Werden standardisierte Parameter verwendet, sollten auch die dafür vorgesehenen Namen genutzt werden.
  - `RETURN`
    Jedes BAPI muss über einen Parameter namens `RETURN` verfügen, mit dem Meldungen an den Aufrufer zurückgegeben werden. Dieser Parameter kann ein Export- oder ein Tabellenparameter sein. Er hat in der Regel den Typ `BAPIRET2`.
  - `TestRun`
    Dieser Importparameter wird in schreibenden BAPIs verwendet, um Testaufrufe durchführen zu können. Ist dieser Parameter nicht initial, führt das BAPI nur die vorgesehenen Prüfungen durch, nimmt aber keine Änderungen an der Datenbank vor.
  - `ExtensionIn` und `ExtensionOut`
    Damit das BAPI ohne Modifikationen erweitert werden kann, sollte es über die Parameter `ExtensionIn` und `ExtensionOut` vom Typ `BAPIPAREX` verfügen. Damit Kundenerweiterungen den Parameter `ExtensionIn` lesen können, sollte zu Beginn des BAPIs ein BAdI (Business Add-in) definiert und aufgerufen werden, dem dieser Parameter übergeben wird. Am Ende des BAPIs sollte ein zweites BAdI definiert und aufgerufen werden, mit dessen Hilfe die Kundenerweiterungen den Parameter `ExtensionOut` füllen können.
- Die Parameternamen sollten so aussagekräftig wie möglich sein.
- Die Parameternamen müssen englisch und dürfen höchstens 30 Zeichen lang sein.
- Die Bestandteile der Parameternamen im Business Object Repository beginnen mit Großbuchstaben, wie z. B. in `TestRun` oder `ExtensionIn`.
- Werte, die semantisch zusammengehören, sollten innerhalb einer Struktur anstelle von mehreren Skalaren übergeben werden.
- Zu jedem Feld, das eine Menge oder einen Währungsbetrag enthält, sollte es ein entsprechendes Feld mit der Mengeneinheit bzw. der Währung geben.
- Für Felder zu Land, Sprache, Maßeinheit oder Währung sollte es auch ein Feld geben, das den passenden ISO-Code enthält.

Transaktionsmodell für BAPIs

Wie in Abschnitt 3.2, »Transaktionaler RFC«, beschrieben, werden schreibende oder ändernde BAPIs über einen synchronen RFC aufgerufen und geben im Parameter `RETURN` eine Erfolgs- oder Fehlermeldung zurück. Damit im Fehlerfall die Änderungen auf dem Zielsystem wieder rückgängig gemacht werden können, rufen BAPIs, die schreibend auf die Datenbank zugreifen, für die Datenbankänderungen einen Verbuchungsbaustein mit dem Zusatz `IN UPDATE TASK` auf. Die Datenbankänderungen werden also nicht sofort beim Aufruf ausgeführt, sondern nur zur Verbuchung aufgezeichnet. Damit die Verbuchung dann auch tatsächlich stattfindet, muss der Client explizit den Funktionsbaustein `BAPI_TRANSACTION_COMMIT` aufrufen. Dieser Funktionsbaustein kapselt ein `COMMIT WORK` und sorgt damit für den Anstoß der Verbuchung auf dem Zielsystem.

BAPIs für die Bestellanwendung

Im Folgenden zeigen wir Ihnen, wie Sie BAPIs zum Anlegen, Ändern, Löschen und Lesen von Kundenbestellungen programmieren. Dabei legen Sie zuerst die benötigten Strukturen im ABAP Dictionary an. Danach schreiben Sie die RFC-Funktionsbausteine und ordnen diese dem Business-Objekttyp als BAPIs zu.

BAPI »CreateFromData«

Konventionen für BAPI-Schnittstelle

Eine Instanz des Business-Objekttyps `Book` soll über das BAPI `CreateFromData` angelegt werden. Die Schnittstelle dieses BAPIs muss einigen Konventionen genügen:

- Die Importparameter des BAPIs stellen die zur Instanzerzeugung notwendigen Daten bereit. Im Fall des Business-Objekts `Order` sind dies die Kopf- und Positionsdaten der Bestellung.
- Das BAPI muss auch über einen Parameter namens `TestRun` verfügen. Wird dieser Parameter mit »X« bewertet, wird das BAPI ganz normal ausgeführt, aber es schreibt keine Daten in den Update Task. Nach dem Aufruf von `BapiService.TransactionCommit` werden die Daten daher nicht in die Datenbank geschrieben.
- Damit die Importparameter des BAPIs ohne Modifikationen erweitert werden können, muss die Schnittstelle den Importparameter `ExtensionIn` bereitstellen.
- Die Schlüsselfelder des neu erzeugten Objekts müssen als Exportparameter zurückgegeben werden.
- Um Warnungen und Fehlernachrichten an den Aufrufer zurückzugeben, muss ein Exportparameter namens `RETURN` zurückgegeben werden. Beim Füllen dieses Parameters müssen Sie einige Regeln beachten, auf die wir im Folgenden eingehen.

Standardnachricht bei Instanzerzeugung

Wurde die neue Instanz erfolgreich erzeugt, muss eine Standardnachricht aus Tabelle `T100` zurückgegeben werden (siehe Tabelle 3.2).

Feld	Inhalt
`TYPE`	S
`ID`	BAPI
`NUMBER`	000
`MESSAGE_V1`	<Objektname>
`MESSAGE_V2`	<Objekt-ID>
`MESSAGE_V3`	<Objekt-ID>
`MESSAGE_V4`	<Referenz-ID>
`SYSTEM`	<System>

Tabelle 3.2 Felder des Parameters »RETURN« im Erfolgsfall

Das Feld `MESSAGE_V1` enthält den Namen des Business-Objekttyps, in diesem Fall `Order`. Der Schlüssel des neu erzeugten Objekts wird in `MESSAGE_V2` zurückgegeben. Gibt es mehr als ein Schlüsselfeld, müssen die Felder aneinandergehängt werden. Reichen die 50 Stellen von `MESSAGE_V2` nicht aus, wird zusätzlich noch das Feld `MESSAGE_V3` verwendet. Ein Referenzschlüssel (z. B. aus einem externen System) wird im Feld `MESSAGE_V4` zurückgegeben.

Fehlermeldungen

Kann das Objekt nicht angelegt werden, wird eine standardisierte Nachricht zurückgegeben (siehe Tabelle 3.3).

Feld	Inhalt
`TYPE`	E
`ID`	BAPI
`NUMBER`	001
`MESSAGE_V1`	<Objektname>
`MESSAGE_V2`	–
`MESSAGE_V3`	–
`MESSAGE_V4`	<Referenz-ID>
`SYSTEM`	<System>

Tabelle 3.3 Felder des Parameters »RETURN« im Fehlerfall

Asynchrone Verbuchung

Bei der Implementierung des BAPIs müssen ebenfalls einige Dinge beachtet werden: Das BAPI muss natürlich ein RFC-Funktionsbaustein sein. Es darf die Erzeugung der Datensätze nicht direkt vornehmen, sondern muss dazu einen Verbuchungsbaustein `IN UPDATE TASK` aufrufen. Dieser Verbuchungsbaustein sollte die ihm übergebenen Daten zunächst einmal in einer internen Tabelle innerhalb der Funktionsgruppe speichern und dann ein Unterprogramm mit dem Zusatz `ON COMMIT` aufrufen, das die eigentliche Verbuchung mit Array-Insert-Techniken vornimmt. Damit wird es möglich, innerhalb einer Transaktion mehrere Objekte performant zu erzeugen. Das Unterprogramm, das die eigentliche Verbuchung vornimmt, wird nur einmal ausgeführt und schreibt alle Datensätze in einem einzigen Datenbankzugriff. Dies ist dann wichtig, wenn das BAPI Massendaten einlesen soll.

Diesen Verbuchungsbaustein haben wir bereits in Listing 3.5 aus Abschnitt 1.3.5, »Verbuchungsbausteine«, programmiert. Listing 3.12 zeigt nun das eigentliche BAPI. Es nimmt die Daten für die neu anzulegende Kundenbestellung in seinen Importparametern entgegen. Fehler- und Erfolgsmeldungen werden in der Tabelle `RETURN` zurückgegeben, deren Zeilen die Struktur `BAPIRET2` haben.

```
FUNCTION z_bapi_order_createfromdata.
*"----------------------------------------------------------
*"*"Lokale Schnittstelle:
*"  IMPORTING
*"     VALUE(IM_ORDERHEADER) TYPE  ZIFPORDER
*"     VALUE(TESTRUN)        TYPE  BAPISFLAUX-TESTRUN
*"                                 DEFAULT SPACE
*"  EXPORTING
*"     VALUE(ORDERID)        TYPE  ZIFPORDERID
*"  TABLES
*"     RETURN STRUCTURE  BAPIRET2
*"     TA_ORDERPOS STRUCTURE  ZIFPORDERPOS
*"----------------------------------------------------------
DATA:
  l_orderid TYPE zifporderid,
  msg_hlp_extkey LIKE sy-msgv1,
  msg1_hlp LIKE sy-msgv1.
* Rückgabeparameter initialisieren
  REFRESH: return.
  CLEAR:   orderid.
  CALL FUNCTION 'Z_IFP_ORDER_CREATE'
    EXPORTING
```

```
    im_orderheader = im_orderheader
    im_testrun     = testrun
    im_commit      = ' '
  IMPORTING
    ex_orderid     = l_orderid
  TABLES
    ta_orderpos    = ta_orderpos
  EXCEPTIONS
    not_authorized = 1
    no_number      = 2
    no_lock        = 3
    OTHERS         = 4.
CASE sy-subrc.
  WHEN 1.
    "Keine Berechtigung
    CALL FUNCTION 'BALW_BAPIRETURN_GET2'
        EXPORTING
            type      = 'E'
            cl        = 'ZIFP'
            number    = 101
            parameter = ''
            field     = ''
        IMPORTING
            return    = return.
    APPEND return.
  WHEN 2.
    "Keine Bestellnummer
    CALL FUNCTION 'BALW_BAPIRETURN_GET2'
        EXPORTING
            type      = 'E'
            cl        = 'ZIFP'
            number    = 103
            parameter = ''
            field     = ''
        IMPORTING
            return    = return.
    APPEND return.
  WHEN 3.
    "Keine Sperre
    CALL FUNCTION 'BALW_BAPIRETURN_GET2'
       EXPORTING
            type      = 'E'
            cl        = 'ZIFP'
```

```
                number    = 104
                parameter = ''
                field     = ''
            IMPORTING
                return    = return.
        APPEND return.
    ENDCASE.
* Abbruch bei Fehler
    IF return-type = 'E'.
      PERFORM final_return_message_create      "BAPI erfolglos
        USING     'E' '' msg_hlp_extkey
        CHANGING  return[].
      RETURN.
    ELSE.
      CLEAR sy-subrc.
    ENDIF.
* im Testlauf Informationsnachricht erzeugen
    IF testrun IS NOT INITIAL.
      CALL FUNCTION 'BALW_BAPIRETURN_GET2'     "Testlauf
          EXPORTING
              type   = 'I'
              cl     = 'ZIFP'
              number = 105
          IMPORTING
              return = return.
    ENDIF.
* Erfolgsmeldung erzeugen
    WRITE: l_orderid TO msg1_hlp.
    PERFORM final_return_message_create     "BAPI erfolgreich
      USING     'S'  msg1_hlp msg_hlp_extkey
      CHANGING  return[].
* Rückgabeparameter füllen
    orderid = l_orderid.
ENDFUNCTION.
```

Listing 3.12 BAPI »Z_BAPI_ORDER_CREATEFROMDATA«

Wurde die Bestellung erfolgreich angelegt, enthält der Exportparameter ORDERID den Schlüsselwert, mit dem die neue Kundenbestellung identifiziert werden kann.

Das BAPI delegiert die Hauptarbeit (Prüfungen und Aufruf des Verbuchers) an den Funktionsbaustein Z_IFP_ORDER_CREATE aus Listing 3.6 in Abschnitt 3.2, »Transaktionaler RFC«. Falls dieser Funktionsbaustein mit einem Fehler zurückkommt, wird eine Fehlermeldung in die interne Tabelle RETURN geschrieben.

Aufbau von Fehlermeldungen

Um die Fehlermeldung aufzubauen, verwendet das BAPI den Funktionsbaustein BALW_BAPIRETURN_GET2. Dieser Funktionsbaustein sorgt dafür, dass das Feld RETURN-Message mit einer Nachricht aus einer Nachrichtenklasse gefüllt wird. Nachrichtennummer und Nachrichtenklasse werden diesem Funktionsbaustein in seinen Importparametern number und cl übergeben. Darüber hinaus werden von diesem Funktionsbaustein die Felder RETURN-PARAMETER, RETURN-ROW, RETURN-FIELD und RETURN-MESSAGE_V1 bis RETURN-MESSAGE_V4 aus den Importparametern PARAMETER, ROW, FIELD und PAR1 bis PAR4 gefüllt.

Ist bei den Prüfungen ein Fehler festgestellt worden, wird im Unterprogramm final_return_message_create (siehe Listing 3.13) eine Fehlermeldung an die Tabelle RETURN gehängt und das BAPI verlassen. Waren die Prüfungen dagegen erfolgreich, wird eine Erfolgsnachricht an die Tabelle RETURN gehängt und der Exportparameter gefüllt, bevor das BAPI verlassen wird.

```
**** Unterprogramm zur Erzeugung der Abschlussnachricht
FORM final_return_message_create
    USING
       value(mess_type)  TYPE bapi_mtype
       value(mess_var2)  TYPE symsgv
       value(mess_var4)  TYPE symsgv
    CHANGING
       return TYPE return_type.
  DATA: return_item TYPE bapiret2.
  IF mess_type = 'S'.
    "Bestellung erzeugt
    CALL FUNCTION 'BALW_BAPIRETURN_GET2'
         EXPORTING
            type   = 'S'
            cl     = 'BAPI'
            number = 0
            par1   = 'Order'
            par2   = mess_var2
            par4   = mess_var4
        IMPORTING
            return = return_item.
    APPEND return_item TO return.
  ENDIF.
  IF mess_type = 'E'.
```

```
    "Bestellung nicht erzeugt
    CALL FUNCTION 'BALW_BAPIRETURN_GET2'
        EXPORTING
            type   = 'E'
            cl     = 'BAPI'
            number = 1
            par1   = 'Order'
            par4   = mess_var4
       IMPORTING
            return = return_item.
    APPEND return_item TO return.
  ENDIF.
ENDFORM.                    "final_return_message_create
```

Listing 3.13 Unterprogramm »final_return_message_create«

Freigabe und Zuordnung

Nachdem Sie das BAPI getestet haben, können Sie es im Function Builder über den Menüpfad **Eigenschaften • Funktionsbaustein • Freigabe • Freigeben** ausgeben. Diesen Menüpfad können Sie allerdings nur dann auswählen, wenn Sie im Function Builder den Änderungsmodus eingestellt haben und sich außerdem auf der Registerkarte **Eigenschaften** befinden.

Anschließend können Sie in Transaktion SWO1 den Funktionsbaustein dem Business-Objekt Z_BUS4500 als API-Methode zuordnen. Dazu wählen Sie im Menü **Hilfsmittel • API-Methoden • Methode einfügen** aus. In den dann folgenden Dialogen selektieren Sie zuerst den Funktionsbaustein und einen Namen für die Methode, danach bestimmen Sie die Parameternamen für die Methode.

Freigabe des BAPIs

Danach geben Sie im Menü über **Bearbeiten • Freigabestatus ändern** zuerst das Business-Objekt und dann die API-Methode frei. Als Resultat verfügt das Business-Objekt nun über ein neues BAPI und wird in Transaktion BAPI angezeigt.

Testen des BAPIs

Mit dem Report ZIFP_TEST_CREATE_BAPI in Listing 3.14 können Sie das BAPI CreateFromData testen. Der Report nimmt die ORDERID einer Lieferantenbestellung vom Anwender in einem Selektionsparameter entgegen. Danach ruft er das BAPI auf und gibt eine Fehler- oder Erfolgsmeldung aus. Im Erfolgsfall muss der Report im Zielsystem den Funktionsbaustein BAPI_TRANSACTION_COMMIT aufrufen, damit die dort nur vorgemerkten Datenbankänderungen auch tatsächlich durchgeführt werden.

```
REPORT zifp_test_create_bapi.
PARAMETERS:
  pa_id  TYPE zifporder-orderid,
```

```
  p_dest TYPE rfcdes-rfcdest VALUE CHECK.
DATA:
  orderheader TYPE zifporder,
  it_orderpos TYPE STANDARD TABLE OF zifporderpos,
  ret         TYPE STANDARD TABLE OF bapiret2,
  waret       TYPE bapiret2,
  orderid     TYPE zifporderid.
AT SELECTION-SCREEN.
  SELECT SINGLE * FROM zifporder
  INTO orderheader
  WHERE
    orderid   = pa_id AND
    type      = 'PO'.
  IF sy-subrc <> 0.
    MESSAGE e001(zifp).
  ENDIF.
START-OF-SELECTION.
  orderheader-type  = 'SO'.
  orderheader-refid = orderheader-orderid.
  SELECT * FROM zifporderpos INTO TABLE it_orderpos
  WHERE
    orderid = pa_id.

  CALL FUNCTION 'Z_BAPI_ORDER_CREATEFROMDATA'
    DESTINATION p_dest
    EXPORTING
      im_orderheader = orderheader
      im_testrun     = space
    IMPORTING
      orderid        = orderid
    TABLES
      return         = ret
      ta_orderpos    = it_orderpos.
  READ TABLE ret WITH KEY type = 'E' TRANSPORTING NO FIELDS.
  IF sy-subrc = 0.
* Fehlerausgabe
    WRITE:/ 'Kundenauftrag konnte nicht angelegt werden.'.
    LOOP AT ret INTO waret.
      WRITE:/
        waret-type,
        waret-id,
        waret-number,
        waret-message.
```

```
    ENDLOOP.
  ELSE.
* Erfolgsmeldung
    CALL FUNCTION 'BAPI_TRANSACTION_COMMIT'
      DESTINATION p_dest.
    WRITE:/ 'Neue Kundenbestellung', orderid.
  ENDIF.
```

Listing 3.14 Testprogramm »ZIFP_TEST_CREATE_BAPI«

BAPI »Change«

Als Nächstes entwickeln Sie das BAPI Change. Dies ist eine instanzabhängige Methode, da es eine bestimmte Instanz eines Business-Objekts ändert. Daher muss das BAPI die Schlüsselfelder des Business-Objekts als Importparameter haben. Diese Importparameter müssen den gleichen Namen und Datentyp wie die Schlüsselfelder des Business-Objekts tragen.

X-Parameter mit Änderungskennzeichen

Für jeden Importparameter mit den zu ändernden Daten sollte das BAPI einen zweiten Importparameter bereitstellen, in dem der Aufrufer angeben kann, welche der übergebenen Daten im ersten Parameter tatsächlich geändert werden sollen. Diese Technik haben Sie bereits in Listing 3.4 in Abschnitt 3.1.3, »Funktionsbausteine zum Löschen und Ändern«, kennengelernt.

Rückgabe im Erfolgsfall

Wurde die Instanz erfolgreich geändert, muss eine Standardnachricht aus der Tabelle T100 zurückgegeben werden (siehe Tabelle 3.4).

Feld	Inhalt
TYPE	S
ID	BAPI
NUMBER	002
MESSAGE_V1	<Objektname>
MESSAGE_V2	<Objekt-ID>
MESSAGE_V3	<Objekt-ID>
MESSAGE_V4	–
SYSTEM	<System>

Tabelle 3.4 Felder des Parameters »RETURN« im Erfolgsfall

Das Feld MESSAGE_V1 enthält den Namen des Business-Objekttyps, in diesem Fall Order. Der Schlüssel des geänderten Objekts wird in MESSAGE_V2 zurückgegeben. Gibt es mehr als ein Schlüsselfeld, müssen die Felder aneinandergehängt werden. Reichen die 50 Stellen von MESSAGE_V2 nicht aus, wird zusätzlich noch MESSAGE_V3 verwendet. Im Gegensatz zum Anlegen einer neuen Instanz muss nun kein Referenzschlüssel im Feld MESSAGE_V4 zurückgegeben werden, da keine neue Objekt-ID erzeugt wird, die mit dem Referenzschlüssel korrelieren müsste.

Rückgabe im Fehlerfall

Kann das Objekt nicht geändert werden, wird eine standardisierte Nachricht wie in Tabelle 3.5 zurückgegeben.

Feld	Inhalt
TYPE	E
ID	BAPI
NUMBER	003
MESSAGE_V1	<Objektname>
MESSAGE_V2	–
MESSAGE_V3	–
MESSAGE_V4	–
SYSTEM	<System>

Tabelle 3.5 Felder des Parameters »RETURN« im Fehlerfall

Weitere Meldungen

Zusätzlich zu diesen beiden standardisierten Fehlermeldungen kann und soll das BAPI, insbesondere im Fehlerfall, weitere detaillierte Meldungen zurückgeben. Dazu kann das BAPI auch die Felder RETURN-PARAMETER, RETURN-ROW und RETURN-FIELD des RETURN-Parameters verwenden, um die Fehlerstelle genau zu kennzeichnen.

Auch dieses BAPI, das in Listing 3.15 dargestellt ist, delegiert die Hauptarbeit an den Funktionsbaustein Z_IFP_ORDER_CHANGE aus Listing 3.4. Löst dieser Funktionsbaustein eine Ausnahme aus, füllt das BAPI den Rückgabeparameter RETURN und bricht die weitere Verarbeitung ab.

```
FUNCTION Z_BAPI_ORDER_CHANGE.
*"----------------------------------------------------------
*"*"Lokale Schnittstelle:
*"  IMPORTING
*"     VALUE(ORDERID)          TYPE  ZIFPORDERID
```

```
*"      VALUE(IM_ORDERHEADER)  TYPE  ZIFPORDER
*"      VALUE(IM_ORDERHEADERX) TYPE  ZIFPORDERX
*"      VALUE(TESTRUN)         TYPE  BAPISFLAUX-TESTRUN
*"                                   DEFAULT SPACE
*"   TABLES
*"       RETURN       STRUCTURE  BAPIRET2
*"       TA_ORDERPOS  STRUCTURE  ZIFPORDERPOS
*"       TA_ORDERPOSX STRUCTURE  ZIFPORDERPOSX
*"------------------------------------------------------------
  DATA:
    l_orderid TYPE zifporderid,
    msg1_hlp LIKE sy-msgv1.

* Rückgabeparameter initialisieren
  REFRESH: return.
  CALL FUNCTION 'Z_IFP_ORDER_CHANGE'
    EXPORTING
      im_orderheader  = im_orderheader
      im_orderheaderx = im_orderheaderx
      im_testrun      = testrun
      im_commit       = ' '
    TABLES
      ta_orderpos     = ta_orderpos
      ta_orderposx    = ta_orderposx
    EXCEPTIONS
      not_authorized  = 1
      no_data         = 2
      no_lock         = 3
      OTHERS          = 4.
  CASE sy-subrc.
    WHEN 1.
      "Keine Berechtigung
      CALL FUNCTION 'BALW_BAPIRETURN_GET2'
          EXPORTING
              type      = 'E'
              cl        = 'ZIFP'
              number    = 101
              parameter = ''
              field     = ''
          IMPORTING
              return    = return.
      APPEND return.
    WHEN 2.
```

```
    CALL FUNCTION 'BALW_BAPIRETURN_GET2'   "Keine Daten
        EXPORTING
            type      = 'E'
            cl        = 'ZIFP'
            number    = 106
            parameter = ''
            field     = ''
        IMPORTING
            return    = return.
    APPEND return.
  WHEN 3.
    CALL FUNCTION 'BALW_BAPIRETURN_GET2'   "Keine Sperre
        EXPORTING
            type      = 'E'
            cl        = 'ZIFP'
            number    = 104
            parameter = ''
            field     = ''
        IMPORTING
            return    = return.
    APPEND return.
ENDCASE.
* Abbruch bei Fehler
IF return-type = 'E'.
  PERFORM final_return_message_change      "BAPI erfolglos
    USING     'E' ''
    CHANGING  return[].
  RETURN.
ELSE.
  CLEAR sy-subrc.
ENDIF.
* im Testlauf Informationsnachricht erzeugen
IF testrun IS NOT INITIAL.
  CALL FUNCTION 'BALW_BAPIRETURN_GET2'     "TestRun
      EXPORTING
          type   = 'I'
          cl     = 'ZIFP'
          number = 105
      IMPORTING
          return = return.
ENDIF.
* Erfolgsmeldung erzeugen
WRITE: orderid TO msg1_hlp NO-GAP.
```

```
  "BAPI erfolgreich
  PERFORM final_return_message_change
    USING     'S'  msg1_hlp
    CHANGING  return[].
ENDFUNCTION.
```

Listing 3.15 Funktion »Z_BAPI_ORDER_CHANGE«

Füllen von »RETURN«

Sowohl im Fehler- als auch im Erfolgsfall fügt das BAPI eine Zeile an den Rückgabeparameter `RETURN` an. Um die Fehlermeldungen in die Rückgabetabelle `RETURN` zu schreiben, verwendet das BAPI das Unterprogramm `final_return_message_change`, das in Listing 3.16 zu sehen ist.

```
**** Unterprogramm zur Erzeugung der Abschlussnachricht
*   (Change)
* schreibt Erfolgs- oder Fehlernachrichten
**********************************************************
FORM final_return_message_change
    USING
       value(mess_type)  TYPE bapi_mtype
       value(mess_var2)  TYPE symsgv
    CHANGING
       return            TYPE return_type.
  DATA: return_item TYPE bapiret2.
  IF mess_type = 'S'.
    "Bestellung geändert
    CALL FUNCTION 'BALW_BAPIRETURN_GET2'
        EXPORTING
            type   = 'S'
            cl     = 'BAPI'
            number = 2
            par1   = 'Order'
            par2   = mess_var2
        IMPORTING
            return = return_item.
    APPEND return_item TO return.
  ENDIF.
  IF mess_type = 'E'.
     "Bestellung nicht geändert
    CALL FUNCTION 'BALW_BAPIRETURN_GET2'
        EXPORTING
            type   = 'E'
            cl     = 'BAPI'
            number = 3
```

```
          par1    = 'Order'
      IMPORTING
          return = return_item.
    APPEND return_item TO return.
  ENDIF.
ENDFORM.                        "final_return_message_change
```

Listing 3.16 Unterprogramm »final_return_message_change«

Testen des BAPIs »Change«

Mit dem Report ZIFP_TEST_CHANGE_BAPI in Listing 3.17 können Sie das Change-BAPI testen. Der Report nimmt die ORDERID der zu ändernden Bestellung und außerdem die neuen Werte für Käufer, Verkäufer und Währung vom Anwender in Selektionsparametern entgegen. Ist ein Selektionsparameter nicht initial, wird das entsprechende Änderungskennzeichen in orderheaderx bzw. ta_orderposx gesetzt und der Inhalt des Parameters nach im_orderheader bzw. ta_orderpos kopiert. Danach wird das BAPI Z_BAPI_ORDER_CHANGE aufgerufen. Enthält die Rückgabetabelle RETURN einen Fehlereintrag, gibt der Report diese Tabelle komplett aus. Im Erfolgsfall ruft er das BAPI BAPI_TRANSACTION_COMMIT auf und schreibt eine Meldung für den Benutzer.

```
REPORT zifp_test_change_bapi.
PARAMETERS:
  pa_id    TYPE zifporder-orderid,
  p_dest   TYPE rfcdes-rfcdest VALUE CHECK.
SELECTION-SCREEN BEGIN OF BLOCK new WITH FRAME
    TITLE text-new.
  PARAMETERS:
    seller   TYPE zifpseller LOWER CASE,
    buyer    TYPE zifpbuyer LOWER CASE,
    currency TYPE zifpcurrency.
SELECTION-SCREEN END OF BLOCK new.
DATA:
  orderheader  TYPE zifporder,
  orderheaderx TYPE zifporderx,
  it_orderpos  TYPE STANDARD TABLE OF zifporderpos,
  it_orderposx TYPE STANDARD TABLE OF zifporderposx,
  wa_orderpos  TYPE zifporderpos,
  wa_orderposx TYPE zifporderposx,
  ret          TYPE STANDARD TABLE OF bapiret2,
  waret        TYPE bapiret2,
  orderid      TYPE zifporderid.
AT SELECTION-SCREEN.
  SELECT SINGLE * FROM zifporder
```

```
  INTO orderheader
  WHERE
    orderid   = pa_id AND
    type      = 'SO'.
  IF sy-subrc <> 0.
    MESSAGE e001(zifp).
  ENDIF.
START-OF-SELECTION.
  IF seller IS NOT INITIAL.
    orderheaderx-seller = 'X'.
    orderheader-seller  = seller.
  ENDIF.
  IF buyer IS NOT INITIAL.
    orderheaderx-buyer = 'X'.
    orderheader-buyer  = buyer.
  ENDIF.
  IF currency IS NOT INITIAL.
    SELECT * FROM zifporderpos INTO TABLE it_orderpos
    WHERE
      orderid = pa_id.
    LOOP AT it_orderpos INTO wa_orderpos.
      wa_orderposx-currency = 'X'.
      APPEND wa_orderposx TO it_orderposx.
      wa_orderpos-currency  = currency.
      MODIFY it_orderpos FROM wa_orderpos.
    ENDLOOP.
  ENDIF.
  CALL FUNCTION 'Z_BAPI_ORDER_CHANGE'
    DESTINATION p_dest
    EXPORTING
      orderid          = pa_id
      im_orderheader   = orderheader
      im_orderheaderx  = orderheaderx
      im_testrun       = space
    TABLES
      return           = ret
      ta_orderpos      = it_orderpos
      ta_orderposx     = it_orderposx.
  READ TABLE ret WITH KEY type = 'E' TRANSPORTING NO FIELDS.
  IF sy-subrc = 0.
* Fehlerausgabe
    WRITE:/ 'Bestellung konnte nicht geändert werden.'.
    LOOP AT ret INTO waret.
```

```
      WRITE:/
        waret-type,
        waret-id,
        waret-number,
        waret-message.
    ENDLOOP.
  ELSE.
* Erfolgsmeldung
    CALL FUNCTION 'BAPI_TRANSACTION_COMMIT'
      DESTINATION p_dest.
    WRITE:/ 'Bestellung geändert'.
  ENDIF.
```

Listing 3.17 Testprogramm »ZIFP_TEST_CHANGE_BAPI«

BAPI »GetList«

Bestellungsliste übergeben

Im Vergleich zu den ändernden BAPIs sind die lesenden BAPIs relativ einfach aufgebaut. Listing 3.18 zeigt das BAPI `GetList` für das Business-Objekt `Order`. Die `GetList`-BAPIs sind instanzunabhängig und liefern eine Liste von Schlüsselwerten für ihre Business-Objekte zurück, die zu den beim Aufruf übergebenen Selektionskriterien passen. Das BAPI `Z_BAPI_ORDER_GETLIST` nimmt eine Referenznummer entgegen und liefert in der Tabelle `TA_ORDERS` eine Liste von Kundenbestellungen mit dieser Referenznummer. Falls die Referenznummer initial ist, wird eine Liste aller Bestellungen zurückgegeben. Im Erfolgs- wie auch im Fehlerfall wird der Rückgabeparameter `RETURN` vom Typ `BAPIRET2` gefüllt.

```
FUNCTION z_bapi_order_getlist.
*"----------------------------------------------------------
*"*"Lokale Schnittstelle:
*"  IMPORTING
*"     VALUE(IM_REFID) LIKE ZIFPORDER-REFID OPTIONAL
*"  EXPORTING
*"     VALUE(RETURN) TYPE  BAPIRET2
*"  TABLES
*"     TA_ORDERS STRUCTURE  ZIFPORDER
*"----------------------------------------------------------
* Rückgabewerte initialisieren
  REFRESH ta_orders.
  CLEAR   return.
  CALL FUNCTION 'Z_IFP_ORDER_GETLIST'
    EXPORTING
      im_ordertype   = 'SO'
```

```
      im_refid       = im_refid
    TABLES
      ta_orders      = ta_orders
    EXCEPTIONS
      not_authorized = 1
      no_data        = 2
      OTHERS         = 3.
  CASE sy-subrc.
    WHEN 0.
      return-type    = 'S'.
    WHEN 1.
      "Keine Berechtigung
      CALL FUNCTION 'BALW_BAPIRETURN_GET2'
          EXPORTING
              type      = 'E'
              cl        = 'ZIFP'
              number    = 101
              parameter = ''
              field     = ''
          IMPORTING
              return    = return.
    WHEN 2.
      CALL FUNCTION 'BALW_BAPIRETURN_GET2'     "Keine Daten
          EXPORTING
              type      = 'E'
              cl        = 'ZIFP'
              number    = 106
              parameter = ''
              field     = ''
          IMPORTING
              return    = return.
  ENDCASE.
ENDFUNCTION.
```

Listing 3.18 BAPI »GetList«

Selektionstabelle

In der Praxis sind GetList-BAPIs oft ein wenig komplexer als dieses einfache Beispiel. Sie erlauben in der Regel die Übergabe einer Selektionstabelle mit den Spalten SIGN, OPTION, HIGH und LOW für ausgewählte Attribute des Business-Objekts. Damit kann der Verwender des BAPIs komplexe Selektionskriterien übergeben, wie es auch für ABAP-Reports durch die Verwendung des Schlüsselworts SELECT-OPTIONS möglich ist. Zumeist haben GetList-BAPIs auch einen Importparameter MaxRows. Ist dieser Parameter beim Aufruf nicht initial, gibt das BAPI nur so viele Zeilen mit Schlüsselwerten zurück, wie in MaxRows angegeben sind.

BAPI »GetDetail«

Bestelldaten nach Bestellnummer selektieren

Das instanzabhängige BAPI GetDetail in Listing 3.19 erwartet eine Bestellnummer als Übergabeparameter. Es selektiert die entsprechenden Daten aus den Datenbanktabellen ZIFPORDER und ZIFPORDERPOS. Falls es dort keine Daten findet, schreibt es eine Fehlermeldung in den RETURN-Parameter. Wird der angeforderte Datensatz gefunden, schreibt das BAPI eine Erfolgsmeldung in den RETURN-Parameter und kopiert die gefundenen Daten in die Rückgabeparameter EX_ORDERHEADER und TA_ORDERPOS.

```
FUNCTION z_bapi_order_getdetail.
*"----------------------------------------------------------
*"*"Lokale Schnittstelle:
*"  IMPORTING
*"     VALUE(ORDERID)       TYPE  ZIFPORDERID
*"  EXPORTING
*"     VALUE(EX_ORDERHEAD) TYPE  ZIFPORDER
*"     VALUE(RETURN)       TYPE  BAPIRET2
*"  TABLES
*"     TA_ORDERPOS STRUCTURE  ZIFPORDERPOS
*"----------------------------------------------------------
* Rückgabeparameter initialisieren
  CLEAR:
    return,
    ex_orderhead.
  REFRESH ta_orderpos.
  CALL FUNCTION 'Z_IFP_ORDER_GETDETAIL'
    EXPORTING
      im_orderid      = orderid
    IMPORTING
      ex_orderhead    = ex_orderhead
    TABLES
      ta_orderpos     = ta_orderpos
    EXCEPTIONS
      not_authorized = 1
      no_data        = 2
      OTHERS         = 3.
  CASE  sy-subrc.
    WHEN 0.
      return-type     = 'S'.
```

```
    WHEN 1.
      "keine Berechtigung
      CALL FUNCTION 'BALW_BAPIRETURN_GET2'
          EXPORTING
              type      = 'E'
              cl        = 'ZIFP'
              number    = 101
              parameter = ''
              field     = ''
          IMPORTING
              return    = return.
    WHEN 2.
      CALL FUNCTION 'BALW_BAPIRETURN_GET2'      "Keine Daten
          EXPORTING
              type      = 'E'
              cl        = 'ZIFP'
              number    = 106
              parameter = ''
              field     = ''
          IMPORTING
              return    = return.
  ENDCASE.
ENDFUNCTION.
```

Listing 3.19 BAPI »GetDetail«

Testen der lesenden BAPIs

Testprogramm

Mit dem Report ZIFP_TEST_READ_BAPIS in Listing 3.20 können Sie das GetList- und das GetDetail-BAPI testen. Der Report fragt eine Referenznummer vom Benutzer ab und ruft damit das BAPI Z_BAPI_ORDER_GETLIST auf. Im Erfolgsfall macht er dann eine Schleife über alle Zeilen der internen Tabelle it_orderhead, die die Schlüsselwerte der Bestellungen enthält. Innerhalb der Schleife ruft er für jede Bestellung das BAPI Z_BAPI_ORDER_GETDETAIL auf. Diese Details werden im Erfolgsfall in der Ausgabeliste ausgegeben; im Fehlerfall wird eine Meldung geschrieben.

```
REPORT  zifp_test_read_bapis.
DATA:
  it_orderhead TYPE STANDARD TABLE OF zifporder,
  wa_orderhead TYPE zifporder,
  it_orderpos  TYPE STANDARD TABLE OF zifporderpos,
  wa_orderpos  TYPE zifporderpos,
  msg_text(80) TYPE c,
```

```
  return       TYPE bapiret2.
PARAMETERS:
  p_dest TYPE rfcdest.
START-OF-SELECTION.
* ORDERID-Liste besorgen
  CALL FUNCTION 'Z_BAPI_ORDER_GETLIST'
    DESTINATION p_dest
    IMPORTING
      return    = return
    TABLES
      ta_orders = it_orderhead.
  IF return-type = 'E'.
    WRITE:/ return-message.
  ELSE.
* alle Bestellungen ausgeben
    LOOP AT it_orderhead INTO wa_orderhead.
      WRITE:/
        wa_orderhead-orderid COLOR COL_KEY,
        wa_orderhead-type,
        wa_orderhead-refid,
        wa_orderhead-buyer,
        wa_orderhead-seller,
        wa_orderhead-orderdate.
* Bestelldetails besorgen
      CALL FUNCTION 'Z_BAPI_ORDER_GETDETAIL'
        DESTINATION p_dest
        EXPORTING
          orderid     = wa_orderhead-orderid
        IMPORTING
          return      = return
        TABLES
          ta_orderpos = it_orderpos.
      IF return-type = 'E'.
        WRITE:/ return-message.
      ELSE.
* Bestelldetails ausgeben
        LOOP AT it_orderpos INTO wa_orderpos.
          WRITE:/
            wa_orderpos-orderid COLOR COL_KEY,
            wa_orderpos-orderpos COLOR COL_KEY,
            wa_orderpos-matid,
            wa_orderpos-mattext,
            wa_orderpos-ordercount,
```

```
          wa_orderpos-price,
          wa_orderpos-currency.
      ENDLOOP.
      ULINE.
    ENDIF.
  ENDLOOP.
ENDIF.
```

Listing 3.20 Testprogramm »ZIFP_TEST_READ_BAPIS«

3.5.3 Business-Objekt »Helpvalues«

BAPIs für Eingabehilfen

Das Business-Objekt Helpvalues stellt zwei BAPIs zur Verfügung, mit denen nach gültigen Werten für Felder von BAPI-Parametern anderer Business-Objekte gesucht werden kann. Diese BAPIs sind hilfreich, wenn ein externes Programm Eingabehilfen im Stil der Wertehilfe (F4-Hilfe) von SAP anbieten möchte. Als Importparameter erwarten diese beiden BAPIs den Namen oder Objekttyp des Business-Objekts, den Namen eines BAPIs dieses Business-Objekts, den Namen eines Parameters in diesem BAPI sowie den Namen eines Felds in diesem Parameter.

Suchhilfen und Trefferlisten

Das BAPI GetSearchhelp liefert mit diesen Informationen eine Liste der Suchhilfen für das gewünschte Feld zurück. Das BAPI GetList gibt mit diesen Informationen und der Angabe einer Suchhilfe eine Trefferliste zurück.

Berechtigungsprüfung

Beide BAPIs prüfen zuvor jedoch durch Aufruf eines Funktionsbausteins, ob der aufrufende Benutzer überhaupt berechtigt ist, sich diese Informationen zu beschaffen. Dieser Funktionsbaustein muss in der Tabelle BAPIF4T hinterlegt sein. Als Selektionskriterium für das Nachschlagen in dieser Tabelle dient den Helpvalues-BAPIs das Datenelement des angefragten Felds.

Möchten Sie nun für das Business-Objekt Order diesen Mechanismus ausnutzen, müssen Sie zuerst einen Funktionsbaustein implementieren, der die Berechtigungsprüfung vornimmt, und diesen Funktionsbaustein dann mithilfe von Transaktion SM30 in die Tabelle BAPIF4T eintragen. Als Kopiervorlage für diesen Funktionsbaustein kann Ihnen jeder Funktionsbaustein dienen, der schon in dieser Tabelle vorhanden ist. Listing 3.21 zeigt den fertigen Funktionsbaustein.

```
FUNCTION z_orderid_f4_authority.
*"----------------------------------------------------------
*"*"Lokale Schnittstelle:
*"  IMPORTING
*"     VALUE(OBJTYPE)  LIKE  BAPIF4F-OBJTYPE
*"     VALUE(METHOD)   LIKE  BAPIF4F-METHOD OPTIONAL
```

```
*"      VALUE(DTEL)      LIKE  BAPIF4F-DTEL OPTIONAL
*"      VALUE(SHLPNAME) LIKE  BAPIF4F-SHLPNAME OPTIONAL
*"      VALUE(TABNAME)  LIKE  BAPIF4F-TABNAME OPTIONAL
*"   EXPORTING
*"      VALUE(RETURN) LIKE  BAPIF4F-RETURN
*"------------------------------------------------------------
  AUTHORITY-CHECK OBJECT 'ZIFPORDER' ID 'ACTVT' FIELD '03'.
  IF sy-subrc = 0.
    MOVE ' ' TO return.
  ELSE.
    MOVE 'X' TO return.
  ENDIF.
ENDFUNCTION.
```

Listing 3.21 Prüfbaustein »Z_ORDERID_F4_AUTHORITY«

Ist die Berechtigungsprüfung erfolgreich, d. h., der Benutzer darf die angeforderten Daten sehen, muss der Exportparameter RETURN initialisiert werden. Im anderen Fall muss er mit 'X' belegt werden.

Registrierung eines Prüfbausteins

Abbildung 3.13 zeigt die Registrierung dieses Funktionsbausteins für das Datenelement ZIFPORDERID. Nach dieser Registrierung können nun die beiden Helpvalues-BAPIs verwendet werden. Dies wird im Folgenden erklärt.

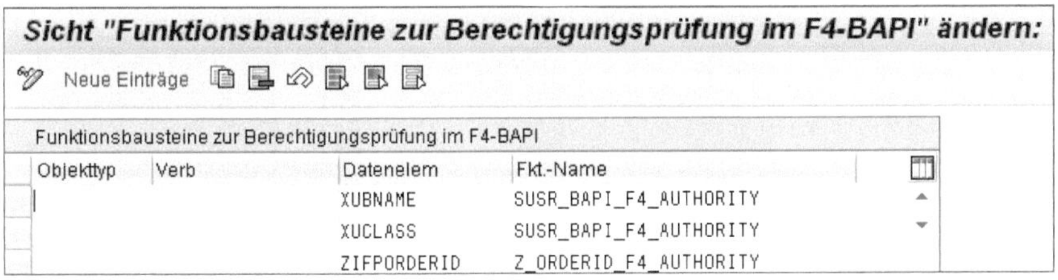

Abbildung 3.13 Registrierung der Prüfbausteine

BAPI »GetSearchhelp«

Abbildung 3.14 zeigt das Ergebnis eines Aufrufs des Helpvalues-BAPIs GetSearchhelp. In den Parametern OBJNAME, METHOD, PARAMETER und FIELD werden der Objektname Order, der BAPI-Name Getdetail, der Parametername ExOrderhead und der Feldname ORDERID übergeben. Im Tabellenparameter SHLP_FOR_HELPVALUES_GET gibt das BAPI die Namen, den Typ (in diesem Fall SH) und den Titel der beiden einfachen Suchhilfen ZIFPORDERA und ZIFPORDERB zurück. Im Tabellenparameter DESCRIPTION_FOR_HELPVALUES werden Informationen über die Suchhilfeparameter zurückgegeben. Diese Informationen könnten z. B. dazu verwendet werden, den Benutzer zwischen den vorhandenen Suchhilfen wählen zu lassen.

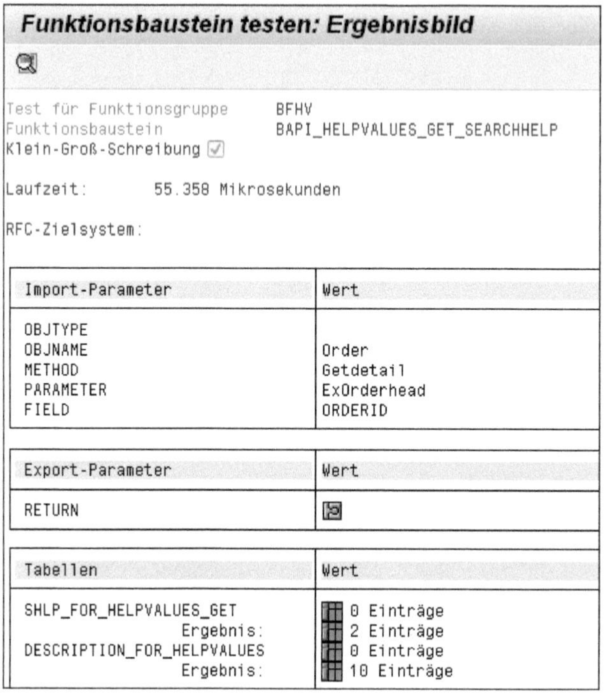

Abbildung 3.14 Ergebnis des BAPIs »GetSearchhelp«

BAPI »Helpvalues«

Abbildung 3.15 zeigt das Ergebnis eines Aufrufs des Helpvalues-BAPIs GetList. Wie zuvor werden in den Parametern OBJNAME, METHOD, PARAMETER und FIELD der Objektname Order, der BAPI-Name Getdetail, der Parametername ExOrderhead und der Feldname ORDERID übergeben. Zusätzlich werden im strukturierten Importparameter EXPLICIT_SHLP der Name und der Typ einer zuvor gefundenen Suchhilfe übergeben.

Das GetList-BAPI wird zweimal aufgerufen. Beim ersten Aufruf wird der Importparameter DESCRIPTIONONLY mit 'X' gefüllt. Es wird dann nur die Tabelle DESCRIPTION_FOR_HELPVALUES ausgewertet. Diese Tabelle enthält die Parameternamen der Suchhilfe und deren Beschreibung. Diese Informationen können verwendet werden, um ein Selektionsbild für den Benutzer darzustellen.

Zwei Aufrufe

In einem zweiten Aufruf wird als Nächstes der Importparameter DESCRIPTIONONLY mit ' ' gefüllt, und die vom Benutzer eingegebenen Selektionskriterien werden in die Tabelle SELECTION_FOR_HELPVALUES übertragen. Diese Tabelle hat den üblichen Aufbau einer Selektionstabelle mit den Spalten SELECT_FLD für den Namen des Selektionsfelds sowie SIGN, OPTION, LOW und HIGH. SIGN kann die Werte »I« (für Include) oder »E« (für Exclude) annehmen. OPTION nimmt einen booleschen Operator (»EQ« für Equal, »LT« für Less

Than, »BT« für Between, »CP« für Contains Pattern usw.) auf. LOW nimmt den vom Benutzer übergebenen Vergleichswert auf. Falls OPTION = »BT« ist, nimmt LOW die untere und HIGH die obere Intervallgrenze auf. Die Tabelle HELPVALUES enthält dann die Liste der gefundenen Werte. Dabei werden die Spalteninhalte der Trefferliste einfach aneinandergehängt. Die Informationen über Position, Offset und Länge einer Spalte finden Sie in der Tabelle DESCRIPTION_FOR_HELPVALUES.

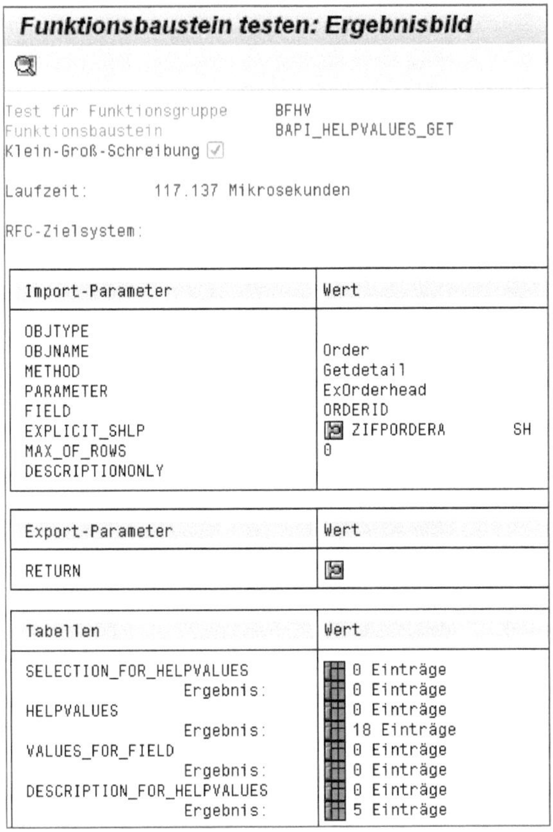

Abbildung 3.15 Aufruf des BAPIs »_HELPVALUES_GET«

Kapitel 4
Remote Function Call mit C/C++

Die Grundlage für die RFC-Programmierung in externen Systemen bildet das SAP NetWeaver RFC Software Development Kit (SDK), das Sie in diesem Kapitel kennenlernen. Dieses SDK gibt es für die wichtigsten Betriebssysteme, und es ist die technische Grundlage für die Java-RFC-Bibliotheken.

In diesem Kapitel lernen Sie, RFC- und BAPI-Clients und -Server mit den Programmiersprachen C und C++ zu schreiben. Mit C/C++ können Sie direkt auf die RFC-Bibliothek zugreifen, die Ihnen im SAP-System zur Verfügung gestellt wird. Dies ist insbesondere dann wichtig, wenn Ihnen auf Ihrer Plattform weder eine Java- noch eine .NET-Umgebung zur Verfügung steht oder wenn Ihre Schnittstelle die maximale Ausführungsgeschwindigkeit benötigt.

Um in der Programmiersprache C/C++ Schnittstellenprogramme für das SAP-System zu schreiben, benötigen Sie einen C/C++-Compiler und das SAP NetWeaver RFC SDK.

4.1 SAP NetWeaver RFC SDK

Mit Release 7.0 EHP 1 wurde das SAP NetWeaver RFC SDK eingeführt und löste das klassische RFC SDK ab. Um neue RFC-Programme in C/C++ zu schreiben, sollten Sie das neuere SDK verwenden.

4.1.1 Inhalte des SAP NetWeaver RFC SDK

Download aus dem SAP Support Portal

Um das SAP NetWeaver RFC SDK herunterzuladen, rufen Sie SAP-Hinweis 2573790 im SAP Support Portal unter *http://service.sap.com/connectors* auf. Hier finden Sie eine Beschreibung und einen Link zum Software Download Center. Im Software Download Center können Sie dann das SAP NetWeaver RFC SDK herunterladen und in ein beliebiges Verzeichnis Ihres Rechners entpacken. Achten Sie darauf, dass Sie die für Ihre Plattform passende Version herunterladen, z. B. für Windows x86 (32 Bit), Windows x86 (64 Bit) oder HP-UX (64 Bit). Das SDK enthält neben der binären RFC-Bibliothek in

Form von Dynamic Link Libraries (DLL) auch Header-Dateien, Linker-Bibliotheken und einige Beispielprogramme. Konkret umfasst es vier Unterverzeichnisse mit folgendem Inhalt:

- **bin**
  Dieses Verzeichnis enthält zwei kompilierte Test- und Beispielprogramme:
  - **startrfc(.exe)**
    ermöglicht den Aufruf eines der beiden Funktionsbausteine EDI_DATA_INCOMING oder EDI_STATUS_INCOMING über RFC
  - **rfcexec(.exe)**
    RFC-Serverprogramm, das von einem SAP-System aus gestartet werden kann, um auf Dateien und Pipes zuzugreifen
- **demo**
  Dieses Verzeichnis enthält Quelldateien in C (Dateiendung **.c**) und C++ (Dateiendung **.cpp**) sowie die dazugehörigen Header-Dateien (Dateiendung **.h**) für Beispielprogramme:
  - **companyClient.c**
    einfacher Client für den Aufruf des Funktionsbausteins BAPI_COMPANY_GETDETAIL
  - **rfcexec.cpp**
    RFC-Serverprogramm, das von einem SAP-System aus gestartet werden kann, um auf Dateien und Pipes zuzugreifen
  - **rfcexec.h**
    Header-Datei zu **rfcexec.cpp**
  - **sflightClient.c**
    Aufruf der Funktionsbausteine BAPI_FLIGHT_GETLIST, BAPI_FLIGHT_GETDETAIL, BAPI_FLBOOKING_CREATEFROMDATA und BAPI_TRANSACTION_COMMIT
  - **startrfc.cpp**
    ermöglicht es, einen der beiden Funktionsbausteine EDI_DATA_INCOMING oder EDI_STATUS_INCOMING über RFC aufzurufen
  - **startrfc.h**
    Header-Datei zu **startrfc.cpp**
  - **stfcDeepTableServer.c**
    Client für den Aufruf des Funktionsbausteins STFC_DEEP_TABLE

- **include**
  Dieses Verzeichnis enthält die Header-Dateien des SAP NetWeaver RFC SDK:
  - **sapdecf.h**
    Header-Datei für die Verwendung des Datentyps `decfloat` (dezimale Fließkommazahlen nach IEEE 754r)
  - **sapnwrfc.h**
    Header-Datei für die Verwendung des SAP NetWeaver RFC SDK
  - **sapucrfc.h**
    Header-Datei mit globalen und speziellen Unicode-Definitionen (früher **sapucx.h** und **sapuc.h**)
- **lib**
  Dieses Verzeichnis enthält die RFC-Bibliotheken und die Importbibliotheken für den Linker. Für die Windows-Plattform sind dies:
  - *sapnwrfc.dll* und *sapnwrfc.lib*
    RFC-Bibliothek und Importbibliothek für Windows
  - *libsapucum.dll* und *libsapucum.lib*
    Bibliothek und Importbibliothek mit der Unicode-Version der Standard-C-Bibliothek für Windows
  - *icudt57.dll, icuuc57.dll* und *icuin57.dll*
    interne Bibliotheken für Codepage-Konvertierungen für Windows

4.1.2 Kompilieren und Linken von C- und C++-Programmen

Sicherlich ist der schwierigste Schritt bei der Entwicklung von C/C++-RFC-Programmen das Einrichten der Schalter für den Compiler und den Linker. Um eine C-Konsolenanwendung unter Nutzung des SAP NetWeaver RFC SDK zu erstellen, müssen folgende Voraussetzungen erfüllt sein: Der Include-Suchpfad muss zur Compile-Zeit auf das Verzeichnis **nwrfcsdk/include** zeigen, und der Library-Suchpfad muss zur Link-Zeit auf das Verzeichnis **nwrfcsdk/lib** gesetzt werden. Außerdem muss die RFC-Bibliothek in das Programm eingebunden werden.

MicrosoftVisual Studio

Sie erfahren im Folgenden, wie Sie die Programme **sflightClient.c** und **startrfc.cpp** mit Microsoft Visual Studio C++ 2022 kompilieren können.

Projekt für »sflightClient.c« anlegen

Wir beginnen zunächst mit dem C-Programm **sflightClient.c** und gehen danach auf das C++-Programm **startrfc.cpp** ein.

1. Starten Sie Microsoft Visual Studio, und erzeugen Sie ein neues Projekt.
2. Wählen Sie als Vorlage **C++ Konsolen-App**, wie Abbildung 4.1 zeigt.

3. Klicken Sie auf **Weiter**, um den Projektassistenten zu starten.
4. Geben Sie im zweiten Schritt »sflightClient« als Projektnamen ein. Legen Sie Ihr Arbeitsverzeichnis (**Ort**) und einen Solution-Namen (**Name der Projektmappe**) fest (siehe Abbildung 4.2).

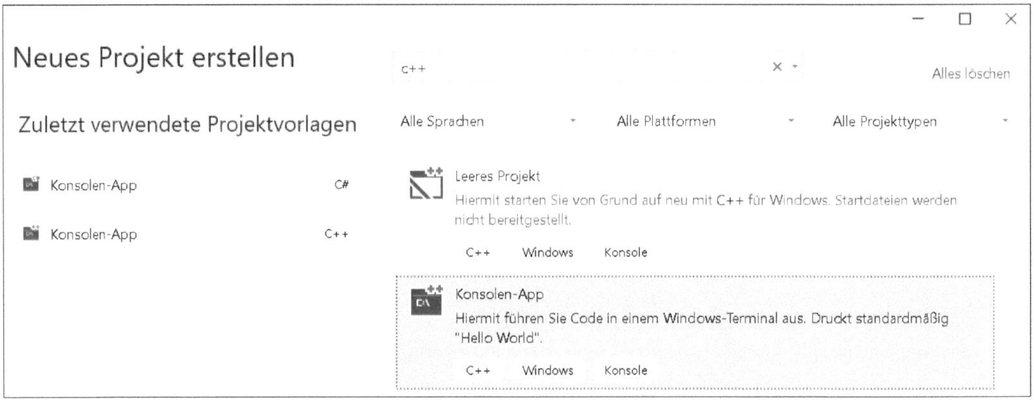

Abbildung 4.1 Anlegen einer Konsolenanwendung

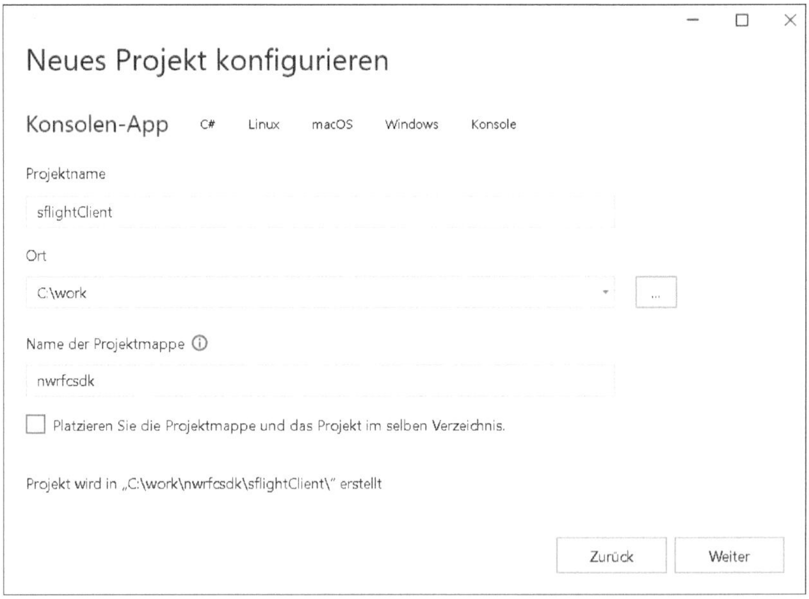

Abbildung 4.2 Projektnamen festlegen

5. Kopieren Sie die Datei **sflightClient.c** aus den Unterverzeichnissen von **nwrfcsdk\demo** in das Projektverzeichnis, und fügen Sie diese Datei als Quelldatei in Ihr Projekt ein.

Nun müssen Sie noch die Schalter für den Compiler und den Linker einstellen:

Schalter für Compiler und Linker

1. Klicken Sie dazu im Solution Explorer mit der rechten Maustaste auf Ihr Projekt, und wählen Sie **Eigenschaften** aus dem angezeigten Kontextmenü aus. Sie sehen dann einen Dialog, in dem Sie die Konfigurationseigenschaften Ihres Projekts ändern können.
2. Sie müssen folgende Änderungen unterhalb von **Konfigurationseigenschaften** vornehmen:
   - **C/C++ • Allgemein**
     Geben Sie hier unter **Zusätzliche Includeverzeichnisse** den Pfad **nwrfcsdk\include** an (siehe Abbildung 4.3). Damit kann der Compiler die benötigten Includes **sapnwrfc.h**, **sapuc.h** und **sapdecf.h** finden.

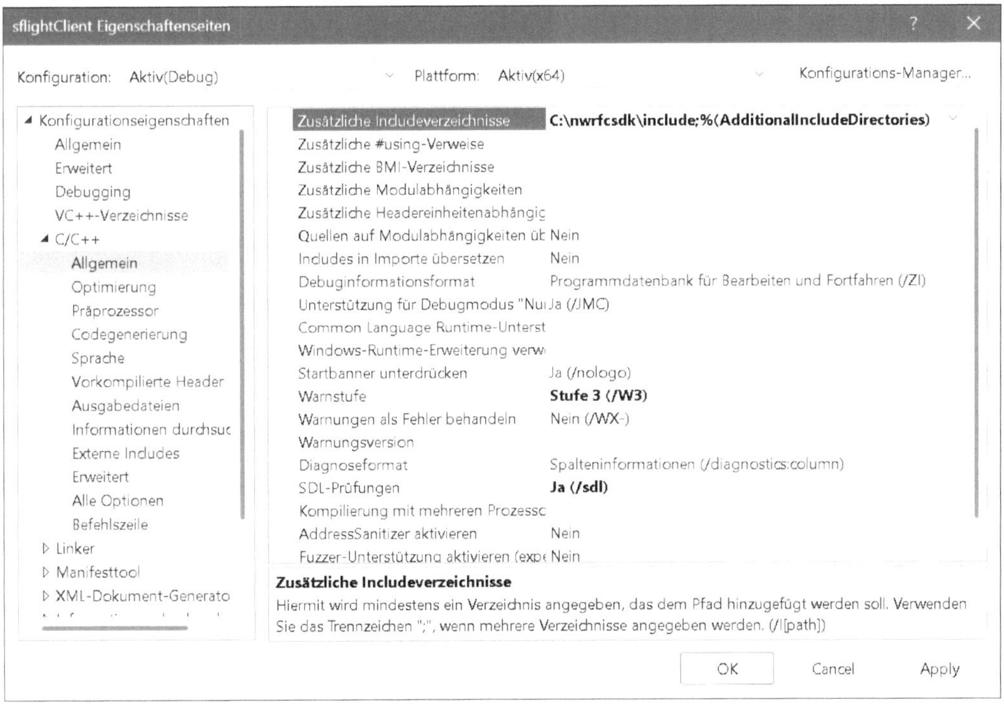

Abbildung 4.3 Angabe der zusätzlichen Include-Verzeichnisse

   - **C/C++ • Präprozessor**
     Geben Sie hier als **Präprozessordefinitionen** »SAPwithUNICODE« an (siehe Abbildung 4.4).

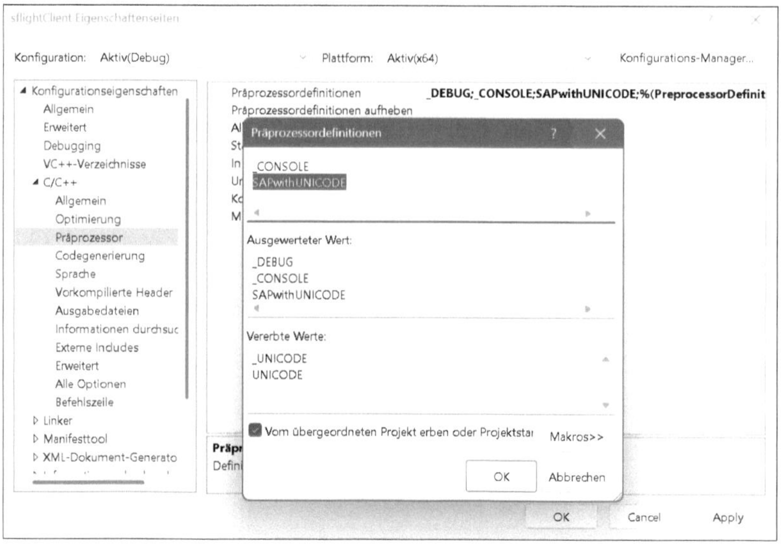

Abbildung 4.4 Angabe des Präprozessorsymbols »SAPwithUNICODE«

- **Linker • Allgemein**
  Geben Sie hier als **Zusätzliche Bibliotheksverzeichnisse** den Pfad **nwrfcsdk\lib** an (siehe Abbildung 4.5). Damit findet der Linker die Bibliotheken **sapnwrfc.lib**, **libsapucum.lib** und **sapdecfICU.lib**.

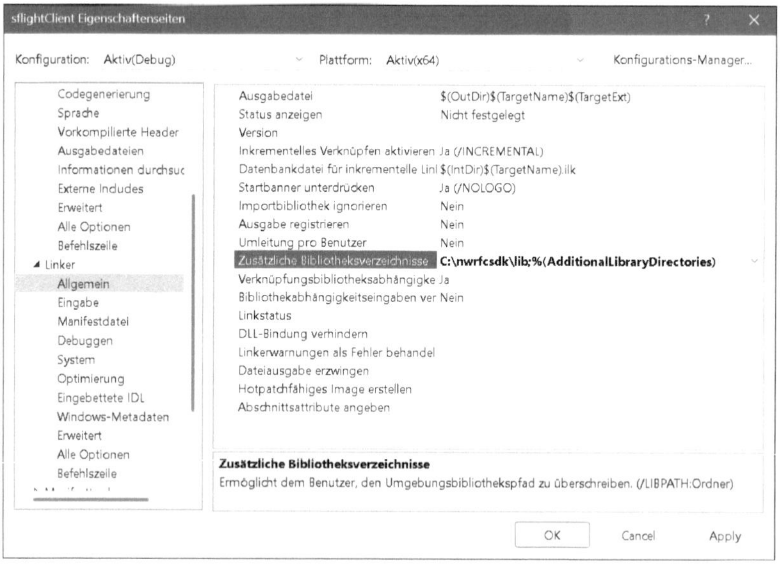

Abbildung 4.5 Angabe des Bibliotheksverzeichnisses

- **Linker • Eingabe**
  Geben Sie hier bei **Zusätzliche Abhängigkeiten** die Bibliotheken *sapnwrfc.lib und libsapucum.lib* an. Damit werden diese Bibliotheken mit Ihrem Programm verlinkt. Abbildung 4.6 zeigt diese Einstellungen.

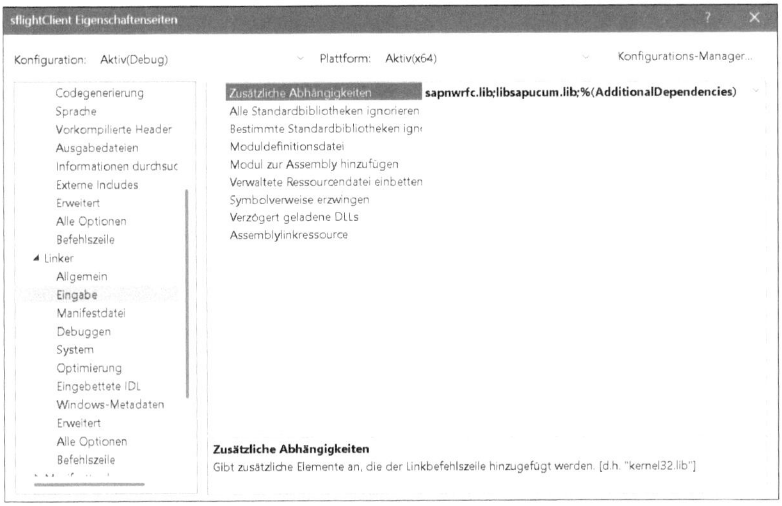

Abbildung 4.6 Linker-Eingaben

- **Debuggen • Umgebungsvariablen**
  Um das Debugging zu unterstützen, müssen Sie hier über eine Pfadvariable bekanntgeben, wo sich die DLL befindet. Erstellen Sie unter **Umgebung** einen neuen Eintrag mit dem Inhalt »PATH=$(PATH);c:\nwrfcsdk\lib« (siehe Abbildung 4.7).

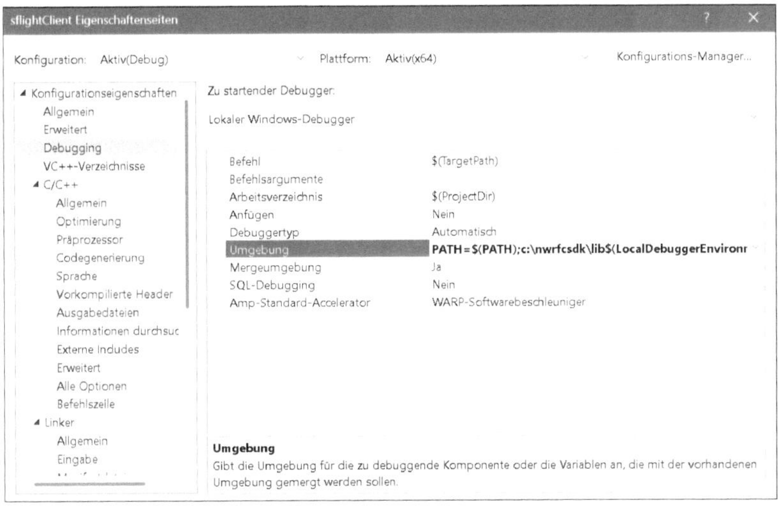

Abbildung 4.7 Angabe der Debugger-Einstellungen

3. Achten Sie darauf, dass Sie diese Einstellungen für alle Konfigurationen (Debug, Release usw.) vornehmen. Danach können Sie über das **Erstellen**-Menü Ihr Projekt kompilieren und binden.

Sie haben nun ein einfaches C-Konsolenprogramm mit dem SAP NetWeaver RFC SDK erstellt, mit dem Sie die SAP-Demo-BAPIs für Flugverbindungen in einem SAP-System aufrufen können. Die Einstellungen für Compiler und Linker können Sie in weiteren Projekten genauso wie in diesem Projekt vornehmen.

[!]

32-Bit-Programme auf 64-Bit-Betriebssystemen

Falls Sie Ihre Programme für die 32-Bit-Version der SAP-NetWeaver-RFC-Bibliothek als 32-Bit-Programme kompiliert haben, müssen Sie die DLLs aus dem **lib**-Verzeichnis des SDK nicht nach **\Windows\System32**, sondern nach **\Windows\SysWOW64** kopieren, damit sie von Ihrem Programm gefunden werden.

C++-Programme kompilieren

Erstellen Sie nun auf dieselbe Weise ein zweites Projekt, um das C++-Programm **startrfc.cpp** zu kompilieren. Kopieren Sie in diesem Fall jedoch die Dateien **startrfc.h** und **startrfc.cpp** in das Projektverzeichnis, und nehmen Sie diese beiden Dateien als Header- bzw. Quelldatei in Ihr Projekt auf. Nun können Sie auch dieses Projekt erstellen und ausführen.

Kompatibilität von C- bzw. C++-Programmen

Sie können die SAP-NetWeaver-RFC-Bibliothek also sowohl aus C- als auch aus C++-Programmen heraus in völlig identischer Weise verwenden. Dies liegt vor allem daran, dass C++ eine Obermenge von C ist und die SAP-NetWeaver-RFC-Bibliothek in C geschrieben wurde. Damit Sie jedoch C-Funktionen in C++-Programmen verwenden können, müssen Sie die C-Funktionen im C++-Programm als `extern "C"` deklarieren. In der Header-Datei **sapnwrfc.h** wird dies automatisch umgesetzt, falls das Präprozessorsymbol `__cplusplus` definiert ist. Dieses Symbol wird von Visual Studio ebenfalls automatisch gesetzt, da die Entwicklungsumgebung an den Dateiendungen der Quelldateien erkennt, dass diese in C++ geschrieben sind.

Um Redundanzen zu vermeiden, sind die folgenden Beispiele in C geschrieben. Falls Sie lieber in C++ programmieren, können Sie den Beispielcode ganz einfach in Methoden Ihrer C++-Klassen kopieren.

4.2 Einfache SAP-NetWeaver-RFC-Clients

In diesem Abschnitt machen Sie sich anhand einfacher SAP-NetWeaver-RFC-Client-Programme mit dem prinzipiellen Aufbau von SAP-NetWeaver-RFC-Clients vertraut. Sie lernen dabei auch, wie Sie mit einfachen, strukturierten und Tabellenparametern umgehen.

4.2.1 Aufbau eines SAP-NetWeaver-RFC-Clients

EinfacherRFC-Client »nwrfcclient.c«

Listing 4.1 zeigt den prinzipiellen Aufbau eines RFC-Clients. Dieser Client ruft nur fünf Funktionen aus der SAP-NetWeaver-RFC-Schnittstelle auf. Zuerst öffnet er mit der Funktion `RfcOpenConnection` eine Verbindung zu einem SAP-System. Dann liest er Metadaten des Funktionsbausteins `RFC_PING` über die RFC-API-Funktion `RfcGetFunctionDesc`. Die notwendigen Strukturen zum Aufruf der Funktion baut sich das Programm mit der Funktion `RfcCreateFunction` auf. Der Funktionsbaustein wird danach über die Funktion `RfcInvoke` aufgerufen. Zum Schluss wird die Verbindung durch einen Aufruf der Funktion `RfcCloseConnection` wieder geschlossen. Nach jedem API-Aufruf prüft das Programm, ob der Aufruf erfolgreich war. Falls nicht, wird in der Funktion `errorHandling` der Fehler ausgegeben, die Verbindung geschlossen und das Programm mit dem Returncode `1` beendet. Im Erfolgsfall endet das Programm mit dem Returncode `0`.

```
#include "sapnwrfc.h"
void errorHandling(RFC_RC rc,
                   SAP_UC description[],
                   RFC_ERROR_INFO* errInf,
                   RFC_CONNECTION_HANDLE connection)
{
  printfU(cU("%s: %d\n"), description, rc);
  printfU(cU("%s: %s\n"), errInf->key,
                          errInf->message);
  if (connection != NULL)
    RfcCloseConnection(connection, errInf);
  exit(1);
}

int mainU(int argc, SAP_UC** argv)
{
  RFC_RC rc = RFC_OK;
  RFC_CONNECTION_PARAMETER login[6];
```

```
  RFC_ERROR_INFO errInf;
  RFC_CONNECTION_HANDLE connection;
  RFC_FUNCTION_DESC_HANDLE rfcPingDesc;
  RFC_FUNCTION_HANDLE rfcPing;

  /* Verbindungsparameter füllen                         */
  login[0].name=cU("ashost");login[0].value=cU("SAP00");
  login[1].name=cU("sysnr");login[1].value=cU("00");
  login[2].name=cU("user");login[2].value=cU("ope");
  login[3].name=cU("passwd");login[3].value=cU("pehnke");
  login[4].name=cU("client");login[4].value=cU("001");
  login[5].name=cU("lang");login[5].value=cU("EN");

  /* Verbindung öffnen                                   */
  connection = RfcOpenConnection(login, 6, &errInf);
  if (connection == NULL)
    errorHandling(rc, cU("Fehler bei der Anmeldung"),
                  &errInf, NULL);
  /* Metadaten der RFC-Funktion lesen                    */
  rfcPingDesc = RfcGetFunctionDesc(
                   connection, cU("RFC_PING"), &errInf);
  if (rfcPingDesc == NULL)
      errorHandling(rc,
                    cU("Fehler beim Lesen der Metadaten"),
                    &errInf, connection);
  /* Strukturen für den Aufruf erzeugen                  */
  rfcPing = RfcCreateFunction(rfcPingDesc, &errInf);
  if (rfcPing == NULL)
      errorHandling(rc,
                    cU("Fehler bei Funktionserzeugung"),
                    &errInf, connection);
  /* RFC-Funktion aufrufen                               */
  rc = RfcInvoke(connection, rfcPing, &errInf);
  if (rc != RFC_OK)
      errorHandling(rc,
                    cU("Fehler beim Aufruf der Funktion"),
                    &errInf, connection);
  /* Verbindung schließen                                */
  RfcCloseConnection(connection, &errInf);
  return 0;
}
```

Listing 4.1 Einfacher RFC-Client »nwrfcclient.c«

Schauen wir uns das Programm in Listing 4.1 im Detail an. Es inkludiert zuerst die Header-Datei **sapnwrfc.h**. Diese Datei enthält die Definitionen der Typen und Konstanten sowie die Deklarationen (Prototypen) der Funktionen in der RFC-API.

Fehlerbehandlung

Danach wird die Funktion `errorHandling` definiert. Diese Funktion hat vier Übergabeparameter:

- `rc`

  Dies ist ein Returncode vom Typ `RFC_RC`. Listing 4.2 zeigt die Definition dieses Datentyps.

```
typedef enum _RFC_RC {
  RFC_OK,             /* OK                                */
  RFC_COMMUNICATION_FAILURE,/* Fehler in Netzwerk       */
  RFC_LOGON_FAILURE,/* Passwort oder Benutzer falsch    */
  RFC_ABAP_RUNTIME_FAILURE, /* ABAP-Kurz-Dump           */
  RFC_ABAP_MESSAGE, /* E-, A- oder X-Message ausgelöst */
  RFC_ABAP_EXCEPTION,/* ABAP-Exception ausgelöst        */
  RFC_CLOSED,     /* Verbindung von Partner geschlossen */
  RFC_CANCELED,       /* nicht mehr verwendet           */
  RFC_TIMEOUT,        /* RFC durch Timeout abgebrochen  */
  RFC_MEMORY_INSUFFICIENT, /* zu wenig Speicher         */
  RFC_VERSION_MISMATCH, /* falsche Version              */
  RFC_INVALID_PROTOCOL /* nicht unterstütztes Format    */
  RFC_SERIALIZATION_FAILURE /* Problem beim Serialisieren*/
  RFC_INVALID_HANDLE,/* ungültiges Handle               */
  RFC_RETRY,          /* noch keine Daten verfügbar     */
  RFC_EXTERNAL_FAILURE,/* Fehler in externem Code       */
  RFC_EXECUTED,       /* Funktion schon ausgeführt      */
  RFC_NOT_FOUND,      /* Funktion nicht gefunden        */
  RFC_NOT_SUPPORTED,/* Operation nicht unterstützt      */
  RFC_ILLEGAL_STATE,/* Operation (noch) nicht möglich   */
  RFC_INVALID_PARAMETER,/* ungültiger Parameter         */
  RFC_CODEPAGE_CONVERSION_FAILURE,/* Fehler bei CP-Umw.*/
  RFC_CONVERSION_FAILURE,/* Fehler bei Datenumwandlung */
  RFC_BUFFER_TOO_SMALL,  /* Buffer-Überlauf             */
  RFC_TABLE_MOVE_BOF,/* Positionierung vor Tabelle      */
  RFC_TABLE_MOVE_EOF,/* Positionierung hinter Tabelle  */
  RFC_UNKNOWN_ERROR, /* unbekannter Fehler              */
} RFC_RC;
```

Listing 4.2 RFC-Returncodes

- description[]

  Dabei handelt es sich um eine Kurzbeschreibung des Fehlers in Form eines Arrays von SAP_UC. Je nach Plattform ist SAP_UC dabei ein char, ein wchar_t oder ein unsigned short und repräsentiert ein Unicode-Zeichen.

- errInf

  Dies ist ein Zeiger auf eine Struktur des Typs RFC_ERROR_INFO mit der Fehlerbeschreibung, wie sie von der API-Funktion zurückgegeben wurde. Listing 4.3 zeigt die Definition dieser Struktur. Die Komponente group dieser Struktur ist ein Mitglied der Enumeration RFC_ERROR_GROUP in Listing 4.4.

```
typedef struct _RFC_ERROR_INFO {
  RFC_RD code;                  // Fehlercode
  RFC_ERROR_GROUP  group;       // Fehlergruppe
  SAP_UC key[128];              // Fehlerschlüssel
  SAP_UC message[512];          // Nachricht
  SAP_UC abapMsgClass[20+1];    // ABAP-Nachrichten-ID
  SAP_UC abapMsgType[1+1];      // ABAP-
  Nachrichtentyp E/A/X
  SAP_UC abapMsgNumber[3+1];    // ABAP-Nachrichtennummer
  SAP_UC abapMsgV1[50+1];       // ABAP-Nachrichtendetail 1
  SAP_UC abapMsgV2[50+1];       // ABAP-Nachrichtendetail 2
  SAP_UC abapMsgV3[50+1];       // ABAP-Nachrichtendetail 3
  SAP_UC abapMsgV4[50+1];       // ABAP-Nachrichtendetail 4
} RFC_ERROR_INFO;
```

Listing 4.3 Struktur »RFC_ERROR_INFO«

```
Typedef enum _RFC_ERROR_GROUP {
    OK,                             // OK
    ABAP_APPLICATION_FAILURE,       // ABAP-
    Exception ausgelöst
    ABAP_RUNTIME_FAILURE,           // ABAP-Laufzeitfehler
    LOGON_FAILURE,                  // Anmeldefehler
    COMMUNICATION_FAILURE,          // Netzwerkproblem
    EXTERNAL_RUNTIME_FAILURE,       // Problem in RFC-Bibl.
    EXTERNAL_APPLICATION_FAILURE    // Problem in ext. Prog
} RFC_ERROR_GROUP;
```

Listing 4.4 Enumeration »RFC_ERROR_GROUP«

- connection

  Dies beschreibt die Verbindung zum SAP-System vom Typ RFC_CONNECTION_HANDLE.

Die Funktion selbst gibt die Kurzbeschreibung des Fehlers, den Returncode, den Fehlerschlüssel und die Fehlermeldung aus. Dazu verwendet sie die Unicode-Variante `printfU` der Standardfunktion `printf`, die in **sapucrfc.h** definiert ist. Nach der Fehlerausgabe schließt die Funktion `errorHandling` gegebenenfalls die Verbindung durch den Aufruf von `RfcCloseConnection` und bricht das Programm unter Rückgabe des Returncodes `1` ab.

Returncode, Fehlerschlüssel, Fehlermeldung

Die Funktion `mainU` enthält das eigentliche Hauptprogramm, das zunächst einmal sechs lokale Variablen definiert:

Lokale Variable

- `rc`
  Diese Variable ist vom Typ `RFC_RC` und dient der Aufnahme des Returncodes von API-Aufrufen.
- `login`
  Dieses Array von `RFC_CONNECTION_PARAMETER`-Strukturen dient der Aufnahme der Verbindungsdaten. Dieser Strukturtyp hat lediglich die beiden Komponenten `name` und `value`.
- `errInf`
  Diese Struktur vom Typ `RFC_ERROR_INFO` wird zur Aufnahme von Fehlermeldungen der API-Funktionen verwendet.
- `connection`
  Das Handle `connection` vom Typ `RFC_CONNECTION_HANDLE` identifiziert die Verbindung.
- `rfcPingDesc`
  Das Handle `rfcPingDesc` vom Typ `RFC_FUNCTION_DESC_HANDLE` identifiziert die Funktionsbeschreibung von `RFC_PING`.
- `rfcPing`
  Das Handle `rfcPing` vom Typ `RFC_FUNCTION_HANDLE` identifiziert die notwendigen Datenübergabestrukturen, die von der SAP-NetWeaver-RFC-Bibliothek zum Aufruf des Funktionsbausteins `RFC_PING` aufgebaut werden.

Nach der Definition der Variablen werden die Verbindungsparameter mithilfe der Funktion `cU` in das Array `login` eingetragen. Die Verbindungsparameter sind der Hostname und die Systemnummer eines ABAP-Applikationsservers sowie Mandant, Benutzername, Passwort und Anmeldesprache zur Anmeldung am SAP-System.

Das Programm übergibt diese Informationen im nächsten Schritt an die Funktion `RfcOpenConnection`, um ein Handle für eine RFC-Verbindung in der Variablen `connection` zu erhalten. Der zweite Parameter von `RfcOpenConnec-`

Funktion »RfcOpenConnection«

tion ist die Länge des login-Arrays. Im Fehlerfall schreibt die Funktion RfcOpenConnection weitere Informationen in die Struktur errorInf, deren Adresse beim Aufruf übergeben wird. Falls connection nach dem Aufruf den Wert »NULL« hat, konnte die Funktion RfcOpenConnection keine Verbindung herstellen.

Funktion»RfcGet-FunctionDesc«

War der Aufruf der Funktion RfcOpenConnection erfolgreich, initialisiert das Programm die Metadaten für den Funktionsbaustein RFC_PING durch einen Aufruf der Funktion RfcGetFunctionDesc. Dabei erfragt die RFC-Bibliothek vom SAP-System die Metadaten des Funktionsbausteins, d. h. die Beschreibung der Parameter des Funktionsbausteins und deren Struktur. War der Aufruf erfolgreich, ist das zurückgegebene Funktionsbeschreibungs-Handle rfcPingDesc ungleich »NULL«.

Danach werden durch einen Aufruf von RfcGetFunction die eigentlichen Datenstrukturen zur Übergabe der Import- und Exportparameter aufgebaut. Dieser Funktion wird das Funktionsbeschreibungs-Handle rfcPing-Dessc übergeben. War dies erfolgreich, ist das zurückgegebene Funktions-Handle rfcPing ungleich »NULL«.

Funktion »RfcInvoke«

Schließlich ruft das Programm den Funktionsbaustein RFC_PING mithilfe der Funktion RfcInvoke auf. Dieser Funktion werden das connection-Handle und das Funktions-Handle rfcPing sowie die Adresse von errInf übergeben. Ist beim Aufruf ein Fehler aufgetreten, ist der Returncode rc ungleich RFC_OK. Nach jedem API-Aufruf überprüft das Programm den Rückgabewert. Im Fehlerfall ruft es errorHandling auf. Diese Funktion gibt den Fehler aus und bricht das Programm mit dem Exitcode 1 ab.

Funktion »RfcClose-Connection«

Zum Schluss wird die RFC-Verbindung durch den Aufruf von RfcClose-Connection wieder geschlossen, und das Programm gibt den Returncode 0 zurück.

Funktion »RfcOpen-Connection«

Um eine Verbindung zu öffnen, verwendet der Client die Funktion RfcOpen-Connection. Diese Funktion nimmt sämtliche Verbindungsparameter im ersten Argument als Array von RFC_CONNECTION_PARAMETER-Strukturen entgegen. Eine solche Struktur enthält in der Komponente name den Namen eines Verbindungsparameters und in der Komponente value dessen Wert. Tabelle 4.1 zeigt die wichtigsten der möglichen Namen, die in der Komponente name verwendet werden können.

Name	Bedeutung
`Client`	SAP-Anmeldemandant
`User`	SAP-Benutzer
`Passwd`	SAP-Anmeldepasswort
`Lang`	SAP-Anmeldesprache
`Trace`	RFC-Trace (0/1 ohne/mit Trace; Voreinstellung = 1)
`Dest`	Destination in **saprfc.ini**
`Mshost`	Hostname des Message-Servers
`Msserv`	Servicename des Message-Servers
`Sysid`	Name des SAP-Systems
`Group`	Logon-Gruppe
`Ashost`	Hostname des SAP-Anwendungsservers
`Sysnr`	Systemnummer des SAP-Anwendungsservers

Tabelle 4.1 Wichtige Verbindungsparameter in der Funktion »RfcOpenConnection«

Datei »saprfc.ini«

Die technischen Verbindungsparameter (`ashost` und `sysnr` bei direkter Verbindung zu einem SAP NetWeaver Application Server bzw. `mshost`, `msserv`, `sysid` und `group` bei der Verwendung von Load Balancing) können Sie auch aus der Datei **saprfc.ini** auslesen lassen. Die Datei **saprfc.ini** muss dabei in demselben Verzeichnis wie das externe RFC-Programm liegen. Alternativ haben Sie die Möglichkeit, in der Umgebungsvariablen `RFC_INI` den vollständigen Pfad zu dieser Datei zu hinterlegen.

Die Datei **saprfc.ini** übernimmt die Rolle von Transaktion SM59 für externe RFC-Programme. Sie speichert die Informationen über RFC-Destinationen. Die Datei kann Informationen zu mehreren RFC-Destinationen speichern. Jeder Eintrag beginnt mit `DEST=<DESTNAME>`, wobei `<DESTNAME>` der frei wählbare Name der Destination ist. In `RfcOpenConnection` geben Sie die Destination aus der Datei **saprfc.ini** im Parameter `dest` an.

Nach dem Eintrag `DEST=<DESTNAME>` folgt für jede Destination in der Datei **saprfc.ini** die Zeile `TYPE=<T>`. Dabei hat `<T>` den Wert »A«, wenn Sie sich mit einem bestimmten SAP NetWeaver Application Server verbinden möchten. Möchten Sie den Lastausgleich nutzen, verwenden Sie für `<T>` den Wert »B«.

Datei »saprfc.ini«

Listing 4.5 zeigt ein Beispiel für die Datei **saprfc.ini**. Im ersten Eintrag mit DEST=BSP wird der Lastausgleich verwendet. Dazu sind Angaben zur SAP-System-ID, zum Message-Server und optional zur Logon-Gruppe notwendig. Diese Angaben werden in den Einträgen R3NAME, MSHOST und GROUP vorgenommen. Der zweite Eintrag mit DEST=BSP_H001 speichert Verbindungsinformationen für einen spezifischen Anwendungsserver. Dazu werden in den Einträgen ASHOST und SYSNR Angaben zum Host und zur Systemnummer des Servers gemacht.

```
/*******************************************************/
/*                        SAPRFC.INI
*******************************************************/
DEST=BSP
TYPE=B
R3NAME=BSP
MSHOST=miniwas
GROUP=PUBLIC
RFC_TRACE=0
ABAP_DEBUG=0
USE_SAP GUI=0
DEST=BSP_H001
TYPE=A
ASHOST=h001
SYSNR=00
RFC_TRACE=0
ABAP_DEBUG=0
USE_SAP GUI=0
```

Listing 4.5 Datei »saprfc.ini«

Hostnamen mit SAP-Router

Wenn zwischen Ihrer Entwicklungsmaschine und dem SAP-System ein oder mehrere SAP-Router stehen, müssen Sie dies in der Angabe der Hostnamen in den Parametern ashost, mshost und gwhost berücksichtigen. Den Hostnamen werden die Hostnamen und Portnummern der SAP-Router in folgender Form vorangestellt:

```
sapinfo ashost=/H/<sapgate1>/S/<port1>/.../H/<host>
```

Ersetzen Sie dabei <sapgate1> durch den Hostnamen oder die IP-Adresse des SAP-Routers, mit dem Ihr Entwicklungssystem zuerst kommunizieren soll, und <port1> durch den TCP-Port, auf dem dieser SAP-Router Anfragen entgegennimmt. Die Sequenz /H/<sapgate> /S/<port> wiederholen Sie für jeden Router, der auf dem Weg von Ihrem Entwicklungssystem zum SAP-System liegt, mit dem Sie kommunizieren möchten.

4.2.2 Einfache Parameter

Verwendung einfacher Parameter

Der Funktionsbaustein RFC_PING definiert überhaupt keine Parameter in seiner Schnittstelle. Er ist lediglich für einen reinen Verbindungstest gedacht. Der nächstschwierigere Fall besteht darin, einen Funktionsbaustein aufzurufen, der in seiner Schnittstelle nur einfache (unstrukturierte) Parameter hat. Dies können Import-, Changing- oder Exportparameter des Funktionsbausteins sein.

RFC-Client mit einfachen Parametern

Als Beispiel für die Verwendung einfacher Parameter zeigt Listing 4.6 Ausschnitte eines RFC-Client-Programms, das den Funktionsbaustein DDIF_FIELDLABEL_GET aufruft. Dieser Funktionsbaustein gibt zu einem Tabellenfeld oder einem Datenelement im ABAP Dictionary einen Feldbezeichner zurück.

```
int mainU (int argc, SAP_UC** argv)
{
  ...
  SAP_UC *temp;
  unsigned int uiLength;
  ...
  /* Importparameter füllen                          */
  rc = RfcSetChars(rfcFunc, cU("TABNAME"),
                   cU("ZIFPORDERID"), 11, &errInf);
  if (rc != RFC_OK)
      errorHandling(rc,
                    cU("Fehler beim Schreiben d. Par."),
                    &errInf, connection);
  /* RFC-Funktion aufrufen                           */
  rc = RfcInvoke(connection, rfcFunc, &errInf);
  if (rc != RFC_OK)
      errorHandling(rc,
                    cU("Fehler beim Aufruf der Funktion"),
                    &errInf, connection);
  /* Exportparameter lesen                           */
  rc = RfcGetStringLength(rfcFunc, cU("LABEL"),
                          &uiLength, &errInf);
  if (rc != RFC_OK)
      errorHandling(rc, cU("Fehler beim Lesen d. Länge"),
                  &errInf, connection);
  temp = mallocU(uiLength + 1);
  rc = RfcGetString(rfcFunc, cU("LABEL"), temp, uiLength+1,
                    &uiLength, &errInf);
```

```
    if (rc != RFC_OK)
        errorHandling(rc, cU("Fehler beim Lesen d. Par."),
                      &errInf, connection);
    printfU(cU("Label: %s\n"), temp);
    ...
}
```

Listing 4.6 RFC-Client mit einfachen Parametern

Vor dem Aufruf des Funktionsbausteins füllt das Programm den Importparameter TABNAME mit dem Namen des Datenelements, für das ein Feldbezeichner ermittelt werden soll. Dazu ruft es einfach die Funktion RfcSetChars auf, der das Funktions-Handle, der Name des Parameters, der Wert des Parameters und die Länge des Parameterwerts übergeben werden. In diesem Fall ist der Wert »ZIFPORDERID«, und dessen Länge beträgt »11«.

[»]

Schreiben in Datencontainer

Das SAP NetWeaver RFC SDK enthält eine Vielzahl von Funktionen mit dem Namen RfcSetXXX, die Daten unterschiedlichen Typs in einen Datencontainer schreiben können. In unserem Fall wird der Datencontainer durch das Funktions-Handle referenziert; es kann aber auch, wie wir später zeigen werden, ein Struktur- oder Tabellen-Handle verwendet werden. Innerhalb des Datencontainers wird auf die Daten über einen Namen zugegriffen, in diesem Fall über den Namen des Exportparameters TABNAME.

Lesen aus Datencontainer

Nach dem Aufruf des Funktionsbausteins liest das Programm den Exportparameter LABEL aus. Wie zum Schreiben in einen Datencontainer gibt es auch zum Lesen aus einem Datencontainer eine Vielzahl von RfcGetXXX-Funktionen, die Daten unterschiedlichen Typs aus einem Datencontainer auslesen können. Da es sich bei unserem Exportparameter um einen String handelt, ermittelt das Programm zunächst mit der Funktion RfcGetStringLength die Länge des Strings und fordert dann mit der Funktion mallocU genügend Speicher an, um den String und einen abschließenden NULL-Character aufnehmen zu können. Danach liest es mit der Funktion RfcGetString den String in den angeforderten Speicherbereich und gibt ihn mit der Funktion printfU aus.

4.2.3 Strukturierte Parameter

RFC-Client mit Strukturparametern

Listing 4.7 zeigt Ausschnitte aus einem SAP-NetWeaver-RFC-Client, der den Funktionsbaustein RFC_SYSTEM_INFO aufruft.

```
int mainU (int argc, SAP_UC** argv)
{
  ...
  RFC_STRUCTURE_HANDLE rfcStruct;
  SAP_UC temp[64];  ...

  /* RFC-Funktion aufrufen                          */
  rc = RfcInvoke(connection, rfcFunc, &errInf);
  if (rc != RFC_OK)
      errorHandling(rc,
                    cU("Fehler beim Aufruf der Funktion"),
                    &errInf, connection);
  /* Exportparameter lesen                          */
  rc = RfcGetStructure(rfcFunc, cU("RFCSI_EXPORT"),
                       &rfcStruct, &errInf);
  if (rc != RFC_OK)
      errorHandling(rc,
                    cU("Fehler beim Lesen d. Struktur"),
                    &errInf, connection);
  memsetU(temp, 0x0, 64);
  rc = RfcGetChars(rfcStruct, cU("RFCSYSID"),
                   temp, 8,&errInf);
  printfU(cU("Name des SAP-Systems %s\n"), temp);
  memsetU(temp, 0x0, 64);
  rc = RfcGetChars(rfcStruct, cU("RFCDBHOST"),
                   temp, 32, &errInf);
  printfU(cU("Datenbank-Hostname   %s\n"), temp);
  memsetU(temp, 0x0, 64);
  rc = RfcGetChars(rfcStruct, cU("RFCSAPRL"),
                   temp, 4, &errInf);
  printfU(cU("SAP-Releasestand     %s\n"), temp);
  ...
}
```

Listing 4.7 RFC-Client mit Strukturparametern

Struktur-Handle

Die mainU-Funktion definiert das RFC-Struktur-Handle rfcStruct vom Typ RFC_STRUCTURE_HANDLE. Dieses Handle verweist auf einen Strukturdatencontainer, aus dem die Daten des Exportparameters RFCSI_EXPORT gespeichert werden. Nach dem Aufruf des Funktionsbausteins erhält der Client dieses Handle über den Aufruf der Funktion RfcGetStructure. Der Client übergibt dieser Funktion das Funktions-Handle und den Namen des Exportparameters. Über dieses Struktur-Handle liest das Programm dann mittels RfcGet-

`Chars` die einzelnen Komponenten der Struktur in den Buffer-Bereich `temp` und gibt sie aus.

Damit `temp` innerhalb von `printfU` auch als nullterminierter String verwendet werden kann, wird dieses Array vor dem Auslesen der Daten mit `memsetU` komplett mit dem Character `0x0` gefüllt. `RfcGetChars` liest nämlich nur so viele Zeichen ein, wie die Zeichenfolge tatsächlich enthält, und fügt kein abschließendes `0x0` hinzu.

4.2.4 Tabellenparameter

Funktionen zur Bearbeitung interner Tabellen

Zuletzt sehen wir uns an, wie Tabellenparameter verwendet werden. Tabelle 4.2 listet die Funktionen des SAP NetWeaver RFC SDK zur Bearbeitung interner Tabellen auf. Ein RFC-Programm liest eine Tabelle aus einem Datencontainer mit der Funktion `RfcGetTable` aus. Die Funktion gibt ein Tabellen-Handle an das aufrufende Programm zurück, das die interne Tabelle eindeutig identifiziert.

Funktion	Verwendung
`RfcGetTable`	Liest das Tabellen-Handle einer internen Tabelle aus einem Datencontainer aus.
`RfcDeleteAllRows`	Entfernt alle Zeilen einer internen Tabelle. Die Tabelle kann weiterverwendet werden.
`RfcDestroyTable`	Löscht eine interne Tabelle und gibt den von ihr belegten Speicherplatz frei.
`RfcAddNewRow`	Fügt eine neue leere Zeile an eine interne Tabelle an und gibt ein Struktur-Handle dafür zurück.
`RfcInsertNewRow`	Fügt eine neue leere Zeile an der aktuellen Zeile ein und gibt ein Struktur-Handle dafür zurück.
`RfcDeleteCurrentRow`	Löscht die aktuelle Zeile einer internen Tabelle.
`RfcMoveToFirstRow`	Setzt die aktuelle Position auf die erste Zeile.
`RfcMoveToLastRow`	Setzt die aktuelle Position auf die letzte Zeile.
`RfcMoveToNextRow`	Setzt die aktuelle Position auf die nächste Zeile.
`RfcMoveToPreviousRow`	Setzt die aktuelle Position auf die vorangegangene Zeile.
`RfcMoveTo`	Setzt die aktuelle Position auf eine bestimmte Zeile.

Tabelle 4.2 Einige Funktionen zur Manipulation interner Tabellen

Funktion	Verwendung
RfcGetCurrentRow	Gibt ein Struktur-Handle der aktuellen Zeile zurück.
RfcGetRowCount	Gibt die Anzahl der Zeilen einer internen Tabelle zurück.

Tabelle 4.2 Einige Funktionen zur Manipulation interner Tabellen (Forts.)

Zeile anhängen mit »RfcAppendNewRow«

Um eine interne Tabelle zu füllen, ruft ein RFC-Programm die Funktion RfcAppendNewRow auf. Diese Funktion alloziert Speicherplatz für eine neue Zeile und gibt ein Struktur-Handle auf diese Zeile zurück. Mit diesem Handle füllt das Programm die einzelnen Komponenten der Zeile.

Zeilenzahl ermitteln

Um eine interne Tabelle zu lesen, ermittelt ein RFC-Programm die Anzahl der Zeilen mit einem Aufruf von RfcGetRowCount. In einer Schleife wird dann für jede Zeile die Funktion RfcGetCurrentRow aufgerufen, die ein Struktur-Handle auf die aktuelle Zeile der internen Tabelle zurückgibt. Vor dem nächsten Schleifendurchlauf setzt der Aufruf von RfcMoveToNextRow den internen Zeilenzeiger der internen Tabelle auf die nächste Zeile.

RFC-Client mit Tabellenparametern

Listing 4.8 zeigt Ausschnitte eines RFC-Clients, der den Funktionsbaustein Z_IFP_ORDER_GETLIST aufruft. Dieser Funktionsbaustein hat den Tabellenparameter TA_ORDERS, dessen Zeilen vom Typ ZIFPORDER sind.

```
int mainU (int argc, SAP_UC** argv)
{
  ...
  RFC_TABLE_HANDLE rfcTab;
  RFC_STRUCTURE_HANDLE rfcStruct;
  SAP_UC temp[11];
  unsigned int uiRowCount;
  unsigned int i;
  SAP_UC temp[64];
  ...
  /* Importparameter füllen                              */
  RfcSetChars(rfcFunc, cU("IM_ORDERTYPE"),
              cU("PO"), 2, &errInf);
  /* interne Tabelle füllen (zur Demo, nicht notwendig)  */

  rc = RfcGetTable(rfcFunc, cU("TA_ORDERS"),
                   &rfcTab, &errInf);
  rfcStruct = RfcAppendNewRow(rfcTab, &errInf);
  rc = RfcSetChars(rfcStruct, cU("ORDERID"),
       cU("0000000001"), 10, &errInf);
```

```
    /* RFC-Funktion aufrufen                              */
    rc = RfcInvoke(connection, rfcFunc, &errInf);
    if (rc != RFC_OK)
        errorHandling(rc,
                      cU("Fehler beim Aufruf der Funktion"),
                      &errInf, connection);
    /* Exportparameter lesen                              */
    rc = RfcGetTable(rfcFunc, cU("TA_ORDERS"),
                     &rfcTab, &errInf);
    if (rc != RFC_OK)
        errorHandling(rc,
                      cU("Fehler beim Lesen der Tabelle"),
                      &errInf, connection);
    rc = RfcGetRowCount(rfcTab, &uiRowCount, &errInf);
    for(i=0; i < uiRowCount; i++)
    {
      rfcStruct = RfcGetCurrentRow(rfcTab, &errInf);
      if(rfcStruct!=NULL)
      {
        memsetU(temp, 0x0, 11);
        RfcGetChars(rfcStruct, cU("ORDERID"),
                    temp, 10, &errInf);
        printfU(cU("ORDERID %s\n"), temp);
      }
      RfcMoveToNextRow(rfcTab, &errInf);
    }
    ...
}
```

Listing 4.8 RFC-Client mit Tabellenparametern

In der mainU-Funktion definiert der Client die Variable rfcTab, die ein Tabellen-Handle für die interne Tabelle TA_ORDERS aufnehmen soll. Die Variable rfcStruct soll ein Struktur-Handle für eine Zeile der zurückgelieferten internen Tabelle aufnehmen.

Interne Tabelle schreiben

Nachdem er ein Funktions-Handle erzeugt hat, holt sich der Client mit RfcGetTable ein Tabellen-Handle auf die interne Tabelle TA_ORDERS. Zu Demonstrationszwecken wird diese Tabelle mit einer Zeile gefüllt. Dazu ruft der Client die Funktion RfcAppendNewLine auf, die das Struktur-Handle für die neue, leere Zeile zurückgibt. Der Client schreibt mit RfcSetChars auf die einzelnen Komponenten dieser Struktur.

Dann ruft der Client den Funktionsbaustein auf und gibt die Zeilen der internen Tabelle aus. Dazu ermittelt er die Anzahl der Zeilen mit einem Aufruf der Funktion RfcGetRowCount und greift in einer Schleife mit der Funktion RfcGetCurrentRow auf die einzelnen Zeilen zu. Am Ende des Schleifenkörpers geht das Programm mit RfcMoveToNextRow zur nächsten Zeile.

Interne Tabelle lesen

4.3 Komplexe SAP-NetWeaver-RFC-Clients

In diesem Abschnitt lernen Sie komplexere SAP-NetWeaver-RFC-Clients kennen. Sie lernen zudem, wie Sie BAPIs aufrufen und tRFC- und qRFC-Clients implementieren können.

4.3.1 Aufruf von BAPIs

Mit den bisher gezeigten Techniken können auch BAPIs aufgerufen werden, da diese als RFC-Funktionsbausteine implementiert sind. Besonderheiten ergeben sich nur aus den speziellen Implementierungsregeln für BAPIs.

Eine dieser Implementierungsregeln ist das Transaktionsmodell für BAPIs, die schreibend auf die Datenbank zugreifen. Wie wir in Abschnitt 3.5.2, »Entwicklung von BAPIs«, erläutert haben, rufen schreibende BAPIs für Datenbankänderungen einen Verbuchungsbaustein mit dem Zusatz IN UPDATE TASK auf. Damit dieser Verbucher auch ausgeführt wird, muss der Client explizit BAPI_TRANSACTION_COMMIT aufrufen.

Transaktionsmodell für BAPIs

Listing 4.9 zeigt Ausschnitte aus dem Quellcode eines RFC-Clients, der das BAPI Order.CreateFromData aufruft. Der Client füllt die Exportparameter mit den Bestelldaten für den Aufruf des Funktionsbausteins Z_BAPI_ORDER_CREATEFROMDATA. Nach dem Aufruf überprüft der Client den Importparameter RETURN. Dieser ist eine interne Tabelle vom Zeilentyp BAPIRET2. Falls kein Fehler aufgetreten ist, ruft er den Funktionsbaustein BAPI_TRANSACTION_COMMIT auf.

BAPI-Client

```
int mainU (int argc, SAP_UC** argv)
{
  ...
  RFC_FUNCTION_DESC_HANDLE bapiOrderCreateDesc;
  RFC_FUNCTION_DESC_HANDLE bapiTransactionCommitDesc;
  RFC_FUNCTION_HANDLE bapiOrderCreate;
  RFC_FUNCTION_HANDLE bapiTransactionCommit;
  RFC_TABLE_HANDLE rfcTab;
```

```
RFC_STRUCTURE_HANDLE rfcStruct;
SAP_UC temp[256];
unsigned int uiRowCount;
unsigned int i;
...
/* Bestellkopf füllen                                  */
rc = RfcGetStructure(bapiOrderCreate,
                     cU("IM_ORDERHEADER"),
                     &rfcStruct, &errInf);
RfcSetNum(rfcStruct, cU("MANDT"), cU("001"),
          3, &errInf);
RfcSetNum(rfcStruct, cU("ORDERID"), cU("0000000001"),
          10, &errInf);
RfcSetChars(rfcStruct, cU("TYPE"), cU("SO"),
            2, &errInf);
RfcSetNum(rfcStruct, cU("REFID"), cU("0000000001"),
          10, &errInf);
RfcSetChars(rfcStruct, cU("BUYER"),
            cU("Buchhandlung Pehnke"),
            20, &errInf);
RfcSetChars(rfcStruct, cU("SELLER"),
            cU("Großhandel Hiller"),
            18, &errInf);
RfcSetDate(rfcStruct, cU("ORDERDATE"),
           cU("20110131"), &errInf);
/* Bestellpositionen füllen                            */
rc = RfcGetTable(bapiOrderCreate,
                 cU("TA_ORDERPOS"),
                 &rfcTab, &errInf);
rfcStruct = RfcAppendNewRow(rfcTab, &errInf);
RfcSetNum(rfcStruct, cU("MANDT"), cU("002"),
          3, &errInf);
RfcSetNum(rfcStruct, cU("ORDERID"), cU("0000000001"),
          10, &errInf);
RfcSetNum(rfcStruct, cU("ORDERPOS"), cU("00001"),
          5, &errInf);
RfcSetChars(rfcStruct, cU("MATID"), cU("4711"),
            4, &errInf);
RfcSetChars(rfcStruct, cU("MATTEXT"),
            cU("ABAP für Anfänger"),
            17, &errInf);
RfcSetInt(rfcStruct, cU("ORDERCOUNT"), 2, &errInf);
```

```
  RfcSetFloat(rfcStruct, cU("PRICE"), 69.90, &errInf);
  RfcSetChars(rfcStruct, cU("CURRENCY"),
              cU("EUR"), 3, &errInf);
  /* RFC-Funktion aufrufen                              */
  rc = RfcInvoke(connection, bapiOrderCreate, &errInf);
  if (rc != RFC_OK)
      errorHandling(rc, cU("Fehler b. Aufruf d. Funktion"),
                    &errInf, connection);
  /* Tabellenparameter RETURN ausgeben                  */
  rc = RfcGetTable(bapiOrderCreate, cU("RETURN"),
                   &rfcTab, &errInf);
  rc = RfcGetRowCount(rfcTab, &uiRowCount, &errInf);
  for(i=0; i < uiRowCount; i++)
  {
    rfcStruct = RfcGetCurrentRow(rfcTab, &errInf);
    if(rfcStruct!=NULL)
    {
      memsetU(temp, 0x0, 256);
      RfcGetChars(rfcStruct, cU("TYPE"),
                  temp, 2, &errInf);
      printfU(cU("TYPE    %s\n"), temp);
      memsetU(temp, 0x0, 256);
      RfcGetChars(rfcStruct, cU("MESSAGE"),
                  temp, 200, &errInf);
      printfU(cU("MESSAGE %s\n"), temp);
    }
    RfcMoveToNextRow(rfcTab, &errInf);
  }
  /* Bestellnummer ausgeben                             */
  memsetU(temp, 0x0, 256);
  RfcGetChars(bapiOrderCreate,
    cU("ORDERID"), temp, 11, &errInf);
  printfU(cU("ORDERID %s\n"), temp);
  /* BAPI_TRANSACTION_COMMIT aufrufen                   */
  RfcInvoke(connection, bapiTransactionCommit, &errInf);
  if (rc != RFC_OK)
      errorHandling(rc, cU("Fehler b. Aufruf d. Funktion"),
                    &errInf, connection);
  ...
}
```

Listing 4.9 BAPI-Client

4.3.2 Transaktionaler RFC-Client

Wie wir in Abschnitt 3.2, »Transaktionaler RFC«, erläutert haben, sollten mit dem bisher besprochenen synchronen RFC keine Funktionsbausteine aufgerufen werden, die Daten in einem SAP-System erzeugen. Falls nämlich ein Aufruf mit einem Kommunikationsfehler fehlschlägt, wissen Sie nicht, ob die Daten im SAP-System erzeugt wurden und ob der Fehler erst bei der Rückmeldung zum Client aufgetreten ist. Um sicherzustellen, dass ein Funktionsbaustein mit den ihm übergebenen Daten auch im Fehlerfall genau einmal aufgerufen wird, verwenden Sie am besten einen transaktionalen RFC (tRFC).

Transaktions-ID

Beim tRFC werden die Export- und Tabellenparameter beim Aufruf zusammen mit einer Transaktions-ID (TID) an die RFC-Bibliothek übergeben. Das SAP-System führt den Funktionsbaustein nur dann aus, wenn die Daten mit der übergebenen TID bislang noch nicht verarbeitet wurden. Wird die TID erstmalig übergeben, wird der Funktionsbaustein ausgeführt; wurde die TID schon einmal verwendet, wird der Funktionsbaustein nicht ausgeführt.

Aufruf der TID

Der Client besorgt sich die TID, die er zusammen mit den Daten für den Funktionsbaustein übergibt, durch einen Aufruf der Funktion `RfcGetTransactionID`. Diese TID wird dann verwendet, um eine Transaktion mit `RfcCreateTransaction` zu starten. Diese Funktion gibt ein Transaktions-Handle zurück. Der Aufruf des Funktionsbausteins erfolgt mit der Funktion `RfcInvokeInTransaction`, mit der nicht nur das Funktions-Handle, sondern auch das Transaktions-Handle übergeben wird. Die Transaktion wird durch den Aufruf von `RfcSubmitTransaction` abgeschlossen, und erst zu diesem Zeitpunkt schickt die SAP-NetWeaver-RFC-Bibliothek die Daten an den Server. War der Aufruf erfolgreich, sollte der Client mit einem Aufruf der Funktion `RfcConfirmTransaction` veranlassen, dass die verwendete TID aus den Datenbanktabellen des SAP-Systems gelöscht wird.

tRFC-Client

Im Folgenden zeigen wir Ihnen einen tRFC-Client, der über Aufrufe des Funktionsbausteins `Z_IFP_ORDER_CREATE` eine Kundenbestellung in ein SAP-System schreibt. Das Programm erwartet auf der Kommandozeile den Namen einer Datei, die die Daten einer Bestellung enthält. Bevor der Client eine TID besorgt und die Daten per tRFC an das SAP-System überträgt, schaut er in der Datei **order.tid** nach, ob die betreffende Datei mit den Bestelldaten bereits einmal übertragen wurde.

TID-Datei

Die Datei **order.tid** speichert den Übertragungszeitpunkt, das Ergebnis der Übertragung und den Namen der Datei mit der Bestellung. Für das Ergebnis der Übertragung gibt es drei Möglichkeiten:

- `CREATED`
  In einem früheren Übertragungsversuch wurde eine TID erzeugt, aber eine der Funktionen `RfcCreateTransaction`, `RfcInvokeIn-Transaction` oder `RfcSubmitTransaction` ist fehlgeschlagen. In diesem Fall führt der Client die Verarbeitung nochmals durch.
- `EXECUTED`
  In einem früheren Übertragungsversuch wurde eine TID erzeugt, und die Daten wurden erfolgreich verarbeitet. In diesem Fall erzeugt der Client eine neue Transaktion mit der TID aus **order.tid** und ruft anschließend `RfcConfirmTransaction`. Er überträgt die Daten nicht noch einmal.
- `CONFIRMED`
  Ein früherer Übertragungsversuch wurde erfolgreich abgeschlossen. In diesem Fall unternimmt der Client gar nichts.

TID-Zustände

Listing 4.10 zeigt ein Beispiel für die Datei **order.tid** mit drei TIDs für die Dateien **order1.dat**, **order2.dat** und **order3.dat**.

```
*** tRFC TID-Management-Datei ***
... C0A89F810CC849AAE89C006A  CONFIRMED  order1.dat
... C0A89F810CC849AAE9B4007E  CREATED    order2.dat
... C0A89F810CC849AAEE0A007F  EXECUTED   order3.dat
```

Listing 4.10 Datei »order.tid« für das TID-Management

Die erste Transaktion wurde erfolgreich durchgeführt, und die TID wurde bestätigt. Für die zweite Transaktion wurde eine TID erzeugt, aber `RfcindirectCallEx` wurde nicht oder fehlerhaft ausgeführt. Bei einem erneuten Aufruf des tRFC-Clients mit `order2` als Kommandozeilenargument überträgt er die Daten mit derselben TID nochmals und bestätigt dann die TID. Die dritte Transaktion wurde zwar ausgeführt, aber die TID noch nicht bestätigt. Bei einem erneuten Aufruf des tRFC-Clients mit `order3` als Kommandozeilenargument überträgt er die Daten nicht nochmals, sondern bestätigt lediglich die TID.

TID-Management

Für das TID-Management muss der Client einige Funktionen definieren. Listing 4.11 zeigt die Header-Datei mit diesen Definitionen. Dort werden die Aufzählungen `TID_RC` und `TID_STATE` definiert. `TID_RC` definiert die Rückgabewerte der beiden TID-Management-Funktionen `update_TID` und `search_TID`.

```
#include <time.h>
#include "sapnwrfc.h"
#define ERROR_OK         0 /* OK                          */
#define ERROR_CONNECT    1 /* Verbindungsfehler           */
```

```
#define ERROR_FAILURE   2 /* anderer Fehler                         */
/* Rückgabewerte vom TID-Management                                  */
typedef enum
{
  TID_OK,               /* OK                                        */
  TID_CREATED_FOUND,    /* TID im Status CREATED gefunden            */
  TID_EXECUTED_FOUND,   /* TID im Status EXECUTED gefunden           */
  TID_CONFIRMED_FOUND,  /* TID im Status CONFIRMED gefunden          */
  TID_ERROR_UPDATE
  /* TID-Status konnte nicht geändert werden                         */
}
TID_RC;
/* TID-Status im TID-Management                                      */
typedef enum
{
  CREATED,                    /* TID erzeugt                         */
  EXECUTED,                   /* Transaktion ausgeführt              */
  CONFIRMED,                  /* TID bestätigt                       */
  ROLLBACK                    /* Transaktion zurückgerollt           */
}
TID_STATE;
#define MAXBUFF               8192
#define LINE_SIZE             256*sizeofR(SAP_UC)
TID_RC search_TID(RFC_TID tid,
  SAP_UC *datafile, SAP_UC *tid_file);
TID_RC update_TID(RFC_TID tid, TID_STATE tid_state,
  SAP_UC *datafile, SAP_UC * tid_file);
```

Listing 4.11 Header-Datei des tRFC-Clients

Die TID-Management-Funktion `search_TID` verwendet der tRFC-Client, um in der Datei **order.tid** nach einer TID für die übergebene Datei zu suchen. Je nach Resultat führt er dann die notwendige Aktion durch und ändert den Zustand der TID über die Funktion `update_TID`. Dieser Funktion übergibt er den neuen Zustand, der ein Mitglied der Aufzählung `TID_STATE` ist.

TID-Management-Funktion »search_TID«

Listing 4.12 zeigt die TID-Management-Funktion `search_TID`. Diese Funktion öffnet die TID-Datei, deren Name als dritter Parameter übergeben wird. Wenn die TID-Datei nicht existiert, wird sie von `search_TID` erzeugt. Danach sucht die Funktion in einer `while`-Schleife nach einem Eintrag für die übergebene Datei. Der Dateiname wird der Funktion als zweiter Parameter übergeben. Wird kein Eintrag gefunden, gibt die Funktion die Meldung `TID_OK` zurück. Wird ein Eintrag gefunden, kopiert die Funktion die gefundene TID in den ersten Übergabeparameter und ermittelt den Status der TID in der TID-Datei. Dieser Status wird dann zurückgegeben.


```
/* nach vorhandener TID für die Datendatei suchen          */
extern TID_RC search_TID(RFC_TID tid, SAP_UC *datafile,
                         SAP_UC *tid_file)
{
  SAP_UC       *ptr, tbuf[MAXBUFF+1];
  TID_RC       tidrc;
  FILE         *fp;
  memsetU (tid, cU('\0'), RFC_TID_LN);
  /* Datei für Suche öffnen   */
  fp = fopenU (tid_file, cU("rb"));
  if (fp == NULL)
  {
    /* TID-Datei erzeugen     */
    fp = fopenU (tid_file, cU("ab"));
    if (fp == NULL)
      return TID_ERROR_UPDATE;
    strcpyU (tbuf,
       cU("*** tRFC TID-Management-Datei ***\n"));
    if (fputsU (tbuf, fp) < 0)
      tidrc = TID_ERROR_UPDATE;
    else
      tidrc = TID_OK;
    fclose(fp);
    return tidrc;
  }
  while ((ptr = fgetsU (tbuf, LINE_SIZE+1, fp)) != NULL)
  {
    if ( memcmpU (tbuf+63, datafile, strlenU(datafile))
         == 0)
      break;
  }
  if (ptr != NULL) /* TID-Eintrag für Datendatei gefunden */
  {
    memcpyU (tid, tbuf+26, RFC_TID_LN);
    if (memcmpU (tbuf+52, cU("CREATED"), 7) == 0)
       tidrc = TID_CREATED_FOUND;
    else if(memcmpU(tbuf+52, cU("EXECUTED"), 8) == 0)
      tidrc = TID_EXECUTED_FOUND;
    else
      tidrc = TID_CONFIRMED_FOUND;
```

```
  }
  else /* Keine TID für diese Datendatei gefunden          */
    tidrc = TID_OK;
  fclose (fp);
  return tidrc;
} /* search_tid */}
```

Listing 4.12 TID-Management-Funktion »search_TID«

TID-Management-Funktion »update_TID«

Listing 4.13 zeigt die TID-Management-Funktion `update_TID`. Die Funktion erwartet als Parameter die TID, den neuen Zustand sowie die Namen der Datendatei und der TID-Datei. Ist der Zustand `CREATED`, schreibt sie die neue TID an das Ende der TID-Datei. Dazu öffnet sie die TID-Datei und ruft die Funktion `write_TID` auf. Bei anderen Zuständen der TID muss die Funktion die TID-Datei zum Ändern öffnen und den Eintrag in einer `while`-Schleife suchen. Wird der Eintrag gefunden, wird der Dateizeiger `fp` an der entsprechenden Stelle positioniert und der neue Zustand mit `write_TID` geschrieben.

```
/* TID-Status in TID-Datei ändern                           */
extern TID_RC update_TID(RFC_TID tid, TID_STATE tid_state,
   SAP_UC *datafile, SAP_UC * tid_file)
{
  SAP_UC       *ptr, tbuf[MAXBUFF+1];
  TID_RC       tidrc;
  long         offset = 0;
  FILE         *fp;
  memsetU (tbuf, cU('\0'), LINE_SIZE/sizeofR(SAP_UC));
  if (tid_state == CREATED)
  {
    /* neue TID ans Ende schreiben                           */
    fp = fopenU (tid_file, cU("ab"));
    if (fp == NULL)
      return TID_ERROR_UPDATE;
    else
    {
      if (write_TID(fp, tid, tid_state, datafile))
        tidrc = TID_ERROR_UPDATE;
      else
        tidrc = TID_OK;
      fclose(fp);
      return tidrc;
    }
```

```
  }
  /* Datei zum Update öffnen                               */
  fp = fopenU (tid_file, cU("rb+"));
  if (fp == NULL)
    return TID_ERROR_UPDATE;
  /* TID suchen                                            */
  while ((ptr = fgetsU (tbuf, LINE_SIZE+1, fp)) != NULL)
  {
    if (memcmpU (tbuf+26, tid, RFC_TID_LN) == 0)
      break;
    offset = offset + strlenU (tbuf)*sizeofR(SAP_UC);
  }

  /* neuen TID-Zustand schreiben                           */
  if ((ptr != NULL) && (fseek (fp, offset, SEEK_SET) == 0) &
      (write_TID (fp, tid, tid_state, datafile) == 0))
    tidrc = TID_OK;
  else
    tidrc = TID_ERROR_UPDATE;
  fclose(fp);
  return tidrc;
} /* update_tid */
```

Listing 4.13 TID-Management-Funktion »update_TID«

TID-Management-Funktion »write_TID«

Listing 4.14 zeigt die TID-Management-Funktion `write_TID`. Die Funktion ermittelt die aktuelle Zeit und schreibt daraufhin die Zeit, die übergebene TID, den übergebenen Zustand und den übergebenen Dateinamen in die TID-Datei. Die TID-Datei wurde zuvor von der aufrufenden Funktion (`update_TID`) geöffnet und an die richtige Stelle positioniert. Der Funktion `write_TID` wird der Dateizeiger als erster Parameter übergeben.

```
/* TID und Datendatei in die TID-Datei schreiben           */
static int write_TID(FILE *fp, RFC_TID tid,
   TID_STATE tid_state, SAP_UC *datafile)
{
  struct tm     *time_ptr;
  time_t        actutime;
  SAP_UC        datetime[25],
                tbuf[MAXBUFF+1];
  memsetU (tbuf, cU('\0'), LINE_SIZE/sizeofR(SAP_UC));
  actutime = time(NULL);
  time_ptr = localtime(&actutime);
```

```
  memcpyU (datetime, asctimeU(time_ptr), 24);
  switch(tid_state)
  {
    case CREATED:
      sprintfU (tbuf, cU("%.*s  %.*s  CREATED    %s\n"),
            24, datetime, RFC_TID_LN, tid, datafile);
      break;
    case EXECUTED:
      sprintfU (tbuf, cU("%.*s  %.*s  EXECUTED   %s\n"),
                24, datetime, RFC_TID_LN, tid, datafile);
      break;

    case CONFIRMED:
      sprintfU (tbuf, cU("%.*s  %.*s  CONFIRMED  %s\n"),
                24, datetime, RFC_TID_LN, tid, datafile);
      break;
    case ROLLBACK:
      sprintfU (tbuf, cU("%.*s  %.*s  ROLLBACK   %s\n"),
                24, datetime, RFC_TID_LN, tid, datafile);
      break;
  }
  if (fputsU (tbuf, fp) < 0)
    return 1;
  else
    return 0;
} /* write_tid */
```

Listing 4.14 TID-Management-Funktion »write_TID«

tRFC-Client

Listing 4.15 zeigt Ausschnitte aus dem Quelltext des tRFC-Clients. Die `mainU`-Funktion deklariert zunächst die notwendigen Variablen. Dazu gehören unter anderem die Namen für die TID-Datei und die Datendatei, der Speicherplatz für die TID und ein Dateizeiger für die Datendatei.

```
#include "tid.h"
...
int mainU(int argc, SAP_UC** argv)
{
  SAP_UC data_file[64];
  SAP_UC tid_file[11] = cU("order.tid");
  RFC_TID tid;
  TID_RC  tid_rc, tid_search_rc;
  FILE   *data_fp;
```

```
  RFC_RC rc = RFC_OK;
  RFC_CONNECTION_PARAMETER login[6];
  RFC_ERROR_INFO errInf;
  RFC_CONNECTION_HANDLE connection;
  RFC_FUNCTION_DESC_HANDLE rfcFuncDesc;
  RFC_FUNCTION_HANDLE rfcFunc;
  RFC_TRANSACTION_HANDLE rfcTrans;
  /* Argumente prüfen                                    */
  if(argc!=2)
  {
      printfU (cU("\nVerwendung: trfc <datei>\n"));
      exit(ERROR_FAILURE);
  }
  strcpyU(data_file,argv[1]);
  /* Datei öffnen                                        */
  data_fp = fopenU (data_file, cU("r"));
  if (data_fp == NULL)
  {
    printfU(cU("\nDatei %s kann nicht geöffnet werden.\n"),
             data_file);
    exit(ERROR_FAILURE);
  }
...
  /* Importparameter setzen                              */
  RfcSetChars(rfcFunc, cU("IM_COMMIT"), cU("X"), 1, NULL);
  /* vorangegangene fehlgeschlagene TID suchen           */
  tid_search_rc = search_TID(tid, data_file, tid_file);
  switch(tid_search_rc)
  {
    case TID_CREATED_FOUND:
    {
      printfU (cU("\n** Vorangegangener tRFC fehlgeschlagen **"));
      printfU (cU("\n   TransID :  %.*s"), RFC_TID_LN, tid);
      printfU (cU("\n   State    :  CREATED\n"));
      break;
    }
    case TID_EXECUTED_FOUND:
    {
      printfU (cU("\n** Vorangegangener tRFC ausgeführt **"));
      printfU (cU("\n   TransID :  %.*s"), RFC_TID_LN, tid);
      printfU (cU("\n   State     :  EXECUTED\n"));
      break;
    }
```

```
  case TID_CONFIRMED_FOUND:
  {
    printfU (cU("\n** voriger tRFC bestätigt **"));
    printfU (cU("\n   TransID :  %.*s"), RFC_TID_LN, tid);
    printfU (cU("\n   State    :  EXECUTED\n"));
    break;
  }
  default:
  {
    printfU (cU("\n** Erster Aufruf des tRFC  **\n"));
    /* neue TID beschaffen                                  */
    rc = RfcGetTransactionID(connection, tid, &errInf);
    if(rc!=RFC_OK)
        errorHandling(rc, cU("RfcCreateTransID"),
                      &errInf, connection);
    printfU (cU("     TID = '%.*s'\n"), RFC_TID_LN, tid);
    /* TID in Datei speichern                               */
    tid_rc = update_TID(tid, CREATED, data_file,
                        tid_file);
  }
}
if (tid_search_rc == TID_OK ||
    tid_search_rc == TID_CREATED_FOUND)
{
  /* Kopfdaten aus der Eingabedatei in order speichern  */
  rc = (RFC_RC) write_file_to_structure(data_fp, rfcFunc);
  if (rc!=RFC_OK)
    errorHandling(rc, cU("write_file_to_structure"),
                  &errInf, connection);
  /* Positionsdaten aus der Eingabedatei in ta_pos
     speichern                                          */
  rc = (RFC_RC) write_file_to_table(data_fp, rfcFunc);
  if (rc!=RFC_OK)
    errorHandling(rc, cU("write_file_to_table"),
                  &errInf, connection);
  fclose(data_fp);
  /* tRFC-Aufruf                                        */
  rfcTrans = RfcCreateTransaction(connection, tid, NULL,
                                  &errInf);
  if(rfcTrans == NULL)
    errorHandling(rc,
            cU("Fehler beim Erzeugen der Transaktion"),
            &errInf, connection);
```

```
    rc = RfcInvokeInTransaction(rfcTrans, rfcFunc, &errInf);
    if (rc != RFC_OK)
      errorHandling(rc,
                  cU("Fehler beim Aufruf der Funktion"),
                  &errInf, connection);
    /* Transaktion abschließen                          */
    rc = RfcSubmitTransaction(rfcTrans, &errInf);
    if (rc != RFC_OK)
      errorHandling(rc,
                  cU("Fehler beim Schließen der Transaktion"),
                  &errInf, connection);
    /* TID-Status in Datei speichern                    */
    tid_rc = update_TID(tid, EXECUTED, data_file, tid_file);
    /* Transaktion bestätigen                           */
    rc = RfcConfirmTransaction(rfcTrans, &errInf);
    if (rc != RFC_OK)
      errorHandling(rc,
                 cU("Fehler beim Bestätigen der Transaktion"),
                 &errInf, connection);
    /* TID-Status in Datei speichern                    */
    tid_rc = update_TID(tid,CONFIRMED, data_file, tid_file);
  }
  /* Verbindung schließen                               */
  RfcCloseConnection(connection, &errInf);
  return 0;
}
```

Listing 4.15 tRFC-Client

Der Client überprüft zunächst die Anzahl der Argumente und kopiert das erste Argument in die Datei data_file. Anschließend versucht er, diese Datei zu öffnen. Wenn alles gut geht, öffnet sich die Verbindung, die Metadaten werden geladen, und die Datencontainer werden initialisiert. Diesen Code haben Sie in den vorangegangenen Listings dieses Kapitels bereits öfter gesehen.

TID wiederverwenden oder neu erzeugen

Danach schaut der Client mit search_TID in der TID-Datei **order.tid** nach, ob die Daten schon einmal verarbeitet wurden, und gibt eine entsprechende Meldung aus. Wurden die Daten noch nie verarbeitet, wird mit RfcGetTransactionID eine neue TID erzeugt. Im Fall der Meldungen TID_OK und TID_CREATED_FOUND liest der Client die Daten aus der Datendatei in den Datencontainer der Funktion. Dann öffnet er mit RfcCreateTransaction eine Transaktion unter Angabe der TID. Innerhalb dieser Transaktion ruft er den

Funktionsbaustein mit RfcInvokeInTransaction auf und schließt dann die Transaktion mit RfcSubmitTransaction ab. Anschließend ändert der Client den Zustand der TID in der TID-Datei auf EXECUTED. Danach bestätigt der Client die TID mit einem Aufruf der Funktion RfcConfirm-Transaction und ändert den Zustand der TID auf CONFIRMED.

»write_file_to_structure« und »write_file_to_table«

Listing 4.16 zeigt die Funktionen write_file_to_structure und write_file_to_table. Diese Funktionen lesen Bestellkopf und Bestellpositionen aus der geöffneten Datei **fp** in den strukturierten Importparameter IM_ORDERHEADER und den Tabellenparameter TA_ORDERPOS des Funktionsbausteins.

```
/* Bestellkopf in Struktur kopieren                        */
RFC_RC write_file_to_structure(
                      FILE *fp, RFC_FUNCTION_HANDLE rfcFunc)
{
  RFC_RC rc = RFC_OK;
  SAP_UC buf[136];
  RFC_STRUCTURE_HANDLE rfcStruct;
  RFC_ERROR_INFO errInf;
  if (fgetsU (buf, 136, fp) != NULL)
  {
    rc = RfcGetStructure(rfcFunc,
                         cU("IM_ORDERHEADER"),
                         &rfcStruct, &errInf);
    RfcSetNum(rfcStruct, cU("MANDT"), buf,
              3, &errInf);
    RfcSetNum(rfcStruct, cU("ORDERID"), buf+3,
              10, &errInf);
    RfcSetChars(rfcStruct, cU("TYPE"), buf+13,
                2, &errInf);
    RfcSetNum(rfcStruct, cU("REFID"), buf+15,
              10, &errInf);
    RfcSetChars(rfcStruct, cU("BUYER"), buf+25,
                50, &errInf);
    RfcSetChars(rfcStruct, cU("SELLER"), buf+75,
                50, &errInf);
    RfcSetDate(rfcStruct, cU("ORDERDATE"), buf+125
               , &errInf);
  }
  else
    rc = RFC_EXTERNAL_FAILURE;
  return rc;
}
/* Bestellpositionen in Tabelle kopieren                   */
```

```
RFC_RC write_file_to_table(
                      FILE *fp, RFC_FUNCTION_HANDLE rfcFunc)
{
  RFC_RC rc = RFC_OK;
  SAP_UC buf[102];
  SAP_UC number[11];
  RFC_TABLE_HANDLE rfcTab;
  RFC_STRUCTURE_HANDLE rfcStruct;
  RFC_ERROR_INFO errInf;
  rc = RfcGetTable(rfcFunc, cU("TA_ORDERPOS"), &rfcTab,
                &errInf);
  while (fgetsU (buf, 102, fp) != NULL)
  {
     rfcStruct = RfcAppendNewRow(rfcTab, &errInf);
     RfcSetNum(rfcStruct, cU("MANDT"),buf,3,&errInf);
     RfcSetNum(rfcStruct, cU("ORDERID"),buf+3,10,&errInf);
     RfcSetNum(rfcStruct, cU("ORDERPOS"),buf+13,5,&errInf);
     RfcSetChars(rfcStruct, cU("MATID"),buf+18,20,&errInf);
     RfcSetChars(rfcStruct, cU("MATTEXT"),buf+38,40,
                 &errInf);
     memcpyU(number,buf+78,10); number[10] = 0;


     RfcSetInt(rfcStruct, cU("ORDERCOUNT"),
               atoiU(number),&errInf);
     memcpyU(number,buf+88,7); number[7]=0;
     RfcSetFloat(rfcStruct, cU("PRICE"),
                 atofU(number),&errInf);
     RfcSetChars(rfcStruct, cU("CURRENCY"),buf+95,5,
                 &errInf);
  }
  return rc;
}
```

Listing 4.16 Funktionen »write_file_to_structure« und »write_file_to_table«

4.3.3 Queued RFC-Client

Die RFC-C-Bibliothek ermöglicht auch die Verwendung von queued RFC (qRFC). Dabei werden mehrere tRFC-Aufrufe in eine Eingangswarteschlange in einem SAP-System gestellt. Damit wird sichergestellt, dass die Aufrufe im Zielsystem in der Reihenfolge abgearbeitet werden, in der sie im Empfängersystem abgesetzt wurden.

Die Verwendung von qRFC funktioniert genauso wie die von tRFC. Sie müssen lediglich bei der Erzeugung der Transaktion mit `RfcCreateTransaction` als dritten Parameter anstelle von `NULL` einen beliebigen Queue-Namen angeben.

Abarbeitung der Eingangswarteschlange

Wie wir in Abschnitt 3.3.2, »qRFC mit Ausgangs- und Eingangswarteschlange«, erläutert haben, erfolgt die Verarbeitung der Funktionsbausteine in der Eingangs-Queue nicht automatisch. Sie müssen dazu den Funktionsbaustein `TRFC_QIN_RESTART` aufrufen oder den QIN-Scheduler verwenden.

4.4 SAP-NetWeaver-RFC-Server

Als C/C++-Programmierer haben Sie auch die Möglichkeit, RFC-Server zu schreiben. Dies sind Programme, die Funktionen bereitstellen, die per RFC aufgerufen werden können. Auch wenn es moderne Alternativen wie OData oder REST gibt, bleibt RFC für Legacy-Systeme relevant, in denen ein Umstieg nicht wirtschaftlich ist, oder für hoch performante oder spezifische Anwendungsfälle, z. B. der Fertigungsindustrie oder in der Echtzeitdatenverarbeitung.

Start eines RFC-Servers

Ein RFC-Server wird entweder beim Aufruf durch den ABAP-Client vom Gateway gestartet, oder er wird unabhängig von einem Client-Aufruf gestartet und registriert sich an einem Gateway. Da der zweite der weitaus häufigere Fall ist, behandeln wir diesen in den folgenden Beispielen.

Serverschema

Listing 4.17 zeigt das Schema eines typischen RFC-Servers. Nach dem Programmstart installiert der Server die von ihm angebotenen Funktionen mit dem API-Aufruf `RfcInstallServerFunction`. Dabei teilt er der SAP-NetWeaver-RFC-Bibliothek den Funktionsnamen einer C-Funktion mit.

Danach registriert er sich mit `RfcRegisterServer` an einem Gateway. Dabei gibt er den Namen des Gateway-Hosts, den Namen des Gateway-Service und eine Programm-ID an, unter der der Server am Gateway eindeutig identifiziert werden kann. Die Funktion `RfcRegisterServer` verbindet den Server mit dem Gateway und gibt im Erfolgsfall ein Handle auf eine RFC-Verbindung zurück.

Schema eines RFC-Servers

In einer Endlosschleife ruft der Server dann die Funktion `RfcListenAndDispatch` auf. Diese Funktion wartet auf eingehende Client-Anfragen. Geht eine Client-Anfrage ein, ruft die RFC-Bibliothek die zuvor mit `RfcInstallServerFunction` installierte Funktion auf. Geht innerhalb des Timeouts, den der Server der API-Funktion mitgeteilt hat, keine Client-Anfrage ein, liefert `RfcListenAndDispatch` den Wert »RFC_RETRY« zurück.

```
int mainU ( int argc, SAP_UC** argv )
{
  RFC_CONNECTION_HANDLE handle;
  RFC_RC rc;
  int timeout = 120;
  rc = RfcInstallServerFunction( ... );
  if( rc != RFC_OK )
  {
    ... Fehlerbehandlung
    return 1;
  }
  handle = RfcRegisterServer( ... );
  if ( handle == NULL )
  {
    ... Fehlerbehandlung
    return 1;
  }
  do
  {
    rc = RfcListenAndDispatch( handle, timeout, ... );
  }
  while( rc == RFC_OK || rc == RFC_RETRY );
  RfcCloseConnection( handle );
  return 0;
}
```

Listing 4.17 Schema eines RFC-Servers

4.4.1 Einfacher RFC-Server

Beispiel für einen RFC-Server

Dieses einfache Schema werden wir in den folgenden Abschnitten in ein funktionierendes Beispiel umsetzen. Der RFC-Server in Listing 4.18 stellt die beiden Funktionen `Z_IFP_ORDER_GETLIST` und `Z_IFP_ORDER_GETDETAIL` bereit. Die eigentlichen Daten liest er aus der Datei **orders.dat** mit den Bestellköpfen und der Datei **orderpos.dat** mit den Bestellpositionen.

```
int mainU(int argc, SAP_UC** argv)
{
  RFC_RC rc = RFC_OK;
  RFC_CONNECTION_PARAMETER rpParm[6], srvParm[3];
  RFC_ERROR_INFO errInf;
  RFC_CONNECTION_HANDLE rpConn, srvConn;
  RFC_FUNCTION_DESC_HANDLE orderGetlistDesc,
                           orderGetdetailDesc;
```

```
unsigned int bRefresh = FALSE;
/* Verbindungsparameter zum Repository füllen         */
rpParm[0].name=cU("ashost");rpParm[0].value=cU("SAP00");
rpParm[1].name=cU("sysnr");rpParm[1].value=cU("00");
rpParm[2].name=cU("user");rpParm[2].value=cU("ope");
rpParm[3].name=cU("passwd");rpParm[3].value=cU("pehnke");
rpParm[4].name=cU("client");rpParm[4].value=cU("001");
rpParm[5].name=cU("lang");rpParm[5].value=cU("EN");
/* Verbindungsparameter zum Gateway füllen            */
srvParm[0].name=cU("gwhost");srvParm[0].value=cU("SAP00");
srvParm[1].name=cU("gwserv");
srvParm[1].value=cU("sapgw00");

rvParm[2].name=cU("program_id");
srvParm[2].value=cU("CSERV");
/* Verbindung zum Repository öffnen                   */
rpConn = RfcOpenConnection(rpParm, 6, &errInf);
if (rpConn == NULL) errorHandling(...);
/* Metadaten der RFC-Funktionen lesen                 */
orderGetlistDesc = RfcGetFunctionDesc(
                     rpConn,
                     cU("Z_IFP_ORDER_GETLIST"), &errInf);
if (orderGetlistDesc == NULL) errorHandling(...);
orderGetdetailDesc = RfcGetFunctionDesc(
                       rpConn,
                       cU("Z_IFP_ORDER_GETDETAIL"),
                       &errInf);
if (orderGetdetailDesc == NULL) errorHandling(...);
/* Verbindung zum Repository schließen                */
RfcCloseConnection(rpConn, &errInf);
/* Serverfunktionen installieren                      */
rc = RfcInstallServerFunction(
       NULL, orderGetlistDesc,
       z_ifp_order_getlist, &errInf);
if(rc != RFC_OK) errorHandling(...);
rc = RfcInstallServerFunction(
       NULL, orderGetdetailDesc,
       z_ifp_order_getdetail, &errInf);
if(rc != RFC_OK) errorHandling(...);  /
* Server am Gateway registrieren                      */
srvConn = RfcRegisterServer(srvParm, 3, &errInf);
if(srvConn == NULL) errorHandling(...);
/* Dispatch-Schleife                                  */
```

```
rc = RFC_OK;
while(rc == RFC_OK ||
      rc == RFC_RETRY ||
      rc == RFC_ABAP_EXCEPTION)
{
  rc = RfcListenAndDispatch(srvConn, 120, &errInf);
  bRefresh = FALSE;
  switch(rc)
  {
    case RFC_RETRY:
      printfU(cU("Warte weitere 120 s.\n"));
      break;
    case RFC_ABAP_EXCEPTION:
      printfU(cU("ABAP-Exception ausgelöst.\n"));
      break;
    case RFC_NOT_FOUND:
      printfU(cU("Unbekannter Funktionsbaustein.\n"));
      bRefresh = TRUE;
      break;
    case RFC_EXTERNAL_FAILURE:
      printfU(cU("Systemfehler.\n"));
      bRefresh = TRUE;
      break;
    case RFC_ABAP_MESSAGE:
      printfU(cU("ABAP-Message.\n"));
      bRefresh = TRUE;
      break;
    case RFC_COMMUNICATION_FAILURE:
      printfU(cU("Netzwerkfehler.\n"));
      bRefresh = TRUE;
      break;
    case RFC_CLOSED:
      printfU(cU("Verbindung geschlossen.\n"));
      bRefresh = TRUE;
      break;
  }
  if(bRefresh)
  {
    srvConn = RfcRegisterServer (srvParm, 3, &errInf);
    rc = errInf.code;
  }
}
```

```
  RfcCloseConnection(srvConn, NULL);
  return 0;
}
```

Listing 4.18 Einfacher RFC-Server

Installation der Funktionen

Direkt nach dem Start verbindet sich der RFC-Server als Client mit einem SAP-System, um von dort die Metadaten der Funktionsbausteine zu lesen, die er selbst bereitstellen möchte. Auf diesem Repository-System müssen daher zumindest die Signaturen der Funktionsbausteine im Function Builder definiert sein. Zur Schnittstelle eines Funktionsbausteins gehören sein Name, die Namen und Typen seiner Parameter sowie die von ihm deklarierten Ausnahmen. Da er auf dem Repository-System nicht ausgeführt wird, darf dort der Code für den Funktionsbaustein fehlen. Die Metadaten-Handles und die Namen der C-Funktionen, in denen der Server die Funktionsbausteine implementiert, übergibt er mit einem Aufruf der Funktion `RfcInstallServerFunction` an die SAP-NetWeaver-RFC-Bibliothek. Im Beispiel von Listing 4.18 implementiert der Server die beiden Funktionsbausteine `Z_IFP_ORDER_GETLIST` und `Z_IFP_ORDER_GETDETAIL` in den C-Funktionen `z_ifp_order_getlist` und `z_ifp_order_getdetail`.

Anmeldung am Gateway

Mit dem Aufruf der Funktion `RfcRegisterServer` meldet sich der Server dann am Gateway an. Dabei übergibt er den Gateway-Host, den Namen des Gateway-Service und eine Programm-ID, die diesen Server im Gateway eindeutig identifiziert. Diese Informationen stellt der Server in einem Array von `RFC_CONNECTION_PARAMETER`-Strukturen bereit. Von der Funktion `RfcRegisterServer` erhält das Programm ein Handle zurück, das die RFC-Verbindung eindeutig identifiziert. Danach geht der Server in eine `WHILE`-Schleife, in der er die Funktion `RfcListenDispatch` aufruft.

Destination vom Typ T

Damit ABAP-Programme die Funktionen des RFC-Servers aufrufen können, müssen Sie in Transaktion SM59 eine Destination vom Typ `T` und vom Untertyp `Registrierung` pflegen. Dabei müssen Sie die Programm-ID genauso angeben, wie sie beim Start des RFC-Servers angegeben wurde. Die Groß- und Kleinschreibung ist dabei wichtig. Außerdem sollten Sie auf alle Fälle bei den Gateway-Optionen das Gateway angeben. Abbildung 4.8 zeigt eine Destination in Transaktion SM59, die zu der Programm-ID `CSERV` in Listing 4.18 passt.

Transaktion SMGW

Nachdem Sie den Server gestartet haben und er sich erfolgreich am Gateway angemeldet hat, können Sie aus der Destinationspflege auch einen Verbindungstest durchführen. In Transaktion SMGW sehen Sie einen Eintrag für den angemeldeten Server, wenn Sie das Menü **Springen • Angemeldete Clients** auswählen.

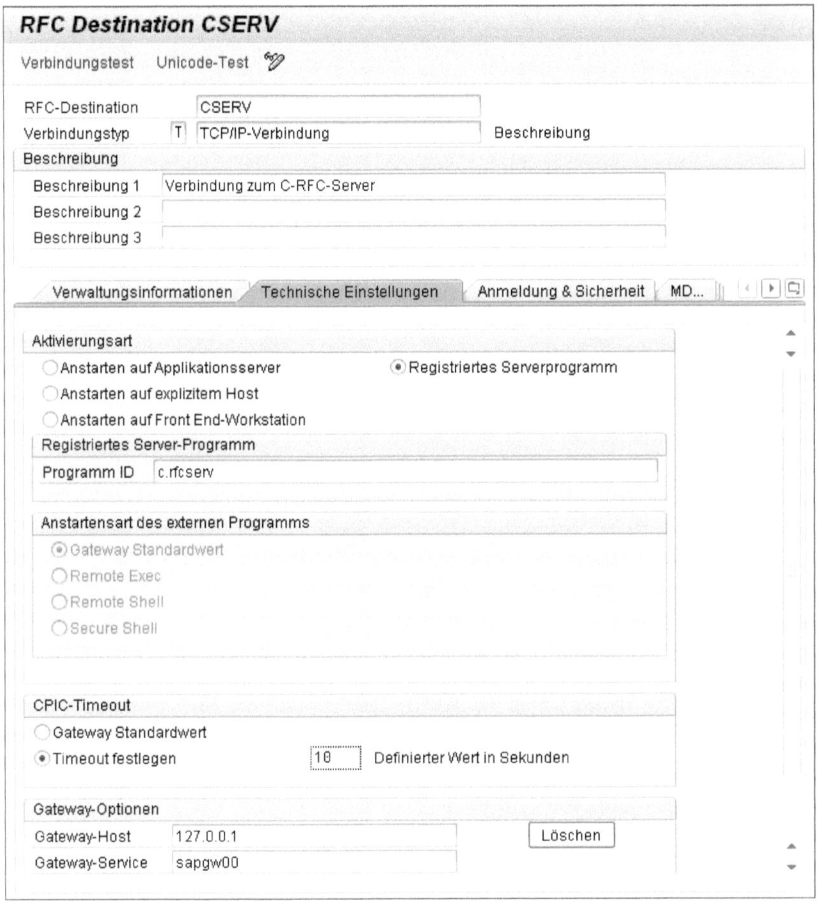

Abbildung 4.8 SM59-Destination für einen registrierten RFC-Server

4.4.2 Implementierung der Funktionen

Die implementierenden C-Funktionen erhalten als einen der drei Parameter ein Funktions-Handle. Aus diesem Datencontainer liest die Funktion die empfangenen Import- und Tabellenparameter aus. Diese Parameter wertet sie aus, berechnet oder liest die angeforderten Informationen aus einer Datei oder einer Datenbank und füllt die Export- und Tabellenparameter mit dem Ergebnis. Falls eine Ausnahme eintritt, teilt die Funktion dies über die Rückgabe des Returncodes `RFC_ABAP_EXCEPTION` mit. Im Erfolgsfall gibt sie den Returncode `RFC_OK` zurück.

Funktion »z_ifp_order_getlist«

Schauen Sie sich zunächst die Funktion `z_ifp_order_getlist` in Listing 4.19 an. Sie liest zuerst die Importparameter `IM_ORDERTYPE` und `IM_REFID` sowie ein Handle auf die zurückzugebende Tabelle `TA_ORDERS` aus dem übergebenen Funktions-Handle aus. Dann öffnet sie die Datei **orders.dat** und erzeugt für jede Zeile in dieser Datei, die den Selektionskriterien entspricht, eine Zeile in der internen Tabelle. Zum Schluss schließt sie die Datei und gibt den Returncode RFC_OK zurück.

```
RFC_RC SAP_API z_ifp_order_getlist(
         RFC_CONNECTION_HANDLE rfcConn,
         RFC_FUNCTION_HANDLE rfcFunc,
         RFC_ERROR_INFO* errInf)
{
  RFC_RC rc = RFC_OK;
  RFC_TABLE_HANDLE rfcTab;
  RFC_STRUCTURE_HANDLE rfcStruct;
  SAP_UC type[2];
  SAP_UC refid[10];
  SAP_UC tbuf[MAXBUFF+1];
  FILE *fp;
  RfcGetChars(rfcFunc, cU("IM_ORDERTYPE"), type, 2, errInf);
  RfcGetChars(rfcFunc, cU("IM_REFID"), refid, 10, errInf);
  RfcGetTable(rfcFunc, cU("TA_ORDERS"), &rfcTab, errInf);
  fp = fopenU (cU("orders.dat"), cU("rb"));
  if (memcmpU(type,cU("  "),2)==0)
    memcpyU(type,cU("SO"),2);
  while(fp && (fgetsU (tbuf,LINE_SIZE_ORDER+3,fp) != NULL))
  {
    if (((memcmpU(tbuf+15,refid,10)==0) ||
         (memcmpU(refid,cU("0000000000"),10)==0)) &&
        ((memcmpU(tbuf+13,type,2)==0)))
      {
        rfcStruct = RfcAppendNewRow(rfcTab, errInf);
        RfcSetNum(rfcStruct, cU("MANDT"), tbuf,
                  3, errInf);
        RfcSetNum(rfcStruct, cU("ORDERID"), tbuf+3,
                  10, errInf);
        RfcSetChars(rfcStruct, cU("TYPE"), tbuf+13,
                    2, errInf);
        RfcSetNum(rfcStruct, cU("REFID"), tbuf+15,
                  10, errInf);
        RfcSetChars(rfcStruct, cU("BUYER"), tbuf+25,
                    50, errInf);

        RfcSetChars(rfcStruct, cU("SELLER"), tbuf+75,
                    50, errInf);
```

```
      RfcSetDate(rfcStruct, cU("ORDERDATE"), tbuf+125,
                 errInf);
    }
  }
  fclose(fp);
  return rc;
}
```

Listing 4.19 Funktion »z_ifp_order_getlist«

Funktion »z_ifp_order_getdetail«

Die Funktion z_ifp_order_getdetail in Listing 4.20 liest ebenfalls zuerst den Importparameter IM_ORDERID und die Handles auf die beiden Exportparameter EX_ORDERHEAD und TA_ORDERPOS aus dem übergebenen Funktions-Handle aus. Danach sucht sie in der Datei **orders.dat** die angeforderte Bestellnummer. Wurde die Bestellnummer gefunden, kopiert die Funktion die Daten in die Struktur EX_ORDERHEAD. Anschließend öffnet sie die Datei **orderpos.dat**, liest die zugehörigen Bestellpositionen und gibt den Wert »RFC_OK« zurück. Findet die Funktion die Bestellung nicht, gibt sie den Wert »RFC_ABAP_EXCEPTION« zurück.

```
RFC_RC SAP_API z_ifp_order_getdetail(
        RFC_CONNECTION_HANDLE rfcConn,
        RFC_FUNCTION_HANDLE rfcFunc,
        RFC_ERROR_INFO* errInf)
{
  RFC_RC rc = RFC_ABAP_EXCEPTION;
  RFC_TABLE_HANDLE rfcTab;
  RFC_STRUCTURE_HANDLE rfcStruct;
  SAP_UC tbuf[MAXBUFF+1];
  SAP_UC number[11];
  SAP_UC orderid[10];
  FILE *fp;
  RfcGetChars(rfcFunc, cU("IM_ORDERID"),
              orderid, 10, errInf);
  RfcGetStructure(rfcFunc, cU("EX_ORDERHEAD"),
                  &rfcStruct, errInf);
  RfcGetTable(rfcFunc, cU("TA_ORDERPOS"),
              &rfcTab, errInf);
  fp = fopenU (cU("orders.dat"), cU("rb"));
  while(fp && (fgetsU (tbuf,LINE_SIZE_ORDER+3,fp) != NULL))
  {
    if(memcmpU(tbuf+3,orderid,10)==0)
    {
```

```
      rc = RFC_OK;
      RfcSetNum(rfcStruct, cU("MANDT"), tbuf,
                3, errInf);
      RfcSetNum(rfcStruct, cU("ORDERID"), tbuf+3,
                10, errInf);
      RfcSetChars(rfcStruct, cU("TYPE"), tbuf+13,
                  2, errInf);
      RfcSetNum(rfcStruct, cU("REFID"), tbuf+15,
                10, errInf);
      RfcSetChars(rfcStruct, cU("BUYER"), tbuf+25,
                  50, errInf);
      RfcSetChars(rfcStruct, cU("SELLER"), tbuf+75,
                  50, errInf);
      RfcSetDate(rfcStruct, cU("ORDERDATE"), tbuf+125,
                 errInf);
      break;
    }
  }
  fclose(fp);
  fp = fopenU (cU("orderpos.dat"), cU("rb"));
  while(fp&&(fgetsU(tbuf,LINE_SIZE_ORDERPOS+2,fp) != NULL))
  {
    if(memcmpU(tbuf+3,orderid,10)==0)
    {
      rfcStruct = RfcAppendNewRow(rfcTab, errInf);
      RfcSetNum(rfcStruct, cU("MANDT"),tbuf,3,errInf);
      RfcSetNum(rfcStruct, cU("ORDERID"),tbuf+3,10,errInf);
      RfcSetNum(rfcStruct, cU("ORDERPOS"),tbuf+13,5,errInf);
      RfcSetChars(rfcStruct, cU("MATID"),tbuf+18,20,errInf);
      RfcSetChars(rfcStruct, cU("MATTEXT"),
                  tbuf+38,40,errInf);
      memcpyU(number,tbuf+78,10); number[10] = 0;
      RfcSetInt(rfcStruct, cU("ORDERCOUNT"),
                atoiU(number),errInf);
      memcpyU(number,tbuf+88,7); number[7]=0;
      RfcSetFloat(rfcStruct, cU("PRICE"),
                  atofU(number),errInf);
      RfcSetChars(rfcStruct, cU("CURRENCY"),
                  tbuf+95,5,errInf);
    }
  }
  fclose(fp);
```

```
  return rc;
}
```

Listing 4.20 Funktion »z_ifp_order_getdetail«

Damit ist der RFC-Server komplett. Um ihn zu testen, können Sie das ABAP-Programm `Z_IFP_ORDERS_READ` aus Listing 4.3 (siehe Abschnitt 3.1.2, »Aufruf per sRFC«) verwenden. Dabei geben Sie im Selektionsbild die zuvor mit Transaktion SM59 erstellte Destination an (siehe Abbildung 4.8 in Abschnitt 4.4.1, »Einfacher RFC-Server«).

4.4.3 Transaktionaler RFC-Server

Transaktionskontrolle

Wenn Sie sicherstellen möchten, dass Daten im Fehlerfall vom Client nochmals an Ihren RFC-Server gesendet werden können, ohne dort doppelt verarbeitet zu werden, müssen Sie tRFC implementieren. Der Ablauf im RFC-Server ist beim transaktionalen RFC etwas komplexer als beim synchronen RFC. Zunächst einmal muss der Server mit einem Aufruf von `RfcInstallTransactionHandlers` der SAP-NetWeaver-RFC-Bibliothek vier Funktionen für das TID-Management bekannt geben. Diese vier Funktionen werden von der SAP-NetWeaver-RFC-Bibliothek zu bestimmten Zeitpunkten aufgerufen:

- `RFC_ON_CHECK_TID`

  Dies ist die erste Funktion, die von der RFC-Bibliothek beim tRFC aufgerufen wird. Diese Funktion muss die übergebene TID permanent speichern und `RFC_OK` zurückgeben, falls die TID noch nicht verwendet wurde. Falls die TID schon verwendet wurde, muss die Funktion einen Wert ungleich »RFC_EXECUTED« zurückgeben.

- `RFC_ON_COMMIT`

  Diese Funktion wird aufgerufen, wenn der Funktionsbaustein ausgeführt wurde. Innerhalb dieser Funktion kann der RFC-Server seine eigenen Datenbankänderungen festschreiben.

- `RFC_ON_ROLLBACK`

  Diese Funktion wird aufgerufen, wenn bei der tRFC-Verarbeitung ein Fehler aufgetreten ist. Innerhalb dieser Funktion sollte der RFC-Server seine eigenen Datenbankänderungen zurücknehmen.

- `RFC_ON_CONFIRM_TID`

  Diese Funktion wird aufgerufen, wenn die gesamte tRFC-Verarbeitung abgeschlossen wurde. Innerhalb dieser Funktion kann der Server die TID löschen.

Beispiel eines tRFC-Servers

Als Beispiel zeigen wir Ihnen einen tRFC-Server, der den Funktionsbaustein Z_IFP_ORDER_CREATE implementiert. Ein tRFC-Client ruft diesen Funktionsbaustein auf, um eine Bestellung an den Server zu schicken. Der Server speichert die Daten in einer Datei. Als Namen für die Datei wählt er **<TID>.dat**, wobei **<TID>** die für die tRFC-Übertragung verwendete TID ist.

Header-Datei des TID-Managements

Listing 4.21 zeigt die Header-Datei für das TID-Management des Servers. Wesentlich sind die beiden Aufzählungstypen TID_RC und TID_STATE sowie die Funktionen check_TID und update_TID. Der Server verwendet den Aufzählungstyp TID_RC für die Rückgabecodes der TID-Management-Funktionen. TID_STATE listet die verschiedenen Zustände auf, in denen eine TID in der TID-Management-Datei gespeichert sein kann. Dies sind die gleichen Zustände wie beim tRFC-Client.

```
#include "sapuc.h"
#define MAXBUFF                 32000
#define LINE_SIZE               256

/* Rückgabewerte vom TID-Management                       */
typedef enum
{
  TID_OK,               /* OK                             */
  TID_FOUND,            /* TID gefunden                   */
  TID_ERROR_UPDATE      /* Fehler beim Update             */
}
TID_RC;
/* TID-Status im TID-Management                           */
typedef enum
{
  CREATED,                /* TID erzeugt                  */
  EXECUTED,               /* Transaktion ausgeführt       */
  CONFIRMED,              /* TID bestätigt                */
  ROLLBACK                /* Transaktion zurückgerollt    */
}
TID_STATE;
TID_RC check_TID(const RFC_TID tid, SAP_UC *datafile,
                 SAP_UC *tid_file);
TID_RC update_TID(const RFC_TID tid, TID_STATE tid_state,
                  SAP_UC *datafile, SAP_UC * tid_file);
```

Listing 4.21 Header-Datei des TID-Managements

Listing 4.22 zeigt die vier Funktionen, die vom tRFC-Server für das TID-Handling bei der SAP-NetWeaver-RFC-Bibliothek mittels der API-Funktion `RfcInstallTransactionHandlers` installiert werden. Die Installation erfolgt beim Start des Programms über den Aufruf in Listing 4.23.

Transaktions-Handling eines tRFC-Servers


```
/* TID_check für tRFC                                    */
RFC_RC SAP_API RfcOnCheckTransaction(
        RFC_CONNECTION_HANDLE rfcHandle, SAP_UC const *tid)
{
  TID_RC tid_rc;
  sprintfU(data_file,65,cU("%.*s.dat"),RFC_TID_LN,tid);
  tid_rc = check_TID(tid, tid_file, data_file);
  if (tid_rc == TID_OK)
    return RFC_OK;
  if (tid_rc == TID_FOUND)
    return RFC_EXECUTED;
  return RFC_EXTERNAL_FAILURE;
}
/* TID_commit für tRFC                                   */
RFC_RC SAP_API RfcOnCommitTransaction(
        RFC_CONNECTION_HANDLE rfcHandle, SAP_UC const *tid)
{
  TID_RC        tid_rc;
  tid_rc = update_TID(tid, EXECUTED, tid_file, data_file);
  if (tid_rc == TID_OK)
    return RFC_OK;
  return RFC_EXTERNAL_FAILURE;
}
/* TID_confirm für tRFC                                  */
RFC_RC SAP_API RfcOnConfirmTransaction(
        RFC_CONNECTION_HANDLE rfcHandle, SAP_UC const *tid)
{
  TID_RC    tid_rc;
  tid_rc = update_TID(tid, CONFIRMED, tid_file, data_file);
  if (tid_rc == TID_OK)
    return RFC_OK;
  return RFC_EXTERNAL_FAILURE;
}
/* TID_rollback für tRFC                                 */
RFC_RC SAP_API RfcOnRollbackTransaction(
        RFC_CONNECTION_HANDLE rfcHandle, SAP_UC const *tid)
{
```

```
  TID_RC tid_rc;
  tid_rc = update_TID(tid, ROLLBACK, tid_file, data_file);
  if (tid_rc == TID_OK)
    return RFC_OK;
  return RFC_EXTERNAL_FAILURE;
}
```

Listing 4.22 Funktionen für das Transaktions-Handling eines tRFC-Servers

```
/* Transaktions-Handler installieren                    */
rc = RfcInstallTransactionHandlers(
       NULL,
       RfcOnCheckTransaction,
       RfcOnCommitTransaction,
       RfcOnRollbackTransaction,
       RfcOnConfirmTransaction,
       &errInf);
if(rc != RFC_OK)errorHandling(...);
```

Listing 4.23 Installation des TID-Managements

Die Funktion RfcOnCheckTransaction ruft die TID-Dateimanagement-Funktion check_TID auf. Diese Funktion öffnet die TID-Datei und sucht die übergebene TID. Wird die TID gefunden (Returncode TID_FOUND), wurden Daten für diese TID vom Server schon einmal verarbeitet. Der Server muss in diesem Fall den Wert »RFC_EXECUTED« zurückgeben. Wird die TID nicht gefunden (Returncode TID_OK), wurde diese TID vom Server noch nicht verarbeitet, und er gibt den Returncode RFC_OK zurück.

Commit

Gibt die Funktion RfcOnCheckTransaction den Wert »RFC_OK« zurück, ruft die RFC-Bibliothek als Nächstes die angeforderten Funktionen auf. Geben alle aufgerufenen Funktionen die Meldung »RFC_OK« zurück, ruft die RFC-Bibliothek zum Abschluss der Transaktion RfcOnCommitTransaction auf. In unserer Implementierung ändert RfcOnCommitTransaction den Zustand der TID in der TID-Datei von CREATED auf EXECUTED. Dazu ruft sie die TID-Management-Funktion update_TID auf.

Rollback

Gibt eine der implementierenden Funktionen einen Returncode ungleich RFC_OK zurück, ruft die RFC-Bibliothek RfcOnRollback-Transaction auf. Der Server muss dort die in der Funktion RfcOnCheckTransaction begonnene lokale Transaktion zurückrollen, also alle vorgenommenen Änderungen rückgängig machen. In unserer einfachen Implementierung ändert der Server den Zustand der TID in der TID-Management-Datei einfach auf ROLLBACK.

Zuletzt ruft die RFC-Bibliothek die Funktion RfcOnConfirmTrans-action auf. Innerhalb dieser Funktion kann der Server die zwischengespeicherte TID und deren Zustand löschen, um permanenten Speicher freizugeben. In unserer Implementierung setzt der Server den Zustand der TID in der TID-Datei auf CONFIRMED.

TID-Datei initialisieren

Der Server definiert vier Funktionen für das Management der TID-Datei. Beim Start ruft er die Funktion init_TID auf (siehe Listing 4.24), um die TID-Datei zu initialisieren. Diese Funktion öffnet die TID-Datei zum Update. Existiert die TID-Datei nicht, wird sie neu erzeugt. Existiert die TID-Datei, sucht die Funktion in einer while-Schleife nach TIDs im Zustand CREATED. Dieser Zustand wird durch den Zustand ROLLBACK ersetzt. Dies ist für das Funktionieren von check_TID in Listing 4.25 wichtig.

```
/* TID-Datei initialisieren                              */
static void init_TID()
{
  FILE          *fp;
  SAP_UC        *ptr, tbuf[MAXBUFF+1];
  RFC_TID       TransID;
  TID_RC        tid_rc;
  /* TID-Datei zum Update öffnen    */
  fp = fopenU (tid_file, cU("rb+"));
  if (fp == NULL)
  {
    /* neue TID-Datei erzeugen       */
    fp = fopenU (tid_file, cU("ab"));
    if (fp == NULL)
    {
      fprintfU(stderr, cU("init_TID\n")); exit(1);
    }
    memsetU (tbuf, cU('\0'), LINE_SIZE);
    strcpyU (tbuf, cU("***   TID-MANAGEMENT  ***\n"));
    if (fputsU (tbuf, fp) < 0)
    {
      fclose(fp);
      fprintfU(stderr, cU("init_TID\n")); exit(1);
    }
  }
  else
  {
    while ((ptr = fgetsU (tbuf, LINE_SIZE+1, fp)) != NULL)
    {
```

```
        /* CREATED durch ROLLBACK ersetzen */
        if (memcmpU (tbuf+52, cU("CREATED"), 7) == 0)
        {
          memcpyU (TransID,   tbuf+26, 24);
          data_file[0] = 0; TransID[24] = 0;
          tid_rc = update_TID(TransID, ROLLBACK,
                              tid_file, data_file);
          if (tid_rc != TID_OK)
          {
            fprintfU(stderr, cU("init_TID")); exit(1);
          }
        }
      }
    }
    fclose(fp);
    return;
  } /* init_TID */
```

Listing 4.24 Funktion »init_TID«

TID prüfen Die Funktion check_TID (siehe Listing 4.25) sucht in der TID-Datei nach der übergebenen TID. Falls sie die TID findet und ihr Zustand ungleich ROLLBACK (d. h. EXECUTED) ist, gibt sie die Meldung TID_FOUND zurück. In diesem Fall gibt die aufrufende Funktion (RfcOnCheckTransaction in Listing 4.22) den Wert »RFC_EXECUTED« an die RFC-Bibliothek zurück, die daraufhin die angeforderten Funktionen kein weiteres Mal aufruft. Findet check_TID die übergebene TID nicht, hängt sie die TID hinten an die TID-Datei im Zustand CREATED an.

```
/* TID prüfen                                            */
extern TID_RC check_TID(const RFC_TID tid,
                        SAP_UC* tid_file, SAP_UC *datafile)
{
  TID_RC         tidrc;
  TID_STATE      tid_state;
  FILE          *fp;
  SAP_UC        *ptr, tbuf[MAXBUFF+1];
  /* zum Update öffnen                                   */
  fp = fopenU (tid_file, cU("rb+"));
  if (fp == NULL)
    tidrc = TID_ERROR_UPDATE;
  /* TID suchen                                          */
  while ((ptr = fgetsU (tbuf, LINE_SIZE, fp)) != NULL)
```

```
  {
    if ((memcmpU (tbuf+26, tid, 24) == 0) &&
        (memcmpU (tbuf+52, cU("ROLLBACK"), 8) != 0))
      break;
  }
  if (ptr != NULL)
  {
    fclose(fp);
    return TID_FOUND;
  }
  /* neue TID hinten anhängen                          */
  tid_state = CREATED;
  if (write_TID(fp, tid, tid_state, datafile))
    tidrc = TID_ERROR_UPDATE;
  else
    tidrc = TID_OK;
  fclose(fp);
  return tidrc;
}/* check TID */
```

Listing 4.25 Funktion »check_TID«

TID-Zustand ändern

Die TID-Management-Funktion `update_TID` (siehe Listing 4.26) sucht in der TID-Datei nach der angegebenen TID, die nicht im Zustand `ROLLBACK` ist. Wenn sie die TID findet, schreibt sie den neuen Zustand der TID in die Datei. Diese Funktion wird von den Funktionen `init_TID`, `RfcOnCommitTransaction`, `RfcOnRollbackTransaction` und `RfcOnConfirmTransaction` verwendet.

```
/* TID-Status in TID-Datei ändern                      */
extern TID_RC update_TID(const RFC_TID tid,
   TID_STATE tid_state, SAP_UC *tid_file, SAP_UC * datafile)
{
  TID_RC          tidrc;
  long            offset = 0;
  FILE           *fp;
  SAP_UC         *ptr, tbuf[MAXBUFF+1];
  /* TID-Datei zum Update öffnen                       */
  fp = fopenU (tid_file, cU("rb+"));
  if (fp == NULL)
    return TID_ERROR_UPDATE;
  /* TID suchen                                        */
  while ((ptr = fgetsU (tbuf, LINE_SIZE+1, fp)) != NULL)
  {
    if ((memcmpU (tbuf+26, tid, 24) == 0) &&
```

```
        (memcmpU (tbuf+52, cU("ROLLBACK"), 8) != 0))
      break;
    offset = offset + strlenU (tbuf);
  }
  /* neuen Status schreiben                              */
  if ((ptr != NULL) &&
      (fseek(fp, offset, SEEK_SET) == 0) &&
      (write_TID(fp, tid, tid_state, datafile) == 0))
    tidrc = TID_OK;
  else
    tidrc = TID_ERROR_UPDATE;
  fclose(fp);
  return tidrc;
} /* update_TID */
```

Listing 4.26 Funktion »update_TID«

Die TID-Management-Funktion write_TID, die von check_TID und update_TID verwendet wird, sieht genauso aus wie beim tRFC-Client in Listing 4.14 (siehe Abschnitt 4.3.2, »Transaktionaler RFC-Client«).

Funktion »z_ifp_order_create«

Dies waren die Funktionen zum Management der TIDs auf dem Server. Die eigentliche Funktionalität zum Schreiben von Bestellungen implementiert der Server in der Funktion z_ifp_order_create (siehe Listing 4.27). Diese definiert zunächst lokale Variablen, unter anderem strid für die Rückgabe der neu erzeugten Bestellnummer und ein Handle für die Importstruktur und die Importtabelle. Sofern der Importparameter IM_TESTRUN ungleich X ist, wird zuerst der Bestellkopf aus der Importstruktur IM_ORDERHEADER in die Datei geschrieben, danach die Bestellpositionen aus der Tabelle TA_ORDERPOS.

```
RFC_RC SAP_API z_ifp_order_create(
         RFC_CONNECTION_HANDLE rfcConn,
         RFC_FUNCTION_HANDLE rfcFunc,
         RFC_ERROR_INFO* errInf)
{
  RFC_RC rc = RFC_OK;
  RFC_TABLE_HANDLE rfcTab;
  RFC_STRUCTURE_HANDLE rfcStruct;
  SAP_UC testrun;
  SAP_UC tbuf[MAXBUFF+1];
  FILE *fp;
  static int id = 0;
  SAP_UC strid[11];
```

```
unsigned int count;
unsigned int i;
RfcGetChars(rfcFunc,cU("IM_TESTRUN"),&testrun,1,errInf);
if(testrun == cU('X'))
  return rc;
RfcGetStructure(rfcFunc, cU("IM_ORDERHEADER"),
                &rfcStruct, errInf);
RfcGetTable(rfcFunc, cU("TA_ORDERPOS"), &rfcTab, errInf);
/* Bestellnummer hochzählen und setzen                  */
id++;
sprintfU(strid,11,cU("%010u"),id);
RfcSetChars(rfcFunc, cU("EX_ORDERID"), strid, 10, errInf);
/* Bestellkopf aus Importparameter wegschreiben         */
fp = fopenU (data_file, cU("a"));
RfcGetNum(rfcStruct, cU("MANDT"), tbuf, 3, errInf);
RfcGetNum(rfcStruct, cU("ORDERID"), tbuf+3, 10, errInf);
RfcGetChars(rfcStruct, cU("TYPE"), tbuf+13, 2, errInf);
RfcGetNum(rfcStruct, cU("REFID"), tbuf+15, 10, errInf);
RfcGetChars(rfcStruct, cU("BUYER"), tbuf+25, 50, errInf);
RfcGetChars(rfcStruct, cU("SELLER"), tbuf+75,50, errInf);
RfcGetDate(rfcStruct, cU("ORDERDATE"), tbuf+125, errInf);
memcpyU(tbuf+3,strid,10);
tbuf[LINE_SIZE_ORDER] = cU('\n');
if(fwriteU(tbuf,1,LINE_SIZE_ORDER+1,fp)<LINE_SIZE_ORDER+1)
    rc = RFC_ABAP_EXCEPTION;
/* Bestellpositionen aus Tabellenparameter wegschreiben */
RfcGetRowCount(rfcTab, &count, errInf);
RfcMoveToFirstRow(rfcTab, errInf);
for(i=0;i<count;i++)
{
  rfcStruct = RfcGetCurrentRow(rfcTab, errInf);
  RfcGetNum(rfcStruct, cU("MANDT"),tbuf,3,errInf);
  RfcGetNum(rfcStruct, cU("ORDERID"),tbuf+3,10,errInf);
  RfcGetNum(rfcStruct, cU("ORDERPOS"),tbuf+13,5,errInf);
  RfcGetChars(rfcStruct, cU("MATID"),tbuf+18,20,errInf);
  RfcGetChars(rfcStruct, cU("MATTEXT"),tbuf+38,40,errInf);
  RfcGetChars(rfcStruct,cU("ORDERCOUNT"),tbuf+78,
              10,errInf);
  RfcGetChars(rfcStruct, cU("PRICE"),tbuf+88,7,errInf);
  RfcGetChars(rfcStruct, cU("CURRENCY"),tbuf+95,5,errInf);
  tbuf[LINE_SIZE_ORDERPOS] = cU('\n');
  fwriteU (tbuf, 1, LINE_SIZE_ORDERPOS+1, fp);
  RfcMoveToNextRow(rfcTab, errInf);
```

```
  }
  fclose(fp);
  return rc;
}
```

Listing 4.27 Funktion »z_ifp_order_create«

Erzeugen einer Bestellung

Damit ist der tRFC-Server komplett. Um ihn zu testen, können Sie das ABAP-Programm `Z_IFP_ORDER_CREATE` aus Listing 4.7 (siehe Abschnitt 3.2, »Transaktionaler RFC«) verwenden. Dabei dürfen Sie nicht vergessen, mit Transaktion SM59 eine passende Destination für Ihren tRFC-Server zu erstellen, die Sie dann im Programm `Z_IFP_ORDER_CREATE` im Selektionsbild angeben.

Kapitel 5
Remote Function Call mit Java

In diesem Kapitel lernen Sie unterschiedliche Möglichkeiten kennen, um RFC-Programme in Java zu schreiben. Wir zeigen Ihnen, wie Sie den SAP Java Connector verwenden, um mit Ihrer On-Premise-SAP-Infrastruktur zu kommunizieren.

In Java gibt es unterschiedliche (und unterschiedlich komfortable) Möglichkeiten, um RFC-Programme zu realisieren. Als grundlegende Möglichkeit bietet SAP den SAP Java Connector an, mit dem Sie auch außerhalb von SAP-Servern und ohne SAP-Entwicklungsumgebung programmieren können (siehe Abschnitt 5.1, »SAP Java Connector«). In Abschnitt 5.2, »RFC-Server«, erklären wir Ihnen die Realisierung von RFC-Servern und zeigen Ihnen, wie man einen eigenen RFC-Server implementiert.

5.1 SAP Java Connector

Der SAP Java Connector (JCo) bildet die Schnittstelle zwischen einem Java-basierten System und dem ABAP-Backend. Der Java Connector bietet beide Richtungen der Kommunikation an: Es ist möglich, sowohl von Java-Anwendungen auf ABAP-Funktionen zuzugreifen als auch aus ABAP-Applikationen auf Java-Anwendungen. Wir verwenden für die in diesem Kapitel gezeigten Beispiel die freie Entwicklungsumgebung Eclipse.

5.1.1 Installation

Die Installation des SAP Java Connectors erfolgt in zwei Schritten:

1. Im ersten Schritt laden Sie den SAP Java Connector vom SAP Support Portal herunter. Nachdem Sie sich unter *https://support.sap.com/en/product/connectors.html* mit Ihrer SAP-Universal ID angemeldet haben, navigieren Sie über **SAP Java Connector • More about SAP Java Connector** zu den Produktdetails des SAP Java Connectors. Wählen Sie im Bereich **Download** die passende Version für Ihr Windows-Betriebssystem aus. Nach dem Download entpacken Sie die heruntergeladene Datei. Auf Ihrer Festplatte befindet sich nun eine Datei mit dem Namen **sapjco3-**

nitel-3.0.<version>. Entpacken Sie diese Datei ebenfalls. Es befinden sich dann die Dateien **sapjco3.jar** und **sapjco3.dll** auf Ihrer Festplatte. Neben diesen beiden Laufzeitdateien beinhaltet die ZIP-Datei zusätzlich die JCo-Dokumentation im Javadoc-Format für den Java Connector.

2. Im zweiten Schritt der Installation fügen Sie die Datei **sapjco3.jar** in den Klassenpfad Ihrer Entwicklungsumgebung ein. Für einen reibungslosen Ablauf wird empfohlen, sowohl die JAR-Datei als auch die Bibliothek **sapjco3.dll** im selben Verzeichnis bereitzustellen.

Windows- und Unix-Bibliotheken

Falls Sie den SAP Java Connector unter Linux bzw. Unix verwenden möchten, laden Sie die entsprechende Version für Ihr Betriebssystem aus dem SAP Support Portal herunter. Sie werden in der Datei fast die gleichen Dateien vorfinden wie unter Windows; der Unterschied besteht lediglich in der Bibliothek. Das Pendant zu **sapjco3.dll** ist unter Linux die Datei **libsapjco3.so**.

5.1.2 Architektur des SAP Java Connectors

Da nun die Installation erfolgreich abgeschlossen ist, befasst sich dieser Abschnitt mit der Verwendung des SAP Java Connectors.

Java Native Interface

Die Architektur des SAP Java Connectors kann prinzipiell in zwei Bereiche unterteilt werden. Zum einen gibt es den reinen Java-Teil, der Ihnen als Entwickler über eine API eine vereinfachte Kommunikation mit dem Backend ermöglicht. Der andere Teil ist ein nativer Layer. Dieser Layer wird über die *Dynamic Link Library* (DLL) bereitgestellt. Bei der Kommunikation zwischen der Java API und der C-RFC-Bibliothek kommt das *Java Native Interface* (JNI) zum Einsatz.

Die Kommunikation zwischen JNI und der DLL ist für Sie als Entwickler jedoch irrelevant. Dies hat den Vorteil, dass Sie sich völlig auf den Java-Teil konzentrieren können und sich nicht um die Realisierung in C sorgen müssen. In Abbildung 5.1 sehen Sie die Kommunikationsmöglichkeiten und die grundlegende Architektur des SAP Java Connectors.

Der SAP Java Connector unterstützt sowohl die Möglichkeit der eingehenden (inbound-/serverseitigen) als auch die der ausgehenden (outbound-/clientseitigen) Kommunikation. In beide Richtungen werden sowohl die herkömmliche RFC-Kommunikation als auch der transaktionale RFC (tRFC) und der queued RFC (qRFC) unterstützt.

Die API ist sehr spartanisch ausgefallen, sodass Sie einige Dinge selbst übernehmen müssen. Dazu gehören z. B. das Zwischenspeichern (Cachen) von Metadaten sowie das Verwalten eindeutiger Verbindungspools.

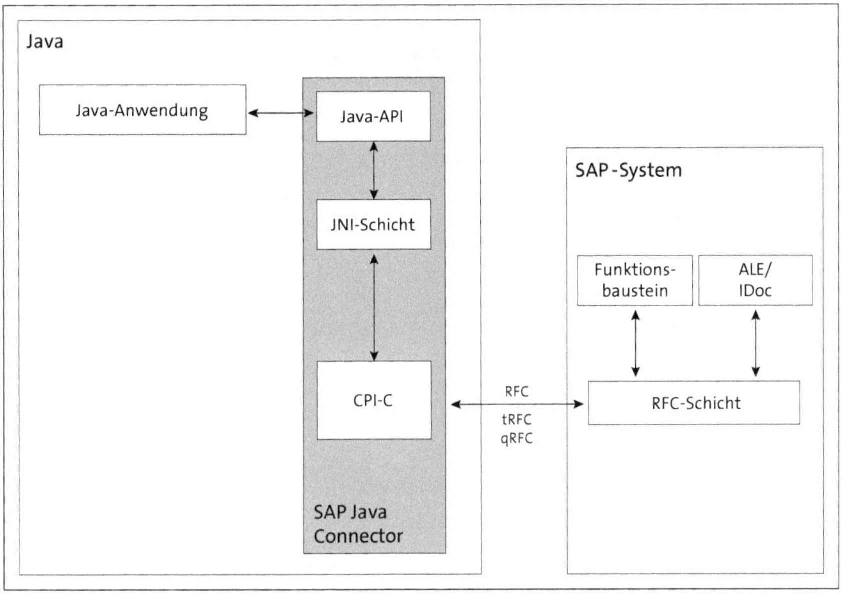

Abbildung 5.1 Architektur des SAP Java Connectors

Noch einmal zurück zur Abarbeitung eines ABAP-Funktionsbausteinaufrufs aus Java: Wie Sie in Abbildung 5.2 sehen können, haben die Entwickler des SAP Java Connectors durchaus darauf geachtet, dass zukünftig möglicherweise weitere Kommunikationsfacetten zwischen dem Java Connector und dem ABAP-Backend denkbar sind.

Middleware-Interface

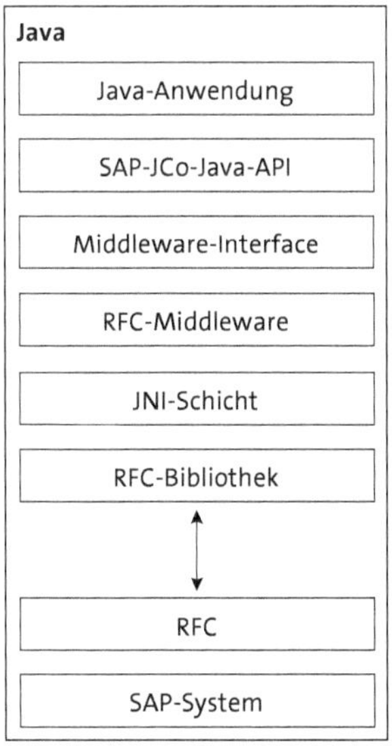

Abbildung 5.2 Kommunikationsbestandteile bei der Verarbeitung eines RFC-Aufrufs

Aus diesem Grund wurde ein Middleware-Interface eingeführt. Dieses Middleware-Interface stellt die Abstraktionsschicht zwischen der JCo-API und der eigentlichen C-RFC-Bibliothek dar. Es ist also durchaus denkbar, dass anstelle des JNI-Aufrufs und der darunterliegenden DLL auch andere Kommunikationsmöglichkeiten verwendet werden könnten, wie z. B. SOAP-Aufrufe. Die Integration anderer Kommunikationsarten anstelle der nativen Kommunikation kann jedoch nur durch SAP selbst erfolgen.

5.1.3 Programmierung mit dem SAP Java Connector

Java-Client

Die Programmierung mit dem SAP Java Connector besteht für einen einfachen synchronen RFC-Aufruf grundsätzlich aus drei Schritten. Abbildung 5.3 stellt die relevanten Klassen aus der JCo-API und deren Kommunikationsschnittstellen in einem Sequenzdiagramm dar. Wie Sie sehen können, wird das Szenario durch die Java-Klasse `JavaClient` initiiert. Der Java-Client kümmert sich im ersten Schritt um den Aufbau der Verbindung zum gewünschten SAP-Backend. Im zweiten Schritt ist es notwendig, einen Funktionsbaustein-Proxy innerhalb des Java-Clients zu erzeugen. Dieser Proxy dient dazu, die Metadaten des gewünschten Funktionsbausteins bereitzustellen. Die Metadaten spielen beim Füllen der Importparameter (Tabellenparameter eingeschlossen) sowie beim Auslesen der Export- und Tabellenparameter eine wichtige Rolle.

Im Folgenden diskutieren wir nun Schritt für Schritt das Sequenzdiagramm aus Abbildung 5.3.

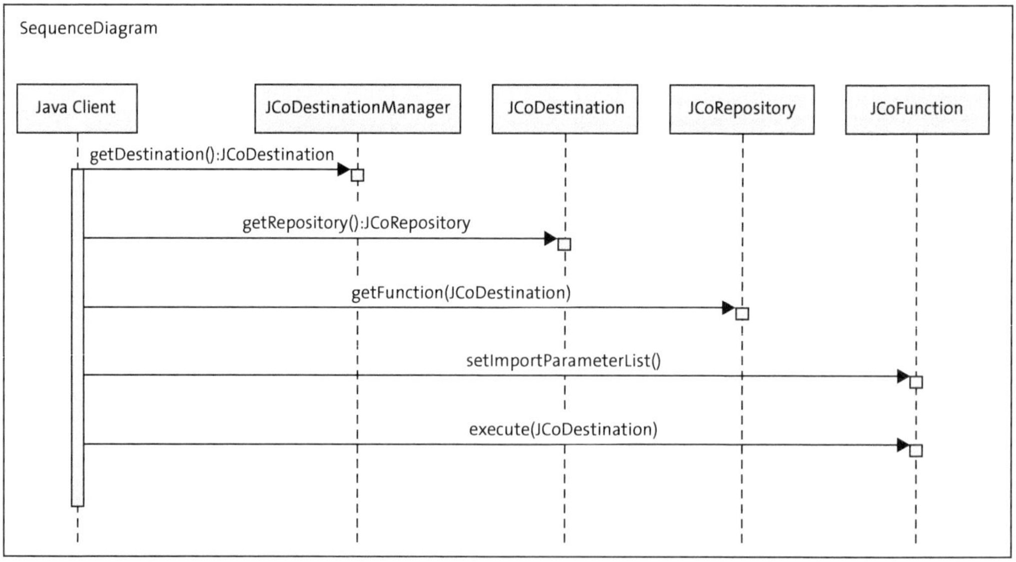

Abbildung 5.3 Abarbeitung eines Funktionsbausteinaufrufs

Verbindungsaufbau

Verbindungsparameter

Um eine Verbindung mit einem ABAP-Backend aufzubauen, wird die Klasse `JCoDestinationManager` verwendet. Die Klasse stellt die Factory-Methode `getDestination` zur Verfügung, mit der Objekte vom Typ `JCoDestination` erzeugt werden. Mittels des erzeugten Objekts werden dem Konnektor die Verbindungsinformationen des Backend-Systems mitgeteilt. Die Methode `getDestination` wird in zwei verschiedenen Ausprägungen bereitgestellt. Die eine Ausprägung erhält lediglich einen String. Dieser enthält den Namen einer Datei, die die Verbindungsparameter umfasst. Die Datei wird durch den SAP Java Connector jeweils im Basisverzeichnis des Projekts gesucht. Die konkrete Angabe eines Verzeichnisses ist standardmäßig nicht möglich, sondern muss über die Implementierung einer eigenen Destinationsinformations-Provider-Klasse realisiert werden. Als Dateiname wird der Bezeichner für die Destination verwendet, als Dateiendung ist zwingend **.jcoDestination** erforderlich. Listing 5.1 zeigt die Erzeugung einer `JCoDestination`-Instanz.

```
public static JCoDestination getJCoDestination(
  String destinationName) throws JCoException {
  JCoDestination lclJCoDestination =
    JCoDestinationManager.getDestination(destinationName);
  return lclJCoDestination;
}
```

Listing 5.1 Erzeugen eines »JCoDestination«-Objekts

Der Aufbau der Property-Datei folgt den bekannten Regeln, die die Klasse `java.util.Property` definiert. Dabei müssen Sie nicht alle Schlüssel der Eigenschaften auswendig kennen. Die Eigenschaften, die vom SAP Java Connector erwartet werden, definiert das Interface `DestinationDataProvider` als Konstanten. Listing 5.2 stellt den Aufbau einer einfachen Konfiguration dar. Die Eigenschaften führen alle das Präfix `jco.client` und sind selbsterklärend.

```
jco.client.client=001
jco.client.user=men
jco.client.passwd=passwort
jco.client.lang=de
jco.client.sysnr=01
jco.client.ashost=192.168.126.128
jco.client.r3name=DEV
```

Listing 5.2 Verbindungsdefinition der Destination »MYDESTINATION.jcoDestination«

Bereitstellen eigener Destination-Provider

In vielen Fällen ist es jedoch nicht sinnvoll und schon gar nicht möglich, Verbindungsdaten unflexibel bei den Binärdateien von Java abzulegen. Im Normalfall möchten Sie über den Ablageort der Verbindungsparameter flexibel bestimmen. Zu diesem Zweck wurde das Interface `DestinationDataProvider` eingeführt. Sollten Sie eine andere Art der Konfiguration Ihrer JCo-Verbindungsdaten wünschen, implementieren Sie einfach dieses Interface. Das Interface definiert die drei Methoden `getDestinationProperties`, `supportEvents` und `setDestinationDataEventListener`.

Session-Management

Zusätzlich zur Methode `getDestination` in der Ausprägung mit nur einem String, der nur der Destinationsbezeichner übergeben wird, wird noch eine weitere Ausprägung angeboten. Diese erhält neben dem Bezeichner der Destination einen zusätzlichen Parameter, den die Java-Dokumentation mit dem Namen `scopeType` beschreibt. Dieser Parameter wird nicht zwingend ausgewertet. Er wird nur dann verarbeitet, wenn eine darunterliegende Infrastruktur für die Verwaltung der Sitzungen angeboten wird. Die Nutzung des Parameters `scopeType` wird über eine Implementierung des Interface `SessionReferenceProvider` verarbeitet. Sie können demnach durchaus ein eigenes Session-Management in Ihrer JCo-basierten Anwendung anbieten. Zur Registrierung Ihrer Implementierung verwenden Sie die Methode `registerSessionReferenceProvider` der Klasse `Environment`. Einfach ausgedrückt, werden über den Parameter `scopeType` Teile der laufenden Java-seitigen Transaktion in kleinere Einheiten unterteilt. Die Nutzung dieser Funktionalität setzt voraus, dass die Infrastruktur eine entsprechende Unterstützung liefert.

Klasse »JCoContext« für zustandsbehaftete Aufrufe

Häufig ist es notwendig, dass Aufrufe mehrerer Funktionsbausteine in einer Transaktionsklammer ausgeführt werden. Der SAP Java Connector bietet dafür die Klasse `JCoContext` an. Zustandsbehaftete Aufrufe sind dadurch gekennzeichnet, dass für die Kommunikation mit dem angegebenen Backend dieselbe Verbindung verwendet wird. Sie müssen jedoch explizit die Kommunikation als zustandsbehaftet markieren. Zu diesem Zweck müssen zum Start der Kommunikation die statische Methode `begin` der Klasse `JCoContext` und zum Abschluss der Kommunikation explizit die Methode `end` aufgerufen werden.

Verbindungstypen für die Kommunikation mit dem Backend

Gepoolte vs. direkte Verbindung

Für den Verbindungsaufbau werden zwei verschiedene Verbindungstypen angeboten. Zum einen ist es möglich, eine sogenannte *direkte Verbindung* aufzubauen, zum anderen können *gepoolte Verbindungen* verwendet werden. Gepoolte Verbindungen haben den Vorteil, dass Verbindungsobjekte vor der Nutzung nicht erst erzeugt werden müssen, sondern aus einem Pool bezogen werden können. Der Nachteil von gepoolten Verbindungen ist allerdings, dass alle Verbindungen mit demselben Benutzer aufgebaut werden. In vielen Systemen werden beide Verbindungsarten verwendet.

Bei einem Katalogsystem etwa, bei dem Kunden Artikel betrachten und kaufen möchten, wird das Laden der Artikelstammdaten aus dem ABAP-Backend über gepoolte Verbindungen durchgeführt, das Absetzen einer Bestellung (Verbuchen der Bestellung im SAP-System) dagegen über eine direkte Verbindung. Somit ist klar ersichtlich, welcher Kunde wann welche Bestellung gesendet hat. Gepoolte Verbindungen werden analog zu direkten Verbindungen über Destinationsdateien erzeugt, wobei die Parameter zusätzlich zu den herkömmlichen Verbindungsinformationen auch Informationen über den Pool beinhalten. In Listing 5.3 fügen wir der in Listing 5.2 eingeführten Konfigurationsdatei drei Eigenschaften hinzu:


```
jco.destination.peak_limit=10
jco.destination.pool_capacity=20
jco.destination.max_get_client_time=100
```

Listing 5.3 Konfigurationsparameter eines Verbindungspools

Die Eigenschaft `peak_limit` legt fest, wie viele Verbindungen für die Destination gleichzeitig aktiv verwendet werden können. Der zweite Parameter `pool_capacity` definiert, wie groß der Pool ist, und `max_get_client_time` gibt an, wie viele Millisekunden der SAP Java Connector warten soll, bis ein Timeout gesendet wird, wenn bereits alle Verbindungen im Pool verwendet werden. Die Nutzung einer gepoolten Destination innerhalb einer Anwendung funktioniert analog zur Programmierung mit direkten Verbindungen.

Factory-Klasse »JCo«

Zentrale Klasse

Neben der reinen Verarbeitung der Daten aus einem SAP-System sind natürlich auch Verwaltungsaufgaben von immenser Bedeutung. Die zentrale Klasse für die Nutzung dieser Funktionen ist die Klasse `JCo`. Sie ist als abstrakte Klasse implementiert und stellt lediglich statische Klassenmethoden zur Verfügung.

Über die bereitgestellten Methoden können für die Java-Connector-Infrastruktur eigene Monitoring-Werkzeuge implementiert und in eigene Anwendungen integriert werden. Genau das werden wir für die Beispielanwendung im Folgenden tun. Im Verlauf dieses Kapitels werden wir noch häufiger auf die Verwendung der `JCo`-Klasse zu sprechen kommen. Fürs

Erste sollen Sie eine Möglichkeit implementieren, um die Konfiguration einer Destination abzufragen.

Monitoring der Destinationen

Dazu implementieren Sie eine Managementklasse, die für alle verwendeten Destinationen die entsprechenden Informationen abruft und zur Verfügung stellt. Für die Arbeit mit Destinationen kann die Klasse `JCoDestinationMonitor` verwendet werden. Sie erhalten eine Referenz auf eine Instanz dieser Klasse durch die Angabe des Destinationsnamens. Die Klasse selbst bietet alle notwendigen Informationen einer Destination an, die Sie benötigen, um zur Laufzeit den Zustand zu einem Backend abzufragen. Listing 5.4 stellt dar, wie diese Informationen über den Aufruf verschiedener Getter-Methoden abgefragt werden können.

```
public void showCurrentConnectionData(String destination) {
  JCoDestinationMonitor destinationMonitor =
    getDestinationMonitor(destination);
  long lastActivity =
    destinationMonitor.getLastActivityTimestamp();
  Date lastActivityAsDate = new Date(lastActivity);
  int maxUsedCount = destinationMonitor.getMaxUsedCount();
  long peakLimit = destinationMonitor.getPeakLimit();
  int poolCapacity = destinationMonitor.getPoolCapacity();
  int pooledConnectionCount =
    destinationMonitor.getPooledConnectionCount();
  int usedConnectionCount =
    destinationMonitor.getUsedConnectionCount();
  //TODO Daten ausgeben;
}
```

Listing 5.4 Abfrage der aktuellen Poolinformationen einer Destination

Information über Poolobjekte

Neben den reinen Poolinformationen könnten auch Informationen über die konkreten Verbindungsobjekte innerhalb des Pools interessant sein. Diese Informationen können Sie über die `JCoConnectionData`-Klasse auslesen. Der SAP Java Connector verwaltet für jede Verbindung zum Backend eine Instanz dieses Typs. Die Instanzen werden über den `DestinationMonitor` verwaltet und können über diesen erfragt werden. Sie erhalten die Liste der aktuellen Verbindungsinformationsinstanzen über den Aufruf der Methode `getConnectionsData`. Diese Methode liefert eine Instanz der Klasse `java.util.List` zurück.

Listing 5.5 stellt das Auslesen dieser Daten dar. Wie Sie sehen, wird mit einem simplen Iterator die Liste wiederholt und jede Instanz einzeln verarbeitet.

```
public void showDestinationData(String destination) {
  JCoDestinationMonitor destinationMonitor =
    JCo.getDestinationMonitor(destination);
  List<?> connectionData =
    destinationMonitor.getConnectionsData();
  for (Iterator iterator = connectionData.iterator();
              iterator.hasNext();) {
    JCoConnectionData currentConnectionData =
      JCoConnectionData) iterator.next();
    //TODO: Daten auslesen/ausgeben
  }
}
```

Listing 5.5 Auflisten der übergebenen Destinationsinformationen

Ausführung der Klasse »JCoFunction«

sRFC

Nachdem die Verbindung mit dem Backend erfolgreich hergestellt worden ist, kann mit dem eigentlichen synchronen Aufruf des Funktionsbausteins begonnen werden. Dazu verwenden Sie die beiden in Kapitel 3, »Remote Function Call mit ABAP«, bereits vorgestellten Funktionsbausteine `Z_IFP_ORDER_CREATE` und `Z_IFP_ORDER_GETDETAIL`.

Der Aufruf eines Funktionsbausteins wird in den folgenden Schritten abgearbeitet:

- Erstellen eines Funktionsstellvertreter-Objekts für den aufzurufenden Funktionsbaustein
- Füllen der Importparameterliste
- Aufruf des Funktionsbausteins und Auswerten der Rückgabewerte

Funktionsstellvertreter-Objekt

Im ersten Schritt ist es notwendig, einen Stellvertreter (Proxy) für den im ABAP-Stack implementierten remotefähigen Funktionsbaustein zu erzeugen. Da der SAP Java Connector eine rein generische API darstellt und keinerlei Unterstützung mittels eines Codegenerators bietet, definiert die JCo-API dafür eine generische Klasse. Die Klasse trägt den Namen `JCoFunction`. Objekte dieses Typs stellen die ABAP-Funktion auf der Java-Seite dar. Somit müssen die Metadaten des Funktionsbausteins, wie sie im ABAP Dictionary definiert sind, bekannt sein. Dies geschieht über ein Objekt der Klasse `JCoRepository`. Wie Listing 5.6 zeigt, dient ein Objekt der Klasse `JCoDestination` als Factory für Repository-Objekte und diese wiederum als Factory für die Erzeugung von `JCoFunction`-Objekten.

```
private JCoFunction createFunction(
  JCoDestination destination,
  String functionName) throws JCoException {

  JCoFunction function =
    destination.getRepository().getFunction(functionName);
Optional<JCoFunction> isFunction = Optional.ofNullable(function);
//    if (function == null)
if(!isFunction.isPresent()){
      throw new RuntimeException(functionName +
        " not defined!");
    else
      return function;
}
```

Listing 5.6 Erzeugen eines Funktionsbaustein-Stellvertreters

Verwendung von »JCoParameterList«

Der zweite Schritt besteht darin, die Importparameterliste des Funktionsbausteins zu füllen. Der Baustein Z_IFP_ORDER_CREATE besitzt in seinen Importparametern die Felder IM_ORDERHEADER als Struktur sowie IM_TESTRUN und IM_COMMIT als skalare Parameter. Darüber hinaus definiert der Baustein einen Tabellenparameter mit dem Namen TA_ORDERS. Wie bereits angesprochen, stellt das JCoFunction-Objekt die Java-seitige Repräsentation des Funktionsbausteins dar, sodass auch über dieses Objekt sowohl der Zugriff auf die Import- als auch auf die Tabellenparameter gewährleistet ist.

Sie erhalten eine Referenz auf die Importparameterliste durch den Aufruf der Methode getImportParameterList. Der Rückgabewert der Methode ist vom Typ JCoParameterList und vom Basis-Interface JCoRecord abgeleitet. Die Basisklasse stellt eine Vielzahl von Methoden mit dem Namen setValue für das Füllen der Importparameter bereit. Die Parameter der Methode folgen der üblichen Java-Konvention für das Setzen von Namen-/Wertpaaren, sodass der erste Parameter der Name des Felds ist und dem zweiten Parameter der typisierte Wert übergeben wird.

ABAP- vs. Java-Datentypen

Dabei müssen Sie darauf achten, dass die korrekten Datentypen verwendet werden, um mögliche Laufzeitfehler zu vermeiden. Tabelle 5.1 gibt Ihnen eine Übersicht über das Mapping zwischen ABAP- und Java-Datentypen. Wie Sie der Tabelle entnehmen können, wird zum Beispiel ein ABAP-Feld vom Datentyp C als String-Datentyp an die setValue-Methode übergeben.

ABAP	Kurzbeschreibung	Java	JCo-Metadaten
B	1-Byte-Integer	Int	TYPE_INT1
S	2-Byte-Integer	Int	TYPE_INT2
L	4-Byte-Integer	Int	TYPE_INT
C	Character	String	TYPE_CHAR
N	numerisches Zeichen	String	TYPE_NUM
P	binär codiertes Dezimalzeichen	BigDecimal	TYPE_BCD
D	Datum	Date	TYPE_DATE
T	Zeit	Date	TYPE_TIME
F	Fließkommazahl	Double	TYPE_FLOAT
X	reine Daten	Byte[]	TYPE_BYTE
G	String mit variabler Länge	String	TYPE_STRING
Y	reine Daten	Byte[]	TYPE_XSTRING

Tabelle 5.1 Mapping der ABAP-Datentypen auf Java-Datentypen

[«]

Feldüberlauf

Bitte beachten Sie, dass bei der Übergabe von Zeichenketten, die die definierte Länge überschreiten, die überzähligen Zeichen des übergebenen Strings abgeschnitten werden. Es erfolgt keine Rückmeldung durch das System. Es ist daher empfehlenswert, dass die Anwendung dies vor dem Aufruf des im eigenen Java-Code entsprechend prüft.

Verarbeiten von komplexen Datentypen

Nachdem die skalaren Parameter gesetzt worden sind, können Strukturen und Tabellen an die Importparameter übergeben werden. Strukturen und Tabellen werden über die im Interface `JCoRecord` definierten Methoden `getStructure` bzw. `getTable` aus der Importparameterliste bzw. Tabellenparameterliste besorgt. Beide Methoden gibt es in zwei Ausprägungen. Einerseits ist es möglich, über den Index das Feld anzusprechen, andererseits kann auch der Feldbezeichner verwendet werden. Für den Funktionsbaustein `Z_IFP_ORDER_CREATE` bedeutet dies, dass der Methode `getStructure` der Wert »IM_ORDERHEADER« übergeben wird. Die in Listing 5.7 dargestellte Methode zeigt, wie die Felder der Struktur mittels der Methode `createOrderHeaderStructure` gefüllt werden.

```
private void createOrderHeaderStructure(
  Orderheader orheader,
  JCoStructure orderheader) {
  orderheader.setValue(IFieldNames.ZIFPORDER_ORDERID,
    orheader.getOrderid());
  orderheader.setValue(IFieldNames.ZIFPORDER_BUYER,
     orheader.getBuyer());
  orderheader.setValue(IFieldNames.ZIFPORDER_SELLER,
    orheader.getSeller());
  orderheader.setValue(IFieldNames.ZIFPORDER_MANDT,
    orheader.getClient());
  orderheader.setValue(IFieldNames.ZIFPORDER_REFID,
    orheader.getRefid());

  orderheader.setValue(IFieldNames.ZIFPORDER_TYPE,
    orheader.getType());
  }
```

Listing 5.7 Füllen der Struktur »IM_ORDERHEADER«

[»]

Domänen von ABAP-Datentypen

Domänen von ABAP-Datentypen sind nicht dazu geeignet, die Wertausprägung eines JCo-Felds einzuschränken. Wird einem domänenbehafteten Feld ein Wert zugewiesen, der außerhalb der Domäne liegt, wird der Funktionsbaustein dennoch mit diesem Wert ausgeführt.

Arbeiten mit der Klasse »JCoTable«

Im Anschluss kann der Tabellenparameter `TA_ORDERPOS` gesetzt werden. Für diesen Zweck implementieren Sie eine Hilfsmethode (siehe Listing 5.8). Die Methode erhält als Aufrufparameter eine Liste von Objekten des selbst definierten Typs `Orderpos` und zusätzlich das ausgelesene Tabellenparameterobjekt. Die Klasse `JCoTable` bietet für das Hinzufügen einer neuen Zeile die Methode `appendRow` an. Nachdem eine neue Zeile hinzugefügt worden ist, können die Felder der neuen Zeile mittels `setValue` mit Werten belegt werden. Der Methode `setValue` werden dabei zum einen der Feldbezeichner und zum anderen der zu setzende Wert als Argumente übergeben. Das selbst definierte Interface `IFieldNames` dient als zentraler Platz für die Definition der String-Konstanten für die Feldbezeichner.

```
private void createOrderPosTbl(
  List<Orderpos> orderposList, JCoTable orderTbl) {
  for (Orderpos orderPos : orderposList) {
    orderTbl.appendRow();
```

```
    orderTbl.setValue(IFieldNames.TA_ORDERPOS_MANDT,
      orderPos.getClient());
    orderTbl.setValue(IFieldNames.TA_ORDERPOS_ORDERID,
      orderPos.getOrderid());
    orderTbl.setValue(IFieldNames.TA_ORDERPOS_ORDERPOS,
      orderPos.getOrderpos());
    orderTbl.setValue(IFieldNames.TA_ORDERPOS_MATID,
      orderPos.getMaterialid());
    orderTbl.setValue(IFieldNames.TA_ORDERPOS_MATTEXT,
      orderPos.getMaterialtext());
    orderTbl.setValue(IFieldNames.TA_ORDERPOS_ORDERCOUNT,
      orderPos.getOrdercount());
    orderTbl.setValue(IFieldNames.TA_ORDERPOS_PRICE,
      orderPos.getPrice());
    orderTbl.setValue(IFieldNames.TA_ORDERPOS_CURRENCY,
      orderPos.getCurrency());
  }
}
```


Listing 5.8 Befüllen des Tabellenparameters »TA_ORDERPOS«

Rückgabewerte des Funktionsbausteins

Nachdem alle Aufrufparameter gesetzt worden sind, kann die Funktion ausgeführt werden. Die Klasse `JCoFunction` bietet für das Ausführen eines sRFC-Aufrufs die Methode `execute` an. Diese Methode erhält als Parameter die Destination, auf der die Funktion ausgeführt werden soll. Nachdem die Funktion erfolgreich auf dem ABAP-Stack verarbeitet worden ist, kann über die Methode `getExportParameterList` auf die Rückgabe des Funktionsbausteins reagiert werden. Für das Auslesen der Werte aus einer Parameterliste bietet das Interface `JCoRecord` für jeden unterstützten Datentyp zwei Ausprägungen einer Getter-Methode an. Es gibt jeweils eine Methode für das Auslesen mittels des Feldindex sowie den Namen des Felds als Aufrufparameter. Dadurch ist es beim Iterieren über alle Felder möglich, einfach über den Feldindex zu arbeiten, wobei beim konkreten Zugriff auf ein spezielles Feld der Feldname verwendet werden kann. Listing 5.9 zeigt den Aufruf der Funktion `Z_IFP_ORDER_CREATE` und die Verarbeitung des skalaren Exportparameters `EX_ORDERID`.

```
try {
  function.execute(destination);
  int orderID = function.getExportParameterList().getInt(
    IFieldNames.EX_ORDERID);
  System.out.println("Bestellung wurde mit der ID " +
    orderID + " erstellt");
```

```
  order.getOrderheader().setOrderid(orderID);
} catch (AbapException e) {
  System.out.println(e.toString());
  return;
}
```

Listing 5.9 Ausführen der Funktion »Z_IFP_ORDER_CREATE«

5.1.4 Verarbeitung von Tabellen und Strukturen

Komplexe Rückgabewerte

Nachdem die Erzeugung einer Bestellung erfolgreich durchgeführt worden ist, lesen Sie im nächsten Schritt die erzeugte Bestellung aus dem ABAP-System aus. Für diesen Zweck wurde der Funktionsbaustein Z_IFP_ORDER_GETDETAIL geschrieben. Sie werden sich dabei weniger um den eigentlichen Aufruf des Funktionsbausteins kümmern als vielmehr um die Verarbeitung der komplexen Rückgabewerte des Funktionsbausteins. Wie bereits zu Beginn des Kapitels beschrieben, definiert der Funktionsbaustein den Exportparameter EX_ORDERHEAD und den Tabellenparameter TA_ORDERPOS.

Analog zum Setzen komplexer Parameter werden komplexe Parameter über die Parameterliste der Funktion zurückgeliefert und über die entsprechende Getter-Methode zur Verfügung gestellt. Für das Abfragen von Strukturen aus der Exportparameterliste bietet das Interface JCoParameterList die Methode getStructure an. Die Methode kann entweder mit dem Index des Felds aufgerufen werden oder mit dem Feldnamen. Nach dem Auslesen des Strukturparameters kann die Struktur weiterverarbeitet werden.

Die in Listing 5.10 dargestellte Methode getOrderHead erhält als Aufrufargument die zu verarbeitende Struktur. Vergleicht man das Interface JCoStructure mit dem Interface JCoTable, sieht man, dass beide das Interface JCoRecord erweitern, sodass das Auslesen der Werte aus der Struktur den gleichen Gesetzmäßigkeiten unterliegt, wie sie bereits bei der Tabellenverarbeitung besprochen wurden. Mittels Getter-Methoden und der Angabe des Felds oder der Angabe des Index kann der Wert typisiert aus der Struktur ausgelesen werden.

```
private Orderheader getOrderHead(JCoStructure orderhead) {
  Orderheader orheader = new Orderheader();
  orheader.setClient(
    orderhead.getInt(IFieldNames.ZIFPORDER_MANDT));
  orheader.setOrderid(
    orderhead.getInt(IFieldNames.ZIFPORDER_ORDERID));
  orheader.setType(
    orderhead.getString(IFieldNames.ZIFPORDER_TYPE));
```

```
  orheader.setRefid(
    orderhead.getString(IFieldNames.ZIFPORDER_REFID));
  orheader.setBuyer(
    orderhead.getString(IFieldNames.ZIFPORDER_BUYER));
  orheader.setSeller(
    orderhead.getString(IFieldNames.ZIFPORDER_SELLER));
  orheader.setOrderdate(
    orderhead.getDate(IFieldNames.ZIFPORDER_ORDERDATE));
  return orheader;
}
```


Listing 5.10 Verarbeiten der Informationen aus der Struktur »EX_ORDERHEAD«

Iteration über Tabellenzeilen

Listing 5.11 stellt die Methode `getOrderPos` vor. Die Methode zeigt dabei, wie das serverseitige Objektmodell auf das clientseitige Objektmodell gemappt wird. Clientseitig werden Order-Positionen als Instanzen der Klasse `Orderpos` gesehen. Die Methode iteriert über die Tabelle, liest über die Getter-Methoden die Werte aus und übergibt sie den entsprechenden Feldern des Java-Modells. Für die Iteration wird eine einfache `for`-Schleife verwendet. Beachten Sie dabei den Aufruf der Methode `setRow`. Die Methode bewirkt beim Aufruf, dass der Cursor jeweils auf die nächste Zeile der Tabelle gesetzt wird.

```
private List<Orderpos> getOrderPos(JCoTable orderposTbl) {
  List<Orderpos> orderPosList = new ArrayList<Orderpos>();
  for (int i = 0; i < orderposTbl.getNumRows(); i++) {
    Orderpos orderpos = new Orderpos();
    orderposTbl.setRow(i);
    orderpos.setClient(
      orderposTbl.getString(IFieldNames.TA_ORDERPOS_MANDT));
    orderpos.setOrderid(
      orderposTbl.getInt(IFieldNames.TA_ORDERPOS_ORDERID));
    orderpos.setOrderpos(
      orderposTbl.getInt(IFieldNames.TA_ORDERPOS_ORDERPOS));
    orderpos.setMaterialid(
      orderposTbl.getString(IFieldNames.TA_ORDERPOS_MATID));
    orderpos.setMaterialtext(
    orderposTbl.getString(IFieldNames.TA_ORDERPOS_MATTEXT));
    orderpos.setOrdercount(
    orderposTbl.getInt(IFieldNames.TA_ORDERPOS_ORDERCOUNT));
    orderpos.setPrice(
      orderposTbl.getDouble(IFieldNames.TA_ORDERPOS_PRICE));
    orderpos.setCurrency(
```

```
      orderposTbl.getString(
        IFieldNames.TA_ORDERPOS_CURRENCY));
    orderPosList.add(orderpos);
  }
  return orderPosList;
}
```

Listing 5.11 Verarbeiten des Tabellenparameters »TA_ORDERPOS«

Iteratoren Neben der Nutzung einer einfachen `for`-Schleife ist es auch möglich, die Klasse `JCoFieldIterator` zu verwenden oder mittels einer `foreach`-Methode über eine `JCoTable`-Instanz zu iterieren. Listing 5.12 stellt die Nutzung beider Möglichkeiten gegenüber. Welche der beiden Arten verwendet wird, bleibt Ihnen selbst überlassen. Die einzige Entscheidungshilfe könnte die Lesbarkeit des Codes sein, denn aus Performancesicht sind die `while`-Schleife und die `foreach`-Schleife identisch. Wie Sie sehen, wird beim Zugriff auf ein Feld die Klasse `JCoField` verwendet. Die Nutzung dieser Klasse im Vergleich zu einem direkten Aufruf der Getter-Methode hat den Vorteil, dass Sie direkt auf die Metadaten und den Wert eines Felds zugreifen können.

```
private void printTable(JCoTable orderposTbl) {
  JCoFieldIterator fieldIter =
    orderposTbl.getFieldIterator();
  while(fieldIter.hasNextField()) {
    JCoField currentField = fieldIter.nextField();
    // Feldinhalt ausgeben
  }
  for (JCoField currentField : orderposTbl) {
    // Tabelleninhalt ausgeben
  }
}
```

Listing 5.12 Verwendung der Klasse »JCoFieldIterator«

Die eigentliche Ausführung des Funktionsbausteins erfolgt über die Methode `execute` auf der `JCoFunction`-Instanz. Die Methode wird in drei verschiedenen Ausprägungen angeboten. Jede Ausprägung stellt jeweils einen Stellvertreter für die drei Kommunikationsarten zwischen Java und ABAP dar.

[»]

Pflichtparameter

Bitte beachten Sie, dass der SAP Java Connector keine Überprüfung der Pflichtparameter von Funktionsbausteinen durchführt. Falls sichergestellt werden muss, dass Pflichtparameter im Aufruf auch tatsächlich gefüllt sind, müssen die Metadaten des Funktionsbausteins ausgelesen und vom Entwickler selbst geprüft werden.

5.1.5 Transaktionaler RFC

Transaktionale RFC-Kommunikation

Der SAP Java Connector bietet neben dem herkömmlichen synchronen Aufruf eines remotefähigen Funktionsbausteins auch die Möglichkeit, einen transaktionalen RFC durchzuführen. Der Unterschied zum synchronen Aufruf eines Funktionsbausteins ist marginal. Er besteht lediglich in der Verwaltung der Transaktions-IDs auf der Seite der externen Java-Anwendung. Zur Erzeugung der Transaktions-ID, die durch das SAP-System zur Verfügung gestellt wird, wird über die Klasse `JCoDestination` die Methode `createTID` angeboten. Das Ergebnis dieses Methodenaufrufs ist die Transaktions-ID als String-Objekt. Da nun die Transaktions-ID und das `JCoFunction`-Objekt vorliegen, kann die Funktion über ihre `execute`-Methode aufgerufen werden; dabei werden die Destination sowie die zuvor erzeugte Transaktions-ID übergeben. Listing 5.13 zeigt die `main`-Methode der Klasse `TRFCDemo`.

```
public static void main(String[] args) {
  try {
    TRFCDemo tRFCDemo = new TRFCDemo();
    JCoDestination currentDestination =
      ConnectionManager.getJCoDestination(
         ConnectionManager.SINGLECONNECTION);
    String transactionID = currentDestination.createTID();
    List<Order> listOfOrders = OrderFactory.createOrders();
    for (Order order : listOfOrders) {
      tRFCDemo.createorder(
        order, transactionID, currentDestination);
    }
    currentDestination.confirmTID(transactionID);
    TRFCHandlerIF transactionIDHandler =
      TRFCFactory.getTIDRegistration ();
    transactionIDHandler.removeTransactionData(
      transactionID);
    } catch (JCoException e) {
      // Funktion mit Transaktionsnummer aufrufen
    }
}
```

Listing 5.13 Erzeugen einer Liste von Bestellungen über tRFC

Der SAP Java Connector bietet für die Verwaltung von Transaktionsnummern auf der Seite der externen Java-Anwendung keinerlei Möglichkeiten zur Verwaltung der verwendeten Transaktionsnummern an. Sie müssen deshalb selbst dafür sorgen, dass nicht korrekt verarbeitete, transaktionale Funktionsbausteinaufrufe entsprechend wiederholt werden.

Verwalten von Transaktionsnummern

In Listing 5.13 wird für die Speicherung von Transaktions-IDs eine Implementierung des Interface `TRFCHandlerIF` verwendet. Die konkrete Implementierung wird über eine Factory-Klasse realisiert, sodass die Verwendung komplett abstrahiert ist. In den Programmierbeispielen, die Sie zu diesem Buch herunterladen können, finden Sie eine Klasse namens `TRFCHashHandler`, die auf der Klasse `java.util.Hashtable` basiert. Die Hash-Tabelle speichert das `JCoFunction`-Objekt mittels der Transaktionsnummer ab. Wie Listing 5.14 zeigt, wird innerhalb der eigentlichen Verarbeitung des Funktionsbausteins eine Instanz des Interface `TRFCHandlerIF` erzeugt. Durch das Speichern des `JCoFunction`-Objekts in der Hash-Tabelle ist es im Fehlerfall möglich, die Funktion unter der Angabe der Transaktions-ID nochmals auszuführen.

```
private void createorder(Order order, String transactionID,
  JCoDestination destination) {
  TRFCHandlerIF transactionIDHandler =
    TRFCFactory.getTIDRegistration();
  try {
    JCoFunction function =
      ABAPTypeHandler.createFunction(destination,
        IFunctionNames.Z_IFP_ORDER_CREATE);
    transactionIDHandler.storeTransactionData(
      transactionID, function);
    // RFC-Aufruf implementieren
}
```

Listing 5.14 Speicherung der Transaktionsnummern

5.1.6 Queued RFC

qRFC-Kommunikation

Zu guter Letzt betrachten wir in diesem Abschnitt die Nutzung des queued RFC (qRFC). Die Programmierung von qRFCs ist der Entwicklung einer tRFC-basierten Verarbeitung sehr ähnlich. Ein qRFC-Aufruf definiert, wie bereits beschrieben, einen asynchronen Verbuchungsprozess. Dies bedeutet, dass der Aufruf eines Funktionsbausteins als qRFC keine Ergebnisse in einer Exportparameterliste zurückerhält, selbst wenn diese im Funktionsbaustein in einen Exportparameter geschrieben wurden. Zudem werden die Aufrufe, die an eine Queue gebunden werden, so lange in die Queue eingereiht, bis diese aktiviert wird. Im Anschluss an die Aktivierung kann die Queue geleert werden. Die eingereihten Aufträge werden dann abgearbeitet.

Wir zeigen Ihnen die Verwendung des qRFC mit dem SAP Java Connector anhand des bereits bekannten Funktionsbausteins Z_IFP_ORDER_CREATE. Dabei liegt das Hauptaugenmerk auf dem Unterschied zum tRFC. Das Programmierbeispiel in Listing 5.15 stellt diese Unterschiede im Code dar.


```
public void createorder(Order order, String transactionID,
  JCoDestination destination) {
  TRFCHandlerIF transactionIDHandler =
    TRFCFactory.getTIDRegistration();
  try {
    // Funktionsobjekt erzeugen
      transactionIDHandler.storeTransactionData
      (transactionID,function);
    // Parameter füllen
    // Aufruf des Funktionsobjekts
    function.execute(destination,transactionID,"EAIQUEUE");
  } catch (JCoException ex) {
    ex.printStackTrace();
  }
}
```

Listing 5.15 qRFC-Verarbeitung des Funktionsbausteins »Z_IFP_ORDER_CREATE«

Nachdem der Funktionsbaustein verarbeitet worden ist, können Sie über Transaktion SMQ2 die gerade erzeugte Queue EAIQUEUE einsehen. Die Transaktion liefert, wie in Abbildung 5.4 gezeigt, eine Übersicht über die aktuellen Queues.

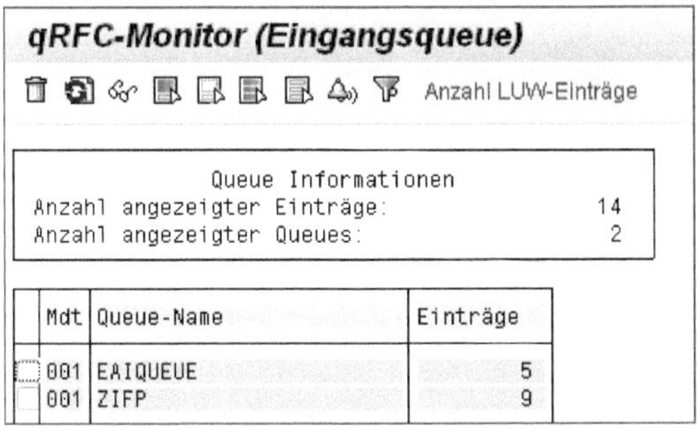

Abbildung 5.4 Übersicht über die im System vorhandenen Queues

Durch einen Doppelklick auf eine Queue können Sie sich deren Inhalt anschauen. Wie Sie Abbildung 5.5 entnehmen können, werden fünf Einträge angezeigt. Es werden also fünf Bestellungen im System erzeugt. Da die Queue noch nicht geschlossen ist, wurden die Funktionsaufrufe noch nicht abgearbeitet. Jeder Eintrag ist einer Transaktions-ID zugeordnet. Mithilfe der [F5]-Taste oder über das Kontextmenü **Bearbeiten • Entsperren** wird die Queue entsperrt, und die Einträge in der Queue werden abgearbeitet.

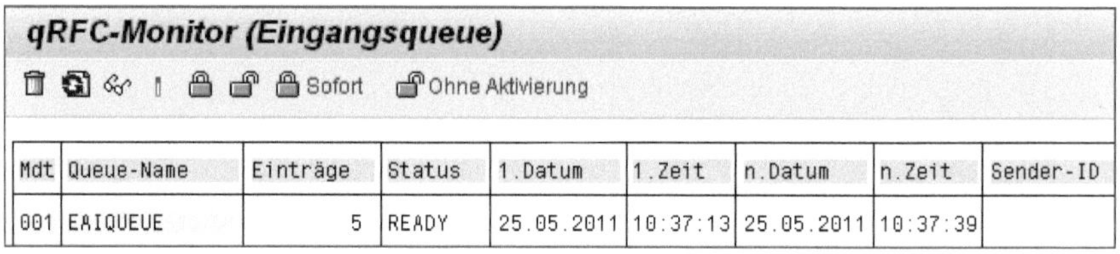

qRFC-Monitor (Eingangsqueue)

Sofort   Ohne Aktivierung

Mdt	Queue-Name	Einträge	Status	1.Datum	1.Zeit	n.Datum	n.Zeit	Sender-ID
001	EAIQUEUE	5	READY	25.05.2011	10:37:13	25.05.2011	10:37:39	

Abbildung 5.5 qRFC-Monitor der Queue »EAIQUEUE«

[»]

TRFC_QIN_ACTIVATE

In unserem Beispiel wird die Queue manuell gestartet. In produktiven Umgebungen ist dies eher selten der Fall. Für einen automatischen Start rufen Sie den Funktionsbaustein TRFC_QIN_ACTIVATE entsprechend in Ihrem Java-Programm auf.

Bei der Ausführung der Funktionsbausteine haben wir bereits die Bedeutung des Repository-Gedankens angesprochen. Repositorys werden für die Bereitstellung der Schnittstellenbeschreibungen der Funktionsbausteine verwendet. Dabei sind sie auch die zentrale Stelle für das Caching dieser Beschreibungen. Metadaten eines Funktionsbausteins werden nicht direkt nach dem Aufruf des Funktionsbausteins gelöscht, sondern so lange gehalten, wie das Repository-Objekt bestehen bleibt. Jedes Repository-Objekt ist genau einer Destination zugeordnet. Im Folgenden beleuchten wir die Arbeit mit Objekten der Klasse `JCoRepository` etwas genauer.

Verwaltung von Repositorys

Für die Arbeit mit den Repository-Objekten erweitern wir die bereits diskutierte Verwaltungsfunktionalität um Aspekte für die Arbeit mit den verwendeten Repositorys. Mögliche Funktionen, die implementiert werden können, sind zum Beispiel das Auslesen der Funktionsbausteinbeschreibungen im Cache oder die Nutzung der Metadaten eines Funktionsbausteins.

Der Zugriff auf die vorhandenen Repositorys kann über mehrere Wege erfolgen. Zum Beispiel kann das Repository über die Destination abgefragt werden, aber auch über die Factory-Klasse `JCo`. In dem hier diskutierten Beispiel werden die Klasse `JCo` und die dort implementierte Methode `getRepository` verwendet. Die Methode erhält als Parameter die ID des Repositorys, das ausgewertet werden soll. Die ID eines Repositorys ist eine Zeichenkette, die automatisch durch den SAP Java Connector erzeugt wird. Die Adressierung eines konkreten Repositorys ist aus diesem Grund eigentlich unmöglich, sodass `getRepository` erst dann aufgerufen werden kann, wenn die ID erfragt wurde. So setzt sich die Arbeit mit dem Repository aus zwei Schritten zusammen: Im ersten Schritt werden die IDs der vorhandenen Repositorys ausgelesen, und im zweiten Schritt wird die Methode `getRepository` aufgerufen.

5.1.7 Metadatenverarbeitung

Neben der reinen Verarbeitung der Daten mittels eines Funktionsbausteins ist die Metadatenbeschreibung der Schnittstelle des Funktionsbausteins für die tägliche Arbeit sehr interessant. Zum Beispiel können Spaltenbezeichnungen eines Tabellenparameters bei der Darstellung der Daten im Frontend verwendet werden. Metadaten werden über das Interface `JCoMetaData` repräsentiert. Zusätzlich bietet die JCo-API das direkt abgeleitete Interface `JCoListMetaData` an. Es kommt immer dann zum Einsatz, wenn die gesamte Schnittstelle benötigt wird, das bedeutet Import-, Export- und Changing-Parameter sowie die Liste der Ausnahmen eines Funktionsbausteins.

Zugriff auf Metadaten

Den Zugriff auf die genannten Objekte erhalten Sie über verschiedene Wege. Zum einen können Sie direkt über die Parameterlistenobjekte des Funktionsbausteins und die dort definierte Methode `getMetaData` auf die Informationen zugreifen oder aber über den Aufruf der Methode `getFunctionTemplate`. Diese Methode liefert ein Objekt vom Typ `JCoFunctionTemplate` zurück. Die Klasse stellt die komplette Metadatenbeschreibung des gesamten Funktionsbausteins bereit und ist die Vorlage für die Erzeugung des konkreten `JCoFunction`-Objekts. Bei Betrachtung wird genau eine Instanz vom Typ `JCoFunctionTemplate` im Repository der Destination gespeichert, solange der Metadaten-Cache nicht invalidiert wird. Dabei stellt das Objekt der `JCoFunctionTemplate`-Instanz des Funktionsbausteins die Schablone für die Erzeugung des Funktions-Proxys dar.

Die Proxy-Klasse definiert für den Zugriff auf die Metadaten die Methoden `getImportParameterList`, `getExportParameterList`, `getChangingParameterList`, `getTableParameterList` sowie die Methode `getFunctionInterfaceList`.

Die vier erstgenannten Methoden liefern dabei konkrete Metadaten des zugrunde liegenden Parameterlistentyps. Die Methode `getFunctionInterfaceList` hingegen liefert alle Metadaten der Parameterlisten insgesamt zurück; eine Unterscheidung, welche Parameterart aktuell ausgelesen wird, wird dabei nicht angegeben. Listing 5.16 zeigt die Verarbeitung der Metadaten aller Funktionsbausteinmetadaten im Cache.

```
public void getCachedMetaDataForRepository(
  String repositoryID) throws JCoException {
  JCoRepository repository =
    JCo.getRepository(repositoryID);
  String[] listOfCachedMetadataFunctions =
    repository.getCachedFunctionTemplateNames();
  for (int i=0;i<listOfCachedMetadataFunctions.length;i++){
    JCoFunctionTemplate functionTemplate =
      repository.getFunctionTemplate(
        listOfCachedMetadataFunctions[i]);
    JCoListMetaData metaDataOfFunction =
      functionTemplate.getImportParameterList();
    int fieldCount = metaDataOfFunction.getFieldCount();
    for(int o = 0; o < fieldCount; o++) {
      String fieldName = metaDataOfFunction.getName(o);
      String description =
        metaDataOfFunction.getDescription(o);
      int fieldLength = metaDataOfFunction.getLength(o);
      // Verarbeitung der Metadaten
    }
  }
}
```

Listing 5.16 Verarbeitung der Metadaten aller Funktionsbausteine im Cache eines Repositorys

5.2 RFC-Server

Nachdem die Entwicklung von externen Java-Client-Anwendungen detailliert beschrieben worden ist, wendet sich der folgende Abschnitt der Programmierung von Java-Connector-Servern zu. ABAP-Anwendungen erhalten dabei die Möglichkeit, externen, in Java vorliegenden Programmcode aufzurufen.

5.2.1 Serverseitiges und clientseitiges Repository

Die Verarbeitung des Aufrufs durch einen ABAP-Client in einem Java-Server wird in ähnlichen Schritten abgearbeitet wie die Kommunikation zwischen einem Java-Client und dem ABAP-Server. Wie Sie bei der Client-Programmierung sehen konnten, werden über ein Repository im ABAP-Stack die Metadaten der Schnittstelle vorgehalten, sodass vor der eigentlichen Verarbeitung des Aufrufs geprüft wird, ob die Schnittstelle durch den Konsumenten eingehalten wird. Damit ist sichergestellt, dass typsichere Daten an die Kommunikationspartner übermittelt werden. Analog sieht die Bereitstellung von Funktionen über einen Java-Server aus. Dies führt dazu, dass ein Repository im Java-Server bereitgestellt werden muss. Das Dilemma liegt dabei darin, dass dies ein sehr komplexer und aufwendiger Entwicklungsschritt ist. Wir gehen in diesem Abschnitt nicht im Detail auf die Implementierung eines eigenen Repositorys ein, sondern diskutieren lediglich die Grundzüge der Repository-Programmierung.

Klassen der JCo-Java-Server-Programmierung

Zur Erstellung eigener Repository-Objekte stellt der SAP Java Connector einige Klassen zur Verfügung. Abbildung 5.6 zeigt ein vereinfachtes Diagramm der für die Repository-Programmierung relevanten Klassen. Im Zentrum steht dabei das Interface `JCoCustomRepository`.

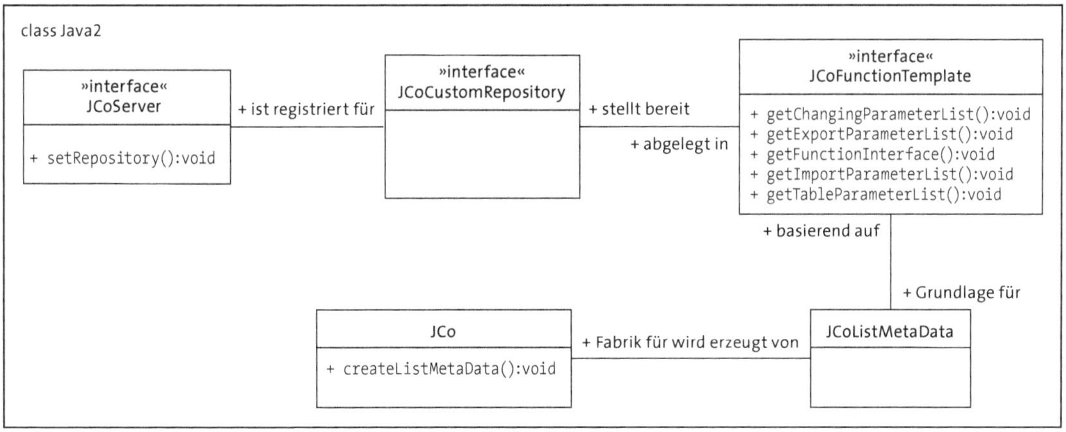

Abbildung 5.6 Übersicht über die für die Repository-Programmierung relevanten Klassen

Das Interface definiert, wie bereits bei der Client-Programmierung angesprochen, eine Vielzahl von Methoden für die Abfrage von Metadaten der Funktionen, die später durch den Server bereitgestellt werden. Da wir ein eigenes Repository implementieren möchten, müssen wir eine Klasse bereitstellen, die das Interface implementiert. Das bedeutet, dass wir alle Funktionen innerhalb des Repositorys beschreiben müssen, die durch das SAP-System aufgerufen werden sollen. Diese Funktionen werden über das Interface `JCoFunction-Template` beschrieben. Das Interface definiert dafür einige Getter-Methoden, die als Rückgabewert eine Liste von Metadaten zurückliefern. Diese Liste wird über das bereits bekannte Interface `JCoListMetaData` dargestellt.

Komplexität der Funktionsbeschreibung

Das Ausprägen einer eigenen Funktionsbeschreibung, wie sie für das Interface `JCoFunctionTemplate` nötig ist, stellt eine Herausforderung dar. Für komplexe Funktionen, die dem SAP-System angeboten werden, müssen jedes einzelne Feld, jede Struktur und jede Tabelle über `JCoListMetaData` und verwandte Metadaten-Interfaces, wie z B. `JCoRecordMetaData`, beschrieben werden. Das Programmierbeispiel in Listing 5.17 stellt eine einfache Implementierung der Methode `getExportParameterList` dar. Die Methode beschreibt die Exportparameter. Sie sehen, dass in der ersten Zeile eine Instanz des Typs `JCoRecordMetaData` zur Beschreibung eines komplexen Typs erzeugt wird.

```
public JCoListMetaData getExportParameterList() {
  JCoRecordMetaData structure =
    JCo.createRecordMetaData("Orderhead");
  structure.add("orderid", JCoRecordMetaData.TYPE_STRING,
                8, 8, 0, 0);
  structure.add("buyer", JCoRecordMetaData.TYPE_STRING,
                50,50,0,0);
  JCoListMetaData exportMetaData =
     JCo.createListMetaData("export");
  exportMetaData.add("Orderhead",
    JCoListMetaData.TYPE_STRUCTURE, structure,
    JCoListMetaData.EXPORT_PARAMETER);
  return exportMetaData;
}
```

Listing 5.17 Implementierung der Methode »getExportParameterList« für das Interface »JCoFunctionTemplate«

Parameter

Das Interface definiert einige Methoden mit dem Bezeichner `add` mit verschiedenen Aufrufparametern. Sie erhalten grundsätzlich folgende Parametereigenschaften:

- **Bezeichner des Parameters**
  An dieser Stelle wird der Name des Parameters definiert, mit dem dieser Parameter später angesprochen wird.

- **Datentyp des Parameters**
  Dabei werden die Datentypen verwendet, die durch die jeweilige Metadatenausprägung angeboten werden. Alle Datentypbezeichner verwenden das Präfix `TYPE_`.
- **Symbollänge des Parameters**
  Diese Symbollänge gibt an, wie viele Zeichen der Parameter enthalten kann.
- **Symbollänge des Parameters für Unicode**
  Diese Symbollänge gibt an, wie viele Zeichen der Parameter bei der Verwendung von Unicode enthalten kann.
- **Offset des internen JCo-Datenpuffers**
  Dabei handelt es sich um die Distanz des Felds vom Beginn der Struktur bei der Nutzung von Unicode.
- **Offset des internen JCo-Datenpuffers bei der Nutzung von Unicode**
  Dies ist die Distanz des Felds vom Beginn der Struktur bei der Nutzung von Unicode.

Metadatenliste

Nachdem die Struktur angelegt worden ist, wird sie der Liste der Metadaten für die Exportparameterliste hinzugefügt. Dazu wird das Interface `JCoListMetaData` verwendet. Die `add`-Methode erhält als Parameter den Namen der Struktur, den Datentyp, das neu erzeugte Strukturobjekt sowie die Art des Parameters. In dem hier geschilderten Beispiel handelt es sich um einen Exportparameter.

Im Anschluss an die Ausprägung der `JCoFunctionTemplate`-Implementierung ist es nun notwendig, die Metadaten im eigenen Repository anzumelden. Dazu stellt das Repository die Methode `addFunctionTemplateToCache` bereit. Den Abschluss der Repository-Programmierung bildet die Registrierung des neuen, autarken Repositorys am Server. Dazu rufen Sie die Methode `setRepository` auf und übergeben eine Instanz des eigenen Repositorys.

5.2.2 Programmierung eines einfachen JCo-Servers

Für die Programmierung eines Java-Servers für ein SAP-System stellt die Java-Connector-API das Interface `JCoServer` und die Factory-Klasse `JCoServerFactory` bereit. Die Factory-Klasse dient dazu, eine Instanz der Implementierung des Interface an den Aufrufer zurückzuliefern. Bei dieser Erzeugung wird versucht, eine Verbindung mit dem SAP-System aufzubauen und den Java-Server entsprechend zu registrieren. Für den Verbindungsaufbau benötigt die Factory-Klasse die Verbindungsinformationen, die von einer Implementierung des Interface `ServerDataProvider` bereitgestellt werden.

JCo-Server starten

Für die Demonstration der Serverprogrammierung erzeugen wir eine Klasse mit dem Namen `EAIServerDemo` und implementieren eine private Hilfsmethode `startServer`. Listing 5.18 stellt die ersten Schritte für das Starten eines synchronen RFC-Servers dar.

```
private void startServer() {
  JCoServer eaiServer;
  try {
      eaiServer = JCoServerFactory.getServer("EAIServer");
  } catch (JCoException ex) {
    throw new RuntimeException(
      "Unable to create server. Error message is:"  +
      ex.getMessage(), ex);
  }
  // register ServerFunctionHandler
  registerServerFunctionHandler(eaiServer);
  eaiServer.start();
  System.out.println(
    "Server successfully started and registered with " +
    server.getProgramID());
}
```

Listing 5.18 Starten des JCo-Servers

Konfiguration der Inbound-Kommunikation

Der Startvorgang des RFC-Servers untergliedert sich in drei Schritte: Im ersten Schritt wird über die Klasse `JCoServerFactory` eine Instanz vom Typ `JCoServer` erzeugt. Die Factory stellt dafür die Methode `getServer` bereit. Die Methode erhält den Bezeichner einer Datei, in der die Verbindungsinformationen für den Registrierungsprozess am SAP-Backend definiert sind. Der Dateiname muss bei dieser Vorgehensweise im Klassenpfad des Java-Servers abgelegt sein und die Dateiendung **.jcoServer** haben. Listing 5.19 zeigt eine exemplarische Konfigurationsdatei. Der Zugriff auf die Bezeichner der Parameter kann auch über das Interface `ServerDataProvider` erfragt werden.

```
jco.server.connection_count=2
jco.server.gwhost=192.168.126.128
jco.server.progid=EAIJAVASERVER
jco.server.gwserv=sapgw01
jco.server.repository_destination=EAIRepository
```

Listing 5.19 Serververbindungs-Konfigurationsdatei

Von besonderem Interesse sind die Einträge `jco.server.progid` und `jco.server.repository_destination`. Der erste Eintrag, `jco.server.progid`, wird als eindeutiger Identifizierer verwendet, mit dem der Server im SAP-System registriert wird. Der zweite Eintrag, `jco.server.repository_destination`, ist ein optionaler Parameter und dient zur Kennzeichnung des Backend-Systems, das für die Bereitstellung des Repositorys und damit für die Bereitstellung der Metadaten der aufzurufenden Funktionen verantwortlich ist.

Serververbindungsparameter

Wie bereits zu Beginn des Kapitels angesprochen, ist die Inbound-Kommunikation analog zur Outbound-Kommunikation aufgebaut. Es ist also notwendig, die Funktionen, die im Java-Server bereitgestellt werden, analog zum ABAP Dictionary auf der ABAP-Seite zur Verfügung zu stellen. Der Parameter `jco.server.repository_destination` bezeichnet daher einfach den Namen einer Konfigurationsdatei, die mit der Endung **.jcoDestination** versehen ist. Den Aufbau dieser Konfigurationsdatei haben Sie bereits in Listing 5.2 (siehe Abschnitt 5.1.3, »Programmierung mit dem SAP Java Connector«) kennengelernt. Beim Aufbau des Servers wird eine Verbindung angegeben, über die der Server die Metadaten für die bereitgestellten Funktionen auslesen kann.

5.2.3 Registrieren eines Funktions-Handlers

Im Anschluss an die Implementierung des Serverprozesses müssen Sie im nächsten Schritt einen sogenannten *Funktions-Handler* implementieren und am Serverprozess registrieren. Der Funktions-Handler verarbeitet die eingehenden Funktionsaufrufe.

Instanz vom Typ »JCoServerFunctionHandle«

Zur Implementierung prägen Sie das Interface `JCoServerFunctionHandle` aus. Dieses Interface definiert lediglich eine Methode mit dem Namen `handleRequest`. Die Aufrufparameter der Methode sind ein Objekt vom Typ `JCoServerContext` und eines vom Typ `JCoFunction`. Das Objekt `JCoServerContext` dient dem Zugriff auf den Ablaufkontext des aktuell eingehenden Aufrufs. Über das Interface können Sie unter anderem auf das Repository und auf Serverinformationen zugreifen. Neben dem Ablaufkontext benötigt die Methode noch die eigentlichen Aufrufparameter. Die Parameter werden dabei analog zur Verarbeitung von ausgehenden Aufrufen über ein `JCoFunction`-Objekt beschrieben. Mithilfe dieses Objekts können Sie auf die Import-, Export- und Tabellenparameter zugreifen, wie Sie es ebenfalls bereits in Abschnitt 5.1.3 kennengelernt haben. Listing 5.20 zeigt die Implementierung der Klasse `EAIJavaOrderCreate`. Diese Klasse dient der Java-seitigen Verarbeitung von Aufrufen des Funktionsbausteins `Z_IFP_ORDER_CREATE`.

```
public class EAIJavaOrderCreate
  implements JCoServerFunctionHandler {
  @Override
  public void handleRequest(
    JCoServerContext arg0, JCoFunction arg1)
    throws AbapException {
    // eingehenden Request verarbeiten
  }
}
```

Listing 5.20 Implementierung eines Funktions-Handlers

Die Implementierung allein reicht jedoch nicht aus. Damit eingehende Funktionsaufrufe verarbeitet werden, müssen Sie die Funktions-Handler am jeweiligen Server registrieren. Die Registrierung einfacher Serverfunktionen wird durch die Klasse `DefaultServerHandlerFactory.FunctionHandlerFactory` angeboten. Durch den Aufruf der Methode `registerHandler` und die Übergabe des Funktionsbezeichners sowie der Instanz des Funktions-Handlers wird auf dem Server bekannt gegeben, wer für die Verarbeitung der eingehenden Aufrufe der Funktion `Z_IFP_ORDER_CREATE` verantwortlich ist. Zum Abschluss wird das erzeugte Factory-Objekt am Server durch die Methode `setCallHandlerFactory` registriert. Das Programmierbeispiel in Listing 5.21 stellt den Registrierungsprozess eines Funktions-Handlers dar.

```
JCoServerFunctionHandler stfcConnectionHandler =
                             new EAIJavaOrderCreate();
DefaultServerHandlerFactory.FunctionHandlerFactory factory =
  new DefaultServerHandlerFactory.FunctionHandlerFactory();
factory.registerHandler("Z_IFP_ORDER_CREATE",
                        stfcConnectionHandler);
server.setCallHandlerFactory(factory);
server.start();
```

Listing 5.21 Registrierung des Funktions-Handlers

Konfiguration einer neuen TCP/IP-Destination

Den Abschluss der Java-Serverprogrammierung stellt die Erzeugung einer TCP/IP-Destination im SAP-System dar. Dazu wechseln Sie über Transaktion SM59 in die Destinationsverwaltung. Nachdem die Transaktion gestartet worden ist, markieren Sie den Eintrag **TCP/IP** und klicken auf **Anlegen**. Im Anschluss geben Sie einen Bezeichner für die RFC-Destination und eine kurze Beschreibung zur einfacheren Identifizierung an. Zusätzlich wählen Sie die Opition **Registriertes Serverprogramm** aus und geben die Programm-ID ein, mit der Sie den Server im SAP-System registriert haben.

In dem hier vorgestellten Szenario ist es die ID EAIJAVASERVER. Abbildung 5.7 zeigt die Konfiguration der Destination.

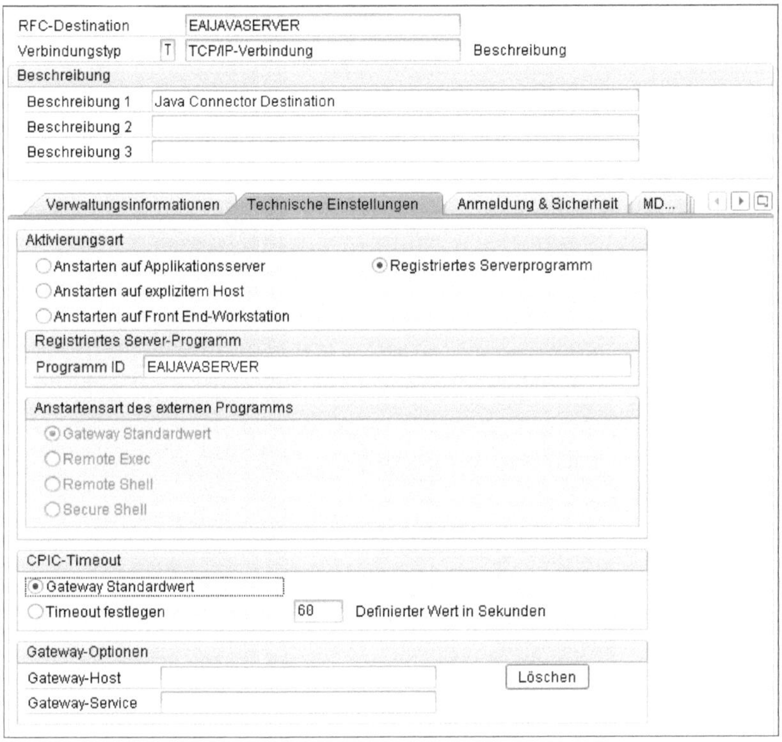

Abbildung 5.7 Konfiguration der Destination »EAIJAVASERVER«

Problematische Fehlerbehandlung

Da nun der Server läuft und entsprechende Anfragen des SAP-Systems verarbeiten kann, stellt sich eine weitere Aufgabe: Das beschriebene Szenario zur Erzeugung von Bestellungen bei einem externen Server ist als blockierender, synchroner Aufruf implementiert. Das SAP-System wird seinerseits blockiert, nachdem es die Funktion auf dem Server aufgerufen hat, bis der Server mit der Abarbeitung fertig ist. Zudem muss sichergestellt werden, dass eine Bestellung auch im Fehlerfall nur einmal auf dem Java-Server erzeugt wird. Um dieses Problem zu lösen, muss die Bestellung in einem transaktionalen RFC-Aufruf angelegt werden. Dies erfordert eine Erweiterung des Servers. Es müssen Funktionen implementiert werden, die den transaktionalen RFC unterstützen.

5.2.4 Verwaltung von Transaktionen

Methoden von »JCoServerTIDHandler«

Die erste Erweiterung, die Sie dem Server hinzufügen, ist die Verarbeitung von transaktionalen Aufrufen nach dem Muster der tRFC-Kommunikation.

Dazu stellt die API `JCoServer` das Interface `JCoServerTIDHandler` bereit. Das Interface bietet folgende Methoden:

- `checkTID`
  Die Methode `checkTID` wird durch das SAP-System aufgerufen, wenn ein RFC-Aufruf als tRFC-Aufruf an den Java-Server übergeben wird. Die Methode erhält als Parameter den Serverkontext und die Transaktions-ID, mit der der Aufruf verarbeitet werden soll.

  Die Methode muss sicherstellen, dass ein Aufruf mit einer übergebenen Transaktions-ID nur einmal ausgeführt wird. Daher ist es enorm wichtig, dass Transaktionsnummern nicht verloren gehen, sodass die Implementierung der Methode meist im Zusammenhang mit dem Speichern der TID in einer Datenbank oder einem anderen persistenten Medium realisiert wird. Neben dem reinen Speichern der TID ist es notwendig, auch den Status der Verarbeitung der Transaktions-ID abzulegen. Dadurch können Sie später leicht ein Monitoring für die Transaktionsnummern implementieren.

  Der Kontrakt dieser Methode definiert, dass ein `boolean`-Parameter an den Aufrufenden zurückgeliefert wird. Für den Fall, dass die übergebene Transaktions-ID bereits einmal verarbeitet wurde, muss der Wert »false« zurückgeliefert werden, sonst der Wert »true«.
- `commit` und `rollback`
  Die Methode `commit` wird aufgerufen, wenn alle RFC-Funktionen, die mit derselben Transaktionsnummer ausgeführt wurden, erfolgreich abgearbeitet wurden. Im Gegensatz dazu steht die Methode `rollback`. Sie wird aufgerufen, wenn eine Transaktion fehlerhaft abgeschlossen wurde.
- `confirmTID`
  Mittels der Methode `confirmTID` wird bestätigt, dass eine Transaktion mit einer spezifischen Transaktionsnummer erfolgreich ausgeführt werden konnte. Die Methode führt dazu, dass die Transaktionsnummer entweder aus dem Persistenzmedium entfernt oder zumindest mit einem entsprechenden Status versehen wird.

Registrierung des TID-Handlers

Vor dem Starten des Servers müssen Sie die Implementierung des Interface `JCoServerTIDHandler` am Server registrieren. Dazu rufen Sie die Methode `setTIDHandler` auf und übergeben eine Instanz der `TIDHandler`-Implementierung. Nachdem der Server gestartet worden ist, kann die Funktion ABAP-seitig mit dem Zusatz `in background task destination 'EAIJAVASERVER'` aufgerufen werden. Der Server wird kontaktiert, und die Methode `checkTID` prüft, ob die Transaktionsnummer bereits verwendet wurde. Liefert die Methode den Wert »true« zurück, wird mit dem Aufruf der Methode `handleRequest` fortgefahren.

[«]

Verarbeitung von bgRFC

Die Verarbeitung von bgRFC-Aufrufen folgt der gleichen Logik wie die Verarbeitung von tRFC-Aufrufen.

Kapitel 6
Remote Function Call mit C#

In diesem Kapitel stellen wir Ihnen die Verwendung des »SAP Connector for Microsoft .NET« vor. Damit können Sie Programme in C# und anderen .NET-Sprachen schreiben, die RFC-Aufrufe ausführen. Sie lernen, RFC-Clients und -Server mit C# zu programmieren und den transaktionalen RFC einzusetzen.

In diesem Kapitel beschreiben wir detailliert die Schnittstellenprogrammierung mit RFC in der Programmiersprache C#. Wir gehen auf die Spielarten des RFC ein und zeigen die Programmierung von RFC-Clients und RFC-Servern mit C#. Dabei wird der *SAP Connector for Microsoft .NET* verwendet, der oft auch als *NCo* bezeichnet wird. Der NCo ist eine Klassenbibliothek, mit der Sie Microsoft-.NET-Programme schreiben können, die per RFC mit SAP-Systemen kommunizieren.

Benötigte Entwicklungsumgebung

Neben dem SAP Connector for Microsoft .NET benötigen Sie als Entwicklungsumgebung ein aktuelles Microsoft Visual Studio. Wir haben die Beispiele mit Microsoft Visual Studio 2022 Community Edition programmiert.

6.1 SAP Connector for Microsoft .NET

NCo herunterladen

Den SAP Connector for Microsoft .NET können Sie unter *https://support.sap.com/en/product/connectors/msnet.html* herunterladen. Es gibt verschiedene Versionen und Kombinationen des Connectors, die jeweils unterschiedliche .NET-Versionen voraussetzen. Bei der NCo Version 3.1 sind es:

- **Compiled with .NET Framework 4.6.2**
  Diese Version läuft auf dem klassischem .NET Framework und ist nur auf Windows verfügbar. Obwohl diese .NET-Version von Microsoft noch unterstützt wird, werden keine neuen Features mehr für sie veröffentlicht.
- **Complied with .NET (formerly .NET Core)**
  Diese Version basiert auf der aktiv weiterentwickelten Version von .NET. Sie läuft auf dem modernen .NET-Framework, das plattformunabhängig ist (für Windows, Linux, macOS).

C++-Laufzeit DLLs

Außerdem werden die *Microsoft C++ Runtime Dynamic Link Libraries* (DLLs) in der Version 14.x benötigt, die in Visual Studio enthalten sind oder separat bezogen werden können.

Neben der NCo-Version muss man zwischen zwei verschiedenen Versionen der Zielplattform wählen:

- x86 (32 Bit)
- x64 (64 Bit)

Achten Sie daher darauf, die richtige Version für Ihre Kombination aus Betriebssystem (32 Bit oder 64 Bit) und .NET-Plattform herunterzuladen.

6.1.1 Installation des SAP Connectors für Microsoft .NET

In den kommenden Beispielen verwenden wir den SAP Connector for Microsoft .NET 3.1, Compiled for .NET (vormals .NET Core) 64 Bit, also die aktuelle Version, die auf der modernen .NET-Plattform aufbaut.

Installation aus ».zip«-Datei

Sie können die heruntergeladene **.zip**-Datei einfach entpacken. Das Installationsverzeichnis enthält eine Installationsanleitung und die notwendigen DLLs **sapnco.dll** und **System.Configuration.ConfigurationManager.dll**, **sapnco_utils.dll** und **ijwhost.dll**. Außerdem gibt es eine API-Dokumentation in Form einer CHM-Datei.

6.1.2 Verwendung des SAP Connectors für Microsoft .NET in Visual-Studio-Projekten

Auswahl der Zielplattform

Um den NCo zu nutzen, müssen dessen Assemblies in Ihrer .NET-Anwendung referenziert werden und zur .NET-Plattform passen. Achten Sie daher besonders auf folgende Punkte:

1. Entscheiden Sie sich für eine Zielplattform (x64 oder x32).
2. Stellen Sie sicher, dass die passende Version der .NET-Laufzeitbibliotheken auf der Maschine installiert ist.
3. Installieren Sie den NCo für die gewünschte Zielplattform.
4. Wählen Sie diese Zielplattform in den Einstellungen des Projekts aus (siehe Abbildung 6.1). Der Hinweis »(.NET Framework)« meint das klassische .NET-Framework. Mit dem Eintrag ohne diesen Hinweis ist das moderne .NET-Framework gemeint.
5. Fügen Sie Ihrem Projekt die Referenzen hinzu: eine Referenz für die Assembly **sapnco.dll**, eine für **sapnco_utils.dll** und **System.Configuration.ConfigurationManager.dll**. Dazu klicken Sie im Projektmappen-

Explorer mit der rechten Maustaste auf den Ordner **Verweise** und wählen im Kontextmenü den Eintrag **Verweis hinzufügen** aus. Wählen Sie dann in der Dialogbox **Verweis hinzufügen (Add COM Referenz)** die Registerkarte **Durchsuchen** aus, und fügen Sie dort die Assemblies aus dem Installationsverzeichnis hinzu. Stellen Sie dann in den Eigenschaften dieser beiden Referenzen den Wert für den Eintrag **Lokale Kopie** auf **Ja** ein (siehe Abbildung 6.2).

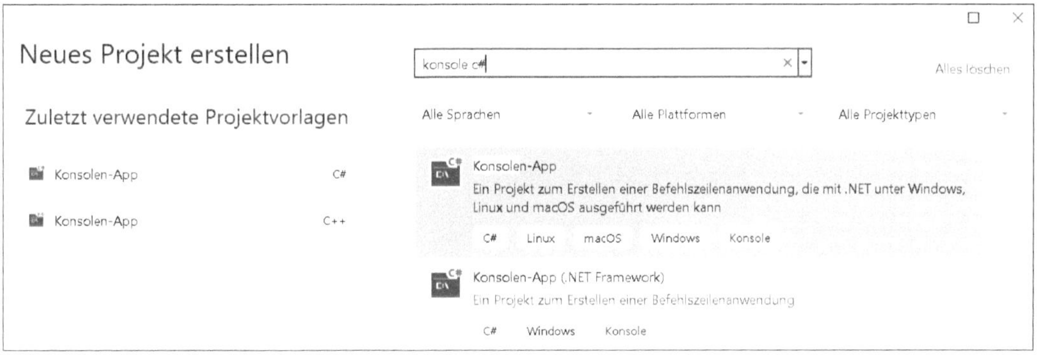

Abbildung 6.1 Auswahl der Plattform

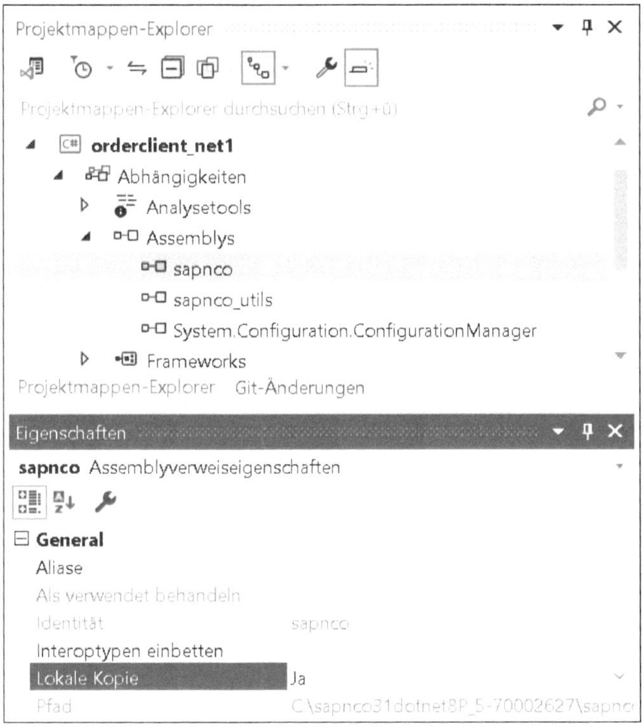

Abbildung 6.2 Verweise einrichten

6. Kopieren Sie nun noch die Assembly **ijwhost.dll** aus dem Installationsverzeichnis in das gleiche Verzeichnis wie das erstellte Binary (die **.exe**-Datei), so wie es in der Datei **installation.txt** dokumentiert ist.

6.2 Einfache RFC-Clients

In diesem Abschnitt werden Sie sich anhand eines einfachen RFC-Client-Programms mit dem prinzipiellen Aufbau von Clients vertraut machen, die den NCo verwenden. Sie lernen, wie der NCo die Destinationen eines Clients verwaltet, wie die Metadaten der aufzurufenden Funktionsbausteine gespeichert werden und wie Sie mit einfachen, strukturierten und tabellenartigen Parametern arbeiten.

6.2.1 Aufbau eines einfachen RFC-Clients

RFC-Client als Konsolenanwendung

Legen Sie in Visual Studio ein neues Projekt vom Typ **Windows-Konsolenanwendung** an, und referenzieren Sie in diesem Projekt auf die Assemblies **sapnco.dll**, **sapnco_utils.dll** und **System.Configuration.ConfigurationManager.dll**, wie in Abbildung 6.2 dargestellt. Achten Sie darauf, in der Build-Konfiguration des Projekts die korrekte Einstellung vorzunehmen. Programmieren Sie dann die Methode `Main` der Klasse `Program` wie in Listing 6.1.

```
using System;
using SAP.Middleware.Connector;
namespace SimpleClient
{
  class Program
  {
    static void Main(string[] args)
    {
      // Verbindungsparameter füllen
      RfcConfigParameters cfgParams =
        new RfcConfigParameters();
      cfgParams.Add("NAME", "NCO_TESTS");
      cfgParams.Add("CLIENT", "001");
      cfgParams.Add("USER", "bcuser");
      cfgParams.Add("PASSWD", "minisap");
      cfgParams.Add("LANG", "EN");
      cfgParams.Add("ASHOST", "localhost");
      cfgParams.Add("SYSNR", "00");
      // Destination beschaffen
      RfcDestination destination =
```

```
        RfcDestinationManager.GetDestination(cfgParams);
     // Metadaten beschaffen
      IRfcFunction rfcFunction =
        destination.Repository.
           CreateFunction("STFC_CONNECTION");
      // Importparameter setzen
      rfcFunction.SetValue("REQUTEXT", "Hello SAP");
      // Funktionsbaustein aufrufen
      rfcFunction.Invoke(destination);
      // Ergebnis anzeigen
      Console.WriteLine(
        "ECHOTEXT: {0}",
        rfcFunction.GetValue("ECHOTEXT")
      );
    }
  }
}
```

Listing 6.1 Prinzipieller Aufbau eines RFC-Clients in .NET

Der Code in Listing 6.1 erzeugt zunächst ein Objekt der Klasse `RfcConfigParameters` und füllt dieses mit den Anmelde- und Verbindungsdaten zu einem SAP-System. Ein Satz von Konfigurationsparametern wird *Destination* genannt. Sie weisen einer Destination einen Namen zu, der im Beispiel von Listing 6.1 `NCO_TESTS` lautet.

»RfcConfig-Parameters«

Der RFC-Client übergibt die Konfigurationsparameter für die Verbindung dann an die Methode `GetDestination` der Klasse `RfcDestinationManager` und erhält von dieser Methode ein Objekt der Klasse `RfcDestination` zurück. Wie wir im nächsten Abschnitt näher besprechen werden, verwaltet der *Destination Manager* sämtliche Verbindungen einer Destination; der Client arbeitet also nicht direkt mit den RFC-Verbindungen und ist auch nicht dafür verantwortlich, sie zu öffnen oder zu schließen.

Destinationen und Destination Manager

Im nächsten Schritt beschafft sich der Client die Metadaten des Funktionsbausteins `STFC_CONNECTION`. Dazu ruft er die Methode `CreateFunction` des Objekts `Repository` auf. Das Repository-Objekt gehört zur Destination. Das Repository-Objekt einer Destination besorgt sich die Metadaten zu Funktionsbausteinen von der ABAP-Plattform, auf die in den Verbindungsdaten der Destination verwiesen wird, und verwaltet diese.

Metadaten

Nun setzt der Client über das zurückgegebene Objekt `rfcFunction`, dessen Klasse die Schnittstelle `IRfcFunction` implementiert, die Importparameter. Dazu ruft er die Methode `SetValue` auf und übergibt Namen und Wert der Importparameter.

Importparameter setzen

Funktionsbaustein aufrufen

Schließlich veranlasst der Client durch Aufruf der Methode `Invoke` des Objekts `rfcFunction`, dass der Funktionsbaustein auf der ABAP-Plattform ausgeführt wird, auf den in der übergebenen Destination verwiesen wird. Der Funktionsbaustein muss also nicht auf dem Server ausgeführt werden, von dem die Metadaten stammen; er kann auch auf einem anderen Server ausgeführt werden.

Exportparameter lesen

Nach dem Aufruf gibt der Client die Namen und Werte des Exportparameters `ECHOTEXT` aus.

6.2.2 Destinationsmanagement

Alle RFC-Destinationen einer .NET-Anwendung werden zentral von der einzigen Instanz der Klasse `RfcDestinationManager`, dem Destination Manager, verwaltet. Dieses Objekt verwaltet die Logon-Daten für alle ABAP-Plattform-Verbindungen, die die Anwendung nutzen will. Die Logon-Daten für einen Server werden durch einen Destinationsnamen identifiziert. Eine .NET-Anwendung hat prinzipiell drei Möglichkeiten, um die Logon-Daten für eine Destination an den Destination Manager zu übergeben:

- Durch die Übergabe eines `RfcConfigParameters`-Objekts, das Sie vorher im Code konfigurieren.
- Durch die Angabe eines Destinationsnamens, der in der Standard-.NET-Konfigurationsdatei der Anwendung konfiguriert wurde. Dies ist die bequemste Option, ist aber nicht sehr sicher, da Sie Passwörter in der Konfigurationsdatei im Klartext ablegen müssen.
- Durch Übergabe eines Objekts, dessen Klasse die Schnittstelle `IDestinationConfiguration` implementiert. Dieses Objekt wird vom Destination Manager bei Bedarf nach den Verbindungsinformationen gefragt, die es dann zur Laufzeit z. B. aus einer Datenbank oder einem LDAP-Verzeichnis lesen kann. Diese Option bietet ein Maximum an Sicherheit und Flexibilität, verursacht aber den meisten Aufwand.

»RfcConfiguration_Parameters«

Listing 6.1 zeigt die erste Variante, die Übergabe eines `RfcConfigurationParameters`-Objekts an die statische Methode `GetDestination` der Klasse `RfcConfigurationManager`. Die Client-Anwendung füllt diese Parameter vor der Übergabe, z. B. im Dialog mit dem Benutzer. Im Listing sind die Parameter hartcodiert, was Sie in produktivem Code jedoch aus Sicherheitsgründen vermeiden sollten.

Konfigurationsdatei

Auch die zweite Variante birgt jedoch noch einige Sicherheitsrisiken. Hier pflegen Sie die Logon-Daten einfach in der Konfigurationsdatei **app.config** der Client-Anwendung, wie dies Listing 6.2 zeigt.

```
<?xml version="1.0"?>
<configuration>
  <configSections>
    <sectionGroup name="SAP.Middleware.Connector">
      <sectionGroup name="ClientSettings">
        <section name="DestinationConfiguration"  type="SAP.
Middleware.Connector.RfcDestinationConfiguration, sapnco"/>
      </sectionGroup>
    </sectionGroup>
  </configSections>
  <SAP.Middleware.Connector>
    <ClientSettings>
      <DestinationConfiguration>
        <destinations>
          <add NAME="NCO_TESTS"
            USER="bcuser" PASSWD="minisap" CLIENT="001"
            LANG="EN" ASHOST="localhost" SYSNR="00"
            POOL_SIZE="5" MAX_POOL_SIZE="10"/>
        </destinations>
      </DestinationConfiguration>
    </ClientSettings>
  </SAP.Middleware.Connector>
</configuration>
```


Listing 6.2 Konfiguration von Logon-Daten in der Konfigurationsdatei »app.config«

Wie Sie sehen, legt der Konfigurationseintrag neben den Logon-Daten und den technischen Verbindungsdaten auch die Anfangs- und Maximalgröße des Verbindungspools für die Destination fest. Die Datei **app.config** liegt im Verzeichnis der Binärdatei. Sobald Sie die Verbindungsdaten in der Konfigurationsdatei gepflegt haben, müssen Sie der Methode `GetDestination` des Destination Managers nur noch den Namen der Destination übergeben:

```
RfcDestination destination =
        RfcDestinationManager.GetDestination("NCO_TESTS");
```

Konfigurationsklasse

Als dritte Variante zur Bereitstellung einer Destination können Sie alternativ eine Konfigurationsklasse schreiben, die die Schnittstelle `IDestinationConfiguration` implementiert. Die Methode `GetParameters` muss auf Anforderung des Destination Managers ein Objekt `RfcConfigParameters` zurückgeben, das die Verbindungsdaten für die Destination enthält, die im Parameter `destinationName` der Methode spezifiziert wurde. Auch die Implementierung in Listing 6.3 ist natürlich sicherheitskritisch, da die Logon-Parameter nicht zur Laufzeit aus einem Verzeichnis gelesen oder vom Benutzer abgefragt werden, sondern hartcodiert sind.

```
public class MyConfig:
  IDestinationConfiguration
{
  public RfcConfigParameters GetParameters(
                              String destinationName)
  {
    if ("NCO_TESTS".Equals(destinationName))
    {
      RfcConfigParameters parms = new RfcConfigParameters();
      parms.Add("NAME", "NCO_TESTS");
      parms.Add(RfcConfigParameters.AppServerHost,
               "127.0.0.1");
      parms.Add(RfcConfigParameters.SystemNumber, "00");
      parms.Add(RfcConfigParameters.User, "bcuser");
      parms.Add(RfcConfigParameters.Password, "minisap");
      parms.Add(RfcConfigParameters.Client, "001");
      parms.Add(RfcConfigParameters.Language, "EN");
      parms.Add(RfcConfigParameters.PoolSize, "5");
      parms.Add(RfcConfigParameters.PeakConnectionsLimit, "10");
      parms.Add(RfcConfigParameters.ConnectionIdleTimeout, "600");
      return parms;
    }
    else return null;
  }
  public bool ChangeEventsSupported()
  {
    return false;
  }
  public event
    RfcDestinationManager.ConfigurationChangeHandler
      ConfigurationChanged;
}
```

Listing 6.3 Implementierung der Schnittstelle »IDestinationConfiguration«

Konfigurationsklasse registrieren

Beim Start der Anwendung müssen Sie eine Instanz Ihrer Konfigurationsklasse anlegen und diese beim Destination Manager registrieren, indem Sie die Methode `RegisterDestinationConfiguration` aufrufen. Anschließend kann

Ihr Code über die Angabe des Destinationsnamens, wie im vorangehenden Fall, auch ein Destinationsobjekt beschaffen. Der Destination Manager ruft bei der erstmaligen Verwendung einer Destination die Methode `GetParameters` Ihrer Konfigurationsklasse auf. Listing 6.4 zeigt den Code dazu.


```
MyConfig config = new MyConfig();
RfcDestinationManager.RegisterDestinationConfiguration(
  config);
RfcDestination destination =
        RfcDestinationManager.GetDestination("NCO_TESTS");
```

Listing 6.4 Konfigurationsklasse verwenden

Konfigurationsparameter für Destinationen

In den bisherigen Listings haben Sie nur einige wenige der vielen möglichen Parameter gesehen, mit denen Sie eine Destination konfigurieren können. Die folgenden Tabellen listen die wichtigsten Parameter auf. In der linken Spalte wird jeweils der Name des Parameters genannt, so wie Sie ihn in der Konfigurationsdatei verwenden. Für diese Strings definiert die Klasse `RfcConfigParameters` jeweils eine Konstante, deren Namen Sie in der zweiten Spalte sehen. Die dritte Spalte enthält eine Beschreibung des Parameters und die vierte seine möglichen Werte.

Logon bei Anwendungsserver

Wenn Sie sich bei einer bestimmten Instanz eines SAP-Systems anmelden wollen, müssen Sie den Hostnamen und die Systemnummer angeben. Den Parameter für die Portnummer bzw. den Servicenamen des RFC-Gateways des Applikationsservers, der in Tabelle 6.1 aufgeführt ist, geben Sie normalerweise nicht an, da er sich aus der Systemnummer eindeutig ergibt.

Name	Konstante	Beschreibung	Mögliche Werte
`ASHOST`	`AppServerHost`	Hostname der ABAP-Plattform	
`ASSERV`	`AppServerService`	Servicename oder Portnummer des RFC-Gateways	z. B. sapgw00, 3300
`SYSNR`	`SystemNumber`	Systemnummer	00–99

Tabelle 6.1 Verbindungsdaten für die Anmeldung an einer ABAP-Plattform

Anmeldung bei Logon-Gruppe

Wollen Sie sich nicht an einem bestimmten Anwendungsserver anmelden, sondern an einem beliebigen Anwendungsserver einer Logon-Gruppe, verwenden Sie die Parameter der Tabelle 6.2.

Name	Konstante	Beschreibung	Mögliche Werte
`MSHOST`	`MessageServer-Host`	Hostname des Message-Servers des SAP-Systems	
`MSSERV`	`MessageServer-Service`	Servicename oder Portnummer des Message-Servers	z. B. sapmsPRD, 3600
`SYSID`	`SystemID`	Systemnummer	z. B. PRD
`GROUP`	`LogonGroup`	Logon-Gruppe, aus der der Anwendungs-server ausgewählt wird	z. B. PUBLIC

Tabelle 6.2 Verbindungsdaten für die Anmeldung an einer Logon-Gruppe

Authentifizierung

Wenn Sie sich anmelden, müssen Sie Mandanten, Sprache, Benutzer und Passwort zur Authentifizierung angeben (siehe Tabelle 6.3). Anstelle eines Benutzers und eines Passworts können Sie auch ein X.509-Zertifikat zur Authentifizierung verwenden. Dieses Zertifikat muss auf dem Server einem Benutzer zugeordnet sein.

Name	Konstante	Beschreibung	Mögliche Werte
`CLIENT`	`Client`	Nummer des Anmeldemandanten	000–999
`LANG`	`Language`	Anmeldesprache	z. B. DE, EN, JA usw.
`USER`	`User`	Benutzername	z. B. bcuser
`PASSWD`	`Password`	Passwort	z. B. minisap
`X509CERT`	`X509Certificate`	Alternativ zur Angabe von Benutzer und Passwort kann auch ein X.509-Zertifikat verwendet werden.	X.509-Zertifikat in Base64-Codierung

Tabelle 6.3 Parameter zur Benutzerauthentifizierung

Verbindungspool-Eigenschaften

Sie können die Eigenschaften des Verbindungspools einer Destination mit den Parametern der Tabelle 6.4 steuern, falls die verwendeten Standardwerte für Ihre Situation ungeeignet sind. Zum Beispiel können Sie den Parameter `POOL_SIZE` auf »10« belassen, aber den Parameter `MAX_POOL_SIZE` auf »15« setzen. Dann kann Ihr Client im Bedarfsfall maximal 15 RFC-Verbindungen gleichzeitig verwenden. Der Verbindungspool schließt jedoch fünf davon sofort wieder, wenn sie nicht mehr verwendet werden.

Name	Konstante	Beschreibung	Mögliche Werte
POOL_SIZE	PoolSize	Maximale Anzahl der RFC-Verbindungen, die im Pool gehalten werden. Es können zwar mehr Verbindungen geöffnet werden; diese werden aber sofort nach der Verwendung wieder geschlossen.	Standard ist 10.
MAX_POOL_SIZE	PeakConnectionsLimit	Maximale Anzahl geöffneter Verbindungen.	Standard ist 10.
POOL_IDLE_TIMEOUT	PoolIdleTimeout	Falls ein Pool eine Weile nicht benutzt wurde, wird er gelöscht.	Zeit in Sekunden; Standard ist 3.600.
MAX_POOL_WAIT_TIME	MaxPoolWaitTime	Falls die maximale Zahl an offenen Verbindungen erreicht wurde, wird bei der Anforderung einer weiteren Verbindung noch so lange gewartet, bevor eine Ausnahme ausgelöst wird.	Zeit in Millisekunden; Standard ist 0.
IDLE_TIMEOUT	ConnectionIDleTimeout	Falls eine Verbindung eine Weile nicht genutzt wurde, wird sie gelöscht.	Zeit in Sekunden; Standard ist 60.
REP_CONN_IDLE_TIMEOUT	Repository-ConnectionIdleTimeout	Wie oben, jedoch nur für Verbindungen, die für Repository-Zugriffe genutzt werden.	Zeit in Sekunden. Wenn nicht angegeben, wird der Wert des Parameters IDLE_TIMEOUT (oder dessen Standard) verwendet.
IDLE_CHECK_TIME	IdleCheckTime	Zeitabstände, in denen der NCo prüft, ob Verbindungen oder Pools weiterhin verwendet werden.	Zeit in Sekunden; Standard ist 60.

Tabelle 6.4 Kontrolle der Eigenschaften des Verbindungspools

Alternativer Repository-Benutzer

Wenn Sie die Metadaten der Funktionsbausteine mit einem anderen Benutzer als mit dem, der anschließend die Funktionsbausteine aufruft, aus dem ABAP Repository auslesen wollen, können Sie die Authentifizierungsdaten für einen alternativen Repository-Benutzer in den Parametern der Tabelle 6.5 angeben. Dadurch können Sie z. B. dem Repository-Benutzer andere Rechte als dem Benutzer geben, der anschließend Anwendungsfunktionen aufrufen wird.

Name	Konstante	Beschreibung	Mögliche Werte
`REPOSITORY_USER`	`RepositoryUser`	Benutzername eines alternativen Benutzers für den Zugriff auf das Repository	–
`REPOSITORY_PASSWD`	`RepositoryPassword`	Passwort des Repository-Benutzers	–
`REPOSITORY_X509CERT`	`RepositoryX509Certificate`	Alternativ zur Angabe von Benutzer und Passwort kann auch ein X.509-Zertifikat verwendet werden.	X.509-Zertifikat in Base64-Codierung

Tabelle 6.5 Zugriff auf das Repository mit einem alternativen Benutzer

6.2.3 Repository und Metadaten

Der NCo liest seit Version 3.0 die Metadaten der Funktionsbausteine nicht zur Designzeit aus einem ABAP Repository, sondern zur Laufzeit. Jedes Destinationsobjekt hat als Member ein Repository-Objekt der Klasse `RfcRepository`. Wenn Sie die Methode `CreateFunction` eines Repository-Objekts aufrufen, erhalten Sie ein Funktionsobjekt für den angegebenen Funktionsbaustein zurück. Das Funktionsobjekt implementiert die Schnittstelle `IRfcFunction`. Über die Methoden dieser Schnittstelle haben Sie sowohl Zugriff auf die Metadaten des Funktionsbausteins als auch auf die Datencontainer, die die Werte der Import- und Exportparameter vor und nach dem Funktionsbausteinaufruf enthalten.

Funktionsbausteine beschreiben

Die Metadaten eines Funktionsbausteins enthalten die Beschreibung seiner Import-, Export- und Tabellenparameter, also deren Namen, deren Typ und die Beschreibung der Typen. Diese Informationen benötigt der NCo, um Datencontainer für die Inhalte der Parameter vor und nach dem Aufruf bereitzustellen. Normalerweise besorgen Sie sich die Metadaten von einem SAP-System, indem Sie das Repository-Objekt eines Destinationsobjekts verwenden, das ja auf diesen Applikationsserver verweist. In extrem seltenen Fällen – etwa wenn Sie einen RFC-Server programmieren wollen, der zur Laufzeit keine Repository-Daten aus einem SAP-System lesen soll oder kann – müssen Sie die Metadaten von Hand in Ihrem Code aufbauen.

Metadaten lesen

Sie werden auch selten die Metadaten eines Funktionsbausteins lesen. Es sei denn, Sie schreiben Entwicklungswerkzeuge und wollen die Struktur unbekannter Funktionsbausteine ermitteln und darstellen. Für diese beiden seltenen Fälle beschreiben wir hier kurz die Klassen der Metadatenobjekte. Prinzipiell gibt es zwei verschiedene Arten von Metadaten:

- *Elementmetadaten* beschreiben Komponenten von Strukturen, Parameter von Funktionsbausteinen und Attribute von Klassen. Sie enthalten z. B. Informationen über den Namen, den Datentyp – etwa CHAR, FLOAT, INT usw. – und die Länge eines Felds.
- *Container-Metadaten* beschreiben zusammengesetzte Typen, wie z. B. Strukturen (als Sammlung von Komponenten), Tabellen oder Funktionsbausteine (als Sammlungen ihrer Parameter und Ausnahmen).

Elementmetadaten

Die Basisklasse für alle Elementmetadatenklassen ist die abstrakte Klasse RfcElementMetadata. Diese Klasse hat drei Unterklassen:

- RfcFieldMetadata beschreibt eine Komponente einer Struktur. Ihre Objekte enthalten Informationen über den Namen, Datentyp, die Länge und Anzahl der Dezimalstellen (abhängig vom Datentyp) und den Offset des Felds innerhalb der Struktur.
- RfcParameterMetadata beschreibt Import-, Export- und Tabellenparameter eines Funktionsbausteins.
- RfcAttributeMetadata beschreibt ein Attribut einer ABAP-Klasse.

Container-Metadaten

Die Basisklasse für alle Container-Metadatenklassen ist die abstrakte generische Klasse RfcContainerMetadata<T>, wobei T eine Unterklasse der Klasse RfcElementMetadata ist. Es gibt vier Unterklassen:

- RfcStructureMetadata:RfcContainerMetadata<RfcFieldMetadata>
  Diese Unterklasse beschreibt eine Struktur. Sie enthält Informationen über den Namen, die Gesamtlänge und die einzelnen Komponenten der Struktur.
- RfcTableMetadata:RfcContainerMetadata<RfcFieldMetadata>
  Diese Klasse beschreibt eine Tabelle.
- RfcFunctionMetadata:RfcContainerMetadata<RfcParameterMetadata>
  Diese Klasse beschreibt einen Funktionsbaustein. Sie enthält allgemeine Informationen zum Funktionsbaustein, seinen Ausnahmen und Parametern.

- `RfcAbapObjectMetadata:RfcContainerMetadata <RfcAttributeMetadata>`
  Diese Klasse beschreibt ein ABAP-Objekt. Objekte dieser Klasse enthalten momentan lediglich die Beschreibung der Attribute von Ausnahmeklassen.

6.2.4 Einfache Parameter

Listing 6.1 zeigt, wie Sie mit einfachen Parametern eines Funktionsbausteins arbeiten können. Unter *einfachen Parametern* verstehen wir Parameter, die nicht weiter strukturiert sind, wie etwa Strings, Zeichenketten oder gepackte Dezimalzahlen. Strukturen und Tabellen sind im Gegensatz dazu keine einfachen Parameter.

»SetValue« Mit der Methode `SetValue()` können Sie den Inhalt eines beliebigen Parameters setzen. Diese Methode wird von der Schnittstelle `IRfcDataContainer` definiert, die Bestandteil der Schnittstelle `IRfcFunction` ist. Diese Methode ist mehrfach überladen. Im ersten Parameter der Methode geben Sie den Namen oder den Index des Parameters an, im zweiten dann den Wert, den Sie setzen wollen. Für den Datentyp des zweiten Parameters haben Sie dabei die Auswahl zwischen fünfzehn verschiedenen Typen, darunter die zehn einfachen Datentypen `byte`, `byte[]`, `char`, `char[]`, `decimal`, `double`, `float`, `int`, `long`, `short` und `string`. In Listing 6.1 haben wir also die Überladung `SetValue(string, string)` verwendet.

»GetValue« Mit der Methode `GetValue()` können Sie den Inhalt eines beliebigen Parameters lesen. Auch diese Methode wird von der Schnittstelle `IRfcDataContainer` definiert. Sie können den Parameter, den Sie lesen wollen, ebenfalls über seinen Namen oder seinen Index identifizieren.

`GetValue()` liefert ein Objekt vom Typ `object` zurück. Zusätzlich zu der generischen Methode `GetValue()` gibt es eine ganze Reihe von `GetXXX`-Methoden, die einen konkreten Datentyp zurückliefern. Für die einfachen Parameter sind dies `GetByte`, `GetByteArray`, `GetChar`, `GetCharArray`, `GetDecimal`, `GetDouble`, `GetFloat`, `GetInt`, `GetLong`, `GetShort` und `GetString`.

»IRfcParameter« NCo bietet Ihnen eine alternative Möglichkeit, um auf die Inhalte von Funktionsbausteinparametern zuzugreifen: Die Schnittstelle `IRfcFunction` definiert einen `string`- und einen `int`-Indexer, die Ihnen `IRfcParameter`-Schnittstellen für den Zugriff auf die Parameter des Funktionsbausteins liefern. Mit diesen Indexern können Sie ganz bequem `foreach`-Schleifen über alle Parameter eines Funktionsbausteins realisieren, wie wir es in Listing 6.5 zeigen. Dieses Listing greift auch auf die Metadaten des Parameters zu, um dessen Namen auszugeben.

```
foreach (IRfcParameter parameter in rfcFunction)
{
  Console.WriteLine("{0}: {1}",
    parameter.Metadata.Name,
    parameter.GetString());
}
```

Listing 6.5 Schleife über alle Parameter eines Funktionsbausteins

»IRfcElement«

Die Schnittstelle `IRfcParameter` umfasst die Schnittstelle `IRfcElement`, die die Methoden `SetValue`, `GetValue` und `GetXXX` definiert, nun jedoch ohne den ersten Parameter zur Identifikation des Funktionsbausteinparameters. Den Code zum Schreiben und Lesen der beiden Parameter in Listing 6.1 könnten Sie alternativ also auch so wie in Listing 6.6 schreiben:

```
rfcFunction["REQUTEXT"].SetValue("Hello SAP");
rfcFunction.Invoke(destination);
Console.WriteLine(
  "ECHOTEXT: {0}",
  rfcFunction["ECHOTEXT"].GetValue()
);
```

Listing 6.6 Verwendung des String-Indexers und der Schnittstelle »IRfcParameter«

Beide Alternativen liefern genau dasselbe Ergebnis und unterscheiden sich auch nicht in der Ausführungsgeschwindigkeit.

6.2.5 Strukturierte Parameter

»GetStructure«

Ausgehend von einem Funktionsbausteinobjekt, das die Schnittstelle `IRfcFunction` implementiert, erhalten Sie über die Methode `GetStructure()` Zugriff auf die Schnittstelle `IRfcStructure` eines strukturierten Funktionsbausteinparameters. Im Parameter der Methode `GetStructure` spezifizieren Sie den Funktionsbausteinparameter über seinen Namen oder seinen Index.

»IRfcStructure«

Über die Schnittstelle `IRfcStructure` können Sie lesend und schreibend auf die Komponenten einer Struktur zugreifen. Diese Schnittstelle umfasst die abstrakte Schnittstelle `IRfcDataContainer`, definiert also insbesondere die Methoden `SetValue`, `GetValue` und `GetXXX`, die Sie im vorangegangenen Abschnitt kennengelernt haben. Im ersten Parameter dieser Methoden geben Sie nun aber den Namen oder den Index einer Strukturkomponente an, nicht den Namen oder den Index eines Funktionsbausteinparameters.

Die einfachen Komponenten einer Struktur lesen und schreiben Sie genau wie die einfachen Parameter eines Funktionsbausteins. Falls eine Strukturkomponente nicht einfach, sondern ihrerseits wieder eine Struktur oder gar eine Tabelle ist, verwenden Sie die Methode GetStructure bzw. GetTable für den Zugriff auf diese Komponente. Listing 6.7 zeigt als Beispiel einen RFC-Client, der den Funktionsbaustein STFC_STRUCTURE aufruft.

```
// Destination beschaffen
RfcDestination destination = RfcDestinationManager.
                               GetDestination("NCO_TESTS");
// Metadaten beschaffen
IRfcFunction function =
  destination.Repository.CreateFunction("STFC_STRUCTURE");
// Importstruktur füllen
IRfcStructure importStructure =
  function.GetStructure("IMPORTSTRUCT");
importStructure.SetValue("RFCFLOAT", 17.0932);
importStructure.SetValue("RFCCHAR1", 'a');
importStructure.SetValue("RFCINT2", (short)17283);
importStructure.SetValue("RFCINT1", (byte)127);
importStructure.SetValue("RFCCHAR4", "hugo");
importStructure.SetValue("RFCINT4", -4367283);
importStructure.SetValue("RFCHEX3", new byte[3]{1, 2, 3});
importStructure.SetValue("RFCCHAR2", "äö");
importStructure.SetValue("RFCTIME", DateTime.Now);
importStructure.SetValue("RFCDATE",
                         new DateTime(1685, 3, 31));
// Funktionsbaustein aufrufen
function.Invoke(destination);
// Exportstruktur lesen und ausgeben
IRfcStructure echoStructure = function.GetStructure
                                          ("ECHOSTRUCT");
Console.WriteLine(
 "RFCFLOAT:\t{0}", echoStructure.GetString("RFCFLOAT")
);
Console.WriteLine(
 "RFCCHAR1:\t{0}", echoStructure.GetString("RFCCHAR1"));
Console.WriteLine(
 "RFCINT2:\t{0}", echoStructure.GetString("RFCINT2"));
...
```

Listing 6.7 RFC-Client mit Strukturparametern

Zunächst setzt der Client die Destinationsdaten und besorgt sich dann ein IRfcFunction-Objekt für den Funktionsbaustein. Über dieses Objekt holt er sich das IRfcStructure-Objekt importStructure für den Importparameter IMPORTSTRUCT des Funktionsbausteins. Er füllt die Komponenten dieser Importstruktur und ruft dann den Funktionsbaustein auf. Anschließend besorgt er sich das IRfcStructure-Objekt echoStructure für den Exportparameter EXPORTSTRUCT und gibt dessen Komponenten aus.

»IRfcField«

Auch hier bietet Ihnen der NCo einen alternativen Zugriff auf die Komponenten einer Struktur. Die Schnittstelle IRfcStructure definiert einen string- und einen int-Indexer zum Zugriff auf die Komponenten der Struktur über eine IRfcField-Schnittstelle. Damit können Sie eine foreach-Schleife über alle Komponenten einer Struktur realisieren, wie in Listing 6.8 gezeigt:

```
foreach (IRfcField field in echoStructure)
{
  Console.WriteLine("{0}: {1}",
    field.Metadata.Name,
    field.GetString());
}
```

Listing 6.8 Schleife über alle Komponenten einer Struktur

Die Schnittstelle IRfcField umfasst die Schnittstelle IRfcElement, die die Methoden SetValue, GetValue und GetXXX definiert, nun jedoch ohne den ersten Parameter zur Identifikation der Strukturkomponente. Den Code zum Schreiben und Lesen der Komponenten in Listing 6.7 könnten Sie alternativ also auch so wie in Listing 6.9 schreiben:

```
importStructure["RFCFLOAT"].SetValue(17.0932);
...
rfcFunction.Invoke(destination);
IRfcStructure echoStructure = function.GetStructure
                                        ("ECHOSTRUCT");
Console.WriteLine(
  "RFCFLOAT: {0}",
  echoStructure["RFCFLOAT"].GetValue());
...
```

Listing 6.9 Verwendung des String-Indexers und der »IRfcField«-Schnittstelle

Performance-unterschied

Beide Alternativen liefern zwar genau dasselbe Ergebnis, die zweite Alternative ist jedoch langsamer, denn das IRfcField-Objekt wird bei jeder Anfrage neu erzeugt, da Strukturen ihre Komponenten direkt als Array von System.Object-Objekten speichern. Funktionsbausteine speichern ihre Parameter jedoch als Array von IRfcParameter-Objekten.

6.2.6 Tabellenparameter

»GetTable«

Listing 6.10 zeigt einen RFC-Client mit Tabellenparametern. Nachdem der Client die Destinationsparameter gesetzt und sich die Metadaten für den Funktionsbaustein STFC_STRUCTURE besorgt hat, greift er mit der Methode GetTable()auf eine IRfcTable-Schnittstelle für den Tabellenparameter RFCTABLE des Funktionsbausteins zu.

```
// Destination beschaffen
RfcDestination destination =
  fcDestinationManager.GetDestination("NCO_TESTS");
// Metadaten beschaffen
IRfcFunction function =
  destination.Repository.CreateFunction("STFC_STRUCTURE");
// Tabelle beschaffen
IRfcTable table = function.GetTable("RFCTABLE");
// Zeilen anhängen
table.Append(3);
// Zeilen/Spalten füllen
for (int i=0; i<table.Count; ++i)
{
  table.CurrentIndex = i;
  table.SetValue(3, i);
}
// Zeilen einfügen
table.CurrentIndex = 1;
table.Insert(2);
for (int i=0; i<2; ++i)
{
  table.CurrentIndex = i;
  table.SetValue(3, -i);
}
// Zeilen löschen
table.CurrentIndex = 1;
table.Delete(2);
// Tabelle ausgeben
for(int i=0; i< table.RowCount; ++i)
{
    table.CurrentIndex = i;
```

```
    Console.WriteLine(
      "Zeile {0}: {1}", i,
      table.GetValue("RFCINT1"));
}
// Tabelle ausgeben, Alternative
foreach(IRfcStructure rfcStructure in table)
{
  Console.WriteLine();
  foreach(IRfcField rfcField in rfcStructure)
  {
    Console.Write("{0}/t", rfcField.GetValue();
  }
}
```


Listing 6.10 RFC-Client mit Tabellenparametern

»Append« Danach hängt der RFC-Client mit der Methode `Append()` drei neue Zeilen an diese Tabelle an. Die Eigenschaft `RowCount` des Tabellenobjekts hat nun ebenso wie die Eigenschaft `Count` den Wert »3«.

»CurrentIndex« Anschließend füllt der Client die vierte Spalte jeder Zeile – d. h. die Spalte mit dem Index »3« – in einer `for`-Schleife mit dem Wert des Schleifenzählers. Dazu setzt der Client innerhalb der Schleife zuerst die Eigenschaft `CurrentIndex` auf den Wert des Schleifenzählers. `CurrentIndex` ist ein Cursor, der auf eine bestimmte Zeile der Tabelle zeigt. Nun kann der Client mit dem `table`-Objekt genauso arbeiten wie mit einer Struktur, da die Schnittstelle `IRfcTable` genau wie die Schnittstelle `IRfcStructure` die Schnittstelle `IRfc-DataContainer` umfasst. Über die Methoden dieser Schnittstelle, der Sie nun schon zum dritten Mal begegnen, können Sie auf die Spalten der aktuellen Zeile zugreifen. Ein Blick ins ABAP Dictionary zeigt, dass die vierte Spalte `RFCINT1` heißt.

»CurrentRow« Anstatt über das `IRfcTable`-Objekt mit der aktuellen Zeile der Tabelle zu arbeiten, können Sie auch über die Eigenschaft `CurrentRow` auf die Schnittstelle `IRfcStructure` der aktuellen Zeile zugreifen. Unter Umständen wird Ihr Code dann besser lesbar.

»Insert« Anstatt mit `Append()` neue Zeilen hinten an die Tabelle anzuhängen, können Sie auch mit `Insert()`neue Zeilen anstelle der aktuellen Zeile einfügen. Die aktuelle Zeile und alle nachfolgenden Zeilen werden dabei hinter die neu eingefügten Zeilen verschoben.

»Clear« und »Delete« Mit `Clear()` entfernen Sie alle Zeilen der Tabelle, mit `Delete()` die aktuelle Zeile. Wenn Sie der Methode `Delete()` noch einen `int`-Parameter mitgeben, werden mehrere Zeilen gelöscht.

Die Schnittstelle `IRfcTable` definiert auch einen `int`-Indexer, mit dem Sie eine einfache `foreach`-Schleife über alle Zeilen der internen Tabelle realisieren oder auch direkt auf eine bestimmte Tabellenzeile zugreifen können. Wenn Sie über diesen Indexer zugreifen, wird die Eigenschaft `CurrentIndex` nicht geändert. Der Client in Listing 6.10 verwendet diesen Indexer am Schluss, um alle Zeilen der internen Tabelle auszugeben.

6.2.7 Ausnahmebehandlung

»Invoke()«

Bislang haben wir uns im vorgestellten Client-Code nicht um Ausnahmen gekümmert. In produktiven Programmen sollten Sie das aber auf alle Fälle tun und die `Invoke()`-Methode in einen `try`-Block mit entsprechenden `catch`-Blöcken einbetten, wie wir es in Listing 6.11 zeigen.

```
try
{
  rfcFunction.Invoke(destination);
}
catch (RfcCommunicationException communicationException)
{
    Console.WriteLine(
      "RfcCommunicationException abgefangen: {0}",
      communicationException.Message);
}
catch (RfcLogonException logonException)
{
  Console.WriteLine(
    "RfcLogonException abgefangen: {0}",
    logonException.PlainText);
}
catch (RfcAbapRuntimeException abapRuntimeException)
{
  Console.WriteLine(
    "RfcAbapRuntimeException abgefangen: {0}",
    abapRuntimeException.PlainText);
}
catch (RfcAbapClassException abapClassException)
{
  Console.WriteLine(
    "RfcAbapClassException abgefangen: {0}",
    abapClassException.PlainText);
  foreach (IRfcAttribute attribute in
             abapClassException.ExceptionObject)
```

```
  {
    Console.WriteLine(
      "Attribut {0} = {1}",
      attribute.Metadata.Name,
      attribute.GetValue());
  }
}
catch (RfcAbapException abapException)
{
  Console.WriteLine(
    "RfcAbapException abgefangen: {0}",
    abapException.Key);
  Console.WriteLine(
     "Nachrichtenparameter:\n" +
     "SY-MSGTY={0}\n" +
     "SY-MSGID={1}\n" +
     "SY-MSGNO={2}\n" +
     "SY-MSGV1={3}",
     abapException.AbapMessageType,
     abapException.AbapMessageClass,
     abapException.AbapMessageNumber,
     abapException.AbapMessageParameters[0]);
}
catch (RfcAbapMessageException abapMessageException)
{
  Console.WriteLine(
    "RfcAbapMessageException abgefangen: {0}",
    abapMessageException.Key);
  Console.WriteLine(
    "Nachrichtenparameter:\n" +
    "SY-MSGTY={0}\n" +
    "SY-MSGID={1}\n" +
    "SY-MSGNO={2}\n" +
    "SY-MSGV1={3}",
    abapMessageException.AbapMessageType,
    abapMessageException.AbapMessageClass,
    abapMessageException.AbapMessageNumber,
    abapMessageException.AbapMessageParameters[0]);
}
```

Listing 6.11 Ausnahmebehandlung

Allgemeine Ausnahmen

Die drei Ausnahmen RfcCommunicationException, RfcLogonException und RfcAbapRuntimeException sollten Sie immer behandeln, da diese drei Probleme unabhängig vom aufgerufenen Funktionsbaustein auftreten können. In Listing 6.11 sind dies die ersten drei catch-Blöcke.

RfcCommunicationException wird ausgelöst, wenn der SAP NetWeaver Application Server nicht erreicht werden kann. RfcLogonException wird ausgelöst, wenn es ein Problem bei der Anmeldung gibt, etwa weil der Benutzer gesperrt oder das Passwort ungültig ist. Eine RfcAbapRuntimeException tritt auf, wenn es ein grundlegendes Problem auf dem Server gibt – z. B. ein Timeout des ABAP-Workprozesses oder eine Division durch null.

Außer diesen Auslösern kann auch der aufgerufene Funktionsbaustein eine Ausnahme auslösen. Dies kann entweder eine klassische Ausnahme oder eine klassenbasierte Ausnahme sein. In beiden Fällen deklariert der Funktionsbaustein die Ausnahmen, die er auslösen kann, auf der Registerkarte **Exceptions** seiner Schnittstellendefinition.

Klassenbasierte Ausnahmen

Will ein Funktionsbaustein klassenbasierte Ausnahmen auslösen, definiert er auf der Registerkarte **Exceptions** die Namen der ABAP-Ausnahmeklassen, die er verwendet. Eine klassenbasierte Ausnahme wird vom NCo durch ein Objekt der Klasse RfcAbapClassException repräsentiert. Dieses Exception-Objekt hat die Eigenschaft ExceptionObject vom Typ IRfcAbapObject. Diese Schnittstelle ist neben IRfcFunction, IRfcStructure und IRfcTable die vierte Schnittstelle, die die Schnittstelle IRfcDataContainer umfasst. Über die Methoden GetValue und GetXXX dieser Schnittstelle erhalten Sie Zugriff auf die Namen und Inhalte von Attributen des ABAP-Ausnahmeobjekts, die möglicherweise noch genauere Informationen zu den ausgelösten Ausnahmen enthalten. Der vierte catch-Block in Listing 6.11 zeigt eine Schleife über diese Attribute.

Die Klasse RfcAbapClassException ist eine Unterklasse von RfcAbapBaseException. Diese Klasse umfasst die Eigenschaft PlainText, die eine Fehlerbeschreibung enthält.

Klassische Ausnahmen

Wenn der Funktionsbaustein klassische Ausnahmen auslösen will, deklariert er auf der Registerkarte **Exceptions** symbolische Namen für die Ausnahmen. Der Funktionsbaustein löst eine klassische Ausnahme namens EXCEPTION_NAME mit der ABAP-Anweisung RAISE EXCEPTION_NAME aus. Der Client sieht diese Ausnahme als RfcAbapException. Verwendet der Funktionsbaustein die MESSAGE-Anweisung mit dem Zusatz RAISING EXCEPTION_NAME, wird clientseitig eine RfcAbapMessageException ausgelöst.

Beide Exceptions sind von RfcAbapClassicException abgeleitet – wie übrigens auch die beiden Klassen RfcLogonException und RfcAbapRuntimeException. Über die Eigenschaften Key, AbapMessageClass, AbapMessageNumber, AbapMessageParameters und AbapMessageType dieser Basisklasse haben Sie Zugriff auf den Ausnahmennamen, die Nachrichtenklasse, die Nachrichtennummer, die Nachrichtenparameter und den Nachrichtentyp. Die beiden letzten catch-Blöcke in Listing 6.11 zeigen den Zugriff auf diese Felder.

Sowohl RfcAbapClassException als auch RfcAbapClassicException sind Unterklassen von RfcAbapBaseException, sodass Sie die Fehlerbeschreibung über die Eigenschaft PlainText erhalten. Die Basisklasse der Ausnahmeklassen RfcAbapBaseException und RfcCommunicationException ist die Klasse RfcBaseException, die wiederum von System.ApplicationException abgeleitet ist. Abbildung 6.3 zeigt die Klassenhierarchie der Ausnahmen im Überblick.

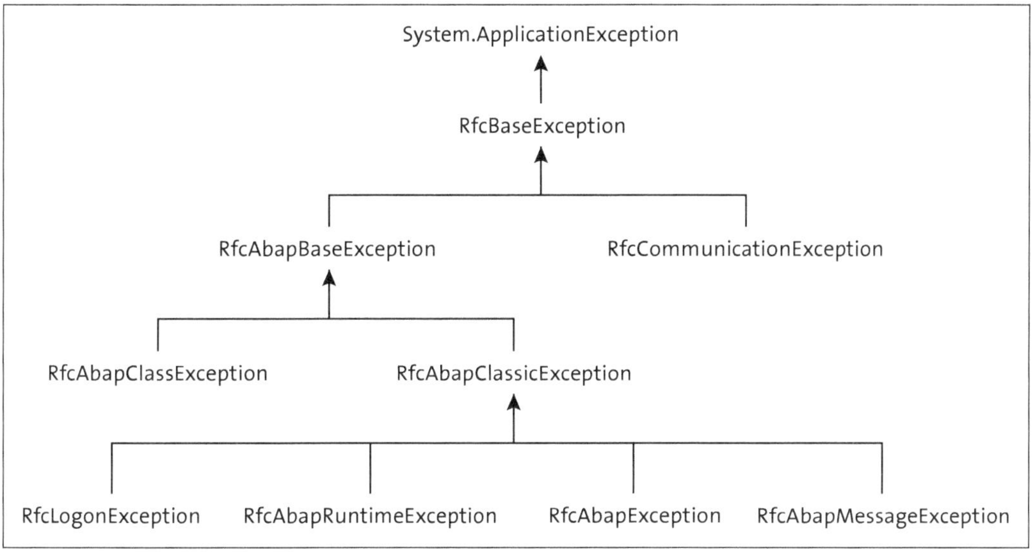

Abbildung 6.3 Klassenhierarchie der Ausnahmen

6.3 Komplexe RFC-Clients

In diesem Abschnitt lernen Sie komplexere RFC-Clients kennen. Sie erfahren im Detail, wie Sie RFC-Sessions verwalten und tRFCs, qRFCs und bgRFCs verwenden.

6.3.1 Aufruf von BAPIs und Session-Management

Mit den bisher gezeigten Techniken können Sie auch BAPIs aufrufen: Dabei müssen Sie die Implementierungsregeln für BAPIs aus Abschnitt 3.5.2, »Entwicklung von BAPIs«, beachten. Insbesondere müssen Sie, wenn Sie schreibende oder ändernde BAPIs aufrufen, nach dem Aufruf des eigentlichen BAPIs zusätzlich noch `BAPI_TRANSACTION_COMMIT` aufrufen.

Die Aufrufe der beiden Funktionsbausteine müssen innerhalb derselben Benutzersitzung erfolgen. Dies stellt eine besondere Herausforderung dar, da der NCo innerhalb der `Invoke`-Methode nach dem Aufruf des Funktionsbausteins den Benutzerkontext auf der ABAP-Seite zurücksetzt, bevor er die verwendete Verbindung wieder an den Verbindungspool der Destination zurückgibt. Wenn Sie zustandslose Funktionsbausteine aufrufen, ist dieses Verhalten des NCo ideal; doch schreibende BAPIs sind eben nicht zustandslos. Daher müssen Sie dem .NET Connector Session Manager mitteilen, dass Sie eine bestimmte Verbindung für eine Reihe von aufeinanderfolgenden Aufrufen verwenden wollen, ohne dass der Benutzerkontext auf der ABAP-Seite zurückgesetzt wird.

»BeginContext« Dazu rufen Sie vor dem ersten `Invoke` die Methode `BeginContext` der Klasse `RfcSessionManager` auf und übergeben dieser Methode das Destinationsobjekt, über das die nachfolgenden Funktionsbausteinaufrufe erfolgen sollen. Dies verknüpft eine Verbindung aus dem Verbindungspool mit dem momentan ausgeführten Thread für dessen exklusive Verwendung.

Bei den nachfolgenden Aufrufen von `Invoke` wird zuerst geprüft, ob eine Verbindung an den aktuellen Thread gebunden ist. Falls ja, verwenden die Aufrufe diese Verbindung und setzen nach dem Aufruf den Benutzerkontext dieser Verbindung auch nicht wieder zurück.

»EndContext« Damit die Verbindung wieder vom Thread gelöst wird, rufen Sie anschließend die Methode `EndContext` der Klasse `RfcManager` auf. Diese Methode löst die Verbindung vom aktuellen Thread und setzt den Benutzerkontext zurück.

Listing 6.12 zeigt dies für den Aufruf des BAPIs `Order.CreateFromData`. Der Client füllt die Exportparameter mit den Bestelldaten für den Aufruf des Funktionsbausteins `Z_BAPI_ORDER_CREATEFROMDATA`. Danach öffnet er mit `BeginContext` einen Aufrufkontext. Innerhalb eines `try`-Blocks ruft der Client den Funktionsbaustein auf und überprüft anschließend den Importparameter `RETURN`. Dieser ist eine interne Tabelle vom Zeilentyp `BAPIRET2`. Falls kein Fehler aufgetreten ist, ruft er den Funktionsbaustein `BAPI_TRANSACTION_COMMIT` auf. Der Aufrufkontext wird im `finally`-Block mit `EndContext` wieder geschlossen. Durch die Platzierung im `finally`-Block stellen Sie sicher, dass der Kontext auch dann geschlossen wird, wenn innerhalb des `try`-Blocks eine Ausnahme aufgetreten ist.

```
// Destination beschaffen
RfcDestination destination =
  RfcDestinationManager.GetDestination("NCO_TESTS");
// Metadaten lesen
IRfcFunction bapiOrderCreate, bapiTransactionCommit;
try
{
    bapiOrderCreate =
      destination.Repository.CreateFunction(
        "Z_BAPI_ORDER_CREATEFROMDATA");
    bapiTransactionCommit =
      destination.Repository.CreateFunction(
        "BAPI_TRANSACTION_COMMIT");
}
catch (RfcBaseException ex)
{
    Console.WriteLine(
      "\nMetadaten konnten nicht geladen werden ({0})",
      ex.Message);
    return;
}
// Bestellkopf füllen
IRfcStructure imOrderHeader =
  bapiOrderCreate.GetStructure("IM_ORDERHEADER");
imOrderHeader.SetValue("MANDT", "001");
imOrderHeader.SetValue("ORDERID", "0000000001");
imOrderHeader.SetValue("TYPE", "SO");
imOrderHeader.SetValue("REFID", "0000000001");
imOrderHeader.SetValue("BUYER", "Buchhandlung Pehnke");
imOrderHeader.SetValue("SELLER", "Großhandel Englbrecht");
imOrderHeader.SetValue("ORDERDATE", System.DateTime.Now);
// Bestellpositionen füllen
IRfcTable imOrderPositions =
  bapiOrderCreate.GetTable("ORDERPOS");
imOrderPositions.Append();
imOrderPositions.SetValue("MANDT", "001");
imOrderPositions.SetValue("ORDERID", "0000000001");
imOrderPositions.SetValue("ORDERPOS", "00001");
imOrderPositions.SetValue("MATID", "4711");
imOrderPositions.SetValue("MATTEXT", "ABAP für Anfänger");
imOrderPositions.SetValue("ORDERCOUNT", 2);
imOrderPositions.SetValue("PRICE", 69.90);
imOrderPositions.SetValue("CURRENCY", "EUR");
```

```
// Aufrufkontext öffnen
RfcSessionManager.BeginContext(destination);
try
{
    // BAPI aufrufen
    bapiOrderCreate.Invoke(destination);
    // Tabellenparameter RETURN ausgeben
    IRfcTable exReturn = bapiOrderCreate.GetTable("RETURN");
    foreach (IRfcStructure exReturnLine in exReturn)
    {
        Console.WriteLine(
          "TYPE: {0}. MESSAGE: {1}",
          exReturnLine.GetValue("TYPE"),
          exReturnLine.GetValue("MESSAGE"));
    }
    // Bestellnummer ORDERID ausgeben
    Console.WriteLine(
      "Bestellnummer {0}",
      bapiOrderCreate.GetValue("ORDERID"));
    // BAPI_TRANSACTION_COMMIT aufrufen
    bapiTransactionCommit.Invoke(destination);
}
Finally
{
    // Aufrufkontext schließen
    RfcSessionManager.EndContext(destination);
}
```

Listing 6.12 Öffnen und Schließen eines Aufrufkontextes

Standardmäßig bindet also die Methode `BeginContext` eine Verbindung aus dem Verbindungspool an den aktuell ausgeführten Thread. Sie können dieses Verhalten jedoch ändern und die Verbindung mit einer beliebigen ID assoziieren, z. B. mit der Session-ID einer HTTP-Session innerhalb eines Webservers.

»ISessionProvider«

Dazu müssen Sie eine Klasse bereitstellen, die die Schnittstelle `ISessionProvider` implementiert, und ein Objekt dieser Klasse mit der Methode `RegisterSessionProvider` der Klasse `RfcSessionManager` registrieren.

Dadurch wird innerhalb von `BeginContext` die Methode `GetCurrentSession()` von `ISessionProvider` aufgerufen. In dieser Methode können Sie einen beliebigen String zurückgeben, der die HTTP-Session eindeutig identifiziert. Der NCo holt sich eine freie Verbindung aus dem Verbindungspool und assoziiert diese mit der Session-ID. Innerhalb der Methode `Invoke()` wird nun ebenfalls mit `GetCurrentSession()` nach der aktuellen Session-ID gefragt und die RFC-Verbindung verwendet, die mit der aktuellen Session-ID assoziiert ist.

6.3.2 Transaktionaler RFC

Wie in Abschnitt 3.2, »Transaktionaler RFC«, besprochen, sollten Sie ändernde Funktionsbausteine über einen transaktionalen RFC (tRFC) aufrufen. Beim tRFC müssen Sie zusätzlich zu den Importparametern des Funktionsbausteins eine Transaktions-ID (TID) übergeben.

Wiederholung im Fehlerfall

Im Fehlerfall können Sie den Aufruf dann mit denselben Daten und derselben TID beliebig oft wiederholen. Aufgrund des in Abschnitt 1.2, »Sicherheit«, beschriebenen Mechanismus können Sie sicher sein, dass die Daten genau einmal verarbeitet werden.

Klasse »RfcTId«

Der NCo repräsentiert TIDs als Instanzen der Klasse `RfcTID`. Diese Klasse hat die Eigenschaft `TID`, die die Transaktions-ID als String repräsentiert, sowie die Eigenschaft `GUID`, die die Transaktions-ID als *Globally Unique Identifier* (GUID) repräsentiert. Die Klasse `RfcTID` hat dementsprechend drei Konstruktoren: Der parameterlose Konstruktor `RfcTID()` erzeugt eine völlig neue TID. Die beiden anderen Konstruktoren – `RfcTID(Guid)` und `RfcTID(string)` – rekonstruieren eine vorher schon einmal erzeugte TID aus deren Repräsentation als GUID bzw. als String.

Klasse »RfcTransaction«

Innerhalb einer Transaktion, die durch eine TID identifiziert wird, können Sie nicht nur einen, sondern beliebig viele Funktionsbausteine aufrufen. Der NCo repräsentiert eine Transaktion durch ein Objekt der Klasse `RfcTransaction`. Auf die TID dieser Transaktion können Sie über die Eigenschaft `TID` zugreifen.

Die Klasse `RfcTransaction` hat mehrere Konstruktoren. Der parameterlose Konstruktor `RfcTransaction()` erzeugt eine völlig neue TID für die Transaktion, während der Konstruktor `RfcTransaction (RfcTID)` eine zuvor rekonstruierte TID wiederverwendet.

Funktionsbaustein mit tRFC aufrufen

Wenn Sie einen Funktionsbaustein mit tRFC aufrufen wollen, gehen Sie folgendermaßen vor:

1. Sie erzeugen eine neue Transaktion mit dem parameterlosen Konstruktor `RfcTransaction()`.
2. Sie speichern die TID und die zu sendenden Daten zusammen mit der TID.
3. Sie füllen die Importparameter der zu rufenden Funktionen.

4. Sie fügen diese Funktionsobjekte zur Transaktion hinzu, indem Sie die Methode `AddFunction(IRfcFunction)` aufrufen.
5. Sie übermitteln die Transaktion an das SAP-System, indem Sie die Methode `Commit(RfcDestination)` aufrufen.

Falls der Commit-Aufruf erfolgreich war, können Sie die vorher gespeicherte TID und die dazugehörigen Daten löschen und dem SAP-System mitteilen, dass die TID nicht länger benötigt wird. Dazu rufen Sie die Methode `ConfirmTransactionID(RfcTID)` des Destinationsobjekts auf.

Falls die `Commit()`-Methode eine Ausnahme auslöst – z. B. wegen eines Netzwerkfehlers –, können Sie die Transaktion nochmals ausführen, sobald Sie den Fehler behoben haben. Dabei gehen Sie genauso vor wie zuvor beschrieben. Allerdings verwenden Sie nun den Konstruktor `RfcTransaction(RfcTID)` und übergeben diesem Konstruktor die alte TID. Sie müssen natürlich auch darauf achten, dass Sie die Importparameter der Funktionsbausteine mit genau denselben Daten füllen. Zu diesem Zweck haben Sie ja die TID und die Daten gespeichert.

tRFC-Client

Sie sind also für das Destinationsmanagement selbst verantwortlich. In Listing 6.13 zeigen wir Ihnen einen tRFC-Client, der über Aufrufe des Funktionsbausteins `Z_IFP_ORDER_CREATE` eine Kundenbestellung in ein SAP-System schreibt.

```
using System;
using System.IO;
using System.Linq;
using SAP.Middleware.Connector;
namespace IFPCSharp.TrfcClient
{
  class Program
  {
    static void Main(string[] args)
    {
      DestinationConfiguration destConfig =
        new DestinationConfiguration();
      RfcDestinationManager.
        RegisterDestinationConfiguration(
          destConfig);
      TidStore tidStore =
        new TidStore("clientTidStore", false);
      bool quit = false;
      try
      {
```

```
    while (!quit)
    {
      Console.Write("Neue Transaktion, alte Transaktion
                    oder beenden? [n/a/b] ");
      String answer = Console.ReadLine().ToLower();
      switch (answer)
      {
        case "n":
          SendNewTransaction(tidStore);
          break;
        case "a":
          ResendOldTransaction(tidStore);
          break;
        default:
          quit = true;
          break;
      }
    }
  }
  finally
  {
    tidStore.Close();
    RfcDestinationManager.
      UnregisterDestinationConfiguration(destConfig);
  }
}
static void SendNewTransaction(TidStore tidStore)
{
  Console.Write("Dateiname der Bestellung? ");
  string dataFileName = Console.ReadLine();
  IRfcFunction orderCreateFunction =
    PrepareFunction(dataFileName);
  // neue Transaktion mit neuer TID erzeugen
  RfcTransaction trans = new RfcTransaction();
  // Daten und neue TID speichern
  File.Copy(dataFileName, trans.Tid.TID);
  tidStore.CreateEntry(trans.Tid.TID);
  // Funktion mit Daten zur Transaktion hinzufügen
  trans.AddFunction(orderCreateFunction);
  // Destination besorgen und Transaktion abschicken
  try
  {
    RfcDestination dest = RfcDestinationManager.
```

6

```
    GetDestination("NCO_ASHOST");
   trans.Commit(dest);
   // TID-Status auf Commited setzen
   tidStore.SetStatus(trans.Tid.TID,
     TidStatus.Committed, null);
   // Wenn bis hierhin kein Fehler auftrat:
   // Transaktion bestätigen und Daten löschen.
   dest.ConfirmTransactionID(trans.Tid);
   File.Delete(trans.Tid.TID);
   tidStore.DeleteEntry(trans.Tid.TID);
  }
  catch (Exception e)
  {
   // TID-Status auf RolledBack setzen
   tidStore.SetStatus(trans.Tid.TID,
     TidStatus.RolledBack, e.Message);
  }
}
static void ResendOldTransaction(TidStore tidStore)
{
  if (tidStore.Size == 0)
  {
   Console.WriteLine("Es gibt keine alten TIDs ...");
   return;
  }
  // eine TID auswählen
  tidStore.PrintOverview();
  string tid = ChooseTid(tidStore);
  if (string.IsNullOrEmpty(tid))
  {
   Console.WriteLine("Die TID existiert nicht.");
   return;
  }
  // alte Daten einlesen
  IRfcFunction orderCreateFunction =
   PrepareFunction(tid);
  // neue Transaktion mit alter TID erzeugen
  RfcTransaction trans =
   new RfcTransaction(new RfcTID(tid));
  // Funktion mit Daten zur Transaktion hinzufügen
  trans.AddFunction(orderCreateFunction);
  // Destination besorgen und Transaktion abschicken
  try
```

```
  {
    RfcDestination dest = RfcDestinationManager.
      GetDestination("NCO_ASHOST");
    trans.Commit(dest);
    // TID-Status auf Commited setzen
    tidStore.SetStatus(trans.Tid.TID,
      TidStatus.Committed, null);
    // Wenn bis hierhin kein Fehler auftrat:
    // Transaktion bestätigen und Daten löschen.
    dest.ConfirmTransactionID(trans.Tid);
    File.Delete(trans.Tid.TID);
    tidStore.DeleteEntry(trans.Tid.TID);
  }
  catch (Exception e)
  {
    // TID-Status auf RolledBack setzen
    tidStore.SetStatus(trans.Tid.TID,
      TidStatus.RolledBack, e.Message);
  }
}
static IRfcFunction PrepareFunction(string dataFileName)
{
  // Metadaten lesen
  RfcDestination dest = RfcDestinationManager.
    GetDestination("NCO_MSERVER");
  IRfcFunction orderCreateFunction =
    dest.Repository.CreateFunction(
      "Z_IFP_ORDER_CREATE");
  // Datei öffnen
  FileStream dataFile = new FileStream(
    dataFileName, FileMode.Open, FileAccess.Read);
  StreamReader reader = new StreamReader(dataFile);
  // Bestellkopf lesen und füllen
  IRfcStructure header =
    orderCreateFunction.GetStructure("IM_ORDERHEADER");
  string line = reader.ReadLine();
  string[] fields = line.Split(new char[] { ';' });
  for(int i=0; i< fields.Count(); i++)
    header.SetValue(i, fields[i]);
  // Bestellpositionen lesen und füllen
  IRfcTable positions =
    orderCreateFunction.GetTable("TA_ORDERPOS");
  while (!reader.EndOfStream)
```

```
        {
          line = reader.ReadLine();
          positions.Append();
          fields = line.Split(new char[] { ';' });
          for (int i = 0; i < fields.Count(); i++)
            positions.SetValue(i, fields[i]);
        }
        dataFile.Close();
        return orderCreateFunction;
      }
      private static string ChooseTid(TidStore tidStore)
      {
        Console.Write("Bitte vorhandene TID auswählen: ");
        string tid = Console.ReadLine();
        try
        {
          // sicherstellen, dass die TID tatsächlich existiert
          string errorMessage = "";
          tidStore.GetStatus(tid, out errorMessage);
        }
        catch (ArgumentException)
        {
          tid = "";
        }
        return tid;
      }
    }
  }
```

Listing 6.13 Beispiel für einen tRFC-Client

Das Programm instanziiert in der Methode `Main()` zunächst eine Instanz der Klasse `DestinationConfiguration` und registriert diese beim `RfcDestinationManager`. Danach instanziiert sie eine Instanz der Klasse `TidStore`, die die TIDs in der Datei **clientTidStore** verwaltet. Den Code für diese Klasse schauen wir uns später an. Schließlich fragt die Methode, ob eine neue Bestellung in einer neuen Transaktion an den Applikationsserver geschickt oder ob eine zuvor fehlgeschlagene Transaktion wiederholt werden soll. Im ersten Fall wird die Methode `SendNewTransaction()` aufgerufen, im zweiten Fall die Methode `ResendOldTransaction()`.

Neue Transaktion

Die Methode `SendNewTransaction()` fragt zunächst nach dem Namen der Datei, in der die neue Bestellung zu finden ist. In dieser Datei sollten der Bestellkopf und jede Bestellposition in einer Zeile stehen und die Felder der Zeile durch Semikolon getrennt sein. Listing zeigt ein Beispiel für solch eine Datei. In der Methode `PrepareFunction()` wird diese Datei gelesen, und die Importparameter eines `IRfcFunction`-Objekts für den Funktionsbaustein `Z_IFP_ORDER_CREATE` werden mit den Bestelldaten aus dieser Datei gefüllt. Danach erzeugt die Methode `SendNewTransaction()` eine neue Transaktion und speichert die Bestelldaten in einer neuen Datei mit dem Namen der neuen TID. Im `TidStore` wir ein neuer Eintrag für die TID mit dem Status **Created** erzeugt. Nun wird das `IRfcFunction`-Objekt der Transaktion hinzugefügt, eine Destination besorgt und die Transaktion mit `Commit()` an den Applikationsserver geschickt. Falls bis hierhin keine Fehler aufgetreten sind, wird der Status der TID im `TidStore` auf `Commited` gesetzt.

```
001;0000000001;SO;0000000001; Englbrecht;Pflugrad;2024-02-14
001;0000000001;00001;4711;Das neue ABAP-Kochbuch;3;89.90;EUR
001;0000000001;00002;4712;SAP-Schnittstellen;7;89.90;EUR
```

Listing 6.14 Kommaseparierte Datei mit einer Bestellung

Danach wird die Transaktion beim Applikationsserver mit `ConfirmTransaction()` bestätigt, die Datei mit den zwischengespeicherten Bestelldaten gelöscht und die TID aus dem `TidStore` entfernt. Falls beim `Commit()` eine Ausnahme auftrat, wird im `catch`-Block der Status der TID im `TidStore` auf `RolledBack` gesetzt. Die zwischengespeicherte Datei wird in diesem Fall nicht gelöscht.

Transaktion wiederholen

Falls der Benutzer in der `Main()`-Methode des Programms angibt, dass er eine alte Transaktion nochmals senden will, wird die Methode `ResendOldTransaction()` ausgeführt. Diese Methode listet zuerst den Inhalt des `TidStore` auf und bittet den Benutzer um die Eingabe einer alten TID. Danach wird eine neue Transaktion mit der alten TID erzeugt und das `IRfcFunction`-Objekt aus der Datei mit dem Namen der alten TID gefüllt. Der Rest der Methode läuft genauso ab wie die Methode `SendNewTransaction()`.

Fehler simulieren

Damit Fehler simuliert werden können, verwendet der Client für das Lesen der Metadaten eine andere Destination als für die Übermittlung der Transaktion. Sie können so z. B. falsche Logon-Daten für die Übermittlungsdestination angeben und auf diese Weise das TID-Management für fehlgeschlagene Transaktionen testen. Listing 6.15 zeigt die Klasse `TidStore` für das TID-Management.

```
using System;
using System.Collections.Generic;
using System.IO;
```

```
using System.Text;
namespace IFPCSharp
{
  public enum TidStatus : byte
  {
    Created = 1,
    Executed,
    Committed,
    RolledBack,
    Confirmed
  };
  class StoreEntry
  {
    internal String tid;
    internal TidStatus status;
    internal int index;
  };
  public class TidStore
  {
    const int REMAINDER_SIZE = 80;
    const int TID_SIZE = 24;
    const int GUID_SIZE = 32;
    static char[] EMPTY_REMAINDER =
      new char[REMAINDER_SIZE];
    readonly int entrySize, idSize;
    readonly char[] empty_id;
    FileStream fs;
    BinaryReader br;
    BinaryWriter bw;
    Dictionary<String, StoreEntry> table;
    Stack<StoreEntry> freeEntries = new Stack<StoreEntry>();
    int slots;
    // Öffnet einen bestehenden TidStore oder erzeugt
    // einen neuen, falls die Datei noch nicht existiert.
    public TidStore(String fileName, bool bgRFC)
    {
      idSize = bgRFC ? GUID_SIZE : TID_SIZE;
      entrySize = idSize + REMAINDER_SIZE;
      empty_id = new char[idSize];
      if (string.IsNullOrEmpty(fileName))
        fileName = "TIDStore.tid";
      try
      {
```

```
    fs = new FileStream(fileName, FileMode.OpenOrCreate,
      FileAccess.ReadWrite);
    br = new BinaryReader(fs);
    bw = new BinaryWriter(fs);
    if (fs.Length < entrySize)
    // Neue leere Store-Datei
    {
      slots = 0;
      bw.Seek(0, SeekOrigin.Begin);
      bw.Write(slots);
      bw.Flush();
    }
    else
    {
      br.BaseStream.Seek(0, SeekOrigin.Begin);
      slots = br.ReadInt32();
    }
    table = new Dictionary<String, StoreEntry>();
    for (int i = 0; i < slots; ++i)
    {
      StoreEntry entry = new StoreEntry();
      entry.index = (int)fs.Position;
      // TID/UID lesen
      char[] tempId = br.ReadChars(idSize);
      if (tempId == null || tempId.Length != idSize)
        throw new IOException(
          "Eintrag an Position " + i + "nicht lesbar.");
      // Status lesen
      entry.status = (TidStatus)br.ReadByte();
      // REMAINDER überspringen
      br.BaseStream.Seek(REMAINDER_SIZE,
       SeekOrigin.Current);
      if (tempId[0] == 0)
      {
        freeEntries.Push(entry);
      }
      else
      {
        entry.tid = new String(tempId);
        table[entry.tid] = entry;
      }
    }
  }
```

```
  catch (Exception)
  {
    if (fs != null)
      fs.Close();
    br = null;
    bw = null;
    throw;
  }
}
public void Close()
{
  lock (this)
  {
    try
    {
      if (fs != null)
        fs.Close();
    }
    catch (Exception) { }
    freeEntries.Clear();
    table.Clear();
  }
}
public TidStatus CreateEntry(String tid)
{
  lock (this)
  {
    if (tid == null || tid.Length != idSize)
      throw new ArgumentException("Invalid TID");
    StoreEntry entry = null;
    table.TryGetValue(tid, out entry);
    if (entry != null)
      return entry.status;
    if (freeEntries.Count > 0)
    {
      entry = freeEntries.Pop();
    }
    else
    {
      entry = new StoreEntry();
      entry.index = (int)fs.Length;
      bw.Seek(0, SeekOrigin.Begin);
      bw.Write(++slots);
```

```
      }
      entry.status = TidStatus.Created;
      entry.tid = tid;
      table.Add(tid, entry);
      bw.Seek(entry.index, SeekOrigin.Begin);
      bw.Write(tid.ToCharArray(), 0, idSize);
      bw.Write((byte)TidStatus.Created);
      bw.Write(EMPTY_REMAINDER, 0, REMAINDER_SIZE);
      bw.Flush();
      return TidStatus.Created;
    }
  }
  public void DeleteEntry(String tid)
  {
    lock (this)
    {
      StoreEntry entry = null;
      if (table.TryGetValue(tid, out entry))
      {
        table.Remove(tid);
        bw.Seek(entry.index, SeekOrigin.Begin);
        bw.Write(empty_id, 0, idSize);
        bw.Flush();
        freeEntries.Push(entry);
      }
    }
  }
  public void SetStatus(String tid, TidStatus tidStatus,
    String errorMessage)
  {
    lock (this)
    {
      StoreEntry entry = null;
      if (!table.TryGetValue(tid, out entry))
        throw new ArgumentException("Invalid TID");
      entry.status = tidStatus;
      bw.Seek(entry.index + idSize, SeekOrigin.Begin);
      bw.Write((byte)tidStatus);
      if (errorMessage != null)
      {
        byte[] err = Encoding.UTF8.GetBytes(errorMessage);
        int result = err.Length < REMAINDER_SIZE ?
          err.Length : REMAINDER_SIZE;
```

```
      bw.Write(err, 0, result);
      if (result < REMAINDER_SIZE) bw.Write((byte)0);
    }
    bw.Flush();
  }
}
public TidStatus GetStatus(String tid,
 out String errorMessage)
{
  TidStatus tidStatus = TidStatus.Created;
  lock (this)
  {
    errorMessage = "";
    StoreEntry entry = null;
    if (!table.TryGetValue(tid, out entry))
      throw new ArgumentException("Invalid TID");
    tidStatus = entry.status;
    if (tidStatus == TidStatus.RolledBack)
    {
      br.BaseStream.Seek(entry.index + idSize + 1,
        SeekOrigin.Begin);
      byte[] err = br.ReadBytes(REMAINDER_SIZE);
      errorMessage = Encoding.UTF8.GetString(err);
    }
  }
  return tidStatus;
}
//  gibt Details eines Eintrags auf der Konsole aus
public void PrintEntry(String tid)
{
  lock (this)
  {
    String error = "";
    TidStatus tidStatus;
    tidStatus = GetStatus(tid, out error);
    Console.WriteLine("TID:  {0}\n", tid);
    Console.WriteLine("Status: {0}\n", tidStatus);
  }
}
//  gibt alle Einträge auf der Konsole aus
public void PrintOverview()
{
  if (table.Count == 0)
```

```
  {
    if (idSize == TID_SIZE)
      Console.WriteLine("Bislang keine tRFC-LUWs
                         empfangen\n");
    else
      Console.WriteLine("Bislang keine bgRFC-LUWs
                         empfangen\n");
    return;
  }
  lock (this)
  {
    string format = "{0,10}  {1,-24}  {2,-20}  {3}";
    if (idSize == GUID_SIZE)
      format = "{0,10}  {1,-32}  {2,-20}  {3}";
    Console.WriteLine("\n" + format, "Index",
      idSize == GUID_SIZE ? "GUID" : "TID",
      "Status", "Fehlermeldung\n");
    string errorMessage = "";
    br.BaseStream.Seek(sizeof(int), SeekOrigin.Begin);
    for (int i = 0; i < slots; ++i)
    {
      char[] temp = br.ReadChars(idSize);
      if (temp[0] == 0)
      {
        br.BaseStream.Seek(1 + REMAINDER_SIZE,
          SeekOrigin.Current);
        continue;
      }
      TidStatus status = (TidStatus)br.ReadByte();
      if (status == TidStatus.RolledBack)
      {
        byte[] byteBuf = br.ReadBytes(REMAINDER_SIZE);
        int result = 0;
        while (result < byteBuf.Length &&
               byteBuf[result] != 0) ++result;
        errorMessage = Encoding.UTF8.GetString(
          byteBuf, 0, result);
      }
      Console.WriteLine(format, i, new String(temp),
        status, errorMessage);
    }
  }
}
```

```
    public int Size
    {
      get
      {
        return table.Count;
      }
    }
  }
}
```

Listing 6.15 Klasse »TidStore« für das TID-Management

TID-Management

Eine beispielhafte Implementierung der Klasse wird von SAP als separater Download auf der Seite **SAP Connector for Microsoft .NET** (*http://s-prs.de/v1032903*) im Bereich **Documentation • Tutorial** bereitgestellt. Der Link führt zu einer Datei namens **dotnet_connector_30_tutorial** und beinhaltet Visual-Basic- und C#-Daten mit Beispielen. Die Klasse in der Datei **TidStore.cs** verwaltet die TIDs in einer Datei. Die Einträge in dieser Datei werden durch Instanzen der Klasse `StoreEntry` repräsentiert. Diese Klasse hat die Eigenschaften `tid`, `status` und `index`, die die TID, den Status der TID und die Position des Eintrags in der Datei enthalten. Neben diesen drei Informationen wird noch eine Fehlermeldung von maximal 80 Zeichen in der TID-Datei gespeichert, falls die TID den Status `RolledBack` hat. Die Eigenschaft `status` ist vom Typ `TidStatus`, eine Enumeration mit den Werten `Created`, `Executed`, `Commited`, `RolledBack` und `Confirmed`.

Die Klasse `TidStore` hat den zweiparametrigen Konstruktor `TidStore(string, bool)`. Der erste Parameter gibt den Namen der TID-Datei an. Falls dieser Parameter `null` oder leer ist, wird **TIDStore.tid** als Dateiname verwendet. Der zweite Parameter entscheidet, ob die TIDs als 24-stellige TIDs oder als 32-stellige GUIDs gespeichert werden sollen. Für tRFCs und qRFCs sind 24-stellige TIDs üblich, für bgRFCs 32-stellige GUIDs.

Freie und belegte TID-Einträge

Der Konstruktor öffnet die angegebene Datei bzw. erzeugt eine neue, falls sie nicht existiert. In der Datei steht zunächst eine binärcodierte Ganzzahl, die die Anzahl der Einträge enthält. Diese Information liest der Konstruktor in die Eigenschaft `slots` ein. Danach folgen die Einträge, die der Konstruktor in einer Schleife einliest. Von jedem Eintrag werden in der Schleife nur die Eigenschaften `tid` und `status` aus der Datei gelesen; die Fehlermeldung wird übersprungen. Außerdem speichert der Konstruktor die Position des Eintrags in der Eigenschaft `index`. Falls `tid` leer ist, ist dieser Eintrag in der Datei noch frei, und der Konstruktor speichert den Eintrag in der Eigenschaft `freeEntries` vom Typ `Stack<StoreEntry>`. Falls `tid` nicht leer ist, wird der Eintrag in der Eigenschaft `table` vom Typ `Dictionary<String, StoreEntry>` gespeichert. `TidStore` verwaltet also freie Einträge im Stack `freeEntries` und belegte Einträge im Dictionary `tables`. Der Schlüssel, der einen Dictionary-Eintrag identifiziert, ist die Eigenschaft `tid`.

Die Methode `Close()` schließt die vom Konstruktor geöffnete TID-Datei wieder. Die Methode `CreateEntry(string)` erwartet eine TID (als 24-stellige TID oder 32-stellige GUID). Sie prüft zunächst, ob diese TID schon existiert. Falls ja, gibt sie deren Status zurück. Falls nein, verwendet die Methode den nächsten freien Eintrag aus dem Stack `freeEntries` oder erzeugt eine neue Instanz der Klasse `StoreEntry`. Diese `StoreEntry`-Instanz wird dann mit der TID und dem `status`-Feld `Created` gefüllt, im Dictionary `table` gespeichert und an der entsprechenden Stelle in der Datei eingetragen. Wurde ein freier Eintrag aus `freeEntries` verwendet, steht die Eintragsstelle in der Eigenschaft `index`; ansonsten ist die Eintragsstelle das Ende der Datei.

Die Methode `DeleteEntry(string)` entfernt den Eintrag aus dem Dictionary `table`, der durch den Übergabeparameter identifiziert wird, legt ihn auf den Stack `freeEntries` und überschreibt die TID in der Datei an der Stelle `index` mit einer leeren TID.

Die Methode `SetStatus(string, TidStatus, string)` setzt den Status des durch den ersten Parameter identifizierten Eintrags. Der Status wird sowohl im Dictionary `table` als auch in der Datei geändert. Gegebenenfalls wird in der Datei noch die Fehlermeldung abgelegt, die im dritten Parameter übergeben wird.

Die Methode `GetStatus(string, out string)` gibt den Status und – im `out`-Parameter – die Fehlermeldung zu einer TID zurück, die im ersten Parameter identifiziert wird.

Die Methode `PrintEntry()` gibt eine TID und deren Status auf der Konsole aus. Die Methode `PrintOverview()` gibt alle TIDs mit Status und gegebenenfalls einer Fehlermeldung auf der Konsole aus.

Für einfache Testszenarien reicht diese Implementierung eines TID-Managements vollkommen aus. Für produktive Programme werden Sie sicher eine Datenbank für das TID-Management verwenden wollen.

6.3.3 Queued RFC

Der NCo ermöglicht auch die Verwendung von queued RFCs (qRFCs). Dabei werden mehrere tRFC-Aufrufe in eine Eingangswarteschlange gestellt, um sicherzustellen, dass die Aufrufe im Zielsystem in der Reihenfolge abgearbeitet werden, in der sie im Empfängersystem abgesetzt wurden.

Die Verwendung von qRFCs funktioniert genauso wie die von tRFCs. Sie müssen lediglich bei der Erzeugung der Transaktion den Konstruktor `RfcTransaction(string)` verwenden und als Parameter einen beliebigen Queue-Namen angeben. Falls Sie eine Transaktion wiederholen müssen, verwenden Sie `RfcTransaction(RfcTID, string)` als Konstruktor.

Eingangs-Queue verarbeiten

Wie in Abschnitt 3.3.2, »qRFC mit Ausgangs- und Eingangswarteschlange«, beschrieben, müssen Sie den Funktionsbaustein `TRFC_QIN_RESTART` aufrufen, damit die Eingangs-Queue verarbeitet wird. Alternativ können Sie den QIN-Scheduler verwenden.

6.3.4 Background RFC

Auch die Verwendung von Background RFCs (bgRFCs), der moderneren Variante von tRFCs und qRFCs, wird vom NCo unterstützt. Die Programmierung mit bgRFCs unterscheidet sich nur in wenigen Punkten von den anderen beiden RFC-Typen.

»RfcBackgroundUnit«

Anstelle der Klasse `RfcTransaction`, die durch eine 24-stellige TID identifiziert wird, benötigen Sie nun eine Instanz der Klasse `RfcBackgroundUnit`, die durch eine 32-stellige GUID identifiziert wird. Die Klasse `TidStore` aus Listing 6.15 berücksichtigt diesen Unterschied im zweiten Parameter des Konstruktors. Wenn Sie dort den Wert »true« übergeben, werden anstelle 24-stelliger TIDs 32-stellige GUIDs gespeichert.

»RfcUnitID«

Der Konstruktor der Klasse `RfcBackgroundUnit` erwartet eine Instanz der Klasse `RfcUnitID`. Deren Konstruktor wiederum müssen Sie einen der beiden Enumerationswerte `RfcUnitType.TRANSACTIONAL` oder `RfcUnitType.QUEUED` mitgeben.

»ConfirmUnitID«

Das Hinzufügen von Funktionen zur Background Unit und das Abschicken der Klasse funktionieren genau wie bei `RfcTransaction`-Objekten mit den Methoden `AddFunction()` und `Commit()`. Um die Klasse beim Applikationsserver zu bestätigen, verwenden Sie nun die Methode `ConfirmUnitID(RfcUnitID)` der RFC-Destination.

»bgRFC-Client«

Listing 6.16 zeigt Ausschnitte aus dem Code für einen bgRFC-Client. Die Unterschiede zum tRFC-Client aus Listing 6.13 sind durch Fettdruck hervorgehoben.

```
namespace IFPCSharp.BgRfcClient
{
  class Program
  {
    static void Main(string[] args)
```

```
{
  ...
  TidStore tidStore = new TidStore(
    "clientTidStore", true);
  ...
  }
}
static void SendNewTransaction(TidStore tidStore)
{
  ...

  // neue Background Unit mit neuer GUID erzeugen
  RfcBackgroundUnit bgUnit = new RfcBackgroundUnit(
    new RfcUnitID(RfcUnitType.TRANSACTIONAL));
  // Daten und neue GUID speichern
  string unitID = bgUnit.UnitID.Uuid.ToString("N");
  File.Copy(dataFileName, unitID);
  tidStore.CreateEntry(unitID);
  // Funktion mit Daten zur Background Unit hinzufügen
  bgUnit.AddFunction(orderCreateFunction);
  // Destination besorgen und Background Unit abschicken
  try
  {
    RfcDestination dest = RfcDestinationManager.
      GetDestination("NCO_ASHOST");
    bgUnit.Commit(dest);
    // GUID-Status auf Commited setzen
    tidStore.SetStatus(unitID,
      TidStatus.Committed, null);
    // Wenn bis hierhin kein Fehler auftrat:
    // Unit bestätigen und Daten löschen.
    dest.ConfirmUnitID(bgUnit.UnitID);
    File.Delete(unitID);
    tidStore.DeleteEntry(unitID);
  }
  catch (Exception e)
  {
    // GUID-Status auf RolledBack setzen
    tidStore.SetStatus(unitID, TidStatus.RolledBack,
                       e.Message);
  }
}
static void ResendOldTransaction(TidStore tidStore)
```

6

```
    {
      ...
      // eine GUID auswählen
      tidStore.PrintOverview();
      string unitID = ChooseTid(tidStore);
      ...
      // alte Daten einlesen
      IRfcFunction orderCreateFunction =
        PrepareFunction(unitID);
      // neue Background Unit mit alter GUID erzeugen
      RfcBackgroundUnit bgUnit =
        new RfcBackgroundUnit(
          new RfcUnitID(new Guid(unitID),
                        RfcUnitType.TRANSACTIONAL));
      // Funktion mit Daten zur Background Unit hinzufügen
      bgUnit.AddFunction(orderCreateFunction);
      // Destination besorgen und Background Unit abschicken
      try
      {
        RfcDestination dest =
         RfcDestinationManager.GetDestination("NCO_ASHOST");
        bgUnit.Commit(dest);
        // GUID-Status auf Commited setzen
        tidStore.SetStatus(unitID, TidStatus.Committed,
                           null);
        // Wenn bis hierhin kein Fehler auftrat:
        // Background Unit bestätigen und Daten löschen.
        dest.ConfirmUnitID(bgUnit.UnitID);
        File.Delete(unitID);
        tidStore.DeleteEntry(unitID);
      }
      catch (Exception e)
      {
        // GUID-Status auf RolledBack setzen
        tidStore.SetStatus(unitID, TidStatus.RolledBack,
                           e.Message);
      }
    }
...
  }
}
```

Listing 6.16 Beispiel eines bgRFC-Clients

6.4 RFC-Server

RFC-Server schreiben

In diesem Abschnitt lernen Sie, RFC-Server mithilfe der SAP-NCo-Bibliothek zu schreiben (siehe Abschnitt 4.4, »SAP-NetWeaver-RFC-Server«). Um einen RFC-Server zu schreiben, folgen Sie den folgenden Schritten, die wir in den weiteren Abschnitten noch im Detail beschreiben.

1. Erzeugen Sie ein `RfcServer`-Objekt, und übergeben Sie diesem die notwendigen RFC-Gateway-Parameter.
2. Registrieren Sie die Serverfunktionen, die Sie implementieren wollen, als .NET-Delegat vom Typ `RfcServerFunction` beim Objekt `RfcServer`. Ein .NET-Delegattyp – in unserem Fall der Typ `RfcServerFunction` – ist ein Typ, der eine Methodensignatur definiert. Die Signatur Ihrer Serverfunktionen muss also in Rückgabe- und Parametertyp mit der vom Delegattyp `RfcServerFunction` definierten Signatur übereinstimmen.
3. Erzeugen Sie ein Objekt `RfcCustomRepository`, das die Metadaten Ihrer Funktionen erhält, oder verwenden Sie das Repository-Objekt eines Destinationsobjekts, das anschließend die Metadaten Ihrer Funktionsbausteine von einem SAP-System liest. Registrieren Sie das Repository-Objekt beim `RfcServer`-Objekt.
4. Implementieren Sie die Schnittstelle `IServerSecurityHandler`, und registrieren Sie ein Objekt der implementierenden Klasse beim Objekt `RfcServer`.
5. Implementieren Sie die Schnittstelle `ISessionProvider`, und registrieren Sie ein Objekt der implementierenden Klasse beim `RfcSessionManager`, falls Sie zustandsbehaftete RFC-Aufrufe realisieren wollen.
6. Implementieren Sie die Schnittstelle `ITransactionIDHandler`, und registrieren Sie ein Objekt der implementierenden Klasse beim `RfcServer`-Objekt, falls Sie tRFC oder qRFC bereitstellen möchten.
7. Implementieren Sie die Schnittstelle `IUnitIDHandler`, und registrieren Sie ein Objekt der implementierenden Klasse beim `RfcServer`-Objekt, falls Sie bgRFC bereitstellen möchten.
8. Starten Sie das `RfcServer`-Objekt.

Wir beginnen mit einem einfachen RFC-Server, der die ersten beiden und den letzten Schritt implementiert.

6.4.1 Serverkonfiguration und Implementierung

Beispiel einfacher RFC-Server

In diesem Abschnitt zeigen wir Ihnen, wie Sie einen einfachen Server schreiben, der synchrone RFC-Aufrufe bedienen kann. Sehen Sie sich zunächst den Code des einfachen RFC-Servers in Listing 6.17 an.

```
using System;
using System.IO;
using SAP.Middleware.Connector;

namespace IFPCSharp.SimpleServer
{
  class Program
  {
    static void Main(string[] args)
    {
      // Server erzeugen
      RfcServer server = RfcServerManager.GetServer(
        "NCO_SERVER",
        new Type[] { typeof(RfcFunctionImpl) });
      // Server starten
      server.Start();
      Console.WriteLine();
      Console.WriteLine("Server gestartet: {0}",
        server.Parameters.ToString());
      Console.WriteLine(
        "Drücken Sie Enter, um den Server zu stoppen");
      Console.ReadLine();
      Console.WriteLine("Server fährt herunter ...");
      // Server herunterfahren
      server.Shutdown(true);
    }
    class RfcFunctionImpl
    {
      [RfcServerFunction(Name = "Z_IFP_ORDER_GETLIST")]
      public static void ZIfpOrderGetlist(
        RfcServerContext serverContext,
        IRfcFunction function)
      {
        Console.WriteLine("Führe Z_IFP_ORDER_GETLIST aus.");
        // Importparameter lesen
        string ordertype =
          function.GetString("IM_ORDERTYPE");
        string refid = function.GetString("IM_REFID");
        if (string.IsNullOrEmpty(ordertype))
          ordertype = "SO";
        // Exportparameter füllen
        IRfcTable orders = function.GetTable("TA_ORDERS");
        FileStream dataFile = new FileStream(
```

```
    "orders.dat", FileMode.Open, FileAccess.Read);
  StreamReader reader = new StreamReader(dataFile);
  while (!reader.EndOfStream)
  {
    string line = reader.ReadLine();
    string[] fields = line.Split(new char[] { ';' });
    if (refid.Equals(fields[3]) ||
        refid.Equals("0000000000") && o
        rdertype.Equals(fields[2]))
    {
      orders.Append();
      for (int i = 0; i < fields.GetLength(0); i++)
      {
        orders.SetValue(i, fields[i]);            }
    }
  }
  dataFile.Close();
}
[RfcServerFunction(Name = "Z_IFP_ORDER_GETDETAIL")]
public static void ZIfpOrderGetdetail(
 RfcServerContext serverContext,
 IRfcFunction function)
{
  Console.WriteLine(
    "Führe Z_IFP_ORDER_GETDETAIL aus.");
  // Importparameter lesen
  string orderid = function.GetString("IM_ORDERID");
  // Bestellkopf füllen
  IRfcStructure header =
    function.GetStructure("EX_ORDERHEAD");
  FileStream dataFile = new FileStream(
    "orders.dat", FileMode.Open, FileAccess.Read);
  StreamReader reader = new StreamReader(dataFile);
  while (!reader.EndOfStream)
  {
    string line = reader.ReadLine();
    string[] fields = line.Split(new char[] { ';' });
    if(orderid.Equals(fields[1]))
    {
      for (int i = 0; i < fields.GetLength(0); i++)
      {
        header.SetValue(i, fields[i]);
      }
```

6

```
              break;
            }
          }
          dataFile.Close();
          // Bestellpositionen füllen
          IRfcTable positions =
            function.GetTable("TA_ORDERPOS");
          dataFile = new FileStream(
            "orderpos.dat", FileMode.Open, FileAccess.Read);
          reader = new StreamReader(dataFile);
          while (!reader.EndOfStream)
          {
            string line = reader.ReadLine();
            string[] fields = line.Split(new char[] { ';' });
            if (orderid.Equals(fields[1]))
            {
              positions.Append();
              for (int i = 0; i < fields.GetLength(0); i++)
              {
                positions.SetValue(i, fields[i]);
              }
            }
          }
          dataFile.Close();
        }
      }
    }
  }
```

Listing 6.17 Einfacher RFC-Server

Der Servercode in Listing 6.17 implementiert die beiden Funktionsbausteine `Z_IFP_ORDER_GETLIST` und `Z_IF_ORDER_GETDETAIL`, die jeweils eine Liste von Bestellungen bzw. die Details zu einer Bestellung zurückgeben. Die Methode `Main()` fragt zunächst vom Server Manager ein `RfcServer`-Objekt über die Methode `GetServer()` ab. Dem ersten Parameter der Methode wird der Name einer Serverkonfiguration aus der Konfigurationsdatei übergeben, dem zweiten Parameter ein Array von Typen, die die Implementierungen der Funktionsbausteine enthalten. Danach wird der Server mit der Methode `Start()` gestartet. Sobald der Anwender die [↵]-Taste drückt, wird der Server mit der Methode `Shutdown()` wieder heruntergefahren.

Optionen zur Serverkonfiguration

Im Folgenden schauen wir uns zuerst die Serverkonfiguration und anschließend die Implementierung der Funktionsbausteine im Detail an. Für die Serverkonfiguration im ersten Parameter der Methode `GetServer()` haben Sie mehrere Möglichkeiten:

- Sie übergeben im ersten Parameter der Methode ein `RfcConfigParameters`-Objekt, dessen Felder die Informationen über die Serverkonfiguration enthalten.
- Sie übergeben im ersten Parameter der Methode den Namen einer Serverkonfiguration. Die Serverkonfiguration wird dann der Konfigurationsdatei entnommen.
- Sie schreiben eine Klasse, die die Schnittstelle `IServerConfiguration` implementiert. Sie erzeugen eine Instanz dieser Klasse und registrieren diese mit der statischen Methode `RegisterServerConfiguration()` beim Server Manager. Nun ruft der Server Manager innerhalb von `GetServer()` die Methode `GetParameters()` des `IRfcServerConfiguration`-Objekts auf. In dieser Methode erzeugen und füllen Sie ein `RfcConfigParameters`-Objekt.

Bestandteile der Serverkonfiguration

Eine Serverkonfiguration wird über einen eindeutigen Namen identifiziert und enthält außerdem Hostnamen, Servicenamen und die Programm-ID für die Registrierung bei einem RFC-Gateway. In der Regel wird auch noch der Name einer RFC-Client-Destination angegeben, über die sich der RFC-Server die Metadaten holt. Listing 6.18 zeigt ein Beispiel einer Konfigurationsdatei, die eine Serverkonfiguration namens `NCO_SERVER` enthält.

```
<?xml version="1.0"?>
<configuration>
  <configSections>
    <sectionGroup name="SAP.Middleware.Connector">
      <sectionGroup name="ClientSettings">
        <section name="DestinationConfiguration"
 type="SAP.Middleware.Connector.RfcDestinationConfiguration, sapnco"/>
      </sectionGroup>
      <sectionGroup name="ServerSettings">
        <section name="ServerConfiguration" type=
"SAP.Middleware.Connector.RfcServerConfiguration, sapnco"/>
      </sectionGroup>
    </sectionGroup>
  </configSections>
```

```
    <SAP.Middleware.Connector>
      <ClientSettings>
        <DestinationConfiguration>
          <destinations>
            <add NAME="NCO_TESTS"
              USER="bcuser" PASSWD="minisap" CLIENT="001"
              LANG="EN" ASHOST="localhost" SYSNR="001"
              POOL_SIZE="5" MAX_POOL_SIZE="10"/>
          </destinations>
        </DestinationConfiguration>
      </ClientSettings>
      <ServerSettings>
        <ServerConfiguration>
          <servers>
            <add NAME="NCO_SERVER" GWHOST="MY_GWHOST"
              GWSERV="MY_SAPGW" PROGRAM_ID="nRfcTestServer"
              REPOSITORY_DESTINATION="NCO_TESTS"
              REG_COUNT="1"/>
          </servers>
        </ServerConfiguration>
      </ServerSettings>
      </SAP.Middleware.Connector>
  </SAP.Middleware.Connector>
</configuration>
```

Listing 6.18 Konfiguration von Serverparametern in der Konfigurationsdatei »App.config«

Konfigurationsdatei

Der Gateway-Host lautet `localhost`, der Gateway-Service ist `sapgw00`, die Programm-ID ist `nRfcTestServer`, und als Client-Destination für das Lesen der Metadaten wird `NCO_TESTS` verwendet. Der Server registriert sich mit einem Thread beim Gateway. Tabelle 6.6 listet die möglichen Parameter für die Serverkonfiguration auf. Dabei enthält die erste Spalte den Namen des Parameters in der Konfigurationsdatei und die zweite Spalte den Namen des Felds der Klasse `RfcConfigParameters`.

Name	Konstante	Beschreibung	Mögliche Werte
GWHOST	GatewayHost	Hostname des RFC-Gateways	
GWSERV	GatewayService	Servicename oder Portnummer des RFC-Gateways	z. B. sapgw00, 3300

Tabelle 6.6 Parameter der Serverkonfiguration

Name	Konstante	Beschreibung	Mögliche Werte
PROGRAM_ID	ProgramID	Programm-ID	00–99
SYS_IDS	SystemIDs	kommaseparierte Liste der System-IDs, von denen Aufrufe akzeptiert werden	
REG_COUNT	RegistrationCount	Anzahl der Registrierungen beim Gateway	Standard: 1
MAX_REG_COUNT	MaxRegistrationCount	Sobald eine Registrierung zustandsbehaftet (stateful) wird, wird eine neue angelegt. Mit diesem Parameter kann die Maximalanzahl beschränkt werden.	Standard: 1
MAX_SHUTDOWN_WAIT_TIME	MaxShutdownWaitTime	Maximale Zeit, die der Server beim Shutdown wartet, bis aktive RFC-Anfragen abgearbeitet sind.	Zeit in Millisekunden; Standard ist 30.000.
SERVER_RESTART_TIMEOUT	ServerRestarTimeout	Falls ein Server abstürzt, versucht das Gateway so lange einen periodischen Neustart, bis diese Zeit erreicht ist.	Zeit in Sekunden; Standard ist –1 (kein Timeout).

Tabelle 6.6 Parameter der Serverkonfiguration (Forts.)

Implementierung der Funktionsbausteine

Die Funktionsbausteine werden als statische Methoden der Klassen implementiert, deren Type-Objekte Sie im zweiten Parameter der Methode GetServer() übergeben haben. Im Fall von Listing 6.17 ist dies lediglich die Klasse RfcFunctionImpl mit den beiden Methoden ZIfpOrderGetList() und ZIfpOrderGetDetail(). Der Name der Methode ist nicht relevant. Wichtig ist jedoch, dass die Methoden mit dem Attribut RfcServerFunction versehen sind, dessen Name-Feld den Namen des Funktionsbausteins enthält, der von der Methode implementiert wird.

Die Methoden haben zwei Parameter. Im ersten Parameter vom Typ RfcServerContext wird ein Kontextobjekt übergeben, das Informationen über das gewünschte transaktionale Verhalten des Servers enthält. In unseren beiden Methoden ignorieren wir dieses Objekt, da wir uns erst später um die Transaktionen kümmern wollen. Der zweite Parameter ist vom Typ IRfcFunction. Über diesen Parameter können Sie auf die Import- und Exportparameter der Funktion zugreifen.

Beide Methoden lesen zuerst die Importparameter aus dem übergebenen Funktionsobjekt, lesen dann die angeforderten Daten aus den Dateien **orders.dat** bzw. **positions.dat** und füllen damit die Exportparameter. Die dazu benötigten Methoden kennen Sie schon aus Abschnitt 6.2, »Einfache RFC-Clients«.

Generischer Funktions-Handler

Wenn Sie die Eigenschaft `Default` des Attributs `RfcServerFunction` auf den Wert »true« setzen, wird diese Funktion für alle Funktionsbausteine aufgerufen, für die Sie keinen expliziten Handler definiert haben. Listing 6.19 zeigt ein vereinfachtes Beispiel dafür.

```
[RfcServerFunction(Default = true)]
public static void GenericHandler(
  RfcServerContext serverContext, IRfcFunction rfcFunction)
{
  Console.WriteLine("Funktionsbaustein {0} wurde gerufen",
                    rfcFunction.Metadata.Name);
  for (int i=0; i<rfcFunction.Metadata.ParameterCount; ++i)
  {
    Console.WriteLine("Parameter {0}",
                      rfcFunction.Metadata[i].Name);
  }
}
```

Listing 6.19 Generischer Funktions-Handler

Ausnahmen auslösen

Wenn Sie Ausnahmen auslösen wollen, erzeugen Sie einfach ein Objekt der Klasse `RfcClassException`, `RfcAbapException` oder `RfcMessageException`, füllen es mit den notwendigen Informationen (z. B. zum `Exception`-Objekt im Falle von `RfcClassException` oder zur Nachricht und den Nachrichtenparametern im Falle von `RfcMessageException`) und lösen dann mit `throw` die Ausnahme aus. Listing 6.20 zeigt ein Beispiel für eine klassenbasierte Ausnahme.

```
IRfcAbapObject exceptionObject =
  serverContext.Repository.GetAbapObjectMetadata("").
    CreateAbapObject();
exceptionObject.SetValue("SOURCE_TYPENAME", "Hallo ABAP");
exceptionObject.SetValue("TARGET_TYPENAME", "Alles klar?");
throw new RfcAbapClassException("Klassenbasierte Ausnahme",
  exceptionObject);
```

Listing 6.20 Klassenbasierte Ausnahme auslösen

6.4.2 Repository-Management

Sobald Sie ein `RfcServer`-Objekt erzeugt haben, müssen Sie ihm mitteilen, wo es die Metadaten für die `IRfcFunction`-Objekte findet. Am einfachsten belegen Sie dazu in den Serverkonfigurationsparametern die Eigenschaft `RepositoryDestination` mit dem Namen einer Client-Destination. Alternativ können Sie dem Server ein Repository auch wie folgt zuweisen:


```
server.Repository = RfcDestinationManager.
  GetDestination("NCO_TESTS").Repository;
```

Für den seltenen Fall, dass Sie Metadaten für Funktionsbausteine zur Verfügung stellen wollen, die nicht im Backend-System vorhanden sind, müssen Sie eine Instanz der Klasse `RfcCustomRepository` erzeugen und die Metadaten für Ihre Funktionsbausteine von Hand anlegen.

6.4.3 Sicherheitsmanagement

»IServerSecurityHandler«

Um den Zugriff auf Ihren Server abzusichern, stellen Sie eine Klasse bereit, die die Schnittstelle `IServerSecurityHandler` implementiert. Sobald diese das `RfcServer`-Objekt erzeugt hat, belegen Sie dessen Feld `SecurityHandler` mit einer Instanz Ihrer Security-Handler-Klasse.

Die Schnittstelle `IServerSecurityHandler` definiert zwei Methoden, `LogonCheck()` und `AuthorizationCheck()`. Die Methode `LogonCheck()` wird immer aufgerufen, wenn ein ABAP-Client-Programm eine neue Verbindung zu Ihrem Server aufmacht. Die Methode `AuthorizationCheck()` wird aufgerufen, bevor einer Ihrer Funktionsbausteine ausgeführt wird.

»LogonCheck()«

In der Implementierung der Methode `LogonCheck()` können Sie unter anderem die System-ID des rufenden Systems (über `RfcServerContext.SystemAttributes.SystemID`) und den Namen des Benutzers (über `RfcSecurityData.UserName`) prüfen. Sie können feststellen, ob die Verbindung über Secure Network Communications (SNC) abgesichert ist (über `RfcSecurityData.Type`) und ob `SncPartnerKey` von einem System stammt, dem Sie vertrauen. Der `SncPartnerKey` ist der Schlüssel des Zertifikats, das für die sichere Übertragung von Autorisierungsinformationen über SNC zwischen RFC-Kommunikationspartnern verwendet wird (siehe Abschnitt 1.2.3, »Sichere Integration externer Systeme«).

»AuthorizationCheck()«

In der Methode `AuthorizationCheck()` können Sie überprüfen, welcher Funktionsbaustein ausgeführt werden soll und ob der Benutzer die Berechtigung dazu hat. Falls Sie außer dem `LogonCheck()` keine zusätzliche Autorisierung vornehmen möchten, können Sie in der Methode `Authorizati-`

onCheck() immer den Wert »true« zurückgeben. Listing 6.21 zeigt eine einfache Implementierung der Schnittstelle IServerSecurityHandler.

```
class SecurityHandler : IServerSecurityHandler
{
  public bool AuthorizationCheck(
    RfcServerContextInfo serverContextInfo,
    RfcSecurityData securityData)
  {
    Console.WriteLine("LogonCheck");
    Console.WriteLine("FunctionName: {0}",
      serverContextInfo.FunctionName);
    Console.WriteLine("User Name: {0}",
      securityData.UserName);
    if (serverContextInfo.FunctionName.Equals("RFC_PING") &&
       securityData.UserName.Equals("BCUSER"))
      return true;
    else
      return false;
  }
  public bool LogonCheck(
    RfcServerContext serverContext,
    RfcSecurityData securityData)
  {
    Console.WriteLine("LogonCheck");
    Console.WriteLine("SystemID: {0}",
      serverContext.SystemAttributes.SystemID);
    Console.WriteLine("User: {0}",
      serverContext.SystemAttributes.User);
    Console.WriteLine("Type: {0}",
      securityData.Type);
    Console.WriteLine("SNC Partner Name: {0}",
      securityData.SncPartnerName);
    Console.WriteLine("SNC Partner Key: {0}",
      securityData.SncPartnerKey);
    Console.WriteLine("Logon Ticket: {0}",
      securityData.Ticket);
    Console.WriteLine("User Name: {0}",
      securityData.UserName);
string SysID = serverContext.SysteAttributes.SystemID;
    if (SysID.Equals("NSP") &&
       securityData.UserName.Equals("BCUSER"))
      return true;
    else
```

```
        return false;
    }
}
```

Listing 6.21 Implementierung von »IServerSecurityHandler«

6.4.4 Session-Management

Wenn Sie auf Ihrem Server den Zustand eines Benutzerkontextes zwischen zwei RFC-Aufrufen speichern wollen, gehen Sie am einfachsten folgendermaßen vor:

1. Implementieren Sie Ihre Funktions-Handler als Instanzmethoden, und speichern Sie den Benutzerkontext in den Instanzvariablen der dazugehörigen Klasse.
2. Markieren Sie die Verbindung als zustandsbehaftet, indem Sie innerhalb Ihrer Methodenimplementierung den Aufruf `context.SetStateful(true)` ausführen.

   In diesem Falle sorgt der NCo für ein entsprechendes Session-Management. Der Aufruf von `SetStateful` weist den NCo an, die Verbindung so lange offen zu halten, bis entweder der rufende ABAP-Client sie schließt oder Sie selbst `context.SetStateful(false)` aufrufen. Die ABAP-Plattform schließt eine Verbindung in folgenden Situationen:

   - Auf der ABAP-Client-Seite wird der Funktionsbaustein `RFC_CLOSE_CONNECTION` aufgerufen.
   - Der interne Modus wird beendet, z. B. indem der Benutzer »/n« in das Befehlsfeld eingibt.
   - Der Dialog-Workprozess oder das RFC-Gateway laufen in einen Timeout.

»STFC_CONNECTION« implementieren

Listing 6.22 zeigt ein Beispiel für eine zustandsbehaftete Implementierung des Funktionsbausteins `STFC_CONNECTION`. Das private Instanzfeld `calls` wird innerhalb der Implementierung bei jedem Aufruf um eins hochgezählt. Im Exportparameter `RESPTEXT` wird dieses Feld zurückgegeben. Vor dem Ende der Methode `StfcConnectionImpl` in Listing 6.22 wird geprüft, ob die Verbindung zustandsbehaftet ist. Ist das nicht der Fall, wird `serverContext.SetStateful(true)` aufgerufen, um die Session als zustandsbehaftet zu markieren.

```
class StfcConnectionImpl
{
  private int calls = 0;
  [RfcServerFunction(Name = "STFC_CONNECTION")]
  public void StfcConnection(
```

```
      RfcServerContext serverContext,
      IRfcFunction function)
    {
      Console.WriteLine(
        "Führe {0} aus", function.Metadata.Name);
      function.SetValue(
        "ECHOTEXT", function.GetString("REQUTEXT"));
      function.SetValue(
        "RESPTEXT", "Aufruf " + (++calls).ToString());
      if(!serverContext.Stateful)
        serverContext.SetStateful(true);
    }
  }
```

Listing 6.22 Zustandsbehaftete Implementierung von »STFC_CONNECTION«

Verbindung testen

Achten Sie darauf, dass der Konfigurationsparameter `REG_COUNT`, zumindest aber der Konfigurationsparameter `MAX_REG_COUNT` größer als eins sein müssen, um mehrere zustandsbehaftete Verbindungen gleichzeitig offen halten zu können. Testen Sie diese Implementierung, indem Sie auf dem SAP-System zwei externe Modi öffnen und den Funktionsbaustein erst einige Male aus dem einen Modus und dann aus dem anderen Modus heraus aufrufen. Sie sehen, dass die Anzahl der Aufrufe für jeden Modus getrennt hochgezählt wird.

»ISessionProvider«

Alternativ zum Session-Management durch den NCo können Sie auch eine Klasse schreiben, die die Schnittstelle `ISessionProvider` implementiert und eine Instanz dieser Klasse mit `RfcSessionManager.RegisterSessionProvider()` beim `RfcSessionManager` registrieren. Die Schnittstelle definiert fünf Methoden:

- `string CreateSession()` wird aufgerufen, sobald der rufende ABAP-Client eine neue Verbindung zum externen Server öffnet. Hier sollten Sie eine neue Session-ID erzeugen und mit dem aktuellen Thread assoziieren.
- `void PassivateSession(String sessionID)` wird aufgerufen, sobald ein RFC-Aufruf abgeschlossen wurde und die Verbindung für diese Session momentan nicht mehr benötigt wird. Hier sollten Sie die Verknüpfung der Session-ID mit dem aktuellen Thread wieder entfernen.
- `void ActivateSession(String sessionID)` wird aufgerufen, sobald ein neuer RFC-Aufruf über eine schon geöffnete Verbindung erfolgt. In dieser Methode sollten Sie die Session-ID wieder mit dem aktuellen Thread verknüpfen.

- `void DestroySession(String sessionID)` wird aufgerufen, sobald eine zustandsbehaftete Session beendet wird.
- `bool IsAlive(String sessionID)` wird vom NCo aufgerufen, um zu prüfen, ob eine bestimmte Session noch immer besteht.

6.4.5 Transaktionaler RFC

»ITransaction-ID-Handler«

Um einen transaktionalen RFC auf Ihrem Server zu realisieren, müssen Sie eine Klasse bereitstellen, die die Schnittstelle `ITransactionIDHandler` implementiert. Sie erzeugen anschließend eine Instanz Ihres Transaktions-Handlers und kopieren eine Referenz auf diese Instanz auf die Eigenschaft `TransactionIDHandler` des `RfcServer`-Objekts.

Methoden von »ITransaction-ID-Handler«

Die Schnittstelle `ITransactionIDHandler` definiert vier Methoden:

- Die Methode `CheckTransactionID` wird aufgerufen, sobald eine neue Transaktion bei Ihrem Server ankommt. Hier überprüfen Sie, ob Sie diese TID schon kennen und in welchem Zustand sie sich befindet. Hier können mehrere Fälle auftreten:
  - Falls sich die TID noch nicht in Ihrem TID-Speicher befindet, speichern Sie diese dort mit dem Zustand `Created` und geben den Wert »true« zurück. Sie geben auch »true« zurück, wenn sich die TID zwar im TID-Speicher befindet, dort aber den Zustand `Created` oder `RolledBack` hat, da Sie in diesem Fall die Transaktion noch nicht durchgeführt haben.
  - Falls sich die TID in Ihrem TID-Speicher befindet und den Zustand `Commited` hat, geben Sie den Wert »false« zurück. Dann ruft der NCo Ihren Funktions-Handler nicht auf, und die Transaktion wird nicht noch ein zweites Mal ausgeführt.
  - Falls Sie momentan nicht auf den TID-Speicher zugreifen können, lösen Sie die Ausnahme `RfcInternalError` aus.
- Die Methode `Commit` wird aufgerufen, sobald der NCo Ihren Funktions-Handler erfolgreich ausführen konnte. Hier sollten Sie alle Datenbankänderungen übergeben und die TID im TID-Speicher auf den Zustand `Commited` setzen.
- Die Methode `Rollback` wird aufgerufen, wenn in Ihrem Funktions-Handler eine Ausnahme ausgelöst wurde. Sie sollten alle Datenbankänderungen zurückrollen und die TID im TID-Speicher auf den Zustand `RolledBack` setzen.
- In der Methode `ConfirmTransactionID` löschen Sie einfach die TID in Ihrem TID-Speicher.

Implementierung In Listing 6.23 zeigen wir eine Implementierung der Schnittstelle `ITransactionIDHandler`, die den TID-Speicher aus Listing 6.15 verwendet.

```
class TidHandler : ITransactionIDHandler
{
  // TID-Speicher
  private static TidStore tidStore =
    new TidStore("serverTidStore", false);
  public bool CheckTransactionID(
    RfcServerContextInfo serverContext, RfcTID tid)
  {
    Console.Write("TRFC: Prüfe TID {0} --> ", tid.TID);
    TidStatus status = tidStore.CreateEntry(tid.TID);
    switch (status)
    {
      case TidStatus.Created:
        Console.WriteLine("Neue Transaktion");
        return true;
      case TidStatus.RolledBack:
        Console.WriteLine(
          "Alte Transaktion (zurückgerollt)");
        return true;
      default:
        Console.WriteLine("Alte Transaktion (bestätigt)");
        return false;
    }
  }
  public void ConfirmTransactionID(
    RfcServerContextInfo serverContext, RfcTID tid)
  {
    Console.WriteLine("Bestätige TID {0}", tid.TID);
    try
    {
      // TIDs mit Status RolledBack nicht löschen
      string error = "";
      TidStatus status = tidStore.GetStatus(
        tid.TID, out error);
      if (status == TidStatus.RolledBack)
        return;
      tidStore.DeleteEntry(tid.TID);
    }
    catch (Exception) { }
  }
```

```
  public void Commit(
    RfcServerContextInfo serverContext, RfcTID tid)
  {
    Console.WriteLine("Commit TID {0}", tid.TID);
    try
    {
      tidStore.SetStatus(
        tid.TID, TidStatus.Committed, null);
    }
    catch (Exception) { }
  }
  public void Rollback(
    RfcServerContextInfo serverContext, RfcTID tid)
  {
    Console.WriteLine("Rollback TID {0}", tid.TID);
    tidStore.SetStatus(tid.TID, TidStatus.RolledBack, null);
  }
  public static void SetError(
    RfcTID tid, String errorMessage)
  {
    try
    {
      tidStore.SetStatus(
        tid.TID, TidStatus.RolledBack, errorMessage);
    }
    catch (Exception) { }
  }
}
```


Listing 6.23 Implementierung der Schnittstelle »ITransactionIDHandler«

Die Methode `SetError()` in Listing 6.23 ist keine Methode von `ITransactionIDHandler`. Sie können sie aber im Fehlerfall aus Ihren Funktions-Handlern aufrufen, falls dort ein Fehler auftritt und Sie die Fehlermeldung zur TID im TID-Speicher speichern wollen.

Innerhalb eines Funktions-Handlers können Sie mithilfe des übergebenen `RfcServerContext`-Objekts herausfinden, ob Sie sich innerhalb einer Transaktion befinden. In diesem Fall hat die Eigenschaft `InTransaction` dieses Objekts den Wert »true«, und die Eigenschaft `TransactionID` enthält eine Referenz auf das `RfcTID`-Objekt, das wiederum die TID enthält.

6.4.6 Queued RFC

Beim queued RFC (qRFC) müssen Sie neben den TIDs auch die verschiedenen Queues managen, in denen die Funktionsbausteine ausgeführt werden. In welcher Queue ein Funktionsbaustein ausgeführt wird, erfahren Sie aus dem übergebenen `RfcServerContext`-Objekt. Dessen Feld `QueueNames` vom Typ `string[]` enthält dann einen Eintrag, nämlich den Namen der qRFC-Queue.

Zusätzlich hat die Eigenschaft `InTransaction` den Wert »true«, und die Eigenschaft `TransactionID` enthält eine Referenz auf das `RfcTID`-Objekt.

6.4.7 Background RFC

Die Implementierung von Background RFCs (bgRFCs) verläuft ganz ähnlich wie die Implementierung von transaktionalen RFCs. An die Stelle der 24-stelligen TIDs treten 32-stellige GUIDs, die die Background Units identifizieren. An die Stelle der Schnittstelle `ITransactionIDHandler` tritt die Schnittstelle `IUnitIDHandler`. Um bgRFCs auf Ihrem Server zu realisieren, müssen Sie also eine Klasse bereitstellen, die die Schnittstelle `IUnitIDHandler` implementiert. Sie erzeugen danach eine Instanz Ihres Unit-ID-Handlers und kopieren eine Referenz auf diese Instanz in die Eigenschaft `UnitIDHandler` des `RfcServer`-Objekts.

Methoden von »IUnitIDHandler«

Die Schnittstelle `IUnitIDHandler` definiert fünf Methoden:

- Die Methode `CheckUnitID` wird aufgerufen, sobald eine neue Background Unit bei Ihrem Server ankommt. Hier überprüfen Sie, ob Sie deren GUID schon kennen und in welchem Zustand sie sich befindet. Hier können mehrere Zustände auftreten:
  - Falls sich die GUID noch nicht in Ihrem GUID-Speicher befindet, speichern Sie diese dort mit dem Zustand `Created` und geben den Wert »true« zurück. Sie geben auch den Wert »true« zurück, wenn sich die GUID zwar im GUID-Speicher befindet, dort aber den Zustand `Created` oder `RolledBack` hat, da Sie in diesem Fall die Background Unit noch nicht durchgeführt haben.
  - Falls sich die GUID in Ihrem GUID-Speicher befindet und den Zustand `Commited` hat, geben Sie »false« zurück. Dann ruft der NCo Ihren Funktions-Handler nicht auf, und die Background Unit wird nicht noch ein zweites Mal ausgeführt.
  - Falls Sie momentan nicht auf den GUID-Speicher zugreifen können, lösen Sie eine `RfcInternalError`-Ausnahme aus.

- Die Methode Commit wird aufgerufen, sobald der NCo Ihren Funktions-Handler erfolgreich ausführen konnte. Hier sollten Sie alle Datenbankänderungen übergeben und die GUID im GUID-Speicher auf den Zustand Commited setzen.
- Die Methode Rollback wird aufgerufen, wenn in Ihrem Funktions-Handler eine Ausnahme ausgelöst wurde. Sie sollten alle Datenbankänderungen zurückrollen und die GUID im GUID-Speicher auf den Zustand RolledBack setzen.
- In der Methode ConfirmUnitID löschen Sie einfach die GUID in Ihrem GUID-Speicher.
- In der Methode GetUnitState sollten Sie den Status der Background Unit zurückgeben. Die möglichen Werte sind in der Enumeration RfcUnitState definiert und lauten »IN_PROCESS«, »COMMITED«, »CONFIRMED«, »ROLLED_BACK« und »NOT_FOUND«.

6.4.8 Zustand des Servers überwachen

Ereignisse von »RfcServer«

Die Klasse RfcServer stellt Ihnen drei Ereignisse zur Verfügung, auf die Sie einen eigenen Ereignis-Handler registrieren können, um Informationen über den Zustand des Servers und über mögliche Probleme zu bekommen.

- public event RfcServerStateChangedEventHandler RfcServerStateChanged
  Auf dieses Ereignis können Sie ein Delegat vom Typ public delegate void RfcServerStateChangedEventHandler(Object server, RfcServerStateChangedEventArgs stateEventData) registrieren. Das Objekt server können Sie nach RfcServer casten. Der Parameter stateEventData gibt Ihnen Informationen über den alten und neuen Zustand des Servers in Form einer RfcServerState-Enumeration, die die Werte »STARTING«, »RUNNING«, »BROKEN«, »STOPPING« oder »STOPPED« annehmen kann.
- public event RfcErrorEventHandler RfcServerError
  Dieses Ereignis wird bei Problemen in tieferen Schichten des Servers ausgelöst, etwa wenn eine Netzwerkverbindung zusammenbricht, ein Benutzer nicht authentifiziert werden kann oder nicht auf den TID-Speicher zugegriffen werden kann. Auf dieses Ereignis können Sie ein Delegat vom Typ public delegate void RfcServerErrorEventHandler(Object server, RfcErrorEventArgs errorEventData) registrieren. Das server-Objekt können Sie auf RfcServer casten. Es enthält eine Referenz auf den Server, bei dem das Problem aufgetreten ist (falls Ihre Applikation mehrere Server hostet). Der Parameter errorEventData gibt Ihnen Zugriff auf die ursprüngliche Ausnahme und den Serverkontext.

- `public event RfcErrorEventHandler RfcServerApplicationError`
  Dieses Ereignis wird ausgelöst, wenn einer Ihrer Funktions-Handler eine Ausnahme auslöst. Auf dieses Ereignis können Sie ein Delegat desselben Typs wie dem des Delegats des `RfcServerError`-Ereignisses registrieren.

Kapitel 7
IDocs und Application Link Enabling

In diesem Kapitel stellen wir Ihnen die Werkzeuge vor, die zur Entwicklung von ALE-Szenarien, in denen Anwendungen ihre Daten in Form von IDocs austauschen, notwendig sind. Sie lernen, wie Sie IDocs definieren, die ALE-Schicht konfigurieren und ALE-Szenarien in ABAP, C/C++, Java und C# implementieren.

In diesem Kapitel beschreiben wir das *Application Link Enabling* (ALE). Bei dieser Integrationstechnologie tauschen die beteiligten Anwendungen ihre Daten in Form von *Intermediate Documents* (IDocs) aus. Die Kommunikation erfolgt asynchron, d. h., der Sender einer Nachricht wartet nicht auf eine direkte Antwort des Empfängers, sondern fährt nach dem Senden des Dokuments mit seiner Arbeit fort.

Wir werden ALE-Szenarien in den Programmiersprachen ABAP (in Abschnitt 7.1, »IDocs«, und Abschnitt 7.2, »Application Link Enabling«), C/C++ (in Abschnitt 7.3, »IDoc-Programmierung mit dem SAP NetWeaver RFC SDK«), Java (in Abschnitt 7.4, »IDoc-Programmierung mit Java und dem SAP Java Connector«) und C# (Abschnitt 7.5, »IDoc-Programmierung mit dem SAP Connector for Microsoft .NET«) entwickeln.

7.1 IDocs

In diesem Abschnitt lernen Sie anhand eines Beispiels, wie Sie die notwendigen Definitionen, Reports und Funktionsbausteine für die IDoc-Kommunikation in SAP-Systemen erstellen können. In dem gewählten Szenario sollen Bestelldaten vom Mandanten 001 in den Mandanten 002 desselben SAP-Systems geschickt werden. In weiteren Abschnitten werden wir dieses Szenario für externe Systeme erweitern.

Vier Realisierungsschritte

Um das Szenario zu realisieren, sind die folgenden Schritte erforderlich:

1. **Definition des IDoc-Typs**
   Zunächst wird in Abschnitt 7.1.1, »Entwicklung von IDocs«, ein IDoc-Typ definiert. Dieser Typ legt die Struktur des IDocs fest, das versendet wird.
2. **Entwicklung eines Reports für den Versand**
   Dieser Report wird in Abschnitt 7.1.2, »Erzeugung von IDocs«, entwickelt, holt die Daten aus den Anwendungstabellen ein, baut das IDoc auf und übergibt es an das ALE-Subsystem zum Versand.
3. **Entwicklung eines Funktionsbausteins für den Empfang**
   Der Funktionsbaustein, den wir in Abschnitt 7.1.3, »Eingangsverarbeitung von IDocs«, entwickeln, nimmt das empfangene IDoc vom ALE-Subsystem entgegen und schreibt die Daten in die Anwendungstabellen.
4. **Customizing des ALE-Subsystems**
   Das ALE-Subsystem muss so eingerichtet werden, dass das ausgehende IDoc über einen transaktionalen RFC an das Empfangssystem weitergeleitet und das eingehende IDoc an den richtigen Funktionsbaustein übergeben wird. Dies zeigen wir in Abschnitt 7.2, »Application Link Enabling«.

In den genannten Abschnitten werden diese vier Schritte detailliert beschrieben, bevor in den darauffolgenden Abschnitten die Realisierung in C/C++, Java und C# erfolgt.

7.1.1 Entwicklung von IDocs

Segmente

IDocs sind Dokumente, die aus einzelnen Zeilen bestehen, die *Segmente* heißen. Der Aufbau eines Segments wird durch seinen Segmenttyp festgelegt. Segmenttypen werden mit Transaktion WE31 definiert. SAP spricht in dieser Transaktion allerdings nicht von Segmenttypen, sondern von Segmenten.

IDoc-Segmente

Für das angesprochene Szenario müssen Sie zwei Segmente definieren: eines für die Kopfdaten und eines für die Positionsdaten einer Bestellung. Um ein Segment zu definieren, das die Kopfdaten für eine Bestellung aufnehmen kann, starten Sie Transaktion WE31 und geben als Namen für den Segmenttyp »Z1ORDHD« an. Die Namen von SAP-Segmenten beginnen mit dem Kürzel »E1«, kundendefinierte Segmente beginnen hingegen mit »Z1«.

Datenelemente

Über den Menüpfad **Bearbeiten • Anlegen** können Sie die einzelnen Feldnamen in der Segmentdefinition definieren. Dazu nehmen Sie in den Spalten

Feldname und **Datenelement** die notwendigen Angaben vor (siehe Abbildung 7.1). Das System vergibt automatisch einen Namen für die Segmentdefinition, in diesem Fall Z2ORDHD000. Der Name für die Definition beginnt mit dem Namen für das Segment und endet mit einer dreistelligen Versionsnummer. Speichern Sie diese Segmentdefinition, und ordnen Sie sie dabei einem Entwicklungspaket zu. Sobald Sie die Definition abgeschlossen haben, können Sie sie über den Menüpfad **Bearbeiten • Freigabe** freigeben.

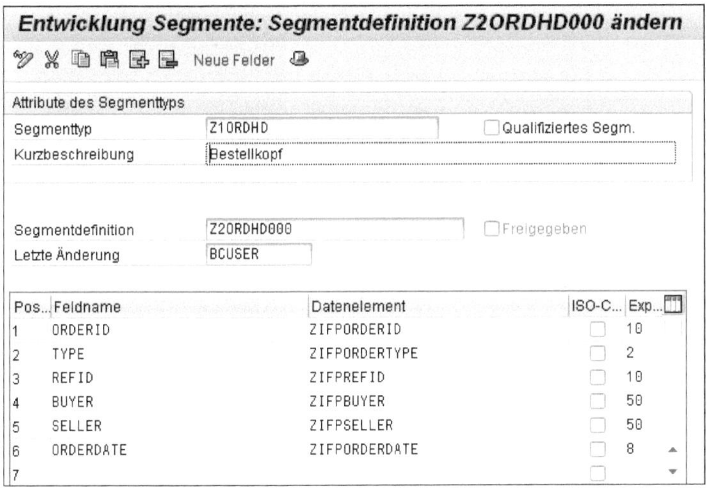

Abbildung 7.1 Version 000 des Segments »Z1ORDHD«

Um Daten für die Positionsdaten in IDocs versenden zu können, müssen Sie zusätzlich das Segment Z1ORDPS definieren (siehe Abbildung 7.2).

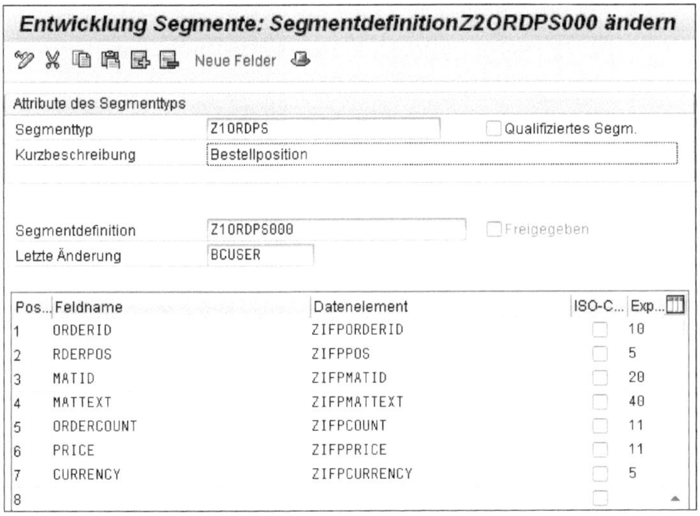

Abbildung 7.2 Version 000 des Segments »Z1ORDPS«

[+]

Versionierung von Segmenten

Noch ein Wort zu den Namenskonventionen, die die Entwicklungsumgebung hier erzwingt: Die Namen von Segmenttypen beginnen immer mit »Z1« (für kundendefinierte Segmente) bzw. »E1« (für SAP-definierte Segmente). Die Namen von Segmentdefinitionen beginnen immer mit »Z2« bzw. »E2«.

Wenn Sie Ihre IDoc-Segmente später in einem SAP-System mit höherer Versionsnummer weiterentwickeln möchten, können Sie dem Segmenttyp eine weitere Version mit einer erweiterten Segmentdefinition hinzufügen. Diese erweiterte Segmentdefinition enthält zusätzliche Felder. Bestehende Felder können nicht entfernt oder geändert werden. Segmenttyp und Version der SAP-Basis legen demnach eindeutig die zugehörige Segmentdefinition fest.

IDoc-Typen

Nach der Definition der Segmente können Sie mit Transaktion WE30 den IDoc-Typ ZORDER01 definieren. Mit IDocs dieses Typs werden Bestellungen transportiert.

IDoc-Typ definieren

Geben Sie im Feld **Objektname** den Namen für den IDoc-Typ ein, belassen Sie die Selektion des Optionsfelds bei **Basistyp**, und folgen Sie dem Pfad **Entwicklungsobjekt • Anlegen** ([F5]). Im folgenden Dialog belassen Sie die Selektion des Optionsfelds bei **Neu anlegen** und geben dann eine Beschreibung für den IDoc-Typ an. Danach können Sie den Basistyp ZORDER01 anlegen. Wählen Sie **Bearbeiten • Segment Anlegen** ([⇧] + [F6]). Geben Sie an, dass es sich um ein Muss-Segment handelt, und bestimmen Sie die minimale und die maximale Anzahl für das Vorkommen dieses Segments im IDoc (siehe Abbildung 7.3).

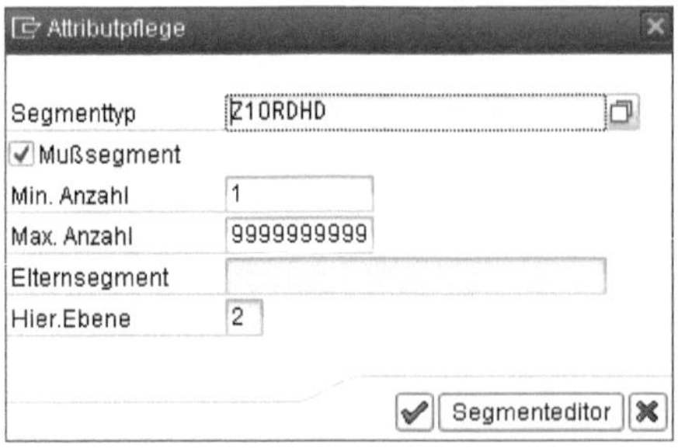

Abbildung 7.3 Attribute des Segments »Z1ORDHD« im IDoc »ZORDER01«

Hierarchische IDoc-Struktur

Wählen Sie dann mit einem Mausklick das soeben eingefügte Segment aus, und fügen Sie das Segment Z1ORDPS als Kind des Segments Z1ORDHD hinzu. Der IDoc-Typ ZORDER01 sieht dann aus wie in Abbildung 7.4.

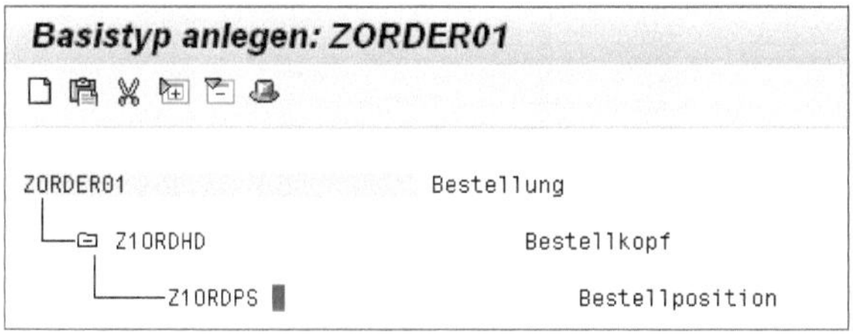

Abbildung 7.4 IDoc-Typ »ZORDER01«

Nach der Definition geben Sie den IDoc-Typ im Einstiegsbild von Transaktion WE31 über **Bearbeiten • Freigabe setzen** frei.

Nachrichtentyp

Der nächste Schritt besteht aus der Definition eines Nachrichtentyps mit Transaktion WE81. Nachrichtentypen legen die Bedeutung einer Nachricht fest, deren Inhalt durch ein IDoc transportiert wird. Dabei können verschiedene Nachrichtentypen durchaus mithilfe desselben IDoc-Typs transportiert werden. Zum Beispiel entsprechen Anfragen nach Stammdaten an verschiedene SAP-Anwendungen unterschiedlichen Nachrichtentypen. Sie werden aber meistens durch den IDoc-Typ ALEREQ01 transportiert. Für die Zwecke der Bestellanwendung legen Sie den Nachrichtentyp ZORDER mit der Kurzbeschreibung »Bestellung« an.

IDoc-Typ für einen Nachrichtentyp

Als letzter Entwicklungsschritt muss diesem Nachrichtentyp ein IDoc-Typ zugeordnet werden. Dies geschieht mittels Transaktion WE82. Ordnen Sie dort dem Nachrichtentyp ZORDER den Basistyp ZORDER01 für Ihr aktuelles SAP-Basis-Release zu. Auch hier können Sie in einem späteren Release eine Zuordnung für einen neuen IDoc-Typ anlegen, der dieselbe Nachricht transportiert. Dieser IDoc-Typ sollte dann natürlich eine Erweiterung des bisherigen Typs sein.

7.1.2 Erzeugung von IDocs

Report zur Datenselektion

Für das Anlegen von IDocs und deren Übergabe an die ALE-Schicht ist die Anwendung verantwortlich. Im einfachsten Fall stellt sie dazu einen Report zur Verfügung, in dem Sie als Anwender die zu versendenden Daten selektieren. Listing 7.1 zeigt einen solchen Report für das Anwendungsbeispiel.

```
REPORT  zifp_send_idoc.
DATA:
  wa_hdr          TYPE zifporder,          " Bestellkopf
  wa_pos          TYPE zifporderpos,       " Bestellposition
  rec_control     TYPE edidc,              " Control-Record
  it_control      TYPE TABLE OF edidc,     " Control-Records
  it_data         TYPE TABLE OF edidd,     " IDoc-Zeilen
  wa_data         TYPE edidd,              " IDoc-Zeile
  wa_idoc_hdr     TYPE z1ordhd,            " IDoc-Daten Kopf
  wa_idoc_pos     TYPE z1ordps,            " IDoc-Daten
                                           " Position
  segnum          TYPE i,                  " Segmentnummer
  psgnum          TYPE i.                  " Eltern-
                                           " Segmentnummer
PARAMETERS:
  pa_ord TYPE zifporderid.
START-OF-SELECTION.
* prüfen, ob überhaupt Empfänger existieren
  CALL FUNCTION 'ALE_MODEL_INFO_GET'
    EXPORTING
      message_type           = 'ZORDER'
    EXCEPTIONS
      no_model_info_found    = 1
      own_system_not_defined = 2
      OTHERS                 = 3.
  IF sy-subrc <> 0.
    MESSAGE ID sy-msgid TYPE sy-msgty NUMBER sy-msgno
            WITH sy-msgv1 sy-msgv2 sy-msgv3 sy-msgv4.
  ENDIF.
* Kontrollsatz erzeugen
  rec_control-mestyp = 'ZORDER'.
  rec_control-idoctp = 'ZORDER01'.
* IDoc aufbauen
  segnum = 1.
  SELECT SINGLE * FROM zifporder INTO wa_hdr
    WHERE orderid = pa_ord AND type = 'PO'.
  MOVE-CORRESPONDING wa_hdr TO wa_idoc_hdr.
  CLEAR wa_data.
  wa_data-segnum = segnum.
  wa_data-psgnum = 0.
  wa_data-segnam = 'Z1ORDHD'.
  wa_data-mandt  = sy-mandt.
  wa_data-sdata  = wa_idoc_hdr.
```

```
  APPEND wa_data TO it_data.
  ADD 1 TO segnum.
  psgnum = wa_data-segnum.
  SELECT * FROM zifporderpos INTO wa_pos
    WHERE orderid = wa_hdr-orderid.
    MOVE-CORRESPONDING wa_pos TO wa_idoc_pos.
    wa_data-segnum = segnum.
    wa_data-psgnum = psgnum.
    wa_data-segnam = 'Z1ORDPS'.
    wa_data-mandt  = sy-mandt.
    wa_data-sdata  = wa_idoc_pos.
    APPEND wa_data TO it_data.
    ADD 1 TO segnum.
  ENDSELECT.
* IDoc verschicken
  CALL FUNCTION 'MASTER_IDOC_DISTRIBUTE'
    EXPORTING
      master_idoc_control            = rec_control
    TABLES
      communication_idoc_control     = it_control
      master_idoc_data               = it_data
    EXCEPTIONS
      error_in_idoc_control          = 1
      error_writing_idoc_status      = 2
      error_in_idoc_data             = 3
      sending_logical_system_unknown = 4
      OTHERS                         = 5.
  IF sy-subrc <> 0.
    MESSAGE ID sy-msgid TYPE sy-msgty NUMBER sy-msgno
            WITH sy-msgv1 sy-msgv2 sy-msgv3 sy-msgv4.
  ENDIF.
  COMMIT WORK.
  WRITE:/ 'IDoc verschickt.'.
```

Listing 7.1 Programm »ZEAI_SEND_IDOC«

Funktionsbaustein »ALE_MODEL_INFO_GET«

Der Report überprüft zunächst, ob überhaupt ein Empfangssystem existiert, das sich für die Nachricht ZORDER interessiert. Dazu verwendet er den Funktionsbaustein ALE_MODEL_INFO_GET und übergibt dem Importparameter message_type den Wert »ZORDER«.

Im Erfolgsfall füllt der Report zuerst einmal die Felder mestyp und idoctp des Kontrollsatzes rec_control mit den Werten »ZORDER« bzw. »ZORDER01«. Anhand dieses Kontrollsatzes ermittelt das ALE-Subsystem die Empfänger aus dem Verteilungsmodell, das im ALE-Customizing angelegt wird. Tabelle 7.1 zeigt einige Felder des Kontrollsatzes. Die Applikation muss dabei nur wenige Felder füllen; der Rest wird vom ALE-Subsystem erledigt.

Feld	Inhalt
MANDT	Mandant
DOCNUM	Nummer des IDocs
DOCREL	SAP-Release des IDocs
STATUS	Status des IDocs
DOCTYP	IDoc-Typ
DIRECT	Richtung der Übertragung (1 = Ausgang, 2 = Eingang)
RCVPOR	Empfängerport
RCVPRT	Partnerart Empfänger
RCVPRN	Partnernummer des Empfängers
SNDPOR	Senderport
SNDPRT	Partnerart Sender
SNDPRN	Partnernummer des Senders

Tabelle 7.1 Komponenten des IDoc-Kontrollsatzes »EDIDC«

Kontrollsegment

Danach baut der Report das IDoc auf. Für jeden selektierten Satz der Tabelle ZIFPORDERHEADER schreibt er eine Zeile in die interne Tabelle it_data. Diese Zeile ist vom Typ EDIDD und enthält Informationen über das Segment sowie die eigentlichen Anwendungsdaten (siehe Tabelle 7.2). Das Feld SEGNAM wird dabei auf »Z1ORDHD« gesetzt, und in das Feld SDATA werden die Daten des Bestellkopfs kopiert.

Feld	Inhalt
MANDT	Mandant
DOCNUM	Nummer des IDocs
SEGNUM	Segmentnummer innerhalb des Dokuments
SEGNAM	Segmentname

Tabelle 7.2 Komponenten eines IDoc-Datensatzes »EDIDD«

Feld	Inhalt
PSGNUM	Nummer des Elternsegments
HLEVEL	Hierarchieebene
SDATA	Anwendungsdaten

Tabelle 7.2 Komponenten eines IDoc-Datensatzes »EDIDD« (Forts.)

Datensegmente

Für jede Bestellung liest der Report alle Positionen dieser Bestellung und schreibt für jede Position eine Zeile in das IDoc. Das Feld SEGNAM wird dabei natürlich auf »Z1ORDPS« gesetzt, und in das Feld SDATA werden die Positionsdaten kopiert. Schließlich übergibt der Report das aufgebaute IDoc an das ALE-Subsystem, indem er den Funktionsbaustein MASTER_IDOC_DISTRIBUTE aufruft.

7.1.3 Eingangsverarbeitung von IDocs

Funktionsbaustein zum Empfang des IDocs

Auf Empfängerseite nimmt ein Funktionsbaustein das IDoc vom ALE-Subsystem entgegen. Der Name dieses Funktionsbausteins sollte Z_IDOC_INPUT_ZORDER sein. Zum Anlegen kopieren Sie am einfachsten den Funktionsbaustein ALE_INPUT_ALEAUD, da er dann sofort die richtige Schnittstelle hat (siehe Listing 7.2).

```
FUNCTION z_idoc_input_zorder.
*"----------------------------------------------------------
*"*"Lokale Schnittstelle:
*"  IMPORTING
*"     VALUE(INPUT_METHOD) LIKE  BDWFAP_PAR-INPUTMETHD
*"     VALUE(MASS_PROCESSING) LIKE  BDWFAP_PAR-MASS_PROC
*"  EXPORTING
*"     VALUE(WORKFLOW_RESULT) LIKE  BDWF_PARAM-RESULT
*"     VALUE(APPLICATION_VARIABLE) LIKE  BDWF_PARAM-APPL_VAR
*"     VALUE(IN_UPDATE_TASK) LIKE  BDWFAP_PAR-UPDATETASK
*"     VALUE(CALL_TRANSACTION_DONE) LIKE BDWFAP_PAR-
*"     CALLTRANS
*"  TABLES
*"      IDOC_CONTRL STRUCTURE  EDIDC
*"      IDOC_DATA STRUCTURE  EDIDD
*"      IDOC_STATUS STRUCTURE  BDIDOCSTAT
*"      RETURN_VARIABLES STRUCTURE  BDWFRETVAR
*"      SERIALIZATION_INFO STRUCTURE  BDI_SER
*"  EXCEPTIONS
```

```
*"      WRONG_FUNCTION_CALLED
*"----------------------------------------------------------
  INCLUDE mbdconwf.         " Konstanten des ALE-Subsystems
  DATA:
    wa_data     TYPE edidd,        " IDoc-Datenzeile
    wa_control  TYPE edidc,        " Kontrolldatensatz
    wa_idoc_hdr TYPE z1ordhd,      " Kopfdaten aus IDoc
    wa_idoc_pos TYPE z1ordps,      " Positionsdaten aus IDoc
    wa_hdr      TYPE zifporder,    " Kopfdaten für DB
    wa_hdr_old  TYPE zifporder,    " Alte Kopfdaten
    wa_pos      TYPE zifporderpos. " Positionsdaten für DB
* Kontrolldatensatz lesen
  READ TABLE idoc_contrl INTO wa_control INDEX 1.
  LOOP AT idoc_data INTO wa_data WHERE
    docnum = wa_control-docnum.
    IF wa_data-segnam ='Z1ORDHD'.
* Bestelldatensatz einfügen oder modifizieren
      wa_idoc_hdr = wa_data-sdata.
      MOVE-CORRESPONDING wa_idoc_hdr TO wa_hdr.
      wa_hdr-refid = wa_hdr-orderid.
      wa_hdr-type  = 'SO'.
* Neuanlage oder Update?
      SELECT SINGLE * FROM zifporder INTO wa_hdr_old
        WHERE refid = wa_hdr-orderid.
      IF sy-subrc EQ 0.
        wa_hdr-orderid = wa_hdr_old-orderid.
      ELSE.
        CALL FUNCTION 'NUMBER_GET_NEXT'
          EXPORTING
            nr_range_nr = '01'
            object      = 'ZIFPORDER'
          IMPORTING
            number      = wa_hdr-orderid
          EXCEPTIONS
            OTHERS      = 1.
      ENDIF.
      MODIFY zifporder FROM wa_hdr.
      IF sy-subrc NE 0.
        EXIT.
      ENDIF.
    ELSEIF wa_data-segnam = 'Z1ORDPS'.
```

```
* Positionsdatensatz einfügen oder aktualisieren
      wa_idoc_pos = wa_data-sdata.
      MOVE-CORRESPONDING wa_idoc_pos TO wa_pos.
      wa_idoc_pos = wa_data-sdata.
      MODIFY zifporderpos FROM wa_pos.
      IF sy-subrc NE 0.
        EXIT.
      ENDIF.
    ENDIF.
  ENDLOOP.
* Rückmeldung schreiben
  IF sy-subrc NE 0.
    idoc_status-status = c_idoc_status_error.
    idoc_status-msgty  = sy-msgty.
    idoc_status-msgid  = sy-msgid.
    idoc_status-msgno  = sy-msgno.
    idoc_status-msgv1  = sy-msgv1.
    idoc_status-msgv2  = sy-msgv2.
    idoc_status-msgv3  = sy-msgv3.
    idoc_status-msgv4  = sy-msgv4.
    workflow_result    = c_wf_result_error.
    return_variables-wf_param   = c_wf_par_error_idocs.
  ELSE.
    idoc_status-status = c_idoc_status_ok.
    idoc_status-msgty  = 'S'.
    idoc_status-msgid  = 'ZIFP'.
    idoc_status-msgno  = 150.
    workflow_result    = c_wf_result_ok.
    return_variables-wf_param   = c_wf_par_processed_idocs.
  ENDIF.

  idoc_status-docnum = wa_control-docnum.
  idoc_status-repid  = sy-repid.
  APPEND idoc_status.
  return_variables-doc_number   = wa_control-docnum.
  APPEND return_variables.
ENDFUNCTION.
```

Listing 7.2 Funktionsbaustein »Z_IDOC_INPUT_ZORDER«

Parameter der Schnittstelle

Die Schnittstelle des Funktionsbausteins hat elf Parameter. Diese Parameter haben folgende Bedeutung:

- `IDOC_CONTRL`
  Diese Tabelle enthält einen Kontrolldatensatz für jedes übergebene IDoc. Von ihr benötigt der Funktionsbaustein die Spalten `Docnum` und `Idoctp`, die die Nummern und IDoc-Typen der übergebenen IDocs enthalten.
- `IDOC_DATA`
  Diese Tabelle enthält die Segmente der IDocs, die an den Funktionsbaustein übergeben wurden. Aus dieser Tabelle sind die Spalten `Docnum`, `Segnam` und `Sdata` relevant, die die IDoc-Nummer, den Segmentnamen und die Anwendungsdaten enthalten.
- `INPUT_METHOD`
  Soll der Funktionsbaustein im Hintergrund ablaufen, ist dieser Parameter initial. Falls der Funktionsbaustein als dialogfähig markiert wurde, d. h., wenn er Eingabebildschirme anzeigt, kann er die Werte »A« oder »E« annehmen. Im ersten Fall soll er alle Eingabebildschirme anzeigen, im zweiten nur dann, wenn ein Fehler auftritt.
- `MASS_PROCESSING`
  Dieser Parameter wird nicht mehr verwendet. Er wurde aus Gründen der Rückwärtskompatibilität mit alten Clients nicht entfernt.
- `IN_UPDATE_TASK`
  Der Funktionsbaustein bewertet diesen Exportparameter mit »X«, wenn er die Verbuchung über Verbuchungsbausteine mit dem Zusatz `IN UPDATE TASK` vornimmt.
- `CALL_TRANSACTION_DONE`
  Der Funktionsbaustein füllt diesen Exportparameter mit »X«, wenn er `CALL TRANSACTION` verwendet, um den IDoc-Status zu schreiben.
- `WORKFLOW_RESULT`
  Über diesen Exportparameter steuert der Funktionsbaustein, ob Ereignisse ausgelöst werden sollen.
- `APPLICATION_VARIABLE`
  Dies ist ein optionaler Parameter, der dem Workflow übergeben werden kann.
- `IDOC_STATUS`
  Diese Tabelle enthält für jedes IDoc, das der Funktionsbaustein verarbeitet hat, einen Eintrag. Das Feld `Status` kann dabei die Werte »53« im Erfolgs- und »51« im Fehlerfall annehmen.
- `RETURN_VARIABLES`
  Diese Tabelle enthält die IDoc-Nummern und die zugehörigen Nummern der verarbeiteten Anwendungsobjekte. Diese Informationen

werden dazu verwendet, um das IDoc mit dem entsprechenden Anwendungsobjekt zu verknüpfen.

- SERIALIZATION_INFO
  Dieser Parameter wird nicht mehr verwendet.

Der Funktionsbaustein Z_IDOC_INPUT_ZORDER geht davon aus, dass ihm nur ein IDoc übergeben wird. Dessen Nummer ermittelt er über READ TABLE aus der Tabelle IDOC_CONTRL. Danach macht er eine Schleife über alle Segmente des IDocs in der Tabelle IDOC_DATA. Je nachdem, ob es sich um ein Segment Z1ORDHD oder Z1ORDPS handelt, nimmt er Änderungen an den Daten der Datenbanktabelle ZIFPORDER oder ZIFPORDERPOS vor. Bei einem Fehler bricht der Funktionsbaustein die Verarbeitung des IDocs ab. Sowohl im Fehler- als auch im Erfolgsfall füllt er zum Schluss die Parameter IDOC_STATUS, RETURN_VARIABLES und WORKFLOW_RESULT.

Registrierung

Nach der Entwicklung müssen Sie den Funktionsbaustein mit Transaktion BD51 als Eingangsbaustein für die ALE-Verarbeitung registrieren. Da er nur ein IDoc verarbeiten kann, setzen Sie dabei den Input-Typ auf »1«. Mit Transaktion WE57 legen Sie dann noch fest, dass der Funktionsbaustein dem **Nachrichtentyp** ZORDER und dem **Basistyp** ZORDER01 für die Eingangsverarbeitung zugeordnet ist (siehe Abbildung 7.5).

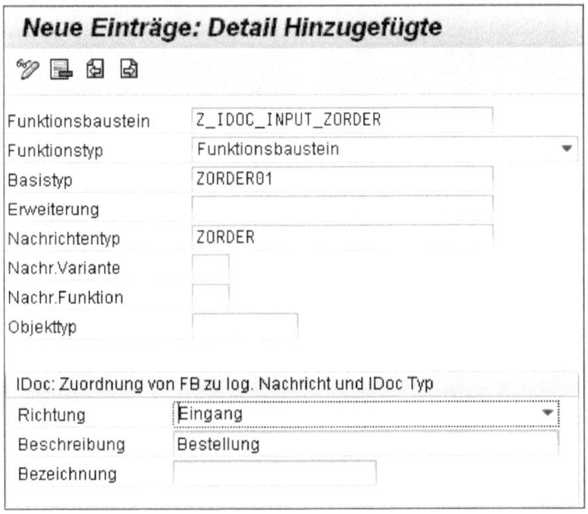

Abbildung 7.5 Transaktion WE57

Vorgangscodes

Damit der Funktionsbaustein tatsächlich für die Eingangsverarbeitung verwendet wird, müssen Sie im empfangenden System noch einen Vorgangscode ZORDER für den Eingang mittels Transaktion WE42 hinzufügen. Wie in Abbildung 7.6 zu sehen ist, wird in diesem Vorgangscode hinterlegt, wie das eingehende IDoc zu verarbeiten ist. Der Vorgangscode wird später im ALE-

Customizing bei der Festlegung der Eingangsparameter für den Nachrichtentyp ZORDER verwendet (siehe Abschnitt 7.2.1, »Konfiguration von ALE«).

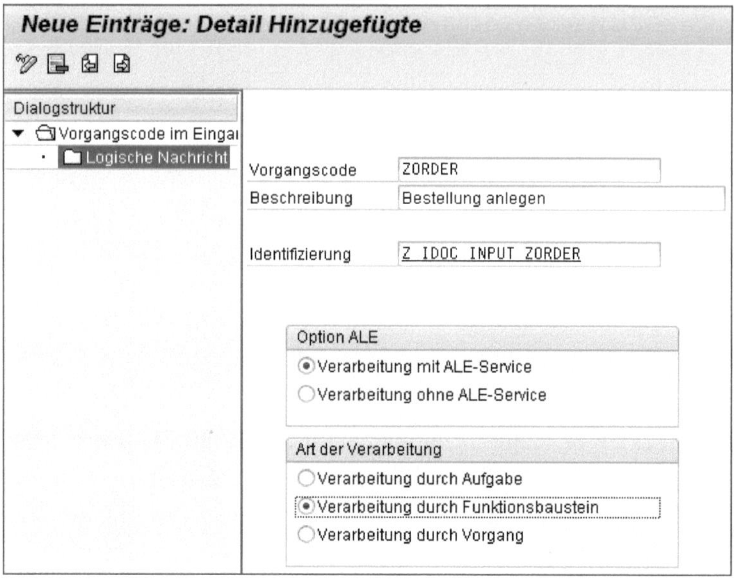

Abbildung 7.6 Transaktion WE42 zur Pflege von Vorgangscodes

7.2 Application Link Enabling

Application Link Enabling (ALE) ist ein Basisdienst innerhalb der ABAP-Plattform, mit dem Anwendungen IDocs versenden und empfangen können. In diesem Abschnitt erläutern wir Ihnen die Konfiguration dieses Subsystems. Wir werden ALE so konfigurieren, dass wir ein IDoc vom Typ ZORDER01 vom Mandanten 001 zum Mandanten 002 senden können.

7.2.1 Konfiguration von ALE

Transaktion SALE

Damit IDocs versendet und empfangen werden können, muss das ALE-Subsystem entsprechend eingerichtet werden. Dazu können Sie Transaktion SALE verwenden, die die notwendigen Schritte in der richtigen Reihenfolge auflistet, dokumentiert und Verknüpfungen zu den benötigten Transaktionen bereitstellt. Abbildung 7.7 zeigt einen Ausschnitt aus der von Transaktion SALE angezeigten Liste.

Schritte der Konfiguration

Folgende Schritte sind erforderlich:

- **Logische Systeme benennen**
  Jedes an ALE teilnehmende System wird durch einen logischen Namen

identifiziert. Diese Namen werden in die Datenbanktabelle TBDLS eingetragen.

- **Mandanten die logischen Systeme zuordnen**
  Jedem Mandanten in einem SAP-System wird ein logisches System zugeordnet. Dies geschieht bei der Pflege der Stammdaten des Mandanten.
- **Zielsysteme für RFC-Aufrufe definieren**
  Im sendenden System müssen Sie mit Transaktion SM59 tRFC-Destinationen für die Zielsysteme anlegen. Hat die tRFC-Destination den gleichen Namen wie das Zielsystem, können im letzten Schritt einige Definitionen automatisch generiert werden.
- **Verteilungsmodell pflegen**
  Hier wird festgelegt, welche Nachrichten vom sendenden System an welche Empfangssysteme verschickt werden. Dieser Schritt wird im sendenden System durchgeführt.
- **Partnervereinbarungen pflegen**
  Schließlich wird festgelegt, wie ausgehende IDocs an die Empfangssysteme geschickt und eingehende IDocs im Empfangssystem verarbeitet werden.

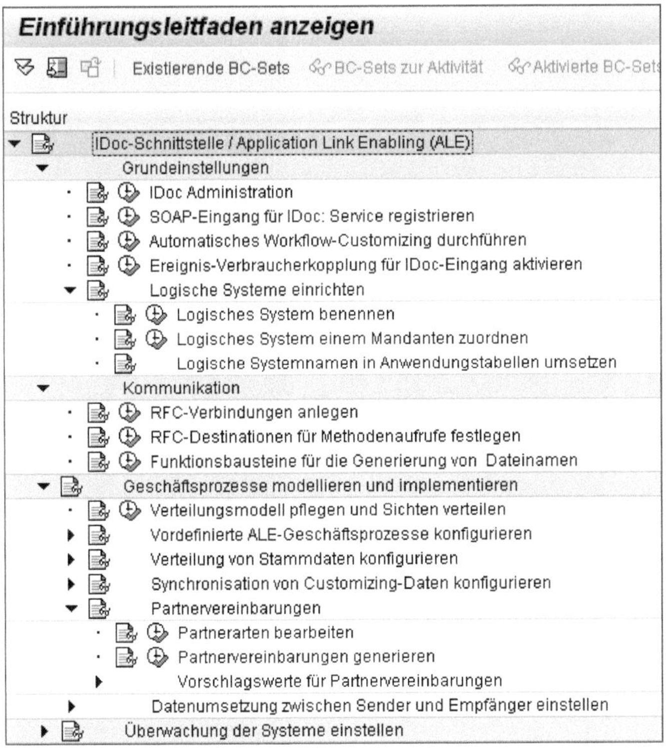

Abbildung 7.7 Transaktion SALE

Logische Systeme benennen

Um die Namen der logischen Systeme in die Datenbanktabelle TBDLS einzutragen, klicken Sie in Transaktion SALE auf den Knoten **Logisches System benennen**. Dies führt Sie in die Tabellenpflege der Tabelle TBDLS. Für jeden der am Szenario beteiligten Mandanten tragen Sie ein logisches System mit einer Bezeichnung ein. Typischerweise wird das logische System des Mandanten <xxx> mit der System-ID <SID> im SAP-System <SID>CLNT<xxx> benannt. Für das vorliegende Szenario benötigen Sie die beiden logischen Systeme AOUCLNT001 und AOUCLNT002.

Logisches System eines Mandanten

Um das logische System einem Mandanten zuzuordnen, klicken Sie in Transaktion SALE auf den Knoten **Logisches System einem Mandanten zuordnen**. Wählen Sie den Mandanten aus, und navigieren Sie in die Detailansicht, um zur Stammdatenpflege zu gelangen. Dort tragen Sie das logische System für den ausgewählten Mandanten ein, wie es Abbildung 7.8 zeigt. Diese Zuordnung eines logischen Systems zum Mandanten müssen Sie sowohl für den sendenden als auch für den empfangenden Mandanten vornehmen.

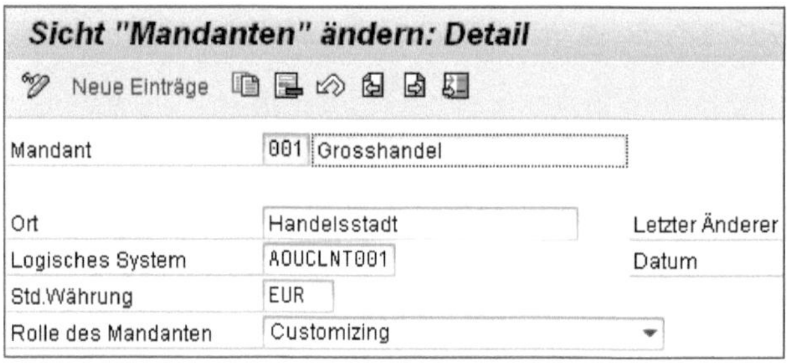

Abbildung 7.8 Logisches System eines SAP-Mandanten

RFC-Destination für den Empfänger

Im dritten Schritt pflegen Sie eine tRFC-Destination für das Empfangssystem. Dazu führen Sie in Transaktion SALE den Knoten **RFC-Verbindungen anlegen** aus. Dies führt Sie in Transaktion SM59, mit der Sie eine neue **RFC-Destination** für das Zielsystem anlegen können (siehe Abbildung 7.9). Die RFC-Destination sollten Sie genauso benennen wie das logische System des Empfängers, damit im nächsten Schritt die Partnervereinbarungen automatisch generiert werden können.

Stellen Sie sicher, dass Sie auf der Registerkarte **Anmeldung & Sicherheit** ein Konto angeben, mit dem eine Anmeldung am Zielsystem möglich ist. Außerdem sollten Sie die tRFC-Optionen unter dem Menüpunkt **Bearbeiten • tRFC-Optionen** pflegen. Wenn es bei der Übertragung des IDocs zum Empfangssystem einen Kommunikationsfehler gibt, plant ALE automatisch einen Hintergrundjob ein, der den Versand des IDocs erneut vornimmt. Bei den tRFC-Optionen können Sie angeben, wie viele Verbindungsversuche das System maximal vornehmen und wie lange zwischen zwei Verbindungsversuchen gewartet werden soll. Sie können die Einplanung dieses Hintergrundjobs aber auch ganz unterdrücken.

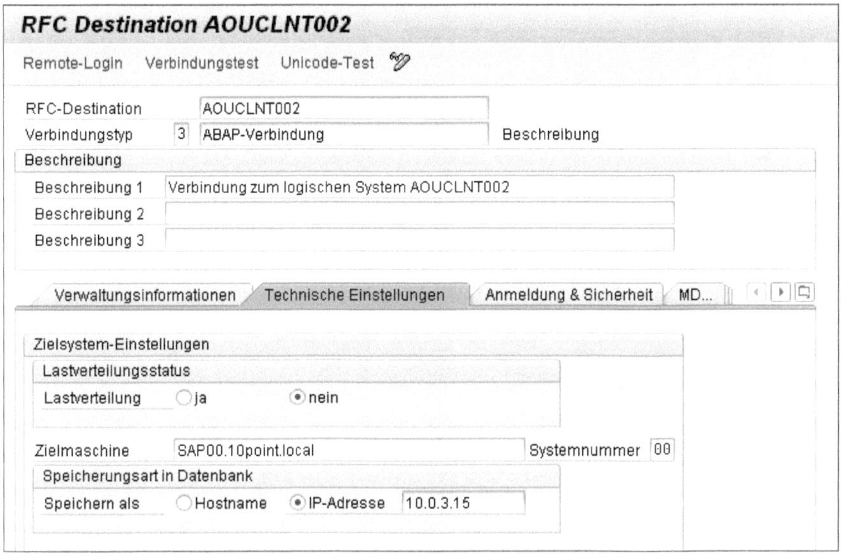

Abbildung 7.9 RFC-Destination für ein logisches System

Verteilungsmodell pflegen

Um das Verteilungsmodell zu pflegen, müssen Sie am Mandanten für das sendende logische System angemeldet sein. Wählen Sie in Transaktion SALE den Knoten **Verteilungsmodell pflegen und Sichten verteilen**. Legen Sie eine neue Modellsicht mit dem Kurztext »Bestellungen« und dem technischen Namen ZORDER an. Fügen Sie in diese Modellsicht einen Nachrichtentyp ein. Legen Sie dabei fest, dass der Sender AOUCLNT001 an den Empfänger AOUCLNT002 den Nachrichtentyp ZORDER schickt. Abbildung 7.10 zeigt das fertige Verteilungsmodell.

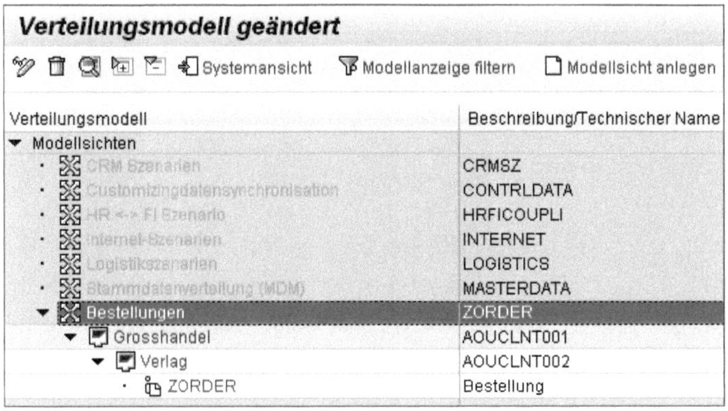

Abbildung 7.10 Verteilungsmodell

Partnervereinbarungen generieren

Vom Verteilungsmodell aus können Sie anschließend über den Menüpfad **Umfeld • Partnervereinbarung generieren** die Partnervereinbarungen erzeugen. Dabei legt das System Partnervereinbarungen für das sendende und empfangende System, einen Port mit der vorher angelegten tRFC-Destination sowie Ausgangsparameter zum Nachrichtentyp ZORDER an.

Partnervereinbarungen prüfen

Sie können den Anlegen-Vorgang kontrollieren, indem Sie im Verteilungsmodell den Menüpunkt **Umfeld • Partnervereinbarung ändern** wählen. Dies führt Sie zu Transaktion WE20 (siehe Abbildung 7.11). Dort sehen Sie, dass unter der Partnerart **Logisches System (LS)** sowohl das Sende- als auch das Empfangssystem eingetragen worden sind. Für das Empfangssystem wurden außerdem Ausgangsparameter für den Nachrichtentyp ZORDER angelegt.

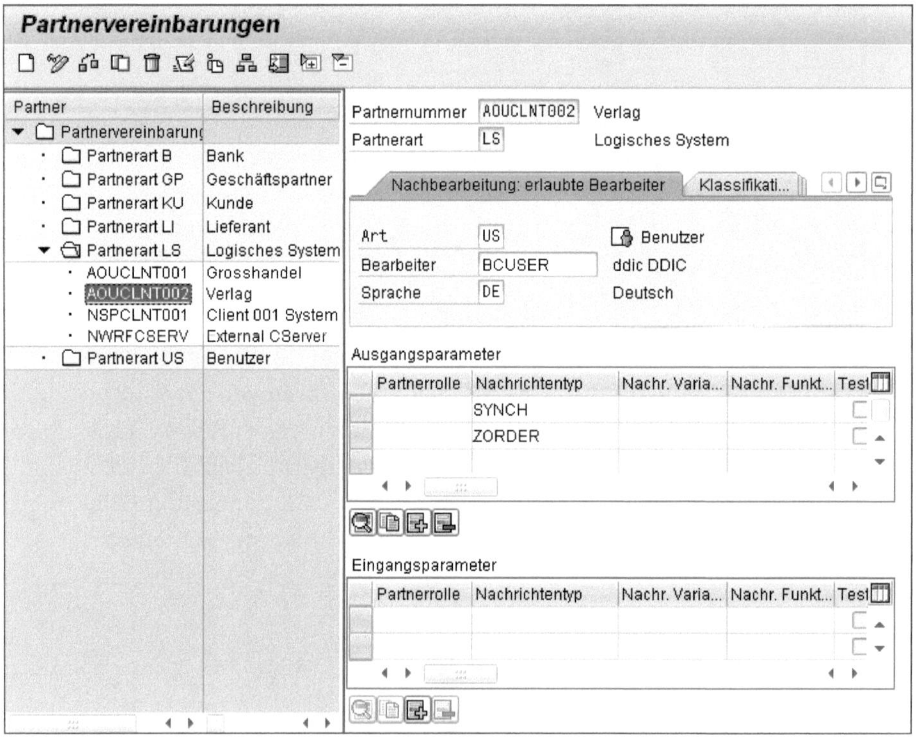

Abbildung 7.11 Partnervereinbarungen

Ausgangsparameter pflegen

Abbildung 7.12 zeigt die Ausgangsparameter für den Nachrichtentyp ZORDER. Dort ist als Empfängerport der generierte Port eingetragen, der seinerseits auf die zuvor angelegte tRFC-Destination verweist. Als Ausgabemodus wurde auf der Registerkarte **Ausgangsoptionen** das Kennzeichen für **IDoc sofort übergeben** gesetzt. Alternativ könnten die IDocs vor dem Übergeben zunächst gesammelt und dann als Paket übergeben werden. Im Eingabefeld **Paketgröße** kann die Anzahl der zu sammelnden IDocs festgelegt werden. Schließlich ist im Feld **Basistyp** auch noch der IDoc-Typ angegeben.

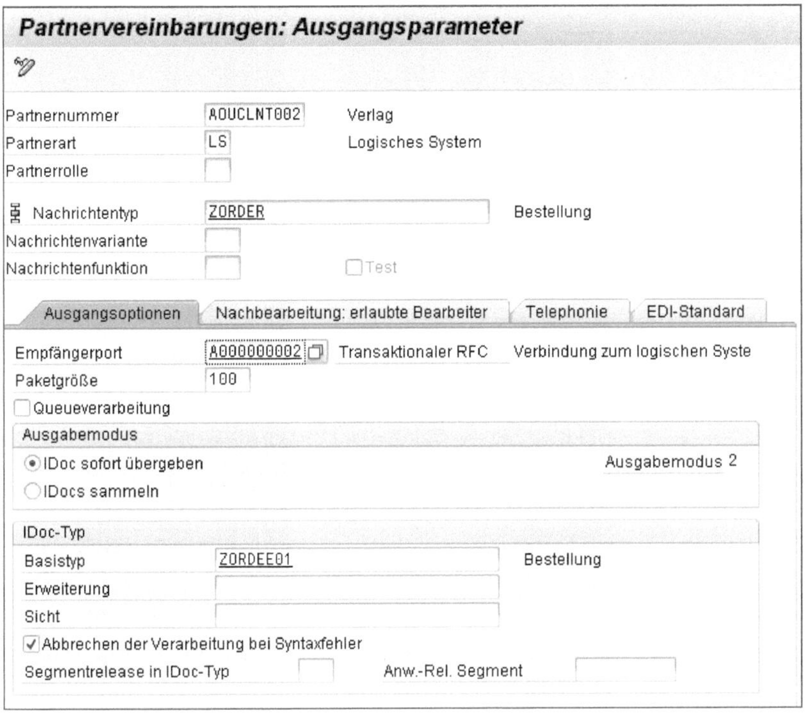

Abbildung 7.12 Ausgangsparameter

Eingangsparameter pflegen

Um die Eingangsparameter zu pflegen, müssen Sie sich am empfangenden System anmelden. Zuerst müssen Sie mit Transaktion WE42 den Vorgangscode `ZORDER` für den Eingang hinzufügen. Wie bereits beschrieben, wird im Vorgangscode hinterlegt, wie das eingehende IDoc zu verarbeiten ist (siehe Abbildung 7.6). Danach rufen Sie Transaktion WE20 zur manuellen Pflege der Eingangsparameter auf. Legen Sie zunächst unter dem Knoten **Partnerart LS** einen Eintrag für das logische System des Senders an.

Fügen Sie dann bei den Eingangsparametern einen Eintrag für den Nachrichtentyp `ZORDER` hinzu. Durch einen Doppelklick auf diesen Eintrag gelangen Sie zur Pflege der Eingangsparameter. Tragen Sie im Feld **Vorgangscode** `ZORDER` ein, d. h. den Vorgangscode, den Sie zuvor mit der Transaktion angelegt haben. Abbildung 7.13 zeigt die konfigurierten Eingangsparameter. Durch einen Doppelklick auf den Vorgangscode sehen Sie, dass er mit dem Funktionsbaustein `Z_IDOC_INPUT_ZORDER` verknüpft ist, der zur individuellen Verarbeitung von eingehenden IDocs dient.

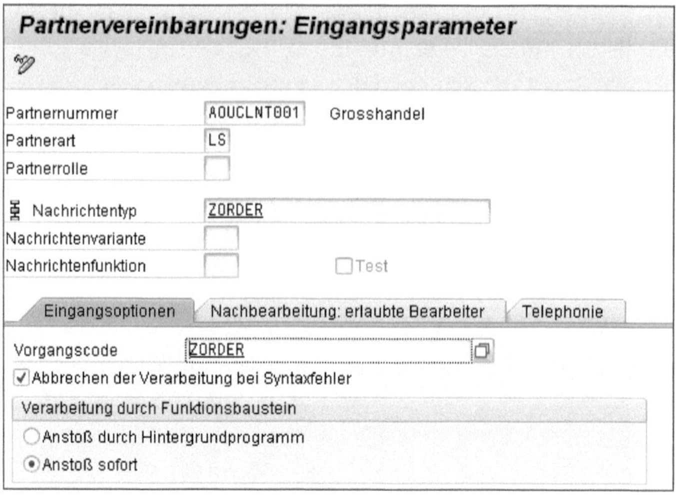

Abbildung 7.13 Eingangsparameter

7.2.2 Test und Monitoring

Szenario testen

Nachdem dieses Szenario fertiggestellt ist, können Sie es testen. Melden Sie sich dazu an dem Mandanten an, der dem sendenden System zugeordnet ist. Führen Sie dann den Report `ZIFP_SEND_IDOC` aus, um Bestellungen an das empfangende System zu verschicken. Sollte der Report einen Fehler melden, können Sie sich mit dem Statusmonitor für ALE-Nachrichten (Transaktion BD87) eine Liste der IDocs anzeigen lassen (siehe Abbildung 7.14).

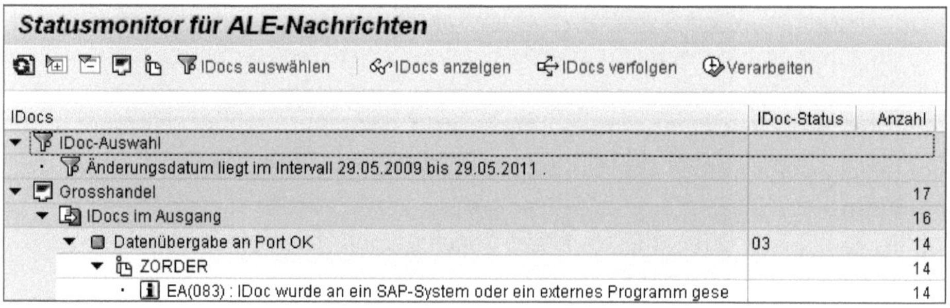

Abbildung 7.14 Statusmonitor für ALE-Nachrichten (Transaktion BD87)

Diese Liste ist nach dem Status der IDocs sortiert. Durch einen Doppelklick auf einen Eintrag zeigt die Transaktion die Liste der dazugehörigen IDocs an. Durch einen Doppelklick auf ein IDoc können Sie sich die Details des IDocs anzeigen lassen (siehe Abbildung 7.15).

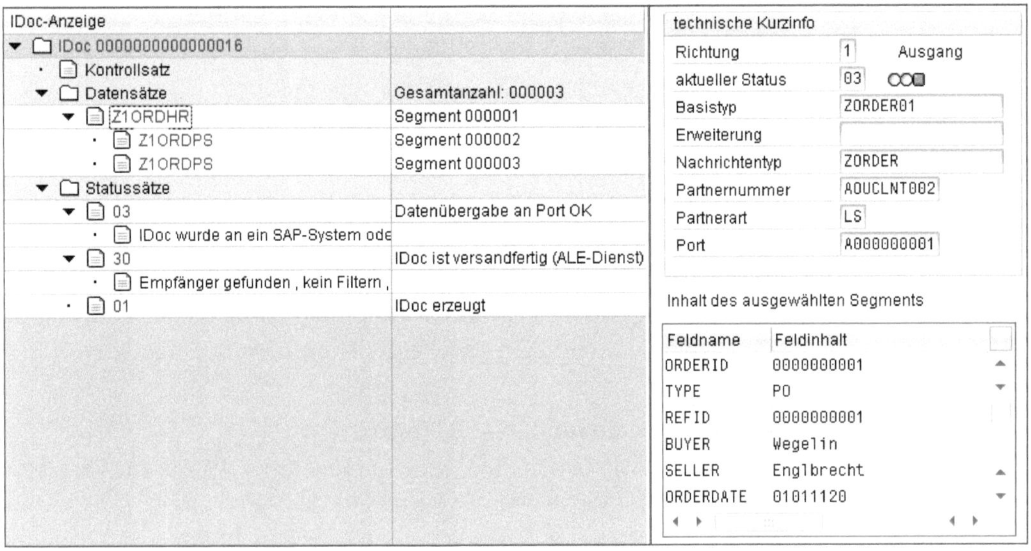

Abbildung 7.15 IDoc im Statusmonitor für ALE-Nachrichten

Nachverarbeitung bei Fehlern

Mit Transaktion BD87 können Sie IDocs auch erneut verarbeiten, nachdem die Fehler beseitigt worden sind. Wenn Sie sich am Mandanten des empfangenden Systems anmelden, sollten Sie dort bei einer fehlerfreien Verarbeitung die übertragenen Daten vorfinden. Auch hier können Sie sich wieder mit Transaktion BD87 eine Liste der empfangenen IDocs anzeigen lassen, Fehler finden und IDocs nach der Fehlerbeseitigung nochmals verarbeiten.

7.2.3 ALE-Schnittstelle für BAPIs

Damit beim Aufruf von BAPIs in einem anderen System auch die ALE-Infrastruktur genutzt werden kann, bietet Transaktion BDBG die Möglichkeit, eine ALE-Schnittstelle für ein BAPI zu generieren und zu pflegen. Im Eingangsbild von Transaktion BDBG geben Sie den Objekttyp und die Methode an, für die Sie eine ALE-Schnittstelle erzeugen lassen möchten.

Schnittstellenobjekte generieren

Die Transaktion erzeugt dann folgende Objekte, die auch in Abbildung 7.16 dargestellt sind:

- **Nachrichtentyp**
  Diesen Nachrichtentyp können Sie in ALE-Szenarien verwenden, um den Aufruf des entsprechenden BAPIs im Zielsystem zu veranlassen.
- **IDoc-Typ**
  IDocs dieses Typs können die Export- und Tabellenparameter des BAPIs aufnehmen und diese zum Zielsystem transportieren. Für den IDoc-Typ

werden die dazugehörigen Segmenttypen automatisch generiert. Nach der Erzeugung müssen Sie sie lediglich freigeben. Der IDoc-Typ wird auch mit dem generierten Nachrichtentyp verknüpft.

- **Funktionsbaustein für den ALE-Ausgang**
  Dieser Funktionsbaustein wird von der sendenden Anwendung aufgerufen. Seine Schnittstelle entspricht der des BAPIs, d. h., die sendende Anwendung ruft diesen Funktionsbaustein fast genauso auf wie das BAPI. Es werden lediglich noch ALE-spezifische Parameter zum Objekttyp und zu den Empfängern mitgegeben. Nach einem erfolgreichen Aufruf gibt der Funktionsbaustein eine Tabelle der Nummern der erzeugten IDocs zurück.
- **Funktionsbaustein für den ALE-Eingang**
  Dieser Funktionsbaustein dient im empfangenden System zur Verarbeitung des eingehenden IDocs. Er extrahiert die Daten aus dem IDoc und ruft das BAPI mit diesen Daten im empfangenden System auf.

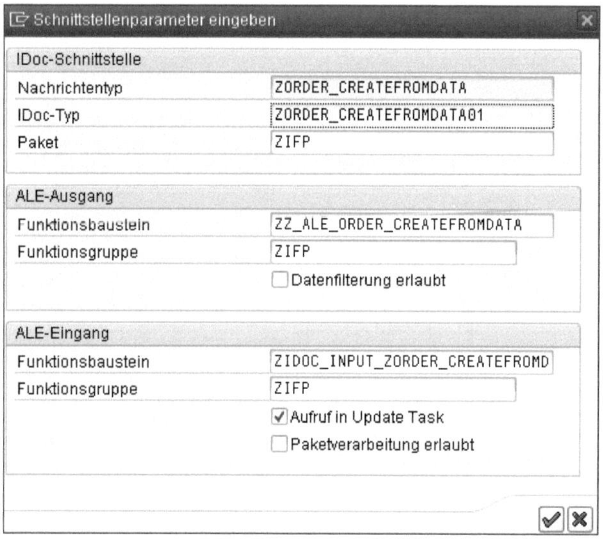

Abbildung 7.16 Erzeugung einer ALE-Schnittstelle für das BAPI »CreateFromData«

Mit dieser ALE-Schnittstelle für BAPIs können Sie die Funktionen nutzen, die ALE für verteilte Prozesse bietet. Allerdings erhalten Sie nicht die Rückgabeparameter des so gerufenen BAPIs, da die Kommunikation asynchron verläuft.

Verteilungsmodell mit BAPI

Um die generierte ALE-Schnittstelle zu verwenden, müssen Sie, wie zuvor, ein ALE-Verteilungsmodell pflegen. In dieses ALE-Verteilungsmodell fügen

Sie nun aber keinen Nachrichtentyp, sondern ein BAPI ein (siehe Abbildung 7.17). Nachdem Sie das Verteilungsmodell gesichert haben, können Sie, wie üblich, die Partnervereinbarungen generieren lassen. Für das Zielsystem wird ein neuer Ausgangsparameter zum generierten Nachrichtentyp erzeugt.

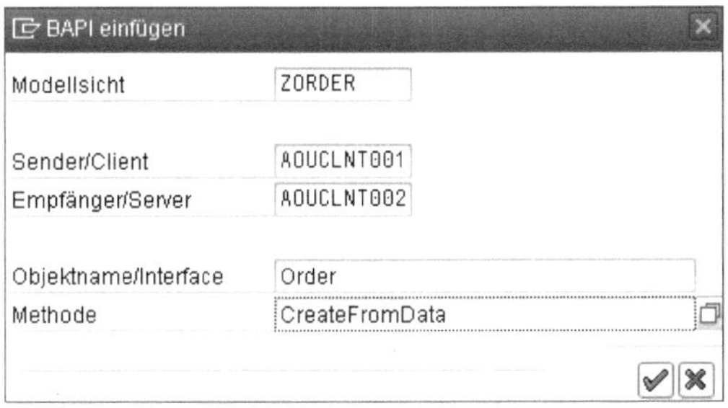

Abbildung 7.17 ALE-Verteilungsmodell für ein BAPI

Eingangsparameter

Im empfangenden System müssen Sie erneut Eingangsparameter für das sendende System zum generierten Nachrichtentyp hinzufügen. Auf der Registerkarte **Eingangsoptionen** verknüpfen Sie den Nachrichtentyp mit dem **Vorgangscode** BAPI, wie es in Abbildung 7.18 dargestellt ist. Dieser Vorgangscode verweist auf den Funktionsbaustein BAPI_IDOC_INPUT1.

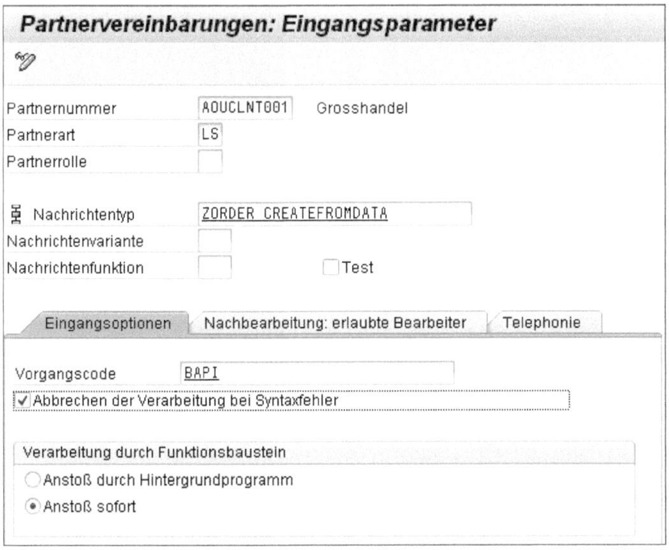

Abbildung 7.18 Eingangsparameter für ein BAPI

Empfänger-ermittlung

Das IDoc wird beim Eingang vom ALE-Subsystem an diesen Funktionsbaustein übergeben. Er schlägt in der Tabelle TBDE den Namen des generierten Funktionsbausteins nach. Als Selektionskriterium dient der Nachrichtentyp. Bei der Generierung der ALE-Schnittstelle hat Transaktion BDBG eine entsprechende Zeile in die Tabelle TBDE eingetragen. An den so ermittelten Funktionsbaustein wird nun das IDoc übergeben, und er ruft, wie schon beschrieben, das BAPI mit den übergebenen Daten auf.

Zielsysteme ermitteln

Listing 7.3 zeigt einen Report, der den generierten Funktionsbaustein verwendet, um Bestellungen in den Zielsystemen zu erzeugen. Um die Zielsysteme zu ermitteln, ruft der Report zunächst den Funktionsbaustein ALE_BAPI_GET_MODEL_DATA auf. In dem zurückgegebenen Tabellenparameter bapi_model_data sind in der Spalte rcvsystem die Empfangssysteme aufgelistet, die sich aufgrund der Verteilungsmodelle für diese Daten aus dem sendenden System interessieren. Mit diesen Informationen baut der Report die interne Tabelle it_receivers auf, die er im anschließenden Aufruf des generierten Ausgangsbausteins übergibt.

```
REPORT  zifp_send_bapi_idoc.
DATA:
  it_model_data TYPE STANDARD TABLE OF bdi_bmodel,
  wa_model_data TYPE bdi_bmodel,
  it_log_system TYPE STANDARD TABLE OF bdi_logsys,
  it_receivers  TYPE STANDARD TABLE OF bdi_logsys,
  wa_receivers  TYPE bdi_logsys,
  orderheader   TYPE zifporder,
  it_orderpos   TYPE STANDARD TABLE OF zifporderpos,
  msg_text(80)  TYPE c.
PARAMETERS:
  pa_id TYPE zifporder-orderid.
AT SELECTION-SCREEN.
  SELECT SINGLE * FROM zifporder
  INTO orderheader
  WHERE
    orderid   = pa_id AND
    type      = 'PO'.
  IF sy-subrc <> 0.
    MESSAGE e001(zifp).
  ELSE.
    orderheader-refid = pa_id.
    orderheader-type = 'SO'.
ENDIF.
START-OF-SELECTION.
  SELECT * FROM zifporderpos INTO TABLE it_orderpos
  WHERE
    orderid = pa_id.
```

```
CALL FUNCTION 'ALE_BAPI_GET_MODEL_DATA'
  EXPORTING
    object                          = 'Z_BUS4500'
    method                          = 'CREATEFROMDATA'
  TABLES
    log_system                      = it_log_system
    bapi_model_data                 = it_model_data
  EXCEPTIONS
    own_logical_system_not_defined = 1
    OTHERS                          = 2.
IF sy-subrc <> 0.
  MESSAGE ID sy-msgid TYPE sy-msgty NUMBER sy-msgno
          WITH sy-msgv1 sy-msgv2 sy-msgv3 sy-msgv4.
ENDIF.
LOOP AT it_model_data INTO wa_model_data.
  APPEND wa_model_data-rcvsystem TO it_receivers.
ENDLOOP.
CALL FUNCTION 'ZZ_ALE_ORDER_CREATEFROMDATA'
  EXPORTING
    imorderheader        = orderheader
  TABLES
    taorderpos           = it_orderpos
    receivers            = it_receivers
  EXCEPTIONS
    error_creating_idocs = 1
    OTHERS               = 2.
IF sy-subrc <> 0.
  MESSAGE ID sy-msgid TYPE sy-msgty NUMBER sy-msgno
          WITH sy-msgv1 sy-msgv2 sy-msgv3 sy-msgv4.
ENDIF.
COMMIT WORK.
```

Listing 7.3 Report zum Testen der ALE-Schnittstelle für ein BAPI

7

7.3 IDoc-Programmierung mit dem SAP NetWeaver RFC SDK

IDoc-Sender und -Empfänger

Um mit C/C++-Programmen ALE-Szenarien realisieren zu können, müssen Sie einen tRFC-Server und einen tRFC-Client schreiben. Der tRFC-Server hat die Aufgabe, den Funktionsbaustein `IDOC_INBOUND_ASYNCHRONOUS` zur Verfügung zu stellen. Dieser Funktionsbaustein empfängt ein IDoc als interne Tabelle. Dieses IDoc kann von der implementierenden C-Funktion bzw. C++-

Methode in eine Datei oder in eine Datenbank geschrieben werden. Der tRFC-Client muss aus einer Datei oder aus den Daten einer Datenbank ein IDoc als interne Tabelle erzeugen und per tRFC an den Funktionsbaustein IDOC_INBOUND_ASYNCHRONOUS schicken.

In diesem Abschnitt zeigen wir Ihnen die IDoc-Programmierung mit dem SAP NetWeaver RFC SDK. Die Arbeit mit diesem SDK haben Sie bereits in Abschnitt 4.2, »Einfache SAP-NetWeaver-RFC-Clients«, Abschnitt 4.3, »Komplexe SAP-NetWeaver-RFC-Clients«, und Abschnitt 4.4, »SAP-NetWeaver-RFC-Server«, kennengelernt.

7.3.1 IDoc-Empfänger

tRFC-Server

Der IDoc-Empfänger ist ein tRFC-Server, der den Funktionsbaustein IDOC_INBOUND_ASYNCHRONOUS als C-Funktion bzw. als C++-Methode implementiert. Listing 7.4 zeigt diese Funktion. Sie schreibt die empfangenen IDoc-Zeilen aus dem Tabellenparameter IDOC_DATA_REC_40 in eine Datei.

```
/* IDOC_INBOUND_ASYNCHRONOUS                              */
RFC_RC SAP_API idoc_inbound_asynchronous(
        RFC_CONNECTION_HANDLE rfcConn,
        RFC_FUNCTION_HANDLE rfcFunc,
        RFC_ERROR_INFO* errInf)
{
  RFC_RC rc = RFC_OK;
  RFC_TABLE_HANDLE rfcTabData;
  RFC_STRUCTURE_HANDLE rfcStruct;
  SAP_UC tbuf[MAXBUFF+1];
  FILE *fp;
  unsigned int count;
  unsigned int i;
  RfcGetTable(rfcFunc, cU("IDOC_DATA_REC_40"),
            &rfcTabData, errInf);
  fp = fopenU (data_file, cU("a"));
  rc = RfcGetRowCount(rfcTabData, &count, errInf);
  rc = RfcMoveToFirstRow(rfcTabData, errInf);
  for(i=0; i < count; i++)
  {
        memsetU(tbuf, cU(' '), 1064);
        rfcStruct = RfcGetCurrentRow(rfcTabData, errInf);
        RfcGetChars(rfcStruct,cU("SEGNAM"),
                    tbuf, 30, errInf);
```

```
        RfcGetChars(rfcStruct,cU("MANDT"),
                    tbuf+30, 3, errInf);
        RfcGetChars(rfcStruct, cU("DOCNUM"),
                    tbuf+33, 16, errInf);
        RfcGetChars(rfcStruct, cU("SEGNUM"),
                    tbuf+49, 6, errInf);
        RfcGetChars(rfcStruct, cU("PSGNUM"),
                    tbuf+55, 6, errInf);
        RfcGetChars(rfcStruct, cU("HLEVEL"),
                    tbuf+61, 2, errInf);
        RfcGetChars(rfcStruct, cU("SDATA"),
                    tbuf+63, 1000, errInf);
        tbuf[1063] = cU('\n');
      if (fwriteU (tbuf, 1, 1064, fp) < 1064)
        rc = RFC_ABAP_EXCEPTION;
      if(i < count - 1)
        rc = RfcMoveToNextRow(rfcTabData, errInf);
   }
   fclose(fp);
   return rc;
} /* idoc_inbound_asynchronous */
```

Listing 7.4 Funktion »idoc_inbound_asynchronous«

ALE-Customizing

Um den Empfänger zu testen, müssen Sie mithilfe von Transaktion SALE das entsprechende Customizing im ALE-Subsystem vornehmen. Zunächst definieren Sie ein logisches System für das externe C/C++-Programm, z. B. `CTSERV`. Dann pflegen Sie eine tRFC-Destination für dieses System. Damit Sie es nachher bei der Generierung der Partnervereinbarungen einfacher haben, sollten Sie die Destination genauso nennen wie das logische System.

Schließlich erstellen oder erweitern Sie in Transaktion BD64 ein ALE-Verteilungsmodell so, dass `ZORDER`-Nachrichten von einem SAP-Mandanten an Ihr externes C/C++-Programm geschickt werden (siehe Abbildung 7.19). Aus dieser Transaktion heraus können Sie auch die Partnervereinbarungen generieren.

Mit dem ABAP-Programm `ZIFP_SEND_IDOC` können Sie nun Ihren IDoc-Empfänger testen. Wenn alles richtig funktioniert, schreibt der Empfänger das von dieser Transaktion gesendete IDoc in eine Datei mit dem Namen <TID>.dat.

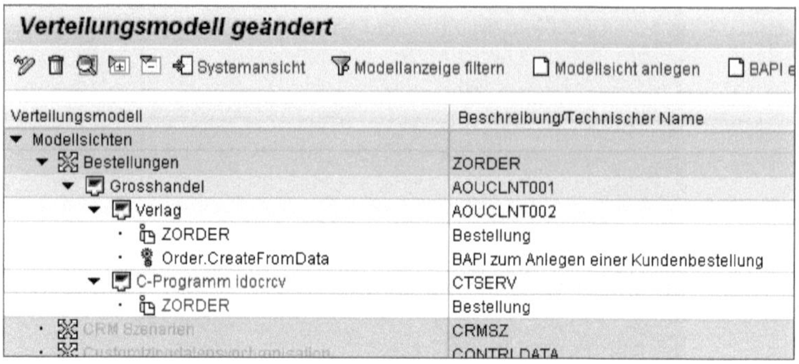

Abbildung 7.19 Erweiterung des ALE-Verteilungsmodells

7.3.2 IDoc-Sender

Der IDoc-Sender sieht genauso aus wie der tRFC-Client, den Sie in Abschnitt 4.3.2, »Transaktionaler RFC-Client«, kennengelernt haben.

IDoc lesen

Die Funktion `read_idoc` in Listing 7.5 liest das IDoc aus einer Datei, deren Name dem Sender als Kommandozeilenargument übergeben wird. Die Funktion liest die Zeilen der Datei und hängt sie an die interne Tabelle `IDOC_DATA_REC_40` an. Danach baut sie den Kontrolldatensatz auf und hängt ihn an die interne Tabelle `IDOC_CONTROL_REC_40` an.

```
/* IDoc in Tabelle IDOC_DATA_REC_40 schreiben              */
RFC_RC read_idoc(FILE *fp, RFC_FUNCTION_HANDLE rfcFunc)
{
  RFC_RC rc = RFC_OK;
  RFC_TABLE_HANDLE rfcTabData;
  RFC_STRUCTURE_HANDLE rfcStruct;
  SAP_UC tbuf[IDOCBUFF+1];
  SAP_UC docnum[16];
  RFC_ERROR_INFO errInf;
  /* IDoc in Tabelle IDOC_DATA_REC_40 schreiben            */
  rc = RfcGetTable(rfcFunc, cU("IDOC_DATA_REC_40"),
                   &rfcTabData, &errInf);
  while (fgetsU (tbuf, 1065, fp) != NULL)
  {
    rfcStruct = RfcAppendNewRow(rfcTabData, &errInf);
    RfcSetChars(rfcStruct, cU("SEGNAM"), tbuf, 30, &errInf);
    RfcSetChars(rfcStruct, cU("MANDT"),
                tbuf+30, 3, &errInf);
    RfcSetChars(rfcStruct, cU("DOCNUM"),
                tbuf+33, 16, &errInf);
    memcpyU(docnum, tbuf+33, 16);
```

```
    RfcSetChars(rfcStruct, cU("DOCNUM"),
                tbuf+33, 16, &errInf);
    RfcSetChars(rfcStruct, cU("SEGNUM"),
                tbuf+49, 6, &errInf);
    RfcSetChars(rfcStruct, cU("PSGNUM"),
                tbuf+55, 6, &errInf);
    RfcSetChars(rfcStruct, cU("HLEVEL"),
                tbuf+61, 2, &errInf);
    RfcSetChars(rfcStruct, cU("SDATA"),
                tbuf+63, 1000, &errInf);
  }
  /* IDOC_CONTROL_REC_40 schreiben                    */
  RfcGetTable(rfcFunc, cU("IDOC_CONTROL_REC_40"),
              &rfcTabData, &errInf);
  rfcStruct = RfcAppendNewRow(rfcTabData, &errInf);
  RfcSetChars(rfcStruct, cU("DOCNUM"), docnum, 16, &errInf);
  RfcSetChars(rfcStruct, cU("DOCREL"), cU("701"),
              3, &errInf);
  RfcSetChars(rfcStruct, cU("IDOCTYP"), cU("ZORDER01"),
              8, &errInf);
  RfcSetChars(rfcStruct, cU("MESTYP"), cU("ZORDER"),
              6, &errInf);
  RfcSetChars(rfcStruct, cU("SNDPRT"), cU("LS"),
              2, &errInf);
  RfcSetChars(rfcStruct, cU("SNDPRN"), cU("CTSERV"),
              2, &errInf);
  return rc;
}
```

Listing 7.5 Funktion »read_idoc«

Damit das IDoc, das von Ihrem IDoc-Sender verschickt wird, im SAP-System auch richtig verarbeitet wird, müssen Sie mit Transaktion WE20 eine Partnervereinbarung für Ihr sendendes System pflegen (siehe Abbildung 7.13).

7.4 IDoc-Programmierung mit Java und dem SAP Java Connector

In diesem Abschnitt wenden wir uns der Programmierung mit der Java-IDoc-Bibliothek zu. Nachdem wir Ihnen die IDoc-Client-Programmierung vorgestellt haben, beleuchten wir nun die Implementierungsschritte, die nötig sind, um IDocs an ein empfangendes Java-System zu senden.

7.4.1 Vorbereitung zur Verwendung der IDoc-Bibliotheken

Für die Programmierung von Java-basierten, IDocs nutzenden Anwendungen ist es zunächst erforderlich, die SAP-IDoc-Bibliothek vom SAP Support Portal herunterzuladen. Dabei gehen Sie so vor, wie in Abschnitt 5.1.1, »Installation«, beschrieben: Nachdem Sie sich unter *https://support.sap.com/en/product/connectors.html* mit Ihrem Benutzer für das SAP Support Portal angemeldet haben, navigieren Sie zu **SAP Java Connector** und wählen unter **SAP Java IDoc Library** den Link **Download SAP Java IDoc Library 3.1.<Version>**. Die in diesem Buch verwendete Bibliothek entspricht Version 3.1.x und ist zu diesem Zeitpunkt die aktuellste Version, die mit dem SAP Java Connector 3.1 und nachfolgenden Implementierungen des SAP Java Connectors zusammenarbeitet. Die Datei trägt für die Windows-Plattform den Namen **sapjidoc31P_3-80004914.zip**.

Aufsetzen der Programmierumgebung

Die Bibliothek ist sowohl für Windows als auch für zahlreiche andere Umgebungen wie Unix oder HP-UX vorhanden. Nach dem Herunterladen und Entpacken der ZIP-Datei befindet sich ein neuer Ordner auf der Festplatte, der die Java-Dokumentation, Beispiele für die Programmierung von IDoc-Client und IDoc-Server sowie ein Java-Archiv mit dem Namen **sapidoc3.jar** beinhaltet. Wenn Sie bereits mit Java-basierten IDoc-Anwendungen gearbeitet haben, werden Sie feststellen, dass es im Gegensatz zu älteren Versionen nur noch eine Bibliothek gibt (statt zwei). Neben dieser Neuerung ist auch eine Vielzahl von Klassen umbenannt und restrukturiert worden.

Wie bereits angedeutet, ist es für die Nutzung der IDoc-Bibliothek notwendig, die Java-Connector-Bibliothek zu verwenden. Die JCo-Bibliothek übernimmt dabei die Kommunikation mit dem Backend, während die IDoc-Bibliothek die Klassen für den Aufbau und die Verarbeitung von IDocs beisteuert. Für die Programmierung setzen Sie daher neben der möglicherweise bereits vorhandenen JCo-Bibliothek zusätzlich das eben angesprochene Java-Archiv **sapidoc3.jar** in den Klassenpfad Ihrer Entwicklungsumgebung.

7.4.2 Client-Anwendung für IDocs

Nachdem Sie Ihr Java-Projekt in Ihrer Entwicklungsumgebung aufgesetzt haben, können Sie mit der Programmierung der ersten IDoc-Anwendung beginnen. Die Anwendung sendet dem Mandanten 002 ein IDoc vom Typ `ZORDER` zu.

Verbindung aufbauen

Zunächst muss, wie bei der herkömmlichen Java-Client-Programmierung, eine Verbindung zum SAP-System aufgebaut werden. Der Verbindungsaufbau ist dabei analog zur reinen Java-Connector-Programmierung, die Sie in

Abschnitt 5.1, »SAP Java Connector«, kennengelernt haben. Das heißt, Sie erzeugen ein neues `JCoDestination`-Objekt über die Factory-Klasse `JCoDestinationManager`. Wie aus dem Sequenzdiagramm aus Abbildung 7.20 ersichtlich ist, wird im nächsten Schritt der Zugriff auf die Metadaten der IDocs instanziiert. Metadaten werden dabei über eine Instanz vom Typ `IDocRepository` beschrieben. Da es sich um ein Interface handelt, muss das Objekt über eine Factory erzeugt werden. Die zentrale Klasse für die Erzeugung aller relevanten Typen ist die Klasse `JCoIDoc`.

Zugriff über Repository-Objekt

Wie aus dem vereinfachten Klassenbild der Klasse `JCoIDoc` in Abbildung 7.20 ersichtlich ist, implementiert die Klasse für die Arbeit mit Repositorys die Methode `getIDocRepository`. Über das Repository-Objekt kann auf die gesamte Metadatenstruktur der IDocs zugegriffen werden. Wie bei der reinen JCo-Programmierung ist auch bei der IDoc-Programmierung das Repository der Ausgangspunkt für die Validierung der angegebenen Ist-Werte gegen die im ABAP-Stack definierten Metadaten. Die Metadaten müssen deshalb auch Ausgangspunkt für die Erzeugung des IDocs sein. IDocs werden in der Java-IDoc-Bibliothek über das Interface `IDocDocument` repräsentiert.

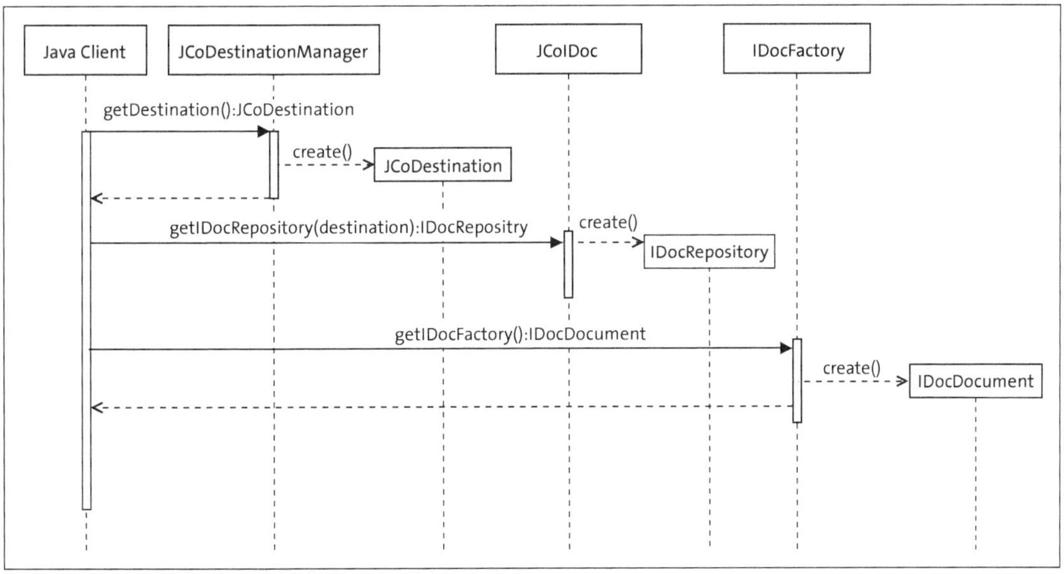

Abbildung 7.20 Kommunikationsabhängigkeiten für die Erzeugung eines Objekts vom Typ »IDocDocument«

Die Erzeugung eines solchen Objekts wird über zwei Schritte ermöglicht. Im ersten Schritt ist es nötig, eine Ausprägung des Interface `IDocFactory` zu erzeugen. Dazu rufen Sie die Methode `getIDocFactory` in der zentralen Factory-Klasse JCoIDoc auf. Die erzeugte Factory-Instanz ist Dreh- und Angelpunkt für die Bereitstellung eines IDoc-Objekts. Das IDoc-Objekt wird repräsentiert durch das Interface IDocDocument. Um eine Instanz dieser Klasse zu erzeugen, rufen Sie die Methode createIDocDocument auf. Die Methode erhält zwei Parameter: Der erste Parameter ist das bereits erzeugte Repository-Objekt, der zweite Parameter gibt den Namen des IDocs an, für das eine Proxy-Repräsentation benötigt wird.

Verarbeiten der Segmente

Nachdem das Proxy-Objekt erzeugt worden ist, können Sie mit der eigentlichen Verarbeitung der IDoc-relevanten Informationen beginnen. Verwenden Sie hier das IDoc mit dem Namen ZOrder, das in Abschnitt 7.1.1, »Entwicklung von IDocs«, eingeführt und diskutiert wurde. Das IDoc besteht aus zwei Segmenten, Z1ORDHD und Z1ORDPS. Segmente werden in der Java-IDoc-Bibliothek als ISegment verarbeitet. Um die einzelnen Segmenttypen mit Daten zu füllen, muss eine Referenz auf das Wurzelsegment der IDoc-Proxy-Repräsentation bezogen werden.

Das Wurzelsegment wird dabei über die Methode getRootDocument besorgt. Da aus der Sicht der Wurzel die Bestellkopfinformationen als Kindelemente zu sehen sind, wird die Methode addChild auf dem Wurzelsegment aufgerufen. Die Methode erhält den Namen des Segments und liefert ein neues ISegment-Objekt zurück. Dieses Objekt kann nun über die Methode setValue mit den entsprechenden Werten gefüllt werden. Die Methode folgt dem Java-Standard und erhält als ersten Parameter den Feldbezeichner und als zweiten Parameter den zu setzenden Wert. Nachdem der Bestellkopf mit Daten versorgt ist, können die Bestellpositionen gesetzt werden. Dazu wird auf dem ISegment-Objekt der Kopfdaten die Methode addChild aufgerufen, und die jeweiligen Werte für die Bestellpositionen werden übergeben.

Senden des IDocs an das ABAP-System

Den Abschluss bildet das Versenden des IDocs. Für das Versenden bietet die zentrale IDoc-Klasse JCoIDoc die Methode send. Die Methode wird in vier verschiedenen Ausprägungen zur Verfügung gestellt. Die Methodenausprägungen können dabei grob in zwei Typen eingeteilt werden: Eine Ausprägung wird verwendet, wenn lediglich ein einziges IDoc an das ABAP-System gesendet werden soll. Die zweite Ausprägung der Methode wird mit einer Liste von IDocs (vom Typ IDocDocumentList) aufgerufen. Allen Methoden ist gemeinsam, dass sie neben den IDoc-Objekten auch die IDoc-Version, ein Objekt vom Typ JCoDestination und die Transaktionsnummer entgegennehmen, mit der das IDoc verarbeitet werden soll. Die Transaktionsnummer wird analog zur JCo-Programmierung über die Methode createTID in der Klasse JCoDestination aufgerufen.

Nachdem auf dem IDoc-Proxy-Objekt die nötigen Informationen des sendenden und des empfangenen Systems gesetzt wurden, kann mittels der

Methode send das IDoc an das ABAP-System übergeben werden (siehe Listing 7.6).

```
public static void main(String[] args) {
  try {
    JCoDestination lcoDestination =
      ConnectionMan-ager.getJCoDestination("MYDESTINATION");
    IDocRepository repository =
      JCoIDoc.getIDocRepository(lcoDestination);
    IDocFactory idocFactory = JCoIDoc.getIDocFactory();
    IDocDocument iDocument =
      idocFactory.createIDocDocument(repository,IDOCNAME);
    //Hinzufügen des root-Segments
    IDocSegment rootSegement = iDocument.getRootSegment();
    //Erzeugen des Bestellkopfsegments
    IDocSegment orderheader =
      rootSegement.addChild(IDOC_ORDER_HEADER);
      orderheader.setValue(ORDER_HEADER_ORDERID , 122);
      orderheader.setValue(ORDER_HEADER_BUYER,
        "Michael Englbrecht");
     orderheader.setValue(ORDER_HEADER_TYPE, "AO");
     orderheader.setValue(ORDER_HEADER_REFID, "2");
    //Hinzufügen eines Bestellungssegments

    IDocSegment orderpos =
      orderheader.addChild(IDOC_ORDER_POS);
    orderpos.setValue(ORDER_POS_ORDERID,"122");
    orderpos.setValue(ORDER_POS_ORDERPOS,1);
    orderpos.setValue(ORDER_POS_MATID, "M1");
    orderpos.setValue(ORDER_POS_MATTEXT,
      "Schrauben und Dübel");
    orderpos.setValue(ORDER_POS_ORDERCOUNT, "23");
    orderpos.setValue(ORDER_POS_PRICE, 12.30);
    orderpos.setValue(ORDER_POS_CURRENCY, "EUR");
    String tid = lcoDestination.createTID();
    iDocument.setMessageType("ZORDER");
    iDocument.setRecipientPartnerNumber("AOUCLNT002");
    iDocument.setRecipientPartnerType("LS");
    iDocument.setSenderPort("SAPBSP");
    iDocument.setSenderPartnerType("LS");
    iDocument.setSenderPartnerNumber("AOUCLNT001");
    JCoIDoc.send(iDocument,IDocFactory.IDOC_VERSION_DEFAULT,
               lcoDestination , tid);
```

7

```
    JcoDestination.confirmTID(tid);
  } catch (JCoException e) {
    e.printStackTrace();
  } catch (IDocMetaDataUnavailableException e) {
    e.printStackTrace();
  } catch(IDocIllegalTypeException e) {
    e.printStackTrace();
  } catch (IDocSyntaxException e) {
    e.printStackTrace();
  } catch (IDocConversionException e) {
    e.printStackTrace();
  } catch(IDocFieldNotFoundException e) {
    e.printStackTrace();
  }
}
```

Listing 7.6 Versenden eines IDocs mit Java

Prüfen der IDoc-Konsistenz

Um die Konsistenz und Syntax des `IDocument`-Objekts zu prüfen, können Sie die Methode `checkSyntax` aufrufen. Falls die Syntax beschädigt bzw. fehlerhaft ist, wird eine Ausnahme vom Typ `IDocSyntaxException` ausgelöst. Daher müssen Sie den Methodenaufruf in einem `try-catch`-Block platzieren. Falls keinerlei Fehler in der Syntax vorhanden sind, kann das IDoc an das SAP-System gesendet werden.

Verarbeitung von IDocument-Objekten

Für sendende sowie für empfangende Java-Systeme ist die Verarbeitung der reinen `IDocument`-Objekte oft nicht ausreichend. In vielen Fällen ist es z. B. notwendig, das empfangene Dokument in ein anderes Format zu überführen und entsprechend weiterzuverarbeiten. Genauso kann es gerade in Infrastrukturen, in denen Nachrichten ausgetauscht werden, vorkommen, dass aus einem Zwischenformat ein `IDocument`-Objekt initialisiert und an das SAP-System übermittelt wird. Die Vergangenheit hat gezeigt, dass besonders hier das XML-Format (Extensible Markup Language) seine Vorteile hat, obgleich andere Formate ähnlich komfortabel sind. Ein möglicher Vorteil der Nutzung von XML ist die einfachere Konvertierung mittels *Extensible Stylesheet Language for Transformations* (XSLT) in unterschiedliche Formate. In heterogenen Landschaften ist dadurch eine komfortable Kommunikation möglich.

XML-basierte Verarbeitung

Für die XML-basierte Verarbeitung bietet die Java-IDoc-Bibliothek als Ausgangspunkt das Interface `IDocXMLProcessor`. Es bietet eine Vielzahl von Methodenausprägungen mit der Bezeichnung `parse` und `render`. Die `parse`-Methoden dienen der Erzeugung von `IDocument`-Objekten bzw. einer Liste von IDocument-Objekten (als IDocumentList-Implementierung); analog verhalten sich die render-Methoden. Sie ermöglichen es, IDocument-Objekte als XML-Darstellungen zu erzeugen.

Sie erhalten die Instanz einer SAP-Implementierung für diese Schnittstelle über die zentrale IDoc-Factory-Klasse IDocFactory. Die benötigte Methode trägt den Namen getIDocXMLProcessor. Das Programmierbeispiel in Listing 7.7 zeigt die Möglichkeit der Speicherung eines IDocs als XML-Dokument.


```
private void processIDoc(IDocDocument document) {
  try {
    IDocFactory idocFactory = JCoI-Doc.getIDocFactory();
    IDocXMLProcessor xmlProcessor =
      idocFactory.getIDocXMLProcessor();
    FileWriter fileWriter =
      new FileWriter("c:\\temp\\bestellung.xml");
    xmlProcessor.render(document, fileWriter);
  } catch (IOException e) {
    e.printStackTrace();
  }
}
```

Listing 7.7 XML-Verarbeitung eines IDocument-Objekts

7.4.3 IDoc-Server

Nachdem Sie ein IDoc versendet haben, stellen wir Ihnen in diesem Abschnitt das Empfangen eines IDocs vor. In unserem Beispiel schreiben Sie das empfangene IDoc als XML-Datei auf die Festplatte. Die Projektkonfiguration in der Entwicklungsumgebung ist ähnlich wie bei der Programmierung eines IDoc-Senders. Im Klassenpfad befinden sich die Bibliotheken des SAP Java Connectors sowie die Java-IDoc-Bibliothek.

Implementierung eines IDoc-Servers

Für die Implementierung des IDoc-Servers erstellen Sie eine Klasse mit dem Namen EAIIDocServer. Sie finden diese Klasse bei den Programmierbeispielen zum Buch im Eclipse-Projekt JCoServerProgrammierung im Paket de.eai.javaserverprg.idoc. Ausgangspunkt ist das Interface JCoIDocServer. Das Interface erbt dabei vom Interface JCoServer. Das bedeutet, dass es möglich ist, eine Java-basierte Infrastruktur aufzubauen, die sowohl eine reine RFC-Kommunikation als auch eine IDoc-basierte Kommunikation mit dem SAP-System ermöglicht. Das Interface JCoIDocServer führt vier neue Methoden in die Java-Connector-Programmierung ein. Es handelt sich dabei um die Methoden getIDocHandlerFactory, getIDocRepository, setIDocHandlerFactory und setIDocRepository.

Zu Beginn der Implementierung wird ein neues JCoIDocServer-Objekt erzeugt. Das Objekt wird mit den Kommunikationsparametern für das SAP-System initialisiert. Wie Sie im Programmierbeispiel in Listing 7.8 sehen können, wird dies über die Factory-Methode getServer auf der Klasse JCoIDoc ermöglicht. Darüber hinaus ist es notwendig, dem Java-Server mitzuteilen, wer welche eingehenden IDocs verarbeiten soll. Dies geschieht über die Registrierung einer Implementierung der Schnittstelle JCoIDocHandlerFactory. In dem hier vorgestellten Beispiel übernimmt dies die Klasse EAIIDocHandlerFactory.

```
public class EAIIDocServer {
  public static void main(String[] args) {
    try {
      JCoIDocServer eaiServer =
        JCoIDoc.getServer("EAIIDocSample");
        eaiServer.setIDocHandlerFactory(
          new EAIIDocHandlerFactory());
        eaiServer.setTIDHandler(new EAITIDHandler());

      EAIIDocErrorListener listener =
        new EAIIDocErrorListener();
      eaiServer.addServerErrorListener(listener);
      eaiServer.addServerExceptionListener(listener);
      eaiServer.setConnectionCount(1);
      eaiServer.start();
    } catch (JCoException e) {
      System.out.println(
        "Problems while starting the IDoc-Server " +
        e.getMessage());
    }
  }
}
```

Listing 7.8 Implementierung eines IDoc-Empfängers in Java

Wie Sie bereits gesehen haben, werden IDocs per tRFC übermittelt. Daher müssen Sie dem Serverobjekt mitteilen, wer im Java-System die Verwaltung von Transaktionsnummern übernimmt. Sie registrieren eine Implementierung des Interface JCoServerTIDHandler. Die Implementierung dieses Interface ist dabei identisch mit der reinen JCo-Serverprogrammierung.

Verarbeitung von eingehenden IDocs

Wie bereits angedeutet, ist ein Java-IDoc-Server in der Lage, unterschiedliche Verarbeiter für eingehende IDoc-Objekte zu implementieren. Die entscheidende Komponente ist dabei eine Implementierung der Schnittstelle JCoIDocHandlerFactory. Die Schnittstelle bietet eine Methode mit dem Namen getIDocHandler. Sie erhält als Aufrufparameter ein Objekt vom Typ JCoIDocServerContext. Der Kontext kann dazu verwendet werden, zu entscheiden, wer die eigentliche Verarbeitung eines IDocs übernimmt. Zum Beispiel kann als Entscheidungskriterium die IDoc-Version aus dem Kontext bezogen werden. Die Methode getIDocHandler liefert Implementierungen der Schnittstelle JCoIDocHandler zurück. Das Interface selbst stellt letztlich die Grundlage für die eigentliche Verarbeitung von IDocs dar und bietet dafür die Methode handleRequest an.

Die Methode erhält zwei Parameter: Der erste Parameter ist vom Typ JCoServerContext, der zweite ist vom Typ IDocDocumentList und stellt eine Liste eingegangener IDocs dar. Das Programmierbeispiel in Listing 7.9 zeigt, wie empfangene IDocs über IDocXMLProcessor als XML-Dokumente gespeichert werden können.

```
public void handleRequest(JCoServerContext serverCtx,
   IDoc-DocumentList idocList) {
  String filepath = "c:\\idocoutput\\";
  FileOutputStream fileOS = null;
  OutputStreamWriter objectOS = null;
  try {
    IDocXMLProcessor xmlProcessor =
      JCoIDoc.getIDocFactory().getIDocXMLProcessor();
    fileOS = new FileOutputStream(filepath +
      serverCtx.getTID()+ "Document.xml");
    objectOS=new OutputStreamWriter(fileOS, "UTF8");
    xmlProcessor.render(idocList, objectOS,
      IDocXMLProcessor.RENDER_WITH_TABS_AND_CRLF);
    objectOS.flush();
  } catch (FileNotFoundException e) {
    e.printStackTrace();
  } catch (UnsupportedEncodingException e) {
    e.printStackTrace();
  } catch (IOException e) {
    e.printStackTrace();
  }
}
```

Listing 7.9 Implementierung der Methode »handleRequest«

7.4.4 Konfiguration für den Versand von IDocs

Im Anschluss an die Implementierung des externen Java-IDoc-Servers muss das SAP-System entsprechend konfiguriert werden. Dazu melden Sie sich an Ihrem SAP-System an und rufen dort Transaktion SALE auf. Zunächst definieren Sie ein logisches System für den soeben vorgestellten Java-Server. Dazu folgen Sie dem Menüpfad **Grundeinstellungen • Logische Systeme einrichten • Logisches System benennen.**

Logisches System und tRFC-Destination

Fügen Sie nun einen neuen Eintrag hinzu. Konfigurieren Sie dann über Transaktion WE20 Ihr gerade eingeführtes logisches System. Im Anschluss starten Sie Transaktion SM59 und pflegen eine tRFC-Destination für den empfangenden Java-Server, wie wir es bei der herkömmlichen JCo-Serverprogrammierung in Abschnitt 5.1, »SAP Java Connector«, gezeigt haben. Benennen Sie auch hier die Destination genauso wie das logische System, damit Sie es bei der Generierung der Partnervereinbarungen einfacher haben.

Verteilungsmodell erweitern

Nachdem Sie die Destination erfolgreich angelegt haben, ändern Sie das Verteilungsmodell, sodass ZORDER-Nachrichten von einem SAP-Mandanten an Ihr externes Java-Programm geschickt werden (siehe Abbildung 7.21). Aus dieser Transaktion heraus können Sie auch die Partnervereinbarung erzeugen.

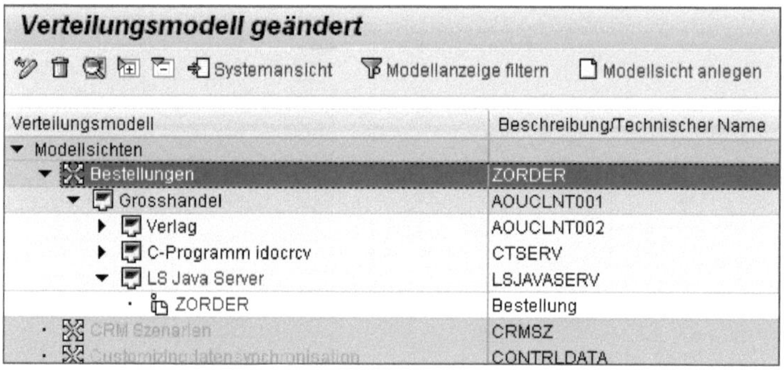

Abbildung 7.21 Erweiterung des ALE-Verteilungsmodells

Abschließend starten Sie Ihren Java-IDoc-Server. Mit dem ABAP-Programm ZIFP_SEND_IDOC können Sie nun Ihren IDoc-Empfänger testen. Wenn alles richtig funktioniert, schreibt der Empfänger das von dieser Transaktion gesendete IDoc in das von Ihnen bei der Programmierung angegebene Verzeichnis.

7.5 IDoc-Programmierung mit dem SAP Connector for Microsoft .NET

In diesem Abschnitt lernen Sie die IDoc-Programmierung mit dem SAP Connector for Microsoft .NET kennen. Dazu müssen Sie einen tRFC-Server und einen tRFC-Client schreiben, wie Sie es in Kapitel 6, »Remote Function Call mit C#«, gelernt haben.

tRFC-Server und -Client 7

Der tRFC-Server muss den Funktionsbaustein `IDOC_INBOUND_ASYNCHRONOUS` implementieren. Dieser Funktionsbaustein empfängt ein IDoc als interne Tabelle, die dann in eine Datei oder Datenbank geschrieben werden muss. Umgekehrt muss der tRFC-Client aus einer Datei oder aus Daten in einer Datenbank ein IDoc als interne Tabelle erzeugen und per tRFC an den Funktionsbaustein `IDOC_INBOUND_ASYNCHRONOUS` schicken.

7.5.1 IDoc-Empfänger

Funktionsbaustein »IDOC_INBOUND_ASYNCHRONOUS«

Listing 7.10 zeigt die Implementierung des Funktionsbausteins `IDOC_INBOUND_ASYNCHRONOUS` als Methode `IdocInboundAsynchronous` einer C#-Klasse `RfcFunctionImpl`. Diese Methode schreibt die empfangenen IDoc-Zeilen aus dem Tabellenparameter `IDOC_DATA_REC_40` in eine Datei mit dem Namen **<tid>.dat**, wobei **<tid>** die Transaktions-ID ist.

```
class RfcFunctionImpl
{
  [RfcServerFunction(Name = "IDOC_INBOUND_ASYNCHRONOUS")]
  public static void IdocInboundAsynchronous(
    RfcServerContext serverContext, IRfcFunction function)
  {
    Console.WriteLine(
     "Führe IDOC_INBOUND_ASYNCHRONOUS aus.");

    // Datei TID.dat zum Schreiben öffnen
    string dataFileName = string.Format(
      "{0}.dat", serverContext.TransactionID);
    FileStream dataFile = new FileStream(
      dataFileName, FileMode.OpenOrCreate,
   FileAccess.Write);
    StreamWriter writer = new StreamWriter(dataFile);
```

```
      // IDoc lesen und in Datei schreiben
      IRfcTable idoc = function.GetTable("IDOC_DATA_REC_40");
      foreach (IRfcStructure record in idoc)
      {
        for (int i = 0; i < record.Count; i++)
        {
          if (i == record.Count - 1)
            writer.WriteLine(record.GetString(i));
          else
            writer.Write("{0};", record.GetString(i));
        }
      }
      writer.Flush();
      dataFile.Close();
    }
  }
```

Listing 7.10 C#-Methode »IdocInboundAsynchronous«

ALE konfigurieren

Um den Empfänger zu testen, müssen Sie, wie in Abschnitt 7.2.1, »Konfiguration von ALE«, beschrieben, das entsprechende Customizing im ALE-Subsystem vornehmen: Sie definieren ein logisches System für das externe C#-Programm, pflegen eine tRFC-Destination für dieses System und erstellen oder erweitern ein ALE-Verteilungsmodell so, dass ZORDER-Nachrichten von einem SAP-Mandanten an Ihr externes C#-Programm geschickt werden. Danach generieren Sie aus dem Verteilungsmodell heraus die Partnervereinbarungen und testen anschließend Ihren IDoc-Empfänger mit dem ABAP-Programm ZIFP_SEND_IDOC.

7.5.2 IDoc-Sender

IDoc lesen

Der IDoc-Sender sieht genauso aus wie der tRFC-Client, den wir in Abschnitt 6.3.2, »Transaktionaler RFC«, implementiert haben. Die Methode PrepareFunction in Listing 7.11 liest das IDoc aus einer Datei, deren Name als Parameter übergeben wird. Die Methode liest die Zeilen der Datei und hängt sie an die interne Tabelle IDOC_DATA_REC_40 an. Danach baut sie den Kontrolldatensatz auf und hängt ihn an die interne Tabelle IDOC_CONTROL_REC_40 an.

```
static IRfcFunction PrepareFunction(string dataFileName)
{
  RfcDestination dest = RfcDestinationManager.
    GetDestination("NCO_ASHOST");
```

```
  IRfcFunction function = dest.Repository.CreateFunction(
    "IDOC_INBOUND_ASYNCHRONOUS");

  FileStream dataFile = new FileStream(
    dataFileName, FileMode.Open, FileAccess.Read);
  StreamReader reader = new StreamReader(dataFile);

  // IDoc lesen und in Tabelle füllen
  IRfcTable records = function.GetTable("IDOC_DATA_REC_40");
  while (!reader.EndOfStream)
  {
    string line = reader.ReadLine();
    records.Append();
    string[] fields = line.Split(new char[] { ';' });
    for (int i = 0; i < fields.Count(); i++)
      records.SetValue(i, fields[i]);
  }

  // Kontrolldatensatz aufbauen
  string docnum = records.GetString("DOCNUM");
  IRfcTable control = function.GetTable(
    "IDOC_CONTROL_REC_40");
  control.Append();
  control.SetValue("DOCNUM", docnum);
  control.SetValue("DOCREL", "702");
  control.SetValue("IDOCTYP", "ZORDER01");
  control.SetValue("MESTYP", "ZORDER");
  control.SetValue("SNDPRT", "LS");
  control.SetValue("SNDPRN", "CSTSERV");

  dataFile.Close();
  return function;
}
```

Listing 7.11 Die Methode »PrepareFunction«

Damit das IDoc, das von Ihrem IDoc-Sender verschickt wird, im SAP-System auch richtig verarbeitet wird, müssen Sie mit Transaktion WE20 eine Partnervereinbarung für Ihr sendendes System pflegen, wie in Abschnitt 7.2.1, »Konfiguration von ALE«, beschrieben (siehe Abbildung 7.13).

7

Kapitel 8
SOAP-Webservices

In diesem Kapitel zeigen wir Ihnen, wie Sie auf der ABAP-Plattform schnell und einfach SOAP-Clients und SOAP-Server in ABAP und Java entwickeln können. Ebenso lernen Sie, wie Sie die SOAP-Services aus C# nutzen.

SOAP, ursprünglich als Akronym für *Simple Object Access Protocol* stehend, ist seit Version 1.2 kein Akronym mehr und wird nur noch als SOAP bezeichnet. SOAP hat sich innerhalb sehr kurzer Zeit als wichtiger Standard der Interprozesskommunikation durchgesetzt und ist auch heute noch, über 20 Jahre nach Veröffentlichung der Version 1.2, von Bedeutung. Das liegt vor allem an seiner hohen Plattformunabhängigkeit und der Nutzung von Internetstandards: Die Nachrichten zwischen zwei Prozessen werden als XML-Nachrichten transportiert, und der Transport erfolgt in der Regel über HTTP. Sowohl XML als auch HTTP sind plattformunabhängig und werden von zahlreichen Plattformen unterstützt, so auch von der ABAP-Plattform.

In diesem Kapitel zeigen wir Ihnen mit vielen Programmierbeispielen, wie SOAP-Komponenten, die in unterschiedlichen Programmiersprachen entwickelt wurden, Nachrichten miteinander austauschen können. Als etablierte und standardisierte Technologie wird SOAP häufig für die Integration mit älteren SAP-Systemen oder bestehenden Enterprise-Anwendungen genutzt.

8.1 Inside-Out-Webservices und -Webclients mit der ABAP-Plattform

Für die Entwicklung von Webservices und Webclients bietet die ABAP Workbench einen Wizard, der Sie in wenigen Schritten schnell zum Ziel führt. Zuerst zeigen wir Ihnen in diesem Abschnitt die Entwicklung eines ABAP-Webservice, den Sie danach aus einem ABAP-Client aufrufen können. Dabei gehen wir nach dem *Inside-Out-Ansatz* vor (auch als *Code-First-Ansatz* bekannt). Bei diesem Ansatz existiert bereits ein Business-Objekt mit BAPIs oder eine Funktionsgruppe mit Funktionsbausteinen, die wir anschließend als Webservice veröffentlichen möchten. Den *Outside-In-Ansatz* (auch bekannt als *Contract-First-Ansatz*), bei dem wir zuerst den Webservice beschreiben und dann die Funktionalität in ABAP bereitstellen, erläutern wir in Abschnitt 8.2, »Outside-In-Webservices und -Webclients mit der ABAP-Plattform«.

8.1.1 SOAP-Webservice mit ABAP

Es ist einfach, auf der ABAP-Plattform einen SOAP-Webservice zu entwickeln. Als Beispiel erstellen wir in diesem Abschnitt einen Webservice, der die Funktionalität des Business-Objekts `Order` aus Abschnitt 1.4, »Überblick über die Schnittstellentechnologien von SAP«, per SOAP bereitstellt. Mit diesem Webservice können Sie Bestellungen anlegen, ändern, suchen und lesen. Wir verwenden dazu Transaktion SE80 anstelle der ABAP Development Tools (ADT) in Eclipse, weil Letztere nur den Outside-In-Ansatz unterstützen und dieser Ansatz zur Anbindung eines Legacy-Systems in der Praxis selten verfolgt wird. Wir werden dabei eine WSDL-Datei (Web Service Description Language) anlegen.

Neun Schritte zum Webservice

Starten Sie daher Transaktion SE80, den Object Navigator. Lassen Sie sich das Paket anzeigen, das Ihren Webservice enthalten soll. Im Kontextmenü des Pakets starten Sie über **Anlegen • Enterprise Service** den Webservice-Wizard, der Sie in den folgenden neun Schritten zum fertigen Webservice führt:

1. **Objekttyp**
   Im ersten Schritt zeigt Ihnen der Wizard eine Übersicht über die Objekttypen an, die Sie anlegen können. Dort haben Sie unter anderem die Auswahl zwischen **Service-Provider** (Webservice) und **Service-Consumer** (Webservice-Client). Hier wählen Sie **Service-Provider** als Objekttyp und klicken dann den Button **Weiter** an, um zum nächsten Bildschirm zu gelangen.
2. **Art des Service-Providers**
   Im nächsten Schritt wählen Sie den Typ des zu generierenden Service-Providers aus. Sie haben die Wahl zwischen **Backend**, **Enterprise Services Repository**, **Vorhandenes ABAP-Objekt (Inside Out)** und **Externe(s) WSDL/Schema**. Wählen Sie hier **Vorhandenes ABAP-Objekt (Inside Out)**, und klicken Sie dann auf den Button **Weiter**.
3. **Service**
   Im Eingabefeld **Service-Definition** geben Sie einen Namen für den Webservice ein, z. B. »ZIFP_ORDER_SERVICE«. Im Eingabefeld **Beschreibung** können Sie eine Kurzbeschreibung eingeben.

4. **Endpunkttyp**
   Im vierten Schritt wählen Sie den Endpunkttyp aus. Hier haben Sie die Wahl zwischen **Funktionsgruppe**, **Funktionsbaustein** und **BAPI**. Für dieses Beispiel wählen Sie den Eintrag **BAPI** aus.
5. **Endpunkt-BAPI**
   Je nach Endpunkttyp, den Sie im vorangegangenen Schritt ausgewählt haben, geben Sie hier den Namen eines Funktionsbausteins, einer Funktionsgruppe oder eines Business-Objekts an. Für dieses Beispiel wählen Sie das BAPI (eigentlich Business-Objekt) `Order`, das Sie in Abschnitt 3.5, »Business-Objekte und BAPIs«, innerhalb der Anwendung `Z` angelegt haben. Wählen Sie **Namen zuordnen**, um die Namen der Funktionsbausteine zuzuordnen. Anfangsbuchstaben werden großgeschrieben und Unterstriche entfernt. 8
6. **BAPI**
   In diesem Schritt wählen Sie die Operationen, die Ihr Webservice anbieten soll. Der Schritt wird nur bei den Endpunkttypen **Funktionsgruppe** und **BAPI** angezeigt, da eine Funktionsgruppe mehrere Funktionsbausteine bzw. ein Business-Objekt mehrere BAPIs enthalten kann. In diesem Beispiel sollen alle vier BAPIs auch als Operationen im Webservice angeboten werden. Zusätzlich legen Sie über den Button **BAPI Commit/Rollback** fest, dass auch die Methoden `TransactionCommit` und `TransactionRollback` des Business-Objekts `BapiService` als Operationen in den Webservice aufgenommen werden sollen. Abbildung 8.1 zeigt diesen Schritt.

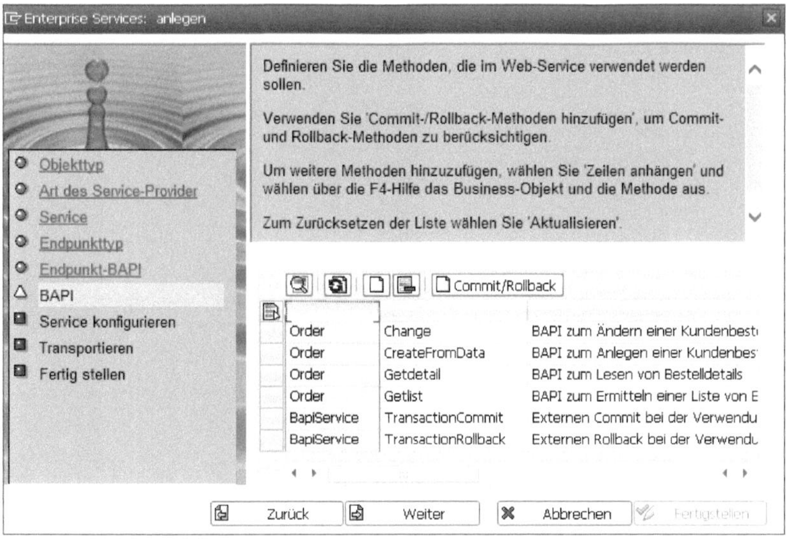

Abbildung 8.1 Operationen des Webservice wählen

7. **Service konfigurieren**
   In diesem Schritt wählen Sie ein Profil für die Sicherheitseinstellungen aus, das Ihren Anforderungen entspricht. In der Drop-down-Liste **Profil** haben Sie die Wahl zwischen vier verschiedenen Profilen:
   - Authentifizierung mit Zertifikaten und Transportgarantie
   - Authentifizierung mit Benutzer und Kennwort, keine Transportgarantie
   - Authentifizierung mit Benutzer, Kennwort und Transportgarantie
   - keine Authentifizierung und keine Transportgarantie
8. **Transportieren**
   Im vorletzten Schritt geben Sie ein Paket und einen Entwicklungsauftrag an.
9. **Fertigstellen**
   Im letzten Schritt wird Ihnen angezeigt, dass Ihr Webservice angelegt werden wird. Klicken Sie auf den Button **Fertigstellen**.

Schnittstelle eines Webservice

Abbildung 8.2 zeigt die externe Sicht auf die Schnittstelle des Webservice. Sie sehen, dass für jedes BAPI eine Operation erzeugt wurde.

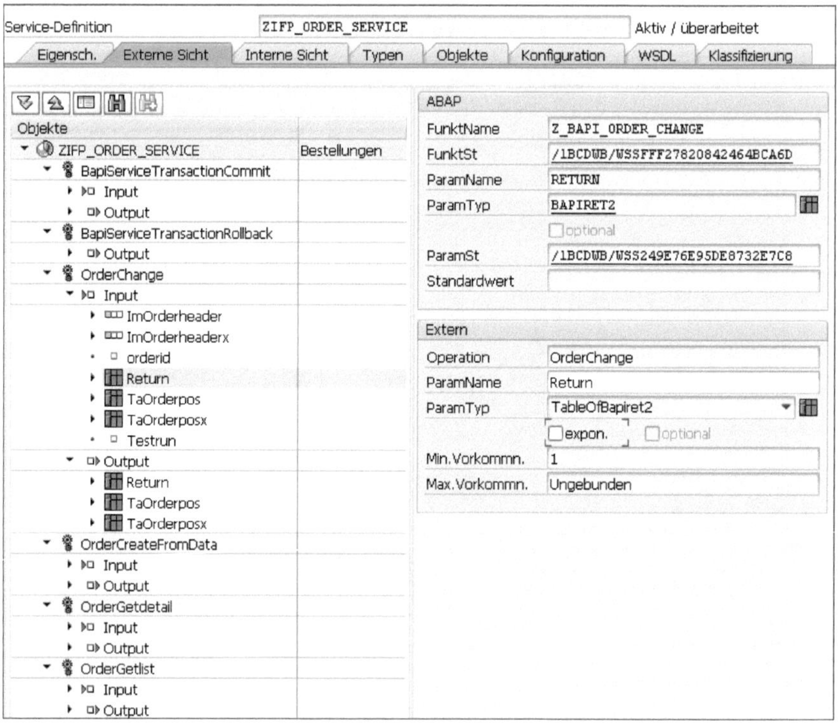

Abbildung 8.2 Serviceschnittstelle des Webservice

Jede Operation hat einen Importparameter namens `Input` und einen Exportparameter namens `Output`. Im Importparameter finden Sie Entsprechungen zu den Import- und Tabellenparametern des Funktionsbausteins, im Exportparameter Entsprechungen zu dessen Export- und Tabellenparametern.

Dass die Tabellenparameter zweimal erscheinen, liegt daran, dass sie bei Funktionsbausteinen sowohl als Import- als auch als Exportparameter dienen können. Wenn Sie in der Strukturübersicht der Serviceschnittstelle auf einen solchen Parameter klicken, sehen Sie rechts die Zuordnung des Parameters von **ABAP** (oben) zum entsprechenden Parameter in der Sicht **Extern** (unten). Über die Auswahl **expon.** können Sie festlegen, ob der Parameter überhaupt in der Serviceschnittstelle erscheinen soll. In Abbildung 8.2 haben wir z. B. den Tabellenparameter `Return` aus dem Input-Parameter herausgenommen, da dieser Tabellenparameter definitiv ein Rückgabeparameter ist.

8

Webservice testen

Wenn Sie mögen, können Sie an dieser Stelle den Webservice aktivieren und anschließend mit der Funktionstaste [F8] testen. Im Testdialog wählen Sie zuerst die Operation aus. Danach wird Ihnen ein Template für ein XML-Request-Dokument generiert, das Sie auch noch editieren können, bevor Sie es ebenfalls mit der Taste [F8] an den Webservice schicken. Wurde die Methode erfolgreich ausgeführt, zeigt Ihnen die Testumgebung das XML-Response-Dokument an.

SOA-Manager

Damit Sie den Service nutzen können, müssen Sie noch einen *Endpunkt* anlegen. Dazu wechseln Sie in die Leseansicht und starten den SOA-Manager über die Tastenkombination [Strg] + [F10]. Der SOA-Manager ist eine Web-Dynpro-Anwendung für das SOA-Management. Klicken Sie auf **Service anlegen**. Es startet ein Wizard, der Sie in vier Schritten durch die Konfiguration des Endpunkts führt.

1. **Service- und Binding-Namen**
   Geben Sie hier einen beliebigen Service- und Binding-Namen ein. Dies sind zwei Schlüsselwerte, die Ihre Endpunktkonfiguration identifizieren. Klicken Sie danach auf **Weiter**.
2. **Provider-Sicherheit**
   Hier können Sie unter verschiedenen Transportgarantie- und Authentifizierungseinstellungen wählen und diese konfigurieren. Für unser einfaches Beispiel wählen Sie **Benutzer-ID und Kennwort** im Bereich **Authentifizierung auf Transportebene**. Klicken Sie dann auf **Weiter**.
3. **SOAP-Protokoll**
   Hier können Sie eine alternative Zugriffs-URL angeben und den Typ des

Identifiable Business Context auswählen. Identifiable Business Contexts sind SAP-proprietäre Konzepte zur Identifizierung der an einem Integrationsszenario beteiligten Sender und Empfänger. Für unser Beispiel geben wir hier nichts ein und klicken auf **Weiter**.

4. **Operationseinstellungen**
   Hier werden nochmals alle Operationen aufgelistet. An dieser Stelle klicken Sie auf **Fertig**. Es wird dann die Liste der Konfigurationen wie in Abbildung 8.3 angezeigt.

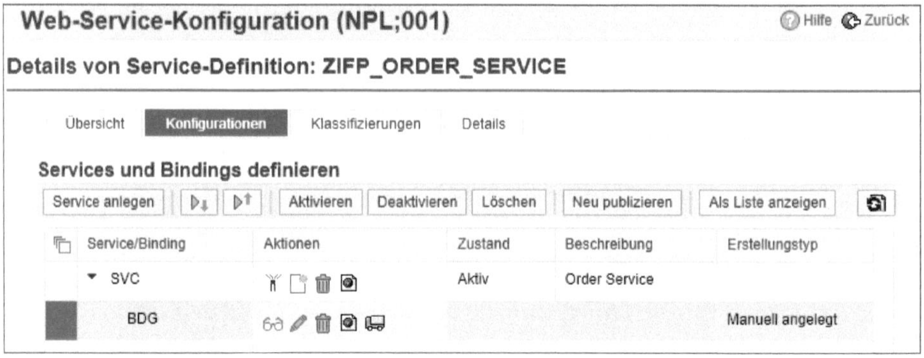

Abbildung 8.3 SOA-Manager

WSDL-Generierung

Wenn Sie im SOA-Manager für den Service auf das Icon (**WSDL-Generierung für Binding öffnen**) klicken, öffnet sich ein Dialog, in dem Sie verschiedene Optionen für die Generierung einer WSDL-Datei (WSDL = Web Services Description Language) wählen können. Jede Kombination von Einstellungen, die Sie in den Drop-down-Listen im oberen Bereich wählen können, definiert ein *Flavor*, das Sie unter einem frei wählbaren Namen speichern können. Dieses Flavor wird auch in der URL der WSDL-Datei als hexadezimale ID benutzt. Ändern sich die Einstellungen, ändert sich auch die URL. Die gültige WSDL-Datei kann über den Dialog direkt heruntergeladen werden.

WSDL-Format/ Bindungsstil wählen

Schließt man den SOA-Manager, kann man auf der Registerkarte **WSDL** ebenso eine WSDL-Datei samt URL einsehen. Über das Drop-down-Menü **SOAP-Style** können Sie zwischen **RPC** und **Dokument** wählen (siehe Abbildung 8.4). Der Unterschied zwischen den WSDL-Formaten bzw. *Bindungsstilen* RPC und Dokument liegt in ihrer Struktur und ihrem Verwendungszweck. Die an dieser Stelle heruntergeladene WSDL-Datei hat jedoch kein `<wsdl:service>`-Element, definiert also keinen Endpunkt, entspricht aber dem zuvor eingestellten Flavor.

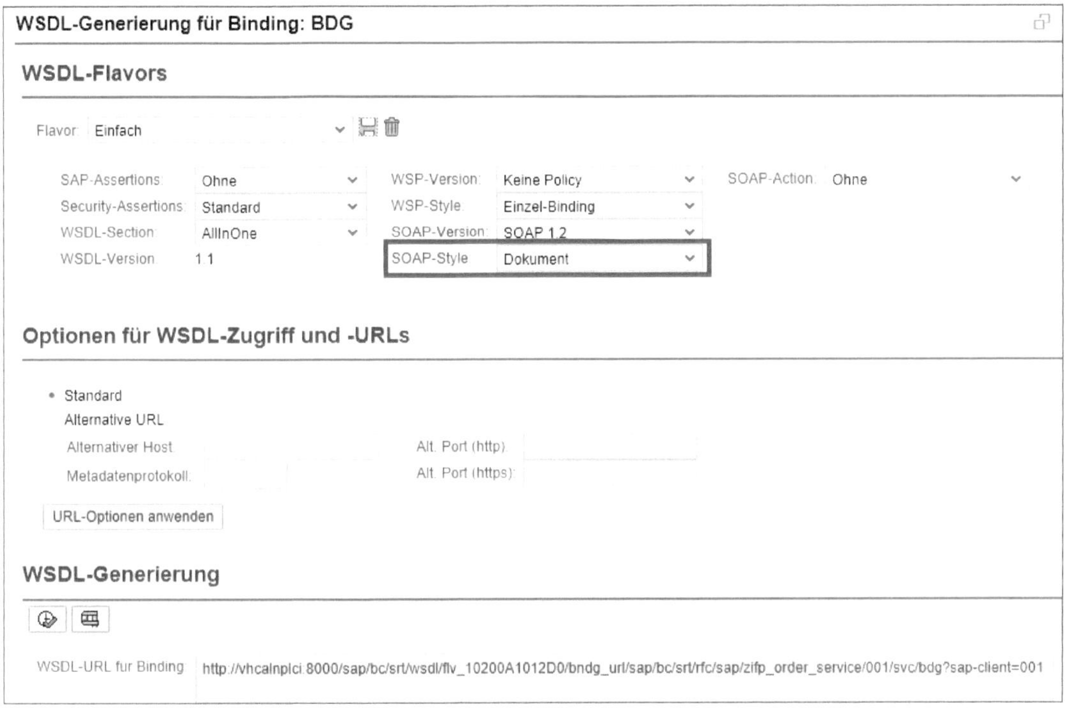

Abbildung 8.4 WSDL-Generierung

Bindungsstile

Innerhalb von SOAP werden zwei verschiedene Bindungsstile verwendet, die zwei unterschiedliche Auffassungen des Datenaustauschs (Versenden von Dokumenten vs. Aufruf von Funktionen) reflektieren.

- Im *Dokument-Stil* werden die Input- und Output-Parameter der Operationen als Dokumente betrachtet, die eine beliebige Struktur haben können. Die ausgetauschten Nachrichten werden als nicht mehr weiter unterteilbar betrachtet; sie bestehen demnach aus nur einem Teil:

  ```
  <wsdl:message name="OrderChange">
  <wsdl:part name="parameters" element="tns:OrderChange" />
  </wsdl:message>
  ```

- Beim *RPC-Stil* wird davon ausgegangen, dass die Input- und Output-Parameter in einzelne, benannte Parameter unterteilt werden können. Die ausgetauschten Nachrichten bestehen demnach aus mehreren Teilen:

```
<wsdl:message name="OrderChange">
<wsdl:part name="ImOrderheader" type="tns:Zifporder" />
<wsdl:part name="ImOrderheaderx" type="tns:Zifporderx" />
<wsdl:part name="TaOrderpos"
         type="tns:TableOfZifporderpos" />
<wsdl:part name="TaOrderposx"
         type="tns:TableOfZifporderposx" />
<wsdl:part name="Testrun" type="n0:char1" />
<wsdl:part name="orderid" type="n0:numeric10" />
</wsdl:message>
```

WSDL-Datei

Grundsätzlich ist eine WSDL-Datei ein XML-Dokument, das den Webservice genau definiert. Es handelt sich dabei also um einen Schnittstellenvertrag. Abbildung 8.5 zeigt Teile der WSDL-Datei für unseren Webservice. Im Element `<wsdl:service>` der WSDL-Datei steht im Kind-Element `<soap:address>` im Attribut `location` der sogenannte *Endpunkt*, also die URL, unter der der Webservice aufgerufen werden kann. Normalerweise schauen Sie sich eine solche WSDL-Datei wahrscheinlich nicht an. Sie benötigen sie hier aber, um den Code für Clients zu generieren, die den Webservice verwenden sollen.

Aufbau der WSDL-Datei

Wie Abbildung 8.5 zeigt, besteht die WSDL-Datei aus fünf Teilen:

❶ **Definition der einfachen und komplexen Datentypen**
Die vom Webservice verwendeten Datentypen werden im XML-Element `<wsdl:types>` in der *XML Schema Definition Language* (XSD) beschrieben.

❷ **Beschreibung der Nachrichtentypen**
Die Beschreibung der Nachrichtentypen erfolgt in den XML-Elementen `<wsdl:message>`. Jede Operation des Webservice hat dabei eine Input- und eine Output-Message, z. B. `OrderChange` und `OrderChangeResponse`. Die Nachrichtendefinitionen beziehen sich auf die vorangegangenen Typdefinitionen in `<wsdl:types>`.

❸ **Beschreibung der Operationen**
Innerhalb von `<wsdl:portType>`-Elementen beschreibt die WSDL-Datei, welche Operationen der Webservice zur Verfügung stellt und welche Input- und Output-Message jeweils von einer Operation erwartet und zurückgeschickt wird.

❹ **Bindungsstil und SOAP-Action**
Im Abschnitt `<wsdl:binding>` wird definiert, an welche SOAP-Actions die Operationen gebunden sind und welchen Bindungsstil die Nachrichten haben. Die SOAP-Action wird beim Aufruf per HTTP im HTTP-Header mitgegeben und hilft dem Webservice dabei, die richtige Operation aus-

zuwählen. Die Bindungsstile wurden im Hinweiskasten »Bindungsstile« erläutert.

❺ **Servicename und URL**
Innerhalb eines `<wsdl:service>`-Elements wird nun der Webservice benannt und die URL angegeben, unter der er per HTTP aufgerufen werden kann (Endpunkt des Webservice).


```
  <?xml version="1.0" encoding="utf-8" ?>
- <wsdl:definitions targetNamespace="urn:sap-com:document:sap:soap:functions:mc-style" xmlns:wsdl="http://schemas.x
   xmlns:xsd="http://www.w3.org/2001/XMLSchema" xmlns:soap="http://schemas.xmlsoap.org/wsdl/soap/"
   xmlns:wsoap12="http://schemas.xmlsoap.org/wsdl/soap12/" xmlns:http="http://schemas.xmlsoap.org/wsdl/http/
   xmlns:mime="http://schemas.xmlsoap.org/wsdl/mime/" xmlns:tns="urn:sap-com:document:sap:soap:functions:mc-
   com:document:sap:rfc:functions">
  + <wsdl:documentation>
  + <wsdl:types> ❶
  + <wsdl:message name="BapiServiceTransactionCommit"> ❷
  + <wsdl:message name="BapiServiceTransactionCommitResponse">
  + <wsdl:message name="BapiServiceTransactionRollback">
  + <wsdl:message name="BapiServiceTransactionRollbackResponse">
  + <wsdl:message name="OrderChange">
  + <wsdl:message name="OrderChangeResponse">
  + <wsdl:message name="OrderCreateFromData">
  + <wsdl:message name="OrderCreateFromDataResponse">
  + <wsdl:message name="OrderGetdetail">
  + <wsdl:message name="OrderGetdetailResponse">
  + <wsdl:message name="OrderGetlist">
  + <wsdl:message name="OrderGetlistResponse">
  - <wsdl:portType name="ZIFP_ORDER_SERVICE"> ❸
    + <wsdl:operation name="BapiServiceTransactionCommit">
    + <wsdl:operation name="BapiServiceTransactionRollback">
    + <wsdl:operation name="OrderChange">
    - <wsdl:operation name="OrderCreateFromData">
        <wsdl:input message="tns:OrderCreateFromData" />
        <wsdl:output message="tns:OrderCreateFromDataResponse" />
      </wsdl:operation>
    + <wsdl:operation name="OrderGetdetail">
    + <wsdl:operation name="OrderGetlist">
    </wsdl:portType>
  - <wsdl:binding name="BDG_soap12" type="tns:ZIFP_ORDER_SERVICE"> ❹
      <wsoap12:binding transport="http://schemas.xmlsoap.org/soap/http" style="document" />
    + <wsdl:operation name="BapiServiceTransactionCommit">
    + <wsdl:operation name="BapiServiceTransactionRollback">
    + <wsdl:operation name="OrderChange">
    + <wsdl:operation name="OrderCreateFromData">
    + <wsdl:operation name="OrderGetdetail">
    + <wsdl:operation name="OrderGetlist">
    </wsdl:binding>
  - <wsdl:service name="SVC"> ❺
    - <wsdl:port name="BDG_soap12" binding="tns:BDG_soap12">
        <wsoap12:address location="http://vhcalnplci:8000/sap/bc/srt/rfc/sap/zifp_order_service/001/svc/bdg" />
      </wsdl:port>
    </wsdl:service>
  </wsdl:definitions>
```

Abbildung 8.5 Bestandteile der WSDL-Datei

SOAP-Dokumente

Obwohl die WSDL-Datei auf den ersten Blick beeindruckend ist, sind die ausgetauschten Dokumente einfach aufgebaut. Wenn Sie im SOA-Manager in der Webservice-Administration auf das Icon (**Web-Service-Navigator für gewähltes Binding öffnen**) klicken, öffnet sich ein Webbrowser-Fenster und zeigt eine Java-Anwendung an, die das WSDL-Dokument liest und eine grafische Benutzeroberfläche zum Testen des Webservice erzeugt. Dieses

Testwerkzeug zeigt Ihnen auch die XML-Dateien an, die per HTTP-POST ausgetauscht werden. Listing 8.1 zeigt das Request-Dokument.

```
<?xml version="1.0" encoding="UTF-8" ?>
<SOAP-ENV:Envelope
  xmlns:SOAP-ENV="http://schemas.xmlsoap.org/soap/envelope/"
  xmlns:xsi="http://www.w3.org/2001/XMLSchema-instance"
  xmlns:xs="http://www.w3.org/2001/XMLSchema">
  <SOAP-ENV:Header>
    <!-- ... -->
  </SOAP-ENV:Header>
  <SOAP-ENV:Body>
    <ns1:OrderGetlist xmlns:ns1='urn:sap...'>
      <ImRefid></ImRefid>
    </ns1:OrderGetlist>
  </SOAP-ENV:Body>
</SOAP-ENV:Envelope>
```

Listing 8.1 SOAP-Request

SOAP-Envelope

Das Wurzelelement ist ein SOAP-Envelope, der einen optionalen SOAP-Header und einen SOAP-Body enthält. Im SOAP-Body sehen Sie die Request-Nachricht `OrderGetList`. Der SOAP-Header enthält SAP-spezifische Informationen über das Management der Sitzung.

Listing 8.2 zeigt die Antwort des Servers. Wiederum ist das Antwortdokument, in diesem Fall `OrderGetlistResponse`, in das SOAP-Body-Element innerhalb des SOAP-Envelope-Elements eingebettet.

```
<?xml version="1.0" encoding="UTF-8" ?>
<soap-env:Envelope
 xmlns:soap.env="http://schemas.xmlsoap.org/soap/envelope/">
  <soap-env:Body>
    <n0:OrderGetlistResponse xmlns:n0="urn:sap... ">
      <Return>
        <Type>S</Type>
        <Id></Id>
        <Number>000</Number>
        <Message></Message>
        <LogNo></LogNo>
        <LogMsgNo>000000</LogMsgNo>
        <MessageV1></MessageV1>
        <MessageV2></MessageV2>
        <MessageV3></MessageV3>
        <MessageV4></MessageV4>
```

```
        <Parameter></Parameter>
        <Row>0</Row>
        <Field></Field>
        <System></System>
      </Return>
      <TaOrders>
        <item>
          <Mandt>001</Mandt>
          <Orderid>0000000040</Orderid>
          <Type>SO</Type>
          <Refid>0000000002</Refid>
          <Buyer>Käufer</Buyer>
          <Seller>Lieferant</Seller>
          <Orderdate>2008-12-19</Orderdate>
        </item>
        <item>
          <Mandt>001</Mandt>
          <Orderid>0000000053</Orderid>
          <Type>SO</Type>
          <Refid>0000000001</Refid>
          <Buyer>Buchhandlung Pehnke</Buyer>
          <Seller>Grosshandel Englbrecht</Seller>
          <Orderdate>2018-01-31</Orderdate>
        </item>
      </TaOrders>
    </n0:OrderGetlistResponse>
  </soap-env:Body>
</soap-env:Envelope>
```


Listing 8.2 SOAP-Response

Sie können den Exportparameter `Return` und die Tabelle `TaOrders` mit zwei Einträgen erkennen. In der Antwort fehlt der SOAP-Header sogar ganz. Wie Sie im Listing z. B. am Element `Orderid` erkennen können, werden ABAP-Felder vom Typ `N` bzw. Dictionary-Felder vom Typ `NUMC` mit führenden Nullen bis zu deren Gesamtlänge aufgefüllt. In einem Request-Dokument mit derartigen Feldern müssen Sie darauf achten, diese selbst mit führenden Nullen aufzufüllen.

8.1.2 SOAP-Webclient mit ABAP

Einen ABAP-Client zu schreiben, der die Operationen des Webservice aufruft, ist ebenfalls nicht schwierig und in drei Schritten erledigt. Zuerst lassen Sie sich eine Proxy-Klasse aus der WSDL-Datei generieren, konfigurieren danach einen logischen Port, der auf den Endpunkt des Webservice zeigt, und schreiben zum Schluss ein Programm, das die Proxy-Klasse instanziiert und deren Methoden verwendet.

Starten Sie dazu Transaktion SE80, den Object Navigator. Lassen Sie sich das Paket anzeigen, das Ihre Proxy-Klasse enthalten soll. Im Kontextmenü des Pakets starten Sie über **Anlegen • Enterprise Service** den Webservice-Wizard, der für Sie die Proxy-Klasse generiert.

Angabe der WSDL-Datei

Im ersten Schritt wählen Sie nun **Service-Consumer** als Objekttyp und klicken dann auf den Button **Weiter**, um zum nächsten Bildschirm zu gelangen. Im zweiten Schritt müssen Sie die Herkunft der WSDL-Datei angeben, die den Webservice beschreibt, für den Sie einen Client-Proxy erzeugen möchten. Hier geben Sie dem Wizard an, ob er die WSDL-Datei aus dem Backend, aus dem Enterprise Services Repository oder aus einer externen WSDL-Datei beziehen wollen. Für den vorliegenden Webservice, der in Abschnitt 8.1.1, »SOAP-Webservice mit ABAP«, erzeugt wurde, wählen Sie hier **Externe(s) WSDL/Schema** an und selektieren im nächsten Schritt die Option **URL**. Geben Sie im nächsten Schritt die URL ein, die Sie zuvor aus dem Browser kopiert haben, als Sie sich die WSDL-Datei in Transaktion SOAMANAGER angeschaut haben. Wenn Sie die WSDL-Datei in einer lokalen Datei gespeichert haben, geben Sie diese an.

Auswahl von Paket und Präfix

Im nächsten Schritt wählen Sie das Paket aus, in dem die generierten Objekte abgelegt werden sollen. Außerdem geben Sie ein Präfix an, das vor alle generierten Objektnamen gestellt werden soll. Wir haben hier als Paket `ZIFP` und als Präfix `ZIFP_` gewählt. Möglicherweise erhalten Sie eine Warnung, dass Ihr Paket keine Verwendungserklärung für das Paket `SAI_TOOLS` hat. Diese Verwendungserklärung können Sie nachträglich noch einfügen, indem Sie im Object Navigator Ihr Paket öffnen, zur Registerkarte **Verwendungserklärungen** gehen und dort eine neue Verwendungserklärung für das Paket `SAI_TOOLS` anlegen. Sie erhalten zudem wahrscheinlich eine Warnung, dass es zu Namenskollisionen und Namensverkürzungen gekommen ist. Sie haben aber die Möglichkeit, die generierten Namen auf der Registerkarte **Namensprobleme** zu ändern, bevor Sie den generierten Proxy aktivieren.

Abbildung 8.6 zeigt den generierten Webservice-Client-Proxy. Sie sehen, dass die generierte Proxy-Klasse `ZIFP_CO_ZIFP_ORDER_SERVICE` sechs Methoden hat, eine für jede Operation des Webservice. Jede Operation verfügt über einen Import- und einen Exportparameter. Die einzelnen Komponenten dieser Parameter entsprechen den Import- und Exportparametern des Webservice.

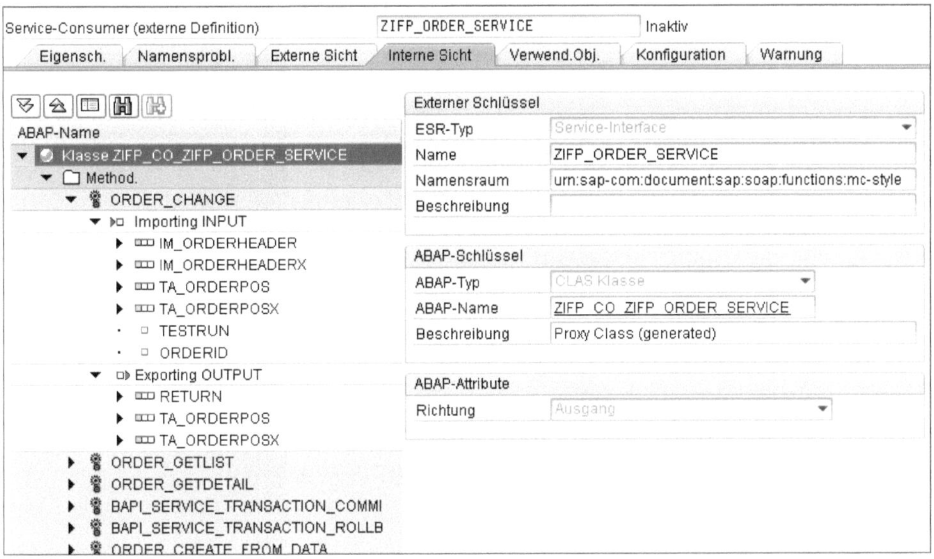

Abbildung 8.6 Generierter Webservice-Client-Proxy

Logische Ports

Bevor Sie den Proxy testen und verwenden können, müssen Sie mit Transaktion SOAMANAGER noch einen sogenannten *logischen Port* für die generierte Klasse anlegen. Die generierte Proxy-Klasse enthält nämlich keine Informationen über die URL, über die der Webservice aufgerufen werden kann. Diese Informationen werden in einem logischen Port hinterlegt, der bei der Instanziierung der Proxy-Klasse im Konstruktor mitgegeben wird. Für eine Proxy-Klasse können Sie in Transaktion SOAMANAGER mehrere Ports anlegen. Damit können Sie flexibel auf verschiedene URLs verweisen, bei denen die gleichen Webservices erreichbar sind. Sie können auf die Übergabe eines Ports bei der Instanziierung verzichten, wenn Sie einen der Ports als Default-Port markieren.

Klicken Sie auf das Icon  (**SOAMANAGER für Konfiguration starten**), um den SOA-Manager zu starten. Klicken Sie im SOA-Manager auf **Anlegen**, und wählen Sie **WSDL-basierte Konfiguration** aus. Es erscheint ein Wizard, der Sie in acht Schritten durch die Konfiguration führt, wobei nur die ersten vier Schritte für unser Beispiel relevant sind.

1. **Name des logischen Ports**
   Geben Sie in das Eingabefeld **Name des logischen Ports** einen beliebigen Namen für den logischen Port ein, den Sie erstellen möchten. Markieren Sie außerdem das Auswahlfeld **Logischer Port ist Standard**, um Ihren Port, den Sie gerade erstellen, als Standardport zu markieren. Geben Sie zusätzlich noch eine kurze Beschreibung für den neuen Port ein. Klicken Sie dann auf **Weiter**.

2. **WSDL-Informationen**
   Hier haben Sie wieder die Wahl, ob Sie auf die WSDL per HTTP zugreifen oder diese aus einer lokalen Datei auslesen möchten. Wählen Sie die erste Möglichkeit, müssen Sie noch die URL der WSDL sowie Benutzer und Passwort für den WSDL-Zugriff angeben. Bei der zweiten Möglichkeit genügt es, wenn Sie den Dateipfad angeben. Klicken Sie dann auf **Weiter**.
3. **Binding-Auswahl**
   Falls die WSDL mehrere Bindings enthält, wählen Sie in diesem Schritt eines der angebotenen Bindings aus und klicken dann auf **Weiter**.
4. **Consumer-Sicherheit**
   Geben Sie hier einen Benutzername und ein Passwort für den Zugriff auf den Webservice an, und klicken Sie dann auf **Weiter**.
5. **HTTP-Einstellungen**
   Hier zeigt der Wizard die URL des Webservice an, und Sie können weitere Angaben zum HTTP-Proxy und zum Binding vornehmen. Klicken Sie anschließend auf **Weiter**.
6. **SOAP-Protokoll**
   Hier können Sie Änderungen zu den Details des SOAP-Protokolls vornehmen und mit einem Klick auf **Weiter** zum nächsten Schritt gehen.
7. **Identifiable Business Context**
   Hier können Sie Angaben zum Identifiable Business Context machen und mit einem Klick auf **Weiter** zum letzten Schritt gehen.
8. **Operationseinstellungen**
   Hier zeigt Ihnen der Wizard nochmals alle Operationen an, und Sie können die Standardeinstellungen zu jeder Operation ändern. Klicken Sie hier auf **Fertig**.

Test des Proxys

Schließen Sie den Dialog und gehen Sie nun zurück in den Object Navigator, um Ihren Proxy zu testen. Klicken Sie in der Anwendungsfunktionsleiste auf **Testen** ([F8]). Geben Sie den Namen des logischen Ports an, den Sie soeben angelegt haben. Geben Sie ebenfalls eine Operation an, die Sie testen möchten, z. B. `ORDER_GETDETAIL`. Wählen Sie **Ausführen** ([F8]), und klicken Sie dann in der Anwendungsfunktionsleiste auf **XML-Editor** ([Strg] + [F2]).

Ersetzen Sie die generierte `orderid` (Bestellnummer) durch eine `orderid`, von der Sie wissen, dass sie im Zielsystem existiert, damit Sie auch sinnvolle Daten zurückbekommen. Klicken Sie nochmals auf **Ausführen** ([F8]); dann können Sie sich die Antwortnachricht anzeigen lassen.

Client-Programm

Nach dem erfolgreichen Test können Sie nun ein Programm schreiben, das den Webservice aufruft. Listing 8.3 zeigt ein ABAP-Programm, das die Methode `order_getlist` der generierten Proxy-Klasse aufruft und die zurückgegebenen Bestelldetails in einer ABAP-Liste ausgibt.

```
REPORT  zifp_test_webservice.
DATA:
  r_proxy TYPE REF TO zifp_co_zifp_order_service,
  output TYPE zifp_order_getlist_response,
  input TYPE zifp_order_getlist,
  wa TYPE zifp_zifporder.
TRY.
    CREATE OBJECT r_proxy
*   EXPORTING
*     LOGICAL_PORT_NAME  =

  CATCH cx_ai_system_fault.
ENDTRY.
TRY.
    CALL METHOD r_proxy->order_getlist
      EXPORTING
        input  = input
      IMPORTING
        output = output.
  CATCH cx_ai_system_fault.
  CATCH cx_ai_application_fault.
ENDTRY.
LOOP AT output-ta_orders-item INTO wa.
  WRITE:/ wa-orderid, wa-type, wa-refid,
          wa-buyer, wa-seller, wa-orderdate.
ENDLOOP.
```

Listing 8.3 ABAP-Programm für einen Webservice-Aufruf

Das Programm erzeugt zuerst ein Objekt der Proxy-Klasse. Da die Methode `order_getlist` keine relevanten Input-Parameter hat, müssen diese vor dem Aufruf auch nicht gefüllt werden. Nach dem Aufruf der Methode wird die interne Tabelle `output-ta_orders-item` mit den Bestellköpfen ausgegeben.

Aufruf eines externen Webservice

Sobald Ihnen eine WSDL-Datei vorliegt, können Sie sich einen ABAP-Proxy für den Aufruf des Webservice generieren lassen, der in der WSDL-Datei beschrieben ist. In der Praxis wird es leider nicht möglich sein, den zuvor für den ABAP-Webservice generierten Proxy wiederzuverwenden, da die

WSDL-Dateien für den ABAP-Service und für den Java-Service subtile und eventuell weniger subtile Unterschiede aufweisen, obwohl beide Services das Gleiche tun. Zum Beispiel könnte der eine WSDL-Generator den Dokumentenbindungsstil bevorzugen und der andere den RPC-Bindungsstil. Der eine Generator setzt Listen als eine Hierarchie von zwei XML-Elementen um (eine für die Liste mit `maxOccurs=1`; das Kindelement für das Listenelement mit `maxOccurs=unbounded`), und der andere Generator verzichtet auf dieses übergeordnete Listenelement. Der Ausgangspunkt für die Entwicklung war nicht die WSDL-Datei, sondern die WSDL-Datei wurde aus dem ABAP- bzw. Java-Code heraus generiert. Den umgekehrten Ansatz, nämlich zuerst die Schnittstellenbeschreibung zu erstellen und dann einen Server-Proxy aus der Schnittstellenbeschreibung für unterschiedliche Programmiersprachen generieren zu lassen, lernen Sie im nächsten Abschnitt kennen.

8.2 Outside-In-Webservices und -Webclients mit der ABAP-Plattform

In diesem Abschnitt erläutern wir die Entwicklung von Webservices und Webservice-Clients nach dem Outside-In-Verfahren (auch als Contract-First-Ansatz bekannt). Dabei beschreiben Sie die Schnittstelle zuerst im Enterprise Services Repository (ESR) oder im Backend Repository und generieren dann daraus Server- und Client-Proxys. Das ESR wird sowohl mit SAP Process Integration (PI, ist eine Komponente von SAP Process Orchestration) als auch direkt mit SAP Process Orchestration ausgeliefert, während das Backend Repository Bestandteil einer jeden ABAP-Plattform ist. Damit Sie im Enterprise Services Repository eine Schnittstelle beschreiben können, müssen Sie diese einer Softwarekomponentenversion zuordnen, die Sie im *System Landscape Directory* (SLD) anlegen und danach in das Enterprise Services Repository importieren müssen. Daher erklären wir Ihnen in den nächsten vier Abschnitten zunächst das System Landscape Directory, danach die Schnittstellen im Enterprise Services Repository, anschließend die Schnittstellen im Backend-Repository und schließlich die Generierung von ABAP-Proxys.

8.2.1 System Landscape Directory

Das SLD speichert Informationen zur System- und Softwarelandschaft eines Unternehmens. Diese Informationen werden auch von anderen Komponenten der ABAP-Plattform verwendet, z. B. vom SAP Solution Manager.

Hier beschreiben wir nur die Funktionen, die das Enterprise Services Repository nutzt.

Softwareprodukte

Das SLD speichert Informationen über Softwareprodukte, deren Hersteller und Versionen. Ein Beispiel für die vielen Softwareproduktversionen, die im System Landscape Directory gespeichert sind, ist SAP SCM 7.0. Die Softwareproduktversion SAP SCM 7.0 ist die Version 7.0 des Produkts SAP Supply Chain Management des Herstellers SAP. Zwischen einem Softwareprodukt und seinen Versionen gibt es eine 1:n-Beziehung.

Softwarekomponenten

Eine Softwareproduktversion umfasst eine oder mehrere Softwarekomponentenversionen. Dabei werden die Softwarekomponenten und ihre Versionen unabhängig von den Softwareprodukten gepflegt. Daher gibt es eine m:n-Beziehung zwischen Softwareproduktversionen und Softwarekomponentenversionen. Oder anders gesagt: Eine Softwarekomponentenversion kann in mehreren Softwareproduktversionen enthalten sein. Zum Beispiel ist die Softwarekomponentenversion `SAP_BASIS` 7.5 in vielen Softwareproduktversionen von SAP enthalten, unter anderem in SAP ERP 6.0 EHP8.

Für unser Szenario legen Sie im SLD die Softwareproduktversion `SP_IFP` 2.0 mit der einzigen Softwarekomponentenversion `SC_IFP` 2.0 an. Starten Sie das SLD im Webbrowser über die URL *http://server:port/sld*, und melden Sie sich dort an. Abbildung 8.7 zeigt den Einstiegsbildschirm nach der erfolgreichen Anmeldung am SLD.

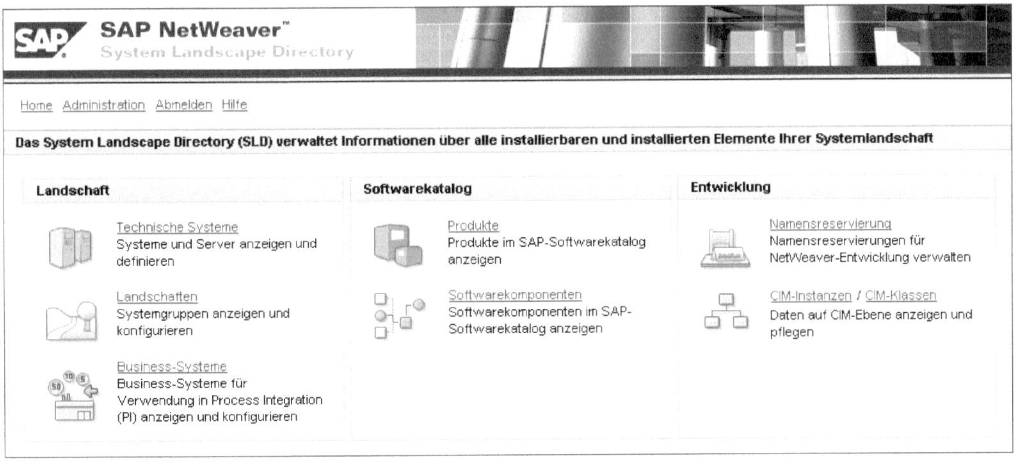

Abbildung 8.7 Einstiegsbildschirm des System Landscape Directorys

Um die Softwarekomponentenversion anzulegen, die Sie nachher im Enterprise Services Repository benötigen, wählen Sie den Link **Produkte** und erzeugen von dort aus zuerst eine neue Softwareproduktversion. Dazu geben Sie den Namen des Herstellers, den Namen des Softwareprodukts und die

Version ein. Anschließend werden Sie aufgefordert, eine Software-Unit und eine Softwarekomponentenversion innerhalb der Produktversion anzulegen.

8.2.2 Service-Interfaces

Datentypen und Nachrichtentypen

Die Softwarekomponentenversion `SC_IFP` 2.0, die Sie zuvor angelegt haben, importieren Sie nun ins Enterprise Services Repository. Danach legen Sie im Enterprise Services Repository die notwendigen Datentypen für die Nachrichten an, die die Operationen der Service-Interfaces austauschen sollen. Dies sind unter anderem Datentypen für Bestellkopf, Bestellposition, Bestellung, Bestellnummer und Bestellreferenz. Als Nachrichtentypen benötigen Sie nun für jede Operation eigene Request- und Response-Nachrichten.

Abbildung 8.8 zeigt als Beispiel den Nachrichtentyp `MT_ORDERCREATE_REQ`. Dieser Nachrichtentyp verweist auf den Datentyp `DT_IFP_ORDER` mit den beiden Komponenten `ORDERHEAD` und `ORDERPOS`, die ihrerseits auf die beiden einfacheren Datentypen `DT_IFP_ORDERHEAD` und `DT_IFP_ORDERPOS` verweisen. Links in Abbildung 8.8 sind weitere Datentypen und Nachrichtentypen aufgelistet.

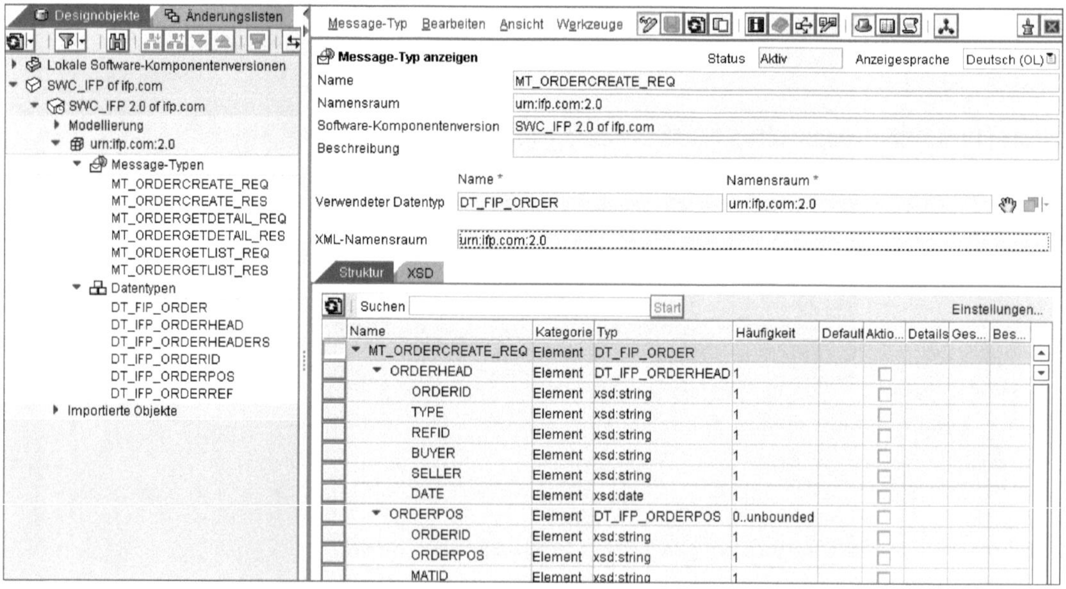

Abbildung 8.8 Nachrichtentyp im Enterprise Services Repository

Service-Interfaces

Um die Arbeiten im Enterprise Services Repository abzuschließen, legen Sie die benötigten Service-Interfaces an. Ein Service-Interface eines Senders

(Client) gehört der Kategorie outbound an, ein Service-Interface eines Empfängers (Server) der Kategorie inbound. Jede einzelne Operation im Service-Interface hat entweder den Modus synchron oder asynchron.

Interface-Patterns

Ein Service-Interface kann einem von vier Interface-Patterns zugeordnet werden:

- **Stateless**
  Die Operationen dieser Interfaces hinterlassen auf dem Server keinen Zustand, der von anderen Operationen desselben Interface in weiteren Aufrufen desselben Clients verwendet werden kann. Dies ist das bei Weitem wichtigste Interface-Pattern.
- **Stateless (SAP-XI-3.0-kompatibel)**
  Diese Interfaces wurden in SAP Process Integration 7.0 (jetzt Teil von SAP Process Orchestration) aus Gründen der Rückwärtskompatibilität zu den Message-Interfaces der SAP Exchange Infrastructure 3.0 eingeführt, die es ab SAP Process Integration 7.0 nicht mehr gibt. Sie haben genau eine Operation mit dem gleichen Namen wie das Interface.
- **Tentative Update & Confirm/Compensate (TU&C/C)**
  Diese Interfaces umfassen vier Arten von Operationen. Tentative-Update-Operationen erzeugen oder ändern Daten auf dem Server vorläufig. Diese Operationen sind synchron. Eine asynchrone `Confirm`-Operation bestätigt die Änderungen und schreibt sie fest. Eine asynchrone `Compensate`-Operation verwirft die Änderungen und macht sie rückgängig.
- **Stateful**
  Die Operationen dieser Interfaces hinterlassen auf dem Server einen Zustand, der von anderen Operationen desselben Interface in weiteren Aufrufen desselben Clients verwendet werden kann. Dieses Pattern wird nur für ganz spezielle technische Zwecke benötigt.

8

Service-Interfaces anlegen

Für das Beispiel legen Sie die beiden Service-Interfaces `SI_IFP_ORDER_IN` und `SI_IFP_ORDER_OUT` mit den beiden Operationen `GetList` und `GetDetail` an. Abbildung 8.9 zeigt die Operation `GetList` des Interface `SI_IFP_ORDER_IN`. Der Message-Typ für die Request-Nachricht ist `MT_ORDERLIST_REQ`, der Message-Typ für die Response-Nachricht ist `MT_ORDERLIST_RES`. Für die beiden Interfaces werden Sie Server- und Client-Proxys in ABAP erzeugen lassen und diese Proxys verwenden, um Webservices (Provider) und Webservice-Clients (Consumer) zu entwickeln.

Das Service-Interface `SI_IFP_ODERCREATE_IN` illustriert das Interface-Pattern **TU&C/C** (siehe Abbildung 8.10).

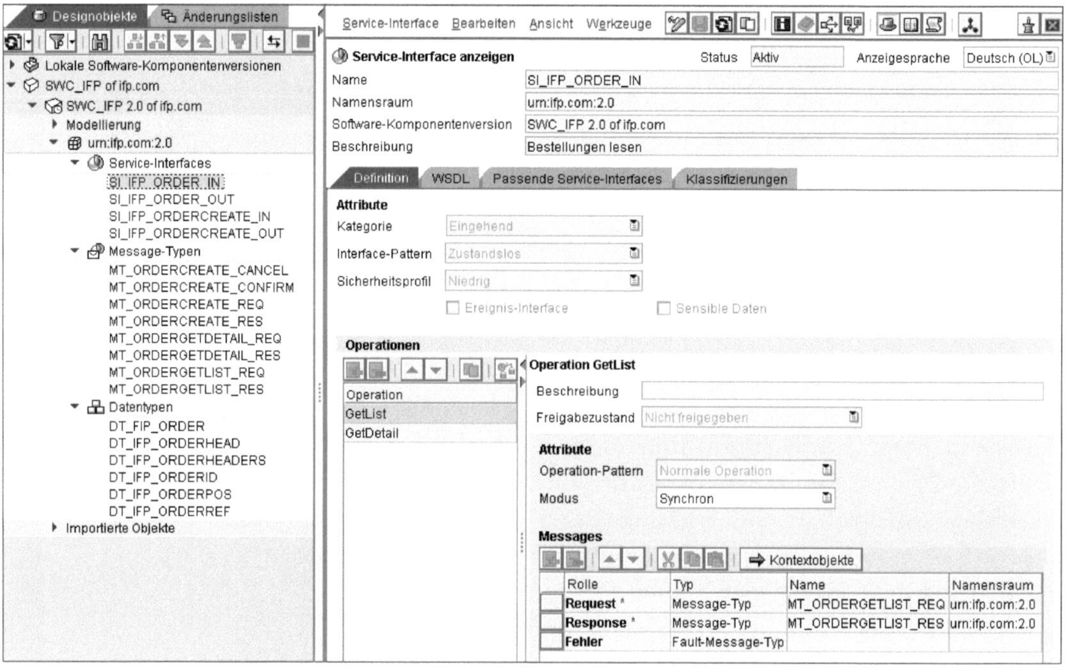

Abbildung 8.9 Service-Interface mit zwei Operationen

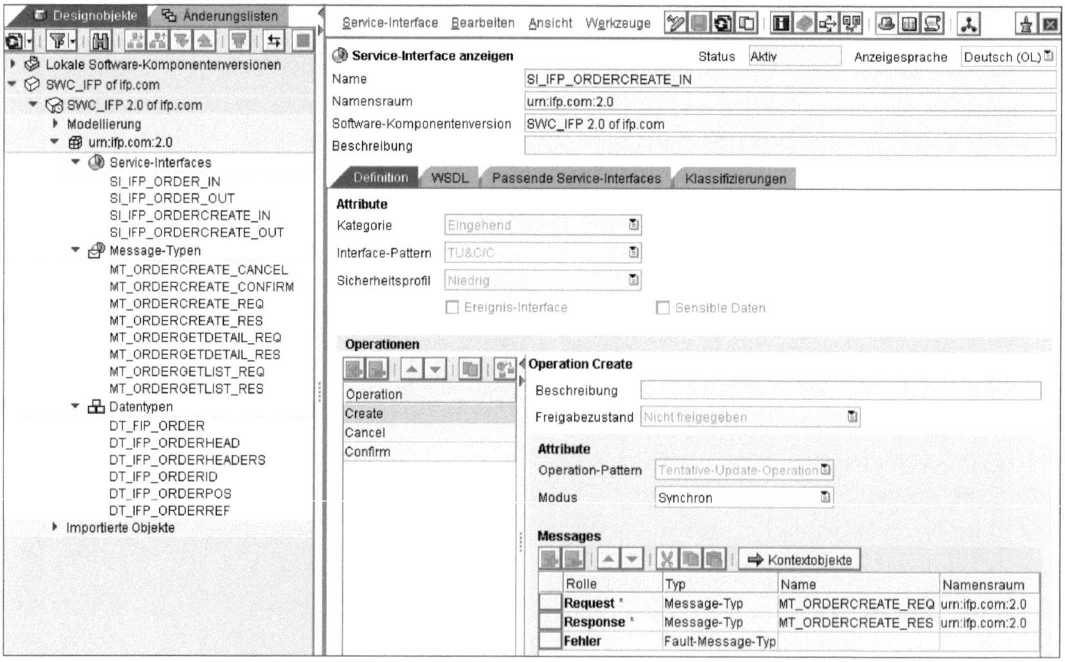

Abbildung 8.10 Service-Interface mit dem Pattern »TU&C/C«

Es verfügt über die synchrone Tentative-Update-Operation `Create`, die eine Bestellung nur vorläufig anlegt. Erst durch die asynchrone Confirm-Operation namens `Confirm` wird diese Bestellung bestätigt. Falls der Client, der mit der Tentative-Update-Operation eine vorläufige Bestellung angelegt hat, diese aber doch wieder stornieren möchte, kann er sie mittels der Compensate-Operation `Cancel` wieder rückgängig machen.

8.2.3 Das Backend Repository

Auch der SAP NetWeaver Application Server ABAP stellt ein Repository für Datentypen, Nachrichtentypen und Service-Interfaces bereit, das sogenannte *Backend Repository*. In diesem Abschnitt beschreiben wir die Möglichkeiten des Backend Repositorys anhand eines einfachen Beispiels:

Namensräume zuordnen

Zuerst legen Sie mit Transaktion SPXNGENAPPL fest, welche Namensräume dem Backend Repository und welche dem Enterprise Services Repository zugeordnet sind. Abbildung 8.11 zeigt beispielsweise, wie der Namensraum `urn:zifp` dem Backend Repository zugeordnet wird. Erst nachdem Sie dem Backend Repository Namensräume zugeordnet haben, können Sie mit dem Enterprise Service Wizard im Object Navigator die weiteren Objekte anlegen.

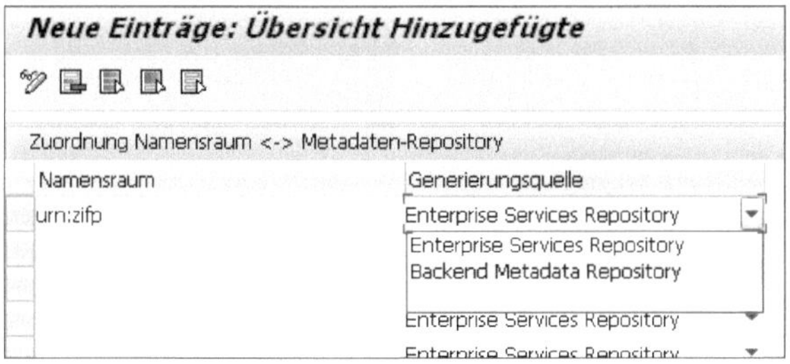

Abbildung 8.11 Namensräume zuordnen

Datentypen anlegen

Wir wollen als einfaches Beispiel ein Service-Interface bereitstellen, das arithmetische Operationen zur Verfügung stellt. Dazu definieren wir zuerst zwei Datentypen für die Operatoren und das Ergebnis der Operation. Legen Sie dazu im Object Navigator ein neues Objekt vom Typ *Enterprise Service* an, indem Sie im Kontextmenü Ihres Pakets den Eintrag **Anlegen • Enterprise Service** auswählen. Wählen Sie anschließend im Enterprise Service Wizard den Eintrag **Datentyp** aus, und bestätigen Sie mit **Weiter**. Wählen Sie nun im nächsten Schritt den Eintrag **Backend** aus, und klicken Sie erneut auf **Weiter**. Vergeben Sie im nächsten Schritt einen Namen für den Datentyp (z. B. »ZIFP_OPERANDS«), wählen Sie den Namensraum `urn:zifp` aus, und bestätigen Sie mit **Weiter**. Im letzten Schritt geben Sie Paket, Workbench-Auftrag und Namenspräfix an und wählen **Fertigstellen**.

Der Datentyp wird nun angezeigt; er ist vom XSD-Typ `xsd:string` und vom ABAP-Typ `String`. Sie können daraus einen komplexen Datentyp machen, indem Sie im Kontextmenü des Datentyps den Eintrag **Zu Complex Content Type wechseln** auswählen und dann über das Kontextmenü weitere Elemente oder Attribute hinzufügen. Fügen Sie auf diese Weise zwei Elemente namens `Operand1` und `Operand2` vom XSD-Typ `xsd:int` hinzu, wie es Abbildung 8.12 zeigt. Speichern und aktivieren Sie Ihren Datentypen, und legen Sie auf die gleiche Art einen zweiten Datentyp namens »ZIFP_RESULT« vom XSD-Typ `xsd:int` an.

Nachrichtentypen anlegen

Legen Sie als Nächstes die beiden Nachrichtentypen `ZIFP_ADD_REQ` und `ZIFP_ADD_RES` an, die auf die beiden Datentypen `ZIFP_OPERANDS` und `ZIFP_RESULT` verweisen, die Sie soeben angelegt haben.

Dazu starten Sie wieder den Enterprise Service Wizard und wählen im ersten Schritt den Eintrag **Message-Typ** aus. Im Proxy-Editor des neuen Message-Typs wählen Sie dann im Kontextmenü den Eintrag **Datentyp setzen • Vorhandenen Datentyp auswählen** aus, um den Datentyp zu setzen.

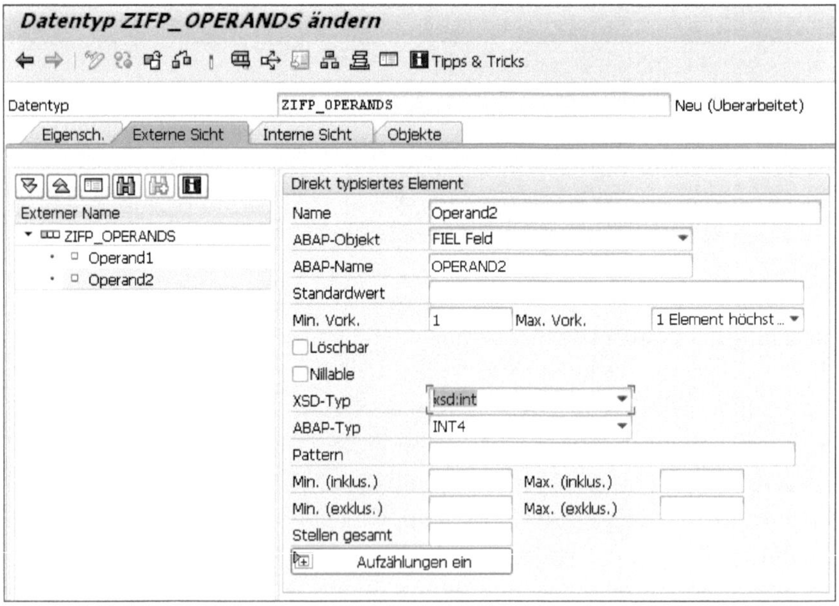

Abbildung 8.12 Datentyp »ZIFP_OPERANDS«

Abbildung 8.13 zeigt das Ergebnis für den Nachrichtentyp `ZIFP_ADD_REQ`.

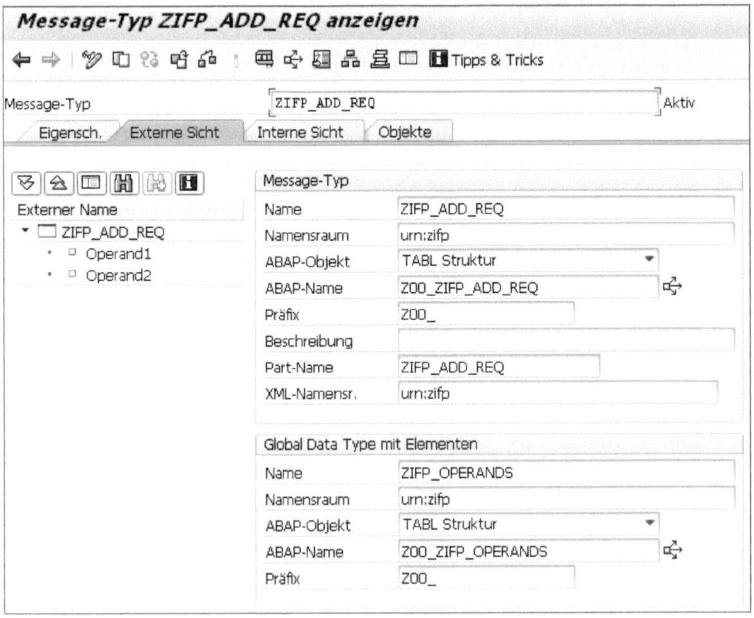

Abbildung 8.13 Nachrichtentyp »ZIFP_ADD_REQ«

Service-Provider anlegen

Nun können Sie einen Service-Provider anlegen. Gehen Sie dazu so vor wie bisher, und wählen Sie im ersten Schritt im Enterprise Service Wizard den Eintrag **Service-Provider**. Vergeben Sie im zweiten Schritt den Namen für den Service-Provider, z. B. »ZIFP_ARITHMETIC_SRV«. Im Proxy-Editor wählen Sie im Kontextmenü den Eintrag **Operation hinzufügen** aus, um eine Operation namens »Add« hinzuzufügen. Im Kontextmenü der neuen Operation wählen Sie **Request setzen • Vorhand. Message-Typ auswäh.**, um den Nachrichtentyp der Request-Nachricht zu setzen. Analog wählen Sie **Response setzen • Vorhand. Message-Typ auswäh.**, um den Nachrichtentyp der Request-Nachricht zu setzen. Abbildung 8.14 zeigt das Ergebnis.

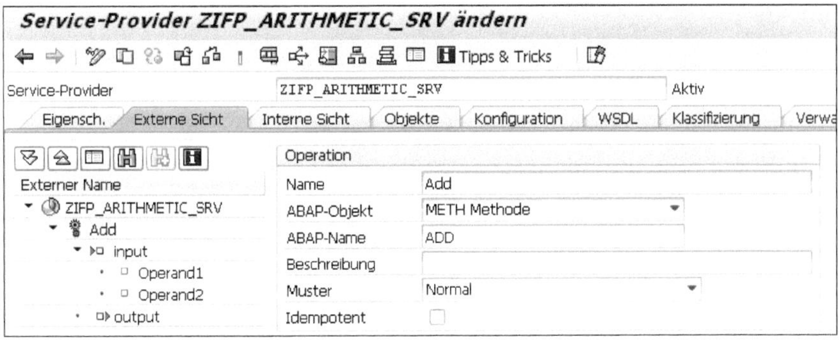

Abbildung 8.14 Service-Provider »ZIFP_ARITHMETIC_SRV«

Service-Provider implementieren

Wenn Sie auf die Registerkarte **Eigensch.** klicken, sehen Sie, dass für den Service-Provider ein ABAP-Interface mit den Methodendeklarationen und eine implementierende Klasse erzeugt wurden. Die Methoden dieser Klasse sind noch leer und müssen als Nächstes implementiert werden. Öffnen Sie dazu die generierte Methode der generierten Klasse, und geben Sie den Code aus Listing 8.4 ein.

```
METHOD z00_ii_zifp_arithmetic_srv~add.
  output-zifp_add_res =
    input-zifp_add_req-operand1 +
    input-zifp_add_req-operand2.
ENDMETHOD.
```

Listing 8.4 Implementierung der Add-Methode

Nachdem Sie alles aktiviert haben, können Sie wieder zurück zu Ihrem Service-Provider gehen, ihn testen und einen Endpunkt dafür anlegen, so wie wir dies schon im Abschnitt 8.1.2, »SOAP-Webclient mit ABAP«, beschrieben haben.

8.2.4 SOAP-Proxys in ABAP

Proxys erzeugen

In diesem Abschnitt erzeugen wir für die eingehende Serviceschnittstelle `SI_IFP_ORDER_IN` einen Server- oder Provider-Proxy und für die ausgehende Serviceschnittstelle `SI_IFP_ORDER_OUT` einen Client- oder Consumer-Proxy. Wir schreiben einen ABAP-Report, der den Consumer-Proxy verwendet, um den Webservice aufzurufen, der durch den Provider-Proxy implementiert wird. Die Proxys können Sie entweder in Transaktion SPROXY erzeugen, oder Sie verwenden Transaktion SE80 (Object Navigator), wie im Folgenden beschrieben.

Provider

Enterprise Service anlegen

Melden Sie sich am Empfangssystem an, und legen Sie dort im Object Navigator (Transaktion SE80) ein neues Paket an. In diesem Paket legen Sie wiederum ein neues Objekt vom Typ **Enterprise Service** an. Dies startet einen Wizard, der Sie in mehreren Schritten zum fertigen Provider-Proxy führt.

Im ersten Schritt nach der Übersicht wählen Sie die Option **Objekttyp Service-Provider**. Im nächsten Schritt selektieren Sie die Option **ESR-Service-Interface (Outside-in)**. Wählen Sie dann das ESR-Interface `SI_IFP_ORDER_IN` aus, und geben Sie ein Paket, ein Präfix und einen Workbench-Auftrag an. Sorgen Sie auch dafür, dass der Webservice sofort freigegeben wird, indem

Sie das Ankreuzfeld **Serv. deployen** auswählen. Markieren Sie das Feld nicht, müssen Sie den Webservice später in Transaktion SOAMANAGER manuell freigeben. Wählen Sie **Fertigstellen und Speichern**, und aktivieren Sie Ihren Proxy. Abbildung 8.15 zeigt das Ergebnis.

Server-Proxy

Es wurde ein Server-Proxy namens ZIFPII_SI_IFP_ORDER_IN erzeugt, der von der Klasse ZIFPCL_SI_IFP_ORDER_IN implementiert wird. Außerdem wurde die Webservice-Definition ZSI_IFP_ORDER_IN angelegt. Da Sie im Service-Interface zwei Methoden definiert haben, verfügt auch der generierte Proxy über zwei Methoden (siehe Abbildung 8.15). Sie sehen die beiden Methoden GET_DETAIL und GET_LIST. Jede dieser Methoden hat einen Importparameter namens INPUT und einen Exportparameter namens OUTPUT. Für die Parameter wurden gemäß den Request- und Response-Message-Typen entsprechende ABAP-Strukturen generiert.

Den Code für die beiden Methoden müssen Sie selbst bereitstellen. Listing 8.5 zeigt dies am Beispiel der Methode GET_LIST.

```
METHOD zifpii_si_ifp_order_in~get_list.
  DATA:
    orders TYPE STANDARD TABLE OF zifporder,
    wa_orders TYPE zifporder,
    wa TYPE zifpdt_ifp_orderhead,
    ordertype TYPE zifpordertype,
    refid TYPE zifprefid.
  ordertype = input-mt_ordergetlist_req-type.
  refid = input-mt_ordergetlist_req-refid.
  IF ordertype IS INITIAL.
    ordertype = 'SO'.
  ENDIF.
  CALL FUNCTION 'Z_IFP_ORDER_GETLIST'
    EXPORTING
      im_ordertype = ordertype
      im_refid     = refid
    TABLES
      ta_orders    = orders.
  LOOP AT orders INTO wa_orders.
    MOVE-CORRESPONDING wa_orders TO wa.
    APPEND wa TO output-mt_ordergetlist_res-orderheader.
  ENDLOOP.
ENDMETHOD.
```

Listing 8.5 Implementierung der Methode »get_list« in der Service-Provider-Klasse

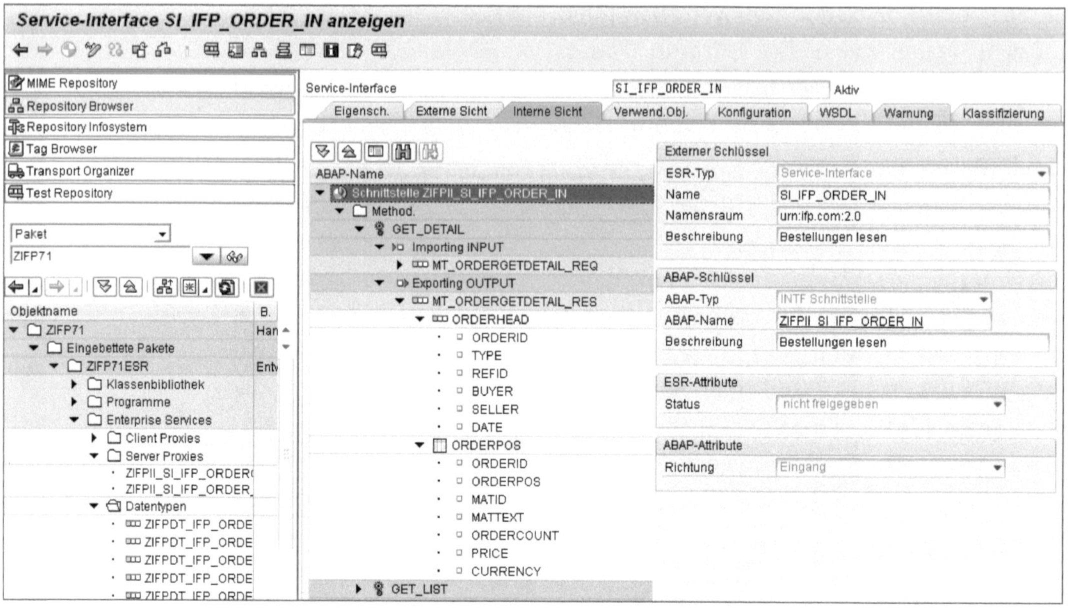

Abbildung 8.15 Generierter Service-Provider

Über Transaktion SOAMANAGER können Sie, wie schon bei der Outside-In-Entwicklung, einen Endpunkt anlegen, die WSDL-Datei generieren und Ihren Webservice testen. Diese WSDL-Datei benötigen Sie, wenn Sie später einen logischen Port für den Consumer anlegen.

Damit ist die Entwicklung des Service-Providers abgeschlossen, und Sie können sich nun dem Consumer zuwenden.

Consumer

Melden Sie sich am Sendesystem an, und legen Sie dort im Object Navigator (Transaktion SE80) in einem Entwicklungspaket ein neues Objekt vom Typ *Enterprise Service* an. Dies startet einen Wizard, der Sie in mehreren Schritten zum fertigen Consumer-Proxy führt.

Service-Consumer

Im ersten Schritt nach der Übersicht wählen Sie die Option **Objekttyp Service-Consumer.** Im nächsten Schritt selektieren Sie die Option **ESR-Service-Interface (Outside-in)**. Wählen Sie das ESR-Interface `SI_IFP_ORDER_OUT` aus, und geben Sie ein Paket, ein Präfix und einen Workbench-Auftrag an. Wählen Sie **Fertigstellen und Speichern**, und aktivieren Sie Ihren Proxy. Abbildung 8.16 zeigt das Ergebnis. Es wurde ein Proxy namens `ZIFPCO_SI_IFP_ORDER_OUT` mit zwei Methoden erzeugt.

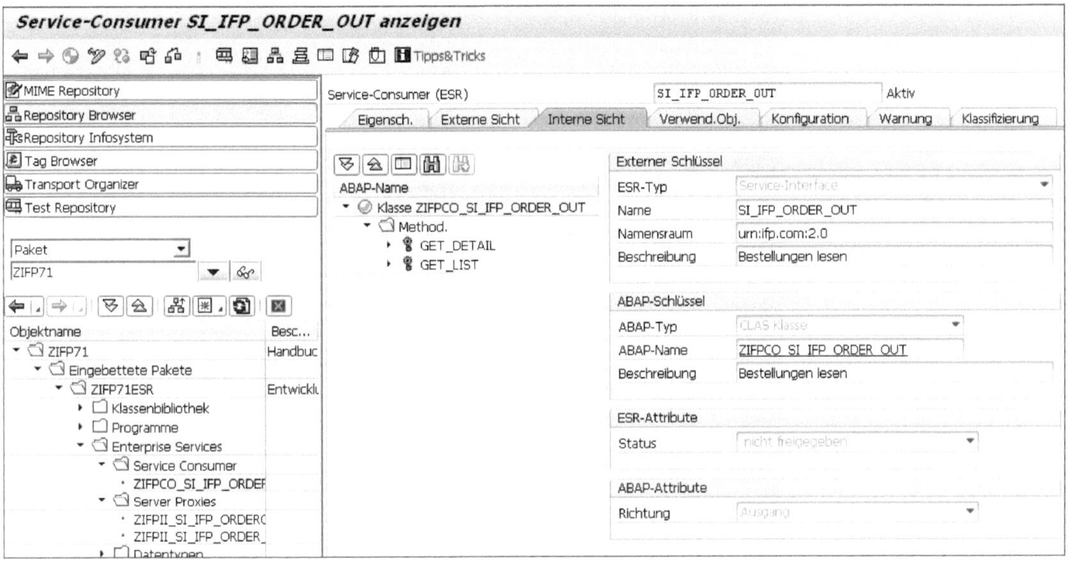

Abbildung 8.16 Consumer-Proxy

Logischer Port

Damit Sie diesen Proxy aus einem ABAP-Programm nutzen können, müssen Sie so wie in Abschnitt 8.1.2, »SOAP-Webclient mit ABAP«, beschrieben, einen logischen Port anlegen.

Consumer-Proxy testen

Sobald Sie den logischen Port angelegt haben, können Sie Ihren Consumer-Proxy in Transaktion SE80 testen. Sie können aber auch gleich den kleinen Test-Report aus Listing 8.6 schreiben. In diesem Report instanziieren Sie den Consumer-Proxy und rufen anschließend die Methode `get_list` auf. Die zurückgegebenen Bestellköpfe geben Sie in einer Schleife aus.

```
REPORT  zifp_test_esr.
DATA:
  rp TYPE REF TO zifpco_si_ifp_order_out,
  input TYPE zifpmt_ordergetlist_res,
  output TYPE zifpmt_ordergetlist_req,
  wa TYPE zifpdt_ifp_orderhead.
START-OF-SELECTION.
  TRY.
      CREATE OBJECT rp
        EXPORTING
          logical_port_name = 'LP00'.
    CATCH cx_ai_system_fault.
  ENDTRY.
  TRY.
      CALL METHOD rp->get_list
```

```
        EXPORTING
          output = output
        IMPORTING
          input  = input.
      LOOP AT input-mt_ordergetlist_res-orderheader INTO wa.
        WRITE:/
          wa-orderid,
          wa-type,
          wa-refid,
          wa-buyer,
          wa-seller,
          wa-date.
      ENDLOOP.
    CATCH cx_ai_system_fault.
    CATCH cx_ai_application_fault.
  ENDTRY.
```

Listing 8.6 Webservice-Consumer in ABAP

Damit sind die ABAP-Szenarien abgeschlossen, und wir wenden uns in den nächsten Abschnitten den Java-Szenarien zu.

8.3 SOAP-Programmierung mit Java

Auch wenn der SAP NetWeaver Application Server Java von SAP noch bis 2030 unterstützt wird, wird er nicht mehr weiterentwickelt. Daher wenden wir uns den im Standard-Java-Umfeld gebräuchlichen Werkzeugen und Standards zu. Wir diskutieren dabei die Verwendung der in Java 21 (Long Term Support, LTS) enthaltenen Mittel. Dabei gehen wir sowohl auf Werkzeuge als auch auf die zu verwendenden Java-Klassen ein. Auch wenn der Fokus von SAP in den letzten Jahren stärker auf RESTful APIs lag, ist die SOAP-basierte Webservice-Entwicklung weiterhin relevant – insbesondere im Enterprise-Umfeld, wo SOAP aufgrund seiner Standardisierung, Sicherheit und Transaktionsunterstützung oft bevorzugt wird.

8.3.1 Jakarta XML Web Services

Jakarta XML Web Services

Java bietet eine Reihe von eigenen Spezifikationen für die Arbeit mit Webservices an. Diese sind unter dem Namen *Jakarta XML Web Services* bekannt und bauen auf den Spezifikationen *Jakarta SOAP with Attachments* und *Jakarta Web Services Metadata* auf.

[«]

Neue Begriffe im Java-Umfeld

Seit Oracle 2017 Java EE an die Eclipse Foundation übergab, wurden viele Begriffe neu definiert. Der Name »Java« wurde in diesem Kontext etwa durch »Jakarta« ersetzt. Java XML Web Services (JAX-WS) heißen demnach nun Jakarta XML Web Services, und aus Java EE wird Jakarta EE.

Neuerungen im Umfeld der Java-Spezifikationen

Diese Spezifikationen beschreiben aber weiterhin das bewährte Programmiermodell, um effizient unter Verwendung von Annotationen Java-Methoden als Webservices bereitzustellen (Service) und über Proxy-Klassen einen Webservice anhand seiner WSDL-Beschreibung konsumieren (Client) zu können. Aktuelle Versionen wie Java 21 enthalten im *Java Development Kit* (JDK) jedoch keine nativen Bibliotheken mehr für SOAP oder REST, wie es noch bis Version 8 der Fall war, da diese seit Java 11 aus dem Standard-JDK entfernt wurden. Dennoch bietet Java 21 eine solide Grundlage. Diese Version baut auf externen Bibliotheken auf, die die genannten Spezifikationen implementieren, wie *Eclipse Metro*, *Apache CXF* oder *Spring Web Services*.

Eclipse Metro galt als Referenzimplementierung, als sich die Spezifikation noch JAX-WS nannte. Sie enthält die aus dem JDK 8 bekannten Werkzeuge und ist umfangreich dokumentiert. Eclipse Metro war daher auch Teil vieler Java-EE-Applikationsserver-Implementierungen verschiedener Hersteller, die es zum Teil noch heute gibt. Da sich der Trend jedoch von schweren, monolithischen Applikationsservern wie *GlassFish* oder *WildFly* hin zu leichtgewichtigen, containerbasierten Lösungen verlagert hat, haben sich die Plattformen verändert. Anstelle eines komplexen Server-Ökosystems wird zunehmend auf Bibliotheken und Frameworks gesetzt, die direkt in die Anwendung und nicht in den Applikationsserver integriert werden. Die neuen Applikationsserver sind zumeist in Containern organisiert und stellen jeweils einen Service da. Damit folgt Java der allgemeinen Entwicklung hin zu modularen und containerfreundlichen Lösungen, die sich leichter in moderne DevOps- und Cloud-Umgebungen integrieren lassen.

Java-Bibliotheken

Was unterscheidet nun die Java-Bibliotheken? Unterschiede gibt es hinsichtlich der Anzahl der Open-Source-Unterstützer, des Releasetakts, des Supports sowie der Leichtigkeit der Anbindung an bestimmte Plattformen, wie Spring, die teils eigene Bibliotheken mitbringen (Spring Web Services). Ebenso unterstützten die verschiedenen Bibliotheken die vielen auf SOAP aufbauenden WS-Standards (*WS-Security*, *WS-Reliable Messaging*, *WS-Policy* oder *WS-Addressing*) in unterschiedlichem Maße. Diese Standards erweitern Aufrufe um nicht-funktionale Aspekte. Der Standard WS-Reliable Messaging etwa stellt eine Art Übertragungsgarantie bereit, bei der sichergestellt wird, dass entsprechende Server die Nachrichten persistieren und dass diese z. B. garantiert in der Reihenfolge versendet und empfangen werden, in der sie gesendet wurden. Die entsprechenden Optionen haben wir bereits in Abschnitt 8.1, »Inside-Out-Webservices und -Webclients mit der ABAP-Plattform«, als eine der vielen Optionen in der SAP-seitigen Serviceentwicklung beschrieben. Und sie sind auch der Grund, warum unterschiedliche Webservice-Bindings für SAP-Systeme eine so große Rolle spielen: Sender und Empfänger müssen die gleichen Standards unterstützen. Diese Aspekte gilt es zu beachten, bevor man eine Bibliothek auswählt.

Webservice-Client- und Server-Programmierung

Die Webservice-Client- und Server-Programmierung mit dem JDK und der separaten Bibliothek hat sich infolge der neuen Spezifikationen von den Grundzügen her nicht geändert. Die WSDL-Datei steht hier nach wie vor im Zentrum. Aus ihr wird mit den Werkzeugen des JDK Java-Code erzeugt. Umgekehrt kann aus Java-Code auch wieder eine WSDL-Datei erzeugt werden. Im Falle von Eclipse Metro sind die Kommandos identisch zu denen aus dem JDK bis Version 11.

Für eine Clientprogrammierung werden Proxy-Klassen mit dem Werkzeug `wsimport` generiert. Dabei handelt es sich um eine einfache Konsolenanwendung, die über eine Vielzahl von Schaltern konfiguriert werden kann. Andere Bibliotheken, wie Apache CXF, bieten ähnliche Werkzeuge für den gleichen Zweck an. Bei Apache CXF heißt das entsprechende Werkzeug etwa `wsdl2java`. Typischerweise werden diese Werkzeuge nicht direkt, sondern als Plug-ins in z. B. Apache Maven genutzt.

[»]

Apache Maven

Maven ist ein Open-Source-Werkzeug zur Organisation von Java-Projekten. Es orientiert sich am typischen Build-Lifecycle von Java-Programmen, die durchlaufen werden: das Auflösen von Abhängigkeiten, das Generieren von Java-Quellcode aus Projektartefakten, das Compiling, das Verpacken, das Testen und das Deployen. Abhängigkeiten zu Bibliotheken werden in Maven per Deklaration beschrieben. Eine umfangreiche Infrastruktur im Internet erlaubt es, diese Deklarationen sekundenschnell herunterzuladen. Ebenso unterstützt Maven Plug-ins, um Aktionen an bestimmten Stellen des Build-Lifecycles auszulösen. So kann man in der Phase »Generieren« beispielweise Java-Quellcode aus WSDL-Dateien mit einem Plug-in generieren lassen.

Der Vorteil ist die direkte Integration in den Build-Lifecycle, um die Proxy-Klassen noch vor dem `Compile`-Schritt in Java aus der WSDL-Datei zu generieren. So werden Änderungen der WSDL so früh wie möglich sichtbar. Außerdem erzwingen diese Plug-ins einen besser wartbaren Code, bei dem z. B. die generierten Klassen separat abgelegt und nicht versioniert werden. Für unser Beispiel haben wir die WSDL-Datei selbst im Flavor »SAP-Standard-WSDL-Repräsentation« gespeichert.

WSDL-Datei erzeugen

Im Folgenden sehen Sie eine typische Anweisung, die auch die Plug-ins ausführen, um die Webservice-Proxy-Klassen aus einer vorhandenen WSDL-Datei zu erzeugen und in ein Paket `de.order` zu schreiben:

```
wsimport -s src -d bin -p de.order zifp_order_service.wsdl
```


Dazu verwenden wir das Werkzeug `wsimport` aus der Eclipse-Metro-Bibliothek. Dies ist ein einfacher Weg, um die Proxy-Klassen zu erzeugen.

Aufgrund der vielen Optionen im Bereich der WS-Standards und der unterschiedlichen Implementierung einiger Hersteller kann das Werkzeug `wsimport` leider nicht immer alle angegebenen WSDL-Dateien verarbeiten. In solchen Fällen können Sie die Generierung entweder über Parameter beeinflussen, das Flavor auf dem Server ändern (wenn möglich) oder die Bibliothek austauschen, z. B. von Eclipse Metro auf Apache CXF.

8.3.2 Implementierung eines Webservice-Clients

Java IDEs

Für die Implementierung eines Webservice-Clients verwenden Sie eine beliebige integrierte Entwicklungsumgebung (IDE). Um das Jahr 2014 herum beherrschte Eclipse den Markt der Java IDEs, und Webservices hatten eine so große Bedeutung, dass diese direkt per Wizard erzeugt werden konnten. Dies hat sich mittlerweile geändert. *IntelliJ*, *Eclipse* und *Visual Studio Code* sind mit vielen anderen Programmiersprachen auf den Markt gekommen, und neue Projekte werden vorrangig über kommandozeilenbasierte Werkzeuge wie *Maven Archetypes*, oder *Spring Initializr* aufgesetzt. Diese Werkzeuge erzeugen Anwendungsgerüste über Projektvorlagen mit nur wenigen Parametern. Für unser Beispiel verwenden wir IntelliJ. Damit lässt sich *Apache Maven* komfortabel und integriert nutzen.

Wir nutzen für unseren Webservice ein Plug-in, das Proxyklassen aus einer WSDL-Datei generiert, bevor der `Compile`-Schritt ausgeführt wird.

Maven-Projekt

Dies demonstrieren wir im Folgenden an einem einfachen Maven-Projekt. Zunächst erzeugen wir ein leeres Maven-Projekt über die IDE, wie in Abbildung 8.17 gezeigt. Das Projekt hat die typische Maven-Verzeichnisstruktur und enthält eine **pom.xml**-Datei. Maven wird über diese Datei gesteuert, was die Standard-Verzeichnisstruktur bedingt, die in Java zum De-facto-Standard geworden ist.

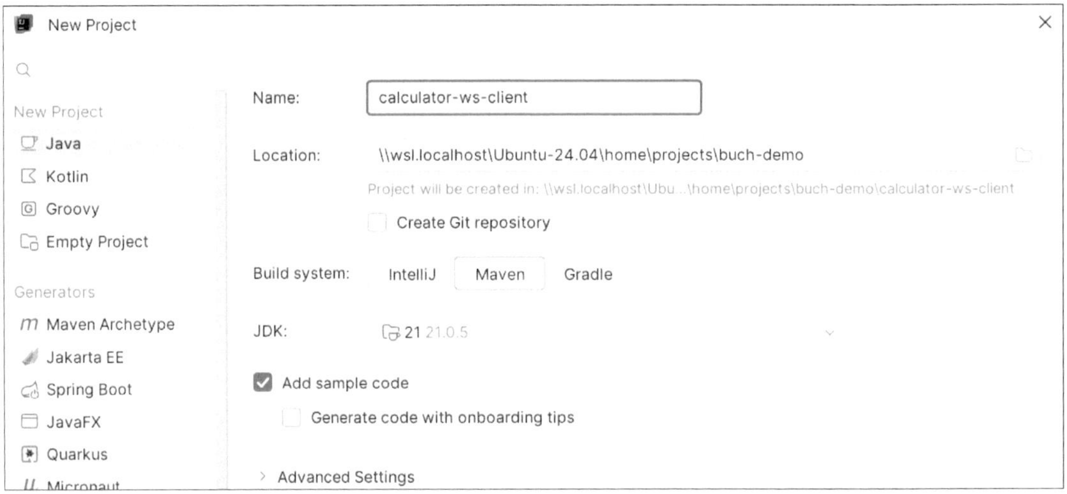

Abbildung 8.17 Java-Projekt-Wizard in IntelliJ

»pom.xml«-Datei

In der pom.xml-Datei definieren wir die Abhängigkeit zur Metro-Bibliothek und fügen ein WSDL-Plug-in zum Generieren der Proxy-Klassen hinzu, wie in Listing 8.7 zu sehen.

```
<project>
    ...
    <dependencies>
        <dependency>
            <groupId>org.glassfish.metro</groupId>
            <artifactId>webservices-rt</artifactId>
            <version>4.0.3</version>
        </dependency>
    </dependencies>

    <build>
        <plugins>
            <plugin>
                <artifactId>maven-compiler-plugin</artifactId>
                <version>3.13.0</version>
                <configuration>
                    <release>8</release>
                </configuration>
            </plugin>
            <plugin>
                <groupId>com.sun.xml.ws</groupId>
                <artifactId>jaxws-maven-plugin</artifactId>
```

```
                <version>3.0.2</version>
                <executions>
                    <execution>
                        <goals>
                            <goal>wsimport</goal>
                        </goals>
                        <configuration>
                            <wsdlFiles><wsdlFile>${project.basedir}/
src/main/resources/META-INF/wsdl/zifp_order_service.wsdl</wsdlFile>
                            </wsdlFiles>
                            <xnocompile>false</xnocompile>
                        </configuration>
                    </execution>
                </executions>
            </plugin>
        </plugins>
    </build>
</project>
```

Listing 8.7 »pom.xml«-Datei eines Maven-Projekts mit Webservice-Import-Plug-in

Maven selbst starten wir über das Kommando `mvn install`, das Sie in der IDE auch auf der Registerkarte **Maven** finden. Der Parameter `install` beschreibt eine Build-Lifecycle-Phase, die das fertige Java-Artefakt des Projekts in unser lokales Maven-Repository ablegt. Das bedeutet, dass alle vorherigen Build-Lifecycle-Phasen durchlaufen werden und damit auch das Plug-in zur Generierung der WSDL-Proxy-Klassen, denn dieses Plug-in wird in der Phase `generate-sources` durchlaufen. Maven beginnt in der ersten Phase zunächst damit, alle deklarierten Abhängigkeiten aus der **pom.xml**-Datei über das Internet aufzulösen, und installiert diese in unser lokales Repository. Dieser Vorgang dauert zu Beginn etwas länger, da Maven selbst Plug-ins zum Compiling und die Abhängigkeiten der Abhängigkeiten noch auflöst. Anschließend wird das WSDL-Plug-in ausgelöst, das Java-Code generiert und in einem **target**-Verzeichnis unter dem Dateinamen **generated-sources** ablegt. Dieses Verzeichnis müssen Sie in IntelliJ markieren, indem Sie mit der rechten Maustaste auf das Verzeichnis klicken und dieses als solches markieren.

Webservice aufrufen

Wir legen nun eine neue Java-Klasse an und können mit der Programmierung eines einfachen Java-Webservice-Clients beginnen, der die generierten Proxy-Klassen nutzt. Die zentrale Klasse, die den Service repräsentiert und die durch den Generator erzeugt wurde, ist die Klasse `OrderService` (siehe Listing 8.8).

```
private void callWebservice() {
    OrderService orderService = new OrderService();

    ZIFPORDERSERVICE service =
                orderService.getOrderServiceBnd();
    BindingProvider bp = ((BindingProvider)service);
    bp.getRequestContext().put(
            BindingProvider.USERNAME_PROPERTY, "user");
    bp.getRequestContext().put(
            BindingProvider.PASSWORD_PROPERTY, "password");

    Holder<TableOfZifporder> taOrders = new Holder<>();
    Bapiret2 bapiret = service.orderGetlist("1", taOrders);

    List<Zifporder> tableOfZifporders =
                taOrders.value.getItem();

    for (Zifporder taOrder: tableOfZifporders) {
        System.out.println("Order ID: " +
                        taOrder.getOrderid());
    }
}
```

Listing 8.8 Aufruf des Webservice in Java

In Listing 8.8 sehen Sie den Aufruf eines Webservice in Java, um eine Liste von Bestellungen aus einem SAP-System abzurufen. Zunächst wird ein `OrderService`-Objekt instanziiert, das als Wrapper für den generierten Webservice-Client dient. Über die Methode `getOrderServiceBnd()` wird eine Instanz des Interface-Typs `ZIFPORDERSERVICE` abgerufen, die die Serviceschnittstelle darstellt.

Authentifizierung

Die Authentifizierung erfolgt über die JAX-WS-Klasse `BindingProvider`. Hier werden Benutzername und Passwort über die Eigenschaften `BindingProvider.USERNAME_PROPERTY` und `BindingProvider.PASSWORD_PROPERTY` im Kontext `RequestContext` der Klasse `BindingProvider` gesetzt.

Anschließend wird der Serviceaufruf `orderGetlist` mit einem `String` sowie einem `Holder`-Objekt vom Typ `TableOfZifporder` durchgeführt. Dies sieht für Java-Entwickler seltsam aus, da unser Ergebnis Teil des Aufrufs ist. JAX-WS hat mit dem `Holder`-Objekt eine Limitierung von Java umgangen: Java erlaubt nur ein Rückgabeobjekt pro Methode, anders als ABAP mit seinen multiplen Export- und Importparametern. Um diese in Java abzubilden, nutzt JAX-WS die Annotation `@WebParam` an der Java-Methode, wie in Listing 8.9 zu sehen.

```
public Bapiret2 orderGetlist(
    @WebParam(name = "ImRefid",
              targetNamespace = "")
    String imRefid,

    @WebParam(name = "TaOrders",
              targetNamespace = "",
              mode = WebParam.Mode.OUT)
    Holder<TableOfZifporder> taOrders);
```

Listing 8.9 Methode »orderGetlist« mit der Annotation @WebParam und dem Mode OUT

Das `Holder`-Objekt wurde generiert, um mehrere Rückgabewerte, die in ABAP-Methoden möglich sind, in einer Java-Methode des Webservice abzubilden. Die Abbildung erfolgt einerseits über den Return-Wert und andererseits über den `OUT`-Parameter in SOAP.

Ergebnis des Aufrufes

Nach dem erfolgreichen Aufruf enthält das `Holder`-Objekt die Daten in Form einer Liste von `Zifporder`-Objekten, die mit der Methode `taOrders.value.getItem()` abgerufen wird. In einer Schleife werden die einzelnen Bestellungen iteriert, und die Bestell-ID `OrderID` jeder Bestellung wird auf der Konsole ausgegeben.

Wenn Sie diesen Code nun mit dem Befehl `mvn install` ausführen, werden jedes Mal die Proxy-Klassen neu generiert und zusammen mit unserem Programm kompiliert, um dann als **.jar**-Datei verpackt im Verzeichnis **target** abgelegt zu werden. Man kann auf diese Art eine Bibliothek bauen, die in Java-Anwendungen verwendet werden kann. Diese Anwendungen würden dann mit unserer Klasse interagieren, die die Webservice-Aufrufe kapselt.

8.3.3 Implementierung eines Webservice-Servers

Um aus dem SAP-System auf einen Java-Webservice zuzugreifen, kann man auf Basis der in Abschnitt 8.3.1, »Jakarta XML Web Services«, beschriebenen Technologien einen Webservice in Java anbieten. Java 21 bietet eine stabile Plattform für den Aufbau von Webservices, die zwei Programmieransätze unterstützt: Contract-First, bei dem eine WSDL-Datei bereits vorliegt, und

Code-First, bei dem mit dem Java-Code gestartet wird. Mit Eclipse Metro können Sie sowohl einen Webservice erstellen, der auf einer WSDL-Datei basiert (Contract-First-Ansatz), als auch einen Webservice ohne vorherige WSDL-Definition erzeugen (Code-First-Ansatz). In diesem Abschnitt zeigen wir für beide Ansätze die erforderlichen Schritte und jeweils ein Codebeispiel.

Outside-In-Ansatz mit Java

Der Outside-In-Ansatz für die Entwicklung von Webservices in Java bedeutet, dass die Definition des Diensts durch eine WSDL-Datei erfolgt, bevor der eigentliche Code geschrieben wird. Ist diese WSDL-Datei geschrieben, kann der Client im SAP-System parallel zur Umsetzung des Webservice-Servers in Java gestartet werden. Dieser Ansatz wird daher in Szenarien bevorzugt, in denen eine klare Spezifikation der Schnittstelle definiert sein muss oder in denen verschiedene Akteure, Abteilungen oder Systeme miteinander integriert werden.

WSDL-Datei

Als Beispiel setzen wir einen Webservice namens `CalculatorService` um, der zwei Zahlen addiert und als Ergebnis eine Zahl zurückliefert. Dieser könnte in unserem Szenario des Buchshops z. B. die zentrale Kalkulation für den Warenkorb übernehmen. Dieser einfache Service kann in WSDL durch einen Service und eine Operation beschrieben werden. Listing 8.10 zeigt den Inhalt der entsprechenden WSDL-Datei. Diese WSDL-Datei könnte von einem SAP-System genutzt werden, um in einem entfernten System Kalkulationen in Java durchzuführen. Die SAP-seitige Implementierung bliebe dabei plattformunabhängig.

```
<?xml version="1.0" encoding="UTF-8"?>
<definitions xmlns="http://schemas.xmlsoap.org/wsdl/"
             xmlns:tns="http://example.com/calculator"
             xmlns:xsd="http://www.w3.org/2001/XMLSchema"
             xmlns:soap="http://schemas.xmlsoap.org/wsdl/soap/"
             name="CalculatorService"
             targetNamespace="http://example.com/calculator">
    <types>
        <xsd:schema targetNamespace="http://example.com/calculator">
            <xsd:element name="add1" type="xsd:int"/>
            <xsd:element name="add2" type="xsd:int"/>
            <xsd:element name="addResponse" type="xsd:int"/>
        </xsd:schema>
    </types>
    <message name="addRequest">
```

```
        <part name="parameters" element="tns:add"/>
    </message>
    <message name="addResponse">
        <part name="parameters" element="tns:addResponse"/>
    </message>
    <portType name="CalculatorPortType">
        <operation name="add">
            <input message="tns:addRequest"/>
            <output message="tns:addResponse"/>
        </operation>
    </portType>
    <binding name="CalculatorBinding"
             type="tns:CalculatorPortType">
        <soap:binding transport=
"http://schemas.xmlsoap.org/soap/http"
    style="document"/>
        <operation name="add">
            <soap:operation
             soapAction="http://example.com/calculator/add"/>
            <input>
                <soap:body use="literal"/>
            </input>
            <output>
                <soap:body use="literal"/>
            </output>
        </operation>
    </binding>
    <service name="CalculatorService">
        <port name="CalculatorPort"
           binding="tns:CalculatorBinding">
            <soap:address
             location="http://localhost:8080/calculator"/>
        </port>
    </service>
</definitions>
```

Listing 8.10 Beispiel einer WSDL-Datei für einen Webservice mit JAX-WS

Betrieb in Servlet-Container

Zur Umsetzung eines Webservices-Servers in Java geht man auf die gleiche Weise vor, wie bei der Umsetzung des Webservice-Clients, d. h., man erzeugt Proxy-Klassen aus der WSDL-Datei. Da unser Webservice in einem einfachen Servlet-Container (z. B. *Apache Tomcat*) betrieben werden soll, führen wir einige zusätzliche Schritte durch. Technisch gesehen erfolgt unsere Bereitstellung über ein Servlet, das als Dispatcher für den Webservice fungiert. Servlet-Container wie der Apache Tomcat nutzen WAR-Projekte (Web Archives). Daher legen wir die WSDL-Datei in dem Verzeichnis **WEB-INF/wsdl/calculator.wsdl** ab und ändern den Artefakttyp in der Datei **pom.xml** auf **WAR**.

Webservice-Klasse

In unserem bereits vorhandenen Maven-Projekt wurden die Proxy-Klassen bereits erzeugt (siehe Abschnitt 8.3.2, »Implementierung eines Webservice-Clients«). Wir können diese beibehalten. Über eine neue Klasse, die Sie z. B. `CalculatorServiceImpl` nennen können und die das Interface `CalculatorPortType` implementiert, können Sie unseren Webservice umsetzen. Dazu wird die Klasse mit der speziellen Webservice-Annotation `@WebService` versehen. Die Methode, die wir anbieten wollen, erhält die Annotation `@WebMethod` (siehe Listing 8.11).

```
package com.example.calculator;

import javax.jws.WebService;
import javax.jws.WebMethod;

@WebService
public class CalculatorServiceImpl implements CalculatorPortType {

     public CalculatorServiceImpl() {}

    @Override
        @WebMethod
    public int add(int a, int b) {
        return a + b;
    }
}
```

Listing 8.11 Implementierung des Webservice in der Klasse »CalculatorServiceImpl«

WAR-Datei erzeugen

Für die Erzeugung der WAR-Datei nutzen wir ein weiteres Plug-in in unserer **pom.xml**-Datei, das die vom Servlet-Container erwartete Verzeichnisstruktur erstellt und das Artefakt in das **target**-Verzeichnis ablegt.

```
...
    <name>calculator</name>
    <packaging>war</packaging>
...
```

```
<plugin>
                <groupId>org.apache.maven.plugins</groupId>
                <artifactId>maven-war-plugin</artifactId>
                <version>3.4.0</version>
            </plugin>
        </plugins>
    </build>
</project>
```

Listing 8.12 Webservice über Maven als Webarchiv verpacken lassen

Die erzeugte WAR-Datei kann nun in einem Servlet-Container installiert werden. Bei Apache Tomcat kann die WAR-Datei dazu z. B. in das **deploy**-Verzeichnis gelegt werden und wird automatisch installiert.

Die URL für den Webservice ergibt sich aus der Serveradresse, dem Namen der WAR-Datei und dem Namen des Webservice:

http://localhost:8080/calculatorservice.war/calculatorservice?wsdl

Inside-Out-Ansatz mit Java

Um in Eclipse Metro einen Webservice in Java mit JAX-WS nach dem Inside-Out-Ansatz zu erstellen, beginnt man mit der Definition der Geschäftslogik direkt in einer Java-Klasse. Im Gegensatz zum Outside-In- bzw. Contract-First-Ansatz, bei dem zunächst eine WSDL-Datei erstellt wird, um die Struktur des Webservice vorzugeben, konzentriert sich der Outside-In-Ansatz darauf, zunächst die Implementierung des Service zu entwickeln. Ein wesentlicher Vorteil dieses Ansatzes liegt in seiner Einfachheit. Sie müssen sich zunächst keine Gedanken über die genaue WSDL-Struktur machen, da diese automatisch auf Basis der Java-Klasse generiert wird. Dies spart Zeit und vereinfacht den Entwicklungsprozess. Ein Nachteil dieser Vorgehensweise ist allerdings, dass die clientseitige Umsetzung auf die Fertigstellung warten muss und die Schnittstelle nicht wie ein Vertrag stabil gehandhabt wird, sondern sich in der Praxis häufig ändern kann.

Maven-Projekt anlegen

Wir beginnen wie im vorangehenden Abschnitt auch zunächst mit einem neuen Maven-Projekt, das wir über eine IDE oder über das Maven-Archetype-Plug-in erzeugen können. In diesem Beispiel nutzen wir Archetype über eine lokale Maven-Installation, damit wir in einer Eingabeaufforderung Maven-Kommandos eingeben können. Über das Maven-Kommando `mvn archetype:generate` generieren wir ein neues Projekt mit dem Namen der `artifactId`:

```
mvn archetype:generate -DgroupId=com.example.web
-DartifactId=java-web-project -DarchetypeArtifactId=maven-archetype-
webapp -DinteractiveMode=false
```

In diesem Verzeichnis werden alle notwendigen Verzeichnisstrukturen sowie die **pom.xml**-Datei angelegt.

»pom.xml«-Datei

Wir bearbeiten die **pom.xml**-Datei, wie im vorangehenden Beispiel, um die Abhängigkeit mit Eclipse Metro einzutragen (siehe Listing 8.7). Das WS-Import-Plug-in benötigen wir nicht. Stattdessen legen wir in Listing 8.13 ein neues Java-Interface mit dem Namen `CalculatorServiceBottomUp` an, um die Kernfunktionalität unseres Webservice zu entwerfen. Dieses Interface stellt unsere Schnittstelle dar. Dies ist wichtig, da dieses Interface mit allen Eingangs- und Ausgangsparametern jeder Methode später durch die Bibliothek übersetzt werden muss. Datentypen fremder Bibliotheken sollten daher vermieden werden, und jeder Typ sollte hier bereits definiert werden. Die Bibliothek muss in der Lage sein, die Typen aus XML in Java umzuwandeln, wenn eine Operation aufgerufen wird. Ebenso muss sie den Java-Code in XML umwandeln können, wenn die Antwort gesendet wird.

```
package com.example.webservice;

public interface CalculatorServiceBottomUp {
   public int add(AddRequestType parameters);
}
```

Listing 8.13 Neues Webservice-Interface »CalculatorServiceBottomUp anlegen«

Klasse zur Implementierung

Wir implementieren in Listing 8.14 außerdem eine Klasse `CalculatorServiceBottomUpImpl` und lassen diese Klasse unser Interface implementieren. Wir markieren diese Klasse mit der Annotation `@WebService`, um anzugeben, dass die Klasse als Webservice verfügbar gemacht werden soll. Die zu veröffentlichten Methoden innerhalb der Klasse werden über die Annotation `@WebMethod` markiert. Über diese Informationen und das starke Typensystem von Java ist es Eclipse Metro möglich, alle anderen erforderlichen Arbeiten automatisch auszuführen.

```
package com.example.webservice;

import jakarta.jws.WebMethod;
import jakarta.jws.WebService;

@WebService
public interface CalculatorServiceBottomUpImpl implements
```

```
CalculatorServiceBottomUp {

   @WebMethod
   public int add(AddRequestType parameters) {
      return parameters.getAdd1() + parameters.getAdd2();
   }
}
```

Listing 8.14 Webservice-Implementierung in der Klasse »CalculatorServiceBottomUpImpl«

Nachdem der Service in der Klasse implementiert wurde, erfolgt die Bereitstellung des Webservice. Moderne Java-EE-Server erkennen die Annotationen automatisch. Falls erforderlich, kann eine **web.xml**-Datei verwendet werden, um den Webservice explizit zu konfigurieren. Wird als Ziel ein Servlet-Container wie Apache Tomcat verwendet, sorgt Eclipse Metro dafür, dass das JAX-WS-Servlet automatisch integriert wird. Listing 8.15 zeigt die optionale Erzeugung eines spezifischen Servlets in der Datei **web.xml**, das den Webservice bereitstellt.

```
<servlet>
    <servlet-name>CalculatorService</servlet-name>
    <servlet-class>com.sun.xml.ws.transport.http.servlet.WSServlet
        </servlet-class>
    <load-on-startup>1</load-on-startup>
</servlet>
<servlet-mapping>
    <servlet-name>CalculatorService</servlet-name>
    <url-pattern>/CalculatorService</url-pattern>
</servlet-mapping>
```

Listing 8.15 Optionale Webservice-Spezifikation

WSDL-Datei

Wenn unser WAR-Archiv in Apache Tomcat installiert ist und wir die Adresse um den Zusatz *?wsdl* erweitern, generiert Eclipse Metro automatisch eine WSDL-Datei, die die Struktur und Funktionen des Webservice beschreibt. Diese Datei ist über den Webbrowser oder andere Tools zugänglich und dient als technische Schnittstellenbeschreibung, die von anderen Entwicklern oder Systemen genutzt werden kann, um den Service zu konsumieren.

Webservice testen

Ein Webservice kann auf verschiedene Weise getestet werden. Tools wie SOAP UI oder Postman bieten die Möglichkeit, SOAP-Anfragen an den Service zu senden und die Antworten zu überprüfen. Dies ist besonders hilfreich, um sicherzustellen, dass der Service korrekt arbeitet und die erwarteten Daten liefert. Alternativ kann auch ein Java-Client generiert werden, der die Kommunikation mit dem Webservice vereinfacht und für Tests verwendet werden kann.

8.4 SOAP-Programmierung mit C#

.NET und Webservice

Dieser Abschnitt widmet sich dem Konsumieren von Webservices unter C# mithilfe von Microsoft Visual Studio 2022 in der Community Edition. .NET liefert eine Vielzahl von Möglichkeiten, um Anwendungen einfach in die .NET-Infrastruktur zu integrieren. Um Webservices zu konsumieren, muss die Visual-Studio-Installation um eine WCF-Komponente (Windows Communication Foundation) erweitert werden. Damit können Webservice-Provider schnell durch entsprechende Attribute markiert und Webservice-Konsumenten über Assistenten im Entwicklungswerkzeug per Generator mit den nötigen Proxy-Klassen versorgt werden.

Webservices konsumieren

Um die im SAP-System angelegten Webservices zu konsumieren, erzeugen Sie ein neues Projekt mit Visual Studio und erstellen Code direkt aus der WSDL-Datei des Webservice.

Starten Sie Visual Studio und fügen Sie ein neues Projekt hinzu, z. B. ein Konsolenprojekt. Nachdem das Projekt angelegt worden ist, können Sie mit der Generierung der Proxy-Klassen beginnen. Dazu wählen Sie das soeben erzeugte Projekt aus und klicken im Kontextmenü auf den Eintrag **Hinzufügen** und dann **Dienstverweis hinzufügen**. Visual Studio öffnet nun einen Dialog für verschiedene Diensttypen, in dem Sie **WCF Webservice** wählen und diese Auswahl mit **Weiter** bestätigen. In der nächsten Maske (siehe Abbildung 8.18) geben Sie in das Feld **URI** die WSDL-URL Ihres Webservice ein. Zur Erinnerung: Sie erhalten die WSDL-URL über Transaktion SOAMANAGER.

Nachdem Sie den Dialog mit **OK** bestätigt haben, versucht Visual Studio, die WSDL-Datei zu laden. Haben Sie auf die Übergabe der Parameter `sap-user` und `sap-password` in der URL verzichtet, werden Sie aufgefordert, den Benutzernamen und das Passwort einzugeben. Nach erfolgreicher Authentifizierung wird die WSDL-Datei geladen. Sie erhalten eine Übersicht über alle Methoden, die durch den Service im SAP-System angeboten werden. Alternativ können Sie auch eine lokal gespeicherte Datei verwenden. Sie können dabei keine Methoden einzeln selektieren, sondern müssen immer alle Methoden des Service generieren lassen.

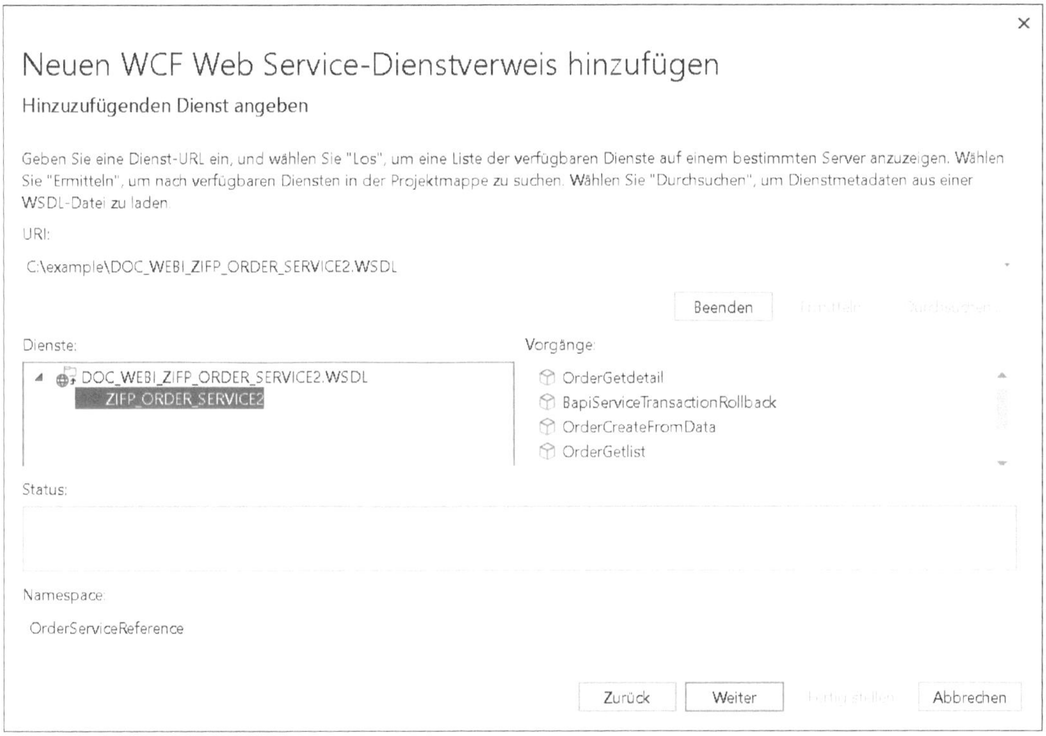

Abbildung 8.18 Hinzufügen einer Servicereferenz

Proxy-Klassen generieren

Zuletzt geben Sie in das Feld **Namespace** den Bezeichner für den Namensraum ein, unter dem die generierten Proxy-Klassen angelegt werden sollen. In dem hier vorgestellten Beispiel verwenden Sie den Namespace `OrderServiceReference`. Klicken Sie auf **Weiter**, um zu dem Schritt **Datentypoptionen festlegen** zu gelangen. Hier können Sie die Voreinstellungen beibehalten und direkt auf **Weiter** klicken, um zu den Client-Optionen zu gelangen.

Dort können Sie beeinflussen, wie die generierte Klasse aussehen wird. Auch hier belassen wir es bei der Voreinstellung. Schließen Sie nun die Generierung der Proxy-Klassen ab, indem Sie auf **Fertigstellen** klicken. Daraufhin wird eine Datei **Reference.cs** generiert, die unseren Webservice in C# beschreibt. Wir nutzen diese Datei, um unseren Webservice-Client zu implementieren.

Die generierte Proxy-Klasse umfasst alle Operationen und Parameterklassen.

Wir instanziieren die Klasse `ZIFP_ORDER_GETLISTClient`. Der nächste Programmierschritt besteht darin, sich gegenüber dem Backend-System zu authentifizieren; dies geschieht hier über den Benutzernamen und das Passwort. Dazu weisen Sie über das Property `ClientCredentials` den Benutzer und das Passwort zu.

[!]

Namenskollisionen vermeiden

Wenn Elemente in der WSDL-Datei verwendet werden, deren Namen mit .NET-Klassen kollidieren, müssen Sie diese Namen ändern. In unserem Beispiel war im `complexType` `Bapiret2` ein Element mit dem Namen `System` angegeben, was zu Syntaxfehlern in der Datei **Reference.cs** führt, weil `System` eine Klasse aus .NET ist. Sie können dies schnell beheben, indem Sie das Element in der WSDL-Datei großschreiben, also `SYSTEM`. Ideal ist diese Lösung nicht, aber sie funktioniert.

Webservices aufrufen

Der Aufruf des Webservice ist danach nur noch Formsache. Sie versorgen die Methode `ZIfpOrderGetlist` noch mit den entsprechenden Aufrufparametern für den Bestelltyp sowie der Referenznummer. Zusätzlich zu den Importparametern wird auch der Tabellenparameter für die Bestellköpfe durch den Webservice-Proxy verlangt. Da es sich bei der Liste der Bestellköpfe um eine Tabelle handelt, übergeben Sie diese als Referenzparameter und geben das Resultat auf der Konsole aus. Das Programmierbeispiel in Listing 8.16 stellt einen Webservice-Client vor.

```
using OrderServiceReference;
using System.ServiceModel;

// 1. Binding konfigurieren
BasicHttpBinding binding = new BasicHttpBinding();
binding.Security.Mode =
BasicHttpSecurityMode.TransportCredentialOnly;
binding.Security.Transport.ClientCredentialType =
HttpClientCredentialType.Basic;
// SOAP 1.1 ist Standard für BasicHttpBinding

// 2. Endpunkt konfigurieren
string serviceUrl = "http://sapdemo-s4-ng.exxcellent.de:8000/sap/bc/
srt/wsdl/flv_10002P111AD1/sdef_url/ZIFP_ORDER_SERVICE2?sap-client=
100";
EndpointAddress endpointAddress = new EndpointAddress(serviceUrl);

ZIFP_ORDER_SERVICE2Client orderClient = new ZIFP_ORDER_
SERVICE2Client(binding, endpointAddress);
orderClient.ClientCredentials.UserName.UserName = "deinBenutzername";
orderClient.ClientCredentials.UserName.Password = "deinPasswort";
```

```
try
{
    // 3. Servicemethode aufrufen
    OrderGetlist listOfOrdersIn = new OrderGetlist();
    listOfOrdersIn.TaOrders = new Zifporder[0];

    OrderGetlistResponse1 response = await
        orderClient.OrderGetlistAsync(listOfOrdersIn);
    for (int i = 0;
         i < response.OrderGetlistResponse.TaOrders.Length; i++)
      {
Console.Write(response.OrderGetlistResponse.TaOrders[i].Orderid);
       Console.Write(" ");
       Console.Write(response.OrderGetlistResponse.
           TaOrders[i].Orderdate);
       Console.Write(" ");
       Console.WriteLine(response.OrderGetlistResponse.
           TaOrders[i].Type);
    }
    // 4. Client schließen
    orderClient.Close();
}
catch (CommunicationException ex)
{
    Console.WriteLine("Fehler: " + ex.Message);
    orderClient.Abort(); // Bei Fehlern den Client abbrechen
}
```

Listing 8.16 Webservice-Konsument mit C#

Binding konfigurieren

Das Beispiel zeigt einen Webservice-Client mit eigener Binding-Definition, um den HTTP-Zugriff auf das SAP-System zu ermöglichen. Über die Einstellung `TransportCredentialOnly` definiert man die HTTP Basic Authentication und indirekt auch SOAP 1.1. Die Übergabe des Benutzernamens und des Passworts erfolgt am Client-Objekt, ebenso wie die der Serveradresse des SAP-Backend-Systems.

[!]

WCF-Client schließen

Wichtig ist es, den WCF-Client mit `client.Close()` sauber zu schließen. Bei Fehlern wird die Methode `client.Abort()` verwendet, um Ressourcen freizugeben.

Ergebnis des Serviceaufrufs

Zum Abschluss starten Sie die Anwendung und erhalten die Liste der Bestellungen aus dem SAP-System zurück (siehe Abbildung 8.19).

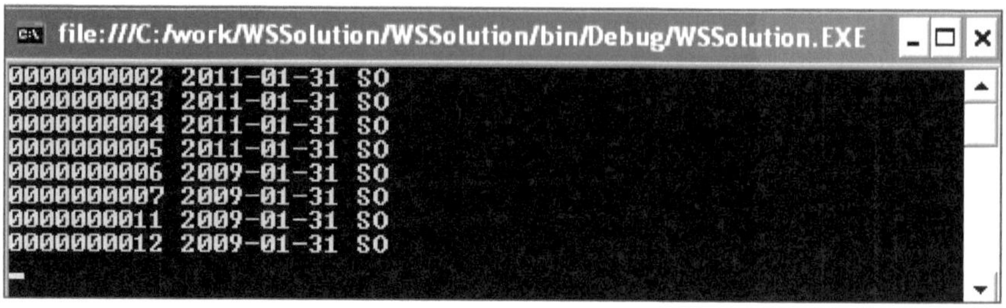

Abbildung 8.19 Liste der Bestellungen per SOAP

Kapitel 9
SAP Gateway und OData

In diesem Kapitel erklären wir, wie Sie OData-Services mit SAP Gateway entwickeln und wie Sie diese Services mit SAPUI5, C# und Java verwenden.

In diesem Kapitel befassen wir uns mit *SAP Gateway*, mit dessen Hilfe Sie Funktionen der ABAP-Plattform das OData-Protokoll veröffentlichen können. Das *OData-Protokoll* ist ein offener Standard, der von Microsoft entwickelt wurde und auf den Webstandards *Atom Syndication* und *Atom Publishing Protocol* basiert.

Wir stellen Ihnen zunächst SAP Gateway und das OData-Protokoll vor. Anschließend entwickeln wir mit der Programmiersprache ABAP einen OData-Service, mit dem wir lesend und schreibend auf Bestellungen und Bestellpositionen aus unserer Beispielanwendung zugreifen können. Schließlich schreiben wir eine Webseite mithilfe der UI-Technologie SAPUI5 sowie ein C#-Konsolenprogramm und ein Java-Programm, um diesen Service zu verwenden.

9.1 SAP Gateway

Vielfalt der Endgeräte

Die stetig wachsende Zahl der Kommunikationsgeräte und damit auch die steigende Zahl potenzieller Zugriffsmöglichkeiten auf die Daten eines SAP-Systems wie SAP S/4HANA machen es für Unternehmen zur Herkulesaufgabe, diese Daten in einem Format bereitzustellen, das sich von allen Endgeräten verarbeiten lässt. Um die Datenübermittlung zu vereinfachen, muss es daher möglich sein, auf die Informationsdienste eines Backend-Systems über eine Standardschnittstelle zuzugreifen. Wie Abbildung 9.1 zeigt, sind die Anforderungen an Informationsinfrastrukturen im Zeitalter von Mobile, Cloud und Social Media derart gewachsen, dass eine Vereinheitlichung der Schnittstellen für die unterschiedlichen Abnehmer unvermeidbar ist. SAP reagierte darauf mit der Bereitstellung des Produkts *SAP Gateway*. Die Lösung verwendet ein Standardprotokoll zur Beschreibung von und zum Zugriff auf Daten. Dieses Protokoll heißt *Open Data Protocol* oder kurz *OData*.

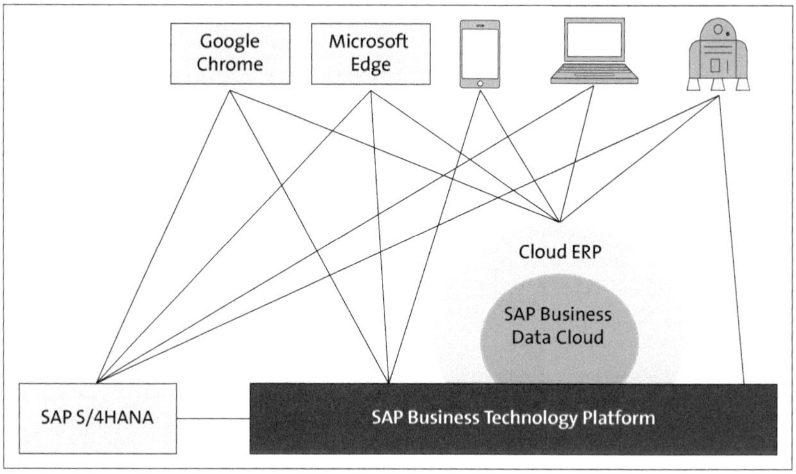

Abbildung 9.1 Vielzahl an Client-Geräten

Installations-optionen

SAP Gateway kann sowohl als *Central Hub* in der *demilitarisierten Zone* (DMZ) eines Unternehmensnetzwerks als auch *embedded*, also eingebettet in das ERP-System, installiert werden. Beide Optionen stellen wir Ihnen in den folgenden Abschnitten vor. Abhängig von Ihrer konkreten Situation und den konkreten Anforderungen im Unternehmen macht SAP Empfehlungen für die Wahl der richtigen Installationsoption über den *SAP Fiori Deployment Options and System Landscape Recommendations*. Sie finden diese Empfehlungen auf der Website von SAP unter der URL *http://s-prs.de/v1032904*.

9.1.1 Embedded Deployment

Beim *Embedded Deployment* werden die Komponenten von SAP Gateway in einem SAP-Business-Suite-System wie SAP S/4HANA installiert (siehe Abbildung 9.2). Ab SAP NetWeaver 7.4 wird die Kernkomponente von SAP Gateway bereits mitausgeliefert, und zusätzliche Komponenten können optional installiert werden.

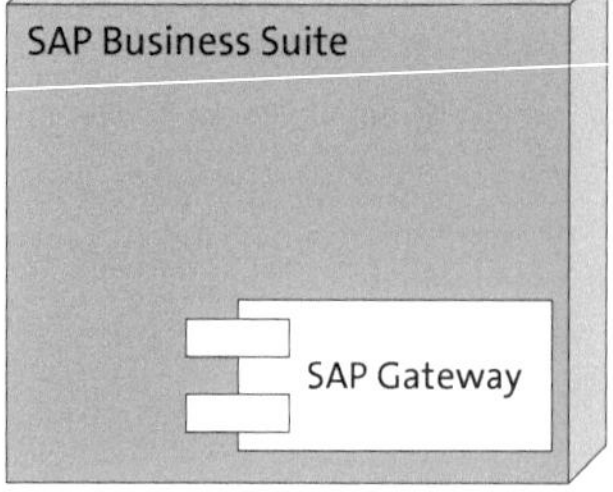

Abbildung 9.2 Embedded Deployment von SAP Gateway

Die Installation von SAP Gateway auf dem SAP-Business-Suite-System bringt den Vorteil mit sich, lokal auf die Metadaten und Geschäftsdaten zugreifen zu können. Dazu muss nicht erst eine Verbindung zwischen dem SAP-Gateway- und dem ERP-System hergestellt werden. Mitunter sind die Kosten für ein solches eingebettetes System geringer.

Releasekompatibilität sicherstellen

Nachteilig kann sich auswirken, dass SAP Gateway anderen Releasezyklen unterworfen ist als die SAP Business Suite. Daher sollten Sie stets darauf achten, dass SAP Gateway und die Ihrer Business Suite zugrunde liegende ABAP-Plattform auf demselben Releasestand gehalten werden. Außerdem kann bei einer eingebetteten Installation das SAP-Gateway-System nur mit dem ERP-System genutzt werden, auf dem es installiert ist, nicht jedoch mit anderen Systemen.

9.1.2 Central Hub Deployment

Installation in DMZ

Beim *Central Hub Deployment* wird ein eigenes System für SAP Gateway installiert (siehe Abbildung 9.3). Dieses Szenario kann auch dann noch sinnvoll sein, falls in Ihrer Landschaft bereits ein SAP-NetWeaver-System auf dem Releasestand 7.4 vorhanden ist. Es ist durchaus denkbar, neben dem SAP-NetWeaver-System mit der Kernkomponente auch noch ein weiteres System mit optionalen Komponenten zu installieren.

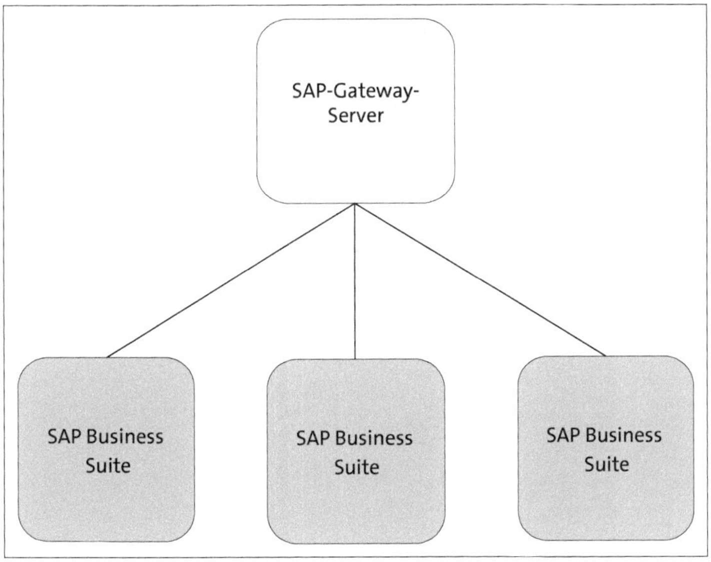

Abbildung 9.3 Central-Hub-Installation von SAP Gateway

Dieses System kann dann entweder vor oder hinter der Firewall etabliert werden. Das bedeutet, dass bei Zugriffen von außen – sei es durch mobile

Anwendungen oder durch internetbasierte Lösungen – ein Central Hub Deployment die beste Lösung ist, da SAP Gateway in der demilitarisierten Zone etabliert werden kann. So können mobile Anwendungen über OData mit Daten aus dem ERP-System versorgt werden, ohne dass weitere Infrastrukturänderungen notwendig wären. Nachteilig bei dieser Art der Installation ist, dass Metadaten und ABAP-Dictionary-Strukturen sowohl in SAP Gateway als auch im ERP-System vorhanden sein müssen.

9.2 OData-Protokoll

OData ist ein offenes, auf HTTP basierendes Protokoll für den Zugriff auf Daten über einen einfachen, definierten Zugriffspfad (die Internetadresse). OData wurde von Microsoft unter der *Open Specification Promise* veröffentlicht. Diese Art der Veröffentlichung macht es für Dritte möglich, dieses Protokoll zu nutzen und zu erweitern, falls die spezifischen Anforderungen eines Anbieters dies erfordern.

HTTP-basiertes Protokoll

Da es sich bei OData um ein HTTP-basiertes Protokoll handelt, ist OData ein idealer Mechanismus für den Zugriff auf Daten über das Internet. OData bietet nicht nur komfortable Möglichkeiten für die Abfrage von Daten, sondern auch zur Manipulation der Daten. Die Navigation erfolgt über *Uniform Resource Identifier* (URI). So können OData-Services bereitgestellt werden, die im Rahmen von responsivem Webdesign integriert werden. Die Daten können bei OData sowohl im *Atom-Syndication-Format*, also XML-basiert, als auch in der *Java Script Object Notation* (JSON) ausgeliefert werden.

Atom-Syndication-Format

Beim Atom-Syndication-Format handelt es sich um ein XML-basiertes Dokumentformat, das für den Austausch von Informationen in Form von *Web-Feeds* entwickelt wurde. Ein Web-Feed kann z. B. eine kurze Schlagzeile (RSS-Feed) im Rahmen einer Nachrichten-Webseite sein, aber auch die komplette Struktur einer Seite beinhalten. OData basiert auf dem Atom-Syndication-Format und stellt eine Erweiterung dieses Standards dar.

9.2.1 Representational State Transfer

OData-Services sind sogenannte *REST-basierte Dienste. Representational State Transfer* (REST) beschreibt ein Programmierparadigma für Webanwendungen. Dabei stellt REST kein Produkt oder ein neues Protokoll dar, sondern beschreibt vielmehr verschiedene Architekturprinzipien. Es ist also ein abstrakter Architekturstil.

REST-Prinzipien

REST wurde durch Roy Fielding in seiner Dissertation »Architectural Styles and the Design of the Network-based Architectures« beschrieben. In dieser Dissertation untersuchte Fielding Architekturmerkmale von verteilten Anwendungen. Die Arbeit definierte dabei fünf Prinzipien, die einen REST-Dienst beschreiben, wobei die genaue Implementierung dem Diensterstel-ler selbst überlassen wird:

- **Adressierbarkeit**
  Ein grundsätzliches Problem beim Auffinden von Informationen ist der Aufbau der Adresse, mit der Informationen eindeutig angesprochen werden können. In webbasierten Lösungen wurde dafür das URI-Konzept eingeführt. Der Aufbau eines URI enthält die Angabe eines globalen Namensraums. Dieser stellt sicher, dass eine Ressource eindeutig identifiziert werden kann.
- **Verwendung von Hypermedia**
  Dieser Grundsatz beschreibt die Verwendung von Verknüpfungen von Inhalten. Durch diese Verknüpfungen können Anwendungen von einer groben zu einer feineren Granularität ihrer Informationen gelangen. Zum Beispiel ist es durch die Verknüpfung möglich, von einem Kunden zu seinen Bestellungen und von dort weiter zu den einzelnen Bestellpositionen einer einzelnen Bestellung zu navigieren. Der Konsument dieser Information muss nichts mehr über die Anwendung wissen, da sich die Verknüpfung der Daten aus den Daten selbst ergibt. So kann es dem Client gleichgültig sein, woher die einzelnen Daten genau gelesen werden, da auch die Adresse der Ressource mitgeliefert wird.
- **Repräsentationen**
  Den REST-Prinzipien folgende Server können jeweils das Format ausliefern, das der Client fordert. Demnach kann eine Anwendung über den gleichen URI eine Beschreibung oder eine Dokumentation abrufen.
- **Zustandslosigkeit**
  REST-basierte Anwendungen sind zustandslos. Das heißt, es ist nicht gewünscht, dass über die Dauer des Requests auf dem Server ein clientspezifischer Status gehalten wird. Vielmehr wird gefordert, dass der Zustand entweder vollständig auf dem Client gehalten wird oder der Server den Zustand bei jedem Response an den Client übermittelt.
- **Operationen**
  REST-basierte Dienste bieten die sogenannten *CRUD-Operationen* an. CRUD steht für Create, Read, Update und Delete. Das HTTP-Protokoll unterstützt z. B. die Methoden `GET`, `POST`, `PUT` und `DELETE`. Dabei können mit `GET` Ressourcen gelesen, mit `POST` erzeugt, mit `PUT` geändert und schließ-

lich mit DELETE gelöscht werden. Dem REST-Paradigma folgende Anwendungen implementieren diese Operationen, sodass ein Aufrufer (eine Anwendung) weiß, welche Operationen auf einer Ressource aufgerufen werden können.

9.2.2 OData-Datenmodell

Datenmodellierung mit OData

OData-Services werden über ein Metamodell, das *Entity Data Model* (EDM), beschrieben. Das Modell dient zur abstrakten Beschreibung der Daten und deren Struktur. Die Implementierung des EDM heißt *Conceptual Schema Definition Language* (CSDL). CSDL ist eine XML-basierte Sprache, mit der die Entitäten, Eigenschaften (engl. *Properties*) und Relationen zwischen Entitäten beschrieben werden können.

Container, Sets und Objekte

Abbildung 9.4 zeigt das Datenmodell, das OData zugrunde liegt. Das EDM definiert einen sogenannten *Entity Container*. Dieser Container dient als zusammenfassendes Element für die darin enthaltenen *Entity Sets*. Diese wiederum beschreiben eine Klammer für die darin enthaltenen *Entity-Objekte*. Eine Entität beschreibt somit letztlich ein einzelnes Datenobjekt zur Laufzeit, wie etwa einen Kunden oder eine Bestellung. Die Struktur einer Entität wird durch einen Datentyp beschrieben, der im Metamodell als *Entity Type* bezeichnet wird.

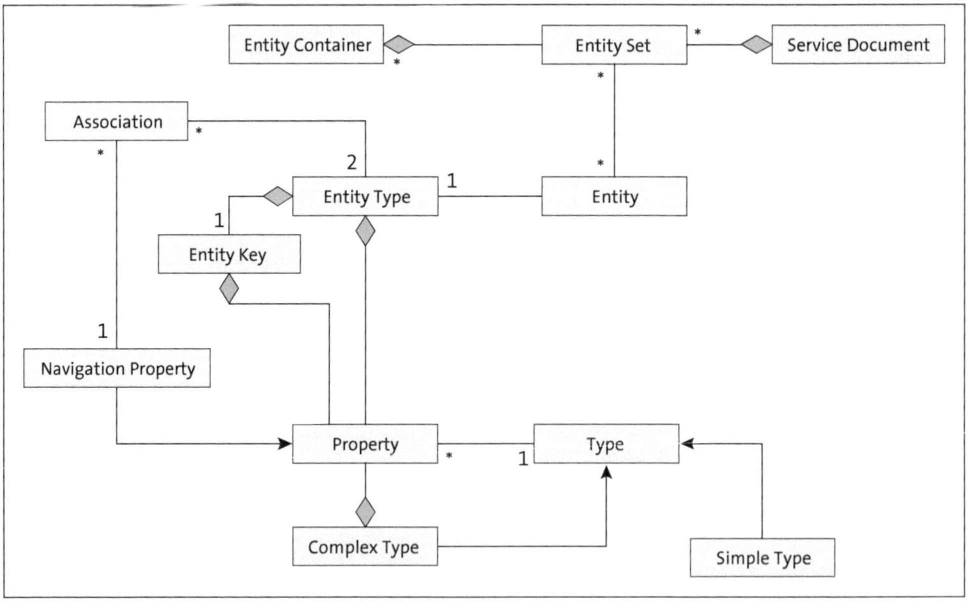

Abbildung 9.4 OData-Metamodell

Entitäten

Eine Entität kann Eigenschaften besitzen. Auch diese Eigenschaften werden bei der Definition mit einem Datentyp versehen. Ein Datentyp kann dabei komplex (*Complex Type*) oder skalar (*Scalar Type*) sein. Eine Entität wird eindeutig über ihren *Entity Key* identifiziert. Es handelt sich dabei also um den Primärschlüssel. Dieser Schlüssel kann aus verschiedenen Eigenschaften zusammengesetzt sein. Mehrere Instanzen einer Entität werden durch ein Entity Set beschrieben. Objektbeziehungen (*Assoziationen*) bilden die Grundlage für *Navigation Properties*. Diese enthalten Links auf andere Entitäten. Eine Navigation kann sowohl uni- als auch bidirektional sein.

OData-Service

Ein OData-Service stellt zwei verschiedene Dokumente bereit, zum einen das *Servicedokument* und zum anderen das *Servicemetadaten-Dokument*. Beide Dokumente werden über einen HTTP-GET-Aufruf vom Server bezogen. Das Servicedokument enthält auf oberster Ebene die Entity Sets, die vom Service bereitgestellt werden. Die Metadaten eines Service sollen es den Clients erleichtern, die Struktur und den Aufbau der Daten des Service zu verstehen und auf der Basis dieser Metadaten auch die Aufrufe des Diensts zu ermöglichen. So ist es z. B. für einen C#-Proxy-Generator möglich, den Aufruf eines OData-Service zu generieren, da der Codegenerator die Metadaten auslesen kann und mit dieser Information den Aufruf des OData-Service – zusammen mit allen notwendigen Proxy-Klassen für die Verarbeitung der Daten – erzeugen kann.

OData-Queries

Query-Optionen

Die OData-Spezifikation sieht zudem vor, über den URI Daten aus dem entsprechenden Backend adressieren zu können. Über den URI können dabei nicht nur komplette Datenkollektionen ausgelesen werden, sondern auch einzelne Entitäten oder auch nur einzelne Eigenschaften von Entitäten. Darüber hinaus können im URI über vordefinierte Query-Optionen Selektionskriterien übergeben werden. Tabelle 9.1 gibt Ihnen eine kurze Übersicht über die Möglichkeiten von OData bei der Auswahl der Daten.

Query	Bedeutung
`$format`	Liefert die Daten in einem anderen unterstützen Format. Geben Sie `json` als Parameter an, können die Daten im JSON-Format ausgelesen werden.
`$top`	Einschränkung der Datenmenge auf eine bestimmte Menge.

Tabelle 9.1 Übersicht der OData-Query-Optionen

Query	Bedeutung
`$skip`	Stellt das Gegenteil von `$top` dar. Dieses Element wird verwendet, wenn Einträge nicht ausgelesen werden sollen. Zum Beispiel liefert `$skip=2` die ersten beiden Datensätze nicht zurück.
`$orderby`	Wie mit SQL definiert man über diesen Parameter, nach welchen Kriterien sortiert wird. Mit dem Zusatz von `desc` oder `asc` geben Sie absteigendes bzw. aufsteigendes Sortieren vor.
`$filter`	Verhält sich wie die `WHERE`-Bedingung in SQL. Sie können dabei sowohl logische als auch arithmetische Operatoren angeben.
`$select`	Über `$select` können Sie die Felder von Entitäten angeben, die ausgewählt werden sollen.
`$inlinecount`	Liefert neben den Daten auch die Anzahl der Datensätze zurück. Dabei wird die Anzahl innerhalb der eigentlichen Daten in einem Feld mit dem Namen `count` zurückgegeben.

Tabelle 9.1 Übersicht der OData-Query-Optionen (Forts.)

Wenn Sie also z. B. von dem OData-Service, den wir in diesem Kapitel entwickeln, eine Liste der Bestellköpfe vom elften bis zum zwanzigsten sehen wollen, müssen Sie folgende URL verwenden:

http://NWASABAP703.WORKGROUP:8000/sap/opu/odata/sap/ZIFP_ORDERS_SRV/Orderheaders?$skip=10&$top=10

Dabei ist *http://NWASABAP703.WORKGROUP:8000/sap/opu/odata/sap/ZIFP_ORDERS_SRV/* die Basis-URL des Service und *Orderheaders* die relative URL für die Bestellköpfe. Daran werden nach dem ? die Query-Optionen und deren Werte, getrennt durch &, angehängt.

Die in Tabelle 9.1 aufgeführten Query-Optionen müssen durch den Entwickler eines OData-Service auf dem entsprechenden System zur Verfügung gestellt werden. In einer Infrastruktur, die auf SAP Gateway basiert, werden diese Query-Optionen durch den Entwickler in einer ABAP-Objects-Methode implementiert und auf SAP Gateway zur Verfügung gestellt.

JSON

Wie bereits erwähnt, unterstützt SAP Gateway auch die Auslieferung des Modells im JSON-Format. JSON stellt ein Format bereit, mit dem es, ähnlich wie mit dem XML-Format, möglich ist, Daten einfach zwischen verschiedenen Systemen auszutauschen. Die semantischen Mittel sind dabei an die Programmiersprache JavaScript angelehnt und entsprechen einer Untermenge der Sprachelemente. Im Gegensatz zu XML reduziert JSON auch den Overhead bei der Definition.

Notationselemente

JSON besitzt zwei Notationselemente:

- Eine Menge von Name-Wert-Paaren. Bei der Angabe der Werte werden verschiedene Datentypen unterstützt.
- Geordnete Listen von Werten/Objekten. Diese sind vergleichbar mit Arrays.

Objektbeschreibung in JSON

Das Programmierbeispiel in Listing 9.1 zeigt den Einsatz von JSON. Das Beispiel beschreibt ein Objekt mit dem Namen company. Das Objekt enthält ein einfaches Attribut mit der Bezeichnung company, dem ein Wert vom Datentyp String zugewiesen wird. Zudem besitzt das Objekt eine Liste von Werten (ein Array) mit dem Namen contacts. Diese Liste enthält zwei weitere Objekte, die jeweils aus zwei String-Werten bestehen.

```
{
  company: {
    name: "eXXcellent solutions",
    info: {
      employees: 180,
      basedin: [Ulm, Darmstadt]
    },
    contacts: [
      {
        lastname: "Pehnke",
        firstname: "Oliver"
      },
      {
        lastname: "Englbrecht",
        firstname: "Michael"
      }
    ]
  }
}
```

Listing 9.1 Einfaches JSON-Dokument

Direkte Verwendbarkeit

Die JSON-Objekte können nach ihrer Definition sowohl in JavaScript-Anwendungen als auch – bei der Nutzung einer entsprechenden API – direkt in

Java oder C# zur Darstellung von Objekten verwendet werden. So können webbasierte Dienste ihre Daten in JSON darstellen, und Clients können diese ohne große Umwandlung direkt in der Anwendung einsetzen. Diese Einfachheit hat sowohl für den Bereitsteller als auch für den Konsumenten der Daten große Vorteile. Der Bereitsteller muss sich keine Gedanken darüber machen, in welchem Spezialformat der Konsument die Daten benötigt; der Konsument auf der anderen Seite verwendet ein Protokoll, das offen und standardisiert ist.

9.3 OData-Services entwickeln

In diesem Abschnitt entwickeln wir mit SAP Gateway und der Programmiersprache ABAP einen OData-Service, der die CRUD-Operationen für Bestellungen über das OData-Protokoll bereitstellt. Bestellkopf (`Orderheader`) und Bestellposition (`Orderposition`) bilden dabei jeweils eigene Entitäten, zwischen denen eine 1-n-Assoziation und eine Navigationsmöglichkeit vom Bestellkopf zu den Bestellpositionen besteht.

Komponenten eines OData-Service

Ein OData-Service in SAP Gateway besteht technisch aus fünf Komponenten (siehe auch Abbildung 9.5):

- **Model-Provider-Klasse**
  Diese Klasse stellt das Objektmodell des OData-Service bereit. Das Objektmodell beschreibt die Struktur der Objekte, die über den OData-Service gelesen, erzeugt und geändert werden können. Sie beschreibt auch die Assoziationen und die Navigationspfade zwischen diesen Objekten.
- **Data-Provider-Klasse**
  Diese Klasse liest, erzeugt, ändert und löscht auf Anforderung der OData-Clients die Objekte zur Laufzeit.
- **Technisches Modell**
  Das technische Modell ist ein Konfigurationsobjekt, das auf die Model-Provider-Klasse verweist und als weitere Attribute eine Versionsnummer und Kurzbeschreibung des Modells enthält.
- **Technischer Service**
  Auch der technische Service ist ein Konfigurationsobjekt. Es verweist auf die Model-Provider-Klasse und auf das technische Modell und enthält als weitere Attribute eine Versionsnummer und Kurzbeschreibung des Service. Durch die Trennung von technischem Service und technischem Modell können mehrere Services dasselbe Modell bereitstellen.
- **OData-Service**
  Dieses Konfigurationsobjekt verweist auf den technischen Service und

macht den Service nach außen über einen ICF-Knoten (Internet Communication Framework) – und damit eine URL – zugänglich.

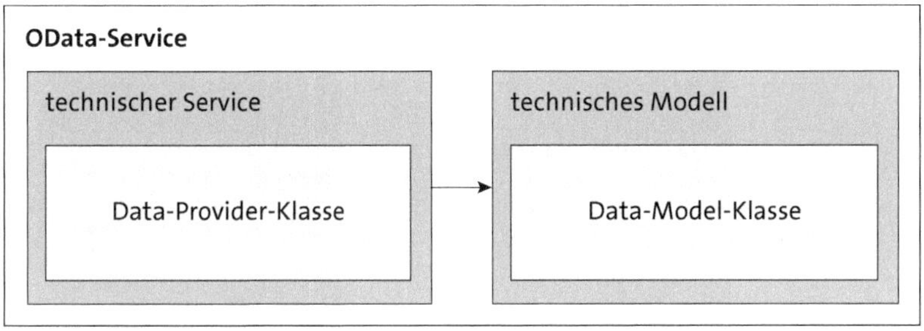

Abbildung 9.5 Komponenten eines OData-Service

Komponentenerzeugung

Sie haben mehrere Möglichkeiten, um diese fünf Komponenten zu erzeugen, die unterschiedlich aufwendig und flexibel sind.

- **Manuelle Erzeugung**
  Sie können die Model-Provider- und die Data-Provider-Klasse von Hand schreiben und das technische Modell und den technischen Service ebenfalls von Hand anlegen. Letzteres erfolgt in Transaktion SPRO im SAP Implementation Guide (IMG) unter **SAP NetWeaver • Gateway • Gateway Service Enablement • Backend OData Channel • Service Development for Backend OData Channel**. Bei diesem Zugang müssen Sie sich mit der OData-API intensiv vertraut machen.
- **Generierung im Object Navigator**
  Sie können im Object Navigator ein technisches Modell anlegen und sich die Model-Provider- und die Data-Provider-Klasse aus vorhandenen RFC-Funktionsbausteinen, BOR-Objekten oder SAP-GUI-Bildschirmen generieren lassen. Anschließend können Sie den technischen Service ebenfalls im Object Navigator erzeugen lassen. Bei diesem Ansatz müssen Sie im besten Fall überhaupt nicht programmieren.
- **Generierung im Gateway Service Builder**
  Sie können das Objektmodell in Transaktion SEGW, dem *Gateway Service Builder*, beschreiben und sich aus dieser Beschreibung die Model-Provider-Klasse ganz und die Data-Provider-Klasse zum Teil generieren lassen. Auch das technische Modell und der Service werden von diesem Werkzeug generiert. Wenn Sie diesen Weg wählen, müssen Sie nur die Datenzugriffe selbst programmieren. In Kapitel 11, »ABAP RESTful Application Programming Model und OData«, zeigen wir Ihnen wie man mit dem ABAP RESTful Application Programming Model unter Verwendung der ABAP Development Tools (ADT) in Eclipse OData-Services für SAP S/4HANA implementiert.

Servicekatalog

Unabhängig davon, welchen der drei Wege Sie wählen, müssen Sie zum Schluss den OData-Service im Servicekatalog mit Transaktion /IWFND/MAINT_SERVICE von Hand anlegen. Wir verwenden in den folgenden Abschnitten den Gateway Service Builder.

9.3.1 Beschreibung des Datenmodells

Starten Sie den Gateway Service Builder mit dem Transaktionscode SEGW, und legen Sie über den Menüpfad **Projekt • Anlegen** (`Strg` + `F5`) oder über einen Klick auf das **Anlegen**-Icon in der Button-Leiste ( ) ein neues Projekt an. Geben Sie dem neuen Projekt einen Namen und eine Beschreibung, und ordnen Sie es einem Entwicklungspaket und beim Speichern einem Änderungsauftrag zu.

Gateway Service Builder

Die Oberfläche des Gateway Service Builders besteht aus drei Bereichen (siehe Abbildung 9.6). Links sehen Sie den Navigationsbereich, in dem Sie die einzelnen Projektkomponenten über das Kontextmenü anlegen und mit einem Doppelklick zum Bearbeiten auswählen können. Im rechten oberen Bereich wird das ausgewählte Objekt angezeigt. Dort können Sie es auch editieren, sofern Sie sich im Editiermodus befinden. Rechts unten werden Fehlermeldungen, Warnungen und Erfolgsnachrichten angezeigt. Im Navigationsbereich sehen Sie unterhalb des Wurzelknotens mit dem Namen Ihres Projekts drei Ordnerknoten, je einen für das Datenmodell, die Implementierung und die generierten Serviceobjekte.

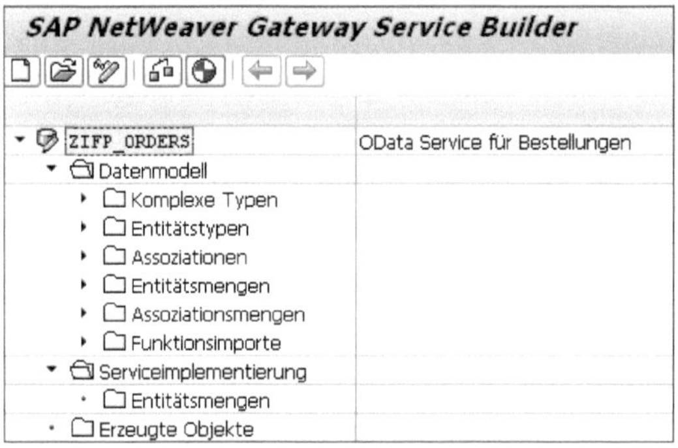

Abbildung 9.6 Gateway Service Builder

Entitätstypen

Wir beginnen im obersten dieser drei Ordner mit der Beschreibung des Datenmodells. Zuerst beschreiben wir die Entitätstypen `Orderheader` und `Orderposition`, danach die Assoziation und den Navigationspfad vom Bestellkopf zu den zugehörigen Bestellpositionen und zum Schluss die beiden Entitätsmengen `Orderheaders` (Bestellköpfe) und `Orderpositions` (Bestellpositionen).

DDIC-Import

Klicken Sie mit der rechten Maustaste auf den Ordner **Datenmodell**, und wählen Sie **Importieren • DDIC-Struktur** im Kontextmenü. Geben Sie dann im Dialog **DDIC-Import** »ZIFPORDER« als ABAP-Struktur an, markieren Sie die Option **Als Entitätst.**, und geben Sie als Objektnamen »Orderheader« ein. Drücken Sie dann die [↵]-Taste, damit die DDIC-Struktur in den Dialog eingelesen und dargestellt wird. Sie können nun auswählen, welche der Felder aus der DDIC-Struktur ignoriert, als Schlüsselfelder oder als Eigenschaftsfelder der neuen Entität aufgenommen werden sollen. Sie können hier auch die Feldnamen festlegen. In Abbildung 9.7 haben wir das Feld `MANDT` ignoriert und einige Knotennamen leicht geändert, damit diese später für den Verwender des OData-Service sinnvoller sind.

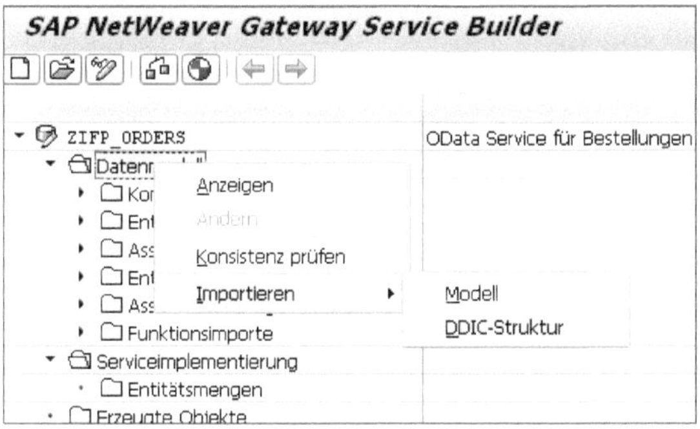

Abbildung 9.7 DDIC-Import

Entitäts-eigenschaften ändern

Bestätigen Sie Ihre Änderungen, indem Sie auf das grüne Häkchen klicken. Klicken Sie dann im Navigationsbereich des Gateway Service Builders doppelt auf die neu angelegte Entität, die im Unterordner **Entitätstypen** angezeigt wird, um einige ihrer Eigenschaften zu ändern. In Abbildung 9.8 haben wir den Namen des Knotens **Zifporder** in **Orderheader** geändert.

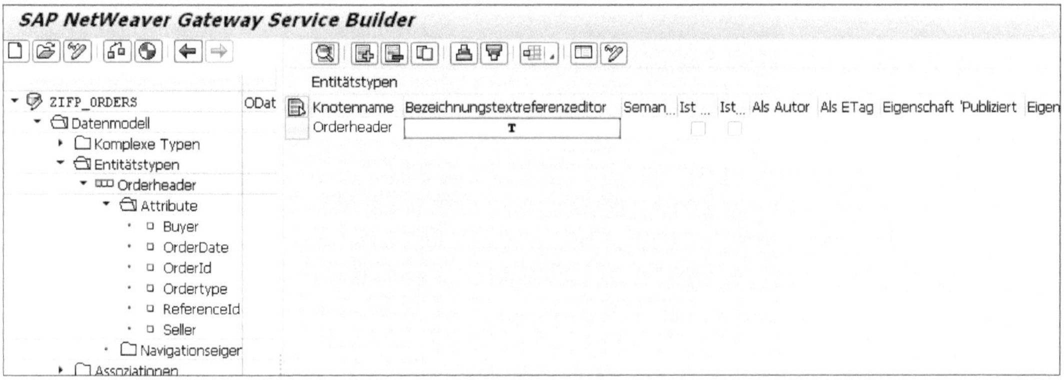

Abbildung 9.8 Eigenschaften des Entitätstyps »Orderheader«

Als weiteren Entitätstyp legen wir die Orderposition durch Import der DDIC-Struktur `ZIFPORDERPOS` auf die gleiche Weise an. Auch hier ignorieren wir das Feld `MANDT` und passen den Knotennamen an.

Assoziationen

Als Nächstes legen wir die Assoziation zwischen den beiden Entitätstypen an. Klicken Sie im Navigationsbereich doppelt auf den Ordner **Assoziationen**, damit diese im rechten oberen Bildschirmbereich angezeigt werden. Klicken Sie auf das grüne Pluszeichen, um eine neue Assoziation hinzuzufügen. Nennen Sie die Assoziation `Orderheader_Orderposition`, wählen Sie als Prinzipalentität `Orderheader`, als Kardinalität der Hauptentität 1, als abhängige Entität `Orderposition`, als Kardinalität der abhängigen Entität N und als Bezeichner `Positions`.

Navigationspfade

Nachdem Sie die Assoziation angelegt haben, können Sie den Navigationspfad von `Orderheader` zu `Orderposition` anlegen. Klicken Sie dazu im Navigationsbereich unterhalb von **Orderheader** doppelt auf den Ordner **Navigationseigenschaften**, und legen Sie im rechten oberen Bildschirmbereich einen neuen Navigationspfad an, indem Sie auf das grüne Pluszeichen klicken. Nennen Sie den neuen Navigationspfad »Positions«, wählen Sie als Beziehungsnamen die soeben angelegte Assoziation `Orderheader_Orderposition` aus, und geben Sie als Bezeichner ebenfalls »Positions« ein.

Entitätsmengen

Nun können Sie die beiden Entitätsmengen `Orderheaders` und `Orderpositions` anlegen. Dazu klicken Sie doppelt auf den Ordner **Entitätsmengen** im Navigationsbereich und anschließend auf das grüne Pluszeichen im rechten oberen Bildschirmbereich. Verweisen Sie von der Entitätsmenge `Orderheaders` auf den Entitätstyp `Orderheader` und bei der Entitätsmenge `Orderpositions` auf den Entitätstyp `Orderposition`. Wählen Sie bei beiden Entitätsmengen die Ankreuzfelder **Anlegbar**, **Aktualisierbar**, **Löschbar** und **Adressierbar** aus, um zu dokumentieren, welche der CRUD-Operationen `Create`, `Update`, `Delete` und `Read` Sie unterstützen wollen.

Funktionsimport

Zum Schluss können Sie noch einen Funktionsimport anlegen. Funktionsimporte sind Funktionen des OData-Service, also Aktionen, die nicht in das CRUD-Schema passen. Zum Anlegen klicken Sie rechts auf den Knoten **Funktionsimporte** im Datenmodell des Service und wählen den Menüeintrag **Anlegen** aus. Vergeben Sie den Namen »MostRecentOrderOfBuyer« als Namen für den Funktionsimport, legen einen Importparameter namens `Buyer` vom Typ `Edm.String` an und legen als Rückgabewert den Entitätstyp `Orderheader` fest. Abbildung 9.9 zeigt diesen Funktionsimport.

Damit ist die Beschreibung des Objektmodells abgeschlossen, und Sie können die Laufzeitobjekte – Model-Provider-Klasse, Data-Provider-Klasse, technisches Modell und technischer Service – generieren lassen und einen OData-Service im Servicekatalog anlegen.

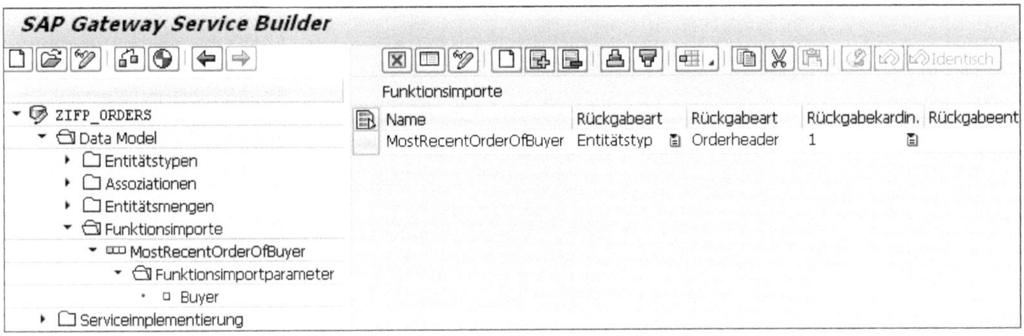

Abbildung 9.9 Funktionsimport

9.3.2 Generierung der Komponenten und Anlegen des OData-Service

Sichern und prüfen Sie Ihr Projekt im Menü mit **Projekt • Sichern** bzw. **Projekt • Prüfung** (Strg + F2). Generieren Sie dann die Laufzeitobjekte durch die Auswahl des Menüeintrags **Projekt • Prüfen** (Strg + F3).

Generierung starten

Im Dialog **Modell- und Servicedefinition** können Sie die Namen der generierten Objekte noch anpassen, bevor Sie auf das grünen Häkchen klicken, um die Generierung zu starten. Bevor der Gateway Service Builder die Objekte generiert, erkundigt er sich noch nach dem Entwicklungspaket und dem Workbench-Auftrag, denen die Objekte zugeordnet werden sollen.

Erzeugte Objekte

Erfolgsnachrichten, Warnungen und Fehlermeldungen während der Generierung werden im rechten unteren Bildschirmbereich angezeigt. Sie sehen die generierten Objekte anschließend im Navigationsbereich im Ordner **Erzeugte Objekte**. Insgesamt erzeugt der Gateway Service Builder in unserem Beispiel sechs Objekte:

- Die *Model-Provider-Klasse* `ZCL_ZIFP_ORDERS_MP` und die davon abgeleitete Klasse `ZCL_ZIFP_ORDERS_MP_EXT`. Die Basisklasse enthält Code, den Sie nicht ändern dürfen, die abgeleitete Klasse enthält Code, den Sie bei Bedarf anpassen können, falls Sie das Objektmodell per Programmierung noch erweitern wollen oder müssen. Dies ist jedoch selten notwendig.
- Die *Data-Provider-Klasse* `ZCL_ZIFP_ORDERS_DP` und die davon abgeleitete Klasse `ZCL_ZIFP_ORDERS_DP_EXT`. Auch hier dürfen Sie die Basisklasse nicht ändern. Für die Implementierung der CRUD-Operationen rufen die Methoden der Basisklasse virtuelle Methoden auf, die Sie in der Unterklasse redefinieren müssen.

- Das *technische Modell* ZIFP_ORDERS:_MDL, das auf die Model-Provider-Klasse ZCL_ZIFP_ORDERS_MP_EXT verweist.
- Den *technischen Service* ZIFP_ORDERS_SRV, der auf die Data-Provider-Klasse ZCL_ZIFP_ORDERS_DP_EXT und das technische Modell ZIFP_ORDERS_MDL verweist.

Als Nächstes können Sie im Servicekatalog einen OData-Service anlegen und dort auch das Servicedokument und das Metadatendokument abrufen.

OData-Service anlegen

Starten Sie dazu Transaktion /IWFND/MAINT_SERVICE, und klicken Sie auf das grüne Pluszeichen, um einen neuen Service hinzuzufügen. Geben Sie im Bereich **Filter** als Systemalias »LOCAL« und als Namen für den technischen Service »ZIFP_ORDERS_SRV« ein, und drücken Sie dann die [↵]-Taste. In der Liste **Service hinzufügen** werden nun alle technischen Services angezeigt, die den Filterkriterien entsprechen. Klicken Sie in dieser Liste auf den Namen des technischen Service, um einen OData-Service anzulegen. Geben Sie im Dialog **Service hinzufügen** ein Entwicklungspaket an. Wie Sie in Abbildung 9.10 sehen, ist in der deutschen Lokalisierung des Dialogs die Auswahloption für den ICF-Knoten **OData-Service** nicht übersetzt worden (wird nicht angezeigt). Das wird uns später beim Anlegen des ICF-Knotens Probleme bereiten, sodass wir uns dazu mit der Anmeldesprache Englisch anmelden müssen.

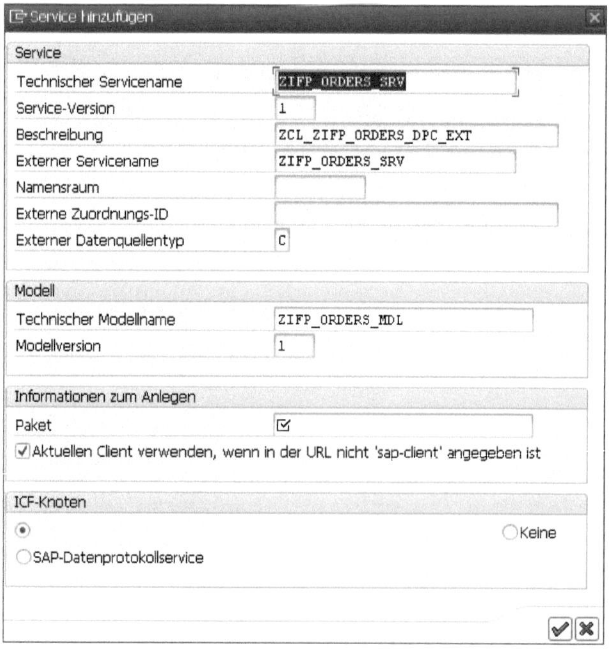

Abbildung 9.10 OData-Service hinzufügen

ICF-Knoten aktivieren

Bestätigen Sie die Eingaben, ordnen Sie einen Workbench-Auftrag zu, und gehen Sie anschließend mit der Funktionstaste [F3] zurück zum Einstiegsbild des Servicekatalogs. Dort ist Ihr Service jetzt zwar eingetragen, aber Sie können den OData-ICF-Knoten wegen des Übersetzungsfehlers nicht aktivieren. Melden Sie sich dazu mit Englisch als Anmeldesprache an, und aktivieren Sie den OData-ICF-Knoten. Dazu wählen Sie im Servicekatalog zuerst Ihren Service und dann im linken unteren Bereich **ICF Nodes** den Knoten **ODATA Standard Mode** aus und klicken dann auf das linke Icon mit dem Streichholz ( ) und der Beschriftung **ICF Node** (siehe Abbildung 9.11).

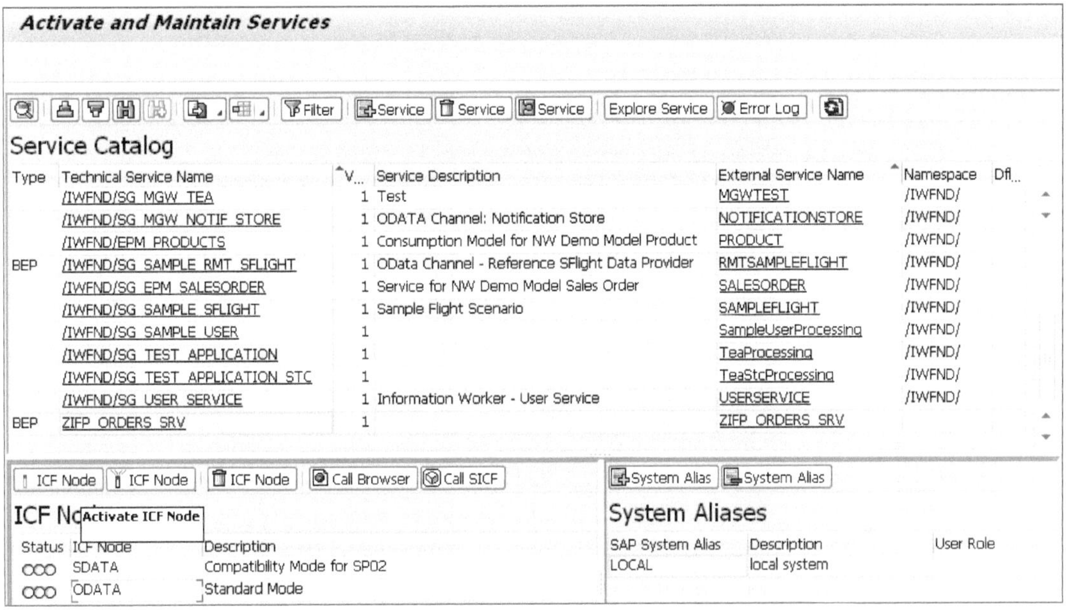

Abbildung 9.11 OData-SICF-Knoten aktivieren

Service-Explorer

Wenn Sie möchten, können Sie sich nun wieder auf Deutsch anmelden und den Servicekatalog aufrufen. Über den Button **Service durchsuchen** können Sie den Service-Explorer starten und sich das Servicedokument, die Metadaten und eine Liste der Entitätsmengen anzeigen lassen.

Dazu selektieren Sie unterhalb des Auswahl-Buttons **ODATA Standardmodus** eine der drei Optionen **Servicedokument abrufen**, **Servicemetadaten abrufen** oder **Entitätsmengen abrufen** und drücken die Funktionstaste [F8]. Abbildung 9.12 zeigt die Servicemetadaten im Service-Explorer. Sie können sich die Metadaten auch in einem Browser anzeigen lassen. Die URL zu den Metadaten finden Sie ganz unten im angezeigten Dokument. Sie lautet in unserem Fall: *http://NWASABAP703.WORKGROUP:8000/sap/opu/odata/sap/ZIFP_ORDERS_SRV/$metadata*

```
  <?xml version="1.0" encoding="utf-8" ?>
- <edmx:Edmx Version="1.0" xmlns:edmx="http://schemas.microsoft.com/ado/2007/06/edmx"
   xmlns:m="http://schemas.microsoft.com/ado/2007/08/dataservices/metadata" xmlns:sap="http://www.sap.com/Protocols/SAPData">
 - <edmx:DataServices m:DataServiceVersion="2.0">
  - <Schema Namespace="ZIFP_ORDERS_SRV" xml:lang="de" sap:schema-version="1" xmlns="http://schemas.microsoft.com/ado/2008/09/edm">
   - <EntityType Name="Orderheader" sap:content-version="1">
    - <Key>
        <PropertyRef Name="OrderId" />
      </Key>
      <Property Name="Buyer" Type="Edm.String" Nullable="false" MaxLength="50" sap:unicode="false" sap:label="Käufer" sap:creatable="false"
        sap:updatable="false" sap:sortable="false" sap:filterable="false" />
      <Property Name="OrderDate" Type="Edm.DateTime" Nullable="false" Precision="7" sap:unicode="false" sap:label="Bestelldatum"
        sap:creatable="false" sap:updatable="false" sap:sortable="false" sap:filterable="false" />
      <Property Name="OrderId" Type="Edm.String" Nullable="false" MaxLength="10" sap:unicode="false" sap:label="Bestellnummer"
        sap:creatable="false" sap:updatable="false" sap:sortable="false" sap:filterable="false" />
      <Property Name="Ordertype" Type="Edm.String" Nullable="false" MaxLength="2" sap:unicode="false" sap:label="Bestelltyp" sap:creatable="false"
        sap:updatable="false" sap:sortable="false" sap:filterable="false" />
      <Property Name="ReferenceId" Type="Edm.String" Nullable="false" MaxLength="10" sap:unicode="false" sap:label="Referenz" sap:creatable="false"
        sap:updatable="false" sap:sortable="false" sap:filterable="false" />
      <Property Name="Seller" Type="Edm.String" Nullable="false" MaxLength="50" sap:unicode="false" sap:label="Lieferant" sap:creatable="false"
        sap:updatable="false" sap:sortable="false" sap:filterable="false" />
      <NavigationProperty Name="Positions" Relationship="ZIFP_ORDERS_SRV.Orderheader_Orderposition"
        FromRole="FromRole_Orderheader_Orderposition" ToRole="ToRole_Orderheader_Orderposition" sap:label="Positions" />
    </EntityType>
   + <EntityType Name="Orderposition" sap:content-version="1">
   + <Association Name="Orderheader_Orderposition" sap:content-version="1" sap:label="Positions">
   - <EntityContainer Name="ZIFP_ORDERS_SRV_Entities" m:IsDefaultEntityContainer="true" sap:supported-formats="atom json xlsx">
      <EntitySet Name="Orderheaders" EntityType="ZIFP_ORDERS_SRV.Orderheader" sap:label="Orderheaders" sap:pageable="false" sap:content-
        version="1" />
      <EntitySet Name="Orderpositions" EntityType="ZIFP_ORDERS_SRV.Orderposition" sap:label="Orderpositions" sap:pageable="false" sap:content-
        version="1" />
    + <AssociationSet Name="Orderheader_Orderposition_AssocSet" Association="ZIFP_ORDERS_SRV.Orderheader_Orderposition"
        sap:creatable="false" sap:updatable="false" sap:deletable="false" sap:content-version="1">
    + <FunctionImport Name="MostRecentOrderOfBuyer" ReturnType="ZIFP_ORDERS_SRV.Orderheader" EntitySet="Orderheaders" m:HttpMethod="GET"
        sap:label="Most recent order of buyer">
    </EntityContainer>
    <atom:link rel="self" href="http://vhcalnplci:8000/sap/opu/odata/sap/ZIFP_ORDERS_SRV/$metadata"
     xmlns:atom="http://www.w3.org/2005/Atom" />
    <atom:link rel="latest-version" href="http://vhcalnplci:8000/sap/opu/odata/sap/ZIFP_ORDERS_SRV/$metadata"
     xmlns:atom="http://www.w3.org/2005/Atom" />
   </Schema>
  </edmx:DataServices>
</edmx:Edmx>
```


Abbildung 9.12 Servicemetadaten

Metadatendokument

Im Metadatendokument werden die Entitätstypen mit ihren Eigenschaften und Navigationspfaden, die Assoziationen und die Entitätsmengen beschrieben, die der OData-Service bereitstellt. Das Servicedokument (dieselbe URL, aber ohne *$metadata*) enthält eine Liste der Entitätsmengen mit ihren Links. Wenn Sie allerdings versuchen, z. B. die Entitätsmenge `Orderheaders` abzurufen, erhalten Sie die Fehlermeldung »Methode 'ORDERHEADERS_GET_ENTITYSET' in Datenanbieterklasse nicht implementiert«. Die Methoden implementieren wir im folgenden Abschnitt.

9.3.3 Implementierung der Data-Provider-Klasse

In der Data-Provider-Klasse `ZCL_ZIFP_ORDERS_DP` wurden insgesamt zehn Methoden definiert, die wir in der abgeleiteten Klasse `ZCL_ZIFP_ORDERS_DP_EXT` redefinieren müssen, um für jeden der beiden Entitätstypen `Orderheader` und `Orderposition` die Operationen für `Query`, `Read`, `Create`, `Update` und `Delete` zu implementieren.

Sie können die Implementierung im Object Navigator vornehmen oder aus dem Gateway Service Builder in die ABAP Workbench abspringen. Dazu folgen Sie im Navigationsbereich des Gateway Service Builders dem Pfad **Ser-**

viceimplementierung • Entitätsmengen • Orderheaders • Operationen, klicken mit der rechten Maustaste auf die entsprechende Operation und wählen im Kontextmenü den Eintrag **Implementierung** aus. Falls die Methode in der Klasse ZCL_ZIFP_ORDERS_DP_EXT schon implementiert wurde, landen Sie direkt im ABAP Editor im Code dieser Methode. Andernfalls landen Sie im Class Builder in der Liste der Methoden dieser Klasse. Dort können Sie die Methoden auswählen und redefinieren, indem Sie auf das Icon (**Redefinieren**) klicken (siehe Abbildung 9.13).

9

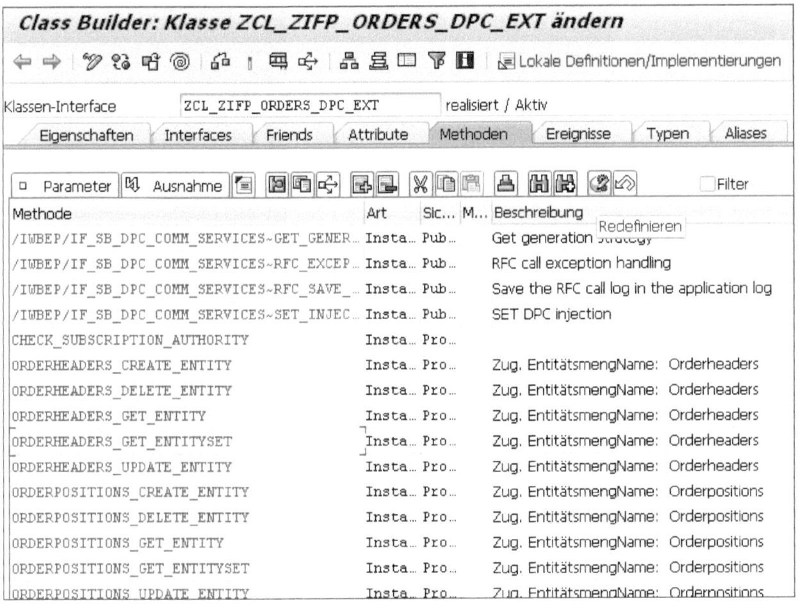

Abbildung 9.13 Ererbte Methode redefinieren

Query-Operation für Bestellköpfe

Fangen Sie am besten mit der Methode ORDERHEADERS_GET_ENTITYSET an. Alles, was Sie dort tun müssen, ist, eine interne Tabelle mit allen Bestellköpfen zu füllen. Sie können das über einen SELECT auf die transparente Tabelle ZIFPORDER oder über einen Aufruf des Funktionsbausteins Z_IFP_ORDER_GETLIST erreichen.

Listing 9.2 zeigt die Implementierung der Methode ORDERHEADERS_GET_ENTITYSET. Der Exportparameter et_entityset ist vom Typ ZCL_ZIFP_ORDERS_MP=>TT_ORDERHEADER, wurde also in der Model-Provider-Klasse definiert und ist einfach eine Standardtabelle mit dem Zeilentyp ZIFPORDER.

```
METHOD orderheaders_get_entityset.
  SELECT * FROM zifporder INTO TABLE et_entityset.
ENDMETHOD.
```

Listing 9.2 Alle Bestellköpfe lesen

Atom-Feed für Bestellköpfe

Wenn Sie nun Ihren Code aktivieren, können Sie mit dem Service-Explorer oder mit einem Browser die Liste aller Bestellköpfe abrufen. Sie müssen einfach an die Basis-URL des OData-Service (*protokoll://<host>:<port>/sap/opu/odata/sap/sap/ZIFP_ORDERS_SRV/*) noch ein *Orderheaders/* anhängen.

[»]

Ausschalten der HTML-Umwandlung

Es kann sein, dass Ihr Browser das zurückgegebene XML-Dokument als Atom-Feed erkennt und in ein HTML-Dokument transformiert. Im Internet Explorer etwa können Sie dies unterbinden, indem Sie im Menü über **Tools • Internet Options** den Dialog **Internet Options** öffnen und dort auf die Registerkarte **Content** wechseln. Klicken Sie dann im unteren Bereich **Feeds and Web Slices** auf die Taste **Settings**, und deaktivieren Sie die Auswahlbox **Turn on feed reading view**.

Abbildung 9.14 zeigt den Atom-Feed der Bestellköpfe im Browser. Das Wurzelelement ist `feed`, als Kindelemente sehen Sie die Atom-Eigenschaften `id`, `title`, `updated` und `author` sowie den relativen Link auf den Feed selbst. Das `id`-Element enthält die vollständige URL des Atom-Feeds.

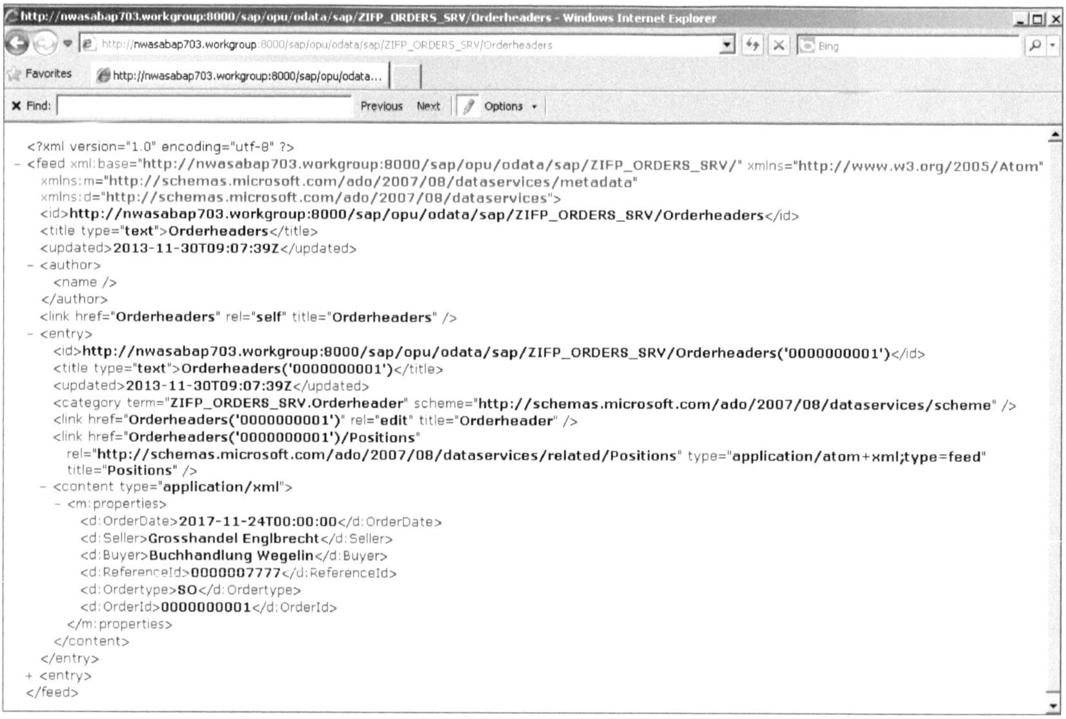

Abbildung 9.14 Atom-Feed der Bestellköpfe

Nach den Atom-Eigenschaften des Feeds folgen mehrere `entry`-Elemente, eines für jeden Bestellkopf. Jedes `entry`-Element beinhaltet die Atom-Eigenschaften `id`, `title`, `updated` und `category`. Auch hier enthält die `id`-Eigenschaft die vollständige URL des Bestellkopfs. Danach folgen zwei Links, einer zum Editieren des Bestellkopfs, einer auf den Feed der Bestellpositionen der Bestellung. Schließlich werden unterhalb des `content`-Elements innerhalb des `properties`-Elements die Eigenschaften des Bestellkopfs angezeigt: `OrderDate`, `Seller`, `Buyer`, `ReferenceId`, `Ordertype` und `OrderId`.

Read-Operation für Bestellkopf

Listing 9.3 zeigt die Implementierung der Methode `ORDERHEADERS_GET_ENTITY`, mit der ein einzelner Bestellkopf gelesen wird. Der Importparameter `it_key_tab` enthält eine Liste der Schlüsselfelder der Entität, die gelesen werden soll, in unserem Fall die `OrderId`. Die Schlüssel sind in der Tabelle als Paare von Schlüsselnamen und Schlüsselwert gespeichert. Die Methode liest also zuerst den Schlüssel und verwendet ihn dann in der `WHERE`-Klausel der `SELECT`-Anweisung. Der Exportparameter `er_entity` ist einfach eine Struktur vom Typ `ZIFPORDER`.

9

```
METHOD orderheaders_get_entity.
  FIELD-SYMBOLS:
    <key> TYPE /iwbep/s_mgw_name_value_pair.

  READ TABLE it_key_tab ASSIGNING <key> INDEX 1.
  SELECT SINGLE * FROM zifporder INTO er_entity WHERE
    orderid = <key>-value.
ENDMETHOD.
```

Listing 9.3 Bestellkopf lesen

Damit Ihnen im Browser ein einzelner Bestellkopf angezeigt wird, hängen Sie *Orderheaders('nnn')/* an die Basis-URL des OData-Service an, wobei *nnn* die zehnstellige Bestellnummer ist. Abbildung 9.15 zeigt den Bestellkopf mit der Nummer »0000000001« im Browser. Sie sehen die URL sowohl in der Titelleiste als auch im Adressfeld. Nun heißt das Wurzelelement `entry` und enthält einen einzigen Eintrag, der genauso aufgebaut ist, wie in Abbildung 9.14 dargestellt.

Query-Operation für Bestellposition

Als Nächstes implementieren wir die Methode `ORDERPOSITIONS_GET_ENTITYSET`. Hier müssen wir berücksichtigen, dass entweder über die URL *Orderpositions/* alle Bestellpositionen oder über die URL *Orderheaders('nnn')/Positions/* nur die Bestellpositionen der Bestellung mit der Bestellnummer *nnn* angefordert werden.

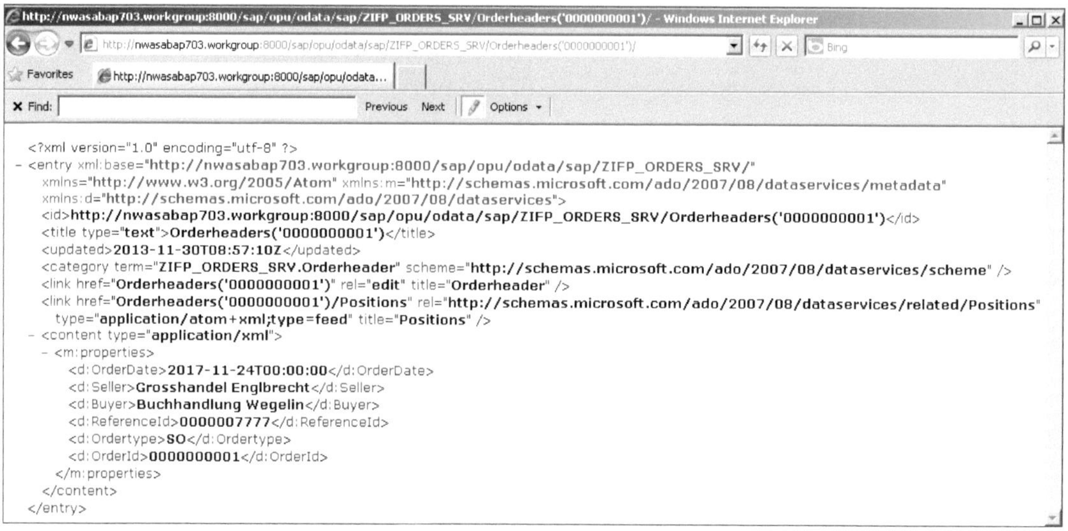

Abbildung 9.15 Bestellkopf mit der Nummer »0000000001« im Browser

Dazu prüft der Code in Listing 9.4 zuerst, ob es im Importparameter `it_navigation_paths` einen Eintrag gibt. Falls ja, dürfen nur die Bestellpositionen der Bestellung zurückgegeben werden, deren Schlüssel in der Tabelle `it_key_tab` übergeben wurde. Andernfalls werden alle Bestellpositionen zurückgegeben.

```
METHOD orderpositions_get_entityset.
  FIELD-SYMBOLS:
    <key> TYPE /iwbep/s_mgw_name_value_pair.

  IF lines( it_navigation_path ) NE 0.
    READ TABLE it_key_tab ASSIGNING <key> INDEX 1.
    SELECT * FROM zifporderpos INTO TABLE et_entityset
      WHERE orderid = <key>-value.
  ELSE.
    SELECT * FROM zifporderpos INTO TABLE et_entityset.
  ENDIF.
ENDMETHOD.
```

Listing 9.4 Bestellpositionen lesen

Read-Operation für Bestellposition

Listing 9.5 zeigt den Code, der nur eine Bestellposition liest. Die einzige Besonderheit besteht darin, dass hier nun zwei Schlüsselwerte zu berücksichtigen sind: die Bestellnummer und die Bestellposition.

```
METHOD orderpositions_get_entity.
  FIELD-SYMBOLS:
   <key_orderid> TYPE /iwbep/s_mgw_name_value_pair,
   <key_orderpos> TYPE /iwbep/s_mgw_name_value_pair.

   READ TABLE it_key_tab ASSIGNING <key_orderid>
     WITH KEY name = 'OrderId'.
   READ TABLE it_key_tab ASSIGNING <key_orderpos>
     WITH KEY name = 'OrderPosition'.

   SELECT SINGLE * from zifporderpos INTO er_entity WHERE
     orderid  = <key_orderid>-value and
     orderpos = <key_orderpos>-value.
ENDMETHOD.
```

Listing 9.5 Bestellposition lesen

Create-Operation für Bestellkopf

Listing 9.6 zeigt den Code zum Anlegen eines Bestellkopfs. Die Methode liest zunächst die übergebenen Daten über die Methode `read_entry_data()` des Importparameters `io_data_provider`. Danach ruft sie den Funktionsbaustein `Z_IFP_ORDER_CREATE` auf, um eine Bestellung ohne Bestellpositionen zu erzeugen. Falls dieser Funktionsbaustein eine Ausnahme auslöst, wird das Objekt `lr_exception` der Klasse `/iwbep/cx_mgw_busi_exception` erzeugt. Objekte dieser Klasse repräsentieren *Business Exceptions*, also Ausnahmen auf der Anwendungsebene. Die Methode `get_msg_container()` dieser Klasse liefert einen Nachrichtencontainer, über den mit `add_message()` eine T100-Nachricht und mit `add_message_text_only()` eine einfache Textfehlermeldung angehängt werden kann.

```
METHOD orderheaders_create_entity.
  DATA:
    lt_orderpos TYPE TABLE OF zifporderpos,
    lv_error TYPE string,
    lr_exception TYPE REF TO /iwbep/cx_mgw_busi_exception,
    lr_msg_cont TYPE REF TO /iwbep/if_message_container,
    lv_subrc type sy-subrc.

  io_data_provider->read_entry_data( IMPORTING es_data = er_entity ).

  CALL FUNCTION 'Z_IFP_ORDER_CREATE'
    EXPORTING
      im_orderheader = er_entity
      im_testrun     = ' '
```

```
        im_commit      = 'X'
      IMPORTING
        ex_orderid     = er_entity-orderid
      TABLES
        ta_orderpos    = lt_orderpos
      EXCEPTIONS
        not_authorized = 1
        no_number      = 2
        no_lock        = 3
        OTHERS         = 4.
    IF sy-subrc NE 0.
      lv_subrc = sy-subrc.
      CREATE OBJECT lr_exception.
      lr_msg_cont = lr_exception->get_msg_container( ).
      CASE lv_subrc.
        WHEN 1.
          lr_msg_cont->add_message(
            iv_msg_type = 'E'
            iv_msg_id = 'ZIFP'
            iv_msg_number = '101' ).
        WHEN 2.
          lr_msg_cont->add_message(
            iv_msg_type = 'E'
            iv_msg_id = 'ZIFP'
            iv_msg_number = '103' ).
        WHEN 3.
          lr_msg_cont->add_message(
            iv_msg_type = 'E'
            iv_msg_id = 'ZIFP'
            iv_msg_number = '104' ).
        WHEN 4.
          lr_msg_cont->add_message_text_only(
            iv_msg_type = 'E'
            iv_msg_text = text-000 ).
      ENDCASE.
      RAISE EXCEPTION lr_exception.
    ENDIF.
  ENDMETHOD.
```

Listing 9.6 Bestellkopf anlegen

Testen mit WFetch

Damit Sie über das OData-Protokoll einen Bestellkopf anlegen können, müssen Sie, wie in Abbildung 9.15, an die Feed-URL *Orderheaders/* per POST ein Orderheaders-Entry-Dokument schicken. Dies ist mit einem einfachen Browser nun nicht mehr möglich. Stattdessen können Sie das Programm *WFetch* verwenden, das von Jaroslav Dunajsky für Microsoft entwickelt wurde und das Sie kostenfrei von Microsoft herunterladen können. Mit WFetch können Sie das HTTP-Verb (`GET`, `POST`, `PUT`, `DELETE`), den HTTP-Header und den HTTP-Body frei wählen.

CSRF Token

Während lesende Zugriffe mit `GET` ohne weitere Sicherheitsmaßnahmen (außer einer Authentifizierung) möglich sind, werden ändernde Zugriffe durch ein sogenanntes *Cross Site Request Forgery Token* (CSRF Token) abgesichert. Der Client fordert dieses Token durch den HTTP-Header `x-csrf-token: Fetch` in einem ersten Lesezugriff an. Im HTTP-Header der Response schickt der Server das angeforderte Token und ein Session-Cookie zurück. Sowohl das CSRF Token als auch das Cookie müssen beim anschließenden ändernden Zugriff zurück an den Server geschickt werden.

Abbildung 9.16 zeigt das Programm WFetch, das einen Bestellkopf liest und dabei ein CSRF Token anfordert.

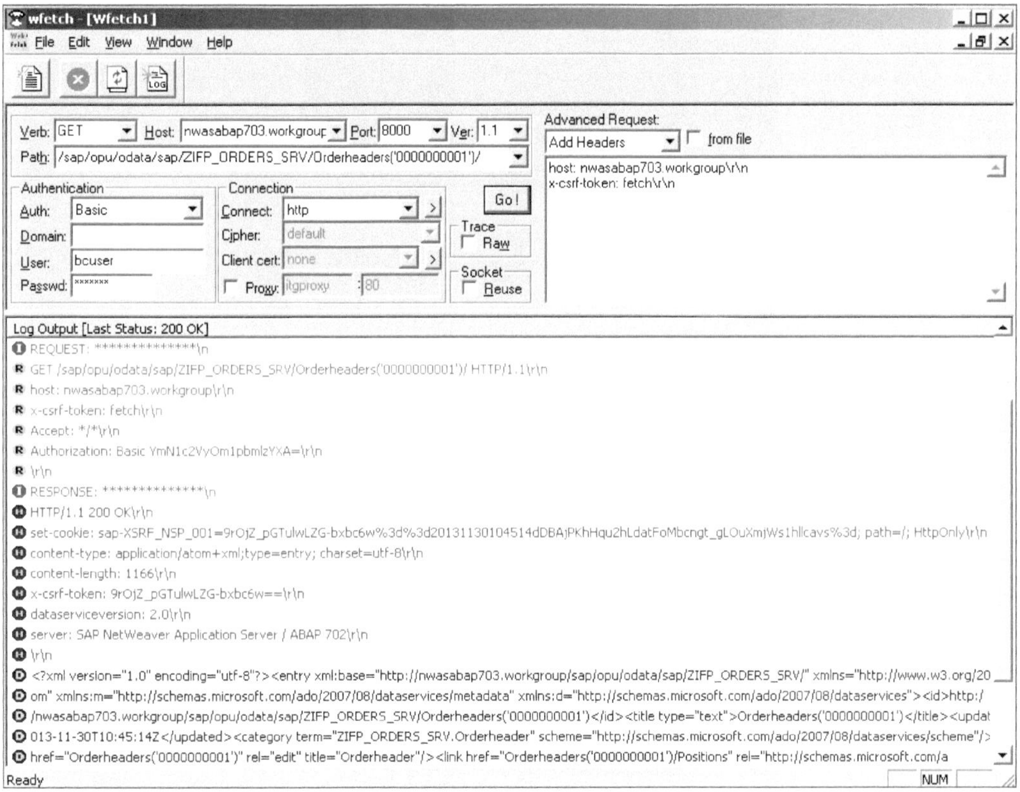

Abbildung 9.16 Bestellkopf mit WFetch mit Anforderung eines CSRF Tokens lesen

Als HTTP-**Verb** ist »GET« eingetragen, als **Host** »nwasabap703.workgroup«, als **Port** »800« und als HTTP-Version (Feld **Ver.**) »1.1«. Der **Path** zum Lesen des Bestellkopfs mit der Nummer »0000000001« lautet */sap/opu/odata/ZIPF_ORDERS_SRV/Orderheaders('0000000001')/*. Bei **Auth.** wurde **Basic** ausgewählt, und Benutzername und Passwort wurden hinterlegt. Als Protokoll wurde **http** ausgewählt. Im Feld **Advanced Request** wurde aus der Drop-down-Liste **Add Headers** ausgewählt, und als Header wurden die beiden Zeilen »host: nwsabap703.workgroup« und »x-csrf-token: fetch« eingetragen.

HTTP-GET ausführen

Sobald Sie auf **Go!** klicken, führt WFetch den HTTP-GET aus. Sowohl den Request als auch die Response sehen Sie im Log im unteren Bildschirmbereich von WFetch. Für uns ist der Inhalt der Header-Felder `set-cookie` und `x-csrf-token` wichtig. Die Inhalte dieser Header-Felder (nach dem Doppelpunkt, ohne das Leerzeichen) kopieren Sie für den HTTP-POST in Abbildung 9.17 in die Header-Felder `cookie` und `x-csrf-token`. Als zusätzliches Header-Feld fügen Sie `content-type` mit dem Inhalt `application/atom+xml;type=entry` hinzu.

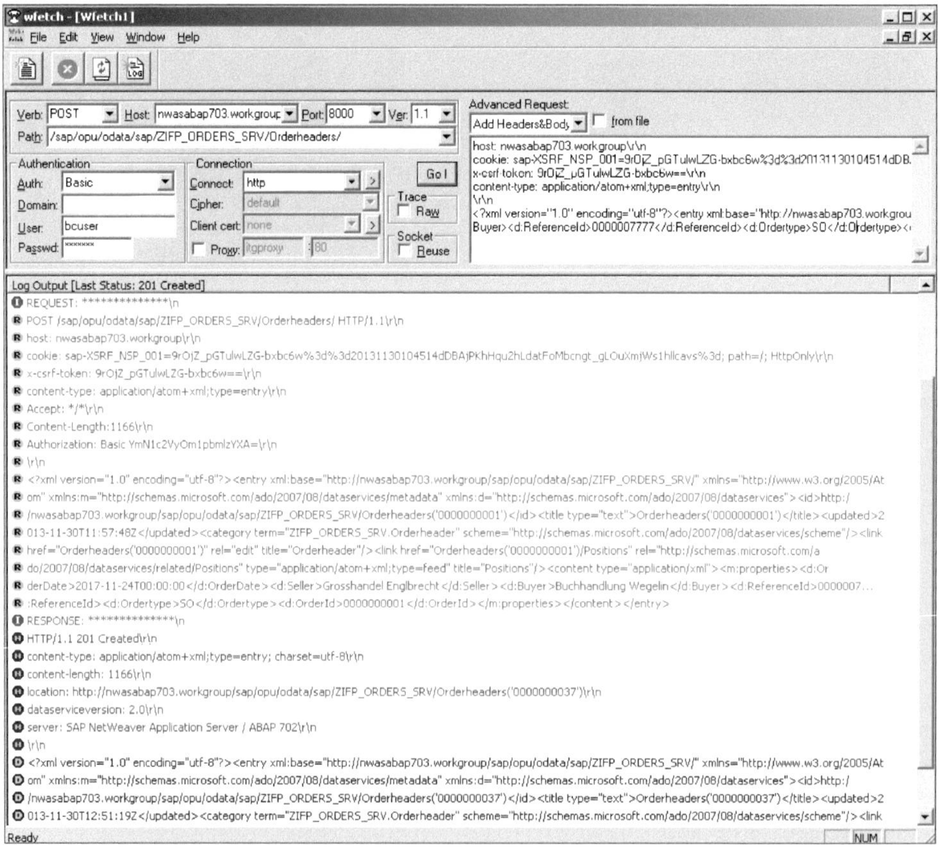

Abbildung 9.17 Bestellkopf mit WFetch mit Angabe eines CSRF Tokens anlegen

Durch eine Leerzeile getrennt, folgt dann der HTTP-Body. Hier können Sie einfach die Antwort aus Abbildung 9.16 kopieren, alle Kindelemente von `entry` außer dem Kindelement `content` löschen und unterhalb von `content` die Attribute für den neuen Bestellkopf eintragen. Achten Sie darauf, dass Sie bei **Advanced Request** nun den Eintrag **Add Header & Body** auswählen.

HTTP-POST ausführen

Wenn Sie nun auf **Go!** klicken, wird der HTTP-POST durchgeführt und ein neuer Bestellkopf angelegt. Der HTTP-Code lautet `201 Created`, und im Body der HTTP-Response wird der neu angelegte Bestellkopf (mit der neuen Bestellnummer) zurückgegeben.


```
METHOD orderpositions_create_entity.
  DATA:
    lt_orderpos TYPE TABLE OF zifporderpos.

  io_data_provider->read_entry_data(
    IMPORTING es_data = er_entity ).
  CALL FUNCTION 'Z_IFP_ORDER_CREATEPOS'
    EXPORTING
      im_orderpos     = er_entity
      im_testrun      = ' '
      im_commit       = 'X'
    EXCEPTIONS
      not_authorized = 1
      no_order       = 2
      no_lock        = 3
      duplicate_pos  = 4
      OTHERS         = 5.
  IF sy-subrc NE 0.
    ...
  ENDIF.
ENDMETHOD.
```

Listing 9.7 Bestellposition anlegen

Create-Operation für Bestellposition

Listing 9.7 zeigt den Code, mit dem Sie eine Bestellposition anlegen können. Er funktioniert analog zum Code zum Anlegen eines Bestellkopfs in Listing 9.6, außer dass nun der Funktionsbaustein `Z_IFP_ORDER_CREATEPOS` aufgerufen wird und der Exportparameter `er_entity` vom Typ `ZIFPORDERPOS` ist. Auch das Testen dieser Methode funktioniert genau wie vorher, nur dass Sie nun die URL *Orderpositions/* verwenden müssen und der HTTP-Body eine Bestellposition enthalten muss.

```
METHOD orderheaders_update_entity.
  DATA:
    lt_orderx TYPE zifporderx,
    lt_orderpos TYPE TABLE OF zifporderpos,
    lt_orderposx TYPE TABLE OF zifporderpos.

  io_data_provider->read_entry_data(
    IMPORTING es_data = er_entity ).
  MOVE:
    'X' TO lt_orderx-buyer,
    'X' TO lt_orderx-seller,
    'X' TO lt_orderx-refid,
    'X' TO lt_orderx-type,
    'X' TO lt_orderx-orderdate.
  CALL FUNCTION 'Z_IFP_ORDER_CHANGE'
    EXPORTING
      im_orderheader  = er_entity
      im_orderheaderx = lt_orderx
      im_testrun      = ' '
      im_commit       = 'X'
    TABLES
      ta_orderpos     = lt_orderpos
      ta_orderposx    = lt_orderposx
    EXCEPTIONS
      not_authorized  = 1
      no_data         = 2
      no_lock         = 3
      OTHERS          = 4.
  IF sy-subrc NE 0.
    ...
  ENDIF.
ENDMETHOD.
```

Listing 9.8 Bestellkopf ändern

Update-Operation für Bestellkopf

Das Ändern eines Bestellkopfs zeigt Listing 9.8. Die Implementierung erfolgt ganz analog zum Anlegen eines Bestellkopfs, nur dass diesmal der Funktionsbaustein Z_IFP_ORDER_CHANGE aufgerufen wird. Wenn Sie die Implementierung testen wollen, müssen Sie wie beim Anlegen eines Bestellkopfs in Listing 9.6 vorgehen, nur dass Sie in WFetch das HTTP-Verb PUT verwenden und als URL *Orderheaders('nnn')/* angeben, wobei *nnn* die Bestellnummer ist. Wenn der Bestellkopf erfolgreich geändert wurde, wird Ihnen als HTTP-Code »201 No Content« zurückgegeben.

Listing 9.9 zeigt den Code zum Ändern einer Bestellposition.

```
METHOD orderpositions_update_entity.
  DATA:
    ls_order TYPE zifporder,
    lt_orderx TYPE zifporderx,
    lt_orderpos TYPE TABLE OF zifporderpos,
    lt_orderposx TYPE TABLE OF zifporderposx,
    ls_orderposx TYPE zifporderposx.

  io_data_provider->read_entry_data(
    IMPORTING es_data = er_entity ).
  MOVE:
    er_entity-orderid TO ls_order-orderid,
    'X' TO ls_orderposx-matid,
    'X' TO ls_orderposx-mattext,
    'X' TO ls_orderposx-ordercount,
    'X' TO ls_orderposx-price,
    'X' TO ls_orderposx-currency.
  APPEND er_entity TO lt_orderpos.
  APPEND ls_orderposx TO lt_orderposx.
  CALL FUNCTION 'Z_IFP_ORDER_CHANGE'
    EXPORTING
      im_orderheader  = ls_order
      im_orderheaderx = lt_orderx
      im_testrun      = ' '
      im_commit       = 'X'
    TABLES
      ta_orderpos     = lt_orderpos
      ta_orderposx    = lt_orderposx
    EXCEPTIONS
      not_authorized  = 1
      no_data         = 2
      no_lock         = 3
      OTHERS          = 4.
  IF sy-subrc NE 0.
    ...
  ENDIF.
ENDMETHOD.
```

Listing 9.9 Bestellposition ändern

Update-Operation für Bestellposition

Der Code funktioniert analog zum Anlegen eines Bestellkopfs in Listing 9.10, und auch das Testen erfolgt wie beim Anlegen eines Bestellkopfs, nur dass Sie nun die URL *Orderpositions(OrderID='nnn',OrderPosition='ppp')/* beim PUT angeben müssen, wobei *nnn* die Bestellnummer und *ppp* die Bestellposition ist.

```
METHOD orderheaders_delete_entity.
  DATA:
    lv_orderid TYPE zifporder-orderid.
  FIELD-SYMBOLS:
    <key> TYPE /iwbep/s_mgw_name_value_pair.

  READ TABLE it_key_tab ASSIGNING <key> INDEX 1.
  lv_orderid = <key>-value.
  CALL FUNCTION 'Z_IFP_ORDER_DELETE'
    EXPORTING
      im_orderid     = lv_orderid
      im_commit      = 'X'
    EXCEPTIONS
      not_authorized = 1
      no_data        = 2
      no_lock        = 3
      OTHERS         = 4.
  IF sy-subrc NE 0.
    ...
  ENDIF.
ENDMETHOD.
```

Listing 9.10 Bestellung löschen

Delete-Operation für Bestellung

Listing 9.10 zeigt den Code zum Löschen einer Bestellung. Wie beim Lesen wird die Bestellnummer aus der Tabelle `it_key_tab` gelesen. Mit dieser Bestellnummer wird dann der Funktionsbaustein `Z_IFP_ORDER_DELETE` aufgerufen. Beim Testen mit WFetch geben Sie das HTTP-Verb `DELETE`, dieselbe URL wie zum Lesen und keinen HTTP-Body an. Auch das Header-Feld `content-type` entfällt.

Delete-Operation für Bestellposition

Listing 9.11 zeigt den Code zum Löschen einer Bestellposition. Wie beim Lesen werden Bestellnummer und Positionsnummer aus der Tabelle `it_key_tab` gelesen. Mit diesen Werten wird dann der Funktionsbaustein `Z_IFP_ORDER_DELETEPOS` aufgerufen. Beim Testen mit WFetch geben Sie als HTTP-Verb `DELETE`, dieselbe URL wie zum Lesen und keinen HTTP-Body an. Auch das Header-Feld `content-type` entfällt.

```
METHOD orderpositions_delete_entity.
  DATA:
    ls_orderpos TYPE zifporderpos.
  FIELD-SYMBOLS:
   <key_orderid> TYPE /iwbep/s_mgw_name_value_pair,
   <key_orderpos> TYPE /iwbep/s_mgw_name_value_pair.

  READ TABLE it_key_tab ASSIGNING <key_orderid>
    WITH KEY name = 'OrderId'.
  READ TABLE it_key_tab ASSIGNING <key_orderpos>
    WITH KEY name = 'OrderPosition'.
  ls_orderpos-orderid = <key_orderid>-value.
  ls_orderpos-orderpos = <key_orderpos>-value.

  CALL FUNCTION 'Z_IFP_ORDER_DELETEPOS'
    EXPORTING
      im_orderid      = ls_orderpos-orderid
      im_orderpos     = ls_orderpos-orderpos
      im_commit       = 'X'
    EXCEPTIONS
      not_authorized = 1
      no_data        = 2
      no_lock        = 3
      OTHERS         = 4.
  IF sy-subrc NE 0.
    ...
  ENDIF.
ENDMETHOD.
```

9

Listing 9.11 Bestellposition löschen

Um die Funktionsimporte zu implementieren, müssen Sie die Methode execute_action redefinieren. Listing 9.12 zeigt dies.

Funktionsimport implementieren

```
METHOD /iwbep/if_mgw_appl_srv_runtime~execute_action.
  DATA:
      ls_parameter TYPE /iwbep/s_mgw_name_value_pair,
      ls_order     TYPE zcl_zifp_orders_mpc=>ts_orderheader,
      lt_orders    TYPE zcl_zifp_orders_mpc=>tt_orderheader.
  CASE iv_action_name.
    WHEN 'MostRecentOrderOfBuyer'.
      READ TABLE it_parameter INTO ls_parameter INDEX 1.
      SELECT  *
        FROM zifporder
```

```
        WHERE buyer EQ @ls_parameter-value
        ORDER BY orderdate DESCENDING
        INTO CORRESPONDING FIELDS OF TABLE @lt_orders
        UP TO 1 ROWS.
      IF sy-subrc EQ 0.
        READ TABLE lt_orders INTO ls_order INDEX 1.
        copy_data_to_ref(
          EXPORTING
            is_data = ls_order
            CHANGING
              cr_data = er_data
        ).
      ENDIF.
  ENDCASE.
ENDMETHOD.
```

Listing 9.12 Funktionsimport implementieren

Der Importparameter iv_action_name enthält den Namen des Funktionsimports, der Importparameter it_parameter die Liste der Parameter als Name-Wert-Paare. In unserem Fall lesen wir mit einer SELECT-Anweisung die neueste Bestellung des angegebenen Bestellers in die interne Tabelle lt_orders aus, kopieren die erste Zeile dieser internen Tabelle in die lokale Struktur ls_order und kopieren diese Daten dann wiederum mit der Methode copy_data_to_ref in ein dynamisch alloziertes Datenobjekt, dessen Referenz wir mit dem Exportparameter er_data zurückgeben können.

9.3.4 Monitoring und Fehlersuche

Wahrscheinlich werden Ihnen beim Entwickeln von OData-Services, genau wie uns, zunächst einige Fehler unterlaufen, die sehr schwer zu lokalisieren sind. Daher geben wir Ihnen in diesem Abschnitt einige Tipps zum Monitoring und zur Fehlersuche.

ICF-Recorder

Mit dem *ICF-Recorder* können Sie die HTTP-Requests und -Responses aufzeichnen, die an den OData-Service geschickt werden bzw. von diesem zurückkommen. Dazu lassen Sie sich zuerst in Transaktion SICF den Servicebaum anzeigen und navigieren zu Ihrem Serviceknoten. Im Menü können Sie nun unter **Bearbeiten • Recorder • Aufzeichnung aktivieren** die Aufzeichnung für diesen Serviceknoten und Ihren Benutzer aktivieren. Dabei haben Sie die Wahl, ob Sie nur den Request oder auch die Response aufzeichnen wollen.

Nach dem Testen können Sie sich die Aufzeichnungen von Request und Response über **Bearbeiten • Recorder • Aufzeichnung anzeigen** anzeigen lassen. Abbildung 9.18 zeigt das Protokoll des C#-Clients, den wir in Abschnitt 9.5, »OData-Services mit C# konsumieren«, verwenden.

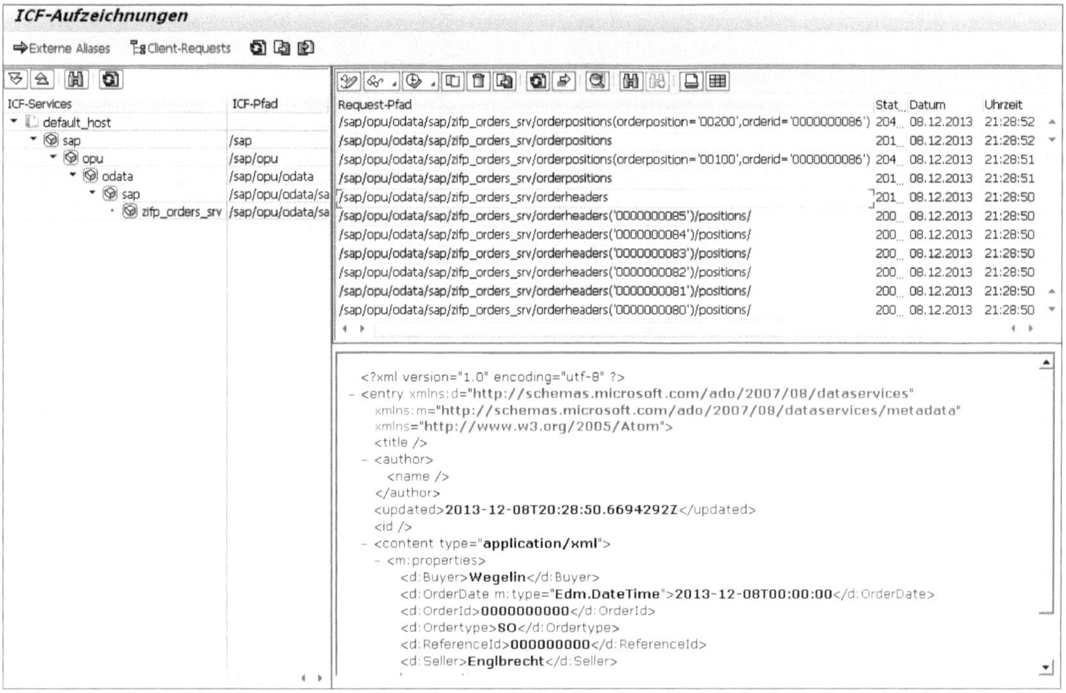

Abbildung 9.18 Bestellkopf im ICF-Recorder anlegen

Fehlerprotokoll

Über Transaktion /IWFND/MAINT_SERVICE können Sie in das Fehlerprotokoll von SAP Gateway abspringen (siehe Abbildung 9.19). Dort sollten Sie zuerst über den Menüpfad **Fehlerprotokoll • Globale Konfiguration** die Auswahl in der Auswahlliste **Fehlerprotokollebene** von **Sicher** auf **Vollständig** ändern, damit Ihnen auch im Fehlerprotokoll die Bodys von Request und Response angezeigt werden.

Das Fehlerprotokoll zeigt im oberen Teil eine Übersicht über die aufgetretenen Fehler. Wenn Sie dort einen Fehler auswählen und auf **Fehlerkontext** klicken, werden im unteren Teil Informationen über den Kontext angezeigt, in dem der Fehler aufgetreten ist. Dort können Sie sich Request- und Response-Daten anzeigen lassen und in das Anwendungsprotokoll abspringen. Im Anwendungsprotokoll können Sie sich auch den Aufruf-Stack anzeigen lassen und, wenn nötig, im betreffenden Code einen Breakpoint für das externe Debugging setzen.

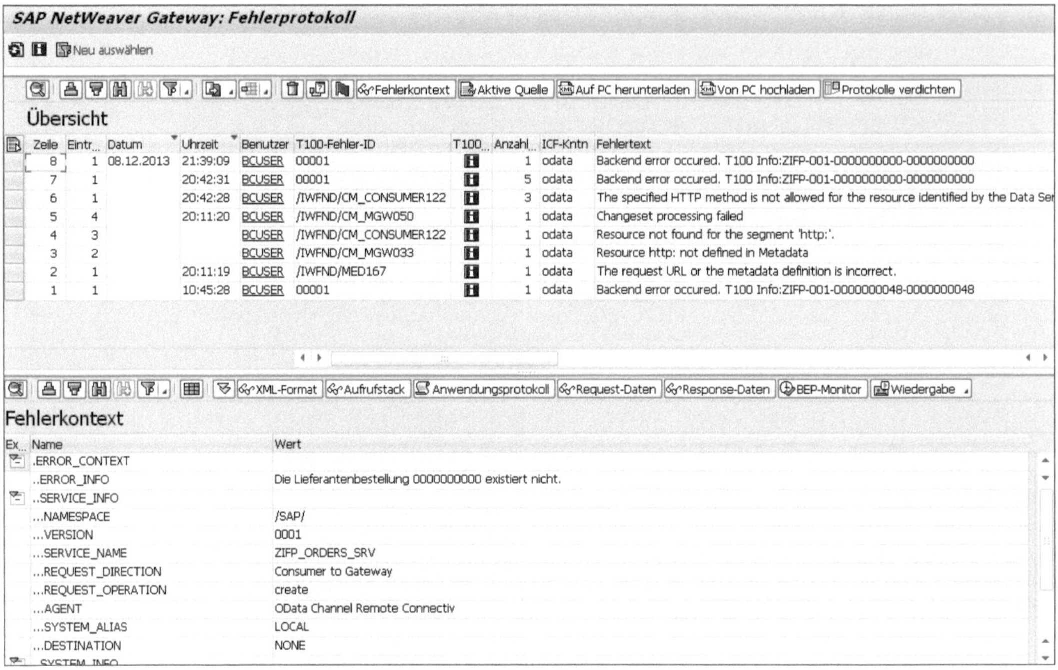

Abbildung 9.19 Fehlerprotokoll in SAP Gateway

9.4 OData-Services mit SAPUI5 konsumieren

Nachdem wir Ihnen gezeigt haben, wie Sie die Daten mit SAP Gateway beschreiben und zugänglich machen, wenden wir uns in den beiden letzten Abschnitten dieses Kapitels der Anzeige der Daten zu. In diesem Abschnitt verwenden wir SAPUI5, ein UI-Framework für die Implementierung von modernen webbasierten Oberflächen.

9.4.1 Überblick über SAPUI5

Serverseitige Integration

Technologien wie Web Dynpro für Java bzw. ABAP oder Business Server Pages (BSP) und HTMLB stellen die klassischen Vertreter der serverseitigen Integration (*Server-side Integration*) im SAP-Umfeld dar. Daten und Anwendungscode werden auf dem Server »zusammengestellt« und an den jeweiligen Client übertragen. Der Client hat dann lediglich die Aufgabe, die erhaltenen Informationen darzustellen. Das Ladeverhalten sowie die Antwortzeiten sind dabei häufig nicht optimal. Besonders im Hinblick auf die Unterstützung verschiedenartiger Clients sind die erwähnten Technologien z. B. oft nicht in der Lage, mit der Entwicklung von Internetbrowsern Schritt zu halten.

Standardbasiertes UI-Framework

Mit SAPUI5 wurde eine UI-Framework implementiert, das heute den De-facto-Standard für die Implementierung von modernen Benutzeroberflächen im SAP-Umfeld darstellt. SAPUI5 bietet Ihnen größtmögliche Offenheit bei der Entwicklung von Webanwendungen. Ist es bei Web Dynpro noch unmöglich, eigene UI-Controls zu implementieren, können Sie dies mit SAPUI5 tun. Im Gegensatz zu Web Dynpro handelt es sich bei SAPUI5 um ein Framework, das auf dem Client ausgeführt wird. Dies stellt einen Paradigmenwechsel für die Implementierung von webbasierten Anwendungen in der SAP-Welt dar. Web Dynpro steht für die serverseitige Integration, während SAPUI5 den clientseitigen Ansatz verfolgt.

Die SAPUI5-Bibliothek stellt sowohl für die Implementierung von Desktop-Anwendungen als auch für die Programmierung von mobilen Anwendungen entsprechende UI-Controls zur Verfügung. Die UI-Controls für mobile Anwendungen sind für die Ausführung auf mobilen Endgeräten optimiert. Es ist aber durchaus auch möglich, auf einem mobilen Gerät entweder einen Mix aus mobilen Controls und nicht mobilen Controls oder nur nicht mobile Controls zu verwenden.

SAPUI5-Laufzeitumgebung

SAPUI5-Anwendungen können dem Endbenutzer durch jeden HTTP-Server zur Verfügung gestellt werden. Somit können SAPUI5-Anwendungen sowohl auf dem SAP NetWeaver Application Server Java als auch auf dem SAP NetWeaver Application Server ABAP installiert werden. SAPUI5-Anwendungen lassen sich auch in der SAP Business Technology Platform (SAP BTP) installieren. Darüber hinaus ist es aber natürlich auch möglich, SAPUI5-Anwendungen, z. B. auf einem Internet Information Server oder einem Tomcat-Webserver, unter der Nutzung von *OpenUI5*, dem Open-Source-Ableger von SAPUI5, bereitzustellen. Grundsätzlich ist die einzige Voraussetzung, dass der Anwendung die SAPUI5-Bibliotheken zur Verfügung gestellt werden.

Entwicklungsumgebung

Für die Entwicklung von SAPUI5-Anwendungen stellt SAP das *SAP Business Application Studio* als Service auf der SAP BTP bereit (siehe Abschnitt 2.4.1). SAP-Kunden, die keinen Zugang zur SAP BTP haben bzw. das SAP Business Application Studio nicht nutzen, können Microsoft Visual Studio Code mit von SAP für die SAPUI5-Entwicklung bereitgestellten Erweiterungen nutzen. In diesem Buch nutzen wir das SAP Business Application Studio für die Implementierung eines SAPUI5-basierten OData-Clients.

Model View Controller

SAPUI5 implementiert ganz klassisch das *MVC-Pattern* (MCV = Model View Controller). Wir gehen davon aus, dass Sie bereits Erfahrung mit diesem Entwurfsmuster haben, und umreißen an dieser Stelle nur kurz dessen Grundpfeiler:

- Das *Model* definiert und enthält die zu verarbeitenden Daten.
- Der *View* stellt die Repräsentationsschicht der Anwendung dar. Er zeigt die zu verarbeitenden Daten an und bietet dem Benutzer die Möglichkeit zur Interaktion mit der Anwendung.
- Der *Controller* implementiert die Datenbeschaffung sowie die Verarbeitung der Benutzerinteraktion.

Die Benutzerinteraktion wird auf dem View durch das Auslösen von Ereignissen (*Events*) durch den Endanwender ausgelöst. Der Controller implementiert für diese Events die entsprechende Verarbeitungslogik (*Event Handler*). Im Event Handler wird, falls nötig, die Kommunikation mit einem Backend-Service ausgeführt. Dieser Service liefert die anzuzeigenden Daten (das Model) zurück. Der Controller stellt nach dem erfolgreichen Aufruf des Service die Daten des Views zur Verfügung.

Datenmodelle

Daten werden bei SAPUI5 in sogenannten *Modellen* gehalten. Es werden folgende Modellarten unterstützt:

- JSON
- OData (V2 und V4)
- XML

Die Daten, die in einem Modell gehalten werden, werden über einen Backend-Service bezogen und in der Anwendung verarbeitet. Der Anwender kann Daten aus einem Modell ändern, neue Datensätze hinzufügen oder bestehende Datensätze löschen.

Datenbindung

Wie bereits angesprochen, ruft der Controller der Anwendung die Dienste im Backend auf. Die gelieferten Daten werden in einem Modellobjekt bereitgestellt und im View für die Bearbeitung durch den Endanwender angeboten. Die Daten des Modells werden an View Controls zur Ein- und Ausgabe gebunden Bei dieser sogenannten *Datenbindung* werden Eigenschaften eines UI-Elements, etwa eines Textfeldes, mit einem Attribut aus dem Modell verbunden. Durch diese Verknüpfung werden Daten aus dem Modell im View erreichbar. Verbindet man z. B. das `text`-Attribut eines Textfeldes mit einem Attribut aus dem Modell, wird der Wert des Modellattributs im Textfeld sichtbar. Dieser Datenfluss ist bidirektional: Gibt der Anwender Daten in das Textfeld ein, werden diese Daten in das Modell übertragen.

One-Way-Binding vs. Two-Way-Binding

Die Übermittlung der Änderungen an einem Modell an das Backend kann entweder aktiv durch den Entwickler über entsprechende Funktionsaufrufe geschehen – man spricht dabei von *One-Way-Binding* – oder aber automatisch durch das Modell durchgeführt werden. Diese Art der Verarbeitung wird *Two-Way-Binding* genannt. SAPUI5 verwendet bei OData standardmäßig das One-Way-Binding. Änderungen werden somit nicht direkt im jeweiligen Backend übernommen, sondern der Entwickler muss die Änderung der Daten über den Aufruf von Methoden auf dem jeweiligen Modellobjekt manuell vornehmen.

9.4.2 Implementierung eines OData-Clients mit SAPUI5

Nach dieser kurzen Einführung in das SAPUI5-Framework wenden wir uns nun der Implementierung einer SAPUI5-Anwendung mit dem SAP Business Application Studio zu. Nach der Anmeldung an der SAP BTP wechseln Sie in den Bereich **Services • Instances and Subscriptions**. Hier sehen Sie eine Liste der im ausgewählten Subaccount verfügbaren Anwendungen (siehe Abbildung 9.20). 9

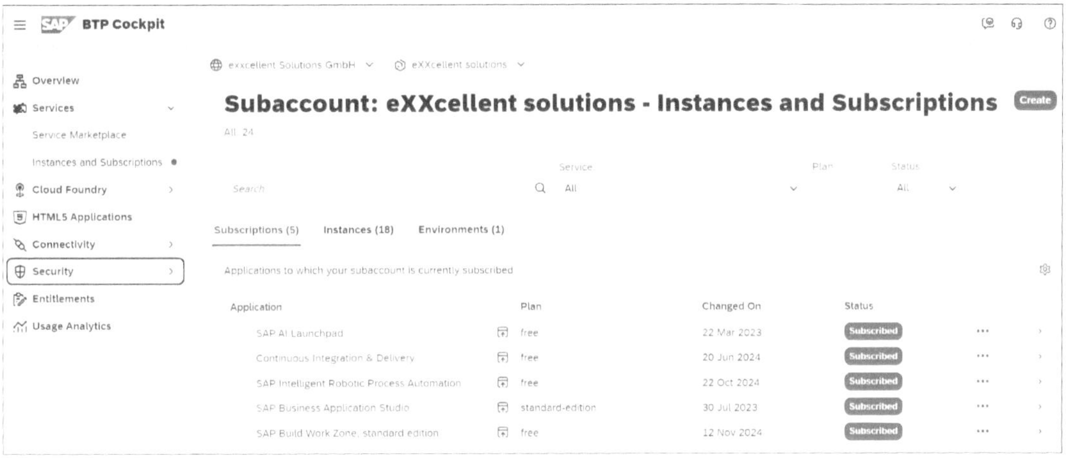

Abbildung 9.20 Die im Subaccount verfügbaren Anwendungen

SAP Business Application Studio starten

Um das SAP Business Application Studio zu starten, klicken Sie auf das Symbol (**Go to Application**). Im Anschluss wird das SAP Business Application Studio gestartet. Nach dem erfolgreichen Start wird Ihnen das in Abbildung 9.21 gezeigte Bild zur Erstellung eines *Dev Space* angezeigt. Ein Dev Space im SAP Business Application Studio dient dazu, Entwicklungsprojekte zu organisieren und zu strukturieren. Ein Dev Space ist technisch gesehen eine virtuelle Maschine, die mit dem Linux-Betriebssystem betrieben wird. SAP bietet unterschiedliche Dev-Space-Typen an. Sie verfügen jeweils über vordefinierte Funktionsumfänge und werden für unterschiedliche Entwicklungsaufgaben und Ziele verwendet. Ein Dev Space kann nicht zwischen

Entwicklern geteilt oder gar zur parallelen Entwicklung verwendet werden. Hierfür wird eine separate zur Verfügung zu stellende Versionskontrollsoftware benötigt.

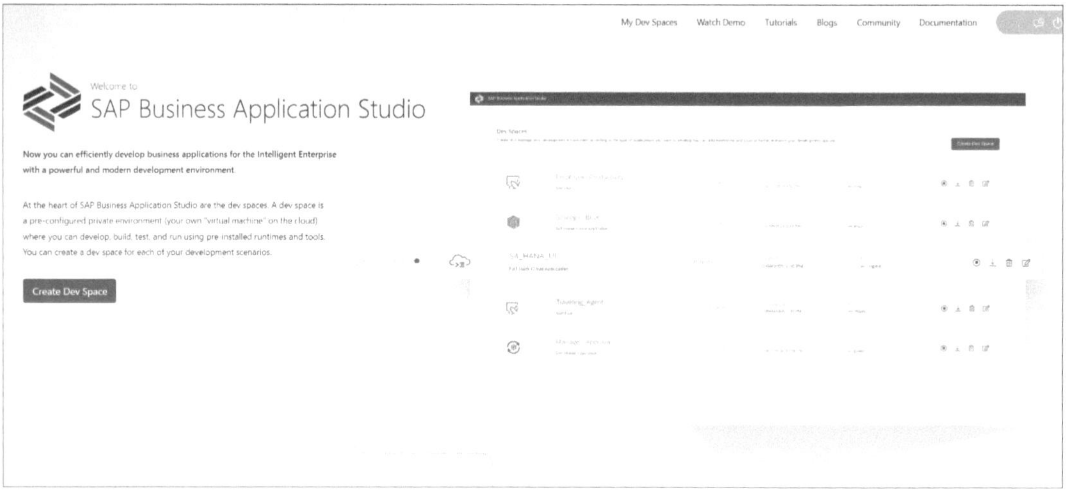

Abbildung 9.21 Startbildschirm des SAP Business Application Studios

Dev Space anlegen

Um einen neuen Dev Space anzulegen, gehen Sie wie folgt vor:

1. Klicken Sie links auf den Button **Create Dev Space**. Sie werden zum entsprechende Bild weitergeleitet.
2. Geben Sie in das links oberen angebotene Eingabefeld »UI5DevSpace« als Bezeichner für unseren neuen Dev Space ein (siehe Abbildung 9.22). Da wir eine SAPUI5-Anwendung implementieren wollen, belassen Sie es bei der Auswahl des Dev-Space-Typs **SAP Fiori**.
3. Die auf der rechten Seite dargestellten und vorausgewählten Werkzeuge sind in dem neu anzulegenden Dev Space für unsere Zwecke ausreichend. Klicken Sie erneut auf **Create Dev Space**.
4. Sie gelangen zu dem in Abbildung 9.23 gezeigten Bild, auf dem Sie den Dev-Space-Anlageprozess verfolgen können.
5. Die Dauer des Startvorgangs eines Dev Spaces kann je nach dessen Größe variieren. Dev Spaces, die bereits eine größere Menge an Projekten beinhalten, benötigen für das Starten länger als, ein noch leerer Dev Space, wie in unserem Fall. Nachdem der Dev Space gestartet ist, ändert sich dessen Status von **STARTING** zu **RUNNING**.

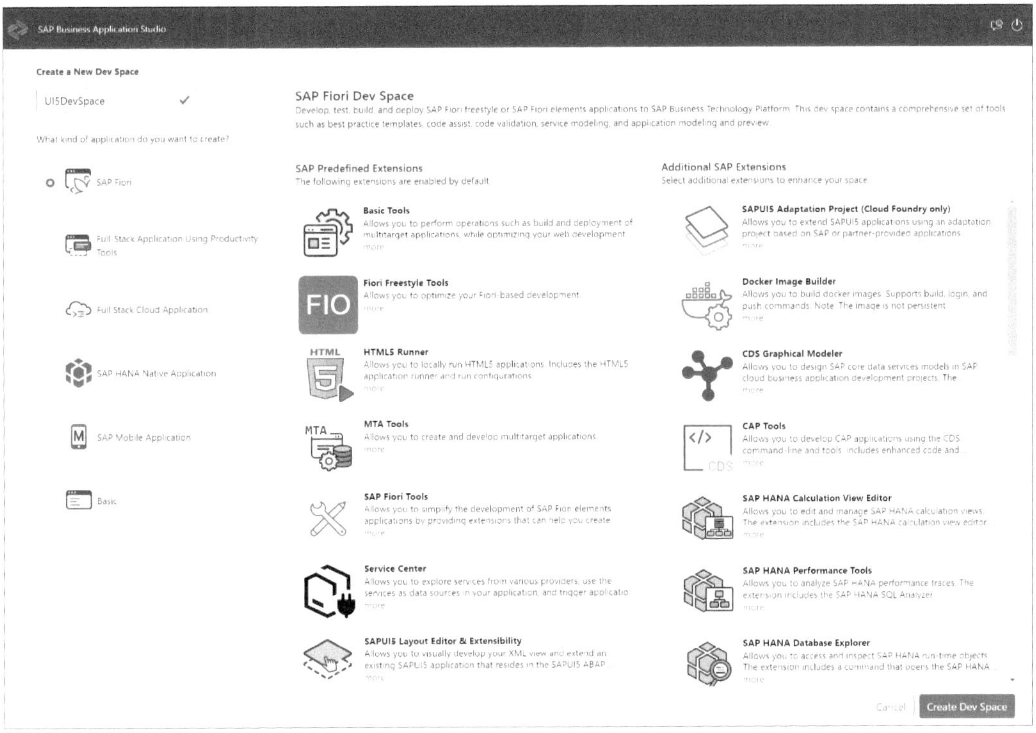

Abbildung 9.22 Anlegen eines Dev Space vom Typ »SAP Fiori«

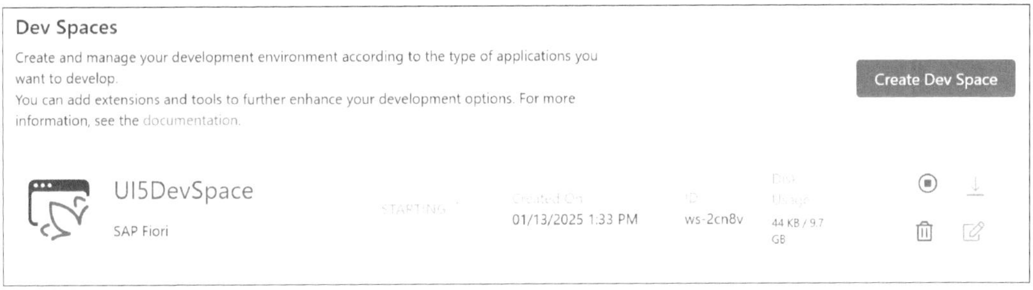

Abbildung 9.23 Startender Dev Space im SAP Business Application Studio

6. Öffnen Sie den Dev Space, indem Sie auf den als Link hervorgehobenen Dev-Space-Name klicken. Sie werden zur Startseite des SAP Business Application Studios weitergeleitet (siehe Abbildung 9.24).

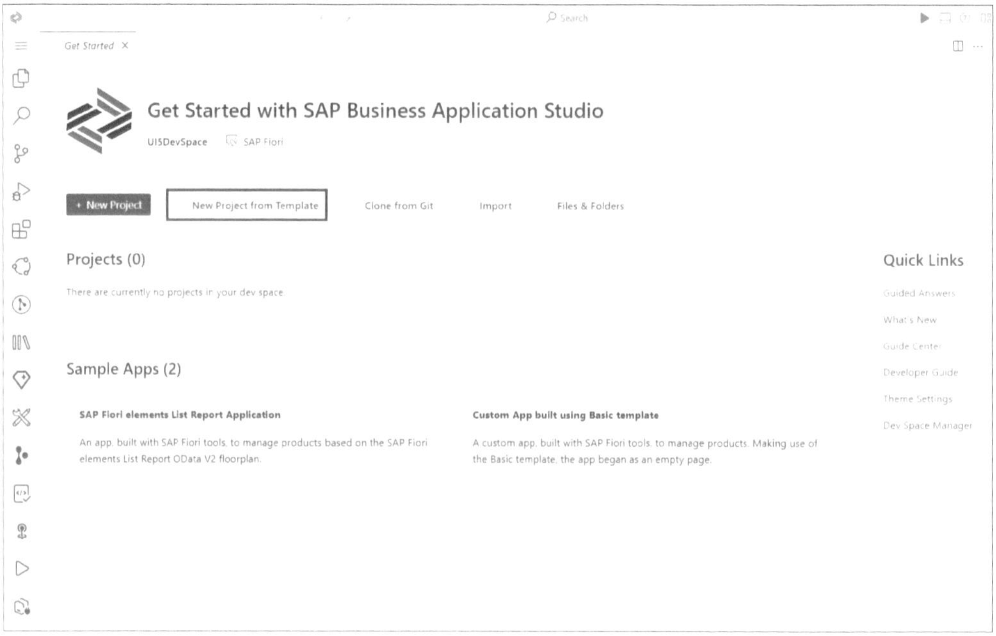

Abbildung 9.24 Startseite des SAP Business Application Studios

Neues Projekt anlegen

Als Nächstes müssen Sie ein neues Projekt für die Entwicklung einer SAPUI5-Anwendung erstellen. Klicken Sie auf den Button **New Project from Template.** Sie gelangen zu dem in Abbildung 9.25 gezeigten Bild zur Auswahl der zu verwendenden Projektvorlage. Es stehen Ihnen drei Vorlagen zur Auswahl:

- Die Vorlage **Basic Multitarget Application** dient zur Erstellung von SAP-Cloud-Anwendungen.
- Die Vorlage **SAPUI5 Adaptation Projekt** wird verwendet, um bestehende SAP-Fiori-Anwendungen zu erweitern.
- Die dritte Vorlage, **SAP Fiori generator**, verwendet man zur Implementierung von SAPUI5-Freestyle- oder SAP-Fiori-Anwendungen.

Da wir eine SAPUI5-Anwendung erstellen möchten, wählen Sie **SAP Fiori generator** aus und klicken im Anschluss auf den Button **Start**. Im nächsten Bild können Sie eine konkrete Projektvorlage auswählen (siehe Abbildung 9.26). Die verfügbaren Vorlagen lassen sich in zwei Kategorien unterteilen: Die Vorlage **Basic** dient zur Implementierung von SAPUI5-Freestyle Anwendungen. Die restlichen Vorlagen werden bei der Implementierung von SAP-Fiori-Anwendungen verwendet. Wählen Sie für unser Projekt die Vorlage **Basic** aus und klicken Sie im Anschluss auf den Button **Next**.

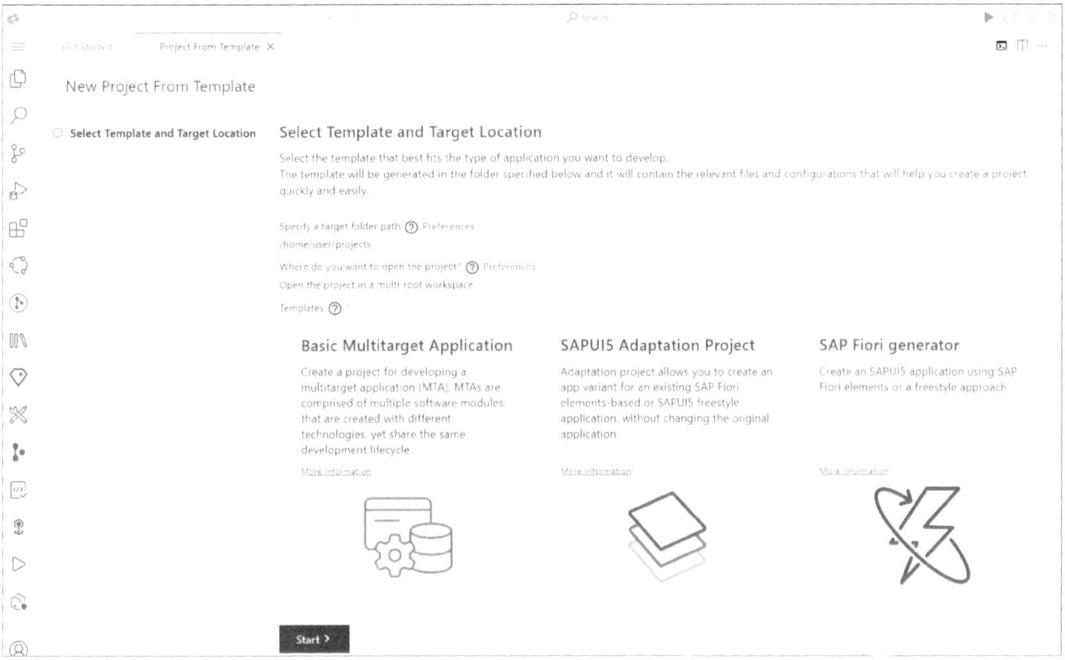

Abbildung 9.25 Verfügbare Projektvorlagen im Dev Space

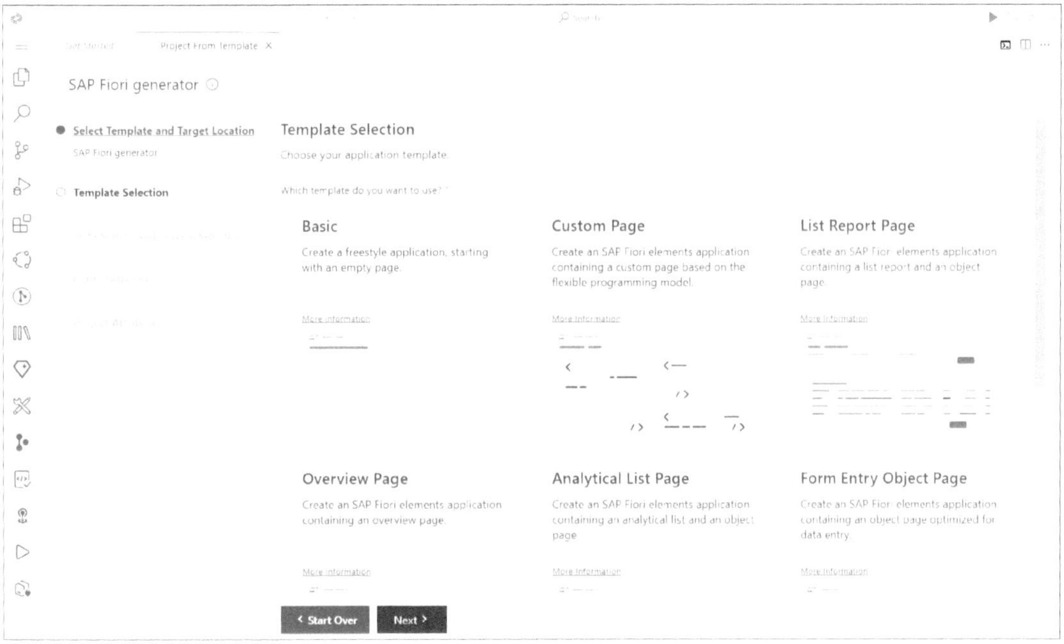

Abbildung 9.26 Projektvorlagen für die SAPUI5- und SAP-Fiori-Anwendungsentwicklung

OData-Service auswählen

Im darauffolgenden Schritt muss OData-Service ausgewählt werden, dessen Daten die Anwendung verarbeiten soll. Wählen Sier dazu in der Auswahlliste **Data source** den Eintrag **Connect to a System** aus. Im Feld **System** wählen Sie die in Abschnitt 2.2.3, »Einführung in den Cloud Connector«, angelegte Destination aus. Nach kurzer Wartezeit geben Sie in den Feldern **Username** und **Password** die Anmeldedaten Ihres SAP-Benutzers ein. Bestätigen Sie diese Eingaben mit ↵. Nach erneuter kurzer Wartezeit können Sie im Auswahlmenü **Service** einen OData-Service auswählen. Abbildung 9.27 zeigt die entsprechenden Eingaben.

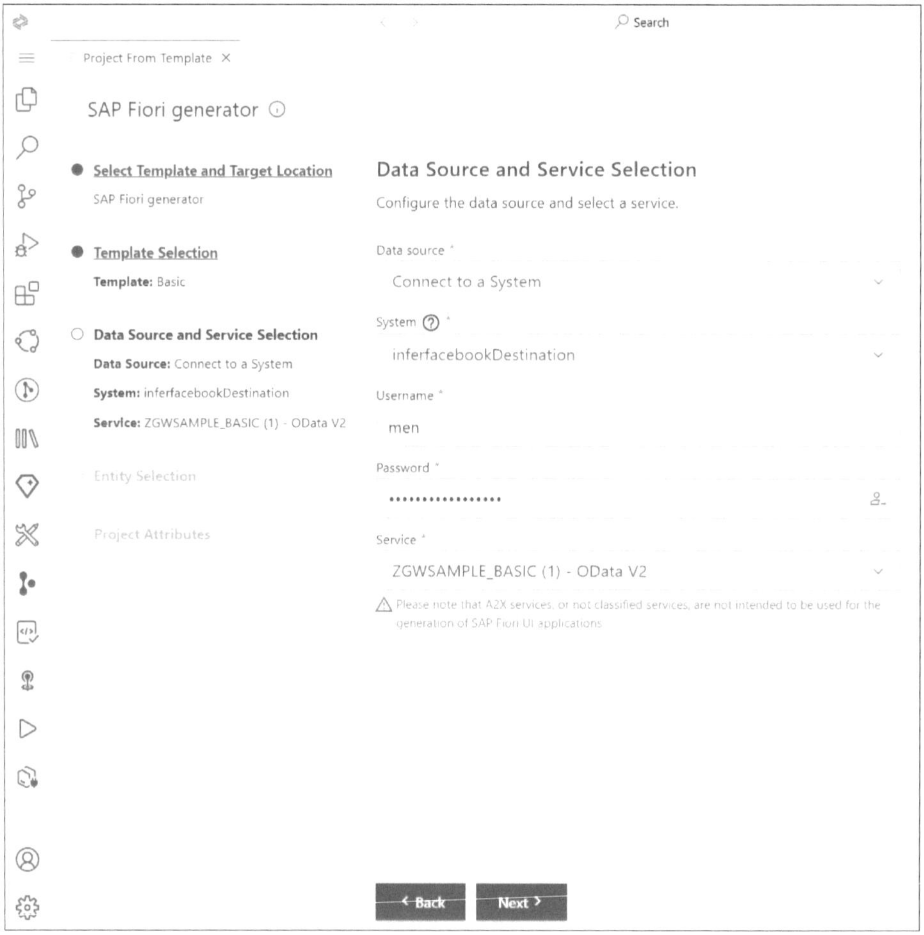

Abbildung 9.27 OData-Service auswählen

View angeben

Nachdem Sie diese Informationen zur Datenquelle der Anwendung eingegeben haben, bestätigen Sie mit **Next**. Im nächsten Bild müssen Sie einen Namen für den View der SAPUI5-Anwendung eingeben. Lassen Sie sich dabei nicht von der irreführenden Überschrift **Entity Selection** irritieren. Geben Sie den View-Namen »OrderDataView« ein und bestätigen Sie mit **Next** (siehe Abbildung 9.28).

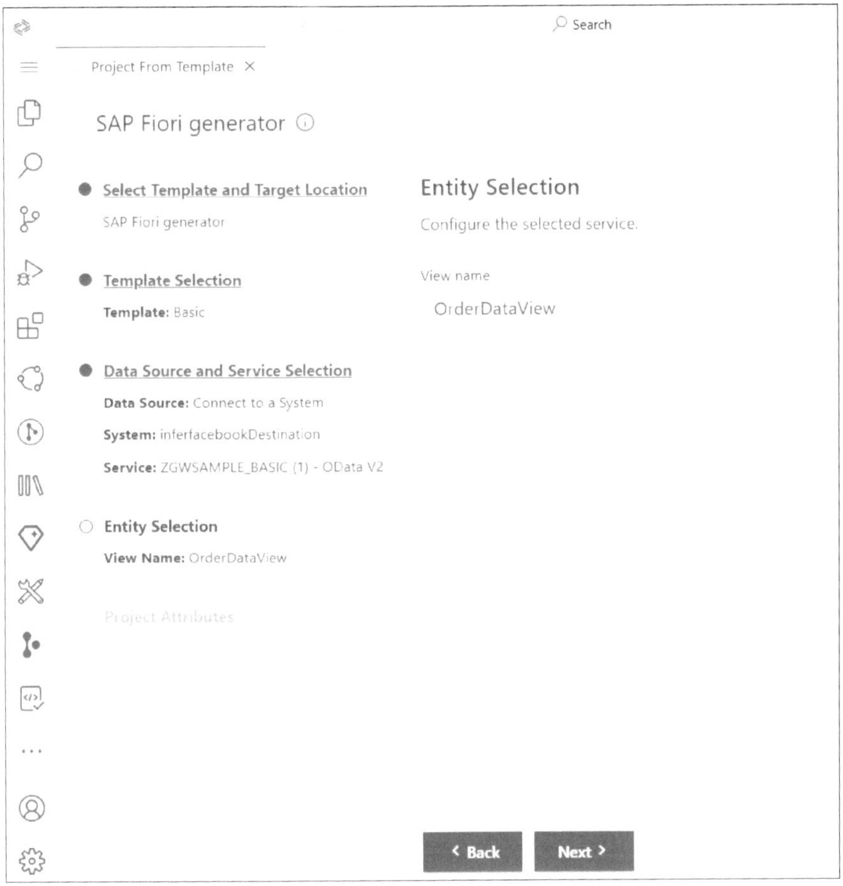

Abbildung 9.28 Eingabe des View-Namens

Projektdetails

Nachdem Sie den View-Namen bestätigt haben, werden Sie gebeten, die Projektdetails anzugeben (siehe Abbildung 9.29). Geben Sie in das Feld **Module name** den Wert »ui5odataexmpale« ein, vergeben Sie im Feld **Application titel** den Anwendungsnamen »Interface programming book« und geben Sie im Feld **Application namepace** den Namensraum »demo.ui5.odata« an. Bei den anderen Feldern können Sie es bei den vorgeschlagenen Werten belassen. Starten Sie nun die Anlage des Projekts mit einem Klick auf den Button **Finish**.

Nachdem alle Projektartefakte generiert wurden, werden Siegefragt, ob Sie das neue Projekt zu Ihrem Workspace hinzufügen möchten (siehe Abbildung 9.30). Bestätigen Sie dies mit einem Klick auf **Add project to workspace**.

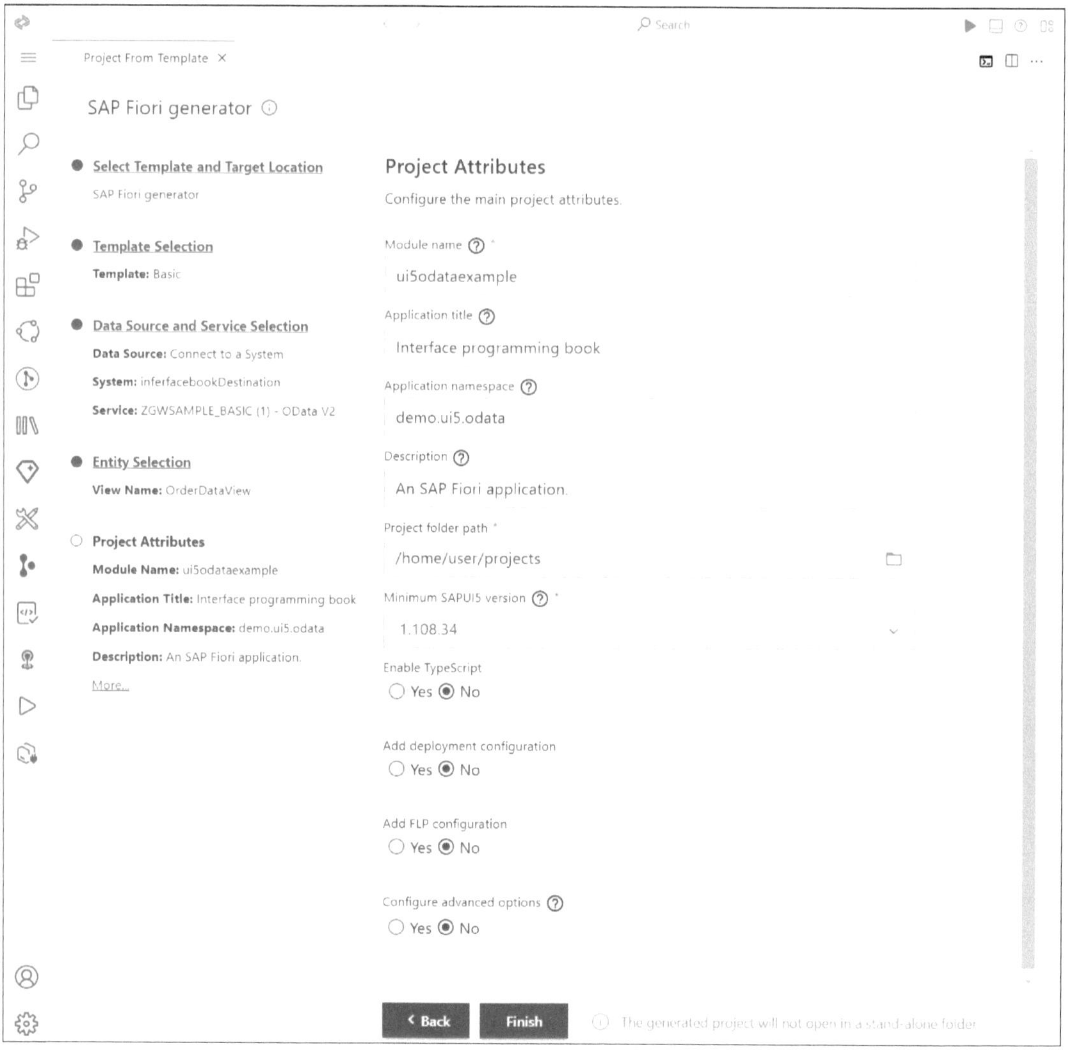

Abbildung 9.29 Eingabe der Projektdetails

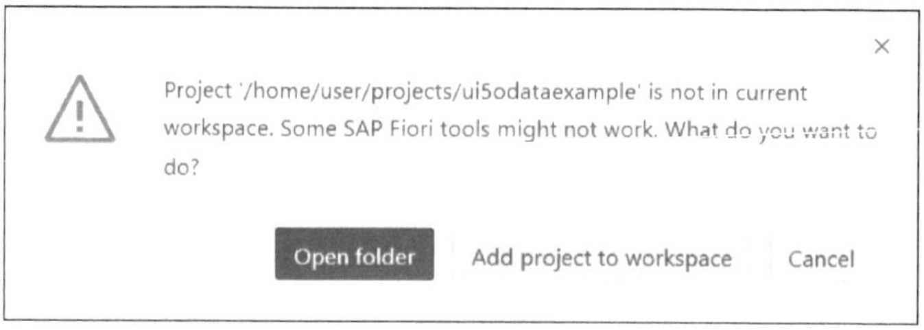

Abbildung 9.30 Hinweis zum Workspace

Fehlerquelle bei der Projekterzeugung

Achten Sie darauf, keine Mausaktionen im Browserfenster durchzuführen, während das Projekt im SAP Business Application Studio generiert wird. Dies führt sehr oft dazu, dass beim Anlegen des Projekts Abhängigkeiten zu anderen, wichtigen Modulen nicht erzeugt werden. Dass das Projekt gerade angelegt wird, erkennen Sie daran, dass in der unteren rechten Ecke des Browserfensters ein entsprechender Hinweis angezeigt wird.

Nachdem das Projekt dem Workspace hinzugefügt wurde, wird das Projekt im Explorer angezeigt. Zusätzlich werden Ihnen hier die Anwendungsinformationen und Projektdetails angezeigt (siehe Abbildung 9.31)

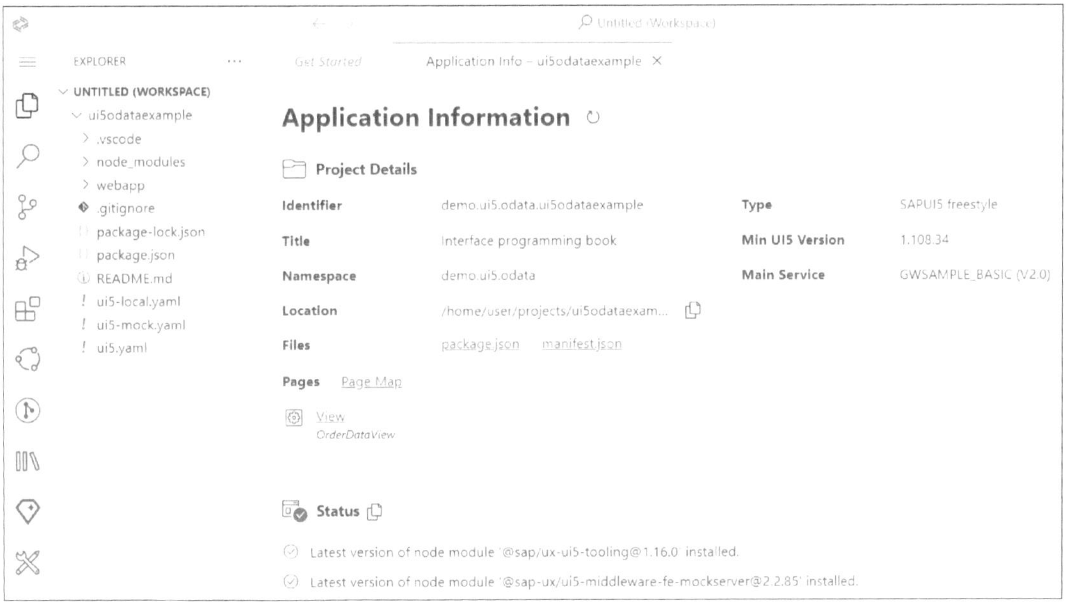

Abbildung 9.31 Informationen zur Anwendung und Projektdetails

Projektstruktur

Bevor Sie mit der Implementierung der Anwendung beginnen, sehen Sie sich die vollständige Projektstruktur in Abbildung 9.32 einmal genauer an. Im Ordner **ui5odataexample** gibt es einen Ordner namens **node_modules**. Das SAP Business Application Studio nutzt *Node.js*. Der Ordner **node_modules** ist ein zentraler Bestandteil von Node.js-Projekten und enthält alle Abhängigkeiten (*Dependencies*), die für das Projekt erforderlich sind.

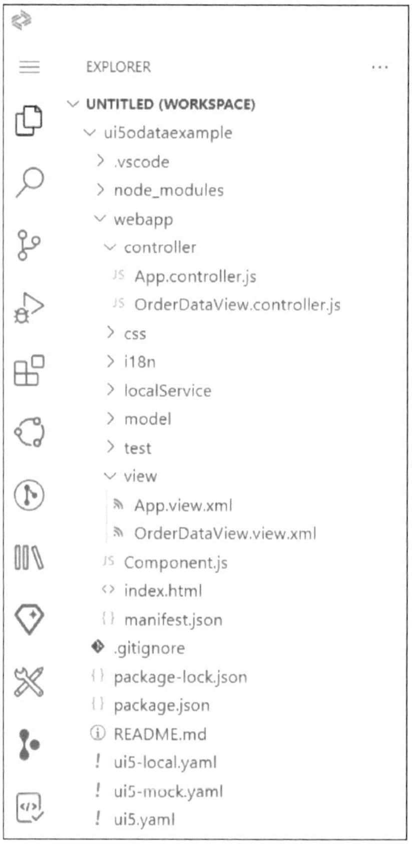

Abbildung 9.32 Struktur eines SAPUI5-Projekts

[»]

Node.js

Node.js ist eine plattformübergreifende Open-Source-Laufzeitumgebung, die es ermöglicht, JavaScript auf Servern auszuführen. Traditionell wurde JavaScript nur im Webbrowser verwendet, um Interaktivität auf Webseiten zu ermöglichen. Node.js hat JavaScript auch für serverseitige Anwendungen nutzbar gemacht.

Der Ordner »webapp«

Der Code zum SAPUI5-Projekt befindet sich im Order **webapp**. Dieser enthält diverse Unterordner und Dateien. Wir werden an dieser Stelle nicht auf alle Unterordner eingehen, sondern nur die für unser Beispiel wichtigen besprechen.

Jede SAPUI5-Anwendung wird als wiederverwendbare *Komponente* implementiert. Diese Komponenten werden über eine Datei namens **Component.js** implementiert. Sie ist dafür zuständig, dass alle für die Ausführung benötigen Sourcen und Abhängigkeiten zur Verfügung gestellt werden und von der Anwendung bzw. durch Code verwendet werden können.

Die Konfigurationsinformationen werden nicht direkt in der Datei **Component.js** hinterlegt, sondern der Komponente über eine Konfigurationsdatei zur Verfügung gestellt. Diese Konfigurationsdatei trägt den Namen **manifest.json** und istebenso Bestandteil des **webapp**-Ordners.

Datenquellen und Modelle

In die Datei **manifest.json** werden im Rahmen der Projekterzeugung viele der im Wizard eingegebenen Informationen geschrieben. Den Inhalt dieser Datei für unser Projekt (im JSON-Format) zeigt Listing 9.13. Sie enthält verschiedene Konfigurationsobjekte auf unterschiedlichen Ebenen. Das Objekt `sap.app` beispielsweise enthält neben einer eindeutigen ID, über die man die SAPUI5-Anwendung in der Anwendungslandschaft identifizieren kann, auch das Konfigurationsobjekt für Datenquellen. Dieses Objekt heißt `dataSources`. WIn unserem Beispiel enthält es den URI des zu verwendenden OData-Services.

9

```
{
    "_version": "1.65.0",
    "sap.app": {
        "id": "demo.ui5.odata.ui5odataexample",
        "type": "application",
        "i18n": "i18n/i18n.properties",
        "applicationVersion": {
            "version": "0.0.1"
        },
        "title": "{{appTitle}}",
        "description": "{{appDescription}}",
        "resources": "resources.json",
        "sourceTemplate": {
            "id": "@sap/generator-fiori:basic",
            "version": "1.17.3",
            "toolsId": "3cc8f998-6ba7-43b1-b231-e11469ddf58a"
        },
        "dataSources": {
            "mainService": {
                "uri": "/sap/opu/odata/iwbep/GWSAMPLE_BASIC/",
                "type": "OData",
                "settings": {
                    "annotations": [],
                    "localUri": "localService/metadata.xml",
                    "odataVersion": "2.0"
                }
```

```
            }
        }
    },
```

Listing 9.13 Konfigurationselemente in der Datei »manifest.json«

Modellkonfiguration

Die in Listing 9.13 definierte Datenquelle wird zur Laufzeit der Anwendung für die Kommunikation mit dem OData-Service verwendet. Die Anwendung greift selbst nicht direkt auf die Datenquelle zu, sondern über ein Modell. Dessen Quellcode kann entweder manuell programmiert oder über eine Konfiguration in der Datei **manifest.json** erzeugt werden. Die automatische Konfiguration über die Datei **manifest.json** ist die empfohlene Variante. Zur Konfiguration solcher Modelle wird hier das Konfigurationsobjekt `models` verwendet. Dieses Objekt befindet sich im Hauptkonfigurationsobjekt `sap.ui5`.

Listing 9.14 zeigt die Konfiguration zweier Modelle. Zunächst wird ein Modell mit der ID `i18n` definiert. Dieses dient zur Bereitstellung sprachabhängiger Texte. Diese werden auf Basis der verwendeten Sprache bereitgestellt. Bei dem zweiten Modell mit einer leeren `Id`-Angabe handelt es sich um das sogenannte *Default-Modell*. Dieses Modell verweist durch die Angabe im Objekt `mainService` beim Attribut `dataSource` auf die in Listing 9.13 definierte Datenquelle.

```
"sap.ui5": {
        "flexEnabled": true,
        "dependencies": {
            "minUI5Version": "1.108.34",
            "libs": {
                "sap.m": {},
                "sap.ui.core": {}
            }
        },
        "contentDensities": {
            "compact": true,
            "cozy": true
        },
        "models": {
            "i18n": {
                "type": "sap.ui.model.resource.ResourceModel",
                "settings": {
                    "bundleName":
                        "demo.ui5.odata.ui5odataexample.i18n.i18n"
                }
```

```
        },
        "": {
            "dataSource": "mainService",
            "preload": true,
            "settings": {}
        }
    },
```

Listing 9.14 Modellkonfiguration in der Datei »manifest.json«

Controller und Views

Wie einleitend bereits erläutert, folgt SAPUI5 dem MVC-Entwicklungsmuster. Dies spiegelt sich auch in der Projektstruktur wider. Views werden im Order **view** und Controller im Ordner **controller** implementiert. Wie in Abbildung 9.32 erkennbar, enthalten beide Ordner jeweils zwei Dateien. Im **view**-Ordner wurde neben der Datei **OrderDataView.view.xml** eine Datei **App.view.xml** angelegt. Zu jedem View wird im **controller**-Ordner ein Controller angelegt. Die Datei **OrderDataView.view.xml** wurde auf Basis unserer Angaben während er Projektanlage erzeugt. Die Datei **App.view.xml** ist der Einstiegspunkt in unsere Anwendung und enthält Basis-Code für die Darstellung des gesamten Anwendungsrahmens. Listing 9.15 zeigt die Implementierung dieser Datei. Das zentrale Objekt in der Implementierung ist die Klasse `sap.m.App`.

```
<mvc:View
    controllerName="demo.ui5.odata.ui5odataexample.controller.App"
    xmlns:html="http://www.w3.org/1999/xhtml"
    xmlns:mvc="sap.ui.core.mvc" displayBlock="true"
    xmlns="sap.m">
    <App id="app">
    </App>
</mvc:View>
```

Listing 9.15 Die Datei »App.view.xml«

Benutzeroberfläche implementieren

Benutzeroberfläche

Als Nächstes wenden wir uns der Implementierung der Benutzeroberfläche, des User Interface (UI), zu. Die Oberfläche soll möglichst einfach sein; aus diesem Grund implementieren wir eine einfache Tabelle zur Darstellung der Bestellköpfe. Hierzu öffnen Sie die Datei **OrderDataView.view.xml** im Code-Editor. Der vom Codegenerator erzeugte Code entspricht dem in Listing 9.16 gezeigten Programmcode.

```
<mvc:View controllerName=
        "demo.ui5.odata.ui5odataexample.controller.OrderDataView"
    xmlns:mvc="sap.ui.core.mvc" displayBlock="true"
    xmlns="sap.m">
    <Page id="page" title="{i18n>title}">
        <content />
    </Page>
</mvc:View>
```

Listing 9.16 Basisimplementierung des Interface »OrderDataViewUser«

Zunächst fügen Sie in die `content`-Aggregation des `Page`-Controls, das die Seite darstellt, ein Tabellen-Control vom Typ `sap.m.Table` ein und definieren zusätzlich das Attribut `items`. Das `items`-Attribut binden Sie an das Entity Set `Ordersheaders` aus dem OData-Service. Zusätzlich fügen Sie, wie Sie Listing 8.14 entnehmen können, eine Toolbar, also eine Funktionsleiste, hinzu.

```
<Page title="{i18n>title}">
       <content>
          <Table items="{ path: '/Orderheaders' }"
                id="idTable">
             <headerToolbar>
               <Toolbar id="idToolbar">
                 <Title text="Bestellungen" level="H2"
                 id="idTitle"/>
               </Toolbar>
             </headerToolbar>
          </Table>
       </content>
</Page>
```

Listing 9.17 Tabelle »Orders« mit den Bestellungen implementieren

Als Nächstes implementieren wir die Spalten der Tabelle `Orders`. Hierzu fügen Sie die `columns`-Aggregation zur Tabelle aus Listing 9.17 hinzu. Wir wollen dabei alle Eigenschaften der Entität `Orderheader` darstellen, die die Spaltenüberschriften der Tabelle repräsentiert. Da wir uns nicht um die Übersetzung der einzelnen Spaltenüberschriften kümmern wollen, greifen wir direkt auf die über die Metadaten gelieferten Informationen zu. Die Implementierung können Sie Listing 9.18 entnehmen.

```
<columns>
  <Column hAlign="Center" minScreenWidth="Tablet" id="col1">
       <Text text="{/#Orderheader/OrderId/@sap:label}" id="txt1"/>
  </Column>
  <Column hAlign="Center" minScreenWidth="Tablet"
          demandPopin="true" id="col2">
       <Text text="{/#Orderheader/OrderDate/@sap:label}"
             id="txt2"/>
  </Column>
  <Column hAlign="Center" minScreenWidth="Tablet"
          demandPopin="true" id="col3">>
        <Text text="{/#Orderheader/Seller/@sap:label}"
              id="txt3"/>
  </Column>
  <Column hAlign="Center" minScreenWidth="Tablet"
          demandPopin="true" id="col4">>
       <Text text="{/#Orderheader/Buyer/@sap:label}"
             id="txt4"/>
  </Column>
  <Column hAlign="Center" id="col5">>
       <Text text="{/#Orderheader/ReferenceId/@sap:label}"
             id="txt5"/>
  </Column>
  <Column hAlign="Center" minScreenWidth="Tablet"
          demandPopin="true" id="col6">>
       <Text text="{/#Orderheader/Ordertype/@sap:label}"
             id="txt6"/>
  </Column>
</columns>
```

Listing 9.18 »columns«-Aggregation implementieren

Den Abschluss der Tabellenimplementierung bildet die Ausprägung der `items`-Aggregation für die Tabellenzeilen. Wir nutzen dabei als Template ein Element vom Typ `sap.m.ColumnListItem`. Dieses Element besitzt eine Aggregation mit dem Namen `cells`. Dieser Aggregation fügen wir für jede Eigenschaft der `Orderheader`-Entität ein entsprechendes UI-Control hinzu. Die Implementierung können Sie Listing 9.19 entnehmen.

```
<items>
    <ColumnListItem  id="cli1">
        <cells>
            <ObjectIdentifier text="{OrderId}" id="c1"/>
```

9

```
            <Text text="{path:'OrderDate'}" id="c2"/>
            <Text text="{Seller}" id="c3"/>
            <Text text="{Buyer}" id="c4"/>
            <Text text="{ReferenceId}" id="c5"/>
            <Text text="{Ordertype}" id="c6"/>
        </cells>
    </ColumnListItem>
</items>
```

Listing 9.19 »items«-Aggregation implementieren

Anwendung testen

Nachdem Sie die Tabellenimplementierung abgeschlossen haben, können Sie die Anwendung testen. Hierzu klicken Sie mit der rechten Maustaste einfach auf den Projektordner **ui5odataexample** aus und wählen im Kontextmenü **Preview Application**. Es öffnet sich ein neues Browserfenster, und Sie werden über ein Pop-up-Fenster nach einem Benutzernamen und einem Passwort gefragt. Hier geben Sie Ihren SAP-Benutzer und das dazugehörige Passwort ein und bestätigen den Dialog. Nachdem unsere Anwendung vollständig geladen wurde, werden die Bestellköpfe aus dem SAP-System dargestellt (siehe Abbildung 9.33).

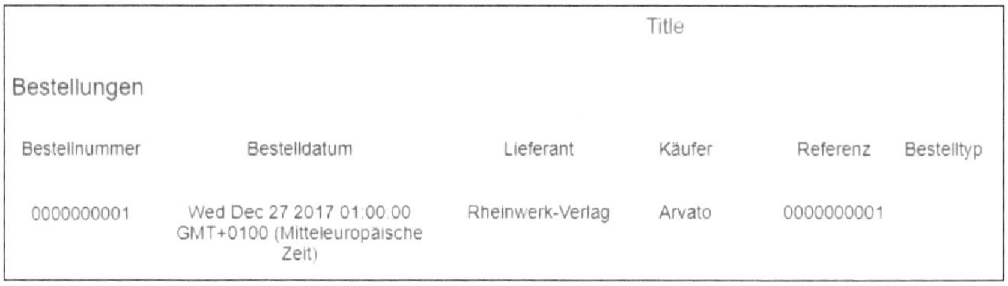

Title

Bestellungen

Bestellnummer	Bestelldatum	Lieferant	Käufer	Referenz	Bestelltyp
0000000001	Wed Dec 27 2017 01:00:00 GMT+0100 (Mitteleuropäische Zeit)	Rheinwerk-Verlag	Arvato	0000000001	

Abbildung 9.33 Daten aus dem SAP-Backend anzeigen

[»]

Pop-up-Blocker

Sollte das in Abbildung 9.33 gezeigte Browserfenster sich nicht öffnen, kann dies an der Verwendung eines Pop-up-Blockers liegen. Akzeptieren Sie in diesem Fall das Anzeigen von Pop-up-Fenstern durch das SAP Business Application Studio. Die Einstellung kann unter Umständen nur für die aktuelle Sitzung gelten, sodass Sie nach dem nächsten Anmelden erneut das Öffnen von Pop-up-Fenstern erlauben müssen.

Cross-Origin Resource Sharing (CORS)

Möglicherweise stellen Sie sich an dieser Stelle die Frage, warum es beim Zugriff aus dem SAP Business Application Studio auf das Backend zu keiner Ausnahme aus der Kategorie *Cross-Origin Resource Sharing* (CORS) kommt. Eine solche Ausnahme wird durch den Browser ausgelöst, wenn ein Konsument auf einen Service zugreift, der nicht vom gleichen System unter der Verwendung des gleichen Protokolls und Ports kommt. Die Antwort darauf ist relativ einfach: Für den Browser greift die SAPUI5-Anwendung nicht auf einen Service auf einem anderen System zu, da das SAP Business Application Studio beim Aufruf der Anwendung den Request auf den OData-Service abfängt und über die Destination leitet, die wir in der SAP BTP angelegt haben. Sie können sich hierzu die Datei **ui5.yaml** im Projektverzeichnis unserer Anwendung anschauen. Wie Sie in Listing 9.20 erkennen können, gibt es eine Middleware-Konfiguration für den Zugriff auf den Pfad **/sap**, und dabei handelt es sich genau um das Präfix des ICF-Wurzelknotens (Internet Communication Framework), unter dem u. a. die OData-Services erreichbar sind *(/sap/opu)*. Wie Sie weiter erkennen können, werden alle Anfragen an diesen URI an die Destination aus der SAP BTP weitergereicht. Durch diese Route stellt CORS kein Problem dar, und wir müssen für die Entwicklung im SAP Business Application Studio und das Testen der Anwendung keinerlei infrastrukturelle Maßnahmen, wie beispielsweise die Installation eines Reverse-Proxys (z. B. des SAP Web Dispatchers) veranlassen.


```
specVersion: "3.1"
metadata:
  name: demo.ui5.odata.ui5odataexample
type: application
server:
  customMiddleware:
    - name: fiori-tools-proxy
      afterMiddleware: compression
      configuration:
        ignoreCertError: false
        ui5:
          path:
            - /resources
            - /test-resources
          url: https://ui5.sap.com
        backend:
          - scp: true
            path: /sap
```

```
        url: https://inferfacebookdestination.dest
        destination: inferfacebookDestination
```

Listing 9.20 Auszug aus der Datei »ui5.yaml«

Bestellung anlegen

Wir wollen die Anwendung so erweitern, dass es dem Anwender im gleichen View möglich ist, eine neue Bestellung anzulegen. Hierzu erweitern wir einerseits den View mit einem Button und weisen dem Event `press` diesen einen Event Handler `onCreatePress` zu. Als Nächstes prägen wir die Funktion `onCreatePress` im Controller des Views aus. Die Funktion erzeugt ein Dialogobjekt auf der Basis eines Fragments. Wir verzichten an dieser Stelle darauf, die Implementierung des Fragments zu zeigen, und verweisen auf die implementierte Lösung, die Sie im Download-Bereich dieses Buchs unter *www.sap-press.de/5955* im Bereich **Materialien** herunterladen können. Nachdem der Dialog instanziiert worden ist, beziehen wir eine Referenz auf das OData-Modell und rufen auf dieser Referenz die Funktion `createEntry` auf. Die Funktion `createEntry` erzeugt ein neues Objekt des übergebenen Entity-Typs und liefert ein `BindingContext`-Objekt zurück. Dieses Objekt binden wir an den Dialog. Listing 9.21 zeigt die Implementierung der `onCreatePress`-Funktion.

```
onCreatePress : function(oEvent) {
        var oView = this.getView();
        //Erstellen eines Dialogs
        var oModel = this.getOwnerComponent().getModel();
        var oBindingContext =
            oModel.createEntry("Orderheaders");
        this._oDialog.bindElement(oBindingContext.getPath());
        this._oDialog.open();
}
```

Listing 9.21 Funktion »onCreatePress« implementieren

Im Dialog selbst lösen wir das Anlegen einer neuen Bestellung ebenfalls durch einen Event Handler aus. Durch die Verwendung des Two-Way-Bindings ist die Implementierung, wie Sie aus Listing 9.22 ersehen können, sehr einfach. Sie rufen lediglich auf dem OData-Modellobjekt die Funktion `submitChanges` auf. Hiermit veranlassen Sie den Aufruf der `createEntity`-Methode für die Entität `Orderheader`.

```
onCreateOrder : function(oEvent) {
       var oModel = this.getOwnerComponent().getModel();
```

```
        var mParameter = {
                success : this._handleCreateOrderSucess,
                error: this._handleCreateOrderError
                        };
                        oModel.submitChanges(mParameter);
}
```

Listing 9.22 Event Handler »onCreateOrder« implementieren

Für das Update und das Löschen von Objekten über den OData-Service liefert das OData-Modell die Funktionen `update` und `remove`. Wir zeigen die Implementierung dieser beiden Funktionen an dieser Stelle nicht, sondern verweisen Sie auf die Beispielimplementierung, die Sie auf der Download-Seite zum Buch herunterladen können.

Funktionsimport aufrufen

Den Abschluss unserer SAPUI5-Implementierung stellt der Aufruf des Funktionsimports `MostRecentOrderOfBuyer` dar. Wir fügen im ersten Schritt einen neuen Button in die Toolbar der Tabelle aus dem View `OrderDataView.view.xml` ein und weisen dem press-Event die Funktion `onGetMostRecentOrderOfBuyer` zu. Nachdem Sie die Änderungen im View gespeichert haben, öffnen Sie den Controller **OrderDataView.controller.js** und fügen eine neue Funktion mit dem Namen `onGetMostRecentOrderOfBuyer` ein. Wie Sie dem Programmierbeispiel aus Listing 9.23 entnehmen können, möchten wir von dem Funktionsimport lediglich statisch für den Käufer Huber die Informationen zur neuesten Bestellung erfragen. Im nächsten Schritt beziehen wir durch die Komponente mittels des Aufrufs `getModel` die Referenz auf das OData-Modell unserer Anwendung und rufen im Anschluss die Funktion `callFunction` auf. Die Funktion erhält als ersten Parameter den Namen des Funktionsimports, der aufgerufen werden soll. Als zweiten Parameter erhält die Funktion ein literales JavaScript-Objekt. Dabei legen wir das HTTP-Verb `GET` sowie zwei Callback-Funktionen fest, die im Erfolgsfall bzw. im Fehlerfall aufgerufen werden sollen. Wie Sie dem Programmierbeispiel entnehmen können, zeigen wir im Erfolgsfall die Informationen in einer einfachen `MessageBox` an.

```
onGetMostRecentOrderOfBuyer: function(oEvent) {
        const buyersName = "Arvato";
        const oModel = this.getOwnerComponent().getModel();
        oModel.callFunction("/MostRecentOrderOfBuyer", {
                method: "GET",
                urlParameters: {
```

```
                Buyer: buyersName
            },
            success: function(oResponse) {
             const dateFormat =
             sap.ui.core.format.DateFormat.getDateInstance({
                pattern: "dd.MM.YYYY"
    });
    const dateFormatted =
    dateFormat.format(oResponse.OrderDate);
    var sFormattedText = "Käufer :" + oResponse.Buyer +
                         "\n Datum: " + dateFormatted +
                         "\n Verkäufer: " + oResponse.Seller;

    MessageBox.show(sFormattedText, {
                       icon: MessageBox.Icon.Information,
                       title: "Zur Information"
                     });          }),
            error: $.proxy(function(oError) {
               var oErrorResponse =
                JSON.parse(oError.responseText);
               this._showErrorMessage(oErrorResponse);
                       }, this)
                  });
            },
```

Listing 9.23 Funktionsimport aus SAPUI5 aufrufen

9.5 OData-Services mit C# konsumieren

In diesem Abschnitt skizzieren wir, wie Sie OData-Services mit C# konsumieren können. Wir verwenden dazu Microsoft Visual Studio 2022 Community Edition mit der Erweiterung *OData Connected Service*. Diese Erweiterung kann stark typisierte C#-Client-Code generieren und vereinfacht so die Entwicklung.

Erweiterung installieren

Um unseren Beispielcode so einfach wie möglich zu halten, entwickeln wir hier eine Konsolenanwendung, mit der wir Bestellungen und Bestellpositionen lesen, anlegen, ändern und löschen können. Installieren Sie dazu die genannte Erweiterung in Visual Studio unter dem Menüpunkt **Erweiterungen**. Wählen Sie hier **Erweiterungen verwalten**. Suchen Sie nach »odata« und klicken Sie auf **Installieren**, um die Erweiterung zu aktivieren (siehe Abbildung 9.34).

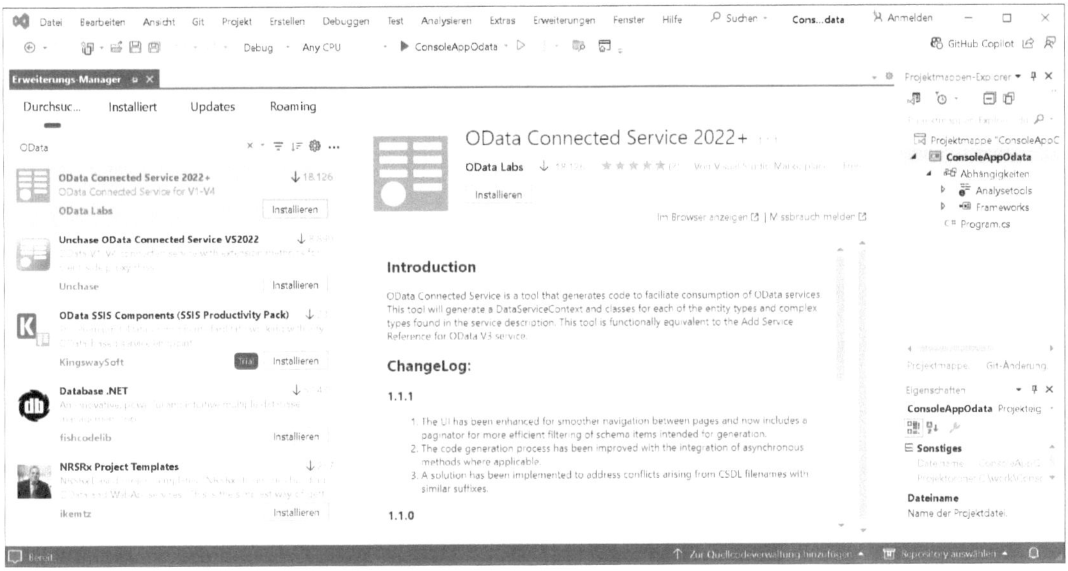

Abbildung 9.34 Erweiterung OData Connected Services installieren

Dienst der Konsolenanwendung hinzufügen

Nach einem Neustart wird Visual Studio die Erweiterung installieren. Sie können nun eine Konsolenanwendung anlegen und dann im **Solution Explorer** mit der rechten Maustaste auf Ihr Projekt klicken. Wählen Sie hier den Kontextmenüeintrag **Hinzufügen** und dann **Verbundener Dienst** aus. Klicken Sie nun auf die Option **OData Connected Service**. Sie werden durch die Konfiguration des Service-Endpunkts geführt:

1. Geben Sie im ersten Schritt die Verbindungsdetails zu Ihrem OData-Service an. Sie können im Feld **Address** eine URL eingeben oder eine lokale XML-Datei mit den Metadaten eines OData- Services auswählen (siehe Abbildung 9.35).

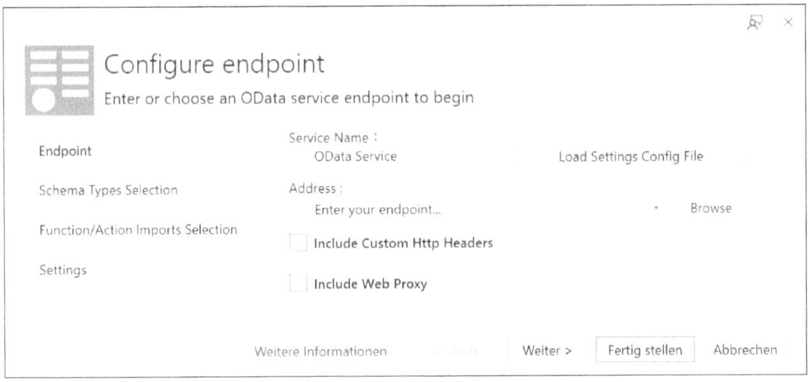

Abbildung 9.35 OData-Endpunkt mit OData Connected Services konfigurieren

Außerdem erlaubt der Dialog die Eingabe eines *Custom HTTP Headers*, also z. B. eines Authentifizierungsschlüssels, sowie die Angabe eines Web Proxys. Klicken Sie anschließend auf **Weiter**.

2. Im zweiten Schritt können Sie die Schema-Typen auswählen, die genutzt werden. Klicken Sie danach auf **Weiter**.
3. Im dritten Schritt sehen Sie *Functions* und *Actions*, also Operationen des OData-Services. Klicken Sie hier ebenfalls auf **Weiter**.
4. Im letzten Schritt können Sie einen Namen für die Datei der generierten Proxy-Klasse angeben. Wir belassen es bei dem Namen **Reference.cs**. Klicken Sie abschließend auf **Fertig stellen**.

Es befindet sich nun eine Klasse `ZIFP_ORDERS_SRV_Entities` in der Datei **Reference.cs**, die die Client-Schnittstelle repräsentiert, um mit dem OData-Service zu interagieren. Sie erbt von der Klasse `System.Data.Services.Client.DataServiceContext`, die Teil vom OData Connected Service ist und OData-Services konsumiert. Diese Klasse verwaltet die Verbindung und erleichtert das Konstruieren von Anfragen und die Durchführung von Änderungen. Da OData-Service einem Standard folgen, ist das Programmiermodell für jeden OData Service gleich.

OData-Client implementieren

Listing 9.24 zeigt einen C#-OData-Client. In der Klasse `Program` deklarieren wir zunächst vier Konstanten:

- für die Basis-URL des OData-Service
- für den Content-Typ, der beim Anlegen und Ändern von Entitäten benötigt wird
- für Benutzernamen und Passwort

Die folgenden vier statischen Eigenschaften `CSRFToken`, `Cookies`, `CredentialCache` und `Request` dienen dazu, das CSRF Token, die Session-Cookies, den Credentials Cache und das HTTP-Request-Objekt zwischen den Methodenaufrufen der Klasse zu speichern. Die Eigenschaft `UpdatePending` dient zur Synchronisation von Threads während des Wartens auf die HTTP-Response des OData-Service.

```
using System.Data.Services.Client;
using System.Net;
using System.Xml.Linq;
using ZIFP_ORDERS_SRV;

namespace IFPGatewayConsole
{
    class Program
```

```
    {
        const string BASE_URL =
"http://nwasabap703.workgroup:8000/sap/opu/odata/sap/ZIFP_ORDERS_SRV/";

        const string CONTENT_TYPE ="application/atom+xml;type=entry";
        const string USER = "bcuser";
        const string PASSWD = "minisap";
        static string CSRFToken = null;
        static CookieCollection Cookies = null;
        static CredentialCache CredentialCache = null;
        static WebRequest Request = null;
        static int UpdatePending = 0;

        static void Main(string[] args)
        {
// Serviceobjekt erzeugen und Event Handler registrieren
            ZIFP_ORDERS_SRV.ZIFP_ORDERS_SRV_Entities service =
              new ZIFP_ORDERS_SRV.ZIFP_ORDERS_SRV_Entities(
                new Uri(BASE_URL)); service.WritingEntity +=
              new EventHandler<ReadingWritingEntityEventArgs>(
                service_WritingEntity);
            service.SendingRequest +=
              new EventHandler<SendingRequestEventArgs>(
                service_SendingRequest);
            // alle Bestellungen lesen
            IAsyncResult asyncResult =
                service.BeginExecute<Orderheader>(
                new Uri("Orderheaders/", UriKind.Relative),
                null,
                null
            );
            IEnumerable<Orderheader> headers =
                service.EndExecute<Orderheader>(asyncResult);

            // Bestellungen und Bestellpositionen ausgeben
            foreach (Orderheader header in headers)
            {
                System.Console.WriteLine(header.OrderId);
                // BeginExecute to fetch positions
                asyncResult = service.BeginExecute<Orderposition>(
                    new Uri($"Orderheaders('{header.OrderId}')/
                        Positions/", UriKind.Relative),
                    null,
```

9

```
            null
        );
        IEnumerable<Orderposition> positions =
         service.EndExecute<Orderposition>(asyncResult);
        foreach (Orderposition position in positions)
        {
            System.Console.WriteLine("    " +
                                    position.OrderPosition);
        }
    }
    // Bestellung anlegen
    Orderheader NewHeader = new Orderheader();
    NewHeader.OrderId = "0000000000";
    NewHeader.ReferenceId = "000000000";
    NewHeader.Ordertype = "SO";
    NewHeader.Buyer = "Pehnke";
    NewHeader.Seller = "Englbrecht";
    NewHeader.OrderDate = DateTime.UtcNow;
    service.AddToOrderheaders(NewHeader);
    SaveChanges(service);
    // Bestellposition zur neuen Bestellung anlegen
    Orderposition NewPosition = new Orderposition();
    NewPosition.OrderId = NewHeader.OrderId;
    NewPosition.OrderPosition = "00100";
    NewPosition.MaterialId = "4711";
    NewPosition.MaterialText = "OData und SAPUI5";
    NewPosition.NumberOfItems = 10;
    NewPosition.Price = (decimal)22.22;
    NewPosition.Currency = "EUR";
    service.AddToOrderpositions(NewPosition);
    SaveChanges(service);
    // Bestellposition ändern
    NewPosition.NumberOfItems = 22;
    service.UpdateObject(NewPosition);
    SaveChanges(service);
    // Bestellpostion wieder löschen
    service.DeleteObject(NewPosition);
    SaveChanges(service);
}
static void service_WritingEntity(
  object sender, ReadingWritingEntityEventArgs e)
{
```

```
        // Datumsdarstellung korrigieren
        if (typeof(Orderheader) == e.Entity.GetType())
        {
            IEnumerable<XElement> elements =
              e.Data.Descendants(
"{http://schemas.microsoft.com/ado/2007/08/dataservices}OrderDate");
            foreach (XElement element in elements)
                element.Value =
                 System.DateTime.Parse(element.Value).ToString(
                    "yyyy-MM-ddT00:00:00");
        }
    }
    static void service_SendingRequest(
      object sender, SendingRequestEventArgs e)
    {
        // Logon-Daten anfügen
        if (CredentialCache == null)
        {
            CredentialCache = new CredentialCache();
            CredentialCache.Add(
             new Uri(BASE_URL), "Basic",
               new NetworkCredential(USER, PASSWD));
        }
        e.Request.Credentials = CredentialCache;
        // Cookies setzen
        if (e.Request is HttpWebRequest httpWebRequest)
        {
            httpWebRequest.CookieContainer
                = new CookieContainer();
            if (Cookies != null)
             httpWebRequest.CookieContainer.Add(Cookies);
             // Client auf 100 setzen
            httpWebRequest.CookieContainer.Add(
                new Uri(BASE_URL),
                new Cookie("sap-usercontext", "sap-client=100")
            );
            // CSRF Token anfordern oder anfügen
            if (CSRFToken == null)
                e.Request.Headers.Add("x-csrf-token", "fetch");
            else
                e.RequestHeaders.Add("x-csrf-token",
                                      CSRFToken);
```

9

```
                // Content-Typ setzen
                if (e.Request.Method != "GET" &&
                    e.Request.Method != "DELETE")
                    e.Request.ContentType = CONTENT_TYPE;
                // Request zwischenspeichern
                if (Request == null)
                    Request = e.Request;
            }
        }
        // Save Changes, threadsafe
        static void SaveChanges(
          ZIFP_ORDERS_SRV.ZIFP_ORDERS_SRV_Entities service)
        {
            Interlocked.Exchange(ref UpdatePending, 1);
            service.BeginSaveChanges(
              new AsyncCallback(save_Callback), service);
            while (UpdatePending == 1)
                System.Threading.Thread.Sleep(500);
        }
        static void save_Callback(IAsyncResult result)
        {
            ZIFP_ORDERS_SRV.ZIFP_ORDERS_SRV_Entities service =
      (ZIFP_ORDERS_SRV.ZIFP_ORDERS_SRV_Entities)result.AsyncState;
            service.EndSaveChanges(result);
            Interlocked.Exchange(ref UpdatePending, 0);
        }
    }
}
```

Listing 9.24 C#-OData-Client

Proxy

In der Methode `Main` wird das Proxy-Objekt `ZIFP_ORDERS_SRV.ZIFP_ORDERS_SRV_Entities` instanziiert. Im Konstruktor wird ihm dabei die Basis-URL übergeben. Danach werden die Event-Handler-Methoden `service_WritingEntity()` und `service_SendingRequest()` für die beiden Events `WritingEntity` und `SendingRequest` registriert. Im Event Handler `service_WritingEntity` können Sie den HTTP-Body noch ändern, bevor ihn der Proxy an den OData-Service schickt. Im Event Handler `service_SendingRequest` können Sie zum HTTP-Request-Objekt noch Header-Felder hinzufügen. Zu den Header-Fehlern gehört, neben den wichtigen Authentifizierungsparametern für Username und Passwort, auch das Feld für den Mandanten (System), der als Cookie mitgegeben wird.

Anschließend werden mit den asynchronen Methoden BeginExecute() und EndExecute alle Bestellköpfe gelesen. Den Methoden geben Sie dazu die URL *Orderheaders/* mit und parametrisieren sie mit dem Typ Orderheaders.

Bestellköpfe lesen

Direkt nach dem Lesen werden über das HTTP-Request-Objekt, das im Event Handler service_SendingRequest für die Eigenschaft Request zwischengespeichert wurde, die Cookies und das CSRF Token ausgelesen und für spätere schreibende Aufrufe zwischengespeichert. Danach werden in einer Schleife alle Bestellnummern ausgegeben. Für jede Bestellnummer werden mit BeginExecute und EndExecute sämtliche Bestellpositionen gelesen, von denen dann in einer inneren Schleife die Positionsnummern ausgegeben werden.

Cookies und CSRF Token speichern

Anschließend wird das neue Bestellkopf-Objekt NewHeader erzeugt, seine Eigenschaften werden gefüllt, und es wird mit AddToOrderheaders() dem Proxy-Objekt übergeben, damit es die neue Entität beim Aufruf der Methode Save() an den OData-Service zur Erzeugung übergibt. Danach wird auf die gleiche Art eine neue Bestellposition angelegt.

Ändernde Zugriffe

Diese Bestellposition wird geändert, und die Änderung wird mit UpdateObject() an das Proxy-Objekt übergeben. Zum Schluss wird die neue Bestellposition mit DeleteObject() gleich wieder gelöscht.

In der Methode service_WritingEntity() kümmern wir uns um einen Fehler bei der Serialisierung eines .NET-Objekts DateTime nach XML. Das Feld OrderDate der Entität Orderheader wird in eine Darstellung konvertiert, die vom OData-Service geparst werden kann.

Bestelldatum korrigieren

In der Methode service_SendingRequest kümmern wir uns um das Setzen der Header-Felder für den Request. Zuerst fügen wir die Logon-Daten für die HTTP-Authentifizierung hinzu. Falls das Session-Cookie schon gelesen wurde, fügen wir diesen als Nächstes hinzu. Falls wir noch kein CSRF Token erhalten haben, fordern wir es an, ansonsten fügen wir es hinzu. Zum Schluss fügen wir, falls notwendig, den Content-Typ hinzu und speichern das HTTP-Request-Objekt in der Eigenschaft Request, damit wir später das CSRF Token und das Session-Cookie daraus lesen können.

Header-Felder setzen

Die Methode Save() haben wir geschrieben, da die Methode SaveChanges() des Proxy-Objekts nur dann funktioniert, wenn wir den Code im Debugger schrittweise durchgehen. Dies liegt wahrscheinlich an einem Fehler bei der Thread-Synchronisation. Daher setzen wir innerhalb der Methode Save() zunächst die Eigenschaft UpdatePending auf den Wert »1«. Danach wird service.BeginSaveChanges() aufgerufen und dabei die Methode save_Callback übergeben. Damit wird der HTTP-POST vom Proxy asynchron in einem neuen Thread ausgeführt und die Methode save_Callback aufgerufen, so-

Änderungen speichern

bald die HTTP-Response angekommen ist. Nach dem Aufruf von `BeginSaveChanges()` warten wir in einer `while`-Schleife so lange, bis `save_Callback` die Eigenschaft `UpdatePending` wieder auf den Wert »0« gesetzt hat. Dies passiert innerhalb der Methode `save_Callback`, sobald die Methode `EndSaveChanges` auf dem Proxy aufgerufen wurde.

9.6 OData-Services mit Java konsumieren

Apache Olingo

Nachdem wir die Nutzung von OData mit C# gezeigt haben, wendet sich dieser Abschnitt dem Konsum von OData-Services mit Java zu. Das Java Development Kit (JDK) und auch SAP bieten für die Nutzung von OData-Services keine API an. Aus diesem Grund ist es notwendig, auf andere Bibliotheken zurückzugreifen. Eine Bibliothek, die sich zum De-facto-Standard für den Konsum von OData mit Java etabliert hat, ist die *Apache Olingo Library*. Aus diesem Grund zeigen wir im folgenden Abschnitt, wie Sie mit Apache Olingo den in diesem Buch besprochenen OData-Service konsumieren.

[+]

Olingo JPA Processor V4

Basierend auf der Apache Olingo Library für OData V4 hat SAP 2017 eine weitere Bibliothek angelegt, die die *Jakarta Persistence API* (JPA) nutzt, um die Programmierung für einen OData Service zu vereinfachen. Dieser Ansatz erlaubt es, mit Annotationen JPA-Entitäten als OData-Entitäten inklusive Standard-Operationen wie Lesen, Filtern, Löschen und Anlegen bereitzustellen und auch die Metadaten automatisch zu generieren. Viele manuelle Programmierschritte für die Standard-Operationen werden so vereinfacht. Lediglich die Randbereiche müssen wie in diesem Kapitel beschrieben programmiert werden.

Apache Olingo stellt Bibliotheken zur Verfügung, mit denen OData-Konsumenten und auch OData-Services implementiert werden können. Apache Olingo bietet neben einer API für die Arbeit mit OData 2 auch eine API für OData 4.

9.6.1 Download und Installation von Apache Olingo

Varianten für OData V2 und V4

Apache Olingo steht in zwei verschiedenen Varianten zum Download bereit. Je nachdem, ob Sie OData-V2- oder OData-V4-konforme OData-Services konsumieren oder anbieten möchten, wählen Sie aus dem Download-Bereich von *http://olingo.apache.org/* die entsprechende Version aus. Da der in Abschnitt 9.3, »OData-Services entwickeln«, implementierte OData-Service ein V2-basierter Service ist, rufen wir aus dem Download-Menü den Eintrag **Download OData 2.0 Java** auf. Nachdem die Seite geladen worden ist, erhalten Sie eine Übersicht über die unterschiedlichen Pakete, die zum Download angeboten werden. Neben der Bibliothek werden auch, wie in Abbildung 9.36, Download-Seite von Apache Olingo. Wählen Sie für den Download **Olingo OData2 Library** aus, und speichern Sie die ZIP-Datei auf der Festplatte.

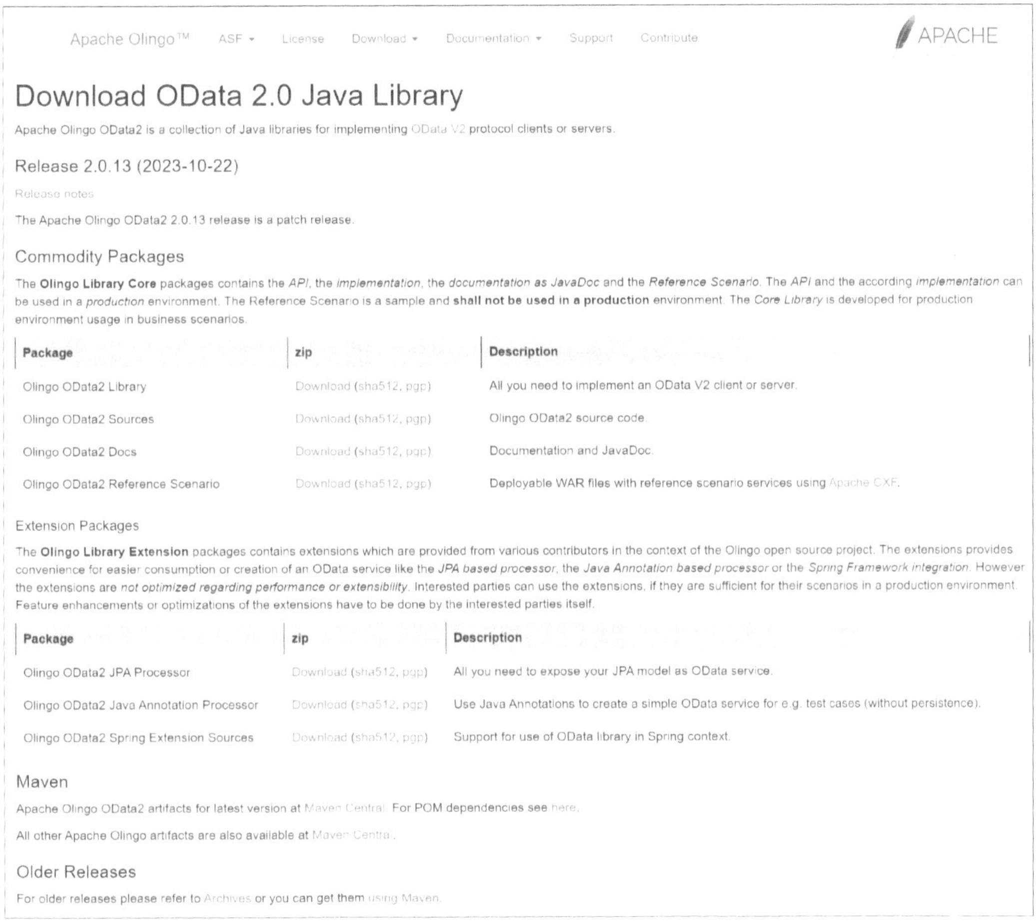

Abbildung 9.36 Download-Seite von Apache Olingo

Nach dem Download entpacken wir die Datei **olingo-odata2-dist-lib-2.0.13-lib.zip**. Im nächsten Schritt starten wir Eclipse und legen dabei ein Standard-Java-Projekt an. Im Rahmen der Projektanlage bietet Ihnen der Assistent die Möglichkeit, benötigte Java-Bibliotheken zum Build-Pfad hinzuzufügen. Fügen Sie die JAR-Dateien aus Tabelle 9.2 als Abhängigkeiten hinzu.

Java-Projekt in Eclipse anlegen

Dateiname	Verwendung
org.apache.olingo-olingo-odata2-core-2.0.13.jar	Core-Klassen von Apache Olingo
org.apache.olingo-olingo-odata2-api-2.0.13.jar	API für die Implementierung
com.google.code.gson-gson-2.9.1.jar	Bibliothek zum Serialisieren und Deserialisieren von Java-Objekten zu JSON-Objekten

Tabelle 9.2 Abhängigkeiten zur Olingo-Bibliothek

Nachdem das Projekt angelegt worden ist, fügen wir eine neue Java-Klasse zum Projekt hinzu. In dem hier vorgestellten einfachen Client nennen wir diese Klasse `SimpleODataClient`. Beim Anlegen der Klasse wählen wir aus, dass eine `main`-Methode angelegt werden soll.

9.6.2 Implementierung eines OData-Clients mit Java

Zunächst implementieren wir eine Hilfsmethode `createAndInitializeHTTPConnection`. Die Methode hat zur Aufgabe, die Verbindung zum Backend aufzubauen und die Verbindung entsprechend mit Header-Parametern, je nach Request-Art, zu initialisieren. Die Methode erhält als Aufrufparameter den Benutzernamen, das Passwort, die vollqualifizierte URL zur angefragten Ressource, den Content-Typ sowie die HTTP-Methode. Zu Beginn der Implementierung werden die Authentifizierungsinformationen aufbereitet und, nachdem die HTTP-Verbindung entsprechend erzeugt wurde, als Header-Parameter mittels der Methode `setRequestProperty` übergeben. Zudem werden der Inhaltstyp, sowie das HTTP-Verb entsprechend gesetzt. Wie Sie Listing 9.25 entnehmen können, liefert die Methode das erzeugte und initialisierte Verbindungsobjekt an den Aufrufer zurück.

[»]

Keine Konstanten

Wir verweisen an dieser Stelle darauf, dass bewusst auf die Verwendung von Konstanten verzichtet wurde, damit das Lesen des Codes fließend ist und gegebenenfalls nicht über die Bezeichner von Konstanten gestolpert wird.

```
private HttpURLConnection createAndInitializeHTTPConnection(
              String username, String password, String absolutUri,
              String contentType, String httpMethod)
                     throws MalformedURLException, IOException
{

 String authorization = "Basic ";
  authorization += new String(
                Base64.getEncoder().encode(
                    ((username + ":" + password).getBytes())));

  URL url = new URL(absolutUri);
  HttpURLConnection connection =
         (HttpURLConnection) url.openConnection();
  connection.setRequestProperty(
         "Authorization", authorization
  );
  connection.setRequestMethod(httpMethod);
  connection.setRequestProperty("Accept", contentType);

  return connection;
}
```

Listing 9.25 Methode »createAndInitializeHTTPConnection« für den Aufbau einer HTTP-Verbindung

Als Nächstes implementieren wir eine zentrale Funktion für das Ausführen von HTTP-Anfragen an das Backend. Diese Methode erhält den Namen `execute`. Wie Sie Listing 9.26 entnehmen können, erhält die Methode neben der URL sowohl den Inhaltstyp als auch das HTTP-Verb als Aufrufparameter. Die Methode `execute` ruft im ersten Schritt die Methode `createAndInitializeHTTPConnection` auf und übergibt dabei die entsprechenden Informationen. Wie Sie dem Listing entnehmen können, werden Benutzername und Passwort als Konstanten übergeben. Nachdem das `HttpURLConnection`-Objekt angelegt und initialisiert worden ist, wird das übergebene HTTP-Verb geprüft. Sollte es sich um eine GET-Anfrage handeln, wird `x-csrf-token` mit dem Wert »Fetch« an das Backend als Header-Parameter übergeben. Dadurch geben Sie an, dass das Authentifizierungs-Token als Teil der Antwort des Backends zurückgeliefert wird. Wir öffnen die Verbindung und führen dadurch die Anfrage an das Backend aus. Nachdem die Anfrage ausgeführt worden ist, prüfen wir das Resultat der Anfrage über die Methode `checkConnectionStatus`. Die Methode prüft lediglich den HTTP-Status unserer Anfrage. Für die konkrete Implementierung verweisen wir auf die Download-Möglichkeit der Sourcen zum Buch. Als Nächstes lesen wir den Header-Parameter x-csrf-token sowie den Parameter set-cookie aus und speichern diese in den Member-Variablen unserer Klassen. Der Header-Parameter set-cookie enthält neben der Session-ID auch das Cookie MYSAPSSO2. Sowohl die x-csrf-token- als auch die Cookie-Informationen werden später für ändernde Zugriffe auf den OData-Service benötigt. Aus diesem Grund speichern wir die Informationen in einer Member-Variablen. Zum Abschluss der Implementierung lesen wir noch das Ergebnis unserer Anfrage aus und liefern dieses an den Aufrufer zurück.

```
private InputStream execute(String relativeUri,
    String contentType, String httpMethod) throws IOException
{
        HttpURLConnection connection =
           createAndInitializeHTTPConnection(
                 USERNAME, PASSWORD,
                  relativeUri, contentType,httpMethod);
        if("GET".equals(httpMethod)){
           connection.setRequestProperty(
                  "X-CSRF-Token", "Fetch");
        }
        connection.connect();
        checkConnectionStatus(connection);
        Map<String, List<String>> headerFields =
           connection.getHeaderFields();
        if("GET".equals(httpMethod)){
             this.xCsrfToken = headerFields.get(
                   "x-csrf-token");
             this.cookies = headerFields.get("set-cookie");
        }
        InputStream content = connection.getInputStream();
        return content;
}
```

Listing 9.26 Methode »execute« für das Ausführen von HTTP-Anfragen

Metadaten lesen

Nachdem die Vorarbeiten soweit geleistet worden sind, implementieren wir die Methode readMetadata. Die Methode hat zur Aufgabe, die Metadaten unseres OData-Service auszulesen. Wie Sie Listing 9.27 entnehmen können, wird die Methode execute aufgerufen. Wir übergeben der Methode dabei den zusammengesetzten Pfad für das Auslesen der Metadaten sowie das Inhaltsformat, das wir zurückerhalten möchten. Da wir Daten lesen, geben wir das HTTP-Verb GET an den Service weiter. Da das Ergebnis vorliegt, konvertieren wir das Ergebnis zu einem Objekt vom Typ Edm. Dies erreichen wir durch den Aufruf der Methode readMetadata, die von der Olingo-Klasse EntityProvider angeboten wird. Das gelieferte Edm-Objekt enthält nun die Metadaten und wird im weiteren Verlauf der Implementierung verwendet.

```
public Edm readMetadata()
              throws IOException, ODataException
{
       InputStream content = execute(
           SERVICE_URI + "/$metadata", "application/xml",
                             "GET");
       return EntityProvider.readMetadata(content, false);
}
```

Listing 9.27 Funktion »readMetadata« implementieren

Die in Listing 9.27 gezeigte Methode kann nun in der main-Methode der Klasse aufgerufen werden. Dabei wird lediglich der Pfad zum Servicedokument des OData-Service mitgegeben. Wie Sie der Dokumentation von Apache Olingo entnehmen können, können Sie über die Klasse Edm auf die entsprechenden Informationen zu dem über den Service verfügbaren Entity Data Model zugreifen.

Entität lesen

Nach dem Lesen der Metadaten können wir nun die CRUD-Methoden des OData-Service nach und nach aufrufen. Wir beginnen dabei mit dem Lesen. Wir implementieren hierzu eine Methode readEntry. Diese Methode liefert an den Aufrufer ein Objekt vom Type ODataEntry zurück. Dieses Objekt kapselt alle Eigenschaften und zusätzlich die dazugehörenden Metadaten der gelesenen Entität. Wie Sie Listing 9.28 entnehmen können, wird in der Methode readEntry unter anderem eine Methode createUri aufgerufen. Diese Methode kapselt lediglich das Erzeugen eines URI aus den übergebenen Bestandteilen, z. B. des URI, um eine konkrete Entität von dem übergebenen Entity Set zu lesen. Nachdem der Service die Daten an den Client zurückgeliefert hat, übergeben wir den Eingabestrom an die Methode readEntry der EntityProvider-Klasse. Die Methode readEntry deserialisiert die gelieferten Informationen zu dem benötigten Objekt vom Typ ODataEntry.

```
public ODataEntry readEntry(Edm edm, String serviceUri,
    String contentType, String entitySetName,
    String keyValue) throws IOException, ODataException
{
    EdmEntityContainer entityContainer =
                       edm.getDefaultEntityContainer();
```

```
    String absolutUri = createUri(serviceUri, entitySetName,
keyValue);
    InputStream content = execute(absolutUri, contentType, "GET");
    return EntityProvider.readEntry(contentType,
        entityContainer.getEntitySet(entitySetName),
        content, EntityProviderReadProperties.init().build()
    );
}
```

Listing 9.28 Methode »readEntry«

Entität anlegen

Um eine Entität anzulegen oder zu ändern, führen wir die Methode `writeEntity` in unsere Klasse ein. Die Methode erhält neben bereits bekannten Aufrufparametern zusätzlich noch ein Objekt vom Typ `Map`. Dieses Objekt enthält die Schlüssel-Wert-Paare der anzulegenden bzw. der zu ändernden Entität. Der Schüssel ist dabei die Eigenschaft der Entität und Value der Wert, den man der entsprechenden Eigenschaft mitgeben möchte. Für das Ändern einer Entität bietet Apache Olingo die Methode `writeEntry` auf der Klasse `EntityProvider` an. Die Methode erhält als Aufrufparameter ein Objekt vom Typ `EdmEntitySet`. Das Objekt repräsentiert das Entity Set, zu dem wir die Entität hinzufügen möchten. Wie Sie dem Code aus Listing 9.29 entnehmen können, wird das Objekt `EdmEntitySet` über den sogenannten `EdmEntityContainer` geliefert. Dieser erhält das `Edm`-Objekt, das die Metadaten enthält. Nachdem das Objekt angelegt worden ist, bildet der Aufruf der Methode `writeEntry` auf dem Entity Provider den Abschluss. Die Methode liefert das angelegte Objekt an den Aufrufer zurück. Dadurch kann beispielsweise direkt die `OrderId` ausgelesen werden.

```
private ODataEntry writeEntity(
     Edm edm, String absolutUri, String entitySetName,
     Map<String, Object> data, String contentType,
     String httpMethod)
          throws EdmException, MalformedURLException,
          IOException, EntityProviderException,
          URISyntaxException
{
     HttpURLConnection connection =
          createAndInitializeHTTPConnection(
                    USERNAME, PASSWORD,
                    absolutUri, contentType,
                    httpMethod);
     EdmEntityContainer entityContainer =
                    edm.getDefaultEntityContainer();
```

```
    EdmEntitySet entitySet =
                 entityContainer.getEntitySet(entitySetName);
    URI rootUri = new URI(entitySetName);
    EntityProviderWriteProperties properties =
         EntityProviderWriteProperties.serviceRoot(rootUri).build();
    ODataResponse response = EntityProvider.writeEntry(
         contentType, entitySet, data, properties);
    Object entity = response.getEntity();
    if (entity instanceof InputStream) {
         byte[] buffer = streamToArray((InputStream)entity);
         connection.getOutputStream().write(buffer);
    }

    ODataEntry entry = null;
    HttpStatusCodes statusCode =
         HttpStatusCodes.fromStatusCode(
              connection.getResponseCode());
    if (statusCode == HttpStatusCodes.CREATED) {
         InputStream content = connection.getInputStream();
         entry = EntityProvider.readEntry(contentType, entitySet,
              content, EntityProviderReadProperties.init().build());
    }
    connection.disconnect();
    return entry;
}
```


Listing 9.29 Methode »writeEntity« für den schreibenden Zugriff auf den OData-Service implementieren

HTTP-Verbindung-anlegen und initialisieren

Wie schon angedeutet, ist es beim ändernden Zugriff auf den OData-Service nötig, das `x-csrf-token` sowie das Cookie auszulesen. Hierzu müssen wir die `createAndInitializeHTTPConnection`-Methode entsprechend anpassen und berücksichtigen auch noch das Löschen sowie das Ändern einer Entität. Wie Sie dem Programmierbeispiel aus Listing 9.30 entnehmen können, wird nun, abhängig von dem übergebenen HTTP-Verb, entschieden, ob das `x-csrf-token` sowie das Cookie mitgeschickt werden sollen.

```
private HttpURLConnection createAndInitializeHTTPConnection(
   String username, String password, String absolutUri,
   String contentType, String httpMethod)
     throws MalformedURLException, IOException
{
  String authorization = "Basic ";
```

```
  authorization += new String(Base64.getEncoder().encode(((
                   username + ":" + password).getBytes())));

  URL url = new URL(absolutUri);
  HttpURLConnection connection =
 (HttpURLConnection) url.openConnection();

  if ("POST".equals(httpMethod) || "PUT".equals(httpMethod) ||
      "DELETE".equals(httpMethod)) {
      connection.setDoOutput(true);
      connection.setRequestProperty("Content-Type", contentType);
      formatToken();
      connection.setRequestProperty("x-csrf-token",
        xCsrfToken.toString());
      String tmpCookie = "";
      for (String cookie : cookies) {
        tmpCookie = tmpCookie + cookie + ",";
      }
      tmpCookie = tmpCookie.substring(0, tmpCookie.length() - 1);
      connection.setRequestProperty("Cookie", tmpCookie);
  }
  connection.setRequestProperty("Authorization", authorization);
  connection.setRequestMethod(httpMethod);
  connection.setRequestProperty("Accept", contentType);

  return connection;
}
```

Listing 9.30 Angepasste Methode »createAndInitializeHTTPConnection«

Anlegen einer Entität testen

Nach der Änderung an `createAndInitializeHTTPConnection` führen wir eine Methode `testCreateOrderHeader` ein. Diese Methode dient dazu, die gerade gemachten Implementierungsschritte zu testen. Die Methode erhält als Parameter lediglich ein Objekt vom Typ `Edm`. Wie Sie dem Programmierbeispiel aus Listing 9.31 entnehmen können, erstellen wir in der Methode ein `Map`-Objekt. Dieses enthält die Schlüssel-Wert-Paare für die anzulegende Entität.

```
private void testCreateOrderHeader(Edm edm) throws Exception {
     Map<String, Object> data =
                          new HashMap<String, Object>();
     data.put("OrderId", "1000");
     data.put("Ordertype", "A");
```

```
    data.put("ReferenceId", "0000000001");
    data.put("Buyer", "Buchshop Online");
    data.put("Seller", "Rheinwerk-Verlag");
    data.put("OrderDate", new
           Timestamp(System.currentTimeMillis()));

    String absolutUri = createUri(SERVICE_URI, "Orderheaders",null);
    ODataEntry createdEntry  = writeEntity(
         edm, absolutUri, "Orderheaders", data, "application/json",
             "POST" );
    System.out.println("Angelegte Entität :\n" +
         formatEntry(createdEntry));
}
```


Listing 9.31 Methode »testCreateOrderHeader«

Update testen

Als Nächstes möchten wir Ihnen noch das Ändern eines Bestellkopfs (Order Header) zeigen. Hierzu Implementieren wir die Methode `testUpdateOrderHeaders`. Wie Sie aus dem Programmierbeispiel aus Listing 9.32 entnehmen können, ist die Implementierung dem Anlegen ähnlich; lediglich beim Aufbau des absoluten URI ist beim Ändern einer Entität die Übergabe des eindeutigen Schlüssels obligatorisch. Zudem verwenden wir als HTTP-Verb `PUT` anstelle von `POST`.

```
private void testUpdateOrderHeaders(Edm edm) throws Exception
{
  Map<String, Object> updateData = new HashMap<String, Object>();
  updateData.put("OrderId", "0000000017");
  updateData.put("Buyer", "Buchshop Online");
  updateData.put("Ordertype", "A");
  updateData.put("ReferenceId", "0000000001");
  updateData.put("Buyer", "Buchshop Online");
  updateData.put("Seller", "Rheinwerk-Verlag");
  updateData.put("OrderDate", new
      Timestamp(System.currentTimeMillis()));

  String absolutUri = createUri(SERVICE_URI, "Orderheaders",
      "'0000000017'");
  writeEntity(edm, absolutUri, "Orderheaders", updateData,
      "application/json", "PUT");
    ODataEntry updatedEntry = readEntry(edm, "application/json",
      "Orderheaders", "'0000000017'");
```

```
    System.out.println(updatedEntry);
}
```

Listing 9.32 Entität mit der Methode »testUpdateOrderHeaders« ändern

Funktionsimport mit Apache Olingo

Zum Abschluss unseres Apache-Olingo-Clients implementieren wir nun den Aufruf des Funktionsimports `MostRecentOrderOfBuyer`. Wir fügen eine neue Methode `callMostRecent` zu unserer Client-Implementierung hinzu und übergeben der Methode neben dem `Edm`-Objekt zusätzlich den Namen des Käufers, für den wir die letzte Bestellung abfragen wollen. Wie Sie dem Programmierbeispiel aus Listing 9.33 entnehmen können, setzen wir zu Beginn die URL des Servicedokuments mit dem Namen des Funktionsimports sowie dem Übergabeparameter `Buyer` zusammen. Als Nächstes rufen wir die Funktion `execute` auf. Die Funktion liefert, wie bereits bekannt, einen `InputStream` mit der Antwort des Servers zurück. Als Nächstes müssen wir nur noch die Antwort entsprechend verarbeiten. Wie Sie Listing 9.33 entnehmen können, lesen wir die Metadaten des Funktionsimports aus dem `edm`-Objekt aus. Da wir nur einen Funktionsimport haben, machen wir dies relativ statisch. Zum Abschluss rufen wir die Funktion `readFunctionImport` auf dem Entity Provider auf und liefern das Ergebnis an den Aufrufer zurück.

```
public ODataEntry callMostRecent(Edm edm, String buyer)
  throws IOException, ODataException
{
  String uri = SERVICE_URI+
    "/MostRecentOrderOfBuyer?Buyer='"+ buyer + "'";
  InputStream content = execute(uri, contentType, "GET");
  EdmFunctionImport functionImport =
   edm.getFunctionImports().get(0);
  return (ODataEntry) EntityProvider.readFunctionImport(
    "application/json", functionImport, content,
      EntityProviderReadProperties.init().build());
}
```

Listing 9.33 Funktionsimport »MostRecentOrderOfBuyer« aufrufen

Fazit

Wie wir Ihnen in diesem Abschnitt gezeigt haben, ist es sehr einfach möglich, über die Apache Olingo Bibliothek einen OData-Service zu konsumieren. SAP bietet hierzu in dessen Java-API-Portfolio allerdings keine eigene API an, sodass Sie an dieser Stelle auf Drittanbieter angewiesen sind. Für das detaillierte Programmierbeispiel laden Sie das zu diesem Buch erhältliche Download-Paket mit begleitenden Programmierbeispielen herunter. Sie finden es auf der Seite *www.sap-press.de/5955* unter **Materialien**.

Kapitel 10
SAP HANA und ABAP Core Data Services

SAP HANA bringt viele Neuerungen und neue Programmiermodelle. Auch in der Schnittstellenprogrammierung gibt es einige Funktionen, die wir Ihnen in diesem Kapitel vorstellen.

SAP HANA ist weit mehr als nur eine In-Memory-Datenbank. Es stellt auch die Grundlage für ein neues Programmiermodell für ABAP bereit und hat damit Einfluss auf die Möglichkeiten der Schnittstellenprogrammierung. In diesem Kapitel zeigen wir Ihnen, wie Sie *Core Data Services* (CDS) auf der ABAP-Seite im Rahmen der Schnittstellenprogrammierung verwenden können. SAP nennt es das SAP S/4HANA Programming Model.

ABAP CDS

ABAP Core Data Services gibt es seit SAP NetWeaver 7.5 SP05. Sie bieten eine Datenbankabstraktionsschicht, die die Definition und das Konsumieren von Datenmodellen vereinfacht. CDS sind eine *Domain Specific Language* (DSL), mit der u. a. Datenbank-SQL-Views erzeugt werden, die Funktionen von SAP HANA, wie Konvertierungen von Währungen oder komplexe Fallunterscheidungen, nutzen.

Wir steigen in diesem Kapitel nicht zu tief in diese Thematik ein, sondern besprechen nur einige Konzepte und Möglichkeiten. Sollten Sie tiefergehende Informationen zur Verwendung von ABAP CDS benötigen, verweisen wir an dieser Stelle auf die Dokumentation und empfehlen die Lektüre des Werks »Core Data Services für ABAP« von Renzo Colle, Ralf Dentzer und Jan Hrastnik (SAP PRESS 2023).

10.1 Einführung in die Programmierung mit ABAP CDS

Mit der Verfügbarkeit der SAP-HANA-Plattform hat sich ein Paradigmenwechsel bei der Entwicklung von Geschäftsanwendungen bei SAP vollzogen. Die Faustregel ist einfach: Tun Sie so viel wie möglich in der Datenbank, um die beste Leistung zu erzielen. Dies gilt auch für die zugrunde liegenden Datenmodelle der Geschäftsanwendungen.

Datenmodellierung

Die Datenmodellierung in ABAP umfasste bisher typischerweise die Organisation der Daten in Datenbanktabellen/-sichten und bietet häufig einige zusätzliche High-Level-Services für die Anwendungen mit geeigneten ABAP-Frameworks. Es liegt nahe, dass einige dieser Dienste idealerweise auch näher an die Daten (Basis) gebracht werden sollten, um Echtzeitunternehmen zu ermöglichen. Dies stellt mehrere Herausforderungen dar. Hochwertige Datenmodelle sollten eine einheitliche Definition und ein einheitliches Format für die Daten bieten. Sie sollten klar und eindeutig, wiederverwendbar und flexibel, sogar erweiterbar sein. Wie können Sie also die Semantik des Datenmodells in der Datenbank erfassen, sodass das Modell leicht von verschiedenen Verbrauchern wiederverwendet werden kann, z. B. von OData-Kunden und von OLAP-Tools (OLAP = Online Analytical Processing)? Wie können Sie das Metamodell existierender Datenmodelle auf Ihre Anwendungen erweitern? Dies ist möglich, wenn Sie ABAP CDS verwenden.

ABAP CDS

Mittels CDS ist es möglich, über eine *Data Definition Language* (DDL) semantische Datenmodelle zu definieren. Die Semantik geht dabei weit über die reine datenbankseitige Definition hinaus. Für die Definition dieser Semantik werden sogenannte Annotationen bereitgestellt. Hierdurch ist es möglich, umfangreiche, semantisch reiche Modelle zu erstellen. CDS bildet die Grundlage für die Implementierung von SAP-Fiori-Anwendungen und damit für die Implementierung moderner Benutzeroberflächen.

Datendefinitionssprache (DDL)

CDS vereinfacht und harmonisiert die Art, wie Sie Ihre Datenmodelle definieren und konsumieren, unabhängig von der Verbrauchstechnologie. Technisch handelt es sich um eine Erweiterung von SQL, die Ihnen eine Datendefinitionssprache (DDL) zur Verfügung stellt, um semantisch reichhaltige Datenbanktabellen/-sichten (CDS-Entitäten) und benutzerdefinierte Typen in der Datenbank zu definieren. Die Verbesserungen umfassen:

- Anmerkungen zur Anreicherung der Datenmodelle mit zusätzlichen (domänenspezifischen) Metadaten
- Assoziationen auf konzeptioneller Ebene, die Joins durch Pfadausdrücke in Abfragen ersetzen
- Ausdrücke, die für Berechnungen und Abfragen im Datenmodell verwendet werden

CDS-Entitäten und ihre Metadaten sind erweiterbar und optimal in das ABAP Dictionary und in die ABAP-Sprache integriert.

Abfragesprache (QL)/ABAP SQL

CDS-Entitäten können in ABAP-Programmen mit der ABAP-SQL-Abfragesprache konsumiert werden. Dieses sogenannte *Open SQL* wurde zu *Enhanced Open SQL* erweitert, um unter anderem CDS-Entitäten zu unterstützen und Limitierungen wie die Join-Anzahl aufzuheben. Die aktuelle Version wird nun als *ABAP SQL* bezeichnet und nähert sich dem Funktionsumfang von SQL auf SAP HANA immer mehr an. In Szenarien, in denen SAP HANA noch nicht eingesetzt wird, können die von der zugrunde liegenden Datenbank unterstützten CDS-Funktionen abgefragt werden, bevor die Open-SQL-Anweisung ausgeführt wird, um alternative Implementierungen zu ermöglichen.

Datenkontrollsprache (DCL)

Die *Data Control Language* (DCL) wird verwendet, um Berechtigungen für CDS-Entitäten in einer modellierten, deklarativen Weise zu definieren. Das CDS-Berechtigungskonzept ermöglicht es, die Berechtigung eines aufrufenden Benutzers für die CDS-Entitäten gemäß dem zugrunde liegenden Datenmodell zu überprüfen und nur die Daten zurückzugeben, zu denen der Benutzer eine Berechtigung hat.

CDS-Berechtigungskonzept

Das CDS-Berechtigungskonzept ist ein neues Konzept, das mit dem klassischen SAP-Berechtigungskonzept koexistiert. Es kann unabhängig oder in Kombination mit dem klassischen Konzept verwendet werden. Während das klassische Berechtigungskonzept auf Berechtigungsobjekten basiert und die Berechtigungen entweder implizit (z. B. beim Aufruf von Transaktionen) oder explizit (über die Anweisung `AUTHORITY-CHECK`) geprüft werden, basiert das CDS-Berechtigungskonzept auf impliziten Prüfungen, die von der ABAP-Laufzeit automatisch durchgeführt werden, wenn auf die CDS-Entität mit Open SQL zugegriffen wird. Das bedeutet, dass die klassischen Berechtigungsprüfungen im Applikationsserver nicht mehr nötig sind, weil sie bereits auf der Datenbank erfolgen.

10.2 ABAP-CDS-Views implementieren

Nach der kurzen Einführung in die Konzepte von ABAP-CDS-Views im vorangehenden Abschnitt wendet sich dieser Abschnitt der Implementierung von CDS-Views und der Bereitstellung dieser Views als OData-Service zu.

ABAP Development Tools

Für die Implementierung von ABAP-CDS-Views verwenden Sie die für Eclipse als Plug-in verfügbaren *ABAP Development Tools* (ADT). Wir gehen an dieser Stelle davon aus, dass Sie Eclipse bereits auf Ihrem Rechner installiert und zudem mit den entsprechenden Plug-ins versehen haben.

Installation der ABAP Development Tools (ADT)

Falls Sie Eclipse noch nicht auf Ihrem Rechner installiert haben, können Sie diese Entwicklungsumgebung von der Seite *http://www.eclipse.org* herunterladen und auf Ihrem Rechner installieren. Gehen Sie anschließend auf die Internetseite *https://tools.hana.ondemand.com*, und klicken Sie auf den ABAP-Link. Sie finden auf dieser Webseite eine Anleitung für die Installation der ABAP Development Tools für die aktuell durch SAP unterstützte Eclipse-Version.

ABAP-Projekt anlegen

Starten Sie nun Eclipse. Um ein ABAP-Projekt anzulegen, gehen Sie wie folgt vor:

1. Wählen Sie im Menü **File • New • Other**.
2. Im daraufhin erscheinenden Dialog geben Sie in das Suchfeld den Begriff »abap« ein, wählen dann in der so eingeschränkten Auswahlliste den Eintrag **ABAP Project** aus und bestätigen den Dialog mit **Next** (siehe Abbildung 10.13).

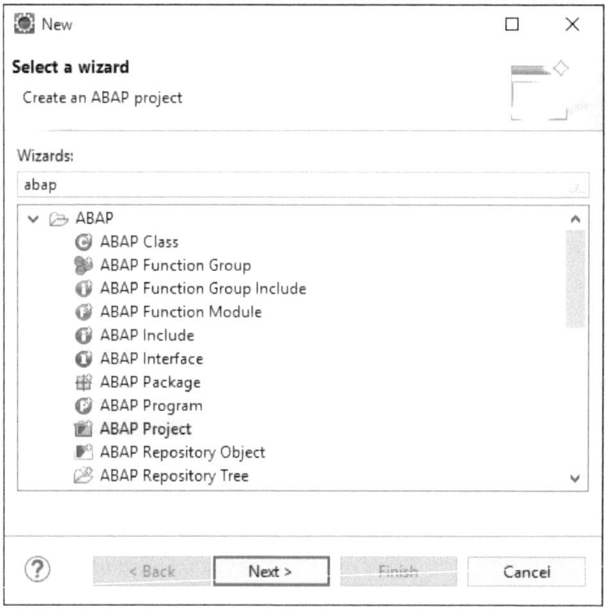

Abbildung 10.1 Auswahl des Projekttyps

3. Im folgenden Dialog werden Ihnen die zur Verfügung stehenden SAP-Systeme angezeigt. Die Liste enthält all jene Systeme, die Ihnen auch im SAP GUI zur Verfügung stehen. Wählen Sie das SAP-System aus, auf dem

Sie die Entwicklung des CDS-Views durchführen möchten, und bestätigen Sie den Dialog mit **Next**.

4. Sie erhalten die für das ausgewählte SAP-System definierten Verbindungsinformationen. Es bestünde die Möglichkeit, die Verbindungsinformationen an dieser Stelle noch zu modifizieren. So wäre es beispielsweise möglich, die Verbindung über Secure Network Communications (SNC) abzusichern. Nachdem Sie etwaige Änderungen durchgeführt haben, bestätigen Sie den Dialog mit **Next**.
5. Es folgt ein Dialog zur Eingabe des Mandanten, des Benutzernamens und des Passworts (siehe Abbildung 10.2). Geben Sie die notwendigen Informationen ein, und bestätigen Sie den Dialog mit **Next**.

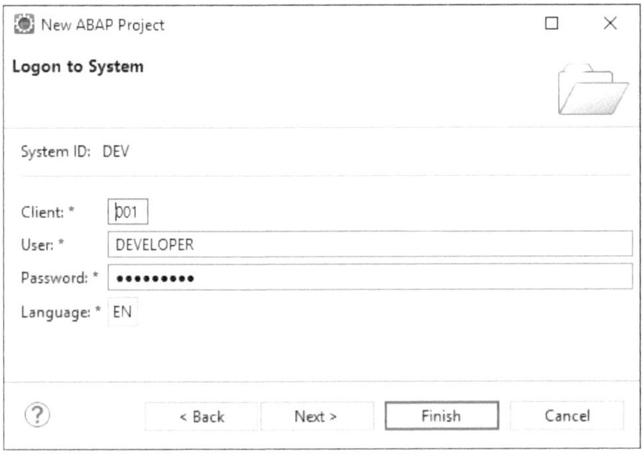

Abbildung 10.2 Eingabe des Mandanten und Benutzers

6. Im letzten Dialogschritt erhalten Sie die Möglichkeit, den Projektnamen sowie Entwicklungspakete, die wir am häufigsten nutzen möchten, auszuwählen. Wir belassen es beim Projektnamen bei dem Vorschlagswert, fügen allerdings zwei Entwicklungspakete hinzu. Hierzu klicken Sie auf den Button **Add** und suchen im daraufhin erscheinenden Auswahldialog nach Ihrem Entwicklungspaket.
7. Im Anschluss wählen Sie dieses aus und bestätigen wiederum den Dialog mit **OK**.
8. Das Paket wird nun, wie in Abbildung 10.3 gezeigt, in der Favoritenliste aufgeführt. Zum Abschluss klicken Sie auf den Button **Finish**.

Nachdem das Projekt angelegt worden ist, werden Sie von Eclipse gefragt, ob Sie zur ABAP-Entwicklungsperspektive wechseln möchten; bestätigen Sie den Dialog, um dorthin zu wechseln.

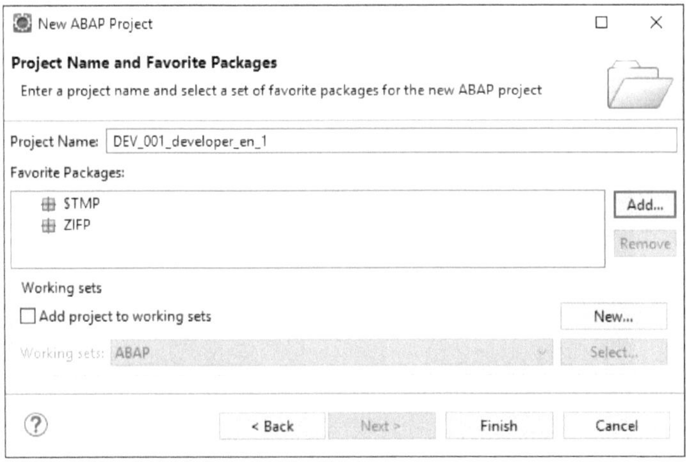

Abbildung 10.3 Entwicklerpaketfavoriten hinzufügen

Project Explorer

Das gerade angelegtes Projekt wird Ihnen nun im **Project Explorer** von Eclipse angezeigt. Wie in Abbildung 10.4 erkennbar, können Sie durch einfaches Expandieren des Eintrags **Favorite Packages** auf Ihr zuvor hinzugefügtes Paket zugreifen.

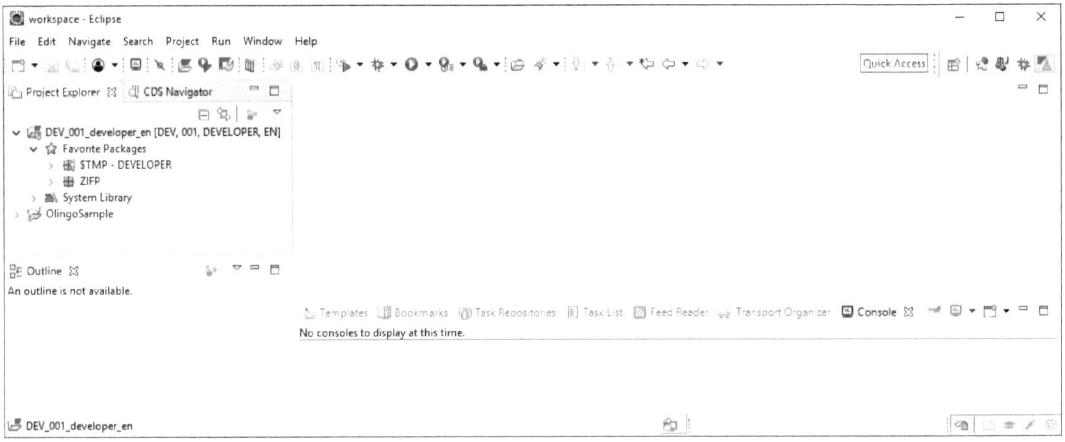

Abbildung 10.4 ABAP-Perspektive von Eclipse

Neuen CDS-View hinzufügen

Um einen neuen CDS-View hinzuzufügen, wählen Sie das Entwicklungspaket aus, dem Sie den View hinzufügen möchten, und rufen im Kontextmenü **New • Other ABAP Repository Object** auf. Es wird Ihnen nun ein Dialog mit einer Vielzahl an Ordnern angezeigt. Um die Auswahl etwas einzuschränken, geben Sie in das Suchfeld den Wert »core« ein (siehe Abbildung 10.5).

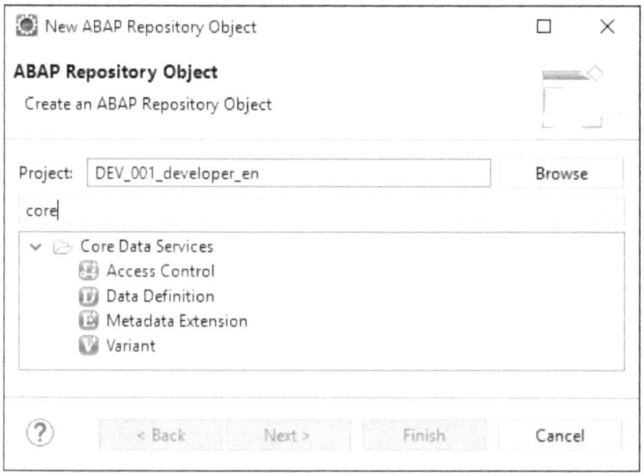

Abbildung 10.5 Auswahl der zur Verfügung stehenden Core-Data-Service-Objekte

Die Auswahl an Repository-Objekten enthält nun lediglich noch jene Objekttypen, die der Kategorie **Core Data Services** zugewiesen sind. Wählen Sie aus dieser Liste den Eintrag **Data Definition** aus, und bestätigen Sie den Dialog mit **Next**.

CDS-View-Details

Im folgenden Dialog geben Sie den Namen des neuen CDS-Views sowie einen Beschreibungstext in die entsprechenden Felder ein. Wie Sie Abbildung 10.6 entnehmen können, nennen wir den CDS-View in diesem Beispiel »ZOrderHeaderView«. Nach der Eingabe bestätigen Sie den Dialog mit **Next**. Im nachfolgenden Dialog wählen Sie einen Transportauftrag aus und verlassen den Dialog wieder mit **Next**.

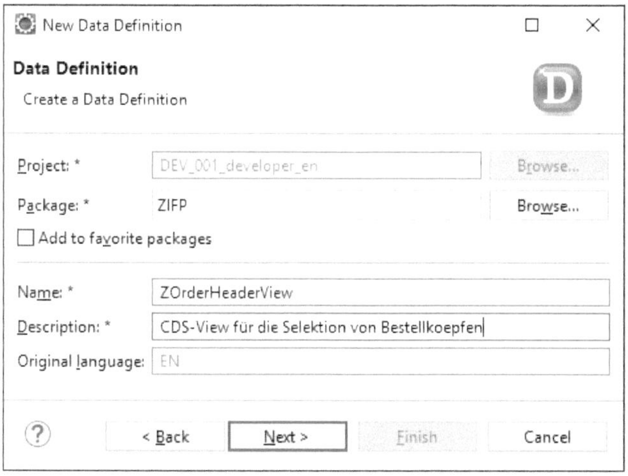

Abbildung 10.6 Anlegen eines neuen CDS-Views

CDS-View-Generator

Den Abschluss der Anlage eines CDS-Views bildet die Auswahl eines Templates, wie in Abbildung 10.7 zu sehen. Die Templates bieten nicht nur eine Dokumentation, sondern sind auch stets eine Referenzvorlage für einen gültigen CDS-View. Sie haben so z. B. eine Vorlage, um Views mit Parametern auszustatten oder Views mit ABAP Managed Database Procedures (AMDP) zu kombinieren. Wählen Sie für unser Beispiel den Eintrag **Define View** aus, und beenden Sie den Assistenten mit einem Klick auf den Button **Finish**.

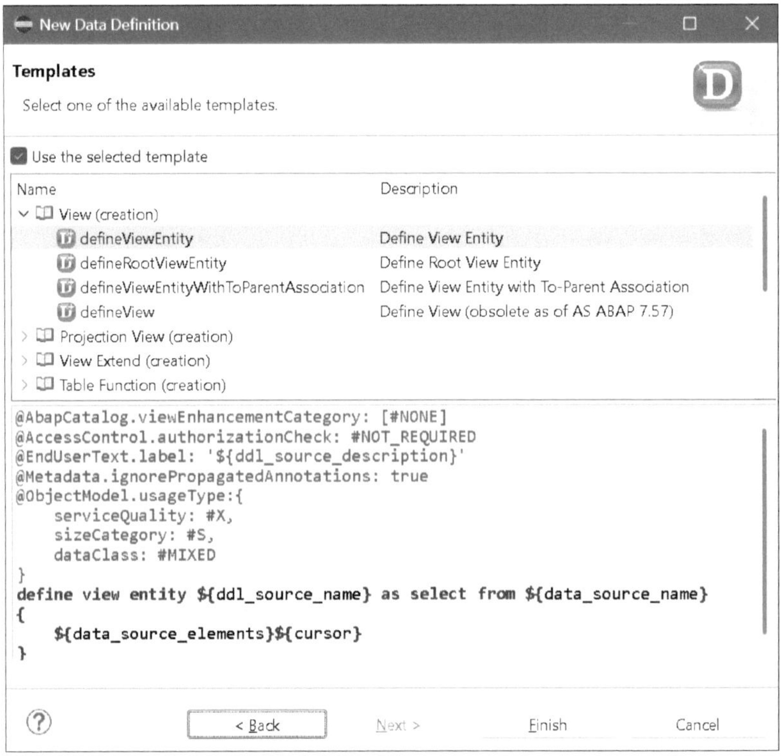

Abbildung 10.7 Auswahl des CDS-View-Entity-Templates

Generierte View-Implementierung

Der Generator legt im Anschluss die in Listing 10.1 gezeigte Implementierung an.

```
@AbapCatalog.viewEnhancementCategory: [#NONE]
@AccessControl.authorizationCheck: #CHECK
@EndUserText.label: 'CDS-View für die Selektion von Bestellkoepfen'
@Metadata.ignorePropagatedAnnotations: true
@ObjectModel.usageType:{
    serviceQuality: #X,
    sizeCategory: #S,
```

```
      dataClass: #MIXED
}
define view entity ZOrderHeaderView as select from data_source_name {

}
```

Listing 10.1 Generierte CDS-View-Entity

Ersetzen Sie nun den Platzhalter data_source_name mit dem Tabellennamen »zifporder«. Zusätzlich geben Sie alle Felder der Tabelle zifporder in der Feldliste des Views an und versehen das Feld orderid mit dem vorangestellten Schlüsselwort key. Sie erhalten die in Listing 10.2 gezeigte View-Implementierung.


```
@AbapCatalog.viewEnhancementCategory: [#NONE]
@AccessControl.authorizationCheck: #CHECK
@EndUserText.label: 'CDS-View für die Selektion von Bestellkoepfen'
@Metadata.ignorePropagatedAnnotations: true
@ObjectModel.usageType:{
      serviceQuality: #X,
      sizeCategory: #S,
      dataClass: #MIXED
}
define view entity ZOrderHeaderView as select from zifporder {
    //zifporder
    key orderid,
    type,
    refid,
    buyer,
    seller,
    orderdate
}
```

Listing 10.2 CDS-View »ZOrderHeaderView«

Aktivierung des CDS-Views

Nach der Anpassung speichern Sie Ihre Änderungen und aktivieren den CDS-View über die Tastenkombination [Strg] + [F3] oder einen Klick auf den Menüpunkt **Edit** und **Activate**. Nachdem die Aktivierung erfolgreich abgeschlossen wurde, testen Sie Ihre Implementierung. Um den View als ABAP-Applikation ausführen zu lassen, drücken Sie die Funktionstaste [F8] oder führen einem Rechtklick auf den CDS-View aus und wählen im Kontextmenü **Open With • Data Preview**. Das Ergebnis wird wie in Abbildung 10.8 gezeigt aufbereitet und dargestellt.

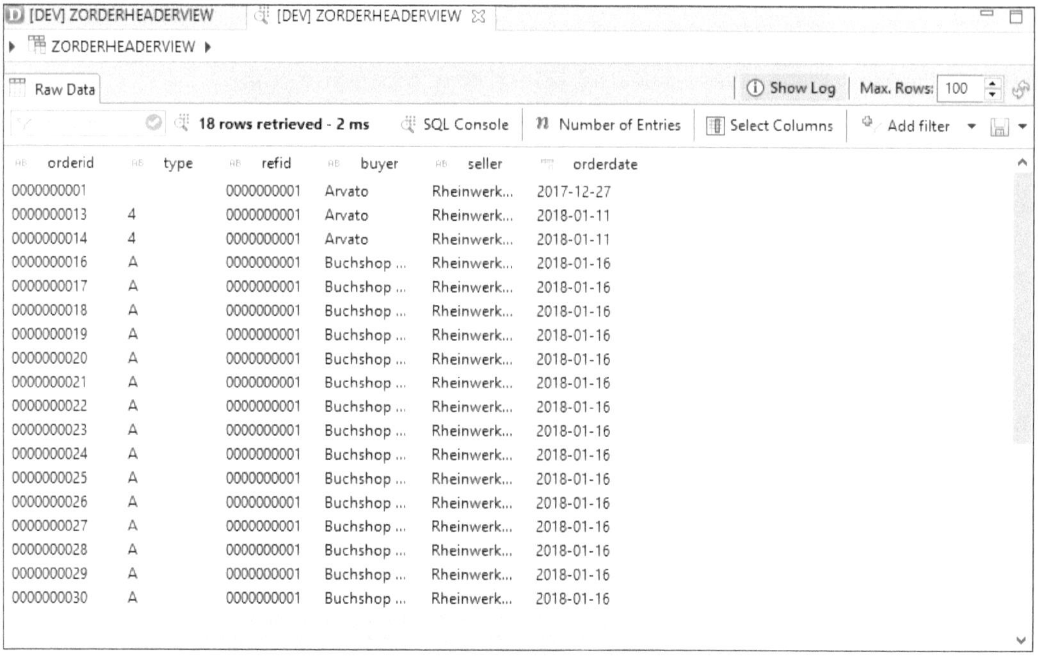

orderid	type	refid	buyer	seller	orderdate
0000000001		0000000001	Arvato	Rheinwerk...	2017-12-27
0000000013	4	0000000001	Arvato	Rheinwerk...	2018-01-11
0000000014	4	0000000001	Arvato	Rheinwerk...	2018-01-11
0000000016	A	0000000001	Buchshop ...	Rheinwerk...	2018-01-16
0000000017	A	0000000001	Buchshop ...	Rheinwerk...	2018-01-16
0000000018	A	0000000001	Buchshop ...	Rheinwerk...	2018-01-16
0000000019	A	0000000001	Buchshop ...	Rheinwerk...	2018-01-16
0000000020	A	0000000001	Buchshop ...	Rheinwerk...	2018-01-16
0000000021	A	0000000001	Buchshop ...	Rheinwerk...	2018-01-16
0000000022	A	0000000001	Buchshop ...	Rheinwerk...	2018-01-16
0000000023	A	0000000001	Buchshop ...	Rheinwerk...	2018-01-16
0000000024	A	0000000001	Buchshop ...	Rheinwerk...	2018-01-16
0000000025	A	0000000001	Buchshop ...	Rheinwerk...	2018-01-16
0000000026	A	0000000001	Buchshop ...	Rheinwerk...	2018-01-16
0000000027	A	0000000001	Buchshop ...	Rheinwerk...	2018-01-16
0000000028	A	0000000001	Buchshop ...	Rheinwerk...	2018-01-16
0000000029	A	0000000001	Buchshop ...	Rheinwerk...	2018-01-16
0000000030	A	0000000001	Buchshop ...	Rheinwerk...	2018-01-16

Abbildung 10.8 Anzeige der Selektion der Bestellköpfe

CDS-View für Bestellpositionen

Damit wir neben den Bestellköpfen auch die Bestellpositionen selektieren können, legen wir einen weiteren View an. Wir gehen dabei genauso wie bei der Anlage des Views für die Bestellköpfe vor. Sie geben dem View den Namen `ZOrderPosView` und passen, nachdem der View erzeugt worden ist, das Coding, wie in Listing 10.3 gezeigt, an.

```
@AbapCatalog.viewEnhancementCategory: [#NONE]
@AccessControl.authorizationCheck: #CHECK
@EndUserText.label: 'CDS-View für die Selektion von
Bestellpositionen'
@Metadata.ignorePropagatedAnnotations: true
@ObjectModel.usageType:{
      serviceQuality: #X,
      sizeCategory: #S,
      dataClass: #MIXED
}
define view entity ZOrderPosView as select from zifporderpos {
 //zifporderpos

 key orderid,
 orderpos,
 matid,
```

```
  mattext,
  ordercount,
  price,
  currency
}
```

Listing 10.3 CDS-View zur Selektion der Bestellpositionen

Mit dem nächsten Schritt wollen wir es ermöglichen, dass zu einem Bestellkopf auch die dazugehörenden Bestellpositionen ausgegeben werden. Hierfür definieren Sie *Assoziationen* in CDS-Views . Dabei verknüpfen Sie eine Assoziationsquelle, in unserem Beispiel den View `ZOrderHeaderView`, mit einem Assoziationsziel, bei uns der View `ZOrderPosView`. Assoziationen werden letztlich als Join-Verknüpfungen abgebildet. Jedoch werden diese Verknüpfungen erst dann tatsächlich ausgewertet, wenn sie verwendet werden. Assoziationen erhalten bei der Definition der Zielverknüpfung auch die Angabe der Beziehung zwischen der Quell- und Zielentität.

Assoziationen

10

Um eine Assoziation zwischen unseren beiden Views herzustellen, passen Sie, wie in Listing 10.4 gezeigt, unseren View `ZOrderHeaderView` an. Wie Sie dem Listing entnehmen können, verwenden wir für die Assoziation das Schlüsselwort `association`, gefolgt von der Angabe der Kardinalität der Assoziation. Die Kardinalität wird in eckige Klammern geschrieben. In unserem Beispiel gehen wir davon aus, dass wir mindestens eine Bestellposition pro Bestellung haben, es aber unendliche viele Bestellpositionen geben kann. Aufgrund dieser Annahme nutzen wir die Kardinalität [1..*].

Assoziation definieren und exponieren

Zusätzlich geben wir der Assoziation unter der Verwendung der Aliasfunktion `as` noch einen Namen. Als Letztes definieren wir den relationalen Zusammenhang zwischen den beiden Assoziationsteilnehmern. Dies geschieht mit einer `on`-Bedingung. Wir verknüpfen so das Feld `orderid` des Quell-CDS-Views mit dem entsprechenden Feld des Ziel-CDS-Views.

```
@AbapCatalog.viewEnhancementCategory: [#NONE]
@AccessControl.authorizationCheck: #CHECK
@EndUserText.label: 'CDS-View für die Selektion von Bestellkoepfen'
@Metadata.ignorePropagatedAnnotations: true
@ObjectModel.usageType:{
      serviceQuality: #X,
      sizeCategory: #S,
      dataClass: #MIXED
}
define view entity ZOrderHeaderView as select from zifporder
association [1..*] to ZOrderPosView as _OrderPositions on
```

```
$projection.orderid = _OrderPositions.orderid
 {
    //zifporder
    mandt,
   key orderid,
    type,
    refid,
    buyer,
    seller,
    orderdate,
    _OrderPositions
}
```

Listing 10.4 Implementierung einer Assoziation

Schließlich müssen wir noch dafür sorgen, dass die Assoziation von außen verwendet werden kann. Denn bis jetzt handelt es sich bei der Definition der Assoziation um ein internes Implementierungsdetail, das keinerlei Verwendung von außen ermöglicht. Das Exponieren erfolgt durch das Hinzufügen der Assoziation in die Feldliste des CDS-Views.

Bestellpositionen anzeigen

Im Anschluss an die erfolgreiche Aktivierung führen wir den CDS-View in Eclipse erneut aus (F8). Nachdem die Ergebnismenge angezeigt worden ist, wählen wir einen Datensatz aus, bei dem wir wissen, dass Bestellpositionen in der Datenbank vorhanden sind, und rufen im Kontextmenü den Menüeintrag **Follow Association** auf (siehe Abbildung 10.9).

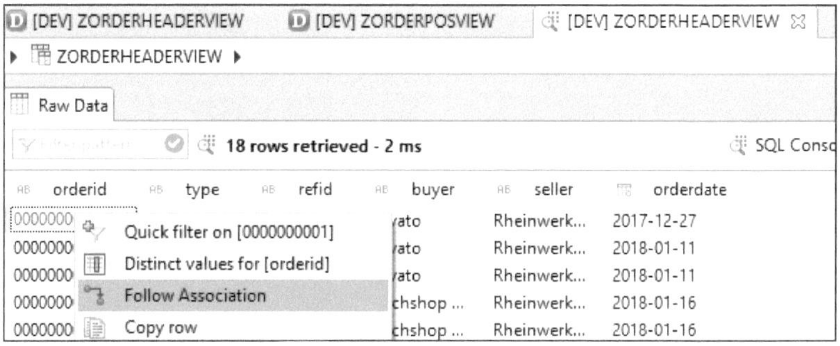

Abbildung 10.9 Auflösen einer Assoziation

Es wird Ihnen nun ein Auswahldialog angezeigt (siehe Abbildung 10.10), in dem Sie die Assoziation `_OrderPositions` auswählen können. Nach der Auswahl wechselt die Anzeige, und Sie erhalten die Bestellpositionen für den entsprechenden Bestellkopf.

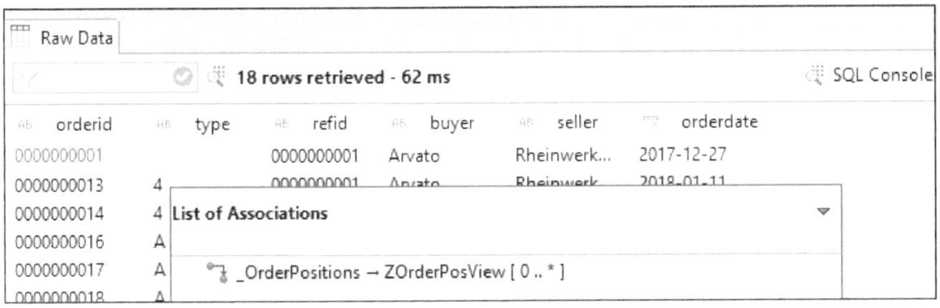

Abbildung 10.10 Liste der verfügbaren Assoziationen

Bereitstellung des CDS-Views als OData-Service

Nach dem Abschluss der Implementierung möchten wir unseren CDS-View als OData-Service bereitstellen. Dies geschieht am einfachsten, indem Sie die Annotation `@OData.publish:true` verwenden. Die Annotation wird dabei vor der eigentlichen View-Implementierung angegeben. Die daraus resultierende Änderung am CDS-View `ZOrderHeaderView` können Sie Listing 10.5 entnehmen.

```
@AbapCatalog.viewEnhancementCategory: [#NONE]
@AccessControl.authorizationCheck: #CHECK
@EndUserText.label: 'CDS-View für die Selektion von Bestellkoepfen'
@Metadata.ignorePropagatedAnnotations: true
@ObjectModel.usageType:{
      serviceQuality: #X,
      sizeCategory: #S,
      dataClass: #MIXED
}
@OData.publish: true
define view entity ZOrderHeaderView as select from zifporder
association [0..*] to ZOrderPosView as _OrderPositions on
zifporder.orderid = _OrderPositions.orderid
 {
    //zifporder
    mandt,
   key orderid,
    type,
    refid,
    buyer,
    seller,
    orderdate,
    _OrderPositions
}
```

Listing 10.5 OData-Annotation

OData-Service generieren

Speichern und aktivieren Sie die Änderungen. Im Anschluss an die erfolgreiche Aktivierung wird vor der OData-Annotation ein Icon mit einem G angezeigt (**Generated Objects**). Führen Sie den Mauszeiger auf dieses Symbol, wird ein Infofeld angezeigt, das Sie darüber informiert, dass die Generierung des CDS-Views als OData-Service erfolgreich abgeschlossen ist (siehe Abbildung 10.11).

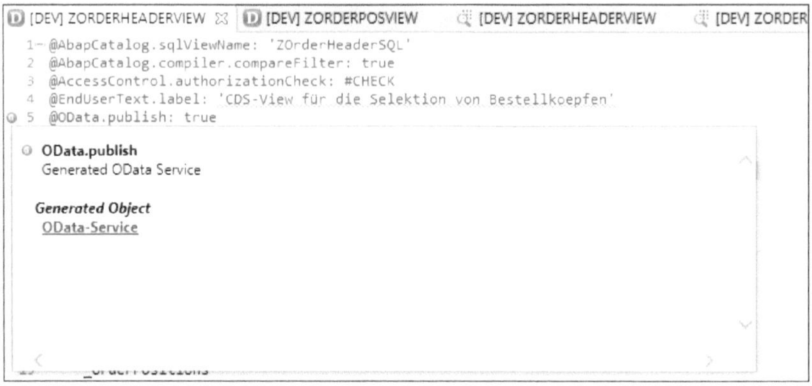

Abbildung 10.11 Als OData-Service generierter CDS-View

10.3 OData-Service registrieren und testen

Transaktion /IWFND/ MAINT_SERVICE

Nach der Aktivierung müssen Sie den OData-Service auf Ihrem System explizit registrieren. Je nach System-Setup geschieht dies entweder direkt auf dem Backend-Server oder auf dem Frontend-Server. Gehen Sie zur Registrierung des Diensts wie folgt vor:

1. Rufen Sie Transaktion /IWFND/MAINT_SERVICE auf.
2. Wählen Sie den Button **Service hinzufügen** aus.
3. Geben Sie im daraufhin erscheinenden Dialog den Alias des Systems ein, auf dem Ihr neu erzeugter OData-Service zu finden ist. Zusätzlich können Sie, damit die Auswahlmenge an Diensten kürzer ist, in das Feld **Technischer Servicename** beispielsweise »Z*CDS« eingeben (siehe Abbildung 10.12).
4. Nach der Eingabe drücken Sie [↵], und der OData-Service `ZORDERHEADERVIEW_CDS` wird in einer Liste angezeigt.
5. Wählen Sie den Eintrag aus, und klicken Sie auf den Button **Ausgewählte Services hinzufügen**.
6. Sie werden nun aufgefordert, ein Paket anzugeben, zu dem Sie die Artefakte hinzufügen möchten. Nachdem Sie ein Paket ausgewählt haben, bestätigen Sie den Dialog mit [↵].

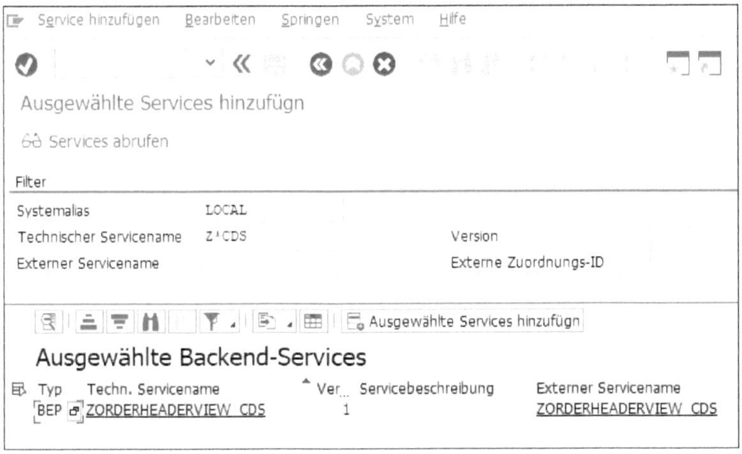

Abbildung 10.12 OData-Service hinzufügen

7. Zum Abschluss müssen Sie noch einen Transportauftrag angeben. Ist dieser angelegt, informiert Sie das System mit einer entsprechenden Erfolgsmeldung, die Sie bestätigen.

Wechseln Sie über die Funktionstaste F3 zum Ausgangsbild von Transaktion /IWFND/MAINT_SERVICE.

Nutzen Sie die Filterfunktion, um unseren OData-Service einfacher zu finden. Er wird wie in Abbildung 10.13 dargestellt angezeigt.

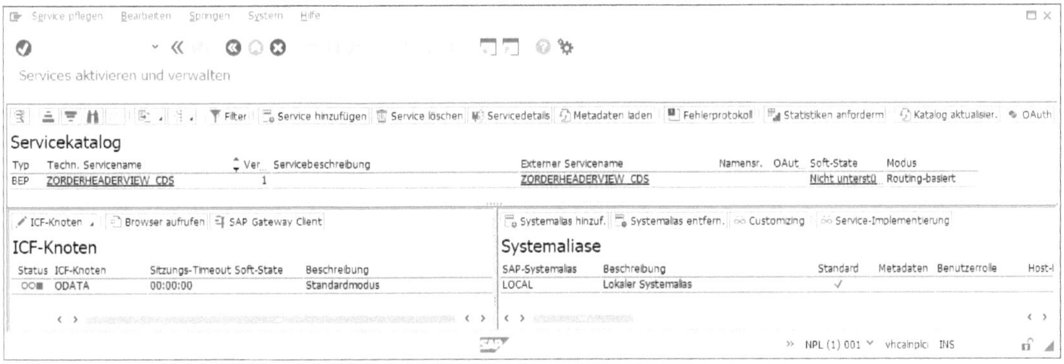

Abbildung 10.13 Registrierter OData-Service

OData-Service testen

Wie bereits in Kapitel 9, »SAP Gateway und OData«, gezeigt, können Sie den OData-Service bequem über den SAP Gateway Client testen. Klicken Sie hierzu in Transaktion /IWFND/MAINT_SERVICE auf den Button **SAP Gateway Client**. Die unter Umständen angezeigte Sicherheitsabfrage bestätigen

Sie mit einem Klick auf den Button **Zulassen**. Nachdem die Transaktion gestartet worden ist, wird in der Adresszeile des SAP Gateway Clients der URI zum Servicedokument unseres Diensts angezeigt. Durch einen Klick auf **Ausführen** oder durch einfaches Bestätigen mit [↵] werden Ihnen das Servicedokument und damit die vorhandenen Entitäten Ihres OData-Service angezeigt. Wie Sie Abbildung 10.14 entnehmen können, werden genau die Entitätsbezeichner im Servicedokument angeboten, die beim Anlegen der CDS-Views verwendet wurden.

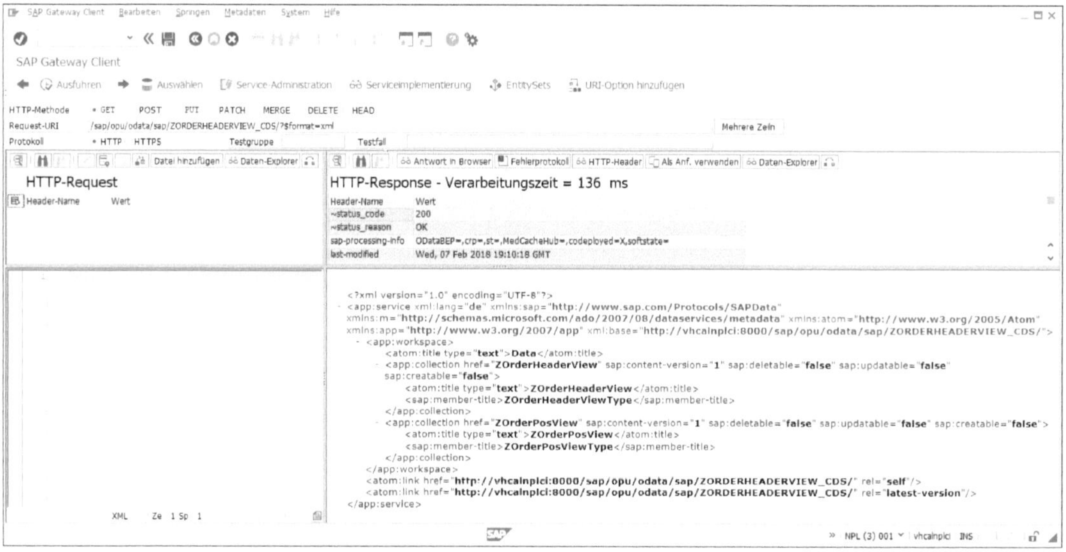

Abbildung 10.14 Servicedokument

Metadaten

Als Nächstes möchten wir uns noch genauer mit den Metadaten des Diensts beschäftigen. Hierzu klicken Sie auf den Button **URI-Option hinzufügen** und wählen aus der daraufhin erscheinenden Liste den Wert »$metadata« per Doppelklick auf den Eintrag aus. Die URI-Option wird an die Servicedokument-URI angehängt. Die Anfrage an den Server setzen Sie mit [↵] ab. Sie erhalten die in Abbildung 10.15 gezeigten Metadaten unseres auf einem CDS-View basierenden OData-Service.

OData-Service testen

Basierend auf dem Wissen der Metadaten, können Sie nun den OData-Service testen. Wählen Sie hierzu den Button **EntitySets**. Sie erhalten, wie in Abbildung 10.16 gezeigt, zwei Entity Sets zur Auswahl. Die Namensgebung beruht dabei auf den Bezeichnungen der CDS-Views.

```xml
<?xml version="1.0" encoding="UTF-8"?>
- <edmx:Edmx xmlns:sap="http://www.sap.com/Protocols/SAPData"
xmlns:m="http://schemas.microsoft.com/ado/2007/08/dataservices/metadata"
xmlns:edmx="http://schemas.microsoft.com/ado/2007/06/edmx" Version="1.0">
  - <edmx:Reference xmlns:edmx="http://docs.oasis-open.org/odata/ns/edmx"
    Uri="http://vhcalnplci:8000/sap/opu/odata/IWFND/CATALOGSERVICE;v=2/Vocabularies(TechnicalName='%2FIWBEP%
    2FVOC_COMMON',Version='0001',SAP__Origin='')/$value">
      <edmx:Include Alias="Common" Namespace="com.sap.vocabularies.Common.v1"/>
    </edmx:Reference>
  - <edmx:DataServices m:DataServiceVersion="2.0">
    - <Schema xml:lang="de" Namespace="ZORDERHEADERVIEW_CDS" xmlns="http://schemas.microsoft.com/ado/2008/09/edm" sap:schema-
      version="1">
      - <EntityType sap:content-version="1" Name="ZOrderHeaderViewType">
        - <Key>
            <PropertyRef Name="orderid"/>
          </Key>
          <Property Name="orderid" sap:label="Bestellnummer" sap:display-format="NonNegative" MaxLength="10" Nullable="false"
            Type="Edm.String"/>
          <Property Name="type" sap:label="Bestelltyp" sap:display-format="UpperCase" MaxLength="2" Type="Edm.String"/>
          <Property Name="refid" sap:label="Referenznummer" sap:display-format="NonNegative" MaxLength="10" Type="Edm.String"/>
          <Property Name="buyer" sap:label="Käufer" sap:display-format="UpperCase" MaxLength="50" Type="Edm.String"/>
          <Property Name="seller" sap:label="Lieferant" sap:display-format="UpperCase" MaxLength="50" Type="Edm.String"/>
          <Property Name="orderdate" sap:label="Bestelldatum" sap:display-format="Date" Type="Edm.DateTime" Precision="0"/>
          <NavigationProperty Name="to_OrderPositions" ToRole="ToRole_assoc_FC3BFA14206F74DE1BEF3F845B155F03"
            FromRole="FromRole_assoc_FC3BFA14206F74DE1BEF3F845B155F03"
            Relationship="ZORDERHEADERVIEW_CDS.assoc_FC3BFA14206F74DE1BEF3F845B155F03"/>
        </EntityType>
      - <EntityType sap:content-version="1" Name="ZOrderPosViewType">
        - <Key>
            <PropertyRef Name="orderid"/>
            <PropertyRef Name="orderpos"/>
          </Key>
          <Property Name="orderid" sap:label="Bestellnummer" sap:display-format="NonNegative" MaxLength="10" Nullable="false"
            Type="Edm.String"/>
          <Property Name="orderpos" sap:label="Bestellposition" sap:display-format="NonNegative" MaxLength="5" Nullable="false"
            Type="Edm.String"/>
          <Property Name="matid" sap:label="Materialnummer" sap:display-format="UpperCase" MaxLength="20" Type="Edm.String"/>
          <Property Name="mattext" sap:label="Materialtext" sap:display-format="UpperCase" MaxLength="40" Type="Edm.String"/>
          <Property Name="ordercount" sap:label="Anzahl" Type="Edm.Int32"/>
          <Property Name="price" sap:label="Preis" Type="Edm.Decimal" Precision="8" sap:unit="currency" Scale="4"/>
          <Property Name="currency" sap:label="Währung" MaxLength="5" Type="Edm.String" sap:semantics="currency-code"/>
        </EntityType>
      - <Association sap:content-version="1" Name="assoc_FC3BFA14206F74DE1BEF3F845B155F03">
          <End Type="ZORDERHEADERVIEW_CDS.ZOrderHeaderViewType" Role="FromRole_assoc_FC3BFA14206F74DE1BEF3F845B155F03"
            Multiplicity="1"/>
          <End Type="ZORDERHEADERVIEW_CDS.ZOrderPosViewType" Role="ToRole_assoc_FC3BFA14206F74DE1BEF3F845B155F03"
            Multiplicity="*"/>
        </Association>
      - <EntityContainer Name="ZORDERHEADERVIEW_CDS_Entities" sap:supported-formats="atom json xlsx" m:IsDefaultEntityContainer="true">
          <EntitySet sap:content-version="1" sap:deletable="false" sap:updatable="false" sap:creatable="false" Name="ZOrderHeaderView"
            EntityType="ZORDERHEADERVIEW_CDS.ZOrderHeaderViewType"/>
          <EntitySet sap:content-version="1" sap:deletable="false" sap:updatable="false" sap:creatable="false" Name="ZOrderPosView"
            EntityType="ZORDERHEADERVIEW_CDS.ZOrderPosViewType"/>
        - <AssociationSet sap:content-version="1" sap:deletable="false" sap:updatable="false" sap:creatable="false"
          Name="assoc_FC3BFA14206F74DE1BEF3F845B155F03"
          Association="ZORDERHEADERVIEW_CDS.assoc_FC3BFA14206F74DE1BEF3F845B155F03">
            <End Role="FromRole_assoc_FC3BFA14206F74DE1BEF3F845B155F03" EntitySet="ZOrderHeaderView"/>
            <End Role="ToRole_assoc_FC3BFA14206F74DE1BEF3F845B155F03" EntitySet="ZOrderPosView"/>
          </AssociationSet>
        </EntityContainer>
        <atom:link xmlns:atom="http://www.w3.org/2005/Atom"
          href="http://vhcalnplci:8000/sap/opu/odata/sap/ZORDERHEADERVIEW_CDS/$metadata" rel="self"/>
        <atom:link xmlns:atom="http://www.w3.org/2005/Atom"
          href="http://vhcalnplci:8000/sap/opu/odata/sap/ZORDERHEADERVIEW_CDS/$metadata" rel="latest-version"/>
      </Schema>
    </edmx:DataServices>
</edmx:Edmx>
```


Abbildung 10.15 Metadaten des OData-Service

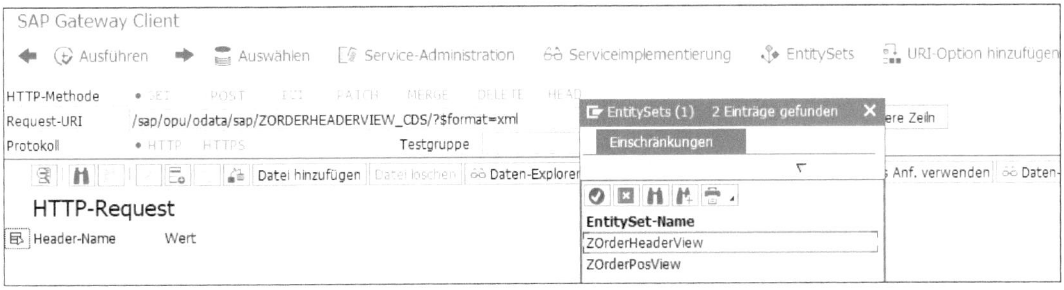

Abbildung 10.16 Verfügbare Entity Sets

10

Wählen Sie den Eintrag **ZOrderHeaderView** aus. Dieser Name wird daraufhin an die URL des Servicedokuments angehängt. Danach führen Sie die Anfrage im SAP Gateway Client mit [F8] oder [↵] aus. Nach der Verarbeitung der Anfrage zeigt der SAP Gateway Client die Antwort des Servers an und listet die gefundenen Datensätze auf.

Einzelne Bestellung ansehen

Da wir an einen bestimmten Datensatz interessiert sind, ändern wir die Anfrage dahingehend ab, dass wir eine konkrete Bestellung adressieren. In unserem Beispiel möchten wir die Bestellkopfdetails der Bestellung mit der Order-ID `'0000000001'` betrachten. Daher geben Sie in das Adressfeld des SAP Gateway Clients den URI »/sap/opu/odata/sap/ZORDERHEADERVIEW_CDS/ZOrderHeaderView('0000000001')« ein und bestätigen die Eingabe mit [↵]. Als Antwort erhalten Sie die in Abbildung 10.17 gezeigte XML-Struktur.


```
<?xml version="1.0" encoding="UTF-8"?>
- <entry xmlns:m="http://schemas.microsoft.com/ado/2007/08/dataservices/metadata"
  xml:base="http://vhcalnplci:8000/sap/opu/odata/sap/ZORDERHEADERVIEW_CDS/"
  xmlns:d="http://schemas.microsoft.com/ado/2007/08/dataservices" xmlns="http://www.w3.org/2005/Atom">
    <id>http://vhcalnplci:8000/sap/opu/odata/sap/ZORDERHEADERVIEW_CDS/ZOrderHeaderView('0000000001')</id>
    <title type="text">ZOrderHeaderView('0000000001')</title>
    <updated>2018-02-07T18:51:48Z</updated>
    <category scheme="http://schemas.microsoft.com/ado/2007/08/dataservices/scheme"
      term="ZORDERHEADERVIEW_CDS.ZOrderHeaderViewType"/>
    <link title="ZOrderHeaderViewType" href="ZOrderHeaderView('0000000001')" rel="self"/>
    <link title="to_OrderPositions" type="application/atom+xml;type=feed" href="ZOrderHeaderView('0000000001')/to_OrderPositions"
      rel="http://schemas.microsoft.com/ado/2007/08/dataservices/related/to_OrderPositions"/>
  - <content type="application/xml">
    - <m:properties>
        <d:orderid>0000000001</d:orderid>
        <d:type/>
        <d:refid>0000000001</d:refid>
        <d:buyer>Arvato</d:buyer>
        <d:seller>Rheinwerk-Verlag</d:seller>
        <d:orderdate>2017-12-27T00:00:00</d:orderdate>
      </m:properties>
    </content>
</entry>
```


Abbildung 10.17 Bestellkopfdetails im SAP Gateway Client

Wie Sie Abbildung 10.17 entnehmen können, liefert der OData-Service neben den Bestellkopfinformationen zusätzlich auch noch die Informationen, dass Sie zu den zugehörenden Bestellpositionen navigieren können. Hierzu stellt uns der Service, basierend auf der im CDS-View implementierten Assoziation, die Navigationseigenschaft `Positions` zur Verfügung. Fügen Sie nun an den in der Adresszeile des SAP Gateway Clients enthaltenen URI die Navigationseigenschaft »/to_OrderPositions« an. Sie erhalten damit den folgenden URI:

/sap/opu/odata/sap/ZORDERHEADERVIEW_CDS/ZOrderHeader-View('0000000001')/to_OrderPositions

Rückantwort des Servers

Bestätigen Sie Ihre Eingabe mit [↵]. So veranlassen Sie, dass der Request an den OData-Service gesendet wird. Nach einer kurzen Wartezeit erhalten Sie die in Abbildung 10.18 gezeigte Rückantwort des Servers.

```
<?xml version="1.0"?>
- <feed xmlns:m="http://schemas.microsoft.com/ado/2007/08/dataservices/metadata"
  xml:base="http://vhcalnplci:8000/sap/opu/odata/sap/ZORDERHEADERVIEW_CDS/"
  xmlns:d="http://schemas.microsoft.com/ado/2007/08/dataservices" xmlns="http://www.w3.org/2005/Atom">
    <id>http://vhcalnplci:8000/sap/opu/odata/sap/ZORDERHEADERVIEW_CDS/ZOrderHeaderView('0000000001')/to_OrderPositions</id>
    <title type="text">ZOrderPosView</title>
    <updated>2018-02-07T18:52:50Z</updated>
  - <author>
      <name/>
    </author>
    <link title="ZOrderPosView" href="ZOrderHeaderView('0000000001')/to_OrderPositions" rel="self"/>
  - <entry>
      <id>http://vhcalnplci:8000/sap/opu/odata/sap/ZORDERHEADERVIEW_CDS/ZOrderPosView(orderid='0000000001',orderpos='00001')
        </id>
      <title type="text">ZOrderPosView(orderid='0000000001',orderpos='00001')</title>
      <updated>2018-02-07T18:52:50Z</updated>
      <category scheme="http://schemas.microsoft.com/ado/2007/08/dataservices/scheme"
        term="ZORDERHEADERVIEW_CDS.ZOrderPosViewType"/>
      <link title="ZOrderPosViewType" href="ZOrderPosView(orderid='0000000001',orderpos='00001')" rel="self"/>
    - <content type="application/xml">
      - <m:properties xmlns:m="http://schemas.microsoft.com/ado/2007/08/dataservices/metadata"
        xmlns:d="http://schemas.microsoft.com/ado/2007/08/dataservices">
          <d:orderid>0000000001</d:orderid>
          <d:orderpos>00001</d:orderpos>
          <d:matid>000000000000001234</d:matid>
          <d:mattext>SAP Schnittstellenprogrammierung</d:mattext>
          <d:ordercount>3</d:ordercount>
          <d:price>79.00</d:price>
          <d:currency>EUR</d:currency>
        </m:properties>
      </content>
    </entry>
  - <entry>
      <id>http://vhcalnplci:8000/sap/opu/odata/sap/ZORDERHEADERVIEW_CDS/ZOrderPosView(orderid='0000000001',orderpos='00002')
        </id>
      <title type="text">ZOrderPosView(orderid='0000000001',orderpos='00002')</title>
      <updated>2018-02-07T18:52:50Z</updated>
      <category scheme="http://schemas.microsoft.com/ado/2007/08/dataservices/scheme"
        term="ZORDERHEADERVIEW_CDS.ZOrderPosViewType"/>
      <link title="ZOrderPosViewType" href="ZOrderPosView(orderid='0000000001',orderpos='00002')" rel="self"/>
    - <content type="application/xml">
      - <m:properties xmlns:m="http://schemas.microsoft.com/ado/2007/08/dataservices/metadata"
        xmlns:d="http://schemas.microsoft.com/ado/2007/08/dataservices">
          <d:orderid>0000000001</d:orderid>
          <d:orderpos>00002</d:orderpos>
          <d:matid>000000000000007899</d:matid>
          <d:mattext>SAP Fiori</d:mattext>
          <d:ordercount>5</d:ordercount>
          <d:price>69.00</d:price>
          <d:currency>EUR</d:currency>
        </m:properties>
      </content>
    </entry>
</feed>
```


Abbildung 10.18 Bestellpositionen zum angegebenen Bestellkopfsatz

10

Kapitel 11
ABAP RESTful Application Programming Model und OData

Ein einheitliches Programmiermodell für die Entwicklung moderner SAP-Anwendungen mit ABAP – on-premise und für die Cloud – bietet viele Möglichkeiten. In diesem Kapitel erfahren Sie, wie sie moderne und wiederverwendbare Lösungen implementieren.

Stabilität, Wartbarkeit, Erweiterbarkeit und Wiederverwendbarkeit sind, neben der Effizienz, wichtige Ziele bei der Entwicklung von Software. Dies gilt selbstverständlich auch für SAP-Lösungen, unabhängig davon, ob es sich um kundenindividuelle oder SAP-Produktentwicklungen handelt, um Erweiterungen oder eigenständige Lösungen. Die in Kapitel 9, »SAP Gateway und OData«, vorgestellten Konzepte und Technologien für die Implementierung eines OData-basierten REST-Service fassen die Leitplanken bei der Entwicklung, also die Vorgaben, wie Funktionen und Modelle zu implementieren sind, noch recht weit. Mit dem *ABAP RESTful Application Programming Model* (RAP) geht SAP neue Wege bei der Implementierung solcher REST-Dienste. Mit einem klar definierten Framework-Design und Werkzeugen sowie, falls gewünscht, einer Übernahme der kompletten Transaktionsverarbeitung durch das Framework, bringt dieses Programmiermodell viele Komponenten mit, die die eingangs erwähnten Ziele verfolgen und deren Einhaltung sicherstellen.

In diesem Kapitel geben wir Ihnen einen Überblick über die Entwicklung von Anwendungen mit dem ABAP RESTful Application Programming Model. Nach einer kurzen Einführung in Abschnitt 11.1 gehen wir in Abschnitt 11.2, »Design des virtuellen Datenmodells«, darauf ein, was ein virtuelles Datenmodell ist und wie dieses aufgebaut wird, und in Abschnitt 11.3 darauf, wie man ein solches virtuelles Datenmodell implementiert. In Abschnitt 11.4 implementieren wir einen RAP-basierten OData-Service. In Abschnitt 11.5 zeigen wir Ihnen, wie leicht man mit dem ABAP RESTful Application Programming Model und unter Verwendung von SAP Fiori Elements eine SAP-Fiori-Anwendung implementieren kann.

11.1 Einführung in das ABAP RESTful Application Programming Model

REST-basierte Webservices

Wie in Abschnitt 9.2.1, »Representational State Transfer«, erläutert, stellt REST aktuell das wohl wichtigste Architekturmuster dar. OData als Protokoll ist hierbei ein wichtiger Pfeiler bei der Bereitstellung von REST-Diensten in einer SAP-Landschaft. Die Implementierung dieser Dienste kann über SAP Gateway erfolgen, allerdings wird dieser Weg im Kontext von SAP S/4HANA von SAP nicht mehr empfohlen. An seine Stelle tritt das ABAP RESTful Application Programming Model. Es wurde entwickelt, um die Entwicklung von REST-basierten Webservices für SAP zu vereinfachen.

Im Wesentlichen bietet das ABAP RESTful Application Programming Model eine umfassende Lösung zur Entwicklung von Webanwendungen, die über RESTful APIs miteinander kommunizieren und sich nahtlos in die SAP-Cloud-Umgebung integrieren lassen. Das Programmiermodell wurde mit SAP Cloud Platform, ABAP Environment 1808 eingeführt (heute *SAP BTP, ABAP Environment*) und mit der ABAP-Plattform 7.54 (1909) auch on-premise zur Verfügung gestellt.

Hauptziele

Eines der Hauptziele des Programmiermodells war die Bereitstellung einer einfachen und effektiven Möglichkeit, RESTful APIs auf der SAP-S/4HANA-Plattform zu entwickeln. Die Plattform unterstützt so schnelle, reaktive Schnittstellen für Frontend- und Backend-Interaktionen. Dabei wird der bestehende ABAP-Stack genutzt, um die Entwicklung in der SAP-Welt zu erleichtern. Weiterhin stell das Design-Paradigma die Implementierung von wiederverwendbaren Artefakten in den Vordergrund und somit eben auch die Reduktion von Redundanzen im System. Mit klar definieren und implementierten Servicekontrakten kann damit ein sowohl vertikal als auch horizontal sauberes System ermöglicht werden.

Architektur

Das ABAP RESTful Application Programming Model besteht grundsätzlich aus drei Hauptbestandteilen, die sich wiederum in einzelne Komponenten untergliedern. Wie Sie Abbildung 11.1 entnehmen können, stellt die Modellierung des Domänenmodells durch das Definieren von Business-Objekten und deren transaktionalem Verhalten die Basis des Modells dar. Das *transaktionale Verhalten* gibt an, ob ein Objekt angelegt, geändert oder gelöscht werden kann. Business-Objekte werden mit ABAP CDS beschrieben (siehe Kapitel 10, »SAP HANA und ABAP Core Data Services«) und folgen somit dem bereits bekannten Paradigma. Dadurch werden auch die bekannten Query-Operationen wie das Sortieren, Gruppieren oder Filtern unterstützt.

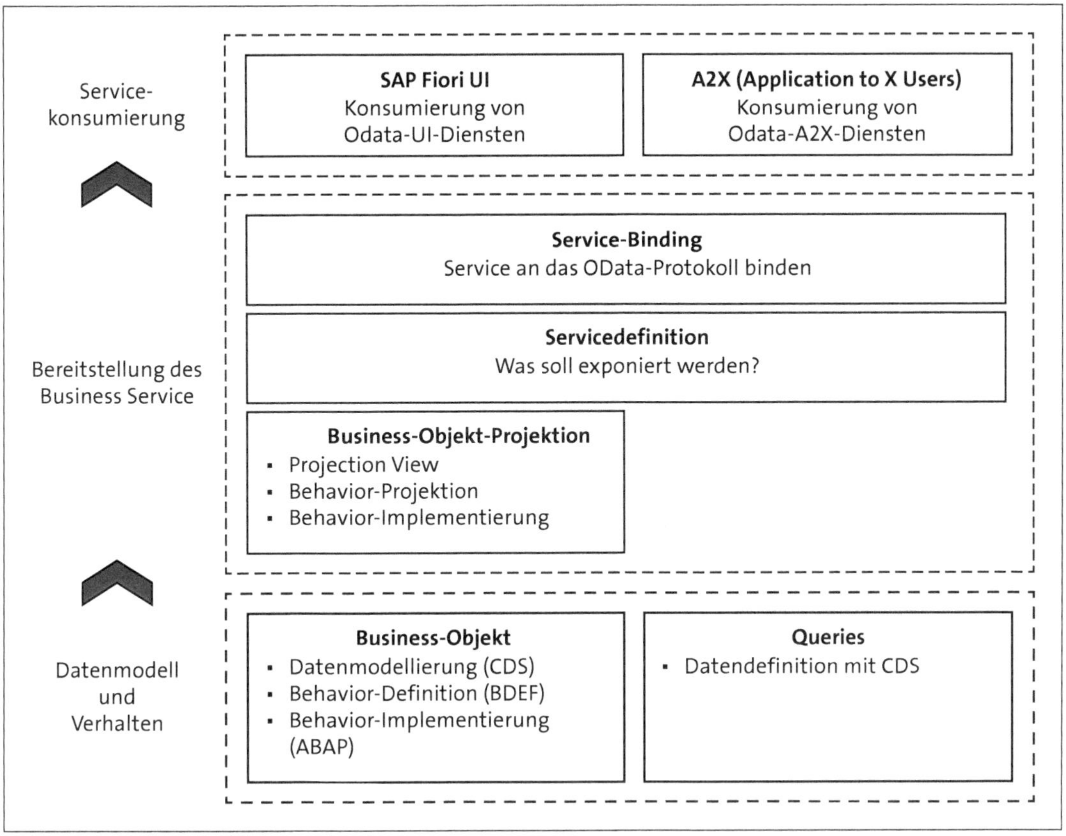

Abbildung 11.1 Artefakte und deren Aufgabe im ABAP RESTful Programming Model

Über die sogenannte *Servicedefinition* wird angegeben, welche Artefakte an den Aufrufer zurückgegeben werden. Hier werden beispielsweise die Entitäten angegeben, die über den Service konsumiert werden können. Oberhalb der Servicedefinition liegt das *Service-Binding*. Denn anders als bei der Implementierung von OData-Diensten mit Transaktion SEGW, bei der man sehr viel über das OData-Protokoll wissen muss, ist das Service Behavior im ABAP RESTful Application Model nicht an ein Protokoll gebunden. Das Binden einer Servicedefinition an ein Protokoll geschieht erst über das Service-Binding. Für eine tiefer gehende Einführung in die Entwicklung mit dem ABAP RESTful Applicatiotion Programming Model empfehlen wir das Buch »ABAP RESTful Applicatiotion Programming Model« von Lutz Baumbusch, Matthias Jäger und Michael Lensch (SAP PRESS 2024).

11.2 Design des virtuellen Datenmodells

Die Modellierung der angesprochenen ABAP-CDS-Views stellt einen wichtigen Aspekte beim Design von wiederverwendbaren und nachhaltigen Lösungen dar. Das dabei verwendete *Virtuelle Datenmodell* (VDM) bildet die Grundlage für den Datenzugriff in SAP S/4HANA, beispielsweise bei der Nutzung von analytischen Anwendungen oder APIs. Virtuelle Datenmodelle enthalten viele semantische Informationen, die durch den Konsumenten bzw. durch das SAP-System selbst verarbeitet und ausgewertet werden kann.

Realisierung durch CDS-Views

In SAP S/4HANA Cloud wird das VDM ebenso wie in der On-Premise-Variante von SAP S/4HANA durch CDS-Views realisiert. Diese CDS-Views, die in ihrer Gesamtheit das VDM bilden, folgen einheitlichen Modellierungs- und Benennungsrichtlinien. Sie repräsentieren Geschäftsdaten, die in Datenbanktabellen gespeichert sind, basierend auf den zugrunde liegenden Geschäftssemantiken und erleichtern so deren Nutzung. Ein Teil der CDS-Views des VDM von SAP ist für die Wiederverwendung durch SAP-Kunden und -Partner verfügbar. Für die Implementierung von kundenindividuellen Lösungen sollten Sie darauf achten, dass Sie sich ebenfalls an die Designregeln von SAP halten. Nur so kann ein sauberes API-Design gewährleistet werden.

Datenbanktabellen

Das VDM setzt sich aus mehreren Schichten zusammen (siehe Abbildung 11.2). Die Datenbanktabellen bilden die unterste Ebene. Views des VDM werden darüber angeordnet und bilden die Zugriffschicht.

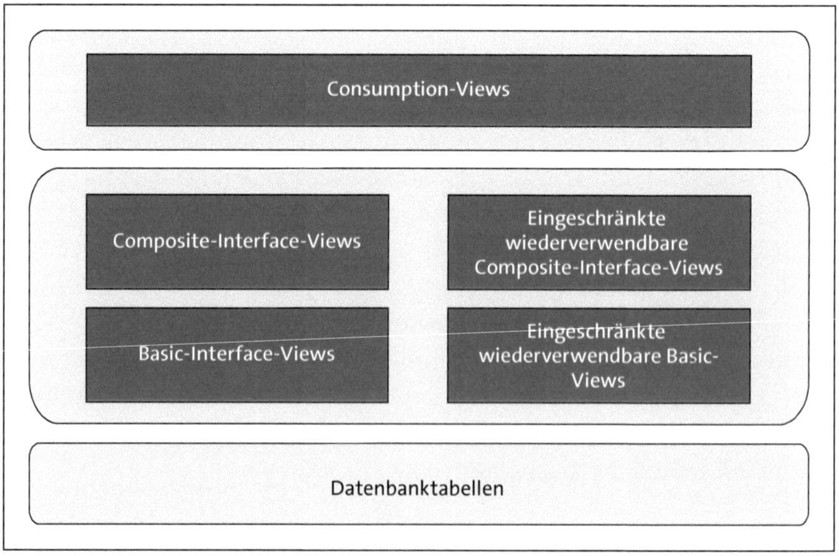

Abbildung 11.2 Schichten des virtuellen Datenmodells

Sie befinden sich in der sogenannten Wiederverwendungsschicht. Im Wesentlichen gibt es zwei View-Typen auf dieser Ebene. Wiederverwendungs-Views und Consumption-Views. Wiederverwendungs-Views lassen sich dabei in Basic-Views und Composite-Views unterteilen.

Wiederverwendungsschicht

Im VDM repräsentiert ein CDS-View in der Wiederverwendungsschicht typischerweise einen Knoten eines Business-Objekts, technischen Objekts oder Konfigurationsobjekts. Ein Beispiel für einen solchen View ist der CDS-View `I_SalesOrder`, der die Wurzel des Business-Objekts »Kundenauftrag« darstellt, während der CDS-View `I_SalesOrderItem` eine Subentität dieses Kundenauftrags abbildet.

Basic-Interface-Views

Basic-Interface-Views basieren direkt auf den Datenbanktabellen und sind die einzigen Views, die direkten Zugriff auf diese Tabellen haben. Sie dienen mehreren Zwecken:

- Die Tabellenspalten in der Datenbankschicht haben häufig schwer verständliche Namen. Auf Ebene der Basic-Interface-Views werden diese in für das Geschäftsverständnis einfachere Begriffe umbenannt, was ihre Handhabung erleichtert.
- Basic-Interface-Views erweitern das Datenmodell der zugrunde liegenden Datenbanktabellen, indem sie zusätzliche Metadaten hinzufügen, wie etwa Annotationen und Relationen zwischen verschiedenen Views. Basic-Interface-Views sind mit der Annotation `@VDM.viewType: #BASIC` versehen.

Composite-Interface-Views

Composite-Interface-Views bauen auf den Basic-Interface-Views auf und können auch anderen Composite-Views zugeordnet werden. Sie haben keinen direkten Zugriff auf die Datenbanktabellen, sondern greifen nur über die Basic-View-Schicht darauf zu. Composite-Interface-Views kombinieren mehrere Basic-Interface-Views oder andere Composite-Interface-Views, um neue semantische Entitäten zu schaffen, die zum Beispiel als analytische Cube-Views genutzt werden können. Diese Views sind mit der Annotation `@VDM.viewType: #COMPOSITE` versehen. Composite-Interface-Views sind ein wichtiges Element für Wiederverwendung.

Konsumentenschicht

Die oberste Ebene des CDS-View-Stacks im VDM wird durch die sogenannten *Consumption-Views* gebildet. Sie basieren auf Wiederverwendungs-Views (also den Basic- oder Composite-Views) und greifen ausschließlich indirekt über diese Schicht auf die Datenbanktabellen zu. Diese Views sind speziell für bestimmte Anwendungszwecke entwickelt worden, wie beispielsweise die Nutzung in einer spezifischen transaktionalen oder analytischen Anwendung. Dabei sind Consumption-Views die einzigen View-Typen im VDM, die für analytische Abfragen genutzt werden können.

Consumption-Views sind durch die Annotation `@VDM.viewType: #CONSUMPTION` gekennzeichnet.

11.3 Implementierung eines virtuellen Datenmodells

Nachdem wir in die Grundlagen des virtuellen Datenmodells eingeführt haben, wenden wir uns nun dessen Implementierung zu. Auf Basis dieser Implementierung wird gemäß der in Abbildung 11.1 dargestellten Architektur der konkrete OData-Service implementiert. Grundlage für die Implementierung sollen die in diesem Buch bereits eingeführten Datenbanktabellen `ZIFPORDER` und `ZIPFODERPOS` sein. Abbildung 11.3 zeigt die Tabelle `ZIPFORDER` in Eclipse.

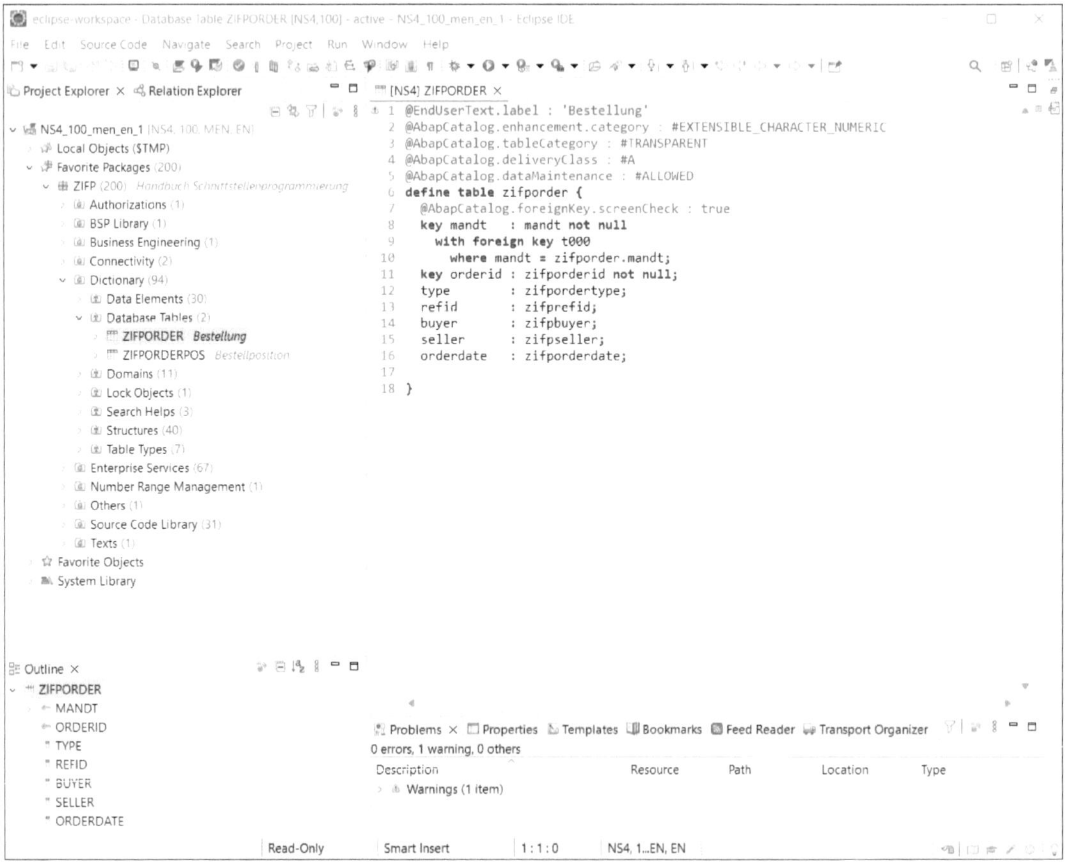

Abbildung 11.3 Die Tabelle »ZIPFORDER« in Eclipse

CDS-View für die Tabelle »ZIFPORDER«

Um einen CDS-View für die Tabelle `ZIFPORDER` anzulegen, wählen Sie die Tabelle im Project Explorer aus und rufen im Kontextmenü den Eintrag **New Data Definition** auf. Im daraufhin erscheinenden Dialog geben Sie in das Feld **Name** den Wert `ZI_IFPORDER` und in das Feld **Description** eine Beschreibung ein (siehe Abbildung 11.4). Das Feld **Referenced Object** beinhaltet bereits die Datenbanktabelle, für die wir einen CDS-View anlegen. Bestätigen Sie diesen Dialogschritt mit **Next**.

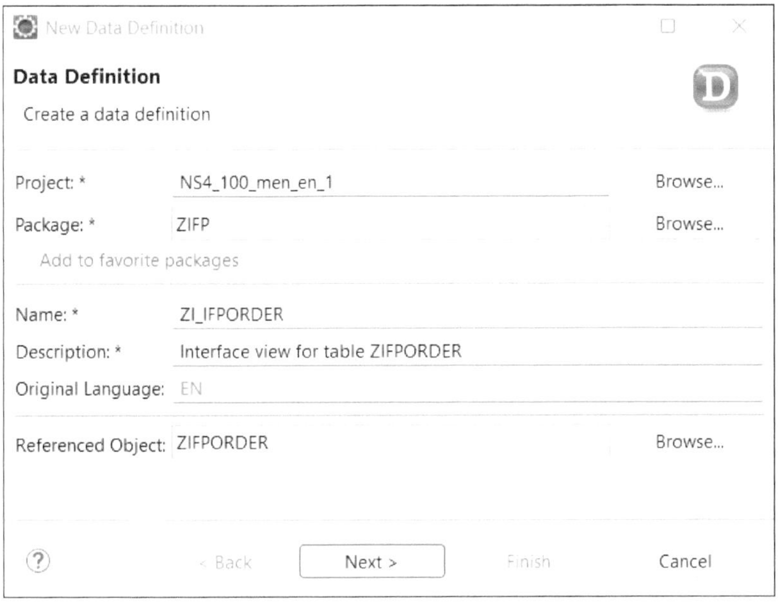

Abbildung 11.4 Anlegen einer neuen Datendefinition

Root-View

Bei der Modellierung des virtuellen Datenmodells erstellt man, wie beschrieben, ein Netz aus zusammenhängenden CDS-Entitäten. In unserem Beispiel beschreibt etwa die anzulegende CDS-Entität `ZI_IFPORDER` die oberste Entität eines Business-Objekts innerhalb eines CDS-Datenmodells. Diese Art von View bezeichnet man auch als *Root-View*. Im nächsten Dialog wählen Sie einen Transportauftrag aus bzw. legen einen neuen an und bestätigen wiederum mit **Next**. Im darauffolgenden Dialogschritt können Sie ein Code-Template auswählen, das für die Anlage des CDS-Views verwendet werden soll. Da wir ein Root-View anlegen wollen, wählen wir den Eintrag **defineRootViewEntity** aus und schließen den Anlageassistenten mit einem Klick auf **Finish** ab.

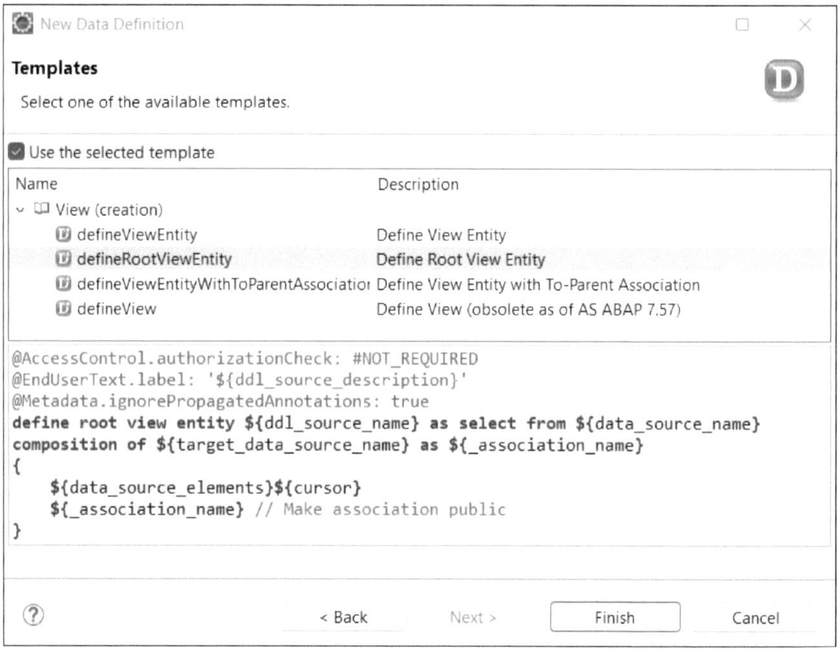

Abbildung 11.5 Auswahl eines Code-Templates

Im Anschluss passen wir den generierten Code so an, dass er dem Code aus Listing 11.1 entspricht.

```
@AccessControl.authorizationCheck: #NOT_REQUIRED
@EndUserText.label: 'Interface view for table ZIFPORDER'
@Metadata.ignorePropagatedAnnotations: true
define root view entity ZI_IFPORDER as select from zifporder
  composition [0..*] of ZI_IFPORDERPOS as _orderpositions

{
    key orderid as Orderid,
    type as Type,
    refid as Refid,
    buyer as Buyer,
    seller as Seller,
    orderdate as Orderdate,
    _orderpositions
}
```

Listing 11.1 Root-View für die Tabelle »ZIFPORDER«

CDS-View für Tabelle »ZIFPORDERPOS«

Nachdem wir den Root-CDS-View für Tabelle ZIFPORDER angelegt haben, wiederholen wir den Vorgang für Tabelle ZIFPORDERPOS. In der durch den Anlegeassistenten generierten Entität müssen Sie noch das Feld price mit dem Währungsfeld currency in Verbindung setzen. Dies geschieht über die Annotation @Semantics.amount.currencyCode. Sie erhalten das in Listing 11.2 gezeigte Ergebnis. Zum Abschluss speichern und aktivieren Sie die Artefakte.

```
@AccessControl.authorizationCheck: #NOT_REQUIRED
@EndUserText.label: 'Orderpositions'
@Metadata.ignorePropagatedAnnotations: true
define view entity ZI_IFPORDERPOS as select from zifporderpos
  association to parent ZI_IFPORDER as _order
  on $projection.Orderid = _order.Orderid
{
    key orderid as Orderid,
    key orderpos as Orderpos,
    matid as Matid,
    mattext as Mattext,
    ordercount as Ordercount,
    @Semantics.amount.currencyCode: 'Currency'
    price as Price,
    currency as Currency,
    _order
}
```

Listing 11.2 CDS-View der Tabelle »ZIPFORDERPOS«

Consumption-View anlegen

Nachdem Sie nun die Basic-Interface-Views für beide Tabellen angelegt haben, können Sie mit der darüberliegenden Schicht fortfahren. Wie im vorangehenden Abschnitt beschrieben, wird der Zugriff auf die Daten für einen konkreten Anwendungsfall nochmals abstrahiert. Dazu dient die Abstraktionsschicht, der Consumption-View. Wie beschrieben, ist der Consumption-View eine für den jeweiligen Anwendungsfall spezifische Sicht auf einen konkreten darunterliegenden View. Diese meist eingeschränkte Sicht (da nicht zwingend alle Felder aus der Projektionsliste eines darunterliegenden Views exponiert werden) nennt man *Projection-View*.

Um den Consumption-View anzulegen, wählen Sie den Basic-Interface-View ZI_IFPORDER im Project Explorer aus und rufen im Kontextmenü den Eintrag **New Data Definition** auf. Im daraufhin angezeigten Dialog geben

Sie in das Feld **Name** den Wert »ZC_IFPORDER« ein und in das Feld **Description** einen Beschreibungstext. Achten Sie darauf, dass im Feld **Referenced Object** der Wert `ZI_IFPORDER` voreingetragen ist. Bestätigen Sie den Schritt mit **Next**.

Im nächsten Schritt wählen Sie einen Transportauftrag aus und bestätigen wiederum mit **Next**. Im darauffolgenden Schritt expandieren Sie, wie in Abbildung 11.6 gezeigt, den Menüeintrag **Projection View** und wählen dann den Eintrag **defineProjectionView** aus. Bestätigen Sie den Schritt mit **Finish**.

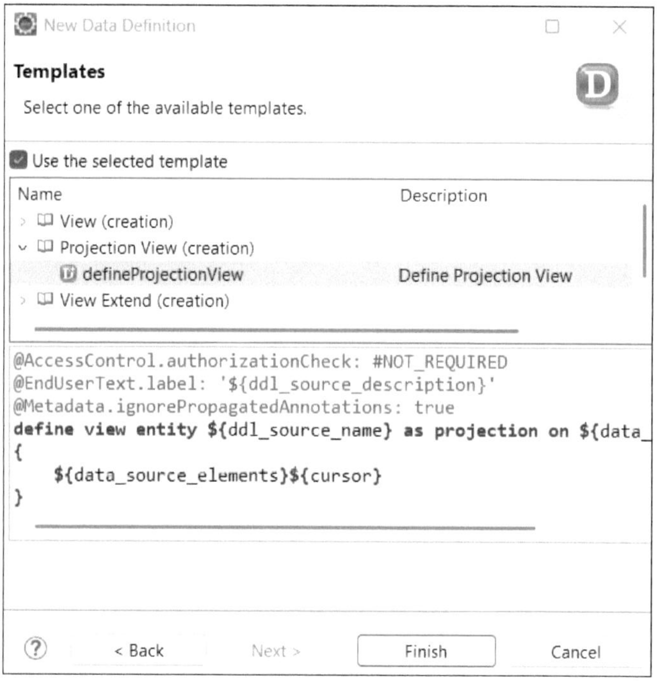

Abbildung 11.6 Anlegen eines Projection-Views

Den generierten Code für den Projection-View `ZC_IFPORDER` erweitern Sie, wie in Listing 11.3 gezeigt.

```
@AccessControl.authorizationCheck: #NOT_REQUIRED
@EndUserText.label: 'Consumption view ZI_IFPORDER'
@Metadata.ignorePropagatedAnnotations: true
define root view entity ZC_IFPORDER
    provider contract transactional_query
        as projection on ZI_IFPORDER
{
```

```
    key Orderid,
    Type,
    Refid,
    Buyer,
    Seller,
    Orderdate
}
```

Listing 11.3 Implementierung des Projection-Views »ZC_IFPORDER«

Projektion für View »ZI_IFPORDERPOS«

Nachdem Sie den Projection-View für den Basic-Interface-View ZI_IFPORDER angelegt haben, wiederholen wir den Vorgang für den Basic-Interface-View ZI_IFPORDERPOS. Dabei verwenden Sie den Bezeichner ZC_IFPORDERPOS für den Projection-View. Nachdem der Code erzeugt ist, passen Sie ihn wie in Listing 11.4 gezeigt an.

11

```
@AccessControl.authorizationCheck: #NOT_REQUIRED
@EndUserText.label: 'Projection view for ZI_IFPORDERPOS'
@Metadata.ignorePropagatedAnnotations: true
define view entity ZC_IFPORDERPOS
    as projection on ZI_IFPORDERPOS as Orderposition
{
    key Orderid,
    key Orderpos,
    Matid,
    Mattext,
    Ordercount,
    Currency
    _order : redirected to parent ZC_IFPORDER
}
```

Listing 11.4 Der Projection-View »ZC_IFPORDERPOS«

Assoziation zwischen den Projection-Views

In der Endausprägung unseres Service soll es möglich sein, von einer Bestellung zu den Bestellpositionen dieser Bestellung zu navigieren, Hierzu müssen wir die beiden Projection-Views in Verbindung bringen. Dies geschieht zunächst über die Herstellung einer Assoziation zwischen dem View ZC_IFPORDER und dem View ZC_IFPORDERPOS. Zusätzlich müssen wir eine Navigationseigenschaft zur Projektionsliste hinzufügen. Der daraus resultierende Code sieht wie in Listing 11.5 aus. Wie man aus dem Programmbeispiel ersehen kann, wurde eine 0..*-Assoziation zwischen den beiden Projection-

Views erstellt und dieser Assoziation der Alias `_orderpositions` zugewiesen. Der führende Unterstrich ist eine Standardnomenklatur. Zusätzlich wurde ans Ende der Projektionsliste der Alias der Navigationseigenschaft angefügt.

```
@AccessControl.authorizationCheck: #NOT_REQUIRED
@EndUserText.label: 'Consumption view ZI_IFPORDER'
@Metadata.ignorePropagatedAnnotations: true
define root view entity ZC_IFPORDER
    provider contract transactional_query
        as projection on ZI_IFPORDER
{
    key Orderid,
    Type,
    Refid,
    Buyer,
    Seller,
    Orderdate,
    _orderpositions: redirected to composition child
        ZC_IFPORDERPOS
}
```

Listing 11.5 Angepasste Implementierung des Project-Views »ZC_IFPORDER«

Die Implementierung des virtuellen Datenmodells ist hiermit so weit abgeschlossen, und wir können mit dem nächsten Schritt, der Implementierung des Business Service fortfahren.

11.4 Business Services implementieren

Servicedefinition und -Binding

Die Implementierung eines OData-Service-Endpunkts wird über zwei Artefakte implementiert. Zunächst ist es notwendig, die sogenannte *Servicedefinition* zu implementieren. Diese Definition eines Service ist vollständig protokollagnostisch und beschreibt lediglich einen Service und die darüber bereitgestellten Business-Entitäten. Damit die Servicedefinition letztlich von einem Konsumenten über ein konkretes Protokoll konsumiert werden kann, muss außerdem ein *Service-Binding* angelegt werden. Dieses Binding ist konkret mit einer Servicedefinition verknüpft und definiert auch das Protokoll, mit dem der Service konsumiert wird.

Binding-Typen

Zum Zeitpunkt der Drucklegung dieses Buchs bietet SAP die in Abbildung 11.7 gezeigten Binding-Typen an. Wie Sie der Abbildung entnehmen können, gibt es für die OData-Versionen 2 und 4 jeweils zwei Auswahloptionen, je eine mit dem Zusatz **UI** und eine mit dem Zusatz **Web API**. Der Zusatz **UI** bedeutet, dass bei Nutzung dieses Binding-Typs nicht nur reine OData-Metainformationen und -Servicedaten ausgeliefert werden, sondern auch Metainformationen für die Erzeugung von Anwendungsoberflächen. Hierauf gehen wir in Abschnitt 11.5, »OData-Services mit SAP Fiori Elements konsumieren«, ein. Bei dem Binding-Typ **InA - UI** kommt das Protokoll **Information Access** (kurz InA) zum Einsatz. Es ermöglicht Anwendungen, Analysen, Planungen und Suchen auf in SAP HANA gespeicherten Daten durchzuführen. Der Typ **SQL – Web API** ermöglicht den Zugriff über das ODBC-Protokoll (Open Database Connectivity).

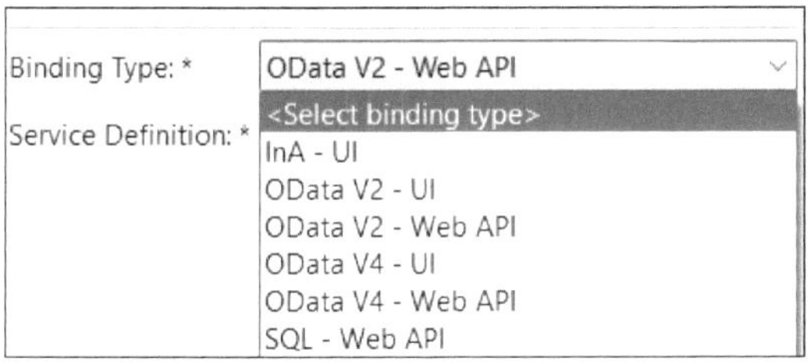

Abbildung 11.7 Auswahl der Binding-Typen

In den folgenden beiden Abschnitten zeigen wir Ihnen zunächst, wie man einen sehr einfachen OData-Service, der lediglich lesenden Zugriff bereitstellt, erzeugt. In den darauffolgenden Abschnitten zeigen wir dann, wie man die Create-, Update- und Delete-Operationen sowie Aktionen bereitstellen kann.

11.4.1 Implementierung einer Servicedefinition

Servicedefinition für View »ZC_IFPORER«

Für die Implementierung der Servicedefinition wählen Sie den Projection-View `ZC_IFPORER` im Project Explorer aus und rufen im Kontextmenü den Eintrag **New Service Definition** aus. Im sich daraufhin öffnenden Assistenten für das Anlegen einer neuen Servicedefinition geben Sie in das Feld **Name** den Wert `ZSD_IFPORDER` ein sowie einen Beschreibungstext in das Feld **Description** (siehe Abbildung 11.8). Achten Sie darauf, dass im Feld **Referenced Object** der Projection-View `ZC_IFPORDER` eingetragen ist. Bestätigen Sie mit **Next**.

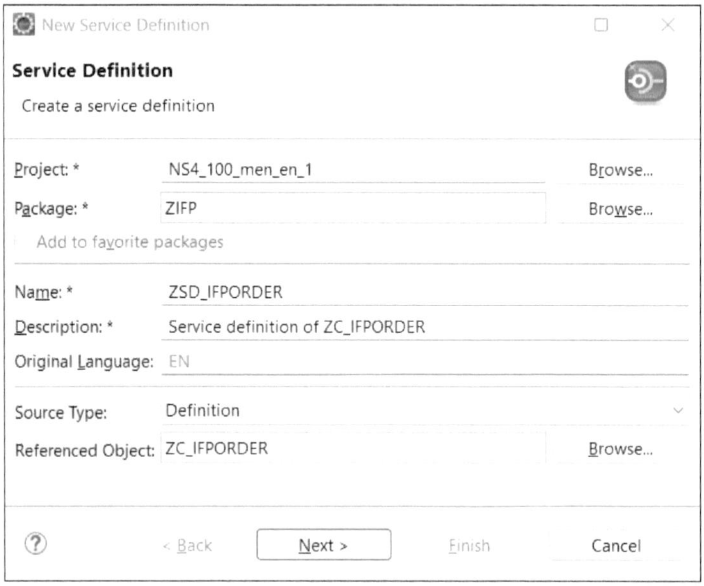

Abbildung 11.8 Anlegen einer Servicedefinition für den Projection-View »ZC_IFPORDER«

Im nächsten Schritt wählen Sie einen Transportauftrag aus und bestätigen mit **Next**. Auch den letzten Dialogschritt bestätigen Sie mit **Finish**.

Aliasse definieren

Nachdem der Codegenerator seine Arbeit erledigt hat, passen Sie den Code wie in Listing 11.6 gezeigt an. Durch die Angabe von `as Orders` kann der Konsument des Service die Entitäten vom Typ `ZC_IFPORDER` über den Bezeichner `Orders` abrufen. Da wir dem Konsumenten nicht nur Zugriff auf die Bestellungen, sondern auch auf die Bestellpositionen ermöglichen wollen, exponieren wir über die Angabe in der zweiten `expose`-Zeile auch die Bestellpositionen und vergeben hierbei das Alias `OrderPositions`.

```
@EndUserText.label: 'Service definition of ZC_IFPORDER'
define service ZSD_IFPORDER {
  expose ZC_IFPORDER as Orders;
  expose ZC_IFPORDERPOS as OrderPositions;
}
```

Listing 11.6 Servicedefinition »ZSD_IFPORDER«

11.4.2 Implementierung eines Service-Bindings

Im Anschluss an die Erzeugung der Servicedefinition können Sie das Service-Binding erzeugen. Hierüber wird die Servicedefinition als OData-Service-Endpunkt bereitgestellt.

Service-Binding

Um ein Service Binding anzulegen, wählen Sie die zuvor erstelle Servicedefinition im Project Explorer aus. Sie finden diese im Order **Business Services • Service Definitions**. Wählen Sie im Kontextmenü den Menüpunkt **New Service Binding**. Geben Sie, wie in Abbildung 11.9 gezeigt, in das Feld **Name** den Wert »Z_IFPORDERSERVICE_1« und in das Feld **Description** einen beschreibenden Text ein. Bei der Auswahlliste **Binding Type** wählen Sie den Eintrag **OData V2 – Web API** aus. Zusätzlich stellen Sie sicher, dass im Feld **Service Definition** die soeben angelegte Servicedefinition `ZSD_IFOORDER` eingetragen ist. Bestätigen Sie den Dialog mit **Next**.

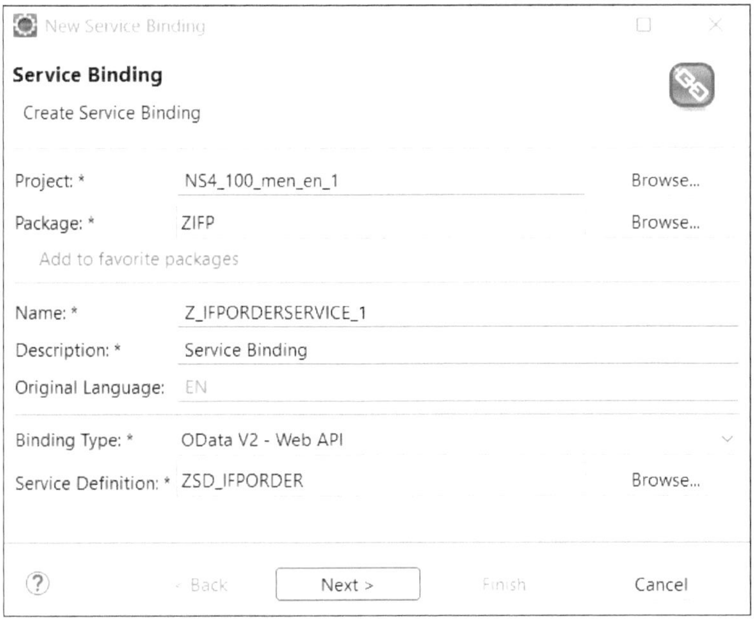

Abbildung 11.9 Anlegen eines Service-Bindings

11

Generiertes Service-Binding

Im darauffolgenden Dialogschritt wählen Sie einen Transportauftrag aus und schließen den Dialog mit **Finish** ab. Sie erhalten das in Abbildung 11.10 gezeigte Service-Binding. Es wurde allerdings noch nicht lokal veröffentlicht. Dies ist auch grundsätzlich sinnvoll, denn je nach vorliegender Infrastruktur wäre eine automatische lokale Veröffentlichung auf dem SAP-System unter Umständen nicht korrekt, nämlich im Falle einer Hub-Architektur. Darüber hinaus können Sie Abbildung 11.10 entnehmen, dass es sich bei dem Service-Binding um einen Endpunkt des Typs **OData Version 2 – Web API** handelt und dass die Servicedefinition `ZSD_IFPORDER` referenziert wird.

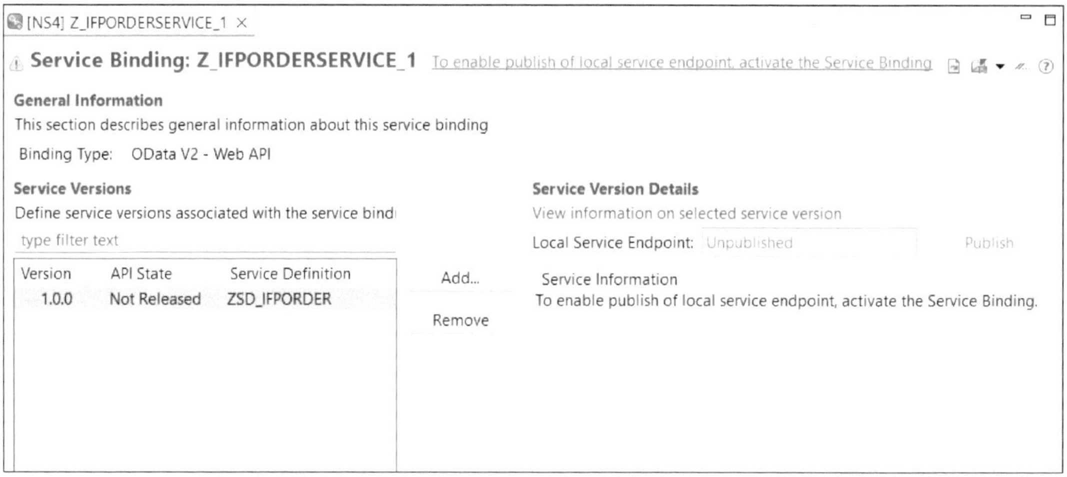

Abbildung 11.10 Nicht veröffentlichtes Service-Binding

Service Binding aktivieren und veröffentlichen

Im nächsten Schritt speichern Sie zunächst das Service Binding und aktivieren es dann über das Symbol (**Activate**) oder die Tastenkombination [Strg] + [F3]. Nach der Aktivierung des Service-Bindings wird der Button **Publish** anwählbar. Klicken Sie darauf, um das Service-Binding als lokalen Service zu veröffentlichen. Nachdem der Service erfolgreich veröffentlicht wurde, sehen Sie das Bild aus Abbildung 11.11.

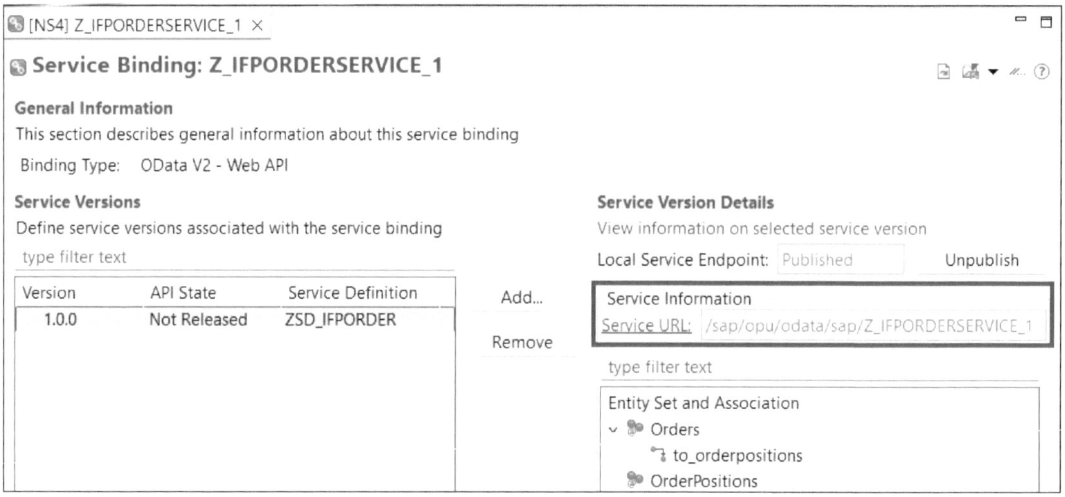

Abbildung 11.11 Veröffentlichter OData-Service

Wie man rechts im Bereich **Service Information** sehen kann, wurde ein entsprechender OData-Service-Endpunkt auf unserem SAP-System angelegt.

Durch einen Klick auf den Link **Service URL** öffnet sich der im SAP-System hinterlegte Standardbrowser. Wie in Kapitel 9, »SAP Gateway und OData«, beschrieben, können wir über die Anpassung der Browser-URL mit dem OData-Service kommunizieren. Der OData-Service kann auch über Transaktion /IWFND/MAINT_SERVICE im SAP GUI eingesehen werden (siehe Abbildung 11.12).

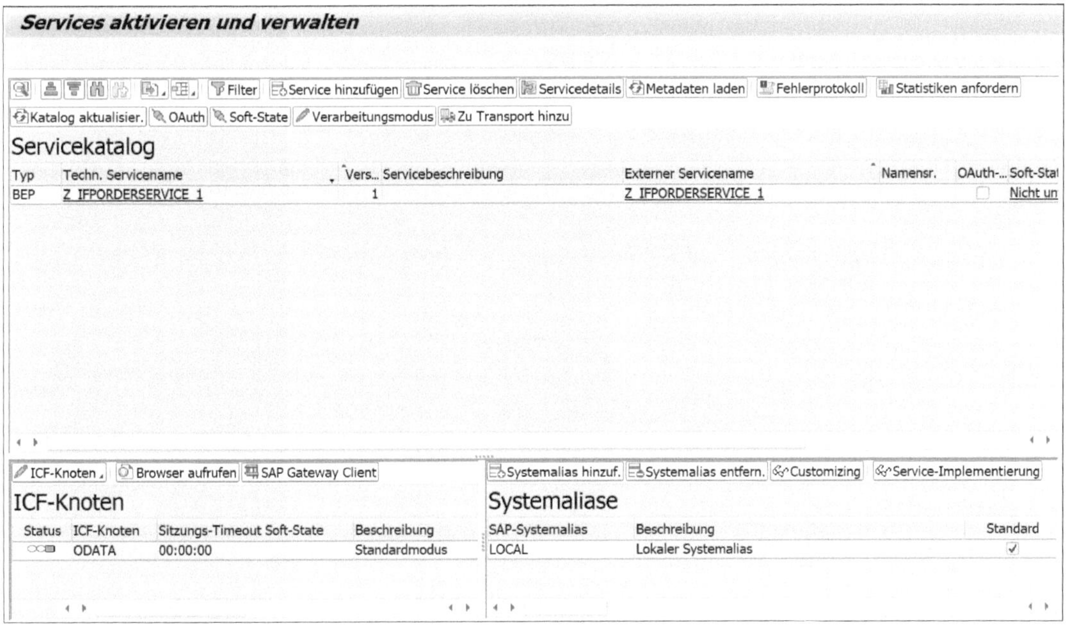

Abbildung 11.12 Der OData-Service in Transaktion /IWFND/MAINT_SERVICE

OData-V4-Service

Ebenso einfach, wie man einen OData-V2-Service erzeugen kann, lässt sich auch einen OData-Service auf Basis der Version V4 anlegen. Hierzu rufen Sie wie zuvor die Servicedefinition `ZSD_IFPORDER` auf und wählen im Kontextmenü wieder **Create New Service Binding**. Im darauffolgenden Dialog geben Sie dem anzulegenden Service-Binding einen Namen, beispielsweise »Z_IFPORDERSERVICE_2«, und wählen als Binding-Typ nun **OData V4 – Web UI** aus. Abbildung 11.13 zeigt das Ergebnis.

Die Veröffentlichung eines V4-basierten OData-Service muss im Moment noch über das SAP GUI in der SAP-Gateway-Service-Administration erfolgen. Diese Anwendung wird über Transaktion /IWFND/V4_ADMIN gestartet. Nach dem Aufruf wird das in Abbildung 11.14 dargestellte Bild angezeigt.

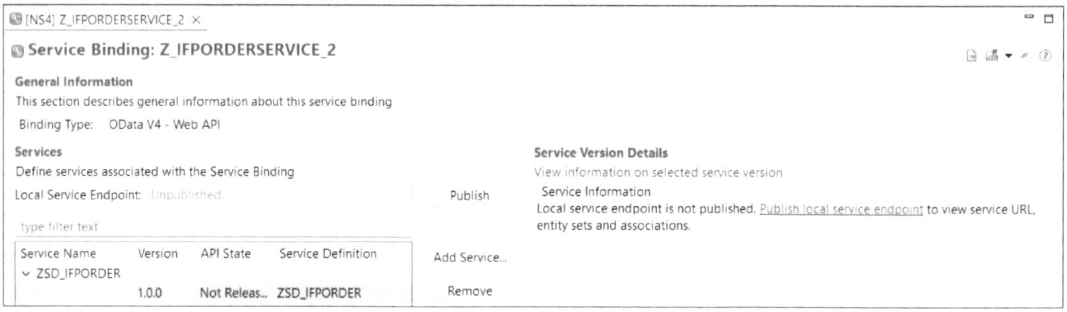

Abbildung 11.13 Nicht veröffentlichtes Service-Binding vom Typ »OData V4 – Web API«

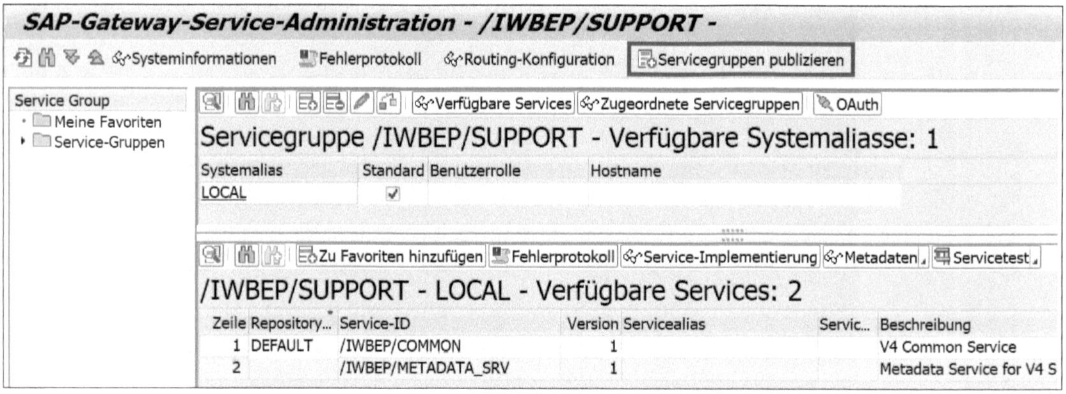

Abbildung 11.14 Administrationsoberfläche für OData-V4-Dienste

OData-Service in SAP Gateway veröffentlichen

Um den OData-Service `Z_IFPORDERSERVICE_2` zu veröffentlichen, klicken Sie auf den Button **Servicegruppe publizieren**. Im Anschluss geben Sie in das Feld **Systemalias** den Wert `LOCAL` ein und klicken auf die Schaltfläche **Servicegruppe abrufen**. Nachdem die verfügbaren Dienste abgerufen wurden, navigieren Sie ans Ende der Liste. Hier finden Sie, wie in Abbildung 11.15 gezeigt, die Servicegruppe für unseren OData-Service `Z_IFPORDERSERVICE_2`.

Zur Veröffentlichung markieren Sie das Auswahlfeld beim Service `Z_IFPORDERSERVICE_2` und klicken auch hier auf die Schaltfläche **Servicegruppe publizieren**. In dem daraufhin angezeigten Dialog geben Sie in das Feld **Beschreib.** einen Beschreibungstext ein und wählen das ✓-Icon (**Weiter**). Im Anschluss wählen Sie einen Customizing-Transportauftrag aus.

Nach dem erfolgreichen Publizieren erhalten Sie eine entsprechende Meldung durch das SAP-System. Wechseln Sie mit F3 zurück ins Ausgangsbild von Transaktion /IWFND/V4_ADMIN. Hier wird Ihnen nun die neue Servicegruppe für unseren OData-Service angezeigt (siehe Abbildung 11.16).

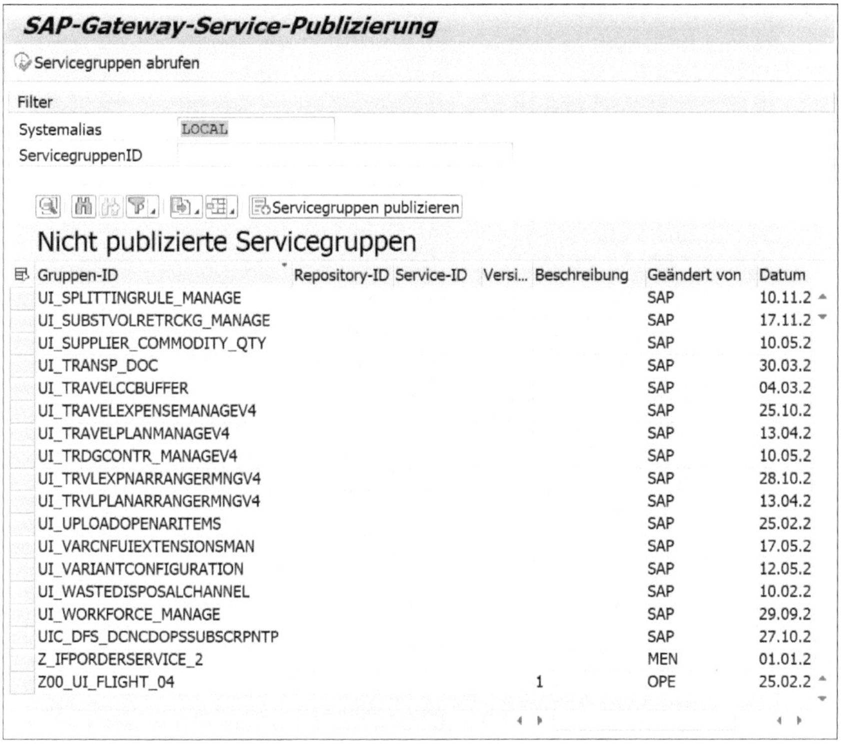

Abbildung 11.15 Verfügbaren Servicegruppen auf dem SAP-System

11

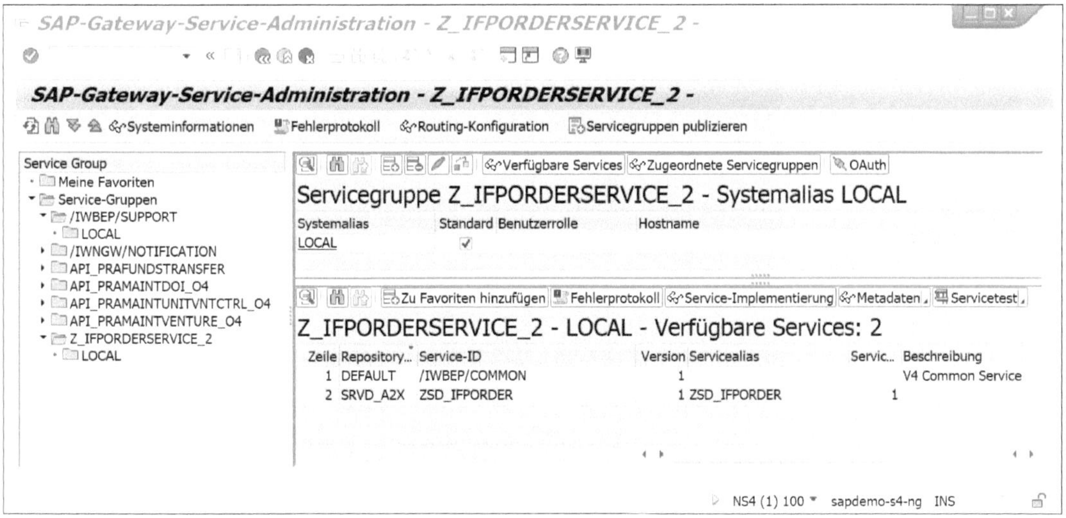

Abbildung 11.16 Die veröffentlichte Servicegruppe »Z_IFPORDERSERVICE_2«

Aufruf in den ABAP Development Tools

Nach der Veröffentlichung können Sie das Service-Binding in den ADT in Eclipse erneut öffnen. Auch hier wird Ihnen der veröffentlichte OData-Service angezeigt (siehe Abbildung 11.17). Wie zuvor schon gesehen, können Sie den OData-Service hier über einen Klick auf **Service URL** direkt aufrufen.

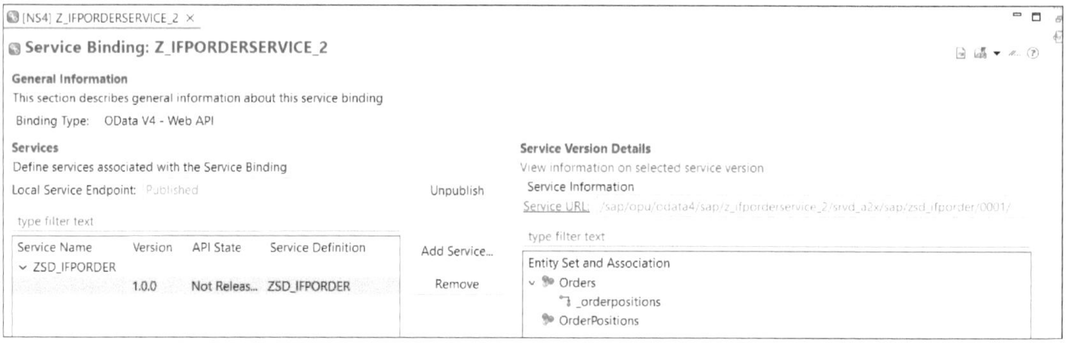

Abbildung 11.17 Die veröffentlichen Servicegruppe in den ABAP Development Tools

Nachdem wir die beiden Service-Bindings erstellt haben, können wir mittels OData-V2 oder OData-V4 auf das virtuelle Datenmodell zugreifen.

11.4.3 Implementierung von Verhalten

In den vorangehenden Abschnitten haben wir darüber gesprochen, wie man einen einfachen Service, der lediglich lesenden Zugriff auf Daten bereitstellt, mit dem ABAP RESTful Application Programming Model erstellt und Konsumenten zur Verfügung stellt. Im nächsten Schritt zeigen wir Ihnen nun, wie man einen Service zur Verfügung stellt, der auch Operationen für das Anlegen, Löschen und Ändern von Daten ermöglicht.

Managed vs. Unmanaged

Das ABAP RESTful Application Programming Model bietet für die transaktionale Verarbeitung von Daten grundsätzlich zwei Verarbeitungsmodi an:

- Einerseits ist es möglich, dass das Framework die Verarbeitung der ändernden Operationen vollständig selbst übernimmt. Hierbei spricht man vom *Managed Scenario*. Hierbei müssen Sie keine ABAP-Methoden für das Anlegen, Ändern und Löschen von Daten implementieren. Die Steuerung der Transaktion obliegt vollständig dem Framework. Man spricht bei diesem Szenario daher auch von einem *Greenfield-Szenario*. Greenfield deshalb, weil es normalerweise dann zum Einsatz kommt, wenn nicht bereits Funktionen für die transaktionale Verarbeitung aus früheren Entwicklungen vorhanden sind und diese wiederverwendet werden sollen. Im Managed Szenario übernimmt man zwar grundsätzlich das Framework die Verarbeitung, allerdings kann der Entwickler definieren, welche Aspekte im Rahmen der Verarbeitung aufgerufen werden.

- Auf der anderen Seite steht das *Unmanaged Scenario*, auch *Brownfield-Szenario* genannt. Bei dieser Implementierungsart implementieren Sie die entsprechenden Methoden und sind für die transaktionale Verarbeitung verantwortlich.

In unserem Beispiel wollen wir uns lediglich auf das Managed Scenario fokussieren. Wir zeigen hier auch keine Spezialfälle.

Verhaltensdefinition anlegen

Der erste Schritt ist das Anlegen einer *Verhaltensdefinition*. Um eine Verhaltensdefinition für das Business-Objekt (den Root-View) `ZI_IFPORDER` bereitzustellen, wählen Sie die entsprechende Datendefinition im Project Explorer aus und wählen im Kontextmenü den Eintrag **New Behavior Definition**. Es erscheint der in Abbildung 11.18 gezeigte Dialog. Die Felder werden durch die ADT bereits vorausgefüllt. Der **Implementation Type** ist standardmäßig auf den Wert **Managed** eingestellt. Es wird also das Managed Scenario verwendet. Bestätigen Sie dies mit **Next** und wählen Sie als Nächstes einen Transportauftrag aus. Bestätigen Sie die Auswahl mit **Finish**.

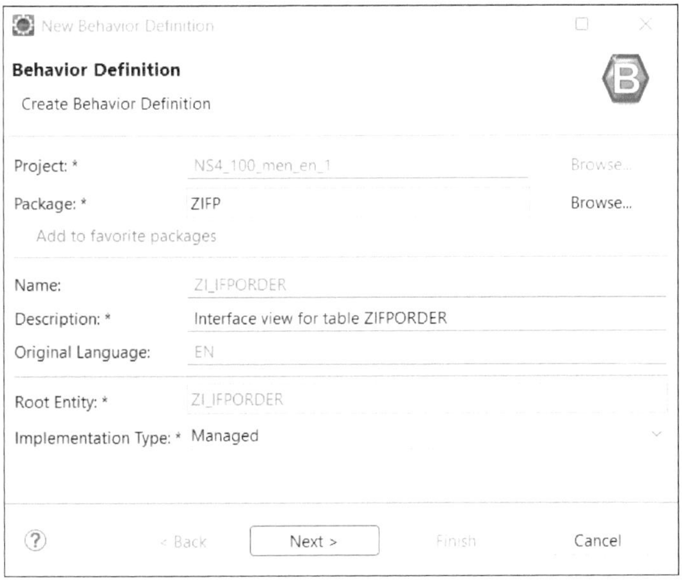

Abbildung 11.18 Anlegen einer Verhaltensdefinition für das Business Objekt »ZI_IFPORDER«

Generierte Verhaltensdefinition

Es wird nun eine neue Verhaltensdefinition für das Business-Objekt `ZIFPORDER` angelegt. Im Project Explorer finden Sie diese im Ordner **Core Data Ser-**

vices • Behavior Definition. Die Verhaltensdefinition enthält die in Listing 11.7 gezeigte Standardimplementierung. In der ersten Zeile wird angegeben, dass das Managed Scenario verwendet wird, man allerdings über die Klasse `ZBP_I_IFPORDER` eigenen Programmcode implementieren könnte. Standardmäßig wird die Klasse beim Anlegen der Verhaltensdefinition nicht mitangelegt, sondern muss von Ihnen erzeugt werden. Wie Sie Listing 11.7 entnehmen können, enthält die Definition standardmäßig auch die Angabe, dass man die Operationen `create`, `update` und `delete` zur Verfügung stellen möchte.

```
managed implementation in class zbp_i_ifporder unique;

define behavior for ZI_IFPORDER //alias <alias_name>
persistent table ZIFPORDER
lock master
authorization master ( instance )
//etag master <field_name>
{
  field ( readonly ) Orderid;
  create;
  update;
  delete;
  association _orderpositions { create; }
}
```

Listing 11.7 Implementierung der Verhaltensdefinition »ZI_IFPORDER«

Klasse »ZBP_I_IFORDER«

Die Klasse `ZBP_I_IFORDER` wird leider nicht automatisch angelegt. Fahren Sie mit dem Mauszeiger über den Klassennamen, wie beispielhaft in Abbildung 11.19 gezeigt, erhalten Sie Unterstützung durch die ADT, um die Klasse anzulegen.

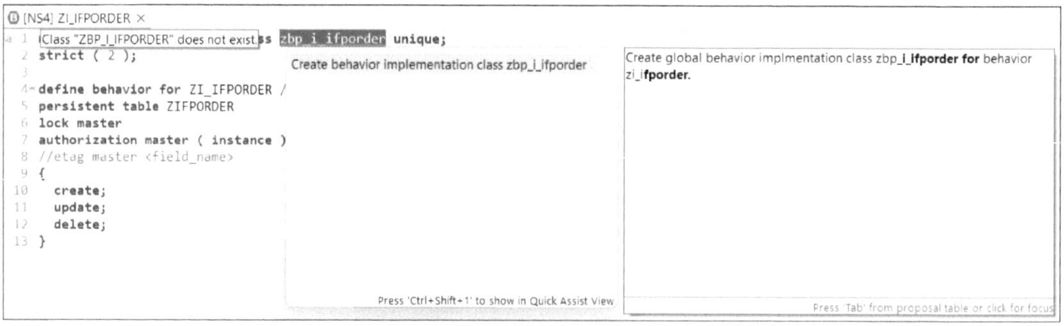

Abbildung 11.19 QuickFix-Hilfe in den ABAP Development Tools

Um die Klasse anzulegen, wählen Sie demnach die Aktion **Create behavior implementation class zbp_i_iforder**. Daraufhin erscheint der in Abbildung 11.20 gezeigte Dialog. Diesen bestätigen Sie mit **Next** und wählen im darauffolgenden Dialog einen Transportauftrag aus. Im Anschluss bestätigen Sie mit **Finish**.

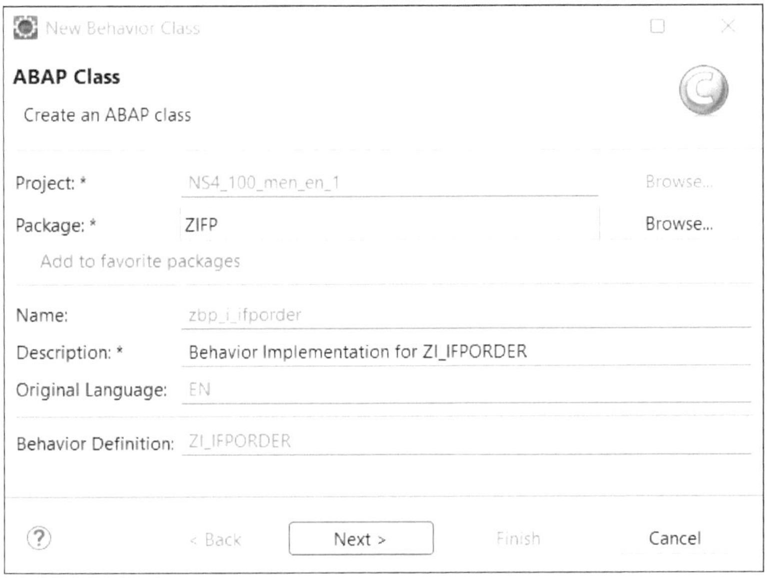

Abbildung 11.20 Anlegen der Verhaltensimplementierung

Nachdem die Verhaltensimplementierung angelegt wurde, können wir diese über (**Aktivieren**) oder die Tastenkombination Strg + F3 aktivieren.

```
CLASS lhc_ZI_IFPORDER DEFINITION INHERITING FROM
    cl_abap_behavior_handler.
  PRIVATE SECTION.

    METHODS get_instance_authorizations FOR INSTANCE AUTHORIZATION
      IMPORTING keys REQUEST requested_authorizations FOR
          zi_ifporder RESULT result.

ENDCLASS.

CLASS lhc_ZI_IFPORDER IMPLEMENTATION.
```

```
  METHOD get_instance_authorizations.
  ENDMETHOD.
ENDCLASS.
```

Listing 11.8 Standardimplementierung

Im Anschluss daran fügen Sie in die Verhaltensdefinition des Business-Objekts ZI_IFPORDER die Verhaltensdefinition für das Business-Objekt ZI_IFPORDERPOS ein. Den für die Verhaltensdefinition von ZI_IFPORDERPOS generierten Code zeigt Listing 11.9.

```
define behavior for ZI_IFPORDERPOS //alias <alias_name>
persistent table ZIFPORDERPOS
lock dependent by _order
//etag master <field_name>
{
  field ( readonly ) Orderid;
  update;
  delete;
  association _order { }
}
```

Listing 11.9 Verhaltensdefinition für das Business-Objekt »ZI_IFPORDERPOS«

11.4.4 Implementierung von Aktionen

Funktionsimport

Die Implementierung von Funktionsimporten, wie in Kapitel 9, »SAP Gateway und OData«, gezeigt, wird auch vom ABAP RESTful Application Programming Model unterstützt. Funktionsimporte werden hier zunächst in der Verhaltensdefinition definiert. Sie werden allerdings nicht Funktionsimporte, sondern *Aktionen* genannt. Zur Laufzeit werden diese Aktionen in den Metainformationen als Funktionsimporte bereitgestellt.

Aktionen definieren

Aktionen gibt es im ABAP RESTful Application Programming Model mit und ohne Entitätsbezug. Listing 11.10 zeigt die Definition zweier Aktionen für das Business-Objekt ZI_IFPORDER. Die Aktion issue_message ist eine Aktion ohne Entitätsbezug. Die Aktion set_to_cancelled ist hingegen eine Aktion mit Bezug zu einer Entität.

```
managed implementation in class zbp_i_ifporder unique;

define behavior for ZI_IFPORDER //alias <alias_name>
persistent table ZIFPORDER
```

```
lock master
authorization master ( instance )
//etag master <field_name>
{
  field ( readonly ) Orderid;
  create;
  update;
  delete;

  static action issue_message;
  action ( features : instance ) set_to_cancelled;

  association _orderpositions { create; }
}
```


Listing 11.10 Definition von Aktionen

Aktionen implementieren

Nachdem man diese Aktionen definiert hat, weisen einen die ADT darauf hin, dass sie noch nicht implementiert sind. Klickt man auf das vor der Codezeile angezeigte Warnsymbol (), erhält man in einem Pop-up-Fenster Unterstützung zur Generierung einer entsprechenden Methode in der Implementierungsklasse. Im Anschluss sollte die Definition und Implementierung der Klasse LHC_ZI_IFPORDER wie in Listing 11.11 aussehen.

```
CLASS lhc_zi_ifporder DEFINITION INHERITING FROM
    cl_abap_behavior_handler.
  PRIVATE SECTION.

    METHODS get_instance_authorizations FOR INSTANCE AUTHORIZATION
      IMPORTING keys REQUEST requested_authorizations
       FOR zi_ifporder RESULT result.
    METHODS get_instance_features FOR INSTANCE FEATURES
      IMPORTING keys REQUEST requested_features
       FOR zi_ifporder RESULT result.

    METHODS issue_message FOR MODIFY
      IMPORTING keys FOR ACTION zi_ifporder~issue_message.

    METHODS set_to_cancelled FOR MODIFY
      IMPORTING keys FOR ACTION zi_ifporder~set_to_cancelled.

ENDCLASS.
```

```
CLASS lhc_zi_ifporder IMPLEMENTATION.

  METHOD get_instance_authorizations.
  ENDMETHOD.

  METHOD get_instance_features.
  ENDMETHOD.
  METHOD issue_message.
  ENDMETHOD.

  METHOD set_to_cancelled.
  ENDMETHOD.

ENDCLASS.
```

Listing 11.11 Implementierung der lokalen Klasse »lhc_ZI_IFPORDER«

Exemplarisch implementieren wir die Methode issue_message wie in Listing 11.12 gezeigt. Wie man hier sehen kann, liefern wir lediglich eine einfache Nachricht an den Aufrufer zurück.

```
METHOD issue_message.
  APPEND new_message(
         id  = 'ZIFP_MSG_Y2122_2'
         number   = 001
         severity = if_abap_behv_message=>
                              severity-information
         v1       = 'Hello message'
         )  TO reported-%other.
  ENDMETHOD.
```

Listing 11.12 Einfache Beispielimplementierung der Methode »issue_message«

Aktionen in der Verhaltensdefinition referenzieren

Damit die Aktionen von den Konsumenten des OData-Service verwendet werden können, müssen sie auch in der Verhaltensdefinition der Consumption-Schicht enthalten sein: Listing 11.13 zeigt die hierzu erweiterte Verhaltensdefinition. Wie man sehen kann, wird über die Anweisung use, gefolgt vom Aktionsbezeichner, die Nutzung der Aktion aus der Basic-Schicht referenziert.

```
projection;

define behavior for ZC_IFPORDER alias IFPOrder
{
```

```
  use create;
  use update;
  use delete;

  use action issue_message;
  use action set_to_cancelled;

  use association _orderpositions { create; }
}

define behavior for ZC_IFPORDERPOS alias IFPOrderPosition
{
  use update;
  use delete;
  use association _order { }
}
```

Listing 11.13 Erweiterung der Verhaltensdefinition »ZC_IFPORDER«

11.5 OData-Services mit SAP Fiori Elements konsumieren

In diesem Abschnitt möchten wir Ihnen einen Überblick über die Implementierung einer SAP-Fiori-Anwendung mittels SAP Fiori Elements und die Konsumierung von OData-Services mit einer solchen Anwendung geben.

11.5.1 SAP Fiori und SAP Fiori Elements im Überblick

SAP Fiori Design Guidelines

Die Implementierung von SAP-Fiori-Oberflächen folgt stets den SAP Fiori Design Guidelines. Die Designvorgaben werden hier beschrieben (*https://experience.sap.com/fiori-design/*). Im Grunde dürfen nur Anwendungen, die diesen Regeln folgen, als SAP-Fiori-Anwendungen bezeichnet werden. Abbildung 11.21 zeigt das Einstiegsbild der Webseite. Zum Zeitpunkt der Drucklegung dieses Buchs werden hier drei verschiedene Design Guidelines für SAP Fiori angeboten:

- Web
- Apple iOS
- Google Android

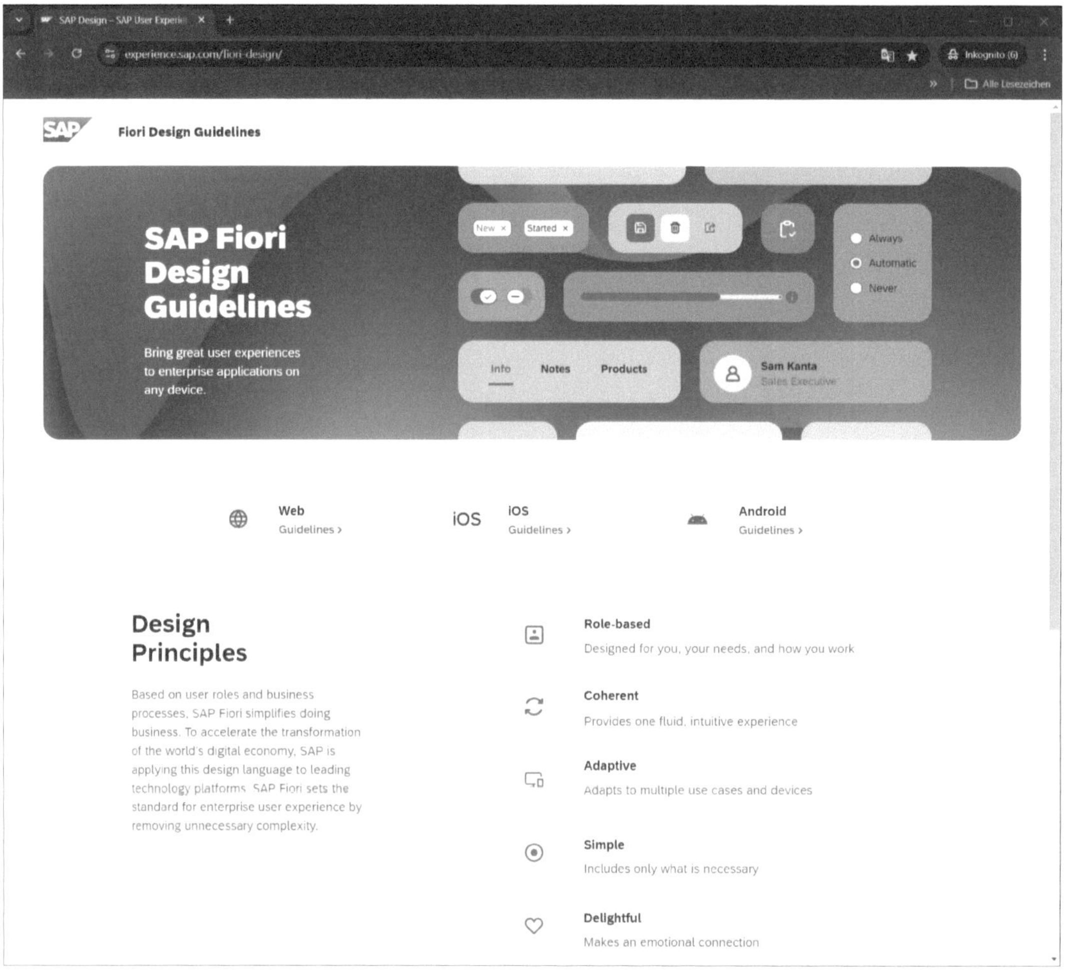

Abbildung 11.21 SAP Fiori Design Guidelines

SAP Fiori Elements

Die Entwicklung von SAP-Fiori-Anwendungen mit SAPUI5, wie in Abschnitt 9.4, »OData-Services mit SAPUI5 konsumieren«, beschrieben, ist zum einen aufwendig, und zum anderen benötigen Sie hierfür Kenntnisse in modernen Technologien zur Entwicklung von Webanwendungen. Dies hat SAP dazu bewegt, andere Wege für die Erstellung solcher Anwendungen bereitzustellen. Das Ergebnis ist *SAP Fiori Elements*.

Diese Technologie basiert auf drei wesentlichen Komponenten:

- OData-Diensten
- Vokabularien
- XML-View-Templates

Metadaten von OData-Services

Die Basis für die Verwendung von SAP Fiori Elements ist stets ein OData-Service. Die Metadaten des OData-Service liefern bereits eine Menge an Informationen, die innerhalb einer SAPUI5- bzw. SAP-Fiori-Anwendung verwendet werden können, beispielsweise die Länge einer Eigenschaft einer Entität oder eine Feldbeschreibung. Diese Metadaten können einfach in einer Anwendung verwendet werden. Zur Laufzeit erhält der Konsument des Diensts die Metadaten über die Datei **metadata.xml**.

SAP Fiori Elements geht aber noch ein Stück weiter. Der Entwickler annotiert Entitäten und Eigenschaften von Entitäten mittels Sprachelementen. Diese Elemente, auch *Terme* genannt, werden in *Vokabularien* beschrieben. Die Verwendung dieser Vokabularien ist über sogenannte *Annotationen* realisiert. Annotationen können auf Serverseite im Rahmen der OData-Service-Entwicklung eingesetzt werden, es gibt aber auch clientseitige Annotationen. Clientseitige Annotationen werden im SAP Business Application Studio oder Visual Studio Code in einer entsprechenden Datei angelegt. Ebenso ist es möglich, beide Optionen miteinander zu kombinieren und damit die serverseitigen Annotationen zu übersteuern oder nur anzureichern.

Verarbeitung der Annotationen

Für die Verarbeitung der Annotationen definiert SAP sogenannte *XML-View-Templates*. Diese Templates definieren in ihrer Struktur, wo und wie welche Annotation visualisiert werden soll. Bei der Erzeugung einer SAP-Fiori-Elements-Anwendung mit dem SAP Business Application Studio oder mit (dem mit entsprechenden Erweiterungen versehenen) Visual Studio Code können Sie ein entsprechendes Projekt anlegen und festlegen, welches SAP-Fiori-Template verwendet werden sollen. Beispiele für solche sogenannten *Floorplans* sind *List Report* (eine Listenanzeige) und *Object Page* (die Detailsicht zu einem Element dieser Liste). Hierbei ist darauf zu achten, dass die Templates zu den Annotationen passen.

Wird die so erstellte Anwendung aufgerufen, werden die Annotationsdatei bzw. die -dateien geladen und die in der Anwendung festgelegten Templates mit den dazu passenden Annotationen verbunden. Abbildung 11.22 zeigt die unterschiedlichen Artefakte von SAP Fiori Elements und deren Zusammenspiel.

Weiterführende Informationen zu SAP Fiori Elements und den Annotationen erhalten Sie unter anderem auf der Dokumentationsseite zu SAPUI5 im Internet unter *http://s-prs.de/v1032905*.

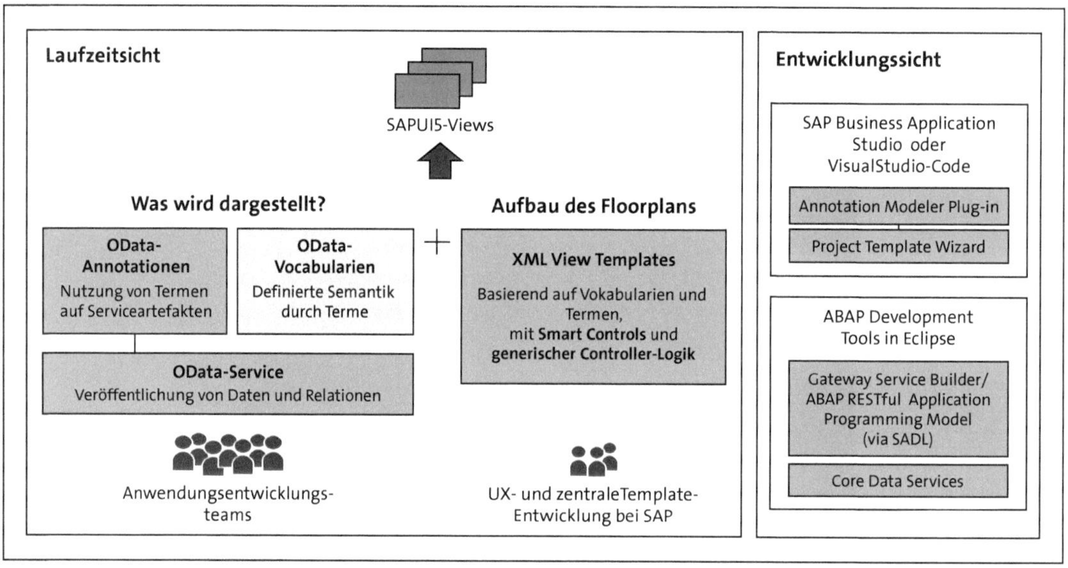

Abbildung 11.22 Architektur von SAP Fiori Elements

11.5.2 Implementierung eines List Reports mit Object Page

Nach dem Kurzüberblick über SAP Fiori und SAP Fiori Elements wenden wir uns nun der Implementierung einer Beispielanwendung als Konsumenten unseres OData-Service zu, die einen List Report und eine Object Page unter Nutzung von SAP Fiori Elements implementiert.

Service-Binding anlegen

Bindungstyp »UI«

In Abschnitt 11.4.2, »Implementierung eines Service-Bindings«, haben wir pro Business-Objekt unserer Beispielanwendung jeweils ein Service-Binding mit reiner OData Web API angelegt. Ein Service-Binding dieses Typs exponiert keine Benutzeroberfläche. Daher legen wir in diesem Abschnitt zunächst ein neues Service-Binding des Typs »UI« an.

Hierzu wählen Sie, wie in Abschnitt 11.4.2 beschrieben, die Servicedefinition `ZSD_IFPORDER` im Project Explorer der ADT aus und rufen im Kontextmenü den Eintrag **New Service Binding** auf. Im Anschluss geben Sie in das Feld **Name** den Wert »Z_IFPORDERSERVICE_3« und in das Feld **Description** einen Beschreibungstext ein (siehe Abbildung 11.23). Da wir ein Service-Binding mit UI erzeugen wollen, wählen Sie im Auswahlmenü **Binding Type** den Wert **OData V2 – UI** aus. Bestätigen Sie den Dialogschritt mit **Next**.

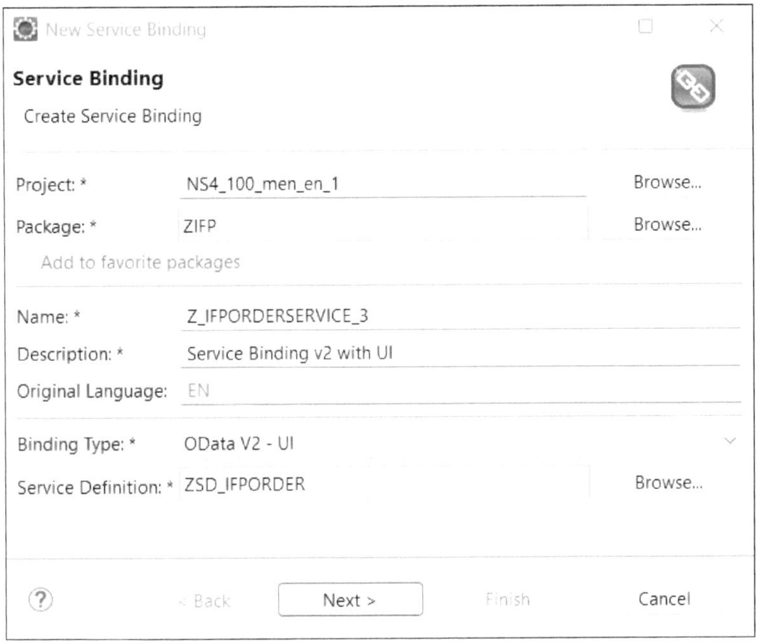

Abbildung 11.23 Anlegen eines Service-Bindings mit Bindungstyp »OData V2 – UI«

Im nächsten Schritt wählen Sie einen Transportauftrag aus und bestätigen mit **Finish**. Nachdem das Service-Binding erzeugt wurde, aktivieren Sie es (über das Icon (**Aktivieren**)) und publizieren es im Anschluss wie in Abschnitt 11.4.2, »Implementierung eines Service-Bindings«, beschrieben.

Vorschau-Funktion

Abbildung 11.24 zeigt das publiziertes Service-Binding vom Typ **OData V2 – UI**. Anders als bei den Service-Bindings, die wir in Abschnitt 11.4.2 angelegt haben, finden Sie hier auf Höhe der veröffentlichten Entitäten und Assoziationen eine Schaltfläche **Preview**. Darüber gelangen Sie zu einer Vorschau der Anwendungsoberfläche. Da es sich bei dieser Ansicht lediglich um eine Vorschau handelt, müssen Sie trotzdem noch ein SAP-Fiori-Elements-Projekt im SAP Business Application Studio bzw. in Visual Studio Code anlegen, um die Anwendung zu implementieren. Hierzu legt man ein Projekt vom Typ **SAP Fiori Elements** im Entwicklungswerkzeug an und passt das generierte Projekt, falls gewünscht, an. Im Anschluss kann die Anwendung auf dem entsprechenden SAP-System veröffentlicht werden.

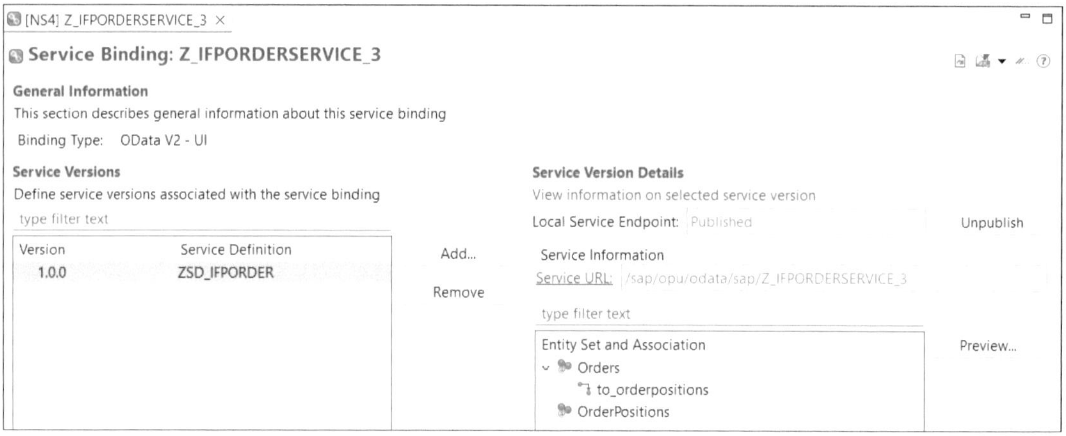

Abbildung 11.24 Publiziertes Service-Binding vom Typ »OData V2 – UI«

Anwendung testen

Für einen ersten Test der Anwendung wählen Sie unter **Service Version Details** das Entity Set **Orders** aus der Liste aus und klicken auf **Preview**. Ihr Standardbrowser öffnet sich, um die Vorschau der Anwendung anzuzeigen (siehe Abbildung 11.25). Wir haben bis jetzt allerdings noch keine UI-relevanten Eigenschaften implementiert. Trotzdem haben wir ohne jeglichen Aufwand bereits eine Standard-Benutzeroberfläche für einen List Report erhalten.

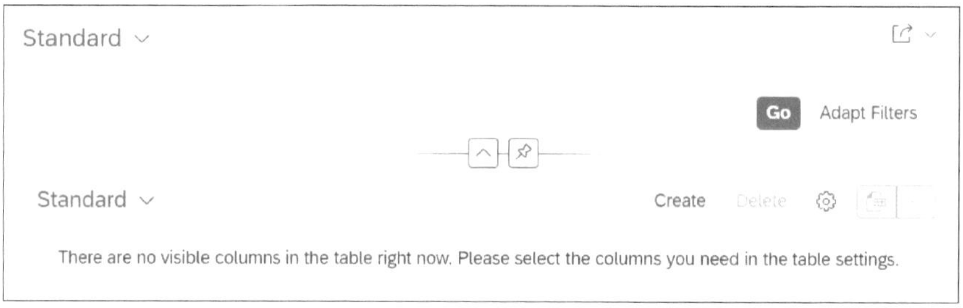

Abbildung 11.25 Vorschau der SAP-Fiori-Elements-Anwendung

Um diese Standardoberfläche weiter zu konfigurieren, klicken Sie auf das ⚙-Icon (**Settings**) und wählen, wie in Abbildung 11.26 gezeigt, alle verfügbaren Spalten aus. Bestätigen Sie diese Auswahl mit **OK**.

List Report mit Daten füllen

Die ausgewählten Spalten werden daraufhin in der Liste auf der Anwendungsoberfläche angezeigt. Um in dieser Liste auch Daten zu sehen, klicken Sie auf den Button **Go**. Nun werden die Bestellungen angezeigt.

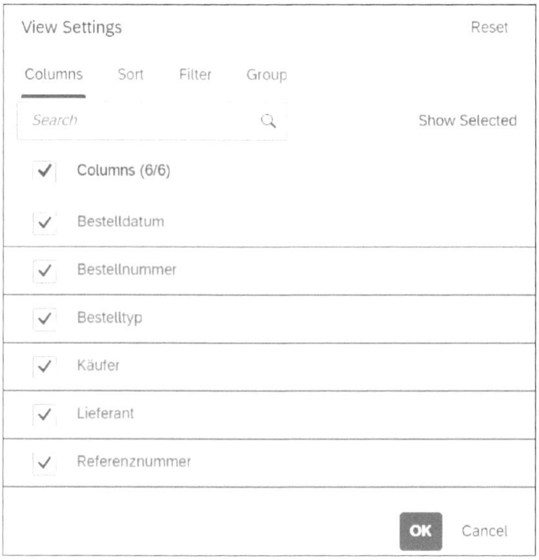

Abbildung 11.26 Feldauswahl für den List Report

Implementierung einer SAP-Fiori-Elements-Benutzeroberfläche

Die im vorangegangenen Abschnitt gezeigte Oberfläche ist schon ein sehr guter Anfang, allerdings möchte sicherlich kein Nutzer jedes Mal aufs Neue die Spalten auswählen, bevor die Daten angezeigt werden. In diesem Abschnitt werden wir daher eine Oberfläche mit SAP Fiori Elements implementieren.

UI-Metainformationen

Hierzu erweitern wir die Implementierung der Entität `ZC_IFPORDER` um entsprechende UI-Metainformationen. Öffnen Sie die Implementierung des CDS-Views `ZC_IFPORDER` aus Abschnitt 11.4.4, »Implementierung von Aktionen«, und erweitern Sie diese, wie in Listing 11.14 gezeigt.

```
@AccessControl.authorizationCheck: #NOT_REQUIRED
@EndUserText.label: 'Consumption view ZI_IFPORDER'
@Metadata.ignorePropagatedAnnotations: true

@UI: {
  headerInfo: {
    typeName: 'Order',
    typeNamePlural: 'Orders',
    title: { value: 'Buyer' },
    description: {value: 'Seller'}
  }
}
```

```
define root view entity ZC_IFPORDER
    provider contract transactional_query
        as projection on ZI_IFPORDER

{
    @UI: { lineItem: [{ position: 10 }]}
    key Orderid,
    @UI: { lineItem: [{ position: 20 }]}
    Type,
    @UI: { lineItem: [{ position: 30 }]}
    Refid,
    @UI: { lineItem: [{ position: 40 }]}
    Buyer,
    @UI: { lineItem: [{ position: 50 }]}
    Seller,
    @UI: { lineItem: [{ position: 60 }]}
    Orderdate,
    _orderpositions
}
```

Listing 11.14 Implementierung der Entität »ZC_IFPORDER«

Wir nutzen hier den Term `headerInfo` für die Überschrift unserer Bestellliste aus dem UI-Vokabular. Über diesen Term geben wir mit `typeNamePlural` an, dass der Text »Orders« über der zur Laufzeit dargestellten Liste als Überschrift angezeigt werden soll. Das Wort ist im Plural anzugeben. Über `typeName` setzen wir das gleiche Wort im Singular. Dieser Text wird den Anwendern im SAP Fiori Launchpad in der Navigationsleiste angezeigt werden, sobald sie einen Listeneintrag ausgewählt haben.

Das Attribut `label` des Ausdrucks `title` verbinden wir mit dem Feld `Orderid` der Entität. Im weiteren Verlauf setzten wir über jedes Feld der Projektionsliste die Annotation `@UI.lineItem`, um es als Spalte innerhalb der Liste zu markieren. Über die Eigenschaft `position` geben wir die Ordnung der Zeilen innerhalb der Liste an. Das Feld mit der Position 10 wird demnach als Erstes angezeigt.

Erneuter Anwendungstest

Nachdem Sie diese Anpassungen am CDS-View durchgeführt haben, speichern und aktivieren Sie diese Änderungen und starten die Anwendung erneut über die Vorschaufunktion. Ihnen wird nun die Listenansicht mit den voreingestellten Spalten angezeigt. Aus Sicht der Schnittstellenimplementierung interessant ist hier die Frage, wie die UI-Metadaten bereitgestellt werden. Hierzu nutzen wir die Entwicklungswerkzeuge des Browsers. Diese kann man in der Regel über die [F12]-Taste oder das Menü des Browsers aufrufen.

Verarbeitung der UI-Metainformationen

Navigieren Sie hier zur Registerkarte **Network** und laden Sie die Anwendung erneut. Sie erhalten nun einen guten Einblick in die verschiedenen Anfragen, die an das SAP-System gestellt werden. Nachdem die Anwendung geladen wurde, suchen Sie nach einem Request an einen OData-Service namens CATALOGSERVICE (zu erkennen in der **Request URL** in Abbildung 11.27). Hierbei handelt es sich um einen Standard-OData-Service des SAP-Systems.

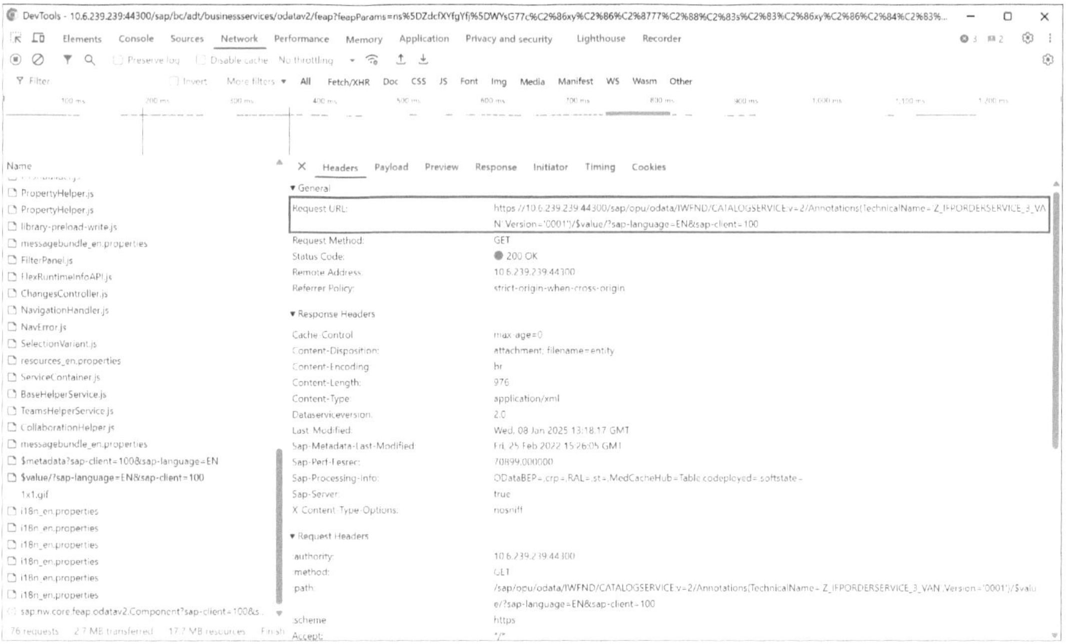

Abbildung 11.27 Auslieferung der UI-Metainformationen

Wählen Sie diesen Eintrag aus (in Abbildung 11.27 markiert) und wechseln Sie auf die Registerkarte **Preview**. Hier sehen Sie die von uns implementierten Annotationen (siehe Abbildung 11.28). Sie werden zwar anders angezeigt, als wir sie implementiert haben, sind jedoch zu erkennen. Was lässt sich hieraus ableiten? Zum einen werden die von uns implementierten UI-Annotationen im Rahmen der Aktivierung im Hintergrund durch das SAP-System weiterverarbeitet. Zum anderen wird der OData-Service CATALOGSERVICE damit beauftragt, SAP-Fiori-Element-Anwendungen mit den nötigen UI-Metainformationen zu versorgen.

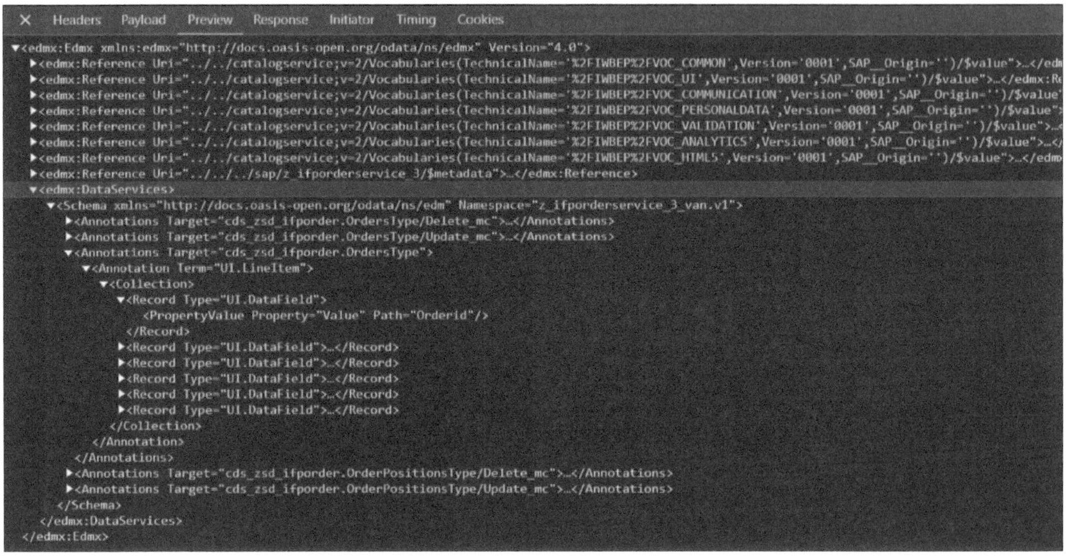

Abbildung 11.28 UI-Metainformationen

Implementierung der Detailansicht

Nach diesem kleinen Exkurs wenden wir uns wieder der Implementierung der Oberfläche unserer Beispielanwendung zu. Wir erweitern die Listendarstellung dahingehend, dass nach Auswahl eines Listeneintrags die Details zum ausgewählten Eintrag auf einer Object Page angezeigt werden. Der geringen Komplexität unseres Beispiels geschuldet, werden wir auf der Detailseite die gleichen Kopfdaten der Bestellung anzeigen wie im Körper der Detailseite. Zusätzlich werden wir in einer Tabelle die Bestellpositionen anzeigen.

Facette

Listing 11.15 zeigt die vollständige Implementierung. Wir implementieren hier drei sogenannte *Facetten*. Jede Facette wird mittels der Eigenschaft `targetQualifier` mit einer Feldgruppe verbunden. Die Feldgruppen ihrerseits besitzen das Attribut `qualifier`, das den referenzierten Bezeichner enthält.

```
@AccessControl.authorizationCheck: #NOT_REQUIRED
@EndUserText.label: 'Consumption view ZI_IFPORDER'
@Metadata.ignorePropagatedAnnotations: true

@UI: {
  headerInfo: {
    typeName: 'Order',
    typeNamePlural: 'Orders',
    title: { label: 'Orderid' }
  }
```

```
}
define root view entity ZC_IFPORDER
    provider contract transactional_query
        as projection on ZI_IFPORDER
{

@UI.facet: [
 {
              purpose: #HEADER,
              type: #FIELDGROUP_REFERENCE,
              importance: #HIGH,
              targetQualifier: 'headerdata'
          },
          {
              purpose: #STANDARD,
              type: #FIELDGROUP_REFERENCE,
              importance: #HIGH,
              targetQualifier: 'detaildata',
              label: 'Details'
          },
            {
              id: 'Buchungen',
              purpose: #STANDARD,
              type: #LINEITEM_REFERENCE,
              label: 'Bestellpositionen',
              position: 50,
              targetElement: '_orderpositions'
            }

 ]

    @UI: {
          lineItem: [
                { position: 10 }
          ],
          fieldGroup:[
                { qualifier: 'headerdata' },
                { qualifier: 'detaildata' }
          ]
         }
    key Orderid,
    @UI: {
          lineItem: [
```

11

```
            { position: 20 }
        ],
        fieldGroup:[
            { qualifier: 'headerdata' },
            { qualifier: 'detaildata' }
        ]
      }
  Type,
  @UI: {
        lineItem: [
            { position: 30 }
        ],
        fieldGroup:[
            { qualifier: 'headerdata' },
            { qualifier: 'detaildata' }
        ]
      }
  Refid,
  @UI: {
        lineItem: [
            { position: 40 }
        ],
        fieldGroup:[
            { qualifier: 'headerdata' },
            { qualifier: 'detaildata' }
        ]
      }
  Buyer,
  @UI: {
        lineItem: [
            { position: 50 }
        ],
        fieldGroup:[
            { qualifier: 'headerdata' },
            { qualifier: 'detaildata' }
        ]
      }
  Seller,
  @UI: {
        lineItem: [
            { position: 60 }
        ],
        fieldGroup:[
```

```
                { qualifier: 'headerdata' },
                { qualifier: 'detaildata' }
            ]
          }
    Orderdate,
    _orderpositions
}
```

Listing 11.15 Erweiterung der Implementierung des CDS-Views »ZC_IFPORDER«

Erneuter Test der Anwendung

Nachdem Sie diese Änderungen gespeichert und aktiviert haben, rufen Sie die Anwendung noch einmal im Vorschaumodus auf. Abbildung 11.29 zeigt das Ergebnis.

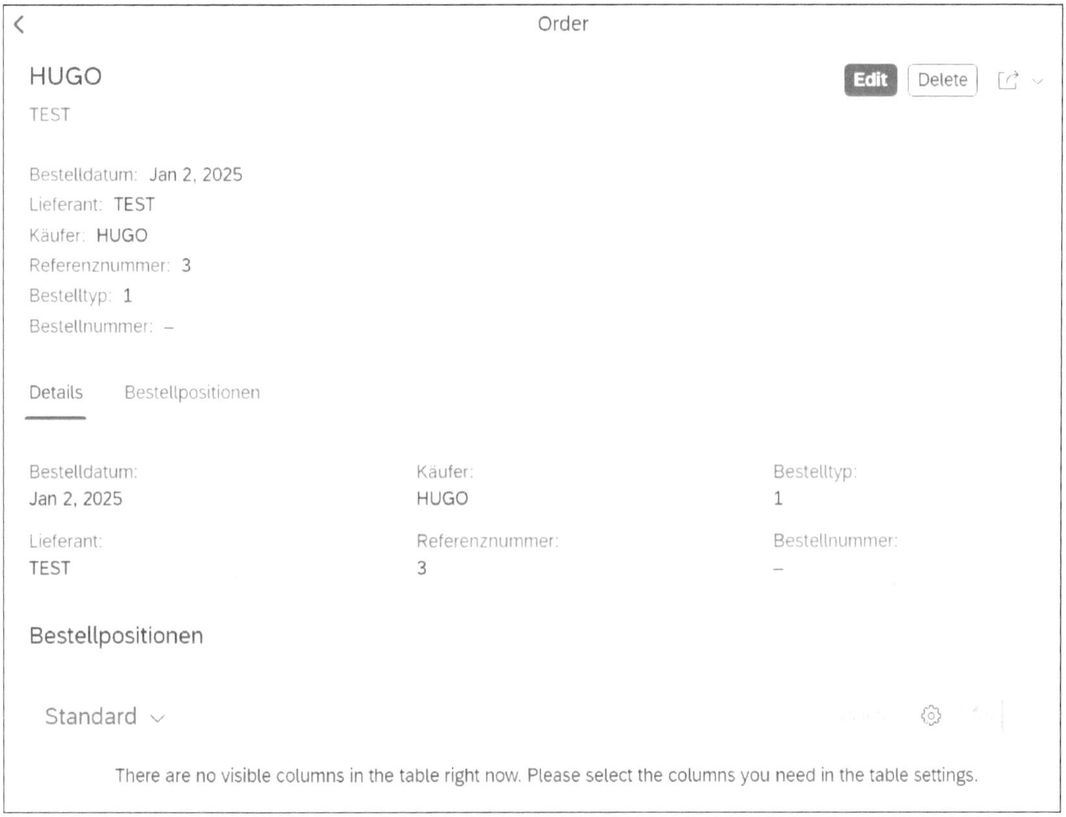

Abbildung 11.29 Die Detailseite einer Bestellung

Im Kopf der Detailseite sehen Sie die Details zur Bestellung. Im Bereich (bzw. in der *Sektion*) **Details** werden ebenfalls die Detailinformationen angezeigt. Neben der Sektion **Details** wird die Sektion **Bestellpositionen** angezeigt. Hier finden Sie eine Listendarstellung ohne weitere Spalten.

Bestellpositionen Da wir in der Anwendung nicht nur die Bestellung, sondern auch die dazugehörenden Bestellpositionen anzeigen lassen wollen, erweitern wir den Consumption-View ZC_IFPORDERPOS um entsprechende Annotationen (siehe Listing 11.16).

```
@AccessControl.authorizationCheck: #NOT_REQUIRED
@EndUserText.label: 'Projection view for ZI_IFPORDERPOS'
@Metadata.ignorePropagatedAnnotations: true
define view entity ZC_IFPORDERPOS
    as projection on ZI_IFPORDERPOS as Orderposition
{

@UI.facet: [
          {
              purpose: #STANDARD,
              type: #FIELDGROUP_REFERENCE,
              importance: #HIGH,
              targetQualifier: 'Details'
          }

 ]

    @UI: {
          lineItem: [
                { position: 10 }
          ],
          fieldGroup:[
                { qualifier: 'Details' }
          ]
         }
    key Orderid,
    @UI: {
          lineItem: [
                { position: 20 }
          ],
          fieldGroup:[
                { qualifier: 'Details' }
          ]
         }
    key Orderpos,
    @UI: {
          lineItem: [
                { position: 30 }
```

```
      ],
      fieldGroup:[
            { qualifier: 'Details' }
      ]
     }
Matid,
@UI: {
      lineItem: [
            { position: 40 }
      ],
      fieldGroup:[
            { qualifier: 'Details' }
      ]
     }
Mattext,
@UI: {
      lineItem: [
            { position: 50 }
      ],
      fieldGroup:[
            { qualifier: 'Details' }
      ]
     }
Ordercount,
@Semantics.amount.currencyCode: 'Currency'
@UI: {
      lineItem: [
            { position: 60 }
      ],
      fieldGroup:[
            { qualifier: 'Details' }
      ]
     }
Price,
@UI: {
      lineItem: [
            { position: 70 }
      ],
      fieldGroup:[
            { qualifier: 'Details' }
      ]
```

```
        }
    Currency
}
```

Listing 11.16 Erweiterung des CDS-Views »ZC_IFPORDERPOS«

Ergebnis in der Anwendungsvorschau

Das Ergebnis der Anpassungen an die CDS-Entität `ZC_IFPORDERPOS` zeigt Abbildung 11.30.

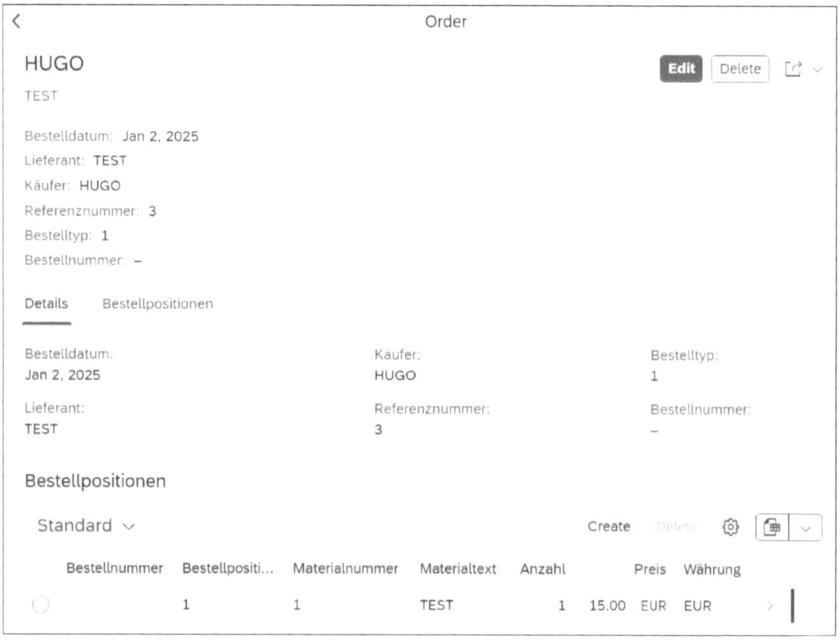

Abbildung 11.30 Anzeige der Bestellpositionen

Wählt man nun in der Liste der vorhandenen Bestellpositionen eine Position aus, wird man zur Detailseite dieser konkreten Position weitergeleitet (siehe Abbildung 11.31). Die Seite bietet auch die Möglichkeit, den aktuellen Datensatz über die Funktion **Edit** zu bearbeiten.

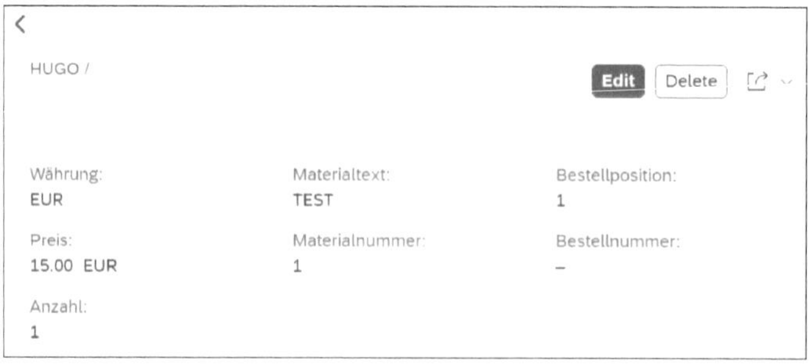

Abbildung 11.31 Detailansicht einer Bestellposition

Kapitel 12
ABAP Channels

ABAP Channels ermöglichen interaktive und kollaborative Szenarien auf der Basis einer ereignisgesteuerten Architektur. Damit kann ein Server bei Änderungen von Daten in einer Benutzersitzung oder durch ein externes Programm aktiv andere Benutzersitzungen oder externe Programme über diese Änderung informieren.

Wenn Webbrowser oder SAP-GUI-Anwendungen auf Ereignisse auf einem ABAP-Server reagieren wollten, mussten sie bis zum Release SAP NetWeaver 7.4 SP05 in regelmäßigen Zeitabständen Anfragen an den Server schicken. Seit diesem Releasestand kann diese ineffiziente Polling-Technik durch Push-Benachrichtigungen von *ABAP Channels* ersetzt werden.

Arten von ABAP Channels

Es gibt zwei Arten von ABAP Channels:

- **ABAP Push Channels**
  Ein *ABAP Push Channel* (APC) ermöglicht die bidirektionale Kommunikation mit einem externen Client – typischerweise einem Webbrowser – über das WebSocket Protocol.
- **ABAP Messaging Channels**
  Ein *ABAP Messaging Channel* (AMC) versendet Nachrichten aus einer Benutzersitzung an andere Benutzersitzungen. Diese können über APC auch an externe Clients weitergeleitet werden.

In Abbildung 12.1 wird eine Nachricht aus der Benutzersitzung 1 über AMC an die Benutzersitzungen 2 (auf demselben Anwendungsserver) und 3 (auf einem anderen Anwendungsserver) und an die beiden Webbrowser 1 und 2 geschickt. Die Webbrowser haben zuvor eine WebSocket-Verbindung zu jeweils einem der beiden Anwendungsserver geöffnet.

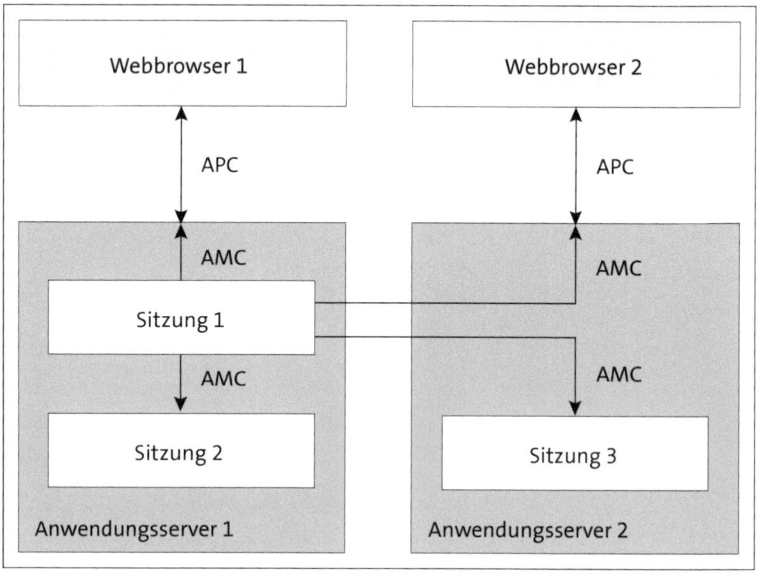

Abbildung 12.1 ABAP Channels

12.1 ABAP Push Channels

WebSocket Protocol

ABAP Push Channels ermöglichen eine bidirektionale Kommunikation zwischen einem Client – typischerweise einem Webbrowser – und einem ABAP-Anwendungsserver über das *WebSocket Protocol*. Das WebSocket Protocol basiert auf dem *Transmission Control Protocol* (TCP) und ist ein Standardprotokoll, das von der Internet Engineering Task Force (IETF) unter der Nummer RFC 6455 verwaltet wird.

Während bei einer reinen HTTP-Verbindung jeglicher Datenaustausch vom Client initiiert wird, genügt es beim WebSocket Protocol, wenn der Client die Verbindung öffnet, ähnlich einem Nachrichtenkanal. Der Server kann anschließend diese offene Verbindung aktiv verwenden und dem Client neue oder geänderte Daten schicken, ohne dass der Client zuvor aktiv werden müsste. Ebenso kann der Client dem Server Nachrichten senden, ohne eine neue Verbindung aufzubauen.

12.1.1 Ein einfacher ABAP Push Channel

ABAP Push Channel anlegen

ABAP Push Channels legen Sie als Repository-Objekte im Object Navigator über das Kontextmenü eines Pakets unter dem Menüpunkt **Connectivity • ABAP Push Channel** an. Dabei müssen Sie einen Namen vergeben. Abbildung 12.2 zeigt den ABAP Push Channel `ZIFP_APC`.

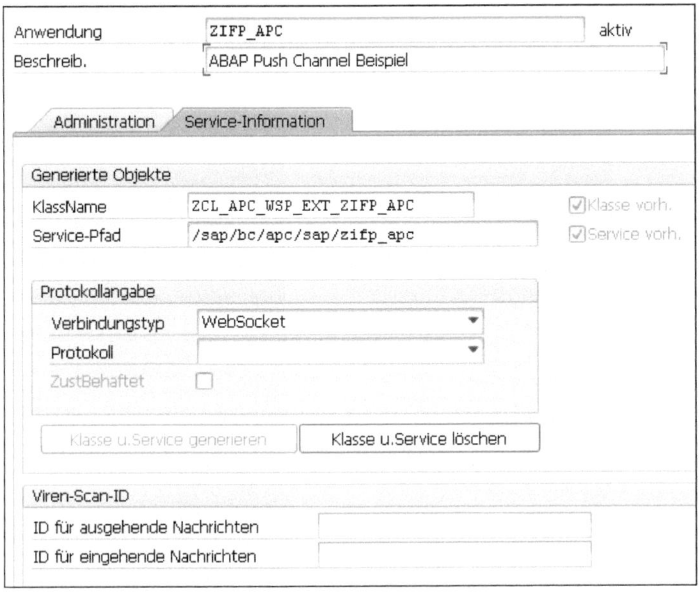

Abbildung 12.2 ABAP Push Channel

Servicepfad

Der Name des ABAP Push Channels legt den *Servicepfad* im Internet Communication Framework (ICF) des ABAP-Servers fest. Dies ist die URL, mit der sich ein WebSocket-Client verbinden kann, um über den ABAP Push Channel Nachrichten auszutauschen. In unserem Beispiel lautet der Servicepfad **/sap/bc/apc/sap/zifp_apc**.

Der ABAP-Code für den ABAP Push Channel befindet sich in einer generierten Klasse, deren Namen Sie frei wählen können. Im Beispiel lautet der Klassenname `ZCL_APC_WSP_EXT_ZIFP_APC`.

Verbindungstypen

Als **Verbindungstyp** können Sie zwischen WebSocket und TCP Socket wählen. Damit legen Sie fest, ob Client und Server über das binäre *TCP Socket Protocol* oder über das darauf aufbauende, zeichenorientierte WebSocket Protocol kommunizieren. Standardmäßig ist **WebSocket** ausgewählt. Als **Protokoll** können Sie statt des Standard-WebSocket-Protocols auch das *Push Channel Protocol* (PCP) von SAP auswählen, das in der Liste als **V10.PCP.SAP.COM** angezeigt wird.

Über das Auswahlfeld **ZustBehaftet** geben Sie an, ob der ABAP Push Channel zustandsbehaftet oder zustandslos ist. Wenn die Option ausgewählt ist, der Kanal also zustandsbehaftet ist, bleibt die APC-Session für die Bearbeitung der empfangenen Nachrichten so lange aktiv, bis die Verbindung geschlossen wird.

APC-Klasse

Nachdem Sie den ABAP Push Channel angelegt haben, klicken Sie auf den Button **Klasse u. Service generieren**, um die beiden Objekte generieren zu lassen. Danach können Sie die generierte Klasse implementieren.

In Abhängigkeit von den gewählten Einstellungen erbt die generierte Klasse von einer dieser Basisklassen:

- `CL_APC_WSP_EXT_STATELESS_BASE`
  WebSocket Protocol, keine Auswahl eines Unterprotokolls, zustandslos
- `CL_APC_WSP_EXT_STATELESS_PCB_B`
  WebSocket Protocol, Auswahl des Push Channel Protocols, zustandslos
- `CL_APC_WSP_EXT_STATEFUL_BASE`
  WebSocket Protocol, keine Auswahl eines Unterprotokolls, zustandsbehaftet
- `CL_APC_WSP_EXT_STATEFUL_PCB_B`
  WebSocket Protocol, Auswahl des Push Channel Protocols, zustandsbehaftet
- `CL_APC_TCP_EXT_STATELESS_BASE`
  TCP Socket Protocol, zustandslos
- `CL_APC_TCP_EXT_STATEFUL_BASE`
  TCP Socket Protocol, zustandsbehaftet

Methoden der APC-Klasse

Alle Klassen haben fünf Methoden, die Sie in der generierten Klasse redefinieren können:

- `on_accept`
  Diese Methode wird aufgerufen, sobald eine WebSocket-Verbindung zum ABAP Push Channel aufgebaut werden soll. Hier haben Sie die Möglichkeit, den Verbindungsaufbau abzulehnen, indem Sie im Exportparameter `e_connect_mode` die Konstante `co_connect_mode_reject` zurückgeben. Die Standardimplementierung der Basisklasse gibt die Konstante `co_connect_mode_accept` zurück und akzeptiert damit den Verbindungsaufbau.
- `on_start`
  Diese Methode wird bei der ersten WebSocket-Anfrage aufgerufen. Sie ist in den Basisklassen nicht implementiert; daher müssen Sie sie in der generierten Klasse redefinieren.
- `on_message`
  Diese Methode wird bei jeder eingehenden Nachricht aufgerufen. Auch diese Methode müssen Sie in der generierten Klasse redefinieren.

- on_close
  Diese Methode wird beim Schließen einer WebSocket-Verbindung aufgerufen.
- on_error
  Diese Methode wird aufgerufen, falls ein WebSocket-Fehler auftritt.

»on_message«-Methode

Listing 12.1 zeigt die Implementierung einer einfachen on_message-Methode. Zunächst wird über den Importparameter i_message_manager das neue Nachrichtenobjekt lr_message erzeugt. Danach wird über den Importparameter i_message die empfangene Nachricht ausgelesen und als Nachricht in das neue Nachrichtenobjekt geschrieben. Dieses neue Nachrichtenobjekt wird anschließend wieder an den Client zurückgeschickt. Diese Klasse implementiert also einen einfachen Echoserver, der eine erhaltene Nachricht einfach wieder zurückschickt.


```
METHOD if_apc_wsp_extension~on_message.
  DATA:
    lr_message TYPE REF TO if_apc_wsp_message.
  TRY.
      " Neues Nachrichtenobjekt erzeugen
      lr_message = i_message_manager->create_message( ).

      " empfangene Nachricht lesen und in neues
      " Nachrichtenobjekt schreiben
      lr_message->set_text( i_message->get_text( ) ).

      " neue Nachricht schicken
      i_message_manager->send( lr_message ).

    CATCH cx_apc_error.
  ENDTRY.
ENDMETHOD.
```

Listing 12.1 »on_message«-Methode einer einfachen APC-Handler-Klasse

12.1.2 Ein einfacher WebSocket-Client

WebSocket-API

Webbrowser können das WebSocket Protocol nutzen, indem sie die vom World Wide Web Consortium (W3C) standardisierte *WebSocket-API* verwenden. Diese API wird von den meisten modernen Browsern unterstützt. Jedoch muss auch die Netzwerkinfrastruktur, insbesondere in Firmennetzwerken, das Protokoll unterstützen. Typische Probleme sind hier Firewall- und Proxy-Einstellungen, Protokoll-Inkompatibilität, Timeouts und Verbindungsunterbrechungen, da die WebSocket-Verbindungen z. B. fälschlicherweise aufgrund von Inaktivität geschlossen werden.

WebSocket-Client

Listing 12.2 zeigt einen einfachen WebSocket-Client. Im `<script>`-Element wird zuerst unter Angabe der URL das neue WebSocket-Objekt `ws` erzeugt. Dann werden die Callback-Funktionen `onopen`, `onmessage`, `onclose` und `onerror` deklariert. In der `onopen`-Funktion wird eine Nachricht an den WebSocket-Server geschickt. Der Server aus Listing 12.1 schickt diese Nachricht unverändert zurück, woraufhin die `onmessage`-Funktion des Clients aufgerufen wird. Diese Funktion zeigt die eingetroffenen Nachrichten des Servers in einer Alert-Dialogbox an.

```
<!DOCTYPE html>
<html>
  <head>
    <meta charset="UTF-8">
    <title>Einfacher WebSocket Client</title>
  </head>
  <body>
    <script>
      // WebSocket-Verbindung öffnen
      var ws = new WebSocket(
        "ws://server.domain:8000/sap/bc/apc/sap/zifp_apc"
      );
      ws.onopen = function() {
        alert("WebSocket geöffnet");
        ws.send("Hallo, Welt");
      };
      ws.onmessage = function (msg) {
        alert(msg.data);
      };
      ws.onclose = function() {
        alert("WebSocket geschlossen");
      };
      ws.onerror = function() {
        alert("WebSocket-Fehler");
      };
    </script>
  </body>
</html>
```

Listing 12.2 JavaScript-Code für einen einfachen WebSocket-Client

Um den Client testen zu können, legen Sie am einfachsten eine Business-Server-Pages-(BSP-)Anwendung an, die Listing 12.1 als Startseite enthält. Denn die WebSocket-Verbindung kann nur geöffnet werden, wenn sich der Client zuvor beim ABAP-Server angemeldet hat.

12.2 ABAP Message Channels

Die Handler-Klasse aus dem vorangehenden Abschnitt kann bislang nur auf WebSocket-Nachrichten vom Client reagieren, diesen aber noch nicht aktiv über Ereignisse auf dem ABAP-Server informieren. Um dies zu ermöglichen, muss er als Konsument eines ABAP Message Channels registriert werden. Doch zuvor zeigen wir Ihnen in diesem Abschnitt, wie Sie über ABAP Message Channels Nachrichten zwischen verschiedenen Benutzersitzungen auf einem SAP-ABAP-System austauschen können.

Publish-/Subscribe-Architektur

Mit ABAP Message Channels stellt SAP eine *Publish-/Subscribe-Architektur* zur Verfügung. Jede ABAP-Benutzersitzung kann die Nachrichten eines AMC subskribieren (d. h. abonnieren), und jede ABAP-Benutzersitzung kann Nachrichten auf diesem AMC publizieren. Dabei spielt es keine Rolle, auf welchem Anwendungsserver die jeweiligen Benutzersitzungen laufen. Ein *AMC Broker* sorgt dafür, dass die publizierten Nachrichten an die Subskribenten weitergeleitet werden. Abbildung 12.3 zeigt ein Beispiel dafür.

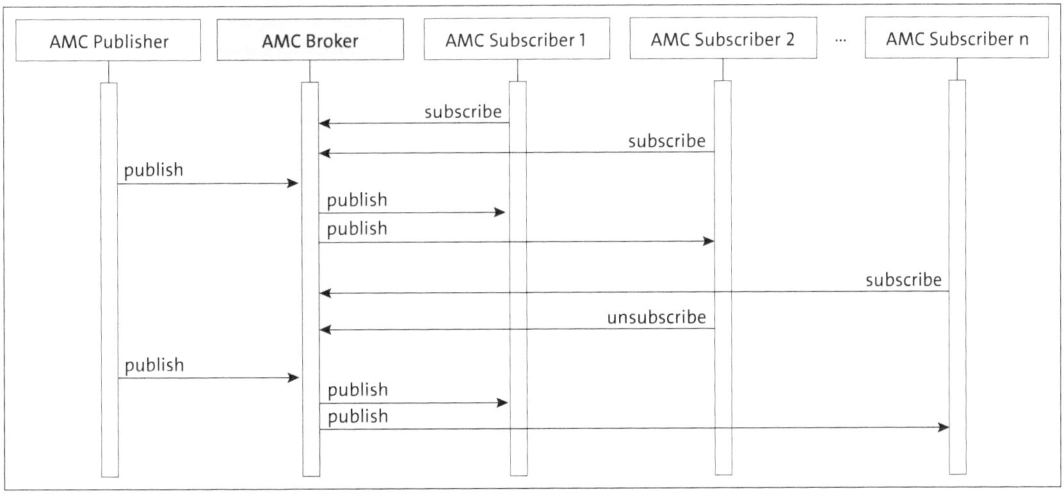

Abbildung 12.3 AMC-Publish-/Subscribe-Architektur

12.2.1 ABAP Message Channels als Repository-Objekte

AMC-Anwendung

Ein ABAP Message Channel ist immer Bestandteil einer *AMC-Anwendung*, die Sie als ABAP-Repository-Objekt in der ABAP Workbench anlegen können. Wählen Sie dazu im Object Navigator über das Kontextmenü eines Pakets den Menüpfad **Connectivity • ABAP Messaging Channel** aus. Vergeben Sie dann einen Namen und eine Beschreibung für die AMC-Anwendung. Auf der Registerkarte **Channels** können Sie nun einen Kanal innerhalb der Anwendung anlegen und dessen Eigenschaften pflegen, so wie dies in Abbildung 12.4 gezeigt wird.

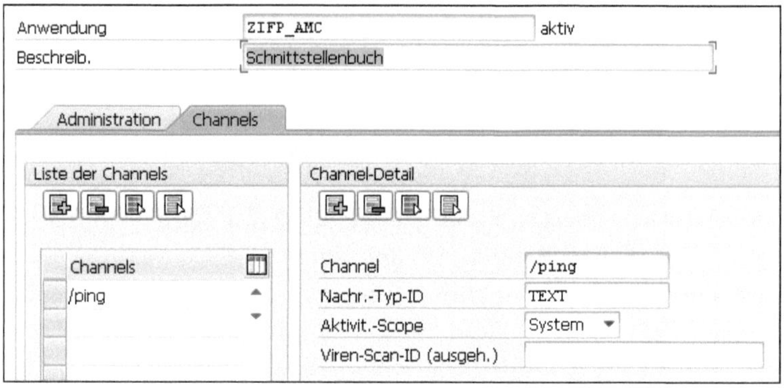

Abbildung 12.4 AMC-Anwendung mit einem »TEXT«-Kanal

Nachrichtentypen

Jeder Kanal ist genau einem von drei Nachrichtentypen zugeordnet, den Sie im Feld **Nachr.-Typ-ID** eintragen. Je nach Nachrichtentyp werden die über diesen Kanal ausgetauschten Nachrichten über unterschiedliche ABAP-Datentypen repräsentiert, und Sendern und Empfängern stehen unterschiedliche Schnittstellen zur Verfügung, um diese Nachrichten zu senden bzw. zu empfangen. Im Einzelnen sind dies die folgenden Datentypen und Schnittstellen:

- TEXT
  - Nachrichtentyp: `STRING`
  - Senderschnittstelle: `IF_AMC_MESSAGE_PRODUCER_TEXT`
  - Empfängerschnittstelle: `IF_AMC_MESSAGE_RECEIVER_TEXT`
- BINARY
  - Nachrichtentyp: `XSTRING`
  - Senderschnittstelle: `IF_AMC_MESSAGE_PRODUCER_BINARY`
  - Empfängerschnittstelle: `IF_AMC_MESSAGE_RECEIVER_BINARY`
- PCP
  - Nachrichtentyp: `IF_AC_MESSAGE_TYPE_PCP`

- Senderschnittstelle: IF_AMC_MESSAGE_PRODUCER_PCP
- Empfängerschnittstelle: IF_AMC_MESSAGE_RECEIVER_PCP

Aktivitätsumfang

Das Feld **Aktivit.-Scope** legt den Aktivitätsumfang des Kanals fest. Hier haben Sie drei Auswahlmöglichkeiten:

- **System**
  Nachrichten werden systemweit, d. h. mandanten- und benutzerübergreifend publiziert.
- **Mandant**
  Nachrichten werden mandantenweit, d. h. benutzerübergreifend an alle Benutzersitzungen in demselben Mandanten publiziert.
- **Benutzer**
  Nachrichten werden nur an Benutzersitzungen desselben Benutzers in demselben Mandanten publiziert.

Berechtigte Programme

Damit ein ABAP-Programm über den Kanal Nachrichten senden bzw. empfangen darf, muss es zuvor in der Tabelle **Attribute für berechtigtes Programm** eingetragen werden. Als berechtigte Programme kommen ABAP-Reports, Funktionsgruppen und Klassen infrage. In der Spalte **Aktivit.** müssen Sie noch angeben, welche Aktivität dieses Programm auf dem Kanal ausführen darf:

- **Senden**
  Das Programm darf über den Kanal Nachrichten versenden.
- **Über Session empfangen**
  Das Programm darf innerhalb einer ABAP-Benutzersitzung über den Kanal Nachrichten empfangen.
- **Über APC WebSocket empfangen**
  Das Programm ist in diesem Fall eine APC-Handler-Klasse und darf Nachrichten über den Kanal empfangen und sie über das WebSocket Protocol weiterleiten.

Diesen Fall werden wir in Abschnitt 12.3, »Kollaborationsszenario mit ABAP Channels«, genauer besprechen. Zuvor implementieren wir in Abschnitten 12.2.2, »AMC-Sender«, und Abschnitt 12.2.3, »AMC-Empfänger«, einfache AMC-Sender- und AMC-Empfängerprogramme, um eine Textnachricht von einer Benutzersitzung zu einer anderen Benutzersitzung zu schicken.

12.2.2 AMC-Sender

Textnachricht verschicken

Der ABAP-Report in Listing 12.3 zeigt einen einfachen AMC-Sender, der eine Textnachricht über den AMC-Kanal aus Abbildung 12.4 verschickt.

```
REPORT zifp_amc_sender.

PARAMETERS:
  pa_msg TYPE string LOWER CASE DEFAULT 'Hallo, Welt!'.
DATA:
  gr_producer_text TYPE REF TO if_amc_message_producer_text,
  gr_amc_error     TYPE REF TO cx_amc_error.

START-OF-SELECTION.
  TRY.
    " Nachrichtenproduzent anlegen
      gr_producer_text ?=
        cl_amc_channel_manager=>create_message_producer(
          i_application_id = 'ZIFP_AMC'
          i_channel_id = '/ping'
      ).

      " Textnachricht verschicken
      gr_producer_text->send( i_message = pa_msg ).

    CATCH cx_amc_error INTO gr_amc_error.
      MESSAGE gr_amc_error->get_text( ) TYPE 'E'.
  ENDTRY.
```

Listing 12.3 Einfacher AMC-Sender

Zunächst legt der Report über den Aufruf der statischen Methode create_message_producer der Klasse CL_AMC_CHANNEL_MANAGER einen Nachrichtenproduzenten vom Typ IF_AMC_MESSAGE_PRODUCER_TEXT an. Danach ruft er die send-Methode des Nachrichtenproduzenten auf, um einen ABAP-String über diesen Kanal zu verschicken.

Falls der Report nicht beim Kanal als sendende Anwendung registriert ist oder ein anderes Problem auftritt, wird ein Fehler vom Typ CX_AMC_ERROR ausgelöst und vom Report angezeigt.

12.2.3 AMC-Empfänger

Empfangendes ABAP-Programm

Damit Sie eine AMC-Nachricht empfangen können, müssen Sie eine Klasse implementieren, die das entsprechende Empfänger-Interface IF_AMC_MESSAGE_REICEIVER_<TYPE> implementiert, wobei <TYPE> für einen der drei Nachrichtentypen TEXT, BINARY oder PCP steht. Im empfangenden Programm legen Sie eine Instanz dieser Klasse an und registrieren diese Instanz beim Kanal. Listing 12.4 zeigt solch ein Programm.

```
REPORT zifp_amc_receiver.

PARAMETERS:
  pa_nr   TYPE i DEFAULT 1,  " Anzahl erwarteter Nachrichten
  pa_wait TYPE i DEFAULT 20. " Wartezeit in Sekunden

DATA:
  gr_consumer  TYPE REF TO if_amc_message_consumer,
  gt_messages  TYPE TABLE OF string,
  gv_message   TYPE string,
  gv_nr        TYPE i, " Anzahl empfangener Nachrichten
  gr_amc_error TYPE REF TO cx_amc_error.

* Implementierungsklasse für die AMC-Empfängerschnittstelle
CLASS lcl_amc_receiver DEFINITION
FINAL
  CREATE PUBLIC.
  PUBLIC SECTION.
    INTERFACES if_amc_message_receiver_text.
ENDCLASS.

CLASS lcl_amc_receiver IMPLEMENTATION.
  METHOD if_amc_message_receiver_text~receive.
* Nachricht in die globale interne Tabelle einfügen
    APPEND i_message TO gt_messages.
    ADD 1 TO gv_nr.
  ENDMETHOD.
ENDCLASS.

START-OF-SELECTION.
  DATA: gr_receiver TYPE REF TO lcl_amc_receiver.

  TRY.
      gr_consumer =
        cl_amc_channel_manager=>create_message_consumer(
          i_application_id = 'ZIFP_AMC'
          i_channel_id = '/ping' ).
      CREATE OBJECT gr_receiver.

      " Empfänger subskribieren
      gr_consumer->start_message_delivery(
        i_receiver = gr_receiver ).
    CATCH cx_amc_error INTO gr_amc_error.
```

12

```
      MESSAGE gr_amc_error->get_text( ) TYPE 'E'.
  ENDTRY.
*
* So lange warten, bis alle Nachrichten empfangen wurden,
* jedoch nicht länger als die Wartezeit.
*
  WAIT FOR MESSAGING CHANNELS UNTIL gv_nr >= pa_nr
       UP TO pa_wait SECONDS.

  IF sy-subrc = 8.
    IF  gv_nr = 0.
      WRITE: 'Time-Out aufgetreten,',
             'keine Nachrichten empfangen.'.
    ELSEIF gv_nr < pa_nr.
      WRITE: 'Time-Out aufgetreten,',
             'nicht alle Nachrichten empfangen.'.
    ENDIF.
  ELSE.
    WRITE: 'Alle Nachrichten empfangen.'.
  ENDIF.
  LOOP AT gt_messages INTO gv_message.
    "Liste der Nachrichten ausgeben
    WRITE: / sy-tabix, gv_message.
  ENDLOOP.
```

Listing 12.4 Einfacher AMC-Empfänger

Empfängerklasse

Der Report definiert eine lokale Empfängerklasse `lcl_amc_receiver`, die die Schnittstelle `IF_AMC_MESSAGE_RECIEVER_TEXT` implementiert. Diese Schnittstelle definiert die Methode `receive`, die beim Empfang von Nachrichten vom AMC Broker aufgerufen wird. Die Implementierung der Methode in der lokalen Klasse `lcl_amc_receiver` schreibt die empfangene Nachricht in die programmglobale interne Tabelle `gt_messages`.

Beim Start ruft das Programm zunächst die statische Methode `create_message_consumer` der Klasse `CL_AMC_CHANNEL_MANAGER` auf, um das Consumer-Objekt `gr_consumer` zu erzeugen. Danach erzeugt das Programm die Instanz `gr_receiver` der lokalen Empfängerklasse `lcl_amc_receiver`. Um den Empfang der Nachrichten zu starten, wird diese Instanz mit der Methode `start_message_delivery` dem Consumer-Objekt übergeben.

Nachrichten empfangen

Danach wartet das Programm über die ABAP-Anweisung `WAIT FOR MESSAGING CHANNELS` so lange auf eingehende Nachrichten, bis entweder alle erwarteten

Nachrichten eingetroffen sind oder der Timeout-Wert »pa_wait« erreicht wurde. Anschließend werden die empfangenen Nachrichten ausgegeben.

12.3 Kollaborationsszenario mit ABAP Channels

Information zu Business-Objekt-Änderungen

In diesem Abschnitt implementieren wir ein Kollaborationsszenario, bei dem WebSocket-Clients über das Anlegen und Ändern von Kundenbestellungen mit den BAPIs Z_BAPI_ORDER_CREATEFROMDATA und Z_BAPI_ORDER_CHANGE informiert werden. Dazu definieren wir zuerst die entsprechenden Ereignisse im *Business Object Repository* (BOR), binden diese Ereignisse an entsprechende Methoden einer AMC-Senderklasse und erweitern die APC-Handler-Klasse so, dass sie die Nachrichten der AMC-Senderklasse an ihre WebSocket-Clients weiterleitet.

Abbildung 12.5 zeigt das Szenario. Zunächst wird die AMC-Publisher-Klasse beim *BOR Event Broker* registriert. Sobald ein WebSocket-Client eine Verbindung zu einem APC-Kanal öffnet, subskribiert der *APC-Handler* Änderungen des AMC Brokers. Wenn nun das Business-Objekt ein Ereignis auslöst, wird es vom Event Broker an den *AMC Publisher* publiziert. Von dort geht es als AMC-Nachricht über den AMC Broker weiter an den APC-Handler, der die Information an den WebSocket-Client weiterleitet. 12

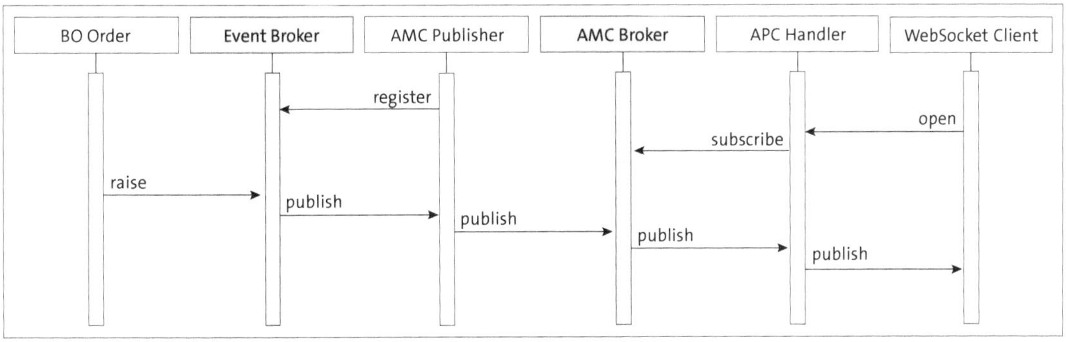

Abbildung 12.5 Kollaborationsszenario

12.3.1 BOR-Ereignisse definieren

Zunächst müssen Sie dafür sorgen, dass unser Business-Objekt Z_BUS4500 für die Bestellung ein Ereignis auslöst, sobald eine Bestellung angelegt oder geändert wird. Dazu müssen Sie zuerst zwei Ereignisse im *Business Object Builder* anlegen und diese dann in den entsprechenden BAPIs auslösen.

Ereignisse anlegen

Zum Anlegen der Ereignisse öffnen Sie im Business Object Builder das Business-Objekt Z_BUS4500 im Änderungsmodus, selektieren den Knoten **Ereig-**

nisse und wählen den Menüeintrag **Bearbeiten • Anlegen** aus, um ein neues Ereignis anzulegen. Legen Sie so die Ereignisse `created` und `changed` an. Ändern Sie über den Menüpfad **Bearbeiten • Freigabestatus • Objektkomponente** den Freigabestatus zuerst in **implementiert** und dann in **freigegeben**. Abbildung 12.6 zeigt die beiden neu hinzugefügten Ereignisse.

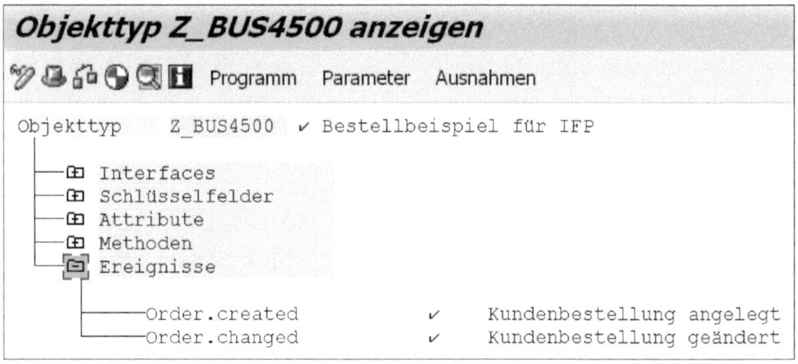

Abbildung 12.6 Ereignisse anlegen

Ereignis auslösen

Damit Sie die beiden Ereignisse in den entsprechenden BAPIs auslösen können, legen Sie zunächst den Verbuchungsfunktionsbaustein `Z_IVP_V_EVENT_CREATE` aus Listing 12.5 an.

```
FUNCTION Z_IFP_V_EVENT_CREATE .
*"----------------------------------------------------------
*"*"Verbuchungsfunktionsbaustein:
*"
*"*"Lokale Schnittstelle:
*"  IMPORTING
*"     VALUE(I_ORDERID) TYPE  ZIFPORDERID
*"     VALUE(I_EVENT) TYPE  SWO_EVENT
*"----------------------------------------------------------
  DATA lv_objkey TYPE swo_typeid.
  WRITE i_orderid TO lv_objkey NO-GAP.
  CALL FUNCTION 'SWE_EVENT_CREATE'
    EXPORTING
      objtype = 'Z_BUS4500'
      objkey  = lv_objkey
      event   = i_event.
ENDFUNCTION.
```

Listing 12.5 Ereignis auslösen

Dieser Verbuchungsbaustein nimmt in den Importparametern `i_orderid` und `i_event` die Bestellnummer und den Namen des Ereignisses (`'created'` oder 'changed') entgegen und ruft den Funktionsbaustein SWE_EVENT_CREATE auf, der dann das Ereignis erzeugt. Dabei wird zusätzlich zu Objektschlüssel und Ereignisname noch der Objekttyp mitgegeben.

Verbuchungsbaustein aufrufen

Diesen Verbuchungsbaustein können Sie nun am Ende der BAPIs Z_BAPI_ORDER_CREATEFROMDATA und Z_BAPI_ORDER_CHANGE mit dem Zusatz IN UPDATE TASK aufrufen und dabei den Importparameter i_event mit 'created' bzw. 'changed' versorgen, so wie dies in Listing 12.6 für das BAPI Z_BAPI_ORDER_CREATEFROMDATA gezeigt wird.

```
* Ereignis auslösen
  CALL FUNCTION 'Z_IFP_V_EVENT_CREATE'
    IN UPDATE TASK
    EXPORTING
      i_orderid = l_orderid
      i_event   = 'created'.
```

Listing 12.6 Verbucher für die Ereignisauslösung aufrufen

Diese beiden Ereignisse werden wir später an eine Methode einer AMC-Senderklasse binden, die das Ereignis als AMC-Nachricht weiterleitet.

12.3.2 AMC-Sender definieren

Das Ereignis, das vom Business-Objekt ausgelöst wird, soll nun über eine statische Methode einer Klasse an den AMC weitergeleitet werden. Damit in Transaktion SWETYPV eine Klasse an ein Ereignis gebunden werden kann, muss diese Klasse das Interface BI_EVENT_HANDLER_STATIC implementieren. Dieses Interface definiert die statische Methode ON_EVENT, die beim Auftreten eines Ereignisses aufgerufen wird.

Ereignis weiterleiten

Listing 12.7 zeigt die Implementierung dieser Methode in der Klasse Z_CL_IFP_FORWARD_EVENT. Zuerst werden die Bestellnummer und der Ereignisname aus den Importparametern sender-instid und event der Methode in den String lv_message eingefügt. Dann wird dieser String über die send-Methode des Nachrichtenproduzenten lr_producer_text verschickt, der zuvor über die Methode create_message_producer der Klasse CL_AMC_CHANNEL_MANAGER erzeugt wurde.

```
METHOD bi_event_handler_static~on_event.
  DATA:
    lr_producer_text TYPE
                      REF TO if_amc_message_producer_text,
    lv_message       TYPE string.
```

```
  TRY.
      " Nachricht aufbauen
      lv_message = |Order { sender-instid } { event }|.
      " Nachrichtenproduzent anlegen
      lr_producer_text ?= cl_amc_channel_manager=>
        create_message_producer(
          i_application_id = 'ZIFP_AMC'
          i_channel_id = '/ping' ).
      " Nachricht verschicken
      lr_producer_text->send( i_message = lv_message ).
    CATCH cx_amc_error.
  ENDTRY.
ENDMETHOD.
```

Listing 12.7 AMC-Nachricht im Ereignisverbraucher versenden

Ereignisverbraucher registrieren

Diese Methode müssen Sie nun noch als Ereignisverbraucher registrieren. Dazu starten Sie Transaktion SWETYPV, mit der Sie Ereignisse von Klassen oder Business-Objekten als Verbraucher an Workprozess-Definitionen, Funktionsbausteine oder Klassenmethoden anbinden können. Wählen Sie in der Transaktion den Button **Neue Einträge** aus, und legen Sie dann für das Ereignis `CREATED` eine neue Ereigniskopplung an, wie in Abbildung 12.7 gezeigt.

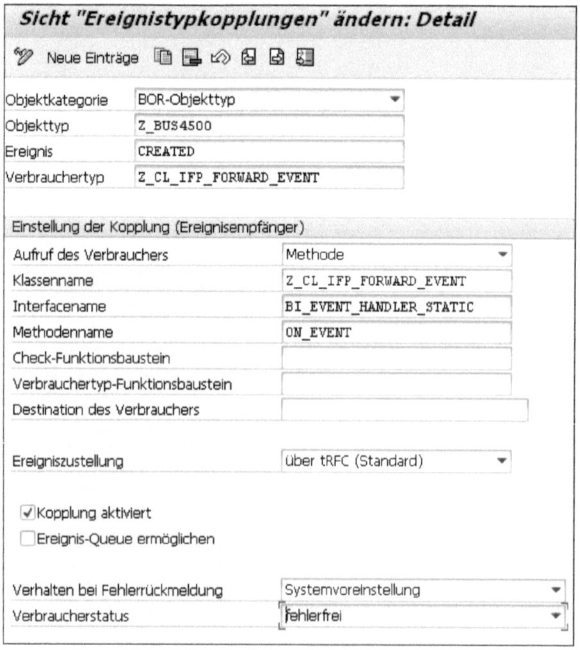

Abbildung 12.7 Ereignis an die »ON_EVENT«-Methode binden

Achten Sie darauf, dass Sie das Kennzeichen **Kopplung aktiviert** aktivieren, denn nur dann wird die Methode aufgerufen, wenn das Ereignis auftritt. Legen Sie für das CHANGED-Ereignis eine weitere Ereigniskopplung auf dieselbe Art und Weise an.

12.3.3 APC-Handler-Klasse festlegen

»on_start«-Methode

Nun müssen Sie nur noch die APC-Handler-Klasse so erweitern, dass sie die AMC-Nachrichten empfängt. Dazu implementieren Sie in der on_start-Methode den Code aus Listing 12.8.

```
METHOD if_apc_wsp_extension~on_start.
  TRY.
* WebSocket-Verbindung an AMC-Kanal binden
      DATA(lr_binding) = i_context->get_binding_manager( ).
      lr_binding->bind_amc_message_consumer(
        i_application_id = 'ZIFP_AMC'
        i_channel_id      = '/ping'
      ).
    CATCH cx_apc_error INTO DATA(lx_apc_error).
      DATA(lv_message) = lx_apc_error->get_text( ).
      MESSAGE lx_apc_error->get_text( ) TYPE 'E'.
  ENDTRY.
ENDMETHOD.
```

Listing 12.8 WebSocket-Verbindung an AMC-Kanal binden

Über den Importparameter i_context besorgt sich der Code über den Aufruf der Methode get_binding_manager einen Binding-Manager und verwendet diesen, um über den Aufruf der Methode bind_amc_message_consumer die Nachrichten des Kanals ZIFP_AMC/ping zu subskribieren.

Sobald nun eine AMC-Nachricht eintrifft, wird die on_message-Methode des APC-Handlers aufgerufen. Auch hier dürfen Sie nicht vergessen, die APC-Handler-Klasse beim AMC-Kanal als berechtigtes Programm zu registrieren, das Ereignisse über APC WebSocket empfangen kann.

Abbildung 12.8 zeigt die für den Kanal /ping der Anwendung ZIFP_AMC berechtigten Programme.

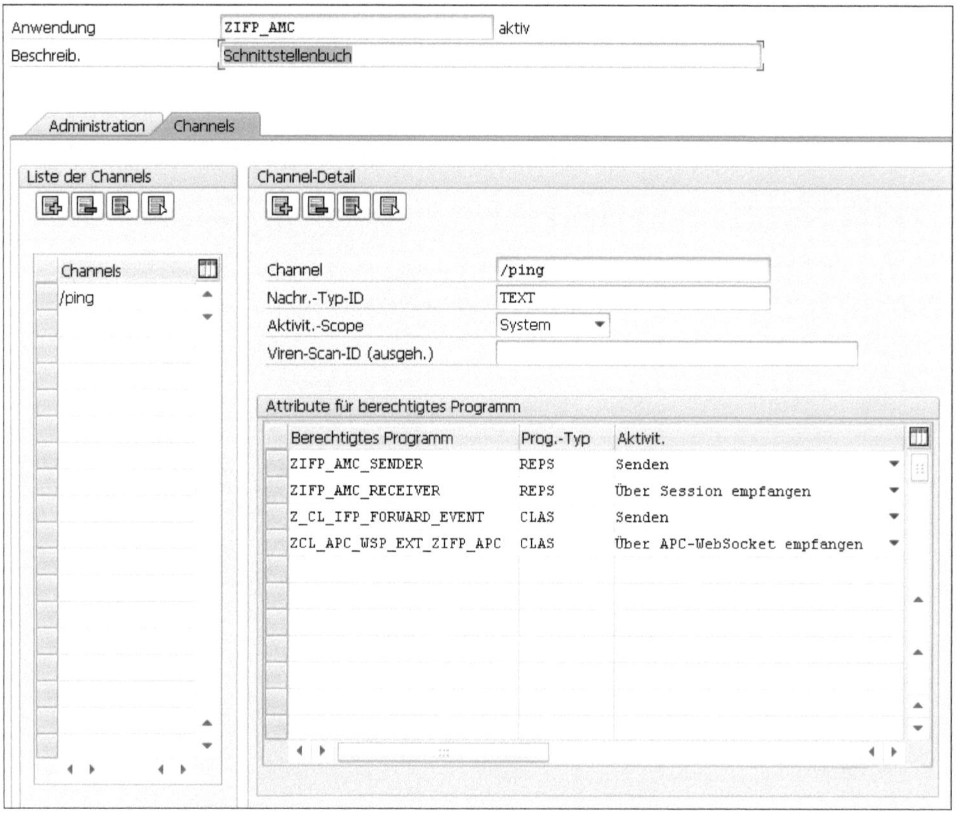

Abbildung 12.8 Berechtigte Programme registrieren

12.3.4 Szenario testen

Nun können Sie das gesamte Szenario testen. Starten Sie dazu zunächst Ihr BSP-Programm mit dem Java-WebSocket-Client aus Listing 12.2. Wie zuvor sollte der Browser nacheinander zwei Alert-Boxen anzeigen. Die erste Alert-Box informiert darüber, dass die WebSocket-Verbindung geöffnet wurde, und die zweite Alert-Box enthält das Echo der Nachricht, die beim Öffnen an den APC-Handler geschickt wurde.

Bestellung anlegen

Starten Sie nun den Report ZIFP_TEST_CREATE_BAPI und kopieren damit eine Bestellung vom Typ PO in eine Bestellung vom Typ SO. Damit wird eine neue Bestellung angelegt und das CREATE-Ereignis des Business-Objekts ausgelöst, das als AMC-Nachricht über den APC Handler bis zum Browser weitergeleitet wird, so wie dies Abbildung 12.9 zeigt.

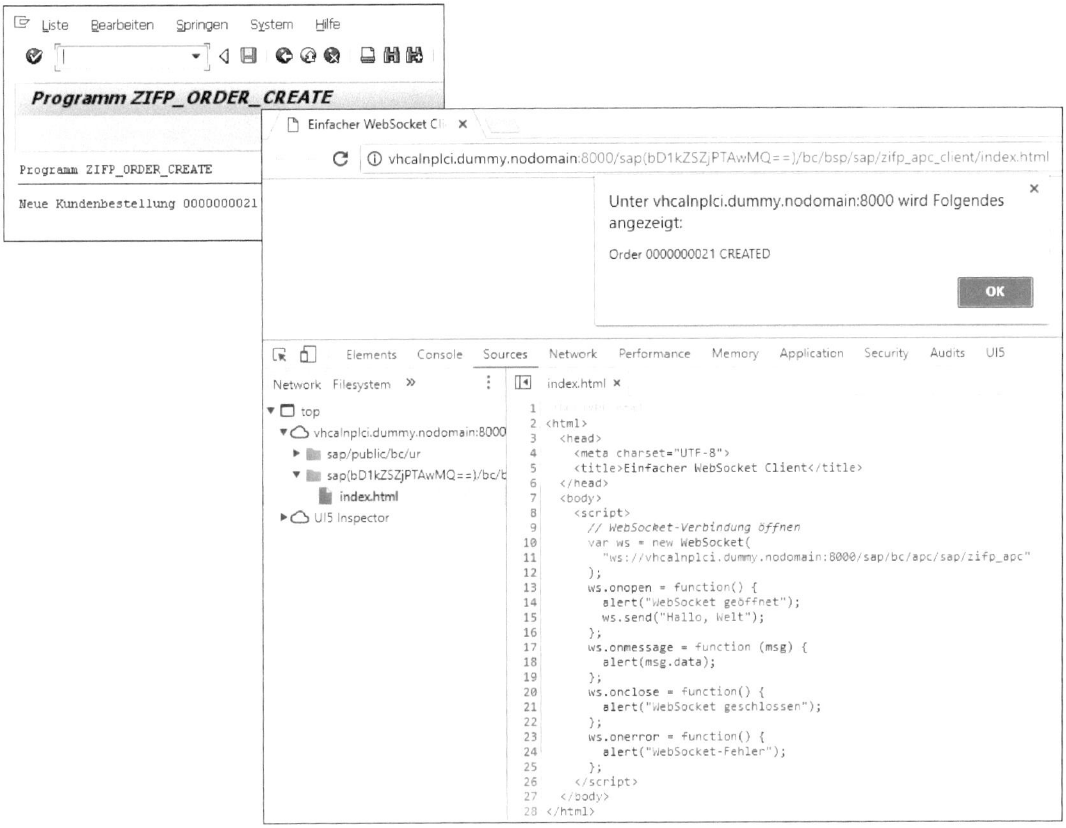

Abbildung 12.9 Weiterleitung eines BOR-Ereignisses an einen WebSocket-Client

12.4 ABAP-Plattform als Push-Channel-Client

Interfaces zur Registrierung als Event Handler

Die ABAP-Plattform kann sich über TCP oder über das WebSocket Protocol als Client mit einem TCP- oder WebSocket-Server verbinden. Um auf die entsprechenden Ereignisse reagieren zu können, muss ein ABAP-Programm eine Instanz einer Klasse bereitstellen, die eine der folgenden beiden Interfaces implementiert:

- IF_APC_WSP_EVENT_HANDLER
  für das TCP Socket und das WebSocket Protocol (ohne Unterprotokoll)
- IF_APC_WSP_EVENT_HANDLER_PCP
  für das WebSocket Protocol mit dem PCP-Unterprotokoll

Zur Instanziierung der eigentlichen Client-Objekte dienen die beiden folgenden Klassen:

- CL_APC_TCP_CLIENT_MANAGER
  für das TCP Socket Protocol mit der Methode create
- CL_APC_WSP_CLIENT_MANAGER
  für das WebSocket Protocol mit den beiden Methoden create_by_url und create_by_destination

Nach dem Senden einer APC-Nachricht können in der Client-Sitzung Nachrichten empfangen werden. Dazu muss die aktuelle Sitzung jedoch in einen Wartezustand gebracht werden, d. h., dass sie aus dem Dialogprozess herausgerollt worden sein muss. Dies kann entweder explizit durch die ABAP-Anweisung WAIT FOR PUSH CHANNELS oder implizit durch das Ende eines Dialogschritts geschehen.

12.4.1 Ein einfacher ABAP-Push-Channel-Client

ABAP-Report als APC-Client

Listing 12.9 zeigt einen einfachen APC-Client, der eine oder mehrere Nachrichten an den APC-Server aus Listing 12.1 schickt und die zurückgeschickten Nachrichten anschließend empfängt und ausgibt.

```
REPORT zifp_apc_client.

PARAMETERS:
  pa_nr   TYPE i DEFAULT 1,  " Anzahl der Nachrichten
  pa_wait TYPE i DEFAULT 20. " Wartezeit in Sekunden

DATA:
  gt_messages  TYPE TABLE OF string,
  gv_message   TYPE string,
  gv_nr        TYPE i,
  gr_apc_error TYPE REF TO cx_apc_error.

CLASS lcl_apc_handler DEFINITION FINAL.
  PUBLIC SECTION.
    INTERFACES if_apc_wsp_event_handler.
ENDCLASS.

CLASS lcl_apc_handler IMPLEMENTATION.
  METHOD if_apc_wsp_event_handler~on_open.
    APPEND 'Verbindung geöffnet!' TO gt_messages.
  ENDMETHOD.

  METHOD if_apc_wsp_event_handler~on_message.
* Nachricht in die globale interne Tabelle einfügen
```

```
    TRY.
        APPEND i_message->get_text( ) TO gt_messages.
        ADD 1 TO gv_nr.
      CATCH cx_apc_error INTO gr_apc_error.
        APPEND gr_apc_error->get_text( ) TO gt_messages.
    ENDTRY.
  ENDMETHOD.

  METHOD if_apc_wsp_event_handler~on_close.
    APPEND 'Verbindung geschlossen!' TO gt_messages.
  ENDMETHOD.

  METHOD if_apc_wsp_event_handler~on_error.
    APPEND 'Fehler!' TO gt_messages.
    LEAVE PROGRAM.
  ENDMETHOD.
ENDCLASS.

DATA:
  gr_apc_handler TYPE REF TO lcl_apc_handler,

  gr_apc_client  TYPE REF TO if_apc_wsp_client,
  gr_apc_request TYPE REF TO if_apc_wsp_client_initial_req,
  gr_apc_msg_mgr TYPE REF TO if_apc_wsp_message_manager,
  gr_apc_message TYPE REF TO if_apc_wsp_message.

START-OF-SELECTION.
  CREATE OBJECT gr_apc_handler.

* APC-Client initialisieren
  gr_apc_client = cl_apc_wsp_client_manager=>
    create_by_destination(
      i_destination   = 'NONE'
      i_event_handler = gr_apc_handler
      i_protocol      = if_apc_wsp_event_handler=>
                          co_event_handler_type
  ).
  gr_apc_request = gr_apc_client->get_context( )->
                     get_initial_request( ).
  gr_apc_request->set_path_and_query(
    i_relative_uri = '/sap/bc/apc/sap/zifp_apc'
  ).
```

12

```
* WebSocket-Verbindung öffnen
  gr_apc_client->connect( ).

* Nachrichten schicken
  gr_apc_msg_mgr ?= gr_apc_client->get_message_manager( ).
  gr_apc_message = gr_apc_msg_mgr->create_message( ).
  DO pa_nr TIMES.
    gr_apc_message->set_text( |Message { sy-index }| ).
    gr_apc_msg_mgr->send( gr_apc_message ).
  ENDDO.

* Nachrichten empfangen
  WAIT FOR PUSH CHANNELS UNTIL gv_nr GE pa_nr
                         UP TO pa_wait SECONDS.
  IF sy-subrc EQ 4.
    WRITE: / 'Kein Handler für APC-Nachrichten registriert!'.
  ELSEIF sy-subrc EQ 8.
    WRITE: / 'Timeout!'.
  ENDIF.
  gr_apc_client->close( ).

  LOOP AT gt_messages INTO gv_message.
    WRITE: / gv_message.
  ENDLOOP.
```

Listing 12.9 Einfacher APC-Client

APC-Handler-Klasse

Das Programm implementiert die lokale APC-Handler-Klasse lcl_apc_handler mit den Methoden on_open, on_message, on_close und on_error, die bei den entsprechenden APC-Ereignissen aufgerufen werden. In der on_message-Methode wird die empfangene Nachricht in die programmglobale Tabelle gt_messages geschrieben.

Client-Initialisierung

Zu Beginn des Hauptprogramms im Ereignisblock START-OF-SELECTION werden eine Instanz dieses Event Handlers sowie ein APC-Client angelegt. Bei der Instanziierung werden der Event Handler und eine Destination aus Transaktion SM59 mitgegeben. Diese Destination dient im Wesentlichen dazu, den Client zu authentifizieren. Anschließend wird der initiale Request des APC-Clients initialisiert. Dieser Request wird beim Öffnen der WebSocket-Verbindung abgesetzt.

Nach der Initialisierung öffnet der Client die WebSocket-Verbindung mit der Methode open. Erst wenn die Verbindung geöffnet ist, kann er einen Message-Manager erzeugen, der Nachrichten erzeugen und über diese Verbindung versenden kann. Anschließend werden in einer DO-Schleife so viele Nachrichten verschickt, wie vom Benutzer im Selektionsparameter pa_nr angegeben wurden.

Nachrichten empfangen

Danach wartet der Client aufgrund der Anweisung WAIT FOR PUSH CHANNELS so lange, bis alle Nachrichten vom Server eingetroffen sind oder die maximale Wartezeit von pa_wait Sekunden verstrichen ist.

Zum Schluss schließt der Client die WebSocket-Verbindung mit der Methode close und gibt die eingegangenen Nachrichten aus. Abbildung 12.10 zeigt die Ausgabe des APC-Clients, wenn drei Nachrichten versendet wurden.

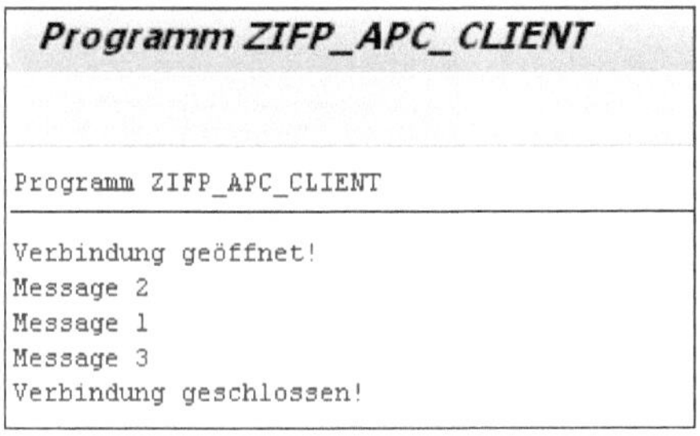

Abbildung 12.10 Ausgabe des APC-Clients

12.4.2 ABAP-Plattform als Detached-Push-Channel-Client

Detached und Attached Client

Ein *Detached-APC-Client* öffnet ebenso wie der im vorangehenden Abschnitt erstellte APC-Client eine Verbindung zu einem APC-Server, trennt diese jedoch sofort wieder (engl. *detach*). Danach kann sich der gleiche oder ein anderer AS ABAP als *Attached-APC-Client* an diese Verbindung anhängen (engl. *attach*). Der AS ABAP, der die Verbindung geöffnet hat, spielt nun als Detached Client die Rolle eines APC-Servers. Damit wird das Szenario unterstützt, dass ein AS ABAP, der als APC-Server arbeiten will, selbst eine APC-Verbindung als Client zu einem anderen Server aufbauen kann.

APC Handler

Auch ein Detached Client benötigt einen APC Handler, bei dem allerdings nur die on_open-Methode aufgerufen wird; daher müssen Sie nur diese Methode implementieren. In der on_open-Methode können Sie sich aus dem Kontextobjekt mit der Methode GET_CONNECTION_ATTACH_HANDLE ein Verbindungs-Handle für den Detached Client besorgen. Mit diesem Handle kann sich ein Attached Client anschließend mit dem Detached Client verbinden. Dabei muss eine Sicherheitsregel festgelegt werden, die definiert, ob entweder nur Sitzungen mit gleichem Mandanten und Benutzer zugelassen werden oder ob nur das aktuelle Programm im gleichen Mandanten als Attached Client agieren kann.

Detached Client instanziieren Zur Instanziierung der Detached-Client-Objekte verwenden Sie andere Klassen als vorher, nämlich die folgenden:

- CL_APC_TCP_CLIENT_CONN_MANAGER
  mit der Methode create für das TCP Socket Protocol
- CL_APC_WSP_CLIENT_CONN_MANAGER
  mit den Methoden create_by_url oder create_by_destination für das WebSocket Protocol

Nachdem Sie die Verbindung mit einem WebSocket-Server definiert haben, können Sie diese mit der Methode connect_and_detach öffnen und sofort wieder abhängen. Dabei wird die Methode on_open der Handler-Klasse ausgeführt, in der Sie sich über das Kontextobjekt ein Verbindungs-Handle für die Verbindung besorgen können.

Attached Client Um einen AS ABAP als Attached Client mit dem Detached Client zu verbinden, können Sie mit der Methode attach der Klassen CL_APC_WSP_CLIENT_CONN_MANAGER oder CL_APC_TCP_CLIENT_CONN_MANAGER Attached-Client-Objekte erzeugen. Dabei müssen Sie das Verbindungs-Handle übergeben. Listing 12.10 zeigt dafür ein Beispiel.

```
REPORT zifp_apc_detached_client.

PARAMETERS:
  pa_nr   TYPE i DEFAULT 1.  " Anzahl der Nachrichten

DATA:
  gr_apc_error TYPE REF TO cx_apc_error,
  gv_handle    TYPE string.

CLASS lcl_apc_handler DEFINITION FINAL.
  PUBLIC SECTION.
    INTERFACES if_apc_wsp_event_handler.
ENDCLASS.

CLASS lcl_apc_handler IMPLEMENTATION.
  METHOD if_apc_wsp_event_handler~on_open.
    TRY.
        gv_handle =
          i_context->get_connection_attach_handle(
            EXPORTING i_connection_security =
              i_context->co_con_security_by_user_id ).
      CATCH cx_apc_error INTO DATA(apc_error).
    ENDTRY.
```

```
  ENDMETHOD.

  METHOD if_apc_wsp_event_handler~on_message.
  ENDMETHOD.

  METHOD if_apc_wsp_event_handler~on_close.
  ENDMETHOD.

  METHOD if_apc_wsp_event_handler~on_error.
  ENDMETHOD.
ENDCLASS.

DATA:
  gr_apc_handler  TYPE REF TO lcl_apc_handler,
  gr_apc_client_d TYPE REF TO if_apc_wsp_client_conn_detach,

  gr_apc_request  TYPE REF TO if_apc_wsp_client_initial_req,
  gr_apc_msg_mgr  TYPE REF TO if_apc_wsp_message_manager,
  gr_apc_message  TYPE REF TO if_apc_wsp_message,
  gr_apc_client_a TYPE REF TO if_apc_wsp_client_conn_attach.

START-OF-SELECTION.
  CREATE OBJECT gr_apc_handler.

* APC-Client initialisieren
  gr_apc_client_d = cl_apc_wsp_client_conn_manager=>
    create_by_destination(
      i_destination    = 'NONE'
      i_application_id = 'ZIFP_APC'
      i_event_handler  = gr_apc_handler
      i_protocol       = if_apc_wsp_event_handler=>
                           co_event_handler_type
  ).
  gr_apc_request = gr_apc_client_d->get_context( )->
                     get_initial_request( ).
  gr_apc_request->set_path_and_query(
    i_relative_uri = '/sap/bc/apc/sap/zifp_apc'
  ).

* WebSocket-Verbindung öffnen und abhängen
  gr_apc_client_d->connect_and_detach( ).
```

12

```
* Attached Client anhängen
  gr_apc_client_a = cl_apc_wsp_client_conn_manager=>
    attach( gv_handle ).

* Nachrichten schicken
  gr_apc_msg_mgr ?= gr_apc_client_a->get_message_manager( ).
  gr_apc_message = gr_apc_msg_mgr->create_message( ).
  DO pa_nr TIMES.
    gr_apc_message->set_text( |Message { sy-index }| ).
    gr_apc_msg_mgr->send( gr_apc_message ).
  ENDDO.

  gr_apc_client_a->close( ).
```

Listing 12.10 Detached- und Attached-APC-Client

TEIL III

SAP-Schnittstellenprogrammierung in der Cloud

Kapitel 13
SAP Cloud Application Programming Model und OData

Die SAP BTP bietet Unternehmen viele Möglichkeiten. Um SAP-Systeme nicht mit kundenspezifischen Entwicklungen zu individualisieren, lässt sich beispielweise auf das SAP Cloud Application Programming Model zurückgreifen.

In Kapitel 2, »Grundlagen der Schnittstellenprogrammierung auf der SAP Business Technology Platform«, haben wir Sie in die SAP Business Technology Platform (SAP BTP) eingeführt. Dieses Kapitel wendet sich nun der Implementierung von Schnittstellen und Lösungen auf der SAP BTP zu. Hierfür bietet SAP mit dem *SAP Cloud Application Programming Model* (CAP) ein Programmiermodell für die Entwicklung von Cloud-Anwendungen z. B. mit JavaScript und Node.js oder Java an.

In diesem Kapitel führen wir in Abschnitt 13.1 in das Framework ein und geben einen kurzen Einblick dessen Aufgaben. In Abschnitt 13.2 zeigen wir, wie man damit einen OData-Service implementiert und über ein SAP-Fiori-Elements-Frontend den Anwendern bereitstellen kann. In Abschnitt 13.3 erfahren Sie, wie man eine CAP-Anwendung auf der SAP BTP deployt und wie man anschließend auf die Artefakte dieser Anwendung zugreifen kann.

13.1 Einführung in das SAP Cloud Application Programming Model

Erweiterungen von SAP S/4HANA Cloud Public Edition

Möchte ein Unternehmen, das SAP S/4HANA Cloud Public Edition einsetzt, die Standardlösung um eigene Geschäftslogik und Benutzeroberflächen erweitern, ist der traditionelle Ansatz, benutzerdefinierte Geschäftslogik direkt auf dem Anwendungsserver zu entwickeln und auszuführen, nicht mehr möglich. In der Vergangenheit wurden SAP-ERP-Lösungen beim Kunden erweitert, indem benutzerdefinierter Code zum ABAP-Anwendungsserver hinzugefügt wurde.

Key-User- und Side-by-Side-Erweiterbarkeit

Trotzdem gibt es auch für SAP S/4HANA Cloud Public Edition noch verschiedene Möglichkeiten, das Standardsystem anzupassen. Mit der *Key-User-Erweiterbarkeit* lassen sich etwa benutzerdefinierte Felder zu einer SAP-Fiori-Benutzeroberfläche (UI) hinzufügen. Damit lassen sich jedoch nur einfache Anpassungen umsetzen. Für komplexere Anforderungen, wie das Hinzufügen benutzerdefinierter Geschäftslogik, ist ein *Side-by-Side-Erweiterungsansatz* erforderlich. Hierbei kann CAP zum Einsatz kommen.

Wie bereits erwähnt, handelt es sich bei der SAP BTP um eine cloudbasierte Entwicklungsplattform, bei der die Geschäftsorientierung im Mittelpunkt steht. Die SAP BTP bietet eine zukunftssichere Cloud- (bzw. Cloud-native) Entwicklungsumgebung, die die Entwicklungserfahrung über SAP-Produkte hinweg harmonisiert. Drei Anwendungslaufzeiten, nämlich die SAP BTP ABAP Runtime, die SAP BTP Cloud Foundry Runtime und die SAP BTP Kyma Runtime, bieten sowohl ABAP- als auch Nicht-ABAP-Entwicklern eine Vielzahl von Möglichkeiten, Anwendungen zu entwickeln und auszuführen.

SAP Build

Für sogenannte *Citizen Developer*, d. h. Fachanwender mit nur geringen Programmierkenntnissen, bietet die SAP BTP außerdem eine Low-Code/No-Code-(LCNC-)Produktsuite, mit der sich Erweiterungen für den Unternehmenseinsatz auf einfach Art und Weise ohne oder mit nur wenig Programmierung erstellen lassen. Diese Suite heißt *SAP Build* und besteht aus drei tief integrierten Produkten:

- SAP Build Apps
- SAP Build Process Automation
- SAP Build Work Zone

Es ist erwähnenswert, dass beide Seiten des Spektrums, Pro-Code und Low-Code, miteinander kombiniert werden können, um Erweiterungen nach einem hybriden Ansatz zu erstellen, bei dem Pro-Code-Entwickler und Citizen Developer in sogenannten *Fusion Teams* zusammenarbeiten, um Erweiterungen zu erstellen.

Clean-Core-Prinzip

In der On-Premise-Variante von SAP S/4HANA und in SAP S/4HANA Cloud Private Edition ist es zwar immer noch möglich, die Standardlösung von SAP (den sogenannten *Core*) weiterzuentwickeln, aber es ist inzwischen bewährte Praxis, diesen Kern »sauber zu halten«. Man spricht in diesem Zusammenhang auch vom *Clean-Core-Prinzip* (siehe Abbildung 13.1). Um den Clean Core zu gewährleisten, verwendet man Application Programming Interfaces (APIs) dieser Kernsysteme und integriert sie in die eigenen Erweiterungsanwendungen. Auf der SAP BTP stehen Ihnen hierzu verschiedene

Entwicklungswerkzeuge, Services und Infrastrukturkomponenten zur Verfügung, um sichere, skalierbare und zuverlässige Cloud-native Anwendungen zu erstellen und zu betreiben. Sie haben Zugang zu Entwicklungswerkzeugen, Services und Infrastrukturkomponenten wie dem SAP Business Application Studio oder der SAP BTP, Kyma Runtime.

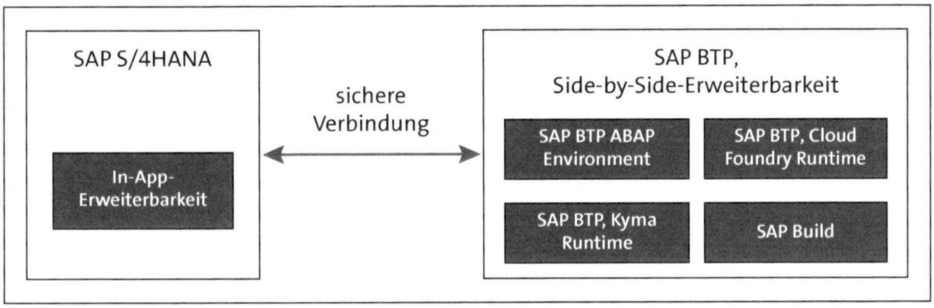

Abbildung 13.1 Side-by-Side-Erweiterbarkeit und Clean-Core-Ansatz

Verwendbare Sprachen und Laufzeitumgebungen

Mit den drei Laufzeiten der SAP BTP stehen unterschiedliche Erweiterungsmöglichkeiten zur Verfügung. Für ABAP-basierte Anwendungen ist das SAP BTP ABAP Environment die einzige Möglichkeit, Erweiterungen zu entwickeln und auszuführen. Hier kommt das im gleichnamigen Kapitel 11 vorgestellte ABAP RESTful Application Programmig Model zum Einsatz. Bei der Erstellung nicht-ABAP-basierter Erweiterungen können Sie verschiedene Technologie-Stacks und auch rein Cloud-native Entwicklungs- und Einsatzszenarien nutzen.

Programmiersprachen wie JavaScript, Java, TypeScript, Go, Python und viele andere können genutzt werden, um benutzerdefinierte Erweiterungen für Unternehmen auf der SAP BTP zu erstellen. Diese Anwendungen können entweder lokal in der Entwicklungsumgebung Ihrer Wahl oder im SAP Business Application Studio auf der SAP BTP entwickelt werden. Die Bereitstellung kann entweder auf der SAP BTP Cloud Foundry Runtime oder der SAP BTP, Kyma Runtime erfolgen.

13.1.1 Das SAP Cloud Application Programming Model im Überblick

CAP ist nicht nur ein weiteres Werkzeug in Ihrem Entwicklungsarsenal, sondern ein umfassendes Framework, das die meisten Probleme, die traditionell mit der Entwicklung von Unternehmensanwendungen verbunden sind, beseitigt. Es umfasst eine Vielzahl von Sprachen, Bibliotheken und Tools für die Erstellung von Diensten und Anwendungen auf Unternehmensniveau. Es führt Entwickler mit bewährten Best Practices und einer

Fülle von sofort einsetzbaren Lösungen durch wiederkehrende Aufgaben der Anwendungsentwicklung.

Komponenten

Wenn Sie in die Welt von CAP eintauchen, werden Sie auf die folgenden Schlüsselkomponenten stoßen, die die Architektur zusammenhalten. Abbildung 13.2 zeigt deren Zusammenspiel:

- **Core Data Services (CDS)**
  CDS ist die Datenmodellierungsinfrastruktur, die auch als Rückgrat des Programmiermodells bezeichnet wird und Ihnen die Mittel zur Erfassung von Servicedefinitionen und Datenmodellen an die Hand gibt. Für Servicedefinitionen und Datenmodelle wird die *Control Definition Language* (CDL) verwendet. Eine ausführliche Dokumentation dieses Sprachumfangs finden Sie in der »Language Reference Documentation« in der offiziellen Dokumentation des Programmiermodells (siehe Abschnitt 13.1.2, »Dokumentation und Informationsquellen«).
- **Service-SDKs**
  CAP stellt Bibliotheken für Java und Node.js zur Verfügung, mit denen Sie Services über synchrone und asynchrone APIs bereitstellen und nutzen können. Die Software Development Kits (SDKs), zu denen diese Bibliotheken gehören, beinhalten auch eine sofort einsatzbereite Integration mit untergeordneten Plattformdiensten, wie z. B. der Authentifizierung und der Bereitstellung von Benutzern beim oder On- und Off-Boarding von Cloud-Nutzern.
- **Entwicklungstools**
  Das SAP Business Application Studio haben Sie bereits in Abschnitt 9.4, »OData-Services mit SAPUI5 konsumieren«, kennengelernt. Es stellt alle erforderlichen Tools für die CAP-Entwicklung bereit und ist entsprechend vorkonfiguriert. Darüber hinaus wird auch die lokale Entwicklung in Visual Studio Code oder Java-spezifischen IDEs von CAP unterstützt.
- **Datenbanken**
  Für die Persistenzschicht Ihrer CAP-Anwendung können Sie zwischen mehreren verfügbaren Datenbankoptionen wählen. *SAP HANA Cloud* ist dabei die erste Wahl. Aber auch andere Technologien wie PostgreSQL oder SQLite (für die lokale Entwicklung) sind möglich.
- **Frontend-Technologien**
  Als Fullstack-Framework ist CAP offen für eine Vielzahl von Frontend-Technologien. SAP Fiori wird vollständig unterstützt, aber auch andere UI-Frameworks wie Vue.js, Angular oder React können auf Ihren Service aufgesetzt werden.

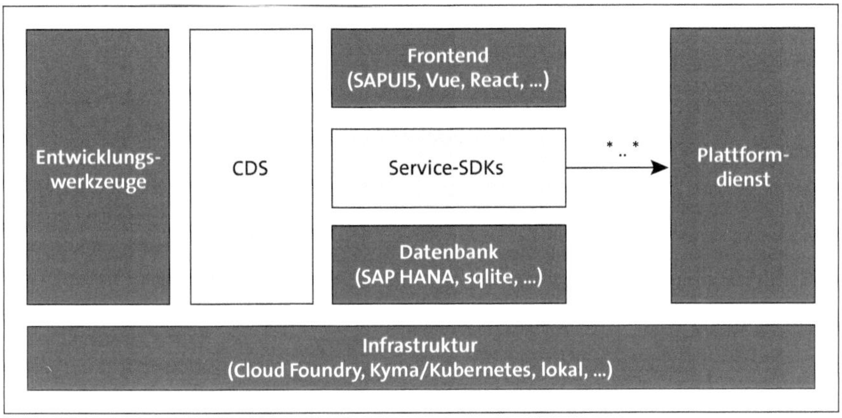

Abbildung 13.2 Komponenten des SAP Cloud Application Programming Models

13.1.2 Dokumentation und Informationsquellen

Offizielle Dokumentation

13

In diesem Abschnitt möchten wir Sie mit einigen wichtigen Informationsquellen vertraut machen, mit denen Sie den Einstieg in CAP finden oder fortgeschrittene Szenarien erkunden können. An erster Stelle steht die offizielle CAP-Dokumentation namens *CAPire*. Sie finden sie unter der Website *https://cap.cloud.sap/docs/*. Abbildung 13.3 zeigt die Einstiegsseite dieser Dokumentation.

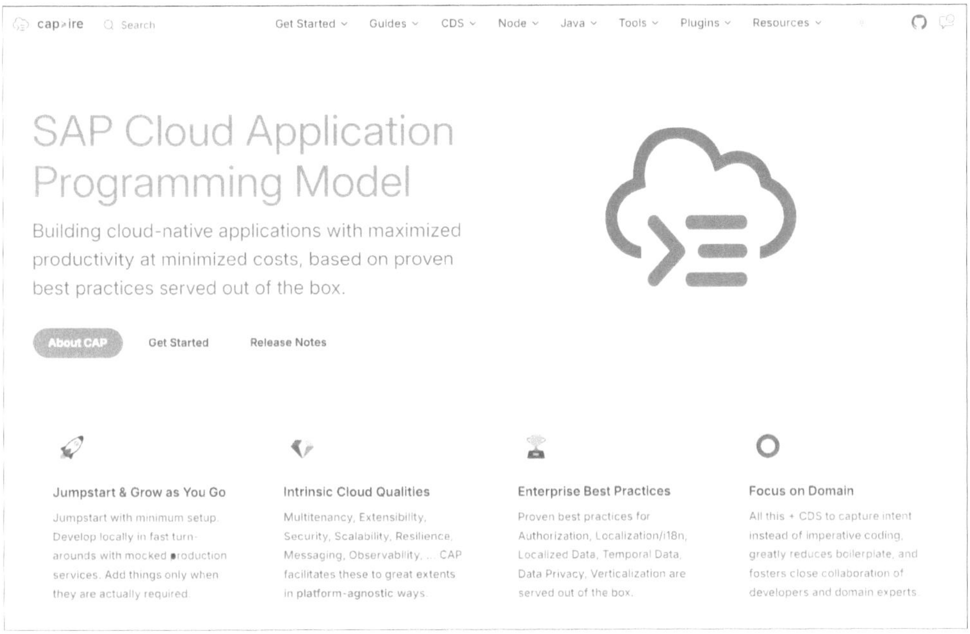

Abbildung 13.3 Einstiegsseite der CAP-Dokumentation

Eine sehr gute Einführung in das Programmiermodell erhält man über den Menüpfad **Get Started • Introduction – What is CAP?** Hier finden Sie unter anderem einen Schnelleinstieg. Darüber hinaus werden alle Aspekte von CAP, sowohl für Node.js als auch für Java, in der Dokumentation beschrieben.

Beispielprojekte auf GitHub

Zahlreiche Beispielprojekte für Anfänger und Fortgeschrittene sind darüber hinaus auf GitHub verfügbar unter *https://github.com/SAP-samples/cloud-cap-samples*. Abbildung 13.4 zeigt den Einstieg in diese Beispiele.

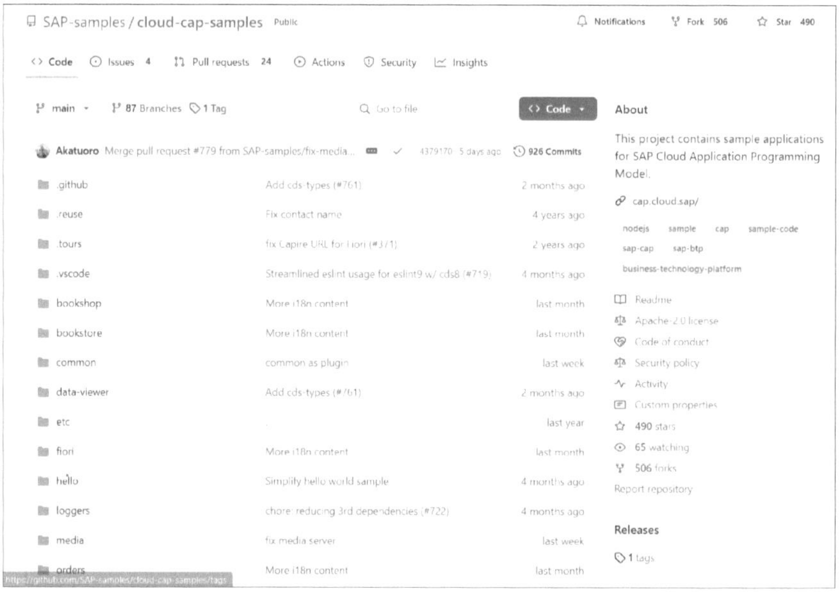

Abbildung 13.4 Codebeispiele zum SAP Cloud Application Programming Model auf GitHub

Bücher

Ausführliche Informationen erhalten Sie in den Büchern »Fullstack-Entwicklung mit SAP« von Rene Glavanovits, Martin Koch, Daniel Krancz und Maximilian Olzinger (SAP PRESS 2025) und »Anwendungsentwicklung auf der SAP Cloud Platform« von Klaus Kopecz (SAP PRESS 2020).

13.2 Eine CAP-Anwendung mit OData-Service entwickeln

Nachdem wir im vorangegangenen Abschnitt in die Grundlagen von CAP eingeführt haben, wendet sich dieser Abschnitt nun dem Aufsetzen der Entwicklungsinfrastruktur und der Entwicklung eines OData-Service unter Verwendung von CAP. Schließlich zeigen wir noch, wie man mit SAP Fiori

Elements eine einfach Anwendungsoberfläche implementieren kann. Der hier implementierte OData-Service kann über die SAP BTP bereitgestellt und entsprechend konsumiert werden. Wir verwenden dazu das SAP Business Application Studio.

13.2.1 Entwicklung im SAP Business Application Studio

SAP Business Application Studio starten

Nachdem wir die nötigen Berechtigungen vergeben haben, wie in Abschnitt 2.3, »Sicherheit«, beschrieben, können Sie das SAP Business Application Studio starten. Hierzu navigieren Sie im SAP BTP Cockpit über **Services • Instances and Subscriptions** zur Übersicht der aktivierten Subskriptionen. Klicken Sie in der Tabelle beim Eintrag **SAP Business Application Studio** auf das Icon (**Go to Application**). Das SAP Business Application Studio wird daraufhin gestartet. Nach dem Start zeigt sich das Bild aus Abbildung 13.5. Diese Seite wird nur beim ersten Start des SAP Business Application Studios angezeigt bzw. solange man noch keinen Dev Space angelegt hat.

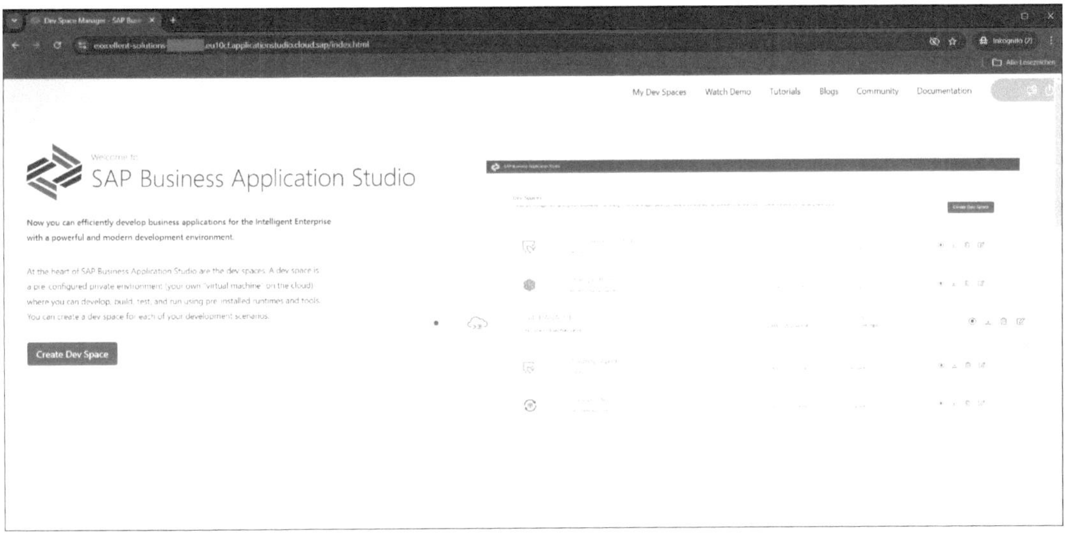

Abbildung 13.5 Initialer Einstiegsbildschirm des SAP Business Application Studios

Dev Space anlegen

Dev Space

Wie Sie es in Abschnitt 9.4.2, »Implementierung eines OData-Clients mit SAPUI5«, bereits im Rahmen der SAPUI5-Entwicklung kennengelernt haben, erfolgt die Entwicklung von Anwendungen und Diensten mit dem SAP Business Application Studio in Dev Spaces. Abhängig vom ausgewählten Dev-Space-Typ wird die Umgebung mit passenden Funktionen und Ansichten vorkonfiguriert.

Um einen Dev Space für die CAP-Entwicklung anzulegen, klicken Sie auf den Button **Create Dev Space** (links in Abbildung 13.5). Es öffnet sich das Bild aus Abbildung 13.6. Geben Sie für unser Beispiel in das Feld **Dev Space name** den Wert »Interfacebook« ein und wählen Sie den für die Entwicklung von CAP-Anwendungen bereitgestellten Dev-Space-Typ **Full Stack Cloud Application** aus.

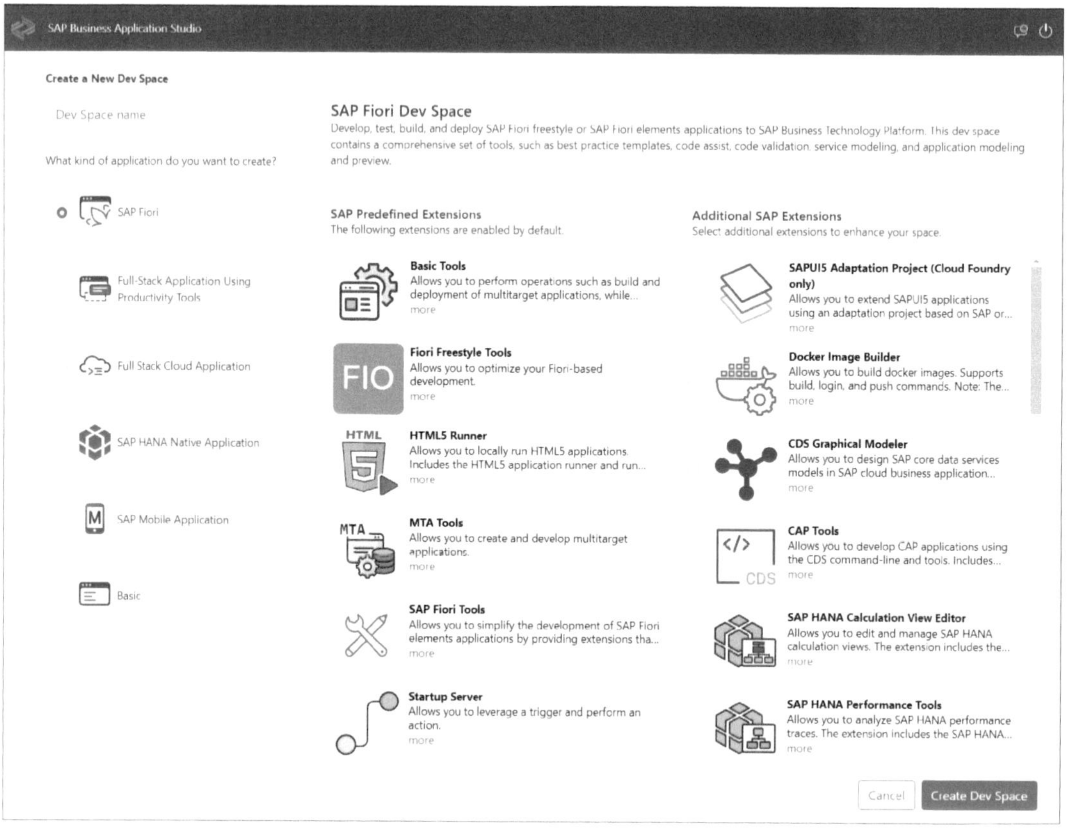

Abbildung 13.6 Anlegen eines Dev Space

Erweiterungen für das SAP Business Application Studio

Wie Sie in Abbildung 13.7 nachvollziehen können, werden einem bei Auswahl dieses Dev-Space-Typs diverse Erweiterungen standardmäßig in seiner Umgebung zur Verfügung gestellt. Insbesondere die Erweiterung **CAP Tools** ist hier für uns relevant. Klicken Sie auch hier noch einmal auf **Create Dev Space**.

Die Ansicht wechselt zu dem in Abbildung 13.8 gezeigten Bild. Der von uns gerade angelegte Dev Space befindet sich im Status **STARTING**. In diesem Status können Sie den Dev Space über die entsprechenden Icons starten und löschen.

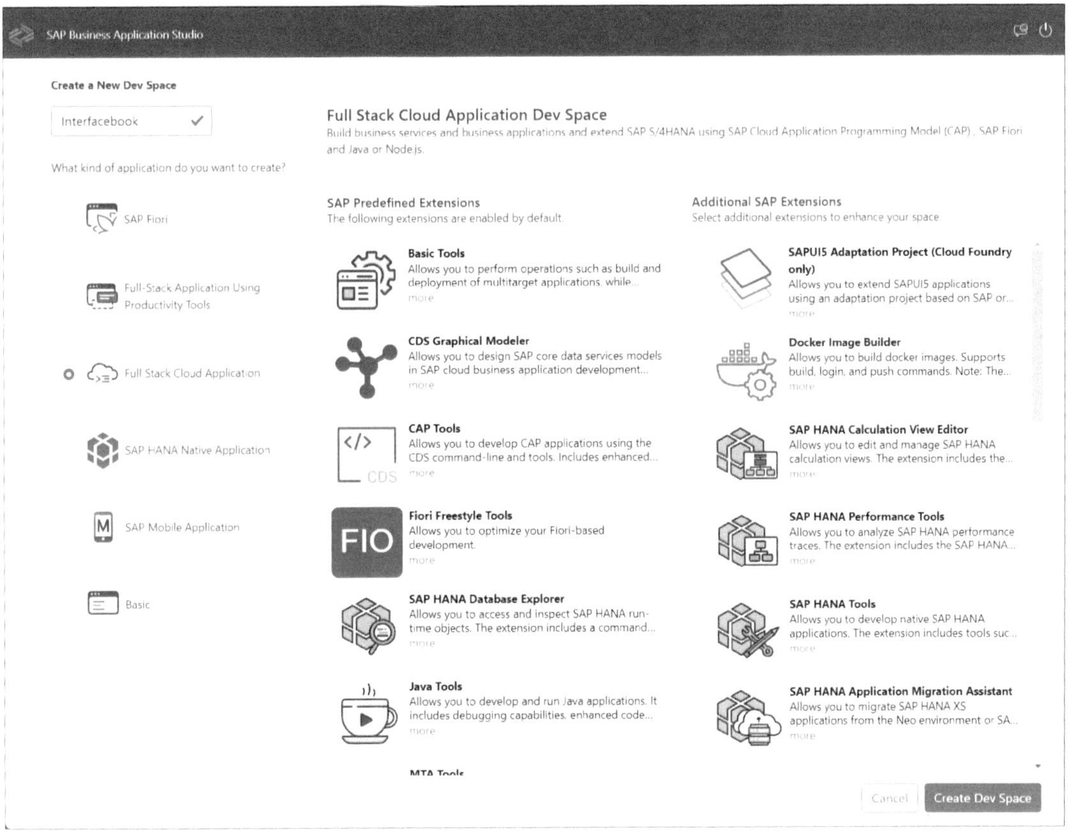

Abbildung 13.7 Anlegen eines Full Stack Cloud Application Dev Space

13

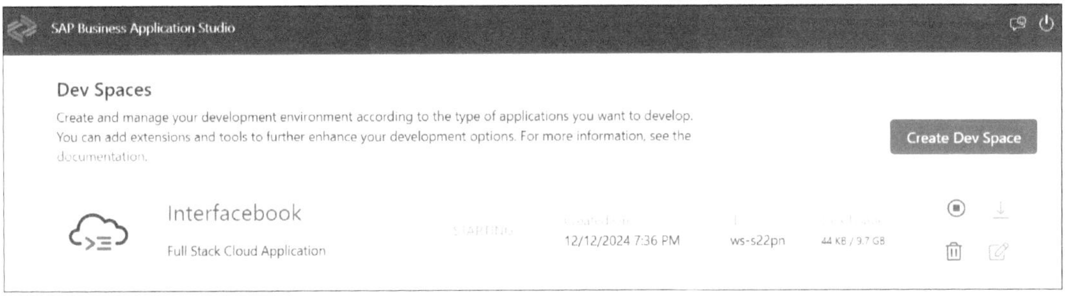

Abbildung 13.8 Im Start befindlicher Dev Space

Ist der Dev Space verfügbar, wechselt der Status von **STARTING** auf **RUNNING**, und der Dev-Space-Bezeichner wird als anklickbarer Link dargestellt. Ebenfalls ist es nun möglich, den Inhalt des Dev Space über den Button [↓] (**Download Dev Space Content**) in gepackter Form auf Ihre lokale Festplatte zu laden.

Einstiegsbild des Dev Space

Klicken Sie auf den Namen des Dev Space, können Sie einige Einstellungen zur Privatsphäre vornehmen. Anschließend gelangen Sie zu dem Bild aus Abbildung 13.9.

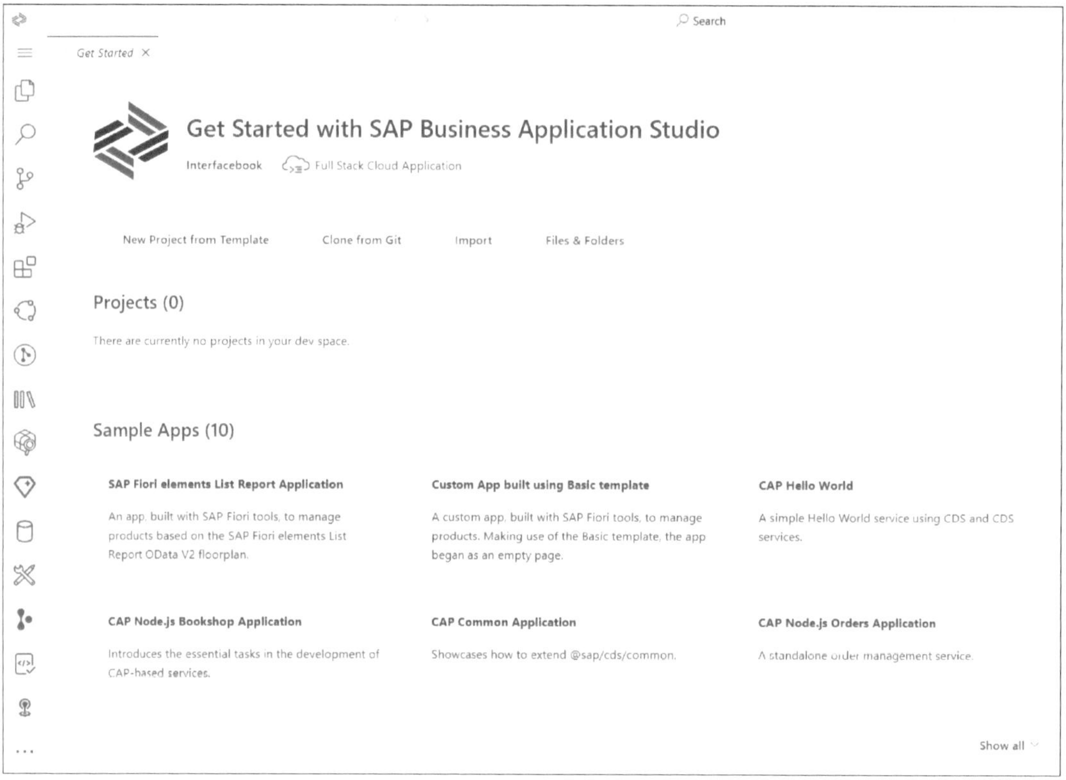

Abbildung 13.9 Einstiegsbild des neuen Dev Space

Projekt anlegen

Klicken Sie hier auf **New Project from Template**. Sie erhalten die in Abbildung 13.10 gezeigte Auswahl an Projektvorlagen.

CAP-Projekt

Als Nächstes wählen Sie die Projektvorlage **CAP Project** aus und bestätigen dies mit einem Klick auf **Start**. Im folgenden Schritt geben Sie die Projektdetails ein und bestätigen Ihre Eingaben mit einem Klick auf **Finish** (siehe Abbildung 13.11).

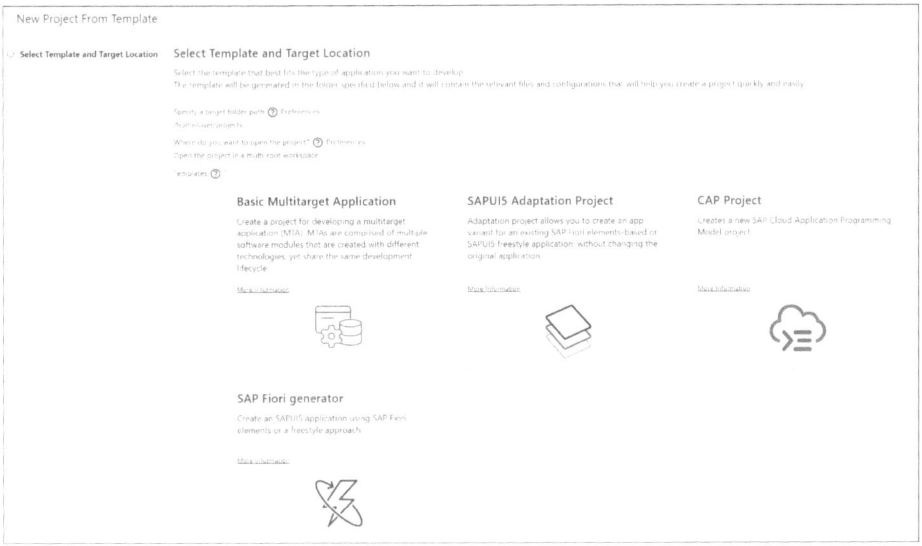

Abbildung 13.10 Übersicht der zur Verfügung stehenden Projektvorlagen

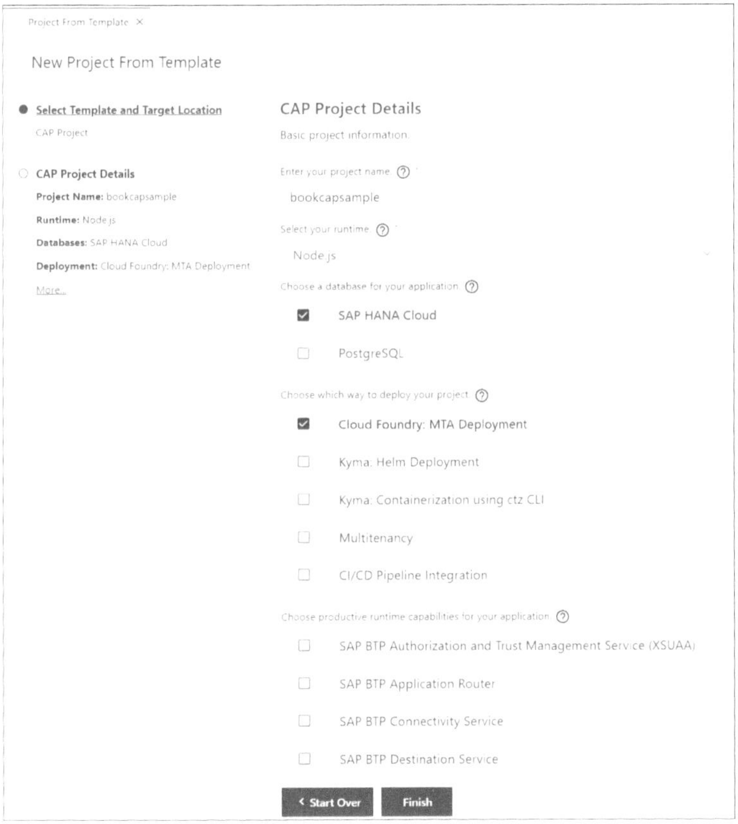

Abbildung 13.11 Konfiguration der Projektdetails

Nachdem das Projekt angelegt ist, wird Ihnen die initiale Projektansicht wie in Abbildung 13.12 dargestellt.

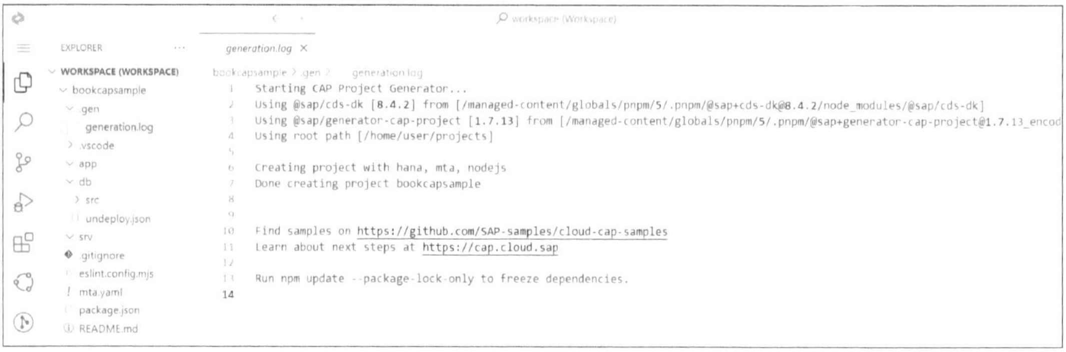

Abbildung 13.12 Generiertes CAP-Projekt im SAP Business Application Studio

Datenmodell implementieren

Datei »schema.cds«

Zu Beginn der Implementierung steht das Definieren des Datenmodells der Anwendung. Das Datenmodell einer CAP-Anwendung wird innerhalb einer Datei namens **schema.cds** angelegt. Hierzu wählen Sie hier den Ordner **db • src** aus und rufen im Kontextmenü **New File** auf. Es wird ein editierbarer Bereich angezeigt, in den Sie einen Dateinamen vergeben können. Hier geben Sie den Wert »schema.cds« ein. Abbildung 13.13 zeigt die neu angelegte Datei in der Projektstruktur. Kopieren Sie den CDS-Code aus Listing 13.1 in diese Datei. Darin werden die Entitäten für die CAP-Anwendung angelegt.

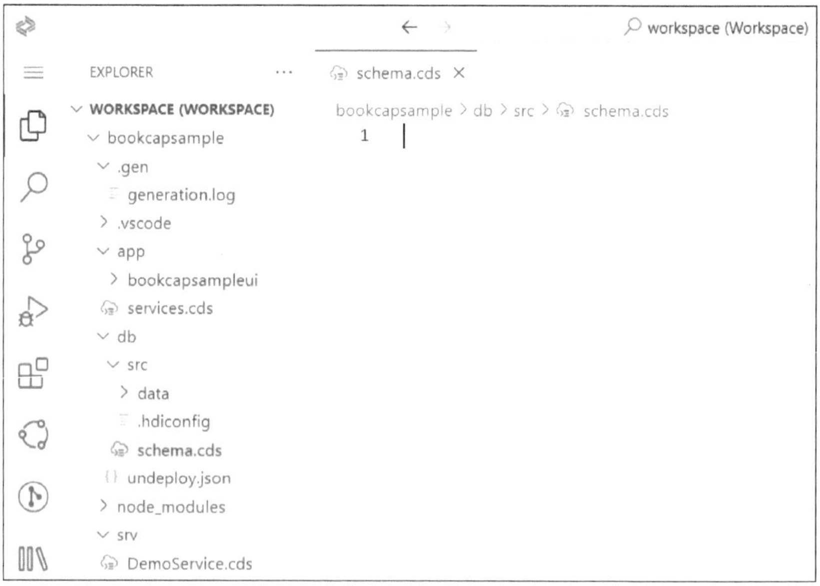

Abbildung 13.13 Neu angelegte »schema.cds«-Datei

```
namespace bookcapsample;

entity Order {
    key orderToDevice : Association to Device;
    key orderToCustomer : Association to Customer;
    amount : Integer;
    orderDate : Date;
}

entity Customer {
    key customerID : Integer;
    firstname : String;
    lastname : String;
    eMail : String;
    optionals : {
        birthday : Date default null;
        gender : String enum {
            male = 'm';
            female = 'f';
            divers = 'd';
        } default null;
    };

    customerToOrders : Association to many Order on
        customerToOrders.orderToCustomer = $self;
}

entity Device {
    key deviceID : UUID;
    name : String;
    price : Decimal (10,2);
    stock : Integer;
    deviceToOrders : Association to many Order on
        deviceToOrders.orderToDevice = $self;
}
```

Listing 13.1 Implementierung der Entitäten in der Datei »schema.cds«

CSV-Dateien für Beispieldaten anlegen

CAP bietet die Möglichkeit an, bereits zur Laufzeit des OData-Service Daten aus CSV-Dateien zu importieren und zu Testzwecken in einem OData-Service zur Verfügung zu stellen. Solche CSV-Dateien lassen sich über ein Befehlsterminal anlegen. Öffnen Sie dazu ein Terminalfenster, indem Sie den Ordner **src** in unserer Projektstruktur auswählen und im Kontextmenü den

Eintrag **Open in Integrated Terminal** wählen. Geben anschließend den Befehl `cds add data` in das Terminalfenster ein (siehe Abbildung 13.14).

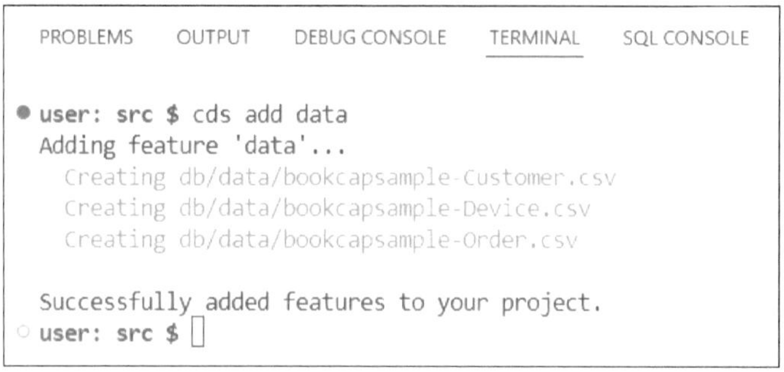

Abbildung 13.14 Generieren einer CSV-Datei mit dem Befehl »cds add data«

Nachdem dieser Befehl ausgeführt wurde, stehen uns entsprechende CSV-Dateien zur Verfügung. Abbildung 13.15 zeigt eine solche CSV-Datei für die Entität `Order`. Sie enthält lediglich die Felder dieser Entität.

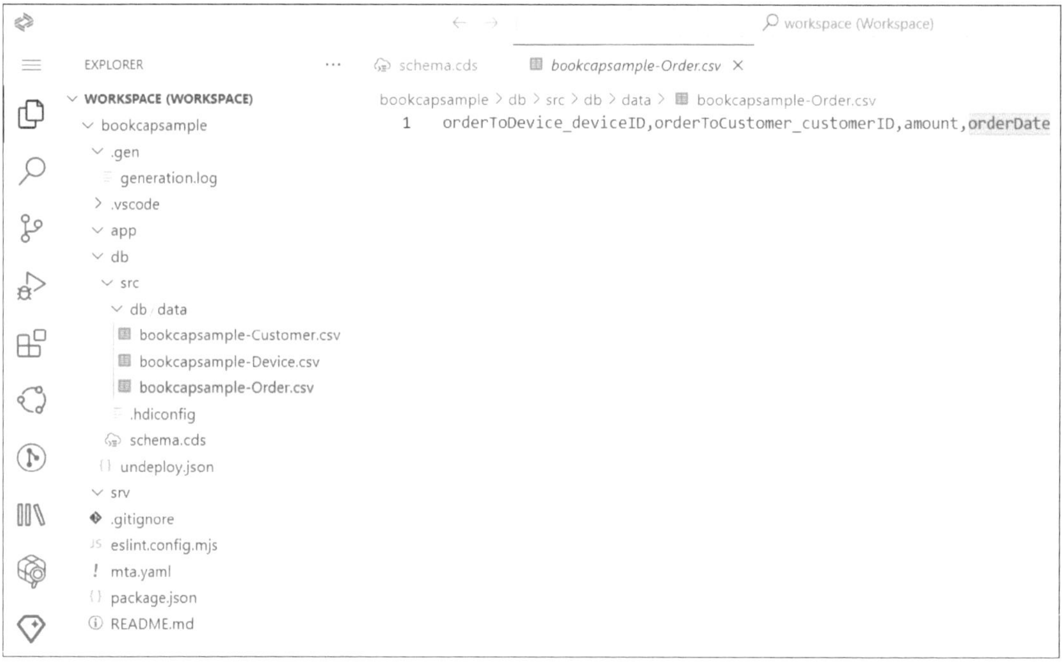

Abbildung 13.15 Generierte CSV-Datei für die Entität »Order«

CSV-Dateien mit Daten befüllen

Die generierten CSV-Dateien können Sie nun mit Testdaten befüllen. Listing 13.2, Listing 13.3 und Listing 13.4 zeigen beispielhafte Testdaten für die jeweiligen CSV-Dateien.

```
orderToDevice_deviceID,orderToCustomer_customerID,amount,orderDate
10d63677-8507-4b24-b595-f2a5fef1458d,10000001,1,2022-01-09
10d63677-8507-4b24-b595-f2a5fef1458d,10000002,1,2022-01-09
ab4fcc95-77b5-4400-8ad3-f7a621bd21bb,10000003,1,2022-01-08
ab4fcc95-77b5-4400-8ad3-f7a621bd21bb,10000002,1,2021-10-13
ab4fcc95-77b5-4400-8ad3-f7a621bd21bb,10000004,1,2021-11-05
92f3f98b-40ca-4e76-b07d-b725fdabdac0,10000005,2,2021-12-16
481c60ba-b8d0-4b2a-8a87-c5cb8a3c7521,10000002,1,2021-12-05
f6196e21-255b-4121-8a4d-8e820fadae64,10000001,1,2021-11-24
f6196e21-255b-4121-8a4d-8e820fadae64,10000004,1,2021-10-03
92f3f98b-40ca-4e76-b07d-b725fdabdac0,10000006,1,2021-11-09
```

Listing 13.2 Inhalt der Datei »Order.csv«

```
deviceID,name,price,stock
10d63677-8507-4b24-b595-f2a5fef1458d,Tintenstrahldrucker Deutsche
Röhren AG,79.99,3
ab4fcc95-77b5-4400-8ad3-f7a621bd21bb,Kühlschrank Deutsche Röhren
AG,569.90,20
92f3f98b-40ca-4e76-b07d-b725fdabdac0,Mikrowellenherd Deutsche Röhren
AG,432.89,10
65672979-d024-4e4c-84b5-cf5db923cc15,Passiermaschine Pahlgruber &
Söhne,229.25,35
3556e62a-0c1e-4c28-88f0-269e835ab0c4,Abfüllmaschine Pahlgruber &
Söhne,329.00,5
481c60ba-b8d0-4b2a-8a87-c5cb8a3c7521,Verkorker Pahlgruber &
Söhne,55.45,17
f6196e21-255b-4121-8a4d-8e820fadae64,Saugblaser ASDF Chemie
AG,39.99,12
```

13

Listing 13.3 Inhalt der Datei »Device.csv«

```
customerID,firstname,lastname,eMail,optionals_birthday,optionals_
gender
10000001,John,Doe,john.doe@gmail.com,1990-05-06,male
10000002,Hans,Lukov,hansLukov34@hotmail.de,1995-02-14,male
10000003,Hannah,Klop,hannahklop@gmail.com,1995-05-14,female
10000004,Svenja,Mueller,Svenja7Mueller@web.de,2002-09-14,female
10000005,Erwin,Winter,erwinWinter@web.de,1977-05-14,male
10000006,Hans,Hauber,Hans.hauber@gmx.de,1995-05-17,male
```

Listing 13.4 Inhalt der Datei »Customer.csv«

UUID-Schlüsselfeld erzeugen

Die Entität `Device` für die mit unserer Anwendung zu bestellenden Geräte verfügt über ein Schlüsselfeld vom Typ Universally Unique Identifier (UUID). Dieser Datentyp kann verwendet werden, um Eigenschaften einer Entität als Schlüsselfeld zu deklarieren. Für die Erzeugung von eindeutigen Schlüsseln dieser Art bietet CAP ebenfalls Unterstützung. Ein entsprechendes Werkzeug kann über das Befehlsterminal mit dem Befehl `cds repl` aufgerufen werden. Im Anschluss kann man den Befehl `cds.utils.uuid()` aufrufen und erhält, wie in Abbildung 13.16 gezeigt, einen Schlüssel, der dem UUID-Format entspricht. Die so generierten Schlüssel können dann in den CSV-Dateien verwendet werden.

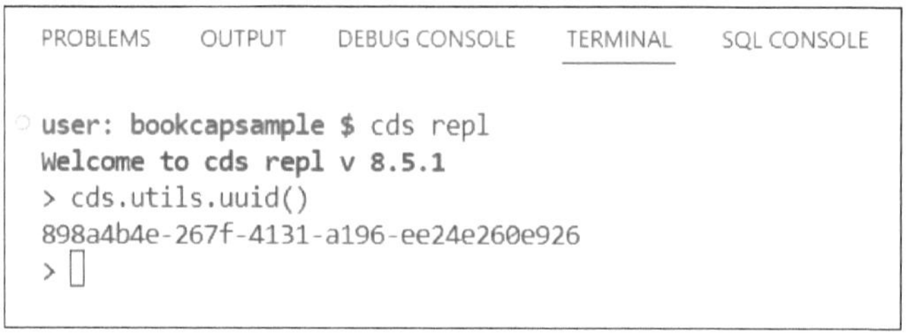

Abbildung 13.16 Generieren eines eindeutigen Schlüssels

13.2.2 Implementierung eines OData-Service

Nachdem wir im vorangehenden Abschnitt das Datenmodell (auch *Domänenmodell* genannt) sowie die Testdaten implementiert und angelegt haben, wenden wir uns in diesem Abschnitt dem Implementieren des OData-Service zu.

Servicedefinition anlegen

Dazu ist es zunächst notwendig, eine Servicedefinition anzulegen. Diese wird in einer Datei im Ordner **srv** unseres Projekts angelegt. Wählen Sie daher den entsprechenden Ordner aus und rufen Sie im Kontextmenü den Eintrag **New File...** auf. Unterhalb des Verzeichnisses **srv** wird daraufhin ein Bereich zur Eingabe eines Dateinamens eingeblendet. Geben Sie hier den Wert »DemoService.cds« ein und drücken Sie die [↵]-Taste. Abbildung 13.17 zeigt die im Moment noch leere Datei zur Servicedefinition.

Füllen Sie diese mit dem CDS-Code aus Listing 13.5. In der ersten Zeile wird angegeben, wie der Service die zu nutzenden Entitäten in der Datei **Schema.cds** findet. Im Anschluss erfolgt die Servicedefinition. Der OData-Service hat den Namen `BookSampleService` und stellt die entsprechenden Entitäten zur Verfügung.

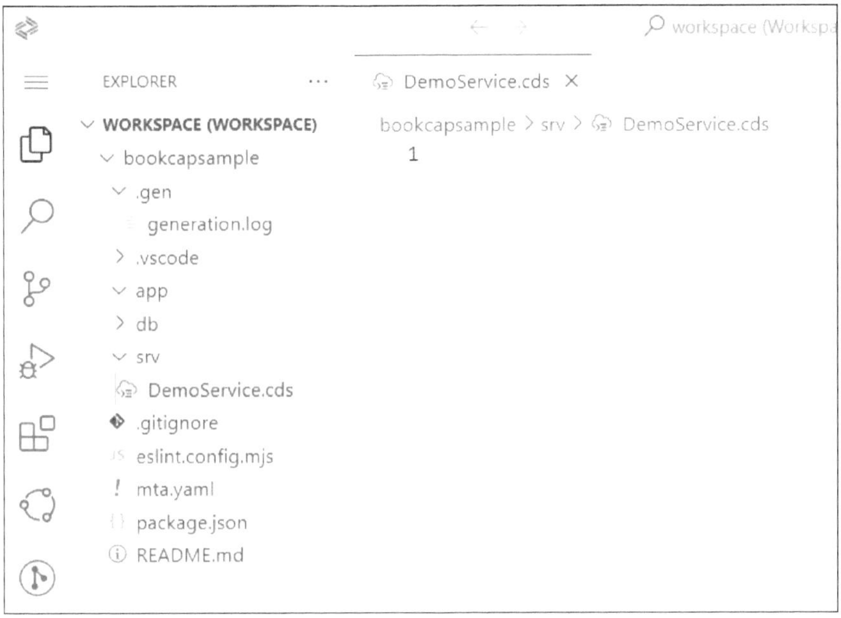

Abbildung 13.17 Die leere Datei zur Servicedefinition

```
using { bookcapsample as demo } from '../db/src/schema';
service BookSampleService {
    @cds.redirection.target
    entity Devices as projection on demo.Device;
    entity Orders as projection on demo.Order;
    entity Customers as projection on demo.Customer;
}
```

Listing 13.5 Servicedefinition für den OData-Service »BookSampleService«

OData-Service testen

Im Anschluss können wir den OData-Service direkt testen. Hierzu wählen Sie den Projektordner **bookcapsample** in der Projektstruktur aus und rufen im Kontextmenü den Eintrag **Open in Integrated Terminal** auf. Das Eingabeterminal öffnet sich. Hier geben Sie den Befehl `cds watch` ein (siehe Abbildung 13.18).

Service-Endpunkte

Mit einem Klick auf **Open in a New Tab** rufen Sie die in Abbildung 13.19 gezeigte Testseite auf. Hier erhalten Sie einen Überblick über die Service-Endpunkte unseres OData-Service. Wie beabsichtigt werden uns hier die drei Entitäten `Devices`, `Orders` und `Customers` angeboten.

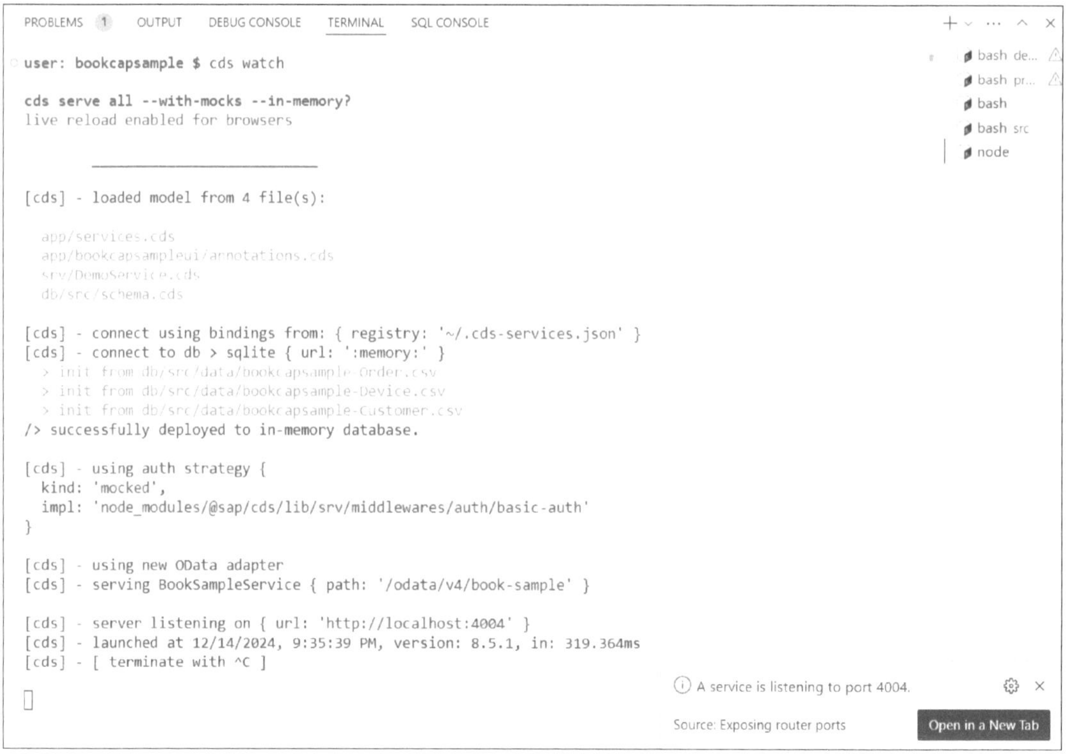

Abbildung 13.18 Terminalausgabe des Startskripts

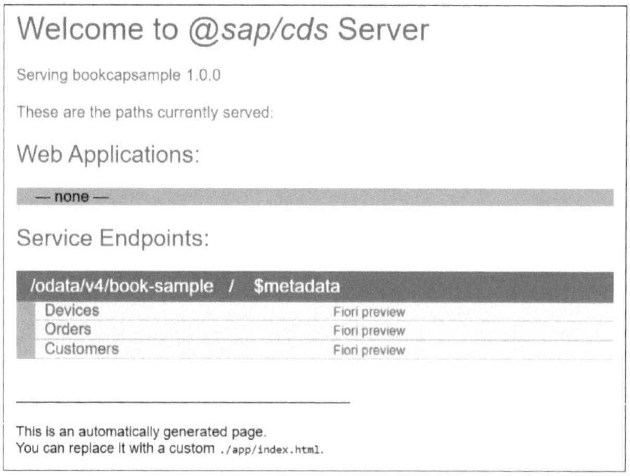

Abbildung 13.19 Testseite mit den drei implementierten Entitäten

Klicken Sie für einen Test auf den Link **Customers**. Daraufhin werden Ihnen die in der Datei **Customers.csv** hinterlegten Daten angezeigt (siehe Abbildung 13.20).

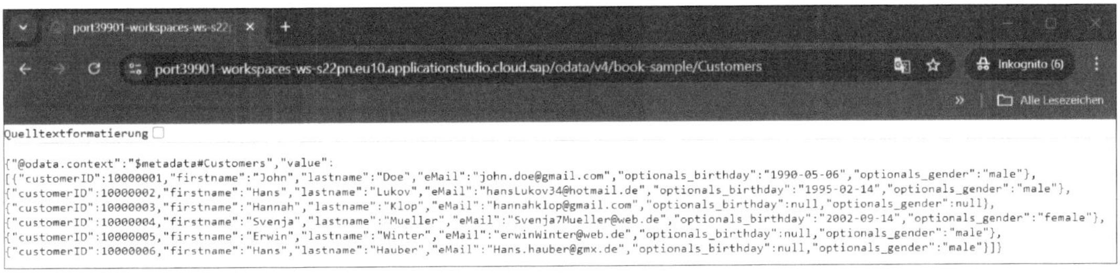

Abbildung 13.20 Anzeige der importierten Beispieldaten

Metadaten

Wie beim OData-Standard üblich, können wir auch die Metadaten des OData-Service abrufen. Hierzu können Sie entweder zurück zur Übersicht in der Testanwendung gehen oder die URL aus Abbildung 13.20 so abändern, dass Sie anstelle von *Customers* den Wert *$metadata* übergeben. Die Metadaten werden Ihnen daraufhin wie in Abbildung 13.21 angezeigt.

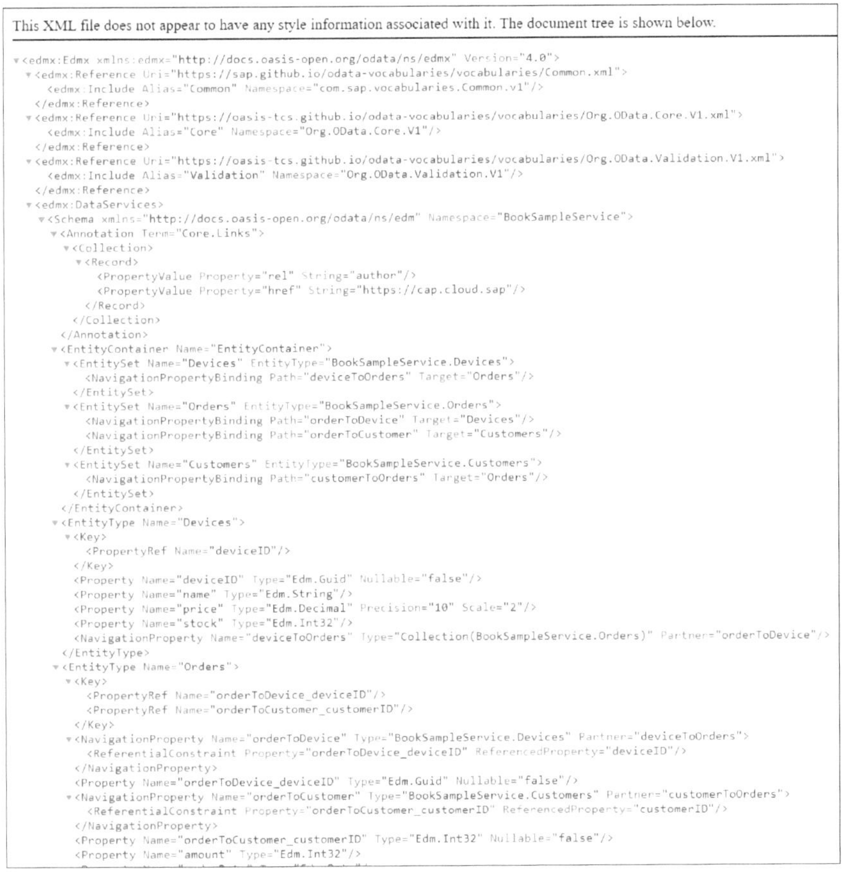

Abbildung 13.21 Die Metadaten des OData-Service

13

Vorschau aufrufen

Wechseln Sie noch einmal zurück zum Einstiegsbild (siehe Abbildung 13.19) der Testanwendung, und klicken Sie auf den Button **Fiori Preview**. Sie erhalten eine Vorschau auf eine SAP-Fiori-Anwendung. Diese basiert auf dem in den SAP Fiori Design Guidelines (siehe Abschnitt 11.5.1, »SAP Fiori und SAP Fiori Elements im Überblick«) definierten Floorplan List Report (siehe Abbildung 13.22).

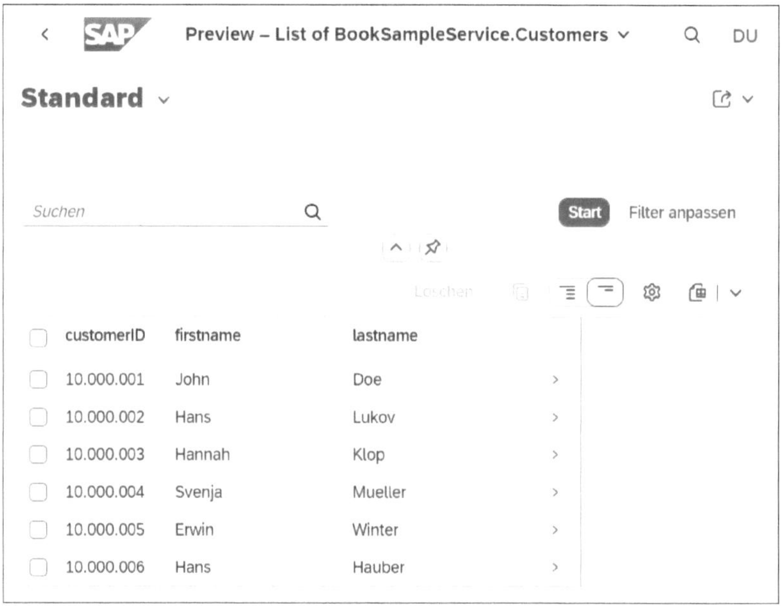

Abbildung 13.22 Vorschau einer List-Report-Anwendung, basierend auf SAP Fiori Elements

13.2.3 Anlegen einer SAP-Fiori-Benutzeroberfläche

Application Generator

Nach der Implementierung des OData-Service können Sie sich der Benutzeroberfläche Ihrer CAP-Anwendung zuwenden. Deren Implementierung erfolgt mittels SAP Fiori Elements. Um die Entwicklungsartefakte anzulegen, nutzen wir den für CAP bereitgestellten *Application Generator*. Dieses Werkzeug erreichen Sie über die *Command Palette* des SAP Business Application Studios. Diese können Sie wiederum mit der Tastenkombination `Ctrl` + `⇧` + `P` aufrufen.

Geben Sie hier, wie in Abbildung 13.23 gezeigt, die Zeichenkette »fiori« in das Eingabefeld ein. Ihnen werden daraufhin verschiedene Werkzeuge angeboten. Wählen Sie den Eintrag **Fiori: Open Application Generator** aus.

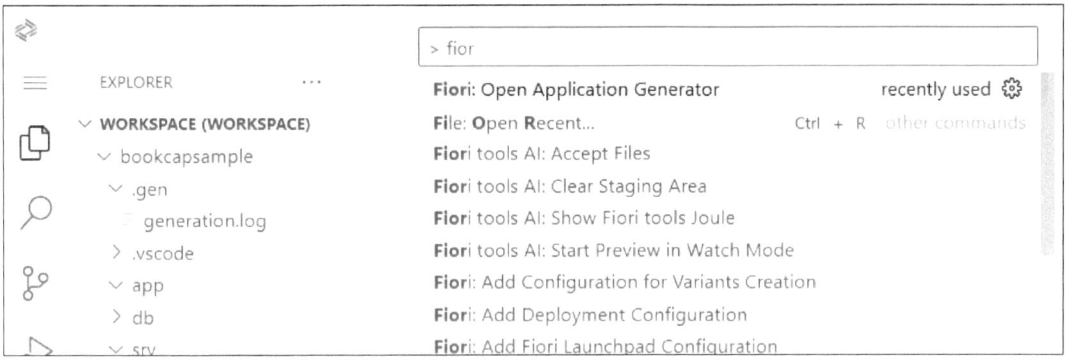

Abbildung 13.23 Nutzen der Kommandozeile im SAP Business Application Studio

Im Anschluss können Sie eine der Vorlagen zur Generierung von SAP-Fiori-Anwendungen auswählen. Wählen Sie das Template **List Report Page** und klicken Sie auf **Next** (siehe Abbildung 13.24). **Vorlage auswählen**

13

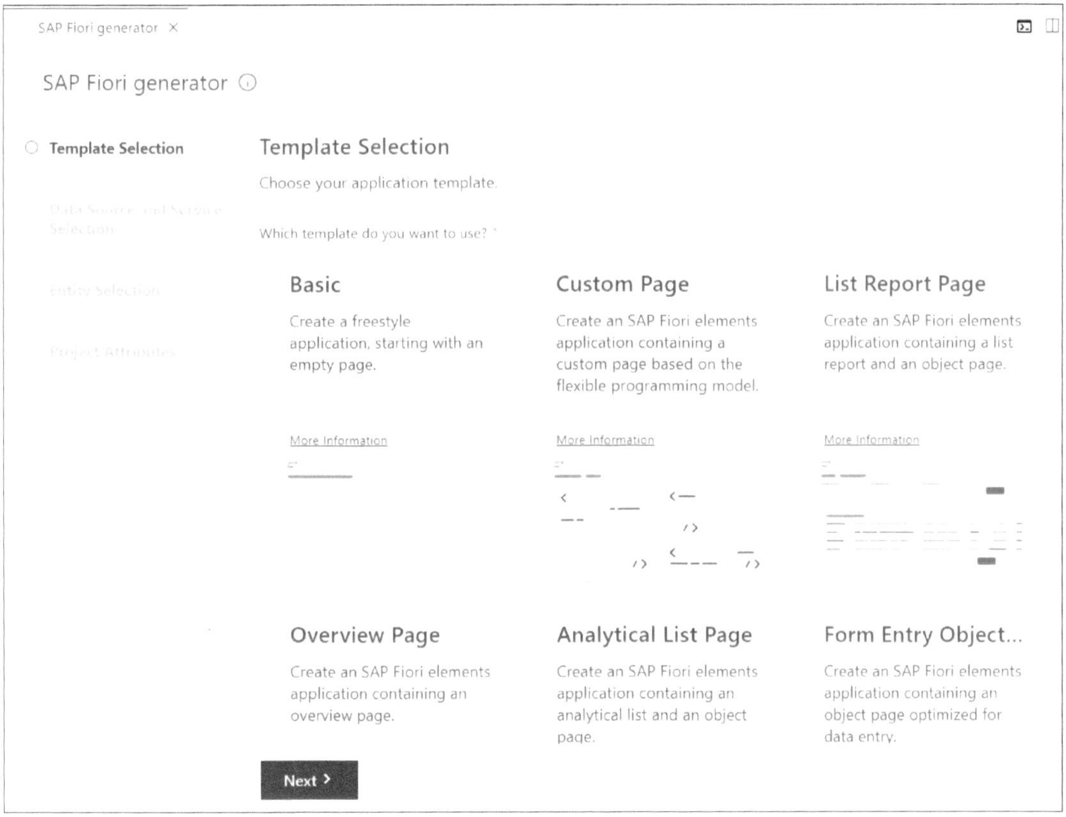

Abbildung 13.24 Template-Auswahl des SAP Fiori Generators

OData-Service auswählen

Im nächsten Schritt (siehe Abbildung 13.25) müssen Sie den Datenservice auswählen. Wählen Sie dazu im Auswahlmenü **Data source** den Eintrag **Use a Local CAP Project**. Als Nächstes wählen Sie im Auswahlmenü **Choose a CAP Project** den Eintrag **bookcapsample** und im Auswahlmenü **OData service** den Service **BookSampleService (Node.js)** aus. Bestätigen Sie die Auswahl mit **Next**.

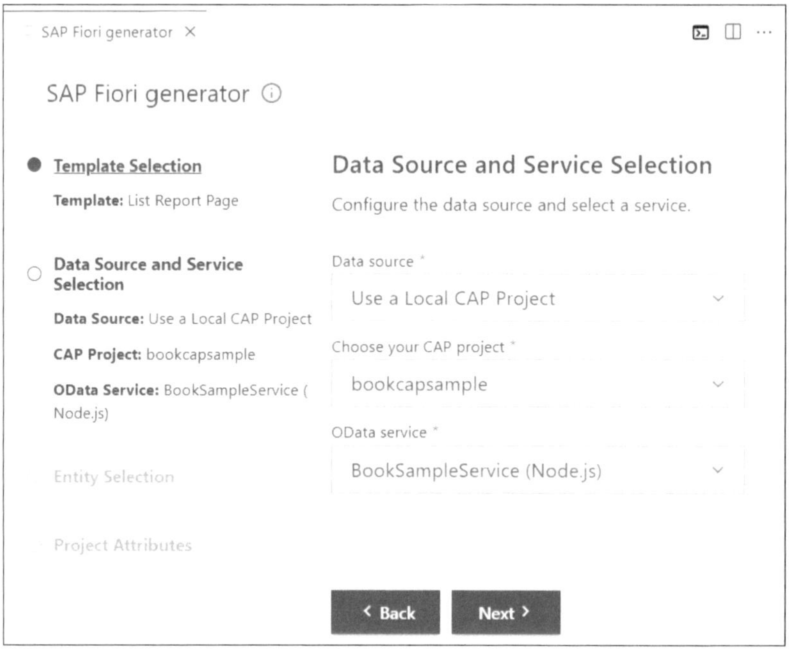

Abbildung 13.25 Auswahl der Datenquelle

Hauptentität

Im nächsten Schritt müssen wir unsere Hauptentität angeben. Die Daten dieser Entität werden später beim Start der Anwendung in der Liste innerhalb des List Reports dargestellt. Für unser Beispiel wählen wir als Hauptentität **Customers** aus und als Navigationseigenschaft **customerToOrders**. Die restlichen Einstellungen belassen wir so, wie in Abbildung 13.26 gezeigt. Unter anderem behalten wir bei der Einstellung **Automatically add table columns to the list page and a section to the object page if none already exists?** den Wert **Yes** bei. Diese Einstellung wird dafür sorgen, dass bereits Code für die Oberflächengestaltung generiert wird. Bestätigen Sie die Auswahl mit **Next**.

Projektdetails

Als Nächstes gelangen wir zur Konfigurationsoberfläche für die Projektparameter. Wir vergeben hier den Projektnamen »bookcampsampleui«. Als Namensraum nutzen wir »de.exxcellent.book« (siehe Abbildung 13.27). Bestätigen Sie erneut mit **Next**.

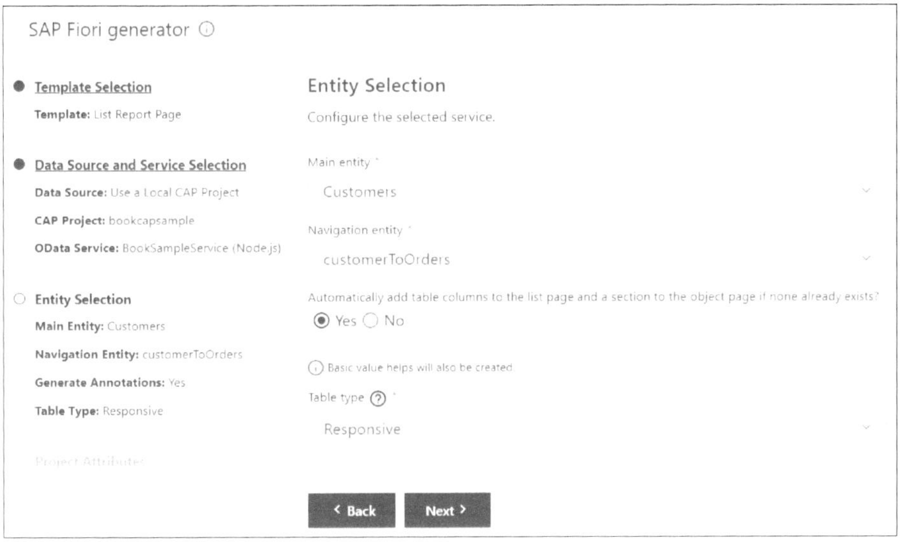

Abbildung 13.26 Auswahl der Entität

13

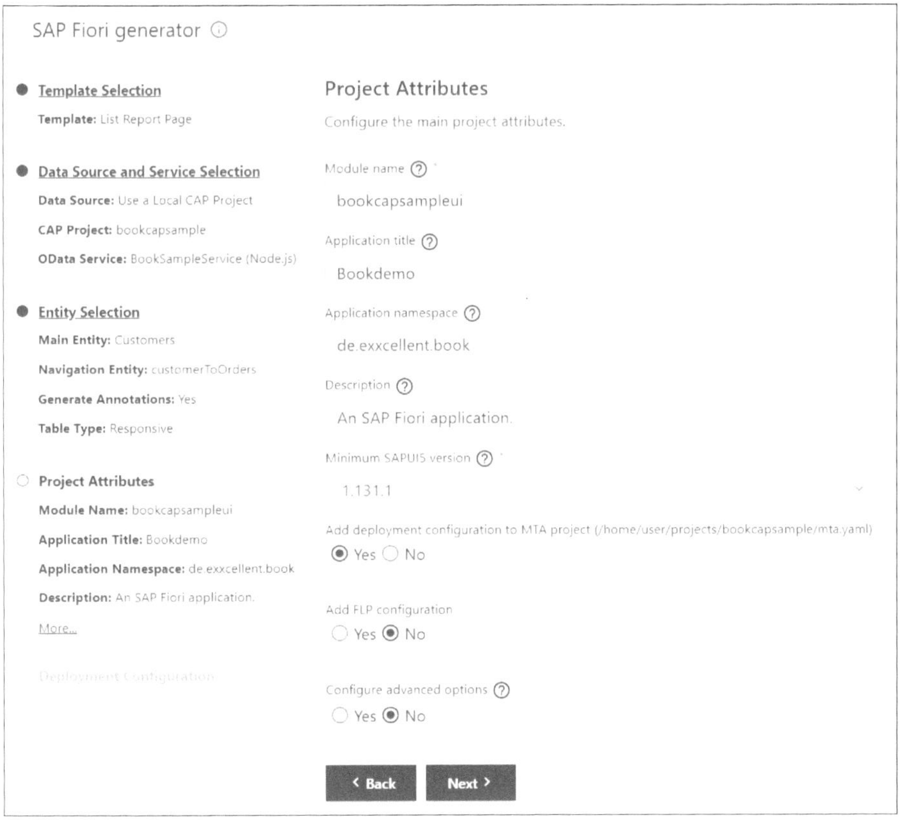

Abbildung 13.27 Projektparameter konfigurieren

Im letzten Schritt wird das Deployment konfiguriert. Wir bleiben auch hier bei der Voreinstellung **Cloud Foundry** (siehe Abbildung 13.28). Starten Sie nun die Projektgenerierung mit einem Klick auf **Finish**.

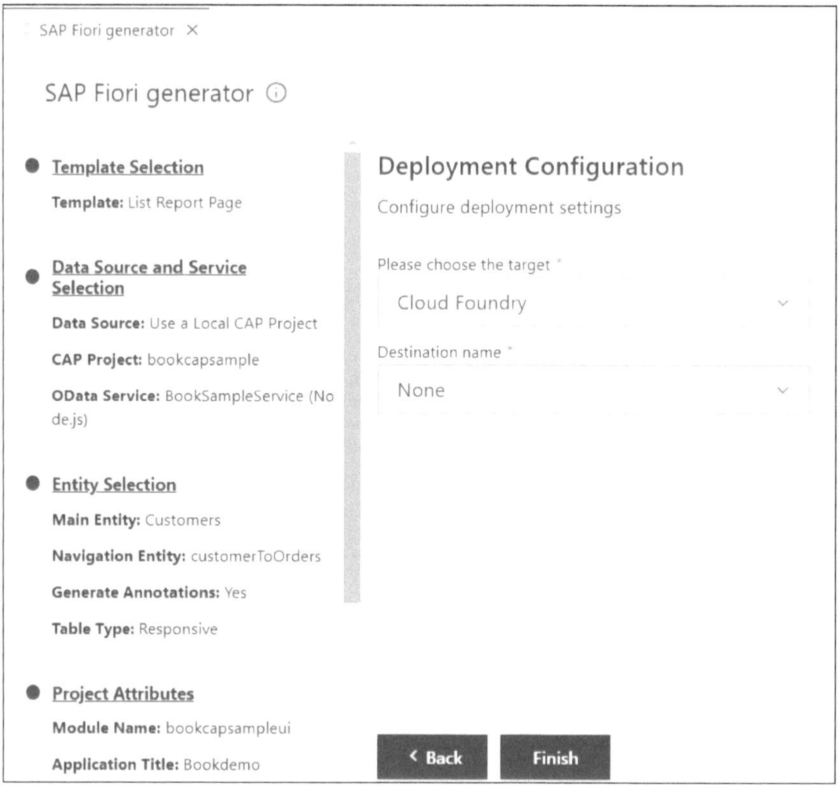

Abbildung 13.28 Deployment-Konfiguration

Generierte Projektstruktur

Im Anschluss an die Projektgenerierung wird Ihnen eine Übersicht wie in Abbildung 13.29 angezeigt. Wie Sie dieser Übersicht entnehmen können, wurde in der Projektstruktur ein Ordner **bookcapsampleui** unterhalb des **app**-Ordners angelegt. Dieser Ordner enthält zwei Unterordner:

- Der Ordner **node_modules** enthält die Node.js-Module, die für die Ausführung und die Arbeit mit den entsprechenden Werkzeugen notwendig sind.
- Der Ordner **webapp** enthält den eigentlichen Anwendungscode.

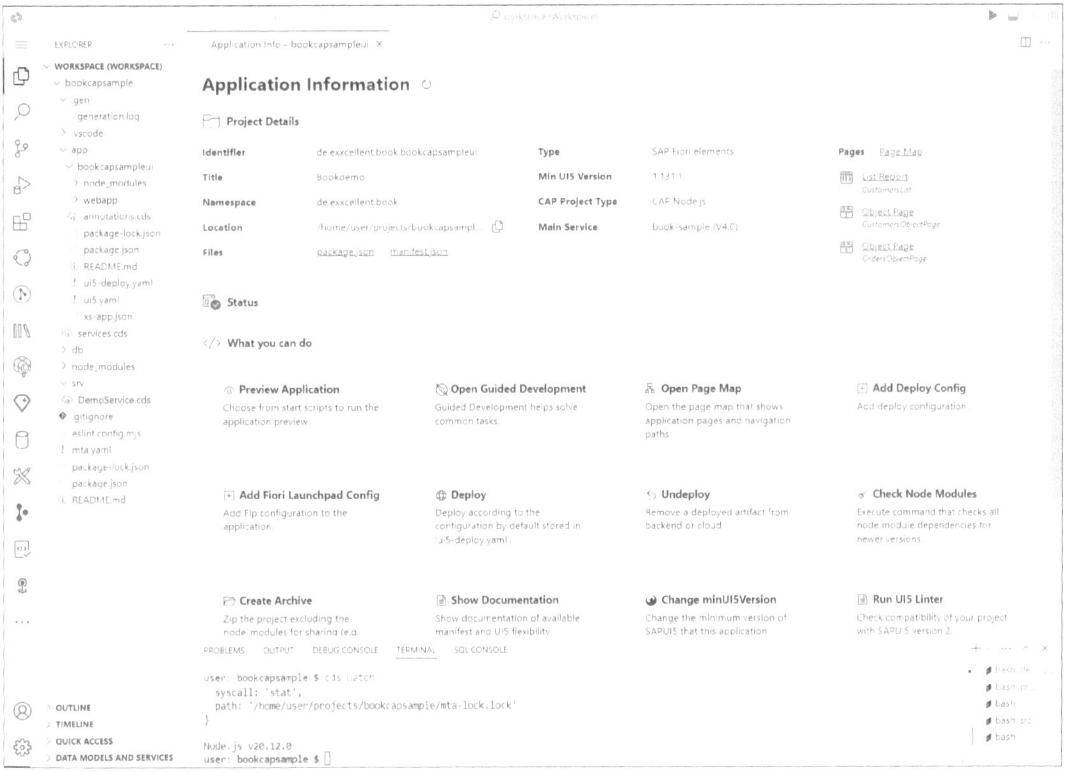

Abbildung 13.29 Anwendungsinformationen zum generierten UI-Projekt

UI-Annotationen

Besonders interessant an dieser Stelle ist die Datei **annotations.cds**. Beim Anlegen des Projekts hatten wir festgelegt, dass bereits UI-Code generiert werden soll. Dieser UI-Code umfasst die CDS-Annotationen von SAP Fiori Elements und wurde in die Datei **annotations.cds** geschrieben. Diese Datei enthält beispielsweise den in Listing 13.6 auszugsweise gezeigten Code. Der Code führt dazu, dass die Felder `customerID`, `firstname`, `lastname`, `eMail` und `optionals_birthday` in einer listenbasierten Darstellung angezeigt werden.

```
UI.LineItem : [
        {
            $Type : 'UI.DataField',
            Label : 'customerID',
            Value : customerID,
        },
        {
            $Type : 'UI.DataField',
            Label : 'firstname',
            Value : firstname,
```

```
        },
        {
            $Type : 'UI.DataField',
            Label : 'lastname',
            Value : lastname,
        },
        {
            $Type : 'UI.DataField',
            Label : 'eMail',
            Value : eMail,
        },
        {
            $Type : 'UI.DataField',
            Label : 'optionals_birthday',
            Value : optionals_birthday,
        },
    ],
```

Listing 13.6 Auszug aus der Datei »annotations.cds«

Anwendung testen

Für einen Test der Anwendung rufen Sie wieder die Testseite unseres Projekts auf. Falls Sie sich nicht mehr sicher sein sollten, wie die Adresse lautet oder ob die Anwendung noch ausgeführt wird, können Sie im Terminal einfach den Befehl `cds watch` eingeben. Die Testseite enthält nun einen Eintrag unter der Überschrift **Web Applications** (siehe Abbildung 13.30).

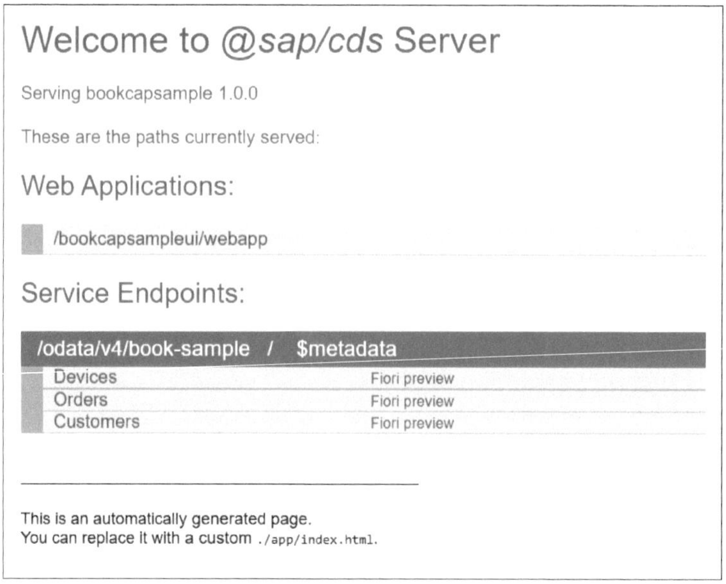

Abbildung 13.30 Testseite der CAP-Anwendung

Wählen Sie den Eintrag **/bookcapsampleui/webapp** auf der Testseite aus. Ihnen wird nun die SAP-Fiori-Anwendung wie in Abbildung 13.31 angezeigt. Nach einem Klick auf **Start** erhalten Sie die Liste der Kunden aus der entsprechenden CSV-Datei. Die generierten Oberflächen folgen dem SAP-Fiori-Standard. Die Spalten der angezeigten Tabelle wurden beispielsweise in der Datei **annotations.cds** beschrieben und werden zur Laufzeit in das SAPUI5-Template für die List-Report-Darstellung übertragen.

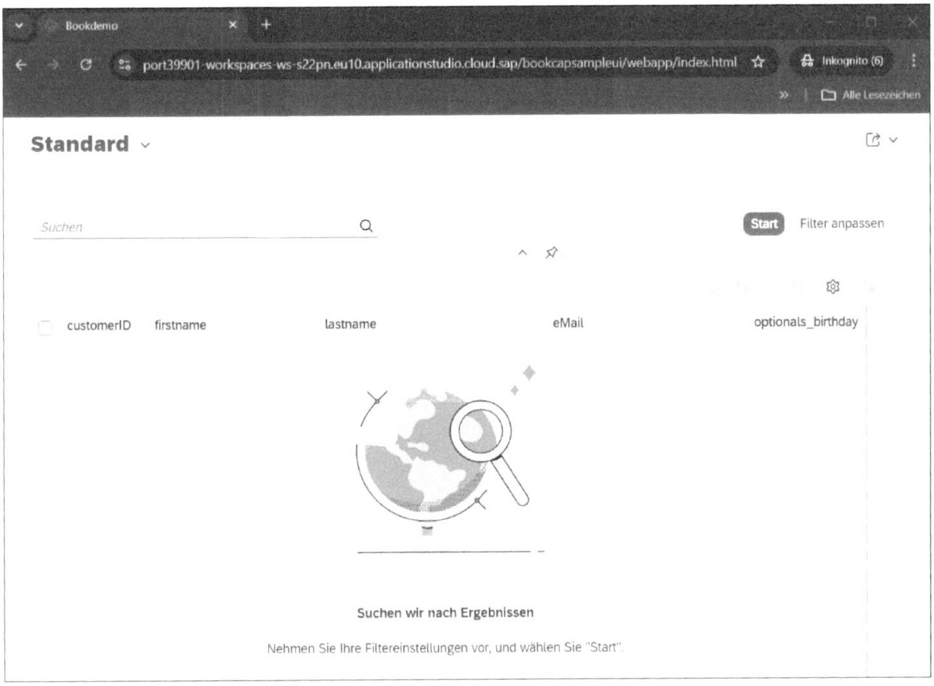

Abbildung 13.31 Generierte SAP-Fiori-Anwendung

Um weitere Details zu einem Datensatz anzuzeigen, klicken Sie auf einen der Datensätze. Die dazugehörenden Details werden nun wie in Abbildung 13.32 gezeigt dargestellt.

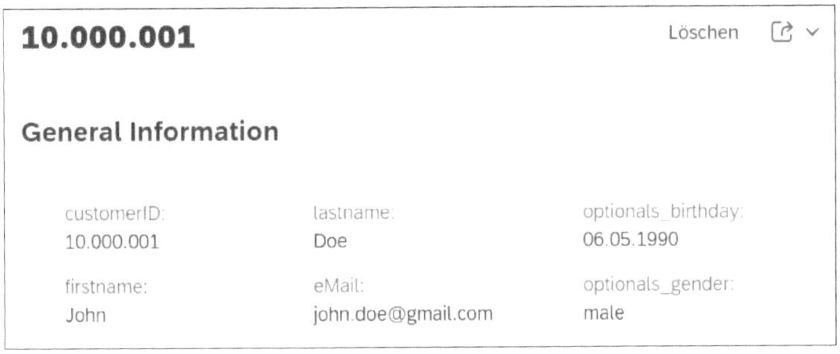

Abbildung 13.32 Details des Kunden John Doe

13

13.2.4 Schreibenden OData-Zugriff erlauben

Bis jetzt hatten wir in unserer Anwendung lediglich lesenden Zugriff auf die Daten. Als Nächstes erweitern wir die Anwendung dahingehend, dass auch neue Daten erfasst und bestehende aktualisiert bzw. gelöscht werden können.

Servicedefinition anpassen

Hierzu öffnen Sie die Datei **DemoService.cds**, die die Servicedefinition enthält. Fügen Sie hier eine Annotationsanweisung hinzu, wie in Listing 13.7 gezeigt. Mit dieser Anweisung geben Sie an, dass für die Entität `Customer` das sogenannte *Draft Handling* aktiv ist. Dadurch ist es nun möglich, neue Datensätze zu erfassen und bestehende zu ändern. Hierbei stellt das Framework durch das Draft-Konzept (dt. Entwurfskonzept) sicher, dass jede Änderung an einer Eigenschaft der Entität gesichert wird. Dadurch wird Datenverlust vorgebeugt.

```
using { bookcapsample as demo } from '../db/src/schema';

service BookSampleService {

    @cds.redirection.target
    entity Devices as projection on demo.Device;
    entity Orders as projection on demo.Order;
    entity Customers as projection on demo.Customer;
}

annotate demo.Customer with @odata.draft.enabled;
```

Listing 13.7 Erweiterung der Servicedefinition zur transaktionalen Verarbeitung der Daten

Anwendung testen

Im Anschluss testen wir die Anwendung erneut. Abbildung 13.33 zeigt die Bearbeitung eines Datensatzes. Bei diesem Datensatz wurde die E-Mail-Adresse geändert. Wie Sie in der Fußzeile der Detailansicht sehen können, wurde die Änderung in einem Entwurf gespeichert. Das Framework bietet sogar die Möglichkeit, zwischen dem Entwurf und der gesicherten Version zu wechseln. Dies ist über die Auswahlliste im Kopf des in Bearbeitung befindlichen Objekts möglich. Aktuell wird in Abbildung 13.33 der Entwurf angezeigt. Über die Schaltfläche **Entwurf** kann das Original angezeigt werden. Sichert man die Änderungen über den Button **Sichern**, wird der Entwurf zum Original.

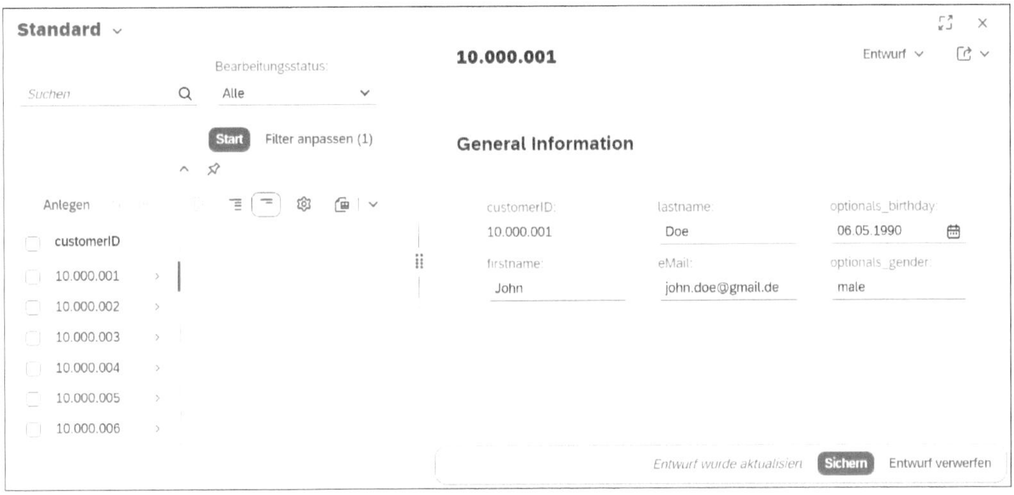

Abbildung 13.33 Entwurfsmodus einer SAP-Fiori-Anwendung

13.3 Deployment einer CAP-Anwendung

Nachdem Sie den Service und die Anwendungsoberfläche implementiert haben, müssen Sie die Anwendung auf der SAP BTP deployen. Eine CAP-basierte Anwendung benötigt eine Laufzeitumgebung auf der SAP BTP. Diese Laufzeitumgebung wird in einem sogenannten *Space* zur Verfügung gestellt. Sie müssen daher sicherstellen, dass in Ihrem SAP BTP Subaccount ein entsprechender Space existiert.

Space anlegen

Zur Verwaltung der Spaces im SAP BTP Cockpit gelangen Sie über den Menüpunkt **Cloud Foundry • Spaces**.

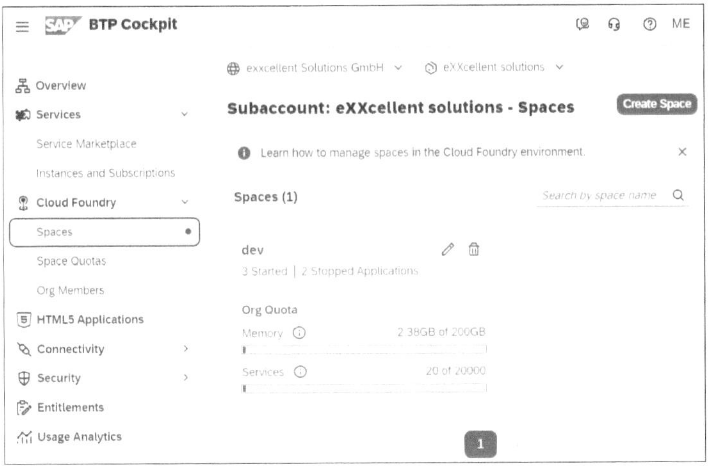

Abbildung 13.34 Cloud Foundry Space auf der SAP BTP

Wie Sie in Abbildung 13.34 sehen können, verfügt der von uns verwendete Subaccount bereits über einen Space namens dev. Falls noch kein Space verfügbar ist, können Sie einen über die Schaltfläche **Create Space** anlegen.

13.3.1 SAP-BTP-Services aktivieren

Datenbankservice

Neben der Laufzeitumgebung nutzen Anwendungen auf der SAP BTP normalerweise Standarddienste, die durch die SAP BTP bereitgestellt werden, so auch unsere Beispielanwendung. Unsere Anwendung persistiert Daten in einer Datenbank. Auf der SAP BTP wir hierzu die SAP-HANA-Datenbank über den Service *SAP HANA Cloud* zur Verfügung gestellt. Um diesen Service zu nutzen, benötigen Sie darüber hinaus noch den Service *SAP HANA Schemas & HDI Container*.

Autorisierungsservice

Genauso wird auch für die Autorisierung der Anwendungsbenutzer ein weiterer SAP-BTP-Service benötig. Der Service *Authorization and Trust Management* wird für die Berechtigung einzelner Benutzer bzw. Benutzergruppen benötigt.

Wie in Abschnitt 2.2.1, »Account-Konzept der SAP BTP«, erläutert, müssen SAP-BTP-Services über Entitlements und Servicepläne lizenziert und bereitgestellt werden. Nachdem sie so im Subaccount verfügbar und durch SAP abrechenbar gemacht wurden, können die Services im Subaccount instanziiert werden.

Service instanziieren

Die Instanziierung eines Service erfolgt im SAP BTP Cockpit über den Menüpfad **Services • Instances and Subscriptions**. Klicken Sie hier auf den Button **Create**. Es öffnet sich ein Dialog, über den Sie zunächst im Feld **Service** den zu instanziierenden Dienst auswählen und dann die benötigten Informationen zu dessen Ausführung eingeben. Abbildung 13.35 zeigt exemplarisch den ersten Dialogschritt für die Anlage einer Instanz des Service SAP HANA Cloud.

Neben der SAP-HANA-Cloud-Instanz legen Sie eine Instanz des Service SAP HANA Schemas & HDI Container sowie eine Instanz des Service Authorization and Trust Management Service an. Nachdem Sie diese drei Instanzen angelegt haben, werden sie wie in Abbildung 13.36 gezeigt, im SAP BTP Cockpit aufgelistet.

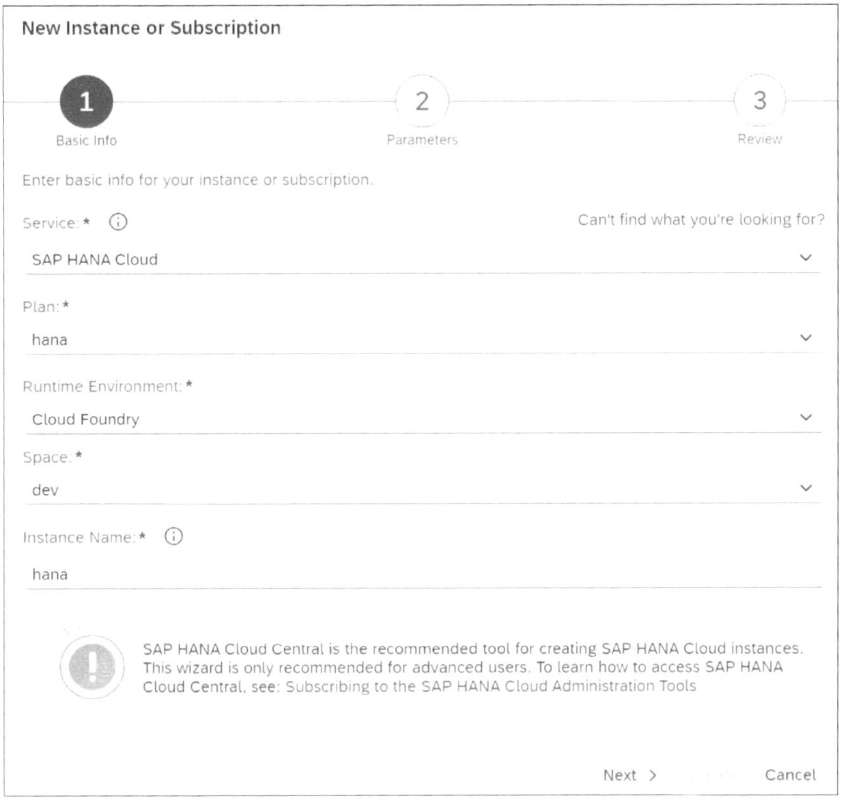

Abbildung 13.35 Anlegen einer SAP-HANA-Cloud-Instanz

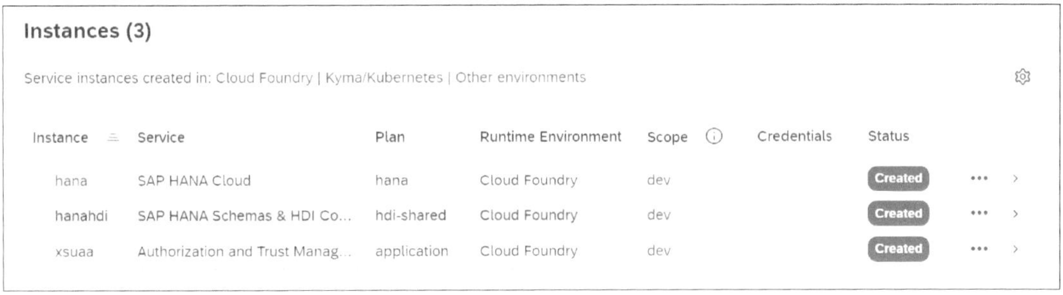

Abbildung 13.36 Serviceinstanzen auf der SAP BTP

Nachdem Ihr SAP BTP Subaccount auf diese Weise vorbereitet wurde, können Sie mit den nächsten Schritten für das Deployment fortfahren.

13.3.2 Anpassungen im Projekt

»cds watch« stoppen

In den weiteren Schritten müssen wir noch ein paar Anpassungen am Projekt durchführen. Zunächst es wichtig, dass der mit `cds watch` gestartete Prozess nicht mehr läuft. Sie können diese Funktion über die Tastenkombination [Ctrl] + [C] im Terminal stoppen. Im daraufhin angezeigten Terminal navigieren Sie zum Wurzelverzeichnis unseres Projekts und geben folgenden Befehl ein (siehe Abbildung 13.37):

```
cds add hana,mta,xsuaa,approuter --for production
```

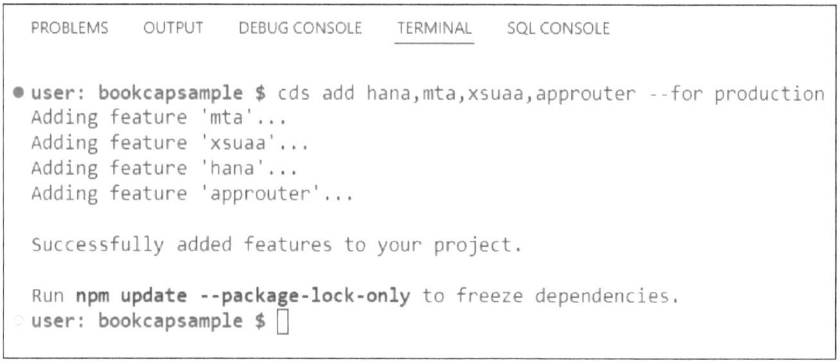

Abbildung 13.37 Eingabe des Befehls zum Stoppen von »cds add«

Da über den Befehl `cds add` einige Abhängigkeiten zu unserem Projekt hinzugefügt wurden, müssen wir sicherzustellen, dass diese Abhängigkeiten zwischen den Modulen stabil bleiben. Rufen Sie dazu den im Terminalfenster vorgegebenen Befehl `npm update --package-lock-only` auf, den Sie in Abbildung 13.37 sehen.

Datei »package.json« erweitern

Damit wir nach dem Deployment die Oberfläche der Anwendung auch benutzen können, müssen wir außerdem die Konfiguration der Datei **package.json** erweitern. Hierzu öffnen Sie die Datei und erweitern die Konfiguration des `cds`-Objekts um den in Listing 13.8 fett hervorgehobenen Code.

```
"cds": {
   "requires": {
      "@capire/db/src/db/data": {
        "model": "bookcapsample"
      },
      "[production]": {
        "auth": "xsuaa",
        "db": "hana"
```

```
        },
    "uaa": {
        "kind": "xsuaa"
    }
    },
    "sql": {
        "native_hana_associations": false
    },
    "hana": {
        "deploy-format": "hdbtable"
    },
    "fiori": {
      "preview": true
    },
    "server": {
      "index": true
    }
}
```

Listing 13.8 Erweiterung der Datei »package.json«

Berechtigungen

Wie in Abschnitt 2.3.2, »Application Roles und Role Collections«, erläutert, nutzen wir zur Berechtigung von Benutzern auf der SAP BTP Role Collections. Diese verweisen wiederum auf Rollen bzw. Role Templates. Anwendungen liefern diese Objekte mit dem Deployment aus. Die Konfiguration erfolgt über die Datei **xs-security.json**.

Wir wollen für unsere Anwendung eine sehr einfache Berechtigungsstruktur festlegen. Die Anwendung kann von jedem Benutzer verwendet werden, der einer Role Collection namens `IFPManager` zugeordnet ist. Aus dieser Anforderung ergibt sich die in Listing 13.9 gezeigte Implementierung der Datei **xs-security.json**. Wir geben hier ein Role Template an, das dann im Rahmen der Role-Collection-Implementierung referenziert wird.

```
{
  "xsappname": "bookcapsample",
  "scopes": [
    {
      "name": "$XSAPPNAME.Manager",
      "description": "Manage permission"
    }
  ],
  "attributes": [],
  "role-templates": [
```

```
    {
      "name": "IFPManager",
      "description": "Full permission",
      "default-role-name": "IFPManager",
      "scope-references": [
        "$XSAPPNAME.Manager"
      ],
      "attribute-references": []
    }
  ],
  "role-collections": [
    {
      "name": "IFPManager",
      "description": "IFP RoleCollection",
      "role-template-references": [
        "$XSAPPNAME.IFPManager"
      ]
    }
  ],
  "oauth2-configuration": {
    "redirect-uris": [
      "https://*.xx.hana.ondemand.com/**"
    ]
  }
}
```

Listing 13.9 Die Konfigurationsdatei »xs-security.json«

[»]

»redirect-uris« aus Listing 13.9

Beachten Sie, dass die unter `redirect-uris` angegeben URL in Listing 13.9 nur ein Platzhalter ist. Ersetzen Sie bei der Implementierung in Ihrer SAP-BTP-Umgebung die beiden xx-Teile mit den korrekten Informationen.

13.3.3 Deployment ausführen

API-Endpunkt identifizieren

Für das Deployment unserer Anwendung auf der SAP BTP müssen wir nun den API-Endpunkt für das SAP-BTP, Cloud Foundry Environment identifizieren. Diesen API-Endpunkt erhalten Sie über das SAP BTP Cockpit. Abbildung 13.38 zeigt den Übersichtsbereich des SAP BTP Cockpits zu unserem Subaccount.

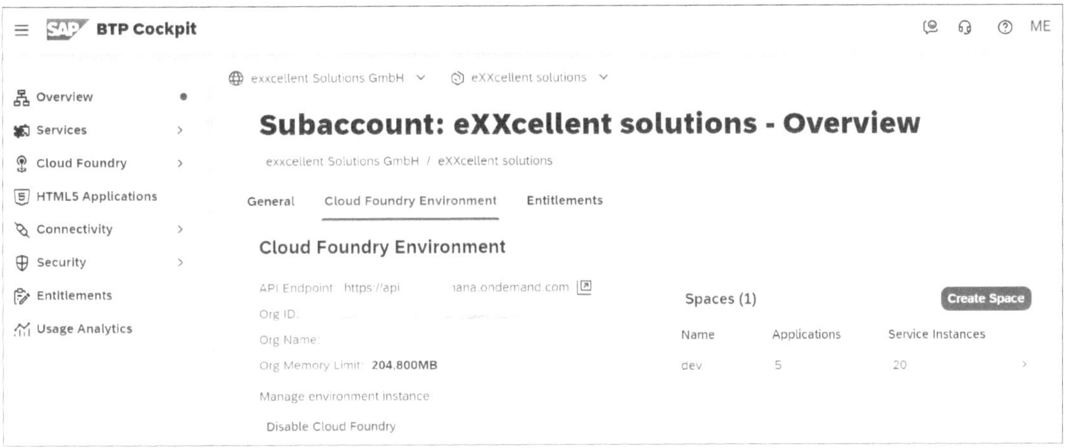

Abbildung 13.38 API-Endpunkt im SAP BTP Cockpit

Am API-Endpunkt anmelden

Für das Deployment müssen Sie an der SAP BTP bzw. am endsprechenden API-Endpunkt angemeldet sein. Hierzu öffnen Sie, falls nicht bereits geschehen, das Terminalfenster und geben den Befehl `cf login` ein, wie in Abbildung 13.39 gezeigt. Die Anmeldung erfolgt am Standard-API-Endpunkt. Geben Sie Ihren Benutzer sowie das Passwort ein.

13

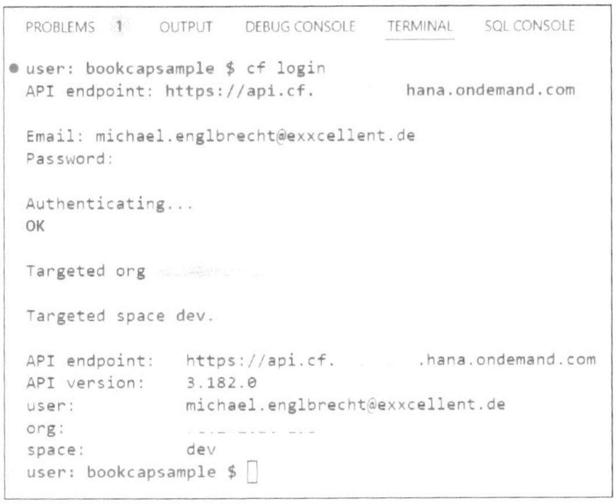

Abbildung 13.39 Anmelden am API-Endpunkt

Archiv erstellen

Für das Deployment erstellen wir nun ein Archiv. Dieses enthält alle relevanten Ressourcen, die im SAP BTP, Cloud Foundry Environment installiert werden sollen. Geben Sie hierzu den Befehl `mbt build -t gen --mtar mta.tar` in das Terminalfenster ein, wie in Abbildung 13.40 gezeigt. Der Befehl erstellt eine Datei namens **mta** im **.tar**-Format und speichert diese Datei im Verzeichnis **gen**.

```
PROBLEMS 1   OUTPUT   DEBUG CONSOLE   TERMINAL   SQL CONSOLE

user: bookcapsample $ mbt build -t gen --mtar mta.tar
[2025-01-14 08:29:55]  INFO Cloud MTA Build Tool version 1.2.18
[2025-01-14 08:29:55]  INFO generating the "Makefile_20250114082955.mta" file...
[2025-01-14 08:29:55]  INFO done
[2025-01-14 08:29:55]  INFO executing the "make -f Makefile_20250114082955.mta p=cf mtar=mta.tar strict=true mode= t=\"gen\"" command...
[2025-01-14 08:29:55]  INFO validating the MTA project
[2025-01-14 08:29:55]  INFO running the "before-all" build...
[2025-01-14 08:29:55]  INFO executing the "npm ci" command...
....
added 429 packages, and audited 430 packages in 4s

61 packages are looking for funding
  run `npm fund` for details

found 0 vulnerabilities
[2025-01-14 08:30:00]  INFO executing the "npx cds build --production" command...
building project [/home/user/projects/bookcapsample], clean [true]
cds-dk [8.6.1], cds [8.6.1], compiler [5.6.0], home [/home/user/projects/bookcapsample/node_modules/@sap/cds]
```

Abbildung 13.40 Erstellen eines Archivs

Deployment starten

Als Nächstes starten Sie das Deployment, indem Sie im Terminalfenster den Befehl `cf deploy gen/mta.tar` ausführen. Der Deployment-Prozess nimmt ein paar Minuten in Anspruch. Währenddessen können Sie im Terminal den aktuellen Stand des Deployments nachvollziehen. Schlägt das Deployment eines Moduls fehl, wird es automatisch noch zwei Mal versucht. Ist das Deployment weiterhin nicht erfolgreich, wird das Modul als »nicht geployt« ausgegeben. Abbildung 13.41 zeigt die Ausgabe eines fehlgeschlagenen Deployments. Die in den Logdateien protokollierten Ausgaben können Sie über den Befehl `cf dmol -i <ID>` in das Projekt laden. Am einfachsten ist es sicherlich, diesen Befehl aus dem Terminalfenster direkt zu kopieren.

```
PROBLEMS 3   OUTPUT   DEBUG CONSOLE   TERMINAL   SQL CONSOLE

user: bookcapsample $ cf deploy gen/mta.tar
Starting application "bookcapsample"...
A step of the process has failed. Retrying it may solve the issue.
Starting application "bookcapsample-srv"...
Proceeding with automatic retry... (1 of 3 attempts left)
Executing task "deploy" on application "bookcapsample-db-deployer"...
Application "bookcapsample" started and available at "7ec24202trial-dev-bookcapsample.            na.ondemand.com"
Application "bookcapsample-srv" started and available at "7ec24202trial-dev-bookcapsample-srv.            .hana.ondemand.com"
Execution of task "deploy" on application "bookcapsample-db-deployer" failed.
Download the application logs via the dmol command and check them for more information.
A step of the process has failed. Retrying it may solve the issue.
Process failed.
Use "cf deploy -i b7696e34-d4af-11ef-b160-eeee0a8712dd -a abort" to abort the process.
Use "cf deploy -i b7696e34-d4af-11ef-b160-eeee0a8712dd -a retry" to retry the process.
Use "cf dmol -i b7696e34-d4af-11ef-b160-eeee0a8712dd" to download the logs of the process.
user: bookcapsample $ cf dmol -i b7696e34-d4af-11ef-b160-eeee0a8712dd
Downloading logs of multi-target app operation with ID b7696e34-d4af-11ef-b160-eeee0a8712dd in org          / space dev as michael.englbrecht@exxcellent.de...
OK
Saving logs to /home/user/projects/bookcapsample/mta-op-b7696e34-d4af-11ef-b160-eeee0a8712dd...
  OPERATION.log
  bookcapsample-app-content_bookcapsample-repo-host.log
  bookcapsample-db-deployer.log
  bookcapsample-srv.log
  bookcapsample.log
OK
user: bookcapsample $ 
```

Abbildung 13.41 Ausgabe des Deployment-Logs und Download der Log-Einträge

Bei einem Deployment, bei dem sowohl die UI-Anwendung als auch der OData-Service und die Datenbankartefakte deployt werden, sieht die Ausgabe des Terminals ähnlich wie in Abbildung 13.42 aus.

```
PROBLEMS 4   OUTPUT   DEBUG CONSOLE   TERMINAL   SQL CONSOLE                bash - bookcapsample

user: bookcapsample $ cf deploy gen/mta.tar
Staging application "bookcapsample-db-deployer"...
Uploading application "bookcapsample"...
Uploading application "bookcapsample-srv"...
Started async upload of application "bookcapsample-srv"
Started async upload of application "bookcapsample"
Application "bookcapsample-db-deployer" staged
Stopping application "bookcapsample-srv"...
Stopping application "bookcapsample"...
Executing task "deploy" on application "bookcapsample-db-deployer"...
Staging application "bookcapsample-srv"...
Staging application "bookcapsample"...
Application "bookcapsample" staged
Application "bookcapsample-srv" staged
Starting application "bookcapsample"...
Starting application "bookcapsample-srv"...
Application "bookcapsample-srv" started and available at "7ec24202trial-dev-bookcapsample-srv.cfapps.us10-001.hana.ondemand.com"
Application "bookcapsample" started and available at "7ec24202trial-dev-bookcapsample.cfapps.us10-001.hana.ondemand.com"
Skipping deletion of services, because the command line option "--delete-services" is not specified.
Process finished.
Use "cf dmol -i 4950396a-d759-11ef-b645-eeee0a970eed" to download the logs of the process.
user: bookcapsample $
```

Abbildung 13.42 Ausgabe eines erfolgreichen Deployments

SAP HANA Cloud in Trial-Umgebung

Beachten Sie, dass bei der Verwendung der Trial-Umgebung der SAP BTP die SAP-HANA-Datenbank jeden Tag neu gestartet werden muss. Die Verwaltung des Datenbankservice, wie beispielsweise das Starten der Datenbank, erfolgt über *SAP HANA Cloud Central*. Um diese Verwaltungsumgebung aufzurufen, klicken Sie im SAP BTP Cockpit auf Ihre Instanz des SAP-HANA-Cloud-Service. Über das Aktionsmenü auf Höhe der Instanz können Sie dort die Datenbank starten. Achten Sie ebenfalls darauf, dass Ihr Benutzer über ausreichende Berechtigungen hierzu verfügt.

Deployte Instanzen

Im Anschluss an das Deployment werden die deployten Instanzen im SAP BTP Cockpit aufgelistet (siehe Abbildung 13.43).

Instances (7)

Service instances created in: Cloud Foundry | Kyma/Kubernetes | Other environments

Instance	Service	Plan	Runtime Environment	Scope	Credentials	Status
bookcapsample-auth	Authorization and Trust Manag...	application	Cloud Foundry	dev	2 bindings	Created
bookcapsample-db	SAP HANA Schemas & HDI Co...	hdi-shared	Cloud Foundry	dev	2 bindings	Created
bookcapsample-destination-s	Destination Service	lite	Cloud Foundry	dev		Created
bookcapsample-html5-srv	HTML5 Application Repository ...	app-host	Cloud Foundry	dev	1 key	Created
hana	SAP HANA Cloud	hana	Cloud Foundry	dev		Created
hanahdi	SAP HANA Schemas & HDI Co...	hdi-shared	Cloud Foundry	dev		Created
xsuaa	Authorization and Trust Manag...	application	Cloud Foundry	dev		Created

Abbildung 13.43 Serviceinstanzen nach dem Deployment

Role Collection

Neben den deployten Laufzeitartefakten erhalten wir damit eine neue Role Collection in unserem SAP BTP Subaccount. Die in der Datei **xs-security.json** angegebene Role Collection wurde wie erwartet angelegt und wird in der Liste der verfügbaren Role Collections angezeigt (siehe Abbildung 13.44). Weisen Sie Ihren Benutzer dieser neuen Role Collection zu. Klicken Sie dazu auf den Button **Edit** und geben Sie im Bereich **User** die E-Mail-Adressen der zu berechtigenden Benutzer ein. Speichern Sie diese Änderungen.

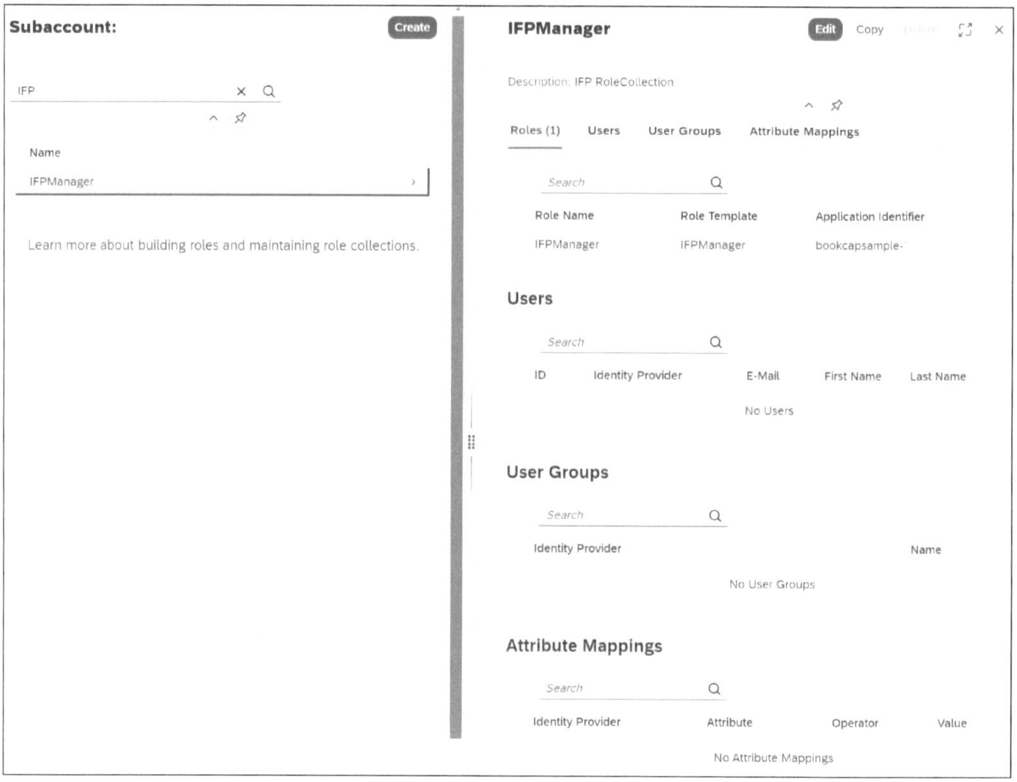

Abbildung 13.44 Die Role Collection »IFPManager«

Weitere Details zu den deployten Anwendungen sehen Sie direkt im **dev**-Space der SAP BTP, Cloud Foundry Environment. Folgen Sie dazu im SAP BTP Cockpit dem Pfad **Cloud Foundry • Spaces** und klicken Sie im Anschluss auf den für das Deployment verwendeten Space **dev**. Sie erhalten die in Abbildung 13.45 gezeigte Liste der deployten Anwendungen.

Details zu einem Service

Weitere Details, wie beispielsweise die URL für den Aufruf der Anwendung bzw. des Service, erhalten Sie mit einem Klick auf den entsprechenden Link. Abbildung 13.46 zeigt beispielsweise die Details zum OData-Service `bookcapsample-srv`. Über diese Ansicht können Sie den Service stoppen, starten oder auch löschen.

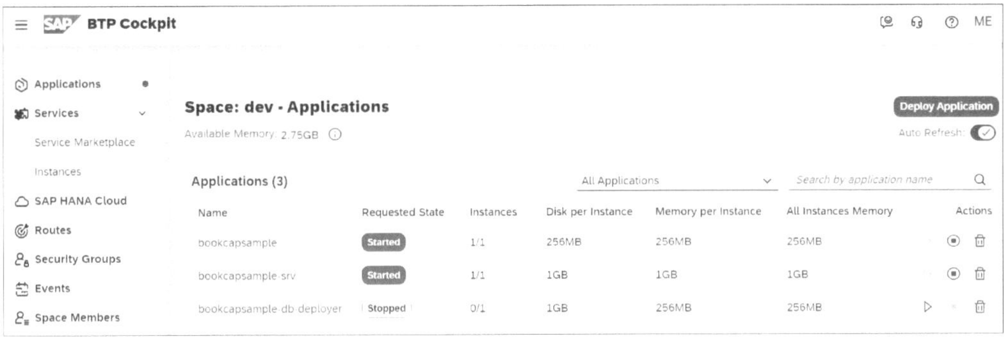

Abbildung 13.45 Anwendungen im »dev«-Space der SAP BTP, Cloud Foundry Environment

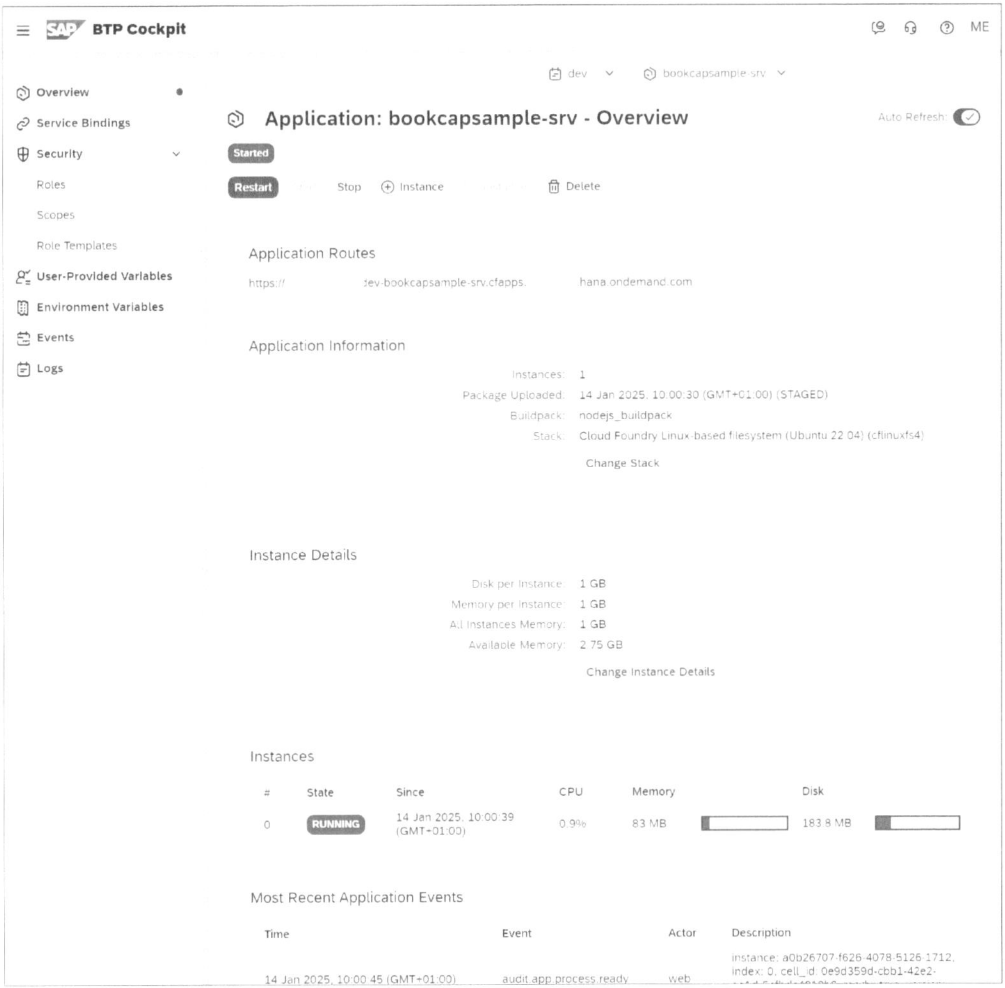

Abbildung 13.46 Details des OData-Service »bookcapsample-srv«

13.3.4 OData-Service testen

OData-Service-Endpunkte

Durch einen Klick auf den Link im Bereich **Application Routes** erreichen Sie die in Abbildung 13.47 gezeigte Liste der OData-Service-Endpunkte.

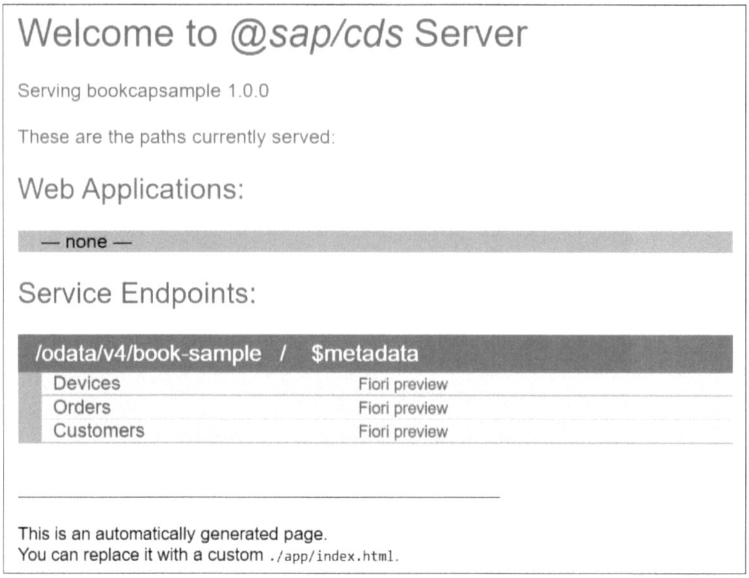

Abbildung 13.47 Übersicht der Service-Endpunkte

Folgt man beispielsweise dem Link **Devices**, erhält man die in Abbildung 13.48 gezeigte Ausgabe (zur besseren Lesbarkeit haben wir hier die Option **Quelltextformatierung** gewählt).

SAP-Fiori-Oberfläche testen

Um die Benutzeroberfläche unserer Anwendung zu testen, wechseln Sie wieder zurück in Ihren Subaccount der SAP BTP. Im Menü wählen Sie unterhalb des Menüpunkts **Cloud Foundry** den Menüpunkt **HTML5 Applications**. Folgen Sie diesem Link, wird eine Liste aller Anwendungen angezeigt, so auch die Anwendung `bookcampsampleui`, die Teil unseres Deployments ist. Über einen Klick auf den Anwendungsnamen erreichen Sie unsere Benutzeroberfläche und können sie im Browser testen.

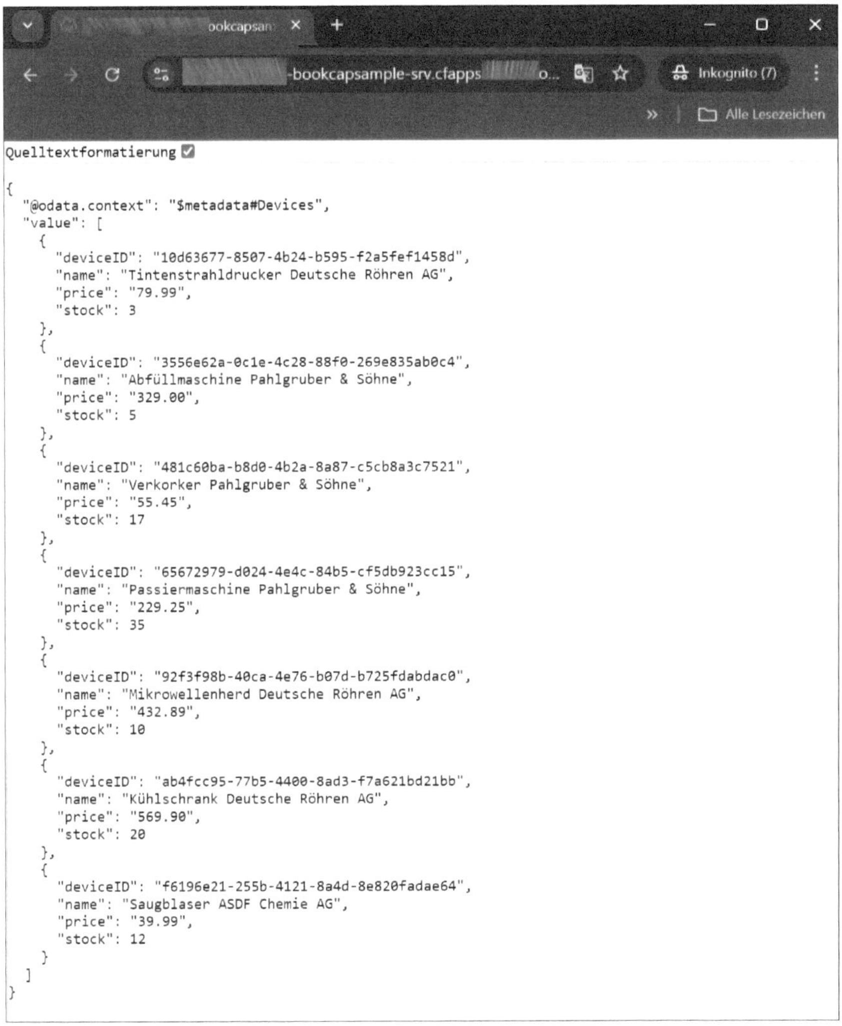

Abbildung 13.48 Anzeige der Daten des OData-Service zur Entität »Devices«

13

Kapitel 14
SAP Business Accelerator Hub

Die Schnittstellenvielfalt von SAP-Produkten bedingt eine gewisse Komplexität bei den Integrationsszenarien in einer heterogenen Systemlandschaft. Hier die Übersicht zu behalten, ist nicht einfach. Mit dem SAP Business Accelerator Hub erleichtert einem SAP den Durchblick im SAP-Schnittstellendschungel.

SAP und auch Partner von SAP bieten viele unterschiedliche Möglichkeiten, um mit SAP-Systemen zu kommunizieren. Es werden Ereignisse ausgelöst, Schnittstellen, Events oder CDS-Views angeboten. In den letzten Jahren stieg die Anzahl dieser Artefakte, und perspektivisch wird sie in einer immer stärker verteilten Infrastruktur noch weiter zunehmen. Die Integrations- und Kommunikationsmöglichkeiten wurden daher über die Zeit immer unübersichtlicher. Im Zweifel werden neue, eigene Möglichkeiten implementiert, um individuelle Lösungen zu schaffen.

Daher stand SAP vor der Aufgabe, eine Dokumentation dieser Schnittstellen in Gänze in einer übersichtlichen Art und Weise bereitzustellen. Mit dem *SAP Business Accelerator Hub* hat SAP eine Möglichkeit geschaffen, sich schneller einen Überblick zu verschaffen, welche Möglichkeiten der Kommunikation mit Systemen, Diensten und Datenbanken es gibt. In Abschnitt 14.1 führen wir in diesen SAP Business Accelerator Hub ein. Wir zeigen Ihnen in Abschnitt 14.2, wie man mit dieser Plattform umgeht und was genau dahintersteckt. In Abschnitt 14.3 erläutern wir, wie man die im SAP Business Accelerator Hub bereitgestellten Schnittstellen konsumiert. In Abschnitt 14.4 zeigen wir Ihnen, wie Sie das Service Center im SAP Business Application Studio nutzen können, um einen Service-Client generieren zu lassen.

14.1 Einführung in den SAP Business Accelerator Hub

Die Produkte von SAP sind ein wichtiger Teil der Geschäftsprozesse in Unternehmen. Dienste, Daten und Funktionen werden durch SAP-Produkte bereitgestellt und durch andere Systeme konsumiert (natürlich auch in entgegengesetzter Richtung). Den Überblick über die Schnittstellen, Geschäftsobjekte und Dienste zu behalten, diese einheitlich zu verwenden sowie für eine nachhaltige Integration zu sorgen und die Verwendung der durch SAP empfohlenen Wege bei der Integration und Kommunikation zu gewährleisten, ist nicht einfach. Die Lösung hierfür ist der SAP Business Accelerator Hub (vormals *SAP API Business Hub*).

Einstiegsseite

Hierbei handelt es sich zunächst um eine von SAP bereitgestellte Webanwendung. Sie ist unter der URL *https://api.sap.com* erreichbar. Abbildung 14.1 zeigt die Einstiegsseite.

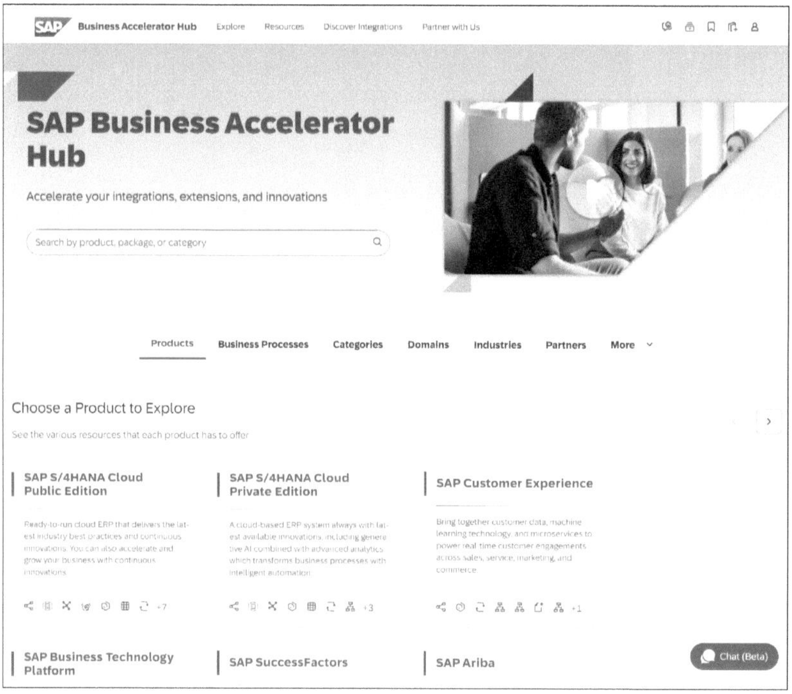

Abbildung 14.1 Einstiegsseite des SAP Business Accelerator Hubs

APIs

Der SAP Business Accelerator Hub bietet eine Vielzahl von Funktionen und Inhalten, die Unternehmen und Entwickler bei der Integration und Weiterentwicklung von SAP-Systemen unterstützen. Ein zentraler Bestandteil des Hubs ist die Sammlung von Application Programming Interfaces (APIs), die von SAP bereitgestellt werden. Diese APIs ermöglichen die Integration von SAP-Anwendungen mit anderen Systemen oder die Entwicklung neuer Anwendungen. Sie decken eine breite Palette von SAP-Produkten ab, darunter SAP S/4HANA, SAP SuccessFactors, SAP Ariba und die SAP Business Technology Platform (BTP).

Weitere Inhalte

Darüber hinaus enthält der Hub *Integrationspakete*, die vorgefertigte Inhalte bieten, um die Verbindung von SAP-Systemen mit anderen Anwendungen – sowohl SAP-eigenen als auch Drittanbieterlösungen – zu beschleunigen. Ein weiteres Feature sind die *Prozesse und Workflows*. Vorlagen für Geschäftsprozesse und Workflows, die mit SAP-Tools erstellt wurden, stehen hier zur Verfügung. Diese Vorlagen ermöglichen eine schnellere Entwicklung und Implementierung individueller Lösungen, die exakt auf die Bedürfnisse der Unternehmen zugeschnitten sind.

Für Entwickler gibt es auch die Möglichkeit, *Erweiterungen und Vorlagen* herunterzuladen und in eigenen Projekten zu verwenden. Diese vorkonfigurierten Inhalte sparen Zeit und bieten eine solide Grundlage für maßgeschneiderte Anwendungen.

Ein weiterer Vorteil des Hubs ist die *Testumgebung*, die es Entwicklern erlaubt, APIs direkt in einer Sandbox-Umgebung zu testen, ohne dass eine vollständige SAP-Installation erforderlich ist. Schließlich stehen umfangreiche *Entwicklerressourcen* zur Verfügung, darunter Dokumentationen, Beispiele und Anleitungen, die den Einstieg erleichtern und die Nutzung der Tools und Inhalte optimieren.

Der SAP Business Accelerator Hub bietet SAP-Kunden und -Partnern somit eine breite Palette an Informationen für verschiedene SAP-Produkte. Abbildung 14.2 zeigt die aktuell im SAP Business Accelerator Hub unterstützten Produkte.

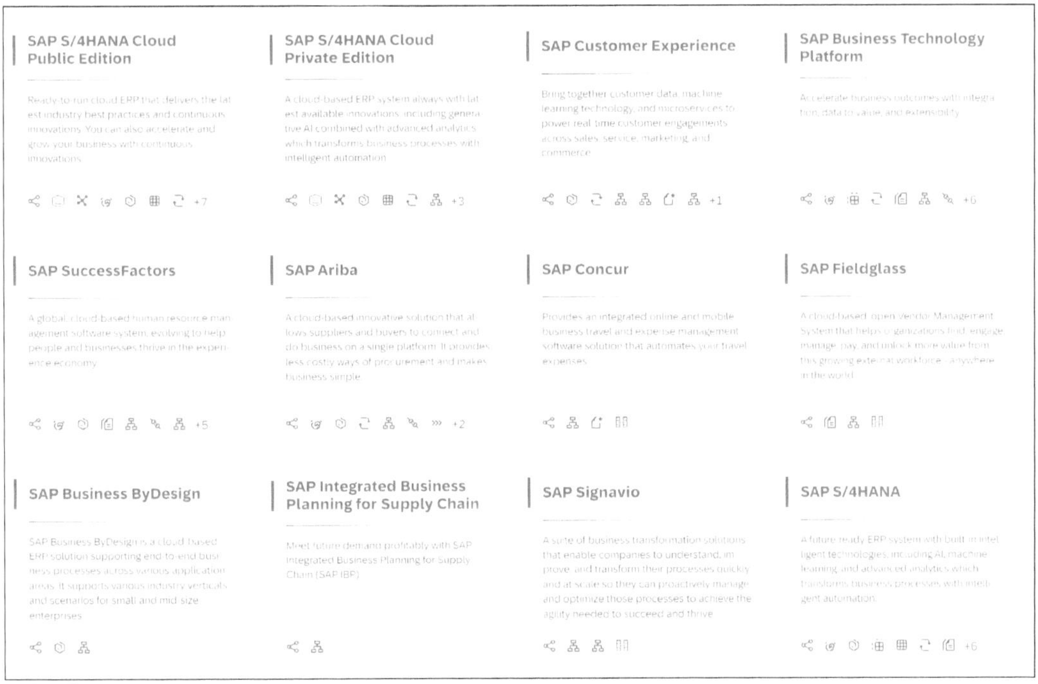

Abbildung 14.2 Unterstützte Produkte im SAP Business Accelerator Hub

Warum mit dem SAP Business Accelerator Hub arbeiten?

Der SAP Business Accelerator Hub bietet zahlreiche Vorteile, die die Entwicklung und Integration von Lösungen erheblich beschleunigen. Durch vorgefertigte APIs, Integrationen und Templates können Entwickler deutlich schneller an ihren Projekten arbeiten. Zudem fördert die Plattform die Kollaboration, indem sie es Partnern, Entwicklern und Unternehmen ermöglicht, gemeinsam zu arbeiten und Inhalte auszutauschen. Ein weiterer Vorteil ist die Flexibilität der Plattform: Sie unterstützt sowohl SAP- als auch Nicht-SAP-Entwickler, was eine Vielzahl von Integrationsmöglichkeiten eröffnet. Darüber hinaus trägt der Hub durch die Bereitstellung vorhandener Inhalte und Werkzeuge zur Kostenersparnis bei, da der Aufwand für die Entwicklung von Grund auf minimiert wird.

Zielgruppe

Die Zielgruppe des SAP Business Accelerator Hubs umfasst vor allem Entwickler, die APIs und Entwicklungsressourcen erkunden und nutzen möchten. Auch Unternehmen profitieren von der Plattform, da sie damit ihre Geschäftsprozesse durch die schnelle Integration und Anpassung von SAP-Systemen optimieren können. Darüber hinaus ist der Hub eine wertvolle Ressource für SAP-Partner, die Erweiterungen oder Lösungen entwickeln und verbreiten möchten. Insgesamt ist der SAP Business Accelerator Hub eine wesentliche Ressource für die Entwicklung und Integration moderner, cloudbasierter Unternehmensanwendungen.

14.2 Mit dem SAP Business Accelerator Hub arbeiten

Suchfunktion

Wie Sie mit dem SAP Business Accelerator Hub arbeiten, möchten wir Ihnen in diesem Abschnitt an einem Beispiel verdeutlichen. Über die Suche auf der Startseite kann nach den dokumentierten Informationen anhand von Produkten, Paketen oder Kategorien gesucht werden. Abbildung 14.3 zeigt das Ergebnis einer Suche nach dem Begriff »business partner«. Wie in Abbildung 14.3 zu erkennen ist, kategorisiert der SAP Business Accelerator Hub Informationen grundsätzlich in folgende Kategorien:

- APIs
- Integrations
- CDS Views
- Build
- Event Objects
- Business Processes
- VPUC
- Analytics

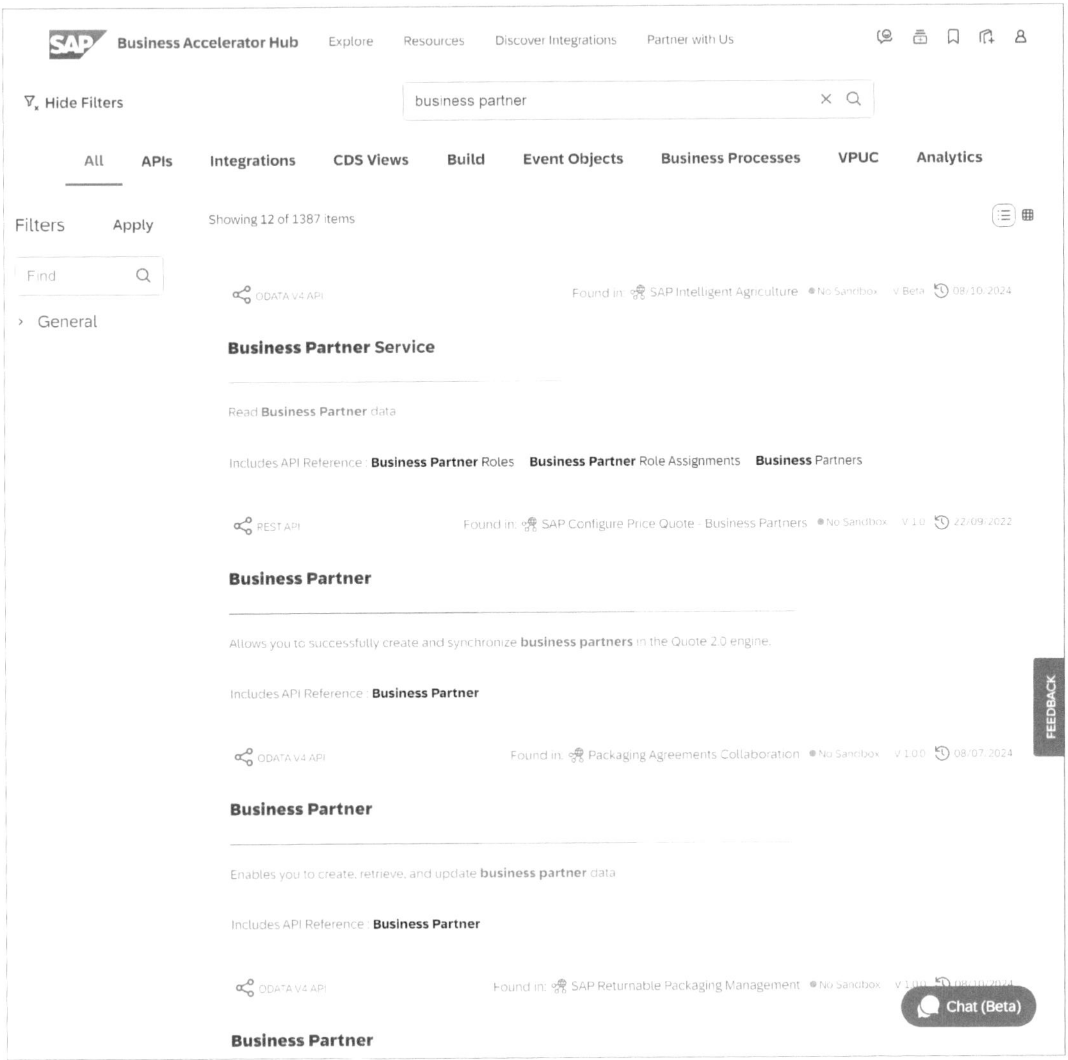

Abbildung 14.3 Ausschnitt aus der Dokumentation zum Suchbegriff »business partner«

Filterfunktion

Über die Filterfunktion auf der linken Seite ist es möglich, die Trefferliste weiter einzuschränken. Wie in Abbildung 14.4 erkennbar, ist es möglich, die Liste nach spezifischen Branchenlösungen, Produkten, Ländern, Herstellern oder Fachbereichen (engl. Lines of Business) zu filtern. Bei der in Abbildung 14.4 gezeigten Liste wurde der Filter beispielsweise auf das Produkt SAP S/4HANA gesetzt.

14

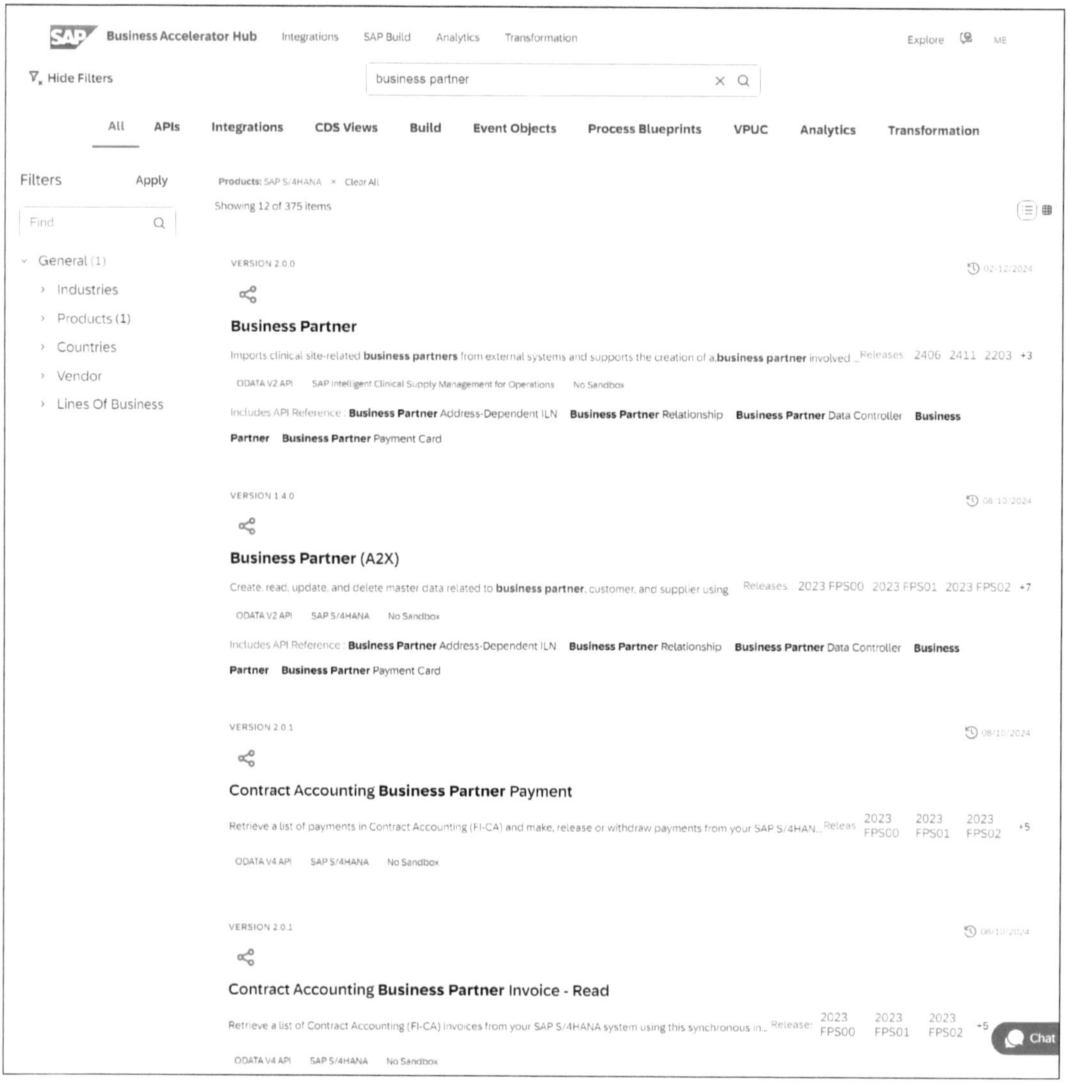

Abbildung 14.4 Nach dem Produkt »SAP S/4HANA« gefilterte Trefferliste

Process Blueprints

Bevor wir uns im Folgenden eine konkrete API genauer ansehen, wenden wir uns zunächst der Registerkarte **Process Blueprints** zu (siehe Abbildung 14.5). Dieser Bereich ist deshalb interessant, weil er eine Übersicht von Geschäftsprozessen zeigt, bei denen der Geschäftspartner eine Rolle spielt. Für diese Geschäftsprozesse werden hier von SAP jeweils Empfehlungen ausgesprochen, wie sie standardkonform umgesetzt werden können. Wählt man beispielsweise den ersten Eintrag **Lead to Cash for Hybrid Deployment**, erhält man detaillierte Informationen über das Lead-to-Cash-Szenario. Für SAP-Kunden ist es ratsam, sich zunächst mit den Standardprozessen und deren Umsetzung zu beschäftigen, bevor eigene, individuelle Schnittstellen implementiert werden.

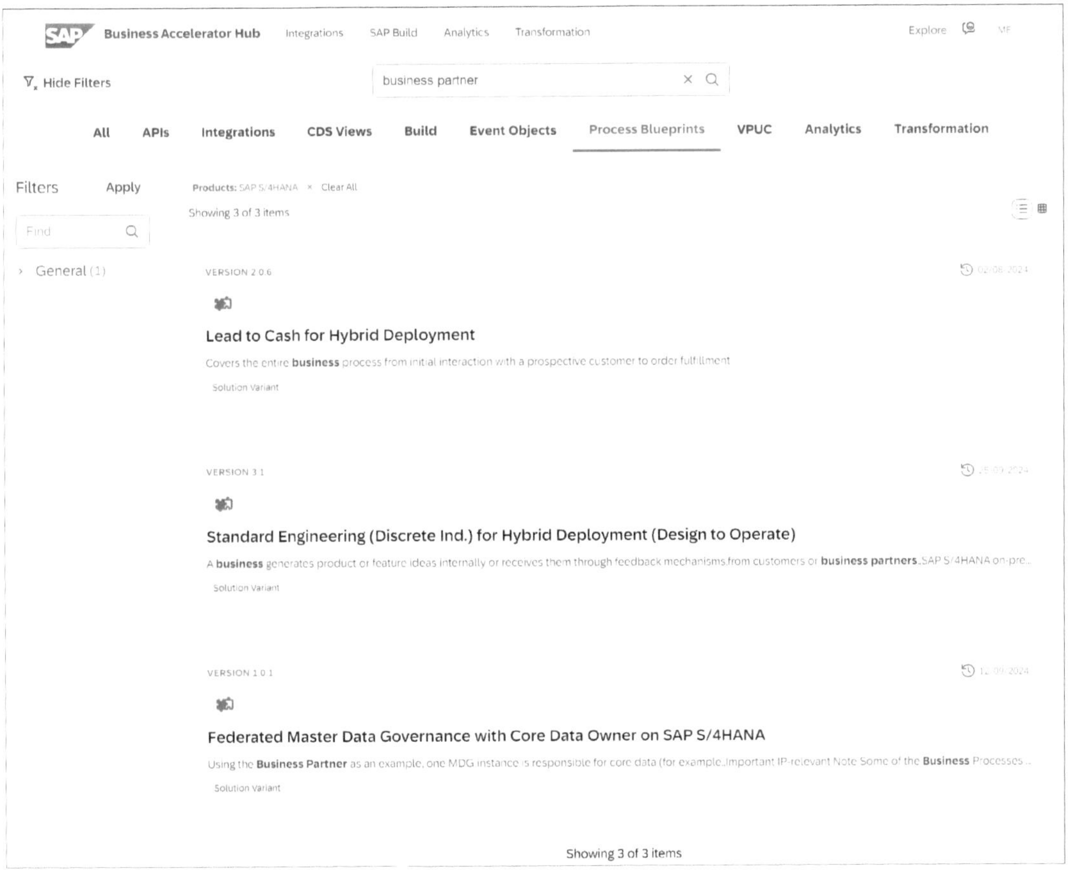

Abbildung 14.5 Vorlagen für die Umsetzung von Geschäftsprozessen

14

Business-Partner-API

Nach diesem kurzen Ausflug in die Geschäftsprozesse im SAP Business Accelerator Hub wählen wir nun den Eintrag **Business Partner (A2X)** aus der in Abbildung 14.4 gezeigten Liste, der zur in Abbildung 14.6 dargestellten Übersichtsseite der *Business-Partner-API* führt. Dieser Dienst mit dem technischen Namen `API_BUSINESS_PARTNER` ermöglicht Benutzern das Erstellen, Anzeigen, Aktualisieren und Löschen von Daten in Bezug auf Geschäftspartner, Lieferanten und Kunden über einen API-Aufruf.

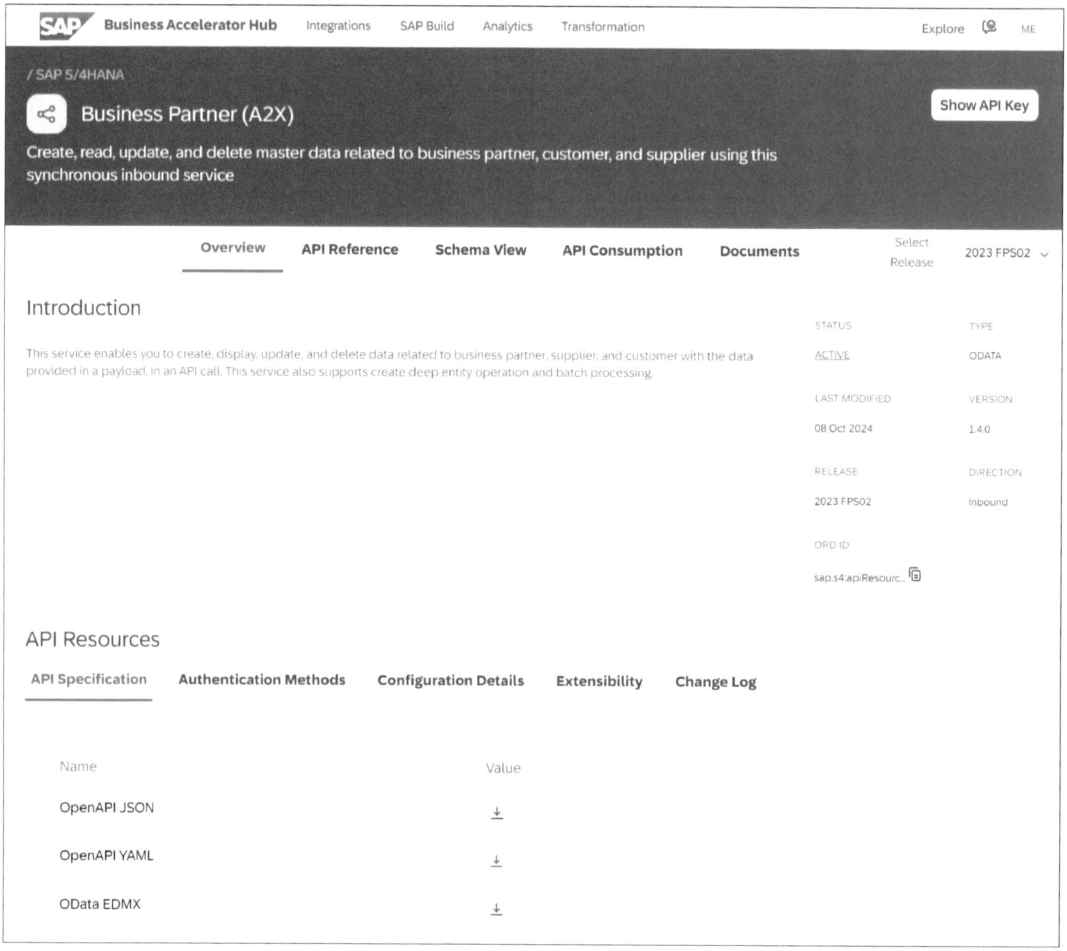

Abbildung 14.6 Übersichtsseite des Service »Business Partner (A2X)«

Dokumentation des Service

Neben einer kurzen Einführung in den Service finden Sie auf dieser Seite im Bereich **API Resources** eine in fünf Bereiche untergliederte Dokumentation des Diensts. Über die *API-Spezifikation* erhalten Sie die Dokumentation zur API. Beispielsweise können Sie hier die OData-Servicemetadaten über den Downloadlink **OData EDMX** beziehen. Der Bereich **Authentication Methods** liefert uns Informationen darüber, welche Authentifizierungsmöglichkeiten der Service bietet bzw. welche verwendet werden müssen.

Wählt man die Registerkarte **Configuration Details** erhält man Informationen dazu, wie der Service konfiguriert bzw. bereitgestellt wird. Abbildung 14.7 zeigt die Konfigurationsdetails. Dieser Service wird in keiner von der SAP bereitgestellten Testumgebung bereitgestellt. Im Eintrag **PRODUCTION**

URL liefert die Dokumentation den Hinweis, wie man auf einem kundeneigenen System auf den Service zugreifen kann.

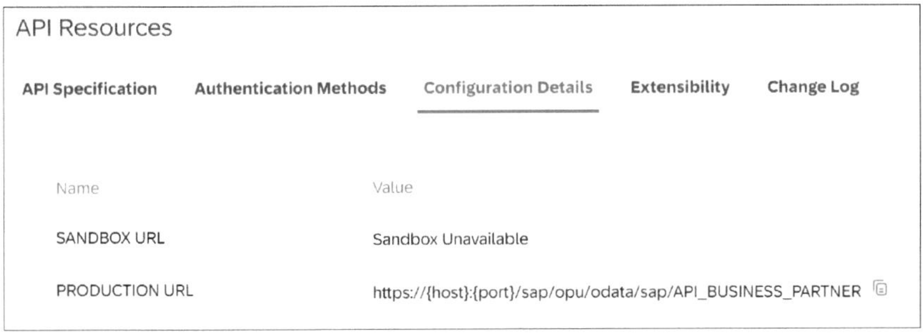

Abbildung 14.7 Konfigurationsdetails des Diensts

Daraus und aus den Konfigurationsdetails ergibt sich, dass der Service `API_BUSINESS_PARTNER` auf dem SAP-S/4HANA-System des Kunden aktiviert und bereitgestellt werden muss, damit man ihn in einem kundeneigenen Integrationsszenario verwenden kann. Abbildung 14.8 zeigt den im SAP-S/4HANA-System aktivierten und bereitgestellten Service in der Transaktion /IWFND/MAINT_SERVICE.

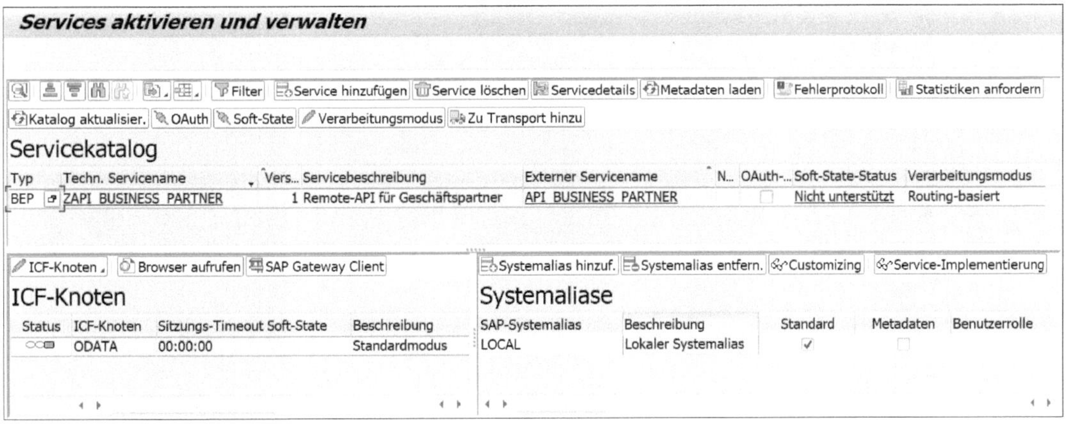

Abbildung 14.8 Aktivierter Dienst API_BUSINESS_PARTNER in einem SAP-S/4HANA-System

API-Referenz

`API_BUSINESS_PARTNER` ist ein sehr umfangreicher Dienst und bietet eine Vielzahl von Möglichkeiten, um mit dem Geschäftspartner-Objekt zu interagieren. Der Bereich **API Reference** im SAP Business Accelerator Hub listet, wie in Abbildung 14.9 dargestellt, die verschiedenen Operationen auf, die auf den unterschiedlichen Entitäten des Service konsumiert werden können. Auf der linken Seite werden die Entitäten des Service in Klarschrift angezeigt. In Abbildung 14.9 ist die Entität **Business Partner** ausgewählt. Neben der Liste werden die bereitgestellten Interaktionsmöglichkeiten dargestellt.

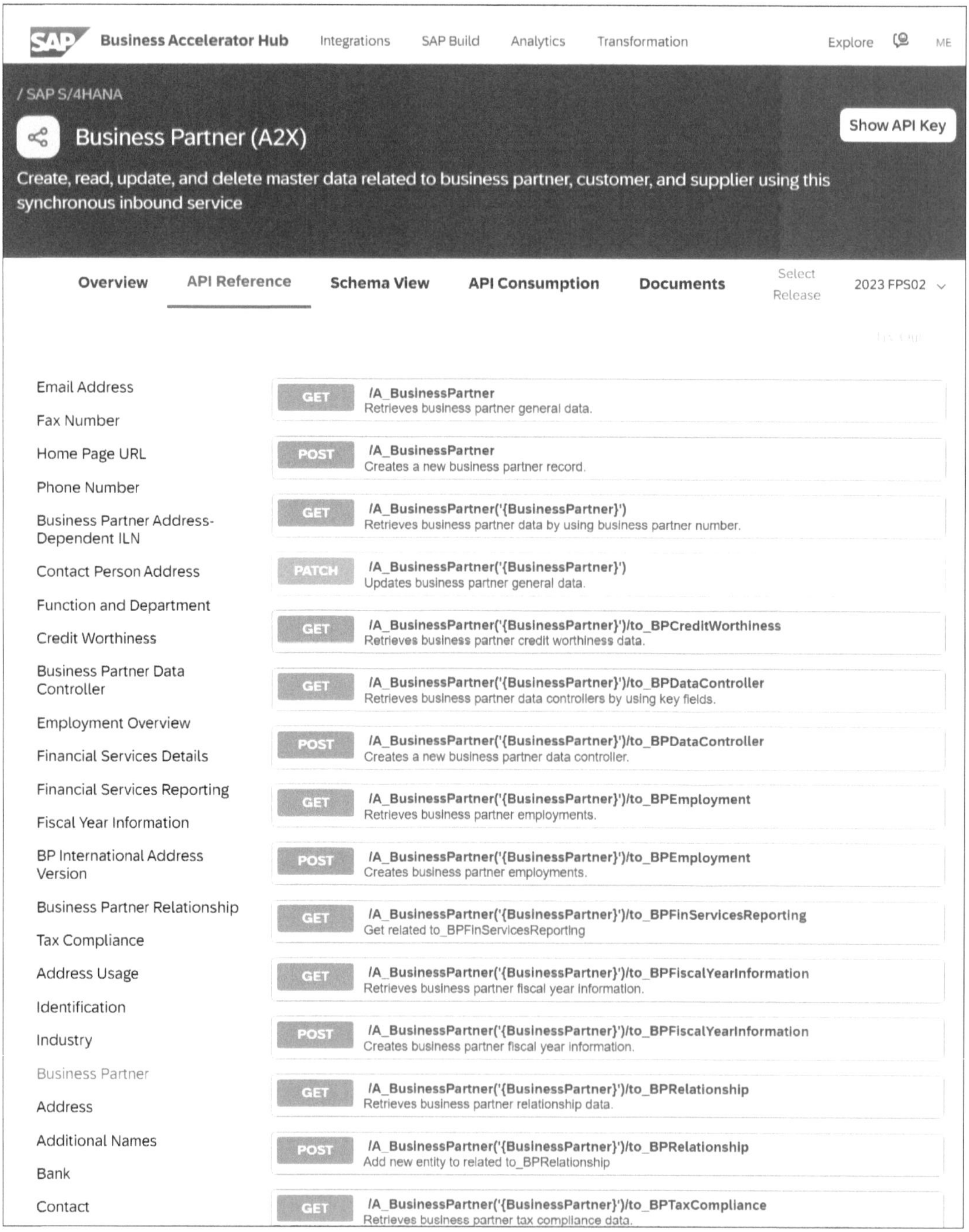

Abbildung 14.9 API-Referenz zum Dienst API_BUSINESS_SERVICE

Test in Transaktion /IWFND/GW_ CLIENT

Auf Basis der in Abbildung 14.9 dargestellten Dokumentation für die Business-Partner-Entität können Sie auf Ihrem SAP-System die dokumentierten Interaktionsmöglichkeiten testen. Den Test können Sie beispielsweise direkt über den Browser oder aber, wie in Abbildung 14.10 gezeigt, über Transaktion /IWFND/GW_CLIENT durchführen. Über diese Transaktion rufen Sie den Gateway Client auf. In das Feld **Request-URI** geben Sie gemäß der Dokumentation die URI »/sap/opu/odata/sap/API_BUSINESS_PARTNER/A_BusinessPartner« ein. Klicken Sie dann auf den Button **Ausführen**. Im Anschluss wird Ihnen die Antwort angezeigt.

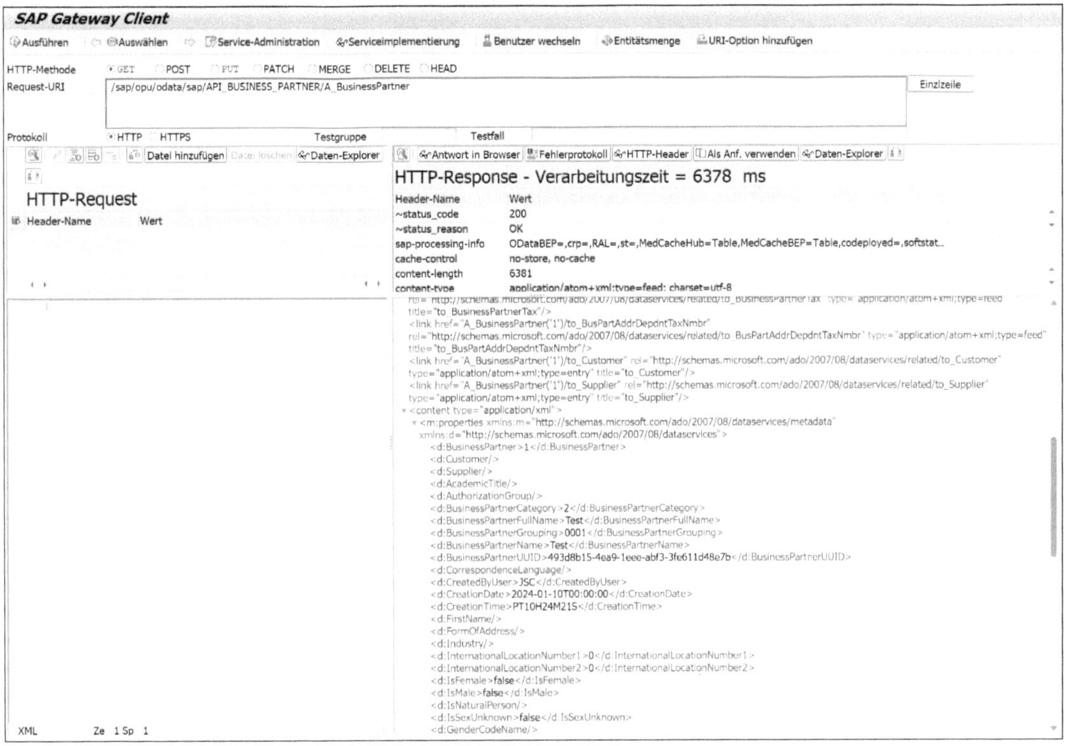

Abbildung 14.10 Auslesen der im SAP-System verfügbaren Business-Partner

14.3 Services konsumieren

Business-Partner-API konsumieren

Nachdem wir uns im vorangegangenen Abschnitt den Dienst **Business Partner (A2X)** etwas genauer angeschaut haben, wenden wir uns in diesem Abschnitt der Konsumierung dieses Diensts zu. Über den Menüeintrag **API Consumption** rufen Sie die Dokumentation der unterschiedlichen Möglichkeiten auf, um mit dem Service in einer Client-Anwendung zu kommunizieren.

Technologien

Wie in Abbildung 14.11 gezeigt, liefert die Dokumentation für den ausgewählten Dienst Informationen zu drei unterschiedlichen Technologien. Im Bereich **ABAP** erhalten Sie Informationen dazu, wie man in SAP S/4HANA Cloud, SAP S/4HANA On-Premise und auf der SAP BTP Interaktionsmöglichkeiten für den Service schaffen kann. Die Dokumentation ist an dieser Stelle allerdings überschaubar. Neben einer allgemeinen Kurzdokumentation finden Sie jeweils einen Link zur entsprechenden Dokumentation für die Generierung von Proxy-Klassen.

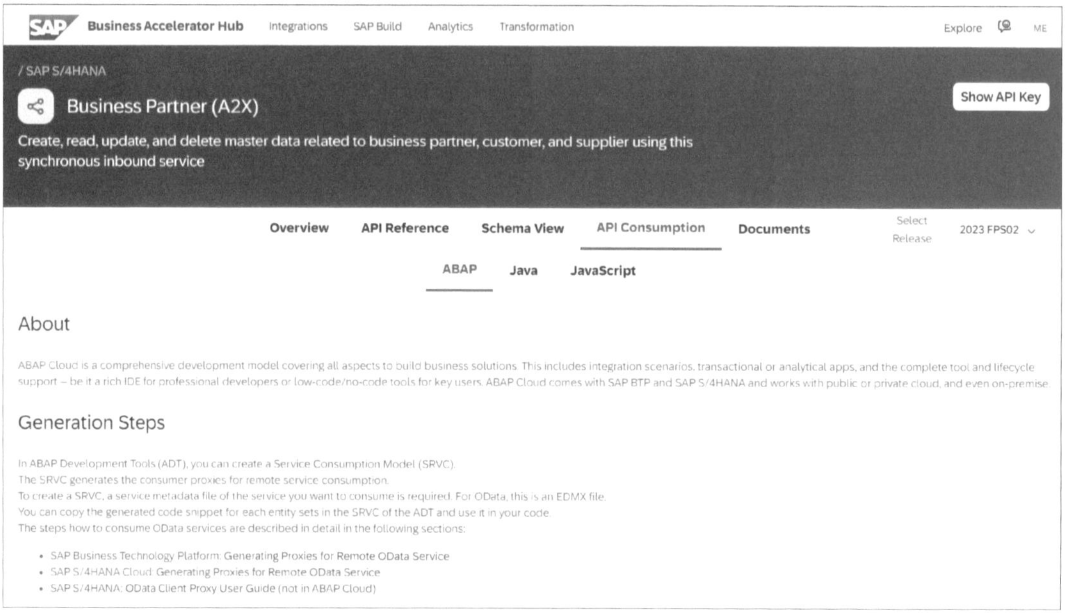

Abbildung 14.11 Konsumentendokumentation

In den Bereichen **Java** und **JavaScript** finden Sie dagegen detaillierte Schrittanweisungen, wie man in der jeweiligen Programmiersprache und mit dem jeweiligen SAP Cloud SDK einen entsprechenden Client implementieren kann. Abbildung 14.12 zeigt beispielsweise die Anleitung für die Verwendung des SAP Cloud SDK für JavaScript.

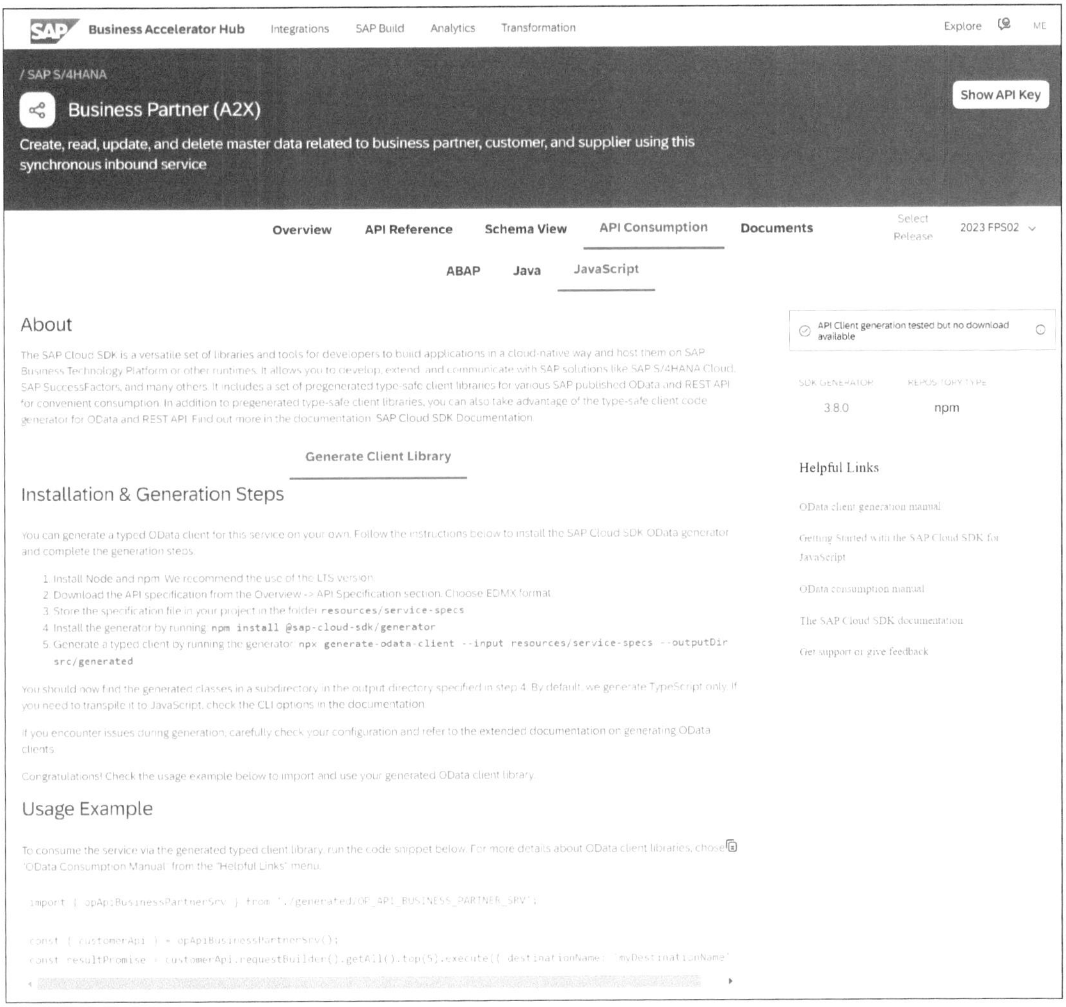

Abbildung 14.12 JavaScript-Dokumentation für die Implementierung eines Clients

14.3.1 Anlegen eines CAP-Projekts

Projekt »businesssapihub«

Für die folgende Implementierung eines Konsumenten der Business-Partner-API nutzen wir das im gleichnamigen Kapitel 13 eingeführte SAP Cloud Application Programming Model (CAP). Starten Sie dazu zunächst den in Abschnitt 13.2.1, »Entwicklung im SAP Business Application Studio«, angelegten Dev Space und legen Sie hier, wie im gleichen Abschnitt beschrieben, ein neues CAP-Projekt an. Vergeben Sie den Projektnamen »businesssapihub«. Abbildung 14.13 zeigt die Projektdetails.

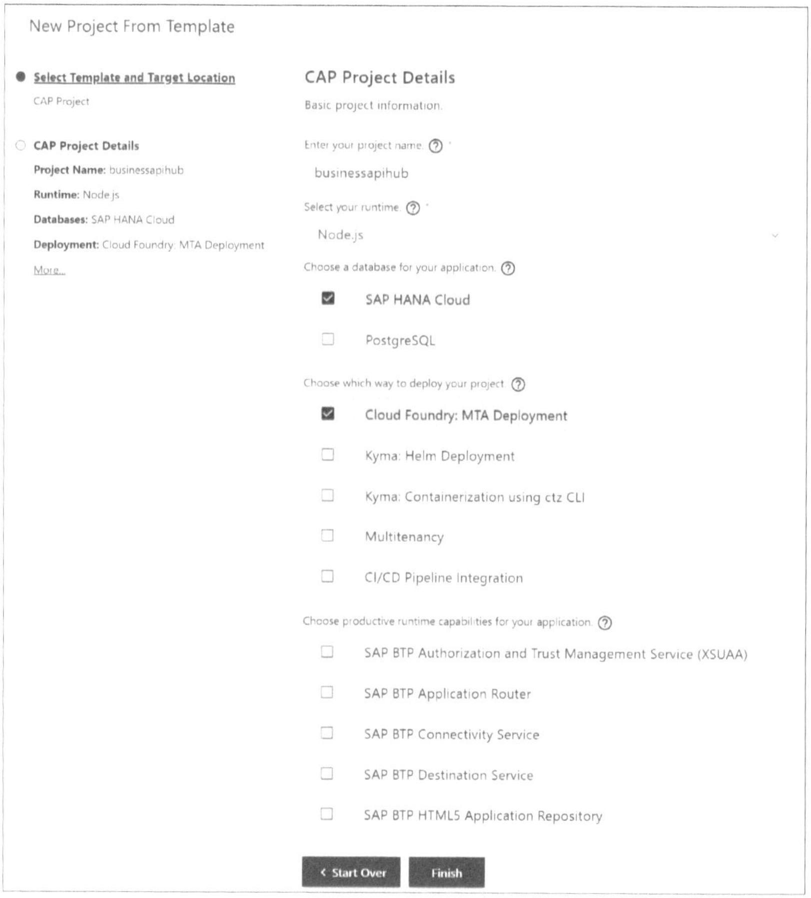

Abbildung 14.13 Anlegen eines neuen CAP-Projekts

CDS-Datei anlegen

Nachdem das Projekt angelegt ist, müssen wir eine CDS-Datei für die Serviceimplementierung anlegen. Hierzu wählen Sie den Ordner **srv** in der Projektstruktur aus und rufen im Kontextmenü den Eintrag **New File** auf. Nennen Sie die Datei »businessapihub.cds«, und bestätigen Sie mit [↵].

Implementierung in TypeScript

Für die Implementierung der eigentlichen Servicefunktion nutzen wir die Programmiersprache *TypeScript*, die auf JavaScript basiert. Wir legen daher als Nächstes und ebenfalls im **srv**-Ordner unseres Projekts eine Datei mit dem Namen »businessapihub.ts« an. Um bereits eine rudimentäre TypeScript-Konfiguration zu erhalten, geben Sie im Anschluss in das Terminal den Befehl `cds add typescript` ein, wie in Abbildung 14.14 gezeigt. Als Ergebnis wird im Projektverzeichnis eine Datei **tsconfig.json** eingefügt. Damit wir die TypeScript-Implementierungsartefakte in unserem CAP-Projekt zur Laufzeit nutzen können, müssen wir noch die TypeScript-Ausführung installieren. Dies geschieht über den Befehl `npm i -g tsx`.

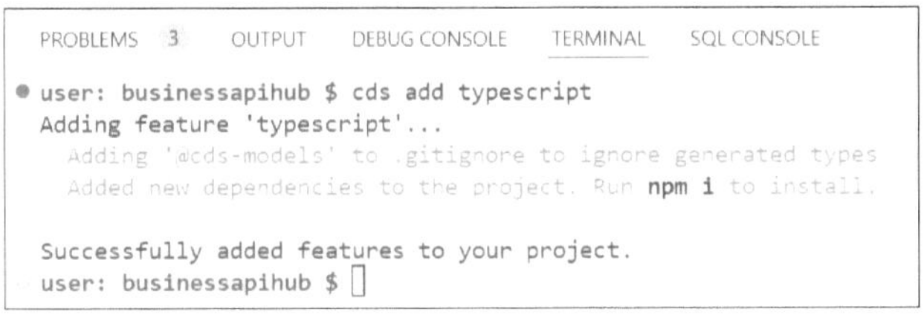

Abbildung 14.14 Hinzufügen von TypeScript über das Terminal

Im Anschluss fügen wir Sie über den folgenden Befehl Abhängigkeiten zu SAP HANA, Multi-Target Applications (MTA) im SAP BTP, Cloud Foundry Environment, dem Authorization and Trust Management Service (XSUAA) und dem SAP Application Router (`approuter`) zu unserer Anwendung hinzu:

```
cds add hana,mta,xsuaa,approuter --for production
```

Was es mit MTA im SAP BTP, Cloud Foundry Environment auf sich hat, erklären wir in Abschnitt 15.2.2, »Nachrichten an SAP Event Mesh senden«.

14.3.2 Generierung der Proxyklassen

SAP Cloud SDK Generator

Damit man einen OData-Service aus der CAP-Anwendung heraus nutzen kann, müssen auf der Client-Seite entsprechende Proxy-Klassen generiert werden. Im *SAP Cloud SDK* wird für diesen Zweck ein Generator angeboten. Diesen fügen Sie über den folgenden Befehl zu unserem Projekt hinzu:

```
npm install @sap-cloud-sdk/generator
```

Abschließend setzen Sie noch den Befehl `npm update --package-lock-only` ab und aktualisieren damit nur die Datei **package-lock.json**, ohne die eigentlichen Pakete in den Dateien **node_modules** oder **package.json** zu verändern.

API-Spezifikation laden

Damit der Generator die Proxy-Klassen generieren kann, müssen Sie die API-Spezifikation aus dem SAP Business Accelerator Hub laden und in unserem Projekt ablegen. Hierfür legen Sie zunächst über die Funktion **New Folder** einen neuen Ordner »resources« in unserem Projekt an. Nachdem dieser Ordner angelegt ist, fügen Sie einen Unterordner mit dem Namen »service-specs« ein.

Nun laden Sie über die URL *https://api.sap.com/api/OP_API_BUSINESS_PARTNER_SRV/overview* die Schnittstellendatei im EDMX-Format auf Ihren lokalen Rechner (siehe Abbildung 14.15). Sobald die Datei sich auf Ihrem lokalen Rechner befindet, kopieren Sie diese per Drag-and-drop in den zuvor im Projekt angelegten Unterordner **service-specs**.

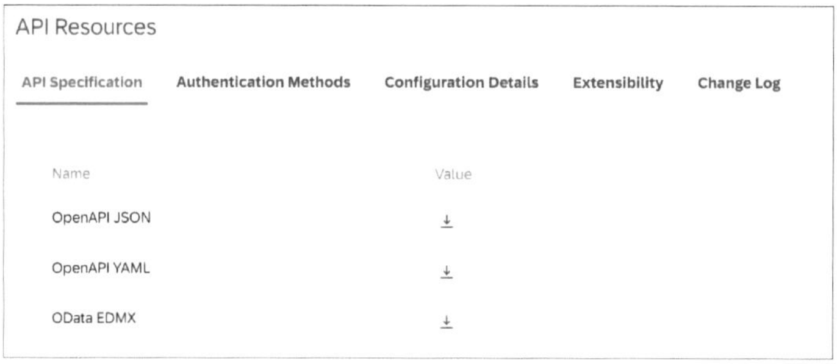

Abbildung 14.15 Schnittstellenbeschreibungen des Service »Business Partner (A2X)«

Proxy-Klasse generieren

Mit dem folgenden Befehl starten Sie nun die Generierung der Proxy-Klasse:

```
npx generate-odata-client --input resources/service-specs --outputDir
src/generated
```

Abbildung 14.16 zeigt den abgesetzten Befehl sowie die Projektstruktur, nachdem die Proxy-Klassen generiert wurden. Wie man in der Projektstruktur erkennen kann, enthält das Projekt nun einen Ordner **src**. In diesem Ordner liegen die Proxy-Klassen.

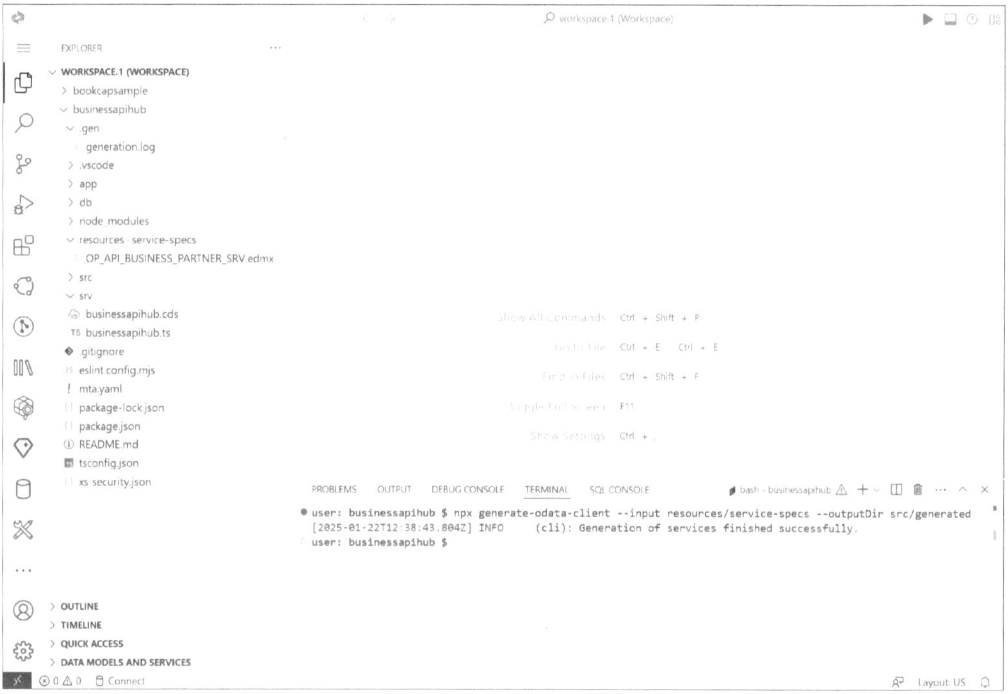

Abbildung 14.16 Projektstruktur nach dem Generieren der Proxy-Klassen

14.3.3 Implementierung des Konsumenten

Serviceschnittstelle

Nachdem die Proxy-Klassen generiert sind, können wir mit der Implementierung der Serviceklassen fortfahren. In unserer Serviceimplementierung möchten wir einen Service mit dem Namen `businesspartner` anbieten. Dieser soll eine Funktion `fetchPartner` bereitstellen. Für die Implementierung öffnen Sie zunächst die Datei **businessapihub.cds**. Im Anschluss implementieren Sie die Serviceschnittstelle wie folgt:

```
service businesspartner {
  function fetchPartner () returns String;
}
```

Nachdem die Schnittstelle so weit ausgeprägt ist, öffnen Sie die Datei **businessapihub.ts** und fügen die Implementierung aus Listing 14.1 ein. Es handelt sich zunächst um eine sehr einfache Implementierung. In der Klasse `businesspartner` stellen wir die Funktion `fetchPartner` zur Verfügung. Die Funktion erhält ein Objekt vom Typ `Request`. Den Typ beziehen wir über die CDS-API. Die Funktion `fetchPartner` liefert im Moment lediglich einen einfachen String an den Aufrufer zurück. 14

```
import { Request } from "@sap/cds"

module.exports = class businesspartner {
    fetchPartner(req: Request) {
        return `Hello from BusinessPartnerAPI!`
    }
}
```

Listing 14.1 Serviceimplementierung

Service starten

Im Anschluss an diese rudimentäre Implementierung wechseln Sie erneut in das Terminal und geben den folgenden Befehl zum Start des Service ein:

```
cds-tsx watch --profile hybrid
```

Nach wenigen Augenblicken wird die Anwendung ausgeführt (siehe Abbildung 14.17), und Sie können den Service über einen Klick auf den Button **Open in a New Tab** in einem neuen Browserfenster nutzen.

Im Browserfenster wird zunächst die in Abbildung 14.18 dargestellte Willkommensseite angezeigt.

Klicken Sie hier auf die Funktion **fetchPartner()**, erhalten Sie die Antwort von unserer Funktionsimplementierung, wie in Abbildung 14.19 gezeigt.

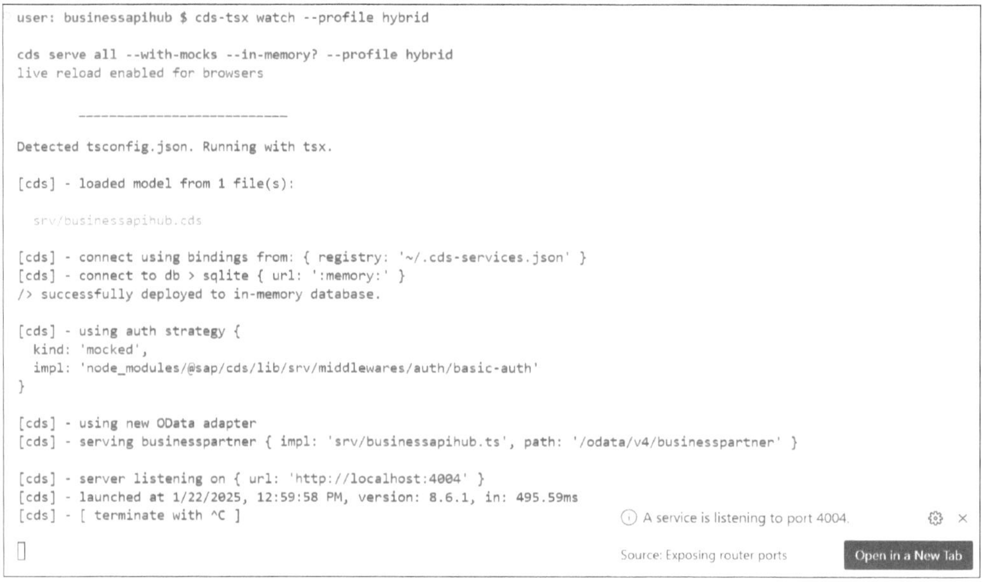

Abbildung 14.17 Terminal mit der ausgeführten Anwendung

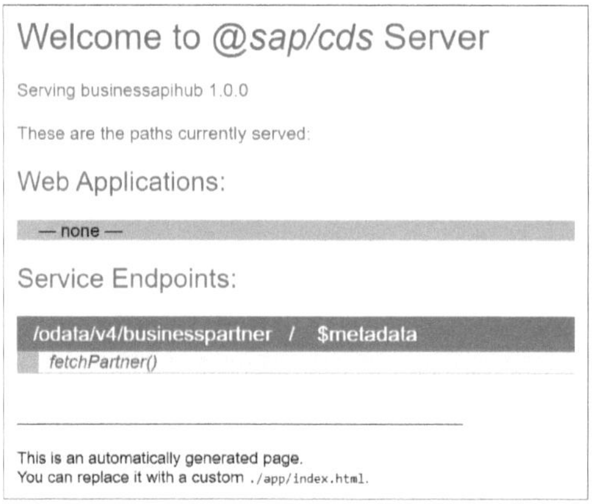

Abbildung 14.18 Willkommensseite des Service

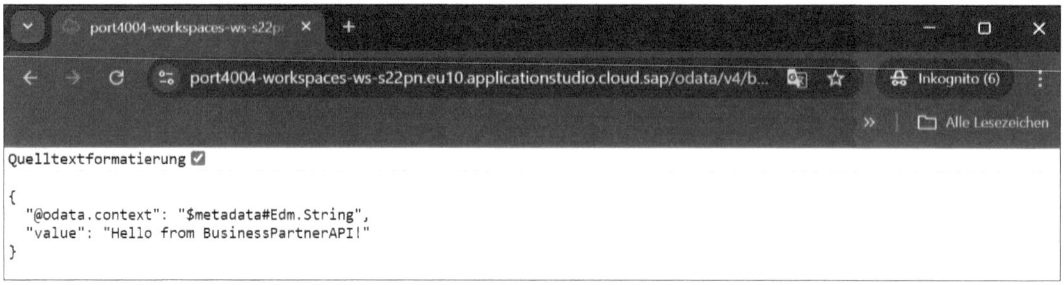

Abbildung 14.19 Antwort der Servicefunktion

Konsumierung über Cloud Connector und Destination

Nachdem wir sichergestellt haben, dass die grundlegende Serviceimplementierung so weit funktionsfähig ist, können wir mit dem nächsten Schritt fortfahren. Wie in Abschnitt 2.2.3, »Einführung in den Cloud Connector«, beschrieben, haben wir zwischen der SAP BTP und unserem SAP-S/4HANA-On-Premise-System eine Verbindung über den Cloud Connector hergestellt. Auf der SAP BTP haben wir hierzu eine Destination mit dem Namen `interfacebookDestination` konfiguriert. Abbildung 14.20 zeigt deren Konfiguration. Diese Konfiguration möchten wir nun in unserer CAP-Anwendung verwenden, um die Business-Partner-API auf unserem SAP-System zu konsumieren.

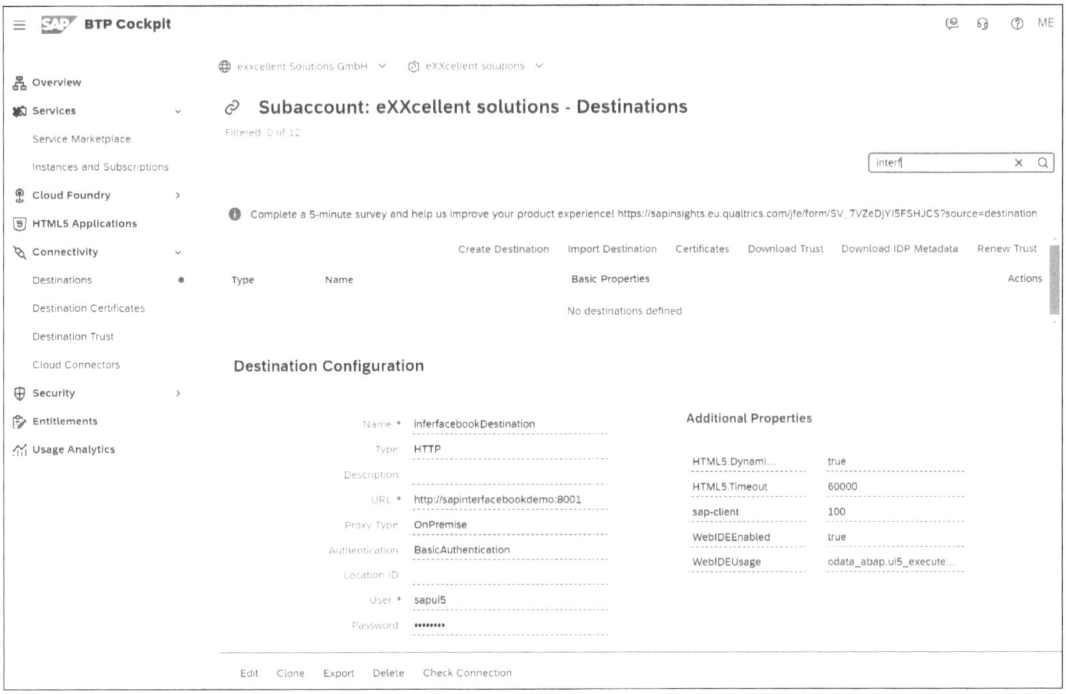

Abbildung 14.20 Konfiguration der Destination »interfacebookDestination«

Business-Partner-API aufrufen

Für den Aufruf der Business-Partner-API erweitern wir die Serviceimplementierung, wie in Listing 14.2 gezeigt. Wir importieren hier zunächst die Klasse `OP_API_BUSINESS_PARTNER_SRV`. Innerhalb der Funktion `fetchPartner` legen wir eine Instanz dieser Klasse an und weisen diese der Variablen `customerAPI` zu. Im weiteren Verlauf rufen wir die Funktion `requestBuilder` auf dem Objekt `customerAPI` auf und setzen einen Request ab.

```
import { Request } from "@sap/cds"
import { opApiBusinessPartnerSrv } from '../src/generated/OP_API_
BUSINESS_PARTNER_SRV'
```

14

```
module.exports = class businesspartner {
    fetchPartner(req: Request) {
        const { customerApi } = opApiBusinessPartnerSrv();
        const resultPromise =
customerApi.requestBuilder().getAll().top(5).execute({
destinationName: 'interfacebookDestination' });

        return `Hello from BusinessPartnerAPI!`
    }
}
```

Listing 14.2 Implementierung des Business-Partner-Clients

Im Anschluss setzen wir erneut eine Anfrage über den noch offenen Browsertab ab. Wir erhalten jedoch keine Antwort durch den Service. Um uns dieses Problem näher zu anzusehen, wechseln wir zurück in das SAP Business Application Studio und schauen uns die Ausgabe im Terminal an. Wie in Abbildung 14.21 zu sehen, erhalten wir eine Fehlermeldung, dass es zwischen unserer Anwendung und dem SAP Destination Service auf der SAP BTP keine Verbindung gibt.

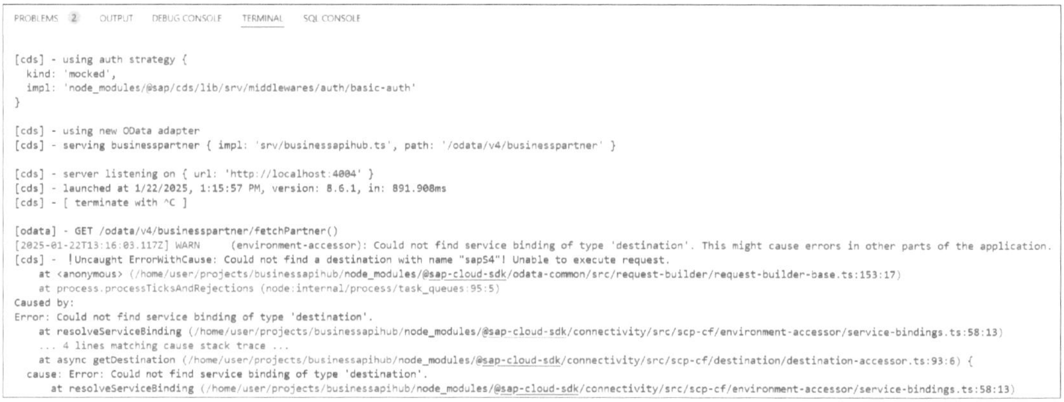

Abbildung 14.21 Fehlermeldung im Terminal

Destination-Service-Binding anlegen

Um den Fehler zu beheben, beenden wir die laufende Session unserer Anwendung mit [Strg] + [C] und geben, wie in Abbildung 14.22 gezeigt, die nötigen Befehle für das Erstellen eines *Destination-Service-Bindings* ein. Mit dem folgenden Befehl legen wir zunächst eine Serviceinstanz mit dem Serviceplan `lite` an:

```
cf create-service destination lite businessapihub-destination
```

Wir geben dieser Instanz den Namen »businessapihub«. Mit dem folgenden Befehl legen wir anschließend einen Serviceschlüssel an:

```
cf create-service-key businessapihub-destination businessapihub-
destination-key
```

Abschließend verbinden wir Serviceinstanz und -schlüssel mit dem folgenden Befehl:

```
cds bind -2 businessapihub-destination: businessapihub-destination-
key
```

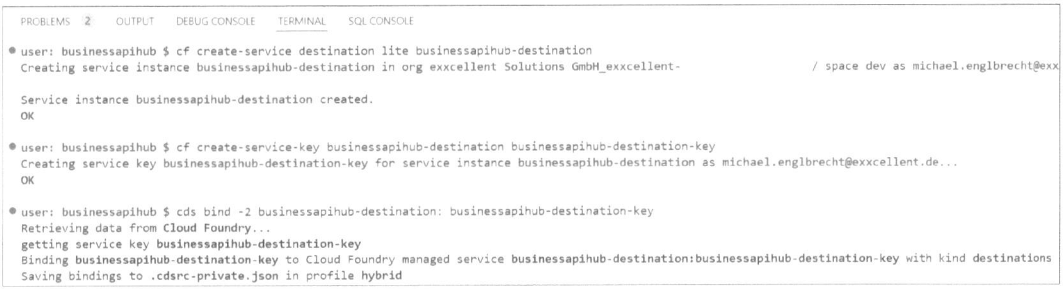

Abbildung 14.22 Erstellen des Destination-Service-Bindings

14

Da der SAP Destination Service lediglich Zugriff auf Verbindungsinformationen ermöglicht und selbst keine Verbindung aufbauen kann, benötigen wir zusätzlich eine Instanz des SAP Connectivity Service. Wie Sie aus Abbildung 14.23 ersehen können, folgt die Erstellung dieser Instanz dem gleichen Muster.

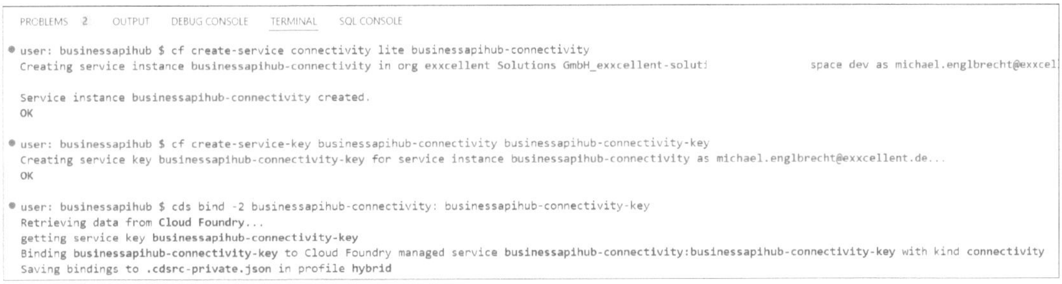

Abbildung 14.23 Erstellen des Connectivity-Service-Bindings

Nachdem wir die Bindings für die beiden Dienste angelegt haben, können wir die Instanzen der beiden Dienste im Cloud Foundry Space dev auf der SAP BTP sehen (siehe Abbildung 14.24). Beide Serviceinstanzen werden hier im Status **Created** angezeigt.

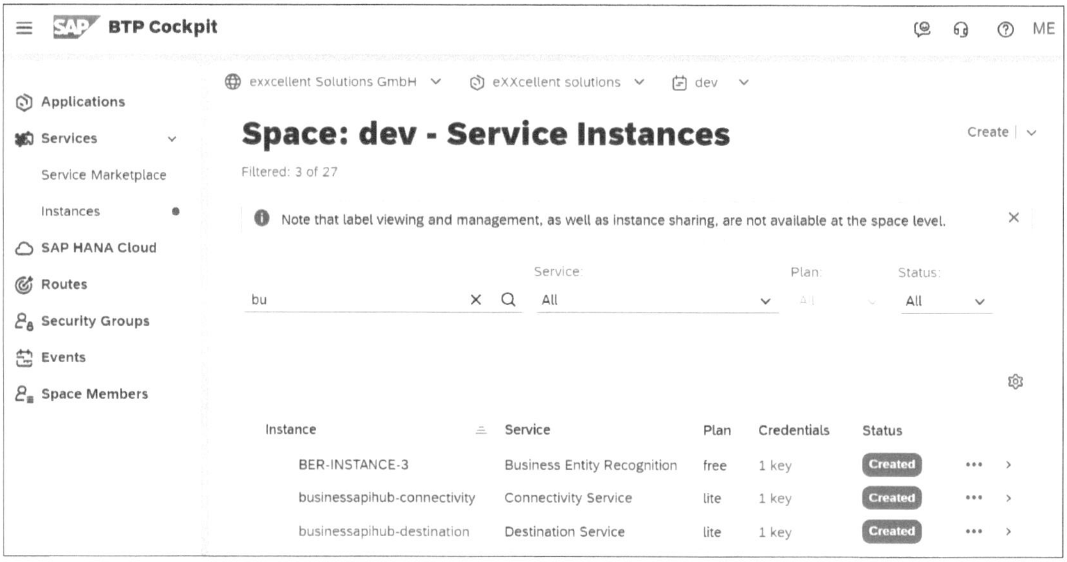

Abbildung 14.24 Serviceinstanzen im Space »dev«

Verbindungsmanagement

Neben der Erstellung der Bindings müssen wir zusätzlich auch das Verbindungsmanagement implementieren. Das SAP Business Application Studio benötigt hierzu die in Listing 14.3 gezeigte Konfiguration in der Datei **package.json**.

```
"requires": {
   "[production]": {
     "auth": "xsuaa",
      "db": "hana"
   },
   "OP_API_BUSINESS_PARTNER_SRV": {
      "kind": "odata-v2",
      "model": "srv/external/OP_API_BUSINESS_PARTNER_SRV",
      "Credentials": {
         "destination": "interfacebook",
         "path": "/sap/opu/odata/sap/API_BUSINESS_PARTNER",
         "requestTimeout": 30000
      }
    }
  }
```

Listing 14.3 Konfiguration des Verbindungsmanagements in der Datei »package.json«

Proxy-Konfiguration

Gemäß SAP-Hinweis 3112360 ist es zusätzlich noch erforderlich, im Wurzelverzeichnis des Projekts eine Proxy-Konfiguration zu hinterlegen. Hierzu legen Sie eine Datei mit der Endung **.env** (ohne Dateinamen) an und fügen die in Listing 14.4 gezeigte Konfiguration ein. Das Attribut `name` enthält den Namen der Destination, die wir für die Kommunikation mit dem Backend nutzen.

```
destination = [{
    "name":"interfacebook",
    "proxyHost":"localhost",
    "proxyPort":8887,
    "url":http://interfacebook.dest
}]
```

Listing 14.4 Proxy-Konfiguration im SAP Business Application Studio

Destinationen neu laden

Im nächsten Schritt laden wir die Destinationskonfigurationen neu. Hierzu öffnen Sie ein Terminal und geben den Befehl `curl http://localhost:8887/reload` ein (siehe Abbildung 14.25).

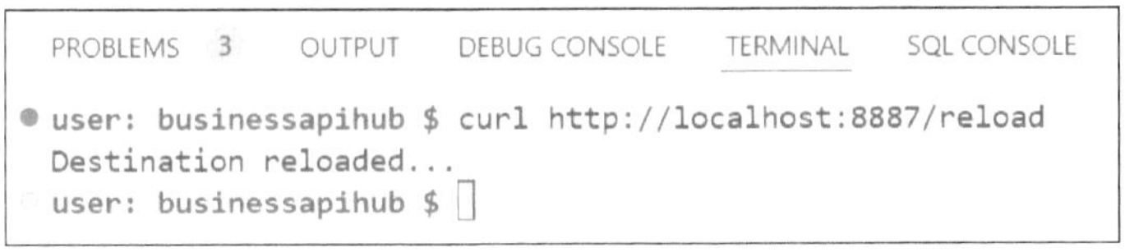

Abbildung 14.25 Neuladen der Destination

Verbindung testen

Um zu testen, ob die Verbindung aus dem SAP Business Application Studio in Richtung des auf dem SAP-S/4HANA-System on-premise implementierten OData-Service korrekt funktioniert, können Sie für die Destination `interfacebook` den folgenden Befehl im Terminal absetzen:

```
curl https://interfacebook.dest /sap/opu/odata/sap/API_BUSINESS_
PARTNER/A_BusinessPartner?%24top=5
```

Abbildung 14.26 zeigt das Ergebnis der Anfrage.

Im Anschluss starten Sie unseren Service im Terminal mit dem folgenden Befehl:

```
cds-tsx watch --profile hybrid
```

Abbildung 14.27 zeigt die Ausgabe des Befehls. Nachdem die Anwendung gestartet wurde, können wir diese über die URL *http://localhost:4004* aufrufen.

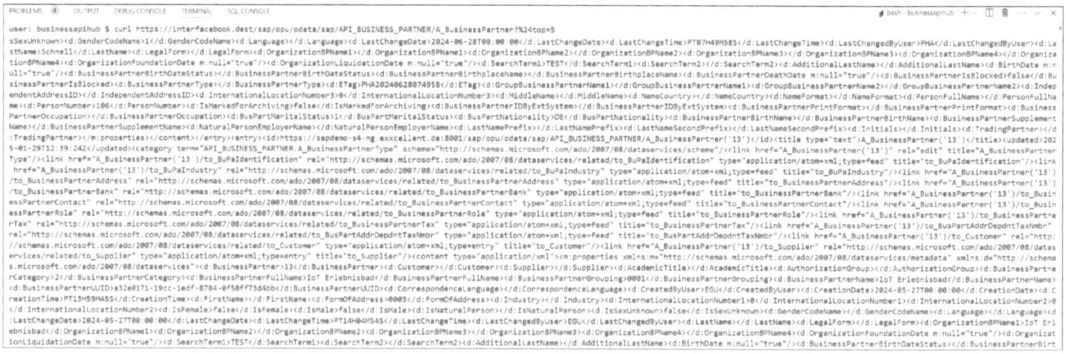

Abbildung 14.26 Ausführung des »curl«-Befehls

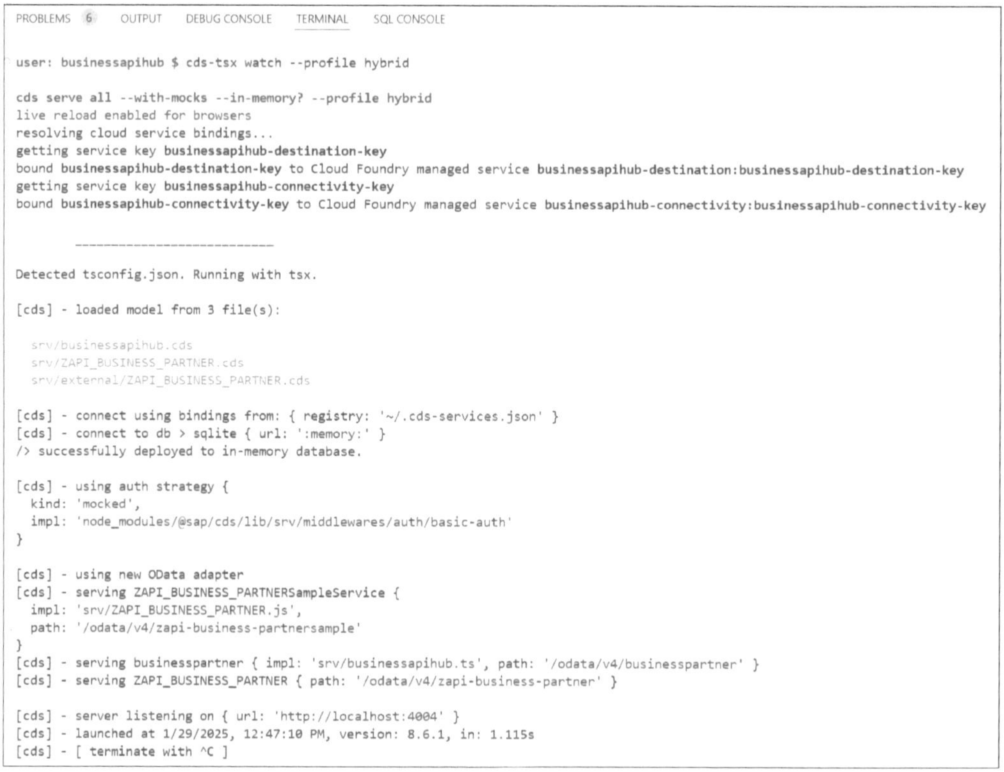

Abbildung 14.27 Ausführung des Service

14.4 Nutzung des Service Centers im SAP Business Application Studio

Neben der Möglichkeit, den im vorangehenden Abschnitt beschriebenen Proxy-Generator zu verwenden, bietet das SAP Business Application Studio zusätzlich die Möglichkeit, einen Client für einen Service generieren zu lassen. Entweder kann dazu direkt ein Client-Projekt angelegt oder die Client-Klasse in ein bestehendes CAP-Projekt eingefügt werden.

»Business Partner (A2X)« in SAP S/4HANA Cloud

In diesem Abschnitt möchten wir diese Möglichkeit zeigen. Wir wollen in diesem Beispiel allerdings keinen Service-Proxy für einen On-Premise-Service verwenden, sondern für den Service **Business Partner (A2X)**, der mit SAP S/4HANA Cloud Public Edition verfügbar ist. Die Details zu diesem Service finden Sie im SAP Business Accelerator Hub unter *https://api.sap.com/api/API_BUSINESS_PARTNER/overview*.

Für diesen Service gibt es eine Sandbox-Implementierung. Das bedeutet, dass man den Service direkt im SAP Business Accellerator Hub ausprobieren kann. Hierzu klicken Sie auf der Übersichtsseite auf den Button **Try out**. Sie gelangen so auf die Testseite *https://api.sap.com/api/API_BUSINESS_PARTNER/tryout* (siehe Abbildung 14.28).

14

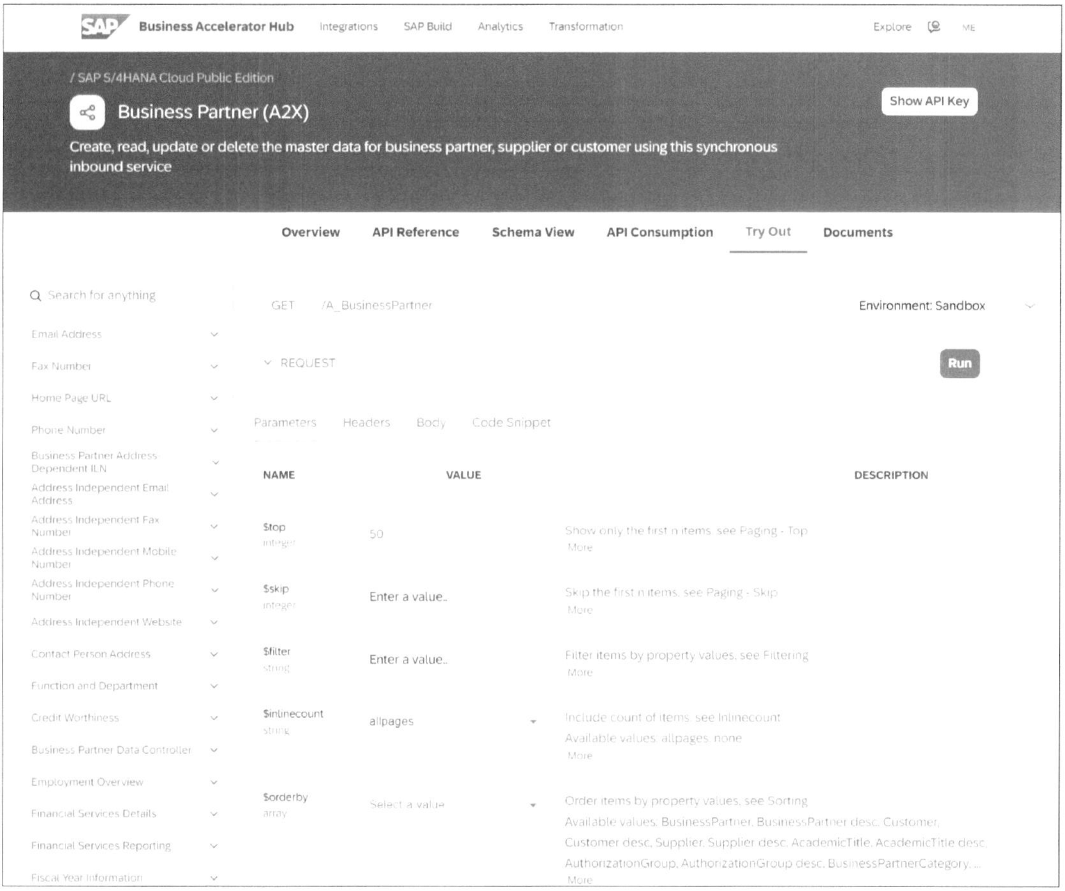

Abbildung 14.28 Einstiegsseite für den Test des Service

Request-Übersicht

Auf der linken Seite werden die durch den Service angebotenen Entitäten aufgelistet. Wählen Sie hier den Eintrag **Business Partner** aus. Sie gelangen zur in Abbildung 14.29 gezeigten Übersicht für den Request.

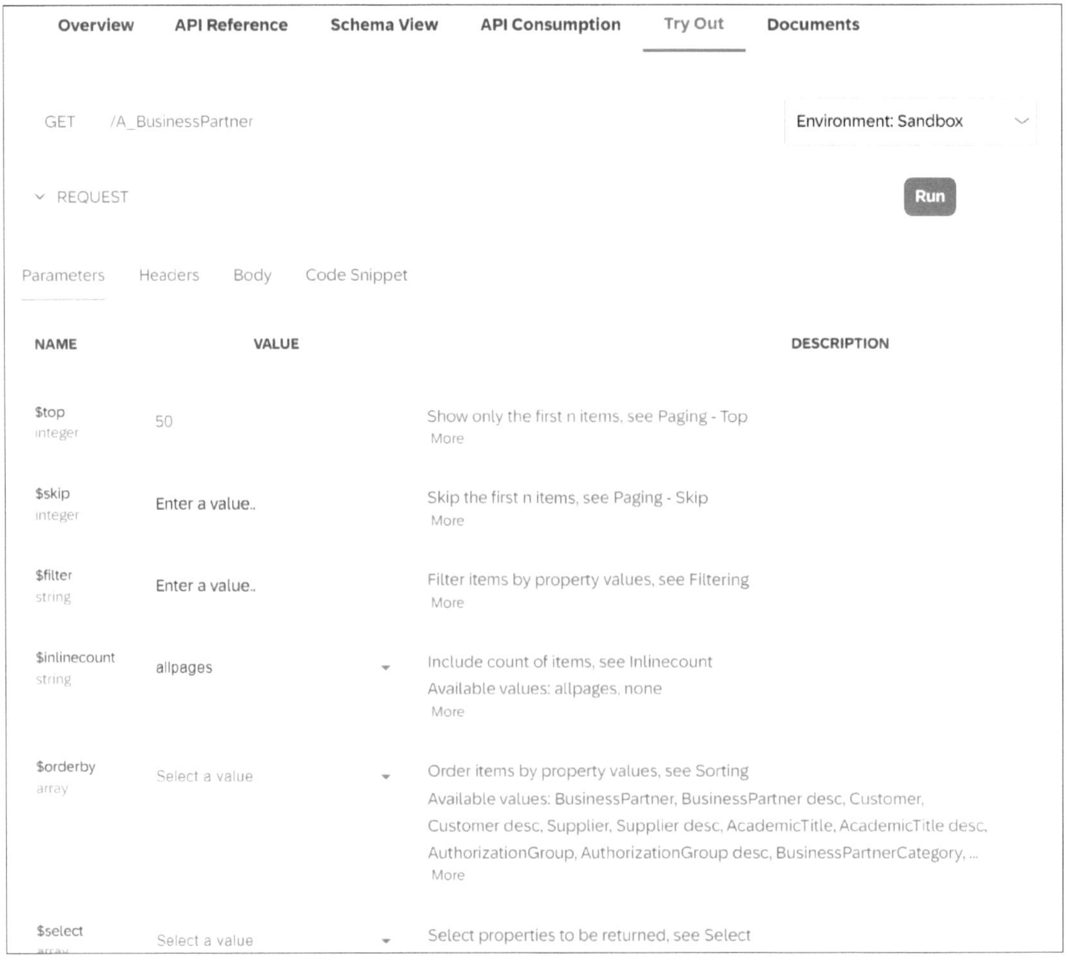

Abbildung 14.29 Request-Übersicht für den Business-Partner

Klicken Sie hier auf den Button **Run**, um den Request auszuführen. Abbildung 14.30 zeigt die Rückantwort des OData-Service. Hier werden die Request-URL sowie die Antwort der Anfrage dargestellt.

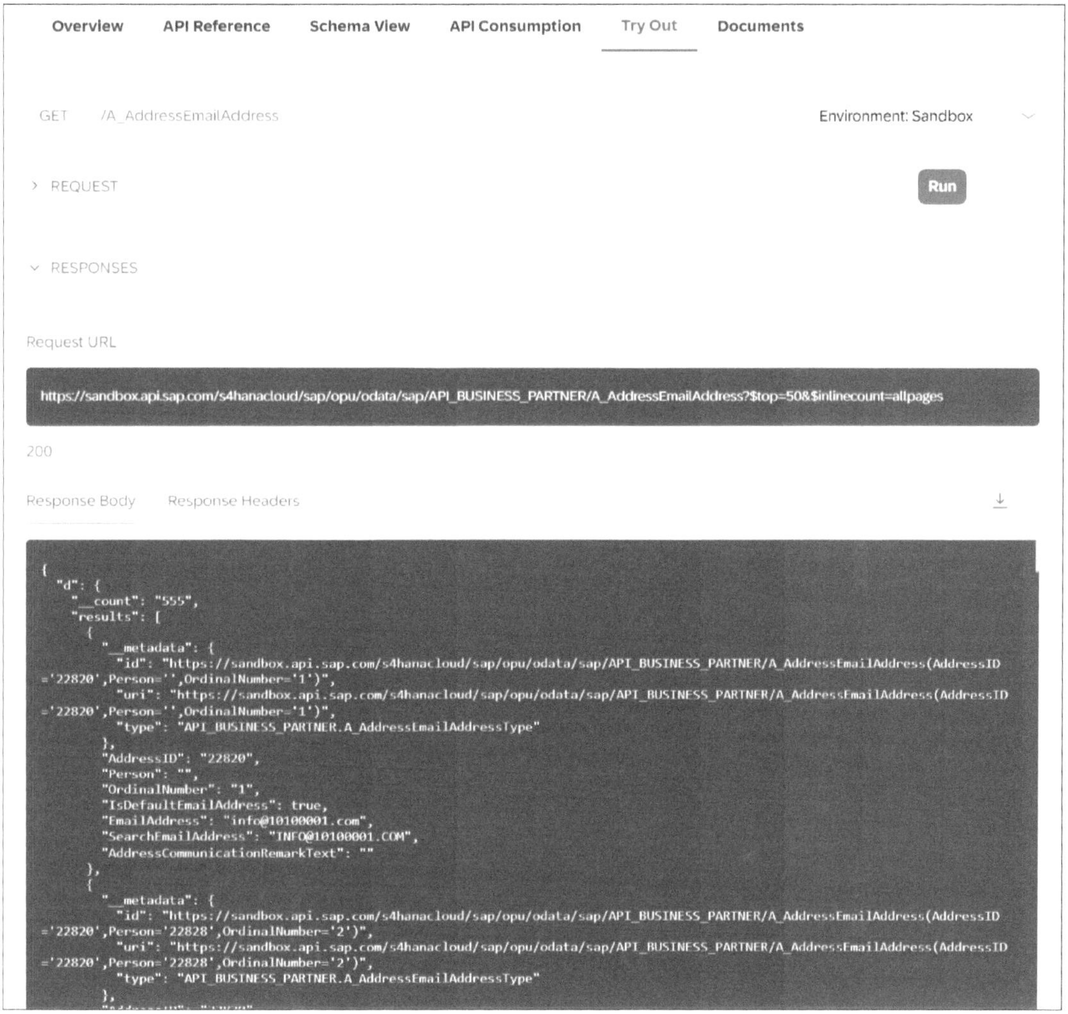

Abbildung 14.30 Antwort der OData-Service-Anfrage

14

Neues CAP-Projekt anlegen

Für die Generierung neuer Client-Proxy-Klassen benötigen wir wieder ein neues CAP-Projekt in unserem SAP Business Application Studio Dev Space. Dieses Projekt legen Sie, wie bereits gezeigt, über den Menüeintrag **New Project from Template** an. Vergeben Sie den Namen »sapbushubdemo« für das Projekt und fügen Sie die standardmäßig sinnvollen Abhängigkeiten zu SAP HANA Cloud, SAP Connectivity Service und SAP Destination Service hinzu (siehe Abbildung 14.31). Im Anschluss klicken Sie auf **Finish**.

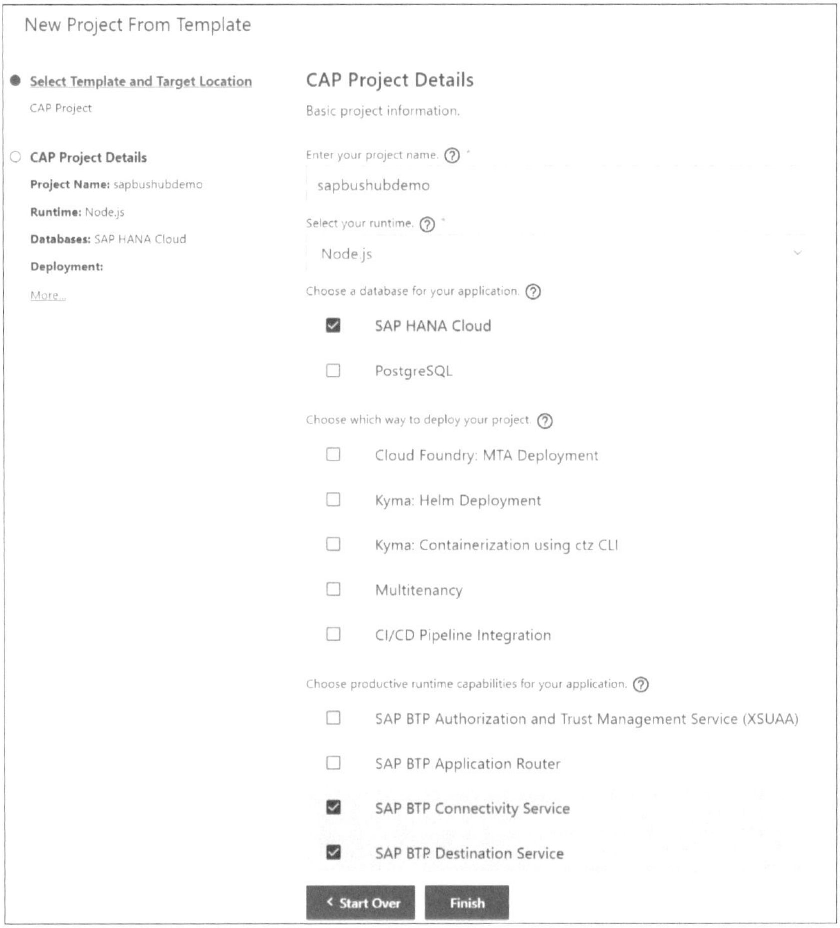

Abbildung 14.31 Anlegen eines neuen CAP-Projekts

Service Center

Für den Zugriff auf Systeme und Schnittstellen bietet das SAP Business Application Studio die Perspektive **SERVICE CENTER**. Über das Icon (**Service Center**) erreichen Sie diese Perspektive. Abbildung 14.32 zeigt den entsprechenden Bereich im SAP Business Application Studio. Über die Optionen **Service**, **Event** und **Business Object/CDS** können Sie vorselektieren, welche Art von Repository-Objekt gesucht wird. Je nach getroffener Auswahl werden im darunterliegenden Bereich unterschiedliche weitere Auswahlmöglichkeiten angeboten.

Provider und Produkt auswählen

Für eine bessere Vergleichbarkeit der Ergebnisse und des Vorgehens verwenden wir auch in diesem Abschnitt den Business-Partner-Service aus den vorangegangenen Abschnitten. Wählen Sie daher die Option **Service** und anschließend aus der Liste der zur Verfügung stehenden Provider (Auswahlmenü **Select a Provider**) den Eintrag **SAP BUSINESS ACCELERATOR HUB** aus. Im Anschluss wählen Sie im Auswahlmenü **Select Product** den Eintrag **SAP S/4HANA Cloud Public Edition** aus. Wir erhalten die in Abbildung 14.33 gezeigte Auswahl an Paketen.

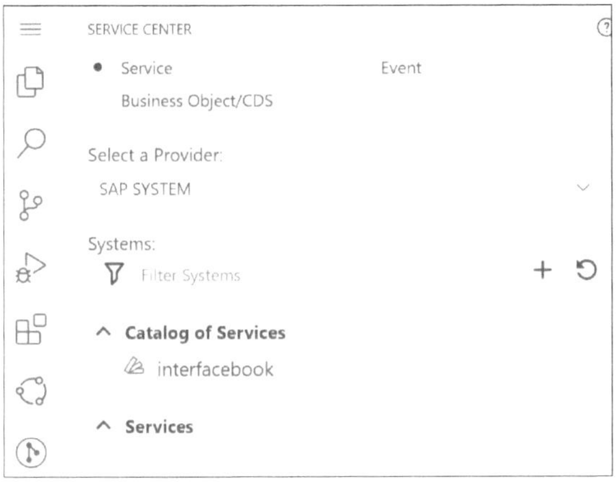

Abbildung 14.32 Service Center im SAP Business Application Studio

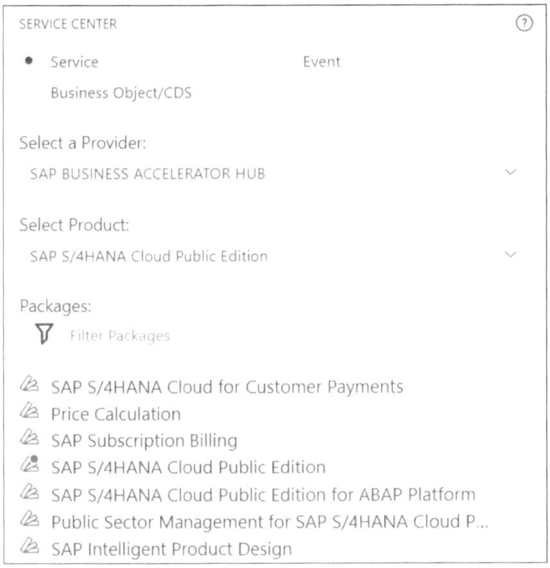

Abbildung 14.33 Auswahlbild im Service Center

Da es unser Ziel ist, einen Service von einem SAP-S/4HANA-On-Premise-System zu konsumieren, wählen Sie unter **Packages** den Eintrag **SAP S/4HANA** aus. Im Anschluss filtern Sie die Liste der verfügbaren Service, wie in Abbildung 14.34 gezeigt, über die Eingabe des Filterbegriffs »busi«. Sie erhalten die in Abbildung 14.34 gezeigte, reduzierte Auswahlliste.

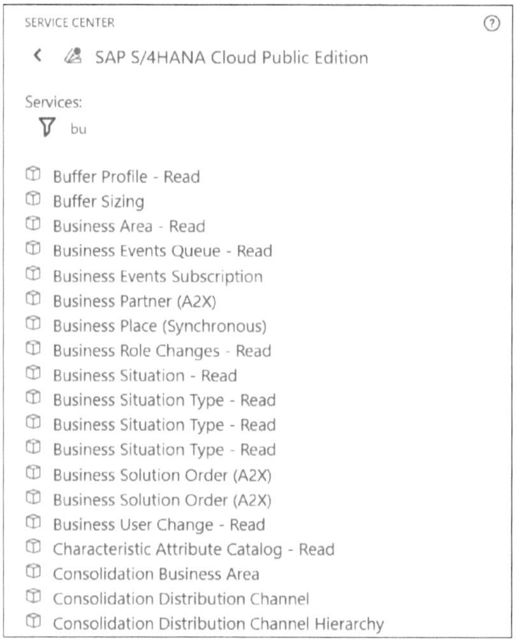

Abbildung 14.34 Gefilterte Serviceliste

Aus dieser Liste wählen Sie den Eintrag **Business Partner (A2X)** aus und erhalten die in Abbildung 14.35 gezeigte Benutzerabfrage. Geben Sie hier Ihren S-User ein und bestätigen Sie die Eingabe. Als Nächstes geben Sie Ihr Passwort ein und bestätigen diese Eingabe ebenfalls.

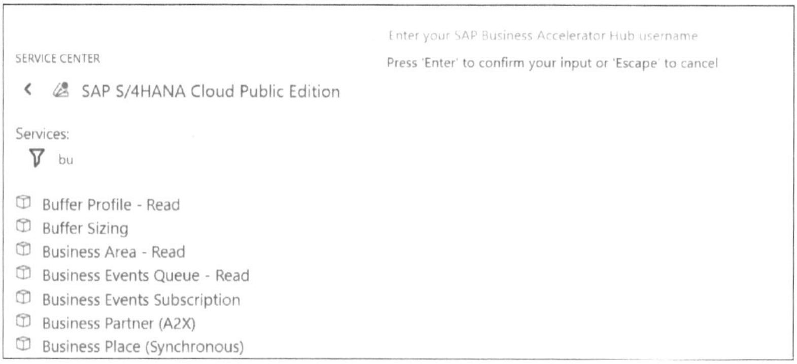

Abbildung 14.35 Abfrage von Benutzernamen und Passwort

[+]

Passwort für den S-User zurücksetzen

Scheinbar gab es zum Zeitpunkt des Schreibens beim Zugriff auf die Dienste *accounts.sap.com* und *account.sap.com* Probleme beim Synchronisieren des Passworts. Dies kann dazu führen, dass die Anmeldung am SAP Business Application Studio fehlschlägt. Uns hat das Zurücksetzen des Passworts für *accounts.sap.com* unter *https://accounts.sap.com/ui/protected/profilemanagement* geholfen. In der SAP Community berichten auch andere Benutzer von diesem Problem. Auch Ihnen half es, das Passwort zurückzusetzen.

Nachdem Sie Ihr Passwort eingegeben haben, erhalten Sie eine Übersicht über die Eigenschaften und Strukturen des Diensts (siehe Abbildung 14.32).

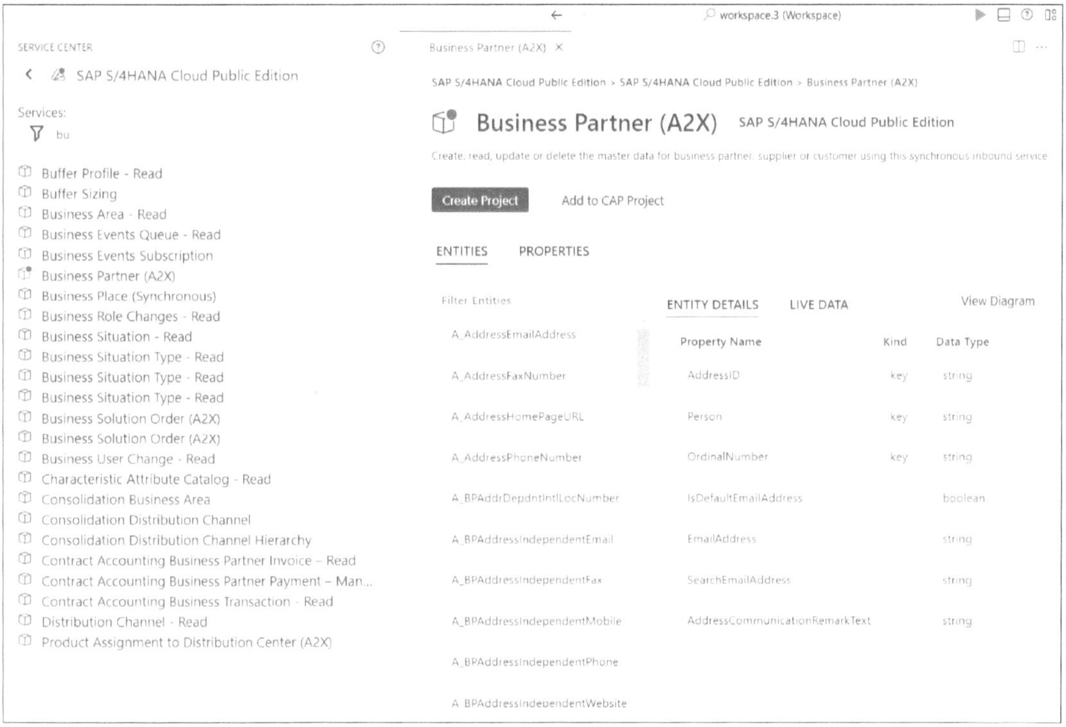

Abbildung 14.36 Übersicht über den Service »Business Partner (A2X)«

14

Service zu CAP-Projekt hinzufügen

Als Nächstes klicken Sie auf den Button **Add to CAP Project**. Im daraufhin erscheinenden Assistenten können Sie das CAP-Projekt auswählen, zu dem Sie die Client-Proxy-Klassen hinzufügen möchten. Nachdem Sie sichergestellt haben, dass hier das zuvor von uns angelegte CAP-Projekt ausgewählt ist, ändern Sie im Bereich **Do you want to add a sample service?** die Auswahl von **No** zu **Yes** und wählen aus der Liste der angebotenen Entitäten die Entität **A_BusinessPartner** aus (siehe Abbildung 14.37). Im Anschluss klicken Sie auf **Add**.

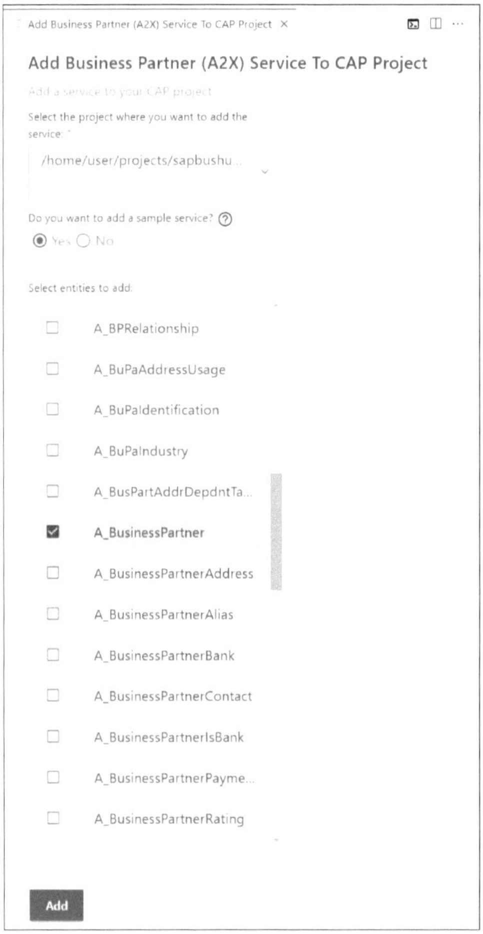

Abbildung 14.37 Projekt und Entität auswählen

Erweiterte Projektstruktur

Nachdem der Generator die entsprechenden Dateien generiert und unserem Projekt hinzugefügt hat, wechseln Sie zurück in die Projektansicht. Wie in Abbildung 14.38 gezeigt liegt in der Projektstruktur nun unterhalb des Ordners **srv** ein Unterordner **external**. Dieser enthält die in der Datei **BusinessPartnerA2X.cds** hinterlegten Entitäten, die durch den Cloud-Service verarbeitet werden, sowie in der Datei **BusinessPartnerA2X.xml** das Entity Data Model des OData-Service. Die Datei **BusinessPArtnerA2X.cds** implementiert den Service, und die Datei **BusinessPartnerA2X.js** enthält die Implementierung des SAP S/4HANA Cloud Service.

Neben den zur Konsumierung des Service generierten Artefakten wurde die Datei **package.json** durch den Generator erweitert. Wie Sie in Abbildung 14.39 sehen können, enthält die Datei nun einen neuen Eintrag im `requires`-Objekt.

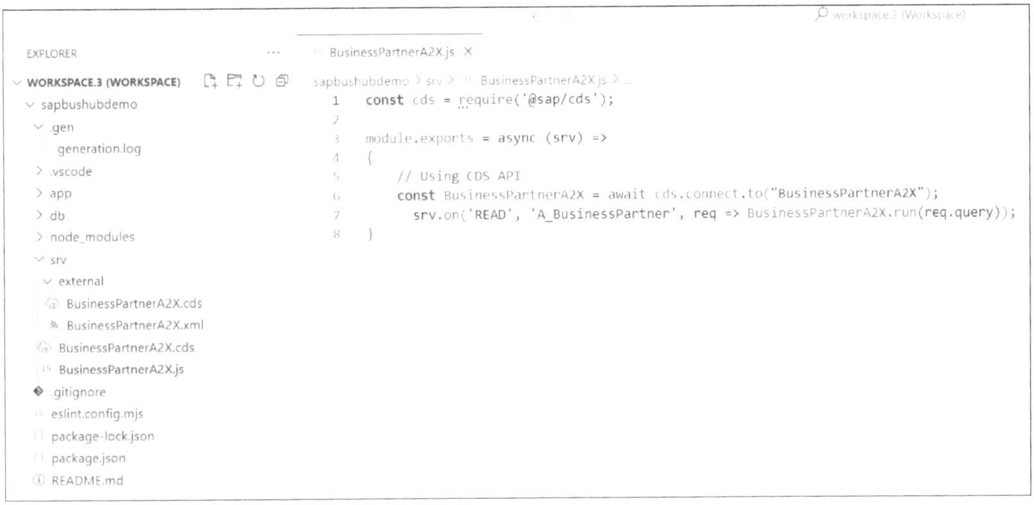

Abbildung 14.38 Neues CAP-Projekt mit Proxy-Klassen

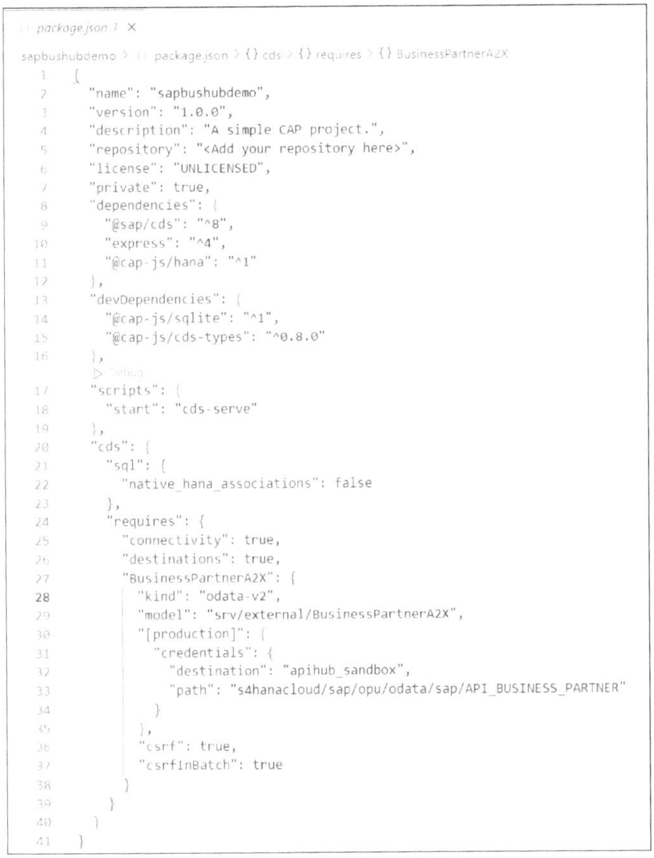

Abbildung 14.39 Die Datei »package.json«

14

Dieser enthält die Konfiguration für unseren Service. Der bei der Eigenschaft `path` angegebene Pfad entspricht der in Abbildung 14.30 dargestellten Pfadangabe. Zusätzlich enthält die Konfiguration die Eigenschaft `destination`. Diese enthält standardmäßig den Eintrag `apihub_sandbox`.

Destination »apihub_sandbox«

Die in der Datei **package.json** angegebene Destination `apihub_sandbox` wird bei der Verarbeitung der OData-Service-Anfrage verwendet und stellt die Verbindung zwischen der Anwendung und SAP S/4HANA Cloud Public Edition her. Hierzu muss die Destination im SAP BTP Cockpit entsprechend angelegt worden sein. Wie eine Destination angelegt wird, haben wir in Abschnitt 2.2.3, »Einführung in den Cloud Connector«, erläutert. Daher zeigen wir an dieser Stelle lediglich die Konfiguration in Abbildung 14.40.

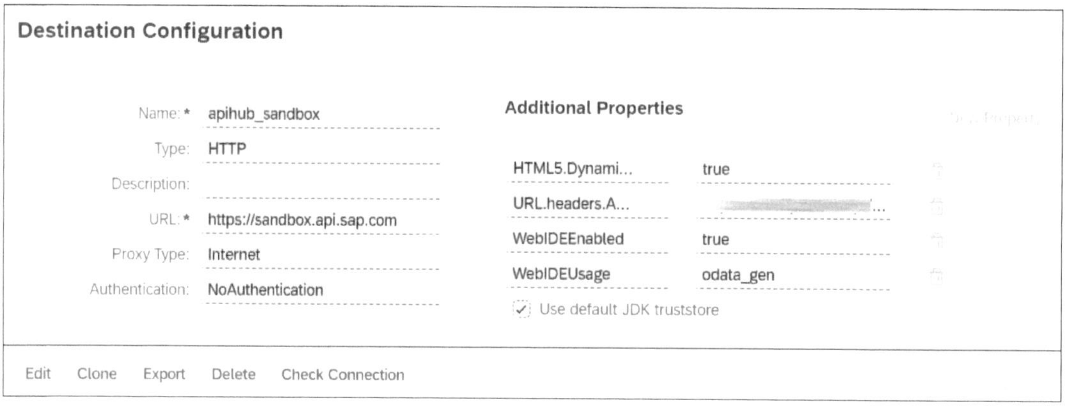

Abbildung 14.40 Konfiguration der Destination »apihub_sandbox«

Die Destination trägt den Namen `apihub_sandbox` und zeigt mit der URL auf den Endpunkt *https://sandbox.api.sap.com*. Der Proxy-Typ ist auf **Internet** eingestellt, und es wird keine Authentifizierung durchgeführt.

API-Schlüssel

Die zusätzlichen Parameter sind Ihnen so weit schon bekannt. Lediglich der Parameter `URL.headers.ApiKey` ist neu. Dieser Parameter enthält den eindeutigen API-Schlüssel (*API Key*) des Benutzers. Diesen API-Schlüssel erhalten Sie im SAP Business Accelerator Hub über die Benutzereigenschaften. Rufen Sie hierzu in Ihrem Benutzermenü den Eintrag **Settings** auf. Sie erhalten im Bereich **API Settings** den für Ihren Benutzer eineindeutigen API-Schlüssel, wie in Abbildung 14.41 gezeigt. Kopieren Sie diesen Schlüssel und geben Sie ihn bei der Eigenschaft `URL.headers.ApiKey` bei der Destination an.

Service testen

Um den Service nun zu testen, rufen Sie in einem Terminal den Befehl `cds watch` auf. Nachdem der Service gestartet wurde, rufen Sie den Service wie gewohnt in einem neuen Browserfenster auf (siehe Abbildung 14.42).

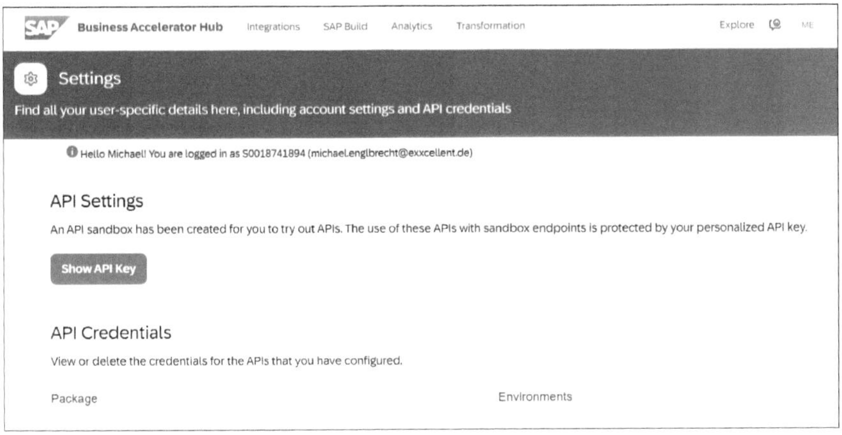

Abbildung 14.41 Benutzerspezifische Einstellungen im SAP Business Accelerator Hub

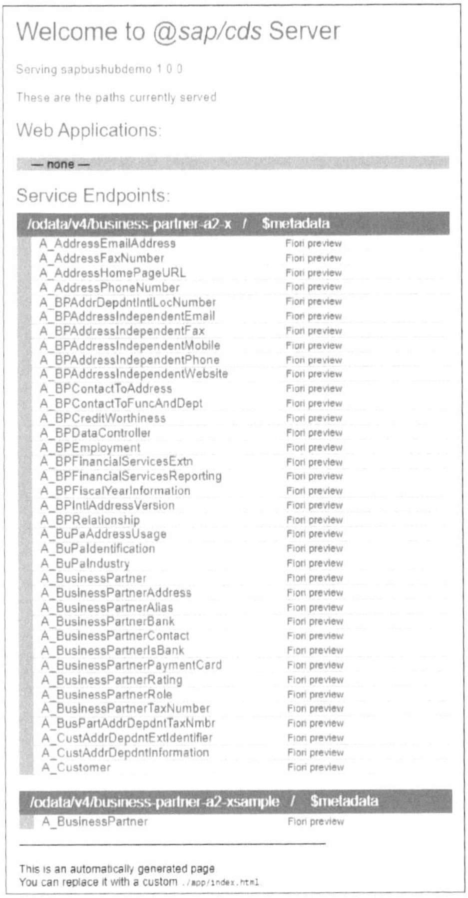

Abbildung 14.42 Seite zum Testen des Service

Um einen Test-Request abzusetzen, rufen Sie hier den Link **A_BusinessPartner** auf. Nach erfolgreicher Verarbeitung der Anfrage wird Ihnen die Rückantwort im Browserfenster angezeigt.

Kapitel 15
Echtzeitkommunikation mit Event-driven Architecture

Mit der fortschreitenden Digitalisierung und der Notwendigkeit, dynamische und agile Geschäftsprozesse zu unterstützen, gewinnt die Echtzeitkommunikation zwischen verteilten Systemen und Anwendungen zunehmend an Bedeutung. SAP Event Mesh und SAP Integration Suite geben Unternehmen Werkzeuge an die Hand, um diese Herausforderungen zu meistern.

Die in diesem Buch bisher beschriebenen Schnittstellentechnologien decken verschiedene Integrationsszenarien ab. Jede Technologie hat dabei andere Stärken, wie in Abbildung 15.1 zu sehen. So stellt Remote Function Call (RFC) beispielsweise einfache, zuverlässige Punkt-zu-Punkt-Verbindungen zwischen zwei Systemen her. Diese sind aber eng gekoppelt, plattformabhängig und müssen individuell erstellt werden.

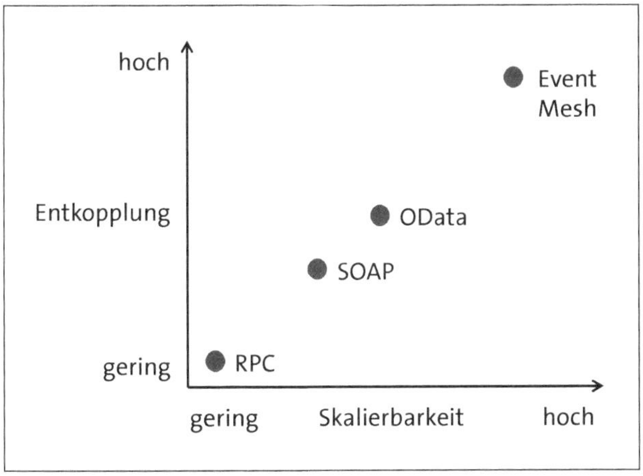

Abbildung 15.1 Schnittstellentechnologien im Vergleich

Mit den HTTP-basierten Webservices und RESTful OData-Services haben sich dank offener Protokolle weitere Schnittstellentechnologien etabliert, die von vielen plattformunabhängigen Konsumenten genutzt werden, jedoch eng gekoppelt bleiben.

Event-driven Architecture

In diesem Kapitel lernen Sie eine weitere Form der Integration kennen, die verspricht, hoch skalierbar und entkoppelt zu sein und dabei auch performant ist. Sie basiert auf der *Event-driven Architecture* (EDA) (deutsch auch *ereignisgesteuerte Architektur*). SAP setzt diese Architektur mit zwei Komponenten um, die wir in diesem Kapitel vorstellen, *SAP Event Mesh* und die *SAP Integration Suite*.

15.1 SAP Event Mesh

Abonnieren von Ereignissen

Um Ihnen die Funktionsweise von SAP Event Mesh zu vermitteln, stellen wir zunächst die EDA vor. Hierbei handelt es sich um ein Software-Architektur-Prinzip, das auf der Kommunikation mit *Ereignissen* (engl. *Events*) beruht. Ein Ereignis ist eine Aktion, eine Beobachtung oder eine Änderung innerhalb eines Systems, die Benachrichtigungen auslöst. Diese Benachrichtigungen werden asynchron an andere Systeme über eine Nachrichtenleitung gesendet. Die Empfänger sind nicht mit dem Sender verbunden, sondern mit dieser Nachrichtenleitung. Konsumenten schreiben sich daher für die Benachrichtigungen zu Ereignissen, die sie interessieren, über die Nachrichtenleitung ein. Es besteht daher keine enge Kopplung zwischen den Systemen. Es ist also nicht definiert, wer der Empfänger der Benachrichtigung ist, und es können auch mehrere Konsumenten dieselbe Nachricht erhalten und einzeln parallel verarbeiten.

Vorteile von EDA

Die asynchrone Kommunikation dieser Architektur hat den Vorteil, dass nicht nur mehrere Konsumenten, sondern auch Ausfälle von Empfängern das System nicht hängen lassen. Die EDA sorgt dafür, dass die Benachrichtigungen zugestellt werden, sobald der Empfänger wieder verfügbar ist. Sie ist auch gut geeignet, um große Datenmengen an verschiedene Systeme zu senden, da nur eine Verbindung zu einem Empfangspunkt im Netzwerk notwendig ist und nicht jedes System mit einem anderen verbunden werden muss.

SAP Event Mesh

Während das EDA-Konzept den Architekturplan definiert, ist SAP Event Mesh eine konkrete technische Infrastruktur, die auf ereignisgesteuerter Kommunikation basiert und die es erlaubt, eine EDA umzusetzen. Eine andere bekannte Umsetzung auf dem Markt ist *Apache Kafka*. Es handelt sich bei SAP Event Mesh um ein Netzwerk von *Event Brokern*, die Ereignisse erzeugen, weiterleiten und zustellen. Die Nachrichtenleitungen nennen sich *Queues*, und Systeme können sich über *Topics* über relevante Ereignisse informieren lassen.

Sender und Empfänger sind nicht direkt miteinander verbunden, was auch eine Erweiterung schnell möglich macht. Wird ein neues System eingebunden, kann es die vorhandenen Benachrichtigungen empfangen. Diese Art der Integration hat folgende Eigenschaften:

- **Entkopplung von Systemen**
  Anwendungen müssen nicht direkt miteinander verbunden sein, um zu kommunizieren.
- **Asynchrone Kommunikation**
  Informationen werden übermittelt, ohne dass die Client-Anwendung auf eine Antwort warten muss.
- **Skalierbarkeit**
  SAP Event Mesh unterstützt komplexe und groß angelegte Umgebungen, in denen mehrere Anwendungen beteiligt sind.

SAP Event Mesh wurde als cloudbasierte Lösung umgesetzt, die es ermöglicht, verschiedene Anwendungen und sowohl SAP- als auch Nicht-SAP-Systeme in einer verteilten Umgebung miteinander zu integrieren. Dies funktioniert ähnlich wie ein neuronales Netz im Gehirn: SAP Event Mesh stellt sicher, dass Ereignisse unabhängig vom Standort der beteiligten Systeme oder Anwendungen sicher und zuverlässig übertragen werden.

Echtzeitkommunikation

Ein Beispiel für den Einsatz von SAP Event Mesh ist die *Echtzeitkommunikation* zwischen Lagerverwaltungssystemen und Logistikpartnern. Angenommen, ein Produkt wird im Wareneingang eines Lagers gescannt. Das Lagerverwaltungssystem sendet dazu eine Benachrichtigung an SAP Event Mesh. SAP Event Mesh verteilt dieses Ereignis in Form einer Benachrichtigung an interessierte Anwendungen, die sich dafür bei SAP Event Mesh registriert haben. Ein möglicher Empfänger könnte beispielsweise ein Transportunternehmen sein, das die Details des Produkts in Echtzeit erhält und daraufhin ein weiteres Ereignis auslöst, die Anlage der Sendung, die dann wieder vom Zustelldienst als Benachrichtigung konsumiert wird, um einen Paketstatus zu aktualisieren. Anders als bei den vielen anderen in diesem Buch beschriebenen Schnittstellen ist keine der Anwendungen dabei direkt mit einer anderen gekoppelt. Auch das Geschäftsziel eines Ereignisses ist nicht vorbestimmt, und keine Anwendung wartet auf das Ergebnis.

15.2 Eine ereignisbasierte Architektur mit SAP Event Mesh einrichten

In diesem Abschnitt beschreiben wir Schritt für Schritt, wie Sie ein SAP-Event-Mesh-Projekt aufsetzen können. Für die folgende Programmierung benötigen Sie eine Subskription für SAP Event Mesh in Ihrem SAP-BTP-

Konto sowie Administratorrechte zur Konfiguration von Diensten und Subskriptionen.

15.2.1 Event Mesh einrichten

SAP Event Mesh aktivieren

Zunächst müssen Sie SAP Event Mesh in der BTP aktivieren. Melden Sie sich als Erstes bei Ihrer SAP-BTP-Subskription an und wählen Sie die entsprechende Sub-Account-Region aus. Navigieren Sie zu **Entitlements**. Fügen Sie den Dienst **SAP Event Mesh** hinzu. Wählen Sie eine passende Serviceplan-Option (z. B. »default« für Standardanwendungen).

Serviceinstanz anlegen

Navigieren Sie nun zu **Services • Instances and Subscriptions** und erstellen Sie eine neue Instanz des Event-Mesh-Diensts. Sie können dabei verschiedene Konfigurationsparameter wie den Speicherplatz und die Anzahl der Warteschlangen (Queues) konfigurieren.

Serviceschlüssel

Öffnen Sie anschließend die Instanz und erstellen Sie einen Serviceschlüssel. Dieser Schlüssel enthält die Zugangsinformationen (URL, Client-ID, Client-Secret) für die Verbindung zu Ihrer Event-Mesh-Instanz. Speichern Sie die Datei mit dem Serviceschlüssel lokal ab.

Subscription für Event-Mesh-Applikation

Damit ist SAP Event Mesh eingerichtet. Öffnen Sie nun den **Event Mesh Administrator**, um eine Subscription für die Event-Mesh-Applikation anzulegen. Wählen Sie dazu die zuvor angelegte Serviceinstanz aus, wechseln Sie auf die Registerkarte **Queues** und legen Sie eine neue Queue an. Fügen Sie dann über **Actions • Create Subscriptions** eine Subscription zur Queue hinzu.

15.2.2 Nachrichten an SAP Event Mesh senden

Node.js als Laufzeitumgebung

Als Nächstes wollen wir eine Node.js-basierte Anwendung bauen, die Benachrichtigungen an die SAP-Event-Mesh-Queue sendet. Node.js ist eine plattformübergreifende JavaScript-Laufzeitumgebung, die große Bedeutung erlangte, um JavaScript-Applikationen ohne Browser laufen zu lassen. Durch die ereignisgesteuerte Architektur von JavaScript und dessen Speichermodell wurde Node.js überall dort eingesetzt, wo auch die Hardware limitiert war, z. B. im Umfeld des Internets der Dinge. Im direkten Vergleich zu Java-Webanwendungen nutzen Node.js-Webanwendungen weniger Speicher pro bestehender Verbindung und skalierten daher sehr gut, weshalb sie oft in Cloud-hosting-Plattformen zu finden sind.

Im SAP-Kontext sind Node.js-Anwendungen eine robuste Wahl für Microservices, um eine schnelle, asynchrone Kommunikation zwischen SAP-Systemen umzusetzen, sowie für kleinere Anwendungen, z. B. für die Echtzeitdatenverarbeitung. Aber auch im SAP Cloud Application Programming Model (CAP) kann man Node.js-Anwendungen als Backend einsetzen. Die Bereitstellung dieser Anwendungen kann über die SAP BTP in der Cloud-Foundry-Umgebung erfolgen. Um in dieser Laufzeitumgebung etwas bereitzustellen, sind im SAP Business Application Studio bereits entsprechende Werkzeuge integriert.

Cloud-Foundry-Deployment-Optionen

Es gibt zwei Möglichkeiten der Bereitstellung:

- **Multi-Target Application (MTA)**
  Über eine **mta.yml**-Datei wird ein Deployment beschrieben, das aus einzelnen Modulen besteht, die in Abhängigkeit voneinander stehen, z. B. eine SAP-HANA-Datenbank, eine SAPUI5-Weboberfläche und ein Java-Backend.
- **Single Application**
  Über eine **manifest.yml**-Datei kann ein einzelner Dienst beschrieben werden, wie eine Node.js-Anwendung.

Für unser Beispiel werden wir eine Node.js-Anwendung als Single Application in einer **manifest.yml**-Datei beschreiben und in der Cloud-Foundry-Umgebung bereitstellen. Dieser Ansatz wird oft für Entwicklertests genutzt, da die **manifest.yml**-Datei weniger komplex ist als die **mta.yml**-Datei.

Vorbereitende Schritte

Führen Sie als Erstes folgende vorbereitende Schritte aus:

1. Legen Sie mit SAP Business Application Studio einen neuen Dev Space vom Typ **Basic** an. (Wie Sie einen Dev Space anlegen, haben wir in Abschnitt 9.4.2, »Implementierung eines OData-Clients mit SAPUI5«, beschrieben.)
2. Legen Sie ein Verzeichnis an, das Sie z. B. »eventmesh-sender« nennen, und führen Sie im Terminal das Kommando `npm init` aus, um den Projektassistenten zu starten.
3. Geben Sie die benötigten Informationen wie den Namen des Projekts und die Version an. Mit diesen Daten wird eine **package.json**-Datei generiert, die eine Node.js-Anwendung beschreibt.
4. Legen Sie eine Datei **manifest.yml** im gleichen Verzeichnis an. Diese Datei dient als Deployment-Deskriptor und enthält alle Informationen dazu, wie unsere Applikation auf der SAP-BTP-Instanz installiert wird.
5. Legen Sie eine weitere Datei **index.js** im gleichen Verzeichnis an, in der wir das Programm schreiben.

Datei »package.json«

In der Datei **package.json** deklarieren wir Abhängigkeiten zu SAP Event Mesh in Form von Bibliotheken, die SAP über das Internet bereitstellt (siehe Listing 15.1).

```
{
        "name": "sender",
        "description": " NodeJS Sender Application",
        "version": "0.0.1",
        "engines": {
                "node": ">=6.9.1"
        },
              "dependencies": {
        "@sap/xb-msg": "^0.9.12",
        "@sap/xb-msg-amqp-v100": "^0.9.48",
        "@sap/xb-msg-env": "^0.9.7",
        "@sap/xsenv": "^3.1.0"
        },
        "scripts": {
                "start": "node index.js"
        }
}
```

Listing 15.1 Inhalt der »package.json«-Datei des Senders

Setzen Sie im gleichen Verzeichnis, in dem auch die Datei **package.json** liegt, das Kommando `npm install` ab, um die Abhängigkeiten herunterzuladen und in ein lokales Verzeichnis **node_modules** zu speichern. Der Paketmanager `npm` sorgt dafür, dass alle Abhängigkeiten zur Version aufgelöst werden.

Domäne, Queue und Messaging-Service konfigurieren

Als Inhalt der Datei **manifest.yml** fügen Sie die Domäne, den Messaging-Service und den Queue-Namen hinzu, wie in Listing 15.2 zu sehen. Da eine YML-Datei mit Einrückungen strukturiert wird, müssen Sie beim Kopieren des Codes genau auf die Schreibweise achten.

```
applications:
  - name: sender
    host: sender-host
    buildpack: 'https://github.com/cloudfoundry/nodejs-
               buildpack'
    memory: 256M
    health-check-type: none
    path: .
    command: node index.js
    services:
      - <REPLACE WITH YOUR MESSAGING SERVICE>
    env:
      SAP_JWT_TRUST_ACL: '[{"clientid":"*","identityzone":"*"}]'
```

```
    SAP_XBEM_BINDINGS: |
      {
        "inputs": {},
        "outputs": {
          "myOutA" : {
            "service": "<REPLACE WITH YOUR MESSAGING
                        SERVICE>",
            "address": "topic:<REPLACE WITH YOUR TOPIC>",
            "reliable": false
          },
          "myOutB" : {
            "service": "<REPLACE WITH YOUR MESSAGING
                        SERVICE>",
            "address": "topic:<REPLACE WITH YOUR TOPIC>",
            "reliable": false
          }
        }
      }
```

Listing 15.2 Inhalt der Datei »manifest.yml« des Senders

Nachrichtenclient

Der eigentliche Code für unseren Nachrichtenclient befindet sich in der Datei **index.js** und implementiert eine Node.js-Anwendung in JavaScript. Listing 15.3 zeigt das entsprechende Coding.

```
"use strict";

import msg from '@sap/xb-msg';
import env from '@sap/xb-msg-env';
import xsenv from '@sap/xsenv';

//---------------------------------------------------------------------
// Basic setup in respect to modules, messaging settings, and
// getting messaging options
//---------------------------------------------------------------------

const service = '<REPLACE WITH YOUR MESSAGING SERVICE>';
const taskList = {
    myOutA: { topic: '<REPLACE WITH YOUR TOPIC>', timerMin: 1,
timerMax: 11 },
    myOutB: { topic: '<REPLACE WITH YOUR TOPIC>', timerMin: 5,
timerMax: 8 }
};
```

```
let counter = 1;

xsenv.loadEnv();

//--------------------------------------------------------------------
// Start messaging client
//--------------------------------------------------------------------

const client = new msg.Client(env.msgClientOptions(service, [],
['myOutA', 'myOutB']));

const getRandomInt = (min, max) => {
    return (Math.floor(Math.random() * (Math.floor(max) -
Math.ceil(min) + 1)) + Math.ceil(min)) * 1000;
};

const initTasks = (tasks, client) => {
    Object.entries(tasks).forEach(([id, task]) => {
        const stream = client.ostream(id);

        const publishMessage = () => {
            console.log(`Publishing message number ${counter}
             to topic ${task.topic}`);

            const message = {
                payload: Buffer.from(`Message Number
                                      ${counter}`)
            };

            if (!stream.write(message)) {
                console.log('Stream is full, waiting for
                            drain...');
                return;
            }

            setTimeout(publishMessage, getRandomInt(task.timerMin,
task.timerMax));
            counter++;
        };

        stream.on('drain', () => {
            setTimeout(publishMessage, getRandomInt(task.timerMin,
task.timerMax));
```

```
        });

        setTimeout(publishMessage, getRandomInt(task.timerMin,
task.timerMax));
    });
};

//-------------------------------------------------------------------
// Messaging client handler methods
//-------------------------------------------------------------------

client
    .on('connected', () => {
        console.log('Connected to messaging service');
        initTasks(taskList, client);
    })
    .on('drain', () => {
        console.log('Stream is ready to continue');
    })
    .on('error', (error) => {
        console.error('An error occurred:', error);
    });

client.connect();
```

Listing 15.3 Inhalt des Node.js-Sender-Programms in der Datei »index.js«

Die Anwendung interagiert mit dem Messaging-Service, um asynchrone Nachrichten an definierte Themen (Topics) zu senden. Das Beispiel simuliert asynchrone Workloads in einem Event-basierten System, indem kontinuierlich Nachrichten an definierte Topics gesendet werden.

Ereignisbasierte Programmierung

Dazu wird ein Client für die SAP-Messaging-Plattform erstellt und konfiguriert, um periodisch Nachrichten zu veröffentlichen. Die Konfiguration erfolgt über eine vordefinierte Aufgabenliste `taskList`, in der jedem Task ein spezifisches Topic und ein Zeitintervall (Min. und Max.) zugewiesen sind. Nach dem Aufbau der Verbindung zum Messaging-Service mit `client.connect()` werden *Streams* für jedes Topic initialisiert. Jeder dieser Streams sendet Nachrichten mit einem ansteigenden Zählerwert `counter`, wobei ein zufälliges Zeitintervall zwischen den Nachrichten eingehalten wird. Wenn ein Stream ausgelastet ist (kein Schreiben möglich), wartet er, bis das `drain`-Event ausgelöst wird, bis er fortzufährt.

Der Code nutzt *Event Listener*, um auf wichtige Zustände des Clients zu reagieren, wie beispielsweise einen Verbindungsaufbau mit `connected`, eine Stream-Entleerung mit `drain` oder einen Fehler `error`.

Deployment in Cloud-Foundry-Umgebung

Um diesen Code nun in der Cloud-Foundry-Umgebung bereitzustellen, rufen Sie ein Terminal auf. Hier wechseln Sie zunächst in das Verzeichnis unseres Projekts. Mit dem Befehl `cf login` melden Sie sich an der **Cloud Foundry Environment** an. Das Terminal fragt dazu den SAP BTP Benutzernamen, das Passwort und den API-Endpunkt ab. Den Endpunkt erhalten Sie in Ihrem Subaccount in der Sektion **Cloud Foundry Environment** unter der Überschrift **API Endpoint**. Nach dem Login können Sie im Projektverzeichnis mit `cf push` den Bereitstellungsprozess anstoßen.

15.2.3 Nachrichten aus SAP Event Mesh empfangen

Nachrichtenempfänger implementieren

Auch für die Entwicklung eines Nachrichtenempfängers in SAP Event Mesh bietet Node.js eine geeignete Basis, da durch das ereignisbasierte Programmiermodell nach einer Verbindung mit SAP Event Mesh fortlaufend auf Ereignisse gewartet werden muss. Typischerweise wird solch ein Microservice für die Verarbeitung von Echtzeitdaten eingesetzt, z. B. für das Aktualisieren von Bestandsinformationen nach einer Bestellung. Die Implementierung des Empfängers unterscheidet sich nur minimal von der Implementierung des Senders:

1. Beginnen Sie wie in Abschnitt 15.2.2, »Nachrichten an SAP Event Mesh senden«, mit der Installation von Node.js und dem Paketmanager `npm`.
2. Legen Sie ein Verzeichnis an, das Sie z. B. »eventmesh-empfaenger« nennen. Legen Sie, wie in Abschnitt 15.2.2 beschrieben, die Dateien **manifest.yml** an und initialisieren Sie das Projekt mit dem Befehl `npm init`.
3. Legen Sie eine leere Datei **index.js** für den Programmcode an

Datei »package.json«

Die angelegte Datei **package.json** erweitern Sie, wie in Listing 15.4 gezeigt, um die Abhängigkeiten zu SAP Event Mesh. Speichern Sie die Datei und rufen Sie dann den Befehl `npm install` im gleichen Verzeichnis auf, in dem auch die Datei **package.json** liegt.

```
{
        "name": "empfaenger",
        "description": "NodeJS Empfaenger Application",
        "version": "0.0.1",
        "engines": {
                "node": ">=6.9.1"
        },
```

```
        "dependencies": {
                "@sap/xsenv": "1.2.8",
                "@sap/xb-msg": ">=0.2.4",
                "@sap/xb-msg-env": ">=0.2.1"
        },
        "scripts": {
                "start": "node index.js"
        }
}
```

Listing 15.4 Datei »package.json« der Node.js-Empfängeranwendung

Datei »manifest.yml«

Die Datei **manifest.yml** beschreibt, ebenso wie in Abschnitt 15.2.2, die Senderdomäne, den Messaging-Service und die Queue (siehe Listing 15.5).

```
applications:
      - name: empfaenger
        host: empfaenger -host
        buildpack: https://github.com/cloudfoundry/nodejs-buildpack
        memory: 256M
        health-check-type: none
        path: .
        command: node index.js
        services:
          - <REPLACE WITH YOUR MESSAGING SERVICE>
        env:
          SAP_JWT_TRUST_ACL: "[{\"clientid\":\"*\",\"identityzone\":\
"*\"}]"
          XBEM_INPUT_X: "inputX"
          RECONNECT_RETRY_MS : 5000
          SAP_XBEM_BINDINGS: >
           {
              "inputs": {
                "inputX": {
                  "service": "<REPLACE WITH YOUR MESSAGING SERVICE>",
                  "address": "queue:<REPLACE WITH YOUR QUEUE>",
                  "reliable": true
                }
              }
            }
```

Listing 15.5 Datei »manifest.yml« der Node.js-Empfängeranwendung

15

Datei »index.js«

Die eigentliche Programmierung für den Nachrichtenempfänger liegt wieder in der Datei **index.js** (siehe Listing 15.6).

```
"use strict";

import msg from '@sap/xb-msg';
import msgenv from '@sap/xb-msg-env';

// Konfiguration
const inputX = process.env.XBEM_INPUT_X;
const reconnectRetryMs = Number(process.env.RECONNECT_RETRY_MS) ||
5000; // Default retry interval

const options = msgenv.msgClientOptions('<REPLACE WITH YOUR MESSAGING
SERVICE>', [inputX], []);

// Start client
// Message Client anlegen für die Event-Mesh-Serviceinstanz
const client = new msg.Client(options);

// Message-Client-Handler-Methoden
client
    .on('connected', () => {
        console.log('Connected to Event Mesh);
    })
    .on('error', (err) => {
        console.error('Error on Event Mesh occurred:', err);
    })
    .on('disconnected', (hadError) => {
        console.warn(`Connection to Event Mesh lost. Retry in
${reconnectRetryMs} ms...`);
        setTimeout(() => client.connect(), reconnectRetryMs);
    });

// Empfangende Stream-Handler-Methoden
client.istream(inputX)
    .on('subscribed', () => {
        console.log(`Subscribed on topic: ${inputX}`);
    })
    .on('ready', () => {
        console.log(`Stream ready on topic: ${inputX}`);
    })
    .on('data', (message) => {
```

```
        const topic = typeof message.source === 'string'
            ? message.source
            : message.source?.topic || 'unknown';

        // Nachricht loggen
        console.log(`Message received from topic "${topic}":
${message.payload.toString()}`);
        message.done();
    });

// Verbindung zu Event Mesh starten
client.connect();
```

Listing 15.6 Datei »index.js« der Node.js- Empfängeranwendung

Wiederverbindung bei Verbindungsverlust

Diese Node.js-Anwendung interagiert mit SAP Event Mesh, um Nachrichten von einem definierten Topic `inputX` zu empfangen. Der Messaging-Client wird zu Beginn aus den Umgebungsvariablen konfiguriert, einschließlich des Topics, das abonniert werden soll, und eines Wiederverbindungsintervalls bei Verbindungsverlust. Sobald der Client verbunden ist, wird ein Input-Stream `istream` für das definierte Topic erstellt, das auf verschiedene Ereignisse wie `subscribed`, `ready` und `data` für eingehende Nachrichten reagiert. Eingehende Nachrichten werden verarbeitet, indem ihre Quelle überprüft und der Inhalt mit der Variablen `payload` in die Konsole geschrieben wird. Nach erfolgreicher Verarbeitung wird die Nachricht mit `message.done()` bestätigt. Bei einer Unterbrechung der Verbindung versucht der Client nach einem definierten Zeitintervall automatisch, sich erneut zu verbinden, sodass die Anwendung robust mit SAP Event Mesh kommuniziert.

15

Die Anwendung können Sie auf die gleiche Weise wie den Sender in der Cloud-Foundry-Umgebung bereitstellen. Nutzen Sie dazu den Befehl `cf push`.

15.3 SAP Integration Suite

Heterogene Systemlandschaften

Anwendungslandschaften sind heute wie damals oft heterogen, weil sie die am besten geeigneten Lösungen aus allen Bereichen einsetzen, z. B. SAP als ERP-System, Salesforce als CRM-System, Mailchimp als Plattform für Marketingautomatisierung und Power BI für Business Analytics. Jede dieser Anwendung an SAP Event Mesh anzubinden, würde erfordern, für jede Anwendung eine Schnittstelle zu schreiben, was Aufwand bedeutet.

Daher bietet SAP die *SAP Integration Suite* an. Dabei handelt es sich um eine Entwicklungsumgebung und Integrationsplattform, die speziell darauf ausgelegt ist, verteilte Geschäftsprozesse und verschiedene Systeme miteinander zu verbinden. Sie bietet eine breite Palette von Werkzeugen und vor allem vorgefertigte Konnektoren, um Datenflüsse und Prozesse zwischen Cloud- und On-Premise-Systemen zu orchestrieren. Mit den verschiedenen Werkzeugen, die in ihrer Gesamtheit Ähnlichkeiten mit einer integrierten Entwicklungsumgebung (IDE) haben, können Prozesse modelliert werden, um Daten von einem System an SAP Event Mesh zu routen oder um die APIs von Systemen unter dem Einsatz der Konnektoren in eine SAP-Landschaft zu integrieren. So kann mit wenig Code eine Systemlandschaft, bestehend aus einer SAP-Anwendung, Salesforce, Power BI und Mailchimp, aufgesetzt werden.

Integration verteilter Systeme

Die SAP Integration Suite ist integrierter Bestandteil der SAP BTP und ermöglicht Unternehmen eine standardisierte und skalierbare Integration, ohne für jede Verbindung eine maßgeschneiderte Lösung entwickeln zu müssen. Die SAP Integration Suite nutzt SAP Event Mesh als technische Infrastruktur und kann als zentrale Drehscheibe für die Integration verteilter Systeme angesehen werden. Dabei wird insbesondere die Datenkonsistenz über alle Geschäftsprozesse der Systeme hinweg sichergestellt, indem Transaktionen und Benachrichtigungen überwacht werden. Die Infrastruktur der SAP Integration Suite wird hochverfügbar betrieben.

Ein typischer Anwendungsfall der SAP Integration Suite wäre etwa gegeben, wenn ein On-Premise-SAP-System eine Benachrichtigung zum Ereignis »Rechnungserstellung abgeschlossen« in SAP Event Mesh veröffentlicht. Die SAP Integration Suite konsumiert dieses Event, wandelt die Daten in das passende Format um und aktualisiert damit ein cloudbasiertes Salesforce-CRM-System. Zeitgleich wird infolge der Benachrichtigung ein Workflow gestartet, der den Druck der Rechnung und die Versandplanung automatisiert.

[»]

Advanced Event Mesh

Obwohl die SAP Integration Suite mit SAP Event Mesh zusammenarbeitet, ist dieses Zusammenspiel durchaus mit Einschränkungen verbunden. Seit 2022 bietet SAP daher *SAP Integration Suite, Advanced Event Mesh* an. Vorteil dieser Variante ist, dass sie es erlaubt, 30-mal größere Nachrichten zu verarbeiten und zu speichern. Ebenso gibt es ein integriertes Event-Management, eine Event-Überwachung sowie eine Unterstützung für Cross-Cloud-, On-Premise und Edge-Deployments.

15.3.1 Open Connectors

Neuartige Integrationsmöglichkeiten mit EDA

Im Rahmen der Programmierung des Event-Mesh-Senders und -Empfängers im vorangehenden Abschnitt haben Sie gesehen, dass kleine JavaScript-Anwendungen mit wenig Code über eine Queue verbunden werden können. Ein typisches Einsatzszenario hierfür ist das Internet der Dinge, wenn Daten von Sensoren weitergeleitet werden, ohne direkt verarbeitet zu werden. Am Beispiel eines Sensors kann man sich auch vorstellen, dass eine RFC-Verbindung (Remote Function Call) für jeden Sensor in ein System weder skalierbar noch wirtschaftlich zu implementieren wäre.

Erst die EDA ermögliche die notwendigen Verbindungen, die über eine Punkt-zu-Punkt-Verbindung hinausgehen. Bei Publish-Subscribe-Verbindungen werden etwa viele Empfänger parallel versorgt, oder es erfolgt eine Aggregation von verschiedenen Ereignissen zu einem neuen bis hin zum *Complex Event Processing*, bei dem man aus Mustern bestimmter Ereignisse (z. B. gescheiterter Anmeldeversuche) neue Informationen erlangt.

Vorteile der SAP Integration Suite

Die genannten Konzepte gibt es bereits seit Längerem. Sie wurden in den 2000er-Jahren über EAI-Patterns (Enterprise Application Integration) ausführlich beschrieben mit vielen konkurrierenden Produkten implementiert, die in Produkten für *Integration Broker* und *Enterprise Service Busses* gipfelten. Dies waren Drittanbieterprodukte, die im einfachsten Fall eine Nachrichtenplattform, Nachrichtentransformation und Routing bereitstellten, ähnlich wie die SAP Integration Suite. Neu bei der SAP Integration Suite ist, dass durch das Cloud-Betriebsmodell und das Zusammenwirken mit SAP Event Mesh ein zugänglicher Weg über die SAP BTP angeboten wird.

Heterogene Standardanwendungen integrieren

Die Integration einer typischen Unternehmenslandschaft mit ihren heterogenen Standardanwendungen in eine ereignisgesteuerte Architektur erfolgte damals wie heute über Adapter, die durch einen Orchestrator in Workflows verbunden werden (siehe Abbildung 15.2). Diese Rolle übernimmt ein Werkzeug der SAP Integration Suite, der *Konnektor* (engl. Connector). SAP liefert eine ganze Sammlung solcher Konnektoren unter dem Begriff *Open Connectors* in der SAP Integration Suite aus. Es handelt sich um vorgefertigte Adapter, die einheitliche Schnittstellen zu über 170 externen Cloud-Anwendungen (wie Salesforce, Google Drive, Slack etc.) bieten.

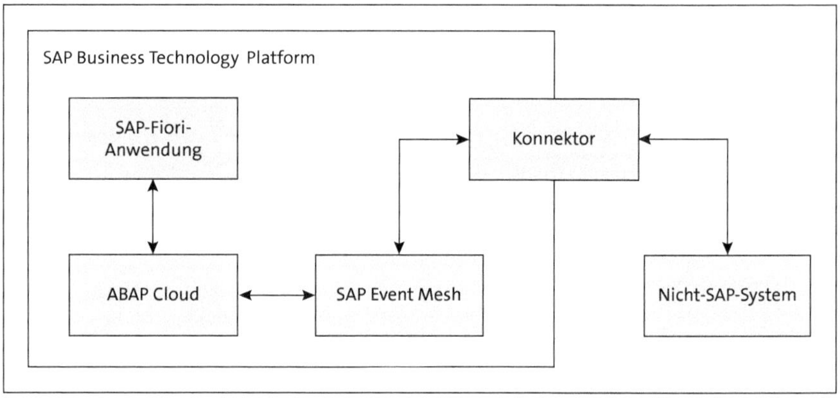

Abbildung 15.2 Integration heterogener Standardanwendungen

15.3.2 Konnektor für einen SOAP-Webservice konfigurieren

In dem folgenden Beispiel zeigen wir, wie ein SOAP-Webservice mithilfe eines solchen Konnektors integriert werden kann – ohne eigenen Code, sondern allein durch Konfiguration.

SAP Integration Suite einrichten

Zunächst müssen Sie dazu die SAP Integration Suite auf der SAP BTP aktivieren und für die Entwicklung vorbereiten.

1. Melden Sie sich an Ihrer SAP-BTP-Subskription an und wählen Sie die entsprechende Subaccount-Region aus.
2. Navigieren Sie zum Menüeintrag **Entitlements**. Fügen Sie hier den Dienst **Integration Suite** hinzu, und wählen Sie einen passenden Serviceplan.
3. Navigieren Sie nun zum Bereich **Services • Instances and Subscriptions** und erstellen Sie über den Button **Create** eine neue Instanz der **Integration Suite**.
4. Sie sehen nun eine neue **Application**. Wechseln Sie hier auf die Registerkarte **Roles** und öffnen Sie den Bereich **Role Collection**. Wählen Sie hier die Role Collections namens `IntegrationProvisioningAdmin`.
5. In dieser Role Collection finden Sie die Rolle `Integration_Provisioner`, die Sie im Bereich **User** Ihrem Benutzer hinzufügen können, indem Sie Ihre E-Mail-Adresse angeben. So erhalten Sie Zugang zur Integrationsentwicklung mit der SAP Integration Suite.

SAP Integration Suite starten

Nachdem Sie den Integration-Suite-Service aktiviert und eingerichtet haben, navigieren Sie erneut in den Bereich **Services • Instances and Subscriptions** und starten die Applikation **Integration Suite**. Sie sehen nun den Startbildschirm, über den Sie sogenannte *Capabilities* hinzufügen können (siehe

Abbildung 15.3). Bei diesen Capabilities handelt es sich um Funktionalitäten, die nach Bedarf hinzugefügt werden können, wie **Cloud Integration**, **API Management**, **Event Mesh** oder **OData Provisioning**. Die Capability **Cloud Integration** unterstützt z. B. einen Ende-zu-Ende-Integrationsprozess, bei dem Nachrichten über Firmen und Organisationsgrenzen hinweg ausgetauscht werden können. Cloud Integration ist mit dem SAP Business Accelerator Hub verbunden und beschreibt auch Konnektoren, die anders als in den bisherigen Kapiteln hier Verbindungen zu Systemen ohne eigene Programmierung versprechen. Wir werden uns eine solche Verbindung nun am Beispiel eines SOAP-Webservice ansehen.

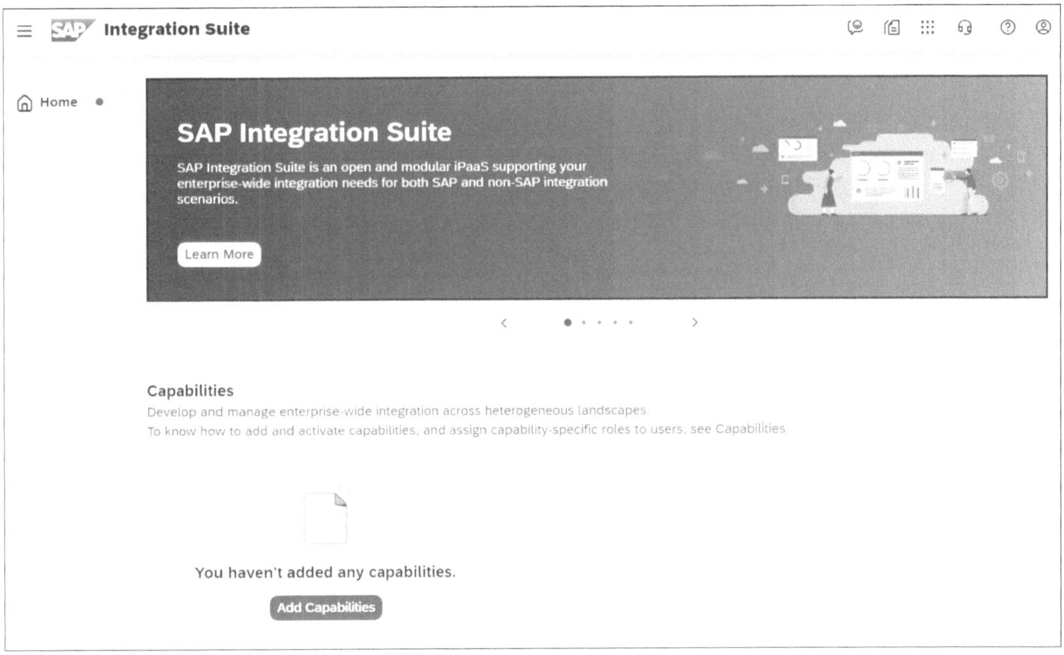

Abbildung 15.3 Startseite der SAP Integration Suite

15

Capability hinzufügen

Klicken Sie auf **Add Capabilities**, wählen Sie **Extend Non-SAP Connectivity** und aktivieren Sie die Capability **Open Connectors**, wie in Abbildung 15.4 zu sehen. Anschließend klicken Sie auf **Next** und bestätigen den Vorgang mit **Activate**.

Die ausgewählte Capability erlaubt es, Adapterinstanzen per Konfiguration anzulegen. Sie vereinfacht so den Zugang zu einem Nicht-SAP-System.

Nach der Aktivierung sehen Sie eine neue Kachel **Extend Non-SAP Connectivity** auf der Integration-Suite-Startseite, die über den Link **Discover Connectors** zu den Konnektoren führt, wie in Abbildung 15.5 zu sehen. Klicken Sie hier auf **Create Connectors**, um die Webanwendung zu starten.

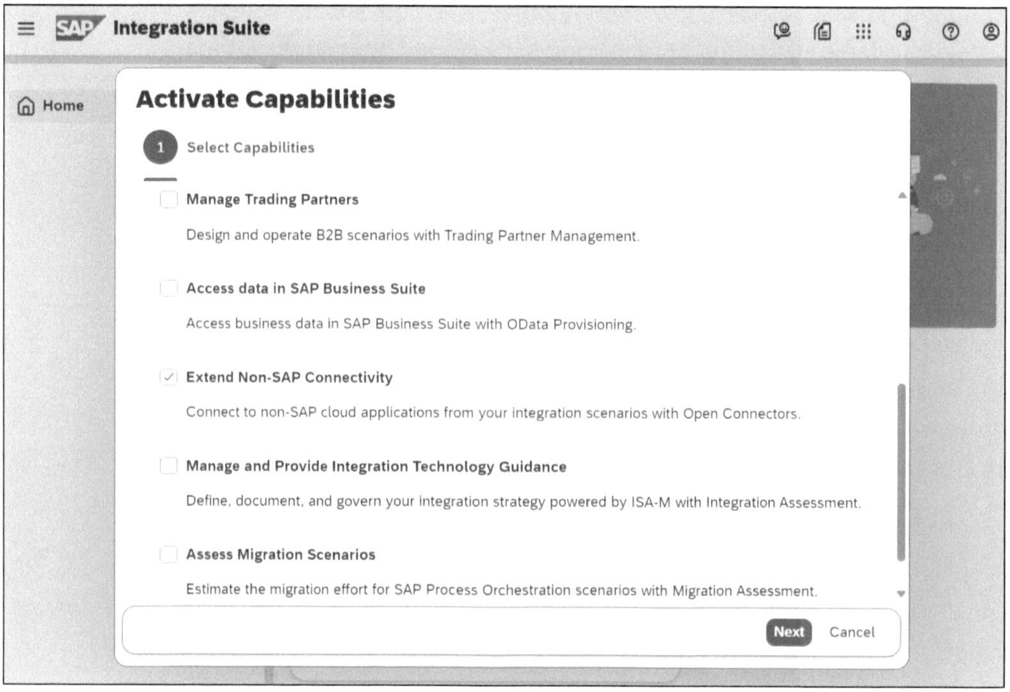

Abbildung 15.4 Aktivieren der Capability »Open Connectors«

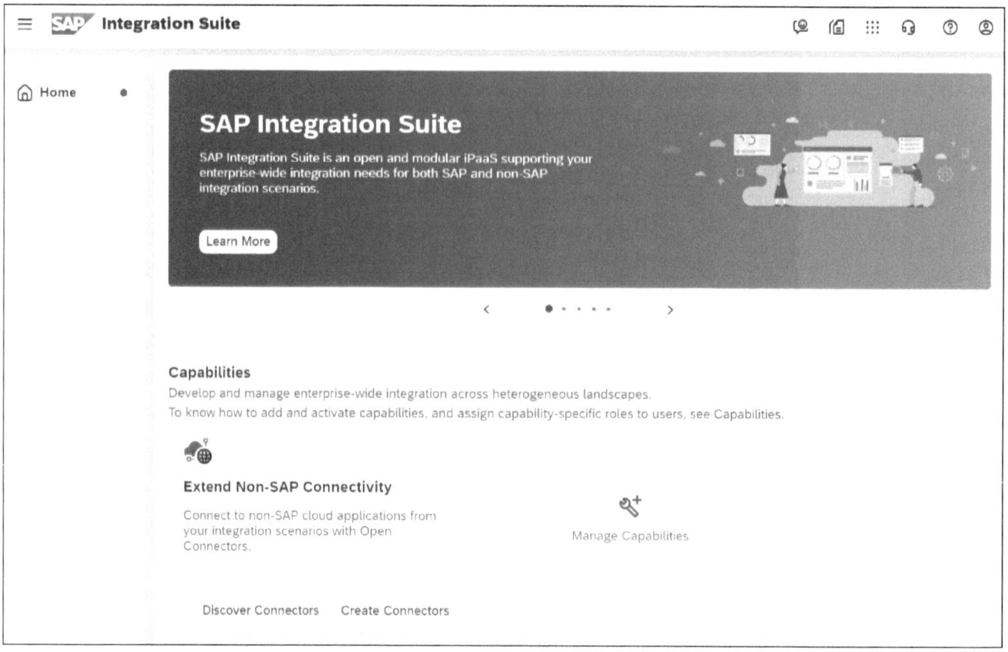

Abbildung 15.5 Aktivierte Capability »Open Connectors«

Konnektor anlegen

In der Webanwendung klicken Sie im Navigationsmenü links auf **Connectors**, um die Übersicht der verfügbaren Konnektoren einzublenden, wie in Abbildung 15.6 zu sehen.

Sie können hier aus Standardadaptern wählen, die über bekannte Protokolle wie Hypertext Transfer Protocol Secure (HTTPS), File Transfer Protocol (FTP), Jakarta Messaging (JMS), Post Office Protocol (POP3), Simple Mail Transfer Protocol (SMTP), Advanced Messaging Queueing Protocol (AMQP) oder Systeme wie SAP Event Mesh angebunden werden. Sie können außerdem aus über 170 Konnektoren für Nicht-SAP-Systeme wie Dropbox, Salesforce, HubSpot, ELSTER oder Stripe wählen, um Zugriff auf die APIs der jeweiligen Applikationen zu erhalten. Des Weiteren stellt die Integration Suite ein *Adapter Development Kit* bereit, um eigene Adapter zu entwickeln und bereitzustellen.

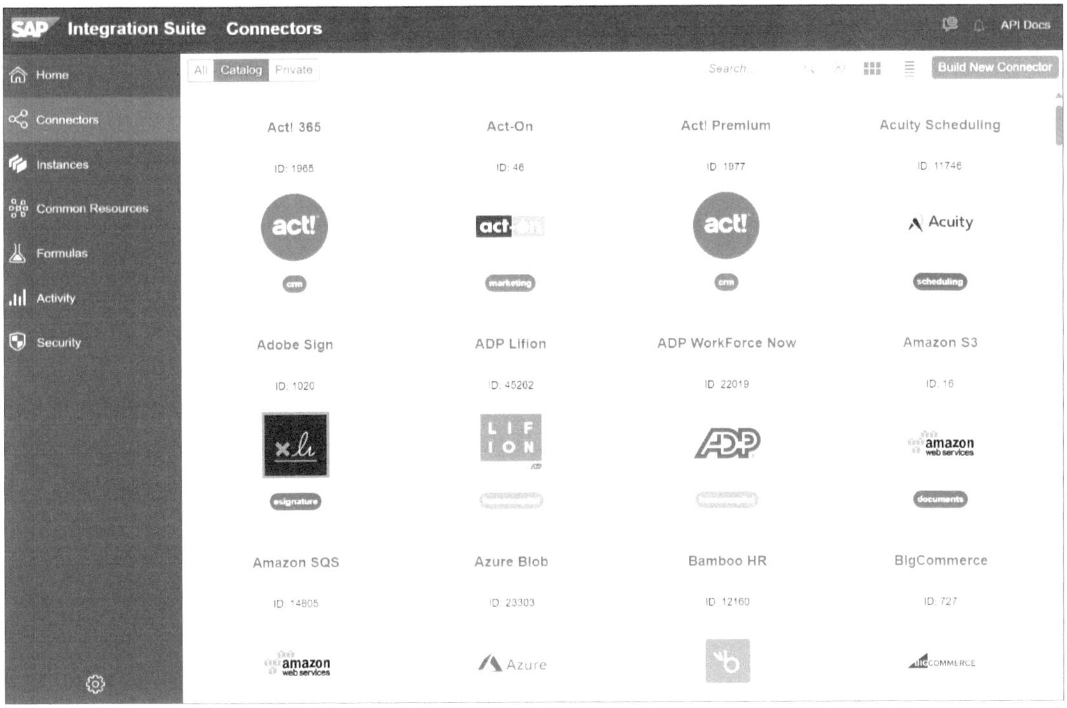

Abbildung 15.6 Übersicht der verfügbaren Konnektoren

Webservice auswählen

Klicken Sie auf **Build New Connector**, um einen generischen SOAP-Webservice anzubinden. Wählen Sie **Import • SOAP** und anschließend die WSDL-Datei aus, die wir in Kapitel 8, »SOAP-Webservices«, erstellt haben. Bestätigen Sie den Vorgang mit einen Klick auf **Continue Import**. Ihnen wird nun eine Liste der Operationen dieses Webservice angezeigt, die wir nutzen können (siehe Abbildung 15.7).

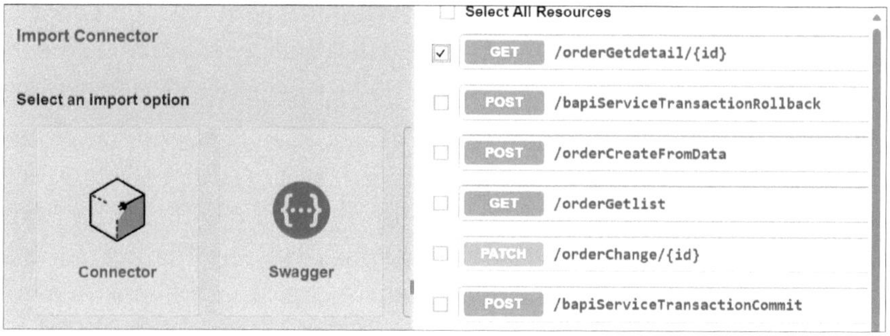

Abbildung 15.7 SOAP-Webservice »ZIFP_Order_Service Connector« in der SAP Integration Suite

REST-API

Wählen Sie die Operationen aus, die Sie benötigen, in unserem Fall **/orderGetdetail/{id}** und bestätigen Sie den Vorgang mit **Import**. Auffällig ist bereits in der Darstellung der Operationen, dass unser SOAP-Webservice innerhalb der SAP Integration Suite als REST-API angeboten wird. Die Transformation passiert innerhalb von Open Connectors zur Laufzeit.

Einstellungsoptionen

Über die verschiedenen Einstellungen des Adapter Development Kits kann das Verhalten des Adapters geändert werden (siehe Abbildung 15.8).

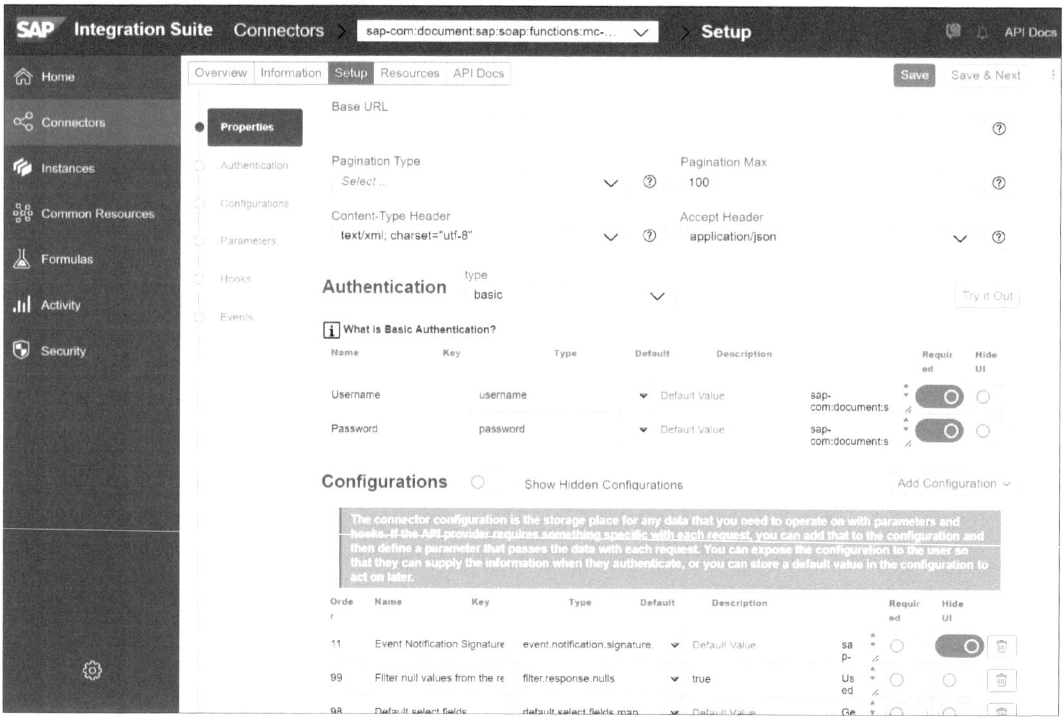

Abbildung 15.8 Konfiguration des Konnektors »ZIFP_Order_Service«

Sie können beispielsweise Authentifizierungsinformationen und Ereignisinformationen festlegen. Klicken Sie auf **Save & Next**, um die ausgewählten Parameter der Operation zu prüfen. Sie können hier nicht nur die Einstellungen nachjustieren, sondern auch ein Programm in JavaScript schreiben, das ausgeführt wird, wenn bestimmte Ereignisse eintreffen. Klicken Sie nun auf **Save**, und Sie sehen unter **API Docs** eine Dokumentation der aus diesem SOAP-Service erstellten REST-API (siehe Abbildung 15.9).

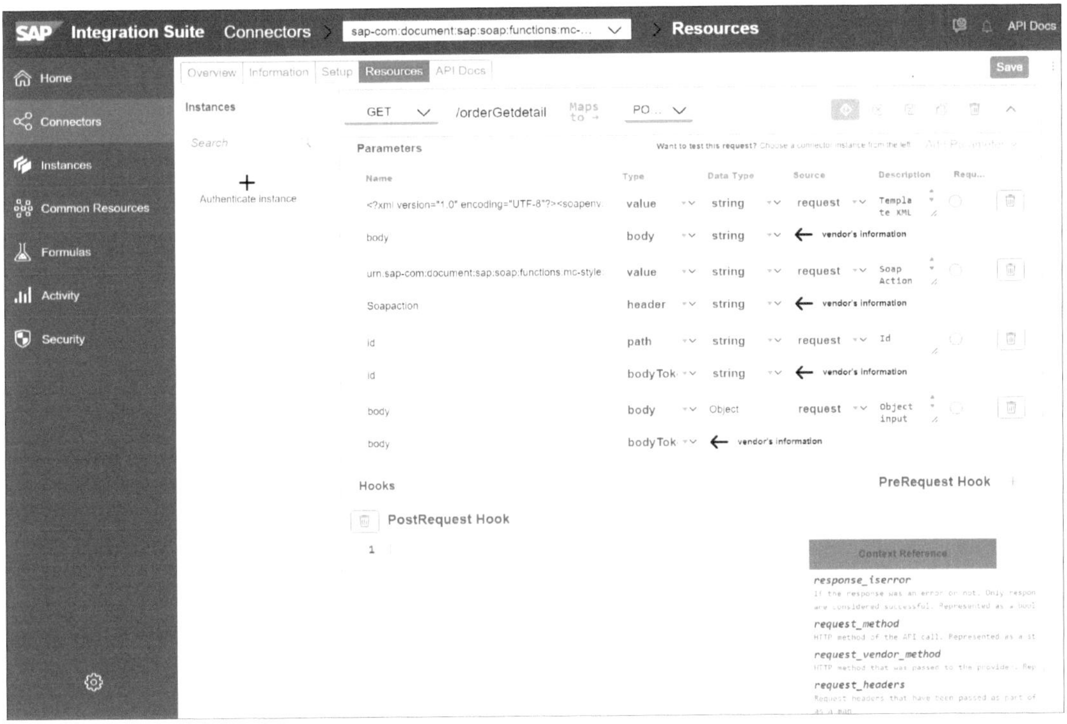

Abbildung 15.9 Konfiguration der Operation

Unter **Overview** können Sie noch einen Namen, ein Icon und eine Beschreibung für ihn angeben.

Webservice instanziieren

Als Nächstes müssen Sie eine Instanz des Webservice erzeugen. Klicken Sie im Menü auf **Instances • Create Instance** (siehe Abbildung 15.10). Sie können nun nach dem Namen suchen, den Sie zuvor unter **Overview** angegeben haben.

Wie in Abbildung 15.10 zu sehen, kann eine Instanz unseres Konnektors erstellt werden. Die angelegte Konnektorinstanz in der SAP Integration Suite (Open Connectors) ist aber kein Service, der nun eigenständig im Hintergrund auf der SAP BTP läuft und periodisch Daten abruft, sondern vielmehr eine vorkonfigurierte Verbindung zu unserem SOAP-Service in Richtung der externen Systeme sowie eine einheitliche API aufseiten der SAP Integration Suite. Über diese API können Daten von Anwendungen der SAP BTP abgerufen werden, wenn aktiv eine Anfrage gesendet wird. Will man automatische zeitgesteuerte Anfragen umsetzen, kann man dies über die Integration Flows in der Capability Cloud Integration tun.

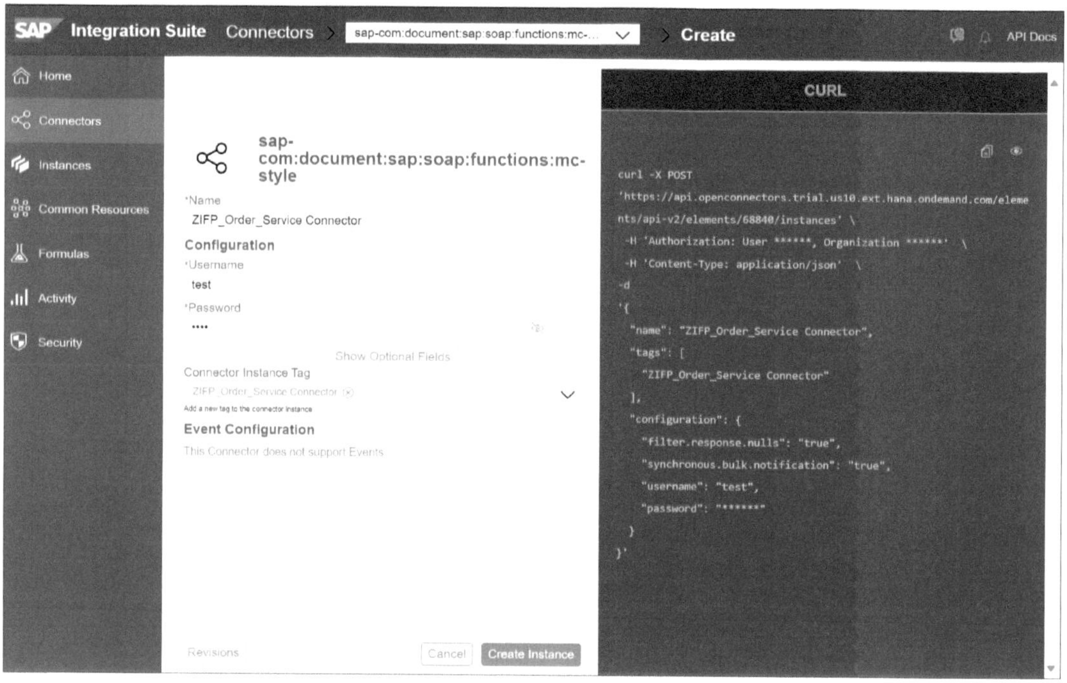

Abbildung 15.10 Eine Konnektorinstanz erstellen

Einheitliche API-Schicht

Mit diesem Szenario wollten wir Ihnen das Konzept der Open Connectors der SAP Integration Suite skizzieren, mit denen eine einheitliche API-Schicht bereitgestellt wird, über die verschiedene Anwendungen einfach auf externe Dienste zugreifen können – unabhängig davon, ob es sich um SOAP-, REST- oder andere APIs handelt.

Noch einfacher als die Konfiguration unseres vorgestellten manuellen Adapters ist die Anbindung über die vorkonfigurierten über 250 fertigen Konnektorvorlagen. Dies ist ein großer Vorteil, da für die Umsetzung von Integrationsszenarien dadurch weniger spezielles Wissen benötigt wird und Betrieb und Skalierung durch die Cloud-Lösung sichergestellt werden. Aus Entwicklungssicht ergeben sich drei wesentliche Vorteile:

- Eine standardisierte REST-API für verschiedene Dienste (auch wenn sie mal SOAP-, mal eine C#-Anwendung ansprechen).

- Eine vereinfachte Authentifizierung mit einmaliger Einrichtung, bei der keine separate Authentifizierung für jede Nutzung nötig ist.
- Eine zentrale Verwaltung, auf die alle Anwendungen im SAP BTP Subaccount zugreifen können, ohne jeweils eigene Integrationen bauen zu müssen.

15.4 Ausblick

Seit die letzte Ausgabe dieses Buchs erschien, sind sieben Jahre vergangen. Da bieten sich ein kurzer Rückblick und eine allgemeine Prognose zur Entwicklung der Schnittstellentechnologien an, um das Buch abzuschließen.

Stabile Schnittstellentechnologien

Die Werkzeuge und Programmiersprachen, die wir in diesem Buch behandeln, darunter Java, C# und JavaScript, haben sich kontinuierlich weiterentwickelt. Das Programmieren von SAP-Schnittstellen sowie der Einsatz standardisierter Schnittstellen wie SOAP und OData haben sich über diese lange Zeitspanne als stabile Konstanten erwiesen.

Neue organisationsübergreifende Szenarien

Die aktuellen Entwicklungen in Richtung einer ereignisgetriebenen Architektur mit SAP Event Mesh und der SAP Integration Suite sowie die Bereitstellung von Schnittstellen in der Cloud über den SAP Business Accelerator Hub erleichtert Integrationsszenarien, die auch über Organisationsgrenzen hinweg funktionieren können. Diese Technologien befinden sich allerdings noch in einer recht frühen Phase der Entwicklung.

Wir gehen davon aus, dass sich diese Entwicklung fortsetzen wird und dass insbesondere der KI-Trend die Integrationsarbeit weiter vereinfachen wird. Künstliche Intelligenz (KI) könnte z. B. das Mapping von Datenstrukturen zwischen Systemen unterstützen. Repetitive Aufgaben werden damit zunehmend entfallen, wie sich bereits bei den Open Connectors andeutet. Es ist daher anzunehmen, dass Entwickler sich zukünftig eher auf die Fachdomänen konzentrieren können und zu Kuratoren und Optimierern werden, statt sich mit technischen Details auseinanderzusetzen.

Literaturhinweise

Michael Englbrecht, Andreas Pflugrad: *Das neue SAPUI5-Handbuch*. 1. Aufl., Bonn: SAP PRESS 2020.

John Mutumba Bilay, Roberto Viana Blanco: *SAP Process Orchestration. The Comprehensive Guide*. Boston: SAP PRESS 2017.

Carsten Bönnen et. al.: *SAP Gateway und OData*. 4. Aufl., Bonn: SAP PRESS 2024.

Renzo Colle, Ralf Dentzler, Jan Hrastnik: *Core Data Services für ABAP*. 3. Aufl., Bonn: SAP PRESS 2023.

Michael Englbrecht: *SAP Fiori. Implementierung und Entwicklung*. 3. Aufl., Bonn: SAP PRESS 2020.

Michael Englbrecht, Andreas Pflugrad: *SAP Fiori – Administration und Konfiguration*. Bonn: SAP PRESS 2025.

Hermann Gahm et. al.: *ABAP-Entwicklung für SAP HANA*. 2. Aufl., Bonn: SAP PRESS 2015.

Horst Keller, Sascha Krüger: *ABAP Objects. ABAP-Programmierung mit SAP NetWeaver*. 3. Aufl., Bonn: SAP PRESS 2006.

Mandy Krimmel, Joachim Orb: *SAP NetWeaver Process Integration*. 2. Aufl., Bonn: SAP PRESS 2010.

Stefan Kühnlein, Holger Seubert: *Native Entwicklung mit SAP HANA*. Bonn: SAP PRESS 2016.

Sabine Maisel: *IDoc-Entwicklung für SAP*. 4. Aufl., Bonn: SAP PRESS 2024.

Dominik Ofenloch, Roland Schwaiger: *Einstieg in Web Dynpro ABAP*. Bonn: SAP PRESS 2009.

Dominik Ofenloch, Roland Schwaiger: *Web Dynpro ABAP. Das umfassende Handbuch*. 2. Aufl., Bonn: SAP PRESS 2014.

Felix Roth, Stefan Stöhr: *BOPF – Business-Objekte mit ABAP entwickeln*. Bonn: SAP PRESS 2017.

Lutz Baumbusch et.al: ABAP RESTful Application Programming Model, 2. Aufl., Bonn: SAP PRESS 2024.

Die Autoren

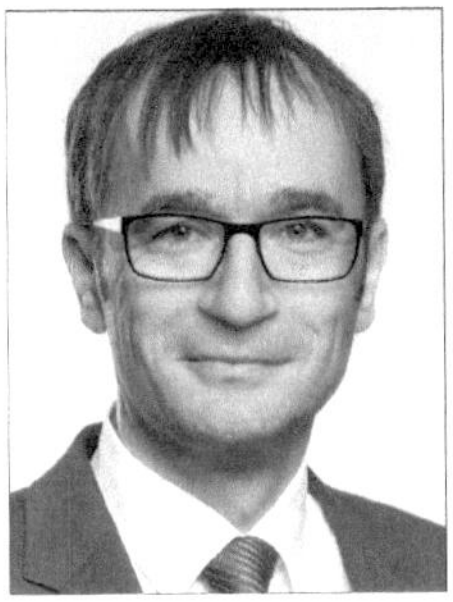

Michael Englbrecht ist Portfolio Manager SAP und Business Manager SAP bei der eXXcellent solutions GmbH in Ulm. Er ist dort für das Leistungsportfolio der eXXcellent solutions GmbH im Bereich SAP verantwortlich. In seiner Rolle als Business Manager SAP ist er gesamtverantwortlich für die Umsetzung von Kundenprojekten sowie die langfristige Betreuung der Kunden. Zuvor war er als Principal Managing Consultant bei der eXXcellent solutions GmbH tätig. Zu seinen Schwerpunkten gehört die Beratung von Unternehmen bei der Integration und Umsetzung von SAP Fiori. Michael Englbrecht arbeitet an der Konzeption, dem Design und der Implementierung von SAP-Fiori- und SAPUI5-Anwendungen mit und berät Kunden bei der Umsetzung der neuen User Experience. Weiterhin gehören die Integration von Systemen in die SAP-Landschaft sowie die Planung und Implementierung serviceorientierter Infrastrukturen zu seinen Themen. Auch in der Beratung bei SAP-Enterprise-Portal-Projekten und im Bereich SAP NetWeaver Knowledge Management and Collaboration verfügt er über langjährige Erfahrung. Michael Englbrecht hat zahlreiche Trainings zu SAP Fiori, SAP User Experience, SAPUI5, ABAP und dem ABAP-Programmiermodell für SAP Fiori, Java-Programmierung, Portalprogrammierung sowie Knowledge Management and Collaboration entwickelt und hält regelmäßig Schulungen zu den Themen. Er studierte Informatik an der FH Augsburg und arbeitete anschließend als Softwareentwickler und Consultant für die MATHEMA AG. Von 2002 bis 2009 war er Senior Consultant bei der AddOn Software GmbH in Neu-Ulm, von 2010 bis 2017 Director NetWeaver Consulting bei der 10 point software GmbH in Dornstadt.

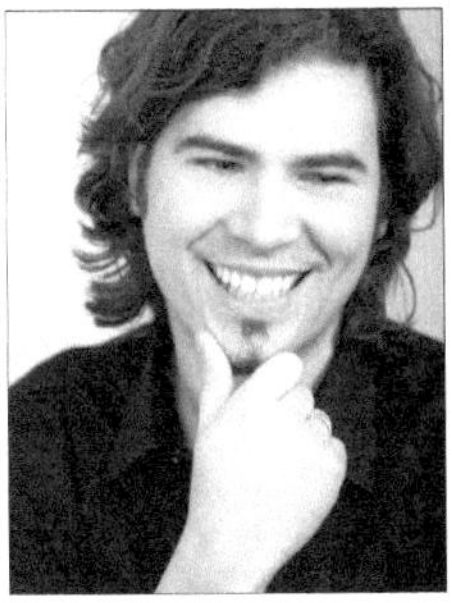

Oliver Pehnke, Dipl.-Ing, ist seit 2005 Entwickler, Architekt und Trainer und in Technologie-Stacks wie Java, Web und SAP zu Hause. Seine Karriere ist geprägt von innovativen Projekten, in denen er robuste, skalierbare und zukunftsfähige Softwarelösungen gestaltet hat. Mit seiner einzigartigen Mischung aus technischem Scharfsinn und der Freude am Entdecken neuer Horizonte – sowohl im Softwarebereich als auch im Leben – ist er ein inspirierender Wegbegleiter für jedes digitale Projekt.

Index

B

G

H

I

J

S

T

X

Z